Advances in Clinical Cardiovascular Imaging Echocardiography & Interventions (ACCI-EI)
A Textbook of Cardiology

Advances in Clinical Cardiovascular Imaging Echocardiography & Interventions (ACCI-EI)
A Textbook of Cardiology

Editors-in-Chief

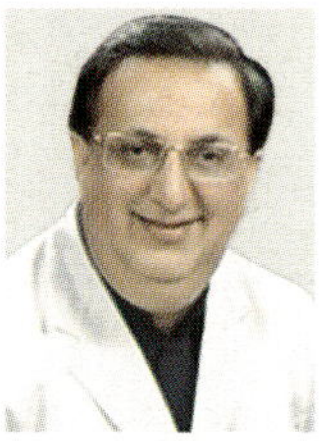

HK Chopra
National President, IAE- 2017
National President, CSI -2015
Chairman, World Wellness Foundation
Country Head, American Heart Association
Sr Consultant Cardiologist, Moolchand Medcity
Chairman, Physician Governing Body, CME, COP
Moolchand Medcity, New Delhi, India

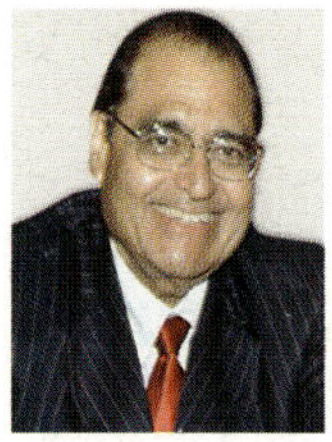

Navin C Nanda
Division of Cardiovascular Disease
Department of Internal Medicine
University of Alabama at Birmingham
Birmingham, Alabama, USA

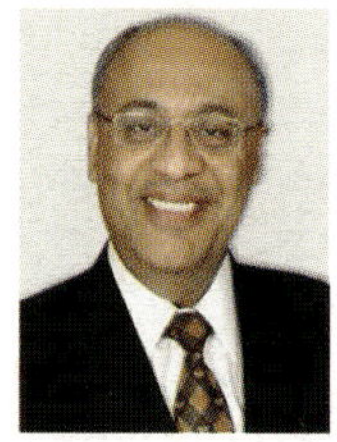

Jagat Narula
Trustee, American College of Cardiology
Director, Cardiovascular Imaging Program
Mount Sinai Cardiovascular Institute
Editor-in- Chief, JACC: CV Imaging
New York, USA

Principal Editors

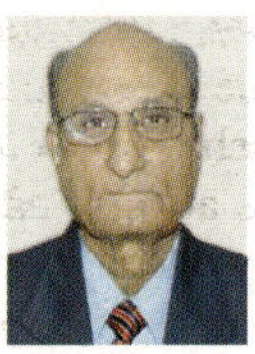

SK Parashar
Director, Non- Invasive Cardiac Laboratory
Metro Hospitals and Heart Institute
Past President, National CSI & IAE
New Delhi, India

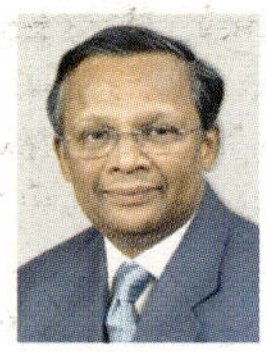

G Vijayaraghavan
Dean Postgraduate Medical Studies
Vice Chairman, Kerala Institute
of Medical Sciences
Past President, IAE
Kerala, India

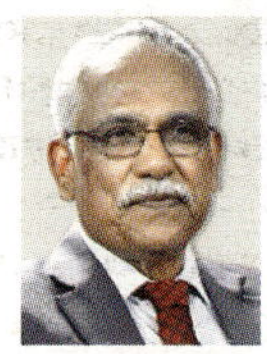

R Alagesan
Retired Professor and
Head of Department of Cardiology
Madras Medical college, Chennai
Past President, IAE

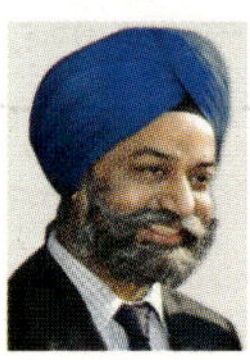

Gurpreet Singh Wander
Professor and Head of Cardiology
Hero DMC Heart Institute
Dayanand Medical College and Hospital
Ludhiana, Punjab, India
Past President, API

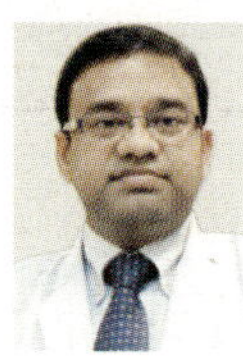

Viveka Kumar
Director, Cath Lab
Senior Consultant Interventional Cardiologist
and Electrophysiologist
Max Superspecialty Hospital
New Delhi, India

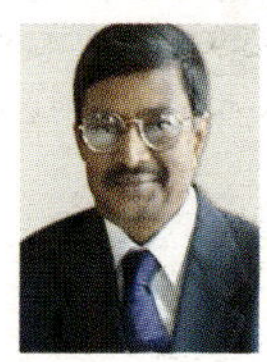

P Krishnam Raju
Sr Consultant Cardiologist
Department of Cardiology
CARE Hospitals, Hyderabad
Past President, IAE

JAYPEE

JAYPEE BROTHERS MEDICAL PUBLISHERS
The Health Sciences Publisher
New Delhi | London | Panama

Jaypee Brothers Medical Publishers (P) Ltd

Headquarters
Jaypee Brothers Medical Publishers (P) Ltd
4838/24, Ansari Road, Daryaganj
New Delhi 110 002, India
Phone: +91-11-43574357
Fax: +91-11-43574314
Email: jaypee@jaypeebrothers.com

Overseas Offices
J.P. Medical Ltd
83 Victoria Street, London
SW1H 0HW (UK)
Phone: +44 20 3170 8910
Fax: +44 (0)20 3008 6180
Email: info@jpmedpub.com

Jaypee-Highlights Medical Publishers Inc
City of Knowledge, Bld. 235, 2nd Floor
Clayton, Panama City, Panama
Phone: +1 507-301-0496
Fax: +1 507-301-0499
Email: cservice@jphmedical.com

Jaypee Brothers Medical Publishers (P) Ltd
Bhotahity, Kathmandu, Nepal
Phone: +977-9741283608
Email: kathmandu@jaypeebrothers.com

Website: www.jaypeebrothers.com
Website: www.jaypeedigital.com

Inquiries for bulk sales may be solicited at: jaypee@jaypeebrothers.com

Advances in Clinical Cardiovascular Imaging, Echocardiography & Interventions (ACCI-EI): A Textbook of Cardiology

First Edition: **2019**

ISBN 978-93-5270-696-9

Printed at: Ajanta Offset & Packagings Ltd., Faridabad, Haryana

Dedicated to

Cardiological Society of India (CSI),
Our parents, our teachers,
All the members of CSI,
Our colleagues, patients, students and our families.

Contributors

AB Gopalamurugan
Senior Consultant Interventional Cardiologist
Chief of Department Percutaneous Valves and Endovascular Interventions
Chennai, Tamil Nadu, India

Abhinav Jain
Consultant
Max Superspecialty Hospital
Saket, New Delhi, India

Adrian Chong
Department of Cardiology
Princess Alexandra Hospital
University of Queensland
Brisbane, Australia

Ahmed K Pasha
Senior Associate Consultant
Division of Hospital Medicine
Mayo Clinic Health System Mankato
Assistant Professor of Medicine
Mayo Clinic School of Medicine and Science
Rochester, Minnesota, USA

Ahmed Y Salama
Division of Cardiovascular Disease
Department of Medicine, University of Alabama
Birmingham, Alabama, USA

Aiman M Smer
Cardiovascular Department
Creighton University School of Medicine
Omaha, Nebraska, USA

Aishwarya Gulati
Dr Gulati Imaging Institute
New Delhi, India

Ajay Garg
Department of Neuroimaging and Interventional Neuroradiology
All India Institute of Medical Sciences, New Delhi, India

Ajay Kumar Sinha
Consultant Intervention Cardiologist
Suraksha Cardiac Care
Paras-HMRI Hospital
Patna, Bihar, India

Ajit Thachil
Consultant Cardiac Electrophysiologist
Lisie Hospital
Kochi, Kerala, India

AK Bali
Senior Consultant Physician
Moolchand Medcity
New Delhi, India

AK Pancholia
Head, Clinical Cardiology
Arihant Hospital and Research Center
Indore, Madhya Pradesh, India

Amit Garg
Consultant
Department of Radiodiagnosis and Imaging
Fortis Escorts Heart Institute, New Delhi, India

Anil Dhall
Director, Cardiovascular Sciences
Venkateshwar Hospital
New Delhi, India

Anil Pareek
President
Medical Affairs and Clinical Research
IPCA Laboratories Ltd.
Mumbai, Maharashtra, India

Anirban Mukherjee
Consultant
Department of Nuclear Medicine
AMRI Hospitals
Kolkata, West Bengal, India

Aniruddha De
Consultant Cardiologist
Department of Noninvasive Cardiology
Apollo Gleneagles Hospital
Kolkata, West Bengal, India

Anjaneyulu V Anne
Consultant Cardiologist
Focus Cardiac Clinic
Hyderabad, Telangana, India

Anjlee M Mehta
Division of Cardiology
University of Texas Health Science Center
San Antonio, Texas, USA

Ankeet Dedhia
Department of Cardiology
Holy Family Hospital and Research Center
Mumbai, Maharashtra, India

Ankit Singh
Department of Cardiology
VMMC and Safdarjung Hospital
New Delhi, India

Ankush Sachdeva
Associate Consultant Cardiology
Fortis Escort Heart Institute
New Delhi, India

Aparna Jaswal
Additional Director Cardiology
Department of Cardiac Pacing and
Electrophysiology
Fortis Escorts Heart Institute
New Delhi, India

Apoorv Mittal
Chief Interventional Cardiologist
Cosmos Hospital, Moradabad, Uttar Pradesh, India

Arif Mirza
Senior Consultant Radiologist
Dr Gulati Imaging Institute
New Delhi, India

Arjun Ravishankar
Indraprastha Apollo Hospital
New Delhi, India

Arnab Banerjee
NH- Rabindranath Tagore International Institute of
Cardiac Sciences (RTIICS)
Kolkata, West Bengal, India

Arti Shah
Cardiovascular and Heart Rhythm Consultants
New York, USA

Arun Chutani
Cardiovascular and Heart Rhythm Consultants
New York, USA

Arun Sharma
Department of Cardiovascular Radiology and
Endovascular interventions
All India Institute of Medical Sciences
New Delhi, India

Ashish Nabar
Jupiter Hospital
Thane, Maharashtra, India

Ashley Pender
Department of Cardiology
Stony Brook Heart Institute, New York, USA

Ashok K Omar
Director, Non-Invasive Cardiology
Fortis Escorts Heart Institute
New Delhi, India

Ashwani Sood
Department of Nuclear Medicine
Postgraduate Institute of Medical Education
and Research (PGIMER)
Chandigarh, India

Atul Karande
Consultant, Echocardiography
CHL Hospitals
Indore, Madhya Pradesh, India

Avani Jain
Intensive Care Unit
Choithram Hospital and Research Center
Indore, Madhya Pradesh, India

Avik Karak
Medical College Hospital
Kolkata, West Bengal, India

Bhagwant R Mittal
Department of Nuclear Medicine
Postgraduate Institute of Medical Education
and Research (PGIMER)
Chandigarh, India

Bharat Bansal
Attending Consultant
Non-Invasive Cardiology
Max Superspecialty Hospital
Saket, New Delhi, India

Bharat Kantharia
Cardiovascular and Heart Rhythm Consultants
New York, USA

Bhargava Mohan
Principal Consultant
Interventional Cardiologist
Max Superspecialty Hospital
Saket, New Delhi, India

Bhargava Prachal
Consultant
Max Superspecialty Hospital
Saket, New Delhi, India

Binoy John
Director and Head
Department of Cardiology and
Interventional Cardiology
Credence Hospital
Thiruvananthapuram, Kerala, India

Bishav Mohan
Dayanand Medical College and Hospital Unit
Hero DMC Heart Institute, Ludhiana, Punjab, India

BP Singh
Professor and Head
Department of Cardiology
IGIMS, Patna, Bihar

Brian Pinto
Chief Cardiologist
Holy Family Hospital and Research Center
Mumbai, Maharashtra, India

Chandramukhi Modi
Consultant Cardiologist, CARE Hospitals
Hyderabad, Telangana, India

Chandramukhi Sunehra
Department of Cardiac Imaging
CARE Hospitals
Hyderabad, Telangana, India

Chandrashekhara SH
Associate Professor
Department of Radiodiagnosis
All India Institute of Medical Sciences
New Delhi, India

Chandril Chugh
Head
Department of Interventional Neurology
MAX Superspecialty Hospital
Saket and Gurugram

Chetan D Patel
Professor
Department of Nuclear Medicine
All India Institute of Medical Sciences
New Delhi, India

Christopher SG Murray
Department of Internal Medicine
Harlem Hospital Center, Columbia University
New York, USA

CK Ponde
Senior Consultant Cardiologist
PD Hinduja National Hospital and MRC
Mahim Hinduja Healthcare Surgical Kar
Mumbai, Maharashtra, India

CN Manjunath
Director
Sri Jayadeva Institute of Cardiovascular Sciences and Research
Bengaluru, Karnataka, India

C Venkata S Ram
Director, Apollo Institute for Blood Pressure Management
World Hypertension League/South Asia Office
Apollo Hospitals, Hyderabad, Telangana, India
Texas Blood Pressure Institute, Dallas
Nephrology Associates, University of Texas
Southwestern Medical School, Dallas, Texas, USA

Debabrata Roy
Senior Consultant Interventional Cardiologist and
Academic Coordinator
NH- Rabindranath Tagore International Institute of Cardiac Sciences
(RTIICS)
Kolkata, West Bengal, India

Debika Chatterjee
Senior Consultant Cardiologist
Rabindranath Tagore International Institute of Cardiac Sciences
Kolkata, West Bengal, India

Devinder Mahal
Dayanand Medical College and Hospital Unit
Hero DMC Heart Institute
Ludhiana, Punjab, India

Dheeraj Arora
Principal Consultant Cardiac Anesthesiology
Medanta Institute of Critical Care and Anesthesiology
Medanta-The Medicity
Gurugram, Haryana, India

E Prabhu
Senior Consultant and Head
Institute of Nuclear Imaging and Molecular Medicine
Chief Coordinator
Institute of Advanced Research in Health Sciences
Academic Officer, Madras Medial College, Chennai
Tamil Nadu Government Multi Superspecialty Hospital
Omandurar Government Estate, Chennai, Tamil Nadu, India

George Koshy
Professor of Cardiology
Government Medical College
Thiruvananthapuram, Kerala, India

GN Mahapatra
Senior Consultant and Head
Department of Nuclear Medicine, SPECT-CT & PET-CT
Seven Hills Hospital
Director West Coast Medical Center, MHADA
Mumbai, Maharashtra, India

Goutam Vaggar
King Edward VII
Memorial Hospital
Mumbai, Maharashtra, India

GS Sainani
Emeritus Director
Department of Medicine
Jaslok Hospital and Research Center
Emeritus Professor of Medicine
Grant Medical College and JJ Hospital
Mumbai, Maharashtra, India

Gulshan Rai
Dayanand Medical College and Hospital Unit
Hero DMC Heart Institute
Ludhiana, Punjab, India

Gurpreet S Gulati
Professor
Department of Cardiovascular Radiology
and Endovascular Interventions
Cardiothoracic Center
All India Institute of Medical Sciences
New Delhi, India

Gurpreet Singh Wander
Professor and Head
Department of Cardiology
Hero DMC Heart Institute
Dayanand Medical College and Hospital
Ludhiana, Punjab, India

G Vijayaraghavan
Dean, Postgraduate Medical Studies
Vice Chairman and Director
Kerala Institute of Medical Sciences
Thiruvananthapuram, Kerala, India

Hala El Marsafawy
Professor of Pediatrics and Pediatric Cardiology
Director Cardiac Catheterization Laboratory
Children Hospital, Mansoura University
President Working Group of Egyptian Pediatric Cardiologists, League from Egyptian Society of Cardiology
Former Director Children Hospital, Mansoura University
Former Dean Faculty of Nursing, Mansoura University
Member SCAI, AEPC

Hanan Fadala
Division of Cardiovascular Disease
Department of Medicine, University of Alabama
Birmingham, Alabama, USA

Hanumanth K Reddy
Adjunct Clinical Professor of Medicine
St Louis University Medical School
St Louis, Missouri, USA

Harmeet Singh
Head, Critical Care
Department of Emergency and Urgent Care
Moolchand Medcity
New Delhi, India

Harshit Gupta
Dayanand Medical College and Hospital Unit
Hero DMC Heart Institute
Ludhiana, Punjab, India

Harsh Mahajan
Padma Shri Awardee
Chief Radiologist
Mahajan Imaging
New Delhi, India

Harsh Wardhan
Head
Department of Cardiology
Primus Superspecialty Hospital
Formerly, Professor
Consultant and Head
Department of Cardiology
RML Hospital and PGIMER
New Delhi, India

Himashu Agarwal
Consultant Interventional Neurology
Max Superspecialty Hospital
Saket, New Delhi, India

HK Chopra
National President, IAE- 2017
National President, CSI -2015
Chairman, World Wellness Foundation
Country Head, American Heart Association
Sr Consultant Cardiologist, Moolchand Medcity
Chairman, Physician Governing Body, CME, COP Moolchand Medcity
New Delhi, India

Hosam Ibrahim
Division of Pediatric Cardiology
Department of Pediatrics
Cairo University, Cairo, Egypt

IB Vijayalakshmi
Professor of Pediatric Cardiology
Superspecialty Hospital-PMSSY
Bengaluru Medical College and Research Institute
Bengaluru, Karnataka, India

I Sathyamurthy
Senior Interventional Cardiologist
Apollo Main Hospitals
Chennai, Tamil Nadu, India

Jabir A
Department of Cardiology
Lisie Heart Institute
Lisie Hospital, Kochi, Kerala, India

Jamshed J Dalal
Director-Cardiac Sciences
Kokilaben Hospital
Mumbai, Maharashtra, India

Jayakeerthi Yoganarasimha
Senior Consultant Electrophysiologist
Vrinchi Hospitals
Hyderabad, Telangana, India

Jimmy George
Department of Cardiology
Lisie Heart Institute
Lisie Hospital, Kochi, Kerala, India

Johann Christopher
Consultant Cardiologist
Director of Cardiac Imaging
CARE Hospitals, Hyderabad, Telangana, India

Jo Joseph
Department of Cardiology
Lisie Heart Institute
Lisie Hospital, Kochi, Kerala, India

JPS Sawhney
Chairperson, Department of Cardiology
Dharma Vira Heart Center
Sir Ganga Ram Hospital
New Delhi, India

Karan Chopra
Consultant, Interventional Cardiology
Venkateshwar Hospital
New Delhi, India

Karishma Walia
Moolchand Medcity
New Delhi, India

Kartik Ganga
Department of Cardiovascular Radiology and Endovascular Interventions
All India Institute of Medical Sciences
New Delhi, India

Kaustubh Mahamine
Associate Consultant
PD Hinduja Hospital and MRC
Mumbai, Maharashtra, India

Kewal Kanabar
Department of Cardiology
Postgraduate Institute of Medical Education and Research
Chandigarh, India

Kewal Krishan
Department of Cardiovascular Surgery
Max Heart and Vascular Institute
Saket, New Delhi, India

Khemendra Kumar
Consultant
Department of Radiodiagnosis and Imaging
Fortis Escorts Heart Institute, New Delhi, India

KK Aggarwal
Padma Shri Awardee
President Heart Care Foundation of India
Immediate National Past President, Indian Medical Association

KK Kapur
Chief, Non-Invasive Cardiac Lab
Indraprastha Apollo Hospital
New Delhi, India

KM Krishnamoorthy
Professor of Cardiology
Sree Chitra Thirunal Institute
Medical Sciences and Technology
Thiruvananthapuram, Kerala, India

KN Srinivasan
Consultant and Interventional Cardiologist
Apollo Main Hospitals
Chennai, Tamil Nadu, India

K Rajeswari
Billroth Hsopitals
Chennai, Tamil Nadu, India

Kumar Hrishikesh
Associate Consultants Cardiology
Asian Institute of Medical Science
Faridabad, Haryana, India

Kushagra Mahansaria
Associate Consultant
Department of Cardiac Sciences
Bhagwan Mahavir MEDICA Superspecialty Hospital
Ranchi, Jharkhand, India

Kushal Madan
Cardiac Rehabilitation Consultant
Dharma Vira Heart Center
Sir Ganga Ram Hospital
New Delhi, India

K Venugopal
Professor and Head
Department of Cardiology
Pushpagiri Institute of Medical Sciences
Tiruvalla, Kerala, India

Liza Thomas
Department of Cardiology
Westmead Hospital
University of New South Wales
Sydney, Australia

Madhu Mary Minz
Senior Consultant Cardiology
Medanta–The Medicity
Gurugram, Haryana, India

Manish Bansal
Associate Director Cardiology
Medanta–The Medicity
Gurugram, Haryana, India

Manish Gaba
Moolchand Medcity
New Delhi, India

Masood Ahmad
Medical Director, Echocardiography Lab
Division of Cardiology, Department of Internal Medicine
University of Texas Medical Branch
Galveston, Texas, USA

Mathew Iype
Additional Professor of Cardiology
Government Medical College
Thiruvananthapuram, Kerala, India

Meera Venkatesh
Director, NAPC, IAEA, Vienna
Ex-Head, Radiopharm Division
BARC, Mumbai, Maharashtra, India

Mitu Minocha
Senior Consultant Non-Invasive Cardiology
Fortis Escorts Heart Institute
New Delhi, India

Mohamed Faher Almahmoud
Division of Cardiology
Department of Internal Medicine
University of Texas Medical Branch
Galveston, Texas, USA

Mohammed Nazir
Dayanand Medical College and Hospital Unit
Hero DMC Heart Institute
Ludhiana, Punjab, India

Mona Bhatia
Director and Head
Department of Radiodiagnosis and Imaging
Fortis Escorts Heart Institute, New Delhi
Convener, Cardiac Imaging, Cardiological Society of India
Chair, International Regional Committee, India Chapter
Society of Cardiovascular CT, USA

Mridul Mahanta
Dayanand Medical College and Hospital Unit
Hero DMC Heart Institute
Ludhiana, Punjab, India

Mrinal Kanti Das
Consultant and Senior Interventional Cardiologist
BM Birla Heart Research Center and CMRI
Kolkata, West Bengal, India

M Srihari Babu
Professor and Head of Medicine
GSL Medical College
Rajahmundry, Andhra Pradesh, India

Mumun Sinha
Department of Cardiovascular Radiology
and Endovascular Interventions
All India Institute of Medical Sciences
New Delhi, India

Mythri Shankar
Lead Consultant - Nuclear Medicine
Aster CMI Hospital
Bengaluru, Karnataka, India

Nagaraja Moorthy
Associate Professor
Department of Cardiology
Sri Jayadeva Institute of Cardiovascular Sciences and Research
Bengaluru, Karnataka, India

Nagendra Chouhan
Associate Director
Interventional Cardiology, Heart Institute
Medanta- The Medcity
Gurugram, Haryana, India

Naman Shastri
Chief Consultant Cardiac Anesthesiologist
SAL Hospital, Ahmedabad, Gujarat, India

Naveen Garg
In-Charge, Non-Invasive Cardiology
BK Hospital
Faridabad, Haryana, India

Navin C Nanda
Division of Cardiovascular Disease
Department of Internal Medicine
University of Alabama at Birmingham
Birmingham, Alabama, USA

Neeraj A Desai
Department of Cardiology
Holy Family Hospital and Research Center
Mumbai, Maharashtra, India

N Chidambaram
Professor of Medicine and Cardiologist
Advisor to VC (Medical Affairs)
Former Dean, Faculty of Medicine
Annamalai University
Chennai, Tamil Nadu, India

Nidhi Goyal
Senior Consultant Radiologist
Dr Gulati Imaging Institute
New Delhi, India

Nikhil Raut
Consultant Cardiologist
HJ Doshi Hindu Sabha Hospital
Mumbai, Maharashtra, India

Nikunj Kotecha
Department of Cardiology
Sanjay Gandhi Postgraduate Institute of Medical Sciences
Lucknow, Uttar Pradesh, India

Niraj Pandey
Department of Cardiovascular Radiology and
Endovascular interventions
All India Institute of Medical Sciences
New Delhi, India

Nisarg Patel
Moolchand Medcity
New Delhi, India

Nitin Aggarwal
Senior Interventional Cardiologist
Rajiv Gandhi Cancer Institute and Research Center
Sri Balaji Action Hospital
New Delhi, India

Nitin Burkule
Consultant Cardiologist
Jupiter Hospital
Thane, Maharashtra, India

NN Khanna
Chairman, Asia Pacific Vascular Society
Past Chairman, National Interventional Council, CSI
President Elect, Indian College of Cardiology
President, International Society of Endovascular Specialist
(ISEVS - Indian Chapter)
Senior Consultant Interventional Cardiology
Senior Consultant Vascular Interventions
Coordinator, Cardiology, Cathlab and Vascular Services
Advisor, Apollo Group of Hospitals
Indraprastha Apollo Hospital
New Delhi, India

N Ramamoorthy
Ex-Associate Director
BARC/DAE, Mumbai
Ex-Director, NAPC
IAEA, Vienna, Austria

Oladimeji Oluwaseye
Indraprastha Apollo Hospital
New Delhi, India

OP Yadava
CEO and Chief Cardiac Surgeon
National Heart Institute
New Delhi, India

Parveen Gulati
Director
Dr Gulati Imaging Institute
New Delhi, India

Pawan K Sharma
Assistant Professor of Medicine
Division of Cardiology
Adjunct Assistant Professor of Radiology
University of Utah School of Medicine
Salt Lake City, Utah, USA

PB Jayagopal
Director and Interventional Cardiologist
Lakshmi Hospital, Palakkad, Kerala, India

PK Mangla
Sr Consultant Pulmonologist
Moolchand Medcity
New Delhi, India

P Krishnam Raju
Senior Consultant Cardiologist
Department of Cardiology
CARE Hospitals
Hyderabad, Telangana, India

Poonam Malhotra
Professor, Cardiac Anesthesia, CTC
All India Institute of Medical Sciences, New Delhi, India

Pranav A Oza
Department of Cardiology
PD Hinduja Hospital
Mumbai, Maharashtra, India

Prashant Bharadwaj
Consultant
Venkateshwar Hospital
New Delhi, India

Prashant Wankhade
Department of Cardiology
Dharma Vira Heart Center
Sir Ganga Ram Hospital
New Delhi, India

Prateek Bajaj
Associate Consultants Cardiology
Asian Institute of Medical Science
Faridabad, Haryana, India

Prateek Sharma
Department of Cardiology
Stony Brook Heart Institute, New York, USA

Preeti Gupta
Assistant Professor
Department of Cardiology
VMMC and Safdarjung Hospital
New Delhi, India

Priya Jagia
Professor
Department of Cardiovascular Radiology and
Endovascular Iinterventions
All India Institute of Medical Sciences
New Delhi, India

PS Soni
Professor and Head
Department of Nuclear Medicine
GGSMC & H, Baba Farid University of Health Sciences, Punjab
Ex-GM & Head, Medical Cyclotron Facility, BRIT/BARC, Mumbai

Puneet Sethi
Senior Consultant Radiologist
Mahajan Imaging
New Delhi, India

R Alagesan
Retired Professor and Head
Department of Cardiology
Madras Medical College, Chennai
Past President, IAE

Raghav Bansal
Associate Consultant, Cardiology
Max Superspecialty Hospital
Saket, New Delhi, India

Raghuveer Kura
Clinical Assistant Professor of Medicine
St Louis University Medical School
St Louis, Missouri, USA

Rahul Kumar
Fortis Escorts Heart Institute
New Delhi, India

Rahul Mehrotra
Associate Director and Head
Non-Invasive Cardiology
Max Superspecialty Hospital
Saket, New Delhi, India

Rahul Nijhara
Department of Radiodiagnosis and Imaging
Fortis Escorts Heart Institute, New Delhi, India

Rajan J Manjuran
Emeritus Professor
Department of Cardiology
Pushpagiri Medical College
Tiruvalla, Kerala, India

Rajat Subhra Ghose
Head, Echocardiography Unit
Ramakrishna Mission Seva Pratishthan Hospital
Kolkata, West Bengal, India

Rajeev Gupta
Preventive Cardiology
Internal Medicine
Eternal Heart Care Center and Research Institute
Mount Sinai New York Affiliate
Jawahar Circle, Jaipur, Rajasthan, India

Rajiv Gupta
Head, CTVS
Dayanand Medical College and Hospital Unit
Hero DMC Heart Institute
Ludhiana, Punjab, India

Rajesh Janardhanan
Professor of Medicine and Medical Imaging
Medical Director, Non-Invasive Cardiac Imaging
Director of Echocardiography
Banner - University Medical Center
Sarver Heart Center
Tucson, Arizona, USA

Rajesh Meena
Senior Consultant Physician
Moolchand Medcity
New Delhi, India

Rajesh Sainani
Honorary Consultant Gastroenterologist
Jaslok Hospital and Research Center
Mumbai, Maharashtra, India

Rajiv Ananthakrishna
Associate Professor
Department of Cardiology
Sri Jayadeva Institute of Cardiovascular Sciences and Research
Bengaluru, Karnataka, India

Raj Kumar
Consultant
Non-Invasive Cardiology
Max Superspecialty Hospital
Saket, New Delhi, India

Rajneesh Malhotra
Department of Cardiovascular Surgery
Max Heart and Vascular Institute
Saket, New Delhi, India

Rakesh Bachloo
Associate Consultant, Non-Invasive Cardiology
National Heart Institute
New Delhi, India

Rakesh Gupta
Director and Chief Cardiologist
JROP Healthcare
Consultant Cardiologist
Max Superspecialty Hospital
New Delhi, India

Ravi Komatireddy
Clinical Assistant Professor of Medicine
University of California
San Diego, California, USA

Ravi Masand
Radiologist
CHL Hospital
Mumbai, Maharashtra, India

Ravina Sharma
Dayanand Medical College and Hospital
Ludhiana, Punjab, India

Ravi Prakash
Consultant, Interventional Cardiology
Moolchand Medcity
New Delhi, India

Ravi R Kasliwal
Chairman, Clinical and Preventive Cardiology
Medanta– The Medicity
Gurugram, Haryana, India

Ravi S Math
Associate Professor of Cardiology
Department of Cardiology
Sri Jayadeva Institute of
Cardiovascular Sciences and Research
Bengaluru, Karnataka, India

Ravi Vishnu Prasad
Associate Professor
Department of Cardiology
IGIMS, Patna, Bihar, India

Raziye E Akdogan
Division of Cardiovascular Disease
Department of Medicine, University of Alabama
Birmingham, Alabama, USA

Reena Anand
Department of Cardiovascular Surgery
Max Heart and Vascular Institute
Saket, New Delhi, India

Rekha Mishra
Consultant Cardiologist
National Heart Institute
New Delhi, India

R Hotchandani
Director and Head
Department of Nephrology, Dialysis and Kidney Tansplant
Moolchand Medcity
New Delhi, India

Richa Kothari
Cardiothoracic Imaging Unit
Narayana Institute of Cardiac Sciences
Naryana Hrudayalaya Health City
Bengaluru, Karnataka, India

Richa Trivedi
NMR Research Center
Institute of Nuclear Medicine and Allied Sciences
New Delhi, India

R Keshava
Fortis Hospitals
Bengaluru, Karnataka, India

Rohin Vinayak
Dayanand Medical College and Hospital
Ludhiana, Punjab, India

Rohit Tandon
Senior Consultant Physician
Dayanand Medical College and Hospital Unit
Hero DMC Heart Institute
Ludhiana, Punjab, India

Rony Mathew
Head of Department - Cardiology
Lisie Heart Institute
Lisie Hospital, Kochi, Kerala, India

Roopali Khanna
Associate Professor, Department of Cardiology
Sanjay Gandhi Postgraduate Institute of Medical Sciences
Lucknow, Uttar Pradesh, India

Roshini Malaney
Department of Cardiology
Stony Brook Heart Institute, New York, USA

R Singhal
Chief Cardiac Electrophysiologist and
Senior Interventional Cardiologist
Heart and General Hospital
Jaipur, Rajasthan, India

RVA Ananth
Consultant Cardiologist
Jeyalakshmi Heart Center
Madurai, Tamil Nadu, India

Sakhalesh Patil
Kerala Institute of Medical Sciences
Thiruvananthapuram, Kerala, India

Sakshi Sachdeva
All India Institute of Medical Sciences
New Delhi, India

Sameer Shrivastava
Director and Head
Department of Noninvasive Cardiology
Fortis Escort Heart Institute
New Delhi, India

Sandeep Bansal
Professor and Head
Department of Cardiology
VMMC and Safdarjung Hospital
New Delhi, India

Sanjeev Kumar
Head of Department-CTVS
AIIMS, Patna, Bihar, India

Sanjeev Kumar
Department of Cardiovascular Radiology
and Endovascular Intervention
All India Institute of Medical Sciences, New Delhi, India

Sanjeev Kumar
Senior Consultant Neurosurgeon
Batra Hospital and Medical Research Center
New Delhi, India

Santanu Guha
Professor and Head
Department of Cardiology
Medical College, Kolkata
Past President, National CSI
Kolkata, West Bengal, India

Satish Govind
Fortis Hospitals
Bengaluru, Karnataka, India

Satish K Parashar
Senior Consultant Cardiologist and
Director, Non-Invasive Cardiac Laboratory
Metro Hospital and Heart Institute
New Delhi, India

Satyavan Sharma
Professor and Head of Cardiology and
Interventional Cardiologist
Bombay Hospital Institute of Medical Sciences
Mumbai, Maharashtra, India

Satyendra Tewari
Professor
Department of Cardiology
Sanjay Gandhi Postgraduate Institute of Medical Sciences
Lucknow, Uttar Pradesh, India

Saumitra Ray
Consultant Interventional Cardiologist
Vivekananda Institute of Medical Sciences, Kolkata, West Bengal, India

Saurabh Mehrotra
Department of Cardiology
Postgraduate Institute of Medical Education and Research
Chandigarh, India

Sayeed Raheem
Batra Hospital and Medical Research Center
New Delhi, India

SC Manchanda
Senior Consultant Cardiologist
Dharma Vira Heart Center
Sir Ganga Ram Hospital
New Delhi, India

SG Prasad
Department of Telemedicine
CARE Hospitals
Hyderabad, Telangana, India

Shafiq Ahmed Zargar
Fortis Escorts Heart Institute
New Delhi, India

Shailendra Bhadoriya
Consultant, Non-Invasive Cardiology
Fortis Escorts Heart Institute
New Delhi, India

Shashank Jain
Department of Radiodiagnosis and Imaging
Fortis Escorts Heart Institute, New Delhi, India

Showkat Hussain Bhat
Attending Consultant
Non-Invasive Cardiology
Max Superspecialty Hospital
Saket, New Delhi, India

Shraddha Ranjan
Department of Cardiology
Medanta- The Medicity
Gurugram, Haryana, India

Simmi Manocha
Associate Director Cardiology
Senior Consultant, Chief-Non-invasive Cardiology
Asian Institute of Medical Sciences
Faridabad, Haryana, India

Simran Kaur
Assistant Professor
Department of Nephrology
Dayanand Medical College and Hospital
Ludhiana, Punjab, India

Simran Sawhney
Department of Medicine
St Stephen's Hospital
New Delhi, India

SKD Bhardwaj
Senior Consultant Cardiologist
Muzaffarnagar, Uttar Pradesh, India

SKM Sarjun Basha
Cardiologist, Peacock Hospital
Tiruttani, Tamil Nadu, India

Smadar Kort
Department of Cardiology
Stony Brook Heart Institute, New York, USA

SN Pathak
Consultant Intervention Cardiologist
Metro Hospital and Heart Institute
New Delhi, India

Somnath Mukhopadhyay
Medical College Hospital
Kolkata, West Bengal, India

Sonia A El-Saiedi
Professor of Pediatric Cardiology
Division of Pediatric Cardiology
Department of Pediatrics
Cairo University, Cairo, Egypt

Soumitra Kumar
Senior Consultant Cardiologist
Fortis Hospital, Rabindranath Tagore International Institute
of Cardiac Sciences, and Sri Aurobindo Seva Kendra
Kolkata, West Bengal, India

S Ramakrishnan
Professor, Department of Cardiology
All India Institute of Medical Sciences
New Delhi, India

Srikant Sharma
Senior Consultant Physician
Moolchand Medcity
New Delhi, India

Shashwat Mishra
National Heart Institute
New Delhi, India

S Shanmugasundaram
Emeritus Professor of Cardiology
The Tamil Nadu Dr MGR Medical University
Cardiologist, Billroth Hospitals
Chennai, Tamil Nadu, India

S Singhal
Director Cardiac Imaging and
Senior Consultant Radiologist
Eternal Heart Care Center
Jaipur, Rajasthan, India

S Sivasankaran
Sree Chitra Tirunal Institute
for Medical Sciences and Technology
Thiruvananthapuram, Kerala, India

SS Iyengar
Consultant Cardiologist
Manipal Hospital
Bengaluru, Karnataka, India

S Santhosh
Consultant Nuclear Medicine Physician
Institute of Nuclear Imaging and Molecular Medicine
Tamil Nadu Government Multi Superspecialty Hospital
Omandurar Government Estate
Chennai, Tamil Nadu, India

Subash Khushu
Head, Division of Radiological Imaging
and Biomedical Engineering
NMR Research Center
Institute of Nuclear Medicine and Allied Sciences
New Delhi, India

Sudhir Wahi
Department of Cardiology
Princess Alexandra Hospital
University of Queensland
Brisbane, Australia

Sulthan R Salih
Department of Cardiology
Pushpagiri Medical College
Tiruvalla, Kerala, India

Suman Singhal
Department of Radiodiagnosis
Eternal Heart Care Center and Research Institute
Mount Sinai New York Affiliate
Jawahar Circle, Jaipur, Rajasthan, India

Suman Singhal
Director Cardiac Imaging
Senior Consultant Radiologist
Eternal Heart Care Center
Jaipur, Rajasthan, India

Sundeep Mishra
Department of Cardiology
All India Institute of Medical Sciences
New Delhi, India

Sunil Aggarwal
Max Superspecialty Hospital
New Delhi, India

Sunil Mangla
Sr Consultant Physician
New Delhi, India

Suparna Rao
Indraprastha Apollo Hospital
New Delhi, India

Surabhi Awasthi
Head, Critical Care
Moolchand Medcity
New Delhi, India

Surendra Chutani
Cardiovascular and Heart Rhythm Consultants
New York, USA

S Venkatesh
Fortis Hospitals
Bengaluru, Karnataka, India

Tamanna Nahar
Section of Cardiology
Department of Internal Medicine
Harlem Hospital Center/Columbia University
New York, USA

Tapan Sinha
Consultant Cardiologist
Kothari Medical Center
Kolkata, West Bengal, India

Tariq Matin
Consultant Intervention Neuroradiology
Narayana Superspecialty Hospital
Gurugram, Haryana, India

Tarun Mittal
Senior Consultant Cardiothoracic Radiologist
Royal Brompton and Harefield Hospital, London
Honorary Senior Clinical Lecturer
Imperial College London, UK

Thirupathi K Reddy
Clinical Assistant Professor of Medicine
Stanford University
Stanford, California, USA

Tinu T Lukose
Department of Nuclear Medicine
Postgraduate Institute of Medical Education
and Research (PGIMER)
Chandigarh, India

Tiny Nair
Head, Department of Cardiology
PRS Hospital
Thiruvananthapuram, Kerala, India

Tony Stanton
Department of Cardiology
Sunshine Coast University Hospital, Birtinya
University of the Sunshine Coast, Sippy Downs
Queensland, Australia

U Ilayaraja
Cardiologist, Billroth Hospitals
Chennai, Tamil Nadu, India

Uma Ravishankar
Senior Consultant and Head
Departent of Nuclear Medicine and Molecular Imaging
Indraprastah Apollo Hospital
New Delhi, India

Upendra Kaul
Padmashiri and Dr BC Roy Awardee
Chairman and Dean Academics
and Research, Batra Heart Center
and Batra Hospital and Medical Research Center
New Delhi, India

V Amuthan
Past President, Indian Academy of Echocardiography
Emeritus Professor of Cardiology
The Tamil Nadu Dr MGR Medical University,
Director of 4D Echocardiography Lab, Jeyalakshmi Heart Center
Madurai
Interventional Cardiologist, Vadamalayan Hospital
Madurai, Tamil Nadu, India

V Anand
Senior Consultant Physician
Moolchand Medcity
New Delhi, India

Vanita Arora
Director and Head
Cardiac Electrophysiology Lab and Arrhythmia Services
Senior Consultant Cardiac Electrophysiologist
and Interventional Cardiologist
Max Healthcare Superspecialty Hospital
Saket, New Delhi, India

Varun Deokate
King Edward VII
Memorial Hospital
Mumbai, Maharashtra, India

Vidyut Jain
Consultant Cardiologist
Choithram Hospital and Research Center
Indore, Madhya Pradesh, India

Vijay Katekhaye
Dev Clinic
Omkar Nagar
Nagpur, Maharashtra, India

Vikas Singh
Consultant Intervention Cardiologist
Daksh Heart Care and 4A Heart Hospital
Patna, Bihar, India

Vimal Raj
Cardiothoracic Imaging Unit
Narayana Institute of Cardiac Sciences
Naryana Hrudayalaya Health City
Bengaluru, Karnataka, India

Vinay Sharma
Senior Consultant
Fortis Escorts Heart Institute
New Delhi, India

Vineeta Ojha
Department of Cardiovascular Radiology
and Endovascular Intervention
All India Institute of Medical Sciences, New Delhi, India

Viveka Kumar
Director, Cath Lab
Senior Consultant Interventional Cardiologist and Electrophysiologist
Max Superspecialty Hospital
New Delhi, India

Vivek Kumar
Consultant
Interventional Cardiology and Electrophysiology
Max Healthcare Superspecialty Hospital
Saket, New Delhi, India

Vivek Lanka
Department of Neuroimaging and
Interventional Neuroradiology
NIMHANS, Bengaluru, Karnataka, India

Vivek Tandon
Principal Consultant Cardiologist
Max Smart Superspecialty Hospital
Saket, New Delhi, India

Wael A Attia
Assistant Professor of Pediatric Cardiology
Division of Pediatric Cardiology
Department of Pediatrics
Cairo University, Cairo, Egypt

Wulan Anggrahini
Indraprastha Apollo Hospital
New Delhi, India

Yatin Mehta
President ISCCM
Chairman, Medanta Institute of Critical Care and Anesthesiology
Medanta-The Medicity
Gurugram, Haryana, India

Foreword

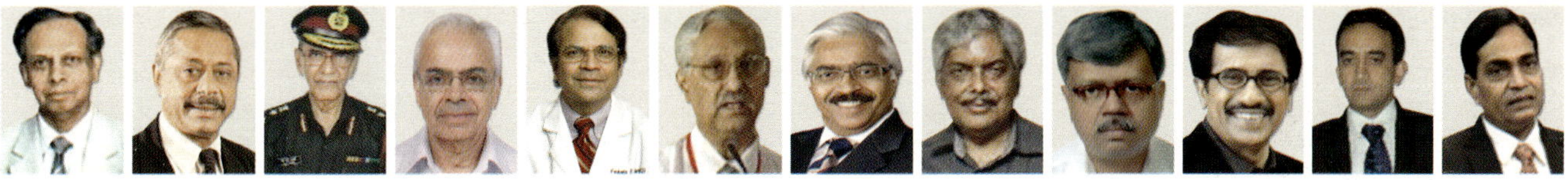

We are honored and have a great pleasure to write the foreword for the state-of-the-art *Advances in Clinical Cardiovascular Imaging, Echocardiography and Interventions (ACCI-EI): A Textbook of Cardiology* being released on the occasion of the inaugural function of 70th Annual Conference of CSI at Mumbai, Maharashtra, India. The textbook on ACCI-EI was long due considering the wealth of data, new strategies which are diagnostically, prognostically and therapeutically imaging based in the clinical practice. It is one of the most needed, comprehensive, illustrative, well-structured book, published with enormous information about advances in cardiovascular imaging, Echocardiography and interventions for better CVD management with morbidity and mortality benefits.

The book is an excellent and outstanding educational initiative by the joint efforts of three Editors-in-Chief, 6 Principal Editors, 15 International Editors, 37 National Editors and over 278 contributing authors. This book comprises 35 sections, 142 chapters, including Basics, Hypertension, Heart Failure, STEMI, CAD, Advances in Echocardiography: Clinical Implications, Emergency Imaging in Chest Pain, Valvular Hear Disease, RHD, Atrial fibrillation, VT Storm, DCMP, HOCM, RCM, Pericardial Effusion, Constrictive Pericarditis, Infective Endocarditis, Pulmonary embolism and DVT, Pulmonary Hypertension, Aortic Disease, Carotid Artery Disease, Vertebral Artery Disease, Peripheral Arterial and Venous Disease, Syncope, Stroke, CHD, Echo in ECMO, Shock, Epidemiological, Nutritional Imaging, Cardiac SOL, Intraoperative Echocardiography in OT, Surgery and Imaging, Echo-oncology, Ethical and Legal Issues, Future Directions. Each chapter addresses a separate and distinct issue of clinical relevance. The chapters are well outlined, organized, well written and referenced. The writing style of every chapter is vivid, concise and practical. There are excellent graphics, tables and figures that present the relevant information. The printing and binding is of excellent quality. This book will represent a milestone for Advances in Clinical Cardiovascular Imaging, Echocardiography and Interventions management strategies in the world.

We congratulate the Editors-in-Chief HK Chopra, Navin C Nanda, Jagat Narula, Principal Editors, International, National Editors and the Contributors, for accomplishing this prodigious achievement of great clinical relevance in Cardiology practice today.

M Khalilullah
Director and Senior Consultant Cardiologist
The Heart Centre
New Delhi, India
Past President, National CSI

C Venkata S Ram
Director, Apollo Institute for Blood Pressure Management
World Hypertension League/South Asia Office
Apollo Hospitals, Hyderabad, Telangana, India
Texas Blood Pressure Institute, Dallas
Nephrology Associates, University of Texas
Southwestern Medical School, Dallas, Texas, USA

Santanu Guha
Professor and Head
Department of Cardiology
Medical College
Past President, National CSI
Kolkata, West Bengal, India

Naresh Trehan
Chairman and Managing Director
Medanta—The Medicity
Gurugram, Haryana, India

Amal K Banerjee
Past President, National CSI
Past President, API
Past President, SAARC CS
Kolkata, West Bengal, India

Shirish (MS) Hiremath
Director, Cath Lab, Ruby Hall
Pune, Maharashtra, India
Immediate President CSI

GS Sainani
Emeritus Director, Department of Medicine
Jaslok Hospital and Research Center
Emeritus Professor of Medicine
Grant Medical College JJ Hospital
Mumbai, Maharashtra, India
Past President, CSI

SC Manchanda
Senior Consultant Cardiology
Dharma Vira Heart Center
Sir Ganga Ram Hospital
New Delhi, India

Ashok Seth
Padma Bhushan and Padma Shri Awardee
Chairman, Fortis Escorts Heart Institute
Past President, National CSI
Vice President, APSC
New Delhi, India

PK Deb
Formerly Chief Cardiologist
ESI PG Institute of Medical Sciences
Past President, National CSI
Kolkata, West Bengal, India

KC Goswami
Professor of Cardiology
All India Institute of Medical Sciences (AIIMS)
New Delhi, India
President Elect CSI-2018
Chairman Scientific Committee
CSICON-2018

K Sarat Chandra
Interventional Cardiologist
Indo-US Super Specialty Hospital
Hyderabad, Telangana, India
President, National CSI

Preface

Echocardiography represents the most widely used and the most cost effective modality in the non-invasive armamentarium of the physician for the assessment of a suspected or known cardiac disorder. The disorder could be primary or secondary to other systemic disease entities or could result as a side effect of therapies and interventions used to manage some of these conditions. The technique has found application not only in the adult, but also in the pediatric patient and the fetus. It also serves as a valuable adjunct in many cardiac and peripheral vascular interventions performed in the cardiac catheterization laboratory and the operating room. The two-dimensional and three-dimensional (more aptly, four-dimensional) modalities together with conventional pulsed, continuous and color Doppler serve to assess all the four cardiac valves for structural abnormalities, all the four cardiac chambers for global and regional function and any intra-cavitary or external mass lesions, the pericardium for any disorders and the proximal great vessels for any pathologies. In addition, all types of congenital cardiac abnormalities including shunt lesions and other more complicated lesions are well evaluated by these techniques. In patients with poor transthoracic acoustic windows, contrast echocardiography and transesophageal echocardiography have come to the rescue of physician and technologist echocardiographers and represent important supplementary techniques. Echocardiography as a modality has still not reached a plateau despite being in vogue for more than half a century and newer refinements in technique with superior quality images and other recent advances such as speckle tracking echocardiography for evaluation of both systolic and diastolic ventricular function, velocity vector imaging, particle velocitimetry, fusion imaging with other non-invasive techniques and artificial intelligence algorithms for cardiac function evaluation are being clinically introduced at a rapid rate. It is therefore important to have a book which will provide a concise state-of-the-art review of echocardiography as it is currently used in the assessment of various cardiac disease entities and more importantly, cover advances which have been recently introduced in the field. This in essence is the aim of this book which covers not only echocardiography, but also other imaging modalities and interventions.

It gives us immense pleasure and a great deal of satisfaction to present to you the enormous contribution by a galaxy of eminent authors of international repute and experts in the field of cardiology, echocardiography, imaging neurology, critical care, pulmonology, in this state of art *Advances in Clinical Cardiovascular Imaging, Echocardiography & Interventions: A Textbook of Cardiology*, despite their extremely busy schedule.

Overall, the book consists of 142 chapters grouped in 35 sections. A majority of chapters deals with echocardiography. These include advances in the usefulness of both two- and three-dimensional echocardiography in the evaluation of left ventricular hypertrophy, mass, diastolic dysfunction, and both left ventricular and left atrial strain.in patients with systemic hypertension. As would be expected, state-of-the-art assessment and recent advances in echocardiography in the diagnosis and management of both systolic and diastolic heart failure, echocardiographic navigation in myocardial infarction with detection of mechanical complications, use of intravascular ultrasound, myocardial perfusion imaging, myocardial viability detection, chest pain evaluation in the Emergency Room, speckle tracking echocardiography, echocardiography in critical care and shock states, management and outcome evaluation, and color flow imaging of coronary arteries are also well covered. The role of echocardiography in the assessment of different types of cardiomyopathy, such as dilated, restrictive and hypertrophic cardiomyopathy, cardiac dyssynchrony, pericardial effusion, oncology, cardiac tamponade and pericardial constriction find good coverage in the book. All types of valvular heart disease encompassing both stenotic and regurgitant lesions, infective endocarditis, prosthetic valve dysfunction, intra-operative echocardiography, heart transplantation, non-cardiac surgery, cardiac structural .interventions such as mitralclip placement, transcatheter aortic valve replacement, rheumatic heart disease, balloon mitral valvuloplasty, incremental value of three/four dimensional echocardiography, pulmonary hypertension, pulmonary embolism, echo based management of patients with atrial fibrillation, including radiofrequency ablation, left atrial appendage closure, syncope work up, ventricular tachycardia storm evaluation are given extensive coverage in the book. The value of echocardiography and ultrasound in patients with aortic syndromes, vertebral artery disease and carotid artery disease with special reference to newer refinements are well described. Last but not least, advances in echocardiographic assessment of all types of congenital heart disease, including neonatal heart failure are fully discussed.

We have made every possible effort to maintain the quality and standard of *Advances in Clinical Cardiovascular Imaging, Echocardiography & Interventions.* We are sure this book will serve as an important reference guide for postgraduate students, fellows, internists, cardiologists, neurologist, critical care, pulmonologist, pediatricians, pedaitric surgeons, cardiovascular surgeons, imaging experts and nutritionists, etc.

Bringing up *Advances in Clinical Cardiovascular Imaging, Echocardiography & Interventions* was a phenomenal task and requires well-structured team efforts with immense dedication, devotion and coordination.

We express our gratitude to all the eminent cardiologists including M Khalilullah, Naresh Trehan, GS Sainani, SC Manchanda, C Venkata S Ram, Amal Kumar Banerejee, Ashok Seth, PK Deb, Santanu Guha, MS Hiremath, K Sarat Chandra, KC Goswami for writing the foreword for this book.

We also express our thanks to each and every member of CSI, manuscript contributors, industry and our Principal Editors SK Parashar, G Vijayaraghavan, R Alagesan, GS Wander, Viveka Kumar, P Krishnam Raju and all the editors for their constant support.

We dedicate this state-of-the-art book to Cardiological Society of India, our teachers, all the members of CSI, our parents, our colleagues, patients, students and our family for being supportive and encouraging throughout in bringing out this *Advances in Clinical Cardiovascular Imaging, Echocardiography & Interventions.*

We also express our thanks to M/s Jaypee Brothers Medical Publishers (P) Ltd. New Delhi, India, for publishing this book so well. We also thank Mr Jitendar P Vij (Group Chairman), Mr Ankit Vij (Managing Director), Ms Chetna Malhotra Vohra (Associate Director—Content Strategy), Nikita Chauhan (Senior Development Editor) and Samina Khan (Executive Assistant to Director, Publishing), for their help, guidance and timely active intervention in composing, designing and editing of the book.

Our sincere thanks to Soban Singh, who worked really hard to keep the record of every minor and finer communication.

Albert Einstein once said

"Learn from yesterday, live for today, hope for tomorrow. The important thing is not to stop questioning".

Navin C Nanda, HK Chopra, Jagat Narula

Preface

The evolution of medicine is going to depend on advances in phenomics and genomics, and artificial intelligence that will allow making the most sense of each and their interaction. Whereas genomics aims at the collective characterization of genes that direct the production of proteins, phenomics is concerned with the measurement of physical and biochemical traits belonging to a given organism as they change in response to genetic and environmental influences. Imaging strategies conveniently identify the physical characteristics, differentiate abnormal traits and will play a role from the bedside to most sophisticated assessment of the evolution of pathology.

Echocardiography represents the most widely used and the most cost effective modality in the non-invasive armamentarium of the physician for the assessment of a suspected or known cardiac disorder. It is expected that ultrasound would be used ubiquitously at the bedside (*dubbed "insonation"*) and be incorporated as the fifth component of the physical examination beyond inspection, palpation, percussion, auscultation. Seeing pathology through imaging would improve interest in physical examination, and should permit appropriate downstream testing and intelligent decision making. Miniaturization of the ultrasound platforms for handheld devices has allowed its renaming to proverbial *"stethoscope"* which literally means looking into the chest (*stethos = chest, Gr.*). Besides a convenient diagnostic acuity, ultrasound serves as a valuable accompaniment during cardiac and peripheral vascular interventional procedures performed in the cardiac catheterization laboratory and the operating room. The 3-dimensional and more aptly, 4-dimensional ensemble with conventional pulsed, continuous and color Doppler serve to assess almost all structural and functional cardiac abnormalities and the proximal great vessel pathology. Echocardiography is the most valued, trusted and used tool in the critical care units. The contrast echocardiography provides enhanced imaging and transesophageal echocardiography provides information from as close as we can get to the heart. Intravascular and intracavitary imaging provide a unique characterization of vascular pathology and assistance in intracardiac manipulation which are less amenable to the use of other more traditionally used laser-based imaging modalities. Echocardiography is constantly being exploited with novel algorithms such as speckle tracking, velocity vector imaging, particle velocitimetry.

Coronary computed tomography imaging has become the fastest growing cardiovascular specialty. A large number of investigations in a short period of time and multiple randomized studies have firmly established it as the primary modality in the assessment of symptomatic and asymptomatic stable coronary disease. It is being proposed as the most cost-effective strategy for the evaluation of patients with no known coronary disease regardless of symptomatic status. Not only does the CT angiography describe the extent of luminal compromise it also allows precise identification of high-risk plaques and calculates fractional flow reserve, and thereby provides a complete anatomic and physiologic characterization of the coronary lesion. A complete assessment of peripheral arteries, entire aorta, including arch and root, and the measurements of valve ring and left ventricular outflow tract also renders it to be an ideal preoperative diagnostic and preparatory strategy for the rampantly increasing transcutaneous aortic valve replacement procedures. Magnetic resonance imaging, on the other hand, provides an ultimate anatomic characterization tool for myocardial alterations, cavity dimensions, structural valvular and congenital anomalies, and large vessel abnormalities. Gadolinium-based enhancements allow definition of interstitial and replacement fibrosis, and the state of myocardial perfusion.

It is therefore important to have a compendium which will provide a concise state-of-the-art review of cardiovascular imaging modalities as currently used in the assessment of various cardiac disease entities and more importantly, cover recent advances pertinent to the field.

It gives us immense pleasure to present to you the enormous efforts of eminent authors and experts from the domain of cardiovascular imaging, neurology, critical care, pulmonology, in this state-of-art *Advances in Clinical Cardiovascular Imaging, Echocardiography & Interventions: A Textbook of Cardiology*. The book comprises 142 chapters grouped in 35 sections and exhaustively discusses the role of various imaging modalities in the context of specific diseases, and comparative roles for each modality. Although various modalities claim to offer one-stop-shop value we have tried to discern as to where we could obtain the maximum benefit. We are sure this book will serve as an important reference guide for fellows and residents, internists, cardiologists, neurologist, pulmonologist, pediatricians, pedaitric surgeons, cardiovascular surgeons, imaging experts, critical care physicians, and nutritionists alike. We also express our sincere gratitude to all the eminent cardiologists who have contributed to this gigantic effort. Our gratitude is also due to Soban Singh, who worked really hard to keep the record of communications.

We dedicate this state-of-the-art book to the Cardiological Society of India and its members, our patients and students who have been our best teachers, and to our family for being supportive and encouraging through the preparation of the text for Advances in Clinical Cardiovascular Imaging, Echocardiography & Interventions.

We sincerely believe that imaging would become a second nature to the physicians. Medical students will learn anatomy and physiology by carrying handheld ultrasound devices in pockets quite as the stethoscopes and with learning to discern organ system abnormalities during their clinical rotations concurrent with their learning of pathology. The later years in the medical school will allow them to use insonation as the examination strategy for the differential diagnosis of a given clinical presentation. Similarly, it is expected that then we will be able to do away with the age-old practice of cadaveric dissection by CT and MR imaging. A medical student would be an imager at graduation from medical school and we insist that to be a good doctor we would need to be a good imager.

Jagat Narula, HK Chopra, Navin C Nanda

International Editors

National Editors

The Scientific Committee of Advances in Clinical Cardiovascular Imaging, Echocardiography & Interventions: A Textbook of Cardiology Express their gratitude and thanks to the following Academic Partners

Platinum Academic Partners

USV Private Limited

Emcure Pharmaceutical Limited
IPCA Laboratories Limited

Gold Academic Partners

Sun Pharmaceutical Industries Limited
Sanofi India Limited

Merck Limited
Three Dots Lifesciences

Silver Academic Partners

Zydus Cadila Healthcare Limited
Eris Lifesciences Private Limited

Torrent Pharma
Nutrabuff Nutraceuticals

Bronze Academic Partners

JB Chemicals & Pharmaceuticals Limited
Supporter:

Micro Labs Limited
Glenmark Pharmaceutical Limited

For rendering unrestricted education grant which made this book possible in its current enhanced form as "Global Education Initiative".

Contents

SECTION 4: ST-ELEVATION MYOCARDIAL INFARCTION AND CORONARY ARTERY DISEASE

SECTION 8: RHEUMATIC HEART DISEASE

SECTION 9: ATRIAL FIBRILLATION

SECTION 10: VENTRICULAR TACHYCARDIA STORM

SECTION 11: DILATED CARDIOMYOPATHY

SECTION 18: PULMONARY HYPERTENSION

SECTION 19: AORTIC DISEASE

SECTION 20: CAROTID ARTERY DISEASE

SECTION 21: VERTEBRAL ARTERY DISEASE

SECTION 22: PERIPHERAL ARTERIAL AND VENOUS DISEASE

SECTION 23: SYNCOPE

SECTION 24: STROKE

SECTION 25: CONGENITAL HEART DISEASE

SECTION 31: INTRAOPERATIVE ECHOCARDIOGRAPHY IN OPERATION THEATER

SECTION 32: SURGERY AND IMAGING

SECTION 33: ECHO ONCOLOGY

SECTION 34: ETHICAL AND LEGAL ISSUES

SECTION 35: FUTURE DIRECTIONS

VIDEO LEGENDS

Video 1: A large myxoma in left atrium.
Video 2: A myxoma in left atrium; smaller compared to Video 1, but producing mitral inflow obstruction.
Video 3: Parasternal long axis view of myxoma attached to anterior mitral leaflet and prolapsing to left ventricular outflow tract.
Video 4: Parasternal short axis view of myxoma shown in Video 3.
Video 5: Myxoma in right atrium producing tricuspid inlet obstruction.
Video 6: A sweep of four-chamber view showing multiple rhabdomyomas in the ventricular septum, apex, and lateral wall of ventricle.
Video 7: Myxosarcoma in left atrium prolapsing into left ventricle. Note the bulky, mobile, heterogeneous mass with the areas of echolucency suggestive of necrosis.
Video 8: Lymphoma in right ventricular outflow tract, producing turbulence in outflow tract.
Video 9: Thickening in free wall and septum due to secondaries from an unknown site.
Video 10: A small thrombus in the left atrial appendage.

**The videos (Chapter 131) are available on www.emedince360.com*

SECTION 1

Basics

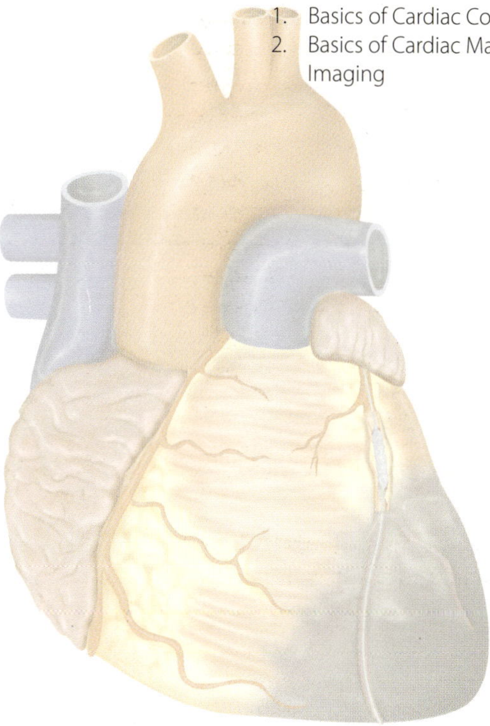

CHAPTER 1

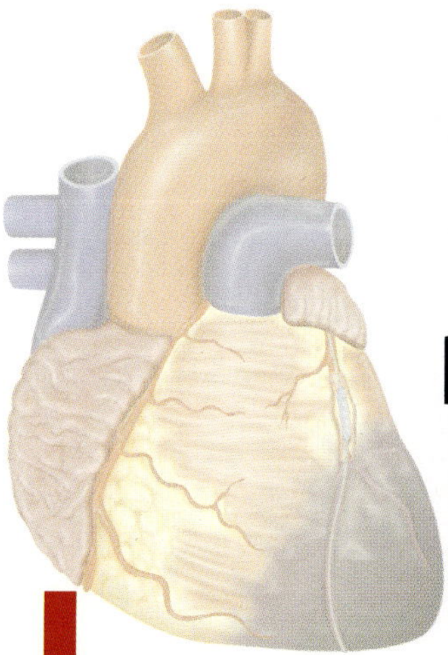

Basics of Cardiac Computed Tomography

Priya Jagia, Kartik Ganga, Arun Sharma

INTRODUCTION

Diagnostic evaluation of cardiac diseases has become very advanced with the advent of cardiac computed tomography (CT). CT is now an indispensable component in the armamentarium of currently available imaging techniques. At present, CT scan can be used as a primary or complementary investigative modality for a variety of cardiac diseases, including ischemic heart disease, congenital heart disorders, aortic and pulmonary artery pathologies, and for pulmonary venous mapping. CT now contributes to screening, diagnosis, treatment optimization, and follow-up of patient with diverse cardiovascular diseases.

BASIC CONCEPTS OF CARDIAC COMPUTED TOMOGRAPHY WITH TECHNICAL DEVELOPMENTS

Technically, a basic CT scanner measures the attenuation of multiple X-ray beams passing through different sequential sections of the body from a multitude of different angles. Using these values, pictures of the internal organs are reconstructed. Classically, CT requires at least 180° of gantry rotation to perform image formation. Initial generation CT scanners required 1–5 seconds (s) to acquire a single slice. Rotation speed of up to 0.3–0.4 s per rotation provided by current generation CT scanners allows for increased temporal resolution.[1] Though, adequate, for most organ systems, it is still not optimal for cardiac CT as heart exhibits a fast complex three-dimensional (3D) motion, which varies from patient to patient and also within the cardiac cycle. For images in cardiac CT to be of diagnostic utility, cardiac CT has to provide images of the heart that are motion free and that correspond to a specific phase of the cardiac cycle. This goal is achieved by synchronizing data acquisition with the cardiac cycle. This synchronization is done using the concurrent acquisition of the electrocardiography (ECG) signal and overcomes the problem of cardiac motion making quantitative data calculation, such as ejection fractions and volumetric assessments possible. In the quest for further reducing scan times and improving temporal resolution, a new concept that simultaneously utilizes two X-ray sources—dual source CT (DSCT)—was introduced. These scanners require only a 90° rotation to acquire sufficient data and hence exhibit a high temporal resolution in the order of 50–60 ms.[2] Moreover, current CT systems are capable of providing a 3D isotropic acquisition, thereby improving spatial resolution for accurate depiction of smaller cardiac structures, including coronaries. The newer third-generation DSCT scanners provide excellent image quality over a wide range of body sizes and heart rates at lower radiation doses than the previous generation CT scanners. Faster gantry rotation time combined with larger Z-axis volume coverage per rotation combine to enable single-heart beat acquisitions in most patients with heart rates of up to 75–80 beats/min.[2] Generally, cardiac CT requires intravenous injection of iodinated contrast agent, with the exception of CT calcium scoring which achieves CT acquisition without contrast. Low contrast protocols described in various studies result in significant reduction in contrast medium requirements, without any

Flowchart 1: Classification and uses of cardiac CT.

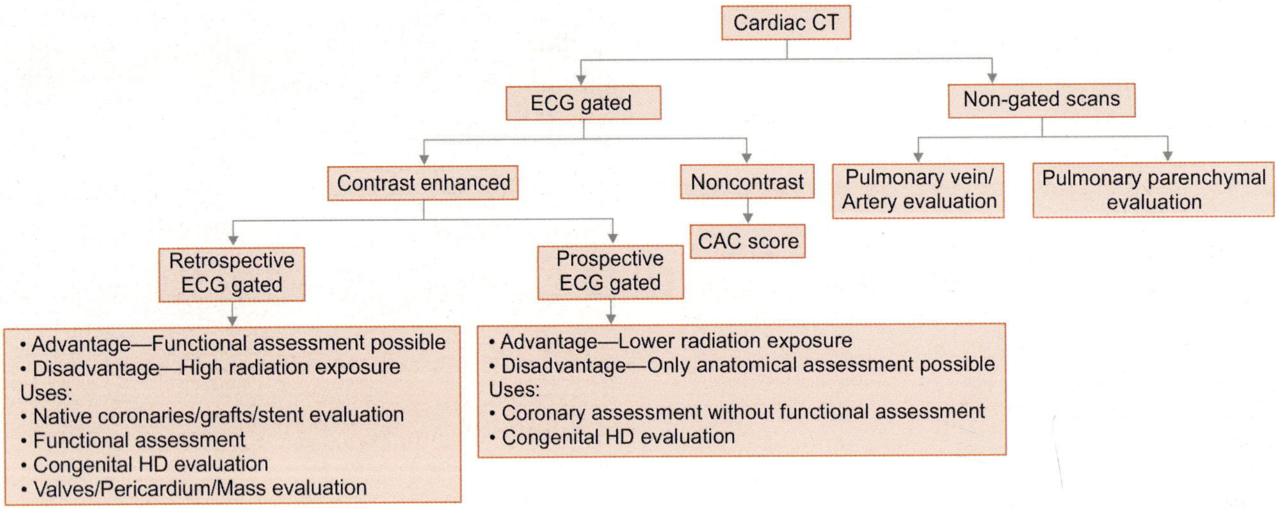

(CT: computed tomography)

difficulties in contrast medium timing or unsatisfactory vessel enhancement.[3] Recent advancements in multislice CT technology have made coronary computed tomography angiography (CTA) a very useful modality in imaging the coronaries with submillisievert doses using very low contrast load, which is of paramount importance in patients with reduced renal functions (Flowchart 1).[4]

Types of Cardiac Computed Tomography (Flowchart 2)

Depending on the area of interest, cardiac CT can be broadly divided into ECG-gated and non-ECG-gated CTs.

Electrocardiography-gated CTs are primarily used for coronary artery assessment. However, they can also be useful in valvular assessment, congenital heart disease (CHD) evaluation, and functional cardiac assessment. *Non-ECG-gated CTs* are useful in morphological assessment of the pulmonary arteries and veins, pericardial assessment, and anatomical assessment of CHD and valves where functional indices are not required.

Gated Cardiac Computed Tomographies

The least amount of cardiac movement is during the end-systole and end-diastole of a particular cardiac cycle. This phase, however, varies with increasing heart rate which narrows the acquisition window. Therefore, motion-free imaging is usually best acquired in these phases. With higher heart rates, however, this dictum no longer applies, and it is advisable to acquire data in all the phases of the cardiac cycle for better visualization of cardiac and coronary morphology. Two gating techniques are utilized: (1) retrospective gating and (2) prospective gating.

Flowchart 2: Acquisition and interpretation of cardiac CT.

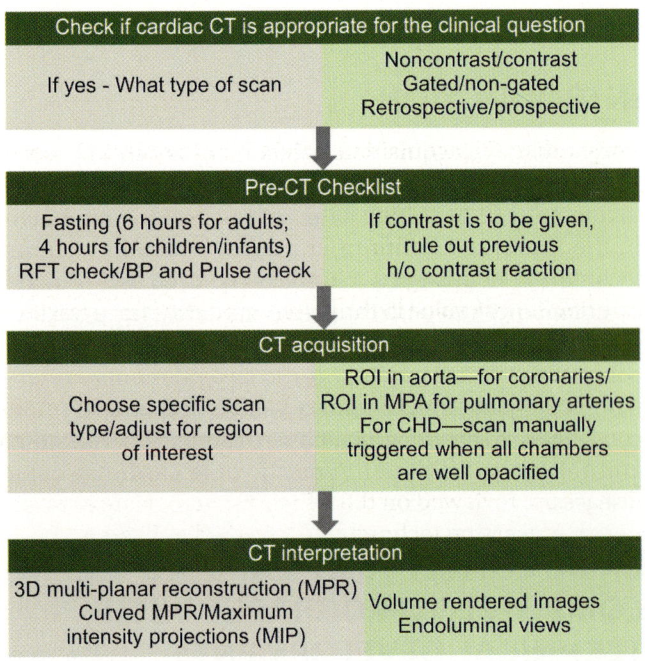

(CT: computed tomography)

Retrospective gating: This is achieved by gating the acquisition with the cardiac cycle with acquisition throughout all the phases of cardiac cycle. Data from several consecutive cardiac cycles is continuously acquired with simultaneous ECG recording, leading to generation of true 3D data set, consisting of overlapping axial imaging slices. Any cardiac phase can, therefore, be reconstructed, but this occurs at the expense of a relatively high radiation dose.[5] Since data from all the cardiac phases are available, ventricular functions (ejection fraction) and volumetric assessment can be performed. This scan is less sensitive to the changes of heart rate during the scan. The images can also be retrospectively analyzed and missed or extra beats can be excluded for analysis during ECG correction.

Prospective gating: This is a sequential CT scan which uses step and shoot technique to overcome the motion of the heart enabling data acquisition in only a certain phase of the cardiac cycle. If only morphological assessment is required, such as only coronary artery imaging, prospectively triggered sequences can be used. Using these sequences, preselection of a fraction of the RR interval width is done, and this allows imaging during a predefined cardiac phase (usually mid-diastole, when there is least cardiac motion—at approximately 75% of the cardiac cycle). With this scan, estimation of the next RR interval is of paramount importance and hence can be performed only in patients with regular heart rates. This type of scan is associated with lower radiation exposure to the patient as compared to retrospectively gated scans but does not allow ventricular functional analysis.[6]

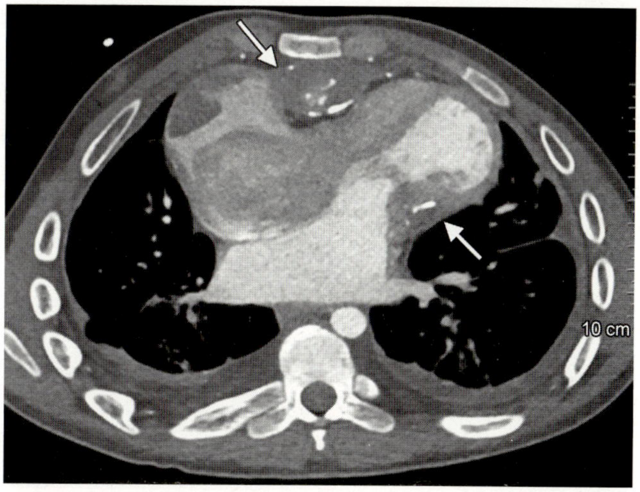

Fig. 1: Axial section showing thickened calcific pericardium causing constriction of bilateral ventricles. Also noted is mild bilateral pleural effusion (arrows).

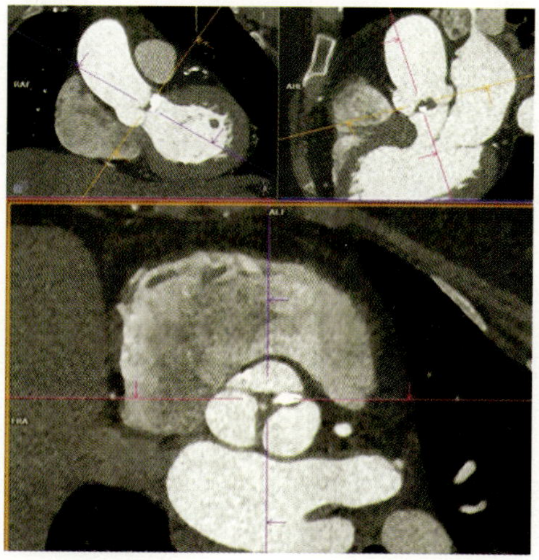

Fig. 2: 3D MPR showing calcified thickened tricuspid aortic valve in three different planes. (3D: three-dimensional; MPR: multiplanar reconstruction)

Acquisition and Interpretation of Cardiac Computed Tomography (Flowchart 2)

For cardiac CT acquisition, injection of contrast is done via an automatic injector which injects the contrast intravenously at a high flow rate (3–5 mL/s in adults and 1–3 mL/s in children/infants). The scan is usually programmed to begin automatically once the contrast reaches its peak value in the vessel of interest (for coronaries and aorta—vessel of interest is the proximal descending thoracic aorta; for pulmonary arteries—vessel of interest is the main pulmonary artery; for CHD evaluation—scan is triggered manually when all the chambers of the heart are optimally opacified). After the data is acquired, the images are reviewed on the CT workstation using a variety of postprocessing techniques (described in Figures 1 to 5) to reach a diagnosis (Table 1).[7,8]

Uses of Gated Cardiac Computed Tomography (Box 1)

Coronary Artery Calcium Scoring

It involves prospectively gated noncontrast cardiac CT acquisition for the assessment of coronary artery calcium (CAC). It identifies and characterizes the location as well as burden of coronary artery disease (CAD) by detecting calcium within plaques. Calcium being defined as areas with greater than 130 HU, these coronary calcifications are usually automatically detected and color-coded. Semi-quantification of coronary calcium is expressed by the Agatston score, which uses the plaque size, density, and a weighting factor to calculate a value ranging from 0 (absence of detectable calcium) to over 1,000 (indicating extensive coronary calcification). An elevated CAC score has consistently been associated with increased mortality and adverse cardiovascular events, independent of other risk factors. CAC score has been found to be superior to well-established cardiovascular risk factor models for predicting silent myocardial ischemia and short-term outcomes.[9] However, the association between CAC score and the extent of coronary atherosclerosis is not linear as severe coronary stenosis can occur at sites with limited calcium deposition and vice versa. *Thus, CAC scoring is better used as a risk stratification tool to identify high-risk asymptomatic patients*

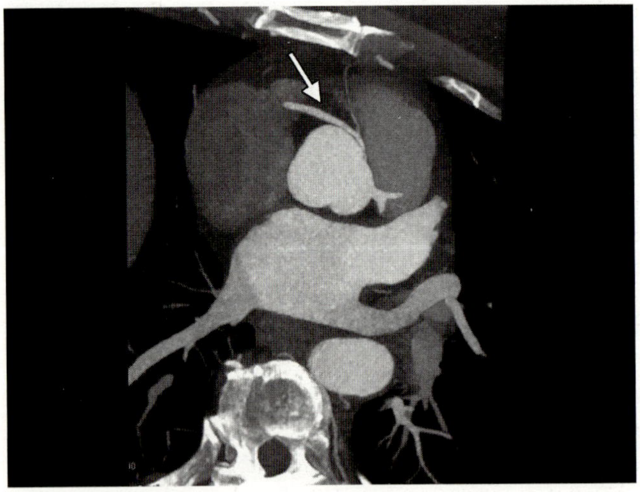

Fig. 3: MIP showing anomalous origin of RCA with interarterial course between aorta and pulmonary artery (arrow). (MIP: maximum intensity projection; RCA: right coronary artery)

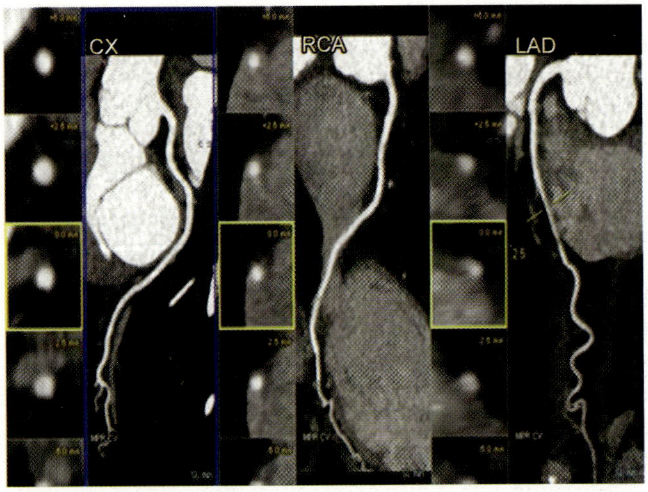

Fig. 5: VRT image of a child with truncus arteriosus showing a common arterial trunk arising from the left ventricle. (VRT: volume-rendered reconstruction)

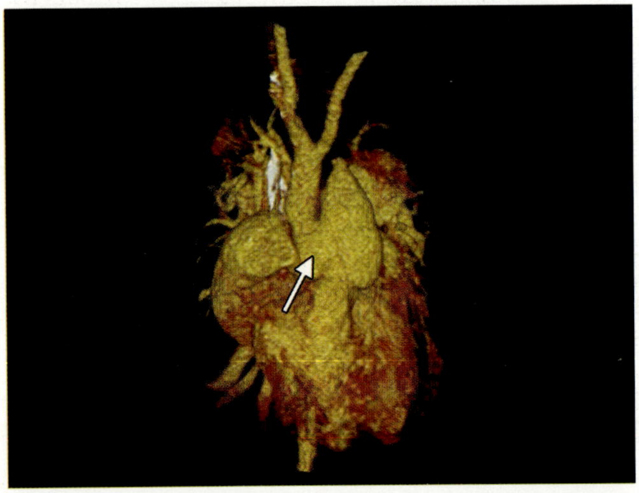

Fig. 4: Curved MPR showing the entire extent of the coronary arterial tree in one image (arrow). (MPR: multiplanar reconstruction)

TABLE 1

Axial data set "Raw" images with thin-section volumetric data (*see* Fig. 1)	3D multiplanar reconstruction (MPR) Thin-section volumetric data with reconstructed sagittal and coronal views (*see* Fig. 2)
Maximum intensity projections (MIP) Thick-section images with accentuated intensity of contrast (Fig. 3)	Curved MPR Displays vessel in a user-determined curved surface as a single image (Fig. 4)
Volume-rendered reconstruction (VRT) 3D illustration of volumetric CT data for display from any desired perspective (Fig. 5)	Endoluminal views VRT technique that simulates an endoscopic examination by locating a point of view from inside hollow structures (Fig. 6)

(3D: three-dimensional; CT: computed tomography)

who might benefit from further investigations rather than being a diagnostic test for obstructive CAD.

Computed Tomography Coronary Angiography for Native Coronaries (Figs. 3 and 4)

Unlike the CAC scan, this scan requires intravenous injection of iodinated contrast. CTCA has a high sensitivity and specificity for diagnosing coronary stenosis. CTCA allows identification of coronary atherosclerotic plaques in the absence of calcium or stenosis, thus permitting visualization of early subclinical atherosclerosis. Studies have demonstrated excellent diagnostic accuracy of CTCA for the detection of coronary stenosis, with a sensitivity of

BOX 1: Appropriate use of cardiac computed tomography.[12,25]

- CAC score assessment of risk in asymptomatic individuals
- Coronary artery evaluation in symptomatic patients with low to intermediate pretest probability of obstructive CAD
- Assessment of bypass grafts and appropriate stents
- Morphological and functional evaluation of ventricles
- CHD evaluation
- Morphological and functional evaluation of valves—pre-/postoperative
- Evaluation of pericardial anatomy
- Assessment of pulmonary veins and arteries
- Characterization of cardiac mass.

(CAC: coronary artery calcium; CAD: coronary artery disease; CHD: congenital heart disease)

86–99%, specificity of 92–98%, and negative predictive value of 92–100%.[10] The high negative predictive value which approaches 100% is the main advantage of this technique. It can provide detailed information on coronary artery anatomy and assess both coronary artery atherosclerosis as well as luminal stenosis. *In view of its high negative predictive value and high sensitivity, CTCA is the most beneficial in symptomatic patients with low to intermediate pretest probability of obstructive CAD.*[11] Moreover, CTCA can be useful for plaque characterization as studies have shown that plaques with spotty calcification, positive remodeling, or those with a lipid-rich core have a higher (95%) risk of rupture.[12] It is also extremely beneficial in identifying the anomalous origin, course, and termination of the coronary arteries (Fig. 4) and is the investigation of choice for the same. CTCA also allows for noninvasive evaluation of hemodynamics in the coronary arterial tree. Using computational fluid dynamics, "three-vessel" fractional flow reserve (CT-FFR) can be calculated from already acquired coronary CTA data with no need for additional imaging or vasodilators. CT-FFR, therefore, can help in assessing the exact area of blockage and its impact on the flow which may guide treatment strategies.[13]

Coronary Computed Tomography Angiography for Graft and Stents

Computed tomography coronary angiography is the recommended investigation of choice for graft patency in postcoronary artery bypass grafting (CABG) patients with acute chest pain. It is also used for the follow-up of asymptomatic patients in whom CABG has been performed more than 5 years ago. Studies have shown a high sensitivity and specificity each ranging more than 95% with positive predictive value of more than 92–94% and negative predictive value to the tune of almost 99%, in the evaluation of stenosis/occlusion of grafts.[14] Patency of coronary stents too can be evaluated with CTCA. However, CTCA is most useful if the diameter of the stent is more than 3 mm. CT has shown high diagnostic accuracy (sensitivity—91%, specificity—91%, positive predictive value—68%, and negative predictive value—98%) for in stent restenosis of stents greater than 3 mm diameter. Thicker stent material and strut thickness may also affect the accuracy of CTCA adversely.[15]

Assessment of Ventricular Volumes, Wall Thickness, and Mass

Magnetic resonance imaging (MRI) is the investigation of choice for functional assessment. But CT may be an equally *accurate investigation with less inter- and intraobserver variability*. This information is exclusively available with retrospectively gated acquisitions. Not only is the cardiac and coronary morphology assessed but cardiac functional assessment can also be performed with a single contrast-enhanced retrospective ECG-gated examination. Ejection fraction, end-systolic and end-diastolic volumes, stroke volumes, and cardiac output can be calculated.[16] Left ventricular regional function can also be displayed on color-coded maps of wall motion and wall thickness for better assessment of wall-motion abnormalities.

Role of Computed Tomography in Congenital Heart Disease (see Fig. 5)

Though echocardiography (ECHO) remains the investigation of choice in these patients, cardiac CT may be used as a problem-solving tool, especially where only morphological information is required. Moreover, *delineation of extracardiac structures*, including pulmonary arteries, aortopulmonary collaterals, and aortic arch anatomy and associated anomalies, may be better evaluated with CT.[17] Simultaneous assessment of the airway and skeletal abnormalities may influence management options. Techniques such as ECG-gated ultrahigh pitch [fast low-angle shot (FLASH) sequences], ECG padding/pulsing (giving full radiation dose only for a part of the cardiac cycle), using prospective ECG gating, help in radiation dose reduction in this population. Moreover, postoperative evaluation of complications is also better done by CT since it facilitates global and rapid simultaneous assessment of the chest and pleural spaces, airways, lung parenchyma, and vasculature.[18]

Evaluation of Valves

Earlier used primarily to identify valvular calcifications, CT can now depict subtle valvular anatomy and also evaluate valve function. It plays a role in both preoperative evaluation and postsurgical assessment. Another advantage of CT is that the coronary arteries can also be simultaneously evaluated in the same study.

For Morphological and Functional Valvular Assessment

Computed tomography offers excellent morphological assessment of valve leaflets, apposition zones, chordae commissures, and papillary annulus muscles during all the phases of the cardiac cycle.[19] In mitral/aortic stenosis, CT helps in anatomical localization of the stenosis (valvular or subvalvular), presence of calcification (*see* Fig. 2), and the ancillary information, such as degree of left atrium (LA) dilation, left ventricle (LV) function, and coronary artery status, which can help in deciding management. CT plays a very important role in preoperative assessment for transcatheter aortic valve implantation (TAVI) (percutaneous aortic valve implantation). It can

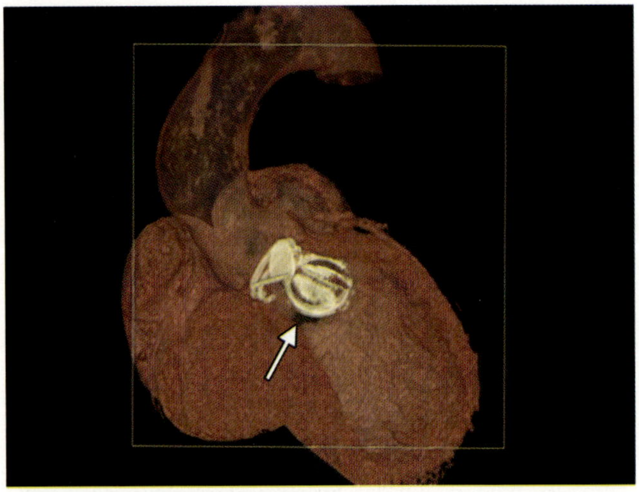

Fig. 6: Endoluminal view showing prosthetic heart valves with tissue discontinuity at the mitral annulus suggesting dehiscence (arrow).

evaluate the aortic root dimensions (for accurate sizing purposes), coronary ostia takeoff as well as LV [specifically left ventricular outflow tract (LVOT)] assessment. CT can also be useful in morphological assessment of the tricuspid valve morphology, especially in the cases, such as Ebstein's anomaly where the displacement of the septal leaflet and redundancy of the anterior leaflet can be depicted in detail. Congenital pulmonary valve abnormalities, such as valvular stenosis or agenesis, can be assessed on CT. Excellent visualization of valve prostheses with minimal streak artifacts can be obtained by CT. Even bioprosthetic valves can be evaluated to assess for leaflet degeneration and dysfunction. Postoperative complications, such as pseudoaneurysms, abscess, paravalvular leaks, and valve dehiscence, can be identified and assessed by CT, providing both anatomic and dynamic information important for redo surgery (Fig. 6).

For Assessment of Valvular Endocarditis

Cardiac CT can demonstrate valvular vegetations, with a sensitivity and specificity of 97% and 88%, far superior to ECHO. On CT, vegetations appear as low-attenuation masses attached to the leaflets.[20] CT is especially helpful in assessing peri- and paravalvular complications, such as abscess, pseudoaneurysm formation, or remote complications, such as septic emboli to the lungs.

Evaluation of Intracardiac Masses

Cardiac CT is often used concomitantly with ECHO and MRI in the evaluation of cardiac masses.[21] Cardiac MRI is the investigation of choice for cardiac masses due to its superior soft-tissue characterization and high temporal resolution. Cardiac CT can be used in patients who cannot undergo an MRI or as an alternative modality. In addition, CT is superior to MRI for the assessment of calcification of the masses. Apart from characterization, CT enables complete evaluation of the chest and lung parenchyma, vascular anatomy, and also allows exclusion of obstructive CAD as a preoperative requisite in older patients.

Pericardial Assessment

Computed tomography enables imaging of the entire pericardium with high spatial and temporal resolution and is an important modality in the diagnostic workup of pericardial diseases (*see* Fig. 1). Moreover, it is the gold standard to visualize calcified pericardium. Although MRI is best suited for pericardial assessment, CT can help in the initial characterization of pericardial effusion (by using HUs to differentiate between transudative and effusive exudate), identifying inflammatory pericarditis (by visualization of enhancing pericardium), assessing constriction (using functional CT), and in characterization of a pericardial mass (enhancement, presence of calcium/fat).[22]

Uses of Nongated Cardiac Computed Tomography

Assessment of Pulmonary Veins: Pulmonary Venous Mapping

Preprocedural CT is helpful for morphological assessment of the pulmonary veins and LA, especially to assess the presence of additional pulmonary veins (e.g. middle lobe vein). This information is vital to the electrophysiologist who is attempting to perform a percutaneous ablation of an arrhythmic focus. Volume- and surface-rendered reconstructions allow for a quick overview of the pulmonary anatomy, thus providing the electrophysiologist with a roadmap prior to the intervention. CT is also useful in identifying postprocedural complications commonly associated with percutaneous ablation, such as pulmonary vein stenosis. For this purpose, however, ECG-gated study is performed for better visualization of the stenosis.[23]

Assessment of Pulmonary Arteries

For evaluation of patients with pathologies of the pulmonary arteries, CT is routinely used.[24,25] Noncontrast study is performed when the assessment of lung parenchyma is the objective. Contrast-enhanced CT may be performed (often with a pulmonary angiography protocol) when chronic thromboembolic pulmonary hypertension (CTEPH) or other parenchymal causes of pulmonary hypertension is suspected. Based on the assessment of pulmonary arteries, heart, parenchyma, and bronchial arteries, the proper etiology of pulmonary hypertension may be identified which helps in planning treatment.

CONCLUSION

Cardiac CT has assumed a wider role in the diagnostic workup of major cardiac pathologies. This has become possible due to continuously evolving technical refinements, such as recent third-generation multislice CT with dual source-dual energy acquisitions, cardiac gating, advanced postprocessing options, and radiation dose reduction strategies. It has now become possible to obtain reproducible functional information in addition to the morphological assessment of cardiac pathologies, thereby influencing the treatment strategies. It is the investigation of choice in emergency settings and in critically ill patients.

REFERENCES

1. Schroeder S, Achenbach S, Bengel F, et al. Cardiac computed tomography: indications, applications, limitations, and training requirements: report of a Writing Group deployed by the Working Group Nuclear Cardiology and Cardiac CT of the European Society of Cardiology and the European Council of Nuclear Cardiology. Eur Heart J. 2008;29(4):531-56.
2. Scheffel H, Alkadhi H, Plass A, et al. Accuracy of dual-source CT coronary angiography: first experience in a high pre-test probability population without heart rate control. Eur Radiol. 2006;16(12):2739-47.
3. Min JK, Lin FY. What makes a coronary CT angiogram nondiagnostic? J Cardiovasc Comput Tomogr. 2008;2(6):351-9.
4. Buechel RR, Husmann L, Herzog BA, et al. Low-dose computed tomography coronary angiography with prospective electrocardiogram triggering: feasibility in a large population. J Am Coll Cardiol. 2011;57(3):332-6.
5. Einstein AJ, Moser KW, Thompson RC, et al. Radiation dose to patients from cardiac diagnostic imaging. Circulation. 2007;116(11):1290-305.
6. Alkadhi H, Leschka S. Radiation dose of cardiac computed tomography—what has been achieved and what needs to be done. Eur Radiol. 2011;21(3):505-9.
7. Lell MM, Anders K, Uder M, et al. New techniques in CT angiography. Radiographics. 2006;26(Suppl 1):S45-62.
8. Anders K, Ropers U, Kuettner A, et al. Individually adapted, interactive multiplanar reformations vs. semi-automated coronary segmentation and curved planar reformations for stenosis detection in coronary computed tomography angiography. Eur J Radiol. 2011;80(1):89-95.
9. Detrano R, Guerci AD, Carr JJ, et al. Coronary calcium as a predictor of coronary events in four racial or ethnic groups. N Engl J Med. 2008;358(13):1336-45.
10. Bax JJ, Schuijf JD. Which role for multislice computed tomography in clinical cardiology? Am Heart J. 2005;149(6): 960-1.
11. Paech DC, Weston AR. A systematic review of the clinical effectiveness of 64-slice or higher computed tomography angiography as an alternative to invasive coronary angiography in the investigation of suspected coronary artery disease. BMC Cardiovasc Disord. 2011;11:32.
12. Taylor AJ, Cerqueira M, Hodgson JM, et al. ACCF/SCCT/ACR/AHA/ASE/ASNC/NASCI/SCAI/SCMR 2010 appropriate use criteria for cardiac computed tomography. A report of the American College of Cardiology Foundation Appropriate Use Criteria Task Force, the Society of Cardiovascular Computed Tomography, the American College of Radiology, the American Heart Association, the American Society of Echocardiography, the American Society of Nuclear Cardiology, the North American Society for Cardiovascular Imaging, the Society for Cardiovascular Angiography and Interventions, and the Society for Cardiovascular Magnetic Resonance. J Am Coll Cardiol. 2010;56(22):1864-94.
13. Norgaard BL, Leipsic J, Gaur S, et al. Diagnostic performance of noninvasive fractional flow reserve derived from coronary computed tomography angiography in suspected coronary artery disease: the NXT trial (Analysis of Coronary Blood Flow Using CT Angiography: Next Steps). J Am Coll Cardiol. 2014;63(12):1145-55.
14. Hamon M, Champ-Rigot L, Morello R, et al. Diagnostic accuracy of in-stent coronary restenosis detection with multislice spiral computed tomography: a meta-analysis. Eur Radiol. 2008;18(2):217-25.
15. Smith SC, Jr., Feldman TE, Hirshfeld JW, Jr., et al. ACC/AHA/SCAI 2005 guideline update for percutaneous coronary intervention: a report of the American College of Cardiology/American Heart Association Task Force on Practice Guidelines (ACC/AHA/SCAI Writing Committee to Update the 2001 Guidelines for Percutaneous Coronary Intervention). J Am Coll Cardiol. 2006;47(1):e1-121.
16. Rizvi A, Deano RC, Bachman DP, et al. Analysis of ventricular function by CT. J Cardiovasc Comput Tomogr. 2015;9(1):1-12.
17. Dillman JR, Hernandez RJ. Role of CT in the evaluation of congenital cardiovascular disease in children. AJR Am J Roentgenol. 2009;192(5):1219-31.
18. Fidler JL, Cheatham JP, Fletcher SE, et al. CT angiography of complications in pediatric patients treated with intravascular stents. AJR Am J Roentgenol. 2000;174(2):355-9.
19. Chen JJ, Manning MA, Frazier AA, et al. CT angiography of the cardiac valves: normal, diseased, and postoperative appearances. Radiographics. 2009;29(5):1393-412.
20. Koo HJ, Yang DH, Kang JW, et al. Demonstration of infective endocarditis by cardiac CT and transoesophageal echocardiography: comparison with intraoperative findings. Eur Heart J Cardiovasc Imaging. 2018;19(2):199-207.
21. Kassop D, Donovan MS, Cheezum MK, et al. Cardiac masses on cardiac CT: a review. Curr Cardiovasc Imaging Rep. 2014;7:9281.
22. O'Leary SM, Williams PL, Williams MP, et al. Imaging the pericardium: appearances on ECG-gated 64-detector row cardiac computed tomography. Br J Radiol. 2010;83(987):194-205.
23. Manghat NE, Mathias HC, Kakani N, et al. Pulmonary venous evaluation using electrocardiogram-gated 64-detector row cardiac CT. Br J Radiol. 2012;85(1015):965-71.
24. Dogan H, de Roos A, Geleijins J, et al. The role of computed tomography in the diagnosis of acute and chronic pulmonary embolism. Diagn Interv Radiol. 2015;21(4):307-16.
25. Halpern EJ. Clinical applications of cardiac CT angiography. Insights Imaging. 2010;1(4):205-22.

CHAPTER 2

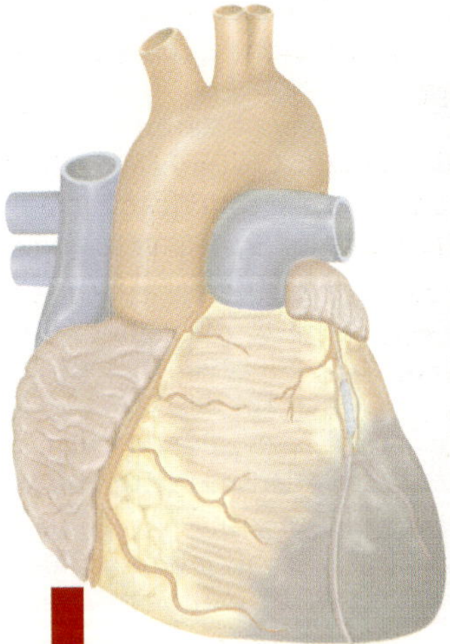

Basics of Cardiac Magnetic Resonance Imaging

Johann Christopher

INTRODUCTION

Magnetic resonance imaging (MRI) works using the principle of nuclear magnetic resonance (MR), that is in the presence of a strong magnetic field (typically 1.5–3.0 T), atoms in the body (hydrogen) are stimulated to emit radio waves. These radio waves are detected by an antenna (coil) placed around, or over, the body part of interest allowing an image of the body to be reconstructed. Extra magnetic fields (gradients) are used to constantly change the magnetic field to allow images of the body to be reconstructed. These fields are created by gradient coils. MRI uses no ionizing radiation and is generally a safe procedure. Contrast in the MR image is primarily due to the inherent magnetic relaxation times within the tissue structure known as the longitudinal relaxation time (T1) and the transverse relaxation time (T2). These two time constants are dependent on the type, and structure, of atoms in the tissue of interest. By altering the timing and strength of the gradient fields during imaging, or through the use of contrast agents, differences in T1 and T2 values between differing tissues can be exploited to produce images.

IMAGING PRINCIPLES

All the signals that are collected under selective applications are registered at the appropriate positions in the spatially encoding space. Once the signals in the *K* space are completely registered, the image of an object is readily obtained by two-dimensional (2D) Fourier transformation of the signal in the *K* space. Electrocardiography (ECG) synchronization helps acquire images of the beating heart without artifacts. Prospective ECG gating uses the preceding R wave as a trigger to acquire a segment of *K*-lines in the *K* space within a short period of time. Retrospective ECG gating continuously acquires data and retrospectively matches the data to the corresponding positions of the ECG gating. This synchronization method is capable of imaging the entire cardiac cycle.

CARDIAC STRUCTURE

Cardiac MRI can assess cardiac structures with adequate spatial resolution and tissue contrast.

Dark Blood and Dark Fat Imaging

This technique uses the double inversion (IR) preparation pulses to null the blood signal and delineates the cardiac structures with the blood darkened. The blood appears dark and the myocardium light in the acquired images. Triple IR is a technique that uses two IR pulses for dark blood preparation, followed by an IR pulse to suppress the fat signal commonly known as the dark fat appearance. Dark blood imaging is routinely used in the assessment of vascular abnormalities, such as congenital intracardiac anomalies, aortic or vascular disease, and myocardial abnormalities, such as nonischemic cardiomyopathy, myocarditis, mediastinal lymphadenopathy (Fig. 1), and cardiovascular tumors.

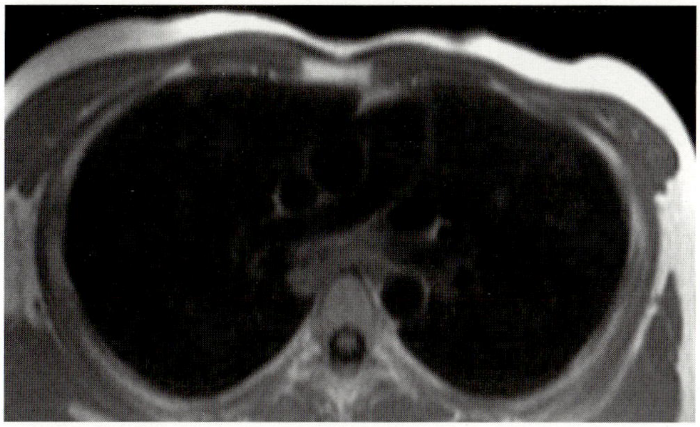

Fig. 1

CARDIAC FUNCTION

Cine MRI is a technique that takes images of the heart in motion throughout the cardiac cycle and displays the cardiac motion in a cine loop fashion. Owing to high tissue contrast between the myocardium and blood, periodic changes of the cardiac chambers and ventricular walls can be readily visualized. This allows accurate quantification of the ventricular function and local wall motion.

White blood imaging: Cine MRI uses a balanced steady-state free precession (bSSFP) technique combined with retrospective ECG gating to assess cardiac function. The bSSFP is a rapid gradient echo (GRE) sequence which ensures high-signal intensity of the images despite very short time to repetition (TR). In addition the bSSFP sequence produces high tissue contrast between the myocardium and blood owing to its unique T1/T2 contrast and inflow effect (Fig. 2A). Cardiac MRI has been considered as a gold standard in the assessment of systolic function of the left ventricle (LV).[1] In addition to volumetric quantification, cine images also allow evaluation of the valvular insufficiency, outflow or inflow tract obstruction, dyssynchrony or asynchrony of the ventricular wall, or mobility of the cardiac tumors.

Ventricular function: Global function of the LV or right ventricle (RV) can be assessed with cine MRI in multiple short-axis views based on Simpson's rule.[2] According to Simpson's rule, ventricular volume at a particular cardiac phase can be estimated by summing the encircled areas of a stack of slices from apical to basal level and multiplying the slice thickness (Fig. 2B). The end-diastolic volume (EDV) and end-systolic volume (ESV) can be obtained, which are then used to compute the stroke volume (SV = EDV – ESV) and ejection fraction (EF = SV/EDV).[3]

The LV mass is quantified by taking the difference between the ventricular volume measured from the epicardial contours and EDV and multiplied by the density of the myocardium (1.05 g/cm^3). The mass-to-volume ratio is a useful index of LV geometric remodeling and is calculated by the ratio of the LV mass divided by the EDV.[4] Accurate quantification of the RV is important for congenital heart disease, such as tetralogy of Fallot, transposition of great arteries, and arrhythmogenic RV dysplasia.[5-7] The RV function estimation, based on Simpson's rule, is recommended due to the complex geometry of the RV. Quantification of regional wall thickening for each myocardial segment is obtained by calculating the ratio of the wall thickness at end-diastole to that at end-systole.

Myocardial T2 and T2* Mapping

Myocardial T2 mapping is a technique used to reconstruct a parametric image based on the T2 value measured in each voxel. The accumulation of water in the myocardium is associated with different types of pathology, such as

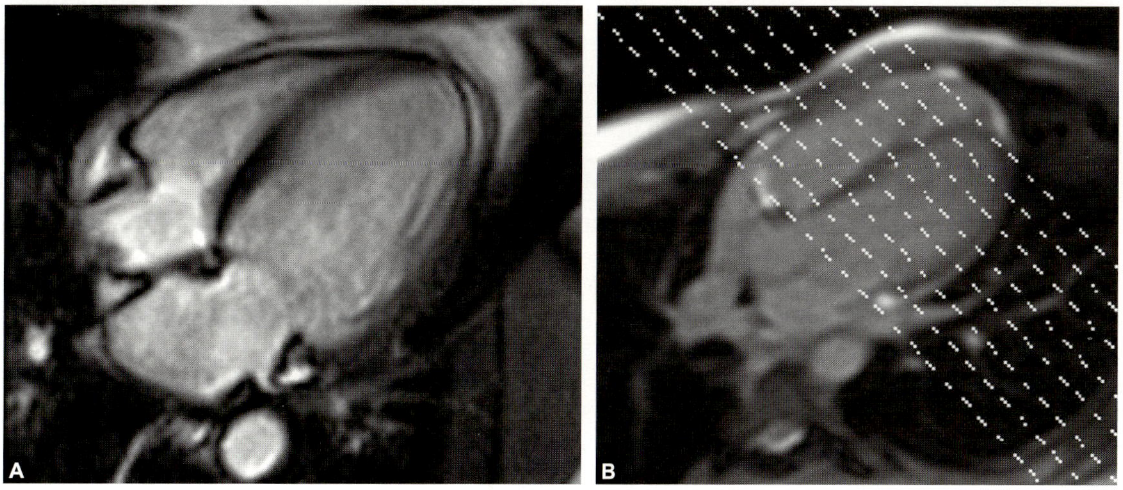

Figs. 2A and B

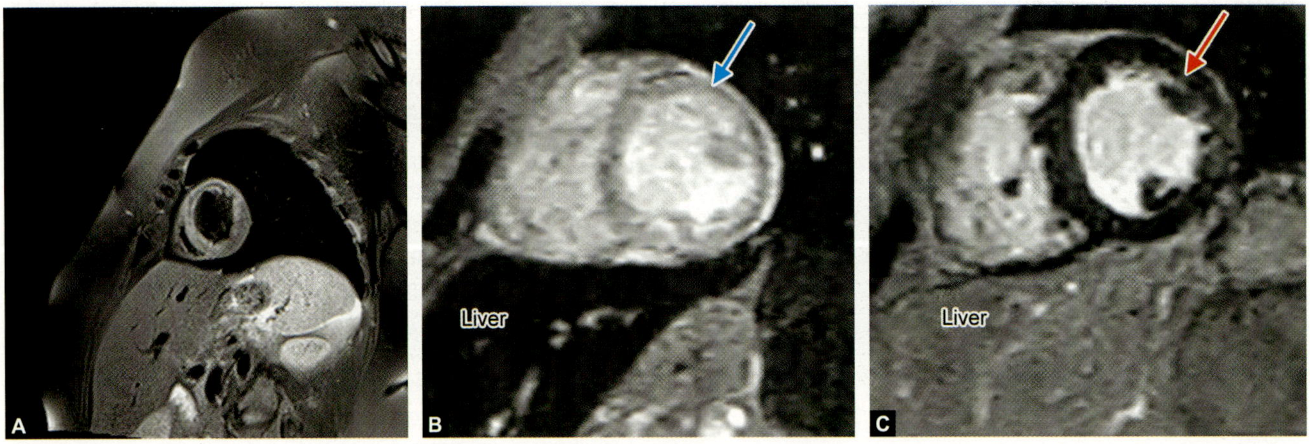

Figs. 3A to C

acute myocardial infarction (Fig. 3A), myocarditis, and graft rejection. Based on the property of a long transverse relaxation time of water protons, myocardial T2 mapping is well suited to detect and quantify myocardial edema in ischemic regions at rest and microvascular obstruction.[8] T2* relaxation is a technique based on the rapid decay of transverse magnetization caused by a local magnetic field inhomogeneity. Myocardial T2* mapping is sensitive to tissue iron content, and so it is specifically utilized in the quantification of iron deposition in the myocardium in patients with thalassemia major (Figs. 3B and C) in order to titrate iron chelation therapy and for prognostication irrespective of liver iron biopsy results and serum ferritin levels.[9]

MYOCARDIAL TISSUE CHARACTERIZATION

Late Gadolinium Enhancement Magnetic Resonance Imaging

Late gadolinium (Gd) MRI images are acquired in the short-axis orientation 15 minutes after the injection of 0.2 mmol/kg of Gd-diethylenetriaminepentaacetic acid using an IR recovery GRE sequence. Gd is a nonradioactive, paramagnetic element in the lanthanide series. Gd is the active element of several nontissue-specific, hyperosmolar contrast agents. Most Gd-containing contrast agents are excreted unchanged almost exclusively by the kidney. For patients with end-stage renal disease (ESRD), the half-life is reduced dramatically to between 1.9 hours and 2.6 hours if hemodialysis follows the administration of Gd.[10] This technique of using Gd has been named delayed enhancement (DE-MRI) and demonstrates nonviable tissue as hyperenhanced or bright. The replacement fibrosis secondary to ischemic injury hyperenhances, and this indicates the lack of functioning myocytes and, therefore, the lack of viability.

The reason for hyperenhancement is likely the greater distribution volume of injured or scarred myocardium compared with that of normal myocardium. This technique is assuming a prominent role in viability assessment as it can be performed in resting conditions without the need to expose the patient to a stressor agent and without the need for ionizing radiation. The high spatial resolution of delayed contrast-enhanced imaging enables precise measures of the extent of myocardial infarct. It is also possible to differentiate ischemic versus nonischemic etiology in heart failure. Ischemic cardiomyopathy is characterized by subendocardial and/or transmural late Gd enhancement (LGE) in comparison, isolated mid-wall or epicardial enhancement is strongly suggestive of a nonischemic cardiomyopathy.[11] Delayed enhancement MRI performed in conjunction with segmental wall motion assessment by resting cine images has helped define several categories of viability. In a seminal study by Kim et al., there was near perfect correlation demonstrated between hyperenhancement on MRI and irreversible damage at pathology.[12] Clinical studies have confirmed that no DE occurs in dysfunctional myocardium that is viable and displays improved contractile function in response to low-dose (5–10 μg/kg/min) dobutamine infusion. In contrast, where there is transmural DE, there is no contractile activity in response to the dobutamine infusion. Territories that have nontransmural necrosis (Fig. 4A) display a diminished contractile response to dobutamine.[13] The transmural extent of infarction predicts improvement in left ventricular function (Figs. 4B and C). In one study of 24 patients the extent of dysfunctional myocardium that was not infarcted or had necrosis comprising less than 25% of left ventricular wall thickness, as established by LGE performed within 1 week of the myocardial infarction, was the best predictor

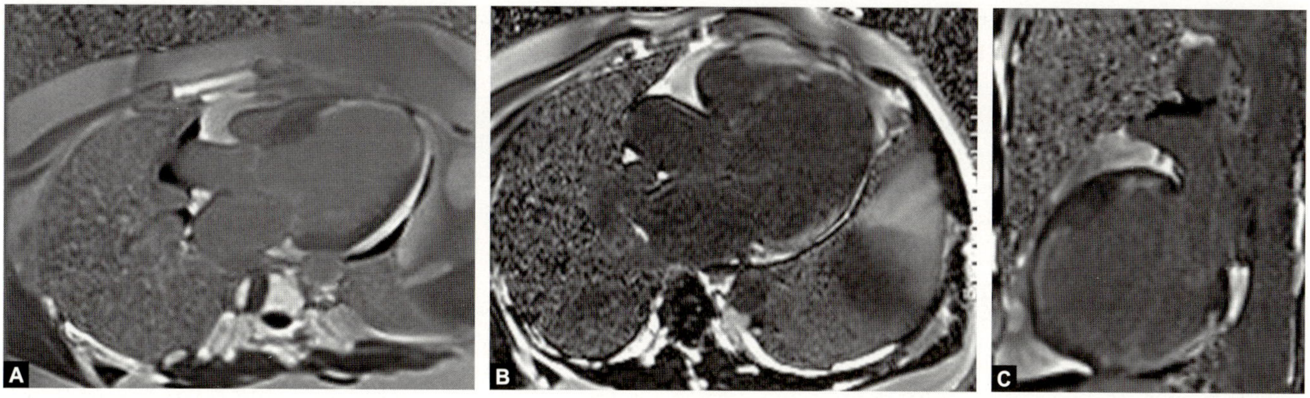

Figs. 4A to C

of global improvement in contractility at 3 months.[14] The degree of recovery of contractile function and the extent of transmural scarring correlates with contractile reserve on dobutamine stress echocardiography for inotropic response.[15] Late Gd enhancement as a marker of scar closely agrees with the finding of matching defects on positron emission tomography viability scanning.[16]

MYOCARDIAL PERFUSION IMAGING

First-pass Contrast-enhanced Magnetic Resonance Imaging

Myocardial perfusion imaging is an imaging technique designed to assess the microcirculation of the myocardium. Myocardial perfusion is usually performed under rest and stress states. In contrast to the rest state, the stress state is induced pharmacologically by a vasodilator, such as adenosine which causes hyperemia of the myocardium and increases perfusion. The technique uses a T1-weighted fast GRE sequence to perform dynamic imaging right after a bolus injection of Gd. A series of dynamic images are acquired during the first pass. When Gd flows into the myocardium, the T1 time shortens and the myocardium is enhanced according to the concentration of Gd. The temporal resolution of first-pass contrast-enhanced MRI is kept at one cardiac cycle. Three to five short-axis slices at the basal, mid, and apical levels are acquired within each heart beat. The ratio of perfusion at stress to that at rest is defined as myocardial perfusion reserve (MPR). In normal myocardium, MPR is above 2, and ischemia is considered if MPR is below 1.5. To ensure complete washout of Gd from the myocardium, the stress and rest tests are separated by a period of 10 minutes. Qualitative assessment is to visualize (eyeballing) perfusion defects based on relatively reduced enhancement in the ischemic myocardium. A dose of Gd (0.1 mmol/kg of body weight) is used to assess perfusion. Artifacts in the subendocardium are common and sometimes can be misdiagnosed as myocardial ischemia. Myocardial perfusion can be assessed quantitatively by analyzing the dynamic change of the signal intensity over time (Fig. 5). The LV myocardium at three short-axis levels is divided into 16 equiangular segments (not including the apical cap) according to the guidelines provided by the American Heart Association.[17] The mean signal intensity in each myocardial segment and LV cavity is measured at each time point to obtain the signal intensity-time curve (SI curve). Myocardial perfusion can be assessed from the SI curves semi-quantitatively or quantitatively. Several studies have demonstrated that semi-quantitative methods reveal strong diagnostic power to detect patients with coronary artery disease.[18] Quantitative analyses of myocardial perfusion involve a two-compartment model.[19] A simple two-compartment model (vascular and interstitial) has been proposed.[20] First-pass contrast-enhanced MRI has been shown to have better diagnostic accuracy in coronary artery disease than the other imaging modalities[21] with exquisite spatial resolution. Transmural perfusion gradient

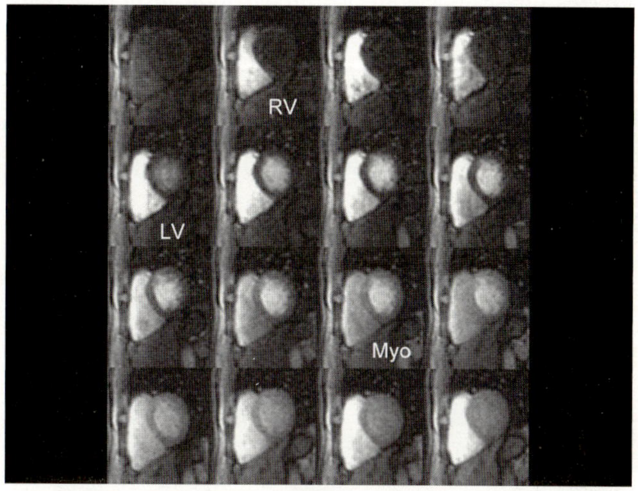

Fig. 5

can be identified from flow-limiting stenosis during global coronary vasodilatation.[22] The applications of perfusion include discrimination of hibernating myocardium by MPR, quantification of severity of atherosclerosis, vasodilator response of patients with hypertrophic cardiomyopathy, and to assess perfusion of residual viable myocardium after percutaneous intervention.[23]

FLOW QUANTIFICATION IMAGING

Phase-Contrast Cine

Phase-contrast cine acquires a series of images within a cardiac cycle with cardiac gating. In addition to magnitude images, phase images are acquired to indicate flow velocity. This is achieved by using a bipolar velocity-encoding gradient added to the cardiac-gated GRE sequence to measure the phase shift caused by the flowing blood. The phase shift is proportional to the flow velocity along the direction of the bipolar gradient. In phase-contrast cine, the flowing blood would appear as a white or black signal intensity (Figs. 6A and B), depending on the direction of the flow relative to the velocity-encoding gradients while the surrounding tissue is gray. The magnitude of the velocity-encoding gradient is adjusted according to the estimated maximal velocity of the target vessel to prevent aliasing artifacts. Phase-contrast technique can also be applied to measure flow velocity in three dimensions. The acquired data can be computed to generate virtual streamlines which represent blood flow within a vessel or cardiac chamber.[24,25] Phase-contrast cine is primarily used for flow quantification of great vessels. The blood flow of a vessel can be determined by the averaged velocity within the vessel lumen multiplied by the lumen area. Regurgitant flow can be determined from the flow–time curve to quantify the severity of valvular regurgitation (Fig. 6C). Phase-contrast cine has been applied to measure pulse-wave velocity of the descending aorta and was found to be associated with the elasticity of the aortic wall.[26] It can be used for indirect estimation of pulmonary hypertension.

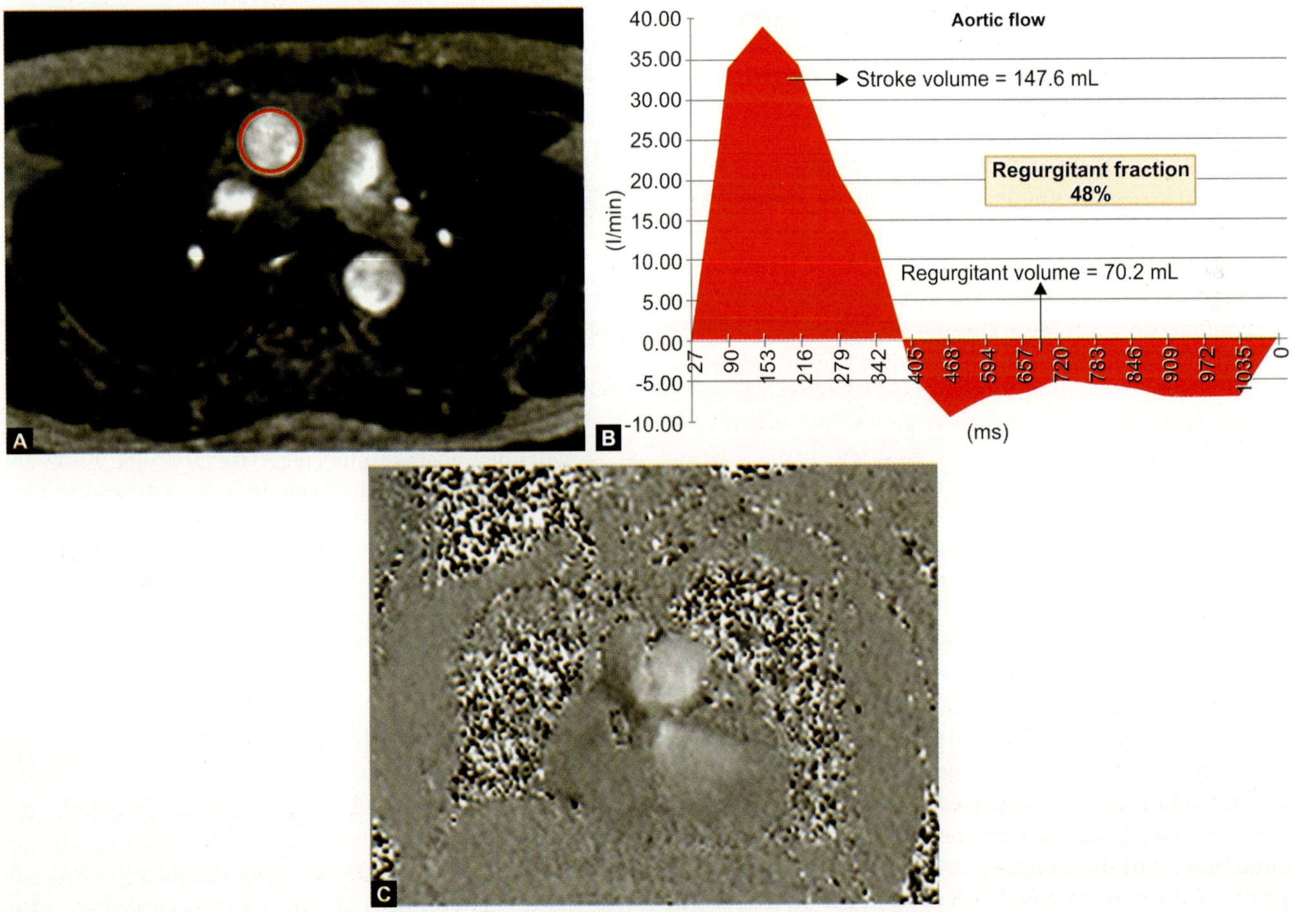

Figs. 6A to C

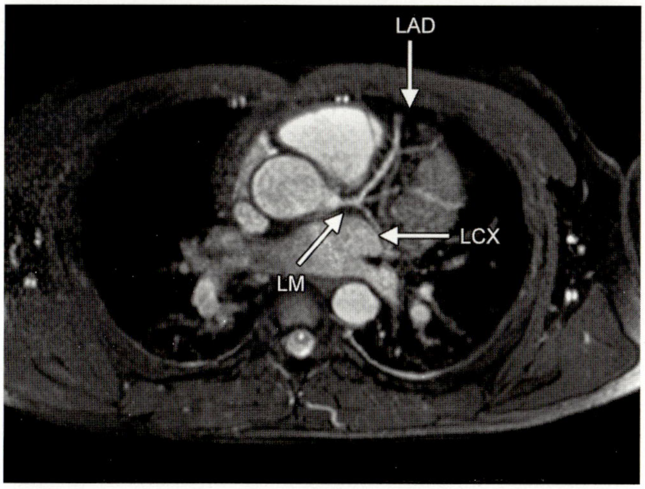

Fig. 7

Coronary Magnetic Resonance Angiography

Coronary MR angiography is a technique to evaluate coronary luminal stenosis. This is challenging because of the small diameter of a coronary artery and the cardiac and respiratory motion. Gd contrast is used to shorten T1 value of blood.[27] With the employment of spoiled GRE sequence using short TR, the vessels will appear bright because of Gd, while the background tissue signal is suppressed due to a saturation effect.[28] A power injector is used to increase contrast concentration and vessel conspicuity.[29] Current imaging technique uses a three-dimensional-GRE sequence with fat-saturation and synchronous ECG and respiratory gating. The scanning of the whole heart takes 5–10 minutes with free breathing. Coronary MR angiography is suitable for identifying coronary artery origins and course (Fig. 7) and morphological abnormalities, such as coronary artery aneurysm or fistula.

CONCLUSION

Magnetic resonance imaging enables the assessment of cardiac structure, function, perfusion, and scar tissue in patients who have diverse cardiac pathologies and is thus, a one-stop shop for the assessment of patients with abnormal cardiac structure or function. MRI is well established in the clinical setting for the assessment of myocardial viability, differentiation of nonischemic cardiomyopathies, multivalvular heart disease for timing of surgery, evaluation of complex structural anomalies in congenital heart disease, and in the evaluation of cardiac tumors. Although this technique is widely accepted in clinical routine, contraindications for MRI, as well as its limited availability, have prevented widespread adoption by the physician community.

REFERENCES

1. Leong DP, De Pasquale CG, Selvanayagam JB. Heart failure with normal ejection fraction: the complementary roles of echocardiography and CMR imaging. JACC Cardiovasc Imaging. 2010;3(4):409-20.
2. Brenner DE, Whitley NO, Houk TL, et al. Volume determinations in computed tomography. JAMA. 1982;247(9): 1299-302.
3. Tseng WY, Liao TY, Wang JL. Normal systolic and diastolic functions of the left ventricle and left atrium by cine magnetic resonance imaging. J Cardiovasc Magn Reson. 2002;4(4):443-57.
4. Gaasch WH, Delorey DE, St John Sutton MG, et al. Patterns of structural and functional remodeling of the left ventricle in chronic heart failure. Am J Cardiol. 2008;102(4):459-62.
5. Nollert G, Fischlein T, Bouterwek S, et al. Long-term survival in patients with repair of tetralogy of Fallot: 36-year follow-up of 490 survivors of the first year after surgical repair. J Am Coll Cardiol. 1997;30(5):1374-83.
6. Jimenez-Juan L, Joshi SB, Wintersperger BJ, et al. Assessment of right ventricular volumes and function using cardiovascular magnetic resonance cine imaging after atrial redirection surgery for complete transposition of the great arteries. Int J Cardiovasc Imaging. 2013;29(2):335-42.
7. Saguner AM, Vecchiati A, Baldinger SH, et al. Different prognostic value of functional right ventricular parameters in arrhythmogenic right ventricular cardiomyopathy/dysplasia. Circ Cardiovasc Imaging. 2014;7(2):230-9.
8. Verhaert D, Thavendiranathan P, Giri S, et al. Direct T2 quantification of myocardial edema in acute ischemic injury. JACC Cardiovasc Imaging. 2011;4(3):269-78.
9. Pennell DJ. T2* magnetic resonance and myocardial iron in thalassemia. Ann N Y Acad Sci. 2005;1054:373-8.
10. Cwajg JM, Cwajg E, Nagueh SF, et al. End-diastolic wall thickness as a predictor of recovery of function in myocardial hibernation: relation to rest-redistribution T1-201 tomography and dobutamine stress echocardiography. J Am Coll Cardiol. 2000;35:1152-61.
11. Joffe P, Thomsen HS, Meusel M. Pharmacokinetics of gadodiamide injection in patients with severe renal insufficiency and patients undergoing hemodialysis or continuous ambulatory peritoneal dialysis. Acad Radiol. 1998;5:491.
12. Lima JA, Judd RM, Bazille A, et al. Regional heterogeneity of human myocardial infarcts demonstrated by contrast-enhanced MRI: potential mechanisms. Circulation. 1995;92:1117-25.
13. Soriano CJ, Ridocci F, Estornell J, et al. Noninvasive diagnosis of coronary artery disease in patients with heart failure and systolic dysfunction of uncertain etiology, using late gadolinium-enhanced cardiovascular magnetic resonance. J Am Coll Cardiol. 2005;45:743.

14. Kim RJ, Fieno DS, Parrish TB, et al. Relationship of MRI delayed contrast enhancement to irreversible injury, infarct age, and contractile function. Circulation. 1999;100:1992-2002.
15. Gerber BL, Rochitte CE, Bluemke DA, et al. Relation between Gd-DTPA contrast enhancement and regional inotropic response in the periphery and center of myocardial infarction. Circulation. 2001;104:998.
16. Choi KM, Kim RJ, Gubernikoff G, et al. Transmural extent of acute myocardial infarction predicts long-term improvement in contractile function. Circulation. 2001;104:1101-7.
17. Cerqueira MD, Weissman NJ, Dilsizian V, et al. Standardized myocardial segmentation and nomenclature for tomographic imaging of the heart. A statement for healthcare professionals from the Cardiac Imaging Committee of the Council on Clinical Cardiology of the American Heart Association. Circulation. 2002;105(4):539-42.
18. Al-Saadi N, Nagel E, Gross M, et al. Noninvasive detection of myocardial ischemia from perfusion reserve based on cardiovascular magnetic resonance. Circulation. 2000;101(12):1379-83.
19. Jerosch-Herold M. Quantification of myocardial perfusion by cardiovascular magnetic resonance. J Cardiovasc Magn Reson. 2010;12:57.
20. Kroll K, Wilke N, Jerosch-Herold M, et al. Modeling regional myocardial flows from residue functions of an intravascular indicator. Am J Physiol. 1996;271(4 Pt 2):H1643-55.
21. Nagel E, Klein C, Paetsch I, et al. Magnetic resonance perfusion measurements for the noninvasive detection of coronary artery disease. Circulation. 2003;108(4):432-7.
22. Lee DC, Simonetti OP, Harris KR, et al. Magnetic resonance versus radionuclide pharmacological stress perfusion imaging for flow limiting stenoses of varying severity. Circulation. 2004;110(1):58-65.
23. Su MY, Lee BC, Wu YW, et al. Perfusion of residual viable myocardium in nontransmural infarct zone after intervention: MR quantitative myocardial blood flow measurement. Radiology. 2008;249(3):820-8.
24. Kilner PJ, Yang GZ, Wilkes AJ, et al. Asymmetric redirection of flow through the heart. Nature. 2000;404(6779):759-61.
25. Frydrychowicz A, Arnold R, Hirtler D, et al. Multidirectional flow analysis by cardiovascular magnetic resonance in aneurysm development following repair of aortic coarctation. J Cardiovasc Magn Reson. 2008;10:30.
26. Yu HY, Peng HH, Wang JL, et al. Quantification of the pulse wave velocity of the descending aorta using axial velocity profiles from phase-contrast magnetic resonance imaging. Magn Reson Med. 2006;56(4):876-83.
27. Kang KW, Chang HJ, Yoo YP, et al. Cardiac magnetic resonance-derived right ventricular outflow tract systolic flow acceleration: a novel index of right ventricular function and prognosis in patients with pulmonary arterial hypertension. Int J Cardiovasc Imaging. 2013;29(8):1759-67.
28. Ruehm SG, Nanz D, Baumann A, et al. 3D contrast-enhanced MR angiography of the run-off vessels: value of image subtraction. J Magn Reson Imaging. 2001;13(3):402-11.
29. Earls JP, Rofsky NM, DeCorato DR, et al. Breath-hold single-dose gadolinium-enhanced three-dimensional MR aortography: usefulness of a timing examination and MR power injector. Radiology. 1996;201(3):705-10.

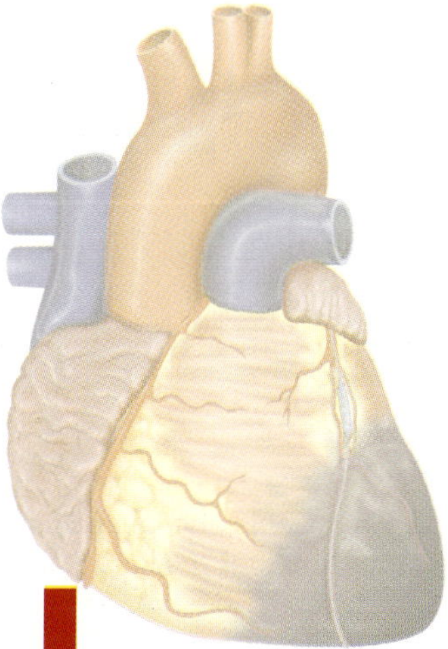

3

CHAPTER

New Cardiac Cameras: Single-photon Emission Computed Tomography and Positron Emission Tomography

PS Soni

INTRODUCTION

Nuclear medicine is an ongoing process undergoing continuous advances in all the instrumentation, clinical software, newer radiopharmaceuticals, faster electronics, basic science research, new technology, etc. Recent advances in technical developments have led to the development of better software techniques for image processing/fusion and, more recently, to the development of multimodality systems, viz. single-photon emission computed tomography/computed tomography (SPECT/CT), positron emission tomography (PET)/CT, and PET/magnetic resonance imaging (MRI). Myocardial perfusion imaging (MPI) is usually performed by standard dual-head scintillation cameras with parallel-hole collimators, typically configured in a 90° detector geometry to acquire the data for 15–20 minutes for each stress and rest. Myocardial perfusion imaging and image reconstruction are done based on standard filtered-back projection (FBP) algorithms. Recently, there was a need to have a small-dedicated cardiac SPECT/CT system instead of bulky conventional SPECT/CT system. This has resulted in the development of a range of dedicated cardiac SPECT/CT systems varying from a simple CT add-on to a conventional SPECT system that can provide low-dose CT images to a full scanner integrated with a SPECT system. Although significant progress in cardiac SPECT system has been achieved, further innovation continues to address challenges in new detectors, better camera resolution, and sensitivity.

DETECTORS

The characteristics of ideal detectors are: (1) high atomic numbers, high density, and intrinsic efficiency; (2) low decay time and good energy resolution; and (3) good intrinsic spatial resolution. Thallium-doped sodium iodide [NaI(TI)] crystal has high intrinsic efficiency for γ-rays of 200 keV, but the energy resolution and intrinsic spatial resolution are only moderate. As a result, there has been an ongoing search for better detectors as well as better detector configurations. Efforts have also been made to make smaller and more compact imaging systems for imaging small organs, such as cardiac, and for preclinical animal imaging[1] and for such type of systems, smaller and improved version of photomultiplier tubes (PMTs) are required for dedicated cardiac system. Conventional Anger gamma camera is having single large crystal with a large number of array of PMTs at the back. The basic detector element of a clinical SPECT system is based on the Anger camera,[2] which offers a spatial resolution of 4–6 mm. A typical gamma camera consists of an array of PMTs coupled with light guide to a large plate of a crystal scintillator material. The coordinate of the photon interaction is determined by positioning circuits from the relative intensity of the light pulse signal simultaneously detected by all of the PMTs. High-resolution images are obtained by choosing high-resolution collimators and photon detectors with high intrinsic position resolving capability. A block diagram of the basic components of a gamma camera is shown in Figure 1. Planner γ-camera is having stationary detector, whereas SPECTs detector rotates around the patient and collects data at different frames.

Search for Faster Scintillators

There are many scintillators available for SPECT and PET systems. NaI(TI) is still the most commonly used scintillator for SPECT applications. In most clinical SPECT systems, NaI(TI) detector is having large field of view (FOV). However, NaI(TI) can be pixelated and used for cardiac and small-animal SPECT systems. Major disadvantages of NaI(TI) are its hygroscopic nature and poor energy resolution. Recently, alternative of NaI(TI), cesium iodide activated with thallium (CsI(TI)), is evaluated, which is having better properties as it is slightly hygroscopic, and efficiency is same as NaI(TI). However, the scintillation light from CsI(TI) has a longer wavelength (λ) that is not as well matched to the conventional PMTs as sodium iodide.[3] However, these photons are detected with high efficiency with photodiodes that can replace bulky conventional PMTs and are being used in many cardiac SPECT systems used for many cardiac SPECT systems. Lanthanum bromide 3 (LaBr 3) is one of the new generations of very promising inorganic scintillation. It has a very high light output with a correspondingly improved energy resolution (6% at 140 keV) and an intrinsic efficiency comparable to NaI(TI). The characteristics of LaBr 3 are most suitable for time-of-flight (TOI) applications in PET scanner. It is also being used as the detector in a recently reported small-animal SPECT system.[4] CsI(TI) scintillators that emit light with longer wavelengths are best suited for multidetectors (pixelated) with sensitive photomultipliers.

Pixelated Multidetectors (With Latest Photomultipliers)

Recently, many new photon transducers, viz. position-sensitive PMT (PSPMT), avalanche photodiode (APD), silicon PMT (SiPMT), are available. Using PSPMT, it is possible to develop smaller and more compact imaging systems. New γ-camera designs have featured pixelated multidetectors, where the FOV is covered by "an array of individual scintillators" (Fig. 2) with a size of typically 2–3 mm instead of "single large crystal", as with a conventional Anger scintillation camera. Dedicated gamma cameras for specific clinical applications, which are based on PSPMTs, are representing a new trend in nuclear medicine.[5] The basic concept of a camera using PSPMT is identical to the Anger camera with the exception of the substitution of PSPMTs for the PMTs. Recently, it has been reported that by coupling a Cs(TI) or NaI(TI) scintillation crystal to a PSPMT, spatial resolution of 2 mm can be achieved.[6]

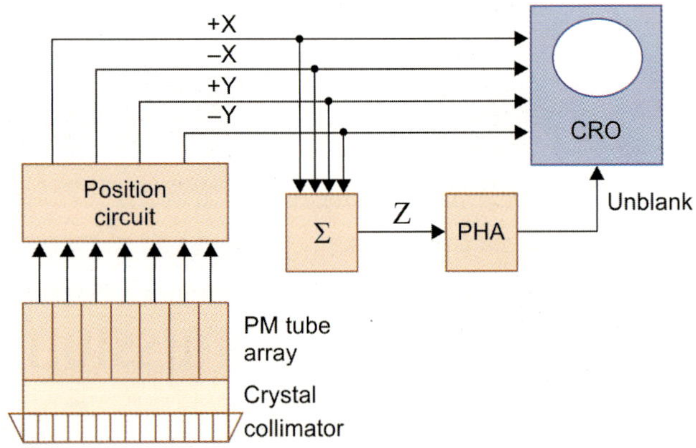

Fig. 1: Block diagram of the basic components of Anger gamma camera and has large thin single crystal and multiple PMTs. (PMT: photomultiplier tube).

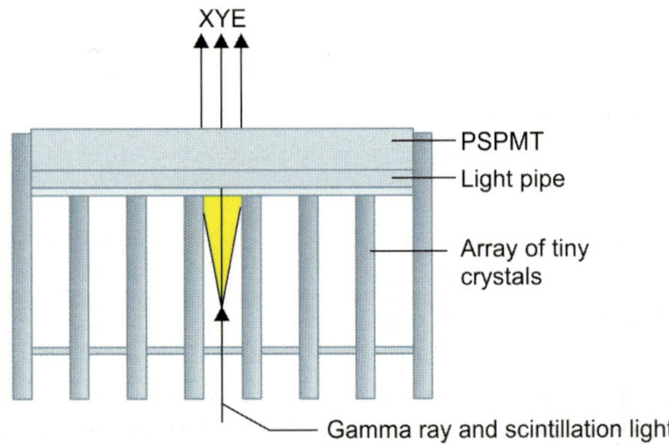

Fig. 2: Pixelated detector: multiple crystals and single PSPMT. (PSPMT: position-sensitive photomultiplier tube).

Semiconductors Detectors

Semiconductors detectors provide direct conversion of absorbed γ-ray energy into an electronic signal.[7] As there is no need for intermediate PMTs, the energy resolution is much better than that of scintillation detectors. Semiconductor cadmium telluride and cadmium zinc telluride (CZT) operate at room temperature and have high stopping power over a wide range of energies. Recently, this material has been used in commercial nuclear medicine imaging devices.[8]

Photomultiplier Tubes for Cardiac Single-photon Emission Computed Tomography System

Conventional PMTs have been used more than from last four decades. Photomultiplier tubes have very large electronic gains[6,10] with relatively low noise. However, their photon conversion efficiency is low, leading to a

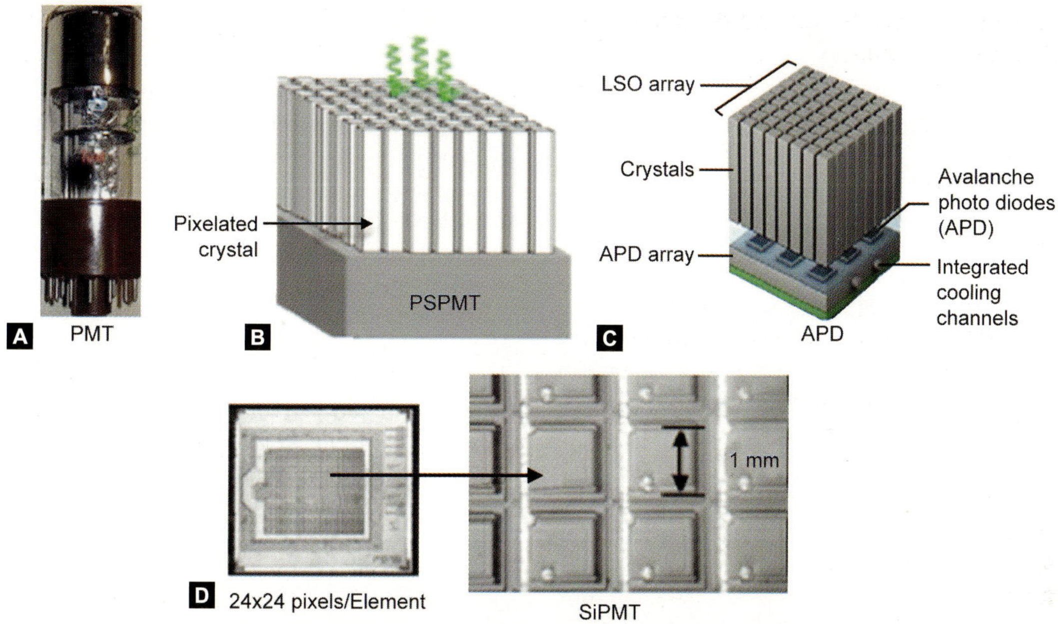

Figs. 3A to D: Conventional PMT. (A) Pixelated crystals PSPMT; (B) Avalanche photodiode; and (C and D) Silicon photomultiplier. (PMT: photomultiplier tube; PSPMT: position-sensitive photomultiplier tube).

significant loss of signal that affects both energy resolution and intrinsic spatial resolution and is affected by magnetic field. In addition, they are bulky as well as very expensive (Fig. 3A). Many new improved versions of commercially PMTs are available; these devices include the PSPMT (Fig. 3B), position-sensitivity avalanche photodiode (PSAPD) (Fig. 3C), and SiPMT (Fig. 3D). In the SiPMT, a large array of Geiger regions is closely packed together. Currently, devices are available with a 24 × 24 arrays of Geiger photodiodes packed into a very small area (1 × 1 mm) and being used in PET/MRI systems. Drawback of PSAPD is that it required liquid nitrogen to keep it cool. Avalanche photodiodes have several advantages over PMTs. They are more rugged, very compact, and not affected by magnetic fields, operate at a lower voltage than PMTs, and have much higher photon conversion efficiency. Position-sensitivity avalanche photodiode is already incorporated into PET/MRI and cardiac SPECT system.

Development of New Cardiac Single-photon Emission Computed Tomography System

Recent advances in nuclear cardiology instrumentation have enabled MPI with improved image quality, faster acquisition, and less radiation dose to the patient by increasing sensitivity and hence resolution. Numbers of factors which help in improving the designing of dedicated cardiac SPECT systems and which are common to all the cardiac cameras are new PMTs, collimators to increase the sensitivity detectors designing and reconstruction techniques. Initial version of FBP or maximum likelihood expectation maximization based on iterative reconstruction (IR) has many limitations. Subsequently, with faster computers, ordered subset expectation maximization has become the reconstruction method of choice, whereby data are grouped into subsets every 60°, allowing more rapid and improved reconstructed image.

MODIFICATION IN DETECTORS DESIGNING

There are new approaches for positioning detectors and controlling their motion during cardiac imaging. These new technologies ease and enable faster acquisitions, the lowering of administered activity by increasing sensitivity of detectors and hence radiation dose, and improved image resolution. Commercially available cardiac-centric SPECT systems based on multiple solid-state detectors are described here.

Digirad Cardius 3 XPO

Digirad, Inc. (Poway, CA) has developed a Cardius XPO camera dedicated to fast cardiac imaging. This system can be configured in two- or three-detector configurations.[9] The Cardius 3 camera and its geometry triple-head configuration (Fig. 4); is having solid-state detectors consisting of pixelated

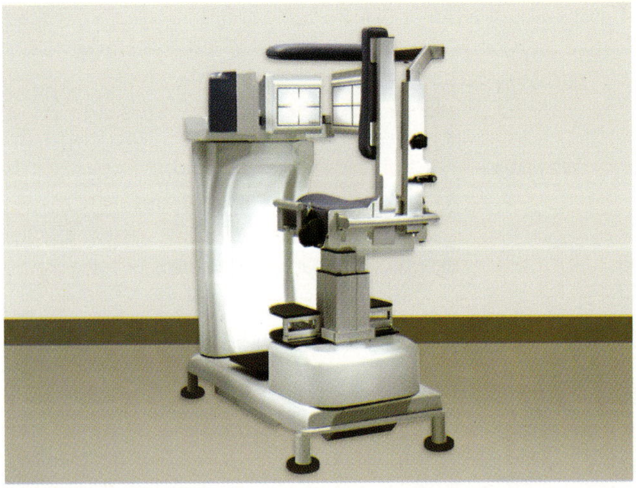

Fig. 4: Digirad Cardius 3 XPO: Upright patient position on the triple-head, pixelated detector camera. Detectors remain fixed while patient is rotated through 202.5° in a rotating chair.

crystals CsI (Tl) and photodiodes. Each detector head is very small and compact than conventional cameras and contains an array of 768 (6.1 × 6.1 × 6 mm thick) CsI(TI) crystals, coupled to individual SiPM. In the three-detector system, the detector heads are positioned at 67.5° angle between heads, which can move in and out to adjust the patient. The patient sits comfortably on a chair with his arms placed on an armrest above the detectors during imaging. Data are acquired by rotating the patient chair by 67.5°, covering a total acquisition arc of 202.5°, and study is completed in around 7.5 minutes. The system performance quality of image to that of a standard dual-headed SPECT camera is almost same, but acquisition time is reduced to 38–50%.[10]

CardiArc (Canton, MI)

CardiArc has developed a dedicated nuclear cardiology SPECT camera in which the detector and collimation are redesigned and optimized specifically for cardiac imaging and have no visibly moving parts and have a single internally moving part which is hidden from the patient,[11] and from outside the detector appears stationary and positioned upright (Figs. 5A and B). This system was originally designed to use arrays of CZT crystals as detectors. However, due to high cost of CZT material, the detector material was changed to NaI (TI) crystals to make it commercially viable. The system is having a high-spatial resolution detector utilizing 3 curved NaI (TI) crystals with graduated grooving technology and an array of 60 PMTs arranged in 3 rows (Fig. 5A). The detector uses a proprietary digital process developed by CardiArc that replaces the conventional Anger logic circuit. Horizontal photon collimation in each slice is accomplished by using a thin, curved, lead sheet with six narrow vertical slots (Aperture Arc) and vertical collimation is achieved by using a series of stationary lead vanes that are stacked vertically between the aperture arc and the NaI (TI) crystals. In this way, data are collected in 1-mm-thick slices using the six vertical apertures to collimate photons so that they are detected continuously across the detector surface with no overlap of data from different apertures. During acquisition, the aperture arc rotates to acquire data from multiple projections providing angular sampling (1,280 angular samples in 0.14° increments over 180°), which is 21 times greater than a conventional camera angular sampling (typically three°). All detector pixels are active simultaneously while photons are detected from multiple angles (Fig. 5B), which provide high-efficiency imaging. The

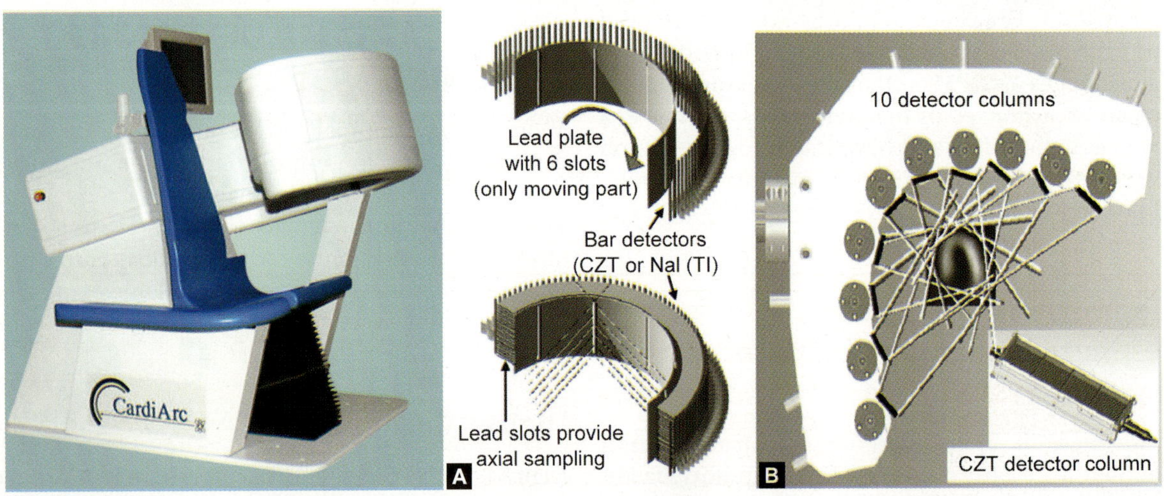

Figs. 5A and B: CardiArc having three-stationary NaI(TI) crystals and PMTs for photon detection. Having rotating aperture arc with six slots for horizontal collimation (A) and 10 detector columns is the only single internal moving part, imaging multiple angles (B). Scanning time is around 2 min and resolution ranges 3.6–7.8 mm. (NaI(TI): thallium-doped sodium iodide; PMT: photomultiplier tube)

movement of the aperture arc is synchronized electronically with the areas of the NaI (TI) crystals that are imaging the photons passing through the individual slots. The aperture arc's weight of approximately 16 kg is much lighter than traditional moving gantries, which facilities precise motion control. The moment of aperture arc ranges approximately 23 cm in order to cover the entire cardiac FOV, and each traverse of the arc takes 10 seconds.

Spectrum Dynamics: D-SPECT

Recently, Spectrum Dynamics, Haifa, Israel (now acquired by Biosensors in March, 2013), has manufactured a solid-state dedicated cardiac system called D-SPECT[12] with semi-stationary detectors, high-sensitivity collimation, and reconstruction optimized specifically for cardiac imaging. The patient is imaged in a semi-upright position with the left arm placed on top of the camera or in the supine position. The design and the principle of its operation are shown in Figure 6A. Acquisition time as short as 2 minutes has been reported.[12] This system uses pixilated CZT detector arrays (Fig. 6B) mounted in nine vertical columns and placed in a 90° gantry geometry (Fig. 6C). Each detector column is fixed in a mechanical mounting, and rotating these multiple columns in synchrony to acquire the data. The photons from a given location are detected at multiple angles by multiple columns as the FOVs of the detectors are swept through the region of interest. Each column consists of an array of 1,024 CZT elements (2.46 × 2.46 × 5 mm thick), arranged in a

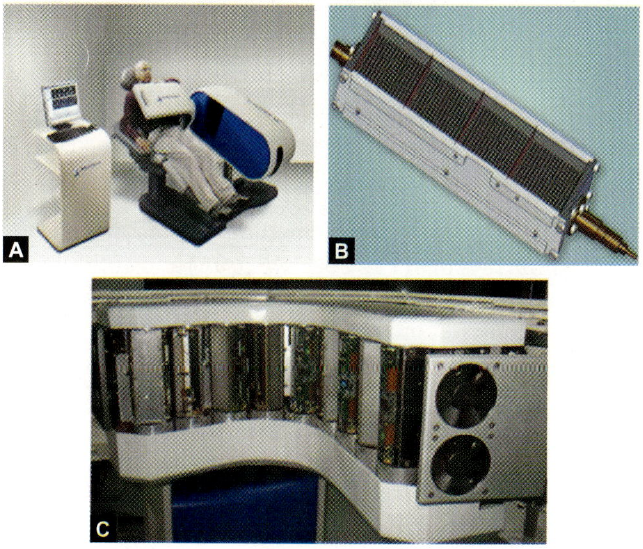

Figs. 6A to C: Photograph of the D-SPECT camera. (A) A single detector column from the D-SPECT camera; and (B and C) The system uses pixelated CZT detector arrays mounted in nine vertical columns and placed in a 90° gantry geometry. (CZT: cadmium zinc telluride)
Source: Courtesy by Spectrum Dynamics, Haifa, Israel.

16 × 64 element array with an approximate size of 40 × 160 mm. Each column is fitted with square, parallel hole, high-sensitivity collimators, such that the dimensions of each hole are matched to the size of a single detector element. All data are collected in list mode. A proprietary Broadview™ IR algorithm was developed.[13] The overall system resolution is 5 mm better than that of the Anger camera systems. Various parameters of D-SPECT were compared with GE Infinia SPECT system.[14] It was found that planer and tomography sensitivity and energy resolution are far superior to conventional Dual-head SPECT system.

GE Healthcare Acylone Discovery NM 539c Ultrafast Cardiac Photomultiplier Tube and Single-photon Emission Computed Tomography System

General Electric Healthcare recently launched the new dedicated Acylone (Figs. 7A and B), ultrafast cardiac solid-state cardiac camera (Discovery NM 530c). Tomographic reconstruction provides optimized image quality based on the "multi-pinhole" design and an array of CZT pixilated detectors.[15] System design enables high-quality imaging of a three-dimensional (3D) volume imaged by all detectors where the patient's heart is to be positioned. Similar to D-SPECT, the CZT improves the energy and spatial resolution, while the use of simultaneously acquired views improves the overall sensitivity and gives complete and consistent angular data needed for both dynamic studies and for the reduction of motion artifacts. Lines of response are acquired simultaneously through a proprietary multi-pinhole collimator with a large number of pinholes and focused collimation enables all views to focus on the area of interest resulting in high-sensitivity capabilities. The combination of CZT with a pinhole collimator has enhanced the image quality. Similar to D-SPECT, it is possible to do simultaneous dual isotope study with 201Tl and ^{99m}Tc.

CARDIAC VIABILITY STUDY WITH PHOTOMULTIPLIER TUBE/COMPUTED TOMOGRAPHY

Positron emission tomography is a noninvasive technique of nuclear medicine imaging that uses short-lived radiopharmaceuticals to detect and assess perfusion and metabolic activity in various organ systems. In other words, it is a diagnostic technique that creates high-resolution two-dimensional/3D tomographic images of the distribution of cyclotron produced positron-emitting radionuclides in the body; the radiolabeled compounds include substrates, ligands, drugs, antibodies, neurotransmitters, and many other molecules that are tracers for specific biological

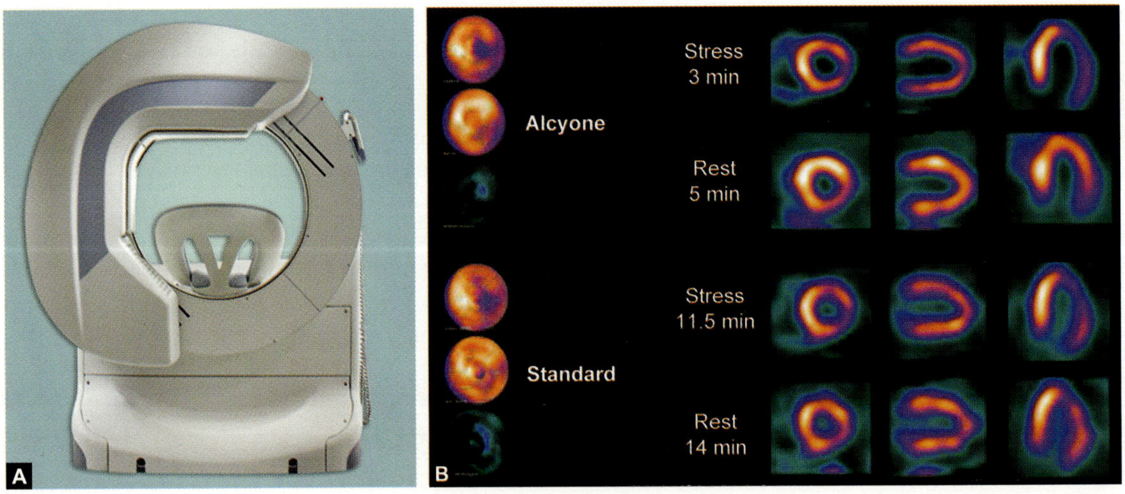

Figs. 7A and B: (A) GE Acylone; Discovery 539c UFC SPECT cardiac camera; and (B) 63 M diagnose lateral wall ischemia having 55% ejection fraction.
Source: Courtesy of GE Healthcare.

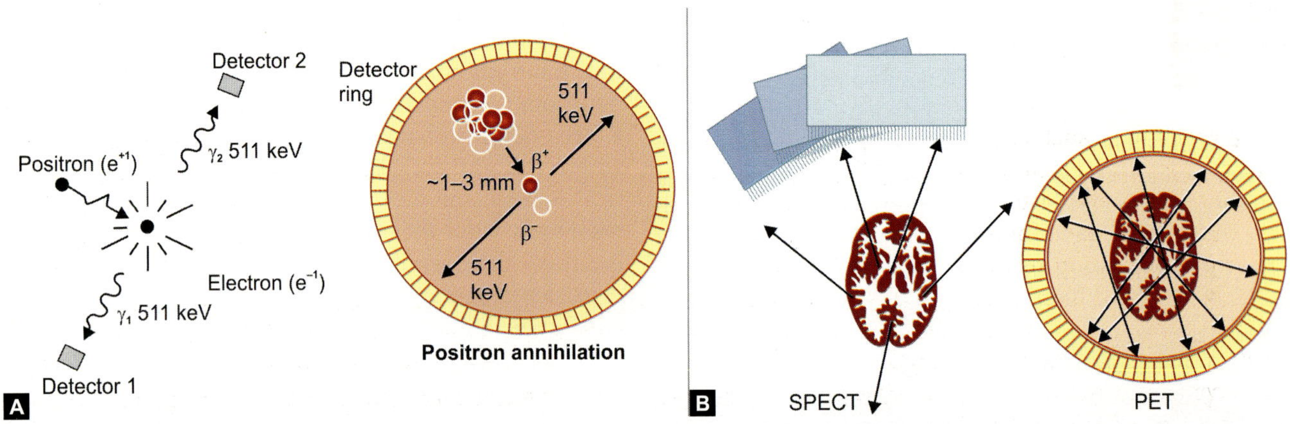

Figs. 8A and B: (A) Positron emission (annihilation) (right); annihilation in PET detector ring (left); and (B) Design of conventional SPECT using a rotating γ-camera at variable angles with collimator and collect data at different frame (left) compared with conventional full ring PET. (SPECT: single photon emission computed tomography; PET: photomultiplier tube)

processes. Thus, the resulting PET images can be considered as images of these biochemical or physiological processes (functional images). It has been proved beyond doubt that cardiac PET has a high diagnostic value in the assessment of myocardial viability in patients with known CAD compared to cardiac SPECT.

Basic Principle of Photomultiplier Tube/ Computed Tomography

The PET images are created by the detection of the emitted photons resulting from radioactive decay (annihilation) process, the radionuclide emits a positron that, after traveling a short distance, encounters an electron from the surrounding environment or body organ. The two particles combine and "annihilate" each other resulting in the emission in nearly opposite directions (180 ± 0.6°) of two gamma rays of 511 keV each (Fig. 8A) and annihilation γ-rays are detected by coincidence circuits at opposite sides of the multiple stationary 360° PET detector rings (Fig. 8B), followed by reconstruction the data.

Photomultiplier Tube Instrument's Design

The imaging of 511 keV photons has been primarily performed with dedicated PET scanners. These devices provide whole body tomographic acquisitions using radionuclides, which have different properties. Thus, a different detector technology was designed specifically for the detection of positrons from the technology used on a traditional gamma camera. Initially, $Bi_4Ge_3O_{12}$ crystal has been commonly used in PET system though it has some

TABLE 1: MPI radiopharmaceuticals for PET and SPECT.

Radionuclides	*Physical; half-life*	*Chemical form*	*Imaging instruments*	*Applications*
		Cyclotron produced		
^{11}C	20 minutes	^{11}C-acetate	PET	MPI, oxygen consumption, hypoxia
^{15}O	2 minutes	$H_2{}^{15}O$	PET	MPI
^{13}N	10 minutes	$^{13}NH_3$	PET	MPI
^{18}F	110 minutes	^{18}F-FDG	PET	MPI viability
		^{18}F-flurpiridaz	PET	New MPI
		^{18}F-MISO	PET	Hypoxia
^{201}Tl	73 hours	Thallous-201 chloride	SPECT	MPI
		Generator produced		
^{82}Ru	76 seconds	Rubidium-82 chloride	PET	MPI
^{68}Ga	68 minutes	^{68}Ga-annexin V	PET	Apoptosis
		Reactor produced radionuclides		
^{99m}Tc	6 hours	^{99m}Tc-teboroxime	SPECT	MPI
^{99m}Tc	"	^{99m}Tc-sestamibi	SPECT	MPI
^{99m}Tc	"	^{99m}Tc-tetrofosmin	SPECT	MPI

of the limitations, such as poor sensitivity and resolution. Furthermore, the recent introduction of multiple rings of detector blocks and faster scintillation crystals (lutetium oxyorthosilicate, gadolinium orthosilicate) has improved the image resolution resulting in a spatial resolution of about 4–6 mm. Addition of CT modality in the same gantry of PET scanner for fusion and attenuation correction further improve the scanner's performance and image quality.[16] The recent trend in PET is toward the use of TOF to improve the image quality further. TOF means the estimation of position of the origin of the photons by estimating the difference between two photons arrival times at the two detectors. The main advantage of TOF-PET is to improve statistical data by reducing rejection of true counts. Initially, the TOF concept was not possible in PET scanner as there was no fast scintillator as well as having high density was available. With the advent of high-density scintillators with high light output and high speed, such as LSO30, the TOF is incorporated in many commercial PET scanners.

CARDIAC IMAGING RADIOPHARMACEUTICALS FOR PHOTOMULTIPLIER TUBE AND SINGLE-PHOTON EMISSION COMPUTED TOMOGRAPHY

Along with the development of cardiac instrumentation in nuclear medicine, the field of radiopharmaceuticals and radiosynthesis is equally important. Radiosynthesis in cyclotron is a complex process, time consuming, and required involvement of scientists from diverse disciplines. Thus, on-site medical cyclotron is required and access to the four radioisotopes ^{15}O, ^{13}N, ^{11}C, and ^{18}F is essential as time is an important factor in radiolabeling. Cardiac study with PET/CT utilizing ^{18}F-fluorodeoxyglucose (^{18}F-FDG) is considered the most sensitive modality for detecting hibernating viable myocardium. It has been found that ^{18}F-FDG cardiac PET has high diagnostic value in the assessment of myocardial viability in patients with known coronary artery disease when compared to cardiac SPECT. Myocardial perfusion imaging RPs used with PET or SPECT instruments are further classified as: (1) cyclotron produced, (2) generator produced, and (3) reactor produced (Table 1). Most SPECT perfusion tracers are reactor produced except 201 Tl, whereas all PET perfusion tracers are either cyclotron or generator produced.

CONCLUSION

Recent developments in nuclear cardiology instrumentation have enabled MPI with improved image quality by using pixelated scintillator and semiconductor detector with elements of new photomultipliers, such as PSPMT, solid-state photon converter PSAPD, and SiPMT instead of conventional PMT. These new technologies enable faster acquisitions, the reducing administered activity and hence radiation dose, and enhance image quality. There are new designs for positioning detectors and controlling their motion during MPI to take care of comforts to patients. These systems also provide significantly higher sensitivity than the conventional SPECT systems so that MPI can be performed faster to improve throughput and patient comfort, since APDs are not affected to magnetic fields and it is being used in PET/MRI and we expect shortly SPECT/MRI will also be a reality based on the semiconductor detector.

REFERENCES

1. Levin CS. Application-specific small field of view nuclear emission imagers in medicine. In: Wernick MN, Aarsvold JN (Eds). Emission Tomography: the Fundamentals of SPECT and PET, 1st edition. San Diego: Elsevier; 2004. pp. 293-334.
2. Anger H. Sensitivity resolution and linearity of the scintillation camera. IEEE Trans Nucl Sci. 1966;13:380.
3. Melcher CL. Perspectives on the future development of new scintillators. Nucl Instrum Methods Phys Res A. 2005;537:6-14.
4. Hammond W, Tekabe Y, Johnson L, et al. Development of high performance mini gamma cameras based on LaBr3 scintillator and H8500 and H9500 PSPMTs and their use in small animal studies. In: Paper presented at 2006 IEEE medical imaging conference. San Diego: Elsevier; 2006.
5. Pani R, Pellegrini R, Soluri A, et al. First results from YAP: Ce Gamma camera for small animal studies. IEEE Trans Nucl Sci. 1996;43(6):3264-71.
6. Wagenaar DJ. CdTe and CdZnTe semiconductor detectors for nuclear medicine imaging. In: Wernick MN, Aarsvold JN (Eds). Emission Tomography: the Fundments of SPECT and PET, 1st edition. San Diego: Elsevier; 2004. pp. 270-92.
7. Darambara DG, Todd-Pokropek A. Solid state detectors in nuclear medicine. Q J Nucl Med. 2002;46:3-7.
8. Madsen MT. Recent advances in SPECT imaging. J Nucl Med. 2007;48(4):661-73.
9. Babla H, Bai C, Conwell R. A triple-head solid-state camera for cardiac single photon emission tomography (SPECT). In: Franks LA, Burger A, James RB, Barber HB, Doty FP, Roehrig H (Eds). Proceedings of the SPIE, vol. 6319; 2005. p. 63190M.
10. Lewin HC, Hyun MC. A clinical comparison of an upright triple-head digital detector system to a standard supine dual-head gamma camera (abstract). J Nucl Cardiol. 2005;12:S113.
11. Slomka PJ, Patton JA, Berman DS, et al. Advances in technical aspects of myocardial perfusion SPECT imaging. J Nucl Cardiol. 2009;16(2):255-76.
12. Sharir T, Ben-Haim S, Merzon K, et al. High-speed myocardial perfusion imaging Initial clinical comparison with conventional dual detector anger camera imaging. J Am Coll Cardiol Cardiovasc Imaging. 2008;1:156-63.
13. Rousso B, Nagler M. Spectrum dynamics LLC, assignee. Multi-dimensional image reconstruction. US patent 7176466. 2007.
14. Erlandsson K, Kacperski K, van Gramberg D, et al. Performance evaluation of D-SPECT: a novel SPECT system for nuclear cardiology. Phys Med Biol. 2009;54(9):2635-49.
15. Garcia EV, Tsukerman L, Keidar Z. 2.05: A new solid state, ultra fast cardiac multi-detector SPECT system. J Nucl Cardiol. 2008;15:S3.
16. Townsend DW. A combined PET/CT scanner: the choices. J Nucl Med. 2001;42:533-4.

SECTION 2

Hypertension

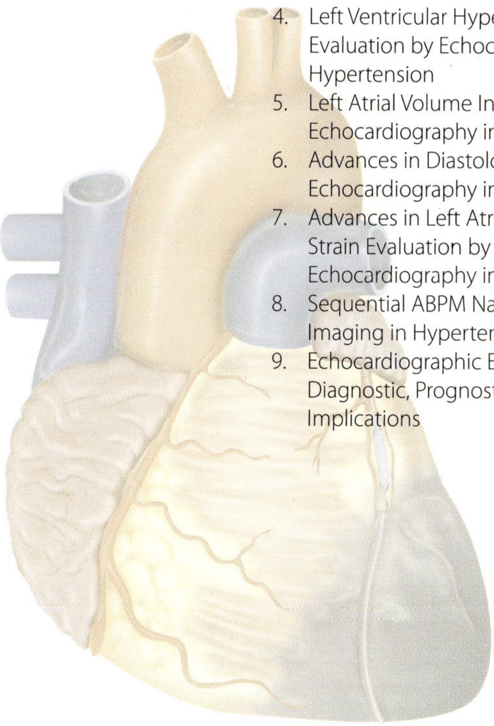

CHAPTER 4

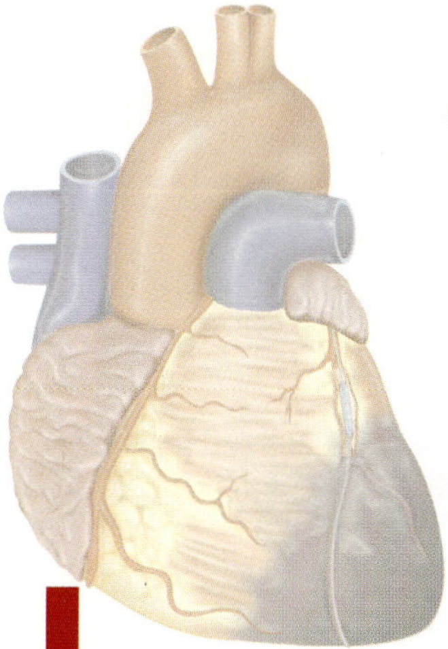

Left Ventricular Hypertrophy Evaluation by Echocardiography in Hypertension

Atul Karande, Manish Bansal, R Hotchandani

INTRODUCTION

Hypertension is currently a major contributor to the global burden of disease. The left ventricle (LV) remains one of the main target organs of hypertension. Echocardiographic measures of structure and function provide prognostic information. Left ventricular mass (LVM) is a well-established measure that can independently predict adverse cardiovascular events and premature death.[1-3] Population-based studies have revealed that increased LVM and left ventricular hypertrophy (LVH), as assessed by two-dimensional (2D) M-mode echocardiography measurements, provide prognostic information beyond traditional cardiovascular disease (CVD) risk factors.[4-6] Left ventricular mass has been stated as a suitable measure for CVD risk stratification and a marker for subclinical disease.[4,7] Moreover, the regression of LVH in patients with hypertension treated with antihypertensive medication has been associated with improved CVD outcomes.[8,9]

DIAGNOSTIC CRITERION

It is essential to have a reliable method for estimation of LVM. Echocardiography offers a reliable, noninvasive, rapidly available, and relatively inexpensive method for estimation of LVM. Regardless of the method used, LVM estimation is derived by converting myocardial volume to mass by multiplying the volume by the myocardial density of 1.05 g/mL.[10] All measurements should be performed at the end of diastole, the frame before mitral valve closure or the frame in the cardiac cycle in which the ventricular dimension is largest.

Linear Method (for Normally Shaped Ventricles)

The linear measurements of LV diastolic dimension (LVDd), septal [interventricular septum (IVS)], and posterior wall (PW) are made from the parasternal long axis or short axis acoustic window with the ultrasound beam directed perpendicular to the LV long axis approximately at the level of the mitral valve leaflet tips (Fig. 1A).[10] M-mode recordings have excellent temporal resolution and may be chosen from 2D images. However, even when directed by 2D guidance, it may not be possible to align the M-mode cursor perpendicular to the long axis of the ventricle.[11] A software has been developed to reconstruct anatomical M-mode images from 2D images (Fig. 1B). This is now available in most of the equipment.

Advantages

- Abundance of published data:
  - Fast and widely used
  - Established prognostic value.
- Fairly accurate in normally shaped ventricles (systemic hypertension, aortic stenosis).

Limitations

Beam orientation frequently off axis

- Based on the assumption that the LV is a prolate ellipsoid with a 2:1 long/short-axis ratio
- Since linear measurements are cubed, small measurement errors in dimensions are also multiplied
- It overestimates LV mass.

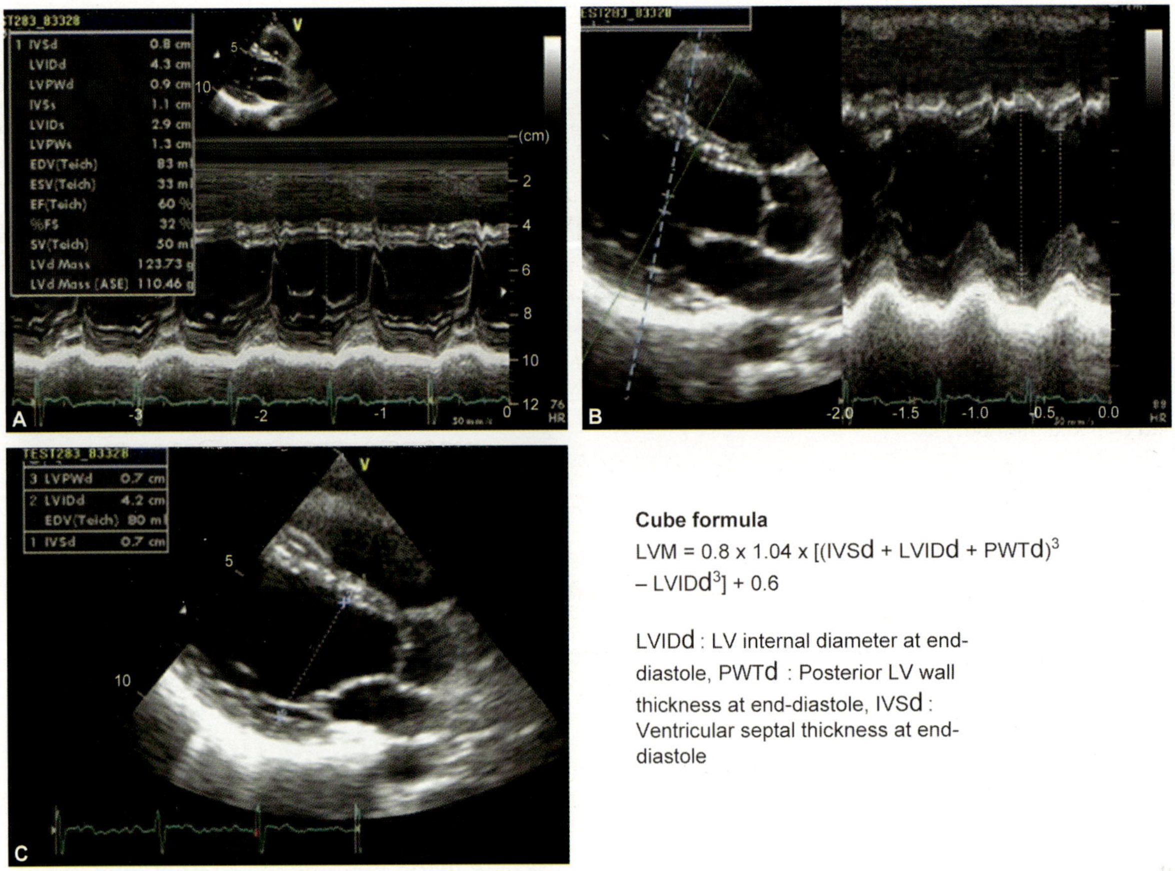

Figs. 1A to C: Linear echocardiographic methods of LVM measurement.

Inaccurate in the Presence of Asymmetric Hypertrophy or Dilated Ventricles

Alternatively, chamber dimension and wall thicknesses can be acquired from the parasternal long-axis view using direct 2D measurements. The use of 2D-derived linear dimensions overcomes the common problem of oblique parasternal images resulting in overestimation of dimensions from M-mode. When 2D measurements are used, the wall thicknesses and linear dimensions should be measured at the level of the LV minor dimension, at the mitral leaflet tips level. Left ventricle internal dimension diastole, IVS diastole, and PW diastole are measured at end-diastole (Fig. 1C).

Advantage

It facilitates orientation perpendicular to the LV long axis.

Limitations

Based on the same geometrical assumptions as M-mode.

- Same limitations as M-mode in patients with abnormal LV geometry
- Impact of harmonic imaging on the mass calculations is not established
- Normal values are less well established.

Normal Values

The upper limits of normal ranges in the American Society of Echocardiography chamber quantification update are more than 95 g/m^2 (>44 g/height 2.7) in women and more than 115 g/m^2 (>48 g/height 2.7) in men.

Two-dimensional Method

The commonly used 2D methods for measuring LVM are based on the area, length formula, and the truncated ellipsoid model (Fig. 2).[12] In the presence of shape distortions, the geometric assumptions in this approach remain problematic. Both methods were validated in the early 1980s in animal models and human autopsies.

Advantages

- Partial correction for shape distortions
- Less dependent on geometrical assumptions than the linear measurements.

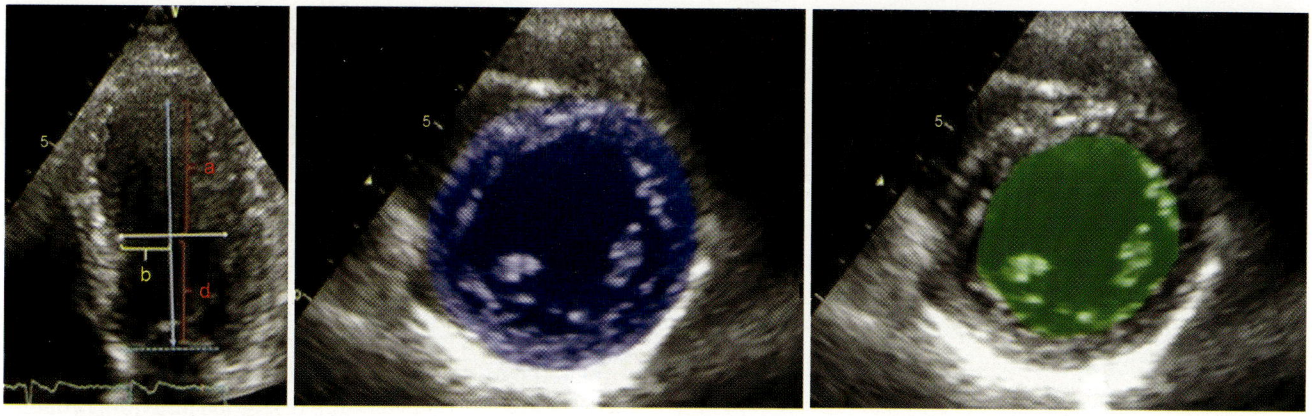

Truncated ellipsoid method:

$$LVM = 1.05\left\{(b+t)^2\left[\frac{2}{3}(a+t)+d-\frac{d^3}{3(a+t)^2}\right]-b^2\left[\frac{2}{3}a+d-\frac{d^3}{3a^2}\right]\right\}$$

Area-length method:

$$LVM = 1.05\left\{\left[\frac{5}{6}A_2(a+d+t)\right]-\left[\frac{5}{6}A_2(a+d)\right]\right\}$$

A_1: Total LV area obtained by tracing the epicardium, A_2: LV cavity area obtained by tracing the endocardium excluding papillary muscles, a: LV extending rom the widest LV to the apex, b: widest LV radius, d: truncated LV extending from widest short axis to the mitral annulus plane, t (mean LV wall thickness) = $\sqrt{(A_1/\pi)}-b$

Fig. 2: 2D echocardiographic methods of LVM measurement.

Limitations

- Good image quality and properly oriented parasternal views are required with no oblique planes
- Cumbersome methodology
- Good epicardial definition is required
- Higher measurement variability
- Less published normative data.

Normal Values[10,13,14]

- *Left ventricle mass (g)*: Men—96-200, women—66-150
- *Left ventricle mass index (g/m²)*: Men—50-102, women—44-88.

Three-dimensional Method (for Abnormally Shaped Ventricles and Ventricles with Asymmetric or Localized Hypotrophy)

The benefit of three-dimensional echocardiography (3DE) is especially to obviate inaccurate geometric assumptions, inherent to two-dimensional echocardiography (2DE). 3DE is a potentially attractive modality for the measurement of LVM, and normal ranges have been developed.[14] The accuracy of 3DE is reportedly similar to cardiac magnetic resonance (CMR) imaging methods.[15-17] However, there are wide limits of agreement which primarily relate to difficulties in tracing accurately the LV epicardial border, particularly in dilated ventricles.[18] Three-dimensional echocardiography underestimates LVM compared with CMR imaging in patients with cardiac disease, yet is more accurate than alternative ultrasound methods.

Advantages

- Higher accuracy than the linear or 2D measurements
- Higher inter-measurement and test/retest reproducibility
- Direct measurement without geometrical assumptions
- Better discrimination of small changes.

Limitations

- Patient's cooperation is required
- Dependent on image quality
- Normal values less well established.

Normal Values[10,13,14]

Left ventricle mass index (g/m²): Men—57-97, women—58-90.

BODY SIZE INDEXATION

Normal values for LVM are derived from the studies of the general population without hypertension or obesity.[9,10] For the comparison of LVM among the subjects of different body sizes, different allometric approaches have been suggested. However, there is controversy about the best method for indexing LVM.[10] Body surface area (BSA) was the first anthropometric variable used to index LVM. It has shown a stronger statistical correlation than height with LVM[19] and better identification of hypertension-related LVH.[20] However, indexing by BSA has been noted to minimize the effect of obesity on LVM, and, therefore, it underestimates the prevalence of obesity-related LVH.[21] Indexation of LVM to height raised to an allometric exponent of 2.7 (LVM/height 2.7), in comparison to BSA or height alone, has shown better predictive value for CVD outcomes, better detection of obesity-related LVH, and less variability of LVM among normal individuals.[22,23] Chirinos et al. demonstrated that indexation to LVM/height 1.7 was the best method, in comparison to BSA and height 2.7, to identify obesity-related LVH.[24] In a population with a low prevalence of obesity, there was no significant difference in the risk attributed to LVH, regardless of the method of indexation.[25] The American Society of Echocardiography and European Association of Cardiovascular Imaging recommend BSA as the preferred method for indexing LVM.[10]

PROGNOSTIC IMPLICATIONS

Left Ventricle Remodeling Patterns and Prognostic Implications

While patients with early hypertensive disease will most likely have normal LV geometry,[26] long-standing or untreated hypertension will result in changes in LV shape, and eventually, a deterioration of systolic function. Broadly, the changes in LV geometry can be classified according to whether LVM is normal or increased and whether ventricular morphology [relative wall thickness (RWT)] is altered (Fig. 3).[13] Relative wall thickness is variably reported as (PW × 2)/LVd or (IVS + PW)/LVd; of which, the former is favored because septal measurements may be confounded by the presence of septal bulge. Relative wall thickness is problematic and not reflective of true LV geometry in patients with asymmetric hypertrophy. The upper limit of normal RWT is 0.42.[10]

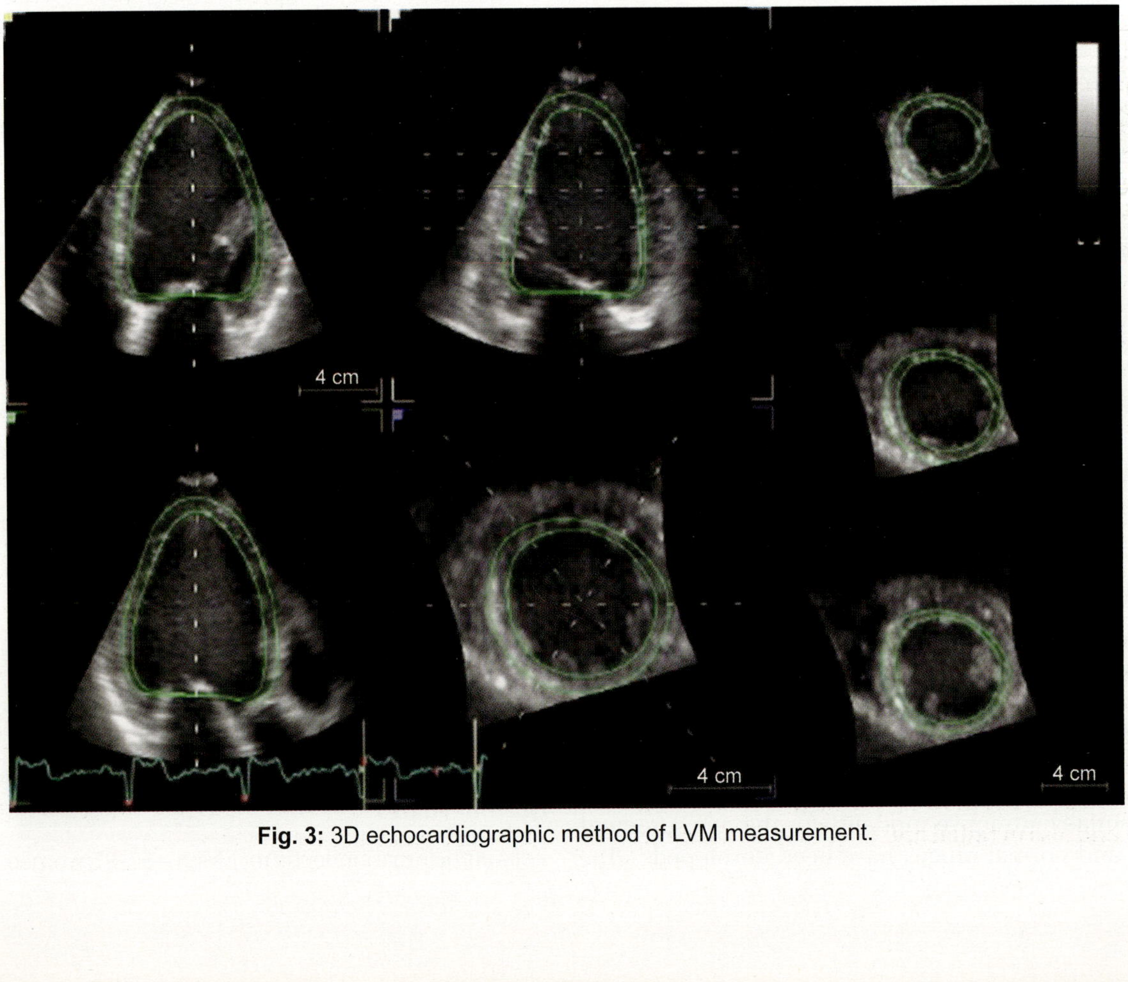

Fig. 3: 3D echocardiographic method of LVM measurement.

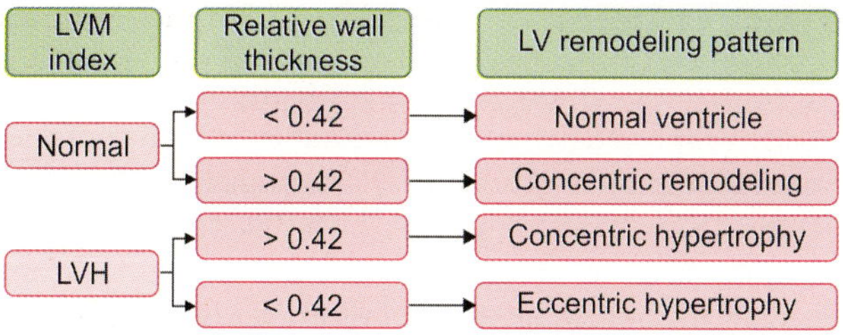

Fig. 4: ASE/EACVI classification of remodeling patterns.

Concentric Left Ventricular Hypertrophy

Concentric LVH, probably most commonly associated with hypertension, is characterized by normal cavity size, uniformly increased LV wall thickness, and increased LVM.[12] Concentric LVH and changes in LV geometry have been shown to affect both men and women, regardless of age,[27] and are also associated with changes in diastolic function, longitudinal and radial myocardial function, and atrial size (Fig. 4).[28-30]

Eccentric Left Ventricular Hypertrophy

In contrast to concentric LVH, eccentric hypertrophy is associated with volume, rather than pressure overload. This is usually due to significant valvular regurgitation or high cardiac index, as is seen in elite athletes. Systemic pressure is normal and peripheral resistance is not increased in patients with eccentric hypertrophy. Echocardiographic findings show increased LV cavity size, normal LV wall thickness, and increased LVM. Patients with eccentric hypertrophy share similar changes in diastolic function and longitudinal and radial function as those with concentric hypertrophy.[27,29,30] Unlike concentric hypertrophy, however, patients with eccentric LVH generally have low normal or mildly impaired systolic function.

Concentric Remodeling

Concentric LV remodeling is a late-stage response of the LV and can be caused by chronic pressure, volume overload, or myocardial infarction. It is most commonly associated with coronary artery disease (CAD), but is also associated with long-standing untreated hypertension.[31] Like eccentric hypertrophy, it is also associated with LV systolic dysfunction. Echocardiographic features show normal or small LV cavity size, usually increased LV wall thickness and normal LVM. Concentric remodeling is also associated with changes in the shape of the LV, which becomes more rounded. This results in dramatic degradation of diastolic function and loss of radial and longitudinal function.[29]

Other Classifications

The limitation of the classical categories is the suboptimal categorization of dilated ventricles.[32] In an attempt to develop a classification that is more inclusive of different physiologic and pathologic remodeling phenotypes, Gaasch and Zile suggested including LV end-diastolic volume as an additional marker to identify LV dilatation.[33] This classification provided incremental prognostic value regarding CVD outcomes in the Cardiovascular Health Study cohort.[34] In another attempt to address the limitations associated with the traditional remodeling classification, Khouri et al. suggested a four-tiered classification of LVH.[32] Dilated LVH and mixed thick and dilated LVH carried the worst prognosis for heart failure or cardiovascular death, and indeterminate hypertrophy had comparable rates to those without LVH.[35]

Prognostic Implication of Left Ventricular Hypertrophy

There is enough evidence indicating association between LVH and increased cardiovascular morbidity and mortality. Levy et al.[36] reported that LVH, quantified by echocardiography, independently predicts cardiovascular morbidity and mortality. The relative risk (RR) for developing CVD was 1.49 in men and 1.57 in women for every 50 g/m^2 increase in the LV mass above normal. This increment was also associated with higher all-cause mortality and cardiovascular mortality. Data from the same cohort also showed that LVH increased the risk of sudden cardiac death, more so in men than women.[37] Hypertensive black adults tend to have higher LV mass and RWT when compared with their Caucasian counterparts.[38] Left ventricular hypertrophy-related cardiovascular risk is higher in black population and women.[39,40] Furthermore, LVH carries more risk than multivessel CAD in this group. Liao et al.[41] showed that among 1,089 African Americans, who had undergone cardiac catheterization and M-mode echocardiography, the attributable RR for all-cause mortality was 2.4 with LVH, 2.0 with reduced ejection fraction, and 1.6 with multivessel CAD. The increase in morbidity and mortality in this group could partly be due to concentric LVH phenotype, which has been independently associated with worse outcomes.[1] Verdecchia et al.[42] showed that for each 29 g/m^2 increase in LV mass, there is a significant independent increase in the risk of stroke in hypertensive patients. In a meta-analysis of 20 studies with 48,545 patients, Vakili et al.[43] found that LVH consistently predicted worse cardiovascular morbidity and all-cause mortality across all groups and population, except end-stage renal disease patients.

THERAPEUTIC IMPLICATIONS

Left Ventricular Hypertrophy Regression

Current evidence suggests that LVH can be targeted through reducing blood pressure (BP) by pharmacotherapy and lifestyle. Nonpharmacological intervention and lifestyle changes aimed at LVH regression include weight loss, aerobic exercise, and low-salt diet.[44,45] All antihypertensive drugs appear to have some effect on LVH regression. While there is no consensus on the best pharmacologic agent, the current evidence favors the drug-targeting renin–angiotensin–aldosterone system (RAAS).[46] Angiotensin receptor blocker seems to have additional class action on LVH regression, independent of BP control. It is not clear whether dual blockage of RAAS with different pharmacological agents will incur incremental benefit in BP control and LV mass reduction. In a meta-analysis, Klingbeil et al.[47] found a significant difference among different medication classes. Overall, LV mass index was decreased by 13% with angiotensin II receptor antagonists, by 11% with calcium channel antagonists, by 10% with angiotensin-converting-enzyme inhibitors, by 8% with diuretics, and by 6% with β-blockers. Recently, the focus has been shifted to downstream pathways and oxidative stress in the pathogenesis of LVH. Previous studies have shown that allopurinol reduces oxidative stress. In a recent randomized, double-blind, placebo-controlled study, allopurinol 600 mg/day was shown to reduce absolute LV mass and LV mass in patients with type II diabetes mellitus.[48]

Left Ventricular Hypertrophy Regression and Outcome

Regression of LVH is independently associated with improved cardiovascular outcome. This has been reported by Levy et al.,[49] HOPE (Heart Outcomes Prevention Evaluation) trial,[50] and Verdecchia et al.[8] in PIUMA (Progetto Ipertensione Umbria Monitoraggio Ambulatoriale) registry. In a meta-analysis, Verdecchia et al. showed the association between LVH regression and lower CVD events.[51] In the LIFE (Losartan Intervention for Endpoint) Echo Study,[52] composite endpoint of cardiovascular death, fatal and nonfatal myocardial infarction, and fatal or nonfatal stroke occurred in 11% of the patients. There was a parallel independent association between LVH regression and lower cardiovascular mortality, all-cause mortality and myocardial infarction. Interestingly, regression or absence of progression of LV mass has been reported to be associated with lower incidence of diabetes mellitus.[53] In addition, LVH regression has been reported to improve LV systolic performance.[54]

CONCLUSION

Left ventricular mass is prognostically important and should be reported in hypertensive patients. In the normally shaped LV, either M-mode or 2DE formulas can be used to calculate LVM. In laboratories that use 3DE routinely, three-dimensional LVM measurement should be considered especially in abnormally shaped ventricles or in individuals with asymmetric or localized hypertrophy. 3DE is the only echocardiographic technique that measures myocardial volume directly, without geometric assumptions about LV shape and distribution of wall thickening. Description of LV geometry, using at the minimum the four categories of normal geometry, concentric remodeling, and concentric and eccentric hypertrophy, should be a standard component of the echocardiography report.

REFERENCES

1. Koren MJ, Devereux RB, Casale PN, et al. Relation of left ventricular mass and geometry to morbidity and mortality in uncomplicated essential hypertension. Ann Intern Med. 1991;114:345-52.
2. Drazner MH, Rame JE, Marino EK, et al. Increased left ventricular mass is a risk factor for the development of a depressed left ventricular ejection fraction within five years: the Cardiovascular Health Study. J Am Coll Cardiol. 2004;43:2207-15.
3. Verma A, Meris A, Skali H, et al. Prognostic implications of left ventricular mass and geometry following myocardial infarction: the VALIANT (VALsartan In Acute myocardial iNfarcTion) Echocardiographic Study. JACC Cardiovasc Imaging. 2008;1:582-91.
4. Levy D, Garrison RJ, Savage DD, et al. Left ventricular mass and incidence of coronary heart disease in an elderly cohort. The Framingham Heart Study. Ann Intern Med. 1989;110:101-7.
5. Gardin JM, McClelland R, Kitzman D, et al. M-mode echocardiographic predictors of six- to seven-year incidence of coronary heart disease, stroke, congestive heart failure, and mortality in an elderly cohort (the Cardiovascular Health Study). Am J Cardiol. 2001;87:1051-7.
6. Verdecchia P, Carini G, Circo A, et al. Left ventricular mass and cardiovascular morbidity in essential hypertension: the MAVI study. J Am Coll Cardiol. 2001;38:1829-35.
7. Devereux RB, Alderman MH. Role of preclinical cardiovascular disease in the evolution from risk factor exposure to development of morbid events. Circulation. 1993;88:1444-55.
8. Verdecchia P, Schillaci G, Borgioni C, et al. Prognostic significance of serial changes in left ventricular mass in essential hypertension. Circulation. 1998;97:48-54.
9. Hatani T, Kitai T, Murai R, et al. Associations of residual left ventricular and left atrial remodeling with clinical outcomes in patients after aortic valve replacement for severe aortic stenosis. J Cardiol. 2016;68(3):241-7.

10. Lang RM, Badano LP, Mor-Avi V, et al. Recommendations for cardiac chamber quantification by echocardiography in adults: an update from the American Society of Echocardiography and the European Association of Cardiovascular Imaging. J Am Soc Echocardiogr. 2015;28: 1-39.e14.
11. Marwick TH, Gillebert TC, Aurigemma G, et al. Recommendations on the Use of Echocardiography in Adult Hypertension: A Report from the European Association of Cardiovascular Imaging (EACVI) and the American Society of Echocardiography (ASE). J Am Soc Echocardiogr. 2015;28:727-54.
12. Lang RM, Bierig M, Devereux RB, et al. Recommendations for chamber quantification. Eur J Echocardiogr. 2006;7:79-108.
13. Fukuda S, Watanabe H, Daimon M, et al. Normal values of real-time 3-dimensional echocardiographic parameters in a healthy Japanese population: the JAMP-3D study. Circ J. 2012;76:1177-81.
14. Muraru D, Badano LP, Peluso D, et al. Comprehensive analysis of left ventricular geometry and function by three-dimensional echocardiography in healthy adults. J Am Soc Echocardiogr. 2013;26:618-28.
15. Jenkins C, Bricknell K, Hanekom L, et al. Reproducibility and accuracy of echocardiographic measurements of left ventricular parameters using real-time three-dimensional echocardiography. J Am Coll Cardiol. 2004;44:878-86.
16. Takeuchi M, Nishikage T, Mor-Avi V, et al. Measurement of left ventricular mass by real-time three-dimensional echocardiography: validation against magnetic resonance and comparison with two-dimensional and M-mode measurements. J Am Soc Echocardiogr. 2008;21:1001-5.
17. van den Bosch AE, Robbers-Visser D, Krenning BJ, et al. Comparison of real-time three-dimensional echocardiography to magnetic resonance imaging for assessment of left ventricular mass. Am J Cardiol. 2006;97:113-7.
18. Shimada YJ, Shiota T. Meta-analysis of accuracy of left ventricular mass measurement by three-dimensional echocardiography. Am J Cardiol. 2012;110:445-52.
19. Gardin JM, Arnold A, Gottdiener JS, et al. Left ventricular mass in the elderly. The Cardiovascular Health Study. Hypertension. 1997;29:1095-103.
20. Ferrara LA, Vaccaro O, Cardoni O, et al. Indexation criteria of ventricular mass and predictive role of blood pressure and body composition. Am J Hypertens. 2005;18:1282-7.
21. Cuspidi C, Giudici V, Negri F, et al. Improving cardiovascular risk stratification in essential hypertensive patients by indexing left ventricular mass to height (2.7). J Hypertens. 2009;27:2465-71.
22. de Simone G, Daniels SR, Devereux RB, et al. Left ventricular mass and body size in normotensive children and adults: assessment of allometric relations and impact of overweight. J Am Coll Cardiol. 1992;20:1251-60.
23. de Simone G, Kizer JR, Chinali M, et al. Normalization for body size and population-attributable risk of left ventricular hypertrophy: the Strong Heart Study. Am J Hypertens. 2005;18:191-6.
24. Chirinos JA, Segers P, De Buyzere ML, et al. Left ventricular mass: allometric scaling, normative values, effect of obesity, and prognostic performance. Hypertension. 2010;56:91-8.
25. de Simone G, Devereux RB, Maggioni AP, et al. Different normalizations for body size and population attributable risk of left ventricular hypertrophy: the MAVI study. Am J Hypertens. 2005;18:1288-93.
26. Krishnamoorthy A, Brown T, Ayers CR, et al. Progression from normal to reduced left ventricular ejection fraction in patients with concentric left ventricular hypertrophy after long-term follow-up. Am J Cardiol. 2011;108:997-1001.
27. Masiha S, Sundstrom J, Lind L. Left ventricular geometric patterns and adaptations to hemodynamics are similar in elderly men and women. BMC Cardiovasc Disord. 2011;11:25.
28. Tsioufis C, Taxiarchou E, Syrseloudis D, et al. Left ventricular mass but not geometry determines left atrial size in the early stages of hypertension. J Hum Hypertens. 2009;23:674-9.
29. Mizuguchi Y, Oishi Y, Miyoshi H, et al. Concentric left ventricular hypertrophy brings deterioration of systolic longitudinal, circumferential, and radial myocardial deformation in hypertensive patients with preserved left ventricular pump function. J Cardiol. 2010;55:23-33.
30. Masugata H, Senda S, Inukai M, et al. Differences in left ventricular diastolic dysfunction between eccentric and concentric left ventricular hypertrophy in hypertensive patients with preserved systolic function. J Int Med Res. 2011;39:772-9.
31. Cameli M, Lisi M, Righini FM, et al. Left ventricular remodeling and torsion dynamics in hypertensive patients. Int J Cardiovasc Imaging. 2013;29:79-86.
32. Khouri MG, Peshock RM, Ayers CR, et al. A 4-tiered classification of left ventricular hypertrophy based on left ventricular geometry: the Dallas Heart Study. Circ Cardiovasc Imaging. 2010;3:164-71.
33. Gaasch WH, Zile MR. Left ventricular structural remodeling in health and disease: with special emphasis on volume, mass, and geometry. J Am Coll Cardiol. 2011;58:1733-40.
34. Zile MR, Gaasch WH, Patel K, et al. Adverse left ventricular remodeling in community-dwelling older adults predicts incident heart failure and mortality. JACC Heart Fail. 2014;2:512-22.
35. Garg S, de Lemos JA, Ayers C, et al. Association of a 4-tiered classification of LV hypertrophy with adverse CV outcomes in the general population. JACC Cardiovasc Imaging. 2015;8:1034-41.
36. Levy D, Garrison RJ, Savage DD, et al. Prognostic implications of echocardiographically determined left ventricular mass in the Framingham Heart Study. N Engl J Med. 1990;322(22):1561-6.
37. Haider AW, Larson MG, Benjamin EJ, et al. Increased left ventricular mass and hypertrophy are associated with increased risk for sudden death. J Am Coll Cardiol. 1998;32(5):1454-9.
38. Kizer JR, Arnett DK, Bella JN, et al. Differences in left ventricular structure between Black and White hypertensive adults: the Hypertension Genetic Epidemiology Network Study. Hypertension. 2004;43(6):1182-8.

39. Havranek EP, Froshaug DB, Emserman CD, et al. Left ventricular hypertrophy and cardiovascular mortality by race and ethnicity. Am J Med. 2008;121(10):870-5.
40. Liao Y, Cooper RS, Mensah GA, et al. Left ventricular hypertrophy has a greater impact on survival in women than in men. Circulation. 1995;92(4):805-10.
41. Liao Y, Cooper RS, McGee DL, et al. The relative effects of left ventricular hypertrophy, coronary artery disease, and ventricular dysfunction on survival among black adults. JAMA. 1995;273(20):1592-7.
42. Verdecchia P, Porcellati C, Reboldi G, et al. Left ventricular hypertrophy as an independent predictor of acute cerebrovascular events in essential hypertension. Circulation. 2001;104(17):2039-44.
43. Vakili BA, Okin PM, Devereux RB. Prognostic implications of left ventricular hypertrophy. Am Heart J. 2001;141(3):334-41.
44. Schmieder RE, Messerli FH, Garavaglia GE, et al. Dietary salt intake. A determinant of cardiac involvement in essential hypertension. Circulation. 1988;78(4):951-6.
45. MacMahon SW, Wilcken DEL, Macdonald GJ. The effect of weight reduction on left ventricular mass. A randomized controlled trial in young, overweight hypertensive patients. N Engl J Med. 1986;314(6):334-9.
46. Sadoshima J, Izumo S. Molecular characterization of angiotensin II-induced hypertrophy of cardiac myocytes and hyperplasia of cardiac fibroblasts. Critical role of the AT1 receptor subtype. Circ Res. 1993;73(3):413-23.
47. Klingbeil AU, Schneider M, Martus P, et al. A meta-analysis of the effects of treatment on left ventricular mass in essential hypertension. Am J Med. 2003;115(1):41-6.
48. Szwejkowski BR, Gandy SJ, Rekhraj S, et al. Allopurinol reduces left ventricular mass in patients with type 2 diabetes and left ventricular hypertrophy. J Am Coll Cardiol. 2013;62(24):2284-93.
49. Levy D, Salomon M, D'Agostino RB, et al. Prognostic implications of baseline electrocardiographic features and their serial changes in subjects with left ventricular hypertrophy. Circulation. 1994;90(4):1786-93.
50. Galzerano D, Tammaro P, Viscovo L, et al. Three-dimensional echocardiographic and magnetic resonance assessment of the effect of telmisartan compared with carvedilol on left ventricular mass: a multicenter, randomized, longitudinal study. Am J Hypertens. 2005;18(12 Pt 1):1563-9.
51. Verdecchia P, Angeli F, Borgioni C, et al. Changes in cardiovascular risk by reduction of left ventricular mass in hypertension: a meta-analysis. Am J Hypertens. 2003;16(11 Pt 1):895-9.
52. Devereux RB, Wachtell K, Gerdts E, et al. Prognostic significance of left ventricular mass change during treatment of hypertension. JAMA. 2004;292(19):2350-6.
53. Okin PM, Devereux RB, Harris KE, et al. In-treatment resolution or absence of electrocardiographic left ventricular hypertrophy is associated with decreased incidence of new-onset diabetes mellitus in hypertensive patients: the Losartan Intervention for Endpoint Reduction in Hypertension (LIFE) Study. Hypertension. 2007;50(5):984-90.
54. Wachtell K, Palmieri V, Olsen MH, et al. Change in systolic left ventricular performance after 3 years of antihypertensive treatment: the Losartan Intervention for Endpoint (LIFE) study. Circulation. 2002;106(2):227-32.

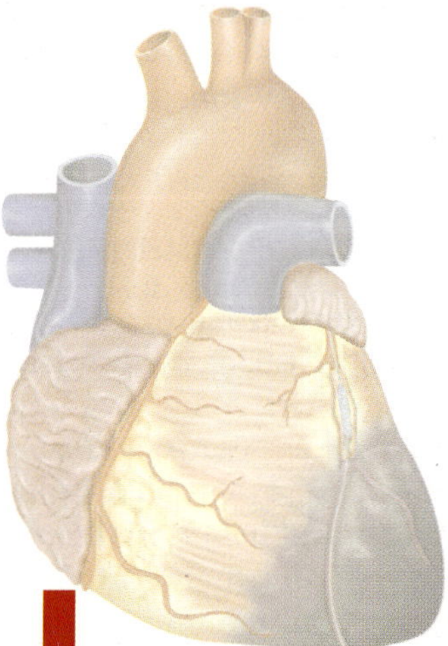

5

CHAPTER

Left Atrial Volume Index Evaluation by Echocardiography in Hypertension

Rohit Tandon, Gurpreet Singh Wander, HK Chopra

INTRODUCTION

Left atrial enlargement (LAE) is considered a high-risk phenotype in hypertensive individuals as it reflects chronicity and magnitude of elevated left ventricular (LV) filling pressure and has causal correlation to new onset atrial flutter (AF), heart failure (HF), stroke, and mortality along with exercise limitation and association with ischemic heart disease (IHD). Evaluation of LA size and function provides a powerful and dynamic morphophysiological marker of cardiovascular disease status that can be used longitudinally to quantify the extent of structural and functional remodeling.

LEFT ATRIAL VOLUME AS AN INDEX OF ATRIAL REMODELING MECHANISMS

Left atrial remodeling is defined as a persistent change in LA size or function, which is time-dependent response of cardiomyocytes to external stressors causing metabolic changes in sources of energy production to fetal glycolysis leading to atrial fibrosis. Even acute short-term trigger, e.g. hypertensive crisis can lead to atrial remodeling albeit reversible. Change in LA volume (LAV) more than 15% compared to baseline, by echocardiography/cardiac magnetic resonance (CMR), is a measure of LA remodeling. Atrial remodeling can be structural seen as atrial dilatation (due to interstitial fibrosis) or functional seen as decreased function with or without alteration in LA size.[1-3]

Recommended technique for LAV measurement: Two-dimensional (2D) volumetric measurements are based on tracings of the blood–tissue interface on apical four- and two-chamber views. At the mitral valve level, the contour is closed by connecting the two opposite sections of the mitral annulus with a straight line. Endocardial tracing should exclude atrial appendage and pulmonary veins. LAV can be calculated using the disc summation technique by adding the volume of a stack of cylinders of height "h" and area calculated by orthogonal minor and major transverse axes (D1 and D2) assuming an oval shape π/4 (h) sigma (D1) (D2) (Figs. 1A and B).

Vyas et al. studied the impact of LA volumetric measurements compared to linear measurements and concluded that in 37% patients, LAE was missed by linear measurements and patients with LAE diagnosed by volume but not by diameter measurements had a lower LV mass index (LVMI) suggesting that volume-based measurements are more sensitive and detect LAE at an earlier stage than diameter-based measurements.

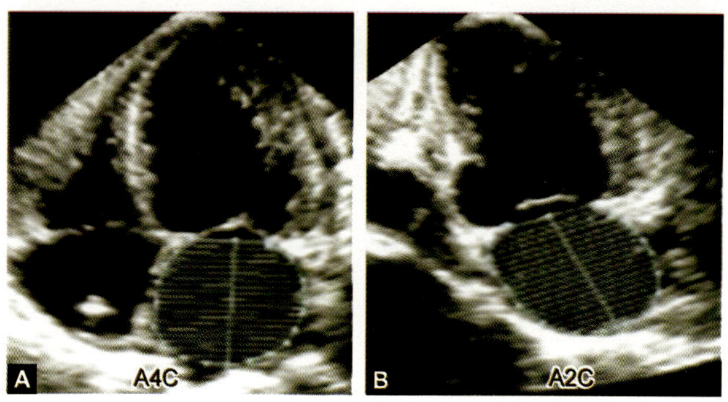

Figs. 1A and B: Biplane method of discs.

TWO-DIMENSIONAL VERSUS THREE-DIMENSIONAL LEFT ATRIAL VOLUMES

The assessment of LA size has evolved from one-dimensional M-mode for LA diameter to 2D biplane area-length Simpson's method for LAV, but insights from cardiac computed tomography (CT) and anatomic studies have indicated that left atrium has a complex shape with an irregular ellipsoid LA-free wall and oblique planar interatrial septal wall; this results in underestimation of LAV by 2D as LA and LV long axes do not appear in the same cutting plane; 2D cutting plane obtained often does not bisect the center of the LA short-axis view, it is not always guaranteed that apical four- and apical two-chamber views are exactly perpendicular to each other. Compared with CMR as standard reference, there were 31-mL and 16-mL underestimations of LAV_{max} and LAV_{min} by 2D echocardiography but only 1-mL underestimation and 0-mL difference by three-dimensional (3D) LAV_{max} and LAV_{min}. These inaccuracies are easily overcome with real-time 3D echocardiography, which has comparable accuracy to CMR (Figs. 2A and B).

Normal LAV index (LAVI) using echocardiography is 22 ± 6 mL/m^2; on the basis of the sensitivity and specificity for predicting cardiac events, the American Society of Echocardiography (ASE) considers LAE as more than 28 mL/m^2 [i.e. 1 standard deviation (SD) from the mean], while identifying LV diastolic dysfunction, an LAVI cut point more than 34 mL/m^2 (i.e. 2 SD) was endorsed.

Left atrial volume measurement is independent of age and gender but is dependent on body size in a proportionate manner, therefore indexing of LAV to body surface area is recommended, and also depends on technique used because echocardiography techniques (2D/3D) tend to slightly underestimate volumes compared to 3D-gated cardiac CT or CMR imaging. Low hemoglobin levels, thyrotoxicosis, and chronic liver/kidney disease are also associated with increased indexed LAV independent of diastolic dysfunction.[4-8]

Minimal or Maximal Left Atrial Volume

Left atrial maximum volume is measured at the end of the ventricular systole just before mitral valve opening; therefore, it is related to increased LA pressure/LAV. Although a large body of data support use of maximal LAV for predicting cardiovascular risk, recent research suggests that minimal LAV may be a more important prognostic indicator. Minimal LAV is measured at end-diastole after being exposed to LV diastolic pressure (therefore accounting for atrial afterload) and is closely related to LA maximal elastance (a load-independent measure of atrial contractility). From the apical four- and two-chamber views, using biplane-modified Simpson's method, LA maximum and minimum volumes are calculated in LV end-systole (just before mitral valve opening) and in LV end-diastole (just after mitral valve closure), respectively, with cutoffs of 22 ± 2.6 mL/m^2 and 11.9 ± 3.2 mL/m^2, respectively, for each LAV. Both LAV_{max} and LAV_{min} increase gradually with the progression of LV diastolic function, the increase in LAV_{min} with worsening diastolic function is more pronounced even in the earlier stages of diastolic dysfunction, whereas increase in LAV_{max} is seen only in the later stages of diastolic dysfunction. Routine echocardiography should, therefore, include the assessment of LAV_{min} for predicting cardiovascular events, especially in patients who already have higher cardiovascular risk profiles. Rational explanation to this could be that while LA maximal volume is related to increased atrial pressure

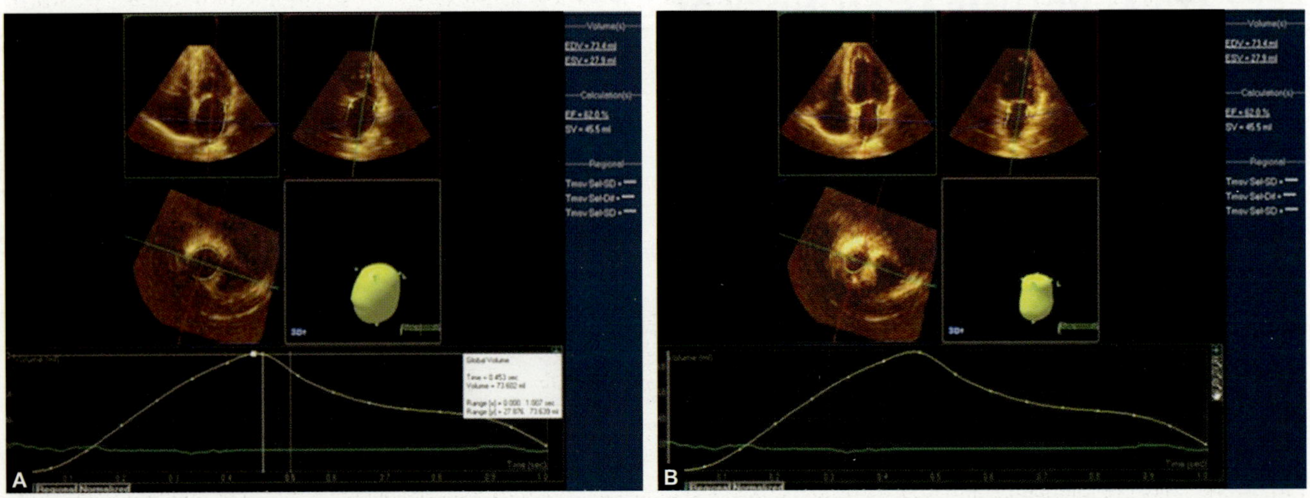

Figs. 2A and B: Real-time three-dimensional echocardiography recordings of maximum (A) and minimum (B) left atrial volumes.

and volume, LA minimum volume is closely related to LA maximal elastance (a load-independent measure of atrial contractility) because it is measured at end-diastole after being exposed to LV diastolic pressure accounting for atrial afterload.[9] The prevalence of LAE in hypertensive populations assessed by volumetric methods ranges from 32% to 68% amongst various studies, and likelihood of having LVH is approximately threefold greater in patients with LAE compared to without.[1]

CLINICAL IMPLICATIONS OF INCREASED LEFT ATRIAL VOLUME

Stroke and LAV, the causal link to enlarged left atrium had been pointed out in 1995 from data of Framingham Heart Study based on linear measurements that for every 10-mm increase in LA size, the relative risk of stroke was 2.4 in men [95% confidence interval (CI), 1.6–3.7] and 1.4 in women (95% CI, 0.9–2.1); the relative risk of death was 1.3 in men (95% CI, 1.0–1.5) and 1.4 in women (95% CI, 1.1–1.7). In 2008, Mayo investigators studied the role of LAV as a biomarker for ischemic stroke and suggested population risk attributable to increased LAVI (LAVI ≥ 28 mL/m^2) was estimated to be 29%. In 2017, the role of LAVI in first-ever acute ischemic stroke was elucidated in a prospective study enrolling patients more than 50 years of age; increased LAVI (LAVI > 28 mL/m^2) was present in most patients (68.4%) with first-ever ischemic stroke; highest prevalence (83.6%) was found in cardioembolic stroke group. LAVI was 32.4 ± 4.0 mL/m^2 for cardioembolic strokes, 29.7 ± 3.4 mL/m^2 for the other stroke subtypes ($p < 0.001$). Optimal cutoff value of LAVI 30 mL/m^2 had 81% sensitivity, and 64% specificity to distinguish cardioembolic strokes from other stroke subtypes. Mortality rate was significantly lower in patients with normal LAV (LAVI ≤ 28 mL/m^2) (n = 4, 4.1%) compared to patients with elevated LAVI (n = 47, 22.2%) ($p < 0.001$) (Fig. 3).

Mortality risk with increased LAV was also studied in a large clinical cohort with normal LV systolic dysfunction. Patients with a severe LAVI had a 42% increased mortality compared with patients with a normal LAVI; mortality risk increased by 0.9% ($p < 0.001$) independently after adjusting for LVMI [hazard ratio (HR), 1.006; 95% CI, 1.004–1.007; $p < 0.001$] with every mL/m^2 increase in LAVI (0.6% in normal LAVI group, 0.9% in concentric remodeling group, 1.5% in eccentric hypertrophy group, and 1.6% in concentric hypertrophy group).

Recent studies have shown the utility of LAV in predicting incident congestive HF (CHF). In a study of older patients with preserved LV systolic function, LAV >32 mL/m^2 was an independent predictor of first CHF. From baseline to within 4 weeks of incident CHF, individuals with preserved ejection fraction had a mean increase of 8 mL/m^2 in LAV, reflecting an additional burden of diastolic dysfunction in the preclinical phase of CHF. Prospective data from the Cardiovascular Health Study also showed an independent association of LAV with incident and prevalent CHF. This association of LAV with prevalent CHF was similar for both systolic and diastolic HF. Tsioufis et al. have shown that in patients with newly diagnosed essential hypertension without LVH, LAV is positively associated with office blood pressure (BP), ambulatory BP, LVMI, and plasma brain natriuretic peptide (BNP) levels. LA minimum volume obtained by 3D echocardiography was found to be the best independent predicting parameter for cardiovascular events (HR: 1.217, 95% CI 1.075–1.378; $p = 0.002$) and had the best correlation with the *E/Em* ratio ($r = 0.40$; $p < 0.001$), followed by LA maximum volume ($r = 0.29$; $p < 0.001$) and LV mass ($r = 0.23$; $p < 0.001$). LA maximum volume enlargement is mainly due to increased filling pressures; increased LA minimum volume also reflects the decreased ejection force of atrial pump. The correlation between LV filling pressures was stronger for minimal than maximal LAV in 70 patients undergoing cardiac catheterization LAV_{min} more than 40 mL/m^2 was sensitive

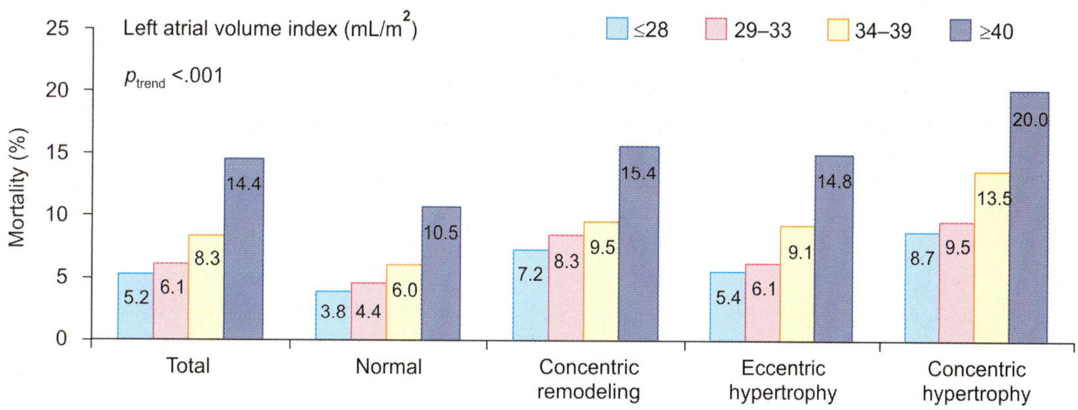

Fig. 3: Mortality prevalence by left atrial volume index in the total cohort and by four distinct left ventricular geometric patterns, including normal, concentric remodeling, eccentric hypertrophy, and concentric hypertrophy.

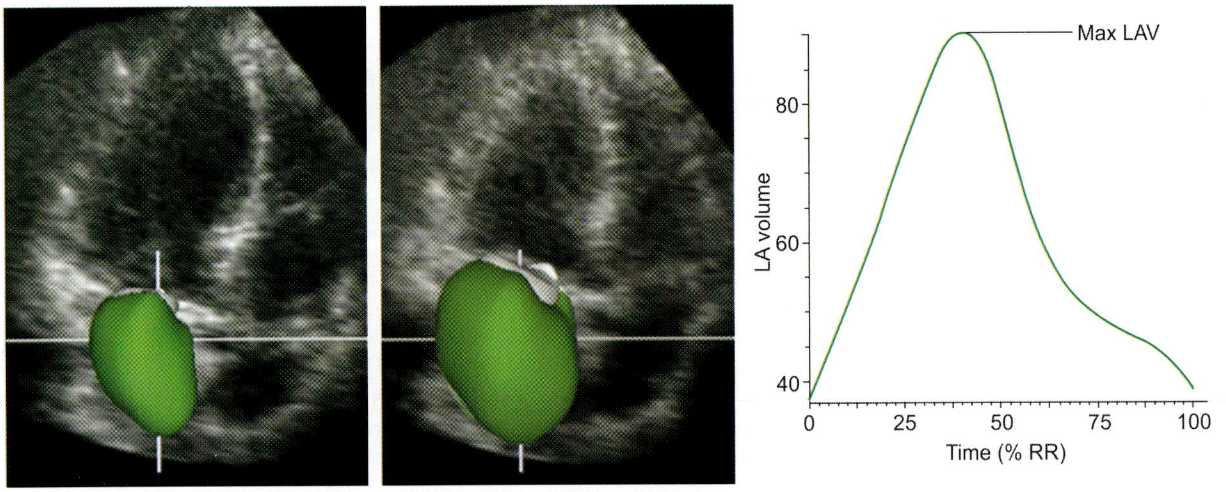

Fig. 4: 3D echocardiography-rendered minimal and maximal LAV and volume-time curve. (3D: three-dimensional; LAV: left atrial volume)

and specific (82% and 98%, respectively) for identifying a pulmonary capillary wedge pressure more than 12 mm Hg. In a prospective study of 574 participants in Olmsted County, minimal LAV was superior for predicting the 3-year risk for developing first AF and was an independent predictor in a model that included clinical variables, body mass index, diastolic dysfunction, and maximal LAV (Fig. 4).

Yoon et al. evaluated LAV and function by strain analysis demonstrating that LA indexed volume more than 34 mL/m^2 and LA strain less than 31% had a twofold and fourfold hazard increase, respectively, for patients with paroxysmal AF to develop persistent AF over a follow-up period of 26 months.

Left atrial volume estimation has been used to document results of interventions, viz. control of traditional cardiovascular risk factors, systemic hypertension, sleep apnea, vascular stiffness, and promoting dietary modification, physical activity for weight loss in addition to pharmacotherapy with vasodilators, such as angiotensin converting-enzyme inhibitor (ACEI) and angiotensin receptor blocker (ARB) aimed at reverse remodeling.[10-15]

The above studies show that LAV is becoming a benchmark of echocardiography measurements as it has proven to be a robust predictive and therapeutic biomarker which is not only the expression of chronic diastolic dysfunction but should be considered as a clinical endpoint for the physicians indicating that a reduction in LAV after any therapeutic intervention reduces the risk of atrial fibrillation, incident HF, and cardioembolic stroke.

CONCLUSION

Left atrial volume index has diagnostic, prognostic and therapeutic clinical implications.

REFERENCES

1. Cuspidi C, Rescaldani M, Sala C. Prevalence of echocardiographic left-atrial enlargement in hypertension: a systematic review of recent clinical studies. Am J Hypertens. 2013;26(4):456-64.
2. Su G, Cao H, Xu S, et al. Left atrial enlargement in the early stage of hypertensive heart disease: a common but ignored condition. J Clin Hypertens. 2014;16(3):192-7.
3. Nikitin NP, Witte KK, Thackray SD, et al. Effect of age and sex on left atrial morphology and function. Eur J Echocardiogr. 2003;4:36-42.
4. Lang RM, Bierig M, Devereux RB, et al. Recommendations for chamber quantification: a report from the American Society of Echocardiography's Guidelines and Standards Committee and the Chamber Quantification Writing Group, developed in conjunction with the European Association of Echocardiography, a branch of the European Society of Cardiology. Eur J Echocardiogr. 2006;7:79-108.
5. Tsang TS, Abhayaratna WP, Barnes ME, et al. Prediction of cardiovascular outcomes with left atrial size: is volume superior to area or diameter? J Am Coll Cardiol. 2006;47:1018-23.
6. Maddukuri PV, Vieira ML, DeCastro S, et al. What is the best approach for the assessment of left atrial size? Comparison of various unidimensional and two-dimensional parameters with three-dimensional echocardiographically determined left atrial volume. J Am Soc Echocardiogr. 2006;19:1026-32.
7. Vyas H, Jackson K, Chenzbraun A. Switching to volumetric left atrial measurements: impact on routine echocardiographic practice. Eur J Echocardiogr. 2011;12:107-11.
8. Badano LP, Pezzutto N, Marinigh R, et al. How many patients would be misclassified using M-mode and two-dimensional estimates of left atrial size instead of left atrial volume? A three-dimensional echocardiographic study. J Cardiovasc Med. 2008;9:476-84.

9. Hoit BD. Left atrial size and function role in prognosis. J Am Coll Cardiol. 2014;63(6):493-505.
10. Benjamin EJ, D'Agostino RB, Belanger AJ, et al. Left atrial size and the risk of stroke and death. The Framingham Heart Study. Circulation. 1995;92:835-41.
11. Biteker M, Kayatas K, Basaran Ö, et al. The role of left atrial volume index in patients with a first-ever acute ischemic stroke. J Stroke Cerebrovasc Dis. 2017; 26(2):321-26.
12. Park SM, Kim YH, Choi JI, et al. Left atrial electromechanical conduction time can predict six-month maintenance of sinus rhythm after electrical cardioversion in persistent atrial fibrillation by Doppler tissue echocardiography. J Am Soc Echocardiogr. 2010; 23(3):309-14.
13. Patel DA, Lavie CJ, Milani RV, et al. Clinical implications of left atrial enlargement: a review. Ochsner J. 2009;9(4):191-6.
14. Caselli S, Canali E, Foschi ML, et al. Long-term prognostic significance of three dimensional echocardiographic parameters of the left ventricle and left atrium. Eur J Echocardiogr. 2010;11(3):250-6.
15. Pritchett AM, Mahoney DW, Jacobsen SJ, et al. Diastolic dysfunction and left atrial volume: a population-based study. J Am Coll Cardiol. 2005;45(1):87-92.

6

CHAPTER

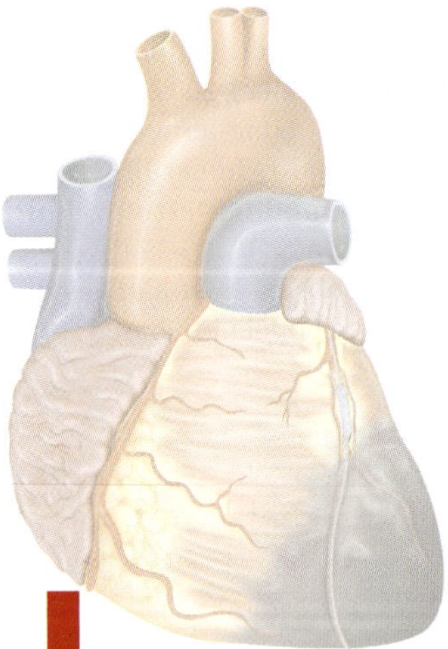

Advances in Diastology by Echocardiography in Hypertension

Aniruddha De

INTRODUCTION

Heart failure (HF) is found in 1–2% of the adult population and increased up to 10% as age advances.[1] 50% of HF cases are heart failure with preserved ejection fraction (EF) (HFpEF) and its incidence is rising. Hypertension (HT) is the major determinant and modifiable risk factor responsible for the pathogenesis and prognosis of patients with HFpEF.[2] Moreover, mortality rate in heart failure in reduced ejection fraction (HFrEF) is slightly higher than for HFpEF patients.[3] In addition to HT, diabetes mellitus, chronic obstructive pulmonary disease, cardiac arrhythmias, coronary artery disease, obesity, dyslipidemia, and arthritis are the major conditions associated frequently with HFpEF. But HT is still the most potent cause of HFpEF and is considered as major cause for diastolic dysfunction (DD).[4] There is no definite treatment available for HFpEF patient in contrast to HFrEF to improve mortality and morbidity.[5] HFpEF is found in 55–90% of patient with HT in contrast to HFrEF where prevalence of HT is 48–82%.[6] The prevalence of HT is 51% in HFpEF and 41% in HFrEF which are observed in a meta-analysis of 31 studies (n = 41,972)[7] and the most frequent comorbidity with HFpEF was found to be HT in the tune of 78% in a recent prospective study.[8] The measurement of left ventricular (LV) diastolic function and LV filling pressure (LVFP) by commonly used and various advanced echocardiographic parameters are the most important tools in any hypertensive patient.

PATHOPHYSIOLOGY MECHANISMS OF LEFT VENTRICULAR DIASTOLIC DYSFUNCTION IN HYPERTENSION (FLOWCHART 1)

Left ventricular DD (LVDD) with impaired LV relaxation and diastolic stiffness with LV hypertrophy (LVH) are the major abnormalities in HFpEF.[9,10] DD is mainly due to ongoing LVH and LV mass is directly proportional to blood pressure (BP) as an adaptive response to increased afterload.[11] Several studies reveal altered myocardial function, cardiomyocyte hypertrophy, stiffness, and fibrosis of myocardium in patient with HFpEF. An elastic protein titin is responsible for cardiac

Flowchart 1: Pathways of LV diastolic dysfunction secondary to hypertension.[48]

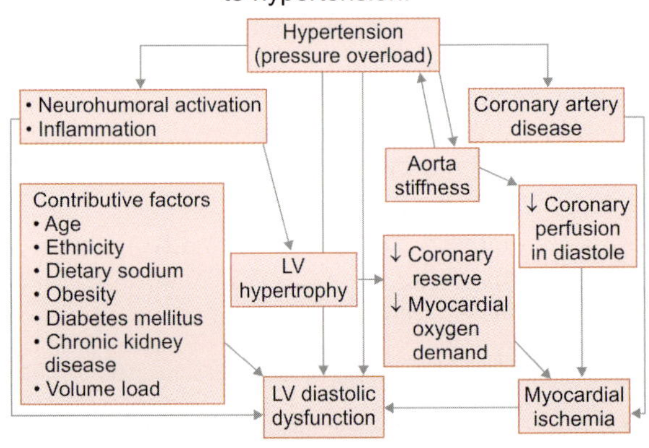

(LV: left ventricular)

stiffness. Moreover, reduced level of protein kinase G (PKG) activity leads to hypophosphorylation of titin, which in turn increase myocardial stiffness in HFpEF.[12-14] In addition, chronic activation of renin-angiotensin-aldosterone system (RAAS), stimulated by HT, is an alternative cause of myocardial fibrosis and LVH. Moreover, LVH of similar extent is found in hypertensive patients with no HF and patient with HFpEF. Hence, severity of LVH is not the sole factor for the development of HFpEF.[15,16] In addition to DD and LVH, various other mechanisms are responsible for the pathogenesis of HFpEF including LV systolic dysfunction, defect in ventricular-arterial coupling, disorder of endothelial function with reduced vasodilator reserve, impaired left atrial (LA) function, pulmonary arterial HT with right ventricular dysfunction. All these factors produced HFpEF a mixed state with complex pathophysiology and heterogeneous phenotypes. Though HT and HFpEF are closely associated with each other, still it is not clearly understood which hypertensive patients will progress to HFpEF. Comorbidities can lead to a systemic inflammatory response and produced oxidative stress in the microvascular endothelium, which reduces bioavailability of nitric oxide (NO) in the myocardium and fall of PKG activity in cardiomyocytes. This in turn produces a proinflammatory state and gradually leads to stiffness of myocardium.[17]

CLINICAL FACTORS INFLUENCING LEFT VENTRICULAR DIASTOLIC FUNCTION IN HYPERTENSION

- *Age:* Aging and HT are intimately related and both are responsible for development LVDD.[18]
- *Ethnicity:* Blacks are more prone to develop DD than whites, which remained statistically significant even after correction of other cardiovascular risk factors and antihypertensive treatment.[19]
- *Dietary sodium intake:* Salt intake may initiate cardiac fibrosis, which is not due to hemodynamic load. Hence, increased salt intake can cause direct action on myocardium.[20]
- *Obesity:* LV diastolic function is impaired in obese compared to lean individuals and the extent of LVDD is proportionate to body mass index.[21]
- *Diabetes mellitus:* LVDD and the consequent higher filling pressures are compounded if diabetes mellitus and systemic HT coexist than the conditions are present alone.[22]
- *Chronic kidney disease:* Worst diastolic function is found in HT with chronic kidney disease, which is not dependent on LV mass and BP.[23]

ASSESSMENT OF LEFT VENTRICULAR DIASTOLIC FUNCTION IN HYPERTENSION BY ECHOCARDIOGRAPHY

Cardiac catheterization is still considered as a gold standard for determination of LVFPs.[24] However, this invasive procedure is not suitable for our routine clinical practice. Advances in Doppler echocardiography are now the most important and commonly used tool to identify LVDD in any clinical setting for the last few years. Several echocardiographic measurements have been used to estimate LV diastolic function, which include mitral valve (MV) inflow velocities (peak E- and A-wave and the E/A ratio), deceleration time (DT) of MV inflow velocity, tissue Doppler velocities (e′ wave and the E/e′ ratio), LA volume index, pulmonary vein velocities (systolic and diastolic wave), measurement of peak tricuspid regurgitation (TR) jet velocity, and isovolumic relaxation time (IVRT). Recent guidelines from the American Society of Echocardiography and the European Association of Cardiovascular Imaging recommended that, in patient with normal LVEF (>50%) and no evidence of myocardial disease, four echocardiographic parameters should be evaluated to find the status of LV diastolic function (e′ velocity, E/e′ ratio, left atrium maximum volume index, and TR systolic jet velocity).[25] Hence, these four variables are ideal and should be used to evaluate the diastolic function for the patient of HT and hypertensive heart disease. However, few advance parameters [e.g. global longitudinal strain (GLS)] can be used in specific situation and have been proposed as close surrogates of LV relaxation with LV and LAFPs.

ADVANCE ECHOCARDIOGRAPHIC PARAMETERS TO EVALUATE DIASTOLIC DYSFUNCTION IN HYPERTENSION

- Longitudinal and circumferential global strain rates are often impaired in patient with HT with LVDD when compared with the individual with normal diastolic function. Longitudinal strain is a strong predictor of cardiovascular morbidity and mortality in patients with HFpEF and reduction in systolic function in patient with LVDD is very important prognostically. Systolic dysfunction and DD are often interrelated and altered the calcium cycling in cardiac myocytes and induce fibrosis. As a result, LV filling will be impaired and will fail to develop optimum LV force by limiting the contraction of myocytes.[26-28]

- Left ventricular global longitudinal diastolic strain rate evaluation during isovolumic relaxation period and early diastole by speckle-tracking echocardiography (STE) correlated well with the time constant of LV relaxation. Diastolic strain is considered a better substitute for e′ to evaluate LVFPs.[29]
- Correlation between DD and LV untwisting rate is also established. Peak observed during untwisting is delayed in DD patient with normal LVEF and volume.[30]
- Normal LV diastolic function become abnormal with exercise in few patients and this subset of patient with HFpEF is prognostically worst. So, diastolic stress test should be performed when DD is absent at rest. An increase in the E/e′ ratio and pulmonary artery systolic pressure with physical exercise is associated with elevation of LV end-diastolic pressure (LVEDP). Diastolic stress test had a sensitivity of 73% and a specificity of 96% if E/e′ ratio is more than 13 for an LVEDP more than 15 mm Hg.[31,32]

Due to technical difficulties, complexities of measurement, and their wide variability, these advance parameters are not routinely used in spite of good results. The real aim is to measure and quantify the LVFP and not to classify the diastolic patterns by echocardiography. Increased LVFP is essential for maintaining the stroke volume initially as a compensatory mechanism but ultimately indicates the prognosis. So, a combination of techniques and maneuvers is needed for the clinical staging of LVDD and filling dynamics not solely by any single parameter.

How to record these echocardiographic parameters?[33]

- *It is recommended to record*:
  - Clinical profile (height, weight, body surface area, relevant history, and physical examination)
  - Heart rate
  - Blood pressure
  - *Echocardiographic findings*: LV wall thickness, regional wall motion abnormality, LV volume, EF
  - Left atrial volume
  - Any rhythm abnormality
  - Morphology of MV for proper evaluation of diastolic function in various and specific clinical conditions.
- Each parameter has its own limitation and signals should be assessed carefully. Suboptimal Doppler signals are not included in final evaluation of LV diastolic function.
- Single normal measurement does not indicate normal diastolic function because several hemodynamic factors affect any particular signal and few measurements may be normal in the presence of DD. Hence, no single parameter should be used alone. Always two or more of the indices should be taken for a given individual. The echocardiographic parameters of DD may not be always correct in normal subject with normal echocardiographic findings.[25]
- The following parameters are routinely used for the evaluation of diastolic function:
  - Transmitral Doppler inflow
  - Tissue Doppler imaging
  - Pulmonary venous Doppler flow.

Transmitral Doppler Inflow (Figs. 1 to 3)

- Normal pattern of LV diastolic filling is recorded with pulsed Doppler [pulse wave (PW)]. Apical four-chamber (4Ch) view with color flow imaging is used for spectral Doppler. Mitral inflow velocities are recorded by PW Doppler after proper alignment.[34,35]
- Sample volume (1–3 mm) is placed at the tip of mitral leaflet and record peak modal velocity in early diastole for peak E wave which corresponds to T wave in electrocardiogram (ECG) and in late diastole for A wave which correspond to P wave in ECG. There should not be any spikes or feathering in optimal waveform. It is recommended that signal gain and filter setting should be kept at minimum level (100–200 MHz).[25]

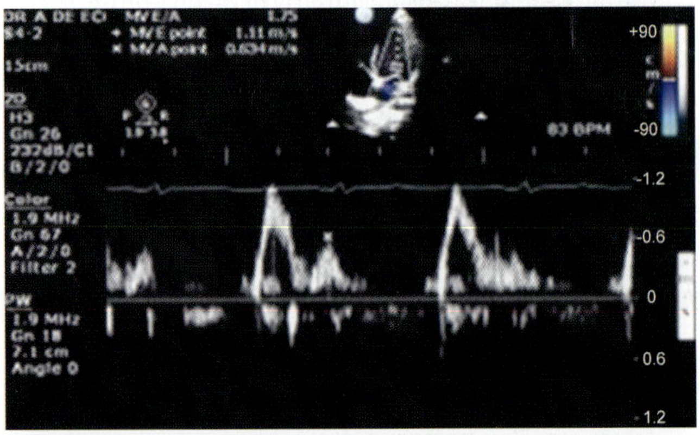

Fig. 1: Mitral inflow: E wave, A wave, and E/A ratio.

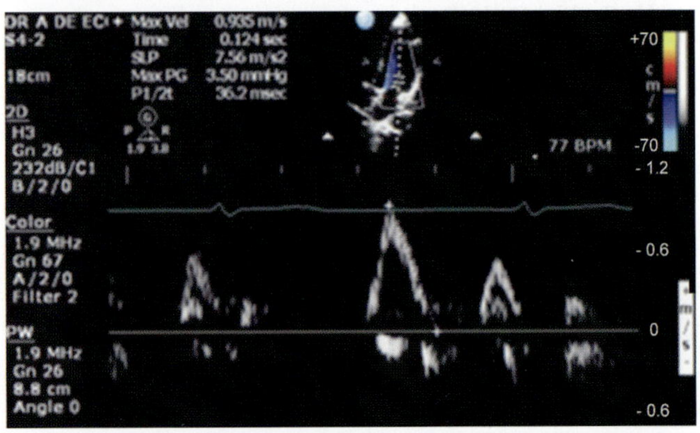

Fig. 2: Slope of E wave for deceleration time.

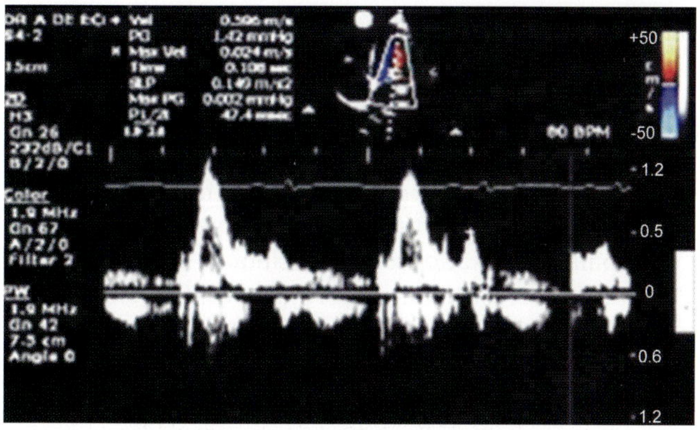

Fig. 3: Mitral inflow A wave duration.

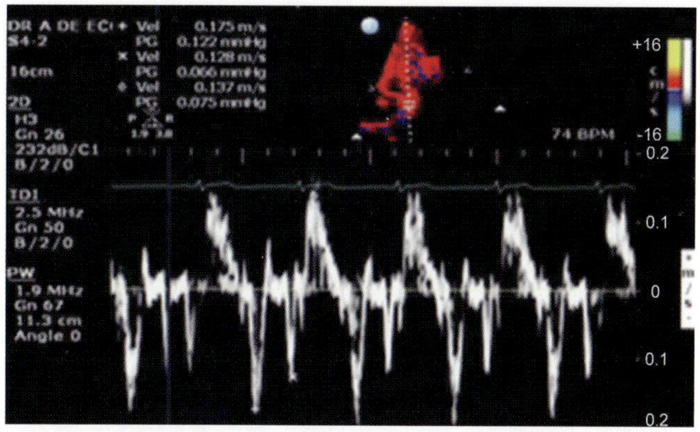

Fig. 5: Lateral mitral annulus tissue Doppler.

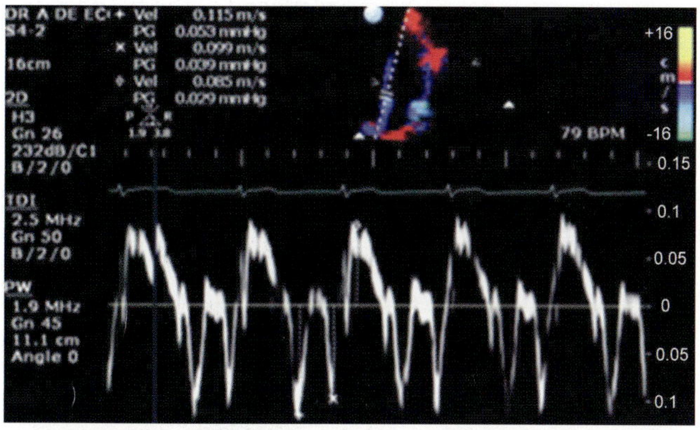

Fig. 4: Septal mitral annulus tissue Doppler.

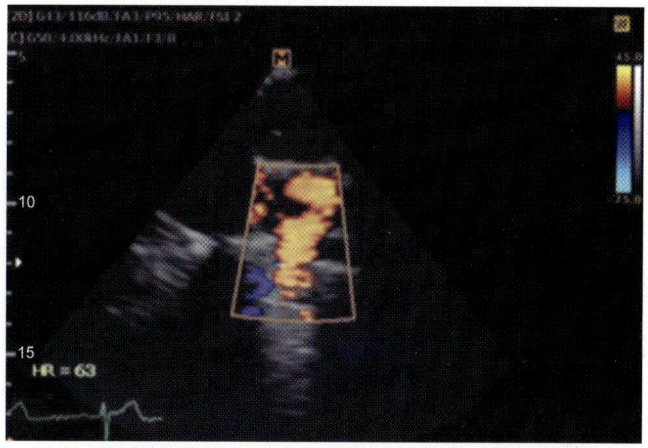

Fig. 6: Right superior pulmonary vein flow.

- Primary measurements are peak E and A velocities, E/A ratio, IVRT, and DT.[25,34]
- Mitral valve A duration (ms) is also measured: Here, sample volume (1–3 mm) is placed at the level of mitral annulus between annulus and leaflet tips. There should not be any spikes or feathering in optimal waveform.[25]
- Mitral inflow patterns are four types: (1) normal, (2) impaired relaxation, (3) pseudonormal, and (4) restrictive pattern.

Tissue Doppler Imaging (Figs. 4 and 5)

- Mitral annular velocities are measured in tissue by PW from the apical 4Ch view.[36-38]
- Sample volume of 5–10 mm by PW Doppler is measured at mitral septal and lateral annulus. Then, average e′ velocity is calculated.[25] Position of sample volume should be kept in the septal and lateral wall within 1 cm from the junction of the mitral leaflet with the walls.
- There should not be any spikes or feathering in optimal waveform. It is recommended that signal gain and filter setting should be kept at minimum level.[25]
- Measure the average of three consecutive cardiac cycles. The measurement should be done at end-expiration. The sweep speed should be kept at 50–100 mm/s.
- Systolic, early (e′), and late (a′) diastolic velocities should be measured.
- E/e′ ratio is an excellent parameter of LVFPs in a patient with HT.
- However, the E/e′ ratio is not a consistent indicator of LVFPs, e.g. normal individual, constrictive pericarditis, severe mitral annular calcification (MAC), and MV disease.

Pulmonary Venous Doppler Flow (Figs. 6 to 8)

- Pulmonary venous flow is evaluated by PW Doppler from apical 4Ch view.[39,40]
- For optimal spectral waveforms, sample volume (1–3 mm) is placed 1–2 cm inside the pulmonary vein.
- There should not be any spikes or feathering in optimal waveform. It is recommended that signal gain and

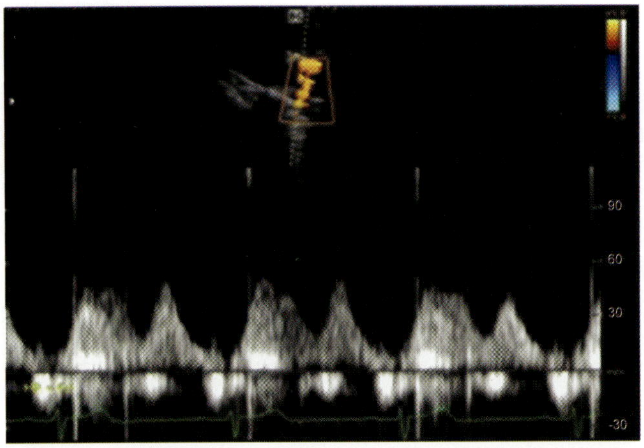

Fig. 7: Pulmonary venous Doppler.

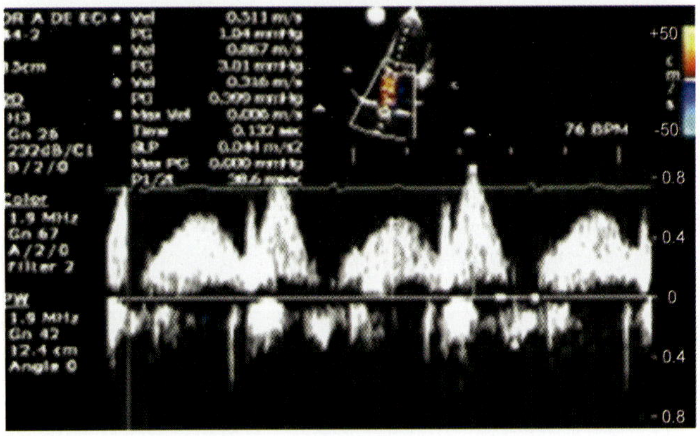

Fig. 8: Peak and duration of Ar velocity.

filter setting should be kept at minimum level (100–200 MHz).[25]

- Peak modal velocity at leading edge of spectral Doppler is measured. Peak S wave is measured at early systole, D wave at early diastole, and peak Ar velocity in late diastole. Then, the S/D ratio and systolic filling fraction are recorded. Another important parameter is (Ar A) measurement, which is calculated by the time difference between Ar duration and mitral A-wave duration.[25]
- Ar velocity, duration, and Ar A duration increased when LVEDP is elevated.
- S—Inward systolic flow: LA relaxation and LV contraction: with mitral annular descent to the apex. D—Forward flow during diastole similar to an E velocity (normal D>> S but older than 60-year S > D). A—Atrial systole, retrograde flow from LA to pulmonary vein (if Ar is increased, then LVEDP is increased).
- *Normal parameters*: Forward flow (systolic and diastolic) and flow reversal during atrial contraction (Ar).
- Reduced flow into the LV during atrial contraction is noted due to increased resistance. Increased resistance is often observed when compliance of LV decreases with subsequent elevation of LVFP. As a result, forward flow into LV is reduced and more back flow of blood into the PV is noted during atrial contraction. Hence, compliance is calculated indirectly by the ratio between forward and back flow. In patient with elevated left atrial pressure (LAP) and low EF, systolic flow is decreased. Higher S/D velocity ratio is observed when there is impaired relaxation of ventricle and low S/D ratio is found with restriction abnormality while evaluating the pulmonary velocity curves.[40]

Diastolic Dysfunction Evaluated Based on the Above Parameters

The four recommended parameters and their values (Flowchart 2):

1. Annular e′ velocity (septal e′ < 7 cm/s, lateral e′ < 10 cm/s)
2. Average E/e′ ratio more than 14
3. Left atrial maximum volume index more than 34 mL/m^2, and
4. Peak TR velocity more than 2.8 m/s.

If a single clinically relevant parameter is available, e.g. lateral e′ or septal e′ velocity, then E/e′ ratio more than 13 at lateral annulus or E/e′ more than 15 at septal annulus is considered abnormal.

If more than 50% of the available variables are not abnormal, then LV diastolic function should be considered normal.

If more than 50% of the available variables are abnormal, then there is LVDD.

If 50% of the available parameters are not matching the values, then study is considered inconclusive.

ADVANCED DIASTOLIC INDICES

- Indices are tissue Doppler imaging or STE.
- Tissue Doppler imaging measures velocities of myocardial tissue by Doppler principle. So, angulation between ultrasound beam and plane of motion should be kept below 15°.
- To achieve high temporal resolution, high frame rate of 100/s is required. Offline analysis was done and evaluated either as color 2D images or reconstructed image as deformation (i.e. strain) curves.
- Speckle-tracking echocardiography actually tracks myocardial "speckles" from frame to frame. The speckles are recognized after filtering out noise as very small structures in the image.
- Myocardial velocity and strain can now be derived from STE. The advantage of this technique is the angle independency and frame rate should be kept at 50–80/s.

Flowchart 2: Practical scheme for diagnosis and graduation of diastolic dysfunction.

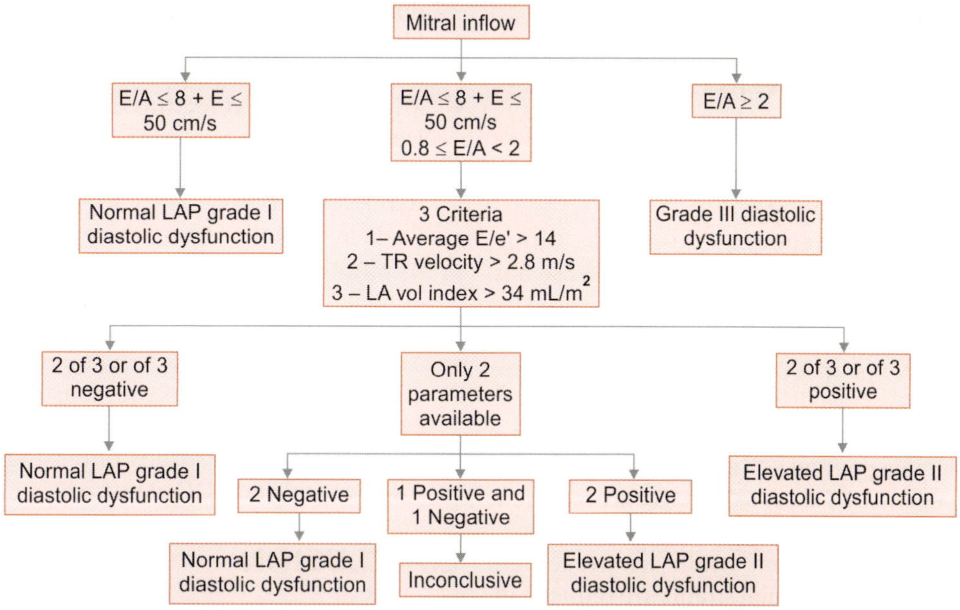

(LAP: left atrial pressure)

Source: Adapted from Nagueh SF, Smiseth OA, Appleton CP, et al. Recommendations for the evaluation of left ventricular diastolic function by echocardiography: an update from the American Society of Echocardiography and the European Association of Cardiovascular Imaging. J Am Soc Echocardiogr. 2016;29:277-314; Nazário Leão R, Marques da Silva P. Diastolic dysfunction in hypertension. Hipertens Riesgo Vasc. 2017;34:128-39.

The same mechanics is applied on velocity vector imaging.[41,42]

VENTRICULAR STRAIN, STRAIN RATE, AND TWIST

- In systolic dysfunction, radial, circumferential, and longitudinal strains are affected. Involvement of twist is also observed.
- In DD, radial and longitudinal strains are only involved, whereas circumferential strain and twist are preserved.
- *Disadvantage*: Still in experimental stage and the software is available in the state-of-art machines.
- Delayed relaxation is observed by STE to recognize ischemic myocardium while evaluating diastolic function.
- This is the basis of diastolic strain where even after recovery from transient myocardial ischemia, delayed relaxation persists for a considerable period of time and can be detected by measurement of strain during diastole.[43,44]

ASSESSMENT OF LEFT VENTRICULAR GLOBAL DIASTOLIC FUNCTION

There are many situations where measurement of DD is a real challenge particularly in patients of HT with MV lesion, chronic constrictive pericarditis, left bundle branch block, and severe MAC, where new parameters are helpful.

- Tissue Doppler echocardiographic time intervals by pulsed Doppler of the mitral annulus.
- Myocardial deformation measurements—estimation of LV twist, untwisting, and relaxation of LV.
- Left atrial function.
- Left ventricular GLS (LV GLS) is usually reduced in patients with HF with normal EF. Hence, LV GLS measurement can estimate LVEDP.[25]

MYOCARDIAL DEFORMATION MEASUREMENTS

- Parameters for deformation are strain rate, which during the IVRT is called strain rates during isovolumetric relaxation (SRIVR) and during E wave is called SRe.
- Consider resting length in deformation measurements but not the velocity measurements.
- Strain rates during isovolumetric relaxation is measured at isovolumic relaxation period. Mitral valve is closed during this period. So, transmitral pressure gradient will not be a problem here and also not affected by any changes in preload.
- Mitral E/SRIVR ratio also may be used as an index of filling pressures. This parameter is applicable where E/e′ ratio falls in the indeterminate range, patient

with normal EF, and also with regional wall motion abnormality.[45,46]

LEFT VENTRICULAR TWIST AND UNTWISTING

Another important cardiac function of left ventricle is twisting and untwisting.

- When we look from the apex of left ventricle during systole, LV apex normally twists counterclockwise but base twists clockwise and potential energy is stored by this process.
- Immediately after systole LV untwists. Intraventricular pressure gradient is created by untwisting. LV torsion is the sum of both apical and basal twist.
- Tissue Doppler imaging and STE are the two parameters used to evaluate twist. LV short-axis images are best view for evaluation. Apical rotation exceeds basal rotation.
- Torsion and circumferential strain are preserved whereas longitudinal and radial strains are reduced in DD. At the initial stage of DD, torsion is reduced.
- Rotation is done by larger subepicardial fibers and the subendocardial torque counteracts this effect. So, the preferential involvement of the subendocardial and subepicardial tissue can lead to a change in twist. Subendocardial function is maximally reduced in diastolic HF.
- In systolic HF, subepicardial and LV midwall tissues are involved. As a result, there is reduction of torsion and circumferential strain.
- In diastolic HF with preserved EF, circumferential strain and torsion are preserved where depressed longitudinal function already exists.
- In normal subjects, both torsion and untwisting are increased during exercise. However, minimal increase of torsion and untwisting occur in a patient of HF due to gross reduction of LV filling during exercise. Twisting stores potential energy, which is released during untwisting at early diastole.[47]

DIASTOLIC STRESS TEST

- In patients presented with dyspnea on exertion, it is essential to evaluate LVFP during exercise if found normal at rest.
- Mitral inflow E, annular e′ velocities, and peak velocity of TR are measured at rest and during exercise.
- Often it is necessary to measure the parameters 1–2 minutes after stoppage of exercise where E and A of mitral inflow velocities fail to merge.
- It is important to note that filling pressures remain elevated even few minutes after cessation of exercise.
- Standard treadmill protocols are followed during diastolic stress test.
- Mitral inflow velocities are recorded by placing pulsed Doppler at the mitral tips.
- Mitral annular velocities are measured by spectral Doppler.
- Peak velocity of TR is measured by continuous wave (CW) Doppler.
- Positive diastolic stress test indicates increased LAP. As a result, velocity of mitral E wave is increased and annular e′ wave is preserved and subsequent increase in the pulmonary artery pressure.
- *Negative diastolic stress test*: Proportionate increase of e′ and mitral E velocities with constant E/e′ ratio during exercise.[36,47,48]
- Hence, major indications of diastolic stress test are dyspnea and early-DD at rest.[47,49]

CONCLUSION

Hypertension is the most common risk factor for LVDD in the general population. Hemodynamic overload, consequent myocardial ischemia, and several other mechanisms are responsible for LVDD because it is the most potent predictor of HF and other cardiovascular events. Advances in Doppler echocardiography are now the most important and commonly used tool to identify LVDD in hypertensive patients for the last decade. Four echocardiographic parameters, annular e′ velocity, average E/e′ ratio, LA maximum volume index, and peak TR velocity are the most important amongst several echocardiographic measurements to estimate LV diastolic function. Advanced echocardiographic parameters are sparing used in specific situation due to technical difficulties and complexities of measurements.

REFERENCES

1. Ponikowski P, Voors AA, Anker SD, et al. ESC Guidelines for the diagnosis and treatment of acute and chronic heart failure: the task force for the diagnosis and treatment of acute and chronic heart failure of the European Society of Cardiology (ESC). Developed with the special contribution of the Heart Failure Association (HFA) of the ESC. Eur J Heart Fail. 2016;37:2129-200.
2. Oktay AA, Shah SJ. Current perspectives on systemic hypertension in heart failure with preserved ejection fraction. Curr Cardiol Rep. 2014;16(12):545.
3. Steinberg BA, Zhao X, Heidenreich PA, et al. Trends in patients hospitalized with heart failure and preserved left ventricular ejection fraction: prevalence, therapies, and outcomes. Circulation. 2012;126(1):65-75.
4. Yancy CW, Jessup M, Bozkurt B, et al. 2013 ACCF/AHA guideline for the management of heart failure: a report of

the American College of Cardiology Foundation/American Heart Association task force on practice guidelines. J Am Coll Cardiol. 2013;62(16):147-239.

5. Teo LY, Chan LL, Lam CS. Heart failure with preserved ejection fraction in hypertension. Curr Opin Cardiol. 2016;31(4):410-6.
6. Nichols GA, Reynolds K, Kimes TM, et al. Comparison of risk of re-hospitalization, all-cause mortality, and medical care resource utilization in patients with heart failure and preserved versus reduced ejection fraction. Am J Cardiol. 2015;116(7):1088-92.
7. Berry C, Doughty RN, Granger C, et al. The survival of patients with heart failure with preserved or reduced left ventricular ejection fraction: an individual patient data meta-analysis. Eur Heart J. 2012;33(14):1750-7.
8. Lund LH, Donal E, Oger E, et al. Association between cardiovascular vs. non-cardiovascular co-morbidities and outcomes in heart failure with reserved ejection fraction. Eur J Heart Fail. 2014;16(9):992-1001.
9. Zile MR, Baicu CF, Gaasch WH. Diastolic heart failure abnormalities in active relaxation and passive stiffness of the left ventricle. N Engl J Med. 2004;350(19):1953-9.
10. Mohammed SF, Borlaug BA, Roger VL, et al. Comorbidity and ventricular and vascular structure and function in heart failure with preserved ejection fraction: a community-based study. Circ Heart Fail. 2012;5(6):710-9.
11. Gradman AH, Wilson JT. Hypertension and diastolic heart failure. Curr Cardiol Rep. 2009;11(6):422-9.
12. Van Heerebeek L, Paulus WJ. Understanding heart failure with preserved ejection fraction: where are we today? Neth Heart J. 2016;24(4):227-36.
13. Linke WA, Hamdani N. Gigantic business: titin properties and function through thick and thin. Circ Res. 2014;114(6):1052-68.
14. Zile MR, Baicu CF, Ikonomidis JS, et al. Myocardial stiffness in patients with heart failure and a preserved ejection fraction: contributions of collagen and titin. Circulation. 2015;131(14):1247-59.
15. Essick EE, Sam F. Cardiac hypertrophy and fibrosis in the metabolic syndrome: a role for aldosterone and the mineralocorticoid receptor. Int J Hypertens. 2011;2011:346985.
16. Lam CS, Roger VL, Rodeheffer RJ, et al. Cardiac structure and ventricular-vascular function in persons with heart failure and reserved ejection fraction from Olmsted County, Minnesota. Circulation. 2007;115(15):1982-90.
17. Paulus WJ, Tschope C. A novel paradigm for heart failure with preserved ejection fraction: comorbidities drive myocardial dysfunction and remodeling through coronary microvascular endothelial inflammation. J Am Coll Cardiol. 2013;62(4):263-71.
18. Dini FL, Galderisi M, Nistri S, et al. Abnormal left ventricular longitudinal function assessed by echocardiographic and tissue Doppler imaging is a powerful predictor of diastolic dysfunction in hypertensive patients: the SPHERE study. Int J Cardiol. 2013;168:3351-8.
19. Kishi S, Reis JP, Venkatesh BA, et al. Race-ethnic and sex differences in left ventricular structure and function: the Coronary Artery Risk Development in Young Adults (CARDIA) Study. J Am Heart Assoc. 2015;4:e001264.
20. Frohlich ED, Varagic J. Sodium directly impairs target organ function in hypertension. Curr Opin Cardiol. 2005;20:424-9.
21. Leggio M, Cruciani G, Sgorbini L, et al. Obesity-related adjunctive systo-diastolic ventricular dysfunction in patients with hypertension: echocardiographic assessment with tissue Doppler velocity and strain imaging. Hypertens Res. 2011;34:468-73.
22. Russo C, Jin Z, Homma S, et al. Effect of diabetes and hypertension on left ventricular diastolic function in a high-risk population without evidence of heart disease. Eur J Heart Fail. 2010;12:454-61.
23. Nardi E, Cottone S, Mulè G, et al. Influence of chronic renal insufficiency on left ventricular diastolic function in hypertensives without left ventricular hypertrophy. J Nephrol. 2007;20:320-8.
24. Verma A, Solomon SD. Diastolic dysfunction as a link between hypertension and heart failure. Med Clin North Am. 2009;93:647-64.
25. Nagueh SF, Smiseth OA, Appleton CP, et al. Recommendations for the evaluation of left ventricular diastolic function by echocardiography: an update from the American Society of Echocardiography and the European Association of Cardiovascular Imaging. J Am Soc Echocardiogr. 2016;29: 277-314.
26. Ballo P, Nistri S, Cameli M, et al. Association of left ventricular longitudinal and circumferential systolic dysfunction with diastolic function in hypertension: a nonlinear analysis focused on the interplay with left ventricular geometry. J Card Fail. 2014;20:110-20.
27. Shah SJ, Aistrup GL, Gupta DK, et al. Ultrastructural and cellular basis for the development of abnormal myocardial mechanics during the transition from hypertension to heart failure. Am J Physiol Heart Circ Physiol. 2014;306:H88-100.
28. Galderisi M. Diagnosis and management of left ventricular diastolic dysfunction in the hypertensive patient. Am J Hypertens. 2011;24:507-17.
29. Kimura K, Takenaka K, Ebihara A, et al. Speckle tracking global strain rate E/E predicts LV filling pressure more accurately than traditional tissue Doppler E/E'. Echocardiography. 2012;29:404-10.
30. Wang J, Khoury DS, Yue Y, et al. Left ventricular untwisting rate by speckle tracking echocardiography. Circulation. 2007;116:2580-6.
31. Burgess MI, Jenkins C, Sharman JE, et al. Diastolic stress echocardiography: hemodynamic validation and clinical significance of estimation of ventricular filling pressure with exercise. J Am Coll Cardiol. 2006;47:1891-900.
32. Shim CY, Kim SA, Choi D, et al. Clinical outcomes of exercise-induced pulmonary hypertension in subjects with preserved left ventricular ejection fraction: implication of an increase in left ventricular filling pressure during exercise. Heart. 2011;97:1417-24.
33. De A. Echocardiographic assessment of diastolic function. J Indian Acad Echocardiogr Cardiovasc Imaging. 2017;1:214-21.

34. Appleton CP, Hatle LK, Popp RL. Relation of transmitral flow velocity patterns to left ventricular diastolic function: new insights from a combined hemodynamic and Doppler echocardiographic study. J Am Coll Cardiol. 1988;12:426-40.
35. Appleton CP, Jensen JL, Hatle LK, et al. Doppler evaluation of left and right ventricular diastolic function: a technical guide for obtaining optimal flow velocity recordings. J Am Soc Echocardiogr. 1997;10:271-92.
36. Waggoner AD, Bierig SM. Tissue Doppler imaging: a useful echocardiographic method for the cardiac sonographer to assess systolic and diastolic ventricular function. J Am Soc Echocardiogr. 2001;14:1143-52.
37. Nagueh SF, Middleton KJ, Kopelen HA, et al. Doppler tissue imaging: a noninvasive technique for evaluation of left ventricular relaxation and estimation of filling pressures. J Am Coll Cardiol. 1997;30:1527-33.
38. Nagueh SF, Sun H, Kopelen HA, et al. Hemodynamic determinants of the mitral annulus diastolic velocities by tissue Doppler. J Am Coll Cardiol. 2001;37:278-85.
39. Jensen JL, Williams FE, Beilby BJ, et al. Feasibility of obtaining pulmonary venous flow velocity in cardiac patients using transthoracic pulsed wave Doppler technique. J Am Soc Echocardiogr. 1997;10:60-6.
40. Klein AL, Tajik AJ. Doppler assessment of pulmonary venous flow in healthy subjects and in patients with heart disease. J Am Soc Echocardiogr. 1991;4:379-92.
41. Urheim S, Edvardsen T, Torp H, et al. Myocardial strain by Doppler echocardiography. Validation of a new method to quantify regional myocardial function. Circulation. 2000;102:1158-64.
42. Amundsen BH, Helle-Valle T, Edvardsen T, et al. Noninvasive myocardial strain measurement by speckle tracking echocardiography: validation against sonomicrometry and tagged magnetic resonance imaging. J Am Coll Cardiol. 2006;47:789-93.
43. Park SJ, Miyazaki C, Bruce CJ, et al. Left ventricular torsion by two-dimensional speckle tracking echocardiography in patients with diastolic dysfunction and normal ejection fraction. J Am Soc Echocardiogr. 2008;21:1129-37.
44. Notomi Y, Lysyansky P, Setser RM, et al. Measurement of ventricular torsion by two-dimensional ultrasound speckle tracking imaging. J Am Coll Cardiol. 2005;45:2034-41.
45. Wang J, Khoury D, Thohan V, et al. Global diastolic strain rate for the assessment of left ventricular relaxation and filling pressures. Circulation. 2007;115:1376-83.
46. Dokainish H, Sengupta R, Pillai M, et al. Usefulness of new diastolic strain and strain rate indexes for the estimation of left ventricular filling pressure. Am J Cardiol. 2008;101:1504-9.
47. Ha JW, Oh JK, Pellikka PA, et al. Diastolic stress echocardiography: a novel noninvasive diagnostic test for diastolic dysfunction using supine bicycle exercise Doppler echocardiography. J Am Soc Echocardiogr. 2005;18:63-8.
48. Nadruz W, Shah AM, Solomon SD. Diastolic dysfunction and hypertension. Med Clin N Am. 2017;101:7-17.
49. Nazário Leão R, Marques da Silva P. Diastolic dysfunction in hypertension. Hipertens Riesgo Vasc. 2017;34(3):128-39.

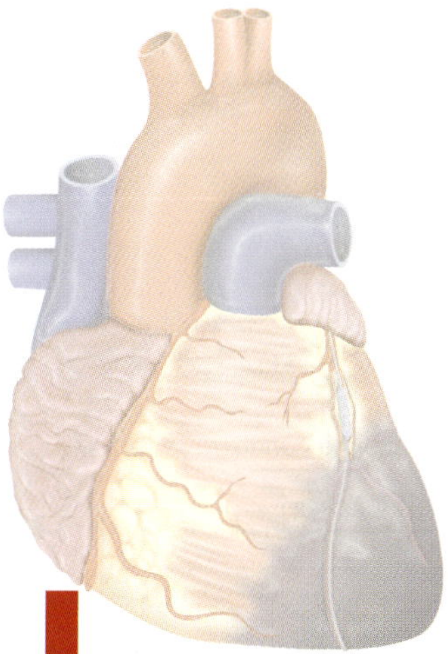

CHAPTER 7

Advances in Left Atrial Strain Evaluation by Echocardiography in Hypertension

KK Kapur, Naveen Garg

INTRODUCTION

Hypertension (HTN) and atrial fibrillations (AFs) both are the most common cardiovascular morbidities and both of these also share common risk factors, such as increasing with age, obesity, smoking, alcohol, diastolic failure, renal pathologies, etc. Both of these conditions are responsible for prothrombotic and hypercoagulation state leading to stroke, myocardial infarction, or other cardiovascular event. Many epidemiological studies had confirmed their intimate relationship in the development of systemic embolic phenomenon. Hypertension is prevalent in about 20–50% of adult population, and AF is prevalent in about 1–2% of general population, but their coexistence ranges from 50% to 90% among adults. Epidemiologic studies have shown that 1.8-fold increased risk of developing new-onset AF is associated with HTN and a 1.5-fold increased risk of progression to permanent AF among hypertensive patients.[1-5] A possible explanation is altered morphology, resulting in increased myocardial fibrosis due to higher pulsatile load on left atrial (LA). This fibrosis leads to microreentry electrical circuits that consequently lead to AF. Significantly, these subtle alterations are undetectable by traditional imaging methods (Fig. 1).

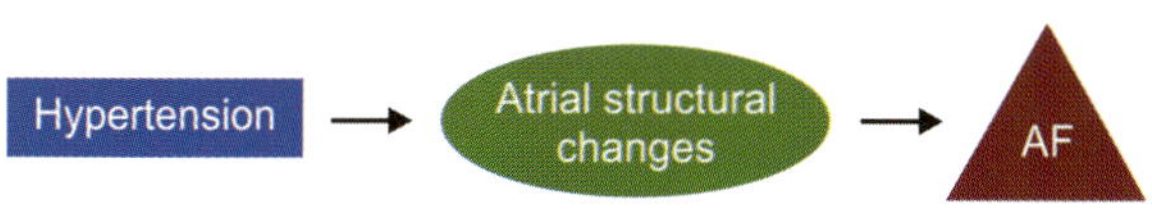

Fig. 1: Depicts hypertension as the cause of atrial structural deformations leading to AF. (AF: atrial fibrillation).

Thus, early diagnosis of LA chamber changes among hypertensive patients had become necessary to predict possible arrhythmias and to initiate suitable therapy. Left atrial strain (LAS) specially measured by novel technology of speckle-tracking echocardiographic (STE) imaging has emerged as a feasible methodology to predict the occurrence of AF.

LEFT ATRIAL FUNCTION

Left atrial function[6-8] has been divided into three phases of cardiac cycle (Figs. 2A and B).

1. *Reservoir:* The LA stores blood from pulmonary venous during left ventricular (LV) contraction and isovolumetric relaxation, from 0.3 seconds to 0.5 seconds.
2. *Conduit:* It transfers blood passively into the LV, during early diastole, from 0.5 seconds to 0.7 seconds.
3. *Pump:* Left atrial actively contracts and contributes between 15% and 30% of LV stroke volume, during the final phase of diastole, from 0.1 seconds to 0.2 seconds (Table 1).

ECHOCARDIOGRAPHIC ASSESSMENT OF LEFT ATRIAL STRAIN

Left atrial strain is the dimensionless index that describes the longitudinal shortening of the atrial fibers as the percentage of their original length and strain rate (SR) is the rate of this shortening. Left atrial strain/strain rate was

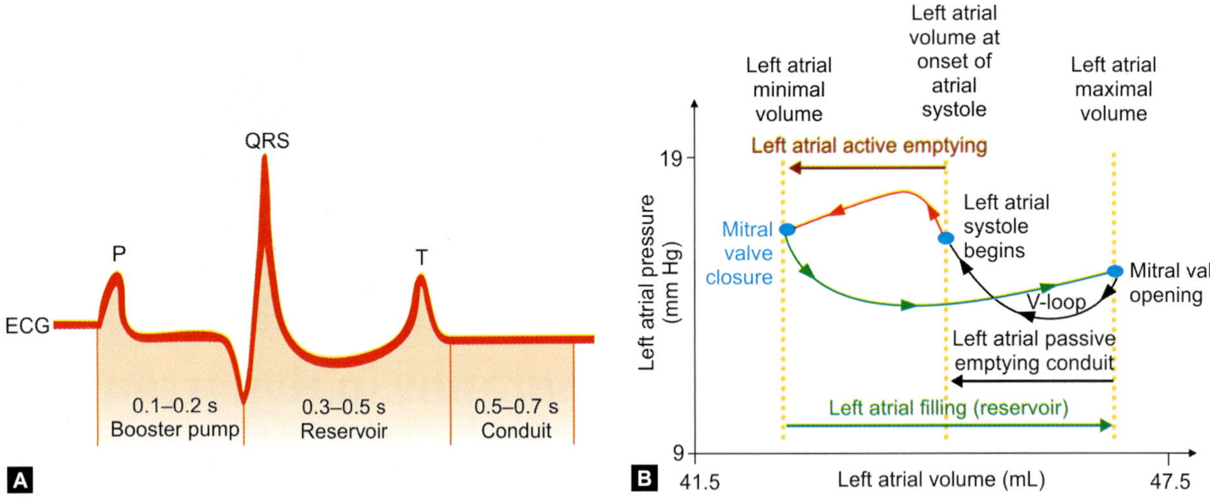

Figs. 2A and B: (A) ECG-gated time sequence of atrial functions; and (B) Pressure–volume curve of LA. A loop signifies atrial contraction or pumping phase and V loop signifies suction produced by ventricles in early diastole or conduit phase. The green curve depicts reservoir phase. (ECG: electrocardiography; LA: left atrium).

earlier assessed by tissue Doppler imaging (TDI); however, with the evident of novel technique of STE, the LAS and SR are more readily assessed by this technique [contraction strain index (CSI)].

Assessment by Tissue Doppler Imaging

Tissue Doppler imaging is obtained in the apical four-chamber (4C) and two-chamber (2C) views with the frame rate of more than 110 frames/s. This requires a narrow image sector angle (usually 30°) should be used to achieve the maximum possible color TDI frame rate, and the atrial walls should be aligned parallel to the Doppler beam using the apical 4C and 2C views. The LA peak tissue strain and SR during the LV systole (S-SR), early (E-SR), and late LV diastole (A-SR) are measured offline as shown in Figure 3. Tissue Doppler imaging measurements are performed at the LA basal, septal, lateral, inferior, and anterior walls from the apical 4C and 2C views.[9,10]

Normal resting SR in the longitudinal direction is 1.0–1.5/s, and normal strain is 10–15%.

Tissue Doppler imaging also allows noninvasive quantification of atrial electromechanical delay. The time distance (PA-TDI) is measured from the onset of the P wave on the electrocardiography (ECG) to the peak of tissue Doppler velocity (a′ wave) as shown in Figure 4. In normal subjects, PA-TDI is shortest at the level of the right atrial wall and is progressively longer from the level of interatrial septum to the lateral LA wall (Fig. 5).[11-17] This can be a suitable parameter for the identification of a potential atrial substrate vulnerable for AF.

TABLE 1: Factors affecting the various atrial functions.

Atrial function	*Factors affecting the function*
Reservoir	• Atrial compliance during ventricular systole • Atrial contractility and relaxation • Descent of left ventricular base • Ventricular end-systolic volume
Conduit	• Atrial compliance • Ventricular compliance
Pump	• Atrial contractility • Atrial preload (venous return) • Atrial afterload (ventricular end-diastolic pressure) • LV compliance

(LV: left atrium)

Lengthening of PA-TDI is found to be associated with AF. Prolonged PA-TDI more than 140 ms is associated with AF.

Limitations

- Tissue Doppler imaging is an angle-dependent and time-consuming technique.
- Cardiac translation movements may affect the results.
- A good temporal resolution is required for LA lateral wall measurements.

TISSUE DOPPLER IMAGING IN HYPERTENSION

On conventional two-dimensional (2D) echocardiography, LA enlargement in patients with HTN was considered as

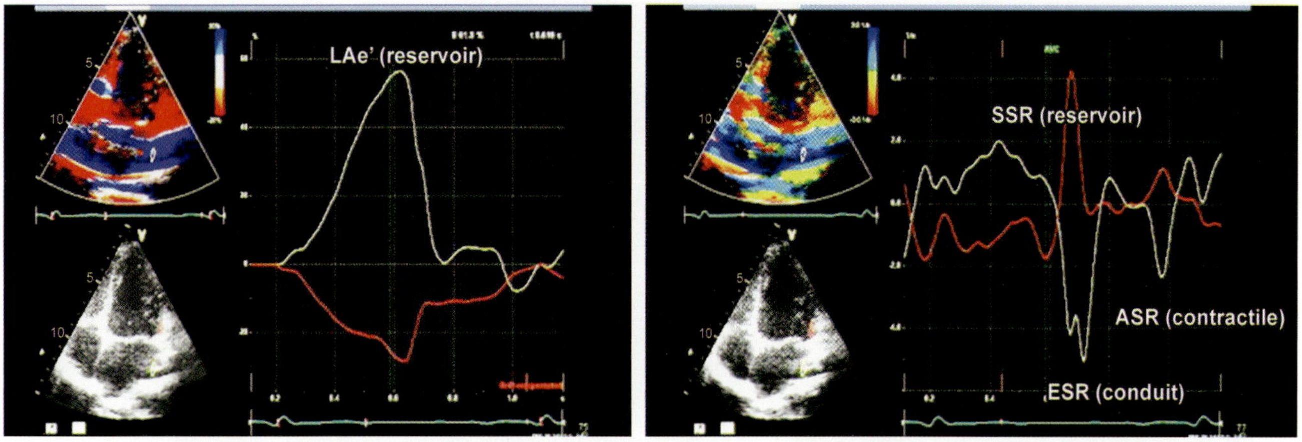

Fig. 3: TDI velocities and strain rate analysis allows the quantification of all three components of LA function: SSR for reservoir function, ESR for conduit function, and late diastolic ASR for contractile function. (ASR: atrial strain rate; ESR: early diastolic atrial strain rate; LA: left atrium; SSR: systolic atrial strain rate; TDI: tissue Doppler imaging).

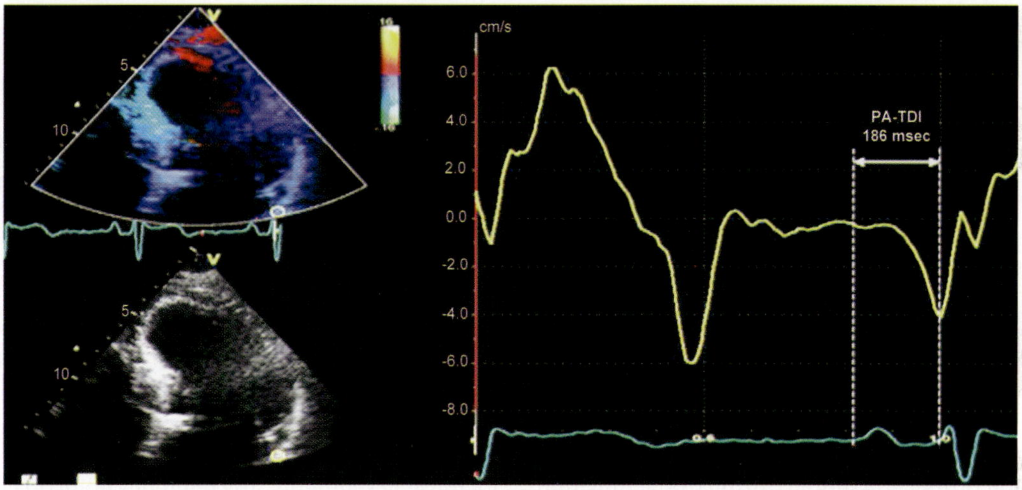

Fig. 4: The time distance between "P" wave of ECG and "a" wave of TDI curve. (ECG: electrocardiography; TDI: tissue Doppler imaging).

a specific substrate for the development of AF. However, LA enlargement is a late event and the assessment of LAS by tissue Doppler allows an early identification of patients who are prone to develop AF even before the changes in LA volume are evident. The earliest decline in the LAS occurs during the conduit phase (early diastole), followed by the changes in atrial strain during the reservoir phase (ventricular systolic) and then later in atrial contractile phase. Thus, the decreased value of strain in conduit phase is the earlier marker of atrial dysfunction which could potentially identify the patients who are likely to develop AF despite the normal LA size, even in patients with mild HTN.[10,18,19]

TWO-DIMENSIONAL SPECKLE STRAIN

Two-dimensional speckle-tracking strain imaging is a new emerging methodology for the assessment of regional myocardial deformations. Movements of the acoustic speckles or kernels are tracked throughout the cardiac cycle, and this allows the assessment of myocardial deformation (shortening or lengthening). Thus, using 2D-STE real-time dynamic LA function can be evaluated. Speckle imaging obviates some of the limitations of TDI. It is nonangle-dependent and less affected by cardiac motion of translation and is thus a fairly robust technique; however, it requires an excellent quality imaging, for accurate and reproducible results. The technical aspects and methodology used for the analysis of LV myocardium is applicable to the LA myocardium.[20]

METHODOLOGY

The LA is imaged in apical 4C and 2C views, which are acquired for three to four consecutive cardiac cycles.

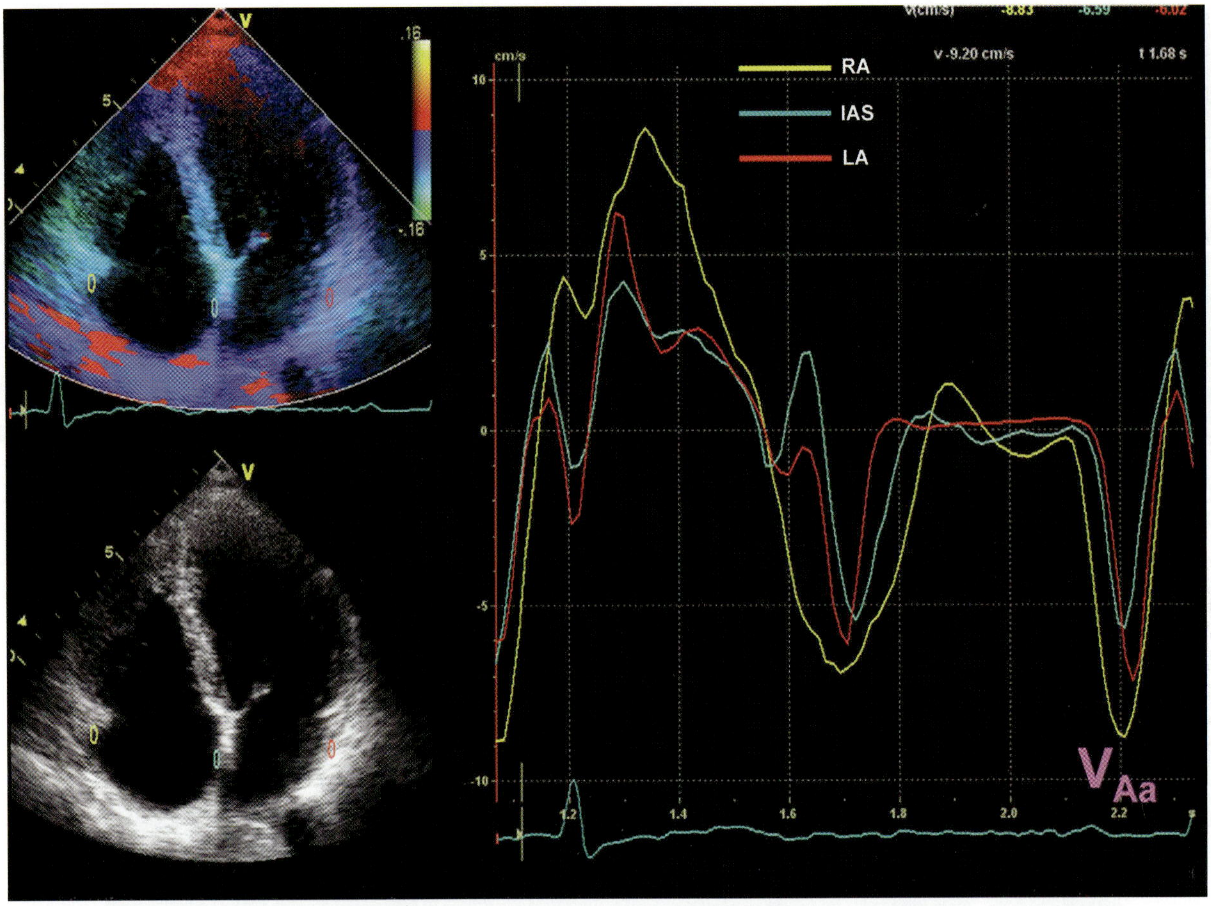

Fig. 5: PA-TDI is longer in LA than in RA (RA < IAS < LA). (IAS: interatrial septum; LA: left atrium; RA: right atrium; PA-TOI: total atrial conduction time assessed by tissue Doppler imaging).

A stable ECG recording is essential during this acquisition. A high-quality 2D view with adequate cardiac delineation and without foreshortening is an important prerequisite. A frame rate of 60–80 Hz with a narrow sector of 30–60° is used during these accusations. Although an LA-specific software is not presently available, the same software dedicated to LV speckle tracking can be used for offline analysis of LA.[21,22] The walls of the LA myocardium are divided into three segments on each side (medial and lateral) using the apical 4C and 2C views. Thus, usually 12 segments of the LA myocardium (six each for apical 4C and apical 2C) are assessed. The nomenclature of these segments is similar to the one used for LV segments (three segments for septal and lateral LA walls in apical 4C and three segments each in apical 2C for anterior and inferior walls). Usually the four superior segments do not generate adequate signals. Therefore, global strain for the LA in apical 4C and 2C actually represents the deformation of the LA myocardium representing middle and annular segments. Thereafter, the speckle-tracking algorithm generates strain and SR curves for these 12 segments. The reference point on ECG is usually taken at the "R" wave of ECG. If other LA contractile indices are computed then apical 3C view is also required, and three segments of inferior–posterior wall are also included giving a total of 15 segments. For these contractile indices, the "P" wave of ECG is used as the reference point (Figs. 6A and B).[23]

LEFT ATRIAL: MECHANICS

During the reservoir phase, LA stretches as it fills up, and the atrial strain reaches a positive peak just before the opening of the mitral valve. This is called peak atrial longitudinal strain (PALS). After the opening of the mitral valve, LA empties into LV, and this is known as conduit phase. During this phase, the strain decreases up to a plateau. During LA contraction, the strain again increases to reach a peak called PACS (peak atrial contraction strain), PACS occurs just after the P wave on surface ECG (Fig. 7).

Global strain is averaged over all the values obtained from the regional strains, which is computed by the software

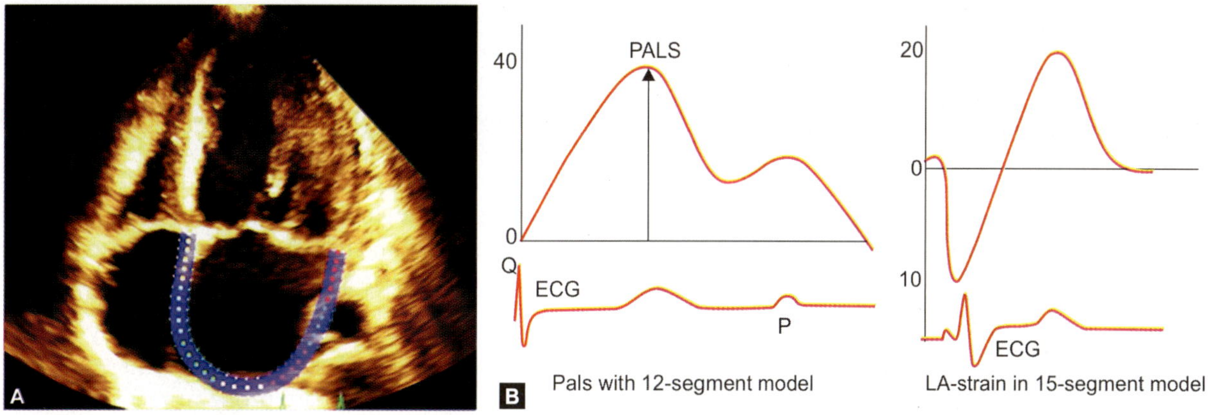

Figs. 6A and B: Computation of LA speckle strain gating with ECG. Strain curve depicts 12-segment model as well as 15-segment model using R wave and P wave of ECG as reference point. (ECG: electrocardiography; LA: left atrium).

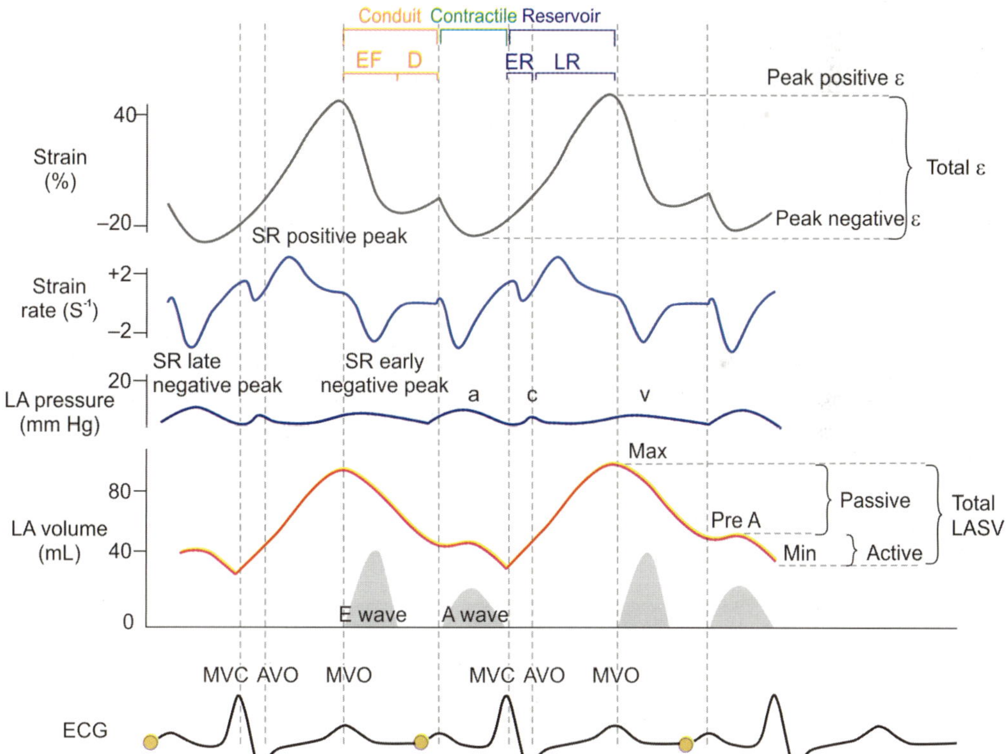

Fig. 7: Depicts strain and LA hemodynamics gated with ECG. (ECG: electrocardiography; LA: left atrium).

automatically. Similarly, time to peak longitudinal strain (TPLS) measured as the average of all 12 segments (global TPLS). LA contraction systolic index CSI was calculated in each LA wall by the formula CSI = (PALS/PACS) × 100 or global CSI = (G-PALS/G-PACS) × 100. It should be noted that both PALS and PACS are positive strain in 12-segment classification where R wave is used, while PACS is negative classification where "P" is used as reference point.

Normal value of PALS is 32.2–53.2% in 12-segment classification. However, the average value of positive and negative strains in 15-segment classification is lower (23.2 ± 6.7% and –14.6 ± 3.5%, respectively) (Figs. 8 and 9).[22,24-30]

POTENTIAL CLINICAL UTILITY

The assessment of LAS by STE is an emerging tool with several potential pathophysiological, diagnostic, therapeutic, and prognostic implications. Two most important applications are in patients with AF and those with diastolic dysfunction (Figs. 10 and 11).

ATRIAL FIBRILLATION

Early diagnosis in patients likely to develop AF: In the evaluation and workup of patients with HTN and diabetes, especially in patients with advanced age (more than 60 years), a reduced PALS is likely to be an early prognostic marker which could identify patients likely to develop AF even before the changes in LA volumes are detected on conventional 2D echocardiography.[31-35] This has important therapeutic implications, as several studies has shown that pharmacological intervention using agents which act on renin–angiotensin system could protect vulnerable patients from developing AF. Low global PALS could therefore identify those patients with HTN and diabetes who are likely to develop AF and thus could be protected from developing this arrhythmia.[36]

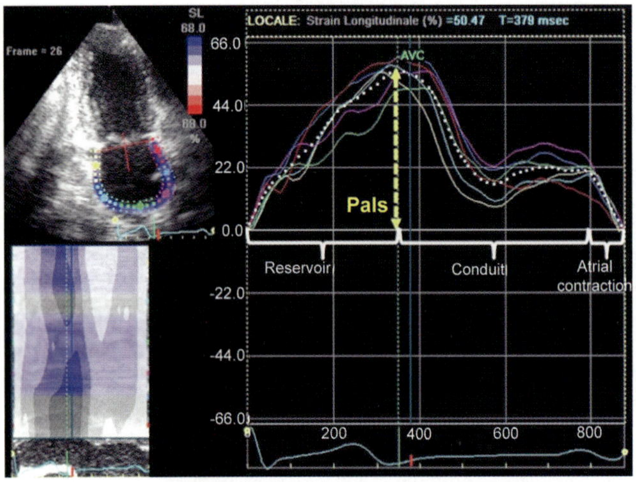

Fig. 8: Figure showing PALS in apical 2C view. Dashed line is average PALS curve. (PALS: peak atrial longitudinal strain; 2C: two chamber).

Prediction of recurrence of AF: A persistently low global PALS in patient who had cardioversion for AF could identify a subset of patients who are prone to recurrences of this arrhythmia.[36-38]

Diastolic Dysfunction in Patients with Heart Failure with Preserved Ejection Fraction

Several elegant studies have shown a good inverse correlation between PALS and invasively evaluated pulmonary capillary wedge pressure (PCWP)/LV filling pressures. This correlation is superior to that obtained by conventional mitral and tissue Doppler. Thus, a simple

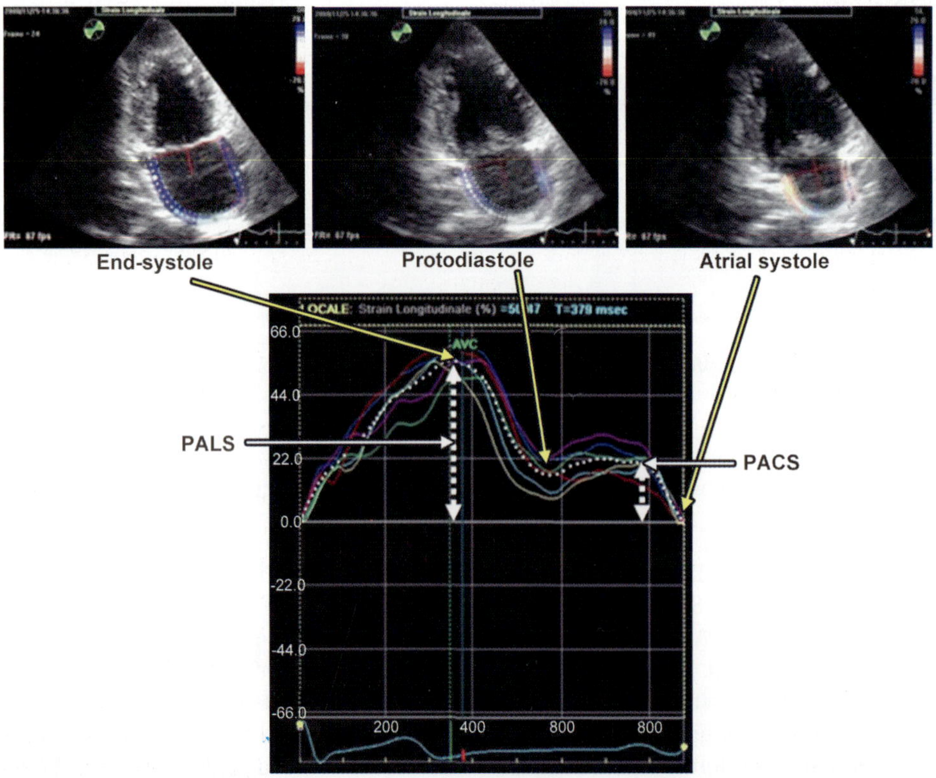

Fig. 9: Strain curves depict PALS and PACS in 12-segment classification. (PACS: peak atrial contraction strain; PALS: peak atrial longitudinal strain).

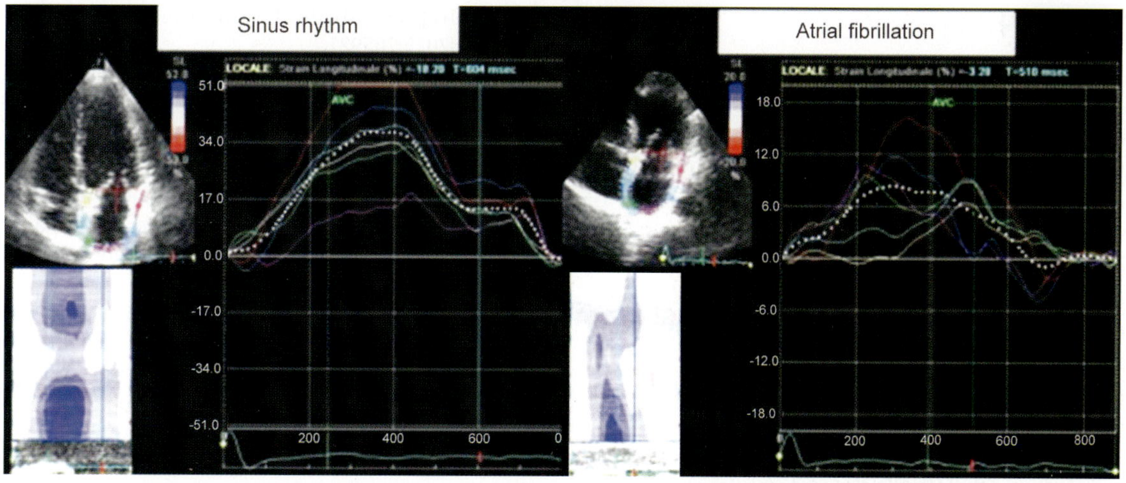

Fig. 10: Figure showing AF patients tend to have low PALS. (AF: atrial fibrillation; PALS: peak atrial longitudinal strain).

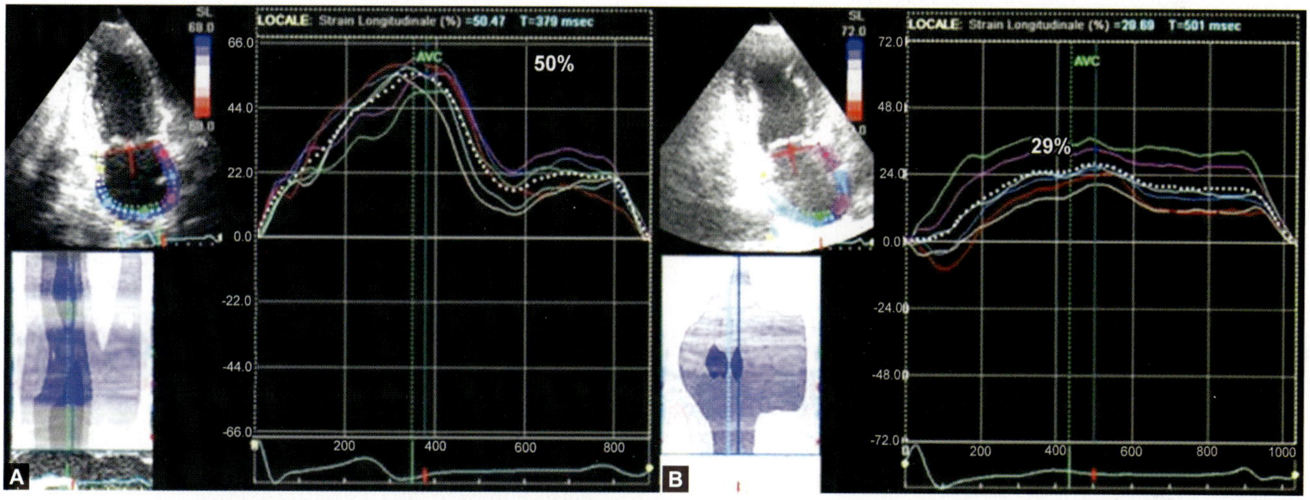

Figs. 11A and B: Hypertensive patients have low PALS: (A) Healthy control; and (B) Hypertension. (PALS: peak atrial longitudinal strain).

easily obtainable index, such as PALS, could accurately and rapidly noninvasively identify patients with elevated filling pressures who are likely to develop HFpEF (heart failure with preserved ejection fraction). In a pioneering study, Singh et al., from Chicago Medical Center, have used LAS measurements for accurate categorization and stratification of diastolic dysfunction because the LAS measurements change progressively with the severity of diastolic dysfunction.[39-46]

Limitations

Assessment of LAS by STE is an emerging technology, which is yet to be standardized and to be recommended for clinical use. There are several challenges and limitations which limit the routine use of this technique:[47]

- A high-quality imaging is a strong prerequisite for accurate and reproducible recording for strain analysis. Suboptimal imaging of LA is likely to show erroneous and often incongruous atrial strain curves.
- A dedicated software for LAS analysis has not yet been developed, and so far only the tracking algorithm of LV strain is being used to provide LAS curves.
- Lack of standardizations and cutoff values of various strains for diagnostic therapeutic and prognostic purposes is a major limitation for the widespread use of this technique.
- Vendor variability among different manufacturers in the computation of the LAS is also an important drawback. This is likely to be adequately addressed in subsequent months.[48]

CONCLUSION

Left atrial strain technology is a technique, which noninvasively assesses deformation of the various LA wall segments either by TDI or more recently using STE. Speckle-tracking echocardiography is being angle independent and more robust is usually preferred. Abnormality of LAS occurs even before the changes in LA volumes and, therefore, is likely to be useful in the early assessment of altered LA mechanics in patients with HTN, diabetes, coronary artery disease, and AF. PALS is the most common well-studied strain, which is readily evaluated by STE. Left atrial strain (PALS) shows a better correlation with LV filling pressures as compared to conventional 2D parameters (such as E/e′, E/A). Thus, computation LAS is likely to be useful in patients with HFpEF. Early detection of altered strain values in patients with HTN could allow therapeutic interventions that could prevent the development of AF and could also identify patients likely to have recurrence after cardioversion. Suboptimal imaging in patients with small acoustic windows as well as lack of standardization, cutoff values, and vender variability are major limitation, which need to be addressed. The assessment of atrial myocardial speckles in three-dimensional (3D-STE) is likely to provide more robust and reproducible strain curves than 2D STE. However, incorporation of 3D technology LAS is yet to be scientifically studied and validated.

REFERENCES

1. Manolisa AJ, Rosei EA, Coca A, et al. Hypertension and atrial fibrillation: diagnostic approach, prevention and treatment. Position paper of the Working Group 'Hypertension Arrhythmias and Thrombosis' of the European Society of Hypertension. J Hypertens. 2012;30(2):239-52.
2. Lip GY. Atrial fibrillation in patients with hypertension trajectories of risk factors in yet another manifestation of hypertensive target organ damage. Hypertension. 2016;68:544-5.
3. Cohen DL, Townsend RR. Blood pressure in patients with atrial fibrillation: Part 2—treatment. J Clin Hypertens (Greenwich). 2017;19(2):212-4.
4. Dzeshka MS, Shantsila A, Shantsila E, et al. Atrial fibrillation and hypertension. Hypertension. 2017;70:854-61.
5. Davis RC, Hobbs FD, Kenkre JE, et al. Prevalence of atrial fibrillation in the general population and in high-risk groups: the ECHOES study. Europace. 2012;14:1553-9.
6. Baysan O, Ocaklı EP, Altuner TK, et al. Atria: a comprehensive evaluation with echocardiography. Heart Vessels Transplant. 2017;1:11-9.
7. Rosca M, Lancellotti P, Popescu BA, et al. Left atrial function: pathophysiology, echocardiographic assessment, and clinical applications. Heart. 2011;97:1982-9.
8. Leischik R, Littwitz H, Dworrak B, et al. Echocardiographic evaluation of left atrial mechanics: function, history, novel techniques, advantages, and pitfalls. Biomed Res Int. 2015;2015:765921.
9. Sirbu C, Herbots L, D'hooge J, et al. Feasibility of strain and strain rate imaging for the assessment of regional left atrial deformation: a study in normal subjects. Eur J Echocardiogr. 2006;7:199-208.
10. Cho KI, Lee HG, Ak SJ, et al. Quantitative assessment of left atrial functional changes in patients with atrial fibrillation by tissue Doppler strain and 2-dimensional strain imaging. Korean Circ J. 2006;36:786-93.
11. Zhang Q, Yip GW, Yu CM. Approaching regional left atrial function by tissue Doppler velocity and strain imaging. Europace. 2008;10:iii62-9.
12. Thomas L, Levett K, Boyd A, et al. Changes in regional left atrial function with aging: evaluation by Doppler tissue imaging. Eur J Echocardiogr. 2003;4:92-100.
13. Shanks M, Valtuille L, Choy JB, et al. Predictive value of various Doppler-derived parameters of atrial conduction time for successful atrial fibrillation ablation. Echo Res Pract. 2015;2(4):99-107.
14. Abou R, Leung M, Tonsbeek AM, et al. Effect of aging on left atrial compliance and electromechanical properties in subjects without structural heart disease. Am J Cardiol. 2017;120:140-7.
15. Biber S, Sieweke JT, Grosse GM, et al. P4318: total atrial conduction time and left atrial strain highly predict occurrence of atrial fibrillation in patients with embolic stroke of unknown source (ESUS) during in-hospital stay. Eur Heart J. 2017;38(Suppl. 1):P4318.
16. Leung M, van Rosendael PJ, Abou R, et al. Left atrial function to identify patients with atrial fibrillation at high risk of stroke: new insights from a large registry. Eur Heart J. 2018;39(16):1416-25.
17. Weijs B, de Vos CB, Tieleman RG, et al. Clinical and echocardiographic correlates of intra-atrial conduction delay. Europace. 2011;13:1681-7.
18. Sahebjam M, Mazareei A, Lotfi-Tokaldany M, et al. Comparison of left atrial function between hypertensive patients with normal atrial size and normotensive subjects using strain rate imaging technique. Arch Cardiovasc Imaging. 2014;2(1):e16081.
19. Kuppahally SS, Akoum N, Burgon NS, et al. Left atrial strain and strain rate in patients with paroxysmal and persistent atrial fibrillation: relationship to left atrial structural remodeling detected by delayed-enhancement MRI. Circ Cardiovasc Imaging. 2010;3:231-9.
20. Donal E, Behagel A. Value of left atrial strain: a highly promising field of investigation. Eur Heart J Cardiovasc Imaging. 2015;16:356-7.
21. Gan GC, Ferkh A, Boyd A, et al. Left atrial function: evaluation by strain analysis. Cardiovasc Diagn Ther. 2018;8(1):29-46.
22. Miglioranza MH, Badano LP, Mihăilă S, et al. Physiologic determinants of left atrial longitudinal strain: a two-dimensional speckle-tracking and three-dimensional echocardiographic study in healthy volunteers. J Am Soc Echocardiogr. 2016;29(11):1023-34.e3.

23. Naveen G, Kapur KK. Strain and strain rate imaging: clinical implications. In: Naveen G, Kapur KK (Eds). CSI: Cardiology Update. New Delhi: Jaypee Brothers Medical Publishers (P) Ltd; 2014.
24. Morris DA, Takeuchi M, Krisper M, et al. Normal values and clinical relevance of left atrial myocardial function analysed by speckle-tracking echocardiography: multicenter study. Eur Heart J Cardiovasc Imaging. 2015;16:364-72.
25. Xu TY, Sun JP, Lee AP, et al. Left atrial function as assessed by speckle-tracking echocardiography in hypertension. Medicine. 2015;94(6):e52.
26. Cacciapuoti F, Paoli VD, Scognamiglio A, et al. Left atrial longitudinal speckle tracking echocardiography in healthy aging heart. J Cardiovasc Echogr. 2015;25(2):40-5.
27. Cameli M, Caputo M, Mondillo S, et al. Feasibility and reference values of left atrial longitudinal strain imaging by two-dimensional speckle tracking. Cardiovasc Ultrasound. 2009;7:6.
28. Cameli M, Lisi M, Focardi M, et al. Left atrial deformation analysis by speckle tracking echocardiography for prediction of cardiovascular outcomes. Am J Cardiol. 2012;110:264-9.
29. Vieira MJ, Teixeira R, Gonçalves L, et al. Left atrial mechanics: echocardiographic assessment and clinical implications. J Am Soc Echocardiogr. 2014;27:463-78.
30. Pathan F, D'Elia N, Nolan MT, et al. Normal ranges of left atrial strain by speckle-tracking echocardiography: a systematic review and meta-analysis. J Am Soc Echocardiogr. 2017;30:59-70.
31. Yoon JH, Moon J, Chung HM, et al. Left atrial function assessed by Doppler echocardiography rather than left atrial volume predicts recurrence in patients with paroxysmal atrial fibrillation. Clin. Cardiol. 2013;36(4):235-40.
32. Sarvari SI, Haugaa KH, Stokke TM, et al. Strain echocardiographic assessment of left atrial function predicts recurrence of atrial fibrillation. Eur Heart J Cardiovasc Imaging. 2016;17:660-7.
33. Obokata M, Negishi K, Kurosawa K, et al. Left atrial strain provides incremental value for embolism risk stratification over CHA2DS2-VASc score and indicates prognostic impact in patients with atrial fibrillation. J Am Soc Echocardiogr. 2014;27(7):709-16.e4.
34. Inaba Y, Yuda S, Kobayashi N, et al. Strain rate imaging for noninvasive functional quantification of the left atrium: comparative studies in controls and patients with atrial fibrillation. J Am Soc Echocardiogr. 2005;18:729-36.
35. Hsu PC, Lee WH, Chu CY, et al. Prognostic role of left atrial strain and its combination index with transmitral E-wave velocity in patients with atrial fibrillation. Sci Rep. 2016;6:17318.
36. Kokubu N, Yuda S, Tsuchihashi K, et al. Noninvasive assessment of left atrial function by strain rate imaging in patients with hypertension: a possible beneficial effect of renin-angiotensin system inhibition on left atrial function. Hypertens Res. 2007;30:13-21.
37. Yasuda R, Murata M, Roberts R, et al. Left atrial strain is a powerful predictor of atrial fibrillation recurrence after catheter ablation: study of a heterogeneous population with sinus rhythm or atrial fibrillation. Eur Heart J Cardiovasc Imaging. 2015;16:1008-14.
38. Salvo GD, Caso P, Lo Piccolo R, et al. Atrial myocardial deformation properties predict maintenance of sinus rhythm after external cardioversion of recent-onset lone atrial fibrillation: a color Doppler myocardial imaging and transthoracic and transesophageal echocardiographic study. Circulation. 2005;112:387-395.
39. Thomas L, McKay T, Byth K, et al. Abnormalities of left atrial function after cardioversion: an atrial strain rate study. Heart. 2007;93:89-95.
40. Georgievska-Ismail L, Zafirovska P, Hristovski Z. Evaluation of the role of left atrial strain using two-dimensional speckle tracking echocardiography in patients with diabetes mellitus and heart failure with preserved left ventricular ejection fraction. Diab Vasc Dis Res. 2016;13(6):384-94.
41. Brecht A, Oertelt-Prigione S, Seeland U, et al. Left atrial function in preclinical diastolic dysfunction: two-dimensional speckle-tracking echocardiography-derived results from the BEFRI trial. J Am Soc Echocardiogr. 2016;29:750-8.
42. Singh A, Addetia K, Maffessanti F, et al. LA strain for categorization of LV diastolic dysfunction. JACC Cardiovasc Imaging. 2017;10(7):735-43.
43. Mondillo S, Cameli M, Caputo ML, et al. Early detection of left atrial strain abnormalities by speckle-tracking in hypertensive and diabetic patients with normal left atrial size. J Am Soc Echocardiogr. 2011;24:898-908.
44. Cameli M, Lisi M, Mondillo S, et al. Left atrial longitudinal strain by speckle tracking echocardiography correlates well with left ventricular filling pressures in patients with heart failure. Cardiovasc Ultrasound. 2010;8:14.
45. Ahmed MK, Soliman MA, Reda AA, et al. Assessment of left atrial deformation properties by speckle tracking in patients with systolic heart failure. Egypt Heart J. 2015;67:199-208.
46. Camelia M, Cicconeb MM, Maiello M, et al. Speckle tracking analysis: a new tool for left atrial function analysis in systemic hypertension: an overview. J Cardiovasc Med. 2014;15:339-43.
47. Rimbaş RC, Dulgheru RE, Vinereanu D. Methodological gaps in left atrial function assessment by 2D speckle tracking echocardiography. Arq Bras Cardiol. 2015;105(6):625-36.
48. Cameli M, Lisi M, Righini FM, et al. Left atrial strain in patients with arterial hypertension. Early effects of arterial hypertension: left atrial deformation analysis by two-dimensional speckle tracking echocardiography. Seman Scholar. 2013;1:31-6.

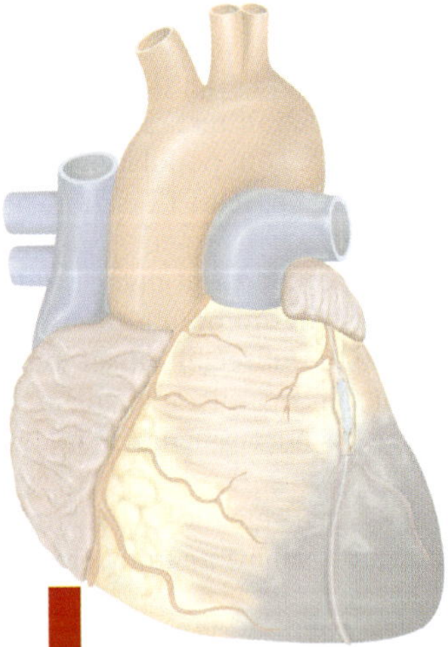

8

CHAPTER

Sequential ABPM Navigation Imaging in Hypertension

AK Pancholia, HK Chopra

HISTORICAL PERSPECTIVE

At the beginning of the twentieth century traditionally, blood pressure (BP) in the office or clinic has been assessed with the auscultatory technique, and was introduced into clinical medicine, which is still existing till date in clinical practice. Although the technique is otherwise accurate but is dependent on observer attention to detail, which is often lacking, and it provides only a momentary measurement of BP. Thus to overcome these methodological limitations, methods for getting automated profiles of BP over 24 hours and measures of BP in the home setting have been developed, what is called ambulatory blood pressure monitoring (ABPM) and home blood pressure monitoring (HBPM), respectively. ABPM in fact is available in one form or another for last 50 years to check the circadian changes in BP and to determine the influence of BP-lowering drugs on the 24 hours profile. In the 1960s, the Remler device, which was capable of measuring BP intermittently during the daytime period, provided clinicians with a new technique for assessing BP. This device has limitations as it is to be operated by the patient, which made measurement of BP impossible during sleep. The next technological advance was the introduction of fully automated devices that could measure BP intermittently at predetermined intervals over the 24 hours period. This class of devices provided a methodology that was applicable not only for research but also for use in routine clinical practice.[1-4]

WHY IS ABPM SUPERIOR TO CONVENTIONAL BP MEASUREMENT?

Traditionally, we use a sphygmomanometer and stethoscope for the office BP measurement but recently, automated office BP measurement has been proposed as an alternative to traditional measurement. Automated office BP is the mean of multiple BP readings recorded with a fully automated device with the patient resting quietly, alone, in the office or clinic.[5] It has several advantages over manual BP, especially in routine clinical practice, by virtually eliminating office-induced increase in BP, improving accuracy, minimizing observer error, and providing a more standardized measurement technique using an automated oscillometric sphygmomanometer.

The mean automated office BP for diagnosing hypertension is similar to the mean awake ambulatory BP and home BP (135/85 mm Hg). Preliminary data suggest that automated office BP is a better predictor of target organ damage, especially compared with routine manual office BP, which correlates poorly with intermediate endpoints, such as left ventricular mass. BP recorded in the patient's home is a significantly better predictor of future cardiovascular (CV) risk than is office BP. In order to avoid reporting bias,[6] a home BP recorder with a memory for storing readings should be used and the patient should take the device to the physician's office to have the mean home BP verified directly from the device's display. More recently,

BOX 1: Advantages of ambulatory blood pressure monitoring.

- Taking of multiple measurements within the 24-hour period;
- Evaluation of blood pressure during daily activities;
- Evaluation of blood pressure during sleep;
- Evaluation of the circadian pattern of blood pressure;
- Evaluation of the means, loads, and variabilities of blood pressure;
- Identification of the "alarm" reaction;
- Attenuation of the placebo effect;
- Evaluation of antihypertensive effect in the 24-hour period;
- Possibility of risk stratification.

Source: O'Brien E, Parati G, Stergiou G, et al. European Society of Hypertension Position Paper on Ambulatory Blood Pressure Monitoring. J Hypertens. 2013;31(9):1731-68.

remote transmissions of home BP readings[7] is becoming available allowing BP readings recorded in the home to be automatically sent to a data collection center via a telephone modem or internet link and from there forwarded to the physician's office. The advantages of ABPM have influenced recommendations for the technique to be used much more widely in clinical practice.[8-11] These advantages may be briefly summarized as follows in Box 1.

DEFINITION OF NORMALITY FOR ABPM

There has been much debate on the definition of diagnostic thresholds for ABPM. According to recent guidelines for the BP measurement, an average daytime ABP of less than 135 mm Hg systolic, and 85 mm Hg diastolic is generally considered normal. This cut-off has been thought to be reasonable because it corresponds approximately to an office BP of 140/90 mm Hg. The threshold value for the average night-time ABP is 120 mm Hg systolic and 70 mm Hg diastolic.[12] However, more recently, a collaborative population-based CV outcome-driven study proposed lower diagnostic thresholds for ABPM. The International Database on Ambulatory BP Monitoring in Relation to Cardiovascular Outcome (IDACO) study[13] was designed as a population based longitudinal follow-up CV outcome study. 24 hours ABPM was performed on 5,682 participants enrolled in the prospective population studies in Denmark (Copenhagen), Belgium (Noorderkempen), Japan (Ohasama), and Sweden (Uppsala). In multivariate analyses, the ABP thresholds were determined, which yielded 10-year CV risks similar to that associated with optimal (120/80 mm Hg), normal (130/85 mm Hg), and high (140/90 mm Hg) BP on office measurement. Over 9.7 years of follow-up, 814 CV endpoint events were recorded. However, one should remember that the ABP value is a continuous variable, and the relationship between CV outcomes and BP is also continuous. Therefore, a critical level cannot be pinpointed, above which the risk suddenly rises.[14]

DAY-NIGHT BLOOD PRESSURE CHANGES

In subjects with normotension or hypertension, a pronounced diurnal rhythm of BP is present. BP usually falls during the first few hours of sleep, and there is a marked rise in the morning coincidently with the transition from sleep to wakefulness. The average difference between waking and sleeping systolic and diastolic BP is 10–20%. In some subjects, the normal nocturnal fall of BP is diminished (as mentioned earlier, in the analysis of Syst-Euro study),[15] the night/day ratio of ambulatory systolic BP was an independent predictor of CV events in the patient group randomized to placebo. It suggests that the mean night-time BP has a better predictive value than the mean daytime BP, although some reports have shown no difference in the predictive power for CV risk between night-time and daytime BP.[16] In the previously mentioned IDACO study analysis, this long-term follow-up prospective cohort study showed that when adjusted for the daytime BP, night-time BP more accurately predicted total and CV mortality than daytime BP.[17] This is the reason why recording ABPM throughout the day is necessary.

CLINICAL INDICATIONS OF ABPM

Clinical indications of ABPM are shown in Box 2.

LIMITATIONS OF ABPM

There are certain limitations of ABPM which has been shown in Box 3.

BOX 2: Clinical indications of ambulatory blood pressure monitoring.

- In excluding white-coat hypertension (evidence strength C)
- In helping with the diagnosis of patients with borderline hypertension (evidence strength D)
- In deciding on treatment for elderly patients (evidence strength A–C)
- In identifying nocturnal hypertension (evidence strength C)
- In assessing patients whose hypertension has been resistant (evidence strength D)
- As a guide to determine the efficacy of drug treatment over 24 hours (evidence strength B)
- In diagnosing and treating hypertension in pregnancy (evidence strength C–D)
- In diagnosing hypotension (evidence strength B–C)

Source: O'Brien E, Parati G, Stergiou G, et al. European Society of Hypertension Position Paper on Ambulatory Blood Pressure Monitoring. J Hypertens. 2013;31(9):1731-68.

BOX 3: Limitations of ambulatory blood pressure monitoring.

- Arms that do not allow appropriate adjustment of the cuff
- Exceedingly high systolic blood pressure
- Clinical conditions associated to movement disorders (Parkinsonism, etc)
- Exceedingly irregular pulses (atrial fibrillation and flutter)
- Auscultatory gap when the auscultatory method is used

INTERPRETATION OF ABPM

It has been shown in Figure 1 and Flowchart 1.

WHITE COAT HYPERTENSION AND WHITE COAT EFFECT

White coat hypertension (WCH) is generally defined as persistently high office BP, with a normal BP outside the office.[18] The alerting reaction to a visit into the physician's office may cause transient elevation in BP. The diagnosis of WCH is important, because it is generally accepted that patients with WCH have relatively low CV risk and are unlikely to benefit from antihypertensive pharmacologic therapy. The Ohasama study[19] also showed that CV morbidity was lower in WCH than in ambulatory hypertension, and was not dissimilar between WCH and clinical normotension in a mixed population of treated and untreated subjects. However, the prognosis is not always benign. Some studies identified that more frequent target organ damage was present in WCH than clinical normotension.[20] In long-term follow-up studies, CV risk was increase in patients with WCH. According to an analysis of the pooled data of four different cohort studies, sustained hypertension may develop in some patients with WCH, and the risk of stroke may increase after a mean follow-up period of 6 years.[21] It could reflect a higher inherent risk in subjects with WCH of developing sustained hypertension in the long run.[22] Therefore, in patients with WCH, long-term follow-up with repeated ABPM or HBPM is necessary. WCH must be distinguished from the "white coat effect" or "white coat phenomenon", which is the term used to describe transient increase in BP that occurs in a medical environment regardless of the ABP status of patients. Measuring BP in the physician's office may trigger an alerting reaction, which causes a rise in BP. The white coat effect is found in many hypertensive patients, whereby the office BP is usually greater than the average daytime ABP. Patients diagnosed with severe hypertension by office BP may have only mild hypertension on ABPM, due to marked white coat effect. It could elicit misinterpretation of the patient's BP status from the physician responsible for the hypertension management. Physicians are likely to identify patients with poorly controlled BP, when in fact they have normal ABP. For correct diagnosis of white coat effect, ABPM and HBPM are very useful in clinical practice "Masked hypertension (MH)" or "reverse white coat hypertension" is defined as having a normal office BP and a high ambulatory or home BP.[23] MH was associated with poor CV outcome in a population based study of untreated elderly patients. After adjustment for CV risk factors, MH was an independent predictor of CV morbidity when compared to normotensive subjects. The Ohasama study with 24-hour ABPM confirmed an excessive risk of events in subjects with MH, compared to subjects with normal office and ABP. When people already have MH, it follows that they should be regarded as being genuinely hypertensive. Identifying MH is substantially important in treated patients. The mechanisms responsible for this phenomenon may be different between treated

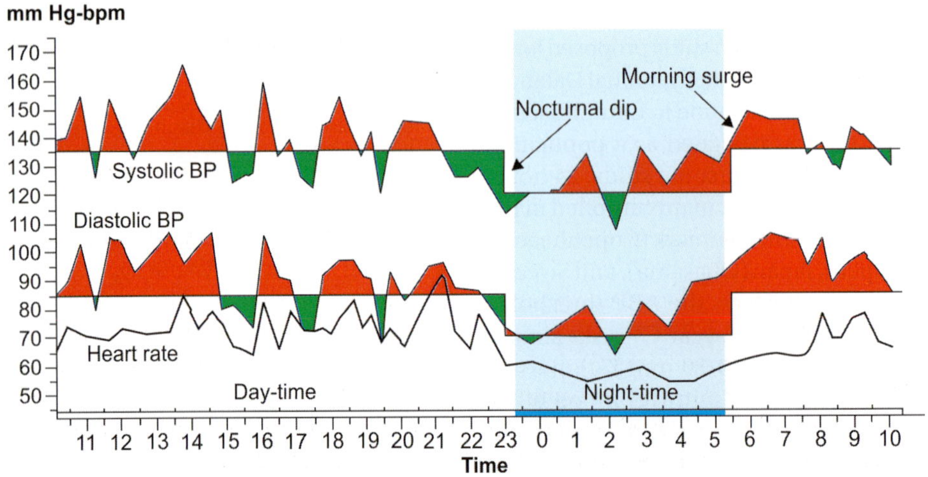

Fig. 1: 24 hours ambulatory blood pressure monitoring data. (BP: blood pressure).
Source: Turner JR, Viera AJ, Shimbo D. Ambulatory blood pressure monitoring in clinical practice: a review. Am J Med. 2015;128(1):14-20.

Flowchart 1: Algorithm for interpretation of ABPM.

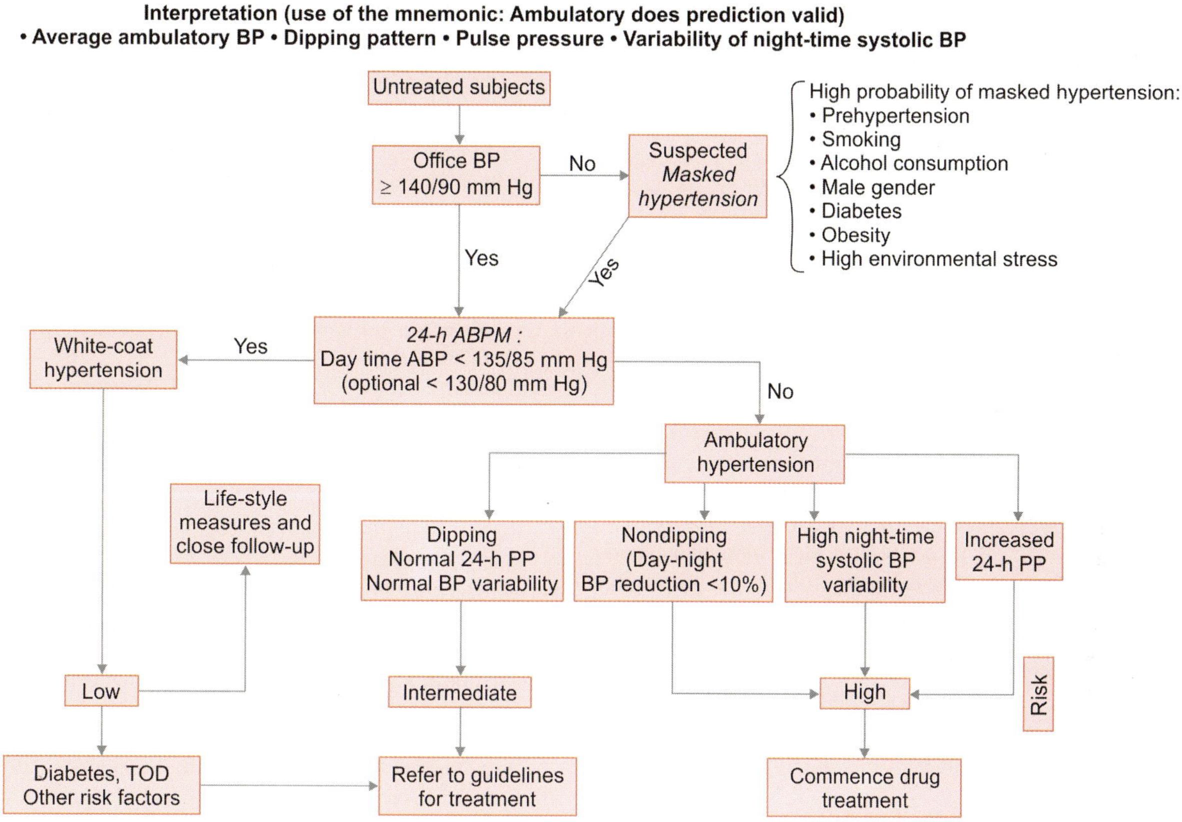

(ABPM: ambulatory blood pressure monitoring; BP: blood pressure; PP: pulse pressure; TOD: target organ damage)
Source: Angeli F, Reboldi G, Poltronieri C, et al. Interpretation of ambulatory blood pressure profile: a approach for clinicians. J Clin Exp Cardiolog. 2013;4(7):e128.

and untreated patients. Drug treatment may elicit a different drop in office BP and ABP attributable to time of administration with respect to the visit and duration of action of drugs. In treated patients, high prevalence of MH may be partly explained by the fact that the office BP is often taken at the time of peak drug effect, whereas ABP or home BP may be taken at its trough, which is particularly evident when short acting drugs are taken. A study showed that the prevalence of MH was present in one-third of treated hypertensive patients in a hypertension clinic. Over 5 years of follow-up, their relative risk for CV events was 2.28, as compared to patients whose office and ABP were adequately controlled.[24] The challenge for clinical practice is how to identify and manage these patients, because the prevalence of MH is estimated to be more than 10% of the general population. MH may be suspected in individuals who have had an increased office BP at some time, in young persons with a normal or high-normal office BP who had early target organ damage, in individuals with a family history of hypertension in both parents, patients with multiple risks for CV disease, and probably diabetic patients.

CONCLUSION

Ambulatory blood pressure monitoring is superior to clinic blood pressure monitoring (CBPM), HBPM for evaluation of total hypertension burden and cardiovascular disease (CVD) inflicted morbidity by various studies. ABPM is the only method by which we can evaluate total hypertension load including the burden of non-nocturnal dipping, reverse dipping, extreme dipping, persistent time elevation, hyperbaric index, double product, morning surge, and evening surge. There is no other method to give us so much of information. The ABPM variables can very well correlated with the biochemical and echocardiographic variables thereby helping in appropriate therapeutic intervention to reduce the hypertension inflicted CVD risk. It has diagnostic, prognostic, and therapeutic implications. With development of digital technology, the patient's inconvenience will be taken care of. It is strongly recommended to have ABPM monitoring at least once in a year in severely hypertensive and subsequently can be monitored by HBPM and CBPM for meticulous hypertension management. If we really want to reduce the rising menace of hypertension inflicted CVD risk and the event rates, we need more ABPM data from our country.

REFERENCES

1. O'Brien E, Fitzgerald D. The history of indirect blood pressure measurement. In: O'Brien E, O'Malley K (Eds). Handbook of Hypertension. Amsterdam: Elsevier; 1991. pp. 1-54.
2. Parati G, Mancia G. History of blood pressure measurement from the pre-Riva-Rocci era to the twenty-first century. In: Birkenhager WH, Reid JL (Eds). Handbook of Hypertension. The Netherlands: Elsevier BV; 2004. pp. 3-32.
3. O'Brien E. Ambulatory blood pressure measurement: the case for implementation in primary care. Hypertension. 2008;51(6):1435-41.
4. O'Brien E. 24-h ambulatory blood pressure measurement in clinical practice and research: a critical review of a technique in need of implementation. J Int Med. 2011;269(5):478-95.
5. Myers MG, Godwin M, Dawes M, et al. Measurement of blood pressure in the office: recognizing the problem and proposing the solution. Hypertension. 2010;55(2):195-200.
6. Myers MG. Reporting bias in self-measurement of blood pressure. Blood Press Monit. 2001;6(4):181-3.
7. Omboni S, Gazzola T, Carabelli G, et al. Clinical usefulness and cost effectiveness of home blood pressure telemonitoring: meta-analysis of randomized controlled studies. J Hypertens. 2013;31(3):455-68.
8. Parati G, Bilo G. Should 24-h ambulatory blood pressure monitoring be done in every patient with diabetes? Diabetes Care. 2009;32 (Suppl 2):S298-304.
9. Dolan E, Stanton A, Thijs L, et al. Superiority of ambulatory over clinic blood pressure measurement in predicting mortality. The Dublin outcome study. Hypertension. 2005;46(1):156-61.
10. Parati G, Bilo G, Mancia G. Prognostic and diagnostic value of ambulatory blood pressure monitoring. In: Oparil S, Weber MA (Eds). Hypertension. Philadelphia: Elsevier; 2005. pp. 305-17.
11. Zaninelli A, Parati G, Cricelli C, et al. Office and 24-h ambulatory blood pressure control by treatment in general practice: the 'Monitoraggio della pressione ARteriosa nella medicina TErritoriale' study. J Hypertens. 2010;28(5):910-7.
12. O'Brien E, Asmar R, Beilin L, et al. European Society of Hypertension recommendations for conventional, ambulatory and home blood pressure measurement. J Hypertens. 2003;21(5):821-48.
13. Kikuya M, Hansen TW, Thijs L, et al. Diagnostic thresholds for ambulatory blood pressure monitoring based on 10-year cardiovascular risk. Circulation. 2007;115(16):2145-52.
14. Kikuya M, Hansen TW, Thijs L, et al. Diagnostic thresholds for ambulatory blood pressure monitoring based on 10-year cardiovascular risk. Blood Press Monit. 2007;12(6):393-5.
15. Staessen JA, Thijs L, Fagard R, et al. Predicting cardiovascular risk using conventional vs. ambulatory blood pressure in older patients with systolic hypertension. JAMA. 1999;282(6):539-46.
16. Bjorklund K, Lind L, Zethelius B, et al. Prognostic significance of 24-h ambulatory blood pressure characteristics for cardiovascular morbidity in a population of elderly men. J Hypertens. 2004;22(9):1691-7.
17. Boggia J, Li Y, Thijs L, et al. Prognostic accuracy of day versus night ambulatory blood pressure: a cohort study. Lancet. 2007;370(9594):1219-29.
18. Verdecchia P. Prognostic value of ambulatory blood pressure: current evidence and clinical implications. Hypertension. 2000;35(3):844-51.
19. Ohkubo T, Kikuya M, Metoki H, et al. Prognosis of "masked" hypertension and "white-coat" hypertension detected by 24-h ambulatory blood pressure monitoring 10-year follow-up from the Ohasama study. J Am Coll Cardiol. 2005;46(3):508-15.
20. Kim HY, Kwack NJ, Park NK, et al. Influences of white-coat hypertension and white-coat effect on the left ventricular mass and diastolic function. Korean Circ J. 1995;25(5):987-97.
21. Verdecchia P, Reboldi GP, Angeli F, et al. Short- and long-term incidence of stroke in white-coat hypertension. Hypertension. 2005;45(2):203-8.
22. Ugajin T, Hozawa A, Ohkubo T, et al. White-coat hypertension as a risk factor for the development of home hypertension: the Ohasama study. Arch Intern Med. 2005;165(13):1541-6.
23. Pickering T, Davidson K, Gerin W, et al. Masked hypertension. Hypertension. 2002;40(6):795-6.
24. Pierdomenico SD, Lapenna D, Bucci A, et al. Cardiovascular outcome in treated hypertensive patients with responder, false resistant, and true resistant hypertension. Am J Hypertens. 2005;18(11):1422-8.

CHAPTER 9

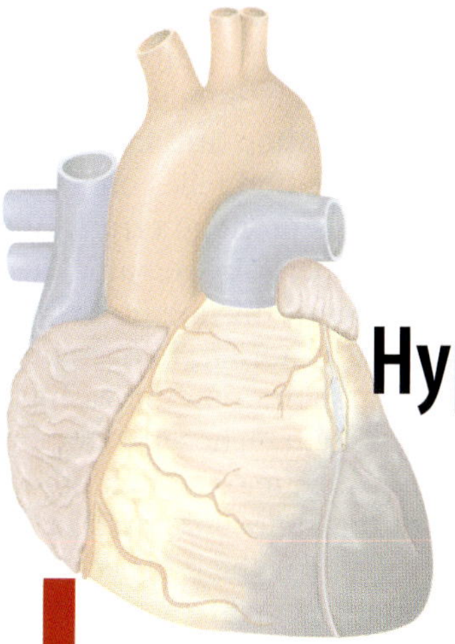

Echocardiographic Evaluation in Hypertension: Diagnostic, Prognostic, and Therapeutic Implications

Manish Bansal, HK Chopra, C Venkata S Ram, Anil Pareek

INTRODUCTION

Hypertension (HT) is currently a major public health problem, directly attributable for more than 7 million deaths per year.[1] Heart, brain, and kidneys are the primary targets for the damage caused by HT which manifests mainly in the form of coronary heart disease, congestive heart failure (HF), stroke, and renal dysfunction. Accordingly, the assessment of the ongoing structural and functional alterations in these organs forms an important component of evaluation of a patient with HT. Echocardiography provides a simple, noninvasive, and relatively inexpensive means to comprehensively assess cardiac abnormalities in HT. Accordingly, echocardiography is recommended as the first-line investigation in the evaluation of patients with HT. It provides a vast amount of information which has considerable prognostic value and has therapeutic implications as well.

ROLE OF ECHOCARDIOGRAPHY IN HYPERTENSION

Detection of left ventricular hypertrophy (LVH) and left ventricular (LV) diastolic dysfunction are the most important objectives of echocardiographic evaluation in a patient with HT. In addition, it also provides information about LV systolic function, aortic size and function, intracardiac hemodynamics, etc. Moreover, among patients who are newly diagnosed to be having HT, echocardiography also helps in excluding coarctation of aorta which is an important secondary cause of HT.

Left Ventricular Hypertrophy

Left ventricular hypertrophy is among the most common cardiac structural abnormalities seen in HT and results from persistently increased afterload on the LV. The pressure overload secondary to elevated blood pressure (BP) and the neurohormonal activation lead to myocyte hypertrophy, collagen deposition, and medial hypertrophy of intramyocardial coronary arteries which together result in myocardial fibrosis. As the myocyte mass increases, the coronary vasodilator reserve becomes impaired due to a relative reduction in coronary blood supply and ongoing myocardial fibrosis.

Detection and Characterization of Left Ventricular Hypertrophy

Traditionally, 12-lead electrocardiogram (ECG) has been used for diagnosing LVH. However, it has been consistently shown that ECG has very low sensitivity (5–10%) for the recognition of LVH. In comparison, echocardiography has much higher sensitivity and is able to detect LVH in nearly 30% of unselected hypertensive adults and in up to 90% of the patients with uncontrolled HT.[2] On echocardiography, LVH is diagnosed by the estimation of LV mass and LV mass index. A number of different methods are available for the estimation of LV mass by echocardiography.[3] The basic principle underlying all these methods is that first LV myocardial volume is calculated by subtracting LV cavity volume from the total LV volume. Then multiplying the LV myocardial volume with myocardial density (1.04) yields LV mass. Traditionally, the linear method has been the most commonly employed method for the estimation of LV mass by echocardiography. Using this method, LV mass is calculated by the following equation:[4]

$$\text{LV mass (g)} = 1.04 \times [(\text{LVIDd} + \text{IVSd} + \text{PWd})^3 - \text{LVIDd}^3] \times 0.8 + 0.6$$

where 1.04 is the myocardial density, and 0.8 is the correction factor. LVIDd, IVSd, and PWd represent the end-diastolic LV internal diameter, interventricular septal thickness, and posterior wall thickness, respectively. These dimensions can be obtained either from M-mode or from two-dimensional (2D) image in the parasternal long-axis view (Fig. 1). However, it should be remembered that M-mode tends to overestimate the true minor axis dimension of the LV; and therefore, the calculated LV mass will be erroneously high. The major advantages of this method are the ease of application and fairly high reproducibility. However, as this method relies only on a single measurement of LV size, it is prone to errors. Any error in obtaining the measurement of LV size gets amplified when calculating LV mass; moreover, this method is not applicable if the LV cavity shape is distorted. To overcome these challenges, 2D echocardiography is now increasingly used for the estimation of LV mass. By 2D echocardiography, LV mass can be calculated using the area–length method, truncated ellipsoid method, or the Simpson's method. Of these the biplane Simpson's method is the most accurate and the easiest to use. This method involves tracing LV epicardial and endocardial borders in apical four-chamber and two-chamber views at end-diastole. The built-in software then automatically calculates LV mass from these tracings. However, it should be noted that most of the data about LVH in HT has been derived from the studies that had used the linear method for the estimation of LV mass. Although 2D echocardiographic methods are more accurate than the linear method for the estimation of LV mass, they also have certain limitations. Three-dimensional (3D) echocardiography is currently the most accurate echocardiographic method for the estimation of LV mass because it does not make assumptions about LV geometry (Fig. 2). Numerous studies have demonstrated superiority of 3D echocardiography over other echocardiographic methods for this purpose.[5-8] However, 3D echocardiography remains underutilized because of the technical challenges.

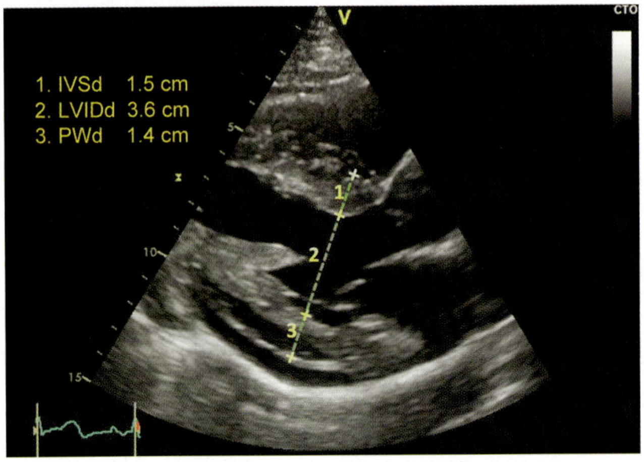

$$\begin{aligned}\text{LV mass (gm)} &= 1.04 \times [(\text{LVIDd} + \text{IVSd} + \text{PWd})^3 - \text{LVIDd}^3] \times 0.8 + 0.6,\\ &= 1.04 \times [(3.6 + 1.5 + 1.4)^3 - 3.6^3] \times 0.8 + 0.6,\\ &= 1.04 \times [274.6 - 46.7] \times 0.8 + 0.6,\\ &= 190.2 \text{ gm}\end{aligned}$$

Fig. 1: Estimation of left ventricular (LV) mass using the linear method. See text for more details. LVIDd, IVSd, and PWd represent the end-diastolic LV internal diameter, interventricular septal thickness, and posterior wall thickness, respectively.

The recent guidelines by the American Society of Echocardiography (ASE) provide age-, gender-, and

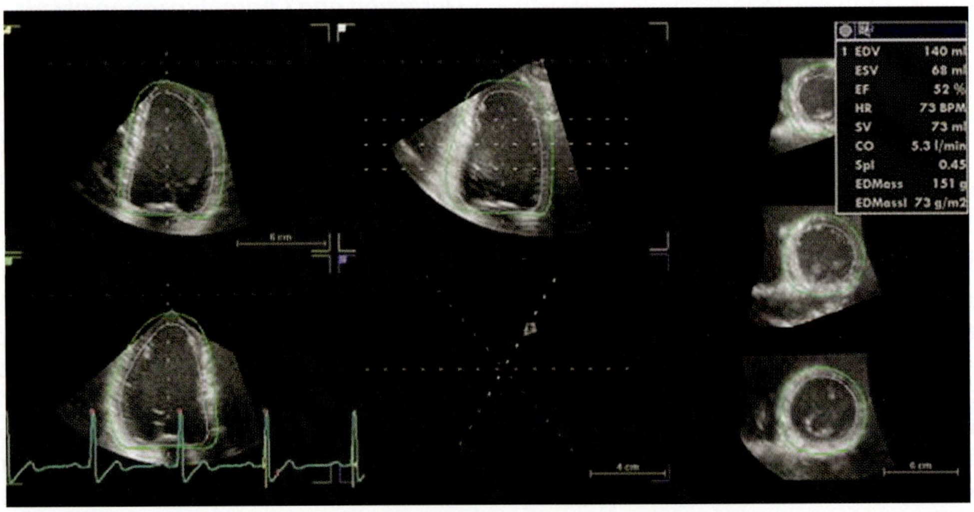

Fig. 2: Estimation of left ventricular mass by three-dimensional echocardiography.

TABLE 1: Normal ranges for LV mass indices.

	Women	*Men*
Linear method:		
• LV mass (g)	67–162	88–224
• LV mass/BSA (g/m^2)	43–95	49–115
• Relative wall thickness	0.22–0.42	0.24–0.42
• Septal thickness (cm)	0.6–0.9	0.6–1.0
• Posterior wall thickness (cm)	0.6–0.9	0.6–1.0
2D method:		
• LV mass (g)	66–150	96–200
• LV mass/BSA (g/m^2)	44–88	50–102

(BSA: body surface area; LV: left ventricular; 2D: two-dimensional)
Source: Adapted from Lang RM, Badano LP, Mor-Avi V, et al. Recommendations for cardiac chamber quantification by echocardiography in adults: an update from the American Society of Echocardiography and the European Association of Cardiovascular Imaging. J Am Soc Echocardiogr. 2015;28:1-39 e14.

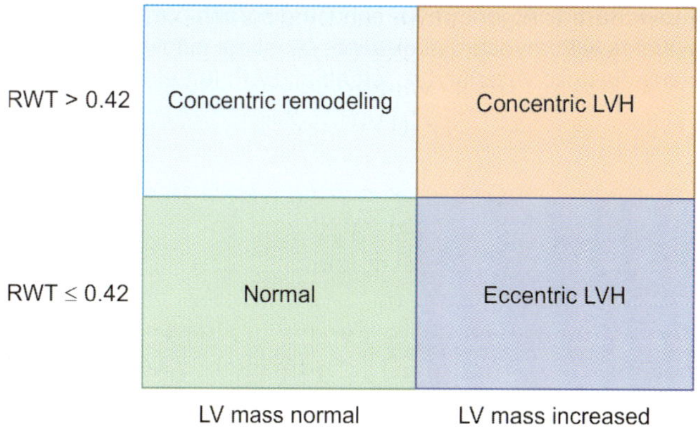

Fig. 3: Different patterns of LV remodeling in hypertension. (LV: left ventricular; LVH: left ventricular hypertrophy; RWT: relative wall thickness).

ethnicity-specific reference ranges for LV mass by different echocardiographic methods.[9] The commonly used threshold values for defining LVH are described in Table 1. It should be noted that regardless of the method used, LV mass needs to be indexed to body surface area to obtain LV mass index which can be used for interindividual or serial comparisons. Some investigators prefer indexing LV mass to height raised to the allometric power of 2.7, instead of body surface area. This approach is more accurate when body composition is disproportionately altered as in obesity or anorexia nervosa.[10]

Pattern of Left Ventricular Hypertrophy

Not only the LV mass but the overall geometry of the LV also has prognostic significance. Based on the relative configuration of LV cavity and LV wall, different geometric patterns of LV remodeling can be recognized (Fig. 3). These include concentric remodeling, concentric LVH, and eccentric LVH.[3] Concentric remodeling refers to a condition in which LV wall thickness is increased relative to the LV cavity size, but the overall LV mass is still within the normal range. Increased wall thickness is ascertained by calculating relative wall thickness (RWT), which is the ratio of double the posterior wall thickness to the LV cavity internal dimension, as shown here:

$$\text{RWT} = \frac{\text{2PWd}}{\text{LVIDd}}$$

Concentric remodeling is diagnosed when RWT is increased (>0.42) but LV mass is normal. It is a precursor to concentric LVH and is an adverse prognostic marker.[11,12]

When both RWT and LV mass are increased, it is described as concentric LVH, which is typical of pressure overload. In contrast, when LV mass is increased but RWT remains normal, it indicates eccentric hypertrophy, which is commonly seen in response to LV volume overload.

Prognostic and Therapeutic Value of Left Ventricular Hypertrophy

Previous studies have shown that LV wall thickness alone does not provide a reliable estimate about cardiovascular (CV) risk, but LV mass index is an independent predictor of incident CV disease.[13] Being a consequence of sustained pressure overload, LV mass is more closely related to mean 24-hour BP than any of the other BP measurements.[14] LV mass is significantly higher in renovascular HT and primary aldosteronism, possibly due to the pathogenic role of renin-angiotensin-aldosterone system in the development of hypertensive LVH.[15,16] LVH is itself a preclinical disease and a risk factor for ischemic heart disease, HF, arrhythmias, stroke, and sudden death. Several studies have demonstrated that LVH is associated with an adjusted relative risk of 1.5–3.5 for CV mortality.[17-19] For example, in the MAVI (MAssa Ventricolare sinistra nell'Ipertensione) study, for each 39 g/m^2 increase in LV mass, there was a 40% rise in the risk of major CV events, and this increment in the risk was independent of several clinical parameters, including age, cigarette smoking, and diabetes.[20] LV mass has also been the most commonly used echocardiographic metric for monitoring response to antihypertensive treatment. LVH regression with treatment is associated with significant benefits in terms of CV event reduction, whereas a failure to regress LVH is associated with worse outcomes.[21,22] It has also been seen that the effect of different antihypertensive drugs on LVH is not alike, and this could underlie their differential impact on CV outcomes in hypertensive subjects. For example, in the Losartan Intervention For Endpoint reduction in hypertension study (LIFE), both atenolol and losartan resulted in a similar reduction in BP. However, the treatment with losartan was associated with a lower risk of CV morbidity and death than treatment with atenolol.[23] A substudy of LIFE later

Flowchart 1: Algorithm for echocardiographic estimation of left atrial pressure and grading left ventricular diastolic function in patients with myocardial disease. (A: mitral inflow late diastolic velocity; E: mitral inflow early diastolic velocity; e′: mitral annular early diastolic velocity; LA: left atrial; LAP: left atrial pressure; TR: tricuspid regurgitation).

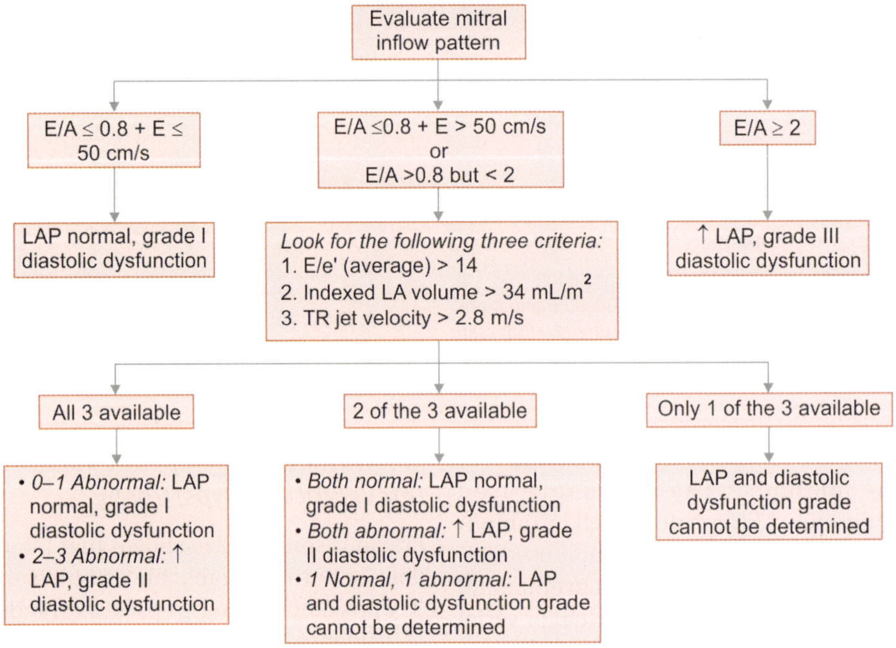

Source: Modified from Nagueh SF, Smiseth OA, Appleton CP, et al. Recommendations for the evaluation of left ventricular diastolic function by echocardiography: an update from the American Society of Echocardiography and the European Association of Cardiovascular Imaging. J Am Soc Echocardiogr. 2016;29:277-314.

showed that losartan resulted in greater reduction in LVH than atenolol, and this could be the reason for greater event reduction with losartan.[24]

Left Ventricular Diastolic Function

As the LV myocardium undergoes hypertrophy and replacement fibrosis in response to chronic pressure overload, it leads to progressive stiffening of LV myocardium. The increasing stiffness of LV myocardium results in the impairment of LV diastolic filling, which is the most common cardiac functional abnormality seen in patients with HT. Clinically, it manifests as exertional dyspnea. As the severity of diastolic dysfunction worsens, there is progressive increase in LV filling pressure culminating into frank diastolic HF. Worsening LV diastolic function also predisposes the patients to atrial fibrillation (AF) by causing left atrial (LA) enlargement and remodeling. Echocardiography is the most useful modality for the assessment of LV diastolic function in clinical practice. A number of echocardiographic parameters have been proposed as measures of LV diastolic function. However, as disagreement among different echocardiographic parameters of LV diastolic function is quite common, an integrative approach combining the most informative parameters needs to be used. The ASE recommends such an algorithm which is based on mitral inflow pattern, early diastolic mitral annular velocity, indexed LA volume, and peak tricuspid regurgitation jet velocity[25] (Flowchart 1). As mentioned above, during the early phase of pathogenesis, LV filling pressure may not be elevated at rest but rises during exercise. In such cases, when the patient presents with exertional dyspnea but the resting echocardiogram shows normal LV diastolic function, diastolic stress test may be required to unmask exercise-induced elevations in LV filling pressure and to explain the patient's symptoms.

Left ventricular diastolic dysfunction not only helps explain patients' symptoms, it has prognostic significance as well. Mitral inflow E/e′ is highly predictive of adverse events in hypertensive heart disease. The PIUMA (Progetto Ipertensione Umbria Monitoraggio Ambulatoriale) study showed that the changes in the mitral inflow E/A ratio were associated with a significant increase in the risk of CV events.[26] In addition, as discussed below, the LA size and function, which have direct relationship with the LV diastolic function, have been shown to be strong predictors of the risk of HF, AF, stroke, and overall CV mortality.[27-37]

Estimation of Left Atrial Size

During ventricular diastole the LA is in direct communication with the LV and is therefore exposed to all pathophysiological

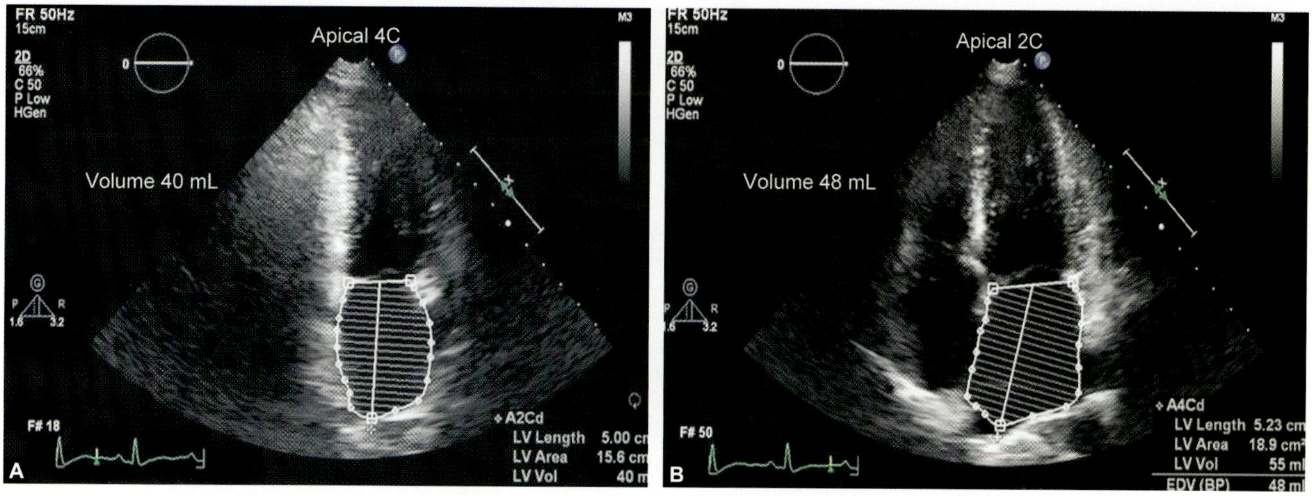

Figs. 4A and B: Measurement of left atrial volume by the biplane Simpson's method.

disturbances impacting LV diastolic function. When LV filling pressure remains chronically elevated, the sustained increase in LA tension leads to LA dilatation, the severity of which correlates with the severity and the chronicity of LV diastolic dysfunction.[28,38,39] Thus the increased LA size is a reflection of long-standing hemodynamic changes and is relatively unaffected by transient, acute changes in LV filling pressures. For this reason the LA size is also considered the glycosylated hemoglobin of LV diastolic function. There are several different echocardiographic measures of LA size, including LA linear dimension, LA area, and LA volume.[3] At present, LA volume estimated using the biplane area-length method or the Simpson's method is the most accepted measure of LA size (Figs. 4A and B).[9] During echocardiography, LA size is conventionally measured at ventricular end-systole when the LA size is maximum. Care should be taken to avoid foreshortening of LA by ensuring that the base of LA is at its largest size. While performing planimetry of LA, confluences of pulmonary veins and LA appendage should be excluded from the measurement. In addition, as the LA size is affected by body size, age, and gender, all LA size measurements should be indexed to body surface area. The indexed LA size does not depend on the age after the childhood. An indexed LA volume >34 mL/m^2 is considered to indicate LA dilatation.

As mentioned above, LA size is a strong predictor of adverse CV outcomes. It increases the risk of AF, stroke, and overall mortality.[27-37] In the Framingham Heart Study, LA size was found to be a strong independent predictor of the risk of nonrheumatic AF in a subset of 1,924 elderly subjects followed up for 7.2 years.[35] Similarly, in yet another study involving elderly subjects with no prior AF, LA volume was independently predictive of the first ischemic stroke and even death.[33] Several other studies have also reported similar findings.

Assessment of Left Atrial Function

Recent data suggest that LA function, in addition to LA size, is also an important determinant of adverse outcomes in various diseases states. For this reason, there has been an increasing interest in the assessment of LA function by echocardiography. Earlier, LA function was assessed by measuring LA size during the different phases of cardiac cycle or by measuring the LA appendage emptying velocity. However, several limitations inherent to these techniques have precluded wider use of LA function assessment in clinical practice. More recently, the advent of speckle-tracking echocardiography has provided a simple means for the assessment of LA function in the form of LA strain, which has now become the most preferred parameter for this purpose (Figs. 5A and B).[40,41] For LA strain measurement, grayscale images are acquired in apical four-chamber and two-chamber views, during breath-hold with a stable ECG recording. The grayscale frame rate should be set between 50 frames/s and 80 frames/s, and the image quality should be optimized to permit clear distinction between LA wall and the surrounding structures. Once the image is optimized, moving images with three consecutive cardiac cycles are recorded for each view. These images are analyzed using one of the proprietary speckle-tracking software to obtain strain curves. The LA strain curves can be generated using either the QRS or the P-wave as the reference point.[40,42] QRS method is used more often, and a typical LA strain curve using this method is shown in Figure 6. From this curve, the peak atrial longitudinal strain (PALS) can be calculated as the peak strain at the end of ventricular systole. PALS represents the reservoir function of the LA and is the most relevant LA strain measurement. PALS averaged for all the analyzed segments in apical four-chamber and two-chamber views is denoted as global PALS. The average

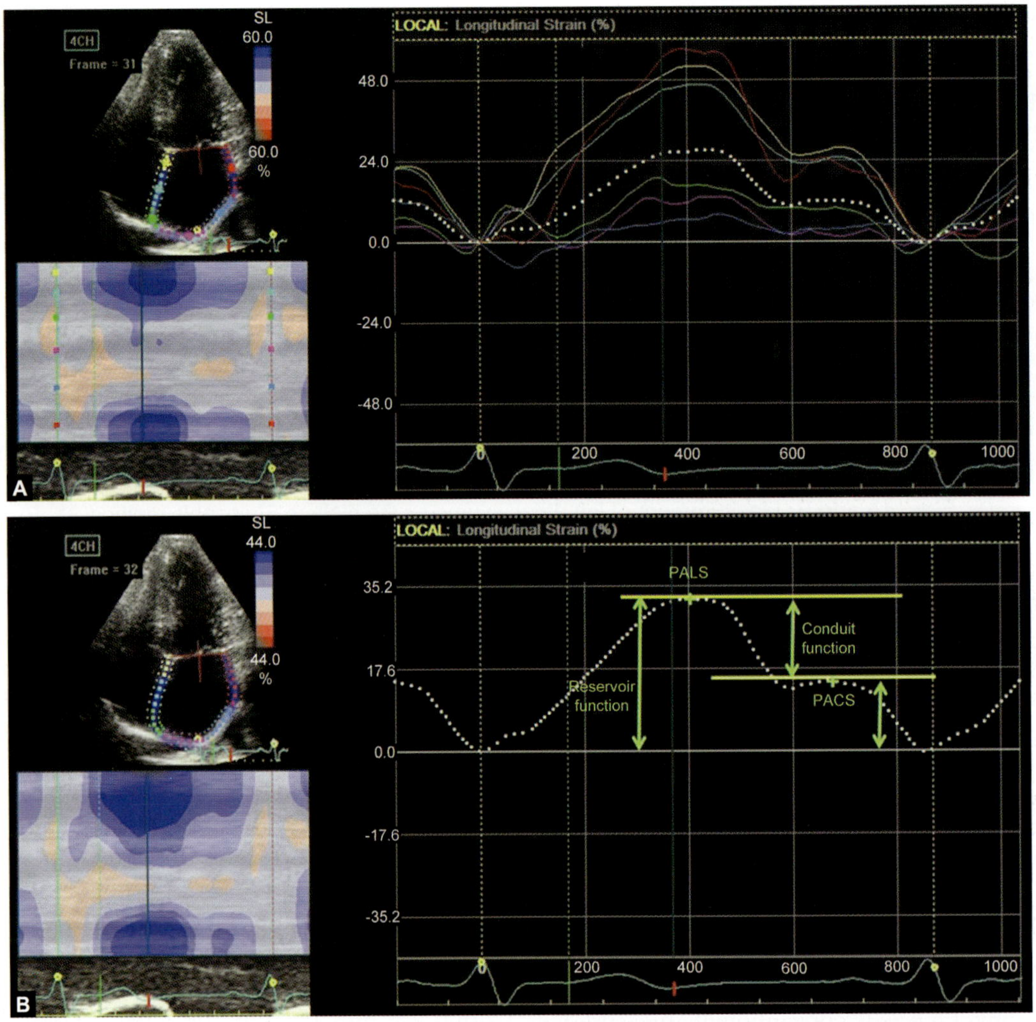

Figs. 5A and B: Measurement of left atrial strain by speckle-tracking echocardiography: (A) The colored curves depict segmental strain, whereas the white-dotted curve depicts the average of all the segments; (B) Left atrial strain waveform using QRS as the reference point. There is an initial positive wave during ventricular systole which is followed by reduction in strain during early rapid filling phase and subsequently during active atrial contraction. (PACS: peak atrial contraction strain; PALS: peak atrial longitudinal strain).

global PALS is normally in the range of 40–45%, and a value of <+ 25% for global PALS is generally considered to indicate reduced LA strain.[43,44] Abnormalities of LA strain have been described in patients with HT,[45-47] and this has been used for understanding the pathophysiology of HT. However, the prognostic value of LA strain in HT is yet to be studied adequately.

Left Ventricular Systolic Function

It is generally assumed that HT primarily results in LV diastolic dysfunction, whereas LV systolic function remains largely preserved, unless the disease is far advanced. However, more recent studies employing newer technologies, such as strain imaging, have shown that LV systolic function is frequently impaired, even during the early stages of disease.[40,48] Conventionally, LV ejection fraction (LVEF) is used as "the measure" of LV systolic function. The biplane Simpson's method is the preferred method for this purpose, though 3D echocardiography provides more accurate estimations as described above. Although LVEF remains largely preserved in most patients with HT, asymptomatic reduction in LVEF is known to occur in these subjects. In a study involving 2,384 initially untreated subjects with HT with no previous CV disease and no symptoms or physical signs of congestive HF, asymptomatic LV systolic dysfunction (defined as LVEF < 50%) was found in 3.6% of the subjects. Such LV systolic dysfunction was more common in male subjects who were smokers and had higher 24-hour ambulatory BP readings and heart rate.

Significantly, LV systolic dysfunction in these patients was found to be a potent and early marker for predicting progression toward HF requiring hospitalization.[49] More commonly, however, LV systolic dysfunction in these patients is covert and is detected when strain imaging is used. Reduction in LV global longitudinal strain (GLS) is common in hypertensive subjects and is associated with increased risk of major adverse cardiac events.[50-54] The association of GLS with adverse cardiac events has been shown to be independent of and incremental to clinical parameters and LVH.[50] Midwall fractional shortening and myocardial performance index are other measures of LV systolic function which can potentially detect LV systolic dysfunction even when LVEF is normal. However, both have their own limitations, with most important being their inability to provide comprehensive information about LV systolic function.

Aortic Root Dilatation

Some earlier reports had suggested that HT predisposes to aortic root enlargement and consequently aortic regurgitation,[55-57] but subsequent studies have reported conflicting findings.[58-61] A more recent study showed that HT predominantly affects the diameter of distal aortic root, primarily supra-aortic ridge, and proximal ascending aorta; and this possibly explains the lack of consistent relationship between HT and aortic root dilatation in the previous studies.[62] Nevertheless, aortic root dilatation in a hypertensive patient is considered to be a marker of increased CV morbidity and mortality.[63] In patients with HT, aortic root enlargement is associated with significantly higher prevalence of LVH, carotid intima-medial thickness, carotid plaques, and microalbuminuria.[63] In addition, it has also been shown to be a useful marker of subclinical LV diastolic dysfunction in these patients.[64]

Other Abnormalities

In all hypertensive patients undergoing echocardiography, it is important to look for the evidence of coarctation of aorta. Although uncommon, coarctation is a treatable cause of HT but is often missed. Similarly, in occasional patient with isolated systolic HT, echocardiography can reveal significant aortic regurgitation to be the actual underlying cause of HT, rather than HT being the primary pathology.

CONCLUSION

Echocardiography is an important diagnostic and prognostic tool in patients with HT. While conventional measures, such as cardiac chamber sizes and LV diastolic function, remain the most important information provided by echocardiography, LV and LA strains help uncover subclinical cardiac dysfunction which is common in these patients. Collectively, all these different echocardiographic measurements aid in facilitating optimum therapeutic decision-making in these patients. In addition, echocardiography is also helpful in monitoring response to therapy and has been a very commonly employed tool in research related to HT.

REFERENCES

1. Guilbert JJ. The world health report 2002—reducing risks, promoting healthy life. Educ Health (Abingdon). 2003;16:230.
2. Victor RG, Kaplan NM. Systemic hypertension: mechanisms and diagnosis. In: Libby P, Bonow RO, Mann DL, Zipes DP (Eds). Braunwald's heart disease: a textbook of cardiovascular medicine, 8th edition. Philadelphia: Saunders; 2008. pp. 1027-48.
3. Lang RM, Bierig M, Devereux RB, et al. Recommendations for chamber quantification: a report from the American Society of Echocardiography's Guidelines and Standards Committee and the Chamber Quantification Writing Group, developed in conjunction with the European Association of Echocardiography, a branch of the European Society of Cardiology. J Am Soc Echocardiogr. 2005;18:1440-63.
4. Devereux RB, Alonso DR, Lutas EM, et al. Echocardiographic assessment of left ventricular hypertrophy: comparison to necropsy findings. Am J Cardiol. 1986;57:450-8.
5. Jenkins C, Bricknell K, Hanekom L, et al. Reproducibility and accuracy of echocardiographic measurements of left ventricular parameters using real-time three-dimensional echocardiography. J Am Coll Cardiol. 2004;44:878-86.
6. Oe H, Hozumi T, Arai K, et al. Comparison of accurate measurement of left ventricular mass in patients with hypertrophied hearts by real-time three-dimensional echocardiography versus magnetic resonance imaging. Am J Cardiol. 2005;95:1263-7.
7. Mor-Avi V, Sugeng L, Weinert L, et al. Fast measurement of left ventricular mass with real-time three-dimensional echocardiography: comparison with magnetic resonance imaging. Circulation. 2004;110:1814-8.
8. Bicudo LS, Tsutsui JM, Shiozaki A, et al. Value of real time three-dimensional echocardiography in patients with hypertrophic cardiomyopathy: comparison with two-dimensional echocardiography and magnetic resonance imaging. Echocardiography. 2008;25:717-26.
9. Lang RM, Badano LP, Mor-Avi V, et al. Recommendations for cardiac chamber quantification by echocardiography in adults: an update from the American Society of Echocardiography and the European Association of Cardiovascular Imaging. J Am Soc Echocardiogr. 2015;28:1-39.e14.
10. de Simone G, Devereux RB, Daniels SR, et al. Effect of growth on variability of left ventricular mass: assessment of allometric signals in adults and children and their capacity to predict cardiovascular risk. J Am Coll Cardiol. 1995;25:1056-62.

11. Berger J, Ren X, Na B, et al. Relation of concentric remodeling to adverse outcomes in patients with stable coronary artery disease (from the Heart and Soul Study). Am J Cardiol. 2011;107:1579-84.
12. Verdecchia P, Schillaci G, Borgioni C, et al. Adverse prognostic significance of concentric remodeling of the left ventricle in hypertensive patients with normal left ventricular mass. J Am Coll Cardiol. 1995;25:871-8.
13. Cuspidi C, Facchetti R, Bombelli M, et al. Differential value of left ventricular mass index and wall thickness in predicting cardiovascular prognosis: data from the PAMELA population. Am J Hypertens. 2014;27(8):1079-86.
14. Parati G, Pomidossi G, Albini F, et al. Relationship of 24-hour blood pressure mean and variability to severity of target-organ damage in hypertension. J Hypertens. 1987;5:93-8.
15. Rizzoni D, Muiesan ML, Porteri E, et al. Relations between cardiac and vascular structure in patients with primary and secondary hypertension. J Am Coll Cardiol. 1998;32:985-92.
16. Rossi GP, Sacchetto A, Pavan E, et al. Remodeling of the left ventricle in primary aldosteronism due to Conn's adenoma. Circulation. 1997;95:1471-8.
17. Levy D, Garrison RJ, Savage DD, et al. Prognostic implications of echocardiographically determined left ventricular mass in the Framingham Heart Study. N Engl J Med. 1990;322:1561-6.
18. Koren MJ, Devereux RB, Casale PN, et al. Relation of left ventricular mass and geometry to morbidity and mortality in uncomplicated essential hypertension. Ann Intern Med. 1991;114:345-52.
19. Muiesan ML, Salvetti M, Rizzoni D, et al. Association of change in left ventricular mass with prognosis during long-term antihypertensive treatment. J Hypertens. 1995;13:1091-5.
20. Verdecchia P, Carini G, Circo A, et al. Left ventricular mass and cardiovascular morbidity in essential hypertension: the MAVI study. J Am Coll Cardiol. 2001;38:1829-35.
21. Devereux RB, Wachtell K, Gerdts E, et al. Prognostic significance of left ventricular mass change during treatment of hypertension. JAMA. 2004;292:2350-6.
22. Fleischmann EH, Schmieder RE. Are all antihypertensive drug classes equal in reducing left ventricular hypertrophy? Curr Cardiol Rep. 2002;4:474-8.
23. Dahlof B, Devereux RB, Kjeldsen SE, et al. Cardiovascular morbidity and mortality in the Losartan Intervention for Endpoint reduction in hypertension study (LIFE): a randomised trial against atenolol. Lancet. 2002;359:995-1003.
24. Devereux RB, Dahlof B, Gerdts E, et al. Regression of hypertensive left ventricular hypertrophy by losartan compared with atenolol: the Losartan Intervention for Endpoint Reduction in Hypertension (LIFE) trial. Circulation. 2004;110:1456-62.
25. Nagueh SF, Smiseth OA, Appleton CP, et al. Recommendations for the evaluation of left ventricular diastolic function by echocardiography: an update from the American Society of Echocardiography and the European Association of Cardiovascular Imaging. J Am Soc Echocardiogr. 2016;29:277-314.
26. Schillaci G, Pasqualini L, Verdecchia P, et al. Prognostic significance of left ventricular diastolic dysfunction in essential hypertension. J Am Coll Cardiol. 2002;39:2005-11.
27. Tsang TSM, Barnes ME, Gersh BJ, et al. Prediction of risk for first age-related cardiovascular events in an elderly population: the incremental value of echocardiography. J Am Coll Cardiol. 2003;42:1199-205.
28. Tsang TSM, Barnes ME, Gersh BJ, et al. Left atrial volume as a morphophysiologic expression of left ventricular diastolic dysfunction and relation to cardiovascular risk burden. Am J Cardiol. 2002;90:1284-9.
29. Benjamin EJ, D'Agostino RB, Belanger AJ, et al. Left atrial size and the risk of stroke and death. The Framingham Heart Study. Circulation. 1995;92:835-41.
30. Bolca O, Akdemir O, Eren M, et al. Left atrial maximum volume is a recurrence predictor in lone atrial fibrillation: an acoustic quantification study. Jpn Heart J. 2002;43:241-8.
31. Di Tullio MR, Sacco RL, Sciacca RR, et al. Left atrial size and the risk of ischemic stroke in an ethnically mixed population. Stroke. 1999;30:2019-24.
32. Tsang TS, Barnes ME, Bailey KR, et al. Left atrial volume: important risk marker of incident atrial fibrillation in 1655 older men and women. Mayo Clin Proc. 2001;76:467-75.
33. Barnes ME, Miyasaka Y, Seward JB, et al. Left atrial volume in the prediction of first ischemic stroke in an elderly cohort without atrial fibrillation. Mayo Clin Proc. 2004;79:1008-14.
34. Tsang TS, Barnes ME, Gersh BJ, et al. Risks for atrial fibrillation and congestive heart failure in patients ≥65 years of age with abnormal left ventricular diastolic relaxation. Am J Cardiol. 2004;93:54-8.
35. Vaziri SM, Larson MG, Benjamin EJ, et al. Echocardiographic predictors of nonrheumatic atrial fibrillation. The Framingham Heart Study. Circulation. 1994;89:724-30.
36. Flaker GC, Fletcher KA, Rothbart RM, et al. Clinical and echocardiographic features of intermittent atrial fibrillation that predict recurrent atrial fibrillation. Stroke Prevention in Atrial Fibrillation (SPAF) Investigators. Am J Cardiol. 1995;76:355-8.
37. Gardin JM, McClelland R, Kitzman D, et al. M-mode echocardiographic predictors of six- to seven-year incidence of coronary heart disease, stroke, congestive heart failure, and mortality in an elderly cohort (The Cardiovascular Health Study). Am J Cardiol. 2001;87:1051-7.
38. Simek CL, Feldman MD, Haber HL, et al. Relationship between left ventricular wall thickness and left atrial size: comparison with other measures of diastolic function. J Am Soc Echocardiogr. 1995;8:37-47.
39. Appleton CP, Galloway JM, Gonzalez MS, et al. Estimation of left ventricular filling pressures using two-dimensional and Doppler echocardiography in adult patients with cardiac disease. Additional value of analyzing left atrial size, left atrial ejection fraction and the difference in duration of pulmonary venous and mitral flow velocity at atrial contraction. J Am Coll Cardiol. 1993;22:1972-82.
40. Mor-Avi V, Lang RM, Badano LP, et al. Current and evolving echocardiographic techniques for the quantitative evaluation of cardiac mechanics: ASE/EAE consensus statement on

methodology and indications endorsed by the Japanese Society of Echocardiography. J Am Soc Echocardiogr. 2011;24:277-313.

41. Rosca M, Lancellotti P, Popescu BA, et al. Left atrial function: pathophysiology, echocardiographic assessment, and clinical applications. Heart. 2011;97:1982-9.
42. Cameli M, Lisi M, Righini FM, et al. Novel echocardiographic techniques to assess left atrial size, anatomy and function. Cardiovasc Ultrasound. 2012;10:4.
43. Cameli M, Caputo M, Mondillo S, et al. Feasibility and reference values of left atrial longitudinal strain imaging by two-dimensional speckle tracking. Cardiovasc Ultrasound. 2009;7:6.
44. Morris DA, Takeuchi M, Krisper M, et al. Normal values and clinical relevance of left atrial myocardial function analysed by speckle-tracking echocardiography: multicentre study. Eur Heart J Cardiovasc Imaging. 2015;16:364-72.
45. Kokubu N, Yuda S, Tsuchihashi K, et al. Noninvasive assessment of left atrial function by strain rate imaging in patients with hypertension: a possible beneficial effect of renin-angiotensin system inhibition on left atrial function. Hypertens Res. 2007;30:13-21.
46. Aung SM, Guler A, Guler Y, et al. Two-dimensional speckle-tracking echocardiography-based left atrial strain parameters predict masked hypertension in patients with hypertensive response to exercise. Blood Press Monit. 2017;22:27-33.
47. Tosun V, Korucuk N, Kilinc AY, et al. Evaluation of atrial electromechanical functions in dipper and nondipper hypertension patients using left atrial strain P-wave dispersion and P terminal force. Echocardiography. 2018;35:1318-25.
48. Geyer H, Caracciolo G, Abe H, et al. Assessment of myocardial mechanics using speckle tracking echocardiography: fundamentals and clinical applications. J Am Soc Echocardiogr. 2010;23:351-69; quiz 453-5.
49. Verdecchia P, Angeli F, Gattobigio R, et al. Asymptomatic left ventricular systolic dysfunction in essential hypertension: prevalence, determinants, and prognostic value. Hypertension. 2005;45:412-8.
50. Saito M, Khan F, Stoklosa T, et al. Prognostic implications of LV strain risk score in asymptomatic patients with hypertensive heart disease. JACC Cardiovasc Imaging. 2016;9:911-21.
51. Hare JL, Brown JK, Marwick TH. Association of myocardial strain with left ventricular geometry and progression of hypertensive heart disease. Am J Cardiol. 2008;102:87-91.
52. Narayanan A, Aurigemma GP, Chinali M, et al. Cardiac mechanics in mild hypertensive heart disease: a speckle-strain imaging study. Circ Cardiovasc Imaging. 2009;2:382-90.
53. Imbalzano E, Zito C, Carerj S, et al. Left ventricular function in hypertension: new insight by speckle tracking echocardiography. Echocardiography. 2011;28:649-57.
54. Kraigher-Krainer E, Shah AM, Gupta DK, et al. Impaired systolic function by strain imaging in heart failure with preserved ejection fraction. J Am Coll Cardiol. 2014;63:447-56.
55. Waller BF, Zoltick JM, Rosen JH, et al. Severe aortic regurgitation from systemic hypertension (without aortic dissection) requiring aortic valve replacement: analysis of four patients. Am J Cardiol. 1982;49:473-7.
56. Puchner TC, Huston JH, Hellmuth GA. Aortic valve insufficiency in arterial hypertension. Am J Cardiol. 1960;5:758-60.
57. Barlow J, Kincaid-Smith P. The auscultatory findings in hypertension. Br Heart J. 1960;22:505-14.
58. Roman MJ, Devereux RB, Cody RJ. Ability of left ventricular stress-shortening relations, end-systolic stress/volume ratio and indirect indexes to detect severe contractile failure in ischemic or idiopathic dilated cardiomyopathy. Am J Cardiol. 1989;64:1338-43.
59. Schlatmann TJ, Becker AE. Pathogenesis of dissecting aneurysm of aorta. Comparative histopathologic study of significance of medial changes. Am J Cardiol. 1977;39:21-6.
60. Roman MJ, Devereux RB, Niles NW, et al. Aortic root dilatation as a cause of isolated, severe aortic regurgitation. Prevalence, clinical and echocardiographic patterns, and relation to left ventricular hypertrophy and function. Ann Intern Med. 1987;106:800-7.
61. Pearson AC, Gudipati C, Nagelhout D, et al. Echocardiographic evaluation of cardiac structure and function in elderly subjects with isolated systolic hypertension. J Am Coll Cardiol. 1991;17:422-30.
62. Kim M, Roman MJ, Cavallini MC, et al. Effect of hypertension on aortic root size and prevalence of aortic regurgitation. Hypertension. 1996;28:47-52.
63. Cuspidi C, Meani S, Valerio C, et al. Ambulatory blood pressure, target organ damage and aortic root size in never-treated essential hypertensive patients. J Hum Hypertens. 2007;21:531-8.
64. Masugata H, Senda S, Murao K, et al. Aortic root dilatation as a marker of subclinical left ventricular diastolic dysfunction in patients with cardiovascular risk factors. J Int Med Res. 2011;39:64-70.

10

CHAPTER

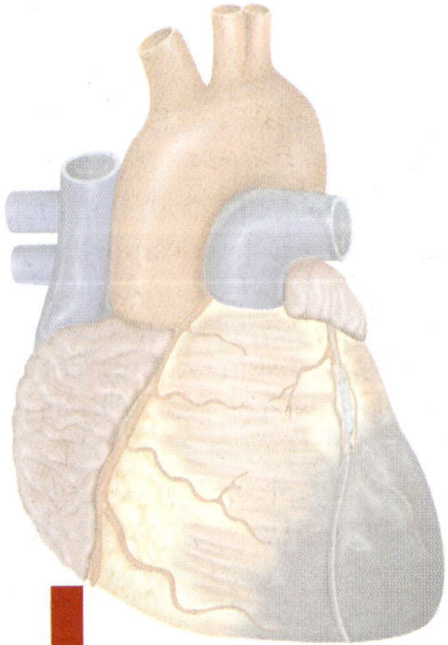

Beta-blocker Effect and Outcome Evaluation by Echocardiography in Hypertension

Jamshed J Dalal, Vijay Katekhaye

INTRODUCTION

Hypertension (HT) is a growing epidemic worldwide. Increased levels of blood pressure (BP) are associated with adverse effects on cardiovascular (CV) system. Along with left ventricular hypertrophy (LVH), a constellation of abnormalities in systolic and diastolic function which manifest as arrhythmias or symptomatic heart failure (HF) is considered as hypertensive heart disease (HHD).[1,2] Echocardiography (ECHO) is the modality of choice to ascertain these cardiac changes in patients with HT. European Society of Hypertension and European Society of Cardiology (ESH/ESC) recommend evaluation by ECHO for suspected LVH, left atrial (LA) dilatation, or concomitant clinical or subclinical systolic or diastolic dysfunction.[3] ECHO assessment in HT is therefore advisable if clinical suspicion of LVH and/or HF, structural heart disease, ischemic heart disease exists. It can also be undertaken for assessing CV risk in certain cases.[4] Role of increased sympathetic neuronal activity is well established in HT and progression of uncomplicated to complicated HT.[5] Beta-blockers (BB) are effective agents in treatment of HT where they lower the sympathetic activity and improve the vagal control.[5,6] Since their introduction in early 1960s, BB still remain one of the widely used agents in HT, HF, and coronary artery disease (CAD).[3,7] Using BB in HT is helpful in reversal of structural and functional cardiac changes in HT. In this chapter, effects of BB use on echocardiographic changes in patients with HT are discussed.

THE ROLE OF ECHO IN HYPERTENSION

It has been suggested that use of ECHO in HT is appropriate in patients with suspected heart disease. However, it may be inappropriate to use ECHO routinely in absence of any specific symptoms or signs and clinical suspicion of heart disease.[4] European Association of Cardiovascular Imaging (EACVI) and the American Society of Echocardiography (ASE) recommend use of ECHO in HT to address the following:

- Measurement of LV mass.
- Left ventricular geometry.
- Tissue characterization.
- Arterial function and ventriculo-arterial matching.

Left Ventricular Mass

It can be determined with following formula using a two-dimensional linear LV measurement.

$$\text{LV mass (g)} = 0.8 \times \{1.04 \times [(\text{LVIDd} + \text{PWTd} + \text{SWTd})^3 - (\text{LVIDd})^3]\} + 0.6$$

Where, LVIDd = LV internal dimension at end diastole; PWTd = LV posterior wall thickness at end diastole; and SWTd = interventricular septal wall thickness at end diastole.

Left Ventricular Geometry

Based on two-dimensional ECHO in M-mode, different LV geometries can be identified with LV mass, LV volume,

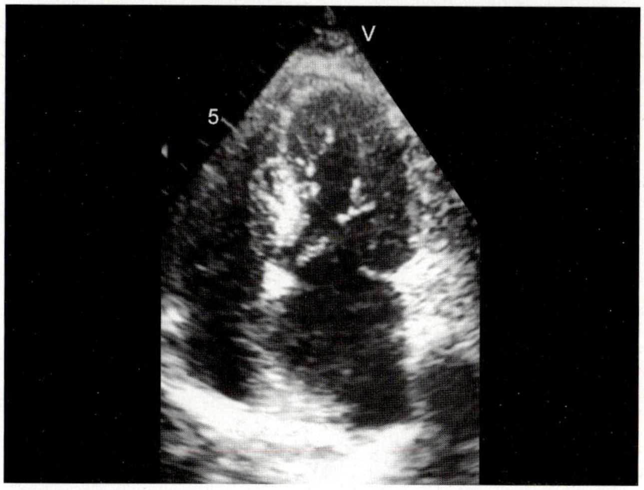

Fig. 1: Concentric left ventricular hypertrophy, a common finding in hypertension.

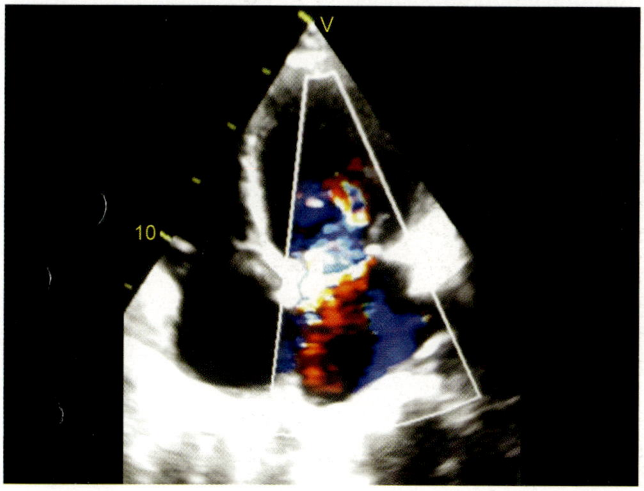

Fig. 2: Dilated left ventricle with mitral regurgitation secondary to hypertension.

and relative wall thickness (RWT) as shown in Table 1. The description of the LV geometry as identified among four categories should be given in every ECHO assessment in patients with HT.[8] Concentric LVH is probably the most frequent abnormality, which occurs mainly due to pressure overload as in HT (Fig. 1). Volume overload results in eccentric hypertrophy and eventually LV dilatation and mitral regurgitation (Fig. 2).

Concentric LVH may be associated with systolic dysfunction but in eccentric hypertrophy, the systolic function is low normal or mildly impaired. Concentric LV remodeling occurs in late-stage and is seen in pressure-volume overload or with associated CAD. In LV remodeling, there can be more severe abnormalities in diastolic function. Impaired relaxation is in the presence of diastolic dysfunction in mild HT in absence of LVH (Table 1).[8]

TABLE 1: LV geometry as assessed by LV mass, LV volume, and RWT.

LV geometry	*LV volume index (mL/m^2)*	*LV mass index (g/m^2)*		*RWT*
Normal ventricle	≤75	Men	≤115	0.32–0.42
		Women	≤95	
Physiological hypertrophy	>75	Men	>115	0.32–0.42
		Women	>95	
Concentric remodeling	≤75	Men	≤115	>0.42
		Women	≤95	
Eccentric remodeling	>75	Men	≤115	<0.32
		Women	≤95	
Concentric hypertrophy	≤75	Men	>115	>0.42
		Women	>95	
Mixed hypertrophy	>75	Men	>115	>0.42
		Women	>95	
Dilated hypertrophy	>75	Men	>115	0.32–0.42
		Women	>95	

(LV: left ventricular; RWT: relative wall thickness)

Tissue Characterization

It can be done with measurement of tissue reflection (density of tissue) and functional changes resulting from changes in myocardial ultrastructure. With ECHO, integrated backscatter is the only marker of tissue density that can be obtained.[8]

Arterial Function and Ventriculo-arterial Matching

The assessments like pulse-wave velocity, wave reflection, wave intensity analysis, aortic assessments for aneurysms or coarctations can be undertaken in during ECHO.[8]

Role of Doppler Evaluation

Color Doppler evaluation of mitral regurgitation, secondary to LV dilatation is an important factor in predicting worsening LV function, and Doppler assessment of the grade of diastolic dysfunction adds another additional physiologic dimension to the ECHO evaluation in patients with HT.

EFFECT OF BETA-BLOCKER IN PRE-EXISTING ECHO FEATURES IN HYPERTENSION

Hypertension involves some degree of LV dysfunction. For an antihypertensive agent, it is important to prevent and/or reduce these secondary cardiac changes in addition to lowering of BP. Treatment of LV dysfunction is therefore an important target for antihypertensive agents. BB have been cornerstone treatment for HT since decades.[9]

Beta-blocker Effect on Systolic Function in Hypertension

Pressure overload associated with HT results in concentric LVH. The increased LV systolic pressure and wall stress result in the addition of new myofibrils along with hypertrophy of cardiac myocytes. Regression of LVH is induced by BB as has been shown by acebutolol.[10] Recently, a Bayesian network meta-analysis demonstrated that fat-soluble selective beta-1 blockers have similar efficacy in reducing LVH when compared to angiotensin-converting enzyme inhibitors or angiotensin receptor blockers but have greater efficacy than diuretics, and calcium channel blockers. Also, beta-1 blockers had highest probability for being most efficacious agents to regress the LVH in HT.[11] This effect is considered usually secondary to reduction in cardiac afterload. Reduction in sympathetic activity aids in regressing LV mass. Less likelihood of peripheral vasoconstriction with use of selective beta-1 blockers also adds to better antihypertensive effect. Overexpression of beta-1 receptor in LVH confirms that selective beta-1 blockers are effective agents for LVH in HT. Also, vasodilatory BB nebivolol has shown antiproliferative effects which is probably secondary to nitric oxide (NO) release and vasodilation at cardiac tissue level.[11]

In uncomplicated HT, nebivolol increased myocardial early diastolic velocity (Em), reduced the ratio between transmitral E velocity and myocardial early diastolic velocity (E/Em ratio), and increased coronary flow reserve (CFR).[12] These changes are seemed to be related to changes in microvascular circulation and release of NO in cardiac tissue. The improvement in CFR observed with nebivolol is especially important because LVH in HT is associated reduced CFR because of endothelial dysfunction, narrowing of the small arteries, rarefaction of microcirculation especially on the subendocardial level and the perivascular fibrosis.[13] Subendothelial function can be assessed by measuring longitudinal shortening. HT with LVH is associated with lower longitudinal velocities and systolic functional reserve at rest as well as at peak stress.[13] Compared to metoprolol, nebivolol has shown to significantly increase the ejection time, the displacement, the flow propagation velocity, and the early diastolic longitudinal velocities without any changes in ejection fraction or the contractile longitudinal reserve.[14] Therefore, it is important to detect reduced functional reserve in HT to predict its progression to HF wherein BB can be of use.

Carvedilol, another selective beta-1 blocker, has shown to lower the LV mass. In comparison to telmisartan (21.97 ± 5.84 g/m^2), the reduction in left ventricular mass index (LVMI) in three-dimensional ECHO was 12.31 ± 3.14 g/m^2 with carvedilol and regression of LVH was seen in 50% and 31% patients from two groups. Benefits in LVH regression was due to reduction in cardiac pressure load. The difference with telmisartan could has arisen because of its greater efficacy in night-time BP reduction and BP reduction during the last 6 hours.[15] However, compared to metoprolol, carvedilol showed higher peak diastolic velocity at rest in anterior descending coronary artery and peak hyperemic diastolic blood flow velocity after dipyridamole treatment. Change in CFR was significantly better with carvedilol than metoprolol suggesting improvements in microvascular function. Interestingly, LVMI was significantly reduced by carvedilol only but not by metoprolol. The differences observed can be attributed to additional alpha-receptor blocking and antioxidant properties of carvedilol.[9]

Beta-blocker Effect on Diastolic Function in Hypertension

In LVH, LV compliance and diastolic filling are known to become abnormal even before the impairment of systolic function. In such a case, slowing of ventricular filling is probably the early marker of heart disease. Diastolic dysfunction is known to be associated directly with the degree of interstitial fibrosis and wall thickness. However,

TABLE 2: Algorithm for diagnosis of LV diastolic dysfunction.

Ratio	Value	Additional evaluation	LAP
E/é	Septal, average or lateral: ≤8		Normal
E/é	Septal, average or lateral: 9–14	LA volume: ≥34 mL/m^2	Increased
		AR-A: >30 ms	
		Valsalva ΔE/A: ≥0.5	
		PAPs: ≥30 mm Hg	
E/é	Septal ≥15		Increased
	Lateral ≥12		
	Average ≥13		

(AR: atrial retrograde velocity; E/A ratio: transmitral ratio between early (E) and late (atrial-A) ventricular filling velocity; E/é: transmitral early diastolic velocity to pulsed tissue Doppler-derived annular early diastolic velocity ratio; LAP: left atrial pressure; PAPs: pulmonary arterial systolic pressure)

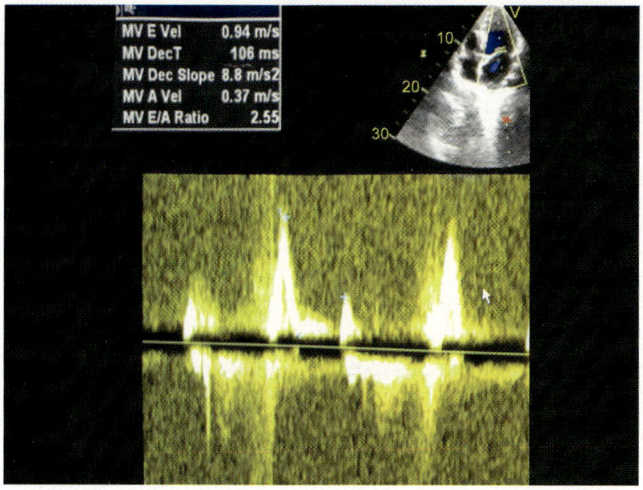

Fig. 3: Diastolic dysfunction judged by mitral Doppler flow, with an E/A ratio of 2.55.

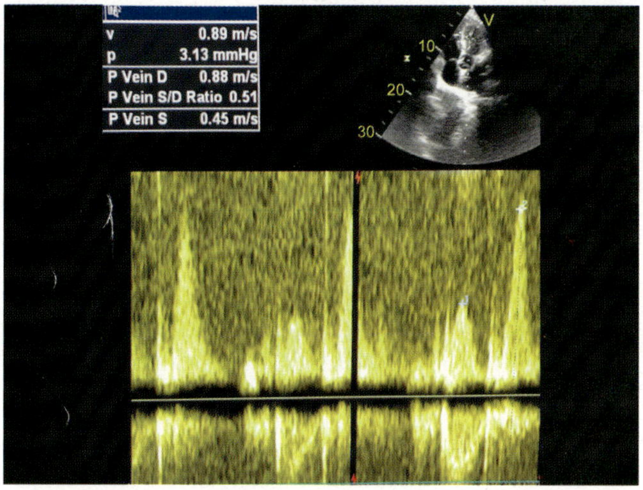

Fig. 4: Diastolic dysfunction judged by pulmonary vein Doppler flow, with an S/D ratio (ratio of peak systolic forward flow velocity/peak diastolic forward flow velocity) of 0.51.

many factors contribute to this which include LV geometry, wall thickness, systolic function, heart rate, age, systolic BP, LV filling pressure, chamber and myocardial stiffness, and myocardial ischemia.[10]

Diagnosis of LV Diastolic Dysfunction

A simple algorithm to diagnose LV diastolic dysfunction[9] in patients with normal ejection fraction is shown in Table 2.

A normal transmitral early diastolic velocity to pulsed tissue Doppler-derived annular early diastolic velocity ratio (E/e′) ratio (<8) indicates normal invasively estimated LA pressure (LAP); an abnormally increased E/e′ ratio corresponds to pathologically elevated LAP. For intermediate range of E/e′ ratio additional findings are needed: increased LA volume, or pulmonary venous flow derived atrial reverse (AR) velocity-transmitral atrial (A) velocity more than 30 ms, or reduction (Δ) of transmitral ratio between early and late ventricular filling velocity (E/A ratio) more than 0.5, or pulmonary arterial systolic pressure (PAPs) more than 35 mm Hg.

Figure 3 shows a Doppler pattern in a patient with HT showing diastolic dysfunction as seen by mitral E/A ratio of 2.55, while Figure 4 shows diastolic dysfunction as judged by pulmonary vein systolic diastolic ratio of 0.51.

Effect of Beta-blocker Treatment

In patients with HT, bisoprolol has shown to improve peak E velocity and the E/A ratio, and reduce peak A velocity, isovolumetric relaxation time (IVRT), and E deceleration time. Though the improvement in LV diastolic parameters was noted, none of the patients had improvement in LV relaxation.[16,17] Bisoprolol also significantly reduced LV mass and LVMI in HT.[17] The improvement in LV dysfunction with BB is achieved via reduction in heart rate and improving LV filling time.

Nebivolol but not metoprolol on the other hand has shown to improve parameters of early diastolic relaxation namely longitudinal early diastolic velocity and flow propagation velocity measured on M-mode ECHO.[14]

In mild to moderate HT, Jurkevicius et al. observed increase in the transmitral early to late diastolic velocity ratio and systolic amplitude of mitral annulus motion with BB treatment. These changes correlated with changes in heart rate. Achievement of heart rate of 57–68 beats per minute was associated with positive improvements in left ventricular diastolic and long axis functions.[18] The role of elevated heart rate in HT has now been established; the heart rate reducing effects of BB may further contribute to their role in the overall management of HT.

PROGNOSTIC ROLE OF ECHO CHANGES WITH BETA-BLOCKERS

Diastolic dysfunction is common in HT and is predictive of development of HF.[19] Ethnicity has important role in development of changes in LV structure and function. African-Caribbean ethnicity has lower probability of diastolic dysfunction but was independently associated with increased LVMI. Despite the prominent hypertrophy in African-Caribbean race, South-Asian ethnicity was associated with increased mortality and worse parameters of diastolic function.[20] African American population, only calcium channel blockers protected against progression of diastolic dysfunction.[21] In asymptomatic HHD, global longitudinal strain (GLS) measured on ECHO predicted major adverse CV events (MACE). GLS in the patients with BB were significantly lower than those without BB. Among various factors, BB use was associated with increased MACE in univariate analysis, but no effect seen in multivariate analysis.[22] This points that the benefit added by antihypertensive treatment in MACE outcome in HHD may be small. However, compared to nonuser of BB, long-term use of BB is associated with more prominent improvement in diastolic function and LVH as well as in reduced risk of new onset of symptomatic HF with preserved ejection fraction, and the elevation of LVMI.[23] In a meta-analysis 12 randomized trials observed 12.6/6.1 mm Hg reductions in blood pressure. The benefit translated to 23% significant reduction in HF risk. The benefit in HF reduction with BB was comparable to other agents as were the outcomes of all-cause mortality, CV mortality, and myocardial infarction.[24]

CONCLUSION

Beta-blockers, though now not occupying the position of first-line drugs in the management of HT, do remain an important part in the overall management of HT; especially when associated with CAD or HF. Their roles in reducing sympathetic effects on the heart, reduction of heart rate, and improvement of both systolic and diastolic HF have been well-established. ECHO is a simple easily available mode of evaluating systolic and diastolic function of the heart. It is effective in picking up early changes of LVH and diastolic dysfunction and is considered almost mandatory in the investigation of HT. Using the early changes detected on ECHO in patients with HT, will allow earlier intervention both with lifestyle modifications and drug therapy. ECHO also helps to easily follow the response to these measures and to adjust the therapy. ECHO will remain an important diagnostic tool in the investigation and management of patients with HT in spite of advances in imaging technology, due to its noninvasive nature, low cost, easy availability, and the important information it provides on systolic and diastolic heart function.

REFERENCES

1. Drazner MH. The progression of hypertensive heart disease. Circulation. 2011;123(3):327-34.
2. Gonzalez-Maqueda I, Alegria-Ezquerra E, Gonzalez-Juanatey JR. (2009). Hypertensive heart disease: a new clinical classification (VIA). [online] Available from https://www.escardio.org/Journals/E-Journal-of-Cardiology-Practice/Volume-7/Hypertensive-heart-disease-a-new-clinical-classification-VIA.
3. Mancia G, Fagard R, Narkiewicz K, et al. 2013 ESH/ESC guidelines for the management of arterial hypertension: the Task Force for the Management of Arterial Hypertension of the European Society of Hypertension (ESH) and of the European Society of Cardiology (ESC). J Hypertension. 2013;31(7):1281-357.
4. Lee JH, Park JH. Role of echocardiography in clinical hypertension. Clin Hypertens. 2015;21:9.
5. Mancia G, Grassi G. The autonomic nervous system and hypertension. Circ Res. 2014;114(11):1804-14.
6. Grassi G. Counteracting the sympathetic nervous system in essential hypertension. Curr Opin Nephrol Hyperten. 2004;13(5):513-9.
7. Frishman WH. A historical perspective on the development of β-adrenergic blockers. J Clin Hyperten. 2007;9(suppl 3):19-27.
8. Marwick TH, Gillebert TC, Aurigemma G, et al. Recommendations on the use of echocardiography in adult hypertension : a report from the European Association of Cardiovascular Imaging (EACVI) and the American Society of Echocardiography (ASE). J Am Soc Echocardiogr. 2015;28(7):727-54.
9. Trimarco B, De Luca N, Cuocolo A, et al. Beta blockers and left ventricular hypertrophy in hypertension. Am Heart J. 1987;114(4 Pt 2):975-83.
10. Xing F, Chen J, Zhao B, et al. Real role of beta-blockers in regression of left ventricular mass in hypertension patients: Bayesian network meta-analysis. Medicine (Baltimore). 2017;96(10):e6290.
11. Galderisi M, D'Errico A, Sidiropulos M, et al. Nebivolol induces parallel improvement of left ventricular filling pressure and coronary flow reserve in uncomplicated arterial hypertension. J Hypertens. 2009;27(10):2108-15.
12. Patrascu N. Assessment of systolic and diastolic cardiac function beyond traditional markers in hypertensive patients. Role of cardiac reserve. Mædica. 2013;8(2):214-9.
13. Vinereanu D, Gherghinescu C, Ciobanu AO, et al. Reversal of subclinical left ventricular dysfunction by antihypertensive treatment: a prospective trial of nebivolol against metoprolol. J Hypertens. 2011;29(4):809-17.
14. Galzerano D, Tammaro P, Del Viscovo L, et al. Three-dimensional echocardiographic and magnetic resonance assessment of the effect of telmisartan compared with carvedilol on left ventricular mass: A multicenter, randomized, longitudinal study. Am J Hypertens. 2005;18(12 Pt 1):1563-9.
15. Xiaozhen H, Yun Z, Mei Z, et al. Effect of carvedilol on coronary flow reserve in patients with hypertensive left-ventricular hypertrophy. Blood Press. 2010;19(1):40-7.
16. Ilgenli F, Kilicaslan F, Kirilmaz A, et al. Bisoprolol improves echocardiographic parameters of left ventricular diastolic function in patients with systemic hypertension. Cardiology. 2006;106(3):127-31.
17. de Teresa E, González M, Camacho-Vázquez C, et al. Effects of bisoprolol on left ventricular hypertrophy in essential hypertension. Cardiovasc Drugs Ther. 1994;8(6):837-43.
18. Jurkevicius R, Sakalyte G, Kavoliuniene A. Effects of beta blockers on left ventricular diastolic function. Acta Cardiol. 2007;62(3):265-70.

19. Kane GC, Karon BL, Mahoney DW, et al. Progression of left ventricular diastolic dysfunction and risk of heart failure. JAMA. 2011;306(8):856-63.
20. Shantsila A, Shantsila E, Gill PS, et al. Predictors of diastolic dysfunction in ethnic groups: observations from the Hypertensive Cohort of The Ethnic-Echocardiographic Heart of England Screening Study (E-ECHOES). J Hum Hypertens. 2018;32(7):477-86.
21. Prendergast HM, Dudley S, Brown M, et al. Antihypertensive medications and diastolic dysfunction progression in an African American population. High Blood Press Cardiovasc Prev. 2014;21(4):269-74.
22. Saito M, Khan F, Stoklosa T, et al. Prognostic implications of LV strain risk score in asymptomatic patients with hypertensive heart disease. JACC Cardiovasc Imaging. 2016;9(8):911-21.
23. Gu J, Fan Y, Bian L, et al. Long-term prescription of beta-blocker delays the progression of heart failure with preserved ejection fraction in patients with hypertension: A retrospective observational cohort study. Eur J Prev Cardiol. 2016;23(13):1421-8.
24. Bangalore S, Wild D, Parkar S, et al. Beta-blockers for primary prevention of heart failure in patients with hypertension. Insights from a meta-analysis. J Am Coll Cardiol. 2008;52(13):1062-72.

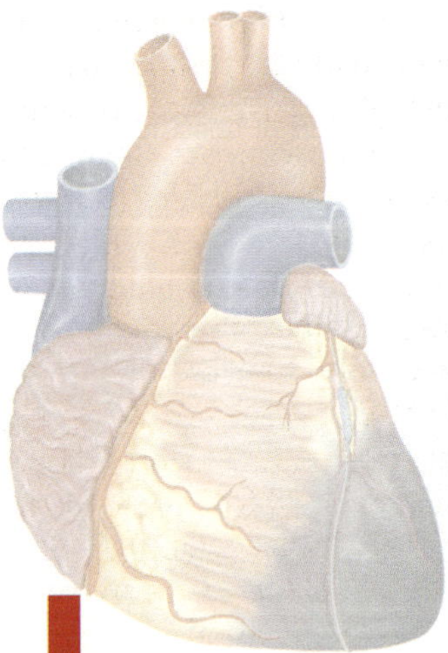

11

CHAPTER

Statin Effect and Outcome Evaluation by Echocardiography

Rahul Mehrotra, Bharat Bansal

INTRODUCTION

Statins [3-hydroxy-3-methylglutaryl coenzyme A (HMG-CoA) reductase inhibitors], have often been hailed as the wonder drugs of our times. Statins work by blocking the enzyme HMG-CoA reductase, the rate-limiting step in cholesterol synthesis. Statins reduce low-density lipoprotein (LDL) cholesterol, total cholesterol, and triglycerides and slightly increase high-density lipoprotein (HDL) cholesterol. Statins may also have anti-inflammatory and other pleiotropic effects. Statins have been shown to lower C-reactive protein levels, but do not affect fibrinogen or several other markers of inflammation. They are the most effective class of drugs for lowering serum LDL concentrations as shown by several large scale trials involving thousands of patients. Based on the evidence accumulated, they are recommended as the first-line agents for patients who require drug therapy to reduce serum LDL. They have been shown to improve survival in patients of established cardiovascular disease (CVD), prevent the progression of atherosclerosis and are also beneficial for primary prevention of CVD in appropriate patient populations. Their efficacy is further supplemented by lack of any serious side effects, as shown by these trials. Although the majority of studies with statins have looked at the measurement of blood values of cholesterol and its relationship with outcomes, few studies have been done to look at the inflammatory markers and other pleiotropic effects. Imaging studies to look at the morphologic effects on the atherosclerotic plaque have also been done with statins. One of the earliest studies done with magnetic resonance imaging (MRI) demonstrated reduction in atherosclerotic plaque volume in thoracic aorta after 6 months' use of simvastatin.[1] This stimulated lot of interest since this indicated reversal of the process of atherosclerosis. Subsequent studies have been done with different statins, doses, and with different imaging modalities like optical coherence tomography (OCT), intravascular ultrasound (IVUS), and in the carotid arteries, by measurement of the carotid intima-media thickness (CIMT). In this chapter we discuss the role of echocardiography based imaging modalities in evaluating the effect and outcomes of statin use.

ECHOCARDIOGRAPHY MODALITIES AND STATIN TRIALS

As discussed above, the majority of trials with statins employed lipid parameters and inflammatory markers for assessing the effects of statins. However, a few of the studies also looked at the plaque morphology and volume in the coronary arteries by IVUS, or in the carotid arteries, by measurement of CIMT. It was widely believed that the effect of statin on atherosclerotic plaque burden could better explain the effect of statins. At one point it was even considered that plaque regression should be considered as the target for statin therapy. The majority of studies employed the use of IVUS and CIMT but a few case reports and small scale studies were also done to indirectly assess the effect of statins on myocardial function by two-dimensional echocardiography, tissue Doppler imaging, and strain imaging. IVUS is an echocardiography based modality in which a miniature transducer is mounted on the tip of a special coronary catheter, attached to the ultrasound equipment. The catheter is advanced through the coronary arteries and gives an image through the vessel, lumen, endothelium, and the vessel wall. The presence of a plaque and its morphology is also delineated clearly by IVUS.[2] It is thus a useful way of looking at the plaques other than by coronary angiography, which only displays the vessel lumen.[3] In the last two decades, a lot of new information related to plaque morphology, vessel remodeling, and vulnerable plaques came out with the use of IVUS.[4] Research studies were also done to look at the changes in plaque morphology after stenting and with the use of drugs, especially statins (discussed below). CIMT is also an ultrasound based technique in which the thickness of the intima and media of the carotid arterial tree is measured in a standardized manner and the presence of visible plaques is characterized. Although most of the atherosclerotic changes occur in the intima, combined thickness of intima and media is measured because of the inability to accurately measure the thickness of intima alone. The ultrasound based measurement of CIMT has been validated in in vitro histologic studies.[5,6] A high frequency linear transducer is used for this purpose and this simple noninvasive tool provides these very useful measurements, which have been extensively studied in different ethnic groups in both genders.[7,8] CIMT is being considered as a marker of risk of CVD along with other parameters and several studies have been done with the use of CIMT for defining its role in evaluating a patient at risk of CAD. The other use of CIMT has been in characterization of plaque morphology (size, volume) and to determine its progression or regression with therapy. We discuss below few major studies where statin effect was studied with the use of these echocardiographic modalities. The ASTEROID (A Study to Evaluate the Effect of Rosuvastatin on IVUS-Derived Coronary Atheroma Burden) study was a prospective multicenter blinded trial which evaluated the effect of very high intensity statin therapy (rosuvastatin 40 mg daily) on IVUS determined coronary atheroma plaque burden after 24 months of use.[8] The patients enrolled were those requiring coronary angiography for a valid clinical indication. At the end of the study, as expected, LDL cholesterol reduced from a mean of 130.4 mg/dL to 60.8 mg/dL (a mean reduction of 53.2%) while mean HDL cholesterol increased from 43.1 mg/dL to 49.0 mg/dL (an increase of 14.7%). The primary efficacy parameters however were the change in percentage atheroma volume (PAV) and the change in nominal atheroma volume in the 10 mm subsegment with the greatest disease severity.[9] The mean change in PAV for the entire vessel was –0.98% [97.5% confidence interval (CI), –1.21% to –0.53%] with a p value of 0.001 vs. baseline. The mean change in atheroma volume in the most diseased 10 mm subsegment was –6.1 mm^3, with a p value of 0.001 vs. baseline. A secondary endpoint change in total atheroma volume showed significant reduction (6.8% median reduction; with a mean reduction of –14.7 mm^3, 95% CI, –15.1 mm^3 to –10.5 mm^3 and a p value of 0.001). In spite of the very high intensity dose of statin used in this trial, the adverse events were infrequent and similar to other statin trials. This study comprehensively demonstrated that the use of a very high intensity statin therapy was safe and resulted in significant reduction in LDL, elevation of HDL cholesterol, and significant reduction of atherosclerotic plaque burden as defined by the prespecified endpoints on IVUS. METEOR trial (Measuring Effects on Intima-Media Thickness: an Evaluation of Rosuvastatin) was also a similar study which measured the effect of 40 mg rosuvastatin on subclinical atherosclerosis as determined by CIMT.[10] It was a double-blind, randomized, placebo controlled study in asymptomatic adults with either a 10-year Framingham risk score of less than 10% or age as the only risk factor coronary heart disease risk factor (mean, 57 tears). In addition, the subjects needed to have modest thickening of CIMT (1.2–3.5 mm) and elevated LDL cholesterol. The outcomes studied were rate of change in maximum CIMT for 12 carotid sites; changes in maximum CIMT of the common carotid artery, carotid bulb, and internal carotid artery sites and in mean CIMT of the common carotid artery sites in the rosuvastatin arm. Rosuvastatin use in 40 mg daily dose in this study resulted in statistically significant reduction in rate of progression of maximum CIMT compared to placebo, over a period of 2 years. As expected based on other trials,[11,12] the mean LDL cholesterol level of 155 mg/dL at baseline reduced to 78 mg/dL (a mean reduction of 49%; p 0.001 vs. placebo group). The change in maximum CIMT for the 12 carotid sites was –0.0014 (95% CI, –0.0041 to 0.0014) mm/y for the rosuvastatin group vs. 0.0131 (95% CI, 0.0087–0.0174) mm/y for the placebo group (p 0.001). The change in maximum CIMT for the rosuvastatin group was –0.0038 (95% CI, –0.0064 to –0.0013) mm/y for the common carotid artery sites, –0.0040 mm/y for the carotid bulb sites (p 0.001), and 0.0039 mm/y for the internal carotid artery sites (p = 0.02). Again, there were infrequent serious adverse cardiovascular events associated. Myalgia was the most common adverse event, occurring in 12.7% and 12.1% of the rosuvastatin and placebo groups, respectively. Although it did not demonstrate plaque regression, this trial demonstrated the efficacy of rosuvastatin in very high dose, for slowing the progression of atherosclerotic plaque burden as determined by CIMT, in asymptomatic, low-risk population without any significant adverse effects. Statins result in improved cardiovascular outcomes in varied population groups is well established now. They do so primarily by their potent LDL cholesterol lowering effects. But this fails to explain their beneficial effects in certain other disease states also.[13,14] These effects of statins are often explained by the certain pleiotropic effects of statins.[15] Besides, statins are known to have myopathy, myalgia, and even rhabdomyolysis as a side effect.[16] Small scale studies have been done to evaluate whether statins have any effect on the left ventricular systolic and diastolic function. In one such study, the authors assessed global and regional systolic function and diastolic function of left ventricle using tissue Doppler and strain imaging.[17] 12 patients who were on statin therapy but without CVD were compared to 16 controls (matched for age, gender, and cholesterol profile) with echocardiography. The authors observed that there was significantly better function noted strain imaging in the control group as compared to the statin therapy group (average global longitudinal strain –19% ± 2.07% vs. –15.91% ± 2.81% p = 0.004). The authors thus concluded that statin therapy was associated with reduced myocardial systolic function as assessed by strain imaging. Although this was a very small scale study, this brought out an interesting facet of studying statin effect by echocardiography. More studies in larger number of subjects on statins are needed to further analyze whether statins have any effect on myocardial function.

CONCLUSION

Although there is no doubt about the efficacy of statin therapy in lowering cardiovascular risk in primary as secondary prevention of CVD, there has been considerable debate about the effect of statins on plaque regression. Imaging modalities, especially echocardiography based, have played a major role in the studies carried out to assess the effect of statins on plaque morphology, volume, and changes with time during statin therapy. The landmark trials done with echocardiography-based imaging modalities like IVUS and CIMT demonstrated either reduced rate of progression, regression or alteration of plaque morphology with the use of statin therapy. In 2015, a systematic review and meta-analysis of virtual histology IVUS studies involving over 800 patients was published.[18] The authors, after extensive analysis concluded that statin therapy had a significant effect on reducing plaque volume and external elastic membrane volume while it did not have any effect on lumen volume, fibro-fatty volume, and necrotic tissue volumes. Studies done with CIMT also have demonstrated similar effect of statin therapy on plaque progression.

Echocardiography-based modalities thus offer a unique, extremely safe, and validated method to assess the effect of statin therapy on plaque composition and volume.

REFERENCES

1. Lima JA, Desai MY, Steen H, et al. Statin-induced cholesterol lowering and plaque regression after 6 months of magnetic resonance imaging-monitored therapy. Circulation. 2004;110(16):2336-41.
2. Sgura FA, Di Mario C. New methods of coronary imaging II. Intracoronary ultrasonography in clinical practice. Ital Heart J Suppl. 2001;2(6):579-92.
3. Görge G, Ge J, von Birgelen C, et al. Intravascular ultrasound—the new gold standard?. Z Kardiol. 1998;87(8):575-85.
4. Glagov S, Weisenberg E, Zarins CK, et al. Compensatory enlargement of human atherosclerotic coronary arteries. N Engl J Med. 1987;316(22):1371-5.
5. Persson J, Formgren J, Israelsson B, et al. Ultrasound-determined intima-media thickness and atherosclerosis. Direct and indirect validation. Arterioscler Thromb. 1994;14(2):261-4.
6. Wong M, Edelstein J, Wollman J, et al. Ultrasonic-pathological comparison of the human arterial wall. Verification of intima-media thickness. Arterioscler Thromb. 1993;13(4):482-6.
7. Kasliwal RR, Bansal M, Desai N, et al. A Study to derive distribution of carotid intima media thickness and to determine its correlation with cardiovascular risk factors in asymptomatic nationwide Indian population (SCORE-India). Indian Heart J. 2016;68(6):821-7.
8. Nissen SE, Nicholls SJ, Sipahi I, et al. Effect of very high-intensity statin therapy on regression of coronary atherosclerosis: the ASTEROID trial. JAMA. 2006;295(13):1556-65.
9. Schoenhagen P, Sapp SK, Tuzcu EM, et al. Variability of area measurements obtained with different intravascular ultrasound catheter systems: impact on clinical trials and a method for accurate calibration. J Am Soc Echocardiogr. 2003;16(3):277-84.
10. Crouse JR, Raichlen JS, Riley WA, et al. Effect of rosuvastatin on progression of carotid intima-media thickness in low-risk individuals with subclinical atherosclerosis: the METEOR trial. JAMA. 2007;297(12):1344-53.
11. Jones PH, Davidson MH, Stein EA, et al. Comparison of the efficacy and safety of rosuvastatin versus atorvastatin, simvastatin, and pravastatin across doses (STELLAR trial). Am J Cardiol. 2003;92(2):152-60.
12. Schuster H, Barter PJ, Stender S, et al. Effects of switching statins on achievement of lipid goals: measuring effective reductions in cholesterol using rosuvastatin therapy (MERCURY I) study. Am Heart J. 2004;147(4):705-13.
13. Rosenhek R, Rader F, Loho N, et al. Statins but not angiotensin-converting enzyme inhibitors delay progression of aortic stenosis. Circulation. 2004;110(10):1291-5.
14. Young-Xu Y, Jabbour S, Goldberg R, et al. Usefulness of statin drugs in protecting against atrial fibrillation in patients with coronary artery disease. Am J Cardiol. 2003;92(12):1379-83.
15. Chia S, Raffel OC, Takano M, et al. Association of statin therapy with reduced coronary plaque rupture: an optical coherence tomography study. Coron Artery Dis. 2008;19(4):237-42.
16. Staffa JA, Chang J, Green L. Cerivastatin and reports of fatal rhabdomyolysis. N Engl J Med. 2002;346(7):539-40.
17. Rubinstein J, Aloka F, Abela GS, et al. Statin therapy decreases myocardial function as evaluated via strain imaging. Clin Cardiol. 2009;32(12):684-9.
18. Banach M, Serban C, Sahebkar A, et al. Impact of statin therapy on coronary plaque composition: a systematic review and meta-analysis of virtual histology intravascular ultrasound studies. BMC Med. 2015;13:229.

12

CHAPTER

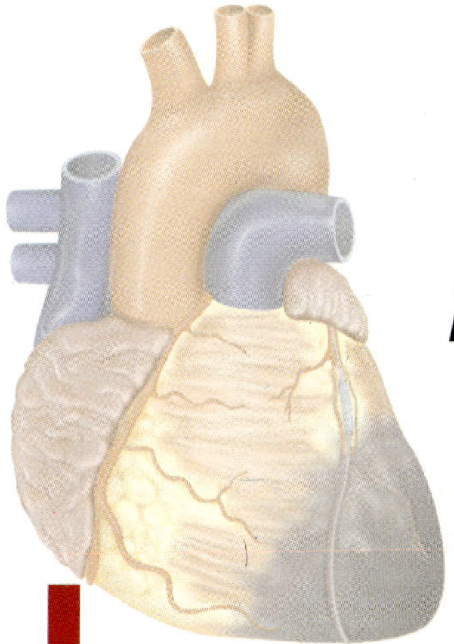

ARNIs Effect and Outcome Evaluation by Echocardiography in Hypertension

Sandeep Bansal, Preeti Gupta, Ankit Singh

INTRODUCTION

Hypertension is an important risk factor and perhaps the most common cause of cardiovascular morbidity and mortality accounting for around 50% cardiovascular deaths.[1] Uncontrolled hypertension can lead to myocardial infarction (MI), stroke, hypertensive heart disease, heart failure, and end-organ damage. Every 10 mm Hg decrease in systolic blood pressure (BP) reduced the risk of major adverse cardiovascular events (MACE) by 20%, of coronary artery disease (CAD) by 17%, of stroke by 27%, of heart failure by 28%, and overall mortality by 13% in a large meta-analysis.[2] Despite the availability of multitude of antihypertensive drugs a vast majority of more than 1 billion hypertensive patients worldwide continue to have uncontrolled BP.[3] BP is regulated by many neurohumoral systems like sympathetic nervous system (SNS), renin-angiotensin-aldosterone system (RAAS), endothelin system, and natriuretic peptide system. The RAAS, the SNS, and the endothelin system play a role in the pathophysiology of cardiovascular diseases.[4] Based on the recognition of its pathophysiological key role across the cardiovascular continuum, the RAAS is one of the most important drug targets for cardiovascular medical therapy.[5] Recently investigators have studied the role of combined inhibition of RAAS and neprilysin (NEP) in management of hypertension.

ROLE OF NATRIURETIC PEPTIDE SYSTEM IN PATHOPHYSIOLOGY OF SYSTEMIC HYPERTENSION

Natriuretic peptides (NPs) are a group of hormones that have a role in maintenance of sodium and fluid balance in body. Additionally, they act to inhibit RAAS, reduce sympathetic drive, and have both antihypertensive and antiproliferative effects.[6,7] NPs also have antifibrosis and antihypertrophic effects and thus prevent cardiac remodeling. Three types of NPs have been identified: atrial NPs (ANP) and B-type NPs (BNP) produced primarily within the heart and C-type NPs (CNP) expressed in the central nervous system, reproductive tract, bone, and endothelium of blood vessels.[8] NEP is a zinc-dependent metallopeptidase that catalyzes the degradation of various peptides including ANP, BNP, and bradykinin, endothelin as well as angiotensin II.[9]

ROLE OF ANGIOTENSIN RECEPTOR-NEPRILYSIN INHIBITOR (ARNI) IN MANAGEMENT OF HYPERTENSION

Since NEP inhibition increases the levels of both NPs as well as vasopressor peptides like endothelin and angiotensin II, therefore its inhibition alone does not have significant antihypertensive effect and has to be combined with

Flowchart 1: Mechanism of action of ARNI.

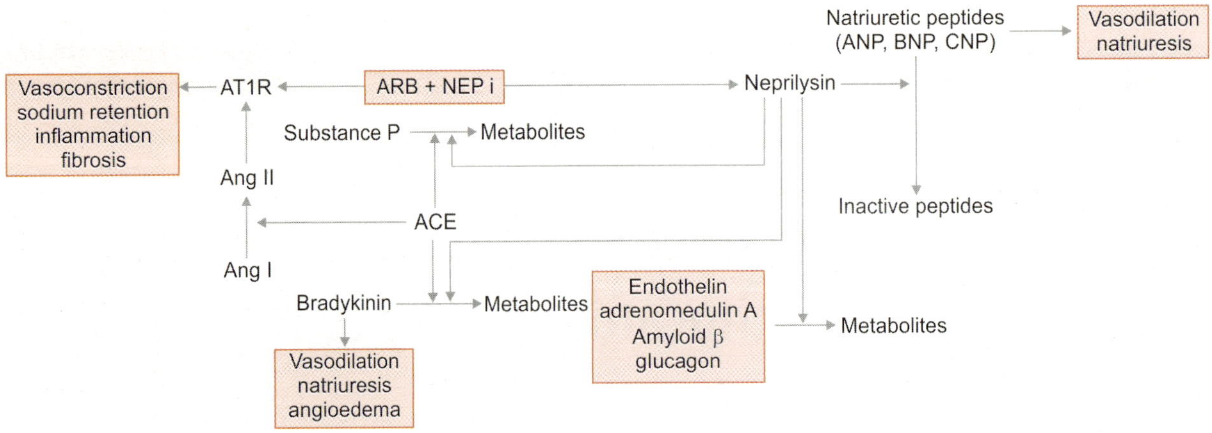

either endothelin or RAAS inhibitors. Drug research was initially focused on combined inhibition of NEP as well as angiotensin-converting enzyme (ACE). Omapatrilat was the first dual vasopeptidase (NEP/ACE) inhibitor which showed greater efficacy in lowering BP than ACE inhibitors and calcium channel blockers[10,11] but induced a three- to four-fold higher incidence of angioedema than enalapril.[12] This high incidence of angioedema was due to excess accumulation of bradykinin due to synergistic inhibition of their degradation by dual NEP/ACE inhibition (Flowchart 1).

To avoid higher rates of angioedema with dual NEP/ACE inhibition, NEP inhibition with angiotensin II type I receptor blockade (ARNI) was studied. LCZ696 is the first-in-class of dual AT1R and neprilysin inhibitors (ARNIs) comprising molecular moieties of valsartan and NEP inhibitor prodrug sacubitril (AHU377) in 1:1 ratio. After ingestion, the drug dissociates into valsartan and sacubitril which is further converted by esterases to active form LBQ657. Both the components of LCZ696 have similar pharmacokinetic properties like elimination half-life (t1/2) for LBQ657 is 9.9–11.1 hours and for valsartan it is 8.9–16.6 hours and time to peak concentration for LBQ657 is 1.9–3.5 hours and for valsartan it is 1.7–2.2 hours.[13] The pharmacodynamics of these two agents is also similar, exemplified by the maximal concentrations of cyclic guanosine monophosphate (cGMP) and RAAS biomarkers being reached in parallel at 4 hours.[14] These properties of LCZ696 allow complementary action of both components and better BP lowering effect.

Clinical Evidence in Favor of ARNI

Earliest studies on ARNI evaluated its role in heart failure. In PARADIGM-HF trial (Prospective Comparison of ARNI with ACEI to Determine Impact on Global Mortality and Morbidity in Heart Failure) apart from a benefit in mortality and hospitalization patients on LCZ697 also had a mean systolic BP which was 3.2 ± 0.4 mm Hg lower than those on enalapril.[15] Joseph L Izzo et al. compared the efficacy of LCZ696 to valsartan, varying doses of valsartan plus NEP and placebo in patients with systolic hypertension. They found that in patients with systolic hypertension LCZ696 is more effective than valsartan for BP reduction and that it caused a greater systolic BP reduction as compared to valsartan in patients more than or equal to 65 years than in those less than 65 years.[16] Ruillope et al. compared varying doses of LCZ696, varying doses of valsartan, 200 mg AHU377 and placebo in double-blinded, randomized 8 weeks study. The average reduction in mean sitting diastolic BP across the doses of LCZ696 versus the appropriate comparator dose of valsartan showed significantly greater reductions with LCZ696.[17]

Nondippers are at high risk of cardiovascular events as compared to dippers.[23] Kario et al. investigated the efficacy of LCZ696 in 389 Asian hypertensive patients classified as dippers and nondippers in a double-blind placebo-controlled study. After 8 weeks of treatment with varying doses of LCZ696 or placebo they found that all doses of LCZ696 provided significantly greater reductions in mean 24 hours and nighttime mean systolic BP and mean diastolic BP versus placebo, with a trend for the greatest benefit observed with higher doses of LCZ696 and in nondippers. These results suggest that ARNI LCZ696 effectively reduces BP throughout the 24 hours period and restores the normal nighttime BP fall in nondippers.[18] Hypertension can be both a cause or a consequence of chronic renal dysfunction and such patients have a poor cardiovascular as well as overall outcome. Ito et al. studied the efficacy and safety of ARNI LCZ696 in Japanese patients with hypertension and renal dysfunction. They found a significant reduction in mean systolic and diastolic BP and urine albumin creatinine ratio after

8 weeks of treatment as compared to baseline.[19] Zhao et al. conducted a meta-analysis comprising of 12 randomized controlled trials to provide further evidence for efficacy and safety of LCZ696 as compared with angiotensin II receptor blockers (ARBs) in patients with hypertension. They found a significant reduction in systolic BP, diastolic BP as well as 24 hours ambulatory BP with LCZ696 as compared to ARBs. In this meta-analysis, LCZ696 was significantly more effective in reducing BP than ARBs, especially in patients who were administered a high dose of LCZ696.[20]

ECHOCARDIOGRAPHY FOR EVALUATION OF HYPERTENSION

Echocardiography is the most commonly used imaging modality used in cardiac patients. In hypertension, it provides information about the pathophysiology and clinical implications since it can detect both hemodynamic and anatomic changes in a quick, reliable, and reproducible manner. It can also detect asymptomatic organ damage, which is a risk factor for cardiovascular events.[21]

Guidelines on Use of Echocardiography in Hypertension

According to 2013 European Society of Hypertension/ European Society of Cardiology (ESH/ESC) Guidelines for the management of arterial hypertension echocardiography is a second-line study.[22] According to Hypertension Canada's 2018 Guidelines[23] routine echocardiographic evaluation of all hypertensive patients is not recommended (Grade D). An echocardiogram for assessment of left ventricular hypertrophy (LVH) is useful in selected cases to help define the future risk of cardiovascular events (Grade C). Echocardiographic assessment of left ventricular (LV) mass and of systolic and diastolic LV function is recommended for hypertensive patients suspected to have LV dysfunction or CAD (Grade D). Patients with hypertension and evidence of heart failure should have an objective assessment of LV ejection fraction (EF) using echocardiogram (Grade D).

Structural Changes due To Hypertension

In long-standing hypertension, myocardial walls become thickened in order to decrease the systolic myocardial wall stress, which leads to increased LV mass and LV hypertrophy. LV hypertrophy prevalence varies with severity of hypertension, ranging from 20% in mild to almost 100% in severe or complicated hypertension.[24] LVH can be easily diagnosed on echocardiography by calculating the LV mass either by two-dimensional (2D) or M mode using Devereux cube formula in a parasternal long axis view.[25]

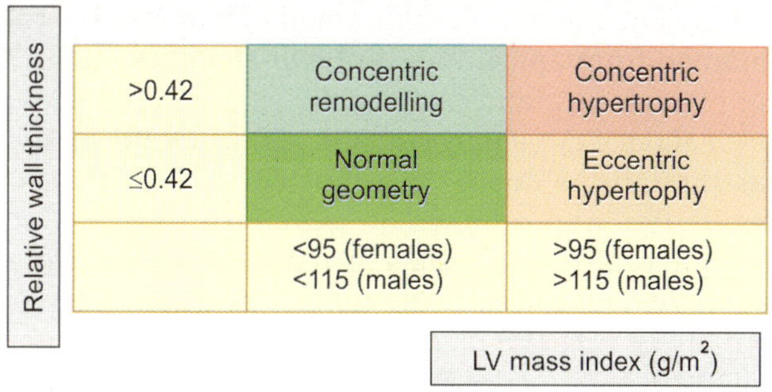

Fig. 1

The limitations are that it is not useful in patients with distorted LV geometry, small errors in measurements get magnified and it cannot detect mild LVH.

Left ventricular mass (g) = $0.8 \times 1.04\ [(LVIDd + PWTd + SWTd)^3 - (LVIDd)^3] + 0.6$

Where, LVIDd: LV internal dimension at end diastole; PWTd: LV posterior wall thickness at end diastole; SWTd: interventricular septal wall thickness at end diastole.

Left ventricular mass can also be measured by 2D echocardiography by area-length method and truncated ellipsoid method.[25] The limitations of this method are related to poor image quality and the temporal resolution of 2D imaging. The limitations of 2D and M mode especially in LV with distorted geometry can be overcome by use of three-dimensional (3D) echocardiography. 3D echocardiography is an attractive modality for the measurement of LV mass and its accuracy is similar to cardiac magnetic resonance (CMR).[26] LV mass is prognostically important and should be reported in hypertensive patients. In the normally shaped LV, either M mode or 2D echocardiography formulas can be used to calculate LV mass.[27] The cutoff points for LV mass indexed to body surface area are 115 g/m^2 for men and 95 g/m^2 for women.[28] Based on the LV mass and relative wall thickness (RWT), patients can be divided into four groups: normal geometry (normal LV mass; RWT ≤0.42), concentric remodeling (normal LV mass; RWT >0.42), concentric hypertrophy (high LV mass; RWT >0.42) and eccentric hypertrophy (high LV mass; RWT ≤0.42) (Fig. 1).[21]

Description of LV geometry using the four categories of normal geometry, concentric remodeling and concentric and eccentric hypertrophy should be a standard component of the echocardiography report.

Left Ventricular Systolic Function in Hypertension

Several echocardiographic indices can be used to estimate the LV systolic function like fractional shortening (FS), stroke volume, EF, and cardiac output. Among them, LVEF calculated by M mode is the most commonly used and has prognostic value in various cardiovascular diseases.

The biplane method of discs (modified Simpson's rule obtained from apical four and two-chamber views) is the most accurate in abnormally shaped ventricles.[29] Calculation of LV volume and EF by 2D echocardiography has limitations due to foreshortening, malrotation, angulation, and reliance on geometric assumptions which may give false results in ventricles with distorted geometry. Transthoracic 3D echocardiography provides a rapid and accurate method for quantifying LV volumes and EF.[30] It has superior reproducibility to 2D, with a closer correlation to CMR-derived volumes.[31] For these reasons, the American Society of Echocardiography (ASE) and European Association of Cardiovascular Imaging (EACVI) recently recommended 3D echocardiography, rather than 2D echocardiography, for the routine assessment of LV volumes and EF.[32] Appropriateness of EF and FS calculation based on measurements performed at endocardial surface has been questioned in patients with LV hypertrophy because LVEF and FS measured at endocardial surface often lead to overestimation of LV systolic performance since they take into account geometric changes that do not accurately reflect the actual contractile function of the myocardium.[33,34] The greatest proportion of ventricular myocardial fibers is located in the myocardial midwall, the region responsible for circumferential LV contraction.[35,36] A variety of parameters have been used to assess LV midwall function and midwall FS (FSmv) has been the most widely used.[27] Study of midwall mechanics has shown it to be superior to indices based on endocardial measurements through better prediction of cardiovascular outcomes and better correlation with patients' clinical status.[37,38]

Tissue Doppler Assessment of Systolic Function

High temporal resolution of tissue Doppler enables accurate determination of myocardial velocity and acceleration even when overall image quality is deficient and endocardial delineation is poor.[39] The main parameter for systolic performance that can be extracted from tissue Doppler evaluation is s'. Among tissue Doppler parameters, s' has shown the best correlation with LVEF and clinical outcomes such as rehospitalization and reduced survival.[40,41] S' measured at septal and lateral mitral annulus in the apical four-chamber view have proved to be useful in detecting LV systolic dysfunction (s' <7 cm/s has 93% sensitivity and 87% specificity in patients with LVEF <45%).[27] Its limitation is that it can also detect passive movement such as swinging or tethering motion along with active myocardial contraction leading to over or underestimation of LV systolic function. Impairment of longitudinal function as assessed by tissue Doppler imaging precedes the depression of LVEF in hypertensive patients, and may be a guide to the presence of fibrosis and early cardiac dysfunction.

LV Systolic Strain

Speckle tracking echocardiography allows to quantitatively measure LV deformation as radial, longitudinal or circumferential strain during systole. Among these, longitudinal strain has been especially focused on because of its clinical significance in patients with heart failure with hypertensive heart disease[42] and its correlation with exercise capacity and prognosis.[43] Longitudinal strain corresponds to the function of the endocardial layer of myocardium, where longitudinal fibers are subjected to the negative impact of early development of fibrosis in hypertensive heart disease.[44] 2D strain has been found to be abnormal in even hypertensive patients with normal EF[45] as well as in prehypertension.[46] Prognostic value of EF in patients with borderline EF is limited and strain imaging can help in risk stratification of such patients and also in detecting the progression of hypertensive heart disease to heart failure.

Diastolic Function in Hypertension

During diastole, LV relaxation and LV filling takes place and a normal diastolic function is required for LV filling without abnormally elevating LV pressure. Several echocardiographic methods can be used to estimate LV diastolic function and filling pressure. The four recommended variables for identifying diastolic dysfunction and their abnormal cutoff values are annular e' velocity: septal e' less than 7 cm/sec, lateral e' less than 10 cm/sec, average E/e' ratio more than 14, LA volume index more than 34 mL/m^2, and peak TR velocity more than 2.8 m/sec. LV diastolic function is normal if three or more of the above variables do not meet the cutoff values and LV diastolic dysfunction is present if three or more of the above parameters meet these cutoff values. The study is inconclusive if two out of four parameters do not meet the cutoff values.[47]

Assessment of Mitral Inflow Pattern

Mitral inflow pattern by pulsed-wave Doppler technique is a useful method of assessment of diastolic function. Mitral inflow measurements should include early peak filling (E velocity), late peak atria filling (A velocity), E/A ratio, deceleration time (DT) of E velocity, and isovolumic relaxation time (IVRT). However, these velocities can be influenced by multiple factors including age, heart rate and rhythm, cardiac output, mitral annular size, and LA function.[48]

Tissue Doppler Assessment of Myocardial Diastolic Function

Measurement of mitral annular diastolic velocity by tissue Doppler imaging reflects the longitudinal relaxation of LV. Early diastolic velocity of mitral annulus (e') has been shown to decline with age and also with pathologic LV hypertrophy.[49] Wang et al.[50] showed that a pulsed-wave e' of 3 cm/s was associated with a 5.3-fold increment of hazard. e' is more useful than transmitral E/A ratio for assessment of LV relaxation as it is a preload independent index. Also since mitral E velocity is influenced by LA pressure and LA relaxation constant, E/e' ratio has been found to better correlate with LV filling pressure and is independent of LA pressure or relaxation properties.[51] E/e' also has prognostic value, with E/e' more than or equal to 15 having been shown to add an independent prognostic value to BNP and EF.[52] All echocardiography reports in patients with hypertension should include specific comments about diastolic function grade, left atrial volume, and about normal versus elevated LV filling pressure based on E/e'.[27]

EVALUATION OF TREATMENT OF HYPERTENSION BY ECHOCARDIOGRAPHY

In hypertension, echocardiography has a role not only in detection of structural and hemodynamic changes, which are markers of increased cardiovascular risk, but it can also be useful in monitoring response of antihypertensive treatment. Some researchers have highlighted the usefulness of echocardiography in monitoring the regression of LV mass and improvement in diastolic filling properties in response to antihypertensive drugs.

Effect on Left Ventricular Hypertrophy

Left ventricular hypertrophy is a marker of end-organ damage and has been demonstrated to be closely associated with adverse events[53] including stroke, renal impairment, LV dysfunction, atrial and ventricular arrhythmias, and sudden cardiac arrhythmia or premature death.[54] LVH has been shown to be reversed by a number of pharmacological or nonpharmacological interventions. In HOPE trial, it was found that ramipril decreases the development and causes regression of electrocardiogram (ECG)-LVH independent of BP reduction, and these changes were associated with reduced risk of death, MI, stroke, and congestive heart failure.[55] In the LIFE trial, investigators found that losartan caused regression of LVH by both ECG and echocardiographic criteria and it was significantly correlated with reduction in the incidence of the primary endpoint cardiovascular death, MI, and stroke. This correlation was independent of treatment method and BP reduction.[56,57] Use of echocardiography to document LVH regression has been difficult to incorporate in routine clinical practice because of the inherent variability in the measurement of LV mass by echocardiography and a significantly larger population has to be examined to overcome the variability of these measurements as compared to CMR. This limitation can be overcome and role of echocardiography may be improved by use of 3D echocardiography, which has been validated against CMR.[58]

Change in Systolic Function

Systolic function as measured by EF is an important prognostic factor in heart failure patients and moderate to severe systolic dysfunction is associated with adverse events. Gonzalez et al. demonstrated that after 9 months treatment with ARNI EF improved by 5–6% and it was associated with improvement in New York Heart Association (NYHA) class.[59] But systolic function is preserved until very late in the course of hypertensive heart disease. Only mild or borderline systolic impairment found with hypertension have not been shown to be consistently associated with adverse events.

Change in Diastolic Function

Diastolic dysfunction is very commonly found in patients with hypertension and is associated with prognosis. Therefore, improvement in diastolic function with treatment will lead to improved outcomes. However, most patients have Grade I diastolic dysfunction and changes in this using mitral E/A are difficult to interpret. After 1 year of treatment with losartan in the LIFE trial, the investigators demonstrated a 3% reduction in left atrial diameter, 9% shortened IVRT, and 10% decrease in atrial filling fraction, and 9% and 7% increase in E/A ratio and mitral valve DT, respectively.[60] Yalsin et al. also demonstrated a decrease in LA volumes and an increase in E velocity and E/A ratio after 6 months treatment with perindopril.[61] Routine reassessment of echocardiograms to examine treatment response in hypertensive subjects is not recommended, due to the limited reproducibility of measurements on an individual patient basis. Follow-up echocardiograms may be of value to assess changes in symptom status.[27]

LIMITATIONS

Although efficacy of ARNI in management of hypertension has been shown in many short-term studies, long-term studies are still lacking. Usefulness of echocardiography for diagnosis and follow-up of hypertensive heart disease and heart failure but its usefulness for follow-up of borderline heart disease is not clear. Many studies have reported the correlation of ACE inhibitors or ARBs treatment with improved echocardiographic indices as well as prognosis in hypertension but such studies with ARNI are still lacking.

CONCLUSION

Angiotensin receptor-neprilysin inhibitor has been found to be useful as an antihypertensive in many studies and it also reverses the deleterious remodeling leading to improved clinical status as well as long-term prognosis. Since long-term safety and efficacy studies are lacking its role in uncomplicated hypertension is not clear. Although echocardiography is not a first-line investigation for hypertension, it is very commonly used because of its easy accessibility, affordability, quick, and reproducible nature. It is also useful as it detects target organ damage and should be used in all patients with suspected hypertensive heart disease. Although not useful for follow-up of uncomplicated hypertension, echocardiography is useful for follow-up of hypertensive heart disease and also for evaluation of treatment effect. Conventional echocardiography has some limitations and newer modalities like 3D echocardiography should be used to overcome these limitations.

REFERENCES

1. Lim SS, Vos T, Flaxman AD, et al. A comparative risk assessment of burden of disease and injury attributable to 67 risk factors and risk factor clusters in 21 regions. 1990-2010: a systematic analysis for the global burden of disease study. 2010. Lancet. 2012;380(9859):2224-60.
2. Ettehad D, Emdin CA, Kiran A, et al. Blood pressure lowering for prevention of cardiovascular disease and death: a systematic review and meta-analysis. Lancet. 2016;387(10022):957-67.
3. Wolf-Maier K, Cooper RS, Kramer H, et al. Hypertension treatment and control in five European countries, Canada, and the United States. Hypertension. 2004;43(1):10-7.
4. Volpe M, Tocci G, Battistoni A, et al. Angiotensin II receptor blocker neprilysin inhibitor (ARNI): new avenues in cardiovascular therapy. High Blood Press Cardiovasc Prev. 2015;22(3):241-6
5. von Lueder TG, Sangaralingham SJ, Wang BH, et al. Renin angiotensin blockade combined with natriuretic peptide system augmentation: novel therapeutic concepts to combat heart failure. Circ Heart Fail. 2013;6(3):594-605.
6. Gardner DG, Chen S, Glenn DJ, et al. Molecular biology of the natriuretic peptide system: implications for physiology and hypertension. Hypertension. 2007;49(3):419-26.
7. Levin ER, Gardner DG, Samson WK. Natriuretic peptides. N Engl J Med. 1998;339(5):321-8.
8. Gardner DG, Chen S, Glenn DG, et al. Molecular biology of the natriuretic peptide system implications for physiology and hypertension. Hypertension. 2007;49(3):419-26.
9. Daniels LB, Maisel AS. Natriuretic peptides. J Am Coll Cardiol. 2007;50(25):2357-68.
10. Mitchell GF, Izzo JL Jr, Lacourciere Y, et al. Omapatrilat reduces pulse pressure and proximal aortic stiffness in patients with systolic hypertension: results of the conduit hemodynamics of omapatrilat international research study. Circulation. 2002;105(25):2955-61.
11. Nawarskas JJ, Anderson JR. Omapatrilat: a unique new agent for the treatment of cardiovascular disease. Heart Dis. 2000;2(3):266-74.
12. Kostis JB, Packer M, Black HR, et al. Omapatrilat and enalapril in patients with hypertension: the Omapatrilat Cardiovascular Treatment vs. Enalapril (OCTAVE) trial. Am J Hypertens. 2004;17(2):103-11.
13. Gu J, Noe A, Chandra P, et al. Pharmacokinetics and pharmacodynamics of LCZ696, a novel dual-acting angiotensin receptor-neprilysin inhibitor (ARNi). J Clin Pharmacol. 2010;50(4):401-14.
14. Bavishi C, Messerli FH, Kadosh B, et al. Role of neprilysin inhibitor combinations in hypertension: insights from hypertension and heart failure trials. Eur Heart J. 2015;36(30):1967-73.
15. McMurray JJ, Packer M, Desai AS, et al. Angiotensin-neprilysin inhibition versus enalapril in heart failure. N Engl J Med. 2014;371(11):993-1004.
16. Izzo JL, Zappe DH, Jia Y, et al. Age and the efficacy of LCZ696, an angiotensin receptor neprilysin inhibitor (ARNI), compared to valsartan in patients with systolic hypertension. J Am Soc Hypertens. 2014;8(4S):e27-34.
17. Ruilope LM, Dukat A, Bohm M, et al. Blood-pressure reduction with LCZ696, a novel dual-acting inhibitor of the angiotensin II receptor and neprilysin: a randomised, double-blind, placebo-controlled, active comparator study. Lancet. 2010;375(9722):1255-66.
18. Kario K, Gotou H, Zhang Y, et al. Blood pressure-lowering efficacy of LCZ696 in non-dipper patients with hypertension. J Am Soc Hypertens. 2014;8(4S):e27-34.
19. Ito S, Satoh M, Tamaki M, et al. Safety and efficacy of LCZ696, a first-in-class angiotensin receptor neprilysin inhibitor, in Japanese patients with hypertension and renal dysfunction. Hypertens Res. 2015;38(4):269-75.
20. Zhao Y, Yu H, Zhao X, et al. The effects of LCZ696 in patients with hypertension compared with angiotensin receptor blockers: a meta-analysis of randomized controlled trials. J Cardiovasc Pharmacol Ther. 2017;22(5):447-57.
21. Lee JH, Park JH. Role of echocardiography in clinical hypertension. Clinical Hypertension. 2015;21:9.
22. Mancia G, Fagard R, Narkiewicz K, et al. 2013 ESH/ESC guidelines for the management of arterial hypertension: the Task Force for the Management of Arterial Hypertension of the European Society of Hypertension (ESH) and of the European Society of Cardiology (ESC). Eur Heart J. 2013;34(28):2159-219.

23. Nerenberg KA, Zarnk KB, Leung AA, et al. Hypertension Canada's 2018 Guidelines for Diagnosis, Risk Assessment, Prevention, and Treatment of Hypertension in Adults and Children. Can J Cardiol. 2018;34(5):506-25.
24. Ruilope LM, Schmieder RE. Left ventricular hypertrophy and clinical outcomes in hypertensive patients. Am J Hypertens. 2008;21(5):500-8.
25. Lang RM, Bierig M, Devereux RB, et al. Recommendations for chamber quantification. Eur J Echocardiogr. 2006;7(2):79-108.
26. Jenkins C, Bricknell K, Hanekom L, et al. Reproducibility and accuracy of echocardiographic measurements of left ventricular parameters using real-time three-dimensional echocardiography. J Am Coll Cardiol. 2004;44(4):878-86.
27. Marwick TH, Gillebert TC, Aurigemma G, et al. Recommendations on the use of echocardiography in adult hypertension: a report from the European Association of Cardiovascular Imaging (EACVI)and the American Society of Echocardiography(ASE). Eur Heart J Cardiovasc Imaging. 2015;16(6):577-605.
28. Enar SC. The role of echocardiography in hypertension. J Clin Exp Cardiolog. 2016,7:12.
29. Schiller NB, Shah PM, Crawford M, et al. Recommendations for quantitation of the left ventricle by two-dimensional echocardiography. American Society of Echocardiography Committee on standards, subcommittee on quantitation of two-dimensional echocardiograms. J Am Soc Echocardiogr. 1989;2(5):358-67.
30. Monaghan MJ. Role of real time 3D echocardiography in evaluating the left ventricle. Heart. 2006;92(1):131-6.
31. Jenkins C, Moir S, Chan J, et al. Left ventricular volume measurement with echocardiography: a comparison of left ventricular opacification, three-dimensional echocardiography, or both with magnetic resonance imaging. Eur Heart J. 2009;30(1):98-106.
32. Lang RM, Badano LP, Tsang W, et al. EAE/ASE recommendations for image acquisition and display using three-dimensional echocardiography. J Am Soc Echocardiogr. 2012;25(1):3-46.
33. de Simone G, Devereux RB, Koren MJ, et al. Midwall left ventricular mechanics. An independent predictor of cardiovascular risk in arterial hypertension. Circulation. 1996;93(2):259-65.
34. de Simone G, Devereux RB, Roman MJ, et al. Assessment of left ventricular function by the midwall fractional shortening end systolic stress relation in human hypertension. J Am Coll Cardiol. 1994;23(6):1444-51.
35. Greenbaum RA, Ho SY, Gibson DG, et al. Left ventricular fibre architecture in man. Br Heart J. 1981;45(3):248-63.
36. Freeman GL, LeWinter MM, Engler RL, et al. Relationship between myocardial fiber direction and segment shortening in the midwall of the canine left ventricle. Circ Res. 1985;56(1):31-9.
37. Zabalgoitia M, Rahman SN, Haley WE, et al. Effect of regression of left ventricular hypertrophy from systemic hypertension on systolic function assessed by midwall shortening (hot echocardiographic study). Am J Cardiol. 2001;88(5):521-5.
38. Wachtell K, Gerdts E, Palmieri V, et al. In-treatment midwall and endocardial fractional shortening predict cardiovascular outcome in hypertensive patients with preserved baseline systolic ventricular function: the losartan intervention for endpoint reduction study. J Hypertens. 2010;28(7):1541-6.
39. Hu K, Liu D, Niemann M, et al. Methods for assessment of left ventricular systolic function in technically difficult patients with poor imaging quality. J Am Soc Echocardiogr. 2013;26(2):105-13.
40. Nikitin NP, Loh PH, Silva R, et al. Prognostic value of systolic mitral annular velocity measured with Doppler tissue imaging in patients with chronic heart failure caused by left ventricular systolic dysfunction. Heart. 2006;92(6):775-9.
41. Ruan Q, Nagueh SF. Usefulness of isovolumic and systolic ejection signals by tissue Doppler for the assessment of left ventricular systolic function in ischemic or idiopathic dilated cardiomyopathy. Am J Cardiol. 2006;97(6):872-5.
42. Mizuguchi Y, Oishi Y, Miyoshi H, et al. Concentric left ventricular hypertrophy brings deterioration of systolic longitudinal, circumferential, and radial myocardial deformation in hypertensive patients with preserved left ventricular pump function. J Cardiol. 2010;55(1):23-33.
43. Stanton T, Leano R, Marwick TH. Prediction of all-cause mortality from global longitudinal speckle strain: comparison with ejection fraction and wall motion scoring. Circ Cardiovasc Imaging. 2009;2(5):356-64.
44. Kang SJ, Lim HS, Choi BJ, et al. Longitudinal strain and torsion assessed by two-dimensional speckle tracking correlate with the serum level of tissue inhibitor of matrix metalloproteinase-1, a marker of myocardial fibrosis, in patients with hypertension. J Am Soc Echocardiogr. 2008;21(8):907-11.
45. Galderisi M, Lomoriello VS, Santoro A, et al. Differences of myocardial systolic deformation and correlates of diastolic function in competitive rowers and young hypertensives: a speckle-tracking echocardiography study. J Am Soc Echocardiogr. 2010;23(11):1190-8.
46. Di Bello V, Talini E, Dell'Omo G, et al. Early left ventricular mechanics abnormalities in prehypertension: a two-dimensional strain echocardiography study. Am J Hypertens. 2010;23(4):405-12.
47. Nagueh SF, Smiseth OA, Appleton CP, et al. Recommendations for the evaluation of left ventricular diastolic function by echocardiography: an update from the American Society of Echocardiography and the European Association of Cardiovascular Imaging. J Am Soc Echocardiogr. 2016;29(4):277-314.
48. Sohn DW, Chai IH, Lee DJ, et al. Assessment of mitral annulus velocity by doppler tissue imaging in the evaluation of left ventricular diastolic function. J Am Coll Cardiol. 1997;30(2):474-80.
49. Rodriguez L, Garcia M, Ares M, et al. Assessment of mitral annular dynamics during diastole by Doppler tissue imaging: comparison with mitral Doppler inflow in subjects without heart disease and in patients with left ventricular hypertrophy. Am Heart J. 1996;131(5):982-7.

50. Wang M, Yip G, Yu CM, et al. Independent and incremental prognostic value of early mitral annulus velocity in patients with impaired left ventricular systolic function. J Am Coll Cardiol. 2005;45(2):272-7.
51. Nagueh SF, Middleton KJ, Kopelen HA, et al. Doppler tissue imaging: a noninvasive technique for evaluation of left ventricular relaxation and estimation of filling pressures. J Am Coll Cardiol. 1997;30(6):1527-33.
52. Dokainish H, Zoghbi WA, Lakkis NM, et al. Incremental predictive power of b-type natriuretic peptide and tissue Doppler echocardiography in the prognosis of patients with congestive heart failure. J Am Coll Cardiol. 2005;45(8):1223-6.
53. Levy D, Garrison RJ, Savage DD, et al. Prognostic implications of echocardiographically determined left ventricular mass in the Framingham Heart study. N Engl J Med. 1990;322(22):1561-6.
54. Verdecchia P, Angeli F, Achilli P, et al. Echocardiographic left ventricular hypertrophy in hypertension: marker for future events or mediator of events? Curr Opin Cardiol. 2007;22(4):329-34.
55. Mathew J, Sleight P, Lonn E, et al. Reduction of cardiovascular risk by regression of electrocardiographic markers of left ventricular hypertrophy by the angiotensin-converting enzyme inhibitor ramipril. Circulation. 2001;104(14):1615-21.
56. Okin PM, Devereux RB, Jern S, et al. Regression of electrocardiographic left ventricular hypertrophy during antihypertensive treatment and the prediction of major cardiovascular events. JAMA. 2004;292(19):2343-9.
57. Devereux RB, Wachtell K, Gerdts E, et al. Prognostic significance of left ventricular mass during treatment of hypertension. JAMA. 2004;292(19):2350-6.
58. Shimada YJ, Shiota T. Meta-analysis of accuracy of left ventricular mass measurement by three-dimensional echocardiography. Am J Cardiol. 2012;110(3):445-52.
59. Gonzalez-Torres L, De Diego C, Centurion R, et al. Angiotensin-neprilysin inhibition further reverses cardiac remodeling as compared to angiotensin inhibition in reduced heart failure patients. Clin Cardiol J. 2018;2(1):6-9.
60. Wachtell K, Bella JN, Rokkedal J, et al. Change in diastolic left ventricular filling after one year of antihypertensive treatment: The Losartan Intervention for Endpoint Reduction in Hypertension (LIFE) Study. Circulation. 2002;105(9):1071-6.
61. Yalcin F, Aksoy FG, Muderrisoglu H, et al. Treatment of hypertension with perindopril reduces plasma atrial natriuretic peptide levels, left ventricular mass, and improves echocardiographic parameters of diastolic function. Clin Cardiol. 2000;23(6):437-41.

13

CHAPTER

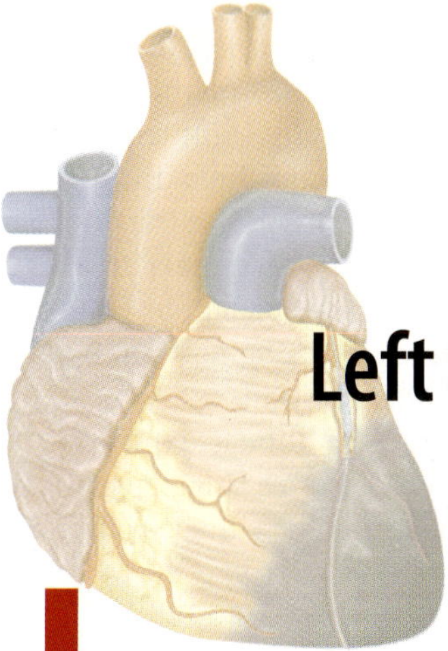

Left Ventricular Hypertrophy and Left Ventricular Mass Index Evaluation by 3D Echocardiography in Hypertension

Mohamed Faher Almahmoud, Masood Ahmad

INTRODUCTION

Left ventricular mass (LVM) is an important clinical parameter with strong predictive value for cardiovascular events and death.[1,2] An increase of LVM above the 95th percentile in patients with left ventricular hypertrophy (LVH) is an independent clinical predictor for cardiovascular mortality and morbidity.[1,2] LVM increases in a variety of cardiovascular diseases such as hypertension, valvular heart disease, heart failure, and following myocardial infarction. Regression of LVM in hypertensive patients reduces the risk of cardiovascular disease in this population.[3] Conventional one-dimensional M-mode or two-dimensional (2D) echocardiographic methods have been used routinely to assess LVM. However, these methods are subjective and limited by the geometric assumptions of the LV shape, image quality, off-axis cuts, and the high variability especially in abnormally shaped ventricles.[4,5] Although alternative methods of assessing LVM, such as cardiac magnetic resonance imaging (CMR) and cardiac computed tomography (CT) are more accurate, they are limited by cost, time needed for scanning and interpretation, and limited availability. Therefore, three-dimensional (3D) echocardiography is a very attractive method for assessing LVM due to its low-cost, ease of use, reproducibility, and wide availability. Real-time (RT) 3D is widely available on many echo scanners. The technique is easy to use clinically with quick acquisition of images. Direct and accurate measurements of LVM are easily obtained from the 3D data sets without geometrical assumptions and modeling algorithms.[6] The American Society of Echocardiography (ASE) recommends 3D echo assessment of LVM, especially in abnormally-shaped ventricles or in patients with asymmetric or localized hypertrophy. However, because of the limited data available on the upper limits of the LVM by 3D echo, the ASE guidelines concluded that at this time there is insufficient information to recommend normal reference values.[7] This chapter discusses the application of echocardiographic methods with particular reference to 3D technique in the assessment of LVM and summarizes the current literature regarding the prognostic implications of LVM measurements in patients with hypertension.

TECHNIQUES FOR LEFT VENTRICULAR MASS MEASUREMENT

Echocardiographic Methods

Several echocardiographic methods can be used to calculate the LVM. All of these methods use the LV end-diastolic diameter (LVID), interventricular septal (IVS), and posterior wall thickness (PWT) at end-diastole, and multiply the calculated volume by the myocardial density (≅ 1.05 g/mL) to obtain LVM. Conventional methods such as M-mode and 2D echocardiography rely on geometric formulas to calculate LV volume, while 3D echo measures LV volume directly. Using the linear M-mode method (either blinded or 2D-guided), LVM is calculated using the Cube formula: $LVM = 0.8 \times 1.04\ [(IVS + LVID + PWT)^3 \simeq (LVID)^3] + 0.6$ g. 2D-based formulas use the truncated ellipsoid and area-length methods to estimate LV volume.[7] The assessment of LVM using M-mode or 2D echocardiography methods has several advantages, including simplicity, low-cost, rapid assessment, wide availability and established prognostic value.[8] However, LVM measurements using these methods suffer from several limitations including wide interobserver variability, poor reproducibility, and geometric assumptions.[5,9] Furthermore, although these methods are recommended for routine follow-up in hypertensive patients to assess regression of LV hypertrophy, they remain limited in measuring LVM in abnormally-shaped hearts.[10] The accuracy of LVM assessment by 3D echocardiography is almost similar to that of CMR with slight overestimation. The use of innermost vs. outermost endocardial contour tracing might explain the differences in measurements, as LVM measurement is higher with inclusion of trabeculae into the LV wall. With a full volume 3D dataset of the LV, it is possible to identify epicardial and endocardial boundaries with user-friendly software. Epicardial and endocardial casts of the LV are measured, and LV volume is calculated by subtraction, which in turn is multiplied by the specific gravity of the myocardium to determine the LVM. This RT 3D technique is easy, accurate, and less time consuming than CMR. Additionally because of its ability to measure LV volume directly, without geometric assumptions, ASE recommends RT 3D especially in abnormally-shaped ventricles or in patients with asymmetric or localized hypertrophy.[7] The 3D technique does have some limitations. Similar to other echocardiographic methods, it depends on the acoustic window for image quality to accurately estimate LV volume. Only few studies have been published about its practical use, feasibility, variability, and prognostic value. Furthermore, limited data regarding the upper limits of LVM measured by 3D echocardiography are currently available.[11]

Cardiac Magnetic Resonance

Left ventricular mass measured by CMR is more accurate and precise than the echocardiographic methods. High resolution 3D images are acquired using breath hold over several cardiac cycles. Myocardial volume is measured directly using endocardial and epicardial boundaries, which is then multiplied by the density of the myocardium to obtain myocardial mass. This technique is highly accurate for LVM measurement. Furthermore, it is not dependent on geometric assumptions, contrast use, or acoustic window quality.[12] However, important limitations prevent its wide usage including high-cost, time required to acquire and analyze the data, as well as contraindications to its use in several patient populations such as those with metal devices, claustrophobia, and severe renal dysfunction.

ADVANCES IN 3D ECHOCARDIOGRAPHY

The early 3D echo techniques were limited by tedious and time-consuming image acquisitions and analysis methods. The development of the fully sampled matrix-array transducers is considered a major breakthrough in the history of RT 3D echocardiography. These transducers allow high-quality RT imaging of the heart in three dimensions. They are composed of $\simeq$ 3,000 piezoelectric elements with operating frequencies ranging from 2 MHz to 4 MHz. RT 3D images can be obtained either as an electrocardiographically triggered multibeat acquisition or as a 3D pyramidal volume data set from a single heartbeat. Multibeat 3D echocardiography provides images of higher temporal resolution. Acquisition is triggered to the R wave over several heartbeats (ranging from two to seven cardiac cycles) that are subsequently stitched together to create a single volumetric data set. Gain and compression controls, as well as the time gain compensation settings, are optimized for quality of 3D images. RT 3D data sets are then obtained with a wide-angled acquisition (93° × 80°) mode in which four wedge-shaped subvolumes (93° × 20° each) are obtained from four different cardiac cycles during held respiration. Commercial software (3DQ-QLab, Philips) is available to analyze the RT 3D data sets. Figures 1 and 2 show the apical 4-chamber, 2-chamber, and short-axis views derived from the 3D data set in a normal subject and in a hypertensive patient, respectively. Using a semiautomated process, epicardial and endocardial borders of the LV are identified. Biplane Simpson's method is used to calculate LV and myocardial volumes. Myocardial volume is multiplied by the specific gravity of the heart muscle to obtain measurements of the LVM, which in turn is divided by the subject's body surface area for calculation of LVM index (LVMI).

VALIDATION OF LVM MEASUREMENTS BY 3D ECHOCARDIOGRAPHY

In Vitro Validation

The accuracy, feasibility, and value of 3D echocardiography have been demonstrated in vivo and in vitro. Table 1 shows a summary of the studies conducted to evaluate LVM using 3D echocardiography. Earlier studies evaluated the feasibility and accuracy of LVM measurement by 3D echocardiography in an in vitro model using sheep, pig and canine hearts, and compared these measurements to the true mass measured by multiplying myocardial volume by the specific density.[13,14] The in vitro results were excellent with a correlation coefficient of 0.995 for the measurements between the two techniques. Sapin et al.

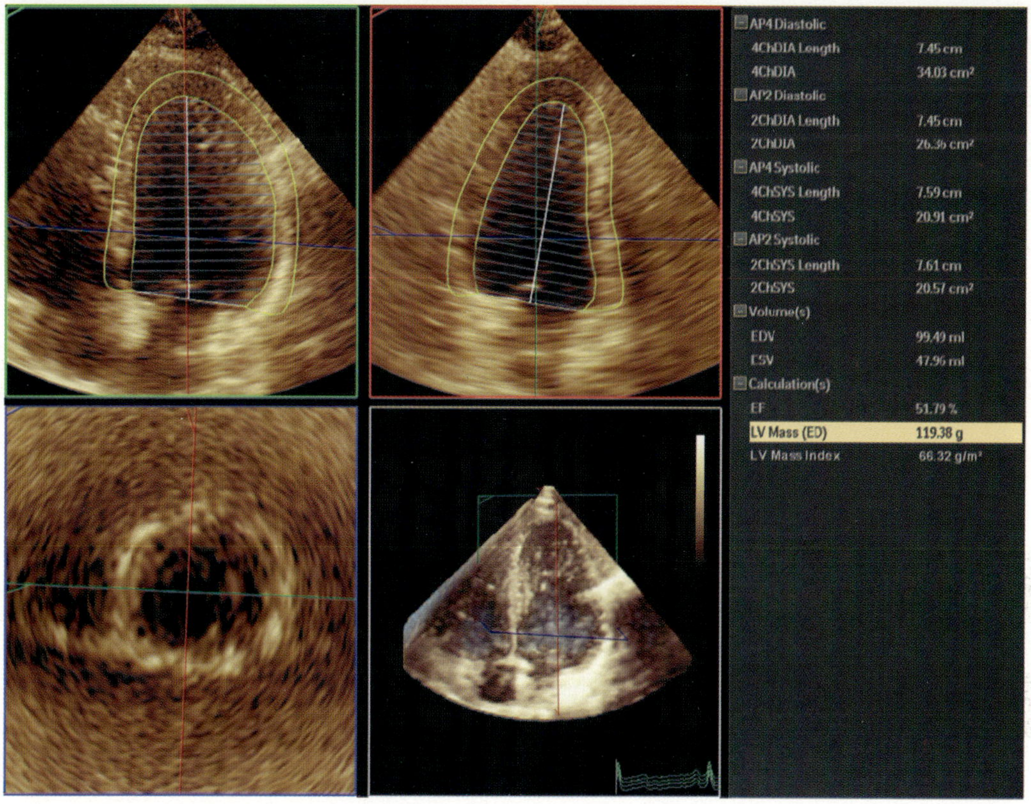

Fig. 1: Example from our laboratory of three-dimensional left ventricular mass (LVM) measurement in a normal heart. Apical four- and two-chamber views are derived from a full-volume dataset of the LV. In a semiautomated process the endocardial and epicardial borders of the LV myocardium are identified and a biplane Simpson's rule calculation applied to obtain both LV and myocardial volume. The myocardial volume is then multiplied by the specific gravity of the heart muscle in order to calculate LVM.

demonstrated in vitro superiority of 3D over conventional 2D echocardiography. 3D provided the best correlation and the lowest standard error in measurements of the true mass when compared to 2D truncated ellipsoid and the area-length models.[13] Rodevand et al. showed superiority of parasternal 3D over conventional 2D methods using porcine heart models.[15] Furthermore, Hubka et al. showed 3D is not only accurate for LVM measurements but for the right ventricular mass and volume evaluations.[16]

In Vivo Validation

Since CMR is the gold standard method for assessing LVM, several in vivo studies compared the accuracy of LVM determination by different 3D echocardiographic techniques with that of CMR (Fig. 3).[17] Gopal et al. showed that in vivo interobserver variability of 3D LVM assessment in systole and diastole was 6.3–12.8% and 7.5% for CMR at end-diastole, and showed better agreement between 3D echocardiography and CMR when compared with M-mode and 2D echocardiography.[14] Jenkins et al. showed that RT 3D is a feasible, reproducible, and an accurate approach to evaluate LVM, unlike M-mode and 2D echocardiography which overestimated LVM measurement compared to CMR.[18] RT 3D assessment of LVM was also compared with CMR by Mor-Avi et al. in 21 patients. They demonstrated better accuracy, improved correlation, and lower interobserver variability by RT 3D when compared to 2D echocardiography.[6]

Validation in Abnormally Shaped Hearts

Several studies used CMR to show superiority of 3D measurement of LVM compared to conventional M-mode and 2D echocardiography in abnormally-shaped hearts. Van den Bosch et al. reported that RT 3D eliminates the geometric assumptions inherent in conventional M-mode and 2D echocardiography which results in inaccurate assessment of LVM in individuals with abnormally-shaped hearts, and demonstrated that LVM measured by RT 3D is feasible, highly accurate, and had low interobserver variability in 20 patients with congenital heart disease.[19] Similar observations by Abramov et al. in hypertensive and heart failure patients with or without low LV ejection fraction,

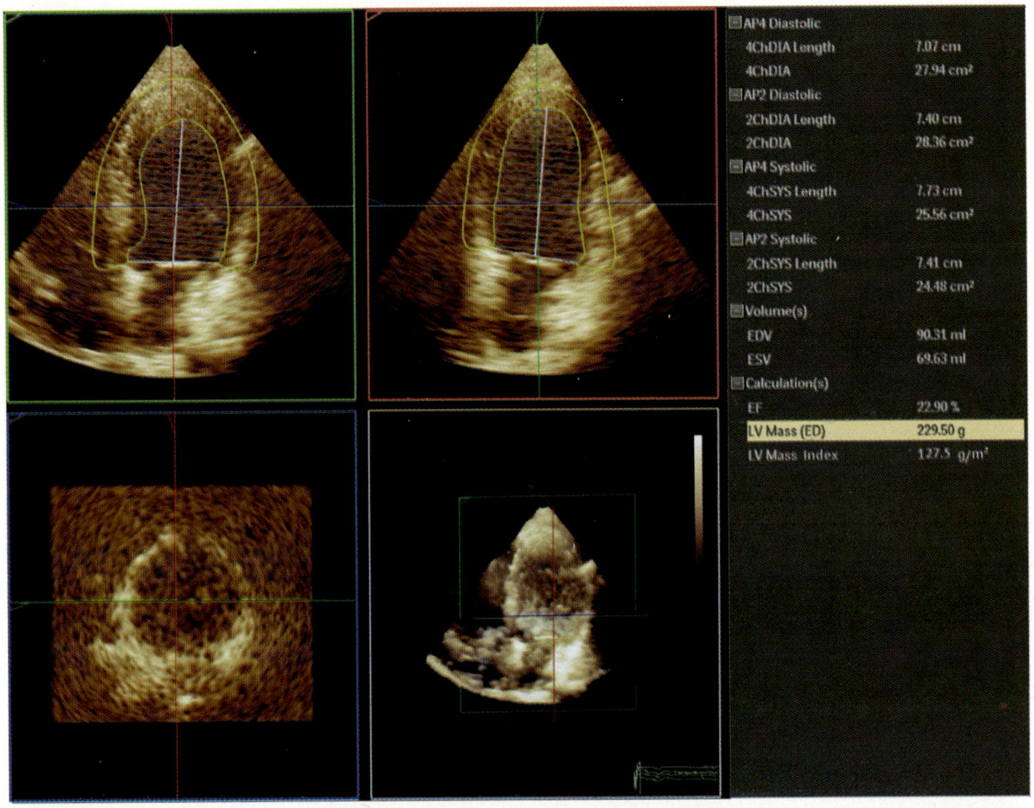

Fig. 2: Example from our laboratory of three-dimensional left ventricular mass (LVM) measurement in a patient with hypertension and LV hypertrophy. Apical four- and two-chamber views have been derived from a full-volume dataset of the LV. In a semiautomated process the endocardial and epicardial borders of the LV myocardium are identified and a biplane Simpson's rule calculation applied to obtain both LV and myocardial volume. The myocardial volume is then multiplied by the specific gravity of the heart muscle in order to calculate LVM.

TABLE 1: Evolution and validation of 3D echocardiography method for LVM assessment.

Author	*Year*	*Objective*	*Conclusion*	*Comments*
Gopal[14]	1994	In vitro and in vivo validation of LVM by 3D echo and comparison with conventional echo methods	Image plane positioning guidance and elimination of geometric assumptions by 3D echo achieve high accuracy for LVM determination in vitro and in vivo	In vitro comparison with the true measured LVM. In vivo validation with CMR
Sapin[13]	1996	3D echo compared to 2D echo for measurement of LVM with anatomic validation in open chest canine model	3D echo is more accurate than standard 2D for measuring LVM	20 open chest dogs had 3D echo and compared to true mass and 2D echo using truncated ellipsoid and the area-length models
Rodevand[15]	1997	Evaluate the potential of LVM determination with new 3D echo method compared with 2D measurements	Postmortem assessment of porcine heart with 3D is accurate and reproducible	3D images were obtained by probe rotation axis, perpendicular and parallel to the ventricular long axis
Hubka[16]	2002	Evaluate the accuracy of 3D surface reconstruction by the piecewise smooth subdivision method in measuring volume and mass in the LV and the more complexly shaped right ventricle	3D echo using freehand scanning combined with surface reconstruction by the piecewise smooth subdivision surface method, enables accurate determination of LV and RV mass and volumes	Comparison with true mass and volume of 15 bovine and 10 porcine hearts in vitro

Contd...

Contd...

Author	Year	Objective	Conclusion	Comments
Kuhl[9]	2003	Evaluate whether LVM determined by M-mode echo is overestimated compared with LVM calculated by 3D echo in patients with normal LV shape	M-mode and 3D echo correlate well for the calculation of LVM with overestimation of LVM by the 1D technique. Normal M-mode LVM values may not apply for 3D echo	25 hypertensive patients, 31 patients with aortic stenosis and 30 control subjects
Jenkins[18]	2004	Whether assessment of LV function with RT 3D could reduce the variation of sequential LV measurements and provide greater accuracy than 2D echo	Real-time 3D reduces test-retest variation of LV volume, EF and LVM measurements	Validation with CMR
Mor-Avi[6]	2004	Fast measurement of LVM with RT 3D comparison with CMR	RT 3D imaging provides the basis for accurate and reliable measurement of LVM	Comparison with 2D echo and CMR
Galzerano[25]	2004	Freehand 3D echo evaluation of the effects of Telmisartan vs. HCTZ on LVM in patients with HTN	Telmisartan 80 mg significantly reduced SBP, DBP and LVMI after 12 months' treatment compared with HCTZ	2D and freehand precordial 3D echo were performed at baseline and after treatment
Lenstrup[36]	2006	Evaluation of different methods of measuring LVM in patients with no known LVH using CMR as the gold standard	LVM measured by 3D echo is highly accurate compared to LVM measured by CMR	Comparison with ECG LVH criteria and 2D echo
Van den Bosch[19]	2006	Assess the feasibility/accuracy of RT 3D echo for LVM measurements in patients with congenital heart disease compared to CMR	LVM of an abnormally shaped LV can be determined with high accuracy and low interobserver variability in patients with good or moderate echocardiographic image quality	20 congenital heart disease patients had RT 3D and CMR
Caiani[37]	2006	Volumetric analysis by RT 3D echocardiography data to quantify LVM and to validate the technique against CMR	Direct 3D model independent LVM measurement from RT 3D images is feasible in the clinical setting and provides fast and accurate assessment of LVM, superior to 2D	RT 3D was feasible in 19 of 21 patients
Chen[22]	2009	RT 3D echo assessment of LV remodeling index in patients with hypertensive heart disease and CAD	LV remodeling index derived from RT 3D echo as a new index for evaluating LV remodeling, superior to LVRI derived from 2D echo	60 subjects had RT 3D echo and 2D echo
Abramov[20]	2010	Compare the assessment of LV size and geometry by 2D echo and 3D echo in normotensive controls and in HF patients with a normal or reduced EF	2D overestimates LVM when compared to 3D echo in patients with HF with both normal and low EF resulting in misclassification of ventricular geometry in many HF patients	42 normotensive patients without cardiac disease, 41 hypertensive patients with normal ejection fraction, and 28 patients with HF and low EF
Avegliano[21]	2015	Validate the use of RT 3D to quantify LVM using CMR as a reference, in a large population with different types of hypertrophic cardiomyopathy	RT 3D is an accurate method for the quantification of LVM in patients with different types of HCM, better agreement with CMR reference values than M-mode measurements	48 patients with HCM had RT 3D echo, M-mode and CMR

Contd...

Contd...

Author	Year	Objective	Conclusion	Comments
Navarini[38]	2017	Evaluate LV mechanics (strain, twist, and torsion) in young patients with HTN compared to healthy controls and assess factors associated with functional measurements	Children with HTN had significantly lower strain indices	53 patients, 26 with HTN and 37 normotensive subjects were enrolled
Lembo[23]	2018	Investigate the ability of 3D echo in identifying a phenotype of LV concentric geometry according to LVM/EDV ratio, possibly detecting early myocardial damage in native hypertensive patients	In HTN patients, 3D derived LVM/EDV ratio identifies a higher prevalence of LV concentric geometry compared to 2D	128 hypertensive patients had both 2D and 3D echo
Meng[24]	2018	Evaluate the changes in LV structure and function in hypertensive patients with CAD before and after PCI using RT 3D echo	3D echo can evaluate the critical parameters in the prognosis of HTN in patients with CAD after PCI accurately and in real-time	280 HTN patients with CAD undergoing PCI and 120 controls

(CAD: coronary artery disease; CMR: cardiac magnetic resonance; 2D: two-dimensional; 3D: three-dimensional; EF: ejection fraction; EDV: end-diastolic volume; HTN: hypertension; HCTZ: hydrochlorothiazide; HF: heart failure; LVM: left ventricular mass; PCI: percutaneous coronary intervention; RT: real-time)

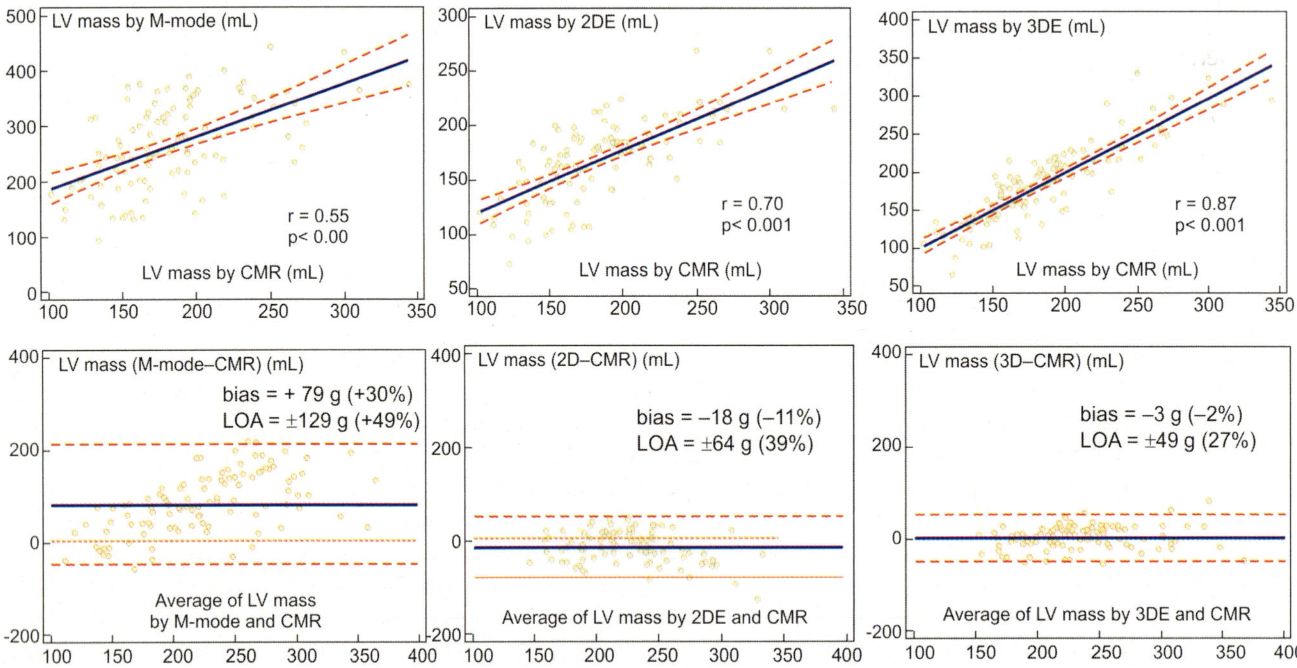

Fig. 3: Comparison between echocardiographic (using M-mode echocardiography, two-dimensional, and three-dimensional echo) and cardiac magnetic resonance measurements of left ventricular mass.

Source: Kusunose K, Kwon DH, Motoki H, et al. Comparison of three-dimensional echocardiographic findings to those of magnetic resonance imaging for determination of left ventricular mass in patients with ischemic and nonischemic cardiomyopathy. Am J Cardiol. 2013;112(4):604-11.

showed that 2D echocardiography overestimates LVM which leads to significant misclassification of ventricular geometry in many hypertensive and heart failure patients.[20] Recently, Avegaliano et al. reported similar overestimation of LVM by M-mode in patients with hypertrophic cardiomyopathy, and superiority of 3D in this clinical setting.[21]

Validation in Hypertensive Patients

Left ventricular mass assessment in hypertensive patients is recommended by the ASE guidelines, and is a very important clinical parameter since the presence of LVH is associated with worse outcomes, and the regression of LVH with improved outcomes. Thus, accurate and reproducible assessment of LVM and LV geometry is of paramount importance. As discussed above, Abramov et al. showed the superiority of RT 3D to 2D echocardiography for assessment of LVM in hypertensive patients.[20] Chen et al. also observed improved evaluation of the LV remodeling index in hypertensive patients by RT 3D compared to 2D echocardiography.[22] Lembo et al. studied the ability of 3D to identify LV concentric geometry according to LVM/end-diastolic volume ratio in hypertensive patients, and found that 3D identified a higher rate of LV concentric geometry in comparison with 2D-derived relative wall thickness (37% vs. 24%, p = 0.03).[23] Meng et al. reported that 3D echocardiography can provide valuable real time information for hypertensive patients with coronary artery disease.[24] Finally, Galzerano et al. demonstrated the value of routine use of 3D echocardiography for follow-up LVM measurements to monitor regression of LVH with antihypertensive medications.[25]

PROGNOSTIC VALUE OF LVM ASSESSMENT

Left ventricular hypertrophy is an independent and a strong predictor of cardiovascular disease in the general population and in patients with hypertension.[3,26-28] LVH was shown to be associated with higher risk of sudden death,[29] myocardial infarction,[30] heart failure,[27] stroke,[28] mortality, and composite major cardiovascular outcomes (Fig. 4).[3] Previous studies also showed higher risk of events as a result of the concentric remodeling associated with long-term hypertension.[31] Furthermore, studies also indicate that antihypertensive treatment may induce regression of LVH and thus improve long-term cardiovascular prognosis.[32,33] Koren et al. compared the risk of cardiovascular events and mortality in a cohort of 280 participants with hypertension. Those with LVH by echo had a greater risk of both cardiovascular events and mortality.[34] Verdecchia et al. demonstrated a 40% higher risk of major cardiovascular outcomes associated with each one standard deviation (SD) increase in LVM in the hypertensive population.[3] In addition, concentric remodeling was associated with higher risk of fatal and nonfatal events compared to normal LV geometry in the hypertensive cohort.[31] Devereux et al. studied the prognostic significance of LVH regression with antihypertensive medications. After 1 year of treatment,

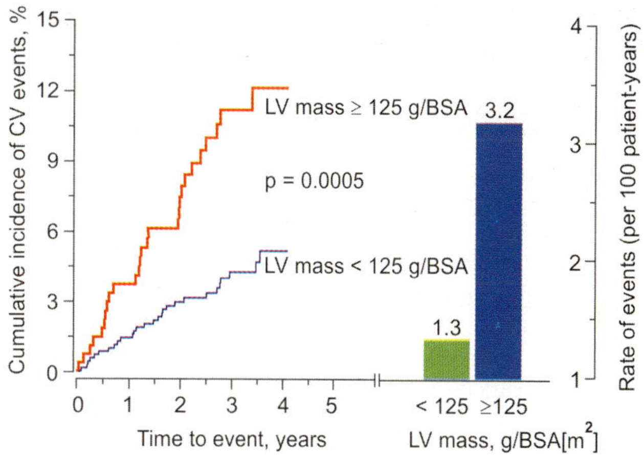

Fig. 4: Cumulative incidence (left) and crude rate (right) of cardiovascular events in subjects with and without left ventricular hypertrophy at echocardiography.
Source: Verdecchia P, Carini G, Circo A, et al. Left ventricular mass and cardiovascular morbidity in essential hypertension: the MAVI study. J Am Coll Cardiol. 2001;38(7):1829-35.

one SD decrease in in-treatment LVMI was associated with a lower risk of composite outcomes of cardiovascular death, myocardial infarction or stroke [Hazard ratio 0.74; confidence interval (CI) 0.65–0.91; p = 0.003].[33] In a meta-analysis of studies reporting echo LVM before and after antihypertensive therapy, Verdecchia et al. showed that LVH regression was associated with 59% reduction in the risk of cardiovascular events compared with persistent or new development of LVH.[35]

CONCLUSION

Left ventricular hypertrophy, as measured by LVMI, is a strong and an independent risk factor for cardiovascular mortality and morbidity. Regression of LVH has a favorable outcome that can be achieved with antihypertensive therapy. Techniques to assess LVH by measuring LVM vary in their accuracy, reproducibility, and availability. While conventional echocardiographic methods (M-mode and 2D echocardiography) are the first diagnostic tools because of their availability, ease of use, and numerous prognostic studies, they suffer from many limitations, especially in abnormally shaped hearts. CMR is considered the gold standard for assessment of LVM because of its accuracy and reproducibility. However, due to economic limitations, this modality is far less accessible in clinical practice compared to echocardiography. 3D echocardiography is a robust, efficient, and a low-cost modality with excellent accuracy and reproducibility of measurements. The technique directly measures LVM with low interobserver variability and without geometric assumptions. Further studies are needed to establish the 3D cut-offs for LVH and their predictive significance.

REFERENCES

1. Ghali JK, Liao Y, Simmons B, et al. The prognostic role of left ventricular hypertrophy in patients with or without coronary artery disease. Ann Intern Med. 1992;117(10):831-6.
2. Levy D, Garrison RJ, Savage DD, et al. Prognostic implications of echocardiographically determined left ventricular mass in the framingham heart study. N Engl J Med. 1990;322(22):1561-6.
3. Verdecchia P, Carini G, Circo A, et al. Left ventricular mass and cardiovascular morbidity in essential hypertension: the MAVI study. J Am Coll Cardiol. 2001;38(7):1829-35.
4. Kuhl HP, Bucker A, Franke A, et al. Transesophageal 3-dimensional echocardiography: in vivo determination of left ventricular mass in comparison with magnetic resonance imaging. J Am Soc Echocardiogr. 2000;13(3):205-15.
5. Missouris CG, Forbat SM, Singer DR, et al. Echocardiography overestimates left ventricular mass: a comparative study with magnetic resonance imaging in patients with hypertension. J Hypertens. 1996;14(8):1005-10.
6. Mor-Avi V, Sugeng L, Weinert L, et al. Fast measurement of left ventricular mass with real-time three-dimensional echocardiography: comparison with magnetic resonance imaging. Circulation. 2004;110(13):1814-8.
7. Lang RM, Badano LP, Mor-Avi V, et al. Recommendations for cardiac chamber quantification by echocardiography in adults: an update from the American Society Of Echocardiography and the European Association of Cardiovascular Imaging. J Am Soc Echocardiogr. 2015;28(1):1-39.
8. Armstrong AC, Gidding S, Gjesdal O, et al. LV mass assessed by echocardiography and CMR, cardiovascular outcomes, and medical practice. JACC Cardiovasc Imaging. 2012;5(8):837-48.
9. Kuhl HP, Hanrath P, Franke A. M-mode echocardiography overestimates left ventricular mass in patients with normal left ventricular shape: a comparative study using three-dimensional echocardiography. Eur J Echocardiogr. 2003;4(4):312-9.
10. Byrd BF 3rd, Wahr D, Wang YS, et al. Left ventricular mass and volume/mass ratio determined by two-dimensional echocardiography in normal adults. J Am Coll Cardiol. 1985;6(5):1021-5.
11. Lang RM, Badano LP, Tsang W, et al. EAE/ASE recommendations for image acquisition and display using three-dimensional echocardiography. Eur Heart J Cardiovasc Imaging. 2012;13(1):1-46.
12. Childs H, Ma L, Ma M, et al. Comparison of long and short axis quantification of left ventricular volume parameters by cardiovascular magnetic resonance, with ex-vivo validation. J Cardiovasc Magn Reson. 2011;13:40.
13. Sapin PM, Gopal AS, Clarke GB, et al. Three-dimensional echocardiography compared to two-dimensional echocardiography for measurement of left ventricular mass anatomic validation in an open chest canine model. Am J Hypertens. 1996;9(5):467-74.
14. Gopal AS, Keller AM, Shen Z, et al. Three-dimensional echocardiography: in vitro and in vivo validation of left ventricular mass and comparison with conventional echocardiographic methods. J Am Coll Cardiol. 1994;24(2):504-13.
15. Rodevand O, Bjornerheim R, Kolbjornsen O, et al. Left ventricular mass assessed by three-dimensional echocardiography using rotational acquisition. Clin Cardiol. 1997;20(11):957-62.
16. Hubka M, Bolson EL, McDonald JA, et al. Three-dimensional echocardiographic measurement of left and right ventricular mass and volume: in vitro validation. Int J Cardiovasc Imaging. 2002;18(2):111-8.
17. Kusunose K, Kwon DH, Motoki H, et al. Comparison of three-dimensional echocardiographic findings to those of magnetic resonance imaging for determination of left ventricular mass in patients with ischemic and non-ischemic cardiomyopathy. Am J Cardiol. 2013;112(4):604-11.
18. Jenkins C, Bricknell K, Hanekom L, et al. Reproducibility and accuracy of echocardiographic measurements of left ventricular parameters using real-time three-dimensional echocardiography. J Am Coll Cardiol. 2004;44(4):878-86.
19. van den Bosch AE, Robbers-Visser D, Krenning BJ, et al. Comparison of real-time three-dimensional echocardiography to magnetic resonance imaging for assessment of left ventricular mass. Am J Cardiol. 2006;97(1):113-7.
20. Abramov D, Helmke S, Rumbarger Lel K, et al. Overestimation of left ventricular mass and misclassification of ventricular geometry in heart failure patients by two-dimensional echocardiography in comparison with three-dimensional echocardiography. Echocardiography. 2010;27(3):223-9.
21. Avegliano GP, Costabel JP, Asch FM, et al. Utility of real time 3D echocardiography for the assessment of left ventricular mass in patients with hypertrophic cardiomyopathy: comparison with cardiac magnetic resonance. Echocardiography. 2016;33(3):431-6.
22. Chen M, Wang J, Xie M, et al. Real-time three-dimensional echocardiographic assessment of left ventricular remodeling index in patients with hypertensive heart disease and coronary artery disease. J Huazhong Univ Sci Technolog Med Sci. 2009;29(1):122-6.
23. Lembo M, Esposito R, Santoro C, et al. Three-dimensional echocardiographic ventricular mass/end-diastolic volume ratio in native hypertensive patients: relation between stroke volume and geometry. J Hypertens. 2018;36(8):1697-1704.
24. Meng Y, Zong L, Zhang Z, et al. Evaluation of changes in left ventricular structure and function in hypertensive patients with coronary artery disease after PCI using real-time three-dimensional echocardiography. Exp Ther Med. 2018;15(2):1493-9.
25. Galzerano D, Tammaro P, Cerciello A, et al. Freehand three-dimensional echocardiographic evaluation of the effect of telmisartan compared with hydrochlorothiazide on left ventricular mass in hypertensive patients with mild-

to-moderate hypertension: a multicentre study. J Hum Hypertens. 2004;18(1):53-9.
26. Oseni AO, Qureshi WT, Almahmoud MF, et al. Left ventricular hypertrophy by ECG versus cardiac MRI as a predictor for heart failure. Heart. 2017;103(1):49-54.
27. Almahmoud MF, O'Neal WT, Qureshi W, et al. Electrocardiographic versus echocardiographic left ventricular hypertrophy in prediction of congestive heart failure in the elderly. Clin Cardiol. 2015;38(6):365-70.
28. O'Neal WT, Almahmoud MF, Qureshi WT, et al. Electrocardiographic and echocardiographic left ventricular hypertrophy in the prediction of stroke in the elderly. J Stroke Cerebrovasc Dis. 2015;24(9):1991-7.
29. Haider AW, Larson MG, Benjamin EJ, et al. Increased left ventricular mass and hypertrophy are associated with increased risk for sudden death. J Am Coll Cardiol. 1998;32(5):1454-9.
30. Verma A, Meris A, Skali H, et al. Prognostic implications of left ventricular mass and geometry following myocardial infarction: the valiant (valsartan in acute myocardial infarction) echocardiographic study. JACC Cardiovasc Imaging. 2008;1(5):582-91.
31. Verdecchia P, Schillaci G, Borgioni C, et al. Adverse prognostic significance of concentric remodeling of the left ventricle in hypertensive patients with normal left ventricular mass. J Am Coll Cardiol. 1995;25(4):871-8.
32. Verdecchia P, Angeli F, Pittavini L, et al. Regression of left ventricular hypertrophy and cardiovascular risk changes in hypertensive patients. Ital Heart J. 2004;5(7):505-10.
33. Devereux RB, Wachtell K, Gerdts E, et al. Prognostic significance of left ventricular mass change during treatment of hypertension. JAMA. 2004;292(19):2350-6.
34. Koren MJ, Devereux RB, Casale PN, et al. Relation of left ventricular mass and geometry to morbidity and mortality in uncomplicated essential hypertension. Ann Intern Med. 1991;114(5):345-52.
35. Verdecchia P, Angeli F, Borgioni C, et al. Changes in cardiovascular risk by reduction of left ventricular mass in hypertension: a meta-analysis. Am J Hypertens. 2003;16(11 Pt 1):895-9.
36. Lenstrup M, Kjaergaard J, Petersen CL, et al. Evaluation of left ventricular mass measured by 3D echocardiography using magnetic resonance imaging as gold standard. Scand J Clin Lab Invest. 2006;66(8):647-57.
37. Caiani EG, Corsi C, Sugeng L, et al. Improved quantification of left ventricular mass based on endocardial and epicardial surface detection with real time three dimensional echocardiography. Heart. 2006;92(2):213-9.
38. Navarini S, Bellsham-Revell H, Chubb H, et al. Myocardial deformation measured by 3-dimensional speckle tracking in children and adolescents with systemic arterial hypertension. Hypertension. 2017;70(6):1142-7.

14

CHAPTER

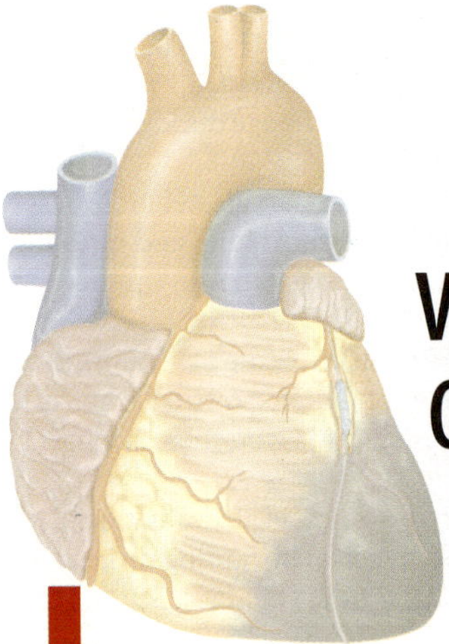

Validation of Chlorthalidone Efficacy and Outcome by Echocardiographic Variables

Harsh Wardhan, Nitin Aggarwal

INTRODUCTION

Chlorthalidone (CTD), the "long lost diuretic", is being reexplored, and increased awareness of its broad evidence-base for improving prognosis in hypertension (HTN) is resurfacing. Lowering of blood pressure (BP) with a diuretic-based regimen has decreased stroke, heart failure (HF), and cardiovascular disease events in several outcome-based clinical trials.[1,2] Most of the studies used the thiazide-like diuretic, CTD, yet 95% of thiazide prescriptions are for hydrochlorothiazide (HCTZ).[3] There is more evidence for CTD reducing cardiovascular events than there is for any of the other thiazide diuretics. The structure of CTD is completely unlike that of the thiazide diuretics, by not possessing the characteristic benzothiadiazine dioxide scaffold.[4] Furthermore, CTD has been shown to inhibit certain carbonic anhydrase (CA) isozymes to a degree that is more than 10,000-fold greater than classic thiazide diuretics such as HCTZ.[4]

DIAGNOSTIC AND EFFICACY ASSESSMENTS

Hypertensive patients with concurrent cardiovascular structural changes such as left ventricular hypertrophy (LVH) have a greater mortality risk than those with HTN alone.[5-7] There is an evidence to suggest that a parallel cardiac and vascular adaptation exists in arterial HTN[8] with a positive relationship between cardiac mass and arterial stiffness.[9] A direct relationship between cardiac mass and BP has been demonstrated, and the main pressure determinants of left ventricular mass (LVM) in essential HTN are systolic BP and pulse pressure (PP).[10-12] Reduced aortic distensibility and compliance may participate in the genesis of cardiac hypertrophy in HTN. Arterial compliance also determines the pulsatile amplitude of the pressure wave and its reduction induces a selective increase in systolic level and PP. Consequently a different response after antihypertensive treatment has been demonstrated in cardiac and arterial changes.[13,14] Left ventricular dimensions were assessed using two-dimensionally directed M-mode echocardiography. Echocardiographic measurements [left ventricular internal dimension (LVID), posterior wall thickness (PWT), and interventricular septum thickness (IVST)] were assessed at the end of diastole, defined as the peak of the R wave of the QRS complex, and in accordance with the recommendations of the American Society of Echocardiography.[15]

PROGNOSTIC IMPLICATION OF LEFT VENTRICULAR HYPERTROPHY

There is robust data indicating association between LVH and increased cardiovascular morbidity and mortality (Table 1). Levy et al.[6] reported that LVH, quantified by echocardiography, independently predicts cardiovascular morbidity and mortality. A total of 3,320 participants, aged more than 40 years and free of cardiovascular disease, were enrolled in the Framingham Heart Study for 4 years. There were total 208 cardiovascular events, 37 cardiovascular

TABLE 1: Prognostic implications of LVH: Data from selected studies.

Authors	*Numbers*	*Design*	*Endpoints*	*Results*
Levy et al.[6]	3,220	Observational. >40 years old subjects from Framingham Heart study with LVH followed up for 4 years	Incidence of CV morbidity, mortality and all-cause mortality	Increased CV morbidity, mortality and all-cause mortality in both men and women
Liao et al.[20]	463	Observational. Black subjects from hospital registry free of angiographic CAD and good echocardiographic images	Incidence of CV mortality among Black men and women	Female sex independently associated with worse outcome as compared with male
Liao et al.[21]	1,089	Observational. Blacks subjects from hospital registry with coronary angiography and M mode echocardiography followed for 5 years	Effect of LVH on survival as compared with multivessel CAD and reduced systolic function	LVH carries worse prognosis than multivessel CAD or reduced EF (attributable risk 2.4 vs. 2 vs. 1.6, respectively)
Verdecchia et al.[22]	2,363	Observational. Hypertensive subjects free of CAD followed for mean of 5 years	Incidence of CVA	LVH independently associated with cerebrovascular accident
Vakili et al.[23]	48,545	Meta-analysis of 20 studies	Association between LVH and cardiovascular morbidity and all-cause mortality	LVH associated with increased CV morbidity and all-cause mortality across all groups except ESRD

(BP: blood pressure; CAD: coronary artery disease; CV: cardiovascular; CVA: cardiovascular accident; ECG: electrocardiogram; ESRD: end-stage renal disease; LVH: left ventricular hypertrophy; NHAHES: National Health and Nutritional Examination Studies)

deaths, and 124 all-cause deaths. The relative risk (RR) for developing cardiovascular disease was 1.49 in men and 1.57 in women for every 50 g/m^2 increase in the LV mass above normal. This increment was also associated with higher all-cause mortality (RR = 1.49 and 2.01 in men and women, respectively) and cardiovascular mortality (RR = 1.73 and 2.12 in men and women, respectively). Hypertensive black adults tend to have higher LV mass odds ratio and relative wall thickness when compared with their Caucasian counterparts.[16-18] In the black population, LVH portends greater cardiovascular risk as compared with other ethnic groups[19] and women fare worse as compared with men in terms of overall mortality and cardiac death.[20] Furthermore, LVH carries more risk than multivessel coronary artery disease (CAD) in this group. Liao et al.[21] showed that among 1,089 African Americans who had undergone cardiac catheterization and M-mode echocardiography, the attributable RR for all-cause mortality was 2.4 with LVH, 2.0 with reduced EF, and 1.6 with multivessel CAD. The increase in morbidity and mortality in this group could be partly due to concentric LVH phenotype, which has been independently associated with worse outcomes. Verdecchia et al.[22] showed that for each 29 g/m^2 increase in LV mass, there is a significant independent increase in the risk of stroke [RR = 1.31; 95% confidence interval (CI): 1.09–1.58] in hypertensive patients. In a meta-analysis of 20 studies with 48,545 patients, Vakili et al.[23] found that LVH consistently predicted worse cardiovascular morbidity and all-cause mortality across all groups and population except end-stage renal disease (ESRD) patients. Mean adjusted risk rates for cardiovascular morbidity and all-cause mortality were 2.3 and 2.5, respectively.

CRITICAL APPRAISAL OF THE VALIDITY OF RELEVANT ARTICLES

Left Ventricular Hypertrophy Regression

Current evidence suggests that LVH can be targeted through reducing BP by pharmacotherapy and lifestyle modifications. However, agents that lower BP do not necessarily have equivalent effects on LV mass, which suggests that additional factors modulate expression of LVH. It is being recognized that neurohormonal and genetic factors play an equally important role in the pathogenesis of LVH. Modulating this factor to target LVH is a promising avenue in the future. All antihypertensive drugs appear to have some effect on LVH regression (Fig. 1). While there is no consensus on the best pharmacologic agent to regress LVH, the current evidence favors the drug-targeting renin-angiotensin-aldosterone system (RAAS) and diuretics. CTD has been employed in four major trials evaluating hard outcomes: the Hypertension Detection and Follow-up Program (HDFP),[24] Multiple Risk Factor Intervention Trial (MRFIT),[25,26]

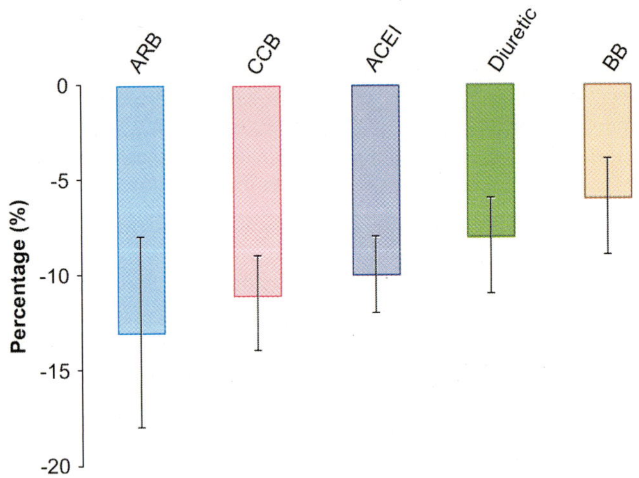

Fig. 1: LVH regression with antihypertensive treatment.
(ACEI: angiotensin-converting enzyme inhibitor; ARB: angiotensin-receptor blocker; BB: beta-blocker; CCB: calcium channel blocker; LVH: left ventricular hypertrophy).

Systolic Hypertension in the Elderly Program (SHEP),[27] and the Antihypertensive and Lipid-Lowering Treatment to Prevent Heart Attack Trial (ALLHAT).[28] In 1979, the HDFP showed that utilizing 25–100 mg of CTD daily as initial HTN therapy leads to a reduction in all-cause mortality as compared with placebo.[29]

In one of the largest trials till date, ALLHAT,[28] a total of 33,357 participants aged 55 years or older with HTN and at least one other coronary heart disease (CHD) risk factor were randomly assigned to receive CTD, 12.5–25 mg/d (n = 15,255); amlodipine, 2.5–10 mg/d (n = 9,048); or lisinopril, 10–40 mg/d (n = 9,054) for planned follow-up of approximately 4–8 years. The trial showed neither amlodipine [representing calcium channel blockers (CCBs), particularly dihydropyridine (DHP) CCBs] nor lisinopril [representing angiotensin-converting enzyme (ACE) inhibitors] was superior to CTD (representing thiazide-type diuretics) in preventing major coronary events or in increasing survival. CTD was superior to amlodipine (by about 25%) in preventing HF, overall, and for hospitalized or fatal cases, although it did not differ from amlodipine in overall cardiovascular disease prevention. CTD was superior to lisinopril in lowering BP and in preventing aggregate cardiovascular events, principally stroke, HF, angina, and coronary revascularization. ALLHAT previously reported that CTD was superior to doxazosin (representing alpha-blockers) in reducing BP and preventing cardiovascular events, particularly HF.

In SHEP[27] and the Systolic Hypertension in Europe trial, in which a thiazide-like diuretic (CTD) or a DHP-CCB was compared with a placebo, major CHD events were reduced by 27% and 30%, and stroke by 37% and 42%, respectively. MRFIT,[25,26] randomly assigned 8,012 hypertensive men to special intervention (SI) or usual care (UC). SI participants could use CTD or HCTZ initially; previous analyses have grouped clinics by their main diuretic used (C-clinics: CTD; H-clinics: HCTZ). After 48 months, SI participants receiving HCTZ were recommended to switch to CTD, in part, because higher mortality was observed for SI compared to UC participants in H-clinics, while the opposite was found in C-clinics. This trial also shows that overall LVH incidence was lower in the SI compared to the UC group and that reductions in BP were associated with a reduced incidence of LVH. It is possible that the differences in LVH between CTD and HCTZ may have occurred as a consequence of improved BP control in participants receiving CTD than HCTZ. Recent analysis of data from the MRFIT showed that the CTD-treated cohort had greater LVH regression than the HCTZ-treated and UC groups. This effect was thought to be secondary to greater reduction in BP with CTD. The Treatment of Mild Hypertension Study (TOMHS)[29] compared the effects of both pharmacological and nonpharmacological approaches with the treatment of HTN on LVH regression. It was a double-blind, placebo-controlled trial involving 844 patients with mild hypertension. The patients were advised weight loss and dietary salt reduction, nutritional-hygienic intervention (NH), or NH intervention and randomized to one of the five classes of antihypertensives: (1) CTD (a diuretic); (2) acebutolol (a β-blocker); (3) doxazosin (an α-antagonist); (4) amlodipine (a calcium channel antagonist); or (5) enalapril (an ACE inhibitor). After a follow-up of 4 years, NH intervention was as effective as NH intervention and pharmacological intervention in reducing LV mass. Interestingly, there was a smaller decrease in BP in the NH intervention only arm (9 vs 13.3 mm Hg). All the groups showed a significant decrease in LV mass from baseline and addition of CTD had modest additional effect on reducing LV mass. In a meta-analysis, Klingbeil et al.[30] identified 80 trials with 146 treatment arms (3,767 patients) and 17 placebo arms, and the data were adjusted for treatment duration and diastolic BP. They found a significant difference among different medication classes ($P = 0.004$). Overall, LV mass index was decreased with (95% CI) by 13% with angiotensin II receptor antagonists, 11% with calcium channel antagonists, 10% with ACE inhibitors, 8% with diuretics, and by 6% with β-blockers (Fig. 1).

Left Ventricular Hypertrophy Regression and Outcome

Left ventricular hypertrophy is an adaptive response by the human heart targeted to maintain cardiac output in the face of increased pressure and/or volume overload. This compensatory response ultimately regresses into a

TABLE 2: LVH regression and outcome: Data from selected studies.

Authors	*Numbers*	*Design*	*Endpoints*	*Results*
Levy et al.[31]	524	Observational. Subjects from Framingham Heart Study with LVH by ERK were followed. Total of 2,660 persons examination	Incidence of CV disease	Improvement in EKG features of LVH result in decrease CV risk
Mathew et al.[32]	8,281	Randomized, double-blinded case control study comparing ramipril and placebo among high-risk patient Followed for 4.5 years	Prevention, progression and regression of LVH CV death, MI and all-cause death in prevention/regression arm vs. persistence/progression arm	Patient treated with ramipril protected against LVH. Reduction of CHF and composite outcome of CV death, MI and all-cause death in prevention/regression arm
Verdecchia et al.[33]	430	Observational. Patient who attended base-line visit and follow-up visit in the setting of PUIMA registry Total 1,217 patients year of follow-up	Incidence of CV disease	Regression of LV mass associated with lesser of cardiovascular risk adjusted for baseline LVH
Verdecchia et al.[34]	1,064	Meta-analysis. Four studies with LVH defined by echocardiogram	LVH regression and CV risk	LVH regression reduced the risk of CV disease
Devereux et al.[35]	941	Prospective, randomized case control study. 50–85 years of patient and electrocardiographically determined LVH randomized to losartan and placebo followed up for 4.8 years	Composite endpoint of CV death, fatal or nonfatal MI and fatal or nonfatal stroke	LVH regression with treatment lowers primary endpoint independent of BP reduction and assigned treatment
Okin et al.[36]	7,998	Prospective Randomized, double-blind study. Hypertensive patient with EKG defined LVH assigned to losartan or atenolol	New onset DM per 1985 WHO criteria	Regression or LV mass progression associated with lower incidence of DM
Wachtell et al.[37]	679	Observational study among participant of LIFF study Follow-up for 3 years	Evaluation LV systolic performance	Regression of LVH with antihypertensive associated with improved stress corrected mid-wall shortening, a marker of systolic performance

(BP: blood pressure; CHF: congestive heart failure; DM: diabetes mellitus; ECG: electrocardiogram; LVH: left ventricular hypertrophy; MI: myocardial infarction; PUIMA: Progetto Ipertensione Umbria Monitoraggio Ambulatoriale)

maladaptive one causing HF. This transition is basically determined by the complex interplay of environmental, neurohormonal, and genetic factors. Over the last two decades, our understating of the pathophysiology of LVH has greatly improved. As a result, attempts to stem or reverse this phenotypic response using pharmacological agents and lifestyle modifications have been fruitful and new novel approaches are being explored. Regression of LVH is independently associated with improved cardiovascular outcome (Table 2). Levy et al.[31] reported reduction in LVH using Cornell voltage criteria was associated with improved cardiovascular outcome in men and women [odds ratio (OR) = 0.46, 95% CI and OR = 0.56, 95% CI, respectively] after adjusting for age and baseline voltage; whereas worsening or no serial change conferred worse outcome. In the same study, the severity of LVH at baseline predicted the outcome in graded manner with the lower quartile associated with lower risk than the highest quartile. In the LVH regression sub-study of the Heart Outcomes Prevention Evaluation (HOPE) trial,[32] LVH prevention or regression significantly reduced primary outcome of cardiovascular death, myocardial infarction and death (12.3% vs 15.4%, $p < 0.006$) and congestive HF (9.3% vs. 15.4%, $p < 0.0001$) when compared with LVH persistence or progression. In both the studies LVH was defined by electrocardiogram criteria which are less sensitive to echocardiography in defining LVH. Regardless, this association holds even when echocardiography is used to define LV mass.

Verdecchia et al.[33] followed 430 patients with serial echocardiography and 24-hour ambulatory BP monitoring from the Progetto Ipertensione Umbria Monitoraggio Ambulatoriale (PIUMA) registry. Total duration of follow-up was 1,217 patients per year. They showed a reduction in LV mass among the patients with essential HTN, predicted lower cardiovascular risk ($p < 0.04$) adjusted for baseline LVH. In the same study, the event rate was lower among the subset of patients with LV mass more than 125g/m^2 with LVH regression than the patients whose LV mass remained persistently elevated (1.58 vs. 6.27 events per 100 person-years; $p = 0.002$). In a meta-analysis, the same group showed association between LVH regression and lower cardiovascular decreased events.[34] A total of 1,064 hypertensive patients from four studies were included in the analysis and showed that LVH regression reduced the risk of subsequent cardiovascular disease ($P = 0.007$) as compared with lack of regression or development of new LVH. In the Life Echo Study, 941 patients aged between 55 years and 80 years with essential HTN and electrocardiographic and echocardiographic evidence were followed for a mean of 4.8 years for composite endpoint of cardiovascular death, fatal, and nonfatal myocardial infarction and fatal or nonfatal stroke.[35] The composite endpoint occurred in 11% of the patients and Cox regression analysis showed a strong association between LVH regression with treatment and composite endpoint ($P = 0.009$) independent of reduction in the BP and assigned treatment. There was a parallel independent association between LVH regression and lower cardiovascular mortality, all-cause mortality and myocardial infarction.

Interestingly, regression or absence of progression of LV mass has been reported to be associated with lower incidence of diabetes mellitus.[36] In addition, LVH regression has been reported to improve LV systolic performance.[37] A total of 679 hypertensive patients with electrocardiogram evidence of LVH from the Losartan Intervention for Endpoint Reduction (LIFE) substudy were followed with a yearly echocardiogram during 3 years of antihypertensive treatment. During this period, the mean BP reduction and LV mass regression were approximately 15% and 17%, respectively, and the stress-corrected mid-wall fractional shortening increased from 97 ± 13 to 105 ± 12% ($P < 0.001$). This improvement was independently inversely related to changes in LVM ($\beta = -0.211$) and relative wall thickness ($\beta = -0.334$). Thus, LVH regression also improved LV systolic function.

CHLORTHALIDONE VERSUS THIAZIDE DIURETICS

Based on analysis of multiple studies, CTD significantly reduced the morality data after a 10.5-year follow-up from MRFIT.[25,26] In March 1980, the CHD mortality of SI clinics using HCTZ was 44% higher than other clinics ($P = 0.23$). From April 1980, the rate of CHD mortality in those clinics decreased by 28% by using CTD as the thiazide diuretic. Obviously, one question that needs to be addressed is why CTD showed better efficacy in reducing cardiovascular events as compared with HCTZ when both agents work in a pharmacologically similar fashion. The answer may be that:

- Chlorthalidone, at the doses studied, is a more potent antihypertensive agent resulting in greater BP lowering and better outcomes.
- Improved metabolic profile: When evaluating the metabolic profile, the CTD group had lower low-density lipoprotein (LDL) and glucose values as compared with the HCTZ group. The lower the LDL levels the greater the chance of reducing cardiovascular events. Similarly, impaired glucose tolerance may also contribute to cardiovascular disease. The trends in glucose values were higher in the HCTZ group compared with the CTD group. The reason for the improved metabolic profile seen in the CTD group is not known.
- Other reasons for improved outcomes with CTD may relate to differences in pharmacokinetic and pharmacodynamic properties between CTD and HCTZ. With regard to pharmacokinetics, the half-life of CTD (45–60 hours) is much longer than the half-life of HCTZ (16–24 hours), and CTD has a larger volume of distribution.
- Chlorthalidone is thought to be 1.5–2 times more potent than HCTZ, with 24-hour ambulatory BP monitoring demonstrating lower BP with CTD during the nighttime hours.[8]

Chlorthalidone: Cellular and Molecular Mechanisms Relevant to Pathogenesis of Cardiovascular Disease

In vitro experiments by Woodman et al.[38] in which CTD was found to reduce epinephrine-induced platelet aggregation and increase angiogenesis much more than bendroflumethiazide, a thiazide diuretic that is widely used in the United Kingdom. If the greater effects of CTD on platelet aggregation and angiogenesis are also obtained in vivo, they could conceivably contribute to greater protection against stroke and myocardial infarction with CTD compared with bendroflumethiazide, and perhaps other thiazides as well. In cultured vascular smooth muscle cells, Woodman et al.[38] also found that CTD reduced expression of messenger ribonucleic acids (mRNAs) for vascular endothelial growth factor C and transforming growth factor-β3 much more than bendroflumethiazide. These proteins have potential to affect a variety of factors that could influence pathogenesis of cardiovascular disease, including interstitial fluid volume balance and cardiac fibrosis and remodeling.[39,40] Thus, the results of Woodman et al. raise the possibility that CTD differs from thiazides with respect to many mechanisms that could theoretically influence a host of cardiovascular outcomes in patients with HTN.

Chlorthalidone: a Strong Inhibitor of Multiple Isoforms of Carbonic Anhydrase

Chlorthalidone inhibits the activity of most CA isozymes much more potently than HCTZ when tested at concentrations within ranges that can be achieved in plasma with suitable oral dosing, the inhibitory potency of CTD against some CA isozymes (e.g. CA VII) is more than 1,000-fold greater than that of HCTZ.[41]

CONCLUSION

Left ventricular hypertrophy is a result of complex interaction among genetic makeup, lifestyle, and environment factors. It represents the end organ dysfunction in HTN and other disease. Multiple studies have shown that LVH is an independent risk factor of increased cardiovascular morbidity and mortality and is of major public health burden. Evidence suggests that targeting LVH regression is possible and results in improved clinical outcomes. Therefore, regression of LVH can be considered surrogate endpoint in the treatment of hypertensive heart disease. Among various drugs, the ones targeting RAAS and diuretics appear to have class actions in reducing LV mass independent of BP control. CTD appears to have meaningful, pleiotropic effects, not necessarily shared by other diuretics, on platelet aggregation, gene transcription, angiogenesis, and vascular permeability. It is also the most potent inhibitor of CA among other diuretics used in the treatment of HTN, reduces platelet aggregation and vascular permeability and promotes angiogenesis much more effectively than other diuretics and also contributes to reductions in the morbidity and mortality associated with essential HTN, so among all diuretics, CTD should continue to be the first-line treatment for essential HTN. Also, because CTD differs from thiazides in many important respects, the use of the vague term "thiazide-like diuretic" should be abandoned.

REFERENCES

1. Dinicolantonio JJ. Hydrochlorothiazide: is it a wise choice? Expert Opin Pharmacother. 2012;1(6):807-14.
2. Ernst ME, Moser M. Use of diuretics in patients with hypertension. N Engl J Med. 2009;361(22):2153-64.
3. Ernst ME, Lund BC. Renewed interest in chlorthalidone: evidence from the Veterans Health Administration. J Clin Hypertens (Greenwich). 2010;12(12):927-34.
4. Kurtz TW. Chlorthalidone: don't call it "Thiazide-Like" anymore. Hypertension. 2010;56(3):335-7.
5. Koren MJ, Devereux RB, Casale PN, et al. Relation of left ventricular mass and geometry to morbidity and mortality in uncomplicated essential hypertension. Ann Intern Med. 1991;114(5):345-52.
6. Levy D, Garrison RJ, Savage DD, et al. Prognostic implications of echocardiographically determined left ventricular mass in the Framingham Heart Study. N Engl J Med. 1990;322(22):1561-6.
7. Ghanem WM, Murin J, Sleiman O, et al. Is left ventricular hypertrophy a risk factor in hypertensive patients? Bratisl Lek Listy. 2002;103(6):215-22.
8. Roman MJ, Saba PG, Pini R, et al. Parallel cardiac and vascular adaptation in hypertension. Circulation. 1992;86(6):1909-18.
9. Bouthier JD, De Luca N, Safar ME, et al. Cardiac hypertrophy and arterial distensibility in essential hypertension. Am Heart J. 1985;109(6):1345-52.
10. Gasowski J, Fagard RH, Staessen JA, et al. INDANA Project Collaborators: Pulsatile blood pressure component as predictor of mortality in hypertension: a meta-analysis of clinical trial control groups. J Hypertens. 2002;20(1):145-51.
11. Jokiniitty JM, Majahalme SK, Kahonen MA, et al. Pulse pressure is the best predictor of future left ventricular mass and change in left ventricular mass: 10 years of follow-up. J Hypertens. 2001;19(11):2047-54.
12. Pini R, Cavallini MC, Bencini F, et al. Cardiovascular remodelling is greater in isolated systolic hypertension than in diastolic hypertension in older adults: the Insufficienza cardiaca negli Anziani residenti (ICARE) a Dicomano Study. J Am Coll Cardiol. 2002;40(7):1283-9.
13. Olsen MH, Wachtell K, Hermann KL, et al. Is cardiovascular remodelling in patients with essential hypertension related to more than high blood pressure? A LIFE substudy. Losartan Intervention for Endpoint-Reduction in Hypertension. Am J Heart. 2002;144(3):530-7.
14. Asmar RG, Pannier B, Santoni JP, et al. Reversion of cardiac hypertrophy and reduced arterial compliance after converting enzyme inhibition in essential hypertension. Circulation. 1988;78(4):941-50.
15. Cheitlin MD, Alpert JS, Armstrong WF, et al. ACC/AHA guidelines for the clinical application of echocardiography. A report of the American College of Cardiology/American Heart Association Task Force on practice guidelines (Committee on Clinical Application of Echocardiography). Developed in collaboration with the American Society of Echocardiography. Circulation. 1997;95(6):1686-744.

16. Devereux BJ, Reichek N. Echocardiographic determination of left ventricular mass in man. Anatomic validation of the methods. Circulation. 1977;55(4):613-8.
17. De Simone G, Daniels S, Devereux R, et al. Left ventricular mass and body size in normotensive children and adults: assessment of allometric relations and impact of overweight. JACC. 1992;20(5):1251-60.
18. Kizer JR, Arnett DK, Bella JN, et al. Differences in left ventricular structure between Black and White hypertensive adults: the Hypertension Genetic Epidemiology Network Study. Hypertension. 2004;43(6):1182-8.
19. Havranek EP, Froshaug DB, Emserman CD, et al. Left ventricular hypertrophy and cardiovascular mortality by race and ethnicity. Am J Med. 2008;121(10):870-5.
20. Liao Y, Cooper RS, Mensah GA, et al. Left ventricular hypertrophy has a greater impact on survival in women than in men. Circulation. 1995;92(4):805-10.
21. Liao Y, Cooper RS, McGee DL, et al. The relative effects of left ventricular hypertrophy, coronary artery disease, and ventricular dysfunction on survival among black adults. JAMA. 1995;273(20):1592-7.
22. Verdecchia P, Porcellati C, Reboldi G, et al. Left ventricular hypertrophy as an independent predictor of acute cerebrovascular events in essential hypertension. Circulation. 2001;104(17):2039-44.
23. Vakili BA, Okin PM, Devereux RB. Prognostic implications of left ventricular hypertrophy. Am Heart J. 2001;141(3):334-41.
24. Hypertension Detection and Follow-up Program Cooperative Group. Five-year findings of the hypertension detection and follow-up program. I. Reduction in mortality of persons with high blood pressure, including mild hypertension. JAMA. 1979;242(33):2562-71.
25. The Multiple Risk Factor Intervention Trial Research Group. Mortality after 10½ years for hypertensive participants in the Multiple Risk Factor Intervention Trial. Circulation. 1990;82(5):1616-28.
26. The Multiple Risk Factor Intervention Trial Research Group. Mortality rates after 10.5 years for participants in the Multiple Risk Factor Intervention Trial. Findings related to a priority hypotheses of the trial. JAMA. 1990;263(13):1795-801.
27. SHEP Cooperative Research Group. Prevention of stroke by antihypertensive drug treatment in older persons with isolated systolic hypertension: final results of the Systolic Hypertension in the Elderly Program (SHEP). JAMA. 1991;265(24):3255-64.
28. ALLHAT Officers and Coordinators for the ALLHAT Collaborative Research Group. Major outcomes in high-risk hypertensive patients randomized to angiotensin-converting enzyme inhibitor or calcium channel blocker versus diuretic: Antihypertensive and Lipid-Lowering Treatment to Prevent Heart Attack Trail (ALLHAT). JAMA. 2002;288(23):2981-97.
29. Neaton JD, Grimm RH Jr, Prineas RJ. Treatment of Mild Hypertension Study: final results. Treatment of Mild Hypertension Study Research Group. JAMA. 1993;270(6):713-24.
30. Klingbeil AU, Schneider M, Martus P, et al. A meta-analysis of the effects of treatment on left ventricular mass in essential hypertension. Am J Med. 2003;115(1):41-6.
31. Levy D, Salomon M, D'Agostino RB, et al. Prognostic implications of baseline electrocardiographic features and their serial changes in subjects with left ventricular hypertrophy. Circulation. 1994;90(4):1786-93.
32. Mathew J, Sleight P, Lonn E, et al. Reduction of cardiovascular risk by regression of electrocardiographic markers of left ventricular hypertrophy by the angiotensin-converting enzyme inhibitor ramipril. Circulation. 2001;104(14):1615-21.
33. Verdecchia P, Schillaci G, Borgioni C, et al. Prognostic significance of serial changes in left ventricular mass in essential hypertension. Circulation. 1998;97(1):48-54.
34. Verdecchia P, Angeli F, Borgioni C, et al. Changes in cardiovascular risk by reduction of left ventricular mass in hypertension: a meta-analysis. Am J Hypertens. 2003;16(11 Pt 1):895-9.
35. Devereux RB, Wachtell K, Gerdts E, et al. Prognostic significance of left ventricular mass change during treatment of hypertension. JAMA. 2004;292(19):2350-6.
36. Okin PM, Devereux RB, Harris KE, et al. In-treatment resolution or absence of electrocardiographic left ventricular hypertrophy is associated with decreased incidence of new-onset diabetes mellitus in hypertensive patients: the Losartan Intervention for Endpoint Reduction in Hypertension (LIFE) Study. Hypertension. 2007;50(5):984-90.
37. Wachtell K, Palmieri V, Olsen MH, et al. Change in systolic left ventricular performance after 3 years of antihypertensive treatment: the Losartan Intervention for Endpoint (LIFE) study. Circulation. 2002;106(2):227-32.
38. Woodman R, Brown C, Lockette W. Chlorthalidone decreases platelet aggregation and vascular permeability and promotes angiogenesis. Hypertension. 2010;56(3):463-70.
39. Machnik A, Neuhofer W, Jantsch J, et al. Macrophages regulate salt-dependent volume and blood pressure by a vascular endothelial growth factor-C dependent buffering mechanism. Nat Med. 2009;15(5):545-52.
40. Bujak M, Frangogiannis NG. The role of TGF-β3 signaling in myocardial infarction and cardiac remodeling. Cardiovasc Res. 2007;74(2):184-95.
41. Temperini C, Cecchi A, Scozzafava A, et al. Carbonic anhydrase inhibitors: sulfonamide diuretics revisited-old leads for new applications? Org Biomol Chem. 2008;6(14):2499-506.

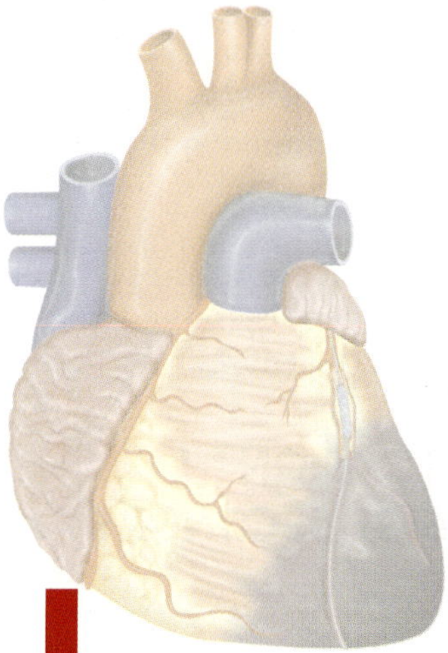

15

CHAPTER

Secondary Hypertension Evaluation: Multimodality Imaging

Simran Kaur, Rohin Vinayak, Ravina Sharma, Gurpreet Singh Wander

INTRODUCTION

Secondary (acquired or remediable) hypertension (HT) constitutes 5–10% of the total hypertensives. Essential (primary) HT though being the most common, evaluation and exclusion of remediable causes can increase the potential for complete control, thus decreasing the long-term morbidities like cardiovascular event, cerebrovascular accidents, and chronic kidney disease (CKD).[1]

WHEN TO SUSPECT SECONDARY HYPERTENSION

Secondary HT should be suspected in cases with onset of HT at age less than 25 (especially with no family history of HT) or older than 55 years, resistant (refractory) HT, with severe end-organ damage (as in grade III or IV retinopathy), recurrent flash pulmonary edema, abdominal bruit (especially with louder diastolic component), specific body habitus or ancillary physical findings, and sudden rise in serum creatinine more than or equal to 30% on initiation of renin-angiotensin-aldosterone system (RAAS) blockers.[1,2]

CAUSES OF SECONDARY HYPERTENSION

The various causes of secondary HT include:

- *Renal parenchymal (80% of secondary HT and 2–6% of all hypertensives)*: CKD, glomerulonephritis, autosomal dominant polycystic kidney disease (ADPKD I and II), autosomal recessive polycystic kidney disease (ARPKD), and reflux nephropathy.
- *Renovascular hypertension (0.5–4%)*: Renal artery stenosis (RAS) due to atherosclerotic disease, fibromuscular dysplasia (FMD-medial, paramedial, intimal or medial hyperplasia), arterial embolus, arteriovenous fistula (congenital/traumatic), segmental arterial occlusion, extrinsic compression of the renal artery (e.g. leiomyosarcomas, pheochromocytoma), and renal compression (e.g. metastatic or retroperitoneal mass).
- *Vascular hypertension*: Due to vascular involvement of vessels other than renal, like in systemic vasculitis (Takayasu arteritis, polyarteritis), coarctation of aorta, vascular occlusion due to endovascular aortic stent graft, etc.
- *Endocrine abnormalities*: Primary hyperaldosteronism (1.4–6%), Cushing syndrome (0.5–1%), pheochromocytoma or paraganglioma (0.3–0.6%), primary hypothyroidism, hyperthyroidism, hyperparathyroidism (HPTH), acromegaly, and renin-secreting tumors.
- *Hereditary or congenital causes*: Multiple endocrinal neoplasia (MEN) 2A, 2B (pheochromocytomas), neuroblastomas, FMD, renal parenchymal diseases (e.g. Alport disease, ADPKD, ARPKD), familial hyperaldosteronism, congenital adrenal hyperplasia, and monogenic primary renal tubular diseases (Gordon's syndrome, Liddle's syndrome, apparent mineralocorticoid excess, Geller's syndrome, HT-brachydactyly syndrome).

- *Lifestyle related*: Obesity and obstructive sleep apnea.
- *Drug-induced (1%)*: Oral contraceptives, steroids, psychiatric medications (buspirone, carbamazepine, clozapine, fluoxetine, lithium, tricyclic antidepressants), sympathomimetic decongestants, diet pills, and illicit drugs like opioids, amphetamines and some Chinese herbs like ginseng. In current times, bodybuilding supplements and anabolic steroid abuse can also be the implicating factor.[1-7]

DIAGNOSIS OF SECONDARY HYPERTENSION

History and Physical Examination

The evaluation begins with detailed history for localization of the possible causes, like paroxysmal spells of headache, sweating, and palpitations in 30–40% cases of pheochromocytoma, proximal muscle weakness in Cushing syndrome, lower limb weakness and cramps in primary hyperaldosteronism, hirsutism and virilization in congenital adrenal hyperplasia, drugs and family history. Thorough clinical examination for features of acromegaly, myxedema, exophthalmos, central obesity, moon face, buffalo hump, and purple striae or bitemporal hemianopia (Cushing disease). Examination for neck, chest, abdominal (coarctation) or renal angle bruit (RAS) and unequal or absent peripheral pulses and differences in BP in all limbs (Takayasu), in upper and lower extremities (coarctation).[1-3] The investigations for possible etiology begin with basic biochemical tests to evaluate renal function (blood urea nitrogen, serum creatinine, electrolytes, urine routine), thyroid profile and cortisol levels, and disease specific special tests. The whole armamentarium of investigations for possible etiologies is beyond the scope of the book. The multimodality imaging for evaluation of some of the major causes of secondary HT will be discussed briefly in this chapter.

Multimodality Imaging

There is a major role of a spectrum of invasive and noninvasive imaging in diagnosis of secondary HT. The diagnosis is facilitated by disease-specific choice of one or more imaging modality, used concurrently or sequentially. The choice of imaging modality is with respect to the various differentials, with careful consideration for the contraindications and potential risks associated with each.

- *Ultrasonography (USG)*: Renal, abdominal, neck, and pelvic.
- *Duplex USG*: Renal vessels and aorta.
- *Computerized tomography (CT) with or without contrast*: Renal, abdominal, and pelvic.
- *Magnetic resonance imaging (MRI)*: Renal, abdominal, and pelvic.
- Conventional or selective vascular angiography.
- Computerized tomography and MR angiography.
- *Nuclear scintigraphy*: Tc99m-dimercaptosuccinic acid (DMSA), captopril renography, and radionuclide voiding cystourethrogram (VCU).

The rational use of one or more of these when collaborated with clinical features, examination and biochemical tests, facilitates in the diagnoses.

APPROACH TO EVALUATION IN MAJOR ETIOLOGIES OF SECONDARY HYPRETENSION

Renal Parenchymal Diseases

The most common cause of secondary HT, can be diagnosed on ultrasound by morphological evaluation of the kidneys (size, shape, echogenicity, corticomedullary differentiation, difference in renal size, scarring), with deranged renal function, proteinuria ± hematuria. CT (with or without contrast) with resolution and reconstruction techniques renders this modality capable of identifying parenchymal characteristics, including malignancy and stones.[8] Diagnostic clues for different renal parenchymal causes are:

- Chronic glomerulonephritis or nephrosclerosis or interstitial diseases—bilaterally small kidneys.
- Polycystic kidney disease: Large lobulated kidney with multiple cysts replacing normal renal parenchyma (with cysts in other organs—liver, pancreas, seminal vesicles, prostate and epididymis). Early detection of renal and hepatic cysts can be done with MRI abdomen in younger age patients with family history of ADPKD.[9] Brain CT or MR angiography can help in diagnosing PKD-related arachnoid cyst and berry aneurysms.[10]
- Reflux nephropathy: Micturating cystourethrography (MCU) and radionuclide cystography for diagnosing reflux. Renal cortical scarring sometimes appreciable on ultrasound, best appreciable on DMSA (for cortical function, activity and scarring).[11]
- Obstructive nephropathy: Renal or ureteric calculi and cortical thinning.
- Chronic pyelonephritic or dysplastic kidney: Unequal size or abnormal shape.
- Ectopic atrophic or solitary kidney.

Renovascular Hypertension

The two most common etiology of RAS according to the age group are atherosclerosis in the elderly and FMD in the younger age group. Atherosclerosis is characterized by progressive luminal stenosis mainly involving the renal arteries, along with other arteries because of its systemic nature. When it affects the renal arteries, it typically involves the proximal segment, within 2 cm from the ostia.[12] FMD affects the middle or distal segment of the renal arteries. It is an idiopathic vascular disorder with a predilection for renal arteries in young adults and occurs more often in females than in males.[13] The median FMD, which is the most common type, has a characteristic "string of beads" appearance of the affected artery, and represents alternating segments of thin and thick portions of the collagen-containing medial layer.[14] RAS can be suspected on renal USG showing unequal kidneys (the one smaller than its counterpart with discrepancy greater than 1.5 cm) and further evaluated using duplex ultrasound. US diagnostic criteria for RAS can be divided into direct signs (seen at the site of stenosis) and indirect signs (which are distal to the stenosis).[15] Direct signs include a peak systolic velocity (PSV) greater than 200 cm/s; a renal artery PSV to prerenal abdominal aorta PSV ratio higher than 3.5:1.0, the lack of a Doppler US signal indicating occlusion and the presence of color artifacts such as aliasing related to turbulence. The flow velocity increases in proportion to the degree of luminal narrowing. Disorderly flow detected at the site of the luminal narrowing manifests as turbulence and/or spectral broadening. Indirect signs of RAS (those distal to the site of stenosis)—include a spectral waveform with a delayed and blunted systolic upstroke known as pulsus parvus et tardus (correlates with an acceleration index lower than 300 cm/s^2, an acceleration time longer than 70 ms, and a loss of early systolic peak). The presence of parvus et tardus waveform has a high specificity (96%) and positive predictive value (92%) for the diagnosis of RAS; however, its sensitivity is only 43%.[15]

Computed tomography angiography using helical, multiple detector scanners and contrast-enhanced CT can provide excellent images of both kidneys, the vascular tree and even the smaller vessels.[16] Three-dimensional phase contrast MRI can evaluate the degrees of RAS, as signal intensity corresponds with flow velocity. Any obstruction in the flow will result in severe dephasing in MR signals and the degree of dephasing correlates with the gradient across the obstruction. Using a combination of the time-of-flight MR angiography with phase contrast sequences can increase the specificity, positive predictive value, and accuracy to 90%, 58%, and 92%, respectively.[17,18] Conventional angiography is the gold standard for diagnosis and gives opportunity for concurrent therapeutic intervention.[1] Radionuclide technetium-99m mercaptoacetyltriglycine (^{99}Tc-MAG3)-captopril renography, based on reduction in ipsilateral renal uptake after administration of captopril, has a high sensitivity and specificity, and it adds a physiologic element to the diagnosis of RAS.[19]

Vascular Hypertension

Steno-occlusion of the aorta can be suspected from basic imaging like chest radiograph showing left ventricular hypertrophy, small aortic arch contour and/or notching of the ribs in coarctation, but confirmation needs CT, MR or conventional angiography for location of the stenotic portion, various collaterals, and other associated anomalies. CT angiography and MR angiography have an advantage of also giving a fair idea of vessel wall thickness.[1,7]

Endocrine Hypertension

Screening tests for hormonal imbalances have a relatively higher probability for diagnosis than other causes of secondary HT.

Primary Hyperaldosteronism

The two principal causes of primary hyperaldosteronism are: adrenal adenoma (35%) and bilateral adrenal hyperplasia (65%). Benign lesions including adenomas are readily diagnosed on precontrast CT or chemical shift MR imaging, when lipid component is evident within the adrenal mass.[20,21] However, when an adrenal incidentaloma is lipid-poor, multiphasic contrast-enhanced CT is usually required. On MRI, adenomas are hypo or isointense in T1 (when compared to the liver) and slightly hyperintense in T2 and demonstrate a sensitivity of 70% and a specificity of 100% for the diagnosis of these tumors very similar to those offered by CT.[22,23]

Cushing Syndrome

After excluding exogenous corticosteroid use (most common cause of Cushing syndrome), pathology can be localized anywhere in the hypothalamic-pituitary-adrenal axis.[24] MRI is helpful in visualizing pituitary in adrenocorticotropic hormone (ACTH)-dependent type (since corticotroph adenoma of the pituitary gland is the cause in 80–85%).[25] In those with ACTH-dependent Cushing syndrome but without a pituitary pathology, or in ACTH-independent Cushing syndrome, adrenal CT to detect incidentaloma can yield results. Patients with excessive ACTH secretion may also have bilateral adrenal cortical hyperplasia with strong enhancement on CT and hypermetabolism in bilateral adrenal cortices on whole body positron emission tomography (PET).[26]

Pheochromocytoma

These are rare tumors originating from the adrenal medulla with rule of "10" applying to them, i.e. 10% are extra-adrenal (called paragangliomas), 10% are bilateral, 10% are multiple, and 10% are malignant. Familial cases are associated with MEN 2A, 2B, von Hippel-Lindau syndrome, and neurofibromatosis (NF) type I.[27,28] Laboratory evaluation needs metanephrine level in a 24-hour urine or plasma sample. On CT, pheochromocytoma shows a varied appearance due to variable fat content, hemorrhage and/or calcifications, but the solid components are usually well-enhanced. Typical MR findings include T1-hypo- and T2-hyperintensities. In false-negative cases, nuclear imaging tests such as metaiodobenzylguanidine scintigraphy (^{123}I-MIBG) or PET may help due to their high diagnostic accuracy.[29]

Thyroid Dysfunction

Thyroid abnormalities (hyper or hypothyroidism) are predominantly diagnosed by biochemical tests, but ultrasound of the neck may help in certain cases of thyroid enlargement (diffuse or heterogeneous) due to thyroiditis. Nuclear scintigraphy with various radiotracers (^{99m}TC, ^{131}I, ^{123}I) can help in evaluation of thyroid functions and metabolic activity.[30]

Hyperparathyroidism

Hyperparathyroidism occurring due to pathologic condition of the parathyroid gland, with adenoma being most common cause of primary HPTH and compensatory hyperplasia following systemic conditions such as CKD, vitamin D deficiency, and malabsorption in the gastrointestinal tract causing secondary HPTH. HT occurs in 40–65% of these patients.[31,32] Parathyroid adenoma or hyperplasia can be suspected if a nodule exceeding 1 cm in size is found in an extrathyroid location on USG or CT. Adenomas being hypervascular are hypoechoic compared to the overlying thyroid gland on gray-scale USG and on multiphase CT. A precontrast scan may discriminate hypodense adenoma from iodine-rich thyroid gland, while an enhanced scan may show a hypervascular nature. Larger lesions may show heterogeneous attenuation or calcifications. Sestamibi scintigraphy helps in diagnosis and localization of adenomatous and hyperplastic parathyroid due to their high avidity and longer retention (clearly noted on delayed images, approximately 2 hours after Sestamibi administration). Plain radiographs may be helpful in assessing skeletal manifestation of HPTH (subperiosteal resorption, rugger-jersey spine, and brown tumors).[33,34]

REFERENCES

1. Elliot JE, Peixoto AJ, Bakris GL. Primary and secondary hypertension. In: Skorecki K, Chertow GM, Marsden PA (Eds). Brenner and Rector's The Kidney, 10th edition. Philadelphia: Saunders; 2016. pp. 1522-66.
2. Richard AM, Nicholls MG. Endocrine cause of hypertension. In: Johnson RJ, Feehally J, Floege J (Eds). Comprehensive Clinical Nephrology, 5th edition. Philadelphia: Saunders; 2016. pp. 478-87.
3. Omura M, Saito J, Yamaguchi K, et al. Prospective study on the prevalence of secondary hypertension among hypertensive patients visiting a general outpatient clinic in Japan. Hypertens Res. 2004;27(3):193-202.
4. Anderson GH, Blakeman N, Streeten DH. The effect of age on prevalence of secondary forms of hypertension in 4429 consecutively referred patients. J Hypertens. 1994;12(5):609-15.
5. Calhoun DA, Jones D, Textor S, et al. Resistant hypertension: diagnosis, evaluation, and treatment: a scientific statement from the American Heart Association Professional Education Committee of the Council for High Blood Pressure Research. Circulation. 2008;117(25):e510-26.
6. Elliott WJ. Drug interactions and drugs that affect blood pressure. J Clin Hypertens (Greenwich). 2006;8(10):731-7.
7. Ahn H, Chun EJ, Lee HJ, et al. Multimodality imaging in patients with secondary hypertension: with a focus on appropriate imaging approaches depending on the etiologies. Korean J Radiol. 2018;19(2):272-83.
8. Glockner JF, Vrtiska TJ. Renal MR and CT angiography: current concepts. Abdom Imaging. 2007;32(3):407-20.
9. Wood CG, Stromberg LJ, Harmath CB, et al. CT and MR imaging for evaluation of cystic renal lesions and diseases. Radiographics. 2015;35(1):125-41.
10. Ong AC. Screening for intracranial aneurysms in ADPKD. BMJ. 2009;339:b3763.
11. Dhandapani R, Vinjamuri S. Radioisotope in diagnostic imaging in nephrology. In: Turner NN, Lameire N, Goldsmith DJ, Winearls CG, Himmelfarb J, Giuseppe Remuzzi (Eds). Oxford Textbook of Clinical Nephrology, 4th edition. Oxford: Oxford University press; 2016.
12. Soulez G, Oliva VL, Turpin S, et al. Imaging of renovascular hypertension: respective values of renal scintigraphy, renal Doppler US, and MR angiography. Radiographics. 2000;20(5):1355-68.
13. Slovut DP, Olin JW. Fibromuscular dysplasia. N Engl J Med. 2004;350(18):1862-71.
14. Olin JW, Sealove BA. Diagnosis, management, and future developments of fibromuscular dysplasia. J Vasc Surg. 2011;53(3):826-36.
15. Granata A, Fiorini F, Andrulli S, et al. Doppler ultrasound and renal artery stenosis: an overview. J Ultrasound. 2009;12(4):133-43.
16. Pellerin O, Sapoval M, Trinquart L, et al. Accuracy of multi-detector computed tomographic angiography assisted by post-processing software for diagnosis atheromatous renal artery stenosis. Diagn Interv Imaging. 2013;94 (11):1123-31.
17. François CJ, Lum DP, Johnson KM, et al. Renal arteries: isotropic, high-spatial-resolution, unenhanced MR angiography with three-dimensional radial phase contrast radiology. 2011;258(1):254-60.
18. Loubeyre P, Trolliet P, Cahen R. MR angiography of renal artery stenosis: value of the combination of three-dimensional time-of-flight and three-dimensional phase-contrast MR angiography sequences. Am J Roentgenol. 1996;167(2):489-94.

19. Vasbinder GB, Nelemans PJ, Kessels AG, et al. Diagnostic tests for renal artery stenosis in patients suspected of having renovascular hypertension: a meta-analysis. Ann Intern Med. 2001;135(6):401-11.
20. Boland GW, Lee MJ, Gazelle GS, et al. Characterization of adrenal masses using unenhanced CT: an analysis of the CT literature. AJR Am J Roentgenol. 1998;171(1):201-4.
21. Sohaib SA, Peppercorn PD, Allan C, et al. Primary hyperaldosteronism (Conn syndrome): MR imaging findings. Radiology. 2000;214(2):527-31.
22. Alexanderson-Rosas E, Berríos-Bárcenas E, Meave A, et al. Novel contributions of multimodality imaging in hypertension: a narrative review. World J Hypertens. 2015;5(2):28-40.
23. Lingam RK, Sohaib SA, Rockall AG, et al. Diagnostic performance of CT versus MR in detecting aldosterone-producing adenoma in primary hyperaldosteronism (Conn's syndrome). Eur Radiol. 2004;14(10):1787-92.
24. Raff H, Sharma ST, Nieman LK. Physiological basis for the etiology, diagnosis, and treatment of adrenal disorders: Cushing's syndrome, adrenal insufficiency, and congenital adrenal hyperplasia. Compr Physiol. 2014;4(2):739-69.
25. Sohaib SA, Hanson JA, Newell-Price JD, et al. CT appearance of the adrenal glands in adrenocorticotrophic hormone-dependent Cushing's syndrome. AJR Am J Roentgenol. 1999;172(4):997-1002.
26. Rockall AG, Babar SA, Sohaib SA, et al. CT and MR imaging of the adrenal glands in ACTH-independent Cushing syndrome. Radiographics. 2004;24(2):435-52.
27. Sukor N. Endocrine hypertension—current understanding and comprehensive management review. Eur J Intern Med. 2011;22(5):433-40.
28. Tischler AS. Pheochromocytoma and extra-adrenal paraganglioma: updates. Arch Pathol Lab Med. 2008;132(8):1272-84.
29. Leung K, Stamm M, Raja A, et al. Pheochromocytoma: the range of appearances on ultrasound, CT, MRI, and functional imaging. AJR Am J Roentgenol. 2013;200(2):370-8.
30. Nachiappan AC, Metwalli ZA, Hailey BS, et al. The thyroid: review of imaging features and biopsy techniques with radiologic-pathologic correlation. Radiographics. 2014;34(2):276-93.
31. Silverberg SJ, Bilezikian JP. The diagnosis and management of asymptomatic primary hyperparathyroidism. Nat Clin Pract Endocrinol Metab. 2006;2(9):494-503.
32. Feldstein CA, Akopian M, Pietrobelli D, et al. Long-term effects of parathyroidectomy on hypertension prevalence and circadian blood pressure profile in primary hyperparathyroidism. Clin Exp Hypertens. 2010;32(3):154-8.
33. Johnson NA, Tublin ME, Ogilvie JB. Parathyroid imaging: technique and role in the preoperative evaluation of primary hyperparathyroidism. AJR Am J Roentgenol. 2007;188(6):1706-15.
34. Chandramohan A, Sathyakumar K, John RA, et al. Atypical ultrasound features of parathyroid tumours may bear a relationship to their clinical and biochemical presentation. Insights Imaging. 2014;5(1):103-11.

SECTION 3

Heart Failure

16

CHAPTER

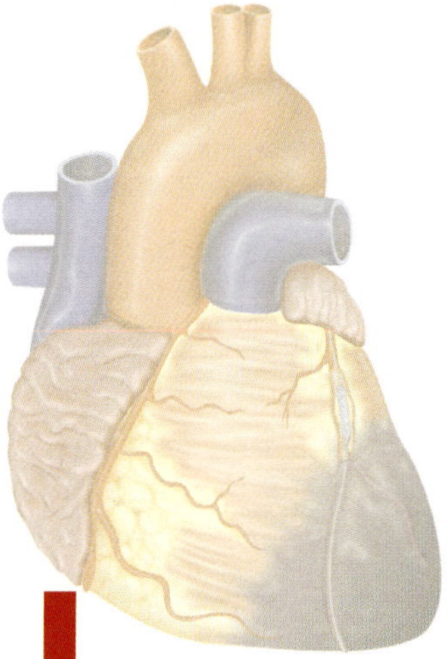

Biomarkers Imaging in Heart Failure

Bhargava Mohan, Abhinav Jain, Bhargava Prachal

INTRODUCTION

"Biomarker" has been defined by the National Institutes of Health (NIH, Bethesda, MD, USA) Director's initiative on biomarkers and surrogate endpoints to be "a characteristic that is objectively measured and evaluated as an indicator of normal biological processes, pathogenic processes, or pharmacologic responses to a therapeutic intervention".[1] Consequently, imaging biomarkers are all those biomarkers, which are determined by imaging techniques. Since there is no exclusivity to that term, examples are found in all methods, e.g. nuchal translucency screening (ultrasound), sizing of adrenocortical incidentalomas (CT scan), BOLD-signal (magnetic resonance imaging—MRI), and renal clearance (single photon emission computed tomography—SPECT). The aspect that distinguishes imaging from mere visualization is quantitation. Imaging (and therefore imaging biomarkers) can be characterized as structural, functional, and molecular. One should distinguish truly molecular information from rather functional or even structural measurements and restrain from thoughtlessly terming everything "molecular imaging" which is the visualization and quantification of a molecular interaction between a molecular probe (MP) and a molecular target. Biomarker imaging is understood as imaging of molecular probes. MPs comprise all kinds of molecules administered to an organism, which carry a signaling moiety. This moiety can, for example, be a radionuclide, a fluorescent chromophore, a paramagnetic core or a gas-filled or gas-producing nanostructure. MPI always leads to an imaging biomarker; but imaging biomarkers do not necessarily require MPI. However, imaging biomarkers require a molecular imaging modality/technique in order to measure them (e.g. magnetic resonance spectroscopy).[2]

BIOMARKERS IN HEART FAILURE

Heart failure (HF) is among the leading causes of death and disability worldwide. Among the challenges in treating this patient population are inadequacies in prediction of disease severity, with a resultant mismatch between risk stratification and intensity of therapy. Identification of biomarkers that allow measurement of the disease on a molecular level has resulted in considerable enthusiasm for their use in prognostication and selection of appropriate therapies.

Classifying Biomarkers in Heart Failure

Biomarkers in HF can be broadly grouped according to their role in HF pathophysiology. The best known subgroup is the neurohormones, including the cardiac natriuretic peptides (NP), the components of the renin-angiotensin-aldosterone system (RAAS), the catecholamines, arginine vasopressin, and endothelium-derived vasoactive peptides including endothelin, adrenomedullin, and the urocortins (Tables 1 and 2).[3]

Imaging Biomarkers in Heart Failure

The American College of Cardiology/American Heart Association (ACC/AHA) practice guidelines for HF have

TABLE 1: Biomarkers in the MORGA-cohorts.

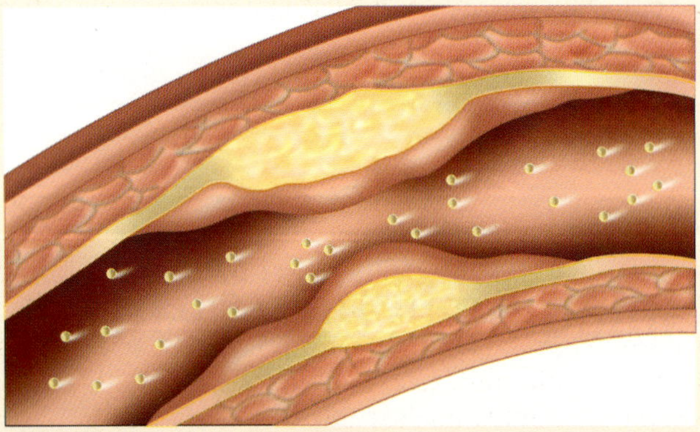

Lipid-related markers	*Markers of vascular function and neurohormonal activity*
Apolipoprotein AI Apolipoprotein B100 Lipoprotein-associated phospholipase A2 • Activity • Mass Paraoxonase- 1	(N terminal pro) B type natriuretic peptide C-terminal provasopressin C-terminal proendothelin-1 Mid-regional proadrenomedulin Mid-regional proatrial natriuretic peptide Tissue inhibitor of metalloproteinase- 1
Renal function markers	*Inflammatory markers*
Creatinine Cystatin-C	C-reactive protein Interleukin-18 Interleukin-1 receptor antagonist Neoprotein
Metabolic markers	*Markers of oxidative stress and antioxidants*
Adiponectin Leptin Insulin Ferritin Glucose *Coagulation markers* D-Dimer	Homocysteine Myeloperoxidase Vitamin B12 Active Vitamin B12
Angiogenesis markers	*Necrosis markers*
Cardiac placental growth factor	Creatine kinase- MB Troponin I

TABLE 2: Biomarkers in heart failure.

Neurohormonal markers	
Cardiac natriuretic peptides	B-type natriuretic peptides (BNP, NT proBNP, pro-BNP) ANP, NTproANP, mid-region pro-ANP C-type natriuretic peptides (CNP, NT proCNP)
Renin-angiotensin-aldosterone system	Plasma renin activity (PRA) Angiotensin II Aldosterone
Adrenergic nervous system	Norepinephrine Epinephrine
Arginine vasopressin (AVP)	AVP Copeptin
Endothelial derived peptides	Endothelin-1, big endothelin Adrenomedulin, mild region pro-adrenomedulin Urocortin I, II, III
Inflammatory markers	C-reactive protein Tumor necrosis factor alpha Fas(APO-1) Interleukins 1, 6, and 18
Oxidative stress markers	Oxidized low-density lipoprotiens Myeloperoxidase Urine biopyrrins Urine and plasma isoprostanes Plasma malondialdehyde Carbonyl proteins
Interstitial matrix remodeling markers	Matrix metalloproteinases (MMPs) Tissue inhibitors of metalloproteinases (TMPs) Propeptide procollagen I Procollagen III
Myocyte injury markers	Cardiac troponins I and T Myosin light-chain kinase I Heart fatty acid binding protein Creatine kinase, creatine kinase MB fraction Ischemia modified albumin
Other/new markers	ST2 Growth differentiation factor 15 Osteoprotegerin Adiponectin Galectin 3 Co-enzyme Q

divided the disorder into four stages, two of which (stages A and B) are in asymptomatic individuals. Cardiac imaging techniques play a pivotal role in defining abnormal myocardial structure and function that appear at and beyond stage B. A phenotypic characterization of HF into heart failure with reduced ejection fraction (HFrEF) or preserved ejection fraction (HFpEF). However, debate exists as to whether these two are really two separate entities or merely represent two different stages in the overall continuum of HF. Cardiac imaging-related HF phenotype might finally have utility in identifying patient subtypes who may benefit from individualized HF therapies. Cardiac imaging as a biomarker can be used for the following purposes:

- Cardiac chamber quantification
- Establishing cause—ischemic versus nonischemic
- To screen for coronary artery disease (CAD)
- Assess myocardial perfusion
- Assess myocardial viability and benefit from revascularization
- Selection of patient for device therapies
- To look for specific causes--sarcoidosis, amyloidosis
- Assessment of heart failure with preserved ejection fraction.

Cardiac Chamber Quantification

Ventricular remodeling occurs due to myocyte hypertrophy, myocyte apoptosis, myofibroblast proliferation, and interstitial fibrosis, which have been measured traditionally as a change in left ventricular (LV) volume, mass and ejection fraction.[4] All four cardiac imaging modalities are used for tracking this process, echocardiography, radionuclide ventriculography, computed tomography, and cardiac magnetic resonance (CMR). Echocardiography remains the predominant imaging technique used in clinical trials, based on broader availability, and cost efficacy. The simultaneous assessment of LV systolic function as well as stress and rest perfusion by gated SPECT imaging provides information for clinical decision making, including the state of LV function, the probability of CAD as the cause of HF, and extent of viability and ischemia. Similarly, the use of contrast-enhanced CMR has emerged as an established marker of myocardial scarring associated with cardiac remodeling. Multiparametric approaches by combining the changes in LV volumes, mass, and ejection fraction (EF) can be helpful in characterizing different patterns of concentric and eccentric LV remodeling and have been used as a prognostic marker for predicting cardiovascular death, myocardial infarction, HF, stroke, or cardiac arrest. Changes in myocardial contractile behavior allow superior characterization of patterns of remodeling leading to use of myocardial deformation parameters such as strain for understanding the mechanistic diversities underlying the development of myocardial dysfunction at the subclinical level and its subsequent progression to clinical HF.[5]

Establishing Cause: Ischemic versus Nonischemic

Imaging techniques can be helpful in distinguishing cause of HF or cardiomyopathy, which may be primarily due to CAD (many of whom have potentially reversible LV dysfunction) from those with idiopathic dilated cardiomyopathy. Among cardiomyopathies with systolic dysfunction (HFrEF), they are generally grouped as ischemic or nonischemic. Nonischemic cardiomyopathy can be further classified as dilated, hypertrophic, restrictive, valvular, and arrhythmogenic.

Coronary Artery Disease as a Cause of Heart Failure

Direct visualization of the coronary arteries either with invasive coronary angiography or noninvasively with CT angiography allows early and direct distinction between ischemic and nonischemic cardiomyopathies, including anomalies.[6] Noninvasive imaging such as echocardiography, nuclear imaging, and CMR provides information about the consequences of CAD on the myocardium (inducible ischemia, such as decreased perfusion or contraction) or myocardial fibrosis/scarring pattern (transmural extent, mural distribution, and pattern). CMR with its high resolution has more often been used to detect fibrosis thereby identifying ischemic versus nonischemic cardiomyopathy.

Assessment of Myocardial Perfusion

Although many patients with nonischemic cardiomyopathy may have perfusion abnormalities detected in myocardial perfusion imaging studies, a normal result in a patient with HFrEF is highly predictive for the absence of CAD. The modest specificity of myocardial perfusion imaging to rule out CAD is explained, in part, by pathologic and CMR studies[6] demonstrating that patients with nonischemic cardiomyopathy may have patchy or larger confluent territories of fibrosis or scarring, manifested as fixed defects on myocardial perfusion studies. Extensive perfusion abnormalities in the setting of LV dysfunction are essentially always associated with CAD rather than with dilated cardiomyopathy, especially when the perfusion defects are segmental.

Myocardial Viability and Assessment for Revascularization

Requirements for myocellular viability include sufficient myocardial blood flow, sarcolemma membrane integrity, intact mitochondria and ionotropic reserve, and preserved glucose or fatty acid metabolism.[7] Because sarcolemma or mitochondria membrane integrity is dependent on preserved intracellular metabolic activity to generate high-energy phosphates, radiotracers that reflect cation flux (e.g. 201 thallium), electrochemical gradients [technetium 99m (Tc99m)-labeled sestamibi or tetrofosmin], or metabolic processes with ^{18}F-labeled fluorodeoxyglucose [(^{18}F) FDG] provide insight into myocardial viability. There are several different protocols. The first and foremost protocol is used to determine the presence and extent of viable, ischemic myocardium, particularly in dysfunctional vascular territories. In the absence of myocardial ischemia, two nuclear imaging protocols are optimized for detection of viable, hibernating myocardium: the first is resting-redistribution thallium SPECT, and the second is resting rubidium-82- or 13N-labeled ammonia perfusion and (^{18}F) FDG metabolism with positron emission tomography (PET). It has been shown that even at a similar mass of viable myocardial tissue (reflected by resting myocardial perfusion studies), the presence of inducible ischemia (reversible defect) is associated with an increased likelihood of functional recovery. For a dysfunctional myocardial region or vascular territory, the probability of functional recovery after revascularization is related to the magnitude of radiotracer uptake, which is a continuous variable; that is, the magnitude of tracer uptake directly reflects the magnitude of preserved tissue viability.[8] Conversely, late gadolinium enhancement (LGE) CMR provides the magnitude of interstitial fibrosis and myocardial scar (extent of transmural and/or nontransmural infarction) and the probability of functional recovery after revascularization. Thus, a dysfunctional territory that does not exhibit LGE or has preserved radiotracer uptake has a high likelihood of improved function after revascularization. In contrast, a territory with evidence of LGE or a severe reduction in radiotracer uptake would represent predominant infarction, and the likelihood of improved function after revascularization would be low. Novel functional strategies using assessment of myocardial deformation with speckle tracking echocardiography can be used readily at the bedside. Several studies have suggested that assessment of peak systolic longitudinal strain after revascularization in patients with acute myocardial infarction can be used for predicting global improvement in LVEF.[9] A meta-analysis of the prognostic value of viability testing and the impact of therapeutic choice on survival demonstrated a significant reduction in the risk of cardiac death during long-term follow-up in patients with evidence of preserved myocardial viability that underwent revascularization.[10] Revascularization conferred no natural history advantage in patients without substantial myocardial viability. Similar findings were observed with ischemic cardiomyopathy patients who underwent LGE CMR. These data suggest that noninvasive imaging of viability and ischemia can potentially play a role in selecting patients for revascularization, with the expectation of improving symptoms, and natural history.[11] The viability substudy of STICH (Surgical Treatment for Ischemic Heart Failure), which consisted of 601 patients, examined whether the presence of viable myocardium as determined by the local participating site (myocardial perfusion SPECT, dobutamine echocardiography, or both) and restoration of coronary flow improved patient outcome.[12] Altered glucose metabolism and myocardial efficiency have also been studied in high-risk patients with HF imaged with PET and have shown that the magnitude of enhanced use of glucose relative to perfusion in PET (termed "mismatch pattern") correlates with the potential for improved HF symptoms after revascularization.[13] Beyond myocardial perfusion and metabolism studies, recent studies have determined the prognostic value of myocardial sympathetic innervation in HF. Results of ADMIRE-HF (AdreView Myocardial Imaging for Risk Evaluation in Heart Failure) showed that for patients with heart to mediastinal ratio (H/M) less than 1.6, 2-year cardiac death, and all-cause mortality were 11.2% and 16.1%, respectively, versus 1.8% and 3.0%, respectively, for those with H/M of more than or equal to 1.6. There was a progressive decline in both cardiac and all-cause mortality from more than 20% in patients with H/M less than 1.10–0% for patients with H/M more than or equal to 1.8.[14]

Assessment of Specific Causes

Cardiac imaging plays important roles in identifying causes that predispose or directly cause HF including structural alterations, congenital or acquired, where there is a disorder of the peripheral vessels, coronary circulation, pericardium, myocardium, endocardium, or cardiac valves.

Selection of Device Therapy

Cardiac resynchronization therapy (CRT) with biventricular pacing has advanced the therapy of HF beyond standard medical therapy. However, 35–50% of patients do not benefit from CRT.[15] One of the goals of recent imaging studies is the ability to predict response to CRT. Guiding placement of the LV lead is essential due to variability of patient response. Potential reasons for lack of response include pacer placement in scar or in regions that are not late activating, both of which are potential targets for imaging. Identifying dyssynchrony as a marker of potential CRT response has been a goal of several imaging studies. The PROSPECT (The Providing Regional Observations to Study Predictors of Events in the Coronary Tree) trial tested 12 echocardiographic markers of dyssynchrony using a blinded core laboratory analysis. Due in part to a lack of reproducibility of the large number of markers tested, the area under the receiver operating characteristic curve for clinical or LV volume response to CRT was only less than or equal to 0.62. Some of these markers measure mechanical dyssynchrony rather than electrical dyssynchrony, and CRT does not necessarily reverse the former.[16] In the TARGET (Targeted Left Ventricular Lead Placement to Guide Cardiac

Resynchronization Therapy) study, 220 patients were randomized to undergo echocardiographically-guided CRT or unguided CRT, and the group with echo-guided LV lead placement demonstrated a significantly higher clinical response and lower rates of combined death and HF hospitalization.[17] Prior CMR studies suggest that scar in the lateral wall is predictive of nonresponse due to lack or poor pacer capture in this location. Strain imaging by CMR can also be used to identify mechanical dyssynchrony and late activating myocardium that is likely to respond well to CRT. A single-center study of 75 patients demonstrated that the combination of mechanical dyssynchrony, pacer placement in the site of latest activation, and absence of scar could predict CRT response with an area under the curve of 0.95.[18] Presently, an EF cutoff of less than or equal to 35% is used as the criterion for implantable cardioverter defibrillator (ICD) placement in patients with New York Heart Association (NYHA) functional classes II and III HF. More precise markers are needed. One potential imaging marker is extent of myocardial scar as identified by CMR. In a study of 137 patients with cardiomyopathy and EF of more than 30%, scar size more than 5% of LV mass increased the risk of death or appropriate ICD discharge similarly to those with an EF less than or equal to 30%. The absence of scar in patients with EF of less than 30% lowered the risk similarly to those with EF of more than or equal to 30%.[19] Retrospective studies in nonischemic cardiomyopathy demonstrate that LGE presence and extent are predictive of cardiovascular death and appropriate ICD therapy.[20] Another potential marker of arrhythmic risk in HF is cardiac innervation as identified by [^{123}I]meta-iodobenzylguanidine. A heart-to-mediastinal ratio of less than 1.6 had a hazard ratio of 3.5 for arrhythmic events in the ADMIRE-HF study.[14] Measurements of mechanical dispersion and global strain using speckle tracking echocardiography after myocardial infarction can aid assessment of risk of arrhythmia.[21]

Imaging Biomarker for Heart Failure with Reduced Ejection Fraction

Quantification of the extracellular matrix (ECM) (surrogate measures of diastolic dysfunction).

Echocardiography

Traditional echocardiographic parameters used to diagnose HFpEF (e.g. E/E′, E/A ratio, LA volume, LV mass) are reliant on assessing the resting functional and structural consequences of fibrosis. Beyond ischemia evaluation, diastolic stress echocardiography may further unmask patients with HFpEF in whom resting filling pressures do not meet current diagnostic criteria but rise with exercise (E/E′ > 15).[22] However, indirect assessment of fibrosis is also possible via echocardiography. Collagen content governs the elasticity of myocardial tissue thereby altering its acoustic impedance, density, and reflectivity in response to ultrasound signals used in echocardiography. Using the pericardium as an internal control, these integrated signals scatter back (IBS) to the imaging probe permitting estimates of regional fibrotic burden.

Cardiac Magnetic Resonance

Cardiac magnetic resonance late gadolinium enhancement (LGE) imaging was initially developed upon an understanding that infarcted (scarred) myocardium is associated with regional increases in collagen content, extracellular volume (ECV) expansion, and a slower washout of extracellular contrast agent. Fibrotic regions appear as areas of high signal intensity compared to "nulled" (black) normal myocardium using inversion recovery CMR sequences. CMR LGE is the accepted gold standard due to its superior spatial resolution and high contrast-to-noise ratio enabling the detection of very small infarcts.[23] Furthermore, focal nonischemic scarring is also seen in dilated cardiomyopathy, aortic stenosis, and sarcoidosis. The pattern of LGE allows discrimination between etiologies (e.g. ischemic versus nonischemic and HFpEF "phenocopies" such as hypertrophic cardiomyopathy (HCM), amyloid, pericardial constriction), provides prognostic information and identifies vulnerable myocardium amenable to targeted therapies. In HFpEF, however, the pattern of fibrosis, at least in the early stages, is typically diffuse and the signal differences between diseased and normal myocardium are less distinct, rendering the LGE technique insensitive. T1 mapping and ECV quantification techniques are promising recent developments in CMR.

Use of Strain Analysis

Remodeling of the ECM compartment alters myocardial tissue mechanics resulting in abnormalities of both diastole and systole in HFpEF. Longitudinal function is typically depressed in HFpEF and can be measured with echocardiography (tissue Doppler) and CMR (velocity-encoded or tissue phase mapping). A more detailed assessment of LV performance can now be made using strain (or deformation) analysis. Simplistically, strain imaging assesses myocardial tissue lengthening, shortening or thickening in orthogonal planes.[24] Regional strain disturbances have demonstrated a strong relation with LV catheter derived relaxation abnormalities and left ventricular end-diastolic pressure (LVEDP) in HCM. Furthermore, the ratio of mitral E wave velocity and global strain rate correctly predicts LVEDP and is more accurate than E/E′ ratios in patients with preserved EF and regional dysfunction.[25] As prognostic biomarkers, strain parameters (global longitudinal peak strain and longitudinal early diastolic strain) are important predictors of adverse outcomes (one-year follow-up) in HFpEF.[26]

Left Atrium Strain and Hemodynamics

A dilated left atrium (LA) is the hemodynamic consequence of chronically elevated LVEDP and provides supportive evidence for HFpEF diagnosis. CMR has already superseded echocardiography for LA volumetric measurement with superior reproducibility. Beyond structural assessment, disturbances in atrial myocardial mechanics have also been observed in HFpEF. LA dysfunction discriminates between HFpEF, hypertensive, and healthy groups.[27] Abnormal measures of LA strain have been noted in the HFpEF antecedent conditions of hypertension and diabetes despite normal LA dimensions, highlighting it as a marker of diastolic dysfunction (DD) in HF.

Metabolic Imaging

Existing nuclear and MRI techniques permit the detection of metabolic derangements of energetic status and substrate utilization (e.g. free fatty acids) implicated in HF. Irrespective of HF etiology, reductions in energy levels (by measuring phosphocreatine) of approximately 70% noted. Using magnetic resonance spectroscopy (MRS), the association between reduced myocardial phosphocreatine: adenosine tri-phosphate ratio (PCr:ATP) and DD has been shown in hypertensive patients and in HFpEF during exercise.[28] Increasing evidence implicates the role of excessive myocardial triglyceride accumulation (steatosis): obesity, diabetes, and pressure overload. Steatosis, as quantified by MRS, is independently associated with echocardiographic measures of DD, strain parameters derived from CMR tagging, and correlates with histology.[29]

Molecular Imaging

Molecular targeting of the key markers implicated in ECM turnover has recently shown good capabilities, mainly in animal models. Targets include MMPs, ECM proteins, the renin-angiotensin axis, and myofibroblasts. Post-infarct studies have already demonstrated the feasibility of assessing collagen deposition and increased probe activity.[30] Hybrid imaging with PET, SPECT, CT or CMR may further improve spatial resolution, which is the current major limitation.

CONCLUSION

Heart failure affects nearly 2.5–5 million population in India. Despite best modalities, the mortality is 50% at 5 years. HFpEF accounts for 50% of heart failure cases and it is grossly underdiagnosed. Imaging modalities as a biomarker have increased the sensitivity. However, no single parameter can provide the precision, and perhaps in the future, weighted algorithms or scoring system using the various available indices of these parameters would give the answer. More emphasis needs to be placed on linking LV remodeling with the underlying cause. The use of LV volumes and EF as surrogate endpoints for trials of novel medical therapies; most previous HF trials have focused on the presence of coronary artery disease established invasively LV systolic dysfunction, by imaging techniques for therapy selection. Combining noninvasive imaging (e.g. scar imaging by CMR and coronary imaging by CTA) to differentiate ischemic from nonischemic cardiomyopathy. Imaging for identifying therapeutic targets in clinical trials remains an area of intense investigation. Especially in the era of devices like CRT and ICD, imaging plays a major role in identifying the responder rates and future studies should focus on identifying multiple parameters, which will improve the selection of patients. Finally, it should be recognized that HF is a disease with large phenotypic variations in cause, clinical features, and natural history. This heterogeneity in presentation is perhaps a reason why several mechanistically sound therapeutic interventions in clinical trials have not shown efficacy. Cardiac imaging provides diverse insights, but the ability to integrate large sets information for identifying specific subtypes of patients with greatest likelihood of response remains a challenging proposition.

REFERENCES

1. Biomarkers Definitions Working Group. Biomarkers and surrogate endpoints: Preferred definitions and conceptual framework. Clin Pharmacol Ther. 2001;69:89-95.
2. Lucignani G. Imaging biomarkers: from research to patient care—a shift in view. Eur J Nucl Med Mol Imaging. 2001;34:1693-7.
3. Blankenberg S, Zeller T, Saarela O, et al. Contribution of 30 biomarkers to 10-year cardiovascular risk estimation in 2 population cohorts: the MONICA, Risk, Genetics, Archiving, and Monograph (MORGAM) biomarker project. Circulation. 2010;121:2388-97.
4. Motiwala SR, Gaggin HK. Biomarkers to predict reverse remodeling and myocardial recovery in heart failure. Curr Heart Fail. 2016;13:207-18.
5. Claus P, Omar AM, Pedrizzetti G, et al. Tissue tracking technology for assessing cardiac mechanics: principles, normal values, and clinical applications. J Am Coll Cardiol Cardiovasc Imaging. 2015; 8:1444-60.
6. McCrohon JA, Moon JC, Prasad SK, et al. Differentiation of heart failure related to dilated cardiomyopathy and coronary artery disease using gadolinium-enhanced cardiovascular magnetic resonance. Circulation. 2003;108:54-9.

7. Gewirtz H, Dilsizian V. Myocardial viability: survival mechanisms and molecular imaging targets in acute and chronic ischemia. Circ Res. 2017;120:1197-212.
8. Dilsizian V. Cardiac magnetic resonance versus SPECT: Are all noninfarct myocardial regions created equal? J Nucl Cardiol. 2007;14:9-14.
9. Huttin O, Coiro S, Selton-Suty C, et al. Prediction of left ventricular remodeling after a myocardial infarction: Role of myocardial deformation: a systematic review and meta-analysis. PLoS One. 2016;11:e0168349.
10. Allman KC, Shaw LJ, Hachamovitch R, et al. Myocardial viability testing and impact of revascularization on prognosis in patients with coronary artery disease and left ventricular dysfunction: a meta-analysis. J Am Coll Cardiol. 2002;39:1151-8.
11. Gerber BL, Rousseau MF, Ahn SA, et al. Prognostic value of myocardial viability by delayed-enhanced magnetic resonance in patients with coronary artery disease and low ejection fraction: impact of revascularization therapy. J Am Coll Cardiol. 2012;59:825-35.
12. Bonow RO, Maurer G, Lee KL, et al. Myocardial viability and survival in ischemic left ventricular dysfunction. N Engl J Med. 2011;364:1617-25.
13. Osterholt M, Sen S, Dilsizian V, et al. Targeted metabolic imaging to improve the management of heart disease. J Am Coll Cardiol Imaging. 2012;5:214-26.
14. Dilsizian V, Chandrashekhar Y, Narula J. Introduction of new tests: low are the mountains, high the expectations. J Am Coll Cardiol Imaging. 2010;3:117-9.
15. Linde C, Ellenbogen K, McAlister FA. Cardiac resynchronization therapy (CRT): clinical trials, guidelines, and target populations. Heart Rhythm. 2012;9:S3-13.
16. Marechaux S, Menet A, Guyomar Y, et al. Role of echocardiography before cardiac resynchronization therapy: New advances and current developments. Echocardiography. 2016;33:1745-52.
17. Khan FZ, Virdee MS, Palmer CR, et al. Targeted left ventricular lead placement to guide cardiac resynchronization therapy: the TARGET study: a randomized, controlled trial. J Am Coll Cardiol. 2012;59:1509-18.
18. Bilchick KC, Kuruvilla S, Hamirani YS, et al. Impact of mechanical activation, scar, and electrical timing on cardiac resynchronization therapy response and clinical outcomes. J Am Coll Cardiol. 2014;63:1657-66.
19. Modesto K, Sengupta PP. Myocardial mechanics in cardiomyopathies. Prog Cardiovasc Dis. 2014;57:111-24.
20. Neilan TG, Coelho-Filho OR, Danik SB, et al. CMR quantification of myocardial scar provides additive prognostic information in nonischemic cardiomyopathy. J Am Coll Cardiol Imaging. 2013;6:944-54.
21. Haugaa KH, Smedsrud MK, Steen T, et al. Mechanical dispersion assessed by myocardial strain in patients after myocardial infarction for risk prediction of ventricular arrhythmia. J Am Coll Cardiol Imaging. 2010;3:247-56.
22. Picano E, Pellikka PA. Stress echo applications beyond coronary artery disease. Eur Heart J. 2014;35:1033-40.
23. Karamitsos TD, Francis JM, Myerson S, et al. The role of cardiovascular magnetic resonance imaging in heart failure. J Am Coll Cardiol. 2009;54:1407-24.
24. Jellis C, Martin J, Narula J, et al. Assessment of nonischemic myocardial fibrosis. J Am Coll Cardiol. 2010;56:89-97.
25. Wang J, Khoury DS, Thohan V, et al. Global diastolic strain rate for the assessment of left ventricular relaxation and filling pressures. Circulation. 2007;115:1376-83.
26. Ohtani T, Mohammed SF, Yamamoto K, et al. Diastolic stiffness as assessed by diastolic wall strain is associated with adverse remodelling and poor outcomes in heart failure with preserved ejection fraction. Eur Heart J. 2012;33:1742-9.
27. Hudsmith LE, Cheng AS, Tyler DJ, et al. Assessment of left atrial volumes at 1.5 Tesla and 3 Tesla using flash and SSFP cine imaging. J. Cardiovasc Mag Reson. 2007;9:673-9.
28. Phan TT, Abozguia K, Nallur Shivu G, et al. HFpEF is characterized by dynamic impairment of active relaxation and contraction of the left ventricle on exercise and associated with myocardial energy deficiency. J Am Coll Cardiol. 2009;54:402-9.
29. Mahmod M, Bull S, Suttie JJ, et al. Myocardial steatosis and left ventricular contractile dysfunction in patients with severe aortic stenosis. Circ Cardiovasc Imaging. 2013;6:808-16.
30. van den Borne SW, Isobe S, Zandbergen HR, et al. Molecular imaging for efficacy of pharmacologic intervention in myocardial remodeling. JACC Cardiovasc. Imaging. 2009;2:187-98.

17

CHAPTER

Advances in Systolic Heart Failure Evaluation by Echocardiography

Rohit Tandon, Mridul Mahanta, Gulshan Rai

INTRODUCTION

Echocardiography evaluation of systolic heart failure has undergone a tremendous shift from M-mode and two-dimensional (2D) volumetric-based quantification to deformation imaging and three-dimensional (3D) volumetric calculations.

With increasing experience and robust data from a large number of patient subsets clinicians are encouraged to accept new terms like heart failure with predominant longitudinal strain dysfunction or heart failure with predominant circumferential strain dysfunction ± dyssynchrony instead of systolic/diastolic heart failure.

Cardinal symptoms of heart failure are not solely dependent on left ventricular systolic functions rather they are more or less reflected upon by left atrial (LA) and right atrial (RA) size, their functions besides of course pulmonary hemodynamics with its resultant effects on right ventricle. This fact is best appreciated in an asymptomatic patient with severe left ventricular dysfunction. Despite severely reduced ejection fraction (EF) normal LA and RA size, right ventricular functions and pulmonary artery pressures render patient asymptomatic. Therefore, this EF paradox needs further explanation especially whenever considering management of systolic heart failure patients because measurement of left ventricular ejection fraction (LVEF) alone gives an incomplete representation of systolic functions since 2D biplane method of discs (2DEF) measurement presents a number of challenges related to image quality, assumptions of left ventricular geometry, and expertise. Carlsson et al. analyzed longitudinal atrioventricular plane displacement with cardiovascular magnetic resonance (CMR) in normal subjects, professional athletes and patients with dilated cardiomyopathy and reduced LVEF (<30%), percentage of stroke volume generated by longitudinal function was similar in all groups at about 60% even though stroke volume was higher in athletes and lower in patients with cardiomyopathy,[1,2] thereby improving upon our understanding that longitudinal contraction is a particular marker of subendocardial function, which may be disproportionately involved in subclinical disease, including myocardial ischemia. Simple measures of longitudinal function, such as mitral annular systolic displacement by M-mode or systolic velocity measured with tissue Doppler have been used previously although they have proven inferior to ejection fraction at least in their prognosticating ability as they represent annular component of longitudinal contraction only. Doppler based indices of systolic functions [myocardial performance index (MPI)] most commonly used for estimating global long-axis ventricular systolic functions are influenced by volume and pressure loading. For the same preload, there is a difference in tissue velocities between acute and chronic cases, i.e. chronic volume overload has a smaller effect on tissue velocities than in acute phase. Pressure loading also influences tissue velocities, increased ventricular pressure as in aortic stenosis leads to decreased tissue velocities. Another impediment is regularity in heart rate and age differences in normal velocities besides their inherent angle dependency.

Two-dimensional strain is an automated and quantitative technique for the measurement of global long-axis function

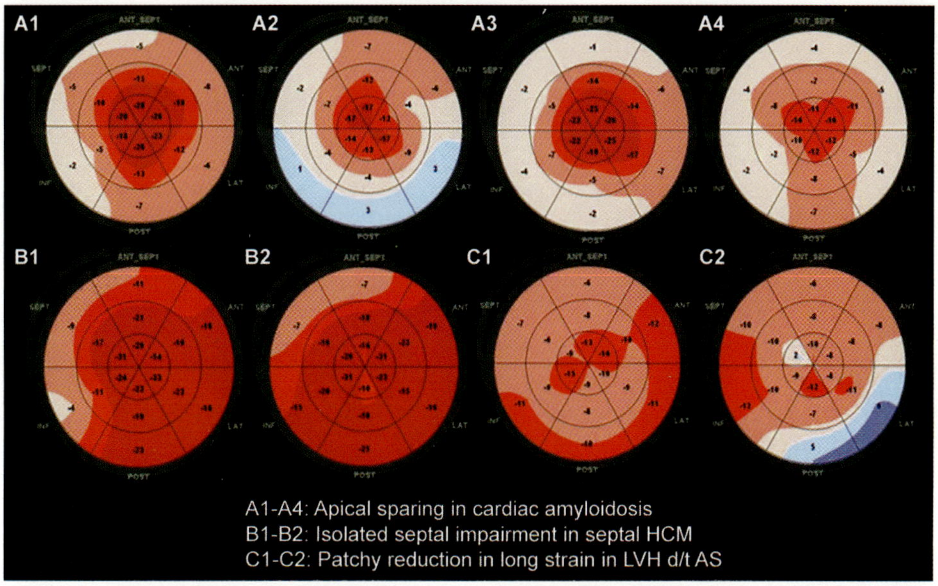

Fig. 1: Patterns of longitudinal strain suggestive of underlying etiology.

from gray-scale images calculated from the mean of 17 cardiac segments. It is more robust than tissue Doppler-derived strain as it does not suffer from angle dependency and is easier to calculate. Global longitudinal strain (GLS) and EF are highly correlated, they measure different aspects of myocardial motion, with EF measuring radial and partly longitudinal function, GLS measures longitudinal function. EF can be derived from GLS using the regression EF = –4.35 × (GLS + 3.9). Using this formula, a cut-off of GLS less than –12% is equivalent to EF 35%, so GLS less than –12% can be recommended as diagnostic cut-off for severe LV dysfunction as an additional parameter in making crucial decisions regarding alternative treatment choices in heart failure patients.[3-8]

Anthracycline usage has 2-year mortality up to 60% due to heart failure. Sawaya et al. showed that unlike LVEF, reduced GLS less than –19% at completion of chemotherapy predicted future LV dysfunction. A relative decrease in GLS of 10–15% is predictive of future cardiotoxicity. In patients receiving trastuzumab, a relative reduction in GLS of over 11% (95% confidence interval 8–15%) was highly predictive of reductions in LVEF. Ali et al. have also demonstrated increased rates of symptomatic HF and cardiac death in those found to have normal LVEF but impaired GLS (less than –17.5%) prior to initiation of anthracyclines (Fig. 1).

In HCMP, hypertrophy and fibrosis progress despite preserved EF. A reduction in strain is associated with fibrosis, increased risk for ventricular arrhythmias, HF, and death as shown by Afonso et al. In cardiac amyloid, LVEF is often not affected early, and diastolic e´ velocities are minimally altered late in the disease process. Reduction in longitudinal strain with relative sparing at the apex may be predictive of cardiac amyloid. In hypertrophied heart, there is little change appreciated in volumetric measurements due to small cavity and stroke volume measurements are not reproducible per se they are dependent on regular heart rate (Fig. 2).

Mansencal et al. reported that there were significant differences in strain, strain rate, and systolic peak velocities between acute and chronic phases in Takatsubo cases. Using speckle tracking to quantitate regional LV systolic function, in the acute phase, systolic dysfunction was circular with similar velocity among basal, mid ventricle, and apical segments and was different from that of patients with left anterior descending (LAD) coronary artery obstruction. Key echocardiographic features in the acute phase is the large area of dysfunctional myocardium extending beyond the territory of a single coronary artery; which presents by symmetrical regional abnormalities, including the midventricular segments in a circumferential pattern peak systolic strain rate is also useful for assessing LV mechanics in this situation because the strain rate seems to be more useful than tissue Doppler velocities in evaluating the LV dynamics during volume loading in patients with depressed LV function.

Left ventricular noncompaction (LVNC) with preserved LVEF has subclinical myocardial dysfunction with impairment of deformation parameters. LV solid body rotation/twist was also described as a potential quantitative functional diagnostic criterion for noncompaction. In one study, a significant increase in longitudinal function from the base to the apex with more preserved longitudinal strain at the level of the apical NC segments was noted. This specific regional deformation pattern may help to distinguish this population of cardiomyopathy from the classical idiopathic DCM. This pattern of myocardial

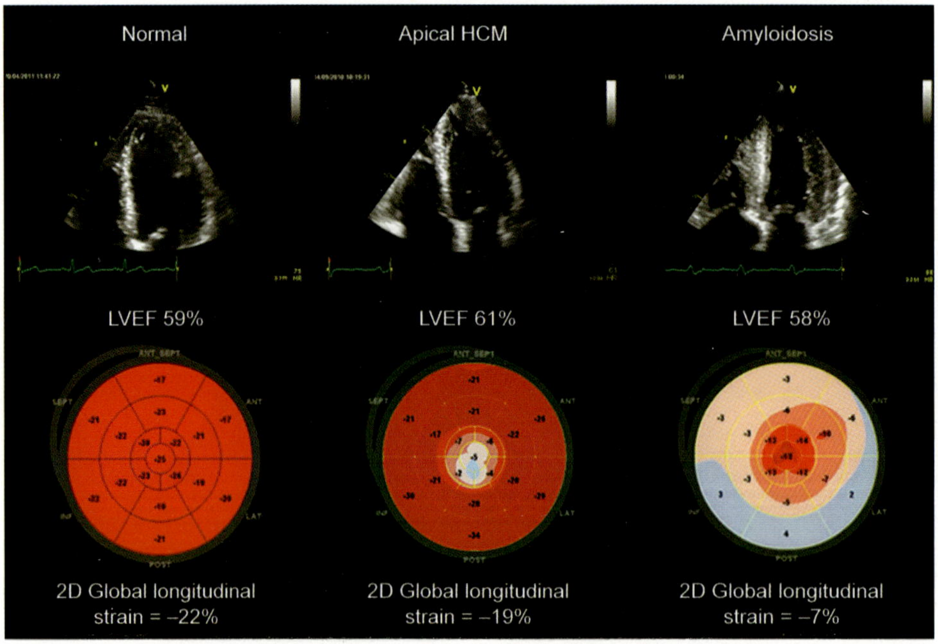

Fig. 2: Heterogeneity in left ventricular myocardial function.

strain with the apex/basal ratio of 1.5 may be related to the shape of the LV and the distribution of noncompacted segments. Sengupta et al. hypothesized that spongy myocardial architecture of the LV apex likely resists to the dilatation and leads to the particular form of ventricular remodeling and causes a synergy in these areas a maximal compacted thickness less than 8 mm is a specific marker that allows the differentiation of pathological trabeculation of noncompaction.[9,10]

Speckle-tracking echocardiography (STE)-based radial strain measurement can be helpful in identifying appropriate site for LV lead placement and may help minimize chances of nonresponse. Cardiac resynchronization therapy (CRT) is likely to result in the greatest benefit when LV lead is implanted adjacent to the most delayed (determined by time to peak radial strain) but nonscarred (segmental radial strain >10%) LV myocardial segment. Increase in GLS after CRT implantation, in addition to the standard echocardiographic measurements, has been shown to predict responders and all-cause mortality at 1-year follow-up (Table 1 and Fig. 3).

Time from QRS (white line) to peak circumferential strain (color dots) in six myocardial segments is calculated in parasternal short axis view in dilated cardiomyopathy patient.

START score: With this score reclassification of patients to identify nonresponders was better than MADIT (Multicenter Automatic Defibrillator Implantation Trial) score especially when speckle tracking measurements were added to it. In this score 1 point is given to left bundle branch block (LBBB) or right ventricular pacing, MR index less than or equal to 40% is assigned a numeric value of 2; use of beta-blocker, blood urea nitrogen (BUN) less than or equal to 30 mg/dL, and LV dimension at end systole (LVDs) less than or equal to 50 mm 3 points; and CS-SD more than or equal to116 ms 4 points. In the multivariable Cox proportional hazard model analysis adjusted for age, sex, ischemic cardiomyopathy, use of loop diuretics, and left ventricular end-diastolic volume

TABLE 1: Potential roles of echocardiography to improve patient response to cardiac resynchronization therapy (CRT).

	Methods most widely supported
Echocardiographic dyssynchrony at baseline	• Pre-ejection delay ≥ 140 ms • IVMD ≥ 40 ms • TDI opposing wall delay ≥ 80 ms • TDE Yu index ≥ 32 ms • Radial strain delay ≥ 130 ms
Echo guided lead positioning to site of latest activation	Speckle tracking radial strain site of latest activation
Echo guided lead positioning to avoid sites of regional scar	Avoid segments with < 10% radial strain amplitude
Atrioventricular and ventricular-ventricular optimization	• Mitral inflow velocity analysis • LV outflow tract time velocity integral

(IVMD: interventricular mechanical delay; LV: left ventricle; TDI: tissue Doppler imaging)

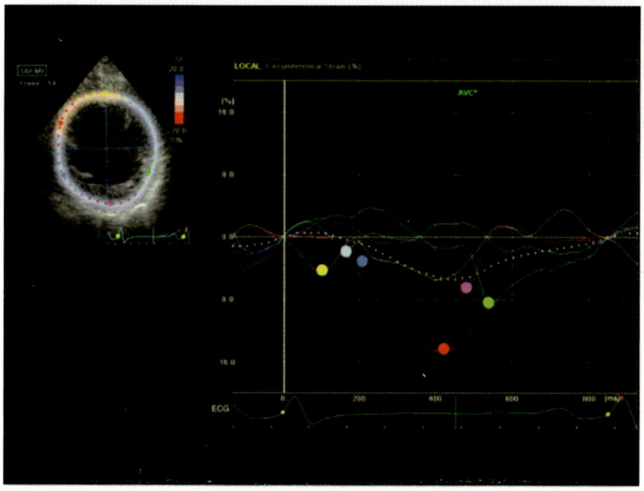

Fig. 3: Time from QRS (white line) to peak circumferential strain (color dots).

more than or equal to 250 mL, a START clinical score less than or equal to 12 was identified as a significant predictor of nonresponders.[11-13]

Resting GLS and stress GLS measured during dobutamine stress echocardiography (DSE) seems superior to other parameters of left ventricular function to assess degree of myocardial impairment and predict outcomes in both patients treated conservatively and those treated surgically. Patients opting conservative management have markedly increased risk of mortality if GLS is less than 9% at rest or less than–10% at stress. These patients should receive particular attention for optimization of heart failure therapy, close clinical and echocardiographic follow-up, and reconsideration for aortic valve replacement. Carasso et al. showed that although longitudinal strain was low in asymptomatic patients with severe aortic stenosis, apical circumferential strain and rotation were supernormal while in symptomatic patients no compensatory circumferential myocardial mechanics was observed. Other investigators suggest that after adjusting for aortic stenosis severity and EF, only basal longitudinal strain (and not GLS) was an independent predictor of symptomatic status as shown by post-TAVR improvement in GLS as a result of basal and mid-segment improvement only. In patients with low flow, low gradient, aortic stenosis with normal EF, both stroke volume index (≤35 mL/m^2) and GLS (<–15%) are independently associated with poor survival. Kusunose et al. studied 395 patients with moderate-severe aortic stenosis (aortic valve area <1.3 cm^2) and found that GLS was an independent predictor of mortality in this population. GLS less than –12% was associated with the lowest survival.[13-15] In a prospective study of young patients (<18 years old) with aortic regurgitation, the only significant predictor of progression of disease on multivariable analysis was GLS, a cut-off value of greater than –19.5% had sensitivity of 77.8% and specificity of 94.1%. Systolic radial strain rate of less than 1.82/s was a good predictor of postoperative left ventricular dysfunction in adult patients. In 129 patients with preserved LVEF (≥50%), LV longitudinal strain was more reduced in symptomatic patients as compared with asymptomatic patients (–14.9 ± 3.0 versus –16.8 ± 2.5%). In chronic severe degenerative mitral regurgitation studies have shown that a reduced baseline GLS signifies a maladaptive preload-related change that is associated with a reduction in left ventricular EF immediately after mitral valve repair. A GLS cutoff of more than –19.9% was a strong independent predictor of long-term left ventricular dysfunction and may become an appropriate indication for intervention in the setting of normal EF. Witkowski and colleagues reported that patients with severe organic MR and LVEF more than 60% who developed LV systolic dysfunction (LVEF < 50%) after surgical mitral valve repair showed more impaired LV global longitudinal strain at baseline compared with patients who had preserved LV systolic function (LVEF ≥50%) after surgery. In patients with dilated cardiomyopathy and functional MR, LV global longitudinal strain often showed worse LV systolic function than suggested by the LVEF, indicating that global longitudinal strain might partially unmask the true impairment in LV contractility. Despite similar LVEF, patients with dilated cardiomyopathy and severe functional MR showed more impaired LV global longitudinal strain compared with patients without functional MR (–9.78 ± 3.78% versus –8.08 ± 3.33%; p = 0.004). Best discriminant parameter to detect a postoperative LVEF reduction of more than 10% in patients of chronic severe mitral regurgitation with speckle tracking was a longitudinal strain rate at the level of the mid isovolumic contraction (IVS) less than –0.80 s-1 (positive predictive value, 90%; negative predictive value, 82.35%).[16-18]

Box chart describing proposed inclusion of GLS in prognosticating DCMP patients is shown in Flowchart 1.

Left atrial size is an important determinant in risk stratification schemes in patients of dilated cardiomyopathy. Left atrial volume index (LAVI) more than 38 mL/m^2 has same prognostic value as of EF in heart failure admissions and need for cardiac transplant (data from MeRGE study). 3D LAV more than 100 mL predicted 1-year adverse cardiovascular outcomes among patients with severe LV dysfunction. Few studies also support the measurement of atrial function to predict cardiovascular outcomes. LA work estimated by left atrial kinetic energy (LAKE) was independently predictive of cardiovascular death and hospitalization for congestive heart failure (CHF) in 243 heart failure patients followed for a median of 3.1 years excluding higher grades of LV diastolic dysfunction (the

Flowchart 1: Proposed inclusion of GLS in prognosticating DCMP patients.

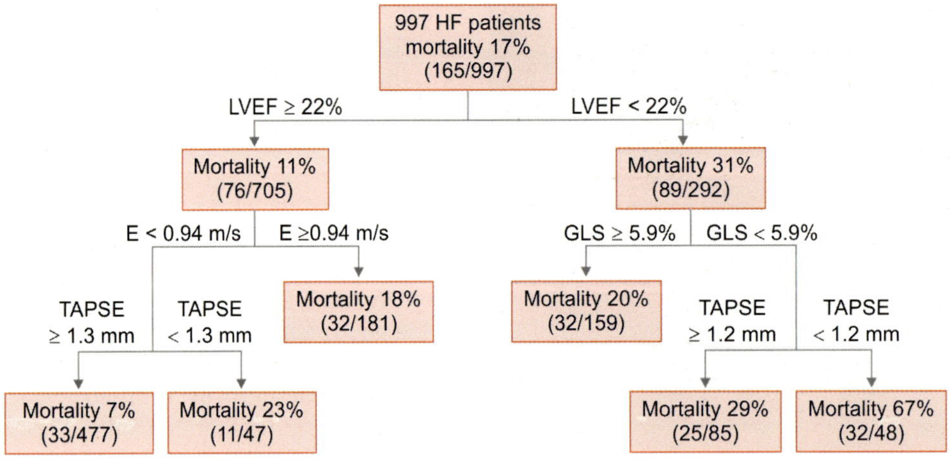

(GLS, global longitudinal strain; LVEF, left ventricular ejection fraction; TAPSE: tricuspid annular plane systolic excursion; DCMP: dilated cardiomyopathy).

Source: Sengeløv M, Jørgensen PG, Jensen JS, et al. Global longitudinal strain is a superior predictor of all-cause mortality in heart failure with reduced ejection fraction. JACC Cardiovasc Imaging. 2015;8:1351-9.

reference value of LAKE derived from 230 controls was 5.4 kdyne/m^2). In HCMP patients, LAVI more than 41 mL/m^2 was an independent predictor of cardiovascular mortality, CHF hospitalization, and cerebrovascular accident (CVA). LAVI more than 32 mL/m^2 was a powerful predictor of all-cause mortality and was incremental to clinical information and LV function in 314 patients with acute myocardial infarctions (AMIs) followed for a mean of 15 months. In addition to clinical variables, baseline LAVI more than 32 mL/m^2 and diastolic dysfunction were independent predictors of 5-year mortality in VALIANT Echo study. LA εs and maximal LAV measured within 48 hours of an AMI were independent predictors of all-cause mortality, reinfarction, and CHF hospitalization after adjusting for clinical and echocardiographic parameters in 320 patients with AMIs followed for a mean of 27 months. Maximal LAV and εs were independent predictors of LA remodeling (≥8 mL/m^2 increase in maximal LAV); in contrast to those without remodeling, those with LA remodeling had worsening of LA εs and SR-S. Le Tourneau et al., prospectively examined 492 patients with chronic organic MR in sinus rhythm and found LAVI more than or equal to 60 mL/m^2 treated medically had increased mortality and more cardiac events (AF and heart failure) than those with LAVI less than 40 mL/m^2. The 5-year survival rates in conservatively managed patients with LAVI more than or equal to 60, 40–59, and less than 40 mL/m^2 were 53 ± 8.6%, 84 ± 4.8%, and 90 ± 3.0%, respectively.[19,20]

Three-dimensional echocardiography shows closer agreement quantification with CMR than 2D echo for estimating LV volumes. In a meta-analysis including 28 studies comparing 3D echo with CMR in 1,198 individuals, 3D echo underestimated the LV end-diastolic volume (LVEDV) by –14 ± 5 mL and the LV end-systolic volume (LVESV) by –7 ± 3 mL, while LVEF was virtually the same among both modalities –0 ± 3%. 2D-derived volumes showed a larger bias, being –33 ± 10 mL for LVEDV and –16 ± 5 mL for LVESV suggesting that LVEF, but not LV volumes, can be used interchangeably among these modalities. Current guidelines recommend 2D biplane Simpson's method for EF calculation and 3D when image quality is adequate for analysis. Bias between 3D echo and CMR has been reported in women, patients with congenital heart disease, ventricular aneurysms or hypertrophic cardiomyopathy. Underestimation of volumes is more pronounced in patients with depressed LVEF, since the true boundary [i.e. endocardial border is less well defined (with reference to noncompacted cardiomyopathy)]. 3D echocardiography proves a very useful tool in asymptomatic regurgitation lesions (stage B and C1) where reproducible measurements of LV size and volumes are quintessential in deciding when to refer the patient for surgery. Three-dimensional transesophageal echocardiography (3DTEE) based annular measurements help in understanding the annular hemodynamics, which have been proven to be different in dilated cardiomyopathy versus ischemic cardiomyopathy. 3D-based systolic dyssynchrony index seems to be promising index in CRT selection as shown by Kleijn et al. in a meta-analysis of 73 studies including more than 5,000 subjects (3,341 patients and 1,832 healthy subjects). 3D systolic dyssynchrony index (SDI) in healthy subjects was 2.7 + 0.9%, heart failure patients in general 9.8 + 3.9% and patients eligible for CRT 10.7+3.6%; thereby concluding that in patients eligible for CRT, SDI more than 9.8% predicted treatment response with a sensitivity of 93% and specificity of 75% and there was 94% feasibility. Although the majority of literature supports using cardiovascular magnetic resonance late gadolinium enhancement (CMR LGE) for quantifying scar.

Delgado et al. used a less than 16.5% radial strain cutoff to relate LV lead position in scar as having a less favorable outcome in ischemic cardiomyopathy patients, which was of additive prognostic value to dyssynchrony and LV lead at site of latest activation.[19] Khan et al. also used radial strain in a group of 140 CRT patients and observed that reverse remodeling response was significantly lower in those patients where low amplitude radial strain was less than 9.8% at site of LV lead placement (62.7% vs. 31.3%, $p < 0.05$) with 92% specificity and 39% sensitivity. These investigators went on to apply the combination of targeting LV lead position to avoiding scarred regions (radial strain <9.8%) while seeking the site of latest activation in the TARGET trial. The targeted LV strategy was associated with more favorable LV reverse remodeling and superior clinical outcomes. So there is growing evidence that avoiding scar is highly advisable when placing LV lead for CRT. A larger experience supports assessing transmural scar by CMR LGE, however, speckle tracking radial strain appears to be able to play a role in determine regions of likely scar.[21,22]

CONCLUSION

We have learnt that recent advances in echocardiography for quantification of systolic functions have now been translated from clinical trials to clinical practice. The modest interobserver and test-retest reproducibility of specific structural and functional parameters with conventional echocardiography has improved over time. These newer echocardiographic modalities provide the best opportunity currently available to demonstrate treatment effects on the myocardium with investigational therapies and provide mechanistic insights for future directions.

REFERENCES

1. Carlsson M, Ugander M, Mosen H, et al. Atrioventricular plane displacement is the major contributor to left ventricular pumping in healthy adults, athletes, and patients with dilated cardiomyopathy. Am J Physiol Heart Circ Physiol. 2007;292:H1452-9.
2. Ersboll M, Valeur N, Mogensen UM, et al. Prediction of all-cause mortality and heart failure admissions from global left ventricular longitudinal strain in patients with acute myocardial infarction and preserved left ventricular ejection fraction. J Am Coll Cardiol. 2013;61:2365-73.
3. Bertini M, Ng AC, Antoni ML, et al. Global longitudinal strain predicts long-term survival in patients with chronic ischemic cardiomyopathy. Circ Cardiovasc Imaging. 2012;5:383-91.
4. Willenheimer R, Cline C, Erhardt L, et al. Left ventricular atrioventricular plane displacement: an echocardiographic technique for rapid assessment of prognosis in heart failure. Heart. 1997;78:230-6.
5. Svealv BG, Olofsson EL, Andersson B. Ventricular long-axis function is of major importance for long-term survival in patients with heart failure. Heart. 2008;94:284-9.
6. Stanton T, Leano R, Marwick TH. Prediction of all-cause mortality from global longitudinal speckle strain: comparison with ejection fraction and wall motion scoring. Circ Cardiovasc Imaging. 2009;2:356-64.
7. Cho GY, Marwick TH, Kim HS, et al. Global 2-dimensional strain as a new prognosticator in patients with heart failure. J Am Coll Cardiol. 2009;54:618-24.
8. Kalam K, Otahal P, Marwick TH. Prognostic implications of global LV dysfunction: a systematic review and meta-analysis of global longitudinal strain and ejection fraction. Heart. 2014;100(21):1673-80.
9. Cai L, Addetia K, Medvedofsky D, et al. Myocardial strain may be useful in differentiating Takotsubo cardiomyopathy from left anterior descending coronary artery ischemia. Int J Cardiol. 2017;230:359-63.
10. Izumo M, Akashi YJ. Role of echocardiography for Takotsubo cardiomyopathy: clinical and prognostic implications. Cardiovasc Diagn Ther. 2018;8(1):90-100.
11. Seo Y, Ishizu T. Incremental value of speckle tracking echocardiography to predict cardiac resynchronization therapy (CRT) responders. J Am Heart Assoc. 2016;5:e003882.
12. Gorcsan J III, Yu CM. ASE Dyssynchrony Writing Group. Echocardiography for cardiac resynchronization therapy: Recommendations for performance and reporting–a report from the American Society of Echocardiography dyssynchrony Writing Group endorsed by the Heart Rhythm Society. J Am Soc Echocardiogr. 2008;21:191-213.
13. Goldenberg I, Klein H. MADIT-CRT Executive Committee. Predictors of response to cardiac resynchronization therapy in the Multicenter Automatic Defibrillator Implantation Trial with Cardiac Resynchronization Therapy (MADIT-CRT). Circulation. 2011;124:1527-36.
14. Dahou A, Bartko PE, Capoulade R, et al. Usefulness of global left ventricular longitudinal strain for risk stratification in low ejection fraction, low-gradient aortic stenosis: results from the multicenter True or Pseudo-Severe Aortic Stenosis study. Circ Cardiovasc Imaging. 2015;8(3):e002117.
15. Nagata Y, Takeuchi M, Wu VC, et al. Prognostic value of LV deformation parameters using 2D and 3D speckle-tracking echocardiography in asymptomatic patients with severe aortic stenosis and preserved LV ejection fraction. JACC Cardiovasc Imaging. 2015;8(3):235-45.
16. de Isla LP, de Agustin A, Rodrigo JL, et al. Chronic mitral regurgitation: a pilot study to assess preoperative left ventricular contractile function using speckle-tracking echocardiography. J Am Soc Echocardiogr. 2009;22(7):831-8.
17. Witkowski TG, Thomas JD, Debonnaire PJMR, et al. Global longitudinal strain predicts left ventricular dysfunction after mitral valve repair. Eur Heart J Cardiovasc Imaging. 2013;14(1):69-76.

18. Pandis D, Sengupta PP, Castillo JG, et al. Assessment of longitudinal myocardial mechanics in patients with degenerative mitral valve regurgitation predicts postoperative worsening of left ventricular systolic function. J Am Soc Echocardiogr. 2014;27(6):627-38.
19. Holt B. Left atrial size and function: role in prognosis. J Am Coll Cardiol. 2014;63(6):493-505.
20. Le Tourneau T, Messika-Zeitoun D, Russo A, et al. Impact of left atrial volume on clinical outcome in organic mitral regurgitation. J Am Coll Cardiol. 2010;56:570-8.
21. Cheung YF. The role of 3D wall motion tracking in heart failure. Nat Rev Cardiol. 2012;9(11):644.
22. Cai Q, Ahmad M. Left ventricular dyssynchrony by three-dimensional echocardiography: current understanding and potential future clinical applications. 2015;32(8):1299-306.

CHAPTER 18

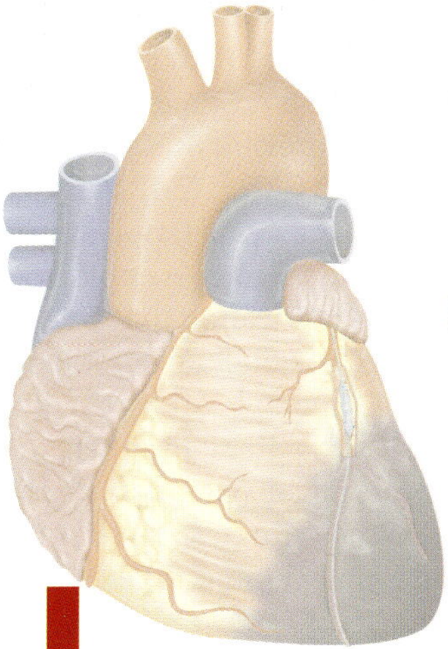

Cardiac Magnetic Resonance Imaging in Ischemic Heart Failure

Mona Bhatia, Khemendra Kumar

INTRODUCTION

Heart failure (HF) is a characterized by breathlessness, fatigue, and ankle swelling which can be accompanied by signs of raised jugular venous pressure, pulmonary crackles, and peripheral edema. Structural or functional abnormality of heart is generally the cause of HF, which leads to reduced cardiac output and/or increased intracardiac pressures at stress or rest. HF assumes more significance as it is associated with significant amount of morbidity, mortality, and financial implications.[1-2] HF currently is rapidly growing into epidemic proportions. Approximately 5.8 million patients in the United States currently suffer from HF, and over 670,000 of them are newly diagnosed with HF each year. HF with sudden cardiac death accounts for more deaths globally than all forms of cancer combined; the 5-year mortality after a diagnosis of HF is approximately 50%.[3]

DIAGNOSTIC CRITERIA

Heart failure is classified into three types depending on the status of the ejection fraction:

1. Reduced ejection fraction (<40%)
2. Mid-range ejection fraction (40–49%)
3. Preserved ejection fraction (>50%).

Suspected HF is diagnosed by the combination of medical history, physical examination, electrocardiogram, chest X-ray, and natriuretic peptide measurement. Transthoracic echocardiography is the first-line imaging investigation.[4] Cardiovascular magnetic resonance (CMR) imaging plays an important complementary role in evaluating the underlying etiology (or etiologies) of the suspected HF.[5]

Imaging in Heart Failure

The main objectives of imaging for HF evaluation revolve primarily around understanding both cardiac structure and function, and, secondarily, in determining the underlying etiology, so that proven medical and invasive therapies may be targeted to appropriate patients. As the prevalence of HF is increasing, there is increased interest regarding the importance of imaging in HF. Dramatic developments have occurred over the recent decades with advancements in imaging modalities, surgical or percutaneous therapies, and medical therapies for HF as well as for the management of the conditions causing HF. To balance the high costs of in-hospital and outpatient HF management, appropriateness of imaging modality is essential.[6] CMR to its credit has multiple studies for evaluation of wall motion abnormality at stress, in patients with HF. CMR has the distinct advantage of ensuring detection of fibrosis, a technique that, in observational studies, helps to identify and differentiate ischemic versus nonischemic cardiomyopathy in HF patients. Recent preliminary reports have also linked fibrosis with clinical outcome.[7]

Coronary Heart Disease and Heart Failure

The effect of coronary artery disease (CAD) on pathophysiology of HF is in the form of reduced systolic function. Following coronary insult, ischemia can produce a rapid and massive increase in the concentration of endogenous catecholamines such as norepinephrine, epinephrine, endothelin, and dopamine in the myocardial interstitial fluid with a deleterious effect on cardiac myocytes, culminating in myocardial apoptosis, fibrosis, and susceptibility to ventricular arrhythmias. Thus, ischemia may contribute to the progression of left ventricular (LV) systolic dysfunction without an obvious clinical ischemic event. Presence and extent of CAD accelerates the progression of HF which in turn explains the higher mortality among ischemic compared with nonischemic HF patients. Acute myocardial infarction (MI) results in loss of functioning myocytes followed by myocardial fibrosis resulting in LV dilatation. The resulting neurohormonal activation and LV remodeling lead to progressive deterioration of the remaining viable myocardium as well.[8]

Pathophysiological Considerations

After the acute coronary occlusion, the time frame of events in the ischemic cascade comprises the reversible changes: myocardial contractile dysfunction (seconds), intracellular edema (20–30 minutes) followed by irreversible injury to myocytes (30–60 minutes), and vascular endothelial cells (60–90 minutes) with cellular necrosis and apoptosis. Postacute coronary insult, progression of necrosis is in wave front manner, beginning from subendocardium and extending up to subepicardium in 3–6 hours, completing transmurally. The jeopardized myocardium or the myocardium at risk is area of myocardium in the territory of the involved artery. Prolonged postischemic contractile dysfunction of the myocardium salvaged by reperfusion is defined as stunned myocardium, which may take days-to-weeks to normalize, though it can be reversed with inotropic agents. Hibernating myocardium is a viable but dysfunctional myocardium secondary to a chronic coronary artery stenosis but is potentially reversible.[9] Chronic ischemia may result in hibernation or stunning of myocardium with further decline in LV function. In a meta-analysis study, there was 80% reduction in mortality in patients who had evidence of viability and underwent revascularization compared to medical treatment. Patient without evidence of viable myocardium had similar mortality rate after revascularization or by medical management.[8] Mitral regurgitation (MR) is one of the complications of CAD. Inferior wall MI is associated with greater severity and incidence of MR. This increased severity and incidence of MR results from changes in the geometry of mitral valvular apparatus. Mild MR is an independent predictor of long-term mortality after MI. All these processes can be interrupted at any time by a sudden coronary occlusion leading to sudden death.[10] Cardiac MR is most commonly indicated for risk stratification in suspected CAD/ischemia in known CAD (34.2%), work-up of myocarditis and cardiomyopathies (32.2%), followed by the assessment of myocardial viability (14.6%).[11] Hypertension or valvular heart disease is no longer the most common cause of HF, as was seen in previous decades. The Framingham Heart Study suggests it is CAD.[12] CMR assesses morphology, function, flow, perfusion, acute tissue injury, and fibrosis in a single setting and hence aids in etiological diagnosis, classification, and risk stratification in HF. CMR is recognized as the gold standard for the measurements of volumes, mass, and EF of both the left and right ventricles. CMR has the potential for a paradigm shift in the noninvasive diagnosis and monitoring of patients with HF. CMR is the preferred imaging method to assess myocardial fibrosis using late gadolinium enhancement (LGE) along with T1 mapping and can be useful for establishing HF etiology. CMR with LGE helps in the differentiation between ischemic and nonischemic pathology. CMR is used for the assessment of extent of myocardial ischemia and viability in patients with HF and CAD (considered suitable for coronary revascularization).

CARDIAC MAGNETIC RESONANCE IMAGING IN ACUTE ISCHEMIA

Cine Imaging

The cine steady-state free-procession sequences acquired in short axis, vertical long axis, and horizontal long axis view, show that the affected segments of myocardium are hypokinetic or akinetic, as one might expect, for a site of myocardial ischemia/infarction. These sequences are used to calculate the ventricular functions and ejection fraction. Valvular regurgitations are also assessed in these sequences.[13]

T2 Imaging for Myocardial Edema Assessment

The territory of the infarct-related artery is at the risk of potentially irreversible damage to the myocardium at risk, if reperfusion does not occur promptly. When myocardial blood flow is promptly restored, the irreversibly damaged myocardial area is significantly smaller than the area at risk. Pathophysiologic model of acute ischemia after coronary occlusion shows a rapid onset of myocardial edema, which can be detected as early as 30 minutes from symptoms onset on T2-weighted images (Fig. 1). T2-weighted sequences can detect the presence and extent of the myocardium at risk and estimate the amount of myocardium that can be salvaged by subtracting the extent of scarred myocardium in the late gadolinium enhanced images from the area at risk on T2-weighted images. The assessment of salvageable

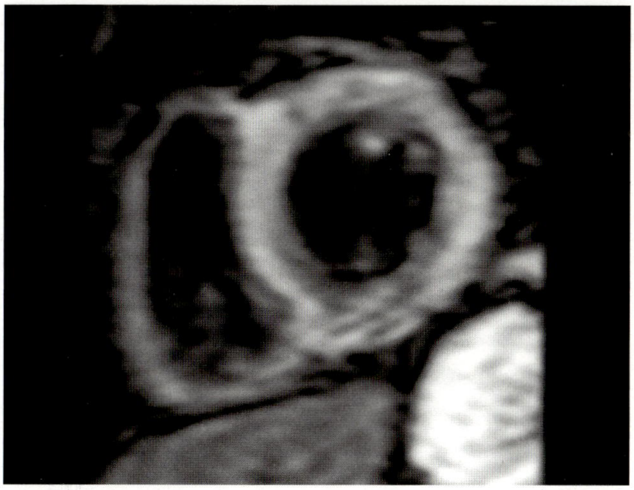

Fig. 1: Short axis T2-weighted cardiovascular magnetic resonance (CMR) image demonstrating myocardial hyperintensity, suggestive of edema in a case of acute myocardial ischemia.

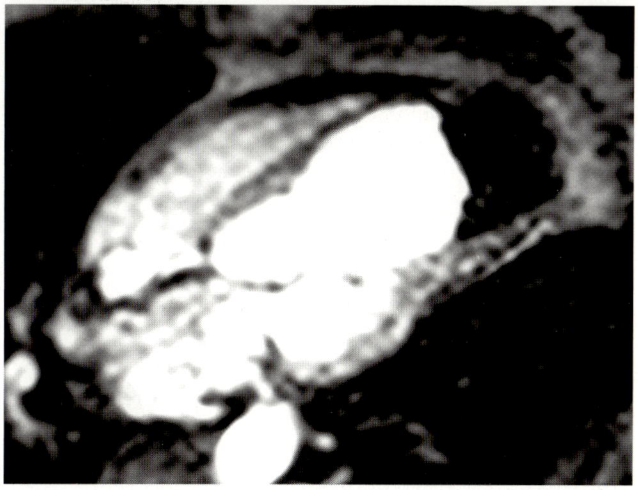

Fig. 2: Four chamber post-gadolinium injection first-pass myocardial perfusion cardiovascular magnetic resonance (CMR) image demonstrating perfusion defect in the left anterior descending artery (LAD) territory with intracavitary nonfilling of the apex on account of an intracavitary thrombus lining an apical aneurysm postmyocardial infarction.

myocardium is reproducible and has been validated against single-photon emission computed tomography (SPECT) and angiographic studies.[14] In a non-negligible proportion of patients with acute coronary syndrome (ACS) (approximately one-third), a "culprit" lesion is not identified by angiogram. T2-weighted sequences can easily allow the detection of the culprit lesion, as an area of increased signal intensity along the distribution territory of a coronary artery. Monney et al. found that MI was identified in 13% of patients with ACS with unobstructed coronaries, as delineated by a localized increase in signal intensity on T2-weighted images in areas of transmural scar.[15] Raman et al. showed that the presence of myocardium at risk on T2-weighted CMR sequences allows the identification of patients who will benefit from an early invasive management. In fact, the presence of myocardial edema has been shown to increase the risk of adverse cardiovascular events, irrespective of revascularization.[16]

Cardiovascular Magnetic Resonance Stress Myocardial Perfusion Imaging

Cardiovascular magnetic resonance myocardial perfusion imaging is performed using extracellular gadolinium (Gd)-based contrast agent. Such agents rapidly diffuse from the vascular space to the extracellular space, so perfusion must be assessed during the first pass into the myocardium, hence, the term "first-pass myocardial perfusion imaging" (Fig. 2). Using a T1-weighted saturation recovery perfusion sequence, perfused myocardium appears bright while hypoperfused myocardium appears dark. However, considerable experience is required to differentiate genuinely hypoperfused myocardium from the common dark rim artifact that occurs at the myocardial/blood pool interface. Typically, three short-axis slice images are planned in the apical, mid, and basal left ventricle, allowing 16 myocardial segments to be assessed. Increasing coverage to image the whole heart would usually require compromise on image resolution, but advanced three-dimensional acceleration techniques and imaging at higher field strengths (where higher baseline signal can be traded for more highly accelerated image acquisition) may overcome this limitation.[17] For stress myocardial perfusion imaging by CMR, physiological stress is usually induced by a vasodilatory agent (adenosine, regadenoson, or dipyridamole), though some centers have developed bespoke equipment to permit physical exercise in the constrained environs of the MR scanner. Traditionally, rest perfusion imaging is performed at least 15 minutes later, and images are compared to look for the presence and reversibility of any perfusion defects. As a consequence, it may be preferable to omit rest perfusion imaging altogether when using this stressor, and comparing stress perfusion images against LGE instead.[17]

Dobutamine Stress CMR Wall Motion Imaging

Cardiovascular magnetic resonance stress wall motion imaging is undertaken using an incremental dobutamine stress protocol similar to that used for stress echocardiography. The ability to plan identical image geometry at each stage of the test and the superior definition of the endocardial border represent key advantages of CMR over echo. However, the temporal resolution of CMR at high heart rates is generally inferior to echo, and image quality may be less favorable in patients with arrhythmia. Patients may also tolerate dobutamine-related symptoms less well in the confined space of the MR scanner, and the management of adverse effects is more complex due to MRI safety concerns.[18]

Early Gadolinium Enhancement

T1-weighted inversion recovery sequences is used for early gadolinium enhancement (EGE) approximately after 1 minute of contrast administration using fixed TI value in the range of 400–500 ms. EGE is helpful in detecting microvascular obstruction (MVO). MVO is the CMR equivalent of the "no-reflow" phenomenon seen at coronary angiography. Low signal in the subendocardial myocardium on EGE imaging is indicative of MVO. Higher signal intensity may be seen in regions of myocardial hyperemia (e.g. myocardial edema).[19]

Late Gadolinium Enhancement

Identical T1-weighted inversion recovery sequence is used as in EGE for late gadolinium enhancement (LGE). LGE imaging is done approximately 10 minutes after contrast administration. In regions where the extracellular volume is increased (e.g. fibrotic tissue or edema) or where cell breakdown has occurred (e.g. acute infarction), the washout of contrast is delayed relative to normal myocardium. LGE exploits this difference in the washout contrast from normal and abnormal myocardium. In LGE sequences, normal myocardial signal is nulled (signal is suppressed and myocardium appears black), by selecting inversion time or a phase-sensitive inversion recovery sequence. Enhancing areas appear white, and the pattern of enhancement varies according to the underlying pathology. Enhancement pattern in ischemic heart disease (IHD) is either subendocardial or transmural, limited to a particular vascular territory involvement (Fig. 3). The high-spatial resolution of LGE imaging allows detection of infarctions involving as little as 1 g of tissue, which results in significantly higher sensitivity than SPECT for the detection of subendocardial infarction.[20]

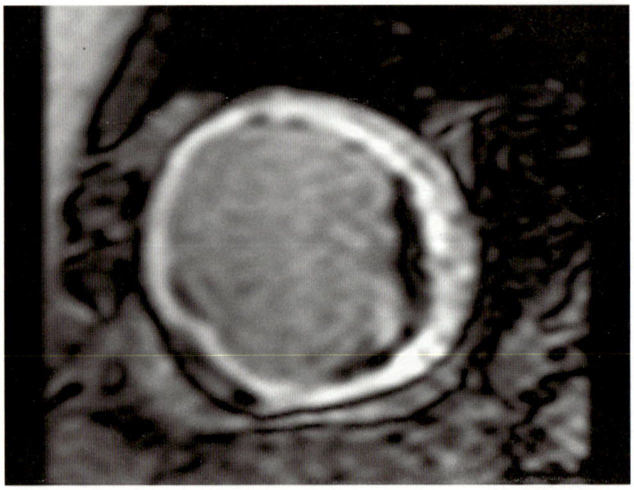

Fig. 3: Short axis post-gadolinium enhanced phase-sensitive inversion recovery cardiovascular magnetic resonance (PSIR CMR) image demonstrating extensive circumferential transmural late gadolinium enhancement consistent with myocardial infarction in the apical left anterior descending artery (LAD) territory with aneurysmal change and intracavitary thrombus in a case of ischemic cardiomyopathy.

CLINICAL APPLICATION OF CARDIAC MITRAL REGURGITATION IN ISCHEMIC HEART DISEASE

Stable Ischemic Heart Disease

As per the 2012 guidelines for the diagnosis and management of patients with stable IHD, pharmacologic stress CMR is a Class IIA recommendation for patients with an intermediate-to-high pretest probability of IHD who are unable to exercise.[21] Stress CMR was recognized as appropriate imaging modality in the evaluation of ischemic etiology and viability of myocardium in HF patients. According to 2013 report, the performance of stress CMR was rated similar to stress echocardiography and SPECT.[22] The 2014 European Society of Cardiology (ESC) guidelines on myocardial revascularization give a class IA recommendation for diagnostic stress MRI testing in patients with intermediate probability of suspected CAD and stable symptoms, and a class IB recommendation for revascularization on prognostic grounds in patients with stable angina or silent ischemia, where there is a large area of ischemia on functional testing.[23] The event rate following a normal dobutamine stress CMR study has been shown to be 1.2% at 1 year which is comparable with the 1.3% annual event rate following a normal dobutamine stress echo. Moderate-to-severe ischemia is defined as 2 of the 16 segments demarcating reversible defects by CMR stress myocardial perfusion imaging (4 of the 32 if the 16 segments are divided into endocardial and epicardial subsegments) or at least three newly dysfunctional segments during dobutamine stress CMR.[24]

Detection of Ischemic Cardiomyopathy

The predominant cause of LV systolic dysfunction in the developed world is IHD.[25] Establishing an ischemic basis to LV dysfunction has important prognostic implications, carrying a higher mortality rate when compared to patients with idiopathic dilated cardiomyopathy.[26] In patients with systolic HF, but without symptoms of angina, studies have suggested that LGE is a sensitive and specific marker of significant CAD. The most recent and largest trial of CMR as a gatekeeper for angiography in HF patients with reduced ejection fraction and without a history of IHD or angina used LGE alongside magnetic resonance imaging of the coronary arteries (MRCA) and reported a diagnostic accuracy of 96% for the detection of significant CAD compared with invasive angiography. High-resolution quantitative CMR myocardial perfusion imaging has also been shown to be feasible in patients with HF.[27]

Viability

Cardiovascular magnetic resonance may be used to assess the probability of recovery of myocardial contractility with revascularization ("viability") in IHD patient. Study by Kim et al. in 2000, undergoing revascularization following LV dysfunction showed that probability of improvement in contractility in LV dysfunction following revascularization is decreased as the transmurality of LGE increases. In the absence of LGE, the likelihood of functional recovery was high (78%). In the 1–50% scar thickness range, revascularization led to functional recovery in 53% of segments (60% recovery in the 1–25% range and 42% recovery in the 26–50% scar thickness range). Where scar thickness exceeded 50%, the chance of functional recovery with revascularization dropped to below 10% overall (10% and 2% chance of recovery in the 51–75% and 76–100% scar thickness ranges, respectively).[28]

A threshold of 50% scar thickness may be adopted as a pragmatic cutoff for viability. In reality, this remains a relatively blunt tool for judging who will and will not benefit from revascularization. By undertaking low-dose dobutamine stress CMR (DSCMR) in those with an intermediate burden of scar by LGE (delayed enhancement of 1–74%), superior accuracy for the prediction of viability has been demonstrated.[29] There have been relatively few trials looking at the relationship between extent of viability on a segmental basis and recovery of LV function. It has been shown that patients with at least 10 viable including normal segments show improved global LV function following coronary artery bypass graft (CABG), whereas patients with fewer such segments do not.[30]

Microvascular Occlusion

Microvascular obstruction is generally seen in a proportion of patients having acute MI following reperfusion therapy of an occluded coronary artery. It is characterized by damage and dysfunction of the myocardial microvasculature with a no-reflow phenomenon within the infarct zone. The pathophysiological mechanisms that result in MVO remain ill-defined, but MVO is likely to result from an interaction of multiple-related pathological processes. In animal models, ischemia causes endothelial damage that narrows the capillary lumen impairing blood flow.[31] The presence of further luminal narrowing of the myocardial capillary bed caused by combined aggregates of fibrin, platelets, and erythrocytes creates an additional mechanical barrier to blood flow. Leucocyte aggregation is also seen at sites of MVO that, as well as causing mechanical obstruction to blood flow, may also impair vasodilatation by triggering oxidative stress pathways. Human studies have shown that microembolization plays an important contributory role in MVO, with distal showers of embolic material causing additional mechanical obstruction and stimulating an inflammatory response.[32] Presence of MVO has been shown to be an independent predictor of poor prognostic outcome following MI, including adverse LV remodeling, subsequent major adverse cardiovascular events and death. Patients with MVO typically demonstrate persistent global LV dysfunction, with less improvement in LV ejection fraction when compared with patients without MVO.[33] MVO typically appears as a central dark focus within an area of early enhancing myocardium signifying a focal absence of contrast enhancement within a site of myocardial infarct.[9] MVO demonstrates similar appearances on both EGE sequences (typically performed between 1 and 3 minutes postgadolinium injection) and LGE sequences (typically performed at 8–10 minutes postgadolinium injection). Myocardial edema demonstrates the potential myocardium at risk. However, areas of MVO represent areas of irreversible MI. Although the appearances of MVO seen on first-pass perfusion, EGE and LGE sequences are broadly similar, there are some important differences. The true area of MVO seen on LGE sequences is smaller than either first-pass perfusion or EGE due to slow diffusion of gadolinium-contrast agent over time around the periphery of the no-reflow site. Therefore, the first-pass perfusion imaging identifies the presence of MVO in a larger proportion of patients than with either EGE or LGE imaging. Importantly, the presence of MVO on LGE is a more accurate prognostic marker than MVO seen on first-pass perfusion or EGE sequences in predicting patients at risk of adverse LV remodeling and future major adverse cardiovascular events.[34] MVO may also be seen following iatrogenic myocardial damage following myocardial ablation therapy for ventricular arrhythmias. Mimickers of MVO on CMR are ventricular thrombus appearing as low signal intensity lesion within the cavity and calcified infarcts in the myocardium. Myocardial thinning is a useful imaging discriminator between these two processes as myocardial thickness should remain preserved in patients presenting acutely following a myocardial infarct with MVO. Myocardial hemorrhage can be seen within the infarct core,

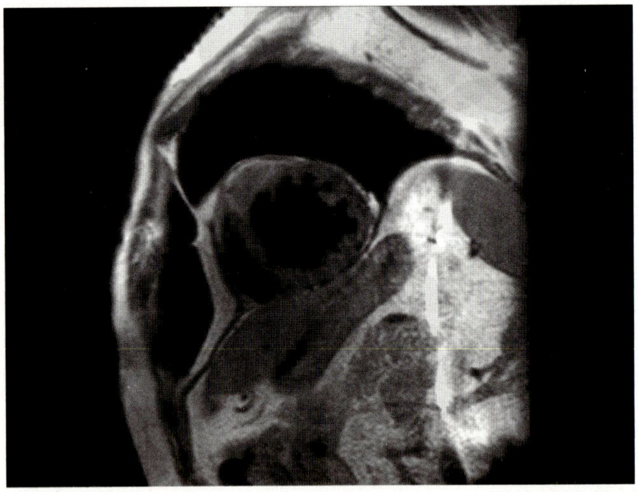

Fig. 4: Short axis T1-weighted image demonstrating intramyocardial T1 hyperintensity in anteroseptal and anterior myocardial wall of left ventricular (LV) cavity consistent with hemorrhage.

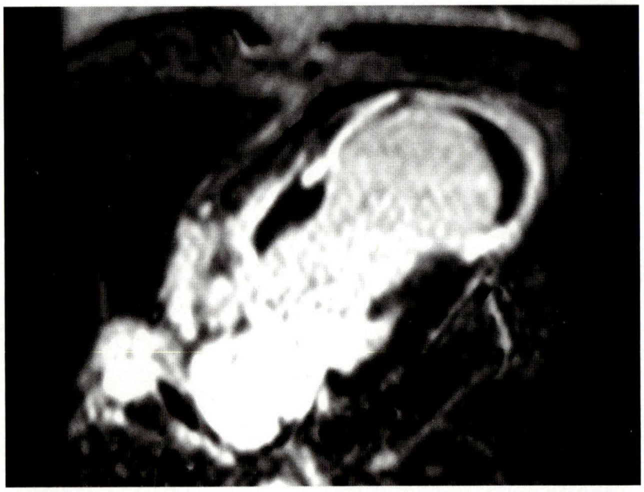

Fig. 5: Four chamber post-gadolinium enhanced phase-sensitive inversion recovery cardiovascular magnetic resonance (PSIR CMR) image demonstrating extensive transmural late gadolinium enhancement consistent with myocardial infarction in the left anterior descending artery (LAD) territory with aneurysmal change in the apex and intracavitary apical thrombus in a case of ischemic cardiomyopathy.

and although MVO and hemorrhage are closely linked, they remain distinct pathological entities (Fig. 4). At sites of MVO, red cell extravasation may be demonstrated in regions of endothelial damage at the myocardial capillary bed. Animal studies have shown that MVO may occur in the absence of myocardial hemorrhage, but myocardial hemorrhage does not occur in the absence of MVO. In addition, although there is concurrence in the anatomical site of both processes, the site of myocardial hemorrhage is typically smaller than the site of MVO.[35]

Complications of Acute Myocardial Infarction

Mechanical complications of acute MI are associated with reduced short and long-term survival.[36] The most encountered mechanical complications include ventricular free wall or septal rupture, papillary muscle infarction or rupture with secondary acute MR, ventricular aneurysm (Fig. 5) and pseudoaneurysm. Right ventricular (RV) involvement may occur in a non-negligible proportion of acute MI, mainly involving the inferior wall (incidence being 24–50%). RV involvement is hemodynamically relevant in up to 25–50% of cases and is usually associated with poorer prognosis. CMR has shown to detect RV involvement in 25% of patients with inferior MI, a percentage that is significantly superior to that detected by ECG and transthoracic echocardiogram (TTE). MR studies have shown that RV MI is usually associated with larger MI, lower left ventricular ejection fraction (LVEF), and lower RV ejection fraction.[37] With its superior spatial resolution and feasibility soon after the acute event, CMR is an extremely promising tool for the identification of early and late MI complications. Post-MI ventricular septal defect (VSD) is associated with 80–90% mortality within few months after acute event; not only is CMR useful to make the diagnosis, but also tissue characterization to look for fibrosis of VSD edges helps identifying the most appropriate time for surgery. Myocardial tissue characterization by CMR also allows to distinguish a true aneurysm, which is characterized by a large neck and typically enhanced aneurysm wall, from pseudoaneurysm, which usually has a small neck, with nonenhanced wall, and represents a contained rupture. A lipomatous metaplasia seen as a high signal intensity area in the cine and postcontrast sequences, is also commonly seen in patients with old MI who underwent surgical myocardial revascularization.[38] LV thrombus is a frequent complication of IHD. The incidence of thrombus is proportionate to poor LVEF, and the scar size. Thrombus typically appears as a nonenhancing structure in early and late contrast enhancement CMR. Detection of thrombus by CMR has shown to be superior to TTE.[39]

CLINICAL APPLICATIONS OF CARDIOVASCULAR MAGNETIC RESONANCE IN ISCHEMIC HEART DISEASE

Acute Coronary Syndromes

Vasodilator stress CMR myocardial perfusion imaging may play a role in the initial investigation of patients presenting with troponin-negative chest pain and a normal electrocardiography (ECG). A normal adenosine stress CMR study has been shown to carry a good prognosis in this group over 1 year follow-up.[40] In those patients who have undergone angiography ± intervention, CMR stress myocardial perfusion imaging may be used to determine the functional significance of residual coronary disease and is safe in the early postinfarct period.[41] CMR may be particularly useful in patients with multivessel disease, prior infarction, and an uncertain culprit vessel. In this setting, edema imaging, and detection of MVO by EGE, may be used to differentiate acute from chronic infarction scar (which could not be differentiated by LGE imaging alone). In addition, comparing the area of infarct scar to the area of myocardial edema by short-tau inversion recovery (STIR) imaging allows for an accurate assessment of the amount of myocardium salvaged by reperfusion and has become an important research tool in trials of primary percutaneous coronary intervention (PCI).[42]

Troponin I Positive with Normal Coronaries

It is recognized that some patients presenting with clinical features suggestive of acute MI demonstrate no obstructive coronary disease at angiography. In this group, CMR has become an important method of determining the cause of myocardial injury. Assomull et al. demonstrated positive diagnoses in 65% of 60 patients with this presentation. Around 11.6% had sustained an MI, possible explanations for which include transient coronary artery occlusion due to emboli or spasm. Notably, 50% of patients received a positive diagnosis of myocarditis, which would support the cessation of otherwise lifelong secondary preventative ACS therapy.[43] Performing CMR early after the index event appears to be important given the regression of myocardial edema over time. In one study, 38% of patients with a chest pain, unobstructed coronary, raised troponin presentation were diagnosed with myocarditis when scanned within 2 weeks, compared with only 14% when scanned at a later stage.[44]

LIMITATIONS OF CARDIOVASCULAR MAGNETIC RESONANCE

Claustrophobia, obesity, poorly controlled arrhythmia, and limited breath-holding capacity may pose challenges, but strategies are available to overcome them. MRI safety concerns may preclude CMR altogether in some patients, hence MR safety for each individual patient particularly in the event of devices and prosthesis, need to be carefully analyzed before embarking in this procedure.

CONCLUSION

There is considerable evidence to support the expectant benefits of CMR for the assessment of patients with known or suspected IHD. Future developments in hardware and software are expected to increase both the breadth of applicability and diagnostic accuracy of the technique.

REFERENCES

1. Peterzan M, Rider O, Anderson L. The role of cardiovascular magnetic resonance imaging in heart failure. Cardiac Fail Rev. 2016;02(02):115.
2. Holdright D, Dayer M, Cowie M. Heart failure: diagnosis and healthcare burden. Clin Med. 2004;4(1):13-8.
3. Patel M, White R, Abbara S, et al. 2013 ACCF/ACR/ASE/ASNC/SCCT/SCMR appropriate utilization of cardiovascular imaging in heart failure. J Am Coll Cardiol. 2013;61(21):2207-31.
4. Garbi M, McDonagh T, Cosyns B, et al. Appropriateness criteria for cardiovascular imaging use in heart failure: report of literature review. Eur Heart J Cardiovasc Imaging. 2014;16(2):147-53.
5. Ponikowski P, Voors A, Anker S, et al. 2016 ESC Guidelines for the diagnosis and treatment of acute and chronic heart failure. Eur Heart J. 2016;37(27):2129-200.
6. Bhatia M. Cardiac MRI: Promise, hope and hype. Cardiol Soc India: Cardiol Update. 2014:1101-7.
7. Gonzalez J, Kramer C. Role of imaging techniques for diagnosis, prognosis and management of heart failure patients: cardiac magnetic resonance. Curr Heart Fail Rep. 2015;12(4):276-83.
8. Gheorghiade M. Navigating the crossroads of coronary artery disease and heart failure. Circulation. 2006;114(11):1202-13.
9. Florian A. Cardiac magnetic resonance imaging in ischemic heart disease: a clinical review. J Med Life. 2011;14;4(4):330-45.
10. Lamas G, Mitchell G, Flaker G, et al. Clinical significance of mitral regurgitation after acute myocardial infarction. Circulation. 1997;96(3):827-33.
11. Wagner A, Bruder O, Lombardi M, et al. European Cardiovascular Magnetic Resonance (EuroCMR) registry--multinational results from 57 centers in 15 countries. J Cardiovasc Magn Reson. 2013;15(S1).
12. DiBianco R, Shabetai R, Kostuk W, et al. A comparison of oral milrinone, digoxin, and their combination in the treatment of patients with chronic heart failure. N Engl J Med. 1989;320(11):677-83.
13. Hundley W, Hamilton C, Thomas M, et al. Utility of fast cine magnetic resonance imaging and display for the detection of myocardial ischemia in patients ot well suited for second harmonic stress echocardiography. Circulation. 1999;100(16):1697-702.
14. Eitel I, Friedrich M. T2-weighted cardiovascular magnetic resonance in acute cardiac disease. J Cardiovasc Magn Reson. 2011;13(1):13.
15. Monney P, Sekhri N, Burchell T, et al. Acute myocarditis presenting as acute coronary syndrome: role of early cardiac magnetic resonance in its diagnosis. Heart. 2010;97(16):1312-8.

16. Raman S, Simonetti O, Winner M, et al. Cardiac magnetic resonance with edema imaging identifies myocardium at risk and predicts worse outcome in patients with Non–ST-segment elevation acute coronary syndrome. J Am Coll Cardiol. 2010;55(22):2480-8.
17. Thompson A, Maredia N. Cardiovascular magnetic resonance imaging for the assessment of ischemic heart disease. Continuing Cardiol Educ. 2017;3(2):56-63.
18. Gebker R, Jahnke C, Manka R, et al. The role of dobutamine stress cardiovascular magnetic resonance in the clinical management of patients with suspected and known coronary artery disease. J Cardiovasc Magn Reson. 2011;13(1):46.
19. Lockie T, Nagel E, Redwood S, et al. The use of cardiovascular magnetic resonance imaging in acute coronary syndromes. Circulation. 2009;119(12):1671-81.
20. Abdelrahman S, Ali M, Salem M, et al. Utility of cardiac MRI in the assessment of myocardial viability: evaluating its role using 3-T machine in correlation with SPECT. Egyptian J Radiol Nucl Med. 2016;47(1):73-81.
21. Qaseem A. Diagnosis of stable ischemic heart disease: Summary of a clinical practice guideline from the American College of Physicians/American College of Cardiology Foundation/American Heart Association/American Association for Thoracic Surgery/Preventive Cardiovascular Nurses Association/Society of Thoracic Surgeons. Ann Intern Med. 2012;157(10):729.
22. Guichard J, Hage F. Guidelines in review: 2015 ACR/ACC/AHA/AATS/ACEP/ASNC/NASCI/SAEM/SCCT/SCMR/SCPC/SNMMI/STR/STS appropriate utilization of cardiovascular imaging in emergency department patients with chest pain: a joint document of the American College of Radiology Appropriateness Criteria Committee and the American College of Cardiology appropriate use criteria task force. J Nucl Cardiol. 2016;23(5):1142-6.
23. Authors/Task Force members, Windecker S, Kolh P, et al. 2014 ESC/EACTS Guidelines on myocardial revascularization: The Task Force on Myocardial Revascularization of the European Society of Cardiology (ESC) and the European Association for Cardio-Thoracic Surgery (EACTS)Developed with the special contribution of the European Association of Percutaneous Cardiovascular Interventions (EAPCI). Eur Heart J. 2014;35(37):2541-619.
24. Shaw L, Berman D, Picard M, et al. Comparative definitions for moderate-severe ischemia in stress nuclear, echocardiography, and magnetic resonance imaging. JACC: Cardiovasc Imaging. 2014;7(6):593-604.
25. Fox K. Coronary artery disease as the cause of incident heart failure in the population. Eur Heart J. 2001;22(3):228-36.
26. Felker G, Shaw L, O'Connor C. A standardized definition of ischemic cardiomyopathy for use in clinical research. J Am Coll Cardiol. 2002;39(2):210-8.
27. Assomull R, Shakespeare C, Kalra P, et al. Role of cardiovascular magnetic resonance as a gatekeeper to invasive coronary angiography in patients presenting with heart failure of unknown etiology. Circulation. 2011;124(12):1351-60.
28. Kim R, Wu E, Rafael A, et al. The use of contrast-enhanced magnetic resonance imaging to identify reversible myocardial dysfunction. N Engl J Med. 2000;343(20):1445-53.
29. Wellnhofer E. Magnetic resonance low-dose dobutamine test is superior to scar quantification for the prediction of functional recovery. Circulation. 2004;109(18):2172-4.
30. Pegg T, Selvanayagam J, Jennifer J, et al. Prediction of global left ventricular functional recovery in patients with heart failure undergoing surgical revascularisation, based on late gadolinium enhancement cardiovascular magnetic resonance. J Cardiovasc Magn Reson. 2010;12(1):56.
31. Schwartz B, Kloner R. Coronary no reflow. J Mol Cell Cardiol. 2012;52(4):873-82.
32. Wu K. CMR of microvascular obstruction and hemorrhage in myocardial infarction. J Cardiovasc Magn Reson. 2012;14(1):68.
33. Weir R, Murphy C, Petrie C, et al. Microvascular obstruction remains a portent of adverse remodeling in optimally treated patients with left ventricular systolic dysfunction after acute myocardial infarction. Circ Cardiovasc Imaging. 2010;3(4):360-7.
34. Mather A, Lockie T, Nagel E, et al. Appearance of microvascular obstruction on high resolution first-pass perfusion, early and late gadolinium enhancement CMR in patients with acute myocardial infarction. J Cardiovasc Magn Reson. 2009;11(1):33.
35. Abbas A, Matthews G, Brown I, et al. Cardiac MR assessment of microvascular obstruction. Br J Radiol. 2015;88(1047):20140470.
36. Kutty R, Jones N, Moorjani N. Mechanical complications of acute myocardial infarction. Cardiol Clin. 2013;31(4):519-31.
37. Baritussio A, Scatteia A, Bucciarelli-Ducci C. Role of cardiovascular magnetic resonance in acute and chronic ischemic heart disease. Int J Cardiovasc Imaging. 2017;34(1):67-80.
38. Flavian A, Carta F, Thuny F, et al. Cardiac MRI in the diagnosis of complications of myocardial infarction. Diagn Interv Imaging. 2012;93(7-8):578-85.
39. Weinsaft J, Kim H, Shah D, et al. Detection of left ventricular thrombus by delayed-enhancement cardiovascular magnetic resonance. J Am Coll Cardiol. 2008;52(2):148-57.
40. Ingkanisorn W, Kwong R, Bohme N, et al. Prognosis of negative adenosine stress magnetic resonance in patients presenting to an emergency department with chest pain. J Am Coll Cardiol. 2006;47(7):1427-32.
41. Greenwood J, Younger J, Ridgway J, et al. Safety and diagnostic accuracy of stress cardiac magnetic resonance imaging vs exercise tolerance testing early after acute ST elevation myocardial infarction. Heart. 2007;93(11):1363-8.
42. Thompson A, Maredia N. Cardiovascular magnetic resonance imaging for the assessment of ischemic heart disease. Contin Cardiol Educ. 2017;3(2):56-63.
43. Assomull R, Lyne J, Keenan N, et al. The role of cardiovascular magnetic resonance in patients presenting with chest pain, raised troponin, and unobstructed coronary arteries. Eur Heart J. 2007;28(10):1242-9.
44. Rajwani A, Stewart M, Richardson J, et al. The incremental impact of cardiac MRI on clinical decision-making. Br J Radiol. 2016;89(1057):20150662.

19

CHAPTER

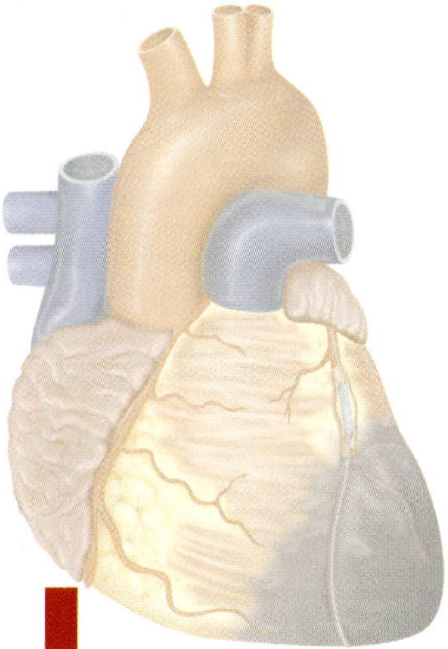

Role of Cardiovascular Magnetic Resonance Imaging in Nonischemic Cardiomyopathy

Mona Bhatia, Amit Garg, Rahul Nijhara, Shashank Jain

INTRODUCTION

Heart failure (HF) is a common disorder, with increasing prevalence, associated with significant morbidity, mortality, and financial impact on healthcare services. The most common causes of HF include ischemic heart disease, hypertension, valvular heart disease, and cardiomyopathies.[1] Early and accurate diagnosis, assessment, risk stratification, and follow-up of HF patients are exceedingly important for appropriate patient management and effective utilization of implantable devices.[2]

DIAGNOSTIC CRITERIA

The key clinical questions that impact patient management in HF include:

- Accurate, reliable, and reproducible ventricular assessment for size and function
- Identification of the cause of HF
- Assessment of myocardial viability
- Assessment of myocardial perfusion
- Evaluation of mechanical dyssynchrony
- Exclusion of potential mimickers of HF such as pericardial diseases, among others.[3]

There are multiple imaging modalities available for assessment of HF. Echocardiography has stood the test of time and remains the modality of choice, on account of being widely available, portable, and easily accessible with a relative low cost.[1] However, poor acoustic windows and operator dependence limit the information and reproducibility of echocardiography.[2] Cardiovascular magnetic resonance (CMR) has over the recent decades emerged as a strong complementary and often superior modality in evaluation of HF patients.[3] CMR has the advantage of excellent spatial and temporal resolution without the risk of ionizing radiation, with the unique capability to assess cardiac structure, function, myocardial tissue characterization, with accurate qualitative and quantitative assessment of myocardial perfusion, and viability, within a single 45–60 minutes study.[2,4] Magnetic resonance spectroscopy (MRS) can further add information on deranged cardiac energetics in HF.[5]

FUNCTIONAL ASSESSMENT OF HEART FAILURE BY CMR

Ventricular Function

Precise left ventricular volumes and ejection fraction (LVEF) are key determinants of prognosis and clinical decision making in HF and are the basis for internal cardioverter defibrillator (ICD), cardiac resynchronization (CRT), and valve replacement therapies.[6-9] Recently, right ventricular (RV) function is a powerful prognosticator.[10-11] CMR is considered the gold standard technique for the measurement of LV and RV volumes, mass, and ejection fraction, without the need of geometrical assumptions as the left ventricle may not be ellipsoidal, in remodeled hearts.[12] Tagging can further assess segmental wall motion, including radial and circumferential strain patterns.[2] In symptomatic HF patients with preserved LV ejection fraction (HFPEF), CMR has the potential for evaluation of diastolic dysfunction.[3,13]

Valve Assessment

Valvular function can be accurately assessed qualitatively from cine imaging and quantitatively from phase contrast velocity mapping with accurate peak velocity and regurgitant volume measurements.[14] Accurate measurements of cardiac output, shunt flow, aortic or pulmonary regurgitation and, indirectly, of mitral and tricuspid regurgitation can be obtained. For stenotic lesions, valve area can be measured by direct planimetry on steady-state free precession (SSFP) cines, whereas peak velocities can be estimated on through plane velocity-encoded images.[15]

MYOCARDIAL STRUCTURE

Different MR sequences are designated to enable tissue characterization. Full quantitative analysis of myocardial T1 and T2 values ("mapping") has been recently developed in an effort to characterize better even noncontrast global changes in the myocardium.[16,17] T1-weighted spin echo techniques are useful for high resolution anatomical as opposed to functional imaging. T2-weighted spin echo and STIR (short Tau inversion recovery) sequences highlight myocardial inflammation or edema with accuracy in detection of acute infarction and myocarditis.[18,19] Intravenous gadolinium-chelated contrast agents further enhance tissue characterization.[20] Following administration of gadolinium-chelated contrast agents, three phases are demonstrable. In the very early (<60 seconds) phase, myocardial segments with a normal blood supply enhance, while areas of ischemia on account of microvascular or epicardial coronary involvement are hypoenhanced. Myocardial perfusion can be evaluated both at rest and with adenosine stress. Over the next phase (1–3 minutes), gadolinium contrast washes out of normal myocardium, but may penetrate areas of inflammation. In the third "late" (10–15 minutes) phase gadolinium contrast accumulates in areas of replacement scar tissue/fibrosis, as a bright signal on T1-weighted inversion recovery scans, while signal from normal myocardium is "nulled" and black. Late gadolinium enhancement (LGE) CMR has excellent spatial resolution for scar detection of 1 g of myocardium even in the sub-endocardium.[21]

Ischemic versus Nonischemic Cardiomyopathy

Cardiovascular magnetic resonance with delayed gadolinium enhancement (DGE) has emerged as an alternative method for differentiating between ischemic

Flowchart 1: Approach to nonischemic cardiomyopathy.

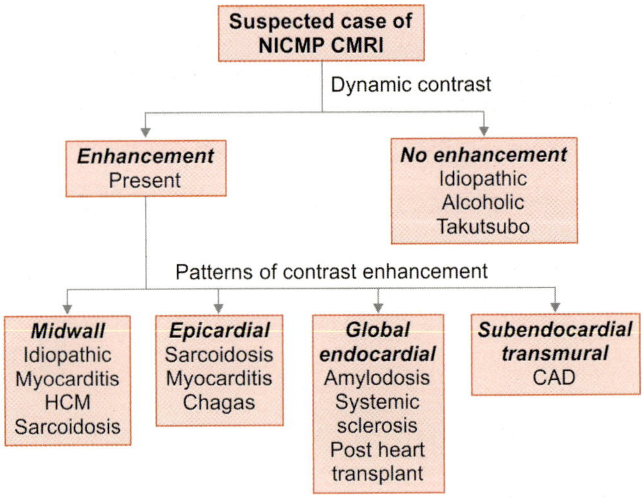

(CAD: coronary artery disease; CMRI: cardiovascular magnetic resonance imaging; HCM: hypertrophic cardiomyopathy; NICMP: nonischemic cardiomyopathy)

and nonischemic cardiomyopathy in the setting of HF.[22] Patients with coronary artery disease (CAD) and myocardial infarction (MI) are expected to have subendocardial or transmural myocardial scar tissue, with a distribution area corresponding to the vascular bed of an epicardial coronary artery. Conversely, patients with nonischemic cardiomyopathy may have no detectable fibrosis or myocardial fibrosis without mural or segmental localization characteristic for CAD (i.e. midwall, subepicardial or patchy distribution).[22] Therefore, the presence, extent, and localization of LGE may distinguish LV dysfunction related to ischemic versus nonischemic cardiomyopathy, for accurate diagnosis and appropriate management of different subtypes of nonischemic cardiomyopathy (Flowchart 1).

Myocardial Iron Evaluation

T2* imaging may be used to measure the myocardial iron concentration, establishing the diagnosis of rare cardiac pathologies related to myocardial iron accumulation in the setting of post-transfusional siderosis, hemochromatosis, or siderosis related to liver disease.[23,24]

Myocardial Viability Assessment

Cardiovascular magnetic resonance today is an extremely robust tool to evaluate myocardial viability. CMR-based assessment of myocardial viability is based on transmural extent of LGE and/or contractile reserve. Viability assessment is extremely important as functional recovery after revascularization is inversely proportional to the transmural extent of MI with cutoff values for minimal thickness of nonenhanced myocardium being 4.5 mm to 5.1 mm in chronic MI for functional recovery after revascularization.[25-27] Microvascular obstruction (MVO) is seen as failure of myocardial tissue reperfusion in the core zone of the MI. MVO has been shown to be a strong and independent predictor of nonviability, adverse myocardial remodeling, and major adverse cardiovascular events after acute MI.[28-30] Low-dose dobutamine stress CMR may be implemented for assessment of contractile reserve of dysfunctional segments as an indicator of tissue viability.[31]

CLASSIFICATION OF CARDIOMYOPATHIES

The current American Heart Association (AHA) classification of cardiomyopathies[32] divides them into:

- Primary, which affect only the heart
- Secondary, a much larger group in which myocardial involvement is part of a systemic (multiorgan) generalized disease process (Box 1).

BOX 1: Primary and secondary cardiomyopathies.

Primary cardiomyopathies

- *Genetic*
  - Hypertrophic (obstructive) cardiomyopathy (HCM or HOCM), arrhythmogenic right ventricular cardiomyopathy/dysplasia (ARVC/D)
  - Isolated ventricular noncompaction
  - Glycogen storage disorders
  - Conduction defects
  - Mitochondrial myopathies
  - Ion channel disorders (e.g. Brugada's, Long QT)
- *Mixed*
  - Dilated cardiomyopathy
  - Restrictive cardiomyopathy
- *Acquired*
  - Inflammatory (myocarditis)
  - Stress induced (Takotsubo)
  - Peripartum
  - Tachycardia induced

Secondary cardiomyopathies

- *Infiltrative*, e.g. amyloidosis
- *Storage*, e.g. hemochromatosis, Fabry's disease
- *Toxicity*, e.g. alcohol, cocaine
- *Endomyocardial*, e.g. endomyocardial fibroelastosis, Loeffler's syndrome
- *Inflammatory*, e.g. sarcoidosis
- *Endocrine*, e.g. diabetes mellitus, thyroid disorders, acromegaly, pheochromocytoma
- Cardiofacial
- *Neuromuscular/neurological*, e.g. Duchenne-Becker, Friedrich's ataxia
- Nutritional deficiencies
- Autoimmune/collagen, e.g. RA, SLE
- Electrolyte imbalance
- *Consequence of cancer therapy,* e.g. anthracyclines, such as doxorubicin, or alkylating agents, such as cisplatin and cyclophosphamide

(RA: rheumatoid arthritis; SLE: systemic lupus erythematosus)

CARDIOVASCULAR MAGNETIC RESONANCE AND SPECIFIC CAUSES OF HEART FAILURE

Using a combination of the above-mentioned techniques, CMR can identify the underlying etiology in the large majority of patients with new-onset HF.

Dilated Cardiomyopathy

Dilated cardiomyopathy (DCM) is characterized by the dilatation and functional impairment of the LV in the absence of significant CAD, with right ventricular involvement seen in a proportion of affected patients.[2] CMR is an ideal technique to assess DCM.[1] Histologically, progressive interstitial fibrosis in DCM demonstrates replacement fibrosis which, unlike in CAD, is mid-wall rather than subendocardial in location due to involvement of the circumferential fiber layer (Fig. 1).[2] The mid-wall and basal anterolateral wall LGE seen in DCM patients is an independent predictor of major adverse cardiac events, in a prospective study of clinically diagnosed DCM patients with normal coronary angiograms.[33,34]

Hypertrophic Cardiomyopathy

Hypertrophic cardiomyopathy (HCM) is characterized by asymmetric wall thickening, myocyte disarray, and interstitial plus replacement fibrosis.[35] CMR enables phenotypical characterization of HCM and is superior to echocardiography in identifying regional hypertrophy (e.g. apical HCM) while estimating maximal wall thickness and overall LV mass. Other features of HCM well evaluated on CMR include systolic anterior motion of anterior mitral valve leaflet with LV outflow tract obstruction, apical microaneurysms, papillary muscle abnormalities, and mitral regurgitation (Fig. 2).[4] LGE-CMR in HCM demonstrates patchy mid-wall scarring in 60–80% patients classically in the areas of maximal wall hypertrophy where microvascular ischemia is a potential mechanism. Other areas of enhancement include LV-RV junctions and nonhypertrophied parts of the ventricle.[36] Fibrosis detected by LGE is a proposed substrate for arrhythmias and is an independent predictor of adverse outcome.[37,38] Hence, LGE may have a role in diagnosing and identifying high-risk patients.[39] CMR distinguishes HF linked to HCM from hypertensive heart disease where there is a concentric

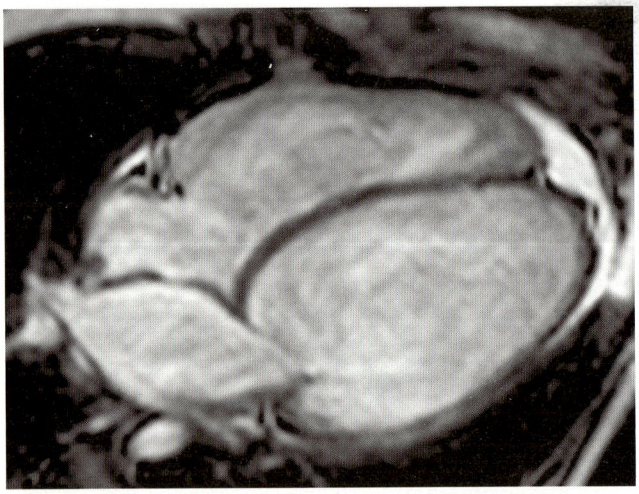

Fig. 1: Four-chamber cardiovascular magnetic resonance (CMR) image demonstrating biventricular dilatation with global myocardial thinning and reduced ejection fraction in a case of dilated cardiomyopathy.

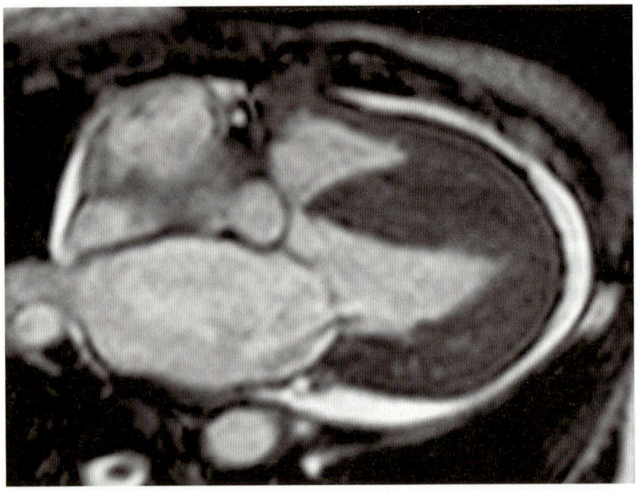

Fig. 2: Four-chamber cardiovascular magnetic resonance (CMR) image demonstrating asymmetric thickening of the interventricular septum with pericardial effusion in a case of hypertrophic cardiomyopathy.

pattern of wall thickening which does not exceed 15 mm, with increased cavity volumes and reduced or normal systolic function. Increased interstitial fibrosis may be seen, however, replacement fibrosis is unusual.[2] Cine-CMR with flow velocity encoding can be utilized to evaluate the flow dynamics and dynamic obstruction of the LV outflow tract.[31]

Arrhythmogenic Right Ventricular Cardiomyopathy

Arrhythmogenic right ventricular cardiomyopathy (ARVC/D) is an inherited condition characterized pathologically by fibrofatty replacement of the ventricular wall, primarily RV, and clinically by life-threatening ventricular arrhythmias, heart failure, and sudden cardiac death.[40] The 2010 revised task force criteria is used for diagnosis of ARVC[41] that includes parameters for regional RV dysfunction, RV volume, and global RV dysfunction. In the early stage, structural changes may be localized to the right ventricle, typically the inflow tract, outflow tract, or apex.[42] Progression to more diffuse RV disease and LV involvement, typically affecting the posterior lateral wall, is common. LGE in the LV myocardium is reliable and useful for LV involvement in ARVC.[43] CMR is extremely well suited to demonstrate regional wall motion abnormalities, thinning and aneurysmal changes in the RV free wall, increased RV and LV volumes, and increased T1 myocardial signal suggesting fatty infiltration.[44] The RV myocardial tissue is thinner with trabeculation which makes detection of RV wall fibrosis difficult. Recent work in genotyped cohorts suggests that about 20% of patients have evidence of LV fibrosis.[31]

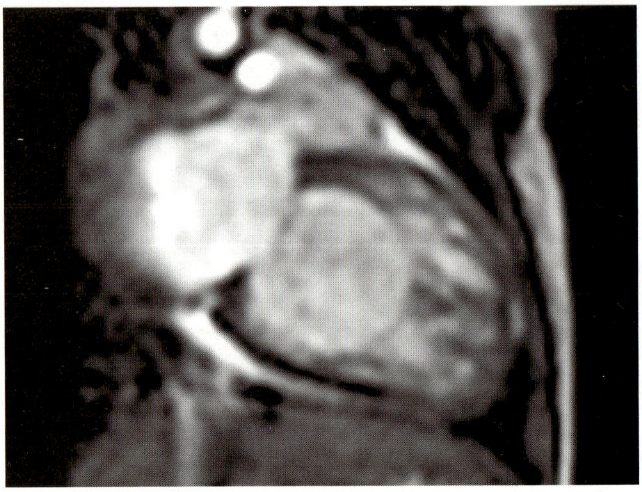

Fig. 3: Two-chamber cardiovascular magnetic resonance (CMR) image demonstrating increased trabeculations with deep intertrabecular recesses in the left ventricular myocardium, consistent with noncompaction.

Left Ventricular Noncompaction

Left ventricular noncompaction (LVNC) is a congenital disorder of endomyocardial embryogenesis due to an arrest in the normal process of myocardial compaction (sensitivity, specificity, and positive and negative predictions of 86%, 99%, 75%, and 99%, respectively) and trabeculated LV mass more than 20% of global LV mass (sensitivity of 94% and specificity of 94%).[9,31] LV noncompaction is characterized by prominent LV trabeculations with deep intertrabecular recesses, resulting in a distinct noncompacted layer lining the LV cavity (Fig. 3).[4] A ratio of noncompacted

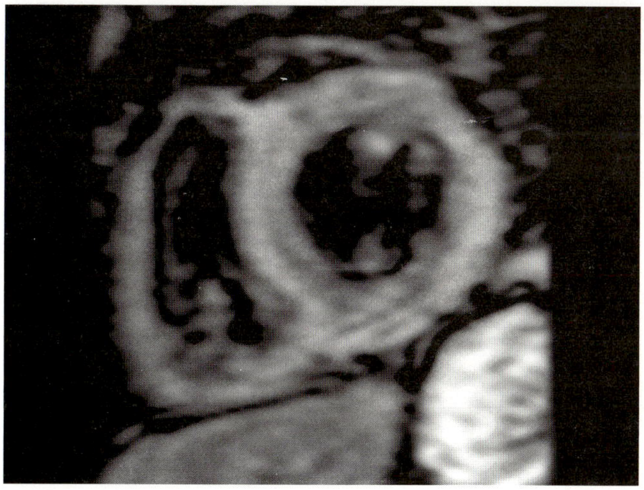

Fig. 4: Short axis T2-weighted cardiovascular magnetic resonance (CMR) image demonstrating myocardial hyperintensity, suggestive of edema in a case of acute myocarditis.

to compacted myocardium greater than 2.3 has a high specificity and sensitivity.[45] Findings are most prominent in the left ventricular apex. LVNC may result in heart failure, malignant arrhythmias, and thromboembolism.[2]

Myocarditis

Myocarditis is an inflammation of the myocardium resulting from a variety of etiologies most commonly viral, but also toxins, drugs, and autoimmune processes.[31] CMR demonstrates myocardial edema in the region resulting from myocardial inflammation with wall motion abnormalities, and patchy myocardial LGE.[31] The typical LGE pattern in myocarditis generally spares the endocardium and involves the mid-myocardial and subepicardial layers (Fig. 4).[46] The lateral free wall is more commonly involved in parvovirus B.[19] LGE in acute myocarditis is often the result of inflammation and edema with enhancement having a sensitivity, specificity, and diagnostic accuracy of 76%, 95.5%, and 85%, respectively.[31]

Takotsubo Cardiomyopathy

Takotsubo cardiomyopathy (stress cardiomyopathy) is a transient left ventricular ballooning with wall motion abnormalities, including apical akinesia in the absence of CAD, usually occurring after emotional stress due to increased circulating catecholamines and sympathetic stimulation.[47] CMR typically demonstrates myocardial edema but no LGE or fibrosis is seen and cardiac function fully recovers over time[1] which helps differentiate it from the acute coronary syndrome (subendocardial enhancement) and myocarditis (patchy subepicardial enhancement).

Amyloidosis

Amyloidosis is an uncommon condition from systemic or organ-specific extracellular deposition of insoluble fibrillar proteins. Cardiac involvement depends on the type of amyloidosis, with up to 50% involvement in primary AL, 10–50% involvement in familial ATTR, and less than 5% in secondary AA types.[31] LGE in amyloidosis has unique sensitivity, specificity, positive predictive, and negative predictive values of 86–88%, 86–90%, 88–95%, and 67–90%, respectively.[48] CMR demonstrates concentric hypertrophy with normal or reduced contractility, thickened atrial walls, interatrial septum, biatrial dilation, pericardial, and pleural effusions. The wash-in and wash-out kinetics of gadolinium are markedly abnormal when amyloid fibrils are accumulated. CMR in amyloidosis demonstrates unique LGE appearances with circumferential enhancement, preferentially involving the subendocardium but sometimes extending transmurally.[49] The blood pool is atypically dark, reflecting high myocardial contrast uptake, and fast blood pool wash-out. Less often there is patchy focal LGE. Characteristic LGE appearances in cardiac amyloidosis is a stronger predictor of mortality compared to electrocardiography (ECG) and echocardiography.[50]

Iron Overload

Myocardial iron deposition can occur due to primary (genetic) hemochromatosis or secondary (transfusion dependent) iron overload.[31] CMR identifies patients at high risk of HF and arrhythmia from myocardial siderosis and is superior to serum ferritin and liver iron in assessing prognosis.[51] CMR is useful to guide treatment and monitor response to iron-chelating agents which differ depending on whether the prime target is extraction of iron from the heart or the liver.

Sarcoidosis

The prevalence of cardiac involvement in patients of sarcoidosis has varied from 5% to 20%.[52] Typically granulomatous changes most commonly affect the LV lateral wall, papillary muscles, RV subendocardial surface, and RV free wall. CMR has characteristic features as LV hypertrophy, septal thinning, LV/RV dilation, systolic dysfunction, and pericardial effusion with areas of acute inflammation on T2-weighted images. LGE-CMR shows replacement fibrosis in mesocardial or subepicardial enhancement with predilection for the basal and lateral segments of the left ventricle (Fig. 5).

Anderson–Fabry Disease

Fabry's disease is an X-linked inherited disorder of lysosomal metabolism with glycosphingolipid deposition in multiple organs.[31] Diagnosis is important as patients respond to enzyme replacement therapy, with improvement in cardiac function and regression of hypertrophy. Cardiac manifestations include LV hypertrophy and fibrosis. LGE is in the mesocardiac and subepicardiac areas of the basal and inferolateral segments of the left ventricle.[31]

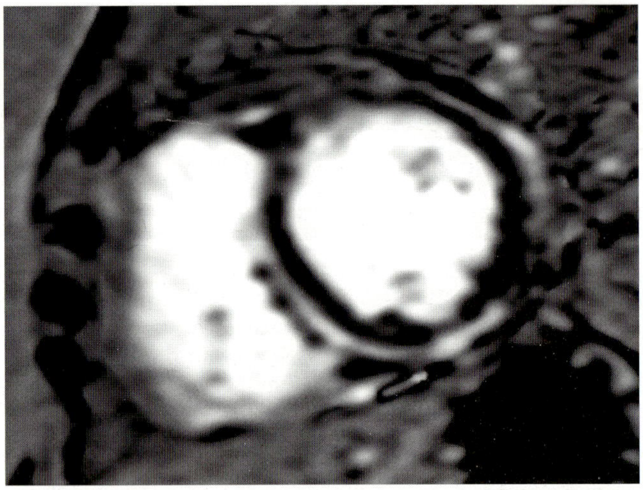

Fig. 5: Postgadolinium-enhanced cardiovascular magnetic resonance (CMR) image depicting mid-wall and epicardial enhancement in a case of nonischemic cardiomyopathy.

Cocaine/Alcohol

Cocaine-induced cardiac toxicity is a result of ischemia (coronary vasospasm) and inflammation (hypersensitivity) to cocaine/adulterants. CMR demonstrates regional LV dysfunction, especially diastolic dysfunction with myocardial edema, and fibrosis both ischemic and nonischemic in pattern. Alcohol also causes dilated cardiomyopathy with LV dilation, reduced wall thickness, and systolic dysfunction.[31]

Hypereosinophilic Syndrome and Endomyocardial Fibrosis

Hypereosinophilic syndrome (HES) with increased eosinophils can be a primary (myeloid or eosinophilic neoplasm), secondary (parasitic infections, i.e. Loeffler's syndrome, or other nonstem cell tumors), or an idiopathic condition. Endomyocardial fibrosis (EMF) is characterized by fibrosis of the apical endomyocardium (Fig. 6). Both HES and EMF on CMR demonstrate subendocardial fibrosis, obliteration of the ventricular apices, occasional thrombus formation in the apices, and restrictive cardiomyopathy.[31]

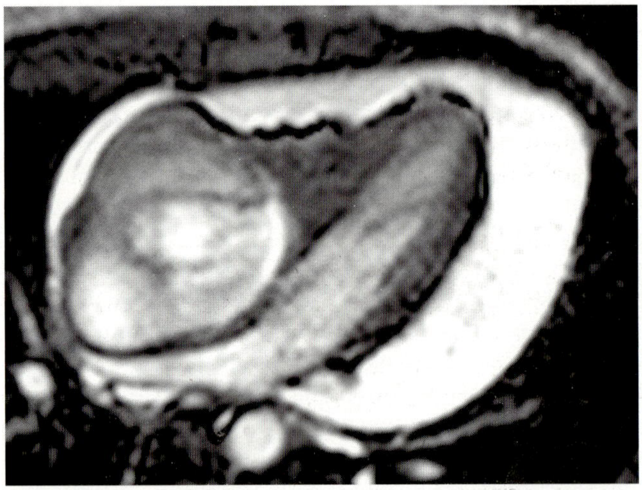

Fig. 6: Four-chamber cardiovascular magnetic resonance (CMR) view depicting right ventricular apical obliteration with dilated right atrium and pericardial effusion in a case of endomyocardial fibrosis.

Secondary Cardiomyopathies

Secondary cardiomyopathy may occur from various causes. CMR may depict nonspecific hypertrophic or dilated cardiomyopathy, and nonspecific LGE fibrosis.[31] Nonspecific findings may be seen in endocrine disorders such as diabetes mellitus, thyroid diseases, pheochromocytoma, and growth hormone excess. HCM or occasionally DCM may be seen in Cushing's syndrome, thiamine deficiency, Duchenne's muscular dystrophy, and chemotherapeutic agents such as doxorubicin.

Other Causes

Valvular Heart Disease

Cardiovascular magnetic resonance cannot only accurately assess the severity of the valve lesion but also its impact on the myocardium, including ventricular volumes, mass, and alterations in systolic function, which may guide planning of correct timing of valve replacement.[1]

Cardiac Masses

Cardiovascular magnetic resonance is excellent for tissue characterization of cardiac masses with precise anatomical, functional, and morphologic information, often allowing the specific diagnosis of the mass, which may manifest as HF, including differentiation from thrombus.[53]

Cardiomyopathy due to Cardiotoxic Chemotherapy

Cancer drug-associated cardiotoxicity as anthracyclines can cause myocardial ischemia, systolic dysfunction, and eventually HF,[54] where CMR can detect and monitor myocardial function, perfusion, and fibrosis.

POSTCARDIAC TRANSPLANTATION

Post heart transplantation, acute cellular rejection with systolic dysfunction, and myocardial edema and cardiac allograft vasculopathy are causes of early and late morbidity and mortality, respectively. CMR can be used for the identification of systolic dysfunction and myocardial edema in cardiac transplant recipients allowing early detection of cardiac rejection.[55] Moreover, LGE-CMR is useful indirectly in the detection of cardiac allograft vasculopathy based on the ability to detect silent myocardial infarctions. Overall, the role of CMR in the transplanted heart is still evolving.

Constrictive Pericarditis

Constrictive pericarditis (CP) is most frequently the result of a long-standing pericardial inflammation, with resultant reduced pericardial compliance. On CMR, normal pericardium appears as a hypointense line usually up to 4 mm thick. CMR can diagnose constrictive pericarditis by providing morphologic evidence of an abnormally thickened pericardium associated with constrictive physiology.[56] On black blood anatomical CMR images, a pericardial thickness of more than 4 mm is suggestive of constriction. The physiologic sequelae of constriction include increased ventricular coupling with early inspiratory flattening of the interventricular septum in diastole and dilation of the inferior vena cava with no or little change in size during respiration. These are demonstrated on real-time free-breathing CMR images.[56]

CONCLUSION

Cardiovascular magnetic resonance is an invaluable tool and is exponentially growing in the evaluation of patients with heart failure. CMR has the unique capability to enabling detailed anatomical and myocardial functional assessment ensuring differentiation of ischemic from nonischemic cardiomyopathy, with additional features in the characterization of nonischemic cardiomyopathy. CMR is neither operator dependent nor limited by the acoustic window, problems commonly faced in echocardiography. CMR should hence be routinely integrated in the diagnostic workup of patients suspected of nonischemic cardiomyopathies for superior diagnosis, prognostication, management, and follow-up.

REFERENCES

1. Karamitsos T, Neubauer S. Cardiovascular magnetic resonance in heart failure. Curr Cardiol Rep. 2011;13(3):210-9.
2. Assomull R, Pennell D, Prasad S. Cardiovascular magnetic resonance in the evaluation of heart failure. Heart. 2007;93(8):985-92.
3. Muzzarelli S, Ordovas K, Higgins C. Cardiovascular MRI for the assessment of heart failure: focus on clinical management and prognosis. J Magn Reson Imaging. 2011;33(2):275-86.
4. Karamitsos T, Francis J, Myerson S, et al. The role of cardiovascular magnetic resonance imaging in heart failure. J Am Coll Cardiol. 2009;54(15):1407-24.
5. Hudsmith L, Neubauer S. Magnetic resonance spectroscopy in myocardial disease. JACC: Cardiovasc Imaging. 2009;2(1):87-96.
6. Bonow R, Carabello B, Chatterjee K, et al. 2008 focused update incorporated into the ACC/AHA 2006 guidelines for the management of patients with valvular heart disease: A report of the American College of Cardiology/American Heart Association Task Force on Practice Guidelines (Writing Committee to Revise the 1998 guidelines for the management of patients with valvular heart disease): endorsed by the Society of Cardiovascular Anesthesiologists, Society for Cardiovascular Angiography and Interventions, and Society of Thoracic Surgeons. Circulation. 2008;118(15):e523-e661.
7. Remme W. Guidelines for the diagnosis and treatment of chronic heart failure. Eur Heart J. 2001;22(17):1527-60.
8. Vardas P, Auricchio A, Blanc J, et al. Guidelines for cardiac pacing and cardiac resynchronization therapy: the Task Force for Cardiac Pacing and Cardiac Resynchronization Therapy of the European Society of Cardiology. Developed in collaboration with the European Heart Rhythm Association. Europace. 2007;9(10):959-98.
9. Zipes DP, Camm AJ, Borggrefe M, et al. ACC/AHA/ESC 2006 Guidelines for management of patients with ventricular arrhythmias and the prevention of sudden cardiac death-executive summary: a report of the American College of Cardiology/American Heart Association Task Force and the European Society of Cardiology Committee for practice guidelines (Writing Committee to develop guidelines for management of patients with ventricular arrhythmias and the prevention of sudden cardiac death): Developed in collaboration with the European Heart Rhythm Association and the Heart Rhythm Society. Circulation. 2006;114(10):1088-132.
10. de Groote P, Millaire A, Foucher-Hossein C, et al. Right ventricular ejection fraction is an independent predictor of survival in patients with moderate heart failure. J Am Coll Cardiol. 1998;32(4):948-54.
11. Ghio S, Gavazzi A, Campana C. Independent and additive prognostic value of right ventricular systolic function and pulmonary artery pressure in patients with chronic heart failure. ACC Curr J Rev. 2001;10(3):56.
12. Karamitsos T, Hudsmith L, Selvanayagam J, et al. Operator induced variability in left ventricular measurements with cardiovascular magnetic resonance is improved after training. J Cardiovasc Magn Reson. 2007;9(5):777-83.

13. Paulus W, Flachskampf F, Smiseth O, et al How to diagnose diastolic heart failure: a consensus statement on the diagnosis of heart failure with normal left ventricular ejection fraction by the Heart Failure and Echocardiography Associations of the European Society of Cardiology: reply. Eur Heart J. 2007;28(21):2686-7.
14. Grothues F, Smith G, Moon J. et al. Comparison of interstudy reproducibility of cardiovascular magnetic resonance with two-dimensional echocardiography in normal subjects and in patients with heart failure or left ventricular hypertrophy. Am J Cardiol. 2002;90(1):29-34.
15. Christiansen J, Karamitsos T, Myerson S. Assessment of valvular heart disease by cardiovascular magnetic resonance imaging: a review. Heart Lung Circ. 2011;20(2):73-82.
16. Piechnik S, Ferreira V, Dall'Armellina E, et al. Shortened Modified Look-Locker Inversion recovery (ShMOLLI) for clinical myocardial T1-mapping at 1.5 and 3 T within a 9 heartbeat breathhold. J Cardiovasc Magn Reson. 2010;12(1):69.
17. Giri S, Chung Y, Merchant A, et al. T2 quantification for improved detection of myocardial edema. J Cardiovasc Magn Reson. 2009;11(1):56.
18. Abdel-Aty H, Zagrosek A, Schulz-Menger J. Delayed enhancement and T2-weighted cardiovascular magnetic resonance imaging differentiate acute from chronic myocardial infarction. ACC Curr J Rev. 2004;13(10):25.
19. Mahrholdt H, Goedecke C, Wagner A. Cardiovascular magnetic resonance assessment of human myocarditis. A comparison to histology and molecular pathology. ACC Curr J Rev. 2004;13(6):25.
20. Kim R, Fieno D, Parrish T, et al. Relationship of MRI delayed contrast enhancement to irreversible injury, infarct age, and contractile function. Circulation. 1999;100(19):1992-2002.
21. Selvanayagam J. Troponin elevation after percutaneous coronary intervention directly represents the extent of irreversible myocardial injury: Insights from cardiovascular magnetic resonance imaging. Circulation. 2005;111(8):1027-32.
22. Mahrholdt H, Wagner A, Judd R, et al. Delayed enhancement cardiovascular magnetic resonance assessment of non-ischaemic cardiomyopathies. Eur Heart J. 2005;26(15):1461-74.
23. Deugnier Y, Brissot P, Loréal O. Iron and the liver: update 2008. J Hepatol. 2008;48:S113-23.
24. Zurlo M, De Stefano P, Borgna-Pignatti C, et al. Survival and causes of death in thalassemia major. Lancet. 1989;334(8653):27-30.
25. Ichikawa Y, Sakuma H, Suzawa N. Late gadolinium-enhanced magnetic resonance imaging in acute and chronic myocardial infarction: Improved prediction of regional myocardial contraction in the chronic state by measuring thickness of nonenhanced myocardium. ACC Curr J Rev. 2005;14(8):34.
26. Knuesel P. Characterization of dysfunctional myocardium by positron emission tomography and magnetic resonance: relation to functional outcome after revascularization. Circulation. 2003;108(9):1095-100.
27. Bhatia M. Evaluation of ischemic heart disease and viability by cardiac MRI. Indian Heart J. 2014;66(1):143-4.
28. Nijveldt R, Hofman M, Hirsch A, et al. Assessment of microvascular obstruction and prediction of short-term remodeling after acute myocardial infarction: Cardiac MR imaging study. Radiology. 2009;250(2):363-70.
29. Nijveldt R, Beek A, Hirsch A, et al. 123 Functional recovery after acute myocardial infarction: a comparison between angiography, electrocardiography and cardiovascular magnetic resonance measures of microvascular injury. J Cardiovasc Magn Reson. 2008;10(Suppl 1):A24.
30. Wu K, Zerhouni E, Judd R, et al. Prognostic significance of microvascular obstruction by magnetic resonance imaging in patients with acute myocardial infarction. Circulation. 1998;97(8):765-72.
31. Wellnhofer E. Magnetic resonance low-dose dobutamine test is superior to scar quantification for the prediction of functional recovery. Circulation. 2004;109(18):2172-4.
32. Anand S, Janardhanan R. Role of cardiac MRI in nonischemic cardiomyopathies. Indian Heart J. 2016;68(3):405-9.
33. Assomull RG, Prasad SK, Lyne J, et al. Cardiovascular magnetic resonance, fibrosis, and prognosis in dilated cardiomyopathy. J Am Coll Cardiol. 2006;48:1977-85.
34. McCrohon J. Differentiation of heart failure related to dilated cardiomyopathy and coronary artery disease using gadolinium-enhanced cardiovascular magnetic resonance. Circulation. 2003;108(1):54-9.
35. Karamitsos TD, Francis JM, Myerson S, et al. The role of cardiovascular magnetic resonance imaging in heart failure. J Am Coll Cardiol. 2009;54:1407-24.
36. Hendel RC, Kramer CM, Patel MR, et al. ACCF/ACR/SCCT/SCMR/ASNC/ NASCI/SCAI/SIR appropriateness criteria for cardiac computed tomography and cardiac magnetic resonance imaging: A report of the American College of Cardiology Foundation Quality Strategic Directions Committee Appropriateness Criteria Working Group, American College of Radiology, Society of Cardiovascular Computed Tomography, Society for Cardiovascular Magnetic Resonance, American Society of Nuclear Cardiology, North American Society for Cardiac Imaging, Society for Cardiovascular Angiography and Interventions, and Society of Interventional Radiology. J Am Coll Cardiol. 2006;48:1475-97.
37. Maron MS. The current and emerging role of cardiovascular magnetic resonance imaging in hypertrophic cardiomyopathy. J Cardiovasc Transl Res. 2009;2:415-25.
38. Bruder O, Wagner A, Jensen CJ, et al. Myocardial scar visualized by cardiovascular magnetic resonance imaging predicts major adverse events in patients with hypertrophic cardiomyopathy. J Am Coll Cardiol. 2010;56:875-87.
39. O'Hanlon R, Grasso A, Roughton M, et al. Prognostic significance of myocardial fibrosis in hypertrophic cardiomyopathy. J Am Coll Cardiol. 2010;56:867-74.
40. Moon JC, McKenna WJ, McCrohon JA, et al. Toward clinical risk assessment in hypertrophic cardiomyopathy with gadolinium cardiovascular magnetic resonance. J Am Coll Cardiol. 2003;41:1561-7.
41. Sen-Chowdhry S. Arrhythmogenic right ventricular cardiomyopathy: C presentation, diagnosis, and management. Am J Med. 2004;117:685-95.

42. Marcus FI. Diagnosis of arrhythmogenic right ventricular cardiomyopathy/dysplasia: proposed modification of the task force criteria. Circulation. 2010;121:1533-41.
43. Sen-Chowdhry S, Syrris P, Prasad SK, et al. Left-dominant arrhythmogenic cardiomyopathy: an under-recognized clinical entity. J Am Coll Cardiol. 2008;52:2175-87.
44. Maksimovic R, Ekinci O, Reiner C, et al. The value of magnetic resonance imaging for the diagnosis of arrhythmogenic right ventricular cardiomyopathy. Eur Radiol. 2006;16:560-8.
45. Petersen SE, Selvanayagam JB, Wiesmann F, et al. Left ventricular non-compaction: insights from cardiovascular magnetic resonance imaging. J Am Coll Cardiol. 2005;46:101-5.
46. Abdel-Aty H. Diagnostic performance of cardiovascular magnetic resonance in patients with suspected acute myocarditis: comparison of different approaches. J Am Coll Cardiol. 2005;45:1815-22.
47. Friedrich MG, Sechtem U, Schulz-Menger J, et al. Cardiovascular magnetic resonance in myocarditis: a JACC white paper. J Am Coll Cardiol. 2009;53:1475-87.
48. Prasad A, Lerman A, Rihal CS. Apical ballooning syndrome (Tako-Tsubo or stress cardiomyopathy): a mimic of acute myocardial infarction. Am Heart J. 2008;155:408-17.
49. Paulus WJ, Tschope C, Sanderson JE, et al. How to diagnose diastolic heart failure: a consensus statement on the diagnosis of heart failure with normal left ventricular ejection fraction by the Heart Failure and Echocardiography Associations of the European Society of Cardiology. Eur Heart J. 2007;28:2539-50.
50. Syed IS, Glockner JF, Feng D, et al. Role of cardiac magnetic resonance imaging in the detection of cardiac amyloidosis. JACC Cardiovasc Imaging. 2010;3:155-64.
51. Austin BA, Tang WH, Rodriguez ER, et al. Delayed hyperenhancement magnetic resonance imaging provides incremental diagnostic and prognostic utility in suspected cardiac amyloidosis. JACC Cardiovasc Imaging. 2009;2:1369-77.
52. Kirk P, Roughton M, Porter JB, et al. Cardiac T2* magnetic resonance for prediction of cardiac complications in thalassemia major. Circulation. 2009;120:1961-8.
53. Sen-Chowdhry S, Syrris P, Prasad SK, et al. Left-dominant arrhythmogenic cardiomyopathy: an under-recognized clinical entity. J Am Coll Cardiol. 2008;52:2175-87.
54. Syed IS, Feng D, Harris SR, et al. MR imaging of cardiac masses. Magn Reson Imaging Clin N Am. 2008;16:137-64.
55. Storkecky S, Suter TM. Insights into cardiovascular side-effects of modern anticancer therapeutics. Curr Opin Oncol. 2010;22:312-7.
56. Estep JD, Shah DJ, Nagueh SF, et al. The role of multimodality cardiac imaging in the transplanted heart. JACC Cardiovasc Imaging. 2009;2:1126-40.

20

CHAPTER

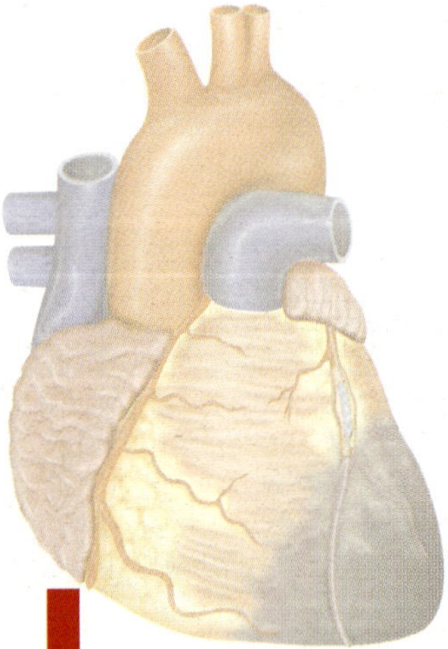

Echocardiography-guided β-blocker Therapy in Heart Failure

Kushagra Mahansaria, Manish Bansal, Ravi R Kasliwal, HK Chopra

INTRODUCTION

Heart failure (HF) is a clinical syndrome caused by structural and/or functional cardiac abnormality, resulting in reduced cardiac output and/or elevated intracardiac pressures. It is characterized by typical symptoms such as breathlessness, ankle swelling, and fatigue, that may be accompanied by certain signs like elevated jugular venous pressure, pulmonary crackles, and peripheral edema;[1] detailed further by the Framingham criteria.[2] Subsequent to the clinical diagnosis, the application of diagnostic investigations, such as echocardiography, can be used for identifying the pathophysiology of the clinical phenotype, together with the provision of prognostic and therapeutic information.[3] Identification of the underlying cardiac problem is crucial for therapeutic reasons, as the precise pathology determines the specific treatment used.[1] HF may be associated with a wide spectrum of LV functional abnormalities, which may range from patients with normal LV size and preserved ejection fraction (EF) to those with severe dilatation and/or markedly reduced EF. In most patients, abnormalities of systolic and diastolic dysfunction coexist, irrespective of EF.[4] An estimated 670,000 new cases of HF are diagnosed annually among USA adults aged more than 45 years, and HF causes or contributes to almost 300,000 deaths each year.[5] Heart failure is primarily a disease of the elderly, with prevalence increasing from 0.9% in patients aged 55–64 years to 17.4% in those more than or equal to 85 years.[6] The lifetime risk of HF at age 55 years is 33% for men and 28% for women.[6] Various demographic trends, including the aging of the population and greater likelihood of survival after acute myocardial infarction, suggest that the prevalence of HF will likely continue to increase. The American Heart Association (AHA) estimates that by 2030, HF prevalence will increase by 25%.[7] The economic impact is significant as well. Cost of HF hospitalizations amount to $29 billion/year in the USA alone[8] and are projected to increase to $69.8 billion by 2030.[7] Although most of the focus in HF is aimed at treatment of affected patients, in 2001, the American College of Cardiology Foundation (ACCF)/AHA revised the HF classification to also include patients who are at high risk for the disease but do not yet have structural cardiac abnormalities or clinical evidence of HF (Stage A) (Fig. 1).[9]

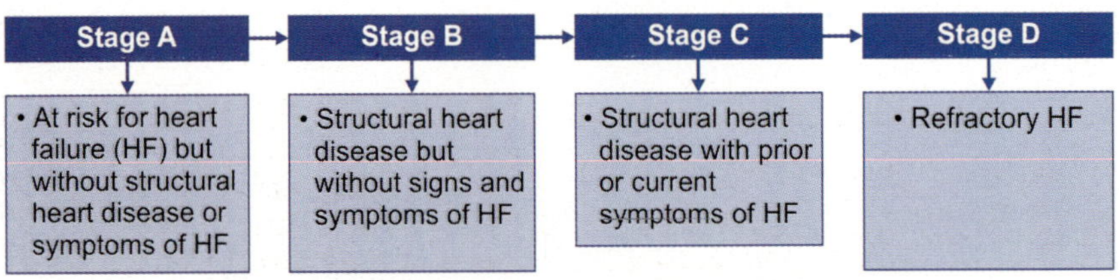

Fig. 1: Stages in the development of heart failure.

In spite of significant advances in the treatment of HF, morbidity, and mortality remain high. Pharmacologic regimens have become increasingly complex, and standard therapy now often consists of multiple drugs. Given these epidemiologic and economic pressures, there is increasing interest in using cardiovascular biomarkers for a personalized medicine approach to more effectively guide diagnosis, risk stratification, and therapy.[8]

DEFINITION OF HEART FAILURE

The main terminology used to describe HF is based on measurement of the left ventricular ejection fraction (LVEF). Those with normal LVEF (typically considered as ≥50%) are classified as HF with preserved EF (HFpEF); those with reduced LVEF (typically considered as <40%) are classified as HF with reduced EF (HFrEF) (Table 1). The 2016 ESC guidelines classified patients with an LVEF in the range of 40–49%, representing a "gray area," as HF with mildly reduced EF (HFmrEF)[1] (Table 1). The 2013 ACC/AHA guidelines classified the same subset at HFpEF-borderline (Table 1). Differentiation of patients with HF based on LVEF is important due to different underlying etiologies, demographics, comorbidities, and response to therapies.[10] It is only in patients with HFrEF that therapies have been shown to reduce both morbidity and mortality.

Apart from the above classification, The ACCF/AHA classification describes stages of HF development based on structural changes and symptoms (Fig. 1). The Killip (Table 2) classification may be used to describe the severity of the patient's condition in the acute setting after myocardial infarction.[11]

TABLE 1: Classification of heart failure according to ejection fraction.

LVEF	Classification	Guideline
≥50%	HFpEF	ESC, ACC/AHA
40–49%	HFmrEF HFpEF-borderline	ESC ACC/AHA
<40%	HFrEF	ESC. ACC/AHA

(ACC: American College of Cardiology; AHA: American Heart Association; ESC: European Society of Cardiology; HFmrEF: heart failure with mildly reduced ejection fraction; HFpEF: heart failure with preserved ejection fraction, HFrEF, heart failure with reduced ejection fraction; LVEF: left ventricular ejection fraction).

TABLE 2: Killip classification.

Killip class	Clinical findings	Hospital mortality
1	No congestion signs	<6%
2	S3. basal rales	<17%
3	Acute pulmonary edema	38%
4	Cardiogenic shock	81%

ROLE OF β-BLOCKERS IN HEART FAILURE

β-blockers in Heart Failure with Reduced Ejection Fraction

All patients with stable, mild, moderate, and severe chronic heart failure from ischemic or nonischemic cardiomyopathies and reduced LVEF, in New York Heart Association (NYHA) class II–IV, (Table 3) should be treated with beta (β)-blockers, unless there is a contraindication (Class I, Level of Evidence A).[1,4,9] In patients with left ventricular systolic dysfunction, with or without symptomatic heart failure following an acute myocardial infarction (AMI), long-term β-blockade is recommended in addition to angiotensin-converting enzyme (ACE) inhibition to reduce mortality (Class I, Level of Evidence A).[1,4,9] β-blockers are also recommended in patients with chronic heart failure and preserved left ventricular function (Class IIa, Level of Evidence C)[1] (Table 4).

Beta-blockers have now been evaluated in more than 20,000 patients with HF who participated in more than 20 published placebo-controlled clinical trials.[12-20] This collective experience indicates that long-term treatment with β-blockers can lessen symptoms, improve clinical status, and enhance the patient's overall sense of well-being.[21-28] β-blockers can also reduce the risk of death and hospitalization.[14,15,20,29] Despite these benefits, β-blockers are underused in patients with heart failure.[30]

Beta-blockers reduce mortality and morbidity in symptomatic patients with HFrEF, despite treatment with an ACEI and, in most cases, a diuretic,[14,15,31-33] β-blockers should be initiated in clinically stable patients at a low

TABLE 3: New York Heart Association (NYHA) classification of stages of heart failure.

NYHA class	Definition
Class I	No limitation of physical activity. Ordinary physical activity does not cause undue fatigue, palpitations, breathlessness
Class II	Slight limitation of physical activity. Comfortable at rest but ordinary physical activity results in undue breathlessness, palpitations or fatigue
Class III	Marked limitation of physical activity. Comfortable at rest but less than ordinary physical activity results in undue breathlessness, palpitations or fatigue
Class IV	Unable to carry on any physical activity without discomfort. Symptoms present at rest. If any physical activity is undertaken, discomfort is increased

TABLE 4: Indications for use of β-blockers in chronic heart failure.

Indication	*Class*	*Level of evidence*
All stable patients with symptomatic HF and reduced LVEF, NYHA functional class II-IV (to prolong survival)	I	A
LV systolic dysfunction without symptoms after AMI	I	A
LV systolic dysfunction without symptoms, no previous MI	I	B
Chronic HF with preserved systolic function (to reduce heart rate)	IIa	C
Acute compensated HF, after AMI	IIa	B
Patient stable after acutely decompensated chronic HF	I	A

(AMI: acute myocardial infarction; HF: heart failure; LV: left ventricle; LVEF: left ventricular ejection fraction; NYHA: New York Heart Association)

dose and gradually up-titrated to the maximum tolerated dose. There is consensus that β-blockers and ACEIs are complementary, and can be started together as soon as the diagnosis of HFrEF is made.[34]

Three β-blockers have been shown to be effective in reducing the risk of death in patients with chronic HF: bisoprolol[14] (selective β-1 blocker) and sustained-release metoprolol (succinate)[32] (selective β-1 blocker) and carvedilol,[31,35] (non-selective α-1, β-1 and β-2 blocker). Placebo-controlled mortality trials with all three drugs[14,15,23,29,31,35,36] have been associated with a long-term reduction in total mortality, cardiovascular mortality, sudden cardiac death and death due to progression of heart failure in patients in functional class II–IV. In these studies, β-blocking therapy also reduced hospitalizations (all, cardiovascular and heart failure-related), improved the functional class and led to less worsening of heart failure than placebo. This beneficial effect has been consistently observed in subgroups of different age, gender, functional class, LVEF and ischemic or nonischemic etiology, diabetics and non-diabetics. Black patients may be an exception, since in the β-blocker Evaluation of Survival (BEST) trial this ethnic group lacked the benefit from β-blocker therapy in heart failure.[37]

In the second Cardiac Insufficiency Bisoprolol Study (CIBIS-2)[14] symptomatic patients in NYHA class III or IV, with LVEF less than or equal to 35%, receiving standard therapy with diuretics and ACE-inhibitors, were randomly assigned to receive bisoprolol or placebo during a mean follow of 1.3 years. The study was stopped early because bisoprolol showed a significant mortality benefit (11.8% vs. 17.3%) [Number Needed to Treat (NNT) for 1.3 year to save 1 life = 18]. There were significantly fewer sudden cardiac deaths among patients on bisoprolol than in those on placebo (3.6% vs. 6.3%). Treatment effects were independent of the severity or cause of heart failure.

In the Metoprolol Randomised Intervention Trial (MERIT-HF)[15] patients with chronic heart failure in NYHA functional class II–IV and ejection fraction less than or equal to 40% were randomly assigned metoprolol CR/XL or placebo. This study was also stopped early after a mean follow-up of 1 year. All-cause mortality was lower in the metoprolol group than in the placebo group (7.2%, per patient-year of follow-up vs. 11.0%) (NNT for 1 year to save 1 life = 28). There was also a 41% reduction in sudden cardiac death and 49% reduction in deaths from worsening heart failure.

In the Carvedilol Prospective Randomised Cumulative Survival (COPERNICUS) study,[20] patients who had symptoms of heart failure at rest or on minimal exertion, clinically euvolemic, and with an EF of less than 25% were randomly assigned to placebo or carvedilol for a mean period of 10.4 months. The study also terminated prematurely after observing a significant reduction in mortality: the cumulative risk for death at 1 year was 18.5% in the placebo group and 11.4% in the carvedilol group (NNT for 10.4 months to save 1 life = 18). As in the previous studies, there was a reduction in hospitalizations and sudden cardiac death.

In the CAPRICORN trial[35] patients with LVEF of less than 40% early after an episode of AMI were randomly assigned to carvedilol or placebo. After a mean follow-up of 1.3 years, all-cause mortality alone was lower in the β-blocker group (12% vs. 15%), although no differences were observed in rehospitalization rate.

Although a reduction in mortality and hospitalization has been demonstrated with several β-blockers in chronic heart failure, a class-effect has not been established. In the BEST Trial[38] patients with chronic heart failure and reduced LVEF were assigned to bucindolol or placebo. The study was stopped prematurely because of lack of differences in total mortality after 2 years of follow-up (33% vs. 30% in the placebo and bucindolol groups, respectively; P = 0.16), although bucindolol was associated with a reduction in cardiovascular mortality and myocardial infarction in non-black patients.[39]

A direct comparison of two different β-blockers (metoprolol vs. carvedilol) has been assessed in the Carvedilol Or Metoprolol European Trial (COMET).[40] In this study patients with chronic HF and reduced LVEF were treated with carvedilol (targeted 25 mg bid) or metoprolol tartrate (targeted 50 mg bid). After a mean follow-up of 58 months all-cause mortality was lower in the carvedilol group (34% vs. 40%) [hazard ratio (HR) 0.83; confidence interval (CI) 0.74–0.93], equivalent to an NNT to save one life = 59.

This suggests that carvedilol is superior to metoprolol in HF patients. Of note is that the formulation of metoprolol was different from the one used in the MERIT-HF trial (tartrate vs. slow release succinate) and the target dose was lower (50 mg/12 h vs. 100 mg/12 h, equivalent to 130 mg/day of tartrate). The COMET trial illustrates that selection of a β-blocker and the dose used may have a significant impact on the outcome of patients with heart failure.

β-blockers in Heart Failure with Preserved Ejection Fraction

There is a paucity of data regarding the possible benefit of β-blockers in patients with HFpEF. Accordingly, the recommended use of β-blockers in these patients is empirical, based mainly on the possible benefit of reducing heart rate and improving myocardial ischemia.

Although controlled studies have been performed with β-blockers in patients with HFpEF, for the most part, these trials have been small or have produced inconclusive results.[41] The sub-analysis of the SENIORS (Study of Effects of Nebivolol Intervention on Outcomes and Rehospitalization in Seniors With Heart Failure) trial showed that the effects of nebivolol were similar between HF patients with EF more than and less than or equal to 35%.[42] The SWEDIC (Results of the Swedish Doppler-echocardiographic study)[43] compared several Doppler echocardiographic indices between HFpEF patients treated with and without carvedilol and concluded that treatment with carvedilol resulted in a significant improvement in E/A ratio in patients with HF due to a LV relaxation abnormality.[43] However, these Doppler echocardiographic indices have many limitations for the assessment of LV diastolic function in subjects with preserved EF.[44,45]

On the other hand, the OPTIMIZE-HF (Organized Program to Initiate Life-saving Treatment in Hospitalized Patients with Heart Failure) registry showed that the use of BBs in HFpEF patients was related to poor outcomes.[46]

β-blockers in Acute Heart Failure

In patients admitted due to acute HF (AHF) β-blockers should be cautiously initiated in hospital, once the patient is stabilized.[1,4,30,47,48] There are no randomized clinical trials with β-blockers in AHF targeted to improve the acute condition.

The Gothenburg Study[49] randomized patients to receive either intravenous metoprolol or placebo after AMI and followed by oral therapy for three months. Patients with new symptoms of heart failure were less frequently found in the metoprolol group, and metoprolol therapy reduced mortality and morbidity. In the COPERNICUS trial, β-blocker therapy started early after acute decompensation of chronic HF was associated with a long-term reduction in mortality.[31] In the CAPRICORN trial patients with HF or left ventricular dysfunction randomized early after AMI also received benefit from β-blocker therapy.[18]

As recommended in the European Society of Cardiology (ESC) Acute Heart Failure Guidelines,[48] patients with acute overt heart failure including more than basal pulmonary rales, β-blockers should be used cautiously. In these patients, if ongoing ischemia and tachycardia are present, intravenous metoprolol can be considered (Class IIb, Level of Evidence C). However, in patients with AMI who stabilize after AHF, β-blockers should be initiated early (Class IIa, Level of Evidence B). In patients with chronic heart failure, β-blockers should be initiated when the patient has stabilized after the acute episode (usually after 4 days) (Class I, Level of Evidence A). Patients, who are already on β-blockers and are admitted due to worsening heart failure, should be continued on this therapy in general unless inotropic support is needed but dose could be reduced if signs of excessive dosages are suspected (bradycardia and hypotension).

ROLE OF ECHOCARDIOGRAPHY IN OPTIMIZING β-BLOCKER TREATMENT IN HEART FAILURE

The initial assessment consists of a clinical diagnosis compatible with complete patient history and physical examination and the assessment of LVEF by echocardiography. As described above, classification of HF into HFrEF and HFpEF is based on estimation of LVEF and this information is critical for therapeutic decision-making as treatment approaches for HFrEF and HFpEF differ markedly. While β-blockers have class I indication in HFrEF, their role in HFpEF is rather limited.

Apart from just LVEF estimation, echocardiography can provide a lot of other important information which is helpful in diagnosing subclinical HF, guiding therapy, and predicting risk of subsequent events.[50-54] Echocardiographic evaluation should address whether LVEF is reduced, LV structure is abnormal, and other structural abnormalities are present that could account for the clinical presentation. This information should be quantified, including numerical estimates of EF measurement, ventricular dimensions, wall thickness, calculations of ventricular volumes, and evaluation of chamber geometry and regional wall motion. Use of echocardiograms in patients with suspected HF improves disease identification and provision of appropriate medical care.[55] Understandably, documentation of LVEF is an HF quality-of-care performance measure.[47]

Right ventricular size and function as well as atrial size and dimensions should also be measured. All valves should be evaluated for anatomic and flow abnormalities. Secondary changes, particularly the severity of mitral and tricuspid valve insufficiency, should be determined. Noninvasive hemodynamic data constitute important additional information. Mitral valve inflow pattern, pulmonary venous inflow pattern, and mitral annular velocity provide data about LV filling and left atrial pressure. The tricuspid valve regurgitant gradient, coupled with measurement of inferior vena cava diameter and its response during respiration, provides estimates of systolic pulmonary artery pressure and central venous pressure. Many of these abnormalities are prognostically important and can be present without manifest HF.

Left Ventricular Filling Pressure

Doppler echocardiography has allowed the establishment of clinically useful cutoffs for prediction of elevated mean left atrial pressure in patients with suspected HF. The most validated technique uses pulsed-wave Doppler to relate the peak velocity of early diastolic transmitral flow to the peak velocity of early diastolic longitudinal motion at the mitral annulus, the so-called E/e' ratio (Figs. 2A and B).[56] When the ratio is significantly elevated and confounders such as mitral valve disease or rhythm disturbance are absent, the clinician can be quite confident that mean left atrial pressure was elevated at the time of the echocardiographic study. In more borderline cases, interpretation can be aided by assessing the effect of load-altering maneuvers on the transmitral flow pattern as well as pulsed-wave Doppler evaluation of pulmonary venous flow.[57] The E/e' ratio can also be determined in serial echocardiographic studies to guide pharmacological intervention and monitor response to therapy in HF patients. In addition, the E/e' ratio is a strong prognostic marker and independently predicts adverse cardiac outcomes in the HF population.[58] This is especially important in guiding initiation/termination of β-blocker therapy in patients presenting with AHF; or, up-titrating β-blocker dosage as per patient's response to echo indices.

The value of LV filling pressure estimation can be understood from the fact that no two patients with HFrEF behave in a similar fashion. For example, while one patient with a dilated LV and poor EF of 25% may be severely symptomatic, another patient with similar LV function who is aggressively treated may be completely asymptomatic. The difference between these two patients largely relates to differences in intravascular volume status and cardiac filling pressures and highlights the clear disconnect between LVEF and clinical symptoms in a given patient. In HFrEF, information from the transmitral flow pattern and E/e' ratio can, therefore, be applied clinically to guide β-blocker as well as to inform prognosis.[59]

Pulmonary Artery Pressure

In addition to estimation of left atrial pressure, Doppler echocardiography has an important application in the estimation of peak systolic pulmonary artery pressure. This is clinically relevant because patients with HF and elevated pulmonary venous pressures often have accompanying elevation of pulmonary artery systolic pressure. This is particularly applicable to hospitalized patients with decompensated HF in whom the degree of pulmonary hypertension helps inform the severity of HF and provides a marker for assessment of response to treatment. The technique uses continuous-wave Doppler interrogation of the tricuspid regurgitant signal (recordable in at least 75% of patients) to determine the instantaneous peak systolic

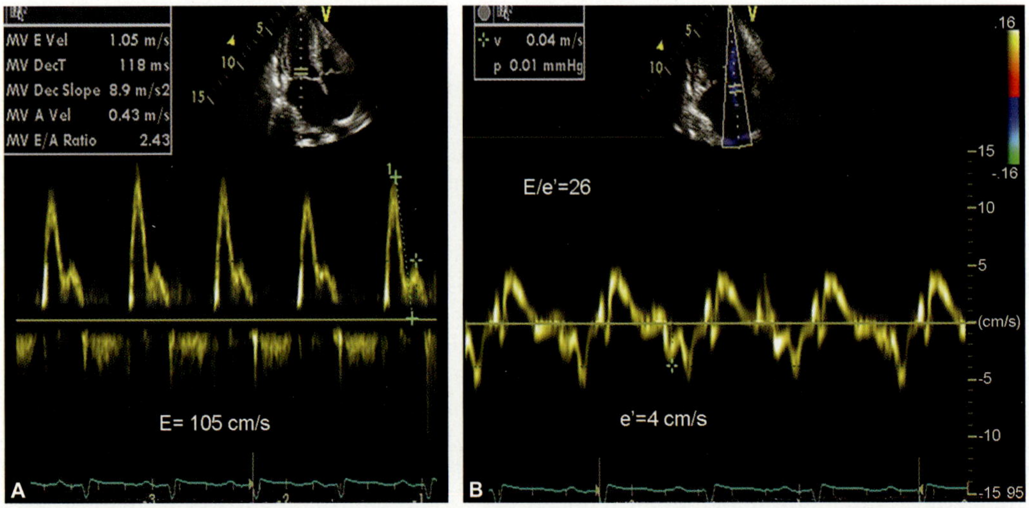

Figs. 2A and B: Estimation of mitral inflow early diastolic velocity (E) to early diastolic medial mitral annular velocity (e') ratio. (A) mitral inflow pattern, (B) mitral annular velocities recorded using tissue Doppler imaging. The mitral E/'e ratio in this patient was 26, suggestive of very high left ventricular filing pressure.

pressure gradient between the right ventricle and the right atrium using the modified Bernoulli equation.[60] By adding an estimation of right atrial pressure, the right ventricular peak systolic pressure can be obtained, which equates to pulmonary arterial systolic pressure in the absence of right ventricular outflow obstruction.

Left Atrial Volume Index

Left atrial volume index (LAVI) increases in proportion to the degree of left atrial pressure elevation and can be viewed as a marker of chronic LV diastolic pressure burden. As such, left atrial dilation is the single most important anatomic feature to implicate a "left heart" cause of a patient's dyspnea, and a diagnosis of HF should be reviewed when the left atrial size is shown to be normal. Outcome studies have demonstrated the strong independent prognostic value of left atrial size for predicting adverse cardiovascular events have been based on 2D echocardiography data.[61]

Role of Echocardiography in Heart Failure with Preserved Ejection Fraction

The clinical importance of being able to estimate cardiac pressures may be most apparent in the subgroup of HF patients who have preserved LV systolic function. LAVI more than 34 mL/m^2 or a left ventricular mass index (LVMI) more than or equal to 115 g/m^2 for males and more than or equal to 95 g/m^2 for females[62-64] are some key structural alterations. Key functional alterations are an E/e' more than or equal to 13 and a mean e' septal and lateral wall less than 9 cm/s.[62-70] Other (indirect) echocardiographically derived measurements are longitudinal strain or tricuspid regurgitation velocity (TRV).[63,68] An overview of normal and abnormal values for echocardiographic parameters related to diastolic function is presented in (Table 5).[71] In addition to the estimation of LV filling pressure, Doppler techniques can be used to characterize the physiology of LV filling, which

TABLE 5: Normal and abnormal values of left ventricular diastolic function.

Parameter	*Normal diastolic function*						*Diastolic dysfunction*		
	20–40 years		*40–60 years*		*>60 years*		*Impaired relaxation*	*Pseudo-normal filling*	*Restrictive filling*
	Male	*Female*	*Male*	*Female*	*Male*	*Female*			
MV-inflow									
MV-E (m/sec)	0.79 ± 0.14	0.84 ± 0.17	0.72 ± 0.16	0.77 ± 0.17	0.67 ± 0.15	0.72 ± 0.17			
MV-A (m/sec)	0.50 ± 0.13	0.51 ± 0.12	0.61 ± 0.15	0.63 ± 0.14	0.73 ± 0.16	0.76 ± 0.16			
DecT (msec)	179.8 ± 46.4	176.7 ± 40.1	186.6 ± 52.8	188.2 ± 39.8	217.5 ± 69.7	201.5 ± 55.7	>220	140–220	<140
DecT (msec)	1.69 ± 0.52	1.72 ± 0.52	1.22 ± 0.31	1.26 ± 0.43	0.96 ± 0.27	0.99 ± 0.31	<1.0	1.0–2.0	>2.0
IVRT (msec)							>110	60–100	<60
Tissue Doppler									
e' septal (cm/s)	11.9 ± 2.7	12.3 ± 2.3	9.8 ± 2.6	9.7 ± 2.5	7.3 ± 2.2	7.9 ± 2.3	<8	<8	<8
e' lateral (cm/s)	16.2 ± 3.6	16.6 ± 3.2	12.6 ± 3.0	12.4 ± 3.0	9.5 ± 2.1	9.7 ± 3.2	<10	<10	<10
e' mean sept-lat (cm/s)	14.0 ± 2.9	14.5 ± 2.4	11.2 ± 2.4	11.1 ± 2.5	8.5 ± 1.9	8.8 ± 2.6			
E/e' septal	6.9 ± 1.7	6.9 ± 1.6	7.8 ± 2.4	8.2 ± 2.2	9.8 ± 3.0	9.7 ± 2.6			
E/e' lateral	5.0 ± 1.3	5.2 ± 1.3	6.1 ± 2.2	6.5 ± 2.3	7.6 ± 2.1	7.9 ± 2.2			
E/e' mean sep-lat	5.8 ± 1.4	5.9 ± 1.3	6.7 ± 2.1	7.2 ± 2.0	8.4 ± 2.2	8.6 ± 2.2		≥13	≥13

(IVRT: isovolumic relaxation time; MV: mitral valve)

is predictive of outcome, independent of other variables.[72] Moreover, the persistence of a restrictive filling pattern, despite medical therapy, is predictive of adverse outcome.[73]

ECHOCARDIOGRAPHY AS A BIOMARKER IN HEART FAILURE?

The ideal candidate biomarker should fulfill some basic pre-requisites: (1) easily defined, safe, and reproducible in each patient; (2) appropriate therapeutic counter measures should be available to reset the abnormal biomarker values toward normal range; (3) the biomarker-triggered therapy change should improve outcome; (4) the biomarker-driven approach should provide an improved benefit and cost-benefit over standard approach.[74] Echocardiography-derived parameters can fulfill the definition of biomarkers. They are simple to measure, and reasonably reproducible in expert hands. They are associated with strong prognostic power, and several have shown independent and incremental prognostic value over standard clinical and biohumoral predictors (e.g., BNP, NT-proBNP, Troponins T and I, etc.). They explore different and complementary aspects of HF pathophysiology including: LV function, RV function, diastolic function, valvular function, and pulmonary hypertension, among others. In today's era of accessible and advanced imaging technology, defining echo parameters for a tailored and personalized HF treatment is no longer a dream and can not only become a rational clinical strategy today, but also serve as a roadmap for future research. It is up to the cardiology and echocardiography community to build the missing evidence required to shift the practice of HF from art of clinicians to evidence-based individualized treatment, guided by a low cost, portable radiation-free imaging technique.[75,76]

REFERENCES

1. Ponikowski P, Voors AA, Anker SD, et al. 2016 ESC Guidelines for the diagnosis and treatment of acute and chronic heart failure: The Task Force for the diagnosis and treatment of acute and chronic heart failure of the European Society of Cardiology (ESC). Developed with the special contribution of the Heart Failure Association (HFA) of the ESC. Eur J Heart Fail. 2016;18(8):891-975.
2. McKee PA, Castelli WP, McNamara PM, et al. The natural history of congestive heart failure: The Framingham study. N Engl J Med. 1971;285(26):1441-6.
3. Nanayakkara S, Kaye DM. Management of heart failure with preserved ejection fraction: A review. Clin Therapeut. 2015;37(10):2186-98.
4. Yancy CW, Jessup M, Bozkurt B, et al. 2013 ACCF/AHA guideline for the management of heart failure: a report of the American College of Cardiology Foundation/American Heart Association Task Force on Practice Guidelines. J Am Coll Cardiol. 2013;62(16):e147-e239.
5. Members WG, Roger VL, Go AS, et al. Executive summary: heart disease and stroke statistics—2011 update: a report from the American Heart Association. Circulation. 2011;123(4):459-63.
6. Bleumink GS, Knetsch AM, Sturkenboom MC, et al. Quantifying the heart failure epidemic: Prevalence, incidence rate, lifetime risk and prognosis of heart failure: the Rotterdam Study. Eur Heart J. 2004;25(18):1614-1619.
7. Heidenreich PA, Albert NM, Allen LA, et al. Forecasting the impact of heart failure in the United States: A policy statement from the American Heart Association. Circ Heart Fail. 2013;6(3):606-19.
8. Fiuzat M, O'Connor CM, Gueyffier F, et al. Biomarker-guided therapies in heart failure: a forum for unified strategies. J Cardiac Fail. 2013;19(8):592-9.
9. Hunt SA, Baker DW, Chin MH, et al. ACC/AHA guidelines for the evaluation and management of chronic heart failure in the adult: Executive summary: A report of the American College of Cardiology/American Heart Association task force on practice guidelines (committee to revise the 1995 guidelines for the evaluation and management of heart failure) developed in collaboration with the International Society for Heart and Lung Transplantation endorsed by the Heart Failure Society of America. J Am Coll Cardiol. 2001;38(7):2101-13.
10. Butler J, Fonarow GC, Zile MR, et al. Developing therapies for heart failure with preserved ejection fraction: Current state and future directions. JACC: Heart Fail. 2014;2(2):97-112.
11. Killip T, Kimball JT. Treatment of myocardial infarction in a coronary care unit: a two year experience with 250 patients. Am J Cardiol. 1967;20(4):457-64.
12. Kenchaiah S, Evans JC, Levy D, et al. Obesity and the risk of heart failure. N Engl J Med. 2002;347(5):305-13.
13. Vaur L, Gueret P, Lievre M, et al. Development of congestive heart failure in type 2 diabetic patients with microalbuminuria or proteinuria: observations from the DIABHYCAR (type 2 DIABetes, Hypertension, CArdiovascular Events and Ramipril) study. Diabet Care. 2003;26(3):855-60.
14. Poole-Wilson PA. The cardiac insufficiency bisoprolol study II. Lancet. 1999;353(9161):1360.
15. Group M-HS. Effect of metoprolol CR/XL in chronic heart failure: metoprolol CR/XL randomised intervention trial in-congestive heart failure (MERIT-HF). Lancet. 1999;353(9169):2001-7.
16. Lechat P, Packer M, Chalon S, et al. Clinical effects of β-adrenergic blockade in chronic heart failure: A meta-analysis of double-blind, placebo-controlled, randomized trials. Circulation. 1998;98(12):1184-91.
17. Packer M, Bristow MR, Cohn JN, et al. The effect of carvedilol on morbidity and mortality in patients with chronic heart failure. N Engl J Med. 1996;334(21):1349-55.
18. Investigators C. Effect of carvedilol on outcome after myocardial infarction in patients with left-ventricular dysfunction: The CAPRICORN randomised trial. Lancet. 2001;357(9266):1385-90.

19. Cleland J, Pennell D, Ray S, et al. Myocardial viability as a determinant of the ejection fraction response to carvedilol in patients with heart failure (CHRISTMAS trial): Randomised controlled trial. Lancet. 2003;362(9377):14-21.
20. Packer M, Fowler MB, Roecker EB, et al. Effect of carvedilol on the morbidity of patients with severe chronic heart failure: Results of the carvedilol prospective randomized cumulative survival (COPERNICUS) study. Circulation. 2002;106(17):2194-9.
21. Fisher ML, Gottlieb SS, Plotnick GD, et al. Beneficial effects of metoprolol in heart failure associated with coronary artery disease: a randomized trial. J Am Coll Cardiol. 1994;23(4):943-50.
22. Colucci WS, Packer M, Bristow MR, et al. Carvedilol inhibits clinical progression in patients with mild symptoms of heart failure. Circulation. 1996;94(11):2800-6.
23. Packer M, Colucci WS, Sackner-Bernstein JD, et al. Double-blind, placebo-controlled study of the effects of carvedilol in patients with moderate to severe heart failure: The PRECISE trial. Circulation. 1996;94(11):2793-9.
24. Lechat P. CIBIS Investigators and Committees. A randomized trial of beta-blockade in heart failure. The Cardiac Insufficiency Bisoprolol Study (CIBIS). Circulation. 1994;90:1765-73.
25. Waagstein F, Hjalmarson A, Swedberg K, et al. Beneficial effects of metoprolol in idiopathic dilated cardiomyopathy. Lancet. 1993;342(8885):1441-6.
26. Krum H, Sackner-Bernstein JD, Goldsmith RL, et al. Double-blind, placebo-controlled study of the long-term efficacy of carvedilol in patients with severe chronic heart failure. Circulation. 1995;92(6):1499-506.
27. Olsen SL, Gilbert EM, Renlund DG, et al. Carvedilol improves left ventricular function and symptoms in chronic heart failure: a double-blind randomized study. J Am Coll Cardiol. 1995;25(6):1225-31.
28. Metra M, Nardi M, Giubbini R, et al. Effects of short- and long-term carvedilol administration on rest and exercise hemodynamic variables, exercise capacity and clinical conditions in patients with idiopathic dilated cardiomyopathy. J Am Coll Cardiol. 1994;24(7):1678-87.
29. MacMahon S, Sharpe N. Randomised, placebo-controlled trial of carvedilol in patients with congestive heart failure due to. Lancet. 1997;349(9049):375-80.
30. Komajda M, The Study Group of Diagnosis of the Working Group on Heart Failure of the European Society of C, Follath F, et al. The EuroHeart Failure Survey programme—a survey on the quality of care among patients with heart failure in EuropePart 2: Treatment. Eur Heart J. 2003;24(5):464-74.
31. Packer M, Coats AJS, Fowler MB, et al. Effect of carvedilol on survival in severe chronic heart failure. N Engl J Med. 2001;344(22):1651-8.
32. Hjalmarson Å, Goldstein S, Fagerberg B, et al. Effects of controlled-release metoprolol on total mortality, hospitalizations, and well-being in patients with heart failure: The metoprolol cr/xl randomized intervention trial in congestive heart failure (MERIT-HF). JAMA. 2000;283(10):1295-302.
33. Flather MD, Shibata MC, Coats AJS, et al. Randomized trial to determine the effect of nebivolol on mortality and cardiovascular hospital admission in elderly patients with heart failure (SENIORS). Eur Heart J. 2005;26(3):215-25.
34. Willenheimer R. CIBIS III Investigators : Effect on survival and hospitalization of initiating treatment for chronic heart failure with bisoprolol followed by enalapril, as compared with the opposite sequence : results of the randomized Cardiac Insufficiency Bisoprolol Study (CIBIS) III. Circulation. 2005;112(16):2426-35.
35. Dargie HJ. Effect of carvedilol on outcome after myocardial infarction in patients with left-ventricular dysfunction: the CAPRICORN randomised trial. Lancet. 2001;357(9266):1385-90.
36. Doughty RN, Whalley GA, Gamble G, et al. Left ventricular remodeling with carvedilol in patients with congestive heart failure due to ischemic heart disease. J Am Coll Cardiol. 1997;29(5):1060-6.
37. Shekelle PG, Rich MW, Morton SC, et al. Efficacy of angiotensin-converting enzyme inhibitors and beta-blockers in the management of left ventricular systolic dysfunction according to race, gender, and diabetic status: A meta-analysis of major clinical trials. J Am Coll Cardiol. 2003;41(9):1529-38.
38. Beta-Blocker Evaluation of Survival Trial Investigators, Eichhorn EJ, Domanski MJ, et al. A Trial of the Beta-Blocker Bucindolol in Patients with Advanced Chronic Heart Failure. N Engl J Med. 2001;344(22):1659-67.
39. Torp-Pedersen C, Køber L, Ball S, et al. The incomplete Bucindolol Evaluation in Acute myocardial infarction Trial (BEAT). Eur J Heart Fail. 2002;4(4):495-9.
40. Poole-Wilson PA, Swedberg K, Cleland JGF, et al. Comparison of carvedilol and metoprolol on clinical outcomes in patients with chronic heart failure in the Carvedilol Or Metoprolol European Trial (COMET): Randomised controlled trial. Lancet. 2003;362(9377):7-13.
41. Aronow WS, Ahn C, Kronzon I. Effect of propranolol versus no propranolol on total mortality plus nonfatal myocardial infarction in older patients with prior myocardial infarction, congestive heart failure, and left ventricular ejection fraction> or= 40% treated with diuretics plus angiotensin-converting enzyme inhibitors. Am J Cardiol. 1997;80(2):207-9.
42. van Veldhuisen DJ, Cohen-Solal A, Böhm M, et al. Beta-blockade with nebivolol in elderly heart failure patients with impaired and preserved left ventricular ejection fraction: Data From SENIORS (Study of Effects of Nebivolol Intervention on Outcomes and Rehospitalization in Seniors With Heart Failure). J Am Coll Cardiol. 2009;53(23):2150-8.
43. Bergström A, Andersson B, Edner M, et al. Effect of carvedilol on diastolic function in patients with diastolic heart failure and preserved systolic function. Results of the Swedish Doppler-echocardiographic study (SWEDIC). Eur J Heart Fail. 2004;6(4):453-61.
44. Yamamoto K, Sakata Y, Ohtani T, et al. Heart failure with preserved ejection fraction. Circ J. 2009;73(3):404-10.
45. Nagueh SF, Smiseth OA, Appleton CP, et al. Recommendations for the evaluation of left ventricular diastolic function

by echocardiography: An update from the American Society of Echocardiography and the European Association of Cardiovascular Imaging. Eur J Echocardiogr. 2016;17(12):1321-60.

46. Hernandez AF, Hammill BG, O'Connor CM, et al. Clinical effectiveness of beta-blockers in heart failure: findings from the OPTIMIZE-HF (Organized Program to Initiate Lifesaving Treatment in Hospitalized Patients with Heart Failure) Registry. J Am Coll Cardiol. 2009;53(2):184-92.
47. Bonow RO, Bennett S, Casey DE, et al. ACC/AHA clinical performance measures for adults with chronic heart failure: a report of the American College of Cardiology/American Heart Association task force on performance measures (writing committee to develop heart failure clinical performance measures) endorsed by the Heart Failure Society of America. J Am Coll Cardiol. 2005;46(6):1144-78.
48. Dickstein K, Members ATF, Cohen-Solal A, et al. ESC Guidelines for the diagnosis and treatment of acute and chronic heart failure 2008: The Task Force for the Diagnosis and Treatment of Acute and Chronic Heart Failure 2008 of the European Society of Cardiology. Developed in collaboration with the Heart Failure Association of the ESC (HFA) and endorsed by the European Society of Intensive Care Medicine (ESICM). Eur J Heart Fail. 2008;10(10):933-89.
49. Herlitz J, Waagstein F, Lindqvist J, et al. Effect of metoprolol on the prognosis for patients with suspected acute myocardial infarction and indirect signs of congestive heart failure (a subgroup analysis of the Göteborg Metoprolol Trial). Am J Cardiol. 1997;80(9S2):40J-44J.
50. Agha SA, Kalogeropoulos AP, Shih J, et al. Echocardiography and risk prediction in advanced heart failure: incremental value over clinical markers. J Cardiac Fail. 2009;15(7):586-592.
51. Grayburn PA, Appleton CP, DeMaria AN, et al. Echocardiographic predictors of morbidity and mortality in patients with advanced heart failure: The Beta-blocker Evaluation of Survival Trial (BEST). J Am Coll Cardiol. 2005;45(7):1064-71.
52. Aurigemma GP, Gottdiener JS, Shemanski L, et al. Predictive value of systolic and diastolic function for incident congestive heart failure in the elderly: the cardiovascular health study. J Am Coll Cardiol. 2001;37(4):1042-8.
53. Chen AA, Wood MJ, Krauser DG, et al. NT-proBNP levels, echocardiographic findings, and outcomes in breathless patients: results from the ProBNP Investigation of Dyspnoea in the Emergency Department (PRIDE) echocardiographic substudy. Eur Heart J. 2006;27(7):839-45.
54. Gardin JM, McClelland R, Kitzman D, et al. M-mode echocardiographic predictors of six-to seven-year incidence of coronary heart disease, stroke, congestive heart failure, and mortality in an elderly cohort (the Cardiovascular Health Study). Am J Cardiol. 2001;87(9):1051-7.
55. Francis C, Caruana L, Kearney P, et al. Open access echocardiography in management of heart failure in the community. BMJ. 1995;310(6980):634-6.
56. Nagueh SF, Middleton KJ, Kopelen HA, et al. Doppler tissue imaging: a noninvasive technique for evaluation of left ventricular relaxation and estimation of filling pressures. J Am Coll Cardiol. 1997;30(6):1527-33.
57. Mottram PM, Marwick TH. Assessment of diastolic function: What the general cardiologist needs to know. Heart. 2005;91(5):681-95.
58. Yu C-M, Sanderson JE, Marwick TH, et al. Tissue Doppler imaging: A new prognosticator for cardiovascular diseases. J Am Coll Cardiol. 2007;49(19):1903-14.
59. Little WC, Oh JK. Echocardiographic evaluation of diastolic function can be used to guide clinical care. Circulation. 2009;120(9):802-9.
60. Yock PG, Popp RL. Noninvasive estimation of right ventricular systolic pressure by Doppler ultrasound in patients with tricuspid regurgitation. Circulation. 1984;70(4):657-62.
61. Tsang TS, Barnes ME, Gersh BJ, et al. Prediction of risk for first age-related cardiovascular events in an elderly population: The incremental value of echocardiography. J Am Coll Cardiol. 2003;42(7):1199-205.
62. Paulus WJ, Tschöpe C, Sanderson JE, et al. How to diagnose diastolic heart failure: a consensus statement on the diagnosis of heart failure with normal left ventricular ejection fraction by the Heart Failure and Echocardiography Associations of the European Society of Cardiology. Eur Heart J. 2007;28(20):2539-50.
63. Lang RM, Badano LP, Mor-Avi V, et al. Recommendations for cardiac chamber quantification by echocardiography in adults: An update from the American Society of Echocardiography and the European Association of Cardiovascular Imaging. Eur Heart J-Cardiovasc Imaging. 2015;16(3):233-71.
64. Dokainish H, Nguyen JS, Bobek J, et al. Assessment of the American Society of Echocardiography-European Association of Echocardiography guidelines for diastolic function in patients with depressed ejection fraction: an echocardiographic and invasive haemodynamic study. Eur J Echocardiogr. 2011;12(11):857-64.
65. Caballero L, Kou S, Dulgheru R, et al. Echocardiographic reference ranges for normal cardiac Doppler data: results from the NORRE Study. Eur Heart J-Cardiovasc Imaging. 2015;16(9):1031-41.
66. Ommen SR, Nishimura R, Appleton CP, et al. Clinical utility of Doppler echocardiography and tissue Doppler imaging in the estimation of left ventricular filling pressures: a comparative simultaneous Doppler-catheterization study. Circulation. 2000;102(15):1788-94.
67. Nishimura RA, Appleton CP, Redfield MM, et al. Noninvasive Doppler echocardiographic evaluation of left ventricular filling pressures in patients with cardiomyopathies: A simultaneous Doppler echocardiographic and cardiac catheterization study. J Am Coll Cardiol. 1996;28(5):1226-33.
68. Nagueh SF, Appleton CP, Gillebert TC, et al. Recommendations for the evaluation of left ventricular diastolic function by echocardiography. Eur J Echocardiogr. 2009;10(2):165-93.
69. Gilman G, Nelson TA, Hansen WH, et al. Diastolic function: A sonographer's approach to the essential echocardiographic measurements of left ventricular diastolic function. J Am Soc Echocardiogr. 2007;20(2):199-209.

70. Cohen GI, Pietrolungo JF, Thomas JD, et al. A practical guide to assessment of ventricular diastolic function using Doppler echocardiography. J Am Coll Cardiol. 1996;27(7):1753-60.
71. Ponikowski P, Voors AA, Anker SD, et al. 2016 ESC Guidelines for the diagnosis and treatment of acute and chronic heart failure: The Task Force for the diagnosis and treatment of acute and chronic heart failure of the European Society of Cardiology (ESC) Developed with the special contribution of the Heart Failure Association (HFA) of the ESC. Eur Heart J. 2016;37(27):2129-200.
72. Collaborators MaRGiEHF. Independence of restrictive filling pattern and LV ejection fraction with mortality in heart failure: An individual patient meta-analysis. Eur J Heart Fail. 2008;10(8):786-92.
73. Pinamonti B, Zecchin M, Di Lenarda A, et al. Persistence of restrictive left ventricular filling pattern in dilated cardiomyopathy: An ominous prognostic sign. J Am Coll Cardiol. 1997;29(3):604-12.
74. Chow SL, Maisel AS, Anand I, et al. Role of biomarkers for the prevention, assessment, and management of heart failure: A scientific statement from the American Heart Association. Circulation. 2017;135(22):e1054-91.
75. Picano E, Vañó E, Rehani MM, et al. The appropriate and justified use of medical radiation in cardiovascular imaging: A position document of the ESC Associations of Cardiovascular Imaging, Percutaneous Cardiovascular Interventions and Electrophysiology. Eur Heart J. 2014;35(10):665-72.
76. Dini FL, Rosa GM, Fontanive P, et al. Combining blood flow and tissue Doppler imaging with N-terminal pro-type B natriuretic peptide for risk stratification of clinically stable patients with systolic heart failure. Eur J Echocardiogr. 2010;11(4):333-40.

21

CHAPTER

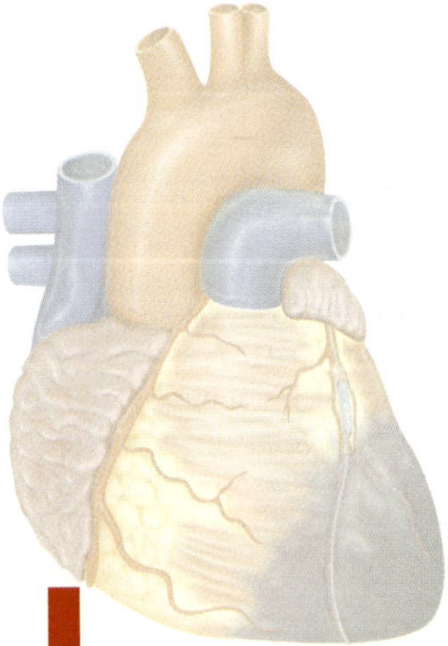

Diuretics Effect and Outcome Evaluation in Heart Failure by Echocardiography

Saumitra Ray, Rajat Subhra Ghose

INTRODUCTION

Heart failure can be defined as a complex clinical syndrome that results from any structural or functional impairment of ventricular filling or ejection of blood and usually manifests with features of fluid retention, dyspnea, fatigue, and exercise intolerance. Heart failure is largely a clinical diagnosis based on a history and physical examination and diagnostic tests are usually supportive. Echocardiography is an easily available imaging modality that can help in establishing a diagnosis of heart failure, determining the etiology, assessing severity of the condition while quantifying and monitoring ventricular performance and evaluating progress and effectiveness of management. It also helps in risk stratification and detection of various complications related to heart failure. Heart failure patients who have undergone echocardiographic examination show better survival rates due to intensified medical treatment and intervention.[1] Various imaging modalities are available to help in determining left ventricular (LV) size and function. Certain imaging techniques, like myocardial strain quantification using speckle tracking imaging, may also determine early LV systolic dysfunction in individuals with preserved ejection fraction. The clinical syndrome of heart failure may be present in those with low LV ejection fraction (LVEF) with or without chamber dilatation, as also in those with preserved LV ejection fraction and normal LV size. In addition to myocardial dysfunction, heart failure can be caused by diseases of the pericardium, endocardium and valvular diseases, as well as in severe anemia and other high output states, and several metabolic, endocrine, nutritional, and multisystem diseases.

While managing patients with heart failure, it is essential to estimate the volume status to guide therapy, most specifically to monitor diuretic use. Volume assessment during the management of heart failure was earlier based on the clinical history and physical examination, which included assessment of jugular venous pressure (JVP). Availability of biomarkers like brain natriuretic peptide (BNP) and N-terminal prohormone of brain natriuretic peptide (NT-proBNP), and echocardiography has helped in increasing accuracy of assessment of volume status in patients being managed for heart failure.

EVALUATION OF THE LEFT VENTRICLE

The initial echocardiography assessment of heart failure would include assessment of LV cavity size, shape and wall thickness, and estimation of LVEF. Cardiac chamber dimensions can be serially measured to look for change in ventricular filling for evaluation of volume status during diuretic therapy. The LV internal diameter at end-diastole (LVIDD), measured serially, can be indicative of volume status in heart failure. Both right ventricular (RV) and LV internal diameters can be measured to monitor response to diuretics. Serial measurements must be made from the same position of the transducer and in the same views so that even small changes can be compared. LVIDD and LVIDS can be measured in the parasternal short-axis (SAX) or long-axis (LAX) view by direct two dimensional (2D) measurements or by M-mode imaging of the LV at the tips of the mitral valve leaflets.

While M-mode method of assessing LVEF (Teichholz method) has been popular in the past (Fig. 1), the current recommendation is to use 2D echocardiography method of disc summation (Biplane Simpson) to eliminate segmental variations in contractility affecting calculation (Fig. 2). However, 3D calculation of LV volumes has less test-retest variability and is the superior method in determining LVEF (Fig. 3).

A recent study followed the outcome of treatment of three separate categories of patients with heart failure: HFpEF (heart failure with preserved ejection fraction - LVEF >40%), HFrEF (heart failure with reduced ejection fraction - LVEF <40%), and HFrecEF (patients in whom LVEF had improved - recovered ejection fraction to >40%).[2] The study showed that there was lower mortality, less frequent hospitalizations, and fewer composite end points with the HFrecEF group.[1] Thus improvement in LVEF, measured by 2D echocardiography following therapy has been proved to improve mortality.

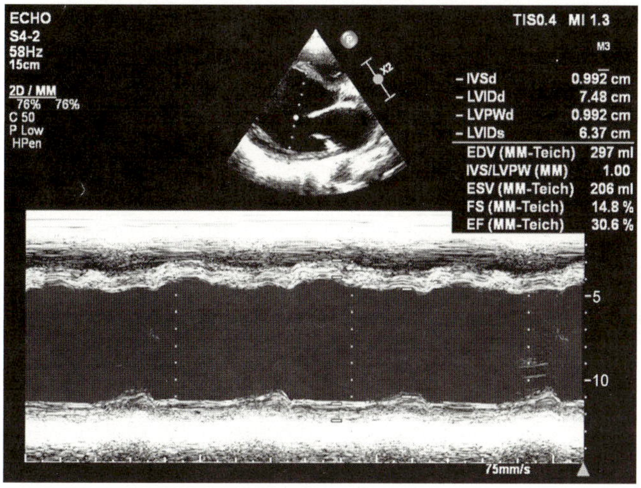

Fig. 1: M-mode method of determining left ventricular ejection fraction (LVEF).

While LVEF is an important prognosticator of outcome in heart failure, it must be understood that a low ejection fraction may not necessarily be associated with heart failure. Intravascular volume status and LV filling pressures are the key determinants of heart failure and can be serially monitored to guide management of heart failure. 2D echocardiography also documents the structural abnormalities that determine the etiology of heart failure including wall motion abnormalities, scarring, myocardial thickness, and associated or causal valvular lesions. Irrespective of the cause of heart failure, whether secondary to LV systolic or diastolic dysfunction or due to structural abnormalities like valve stenosis or regurgitation, breathlessness in heart failure is determined by the pathophysiology of elevation of left atrial pressure (LAP) and a resultant increase in pulmonary venous pressure. Doppler interrogation of the mitral valve flow coupled with determination of the mitral annular velocities in diastole by tissue Doppler imaging (TDI) is fairly reliable in assessing mean LAPs. Because of easy availability, reasonably low cost, and essentially noninvasive nature, this modality of evaluating LAPs is now routinely used to aid in the management of heart failure. Assessment of LV filling pressures and mean LAPs by echocardiography correlates well with pulmonary capillary wedge pressures determined by invasive techniques.

Recommendations for Noninvasive Cardiac Imaging in Heart Failure[3]

A 2D echocardiogram with Doppler should be performed for initial evaluation of heart failure (Class of Recommendation 1; Level of Evidence C).

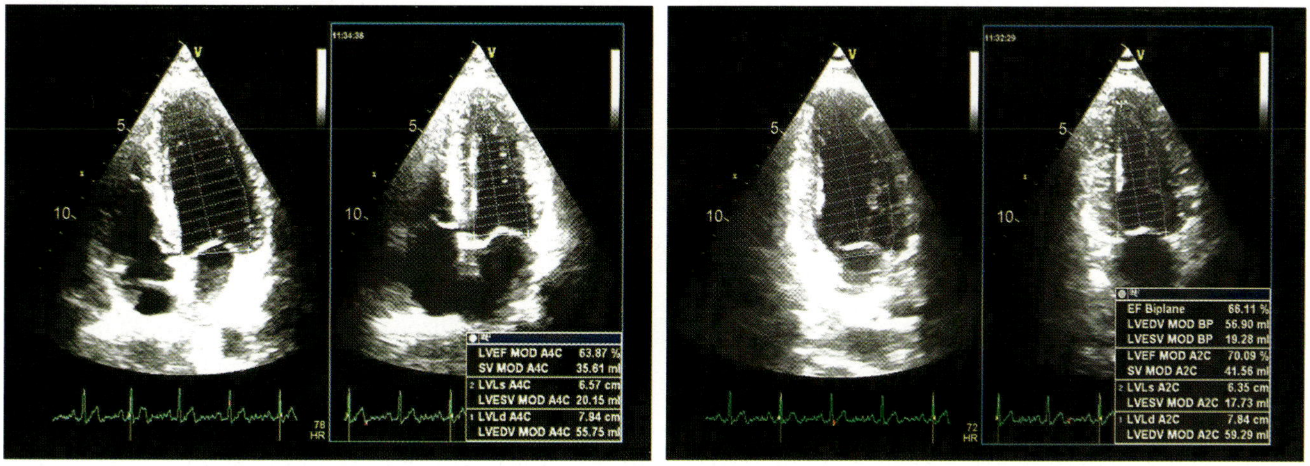

Fig. 2: Biplane Simpson method of evaluation of left ventricular (LV) ejection fraction.

Repeat measurement of EF is useful in patients with heart failure who have had a significant change in clinical status or received treatment that might affect cardiac function or for consideration of device therapy (Class of Recommendation 1; Level of Evidence C).

Recommendations for Use of Diuretics in Heart Failure[3]

Diuretics are recommended in patients with HFrEF, who have evidence of fluid retention to improve symptoms, unless contraindicated. (Class of Recommendation1; level of Evidence: C).

Technique of Determining Left Ventricular Filling Pressure

Echocardiography guidelines to determine LV filling pressures based on the Doppler variables that are evaluated must be considered in the light of the relevant clinical background and with regard to presence of symptoms of heart failure. It is also important to understand the pathophysiological basis of each variable and an understanding of situations in which a certain variable may not hold good. Often no single parameter is helpful in coming to a conclusion, and it becomes necessary to integrate multiple variables to determine presence of raised LAP.

Elevated LV filling pressure has been shown to be associated with adverse outcomes in patients with advanced heart failure.[4] While evaluating a patient with heart failure a preliminary 2D echocardiography imaging may demonstrate common features of left atrial enlargement with or without LV dilatation or hypertrophy and dysfunction. Pulsed wave Doppler interrogation of the mitral flow, with the sample volume placed at the tips of the mitral leaflets in diastole, shows a spectral display of LV filling with an early filling (E) and a late diastolic filling (A) waves in patients in sinus rhythm. A normal filling pattern typically shows E/A greater than 0.8. An E/A ratio is less than 0.8 in early diastolic dysfunction in the younger individual and is classified as Grade 1 LV diastolic dysfunction and is usually associated with normal mean LAPs (Fig. 4).[5] However, such a pattern is usually seen in healthy elderly subjects due to increased LV myocardial stiffness.

With increasing LV filling pressures and rising LAPs, as occurs in heart failure, the LV filling is altered toward normal pattern and typically the E/A ratio is between 0.8 and 2.0, thus being termed "pseudo-normalization". It is important to be able to distinguish pseudonormal (grade 2 LV diastolic dysfunction) from normal filling pattern in identifying patients with raised atrial pressures in heart failure.

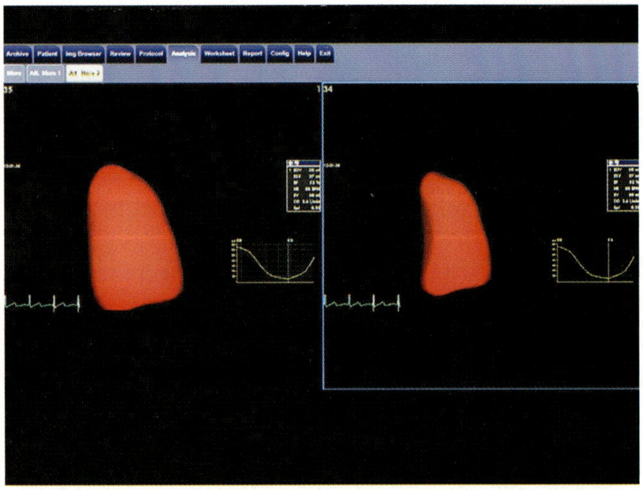

Fig. 3: Three-dimensional (3D) determination of left ventricular (LV) volumes and left ventricular ejection fraction (LVEF).

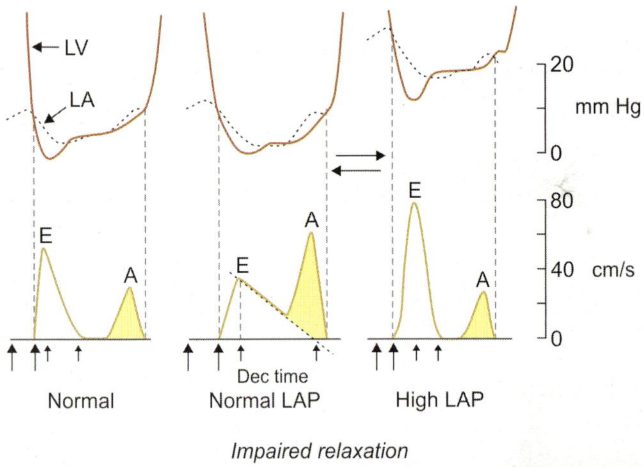

Fig. 4: Normal mean left atrial pressures.

Confirmation of a raised LA pressure can be established by reducing preload and observing the change in LV filling pattern on pulsed-wave (PW) Doppler spectral tracing. This is done by making the patient perform a Valsalva maneuver and recording the mitral flow pattern in the late Valsalva strain phase, i.e. 10 seconds after forced expiration with the nose and mouth closed. This causes the E/A ratio to diminish by 50% in a patient with grade 2 LV diastolic dysfunction. Such reduction of E/A ratio and alteration of filling pattern is seen after successful diuretic therapy, suggesting normalization of mean LAPs. In addition, mitral E deceleration time (DT) less than 130 ms is suggestive of elevated LA pressure in heart failure with reduced LVEF; this parameter has high accuracy both in sinus rhythm and in atrial fibrillation. Failure to reverse an E/A ratio and DT after therapy suggests an adverse prognosis. In dilated ventricles with reduced LVEF color flow Doppler derived flow propagation velocity (Vp) of less than 45 cm/s is suggestive of presence of diastolic dysfunction. E/Vp more than or equal to 2.5 predicts PCWP more than 15 mm Hg with reasonable accuracy in patients with depressed EFs.

Assessing mitral annular velocities during the early diastolic phase (e') (using TDI with PW sample volume placed on the medial and lateral annulus) and determining the average E/e' ratio is now routinely used to evaluate elevated LAP. The variables used to support a diagnosis of raised LA pressure, as per expert consensus[6] are:

- Septal e' less than 7 cm/s or Lateral e' less than 10 cm/s
- Average E/e' more than 14
- Tricuspid regurgitation (TR) peak velocity more than 2.8 m/s
- LA volume index more than 34 mL/m^2.

In patients with normal ejection fraction, presence of more than half of the above four variables indicates LV diastolic dysfunction. This method of assessing LAPs is useful in monitoring treatment of patients with heart failure. Reduction in E/e' ratio to less than 13 can be documented after successful diuretic therapy (Figs. 5A to D).

The American Society of Echocardiography (ASE) guidelines on monitoring diuretic therapy suggests the use of the following algorithm to distinguish normal from raised LAP:[5]

- E/e' less than 8; normal LVEF = normal LAP
- E/e' more than'13; normal LVEF = increased LAP
- E/A more than 2; DT less than 150 ms; depressed LVEF = increased LAP
- E/A less than 1 and E less than 50 cm/s; depressed LVEF = normal LAP.

While E/e' ratio does predict elevated LA pressures, it is not yet recommended to monitor LAP of patients with acute decompensated heart failure with reduced LVEF, as studies show that it does not predict LAPs and cannot be used to guide therapy in this clinical situation.

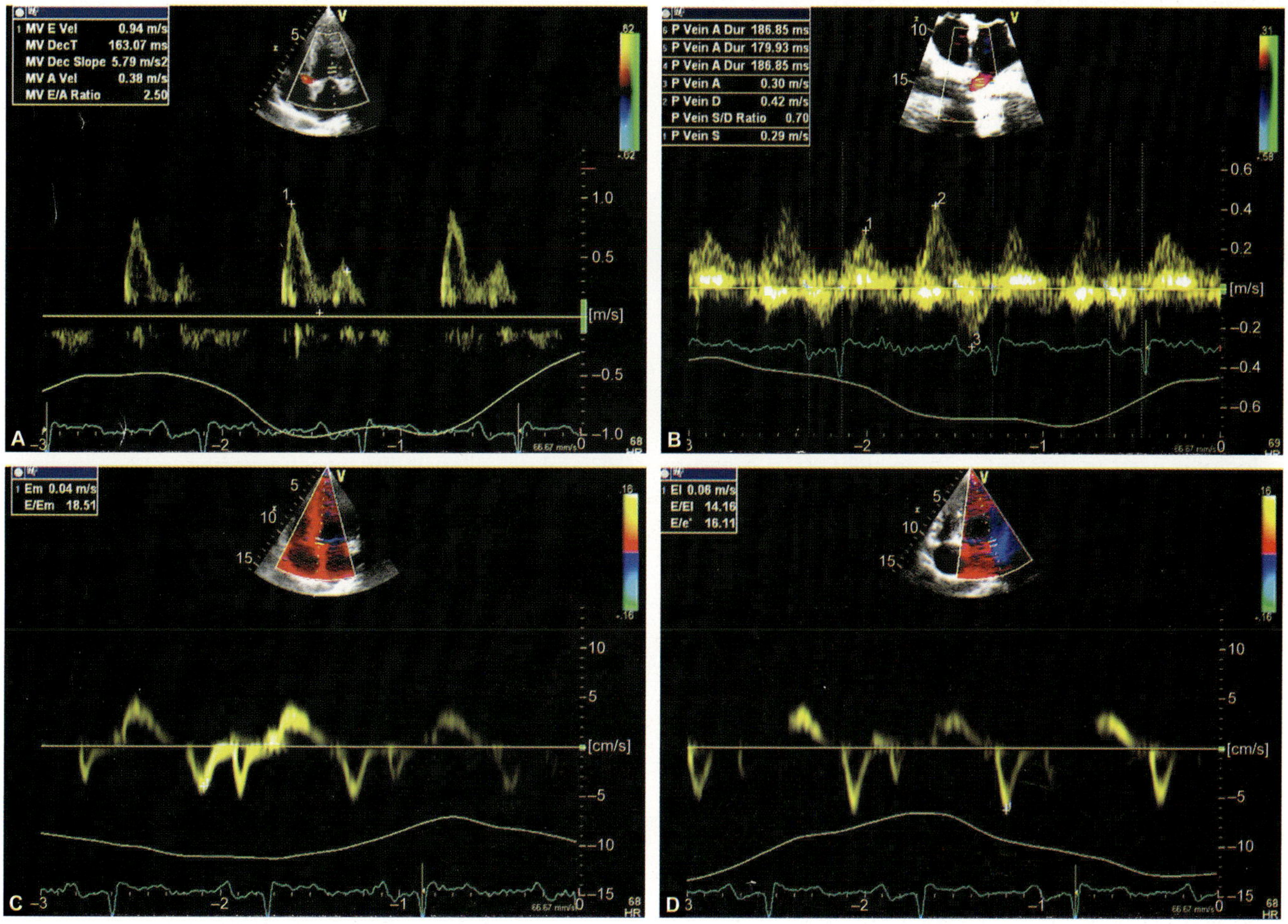

Figs. 5A to D: Doppler study of a patient with heart failure with preserved ejection fraction (HFpEF): (A) PW Doppler at mitral valve; (B) PW Doppler in pulmonary vein; (C) e' at septal mitral annulus; (D) e' at lateral mitral annulus.

Evaluation of Left Ventricular Filling in Presence of Atrial Fibrillation

Atrial fibrillation is often present in patients with heart failure and is commonly associated with an enlarged left atrium and an absence of the late LV filling' A' wave , thus making assessment of LV filling pressures more difficult. Doppler measurements that are abnormal in presence of atrial fibrillation[6] with depressed LVEF are:

- Peak acceleration of mitral E velocity of more than or equal to 1,900 cm/s^2,
- Isovolumetric relaxation time (IVRT) less than or equal to 65 ms,
- DT of pulmonary venous diastolic velocity less than or equal to 220 ms,
- E/mitral Vp more than or equal to 1.4
- E/e' ratio more than or equal to 11
- TE-e (The time interval between onset of mitral E and annular e' velocity)
- IVRT/TE-e'.

Determination of Pulmonary Arterial Pressures

Raised pulmonary artery pressure is associated with increased mortality. Elevation of mean LA pressures in heart failure leads to elevation of pulmonary venous pressures, which in turn results in elevated pulmonary arterial pressure (PAP). This is easily documented by estimating RV peak systolic pressures from assessment of peak TR pressure gradient, provided there is no RV outflow tract (RVOT) obstruction or pulmonary valve stenosis. TR velocity less than 2.8 m/s is considered normal and above 3.4 m/s is suggestive of raised peak pulmonary arterial systolic pressure (PASP). Using the Bernoulli's equation, pressure gradient = 4 × square of the velocity, the peak TR velocity is used to determine RV to right atrial pressure (RAP) gradient. This pressure gradient is then added to the estimated RAP. The RAPs, which are often elevated in heart failure, are first evaluated by measuring the inferior vena cava (IVC) diameter[7] and its collapsibility during normal inspiration (or augmented by a sniff). A useful guide for calculating RA pressure is shown in Table 1.

For convenience of use, average values of 3 mm Hg, 8 mm Hg or 15 mm Hg, respectively, may be added for the three mentioned categories, to the tricuspid regurgitation gradient to get a value of the PASP [Recent the European Society of Cardiology (ESC) guidelines, however, suggest just using max TR velocity only, without adding RA pressure, as IVC assessment may not always be very accurate].

TR velocity-time integral (VTI) can be also used to evaluate the mean RV-RA pressure gradient and to calculate mean PAP (mPAP), by adding the RA pressure.

TABLE 1: Guide to calculate right atrial pressure.

Inferior vena cava diameter	Mean right atrial pressure
<21 mm and showing >50% collapse	0–5 mm Hg
>21 mm and showing <50% collapse or <21 mm and showing > 50% collapse	5–10 mm Hg
>21 mm and showing <50% collapse	10–20 mm Hg

If a definite envelope of a TR spectral display cannot be obtained, an estimate of the mPAP may be made by adding the RA pressure to the peak pulmonary regurgitation pressure gradient.

The pulmonary regurgitation end diastolic gradient can also be measured and added to the estimated RAP to determine pulmonary arterial diastolic pressure (PADP).

RVOT acceleration time (ATRVOT), obtained by placing the sample volume just proximal to the pulmonary valve, and has also been used to calculate mPAP by the formula

mPAP = 90–(0.62 * ATRVOT).

RV systolic pressure is calculated as the sum of estimated RA pressure and the derived peak TR gradient. Following diuretic therapy in heart failure the TR gradient diminishes with concomitant reduction in IVC size and collapsibility.

Importance of Inferior Vena Cava Measurement in Heart Failure

Distension of IVC is associated with an increased RAP.[7] There is plenty of evidence showing that raised RAP is an adverse risk factor in left heart failure. Raised JVP was independently associated with the risk of hospitalization and death from heart failure in the SOLVD (Studies of Left Ventricular Dysfunction) treatment trial.[8] Measuring the IVC and its collapsibility by echocardiography is perhaps more sensitive than clinical estimation of JVP. In patients with left heart failure associated RV systolic dysfunction (reflected in a raised RA pressure) is a risk factor for mortality.[9] Finally, RAP is often elevated in patients with chronic heart failure and raised LV filling pressure in both HFpEF and HFrEF (Fig. 6).[10]

Evaluation of Right Ventricle Systolic Function

The right ventricle is more sensitive to after load than the left ventricle. Raised pulmonary pressures secondary LV failure can lead to RV dysfunction. Echocardiographic evaluation of right heart is essential in the management of right heart failure. Commonly and reliably used parameters of RV function in clinical practice are *T*ricuspid *A*nnular

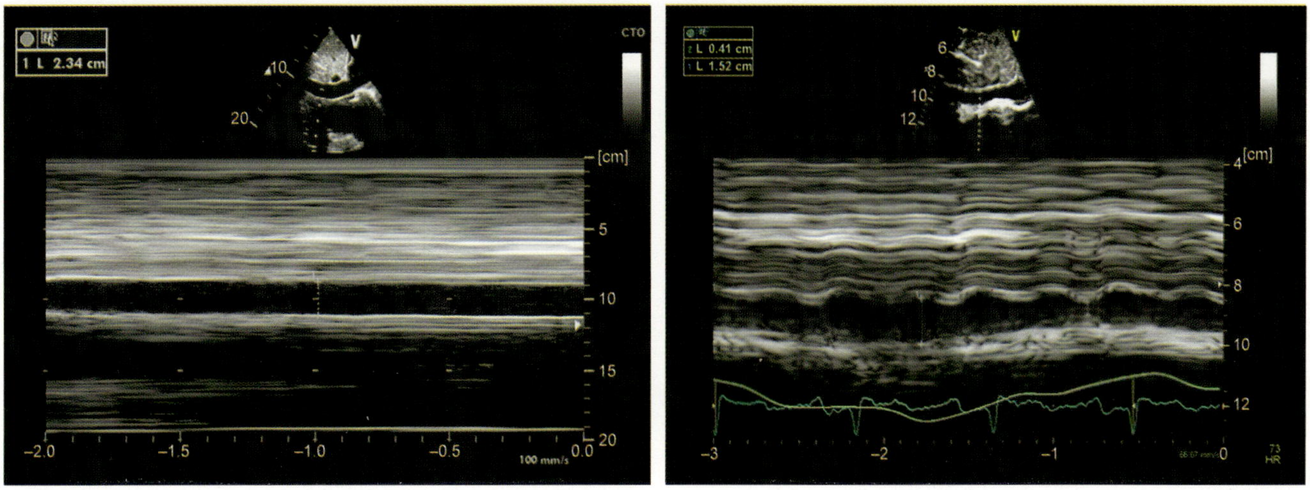

Fig. 6: Change in inferior vena cava (IVC) collapsibility after diuretic therapy in the same patient. The left panel shows a bedside portable echocardiography documentation of a dilated noncollapsing IVC (23 mm). The right panel shows a nondilated IVC showing more than 50% inspiratory collapse following diuretic therapy.

*P*lane *S*ystolic *E*xcursion (TAPSE), RV S' and *F*ractional *A*rea *C*hange (FAC).

Tricuspid annular plane systolic excursion (TAPSE) determines the systolic apical displacement of the lateral tricuspid annulus by M-mode, with the cursor passing through the LV apex and lateral annulus in the apical four chamber view. TAPSE is less preload dependent than other parameters of RV function. Alternatively, measuring the velocity of motion of the tricuspid valve lateral annulus (RV S') toward the RV apex using TDI is also an indicator of RV function.

Features highly specific for RV dysfunction are:

- TAPSE less than16 mm
- RV S' less than10 cm/sec

Both parameters can be used to serially monitor RV systolic function. RV internal diameter in diastole (RVIDD) and FAC can also be measured in follow-up studies during diuretic therapy in heart failure.

CONCLUSION

In summary, the key to monitor effect and outcome of diuretic therapy in heart failure by echocardiography is to comprehensively evaluate volume status and the resultant intracardiac pressure changes that occur in relation to it. Reduction of preload improves LV function and reduces mean LAPs along with abatement of features of heart failure. Transmitral flow patterns coupled with tissue Doppler quantification of mitral annular velocities are now routinely used to determine LAPs. Evaluation of PAPs and its effects on RV size and function is also an effective guide to therapy. Associated reversible features like secondary mitral regurgitation and presence of fluid in pleural, pericardial, and peritoneal cavities along with features of hepatic venous congestion can also be serially monitored on echocardiography. Importantly, all the above echocardiographic parameters and techniques have to be integrated with a thorough clinical evaluation to be an effective guide to the management of heart failure.

REFERENCES

1. Tribouilloy C, Rusinaru D, Mahjoub H, et al. Impact of echocardiography in patients hospitalized for heart failure: A prospective study. Arch Cardiovasc Dis. 2009;101:465-73.
2. Kalogeropoulos AP, Fonarow GC, Georgiopoulou V, et al. Characteristics and outcomes of adult outpatients with heart failure and improved or recovered ejection fraction. JAMA Cardiol. 2016;1(5):510-8.
3. Yancy CW, Jessup M, Bozkurt B, et al. 2013 ACCF/AHA guideline for the management of heart failure: Executive summary. J Am Coll Cardiol. 2013;62(16).
4. Drazner MH, Prasad A, Ayers C, et al. The relationship of right- and left-sided filling pressures in patients with heart failure and a preserved ejection fraction. Circ Heart Fail. 2010;3:202-6.
5. Porter TR, Shillcutt SK, Adams MS. Guidelines for the use of echocardiography as a monitor for therapeutic intervention in adults: A report from the American Society of Echocardiography. J Am Soc Echocardiogr. 2015;28(1):40-56.
6. Nagueh SF, Smiseth OA, Appleton CP. Recommendations for the evaluation of left ventricular diastolic function by echocardiography: An update from the American Society of Echocardiography and the European Association of Cardiovascular Imaging. J Am Soc Echocardiogr. 2016;29:277-314.

7. Kircher BJ, Himelman RB, Schiller NB. Noninvasive estimation of right atrial pressure from the inspiratory collapse of the inferior vena cava. Am J Cardiol. 1990;66:493-6.
8. Drazner MH, Rame JE, Stevenson LW, et al. Prognostic importance of elevated jugular venous pressure and a third heart sound in patients with heart failure. N Engl J Med. 2001;345:574-81.
9. Meyer P, Filippatos GS, Ahmed MI, et al. Effects of right ventricular ejection fraction on outcomes in chronic systolic heart failure. Circulation. 2010;121:252-8.
10. Campbell P, Drazner MH, Kato M, et al. Mismatch of right- and left-sided filling pressures in chronic heart failure. J Card Fail. 2011;17:561-8.

22

CHAPTER

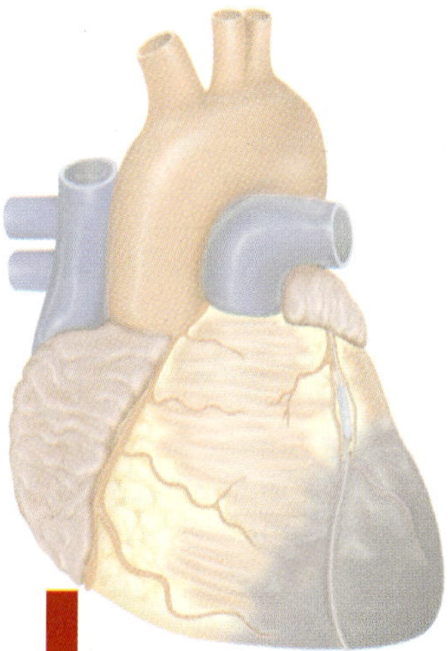

Device Intervention in Heart Failure

Raghav Bansal, Viveka Kumar

INTRODUCTION

Despite all the advances in the field of cardiology, heart failure remains a common and perplexing problem worldwide constantly demanding novel management strategies. With prolonged longevity and aging population the incidence and prevalence of heart failure continue to be on a rise. Approximately 20 million people worldwide are affected with heart failure.[1] End-stage heart failure along with sudden cardiac death are the final common pathways of almost all the cardiovascular diseases and have gained the focus for intervention in the past two decades. Traditionally, the prognosis of heart failure is dismal with a 5-year and 10-year survival of approximately 50% and 15%, respectively.[2] Although with the improvements in medical therapy, the morbidity and mortality rates continue to fall, the improvements have been rather slow leaving behind a substantial burden which needs to be addressed with other therapies. Inadequacy of drug therapy is further highlighted by the fact that there has been only one addition to the list of drugs decreasing heart failure mortality in the past two decades in the form of angiotensin II receptor blocker neprilysin inhibitor. Also, drug therapies are more effective in initial phases of heart failure and continue to be ineffective in difficult cases with refractory or end-stage heart failure. Approval of cardiac resynchronization therapy (CRT) by United States-Food and Drug Association (US-FDA) in 2001 has initiated a new era of device therapy in heart failure in the new millennium. A timeline for effective heart failure therapies has been presented in Figure 1. With expanding application of CRT and implantable cardioverter defibrillator (ICD) in the past two decades and introduction of newer device therapies for monitoring and management of heart failure, device intervention is expected to carry a significant promise in heart failure management in the near future.

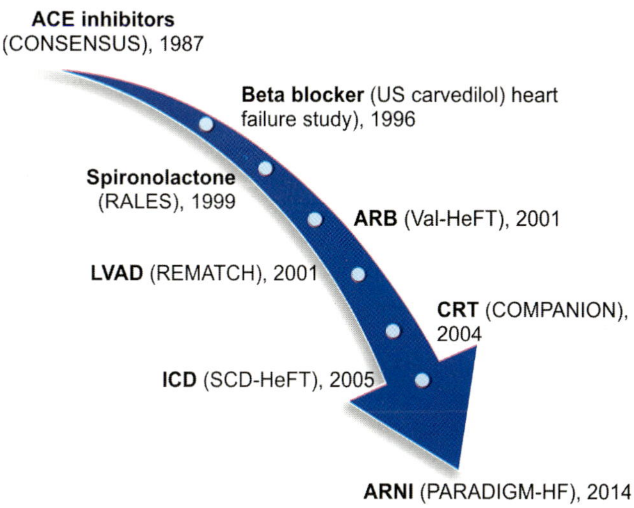

Fig. 1: Evolution of mortality reducing therapies in heart failure over the past three decades with the name of the breakthrough trial in the parenthesis along with the year published. In the twenty-first century, device therapies have come into play with only one single addition of a drug to the list in the form of ARNI. (ACE: angiotensin converting enzyme; ARB: angiotensin receptor blocker; LVAD: left ventricular assist device; CRT: cardiac resynchronization therapy; ICD: implantable cardioverter defibrillator; ARNI: angiotensin receptor neprilysin inhibitor).

DEVICE INTERVENTION IN HEART FAILURE

Cardiac Resynchronization Therapy

Ventricular dyssynchrony as a target of heart failure therapy: Abnormalities of electrical conduction including bundle branch blocks are commonly seen in heart failure states especially in association with reduced ejection fraction. Bundle branch blocks cause ventricular dyssynchrony which in turn leads to significant mechanical disadvantage to the failing heart. Ventricular dyssynchrony is usually defined as a QRS duration of more than 120 msec on the surface electrocardiogram (ECG) and has been showed to be consistently associated with increased mortality in heart failure across many studies. Conduction delays lead to dyssynchronous activation and contraction of ventricular walls leading to less forceful contraction and also impaired left ventricular (LV) filling due to paradoxical septal motion. Another important effect is worsening of mitral regurgitation which contributes to worsening of heart failure. Ventricular dyssynchrony can be addressed with pacing therapy with simultaneous pacing leads placed in right ventricle and the coronary sinus. This form of pacing therapy is known as CRT. After the promising initial experience in observational trials conducted in 1990s, randomized controlled trials were conducted and solidified the use of CRT.

Evidence for use of CRT: Initial CRT trials enrolled sick heart failure patients with New York Heart Association (NYHA) class III and IV symptoms and on drug therapy. Although small in sample size, Multisite Stimulation in Cardiomyopathy (MUSTIC) trials were the first randomized controlled trials for the use of CRT.[3] They included NYHA class III patients with left ventricular ejection fraction (LVEF) less than 35% and QRS duration more than 150 msec as a marker of ventricular dyssynchrony. MUSTIC trials demonstrated benefit in terms of improved quality of life and 6 minute walk distance in the CRT arm and paved the way for further trials. The Multicenter InSync Randomized Clinical Evaluation (MIRACLE) trial then demonstrated the same benefit with a larger sample size and inclusion of patients with QRS duration more than 130 msec in a double-blinded manner.[4] Cardiac Resynchronization in Heart Failure (CARE-HF) trial was the first of its kind to evaluate the morbidity and mortality benefit of CRT without an ICD in NYHA class III and IV symptoms.[5] 819 patients with LVEF less than 35% and evidence of dyssynchrony (QRS duration more than 150 msec or 120–150 msec with echocardiographic evidence of ventricular dyssynchrony) were randomized to either CRT or optimal medical therapy. CRT reduced the all-cause mortality and heart failure hospitalization by 46%. Comparison of Medical Therapy, Pacing, and Defibrillation in Heart Failure (COMPANION) trial further confirmed these findings and first time demonstrated the superior impact of CRT-D (combination of biventricular pacing and defibrillator) at reducing mortality in NYHA class III and IV heart failure patients.[6]

After solidifying role in NYHA class III and class IV patients, CRT was further tested in heart failure patients with milder symptoms (NYHA class I and class II symptoms). Multicenter Automatic Defibrillator Implantation Trial with Cardiac Resynchronization Therapy (MADIT-CRT) was the largest trial to test the hypothesis of prophylactic benefit of CRT in mild heart failure symptoms.[7,8] The trial enrolled 1,820 patient with LVEF less than 30% and QRS duration more than 130 msec with both ischemic and nonischemic causes. There was significant benefit in terms of 41% reduction in heart failure events in the combined CRT and ICD group as compared to ICD only group; and both ischemic and nonischemic subgroups maintained benefit on subgroup analysis. Another interesting finding from the trial was that CRT was uniformly more effective in patients with QRS duration more than 150 msec and in patients with left bundle branch morphology on ECG.[9]

Since CRT targets ventricular dyssynchrony, it has been postulated that it may benefit heart failure patients with significant dyssynchrony on echocardiogram even with a narrow QRS complex on ECG. However, Echocardiography Guided Cardiac Resynchronization Therapy trial failed to demonstrate such benefit even in heart failure patients with NYHA class III and class IV symptoms.[10] Thus, till date, significant ventricular dyssynchrony on ECG (QRS duration more than 130 msec) remains an essential criterion for CRT implantation irrespective of the echocardiographic evidence of dyssynchrony.

Cardiac resynchronization therapy—current indications and recommendations: According to the latest American guidelines CRT is indicated with a class I recommendation in heart failure patients with LVEF less than 35% who continue to be symptomatic despite optimal medical therapy and have a QRS duration of more than 150 msec with left bundle branch block (LBBB) morphology.[11] The patients with non-LBBB morphology with QRS duration more than 150 msec and those with LBBB and QRS duration 120–150 msec constitute class IIa recommendation for CRT. There is no role of CRT in patients with QRS duration less than 120 msec suggesting that evidence of electrocardiographic dyssynchrony is the key to success of CRT. The European guidelines are similar except the fact that LBBB morphology with QRS duration more than 130 msec in heart failure patients constitutes a class I indication.[12] There has been a transition of recommendation of CRT from sicker patients to healthier patients. It should be emphasized that patients with early stages of heart failure who are appropriate candidates for CRT benefit the most with the therapy. An ad-hoc analysis of MADIT-CRT trial suggested that patients with baseline LVEF of more than 30% benefited more with CRT in terms of reverse remodeling and cardiovascular outcomes as compared to the group with lesser ejection fraction. Thus CRT should be considered before the setting in of end-stage heart failure. According to the current guidelines, CRT upgradation is also recommended prophylactically in patients who require chronic right ventricular pacing and have an LVEF of less than 35% even before the setting in of heart failure.

Limitations of CRT: The success rate of CRT implantation procedure is more than 95% in contemporary clinical practice. But still, there are a number of patients (approximately 25%) who do not respond to CRT therapy. The nonresponder rate can be brought down with carefully selecting the patients. Also, optimal lead placement with device programming plays a role in improving the outcomes. Improvement may be lower in patients with significant ventricular scarring as found in ischemic heart disease. Thus, outcomes may be slightly better in patients with nonischemic dilated cardiomyopathy.

Implantable Cardioverter Defibrillator

Sudden cardiac death (SCD) in heart failure: Heart failure patients with severe ventricular dysfunction are at a significantly increased risk (upto six times) of SCD as compared to the general population. SCD remains a leading cause of death in heart failure patients, especially in stable patients with class I and II symptoms. The overall risk of SCD in patients with class I and II symptoms is lower than patients with class III or IV symptoms. However, the proportion of SCD contributing to the total mortality is higher in patients with better functional capacity.[13] Similarly, although the risk of SCD increases with worsening LVEF, the proportion of total mortality contributed by SCD is higher in patients with LVEF more than 30% as compared to those with LVEF less than 30%.[13] The most common cause of SCD is ventricular tachyarrhythmia and fibrillation which is preventable by ICD implantation. The current discussion provides the rationale for prophylactic use of ICD to prevent SCD and hence improve outcomes in heart failure. However, it remains important to strike the sweet spot between extremely sick and healthy patients to derive maximum benefit out of ICD implantation. Very sick class IV patients with poor expected survival will eventually die of pump failure even if SCD is prevented with an ICD. On the other hand, the absolute risk of SCD in class I patients with LVEF more than 35% is so low that it may not be cost-effective to implant ICD in all of these patients. The patients who have already survived a sudden cardiac arrest definitely are at a very high-risk of a repeat event and clearly deserve an ICD as proved in various secondary prevention trials [Antiarrhythmics Versus Implantable Defibrillators (AVID), Canadian Implantable Defibrillator Study (CIDS), and Cardiac Arrest Study Hamburg (CASH).[14] Another aspect deserving attention is the greater risk of arrhythmic events and SCD in patients with ischemic heart disease as compared to nonischemic LV dysfunction. Thus, in contrast to CRT therapy, ICD may be less effective in patients with nonischemic dilated cardiomyopathy.

Evidence for use of ICD: MADIT-II trial prospectively randomized postmyocardial infarction (post-MI) patients with LVEF less than 30% to ICD therapy vs. no ICD therapy after exclusion of class IV patients.[15] There was a significant 31% relative risk reduction for all-cause mortality over a 20-month follow-up. The benefit of ICD therapy emerged only after a follow-up of 9 months in this trial indicating importance of timing of device therapy in such patients. MADIT-II was the landmark trial cementing the role of ICD in patients with post-MI-LV dysfunction. However, doubts persisted regarding the use of ICD therapy in patients with nonischemic LV dysfunction. Defibrillators in Nonischemic Cardiomyopathy Treatment Evaluation (DEFINITE) trial (prophylactic defibrillator implantation in patients with non-ischemic dilated cardiomyopathy trial) enrolled patients with nonischemic LV dysfunction patients with high-risk of arrhythmia.[16] High-risk features included LVEF less than 35% and at least one documented episode of nonsustained ventricular tachycardia (NSVT) or 10 premature ventricular complexes per hour over a 24-hour holter ECG monitoring. Although the study reported an incredible 80% reduction in SCD and a trend toward improvement in all-cause mortality, the study was underpowered and did not show significant improvement in the primary outcome (all-cause mortality). Sudden Cardiac Death-Heart Failure trial forms the most robust evidence of the current guideline recommendations. This trial recruited patients with class II and III heart failure with LVEF less than 35% and randomized them into three arms—ICD arm, amiodarone arm, and placebo.[17] The trial included both nonischemic and ischemic LV dysfunction patients in equal numbers. The trial noted a significant 23% reduction in all-cause mortality in ICD arm with no benefit of amiodarone compared to the placebo. Also, on subgroup analysis both ischemic and nonischemic subsets demonstrated benefit with an ICD in a similar manner. However, in a recent trial [Danish Study to Assess the Efficacy of ICDs in Patients with Nonischemic Systolic Heart Failure on Mortality (DANISH) trial], all-cause mortality did not improve with ICD implantation in nonischemic LV dysfunction patients over a follow-up of 5.6 years, even when there was a significant improvement in the secondary end point of SCD.[18] This trial has stirred a controversy regarding the utility of ICD implantation in nonischemic dilated cardiomyopathy patients. Better stratification according to SCD risk is warranted in future to identify the subset of patients who will benefit the most and hence improve the yield of the therapy. At present, guidelines recommendations remain unchanged, as an updated meta-analysis after DANISH trial was still able to demonstrate mortality benefit with ICD implantation in nonischemic dilated cardiomyopathy patients.

Implantable cardioverter defibrillator—current recommendations: Both the American and European guidelines give a similar class I recommendation of ICD implantation in heart failure patients with LVEF less than 35% with class II or class III symptoms and an expected survival of more than 1 year.[11,12] Post-MI patients with LV dysfunction need to be at least 40 days post-MI before they become eligible for an ICD implantation. Patients who require prophylactic ICD implantation and have a QRS duration more than 150 msec or have a high requirement of right ventricular pacing should ideally undergo combination device (CRT-D) implantation.

Implantable Devices to Monitor Heart Failure

A greater part of heart failure morbidity is related to recurrent hospitalizations due to acute heart failure episodes. However, it is difficult to clinically predict episodes before they happen and often patients present only after going into overt heart failure. As our devices get smarter, we rely progressively lesser on our clinical skills. This domain of device use in heart failure allows to assess physiologic information before decompensation develops in chronic stabilized heart failure patients. Thus, picking an episode of decompensation early will allow to modify treatment and thus prevent an episode of decompensation which is a significant source of morbidity.

DEVICE-BASED HEART FAILURE DIAGNOSTICS

Heart rate variability is a marker of balance of autonomic activity in the body. Heart rate variability can be easily monitored with the current generation electronic implantable devices including CRT and ICD. In a study, a decrease in heart rate variability (which is a marker of increased sympathetic tone) was noted over the preceding weeks in patients admitted with acute heart failure decompensation episode.[19] Thus it may be used to predict earlier detection of acute decompensation of heart failure.

Thoracic impedance is another parameter which can be monitored by the current generation pacemaker devices and can give information regarding the fluid status of the lungs. The fluid status in turn predicts the volume loading of the left ventricle which may help predict acute decompensation before overt heart failure occurs. The clinical surrogate of fluid status in current practice is daily weight monitoring. Monitoring of thoracic impedance was found to be superior to daily weight monitoring for assessing fluid status and helped predict worsening of heart failure earlier in a contemporary study.[20]

The device-based monitoring systems may prove to be more effective when applied with addition of telemetry systems leading to day to day home-based monitoring. Combined use of these diagnostics was tested in Program to Access and Review Trending Information and Evaluate Correlation to Symptoms in Patients with Heart Failure (PARTNERS-HF) trial where, they were effective in prediction of an acute heart failure event within a month.[21] However another trial, Diagnostic Outcome Trial in Heart Failure demonstrated an unexpected increase in outpatient visits and hospitalizations in the group stratified to device monitoring strategy.[22] There remains a lacuna in terms of testing device monitoring in large randomized controlled trials before incorporating device monitoring into clinical practice.

IMPLANTABLE HEMODYNAMIC MONITORS

CardioMEMS heart sensor is an implantable device placed in the distal pulmonary artery allowing ambulatory monitoring of systolic, diastolic, and mean pulmonary artery pressures. Pulmonary pressure gives a direct assessment of LV filling pressure and helps predict heart failure. CardioMEMS device was shown to improve outcomes by reducing heart failure hospitalizations by as much as 37% in patients with class III heart failure in CHAMPION (CardioMEMS heart sensor allows monitoring of pressure to improve outcomes in NYHA class III heart failure patients) trial.[23] CardioMEMS remains the only implantable device which is US-FDA approved for use in heart failure monitoring. However, the device remains unpopular and is rarely used in the contemporary clinical practice.

NOVEL INNOVATIVE DEVICE THERAPIES FOR HEART FAILURE ON THE HORIZON

Cardiac contractility modulation (CCM): Its device sends nonexcitatory electrical signals to the myocardium during the absolute refractory period. This improves the calcium handling by the myocytes due to alteration in the ion channels. CCM targets the Achilles heel of the CRT devices which is the essential requirement of eletrocardiographic dyssynchrony. CCM may be effective in heart failure patients with narrow QRS and also in patients who have a higher LVEF. In a recent trial, CCM was found to be safe and efficacious with improvement in exercise tolerance and reduction in heart failure hospitalizations in patients with class III and IV heart failure patients with LVEF of 25–45% and QRS duration less than 130 msec.[24] Thus, CCM holds promise and may also show improvement in hard endpoints in larger randomized trials in near future.

Vagal nerve stimulation (VNS): Heart failure is chronic state of sympathetic activation. VNS device stimulates cervical preganglionic neurons in the vagus nerve. In preliminary trials, it has shown to decrease inflammation and fibrosis in the heart. It also prolongs the epicardial action potential and lowers the electrical dispersion thus leading to a decreased propensity to heart failure. However, in the Increase of Vagal Tone in Heart Failure (INNOVATE-HF) trial, VNS failed to improve mortality or heart failure events in class III chronic heart failure patients with LVEF less than 40%.[25]

Spinal cord stimulation and baroreceptor activation therapy: The stimulation of spinal cord at T1-4 level and carotid sinus baroreceptor stimulation have been proposed to beneficially modulate autonomic tone leading to improvement in heart failure outcomes. However, similarly to VNS, the initial experience with both these therapies has been largely disappointing.

Interatrial shunt device: This is one of the latest addition to the list of device therapies carrying significant promise. It is based on the rationale of creating a controlled interatrial shunt for relieving the elevated left atrial pressure in heart failure and thus providing symptomatic relief. This is one of the first device therapy which is applicable in the no man's land of heart failure with preserved ejection fraction. Recently, in Reduce Elevated Left Atrial Pressure in Patients With Heart Failure trial, which is a phase II trial presented at the 2018 European Society of Cardiology Congress, the device was found to be safe and effective at reducing the pulmonary capillary wedge pressures during exercise.[26] Long-term studies with clinical hard endpoints as outcomes are awaited for further scrutinizing the role of interatrial shunt device.

CONCLUSION

With a dismal prognosis of heart failure and slow paced advancement in effective pharmacological therapy, device therapy is slowly gaining more and more importance in the management of heart failure. CRT and ICD form the cornerstone of management of heart failure with reduced ejection fraction for improving outcomes. Thus, they have been rightly included in the current guidelines. However, the uptake of device therapy in the current clinical practice is dismal, especially in the Indian subcontinent due to the cost and availability issues. There remains a large untapped potential of device therapy for improving the outcomes in heart failure patients. Device-based monitoring is slowly creeping into the management system with CRT and ICD based systems being increasingly incorporated. But, the area still remains largely unexplored and requires significant work before application in to the routine clinical practice. A number of new device therapies are on the horizon. Cardiac contractility modulation and interatrial shunt device specifically hold promise and may change the landscape of management for heart failure patients.

REFERENCES

1. Bui AL, Horwich TB, Fonarow GC. Epidemiology and risk profile of heart failure. Nat Rev Cardiol. 2011;8:30-41.
2. Matiba M, Matsui S, Hirakawa T, et al. Long-term prognosis of patients with congestive heart failure. Jpn Circ J. 1990;54(1):57-61.
3. Cazeau S, Leclercq C, Lavergne T, et al. Effects of multisite biventricular pacing in patients with heart failure and intraventricular conduction delay. N Engl J Med. 2001;344:873-80.
4. Abraham WT, Fisher WG, Smith AL, et al. Cardiac resynchronization in chronic heart failure. N Engl J Med. 2002;346:1845-53.
5. Cleland JGF, Daubert JC, Erdmann E, et al. The effect of cardiac resynchronization on morbidity and mortality in heart failure. N Engl J Med. 2005;352:1539-49.
6. Bristow MR, Feldman AM, Saxon LA. Heart failure management using implantable devices for ventricular resynchronization: Comparison of Medical Therapy, Pacing, and Defibrillation in Chronic Heart Failure (COMPANION) trial. J Card Fail. 2000;6:276-85.
7. Moss AJ, Hall WJ, Cannom DS, et al. Cardiac resynchronization therapy for the prevention of heart failure events. N Engl J Med. 2009;361:1329-38.
8. Tang AS, Wells GA, Talajic M, et al. Cardiac-resynchronization therapy for mild-to-moderate heart failure. N Engl J Med. 2010;363:2385-95.
9. Zareba W, Klein H, Cygankiewicz I, et al. Effectiveness of cardiac resynchronization therapy by QRS morphology in the Multicenter Automatic Defibrillator Implantation Trial–Cardiac Resynchronization Therapy (MADIT-CRT). Circulation. 2011;123:1061-72.
10. Ruschitzka F, Abraham WT, Singh JP, et al. Cardiac-resynchronization therapy in heart failure with a narrow QRS complex. N Engl J Med. 2013;369:1395-405.
11. Yancy CW, Jessup M, Bozkurt, B, et al. ACCF/AHA Guideline for the Management of Heart Failure. J Am Coll Cardiol. 2013;62(16):e147-e239.

12. Ponikowski P, Voors AA, Anker SD, et al. ESC Guidelines for the diagnosis and treatment of acute and chronic heart failure: The task force for the diagnosis and treatment of acute and chronic heart failure of the European Society of Cardiology (ESC). Eur J Heart Fail. 2016;18(8):891-975.
13. Cleland JG, Chattopadhyay S, Khand A, et al. Prevalence and incidence of arrhythmias and sudden death in heart failure. Heart Fail Rev. 2002;7:229-42.
14. Myerburg RJ, Reddy V, Castellanos A. Indications for implantable cardioverter-defibrillators based on evidence and judgment. J Am Coll Cardiol. 2009;54:747-63.
15. Moss AJ, Zareba W, Hall J, et al. Prophylactic implantation of a defibrillator in patients with myocardial infarction and reduced ejection fraction. N Engl J Med. 2002;346:877-83.
16. Kadish A, Dyer A, Daubert JP, et al. Prophylactic defibrillator implantation in patients with nonischemic dilated cardiomyopathy. N Engl J Med. 2004;350:2151-7.
17. Bardy GH, Lee KL, Mark DB, et al. Amiodarone or an implantable cardioverter-defibrillator for congestive heart failure. N Engl J Med. 2005;352:225-37.
18. Køber L, Thune JJ, Nielsen JC, et al. Defibrillator implantation in patients with nonischemic systolic heart failure. N Engl J Med. 2016;375:1221-30.
19. Adamson P, Smith A, Abraham W, et al. Continuous autonomic assessment in patient with symptomatic heart failure. Circulation. 2004;2389-94.
20. Abraham WT, Compton S, Haas G, et al. Intrathoracic impedance vs daily weight monitoring for predicting worsening heart failure events: results of the Fluid Accumulation Status Trial (FAST). Congest Heart Fail. 2011;17:51-5.
21. Whellan DJ, Ousdigian KT, Al-Khatib SM, et al. Combined heart failure device diagnostics identify patients at higher risk of subsequent heart failure hospitalizations: results from PARTNERS-HF (Program to Access and Review Trending Information and Evaluate Correlation to Symptoms in Patients With Heart Failure) study. J Am Coll Cardiol. 2010;55:1803-10.
22. Van Veldhuisen DJ, Braunschweig F, Conraads V, et al. Intrathoracic impedance monitoring, audible patient alerts, and outcome in patients with heart failure. Circulation. 2011;124:1719-26.
23. Abraham WT, Stevenson LW, Bourge RC, et al. Sustained efficacy of pulmonary artery pressure to guide adjustment of chronic heart failure therapy: Complete follow-up results from the CHAMPION randomised trial. Lancet. 2016;387:453-61.
24. Abraham WT, Kuck KH, Goldsmith RL, et al. A Randomized Controlled Trial to Evaluate the Safety and Efficacy of Cardiac Contractility Modulation. JACC Heart Fail. 2018;6(10):874-83.
25. Gold MR, Van Veldhuisen DJ, Hauptman PJ, et al. Vagus Nerve Stimulation for the Treatment of Heart Failure: The INOVATE-HF Trial. J Am Coll Cardiol. 2016;68(2):149-58.
26. Feldman T, Mauri L, Kahwash R, et al. Transcatheter Interatrial Shunt Device for the Treatment of Heart Failure With Preserved Ejection Fraction (REDUCE LAP-HF I [Reduce Elevated Left Atrial Pressure in Patients With Heart Failure]). Circulation. 2017;137:364-75.

23

CHAPTER

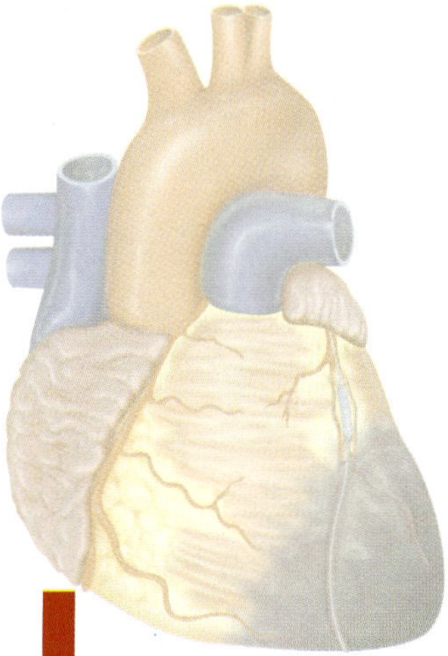

Radionuclide Imaging of Cardiac Autonomic Innervation: MIBG

Pawan K Sharma, HK Chopra, AK Bali

INTRODUCTION

The autonomic system of the heart is innervated with sympathetic and parasympathetic fibers. The sympathetic system works in conjunction with circulating catecholamine mediators, norepinephrine (NE) to regulate cardiac output at rest and during periods of increased cardiovascular demand. Various cardiac diseases can cause impairment of cardiac autonomic function which reflects the severity of the condition and the pathological impairment that can worsen patient outcome. Imaging with radionuclide tracers can assess the molecular process involved in the cardiac autonomic function. Sympathetic nerves follow the coronary arteries in the subepicardium before penetrating the myocardium. The principal chemical mediator of sympathetic function is NE.[1,2] Parasympathetic fibers in the heart are scarce in comparison to sympathetic fibers. Parasympathetic fibers innervate the atria, sinoatrial and atrioventricular nodes but are scarce in the ventricle (mostly the inferior wall). The major chemical mediator of parasympathetic function is acetylcholine. Most of the human clinical experience about autonomic radionuclide imaging is of the sympathetic system. The parasympathetic imaging studies are limited mostly to animal studies. Although, I-123 MIBG (metaiodobenzylguanidine) has been extensively used for cardiac autonomic imaging in Japan, for many years, the approved indication for I-123 MIBG in USA was for the detection, localization, staging, and follow up of neuroendocrine tumors, and their metastasis including pheochromocytoma and carcinoid tumors. In March 2013, the United States-Food and Drug Administration (US-FDA) approved I-123 MIBG for the assessment of myocardial sympathetic innervation in the evaluation of patients with New York Heart Association (NYHA) class II-III heart failure and left ventricular ejection fraction (LVEF) less than and equal to 35%.

PHYSIOLOGY OF I-123 METAIODOBENZYLGUANIDINE IMAGING

The cardiac sympathetic nerve function is assessed by studying the kinetics of the sympathetic neurotransmitter, NE, at the synaptic junction which is the junction of cardiac presynaptic sympathetic nerve and cardiac myocyte (Fig. 1).[3] Most radiotracers image presynaptic anatomy and function. NE is produced in the presynaptic sympathetic nerve terminal and is stored at high concentrations in presynaptic vesicles. In response to a stimulus, the NE containing vesicles are released into the synaptic space and bind to postsynaptic alpha- and beta-adrenergic receptors on the cardiac myocytes, resulting in various cardiac stimulatory effects. NE in the synaptic cleft can also attach to presynaptic adrenergic receptors. Presynaptic beta-2 receptors facilitate the release of NE from the storage granules into the synaptic cleft. Presynaptic alpha-2 receptors inhibit NE release from the storage granules.[4,5] Termination of the sympathetic response occurs when there is no free NE. The NE that is not bound by the presynaptic or postsynaptic receptors is actively taken back into presynaptic storage granules and this occurs through 2 systems known as:

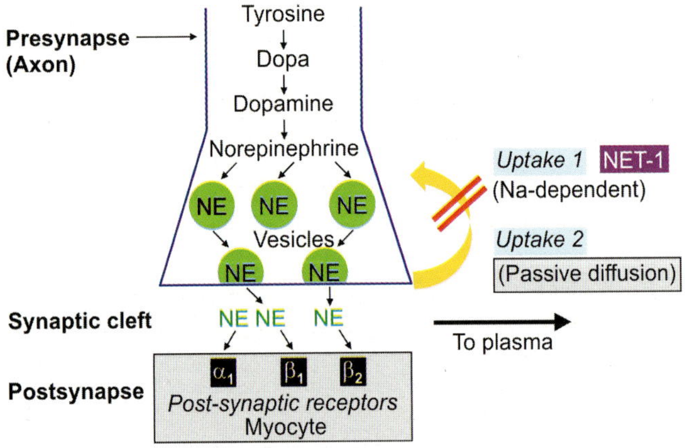

Fig. 1: Physiology of the myocardial sympathetic nerve terminal. (NE: norepinephrine; NET: norepinephrine transporter).
Adapted from: Travin MI. Cardiac autonomic imaging with SPECT tracers. J Nucl Cardiol. 2013;20:128-43.

- Norepinephrine uptake-1 transporter *(Uptake-1 or NET-1)*
- Norepinephrine uptake-2 transporter *(Uptake-2 or NET-2)*

The NET-1 is the main transporter protein-mediated system which is also sodium, energy, and temperature-dependent process, for storage and/or catabolic disposal. Some synaptic NE is also taken up by non-neuronal postsynaptic cells, probably by sodium-independent passive diffusion (i.e. the "NET-2" system).[6,7]

In early heart failure, circulating NE is mildly increased resulting in maintained (normal levels of) NE and I-123 MIBG uptake into the presynaptic nerves. As the circulating NE levels increase with worsening heart failure, the NET-1 transporter cannot keep up with the volume of NE in the synaptic cleft. This results in excessive stimulation of the postsynaptic receptors on the myocyte and gradual desensitization of those receptors.[8] Excess NE in the synaptic cleft activates presynaptic beta-receptors which facilitate the loss of NE from the storage granules, gradually depleting NE stores in the presynaptic nerve terminal. Concomitantly, I-123 MIBG must compete for uptake with the excess NE in the synaptic cleft for uptake by the NE transporter, reducing the amount of I-123 MIBG accumulation in the presynaptic nerve terminal. In addition, the rate of NE and I-123 MIBG washout from the presynaptic sympathetic nerve increases in response to presynaptic beta-receptor activation. As the heart failure becomes severe, presynaptic nerve terminals can be damaged and replaced by fibrosis, further reducing both the uptake and retention of I-123 MIBG. I-123 MIBG is the preferred radionuclide tracer used for cardiac neuronal imaging and is marketed as Adreview (GE Healthcare).[9] I-123 MIBG is an analog of guanethidine, a false neurotransmitter that is structurally similar to the sympathetic neurotransmitter NE. ^{123}I emits predominantly gamma photons with energies of 159 keV (83% abundance). A small fraction (<3%) of I-123 decays into high-energy photons (346, 440, 505, 529, 539 keV), which make imaging for I-123 MIBG difficult on a conventional Anger camera. Unlike NE, I-123 MIBG is not catabolized by monoamine oxidase (MAO) or catechol-o-methyltransferase, allowing it to localize in myocardial sympathetic nerve endings to a higher cytoplasmic concentrations than NE. It has a half-life of 13.2 hours. Therefore, it is well-tolerated and easily imaged with a SPECT camera.[10-12] The estimated effective radiation dose from I-123 MIBG imaging in adults is 0.507 mSv per mCi. The total body effective dose from 10 mCi of I-123 is approximately 5.07 mSv. The urinary bladder is the critical organ for I-123 MIBG. Hydration before and after dosing is encouraged. Patients should be encouraged to void frequently for 48 hours after dose administration to facilitate excretion of I-123 MIBG and thus, minimize the radiation dose to the bladder.[9] Since I-123 MIBG is largely excreted by the kidneys, patients with severe renal impairment may have increased radiation exposure and decreased quality of I-123 images (Box 1). I-123 accumulates in the thyroid, causing an increased long-term risk of thyroid neoplasia. In order to minimize this risk, it is recommended to administer a thyroid blocking agent, such as potassium iodide oral solution, Lugol's solution, or potassium perchlorate, at least 1 hour prior to I-123 MIBG dose.[9]

BOX 1: Properties of I-123 metaiodobenzylguanidine.

- Analog of guanidine
- Predominantly emits gamma photons energy 159 keV (83%)
- Less than 3% decays into gamma photon with high energy (346, 440, 505, 529, 539 keV)
- Half-life 13.2 hours
- Not catabolized by monoamine oxidase (MAO) or catechol-o-methyltransferase (COMT)
- Effective radiation dose emitted in adults is 0.507 mSv per mCi of I-123 MIBG
- Critical organ: Urinary bladder
- Excretion by kidneys.

I-123 IMAGING PROTOCOL

Medications interfering with catecholamine uptake, such as various antidepressants, antipsychotics and some calcium channel blockers should be held for 24 hours before tracer injection and imaging. Intravenous injection of I-123 MIBG is performed at rest. Tracer dosage has not been formally established. A dose of 3–5 mCi (111–185 MBq) over a 1-minute period is generally sufficient for planar image analysis. Since it may be difficult to obtain satisfactory single-photon emission computed tomography (SPECT) images in patients with severe cardiac dysfunction, a dose of 10 mCi (370 MBq) is used for protocols involving both planar and SPECT imaging. Based on the half-life of 13.2 hours, breastfeeding should be stopped for 48 hours after I-123 MIBG injection.[4]

Planar and SPECT images are obtained approximately 15 minutes after tracer administration (early) and again 3–5 hours later (delayed) using a standard single or multiple-head gamma camera. A low energy, high resolution collimator can be used. However, the high-energy photons (3%) resulting from the decay of I-123 can scatter or penetrate the lead collimator septa, producing degradation of image quality. Medium-energy collimators may be preferred for higher quality images, but usually they are limited in their availability. Only the delayed images can be used for most of the interpretation and analysis as it represents actual neuronal uptake. The tracer washout between early and delayed planar images may also provide important additional information.[13,14] Planar images are obtained in the anterior view for 10 minutes using an energy window of 159 keV $\pm$ 20%. SPECT images are obtained using the same energy window by way of a 180° circular acquisition from 45° right anterior oblique to 45° left posterior oblique, using a total of 60 stops (30 stops per head if done with a dual-headed camera at 30 seconds per stop).

INTERPRETATION OF I-123 MIBG IMAGES

Interpretation of I-123 MIBG images consists of:

- Assessment of global tracer uptake on planar images [heart mediastinal ratio (HMR)]
- Tracer washout between early and delayed planar images (washout)
- Regional uptake on tomographic images.

The standard measure of global I-123 MIBG uptake is the HMR, derived through assessment of per pixel activity in a region of interest over the heart in reference to a background area in the upper mediastinum. A normal value for HMR is 2.2 $\pm$ 0.3, with a ratio of less than 1.6 (two standard deviation below the mean) considered to be abnormal and correlate with increased patient risk.[15] The early HMR is obtained from initial 15 minute images. The late HMR is obtained on 4 hour delayed images. The late HMR is the most useful prognostic parameter.[16] In the anterior planar view, a region of interest (ROI) is drawn around the heart, including the cavity. A second ROI, 7 × 7 inch dimension is drawn in the upper mediastinum, positioned in the midline in the region of lowest activity (i.e. nonspecific background). Care must be taken to avoid the thyroid gland. Average counts per pixel in the heart are divided by average counts per pixel in the mediastinum to derive the HMR (Figs. 2 and 3).

$$\text{HMR} = \frac{\text{Average counts per pixel in the heart}}{\text{Average counts per pixel in the mediastinum}}$$

I-123 MIBG washout (compensated for radioactive decay) may reflect turnover of catecholamines attributable to the sympathetic drive, and measures the ability of myocardium to retain MIBG. A normal value is 10% $\pm$ 9%, with sicker patients having higher values.[14,17] Washout may correlate with increased sympathetic tone.

Washout rate (WR) is defined as:

$$\frac{(\text{H/M})\ \text{early} - (\text{H/M})\ \text{late}}{(\text{H/M})\ \text{early}} \times 100\ (\%)$$

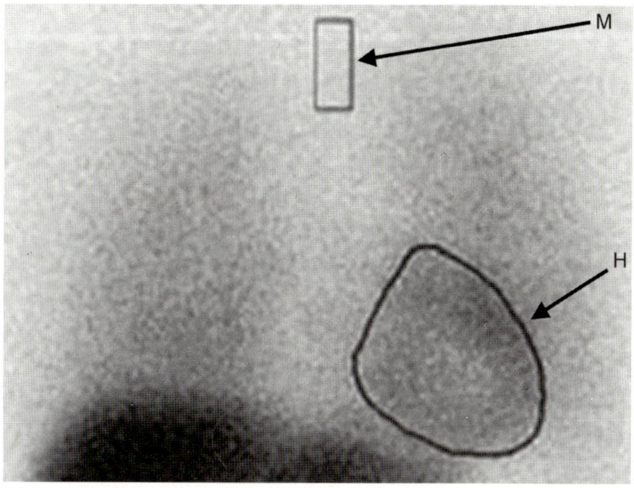

Fig. 2: Derivation of heart-to-mediastinum ratio (HMR).

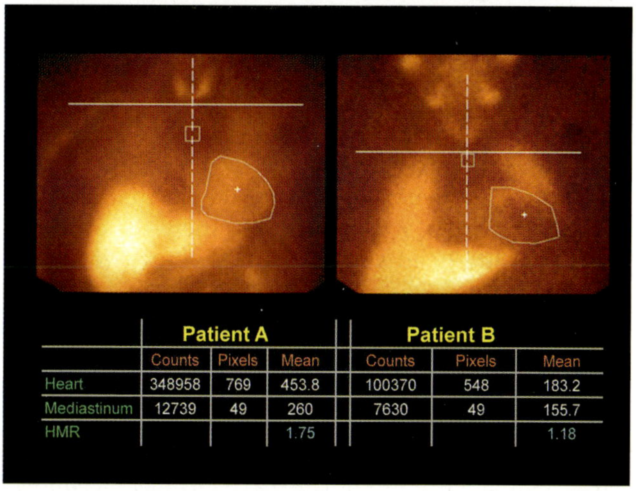

	Patient A			Patient B		
	Counts	Pixels	Mean	Counts	Pixels	Mean
Heart	348958	769	453.8	100370	548	183.2
Mediastinum	12739	49	260	7630	49	155.7
HMR			1.75			1.18

Fig. 3: Examples of normal and abnormal planar cardiac I-123 MIBG images. Normal (patient A) and abnormal (patient B) heart-to-mediastinum ratio (HMR).

Adapted from: Soman P, Travin MI, Gerson M, et al. I-123 MIBG Cardiac Imaging. J Nucl Cardiol. 2015;22:677-85.

I-123 MIBG SPECT imaging can provide measures of LVEF and chamber size, and information regarding the regional uptake of I-123 MIBG in the ventricular walls. A severely decreased MIBG uptake in a large regional area on delayed SPECT imaging predicted ventricular arrhythmias causing appropriated implantable cardioverter defibrillator (ICD) discharge as the primary endpoint. The MIBG SPECT may also help risk stratify the patients at risk for arrhythmic death and, thereby needing ICD appropriately. In this study, a different criteria of denervation as a MIBG defect size was used rather than previously reported HMR and/or WR.[18] Since MIBG uptake can be significantly decreased in many patients with severe HF, it is often difficult to reconstruct SPECT images. Therefore, a standardized criteria showing decreased MIBG uptake or MIBG defect may be required in the future.

I-123 MIBG NEURONAL IMAGING IN CONGESTIVE HEART FAILURE

In congestive heart failure (CHF), initially there is increased sympathetic response as a compensation for decreased cardiac output, but as CHF progresses this response leads to deleterious neurohormonal and myocardial structural changes that worsen the prognosis and increase the likelihood of arrhythmias and cardiac death. There is increased washout of I-123 MIBG as a result of competition for the uptake-1 process by increased circulating NE, and decreased HMR as CHF becomes more advanced with loss of sympathetic neurons and/or impaired uptake-1 function.[19]

Effect of Heart to Mediastinum Ratio

It has been shown that a decreased I-123 MIBG HMR predicts poor prognosis in patients with advanced CHF.[20-22] In patients with severe CHF and mean LVEF of 22%, the HMR less than 1.2 had a 12-month survival of 40% compared with 100% for patients with a higher ratio. Multivariate analysis showed that HMR was a better predictor of outcome than LVEF and heart size.[23] In progressively worsening of CHF, the prognosis worsens as the HMR gets lower.[24] The HMR predicts outcome for CHF of both ischemic and nonischemic origin.[16] In a retrospective study of 290 CHF patients over 2 years, the LVEF and HMR were the only significant predictors of major cardiac events such as cardiac death, need for transplant, and potentially fatal arrhythmias.[25] HMR was helpful in risk stratifying patients who had LVEF less than 35%. The event rate was less than 5% for those who had HMR more than and equal to 2.18, to more than 50% for those who had HMR less than and equal to 1.45. At the same time, patients with a higher LVEF of 35–49%, who had HMR less than and equal to 1.45 had an event rate of more than 10%.

The multicenter, international, AdreView Myocardial Imaging for Risk Evaluation in Heart Failure (ADMIRE-HF), AdreView = I-123 MIBG study looked at 961 patients with NYHA Class II-III CHF and LVEF less than and equal to 35% who underwent rest and delayed I-123 MIBG imaging.[15]

Primary goal was to study the effect of an HMR less than 1.6 on the 4-hour delayed planar image on the occurrence of progression of CHF, a potentially life-threatening arrhythmia, and/or cardiac death over a 2-year follow-up. In patients with HMR more than and equal to 1.6, there were only two cardiac deaths, indicating that in such patients with advanced CHF a normal HMR predicted a less than 1% yearly risk of cardiac death.[26] A multivariate analysis substudy showed that HMR was a predictor of both cardiac and all-cause death independent of other clinical and image variables, including age, LVEF, and brain natriuretic peptide (BNP).[27]

Effect of Washout Ratio

Similarly, increased I-123 MIBG washout may help in identifying patients with worse prognosis in patients with CHF. It has been noted that in CHF and LVEF less than 40%, over a 4-year period, patients with tracer washout more than and equal to 27% had a 35% cardiac death rate compared with 0 deaths in patients with normal washout.[14] The high washout is associated with greater than three-fold increase in hospital admissions for CHF and also predicts sudden cardiac death[28] (Fig. 4).

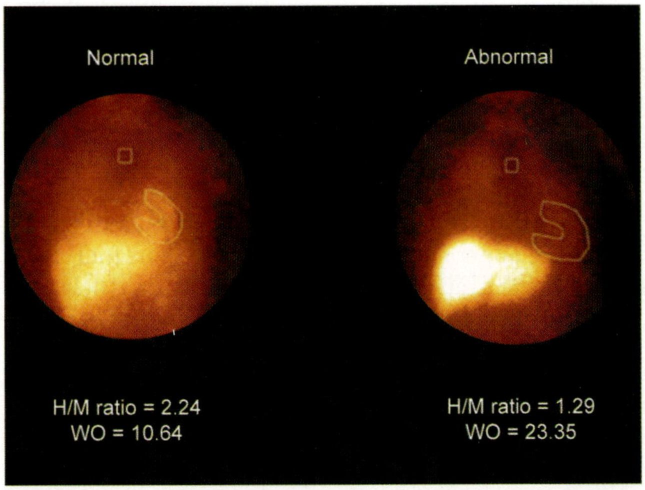

Fig. 4: Planar cardiac I-123 MIBG images showing normal HMR and normal washout ratio (normal) and low HR with high washout ratio (abnormal).

POTENTIAL ROLE OF I-123 MIBG IN GUIDING THERAPY FOR CONGESTIVE HEART FAILURE

I-123 MIBG images improve after institution of beta-blocker therapy associated with decreased ventricular volumes, improved LVEF and symptom relief.[29-31] Various other medications that do not directly influence cardiac sympathetic function, i.e. angiotensin-converting enzyme inhibitors (ACEI), angiotensin receptor blocking (ARB) agents, spironolactone and amiodarone also lead to improvements in I-123 MIBG image findings.[32-34] I-123 MIBG imaging may be useful as an indication of whether or not medical therapy is working satisfactorily, and could therefore help determine whether higher risk and more expensive device therapies or cardiac transplantation are needed.[35] It has also been shown that in severe cardiomyopathy, a worsening HMR after 6 months of optimal therapy had the highest independent predictive value for cardiac death.[36]

I-123 MIBG IMAGING AND VENTRICULAR ARRHYTHMIAS

I-123 MIBG imaging can help identifying patients who would benefit from an ICD. Studies have also shown that a reduced HMR (<1.54) is associated with increased likelihood of an ICD discharge, with a positive-predictive value of 71% and a negative-predictive value of 17%.[37] In ADMIRE-HF study, arrhythmic events were more common in patients with HMR less than 1.60 (10.4%) than those with HMR more than and equal to 1.6 (3.5%, P > 0.01).[26]

These studies show that cardiac neuronal hormonal imaging provides better predictive potential for SCD in CHF patients than the standard LVEF and NYHA class. It can potentially also identify patients with LVEF more than and equal to 35% who are in fact at high-risk of SCD and may need ICD.

I-123 MIBG IMAGING AND ISCHEMIC HEART DISEASE

The sympathetic nerves follow the course of coronary arteries before penetrating the myocardium. Therefore, myocardial ischemia or infarction can disrupt the sympathetic innervation and affect the myocardium distal to the site of injury. In addition, cardiac sympathetic nervous system is more sensitive to ischemia than myocytes, and takes longer to recover. As a result of early revascularization, the myocardium can be perfused and viable, but denervated myocardium which still has not recovered may show supersensitivity that predisposes to arrhythmias. The presence of post MI I-123 MIBG/201 Tl imaging mismatches correlated with electrophysiological abnormalities of prolonged QTc intervals and delayed depolarization on signal averaged ECG, both considered to predispose to lethal arrhythmias.[38] I-123 MIBG imaging showing persistent myocardial denervation can guide post-MI-ICD patient selection.

I-123 MIBG IMAGING AND DIABETES MELLITUS

Diabetes is a complex disease affecting various organs with increased morbidity and mortality if associated with autonomic dysfunction. Some patients with type II DM have no evidence of organic heart disease but I-123 MIBG imaging can help identify high-risk patients with autonomic dysfunction. A combination of decreased HMR on delayed I-123 MIBG image and an abnormality on heart rate variability (HRV) predicted cardiac events, whereas abnormal delayed HMR alone is an independent predictor of all-cause mortality.[39] Neuronal imaging may have a role in identifying patients with subclinical ischemic coronary disease who may benefit from more aggressive management. Neuronal imaging may also help identifying patients with autonomic dysfunction at higher risk for lethal arrhythmias who may benefit from early intervention.

I-123 MIBG IMAGING IN PATIENTS RECEIVING CHEMOTHERAPY

It has been shown that as the cumulative dose of doxorubicin increases, the LVEF decreases. This decrease in LVEF has been associated with decreased uptake of I-123 MIBG.[40] The role of I-123 MIBG imaging in patients with chemotherapy appears promising, but needs further investigation. It also needs to be shown if it is cost-effective and how it would add to currently used monitoring techniques.

CONCLUSION

Cardiac neuronal system plays an important role in the regulation of cardiac function. Patients with abnormal cardiac neuronal function are at increased risk of cardiac arrhythmias and sudden death. The autonomic imaging of the heart may help in identifying high-risk patients earlier in the course of the disease and, thereby, guide therapy. But, large randomized trials are needed to show that these imaging have significant benefit and cost-effectiveness over the existing monitoring modalities.

REFERENCES

1. Carrio I. Cardiac neurotransmission imaging. J Nucl Med. 2001;42:1062-76.
2. Zipes DP. Autonomic modulation of cardiac arrhythmias. In: Zipes DP, Jalife J (Eds). Cardiac Electrophysiology: From Cell to Bedside, 2nd edition. Philadelphia: W.B. Saunders Company; 1995. pp. 441-2.
3. Travin MI. Cardiac autonomic imaging with SPECT tracers. J Nucl Cardiol. 2013;20:128-43.
4. Flotats A, Carrio I. Cardiac neurotransmission SPECT imaging. J Nucl Cardiol. 2004;11:587-602.
5. Verrier RL, Antzelevich C. Autonomic aspects of arrhythmogenesis: The enduring and the new. Curr Opin Cardiol. 2004;19:2-11.
6. Bengel FM, Schwaiger M. Assessment of cardiac sympathetic neuronal function using PET imaging. J Nucl Cardiol. 2004;11:603-16.
7. Sisson JC, Wieland DM. Radiolabelled meta-iodobenzylguanidine pharmacology: Pharmacology and clinical studies. Am J Physiol Imaging. 1986;1:96-103.
8. Bohm M, La Rosee K, Schwinger RH, et al. Evidence for reduction of norepinephrine uptake sites in the failing human heart. J Am Coll Cardiol. 1995;25:146-53.
9. Healthcare G. AdreviewTMIobenguane I-123 Injection Prescribing Information. 2013.
10. Hattori N, Schwaiger M. Metaiodobenzylguanidine scintigraphy of the heart. What have we learned clinically? Eur J Nucl Med. 2000;27:1-6.
11. Kline RC, Swanson DP, Wieland DM, et al. Myocardial imaging in man with I-123 metaiodobenzylguanidine. J Nucl Med. 1981;22:129-32.
12. Wieland DM, Brown LE, Rogers WL, et al. Myocardial imaging with a radioiodinated norepinephrine storage analog. J Nucl Med. 1981;22:22-31.
13. Somsen GA, Verberne HJ, Fleury E, et al. Normal values and within-subject variability of cardiac I-123 MIBG scintigraphy in healthy individuals: Implications for clinical studies. J Nucl Cardiol. 2004;11:126-33.
14. Ogita H, Shimonagata T, Fukunami M, et al. Prognostic significance of cardiac (123)I metaiodobenzylguanidine imaging for mortality and morbidity in patients with chronic heart failure: A prospective study. Heart. 2001;86:656-60.
15. Jacobson AF, Lombard J, Banerjee G, et al. 123I-mIBG scintigraphy to predict risk for adverse cardiac outcomes in heart failure patients: Design of two prospective multicenter international trials ADMIRE-HF study. J Nucl Cardiol. 2009;16:113-21.
16. Wakabayashi T, Nakata T, Hashimoto A, et al. Assessment of underlying etiology and cardiac sympathetic innervation to identify patients at high risk of cardiac death. J Nucl Med. 2001;42:1757-67.
17. Morozumi T, Kusuoka H, Fukuchi K, et al. Myocardial iodine-123-metaiodobenzylguanidine images and autonomic nerve activity in normal subjects. J Nucl Med. 1997;38:49-52.
18. Boogers MJ, Borleffs JW, Henneman MM, et al. Cardiac sympathetic denervation assessed with 123-iodine metaiodobenzylguanidine imaging predicts ventricular arrhythmias in implantable cardioverter-defibrillator patients. J Am Coll Cardiol. 2010;55:2769-77.
19. Chen GP, Tabibiazar R, Branch KR, et al. Cardiac receptor physiology and imaging: An update. J Nucl Cardiol. 2005;12:714-30.
20. Merlet P, Benvenuti C, Moyse D, et al. Prognostic value of MIBG imaging in idiopathic dilated cardiomyopathy. J Nucl Med. 1999;40:917-23.
21. Anastasiou-Nana MI, Terrovitis JV, Athanasoulis T, et al. Prognostic value of iodine-123 metaiodobenzylguanidine myocardial uptake and heart rate variability in chronic congestive heart failure secondary to ischemic or idiopathic dilated cardiomyopathy. Am J Cardiol. 2005;96:427-31.
22. Arimoto T, Takeishi Y, Niizeki T, et al. Cardiac sympathetic denervation and ongoing myocardial damage for prognosis in early stages of heart failure. J Cardiac Fail. 2007;13:34-41.
23. Merlet P, Valette H, Dubois-Rande J, et al. Prognostic value of cardiac metaiodobenzylguanidine in patients with heart failure. J Nucl Med. 1992;33:471-7.
24. Nakata T, Miyamoto K, Doi A, et al. Cardiac death prediction and impaired cardiac sympathetic innervation assessed by MIBG in patients with failing and non failing hearts. J NuclCardiol. 1998;5:579-90.
25. Agostini D, Verberne HJ, Burchert W, et al. I-123-mIBG myocardial imaging for assessment of risk for a major cardiac event in heart failure patients: Insights from a retrospective European multicenter study. Eur J Nucl Med Mol Imaging. 2008;35:535-46.
26. Jacobson AF, Senior R, Cerqueira MD, et al. Myocardial iodine-123 meta-iodobenzylguanidine imaging and cardiac events in heart failure: Result of the prospective ADMIRE-HF (AdreView Myocardial Imaging for Risk Evaluation In Heart Failure) study. J Am Coll Cardiol. 2010;55(20):2212-21.
27. Travin M, Anathassubramaniam K, Henzlova MJ, et al. Imaging of myocardial sympathetic innervation for prediction of cardiac and all-cause mortality in heart failure: Analysis from the ADMIRE-HF trial. Circulation. 2009;120:S350.
28. Kioka H, Yamada T, Mine T, et al. Prediction of sudden death in patients with mild-to-moderate chronic heart failure by using cardiac iodine-123 metaiodobenzylguanidine imaging. Heart. 2007;93:1213-8.
29. Lotze U, Kaepplinger S, Kober A, et al. Recovery of the cardiac adrenergic nervous system after long-term beta-blocker therapy in idiopathic dilated cardiomyopathy: Assessment by increase in myocardial 123I-metaiodobenzylguanidine uptake. J Nucl Med. 2001;42:49-54.
30. Gerson MC, Craft LL, McGuire N, et al. Carvedilol improves left ventricular function in heart failure patients with idiopathic dilated cardiomyopathy and a wide range of sympathetic nervous system function as measured by iodine 123 metaiodobenzylguanidine. J Nucl Cardiol. 2002;9:608-15.
31. Merlet P, Pouillart F, Dubois-Rande J, et al. Sympathetic nerve alterations assessed with 123I-MIBG in the failing human heart. J Nucl Med. 1999;40:224-31.

32. Takeishi Y, Atsumi H, Fujiwara S, et al. ACE inhibition reduces cardiac iodine-123-MIBG release in heart failure. J Nucl Med. 1997;38:1085-9.
33. Kasama S, Toyama T, Kumakura H, et al. Spironolactone improves cardiac sympathetic nerve activity and symptoms in patients with congestive heart failure. J Nucl Med. 2002;43:1279-85.
34. Toyama T, Hoshizaki H, Seki R, et al. Efficacy of amiodarone treatment on cardiac symptom, function, and sympathetic nerve activity in patients with dilated cardiomyopathy: Comparison with beta-blocker therapy. J Nucl Cardiol. 2004;11:134-41.
35. Merlet P, Benvenuti C, Moyse D, et al. Prognostic value of MIBG imaging in idiopathic dilated cardiomyopathy. J Nucl Med. 1999;40:917-23.
36. Matsui T, Tsutamoto T, Maeda K, et al. Prognostic value of repeated 123I-metaiodobenzylguanidine imaging in patients with dilated cardiomyopathy with congestive heart failure before and after optimized treatments-comparison with neurohormonal factors. Circ J. 2002;66:537-43.
37. Arora R, Ferrick KJ, Nakata T, et al. 1-123 MIBG imaging and heart rate variability analysis to predict the need for an implantable cardioverter defibrillator. J Nucl Cardiol. 2003;10:121-31.
38. Simoes MV, Barthel P, Matsunari I, et al. Presence of sympathetically denervated but viable myocardium and its electrophysiologic correlates after early revascularised, acute myocardial infarction. Eur Heart J. 2004;25:551-7.
39. Nagamachi S, Fujita S, Nishii R, et al. Prognostic value of cardiac I-123 metaiodobenzylguanidine imaging in patients with non-insulin-dependent diabetes mellitus. J Nucl Cardiol. 2006;13:34-42.
40. Valdés Olmos RA, ten Bokkel Huinink WW, ten Hoeve RF, et al. Assessment of anthracycline-related myocardial adrenergic derangement by [123I] metaiodobenzylguanidine scintigraphy. Eur J Cancer. 1995;31A:26-31.

24

CHAPTER

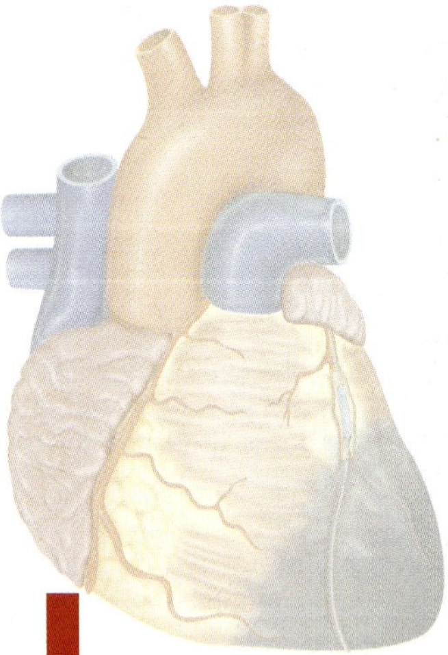

Cardiac Radionuclide Imaging to Assess Patients with Heart Failure

GN Mahapatra

INTRODUCTION

Heart failure (HF) is a major worldwide health problem and represents a common disease affecting approximately 5 million patients in the United States. The incidence of HF is increasing day by day, and it remains the only area in cardiovascular disease where in hospitalization rates and associated mortalities have worsened in the past 25 years. Several conditions play an important role in the development and progression of HF including abnormalities in myocardial blood flow and sympathetic innervation. The focus is on three aspects: (1) the value of nuclear imaging to distinguish ischemic from nonischemic etiologies, (2) risk stratification of patients with HF with the evaluation of candidates for specific treatment strategies, and (3) the role of cardiac neuronal imaging in patients with HF. Distinguishing ischemic from nonischemic cardiomyopathy (NICM) is important because patients with ischemic cardiomyopathy can potentially have dramatic improvement with revascularization. Nuclear imaging represents the only imaging modality with sufficient sensitivity to assess myocardial blood flow and sympathetic innervation of the failing heart. Although nuclear imaging with single-photon emission computed tomography (CT) (SPECT) is most commonly used for the evaluation of myocardial perfusion, positron emission tomography (PET) detects the gold standard technique in the assessment of myocardial viability as well as allows absolute quantification of myocardial blood flow beyond the assessment of relative myocardial perfusion. Both techniques can be used for the evaluation of diagnosis, treatment options, and prognosis in HF patients. In addition to myocardial blood flow, cardiac sympathetic innervation represents an another important parameter in patients with HF. Cardiac neuronal imaging of metaiodobenzylguanidine (MIBG) iodine (I)-131 or I-123 is particularly helpful in risk stratification of patients with HF. This nuclear imaging modality can be used to monitor the response to therapy as dysfunctional MIBG uptake may show improvement with pharmacological treatment. A large number of studies have shown that an abnormal myocardial sympathetic innervation as assessed with I-123 MIBG imaging is associated with increased mortality and morbidity rates in patients with HF. Moreover, cardiac I-123 MIBG imaging can be used to risk stratify patients for ventricular arrhythmias or sudden cardiac death. Furthermore, novel nuclear imaging techniques are developed that may provide more detailed information for the detection of HF in an early phase as well as for monitoring the effects of new therapeutic interventions in patients with HF (Figs. 1 and 2).

POTENTIALITIES OF NUCLEAR IMAGING PROCEDURES IN HEART FAILURE

Myocardial perfusion imaging (MPI) represents the mainstay of cardiovascular radionuclide applications for the diagnostic and prognostic workup of patients with coronary artery disease (CAD) and HF. In addition, sympathetic innervation imaging is increasingly used in patients with HF predominantly for risk stratification.

Several technical advances have been introduced that contribute to the current trend toward molecular targeted

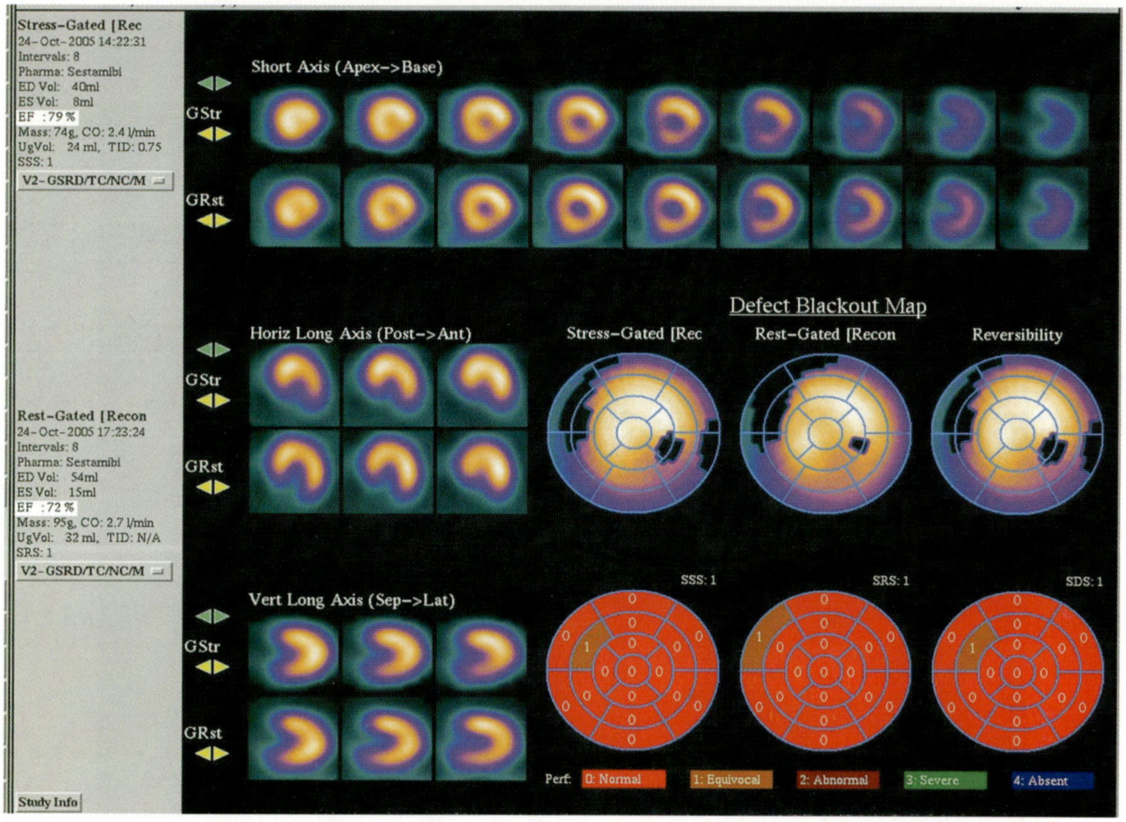

Fig. 1: Normal stress gated SPECT. MPI scan showing uniform stress perfusion pattern involving all the defined myocardial segments. (MPI: myocardial perfusion imaging; SPECT: single photon emission computed tomography).

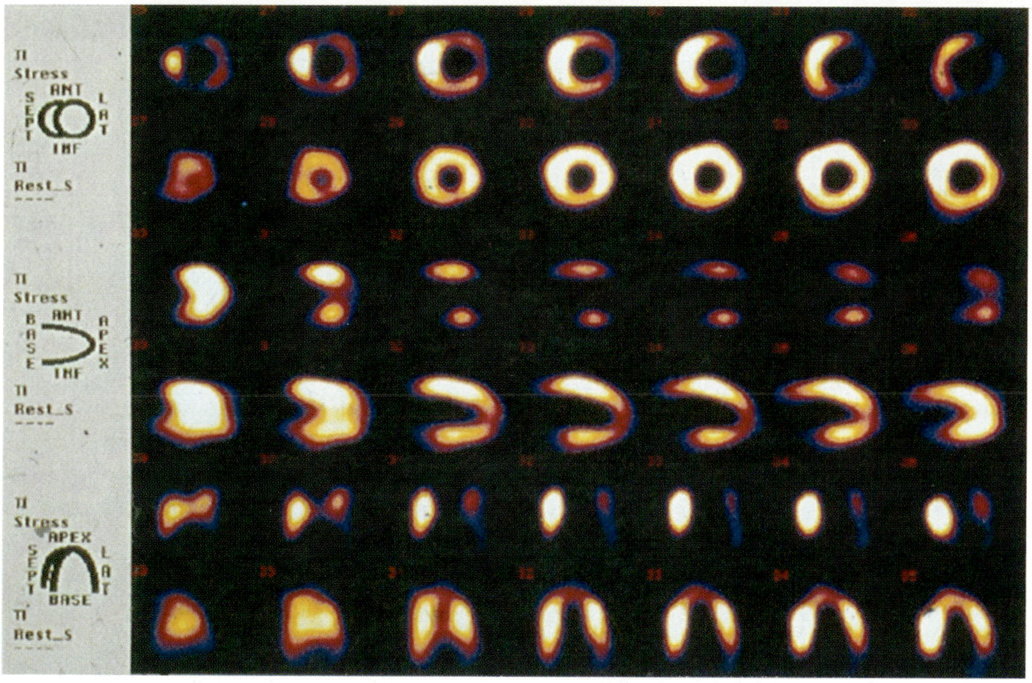

Fig. 2: Stress thallium myocardial perfusion scan showing a large area of stress perfusion defect involving anterolateral myocardial segments which shows fair amount of reperfusion in resting image suggestive of anterolateral myocardial ischemia.

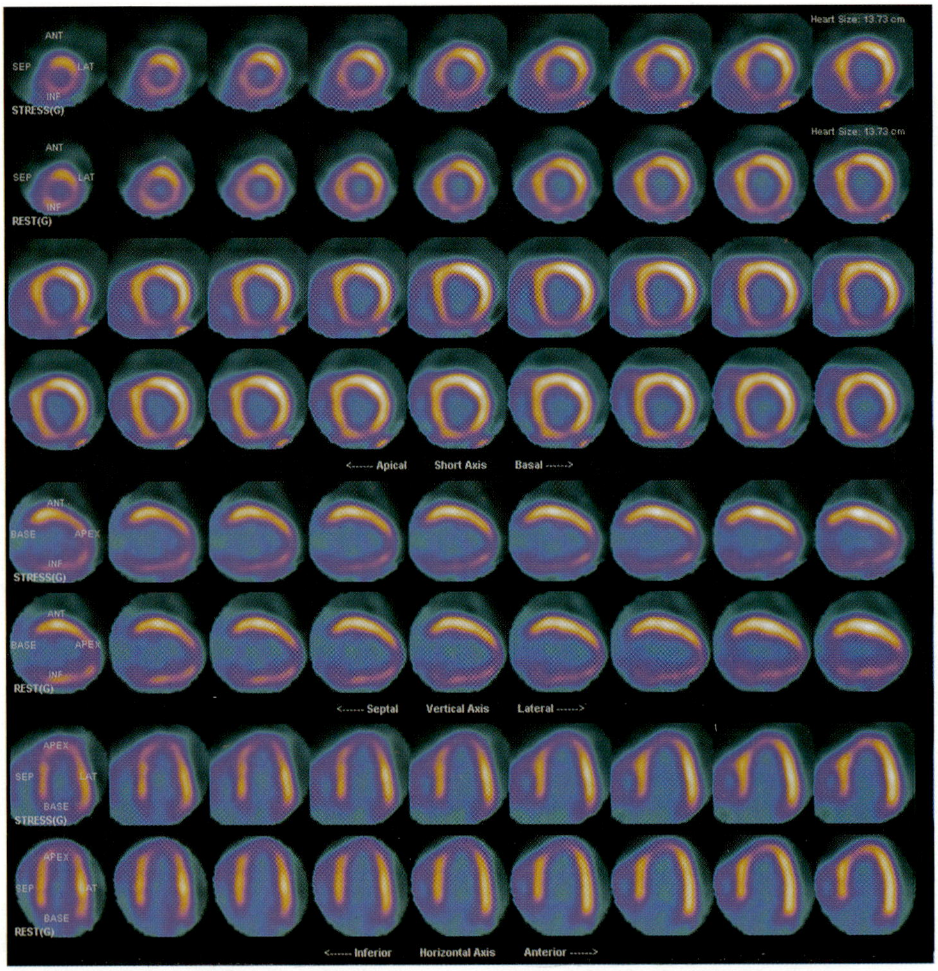

Fig. 3: Rest-dipyridamole stress Rb-82 myocardial perfusion scintigraphy showing dilated left ventricle with uniform stress perfusion pattern showing strong diagnostic information of nonischemic cardiomyopathy with heart failure. (Rb: rubidium).

imaging in clinical cardiology. The availability of high-end scanner systems with improved detection of sensitivity and image resolution allow the detection of weak signal coming from tissue-specific molecular targeted tracers. The availability of PET system has substantially increased in the recent years due to its success in oncology. Moreover, an increasing number of molecular targeted radiotracers is now being introduced which may extend the current possibilities for molecular imaging of biologic processes. Finally, it is important to note that molecular targeted imaging is of growing interests as nuclear systems are increasingly integrated with CT systems into SPECT-CT or PET-CT hybrid imaging devices, which facilitate localization of a molecular signal by fusion with high-resolution morphologic image. Potentially, these dedicated nuclear imaging techniques having their superior detection sensitivity can play an important role in an evaluation of patients with HF by providing valuable information on several biological processes of the failing heart, including myocardial blood flow and sympathetic innervation of the myocardium (Fig. 3).

Use of Radionuclide Imaging to Differentiate Ischemic from Nonischemic Heart Failure

Standard stress or pharmacological stress gated SPECT MPI or resting SPECT with F-18 fludeoxyglucose (FDG) PET study is based on its excellent diagnostic capabilities for the detection of CAD, and ischemia is being used for initial evaluation to determine HF etiology. Present data suggests excellent negative-predictive value with normal imaging findings indicating the likely absence of CAD. There are some frequent false-positive MPI study results in NICM, including thinned walls that appear to have less tracer uptake owing to partial volume effect, soft tissue attenuation from blood pool in large hearts, scar, or fibrosis that may occur in the settings of NICM particularly of hypertrophic cardiomyopathy (HCM) and extensive small vessel or microvascular CAD not appreciated in coronary angiogram. In general, defects in ischemic cardiomyopathies are more extensive and severe than in NICM. A prevailing view among practicing cardiac physicians is that radionuclide MPI can usually exclude CAD in patients with HF, but that perfusion defects often do not indicate CAD, and at the same time, with a normal scan with frequent concerns for the potential occurrence of "balanced ischemia;" in which, ischemia of equivalent severity and all coronary territories lead to the absence of relative perfusion defect. Ancillary markers, such as transient ischemia dilatation of LV cavity, can potentially identify the situation of balanced ischemia in higher risk patients. Alternatively, quantitative blood flow technics, such as coronary flow reserve (CFR) using cardial PET with rubidium-82 or nitrogen-13 ammonia. Abnormal CFR measurements can also potentially identify patients without known heart disease but who are at risk for developing clinical HF. Although CFR abnormalities may identify early nonclinical CAD that may progress to obstructive disease, many patients with nonischemic HF on cardiomyopathy have CFR abnormalities due to disease in the microvasculature. Such disease although nonamenable to revascularization predicts worsened outflow.

Use of Radionuclide Imaging to Evaluate Benefit from Revascularization

Once CAD is established as the probable cause of HF, radionuclide imaging is the choice of noninvasive techniques used to predict whether a patient is likely to benefit from revascularization procedure. The use of radionuclide imaging to access viability began with delayed thallium-201 (Tl-201) or reinjection Tl-201 or augmented intravenous nitroglycerin drip on patients with severe coronary stenosis showing redistribution defects even without stress imaging being performed. Over the years, there have been numerous investigations of the best radionuclide techniques for assessing viability-combined TC-99m sestamibi/tetrofosmin, and F-18 FDG study in a single-day or two-day protocol has been the mainstay of day-to-day nuclear cardiology practice (Figs. 4 and 5).

Radionuclide Imaging in Patients not Amenable to Revascularization

Many patients with HF cannot benefit from revascularization, particularly those with CAD having past history of old myocardium infarction with less than 15% of viable myocardium estimated by our various nuclear imaging procedures. Patients having non-CAD particularly of NICM, radionuclide imaging though differentiates nonischemic from ischemic variety, still nonischemic patients cannot be benefitted following revascularization (Fig. 6).

Radionuclide Imaging of Cardiac Autonomic Innervation

The heart is an organ with a dense distribution of sympathetic nerve. The sympathetic nervous system plays important role in controlling the heart rate, blood pressure, capacity to cause myocardial contraction/dilatation and

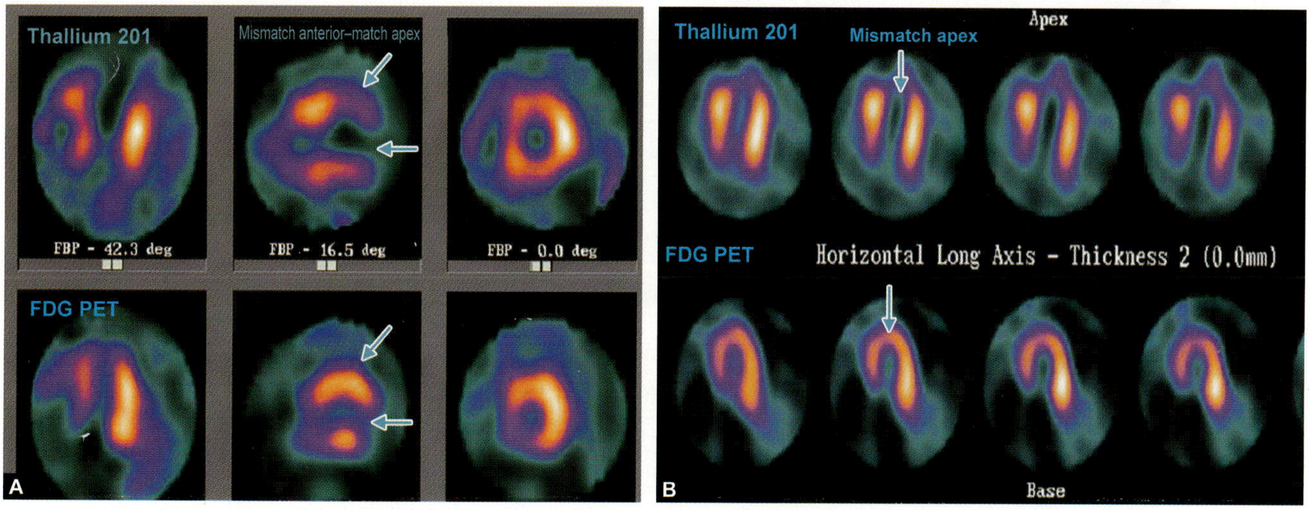

Figs. 4A and B: (A) Dual isotope myocardial imaging shows a resting defect involving part of anterior and apical myocardial segments which shows adequate metabolism involving anterior segments only. However, apical segment seems to have no metabolism suggesting scarred myocardium as evidenced from F-18 FDG metabolism study. (B) Resting myocardial perfusion imaging with thallium-201 perfusion showing an apical defect which shows an adequate metabolism with F-18 FDG metabolism.

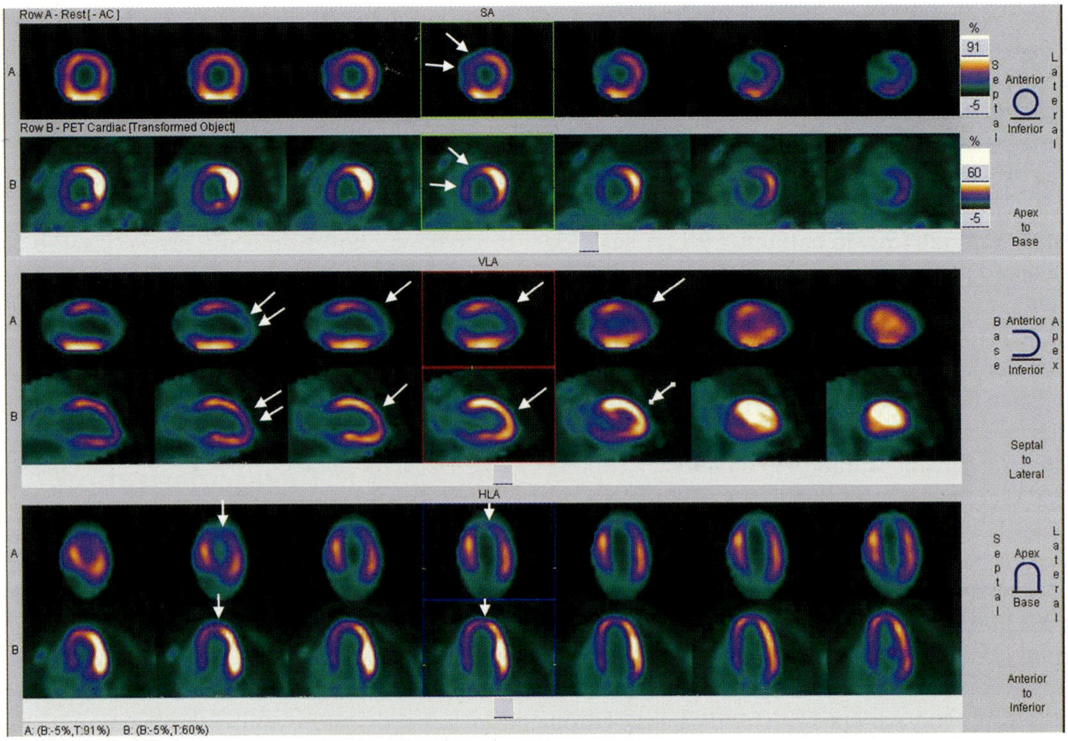

Fig. 5: Resting myocardial perfusion image shows multiple perfusion defects seen in anterior, septal, and apical myocardial segments (first row of images), which shows significant evidence of hibernating myocardium involving anterior and apical myocardial segments in the form of mismatch defects without any evidence of hibernating myocardium in septal segment in the form of match defect (scarred myocardium).

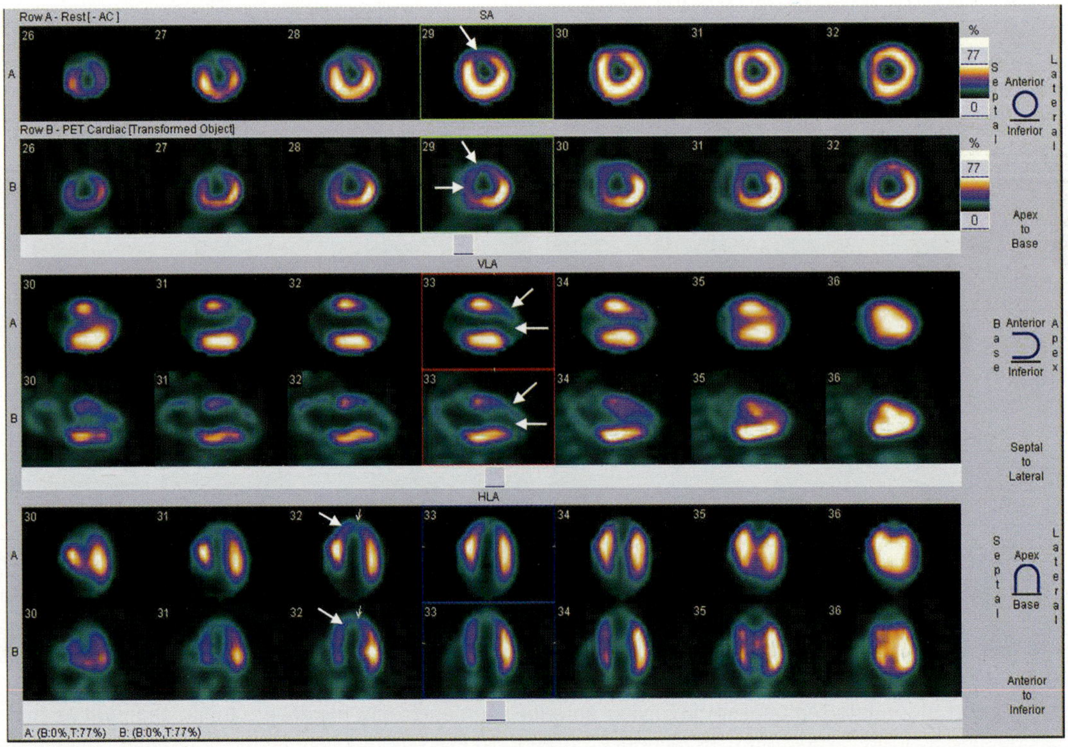

Fig. 6: Resting myocardial perfusion image shows multiple perfusion defects in anteroseptal and apical myocardial segments (first row of images) without any evidence of hibernating myocardium in the form of match defects on FDG images (second row).

coronary tone. Hyperactivity of cardiac sympathetic nerves is known to cause exacerbation of myocardial ischemia, exacerbation of HF, and induction of severe arrhythmia, and sympathetic functional disorder has important clinical significance in heart diseases. I-123 MIBG myocardial scintigraphy is one of the few methods available for objective evaluation of cardiac sympathetic function at the clinical level and provides an abundance of information useful for the evaluation of various heart diseases.

Imaging Methods of Metaiodobenzylguanidine

Metaiodobenzylguanidine an analog of norepinephrine was developed as sympathetic nerve imaging agent. Before conducting the examination, it is necessary to know whether the patient has taken drug that have an influence on accumulation of MIBG. Regarding reserpine and tricyclic antidepressant agents, it is necessary to establish drug withdrawal for an appropriate period taking into account their blood half-life. As I-123 has a short half-life of 13 hour and is a nuclide that emits only gamma rays, it does not necessarily require the blockage of thyroid accumulation. MIBG 111 MBq is intravenously administered at rest, and the early and delayed images are obtained 15–30 minutes later and from 3 hours to 4 hour later, respectively. It is desirable to prepare a gamma camera with sufficient visual field to cover most of the chest, and more than two detectors. In addition, it is necessary to use a collimator for low energy or I-123 only and to set the energy window to 159 keV ± 10%. Planar images have been used in many ways for the evaluation of cardiac sympathetic function, while SPECT images are advantageous for evaluating abnormalities in local distribution in myocardium. Practically, both of the above images are used in combination. In the case of planar images, the anterior view is imaged for roughly 3–5 minutes, using a 128 × 128 or 256 × 256 matrix. If possible, further views in two directions are obtained at a left anterior oblique angle of 35–40° and at a 70° to the left lateral plane. The SPECT images are collected using a 64 × 64 matrix over a 360° range or over 180° from the right anterior oblique plane to left posterior oblique plane.

Analysis and Interpretation of Metaiodobenzylguanidine Images

The most common indices are the heart-to-mediastinum ratio (H/M ratio) and the washout rate obtained from the anterior planar images. These indices represent simple semiquantitative measures, but have been widely used resulting in many reports which support its usefulness in severity and prognosis evaluation for HF. Regions of interest (ROIs) are set in the heart (H) and the mediastinum (M) to obtain the mean count in each ROI after which the H/M ratio is calculated. Based on the resulting ratio the degree of accumulation in the heart is evaluated. It is desirable to set the mediastinal ROI as much as possible at an upper site that is unaffected by the thyroid gland and the cardiac ROI so as to surround the entire heart. The washout rate is an index that indicates the rate at which MIBG is washed out between the early image and the delayed image via comparison with the cardiac count in the early image. In this calculation, the mediastinal count is subtracted from the cardiac count as a background correction, in principle. A correction for decay due to the half-life of I-123 may be performed, as required. The accumulation on the early MIBG image reflects the distribution of cardiac sympathetic nerves and the uptake function at the nerve endings, while the washout rate is an index of the degree of sympatheticotonia. The delayed image is a result of washout from the early image and thus is considered to contain combined information regarding both the accumulation on the early image and the washout rate.

$$\text{Washout rate}(\%) = \frac{\text{Early imgae (H-M)} - \text{Delayed image (H-M)}}{\text{Early image (H-M)}} \times 100$$

Regarding the SPECT images, a method is available for visually scoring the degree of accumulation by division into segments, which is similar to that used in MPI. The rate of uptake of MIBG in the myocardium is as low as 1–2%, and the image quality is inferior compared with Tl-201 images. In some cases, substantial accumulation of MIBG may occur in the liver, which overlaps the myocardial inferoposterior wall and scattering from the lung field to the lateral wall then exerts a considerable influence on the image, requiring careful interpretation (Fig. 7).

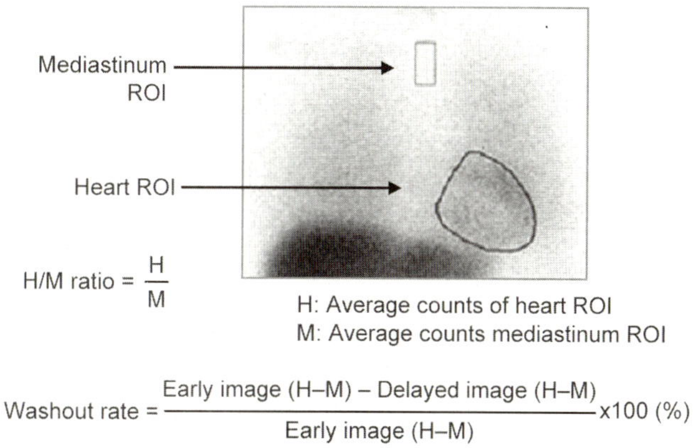

Fig. 7: MIBG parameters.

CLINICAL APPLICATION

Metaiodobenzylguanidine in Ischemic Heart Diseases

Sympathetic nerve ending is easily damaged by ischemia in comparison to myocardial cells, and sympathetic function disorders are known to persist for a certain period even after the alleviation of ischemia. As a result, the potential exists for the use of MIBG to detect ischemia with extreme sensitivity providing images that memorize transient ischemia. Myocardial perfusion imaging (MPI) as a nuclear cardiological examination has been used in many ways for ischemic heart diseases, and sufficient evidence regarding the usefulness of this method had been established. However, in some cases, pathological conditions are difficult to evaluate precisely via perfusion imaging alone, and MIBG may then be effective. In this group of patient, MIBG shows a decreased or reduced accumulation in the involved myocardium on the delayed image, and increased washout is usually observed in the involved regions of myocardium, and the abnormal findings become more marked.

Vasospastic Angina

In vasospastic angina the practice of MPI during nonseizure results in normal accumulation and ordinary exercise loading rarely induces coronary spasms. Accordingly, the ability of MPI to diagnose this disease is not clinically satisfactory. According to a report by Taki et al.,[41] a small proportion of case of vasospastic angina shows abnormal early MIBG images, while a high percentage shows increased washout in the region of the culprit coronary artery on delayed images indicating a clearly abnormal accumulation. In other words, delayed images are highly useful for diagnosis. Taki et al. found the positive and negative accuracy rate to be favorable at 83% and 81%, respectively. Sakata et al.[42] reported MIBG to be more useful than stress myocardial perfusion SPECT in the prediction of cardiac events in patients with vasospastic angina having no dominant coronary stenosis.

Unstable Angina

A loading test is not indicated for unstable angina, although MPI at rest is unable to diagnose this disease in many cases. MIBG makes it possible to identify culprit coronary artery with a high probability via findings at rest, and it is of diagnostic value. In a study by Tsutsui et al.,[43] MIBG was demonstrated to have the ability to diagnose the culprit coronary artery in this disease with the sensitivity of 71% and a specificity 78%.

Evaluation of Risk Areas in Acute Coronary Syndrome

Recently percutaneous coronary intervention (PCI) has been generally conducted for acute coronary syndrome in emergency situations. ^{99m}Tc agents are highly retained in the myocardium and exhibit almost no redistribution as is observed in the case of Tl-201. Thus intravenous injection of such an agent prior to the practice of PCI enables evaluation of the state myocardium perfusion before reperfusion treatment, even if the imaging is conducted after the completion of PCI (this is referred to as freeze image). The defect range indicated on the image obtained via this method is called the risk area (i.e. the area at risk of infarction, if not treated appropriately) and is clinically important. A second MPI procedure conducted in the subacute phase makes it possible to quantitatively measure the infarcted myocardium. The difference between the risk area and the infarcted area corresponds to the myocardium rescued by PCI. While evaluation of risk area by means of ^{99m}Tc agents is an excellent method with high objectivity, it is not necessarily easy to conduct nuclear medical examinations in emergency during the acute phase. MIBG memorizes ischemia and thus reveals a wider range of defects compared with MPI; if used in the subacute phase, this results in a mismatch between two methods. It has been reported that the range of defects for MIBG corresponds more closely to the risk area obtained using ^{99m}Tc agents[44] and that MIBG is useful in evaluating the risk area in acute coronary syndrome.

Non-Q Wave Myocardial Infarction

About 30–50% of cases of myocardial infarction are considered to be non-Q wave infarction. In general, in such cases, myocardial disorders are slight, and cardiac functions are maintained compared with the cases of Q wave infarction. However, no difference in prognosis has been reported between these, and non-Q wave infarction has been reported to have a rather high risk of leading to sudden cardiac death. For non-Q wave infarction, the detection rate via MPI is regarded to be roughly 50%, while it is also reportedly possible to identify the culprit coronary lesions using MIBG in nearly all cases. According to a reported comparative investigation into "Q" wave infarction and non-"Q" wave infarction, ^{99m}Tc-sestamibi (MIBI) myocardial perfusion SPECT and MIBG SPECT,[45] MIBI defects in non-Q wave infarction were significantly smaller than those in Q wave infarction, while MIBG defects showed no difference between these two types of infarction. In addition, the size of MIBG defects in Q wave infarction was proportional to that of MIBI defects, while such a tendency was not observed in non-Q wave infarction. In other words, in non-Q wave infarction, a wide mismatch area is recognized between perfusion SPECT and MIBG SPECT. This mismatch area is said to be denervated but viable and is considered to be in an unstable state which easily results in lethal arrhythmia. This situation may be one of reasons for many cases of cardiac sudden death in non-Q wave infarction.

Heart Failure

It has been reported that increased washout rate and the decreased H/M ratio on delayed MIBG image become marked with an increase in hypofunction in left ventricle in the cases of HF, regardless of the underlying diseases. Similar results have been reported from the studies on dilated cardiomyopathy (DCM),[46] HCM,[47] valvular heart disease, pulmonary hypertension, amyloidosis, and diabetes. As described above, the relationship between cardiac hypofunction and abnormal MIBG indices has been revealed in various diseases, and MIBG is thus useful for the severity evaluation of HF.

Cardiac Neuronal Imaging Using Positron Emission Tomography

Positron emission tomography is a highly specific tool for quantifying physiologic events. Compared with SPECT and conventional scintigraphy, it has higher spatial and temporal resolution, and attenuation correction is readily available and established. In addition, many autonomic PET tracers more closely resemble the endogenous neurotransmitter than I-123 MIBG used for SPECT imaging, and the variety of available tracers may allow for more detailed analysis of neuronal signaling. For practical application, specific activity and radiochemical purity are critical factors. These may expose myocardium to unlabeled catecholamine, which compete with the labeled tracer and may not only limit image quality but also cause pharmacologic action via adrenoceptor activation.

^{11}C-Hydroxyephedrine

^{11}C-Hydroxyephedrine (HED) is most widely used PET tracer for cardiac neuronal imaging. In healthy heart, there is an even distribution of HED over the left ventricle making it a valuable tracer for detecting specific regional defects of presynaptic sympathetic system in disease.[48] Denervation studies in animal model and in human heart transplantation patients have shown that HED has high affinity for the presynaptic neuronal catecholamine transporter [norepinephrine transporter (NET) also known as uptake-1], and there exists negligible nonspecific binding. In addition, HED is not metabolized by monoamine oxidase (MAO) or catechol-*O*-methyltransferase. Recently, it has been confirmed that HED retention is dependent on NET density of the heart. When desipramine is used as a specific inhibitor of the uptake-1 system after HED administration, gradual HED washout may be seen; thus, it has been suggested that HED retention is actually dependent on continuous release and reuptake.

^{11}C-Epinephrine

Epinephrine also functions as true neurotransmitter but only to small extent. Epinephrine may be enzymatically labeled to ^{11}C, producing ^{11}C-epinephrine (EPI). Unlike HED is degraded by MAO; however, its storage in the vesicle is very efficient causing its slow clearance from the heart. Therefore, EPI reflects the whole cascade of uptake, metabolism and storage of neurotransmission, while the primary target for HED is the uptake-1 system. It has been suggested that these properties make it superior as a ligand truly tracing neuronal dysfunction in heart.

^{11}C-Phenylephrine

Phenylephrine is commonly used as nasal decongestant. It may be labeled with ^{11}C, thus making it a PET tracer, ^{11}C-phenylephrine (PHEN). It is metabolized by MAO forming radiolabeled metabolite of PHEN, ^{11}C-methylamine. The metabolite rapidly diffuses out of the nerve terminals. PHEN is gradually washed from myocardium having a half-life of 60 minutes. The importance of vesicular leakage as a contributor to PHEN washout in addition to MAO metabolism has been emphasized.

^{18}F-Flurodopamine

Dopamine may be labeled with ^{18}F-fluroine to obtain ^{18}F-flurodopamine which has been used in humans to assess cardiac and extracardiac sympathetic innervation using PET. In humans, ^{18}F-flurodopamine scanning visualized sympathetic innervation in the heart, renal cortex, and thyroid gland. Its early clinical application was mainly for the identification of abnormalities in neuronal transmission in patients suffering from neurological diseases.* The half-life of ^{18}F-flurodopamine is 110 minutes, which enables PET scanning for longer periods of time as compared with ^{11}C-labeled compounds. After tracer injection, sympathetic nerve terminals take up ^{18}F-flurodopamine via uptake-1, after which it is rapidly internalized into vesicles and beta-hydroxylated, forming radiolabeled nuclear extract (NE). During sympathetic neurotransmission, labeled NE is released similar to the endogenous NE. ^{18}F-flurodopamine uptake may be blocked with desipramine. Owing to the nature of the radiolabel and the similarity of the metabolic pathways compared with the endogenous NE, ^{18}F-flurodopamine may be used to assess the uptake and clearance of NE; however, the production of ^{18}F-flurodopamine is relatively difficult and, furthermore, owing to the complex fate of dopamine in plasma and the heart, it is not widely used as the tracer of choice in assessing cardiac neuronal function.

IN CORONARY ARTERY DISEASE

Myocardial ischemia and infarction result in nerve injury. This may be followed by sympathetic nerve sprouting and regional hyperinnervation, leading to environmental changes favorable to electrical imbalance. It has been observed that after myocardial infarction, beta-adrenoceptor density is decreased as measured with ^{11}C-CGP12177.[49] In humans, chronic CAD caused reduction in HED uptake in patients with CAD but without myocardial infarction. Furthermore, the decrease in HED uptake is most prominent in regions of significant coronary stenosis. After myocardial infarction, there is an abnormal distribution of HED, showing impaired sympathetic activity in the heart when compared with HED distribution in healthy subjects. These defects remained same after 8 months, showing no reinnervation process in these patients. Thus, though there is unarguable evidence of dysinnervation after ischemic insult, there is no clinical evidence as to whether this affects the prognosis of these patients, and further studies are warranted to determine the clear-cut clinical value of the innervation in ischemic heart disease.

IN HEART FAILURE

Heart failure as such is an end-stage form of several cardiac diseases. It is associated with neurohormonal activation causing impaired neurotransmission. Neuronal cardiac imaging with PET is attractive method to study the failing heart, since the sympathetic involvement in HF is extensive. A study employing ^{11}C-CGP12177 showed that in patients with idiopathic DCM, there is significant reduction in amount of left ventricular beta-adrenoceptor. These PET results were comparable with results obtained from cardiac biopsies in the same study. Furthermore, Choudhary et al. presented a similar reduction of beta-adrenoceptor density in both primary and secondary left ventricular hypertrophy with sustained systolic function.[50] Various other studies have also presented results of reduced HED uptake in HF caused by end-stage coronary disease or DCM. Hartmann et al. found that there are significant regional reductions in HED uptake in apical and inferoapical segments in these patients. In another study, patients with end-stage heart disease were scanned with HED before heart transplantation, and after surgery, the diseased heart was investigated for uptake-1 density and NE content. They found to have significant correlation of uptake-1 and NE content with HED uptake, but not with uptake-1 affinity. According to these results, they concluded that in DCM, there is the loss of neurons or downregulation of uptake-1 in humans; furthermore, in the technical perspective, they showed that PET imaging with HED is valid in human HF imaging.

CONCLUSION

Heart failure is a major problem in day-to-day clinical cardiology practice having a high prevalence, morbidity, mortality and is expected to become more widespread in the near future. Radionuclide imaging plays an important role in evaluating these patients and giving substantial information toward the diagnosis and further treatment planning. MPI with SPECT as well as PET radiotracers is commonly used to differentiate ischemic from nonischemic etiology of HF and cardiomyopathy. Further developments in measuring quantitative blood flow promises to provide more accurate determination of HF etiology. MPI or PET myocardial viability has been established as a gold standard for the assessment of myocardial viability and identification of patients likely to benefit from revascularization. In patients with HF who are not the candidates for revascularization, myocardial remodeling often leads to poor patient's outcome. Newer nuclear tests of myocardial shape of dys-synchronous contraction or relaxation can risk stratify patients and may help cardiac resynchronization therapy (CRT) therapy. New molecular imaging techniques promise to better understand underlying pathophysiology, such as in the absence of significant area of resting perfusion, defect in a MPI scan with an area of absence of either I-123 MIBG uptake or ^{11}C-HED uptake which is otherwise known as *autonomic perfusion mismatch* indicates significant amount of sympathetic denervation which warrants immediate CRT therapy.

REFERENCES

1. Paulus WJ, Tscöpe C, Sanderson JE, et al. How to diagnose diastolic heart failure: a consensus statement on the diagnosis of heart failure with normal left ventricular ejection fraction by the Heart Failure and Echocardiography Associations of the European Society of Cardiology. Eur Heart J. 2007;28:2539-50.
2. Cohn JN, Ferrari R, Sharpe N. Cardiac remodeling—concepts and clinical implications: a consensus paper from an international forum on cardiac remodeling. Behalf of an International Forum on Cardiac Remodeling. J Am Coll Cardiol. 2000;35:569-82.
3. Gheorghiade M, Sopko G, De Luca L, et al. Navigating the crossroad of coronary artery disease and heart failure. Circulation. 2006;114:1202-13.

4. Taylor AL, Ziesche S, Yancy C, et al. Combination of isosorbide dinitrate and hydralazine in blacks with heart failure. N Engl J Med. 2004;351:2049-57.
5. Udelson JE, Shafer CD, Carrio I. Radionuclide imaging in heart failure: assessing etiology and outcomes and implications for management. J Nucl Cardiol. 2002;9:S40-52.
6. Iskandrian AS, Hakki AH, Kane S. Resting thallium-201 myocardial perfusion patterns in patients with severe left ventricular dysfunction: differences between patients with primary cardiomyopathy, chronic coronary artery disease, or acute myocardial infarction. Am Heart J. 1986;111:760-7.
7. Mody VF, Brunken RC, Warmer Stevenson L, et al. Differentiating cardiomyopathy of coronary artery disease from nonischemic dilated cardiomyopathy utilizing positron emission tomography. J Am Coll Cardiol. 1991;17:373-83.
8. Danias PG, Ahlberg AW, Clark BA III, et al. Combined assessment of myocardial perfusion and left ventricular function with exercise technetium-99m sestamibi gated single-photon emission computed tomography can differentiate between ischemic and nonischemic dilated cardiomyopathy. Am J Cardiol. 1998;82:1253-8.
9. Prakash R, deKemp RA, Ruddy TD, et al. Potential utility of rubidium 82 PET quantification in patients with 3-vessel coronary artery disease. J Nucl Cardiol. 2004;11:440-9.
10. Herzog BA, Husmann L, Valenta I, et al. Long-term prognostic value of 13 N-ammonia myocardial perfusion positron emission tomography. J Am Coll Cardiol. 2009;54:150-6.
11. Ziadi MC, deKemp RA, Williams KA, et al. Impaired myocardial flow reserve on rubidium-82 positron emission tomography imaging predicts adverse outcomes in patients assessed for myocardial ischemia. J Am Coll Cardiol. 2011;58:740-8.
12. Mori T, Yamabe H, Yokota Y, et al. Clinical significance of dipyridamole Tl-201 emission computed tomography perfusion abnormality for evaluating pathophysiological and pathological aspects in hypertrophic cardiomyopathy. Jpn Circ J. 1988;52(2):111-8.
13. Von Dohlen TW, Prisant LM, Frank MJ. Significance of positive or negative thallium-201 scintigraphy in hypertrophic cardiomyopathy. Am J Cardiol. 1989;64(8):498-503.
14. Camici P, Chiriatti G, Lorenzoni R, et al. Coronary vasodilation is impaired in both hypertrophied and nonhypertrophied myocardium of patients with hypertrophic cardiomyopathy: a study with nitrogen-13 ammonia and positron emission tomography. J Am Coll Cardiol. 1991;17(4):879-86.
15. Choudhury L, Elliott P, Rimoldi O, et al. Transmural myocardial blood flow distribution in hypertrophic cardiomyopathy and effect of treatment. Basic Res Cardiol. 1999;94(1):49-59.
16. Iskandrian AS, Hakki A, Kane SA, et al. Rest and redistribution thallium-201 myocardial scintigraphy to predict improvement in left ventricular function after coronary arterial bypass grafting. Am J Cardiol. 1983;51:1312-6.
17. Kiat H, Berman DS, Maddahi J, et al. Late reversibility of tomographic myocardial thallium-201, defects: an accurate marker of myocardial viability. J Am Coll Cardiol. 1988;12:1456-63.
18. Tillisch J, Brunken R, Marshall R, et al. Reversibility of cardiac wall-motion abnormalities predicted by positron tomography. N Engl J Med. 1986;314:884-8.
19. Marcassa C, Galli M, Cuocolo A, et al. Rest-redistribution thallium-201 and rest technetium-99m-sestamibi SPECT in patients with stable coronary artery disease and ventricular dysfunction. J Nucl Med. 1997;38:419-24.
20. Kauffman GJ, Boyne TS, Watson DD, et al. Comparison of rest thallium-201 imaging and rest technetium-99m sestamibi imaging for assessment of myocardial viability in patients with coronary artery disease and severe left ventricular dysfunction. J Am Coll Cardiol. 1996;27:1592-7.
21. Botvinick EH, Frais MA, Shosa DW, et al. An accurate means of detecting and characterizing abnormal patterns of ventricular activation by phase image analysis. Am J Cardiol. 1982;50:289-98.
22. Altumairi A, Rossin R, Shokeen M, et al. Biodegradable dendritic positron-emitting nanoprobes for the noninvasive imaging of angiogenesis. Proc Natl ACAD Sci USA. 2009;106:685-90.
23. Weber KT. Extracellular matrix remodeling in heart failure: a role for de novo angiotensin II generation. Circulation. 1997;96:4065-82.
24. Flotats A, Carrio I, Agostini D, et al. Proposal for standardization of 123I-metaiodobenzylguanidine (MIBG) cardiac sympathetic imaging by the EANM Cardiovascular Committee and the European Council of Nuclear Cardiology. Eur J Nucl Med Mol Imaging. 2010;37:1802-12.
25. Somsen GA, Verberne HJ, Fleury E, et al. Normal values and within subject variability of cardiac I-123 MIBG scintigraphy in healthy individuals: Implications for clinical studies. J Nucl Cardiol. 2004;11:126-33.
26. Simoes MV, Barthel P, Matsunari I, et al. Presence of sympathetically denervated but viable myocardium and its electrophysiologic correlates after early revascularized, acute myocardial infarction or phenol application. Circulation. 1988;78:1008-19.
27. Kasama S, Toyama T, Hatori T, et al. Evaluation of cardiac sympathetic nerve activity and left ventricular remodeling carvedilol. Eur Heart J. 2007;28:989-95.
28. Drakos SG, Athanasoulis T, Malliaras KG, et al. Myocardial sympathetic innervation and long-term left ventricular mechanical unloading. J Am Coll Cardiol Imaging. 2010;3:64-70.
29. Shah AM, Bourgoun M, Narula J, et al. Influence of ejection fraction on the prognostic value of sympathetic innervation imaging with iodine-123 MIBG in heart failure. J Am Coll Cardiol Imaging. 2012;5:1139-46.

SECTION 4

ST-elevation Myocardial Infarction and Coronary Artery Disease

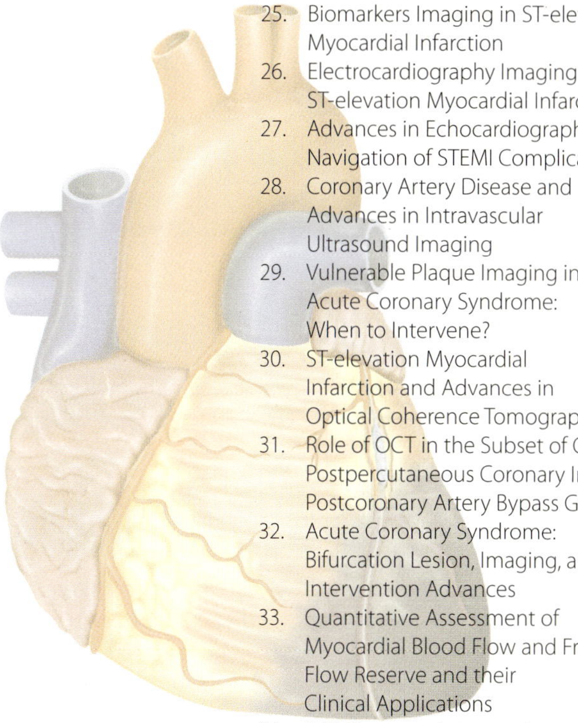

25

CHAPTER

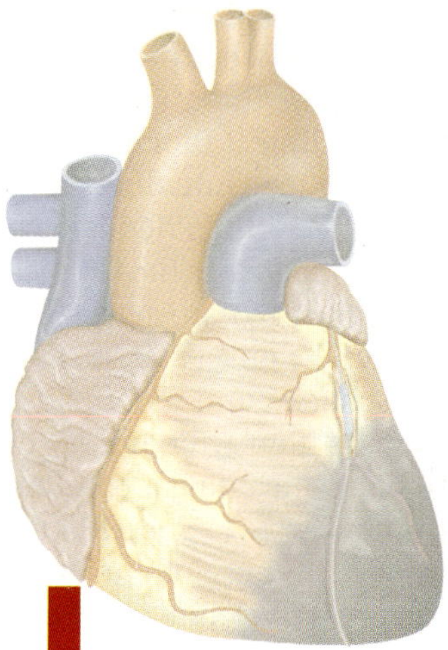

Biomarkers Imaging in ST-elevation Myocardial Infarction

Ajay Kumar Sinha, Sanjeev Kumar, Vikas Singh

INTRODUCTION

A biomarker is defined as a characteristic that is objectively measured and evaluated as an indicator of normal biological processes, pathogenic processes, or pharmacologic responses to a therapeutic intervention. Patient presenting in emergency department with symptoms suggestive of acute coronary syndrome (ACS) needs to be categorized as the low-risk or high-risk from diagnostic, prognostic, and management point of view. Research of ideal biomarkers in ACS has been accelerating at a remarkable pace. Biomarkers play an important role in the diagnosis of ACS, especially in unstable angina and non-ST segment elevation myocardial infarction (NSTEMI). In ST-segment elevation myocardial infarction (STEMI), the main focus of interest has been on the shortening of time from onset of symptoms to treatment. Biomarkers in STEMI have been categorized as markers of myocardial necrosis, hemodynamic stress, inflammation, vascular damage and accelerated atherosclerosis. Thus, there is knowledge regarding associated pathways and/or consequences of the disease, which may be helpful to understand the disease process and identify potential therapeutic targets. Cardiac troponins and creatine kinase appear to be the most sensitive and specific markers of myocardial injury. Recent studies have revealed several novel biomarkers. Elevated levels of C-reactive protein (CRP) and interleukin-6 (IL-6) are strong independent markers of increased mortality among patients with ACS. However, the ideal biomarkers that offer early detection, risk stratification, selection of therapy, monitoring disease progression, and treatment efficacy remain to be elucidated.

ACUTE CORONARY SYNDROME: THE PROBLEM AREAS

Patients with ACS are subdivided into the following two major categories based on the twelve-lead electrocardiogram (ECG): those with new ST-elevation on the ECG that is diagnostic of acute STEMI and those who present with ST-segment depression, T-wave changes, or no ECG abnormalities [non-ST elevation ACS (NSTEACS)]. The latter encompasses both unstable angina (UA) and NSTEMI.[1] This group comprises a growing number of patients with ACS and is emerging as a major public health problem worldwide, especially in Western countries, Asia and other developing countries.[2-3] ECG is the most readily available tool for identifying patients with STEMI. Establishing the correct diagnosis in patients without ST-segment elevation, however, can be more challenging. The ECG is often nondiagnostic for acute chest pain, and in fact, the sensitivity of the baseline ECG for detecting acute myocardial infarction (AMI) is 50-60%. About 33% of patients with ACS have no chest pain.[4] Approximately half of patients with acute chest pain who have initial diagnostic findings of ACS and are admitted to the hospital are later found not to suffer from ACS.[5] Misdiagnosis has been reported to be the main cause of treatment delays.[6] These imperfect strategies result in costly and inappropriate management decisions.

BIOMARKERS IN STEMI

Elevated cardiac biomarkers are an important indicator of risk in clinically validated models, such as the Global Registry of Acute Coronary Events (GRACE) and Thrombolysis in Myocardial Infarction (TIMI) risk scores, whose use is recommended by international guidelines.[7] However clinicians do not routinely use these models in practice, partly because we lack compelling evidence that their use improves care. The most important biomarker is troponin, which has evolved as the foundation of diagnosis for AMI and, in its high-sensitivity fourth-generation iteration, plays an even more important role in the evaluation of chest pain.

Beyond troponin, other biomarkers figure selectively in clinical care. Creatinine, measured routinely for other reasons, is an important marker of risk for ischemic events. And although significantly impaired renal function indicates higher risk for ischemic cardiac events that would warrant aggressive management, it also identifies risk of contrast nephropathy that increases the threshold for coronary angiography. Natriuretic peptides also indicate risk for both short- and long-term mortality, whereas CRP elevation predicts longer term mortality. A list of various biomarkers, which may be of use in detection and managing ACS patients as well as underscoring the pathophysiology, is summed up in /Box 1 and Figure 1.

Cardiac Troponin

In recent years, troponin has become gold standard in detection of ACS. Several well-designed studies have shown that cardiac troponin (cTnI and cTnT) to be the most diagnostically sensitive and specific biomarker of myocardial injury.[7-9] Moreover, on the basis of improved sensitivity and superior tissue specificity compared to other biomarkers of necrosis, cTn is recommended for the diagnosis of AMI by the National Academy of Clinical Biochemistry (NACB) Laboratory Medicine Practice Guidelines and the International Committee of Experts in Epidemiology, Pathology, Clinical, and Laboratory Medicine. The kinetics of cTnI and cTnT are similar; cTnI and cTnT are detectable in the serum within 4-2 hours after the onset of AMI, and depending on the duration of ischemia and reperfusion status, peak values occur 2-48 hours from symptom onset (Fig. 2).[10] Therefore, serial sampling, including a baseline sample and follow-up examination 8–12 hours after symptom onset is recommended.[11] Because of the tissue specificity of cTn, any reliably-detected concentration of cTn in the peripheral circulation is abnormal and indicative of

BOX 1: Various biomarkers underscoring different facets of the pathophysiology and outcomes.

Inflammation
- C-reactive protein
- Myeloperoxidase
- Matrix metalloproteinase
- Soluble CD40 ligand

Platelet activation
- Soluble CD40 ligand

Vulnerable plaque
- Pregnancy-associated plasma protein-A
- Myeloperoxidase placental growth factor matrix metalloproteinase

Myocardial necrosis
- Creatine phosphokinase and isoenzymes
- Troponin I and T
- Fatty acid binding protein

Ischemia
- Ischemia modified albumin

Pump failure
- Brain natriuretic peptide
- N-terminal probrain natriuretic peptide

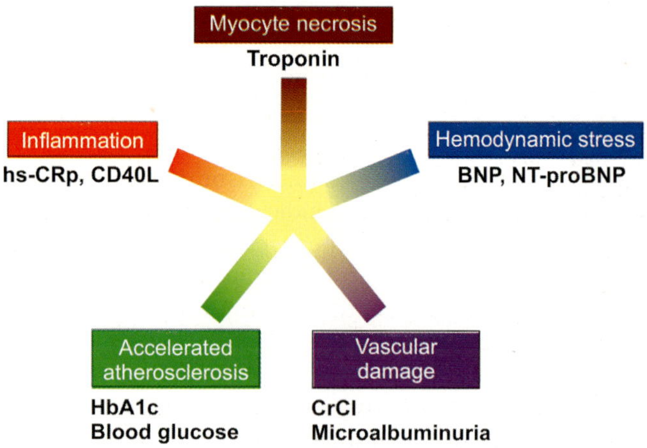

"The highlighted markers are established and rest are emerging"
Fig. 1

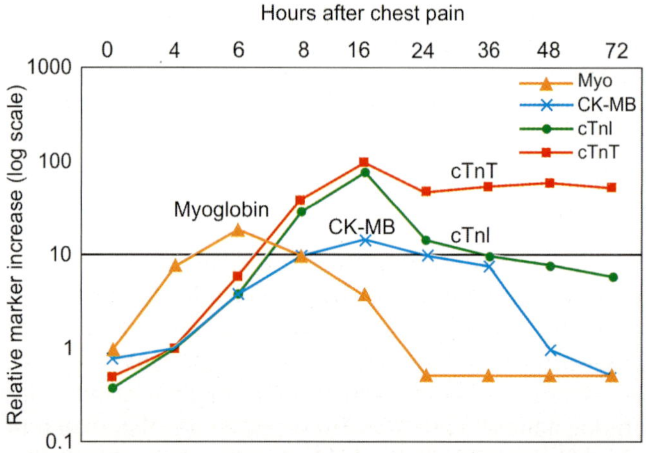

Fig. 2: Temporal release of various biomarkers after chest pain in ST-segment elevation myocardial infarction.

myocardial injury.[12] Moreover, several studies showed that patients presenting with an increased cTn concentration had a poor prognosis compared to those without detectable cTn.[13] Although cTnI is cleared more quickly from the circulation than cTnT, both isoforms remain elevated in the serum for several days after injury, allowing for diagnostic confirmation, even in patients presenting with delayed symptoms. Because of the long half-lives, one of the disadvantages is that neither cTnI nor cTnT assays can be used for detection of re-infarction after an index event. Moreover, an elevated cTn without clinical evidence of STEMI should prompt a search for other possible myocardial injuries, including cardiac trauma, congestive heart failure, and hypertension, as an elevated cTn does not indicate its mechanism.

Creatine Kinase

The creatine kinase-myocardial band (CK-MB) is the next best marker of STEMI. In the early days, the elevated serum levels of CK-MB, the cardiac-specific isoform of CK, was used for the diagnosis of myocardial necrosis. This measure satisfied one component of the diagnostic criteria for myocardial infarction (MI), as proposed by the World Health Organization, and was later extended for monitoring trends and determinants in a cardiovascular disease study.[14] CK-MB is predominantly found in the myocardium. Elevation of CK-MB occurs 4–6 hours after the onset of AMI and remains for 48–72 hours (Fig. 2). Similar to cTn, serial testing of CK-MB has been suggested to increase the sensitivity and specificity in detecting myocardial injury.[15] Although some studies have suggested serial measurement of CK-MB to qualitatively estimate the infarct size, many studies have revealed that a single measurement of plasma cTn can be used as a convenient, cost-effective, and noninvasive method.[16,17]CK-MB is relatively sensitive, but the specificity is in doubt as CK-MB is elevated in any condition following acute or chronic muscle injury, or in patients undergoing a surgical procedure.[18] Furthermore, CK is present in skeletal muscle, intestine, diaphragm, uterus, and prostate, and thus the specificity of CK-MB is impaired in the setting of injury to these organs.[19]

Myoglobin

The NACB Laboratory Medicine Practice Guidelines have recommended myoglobin in addition to cTn for the diagnosis of STEMI patients who present within 6 hours of onset of symptoms. The serum myoglobin level rises faster than CK-MB and cTn, reaching twice normal values with 2 hours and peaking within 4 hours of AMI symptom onset (Fig. 2). Myoglobin achieves its maximal diagnostic sensitivity within 5 hours of symptom onset.[20] The disadvantage of using myoglobin alone is that it has poor specificity for STEMI in patients with concurrent trauma or renal failure.

Natriuretic Peptides

Brain natriuretic peptide (BNP) and its prohormone, N-terminal pro-BNP (NT-proBNP), are neurohormones secreted from cardiac ventricles in response to ventricular wall stress.[21] BNP, an established biomarker for patients with heart failure, and NT-proBNP are elevated in patients with STEMI and can identify STEMI patients who are at higher risk for adverse cardiovascular events, including heart failure and death.[22-24] The utility of BNP and NT-proBNP as diagnostic biomarkers for STEMI is based on the premise that increases in the diameter of and pressure within the left ventricle during remodeling after a transmural infarction, or as a consequence of prior ischemic damage is responsible for increased hemodynamic stress.

EMERGING BIOMARKER OF STEMI

Some cardiac biomarkers do not require myocardial cell death for release, and are thus referred to as myocardial ischemia biomarkers. These include biomarkers of inflammation and platelet activation. As the prototypical acute phase reactants, CRP and IL-6 have been the focus of investigations for the diagnosis of STEMI. A landmark study by Liuzzo et al.[25] showed that patients presenting with UA who had elevated levels of CRP and serum amyloid A had a higher rate of death, AMI, and the need for revascularization compared with patients without elevated levels. The Fragmin and Fast Revascularization during Instability in Coronary Artery Disease II trial study group showed that the circulating level of IL-6 is a strong independent marker of increased mortality and is useful in directing subsequent care.[26] However, the best timing for measurement of CRP and IL-6 for diagnosis and risk stratification of STEMI remains uncertain.

The other inflammatory biomarkers under investigation for the diagnosis and prognosis of STEMI are monocyte chemoattractant protein-1 (MCP-1), IL-18 and IL-10.[27] The MCP-plasma concentration is associated with different cardiovascular risk factors, and a greater risk of developing a cardiovascular event in the future. A prospective study has reported that the serum IL-18 level is a strong independent predictor of death from cardiovascular causes in patients with coronary artery disease. IL-10 and other inflammatory biomarkers, including macrophage inhibitory cytokine- and soluble tumor necrosis factor receptors (sTNFR1/sTNFR2), have shown promise in the prediction of the incidence of coronary artery disease, but these makers require further study for possible application in STEMI risk stratification.

Finally, there are some new groups of biomarkers that may become useful for the diagnosis of STEMI. Most of these biomarkers are still under intense investigation. Most of the prospective studies have demonstrated that these markers were of prognostic value for STEMI. Some of the emerging markers are:

- *Biomarkers of oxidative stress:* Elevated levels of lipoprotein-associated phospholipase A-2, secretory phospholipase A2, oxidised low-density lipoprotein and myeloperoxidase are reported to have a significant association with the risk of death or MI in ACS patients.
- *Biomarkers of tissue necrosis*: Fatty acid binding proteins (FABPs), free fatty acid unbound to albumin (FFAu), and ischemia modified albumin appear to play an important role in the diagnosis of STEMI. Elevated levels of heart-type FABP have been demonstrated as early as 1.5 hours after the onset of infarction, peaks at 4-6 hours and returns to baseline within 24 hours. Heart-type FABP has been proposed to be an early marker of ACS even before troponin. FFAu is increased in 100% of MI patients on admission, whereas only 22% of these patients have increased cTn at presentation. These markers may have an important role in certain clinical settings in the future, and their precise role is currently unknown.

LIMITATIONS OF DIAGNOSTIC BIOMARKERS IN STEMI

An ideal marker is one in which there is a specific easily measurable increase that clearly aligns with a diagnosis or a predictable outcome. cTn appears to be the most sensitive and specific biomarker among all other diagnostic biomarkers for STEMI. However, there is a consensus that a single measurement of cTn on arrival of the patient to the hospital is insufficient because a single measurement of cTn will not detect 10-15% of at-risk patients.[28]

Most importantly, the rapid and correct diagnosis of ACS, specifically UA or NSTEMI, is a challenging and demanding issue. Point-of-care testing plays a crucial role in the context of the diagnosis and management of ACS. American Heart Association/American College of Cardiology, UA/NSTEMI Guidelines have increased the need for rapid testing for cardiac biomarkers through a reduction in laboratory test turnaround time.[29] Saliva-based nano-biochip using 21 biomarkers exhibited a significant diagnostic capability for AMI patients and has been proposed as a screening method for cardiac events in prehospital stages.[30]

NEW DEVELOPMENT IN BIOMARKER DISCOVERY

The pathophysiologic changes in STEMI are influenced by many factors, including genetic and environmental factors. The complete sequencing of human genome and recent advances in genomic, transcriptomic, proteomic, lipidomic, metabolomic and bioinformatics technologies offer tremendous opportunities for novel biomarker discovery. These high-throughput technologies are emerging as powerful platforms for more global approaches to discover pattern-based unique molecular fingerprints or signatures of STEMI.

At the genomic level, various global genomic technologies can be applied to study genetic variation, gene mutation, gene mapping, and epigenetic regulation. At the transcriptomic level, microarray technologies can be used to study the quantity of RNA and alternative splicing. With advances in proteomic technologies, the approach of biomarker identification now shifts from a large scale epidemiologic association to an association between disease phenotype and specific proteomic patterns.

Using multimarker strategy could allow risk stratification and provide prognostic information in patients with ACS. A multimarker study combining baseline levels of cTnI, CRP, and BNP among patients with NSTEMI identified a six- to three-fold gradient of mortality risk between those without elevation of any marker and those in whom all three markers were elevated. Moreover, combined analysis of 10 biomarkers in 3,209 participants attending the sixth examination cycle of the Framingham Heart Study showed that persons with high multimarker scores had a risk of death four times as great and a risk of major cardiovascular events almost two times as great as persons with low multimarker scores.[31]

The *diagnostic sensitivity* of myocardial necrosis markers, such as CK-MB, cardiac troponins, and myoglobin for the earliest stage of STEMI, remains insufficient. A *new biomarker of plaque vulnerability* (*receptor for advanced glycation end-products, S100A12*) was compared with other biomarker at the earliest stage of STEMI. At optimal cut-off value of 161.7 ng/mL, S100A12 discriminated STEMI from non-AMI with 81.6% sensitivity, 81.7% specificity. The diagnosis sensitivity of S100A12, myoglobin, troponin T, and CK-MB for STEMI upon admission (98 min after onset) was 85.2%, 72.3%, 61.1% and 42%, respectively. Plasma S100A12 diagnosed the early stages of STEMI more accurately than myoglobin, troponin T and CK-MB.

Several studies demonstrated the usefulness of inflammatory biomarkers in risk stratification of STEMI. The study assessed the prognostic potential of a new biomarker, neutrophil to platelet ratio (NPR). After adjusting for age, left ventricular ejection fraction (LVEF), hemoglobin and serum creatinine at admission and anterior AMI, NPR was found to be an independent predictor of short-term, all-cause, and long-term mortality. The neutrophil to platelet ratio at admission was an independent predictor of short- and long-term mortality in STEMI patients undergoing pPCI.[33]

MicroRNAs (miRNAs) are endogenous, 21- to 23-nucleotide-long RNA molecules that post-transcriptionally regulate target genes. The field of miRNAs as biomarkers is about to mature. Whether the sparse concentrations of miRNAs present in the circulation exert a functional role is an interesting, yet even more challenging question,[34] the answer to which will come in future.

Admission levels of macrophage migration inhibitory factor predicted infarct size following STEMI. It remains unknown whether MIF alone or in combination with other conventional biomarkers predict adverse outcomes in STEMI patients.[35] Cytochrome C seems to represent a biomarker of mitochondrial dysfunction that may provide prognostic information complementary to those carried by troponin.

The development of left ventricular remodeling (LVR) is associated with heart failure and mortality in patients surviving acute STEMI. It is, however, unclear whether the combination of routine biomarkers improves risk stratification for LVR after STEMI.[36]

Peak concentrations of N-terminal pro-B-type natriuretic peptide, high-sensitivity cardiac troponin T, aspartate aminotransferase, alanine transaminase, high-sensitivity CRP, and lactate dehydrogenase have significant ability to distinguish patients who develop LVR from those who do not. Importantly, the combination of all biomarkers provided incremental prognostic information for LVR when compared with single-biomarker testing. Combined sampling of these routinely available biomarkers could facilitate the identification of patients at increased risk of LVR that might benefit from more intensive postinfarction care. However, considering the lack of randomized trials evaluating a biomarker-guided treatment strategy, this issue awaits further validation and research.

In addition to these routine assays, several more specialized blood biomarkers are associated with risk following ACS, including two recent examples: mid-regional proadrenomedullin and mid-regional proatrial natriuretic peptide. Although frequently predictive of events, these newer biomarkers have not yet been shown to be of sufficient value to add meaningfully to available risk markers or utility to clinical decisions.

Some patients with low levels of troponin are at high-risk whereas others with high levels of troponin are at low-risk, depending on clinical factors. This highlights the need for accurate risk stratification using multivariable models, including clinical and biomarker parameters, and clinical judgment.

An accurate estimation of biomarker release as a surrogate marker of infarct size and a powerful assessment of conditioning treatments. This biomarker kinetic modeling approach identified CK-MB as the most accurate biomarker in determining infarct size and supports the development of limited sampling strategies that estimate total biomarker amount released with a lower number of samples. It will certainly be a useful add-on to future studies in the field of STEMI and cardioprotection.

Thus, depending on the intended use of biomarker information, time-updated modeling may be important. There will continue to be discoveries of new biomarkers that relate to AMI and subsequent risk, but few of these will make it into clinical use.

CONCLUSION

There has been a long march of biomarkers in STEMI from bench to bedside. These need to be offered on routine clinical platform and provide high sensitivity and specificity and thus impact a cost-effective therapeutic decision making which is extremely important in a country like ours.

As the number of cardiovascular biomarkers grows, it is critical to understand each one's specific strengths and limitations. Furthermore, it is critical that all biomarkers are not used as stand-alone tests. They must be interpreted in their appropriate clinical context and do not replace other parts of the examination such as physical examination or imaging modalities. Despite the large number of existing and novel biomarkers for cardiovascular disease, no one marker has enough sensitivity and specificity to be evaluated in isolation. Therefore a multi-biomarker strategy is likely to be the most useful for clinical decision-making. In fact, most patients have multiple processes occurring simultaneously and these biomarkers can help detect distinct points in the pathway of development of STEMI, with cardiac troponin being at the center of the proceedings for now (Fig. 3).

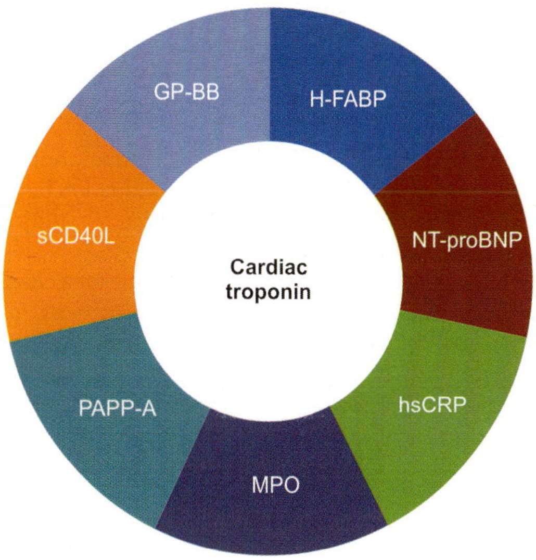

Fig. 3: Multimarker strategy with cardiac troponin in the center.

REFERENCES

1. Wiviott SD, Braunwald E. Unstable angina and non-ST-segment elevation myocardial infarction: part I. Initial evaluation and management, and hospital care. Am Fam Physician. 2004;70:525-32.
2. Boden WE, McKay RG. Optimal treatment of acute coronary syndromes—an evolving strategy. N Engl J Med. 200;344:939-42.
3. Yarlagadda RK, Boden WE. Cardioprotective effects of an early invasive strategy for non-ST-segment elevation acute coronary syndromes: are we all becoming "interventional" cardiologists? J Am Coll Cardiol. 2002;40:95-8.
4. Murray CJ, Lopez AD. Alternative projections of mortality and disability by cause 990-2020: Global Burden of Disease Study. Lancet. 997;349:498-504.
5. Panteghini M. Acute coronary syndrome: biochemical strategies in the troponin era. Chest. 2002;22:428-35.
6. Canto JG, Shlipak MG, Rogers WJ, et al. Prevalence, clinical characteristics, and mortality among patients with myocardial infarction presenting without chest pain. JAMA. 2000;283:3223-9.
7. Storrow AB, Gibler WB. Chest pain centers: diagnosis of acute coronary syndromes. Ann Emerg Med. 2000;35:449-6.
8. Dadkhah S, Sharain K, Sharain R, et al. The value of bedside cardiac multibiomarker assay in rapid and accurate diagnosis of acute coronary syndromes. Crit Path Cardiol. 2007;6:76-84.
9. Rusnak RA, Stair TO, Hansen K, et al. Litigation against the emergency physician: common features in cases of missed myocardial infarction. Ann Emerg Med. 1989;8:029-34.
10. Keller T, Zeller T, Peetz D, et al. Sensitive troponin I assay in early diagnosis of acute myocardial infarction. N Engl J Med. 2009;36:868-77.
11. Reichlin T, Hochholzer W, Bassetti S, et al. Early diagnosis of myocardial infarction with sensitive cardiac troponin assays. N Engl J Med. 2009;36:858-67.
12. Kavsak PA, Wang X, Ko DT, et al. Short- and long-term risk stratification using a next-generation, high-sensitivity research cardiac troponin I (hs-cTnI) assay in an emergency department chest pain population. Clin Chem. 2009;55:809-5.
13. Boden WE, Shah PK, Gupta V, et al. Contemporary approach to the diagnosis and management of non-ST-segment elevation acute coronary syndromes. Prog Cardiovasc Dis. 2008;50:3-5.
14. Evaluation of a bedside whole-blood rapid troponin T assay in the emergency department. Rapid Evaluation by Assay of Cardiac Troponin T (REACTT) Investigators Study Group. Acad Emerg Med. 1997;4:1018-24.
15. Jaffe AS, Ravkilde J, Roberts R, et al. It's time for a change to a troponin standard. Circulation. 2000;102:1216-20.
16. Bonaca MP, Morrow DA. Defining a role for novel biomarkers in acute coronary syndromes. Clin Chem. 2008;54:424-3.
17. Tunstall-Pedoe H, Kuulasmaa K, Amouyel P, et al. Myocardial infarction and coronary deaths in the World Health Organization MONICA Project. Registration procedures, event rates, and case-fatality rates in 38 populations from 2 countries in four continents. Circulation. 1994;90:583-62.
18. Gibler WB, Lewis LM, Erb RE, et al. Early detection of acute myocardial infarction in patients presenting with chest pain and nondiagnostic ECGs: Serial CK-MB sampling in the emergency department. Ann Emerg Med. 1990;9:359-66.
19. Chia S, Senatore F, Raffel OC, et al. Utility of cardiac biomarkers in predicting infarct size, left ventricular function, and clinical outcome after primary percutaneous coronary intervention for ST-segment elevation myocardial infarction. JACC Cardiovasc Interv. 2008;1:415-23.
20. Tzivoni D, Koukoui D, Guetta V, et al. Comparison of Troponin T to creatine kinase and to radionuclide cardiac imaging infarct size in patients with ST-elevation myocardial infarction undergoing primary angioplasty. Am J Cardiol. 2008;101:753-7.
21. Apple FS, Murakami M, Panteghini M, et al. International survey on the use of cardiac markers. Clin Chem. 2001;47:587-8.
22. Selker HP, Zalenski RJ, Antman EM, et al. An evaluation of technologies for identifying acute cardiac ischemia in the emergency department: executive summary of a National Heart Attack Alert Program Working Group Report. Ann Emerg Med. 1997;29:13-87.
23. de Winter RJ, Lijmer JG, Koster RW, et al. Diagnostic accuracy of myoglobin concentration for the early diagnosis of acute myocardial infarction. Ann Emerg Med. 2000;35:3-20.
24. de Lemos JA, McGuire DK, Drazner MH. B-type natriuretic peptide in cardiovascular disease. Lancet. 2003;362:36-22.
25. de Lemos JA, Morrow DA, Bentley JH, et al. The prognostic value of B-type natriuretic peptide in patients with acute coronary syndromes. N Engl J Med. 2001;345:1014-21.
26. Morita E, Yasue H, Yoshimura M, et al. Increased plasma levels of brain natriuretic peptide in patients with acute myocardial infarction. Circulation. 1993;88:82-9.
27. Jernberg T, Stridsberg M, Venge P, et al. N-terminal pro brain natriuretic peptide on admission for early risk stratification of patients with chest pain and no ST-segment elevation. J Am Coll Cardiol. 2002;40:437-45.
28. Pietila K, Hermens WT, Harmoinen A, et al. Comparison of peak serum C-reactive protein and hydroxybutyrate dehydrogenase levels in patients with acute myocardial infarction treated with alteplase and streptokinase. Am J Cardiol. 1997;80:1075-7.
29. Ueda S, Ikeda U, Yamamoto K, et al. C-reactive protein as a predictor of cardiac rupture after acute myocardial infarction. Am Heart J. 1996;3:857-60.
30. Hamm CW. Cardiac biomarkers for rapid evaluation of chest pain. Circulation. 2001;04:454-6.
31. Braunwald E, Antman EM, Beasley JW, et al. ACC/AHA 2002 guideline update for the management of patients with unstable angina and non-ST-segment elevation myocardial infarction—summary article: a report of the American College of Cardiology/American Heart Association Task Force on Practice Guidelines (Committee on the Management of Patients With Unstable Angina). J Am Coll Cardiol. 2002;40:366-74.
32. Cheng M, Naijing G, Xiaolin Z, et al. Journal of the American College of Cardiology. 2017;70(16 Supplement):C182-C3.

33. Abdulhadi B, Naranjo M, Krishnamoorthy P, et al. White blood cell count to platelet ratio: a novel biomarker for predicting outcomes in patients on circulatory support devices. J Am Coll Cardiol. 2018;71(11 Supplement):A810.
34. Zampetaki A, Willeit P, Tilling L et al. J Am Coll Cardiol. 2012;60(4):290-9.
35. Deng X, Wang X, Yu H, et al. J Am Coll Cardiol. 2018;71(11 Supplement):A240.
36. Reinstadler SJ, Feistritzer H-J, Reindl M, et al. Combined biomarker testing for the prediction of left ventricular remodelling in ST-elevation myocardial infarction. Open Heart. 2016;3:e000485.
37. Ternant D, Ivanes F, Prunier F, et al. Revisiting myocardial necrosis biomarkers: assessment of the effect of conditioning therapies on infarct size by kinetic modelling. Scientific Reports. 2017;7(10709).

26

CHAPTER

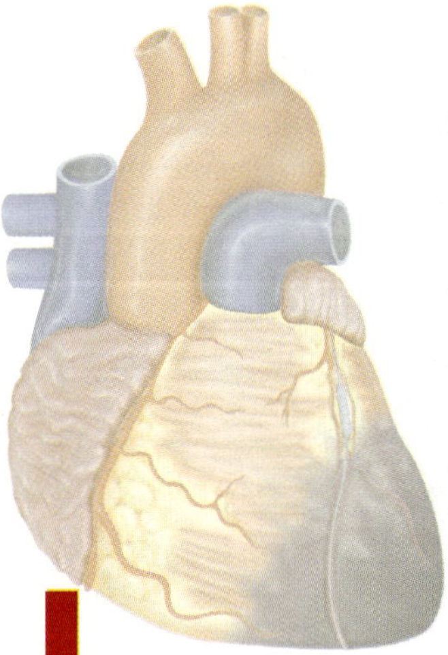

Electrocardiography Imaging in ST-elevation Myocardial Infarction

Apoorv Mittal, HK Chopra, V Anand, Manish Gaba

INTRODUCTION

Coronary heart disease is a major cause of death and disability in developed countries and the world.[1] Unstable coronary disease [acute coronary syndrome (ACS)] is characterized by plaque rupture or erosion with associated thrombosis and is divided into ST-elevation myocardial infarction (STEMI), non-ST elevation myocardial infarction (NSTEMI) and unstable angina (Fig. 1).[1] Out of which STEMI is a true medical emergency. In patients with acute STEMI, the ECG evolves through a typical sequence (Figs. 2A to E).[1] STEMI in ECG[1] can be defined as new ST-elevation at the J-point in two contiguous leads of more than 0.1 mV in all leads other than leads V2-V3. For leads V2-V3, the following cut points apply: more than and equal to 0.2 mV in men more than and equal to 40 years, more than and equal to 0.25 mV in men less than 40 years or more than and equal to 0.15 mV in women. Other conditions which are treated as a STEMI are: (1) New or presumed new left bundle-branch block (LBBB) and (2) Isolated posterior myocardial infarction (MI). The presence of reciprocal ST-depression helps confirm the diagnosis. The early and accurate identification of the infarct-related artery on the ECG can help predict the amount of myocardium at risk and guide decisions regarding the urgency of revascularization in STEMI.

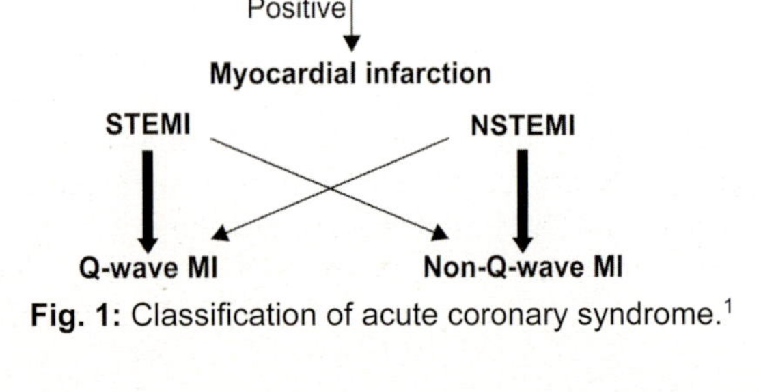

Fig. 1: Classification of acute coronary syndrome.[1]

MYOCARDIAL DISTRIBUTION OF CORONARY ARTERIES

Myocardium is usually supplied by three coronary arteries, although there are several variations in the number, origin, course and distribution of coronary arteries. Major contribution to left ventricular (LV) myocardial blood flow is by left anterior descending (LAD) coronary artery (50%), rest is equally contributed by right coronary artery (RCA), and artery (LCx) left circumflex. In addition, most of the right ventricle is supplied by RCA. The need for a rapid reperfusion therapy is largely determined by how close the occlusion site is to the origin of the coronary artery, which corresponds to the area of ischemic myocardium. Each artery contributes its blood supply to specific regional areas in the heart. The coronary arteries and their relation with ECG is shown in Figure 3[2] and the arterial supply with relation to conducting

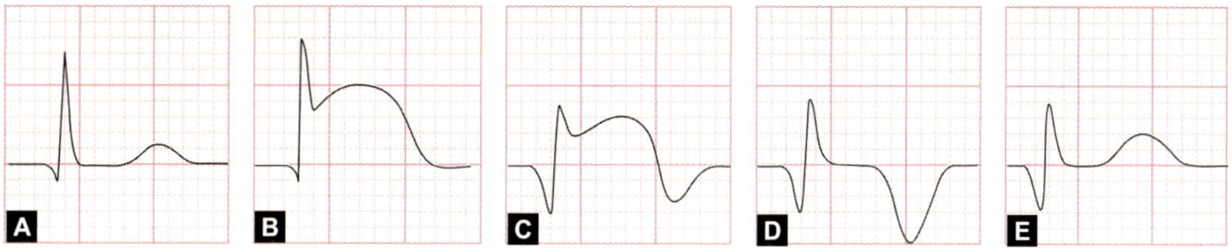

Figs. 2A to E: Typical sequence of ECG evolution in STEMI.[1]

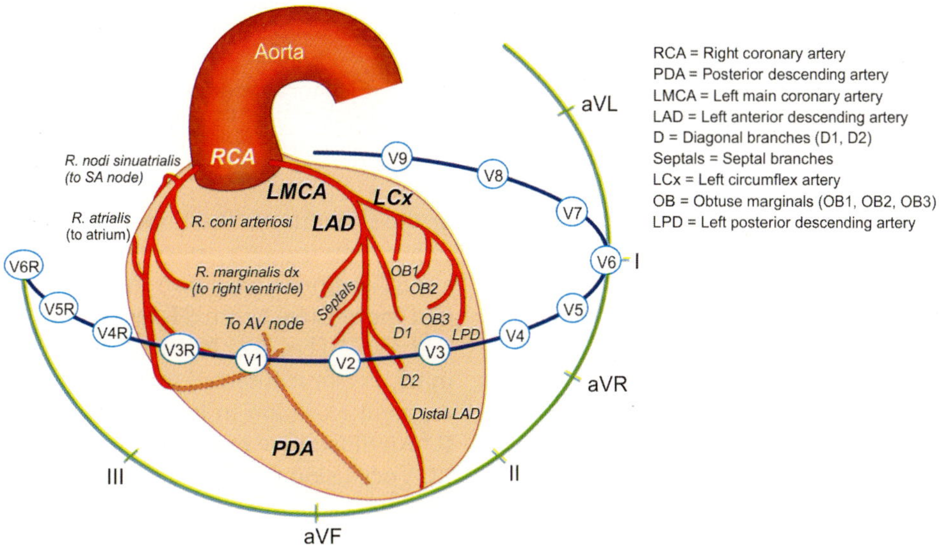

Fig. 3: The coronary arteries and their relation to the ECG leads.[2]

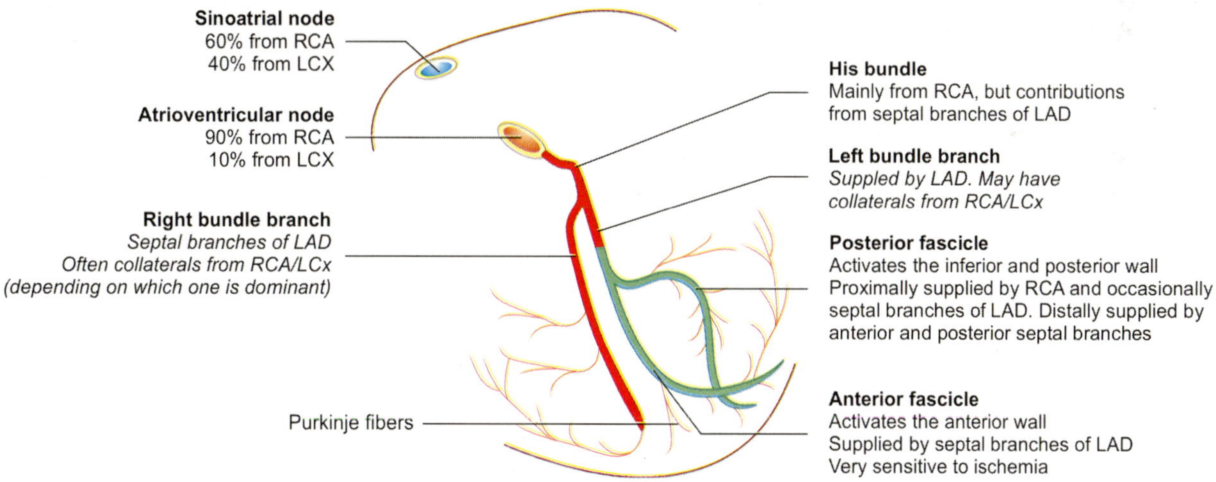

Fig. 4: The arterial supply of the conduction system.[2]

system is shown in Figure 4.[2] The LAD travels along the anterior interventricular groove toward the apex of the heart. The major branches of LAD are septal and diagonal branches. The septal branches arise perpendicularly from the LAD and pass into the interventricular septum. The diagonal branches of the LAD course over the anterolateral aspect of the heart. Considerable variations exist in the number and size of the diagonal branches as shown in Figures 2A to E.[2] In most (80%) patients, the LAD courses around the apex of the left ventricle and terminates along the diaphragmatic aspect of the left ventricle. In the remaining patients, the LAD terminates either at or before the cardiac apex. In these patients, the LV apical portion is supplied by the posterior descending branch (PDA) of the RCA or LCX, which is larger and longer than usual.[3] The LCx artery passes within the left atrioventricular groove toward the inferior interventricular groove. The LCx artery is the dominant vessel in 15% of patients, supplying the left PDA from the distal continuation of the LCx.[3] In the remaining patients, the distal LCx varies in size and length, depending on the number of posterolateral branches supplied by the distal RCA. The major branches of LCx are obtuse marginals, which vary from one to three in number and supply the lateral free wall of the left ventricle as shown in Figure 3.[2] The RCA after originating from the right anterior aortic sinus, courses along the right atrioventricular groove toward the crux. The conus artery arises at the right coronary ostium and is usually the first branch of the RCA. The second branch of the RCA is usually the sinoatrial node artery. This vessel arises from the RCA in about 60% of patients, and from the LCx artery in under 40%, and from both arteries with a dual blood supply in the remaining cases. The mid portion of the RCA usually gives rise to one or several medium-sized acute marginal branches which supply the anterior wall of the right ventricle. The RCA divides at the crux into a PDA and one or more right posterolateral branches as shown in Figure 3.[2]

CORONARY ARTERY DOMINANCE

The right dominant circulation is defined as RCA supplying the PDA and at least one posterolateral branch. This type is present in around 85% of patients. The nondominant RCA is seen in 15% of patients. One half of these patients have left dominant circulation which is defined as distal LCx supplying a left PDA and left posterolateral branches. In these cases, the RCA is very small, ends before reaching the crux, and does not supply any blood to the LV myocardium. The remaining patients have balanced or codominant circulation.[3]

BASIS OF ECG CHANGES

The ECG is a key investigation in diagnosing acute STEMI. During acute transmural ischemia, one of the important determinant of the site of coronary artery occlusion is the direction of the vector of ST-segment deviation.[4] The injury vector is always oriented toward the injured area. The lead facing the injury vector head shows ST-segment elevation and the lead facing the vector tail (opposite leads) shows ST-segment depression.

ACUTE INFERIOR WALL MYOCARDIAL INFARCTION

Inferior wall myocardial infarction (IWMI) may be caused by occlusion in the course of either the RCA (in 80% of the cases)

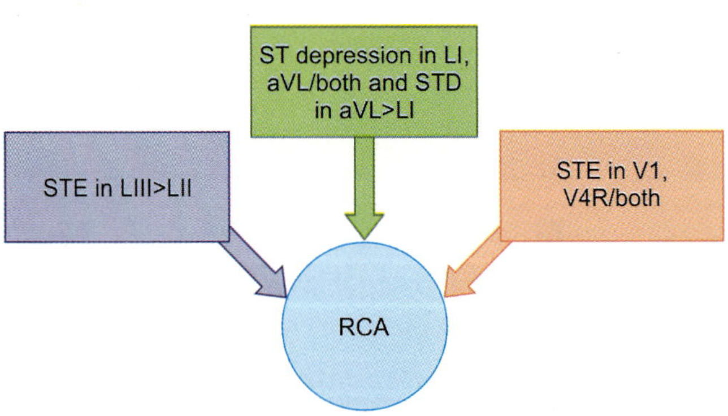

Fig. 5: Electrocardiography predictor of right coronary artery in IWMI.[3]

or the LCx artery. The important features favoring RCA rather than the LCx artery as the culprit artery in IWMI are ST-segment elevation in lead III more than lead II and more than 1 mm ST-segment depression in leads I and aVL[5,6] (Fig. 5).[3] In IWMI caused by RCA occlusion, injury vector is directed toward right (lead III), hence ST-segment elevation in lead III is greater than that in lead II.[6] An illustrative example of a patient with IWMI due to RCA occlusion is shown in Figures 6A and B.[3] One of the important clues that suggests proximal occlusion of the RCA with associated right ventricular infarction in a case of IWMI is the additional finding of ST-segment elevation in lead V1.[7] Conversely, IWMI due to LCx occlusion produces an ST-segment vector directed toward the left (lead II). In this case, ST-segment elevation in lead III is not greater than that in lead II, and there is an isoelectric or elevated ST-segment in lead aVL[8,9](Fig. 7). Associated ST-segment depression in leads V1 and V2 in a case of IWMI suggests concomitant posterior wall MI, which is usually caused by LCx occlusion but may also be seen in dominant RCA occlusion.[10,11]

RIGHT VENTRICULAR MYOCARDIAL INFARCTION

When RCA occlusion occurs proximal to the right ventricular (RV) branch, the right ventricle will be in jeopardy and subsequently infarcted. This concept is the basis for using the ECG findings of RV infarction as an indicator of proximal RCA occlusion.[12] Hence, right ventricular myocardial infarction (RVMI) is always associated with occlusion of the proximal RCA. As discussed before, ST-segment elevation in lead V1 in association with ST-segment elevation in inferior leads (with greater elevation in lead III than in lead II) is highly correlated with the presence of RVMI[5,13] (Fig. 5). ST-segment elevation of more than 1 mm in lead V4R with an upright T wave in that lead is the most sensitive ECG sign of RVMI. This sign is rarely seen more than 12 hours after

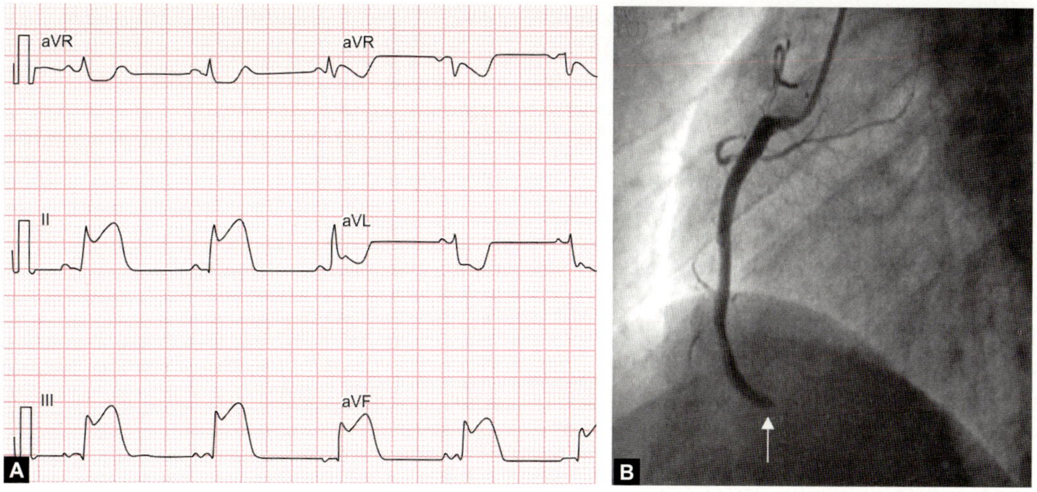

Figs. 6A and B: Inferior wall myocardial infarction-ECG showing ST-elevation in inferior leads with ST-elevation in lead III more than II and ST-depression in LI and aVL suggestive of RCA occlusion.

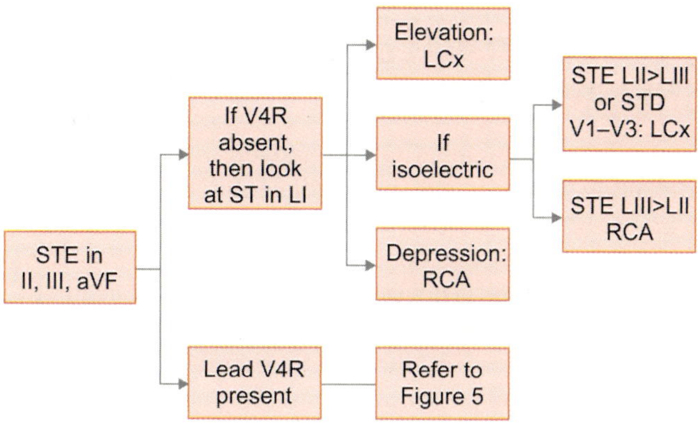

Fig. 7: Algorithm for predicting infarct-related artery in IWMI.[8,9]

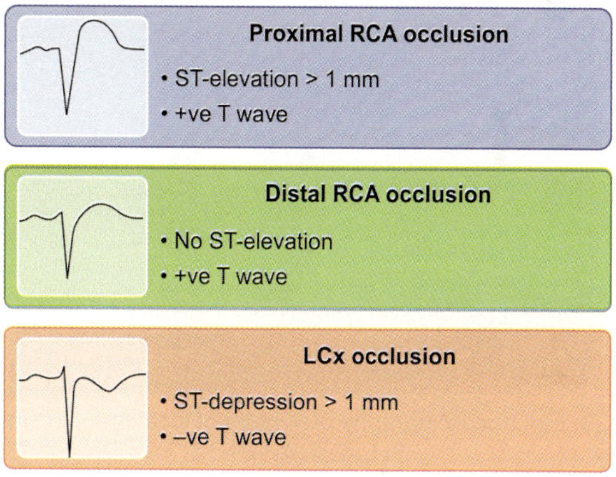

Fig. 8: ST-T changes in lead V4R to predict infarct related artery.[15]

the infarction.[12,13] Lead V4R is helpful in differentiating proximal versus distal RCA occlusion versus LCx occlusion by noting the presence or absence of convex upward ST-segment elevation in V4R and by identifying whether the T wave is positive or negative in V4R (Fig. 7).[15] A QS or QR pattern in leads V3R and/or V4R also suggests right ventricular myocardial necrosis but has less predictive accuracy than ST-segment elevation in these leads (Fig. 8).[16]

ANTERIOR WALL MYOCARDIAL INFARCTION

The amount of LV myocardium at risk of infarction in a case of anterior wall myocardial infarction (AWMI) depends largely on the site of occlusion in the course of LAD. Therefore, knowing the site of LAD occlusion with the help of ECG criteria in the emergency room is of immense help to the treating physician to decide about the plan of further management. Knowing that the occlusion is proximal or distal to first diagonal (D1) or first septal (S1) may be crucial for deciding on the best approach to treatment. LAD occlusion may lead to a very extensive AWMI, or only septal, apical-anterior or mid-anterior MI depending on the location of occlusion.[17] Proximal LAD occlusion has been documented as an independent predictor of worse outcome related to increased mortality and recurrent MI,[18,19] and distal LAD occlusion is considered to have a favorable outcome.[19] Precordial lead (V1-V6) ST-segment elevation in patients with symptoms suggestive of ACS indicates STEMI due to LAD occlusion.[20-24] During acute AWMI, the maximal ST-segment elevation is best recorded in V2 or V3;[25] V2 is the most sensitive lead to record ST-segment elevation (sensitivity 99%) and to identify the culprit lesion at the LAD. Lead V1 captures electrical phenomena from the right paraseptal area, which has dual blood supply by the septal branches of the LAD and by a coronal branch of the RCA. This is the reason why patients with AWMI usually have no ST-segment elevation in V1. The location of occlusion in the course of LAD, whether proximal or distal, can be identified by noting the changes in ST-segment of various leads of surface ECG.[26-] Indicators of proximal LAD occlusion on surface ECG are ST-segment elevation in V1-V3 and in lead aVL with added finding of ST-segment depression of more than 1 mm in lead aVF (Fig. 9).[6,18,26] The most powerful predictors of proximal LAD occlusion include ST-segment elevation in aVL or aVR, concomitant ST-segment depression in inferior leads, ST-segment depression in V5, and disappearance of pre-existent septal Q waves in lateral leads.[18,26,30-33] ST-segment elevation in leads V1, V2 and V3 without significant inferior ST-segment depression suggests occlusion of the LAD beyond the origin of the first diagonal branch.[18] ST-segment elevation in leads V1, V2 and V3 with concomitant elevation in the inferior leads suggests LAD occlusion distal to the origin of the first diagonal branch, in a vessel that wraps around the apex to supply the inferoapical region of the left ventricle. New right bundle-branch block with a Q wave preceding the R wave in lead V1 is a specific but insensitive marker of proximal LAD occlusion in association with AWMI (Fig. 9).[18] An illustrative example of a patient with AWMI due to proximal LAD occlusion is shown in Figures 10A and B. Nevertheless, it is better to have an algorithm based on deviations of ST-segment in 12-lead ECG rather than to assess the ECG criteria separately. An easy to-use, simple, and accurate algorithm (Fig. 11)[34] has been proposed by Fiol et al.[34] based on the evaluation of ST-segment changes in 12-lead ECG which predicts the site of occlusion in LAD in patients with AWMI. This algorithm (Fig. 11)[34] correlated well with angiographic findings.

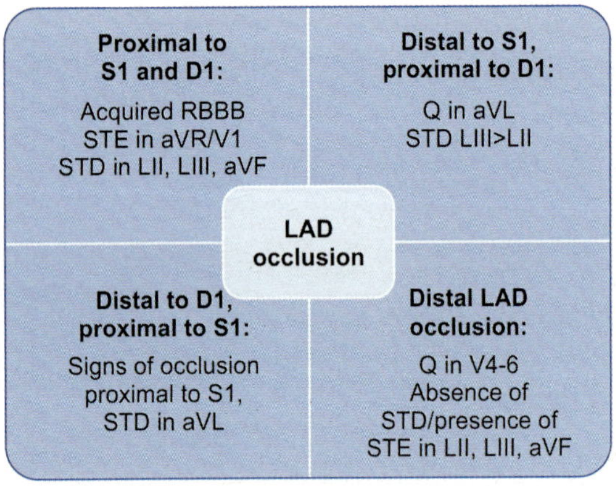

Fig. 9: Electrocardiography predictors of location of occlusion in LAD in AWMI.[18]

POSTERIOR WALL MYOCARDIAL INFARCTION

The standard 12-lead ECG is a relatively insensitive tool for detecting posterior wall myocardial infarction (PWMI).[35,36] This is due to the absence of standard leads facing the posterior wall of LV. In up to 50% of patients with PWMI, ST-segment elevation is not seen on the standard 12-lead ECG. During acute inferior infarction, ST-segment elevation in the posterior chest leads V7 through V9 identifies those patients with concomitant posterior wall involvement. PWMI can be

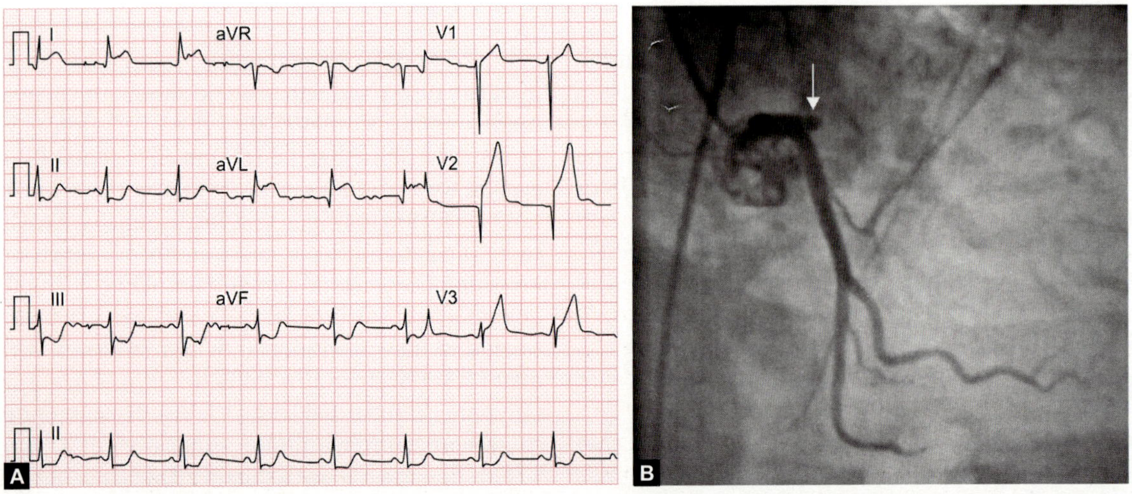

Figs. 10A and B: Anterior wall myocardial infarction. (A) ECG showing ST elevation in leads V2, V3, I, aVL and ST-depression in inferior leads suggestive of proximal LAD occlusion. (B) Left coronary angiogram of the same patient confirming the site of occlusion (arrow) in the proximal LAD.

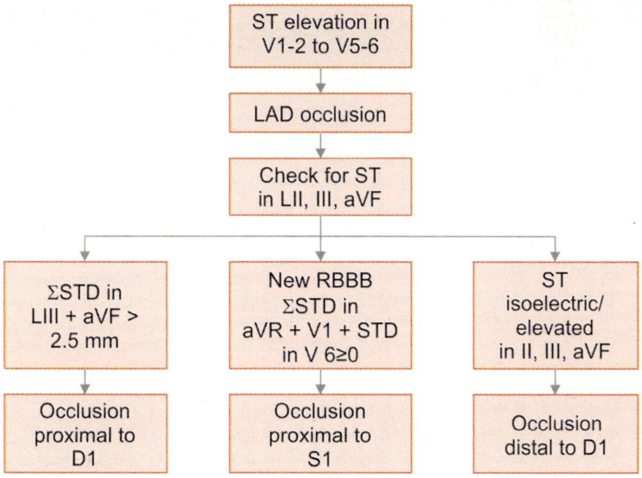

Fig. 11: Algorithm to precisely locate the site of LAD coronary artery occlusion in the case of evolving AWMI.[34]

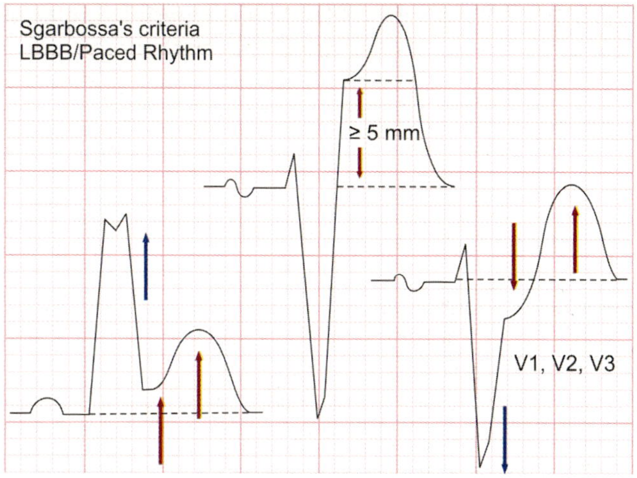

Fig. 12: Three criteria used to diagnosed MI in LBBB also known as Sgarbossa's criteria.[37]

caused by lesions in the RCA or LCx which may be indirectly recognized by reciprocal ST-depression in precordial leads V1-V3. Similar ST changes can also be the primary ECG manifestation of anterior subendocardial ischemia. Posterior inferior wall infarction with reciprocal changes can be differentiated from primary anterior wall ischemia by the presence of ST-segment elevations in posterior leads, although these are not routinely recorded. Patients with an abnormal R wave in V1 (0.04 in duration and/or R/S ratio more than and equal to 1 in the absence of pre-excitation or right ventricular hypertrophy), with inferior or lateral Q waves, have an increased incidence of isolated occlusion of a dominant LCx without collateral circulation. These patients have a lower ejection fraction, increased end-systolic volume, and higher complication rate than patients with IWMI caused by isolated RCA occlusion.[3]

ACUTE MI WITH LBBB OR VENTRICULAR PACED RHYTHM

A new left bundle-branch block (LBBB) or presumably new LBBB in a patient with symptoms consistent with MI should be treated like a STEMI. LBBB or ventricular paced rhythm is associated with ST changes as part of the ECG pattern (discordant changes). Certain ST changes can be used to diagnose acute myocardial infarction in the setting of LBBB mainly called "concordant changes". The three criteria used to diagnose infarction in patients with LBBB also known as Sgarbossa's criteria are: (1) Concordant ST-elevation more than 1 mm in leads with a positive QRS complex (score 5), (2) Concordant ST-depression more than 1 mm in V1-V3 (score 3), and (3) Excessively discordant ST-elevation more than 5 mm in leads with a negative QRS complex (score 2) (Fig. 12). Third criterion is sensitive, but not specific for ischemia in LBBB. It is however, associated with a worse prognosis, when present in LBBB during ischemia. A total score of more than and equal to 3 has a specificity of 90% for diagnosing MI.

EXTENSIVE STEMI WITH "TOMBSTONE" MORPHOLOGY

Electrocardiography (ECG) demonstrating extensive STEMI with "tombstone" morphology has following features: (1) persistent gross ST-elevation in anterior or inferior leads, (2) Early Q wave formation in aVL, and (3) Reciprocal ST-depression in inferior leads in AWMI (Fig. 13)[38] and anterior leads in IWMI. This ECG pattern is seen in proximal LAD occlusion in AWMI and proximal RCA occlusion in IWMI. This pattern is indicative of a large territory infarction with a poor LV ejection fraction and high likelihood of cardiogenic shock and death.[38]

ACUTE MI WITH DE WINTER'S T WAVE

The ECG pattern suggesting de Winter's T wave has following features: ST-depression in V2-5, which slopes upward and joins the ascending limb of the T wave suggesting of de Winter ECG pattern with prominent, "rocket-shaped" T waves in the precordial leads V2-5 with subtle ST-elevation in aVR (Fig. 14).[39] This ECG pattern is now recognized as an anterior STEMI equivalent (~2% of LAD occlusions)[39]and should be treated identically to anterior STEMI, with urgent percutaneous coronary intervention or thrombolysis.

LIMITATIONS OF ELECTROCARDIOGRAM

Assessment of the site of occlusion of a coronary vessel is most reliable in case of a first episode of MI and is impaired

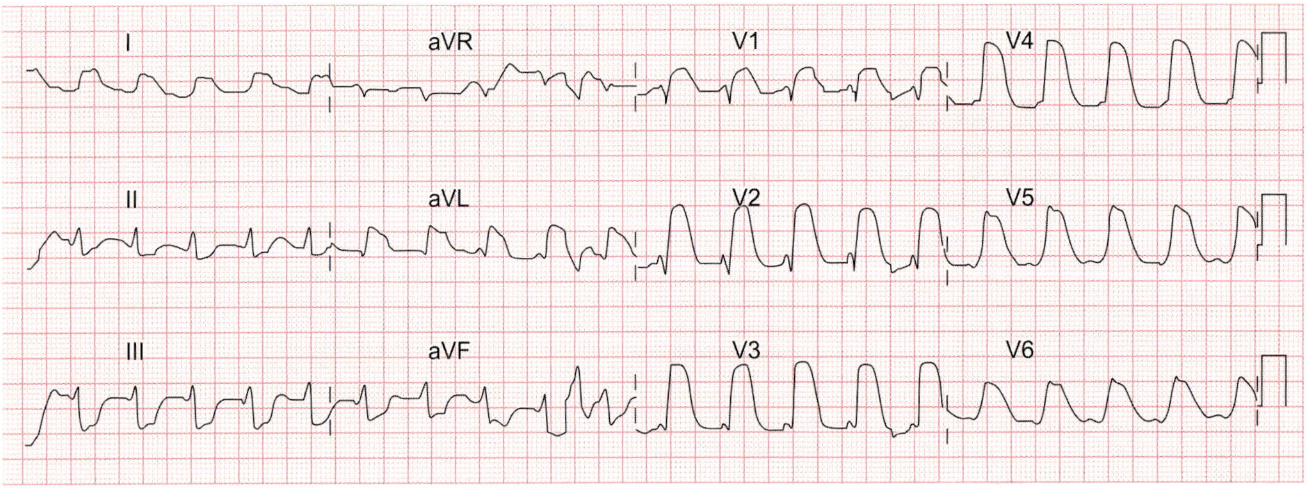

Fig. 13: Twelve lead ECG demonstrating extensive AWMI with "Tombstone" morphology.[38]

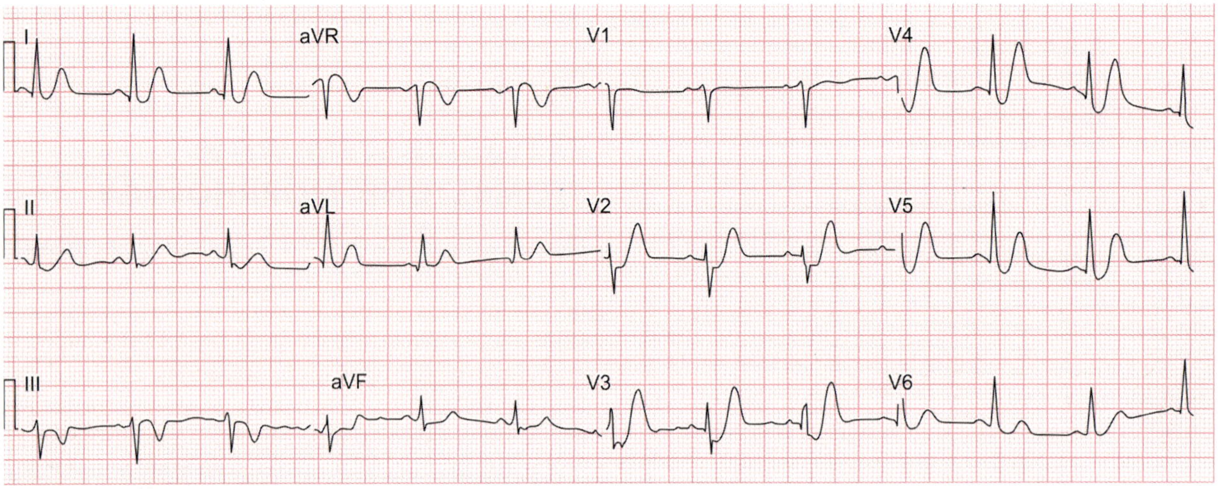

Fig. 14: Twelve lead ECG demonstrating De Winter's T waves suggestive of acute AWMI.[39]

by multivessel disease, an old MI, collateral circulation and when ventricular activation is altered as in pre-existent left bundle branch block, pre-excitation and paced rhythm. The ST-deviation changes with the window period. Hence, these criteria are not so reliable in patients presenting late after the onset of symptoms. The ST-deviation may also change with anteroposterior diameter of the chest and various other extracardiac conditions including chronic obstructive pulmonary disease. These and other criteria proposed for localization of the site of coronary occlusion based on the initial ECG still require additional validation in larger populations. Current and future criteria will always be subject to limitations and exceptions based on variations in coronary anatomy, the dynamic nature of acute ECG changes, the presence of multivessel involvement and the presence of ventricular conduction delays. For example, in some cases, ischemia can affect more than one region of the myocardium (e.g. inferolateral). Not uncommonly, the ECG will show the characteristic findings of involvement in each region. Sometimes, however, partial normalization can result from cancellation of opposing vectorial forces.

CONCLUSION

Despite several limitations described above, the ECG is helpful in diagnosis of acute STEMI and also in identifying the location of occlusion of the coronary arteries in acute STEMI, thereby helping to predict the amount of myocardium at risk and guide decisions regarding the urgency of revascularization. It is better to apply an easy to use, sequential algorithm based on deviations of ST in 12-lead ECG rather than to assess the ECG criteria separately.

REFERENCES

1. O' Gara, Deborah DA, Donald EC, et al. ACCF/AHA Guideline for the management of ST-Elevation myocardial infarction. Circulation. 2013; e362-425.
2. Araz R. Classification of acute coronary syndrome. Guide to ECG Interpretation. www.ecgwaves.com: 2017.
3. Reddy CS, Rajasekhar D, Vanajakshamma V, et al. Electrocardiographic localization of infarct related coronary artery in acute ST elevation myocardial infarction. J Clin Sci Res. 2013;2:151-60.
4. Zimetbaum PJ, Krishnan S, Gold A, et al. Usefulness of ST-segment elevation in lead III exceeding that of lead II for identifying the location of the totally occluded coronary artery in inferior wall myocardial infarction. Am J Cardiol. 1998;81:918-9.
5. Zimetbaum PJ, Josephson ME. Use of ECG in acute myocardial infarction. N Engl J Med. 2003;348:933-40.
6. Wellens HJ. Determining the size of the area at risk, the severity of ischemia, and identifying thesite of occlusion in the culprit coronary artery. In: Wellens HJ, Gorgels AP, Doevendans PA (Eds). The ECG in Acute Myocardial Infarction and Unstable Angina: Diagnosis and Risk Stratification, 2nd edition. Dordrecht: Kluwer Academic Publishers; 2003. pp. 5-42.
7. Herz I, Assali AR, Adler Y, et al. New electrocardiographic criteria for predicting either the right or left circumflex artery as the culprit coronary artery in inferior wall acute myocardial infarction. Am J Cardiol. 1997;80:1343-5.
8. Bairey CN, Shah K, Lew AS, et al. Electrocardiographic differentiation of occlusion of the left circumflex versus the right coronary artery as a cause of inferior acute myocardial infarction. Am J Cardiol. 1987;60:456-9.
9. Bayes de Luna A, Goldwasser D, Fiol M, et al. Surface electrocardiography. In: Fuster V, Walsh RA, Harrington RA (Eds) Hurst's the Heart, 13th edition. New York: McGraw Hill; 2011. pp. 350-8.
10. Hasdai D, Birnbaum Y, Herz I, et al. ST segment depression in lateral limb leads in inferior wall acute myocardial infarction: Implications regarding the culprit artery and the site of obstruction. Eur Heart J. 1995;16:1549-53.
11. Wellens HJ. The ECG in localizing the culprit lesion in acute inferior myocardial infarction: a plea for lead V4R? Europace. 2009;11:1421-2.
12. Braat SH, Brugada P, Wellens HJ, et al. Value of lead V4R for recognition of the infarct coronary artery in acute inferior acute myocardial infarction. Am J Cardiol.1984;53:1538-41.
13. Lopez-Sendon J, Coma-Canella I, Alcasena S, et al. ECG findings in acute right ventricular infarction: sensitivity and specificity of electrocardiographic alterations in right precordial leads V4R, V3R, V1, V2, and V3. J Am Coll Cardiol. 1985;6:1273-9.
14. Klein HO, Tordjman T, Ninio R, et al. The early recognition of right ventricular infarction: diagnostic accuracy of the electrocardiographic V4R lead. Circulation. 1983;67:558-65.
15. Wellens HJ. The value of the right precordial leads of the electrocardiogram. N Engl J Med.1999;340:381-3.
16. Antman EM. ST-segment elevation myocardial infarction: pathology, pathophysiology, and clinical features. Braunwald's heart Disease, 9th edition. Philadelphia: Elsevier Saunders; 2012. pp. 1087-110.
17. Bayés de Luna A, Wagner G, Birnbaum Y, et al. International Society for Holter and Noninvasive Electrocardiography: A new terminology for left ventricular walls and location of myocardial infarcts that present Q wave based on the standard of cardiac magnetic resonance imaging: a statement for healthcare professionals from a committee appointed by the International Society for Holter and Noninvasive Electrocardiography. Circulation. 2006;114:1755-60.
18. Engelen DJ, Gorgels AP, Cheriex EC, et al. Value of the electrocardiogram in localizing the occlusion site in the left anterior descending coronary artery in acute anterior myocardial infarction. J Am Coll Cardiol. 1999;34:389-95.
19. Karha J, Murphy SA, Kirtane AJ, et al. TIMI Study Group: Evaluation of the association of proximal coronary culprit artery lesion location with clinical outcomes in acute myocardial infarction. Am J Cardiol.2003;92:913-8.
20. Bayés de Luna A (Ed). Clinical Electrocardiography: A Textbook, 2nd edition. Armonk: Futura Publications; 1998. pp. 867-8.
21. Wellens HJ, Gorgels AM, Doevendans PAFM (Eds). The ECG in the acute myocardial infarction. Boston: Kluwer Academic Publishers; 2003.
22. Sclarowsky S (Ed). Electrocardiography of acute myocardial ischaemia. London: Martin Dunitz; 1999.
23. Fiol M, Cygankiewicz I, Guindo J, et al. Evolving myocardial infarction with ST-elevation: Ups and downs of ST in different leads identifies the culprit artery and location of the occlusion. Ann Noninv Electrocardiol. 2004;9:180-6.
24. Aldrich HR, Hindman NB, Hinoara T, et al. Identification of optimal electrocardiographic leads for detecting acute epicardial injury in acute myocardial infarction. Am J Cardiol. 1987;59:20-3.
25. Birnbaum Y, Sclarovsky S, Solodky A. Prediction of the level of left anterior descending coronary artery obstruction during anterior wall acute myocardial infarction by the admission electrocardiogram. Am J Cardiol. 1993;72:823-6.
26. Tamura A, Kataoka H, Mikuriya Y, et al. Inferior ST segment depression as a useful marker for identifying proximal left anterior descending artery occlusion during acute anterior myocardial infarction. Eur Heart J. 1995;16:1795-9.
27. Sapin PM, Musselman DR, Dehmer GJ, et al. Implications of inferior ST-segment elevation accompanying anterior wall acute myocardial infarction for the angiographic morphology of the left anterior descending coronary artery morphology and site of occlusion. Am J Cardiol. 1992;69:860-5.
28. Kim TY, Alturk N, Shaikh N, et al. An electrocardiographic algorithm for the prediction of the culprit lesion site in acute anterior myocardial infarction. Clin Cardiol. 1999;22:77-83.
29. Senaratne MP, Weerasinghe C, Smith G, et al. Clinical utility of ST-segment depression in lead aVR in acute myocardial infarction. J Electrocardiol. 2003;36:11-6.

30. Birnbaum Y, Sclarovsky S, Solodky A. Prediction of the level of left anterior descending coronary artery obstruction during anterior wall acute myocardial infarction by the admission electrocardiogram. Am J Cardiol. 1993;72:823-6.
31. Yotsukura M, Toyofuku M, Tajino K. Clinical significance of the disappearance of septal Q waves after the onset of myocardial infarction: correlation with location of responsible coronary lesions. J Electrocardiol. 1999;32:15-20.
32. Tamura A, Kataoka H, Mikuriya Y. Electrocardiographic findings in a patient with pure septal infarction. Br Heart J. 1991;65:166-7.
33. Vasudevan K, Manjunath CN, Srinivas KH, et al. Electrocardiographic localization of the occlusion site in left anterior descending in acute anterior myocardial infarction. Indian Heart J. 2004;56:315-9.
34. Fiol M, Carillo A, Cygankiewicz I et al. A new electrocardiographic algorithm to locate the occlusion in left anterior descending coronary artery. Clin Cardiol. 2009;32:E1-6.
35. Perloff JK. The recognition of strictly posterior myocardial infarction by conventional scalar electrocardiography. Circulation. 1964;30:706-18.
36. Movahed A, Becker LC. Electrocardiography changes of acute lateral wall myocardial infarction: a reappraisal based on scintigraphic localization of the infarct. J Am Coll Cardiol. 1984;4:660-6.
37. Sgarbossa EB, Pinski SL, Barbagelata A, et al. Electrocardiographic diagnosis of evolving acute myocardial infarction in the presence of left bundle-branch block. GUSTO-1 (Global Utilization of Streptokinase and Tissue Plasminogen Activator for Occluded Coronary Arteries) Investigators. N Engl J Med. 1996;334:481-7.
38. Guo XH, Yap YG, Chen LJ, et al. Correlation of coronary angiography with "tombstoning" electrocardiographic pattern in patients after acute myocardial infarction. Clin Cardiol. 2000;23:347-52.
39. De Winter RJ, Verouden NJW, Wellens HJJ, et al. A new ECG sign of proximal LAD occlusion. N Engl J Med. 2008;359:2071-3.

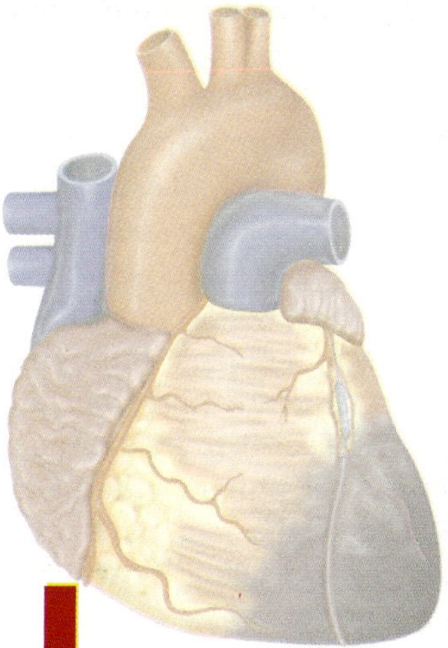

27

CHAPTER

Advances in Echocardiographic Navigation of STEMI Complications

Santanu Guha, Somnath Mukhopadhyay, Avik Karak

INTRODUCTION

A broad range of complications occurs after acute myocardial infarction (AMI), some of which are life-threatening. Usually, these are mechanical and electrical. Echocardiography is the mainstay of noninvasive diagnosis for the mechanical complications which range from cardiogenic shock due to the loss of critical mass of myocardium to development of left ventricular (LV) thrombus, ventricular septal rupture, free wall rupture, papillary muscle rupture, dynamic left ventricular outflow tract (LVOT) obstruction, and right ventricular (RV) infarction.

LEFT VENTRICULAR THROMBUS

Previous studies showed that 1.5–3.6% of AMIs are complicated by systemic embolism[1] and mural thrombus of LV is most often responsible. The risk varies with location and size of myocardial infarction (MI). Gruppo Italiano per lo Studio della Sopravvivenza nell'Infarto (GISSI)-3 database revealed prevalence of 5.1% of LV thrombus in postfibrinolytic AMI group by predischarge transthoracic echocardiography. Anterior wall MI has higher risk of developing this complication compared to other locations (11.5% vs. 2.3%).[2]

The most common location of LV thrombus is apex which is often akinetic. Two-dimensional (2D) echocardiography is most frequently used imaging modality and for the detection and apical view is the best window to visualize the LV thrombus. It is usually appeared as nonhomogeneous echodensity with a margin distinct from the underlying dyskinetic or akinetic LV apex.[3] This characteristic appearance differentiates it from chordate tendineae or artifacts. A protruding or freely mobile thrombus is the predictor of systemic embolization.[4] Contrast echocardiography is particularly helpful in cases of poor acoustic window or and in prominent LV muscle bands or trabeculations. Contrast echocardiography has superior sensitivity and accuracy in detecting thrombus when compared to noncontrast echocardiography.[5]

Systemic anticoagulation is recommended in patients with LV thrombus after an acute MI to reduce the risk of embolization (Fig. 1).[6]

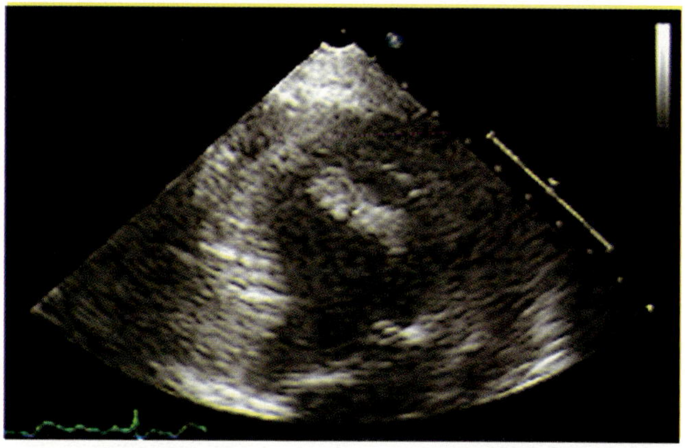

Fig. 1: Organized thrombus in the LV.

POSTINFARCTION VENTRICULAR SEPTAL RUPTURE

Ventricular septal rupture (VSR) is not a common complication occurring in less than 1%. However, the incidence is higher in cardiogenic shock [3.9% in the Should We Emergently Revascularize Occluded Coronaries for Cardiogenic Shock (SHOCK)] Trial Registry and randomized SHOCK Trial).[7] VSR typically presents with holosystolic murmur with a thrill in precordium and progressive hemodynamic deterioration. Apically located VSRs are most commonly associated with an anterior wall MI, whereas an inferior wall MI is associated with VSRs in the posterobasal region. A postinfarction VSR should be suspected in presence of severe wall motion abnormalities of the distal ventricular septum. Color Doppler imaging typically demonstrates a shunt from the LV to RV. Continuous wave (CW) Doppler interrogation corresponds to the pressure gradient between the LV and the RV, and can therefore estimate RV systolic pressure (RV systolic pressure = systolic blood pressure - pressure gradient between LV and RV; in the absence of LVOT or aortic valve obstruction). In addition CW, Doppler assessment may reveal a nearly continuous shunt through VSR except during early diastole. This diastolic left to right shunt is secondary to an elevated LV diastolic pressure in the setting of acute MI. The magnitude of the left to right shunt and the intensity of the systolic murmur are inversely proportional to the size of the infarct and directly related to the preserved residual LV systolic function (Fig. 2).[8]

LEFT VENTRICULAR FREE WALL RUPTURE

This complication is the second most common cause of mortality following cardiogenic shock, in patients of AMI. Incidence is estimated to be around 6% (2.7% in SHOCK Trial Registry), but it can account for 15% in-hospital mortality after an AMI.[7] The most frequent and catastrophic presentation of free wall rupture is electromechanical dissociation due to cardiac tamponade. However, it can present in a more stuttering manner also. In such patients, early diagnosis and prompt surgical intervention are necessary. Echocardiography is the diagnostic modality of choice. Appearance of pericardial effusion in a patient of sudden hemodynamic compromise after an AMI should suggest the diagnosis. Enlarging pericardial effusion with echodense structures (thrombus) are characteristically noted. When this is seen in the background of hemodynamic compromise, it has greater than 98% specificity for free wall rupture.[9] Echocardiography is useful in locating the point of rupture, which is typically at the junction of normal and infracted myocardium.

Myocardial scar formation thinning with subsequent expansion of LV may lead to LV apical aneurysm. In some patient, either the rupture occurs over time or the perforation is incomplete, leading to the development of pseudoaneurysm. These remain somewhat contained within a limited segment of pericardium and are commonly in the inferolateral or inferoposterior walls. Echocardiography can demonstrate a pseudoaneurysm cavity that communicates with the LV chamber via a narrow neck (diameter of entry site less than half of maximal diameter of the pseudoaneurysm) and frequently contains thrombus. Color Doppler imaging can detect characteristic to and fro blood flow through the site of rupture (Figs. 3 to 5).

ACUTE MITRAL REGURGITATION AND PAPILLARY MUSCLE RUPTURE

Prevalence of mitral regurgitation (MR) is up to 50% with AMI. Presence of MR portends a worse short-term

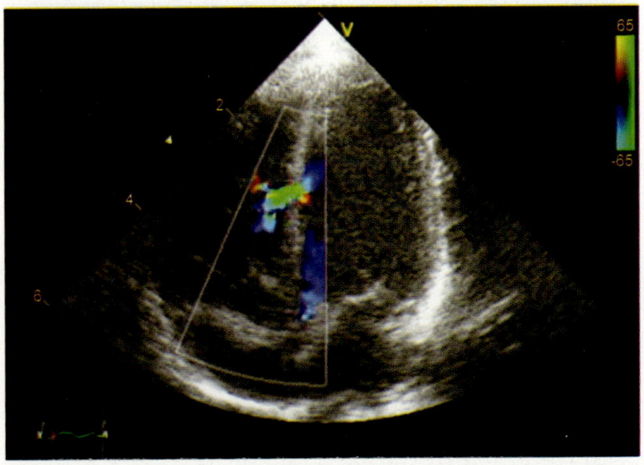

Fig. 2: Ventricular septal rupture.

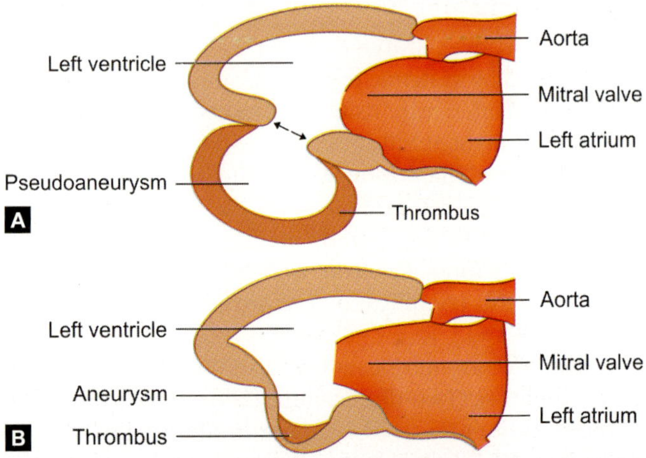

Figs. 3A and B: (A) Showing pseudoaneurysm after MI, (B) Showing true aneurysm.

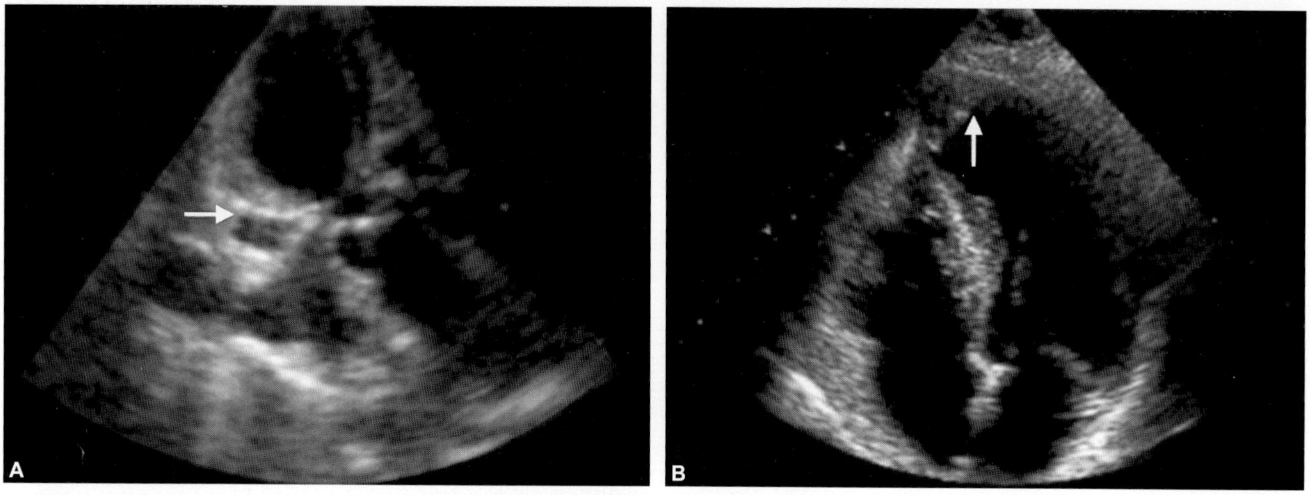

Figs. 4A and B: (A) Apical three-chamber view of inferior wall MI showing basal posterior pseudoaneurysm; (B) Apical four-chamber view showing LV thrombus.

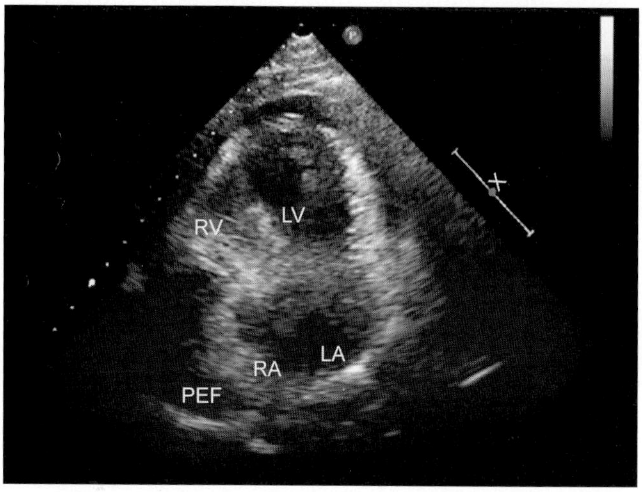

Fig. 5: Left ventricular free wall rupture.

and long-term prognosis.[10,11] Acute MR in AMI can be caused by several mechanisms like: (1) dilatation of mitral annulus secondary to LV dilatation, (2) papillary muscle displacement or dysfunction due to proximity of the insertion of the papillary muscle to the infracted myocardium, and (3) papillary muscle or chordal rupture.[3]

Most cases of MR are transient and asymptomatic. But, papillary muscle rupture is rare and life-threatening. Previous studies showed that papillary muscle rupture complicates approximately 1–3% of AMIs with a mortality of 80% when treated with medical therapy alone.[12] The classic presentation is acute pulmonary edema and cardiogenic shock after 3–5 days of AMI.[13] A new holosystolic murmur is found in physical examination, but the intensity of the murmur does not necessarily correlate with the severity. Rapid equalization of pressure between LV and LA may reduce the intensity and duration of the murmur.

Again, echocardiography plays an important role in diagnosing the presence and etiology. It can also rule out other causes of systolic murmur after MI. Common 2D features include a flail mitral leaflet with severed chordate or papillary muscle head moving freely within the left heart. Complete transection of the papillary muscle is rare, whereas rupture of the tip is more common.[14] Rupture of the posteromedial papillary muscle is 6–10 times more common (because of single coronary artery supply) than anterolateral papillary muscle (having dual coronary artery supply).[3] LV function is often found hyperdynamic due to sudden reduction in afterload, and regional wall motion abnormalities may be subtle or unrecognized.[13] Color Doppler imaging typically reveals eccentric MR which may lead to underestimation of the degree of MR. Usually, transthoracic windows are found poor as the patient is in respiratory distress or hemodynamic compromise and a transesophageal echocardiography (TEE) may be required for diagnosis. Afterload reduction and prompt surgery is the mainstay of treatment (Figs. 6A and B).

LEFT VENTRICULAR OUTFLOW TRACT OBSTRUCTION

In recent years, dynamic LVOT obstruction has been increasingly recognized as a complication of acute anterior wall MI.[15-18] Compensatory hyperdynamic contraction of the basal inferolateral and inferior segments, in the setting of anteroapical MI and LV apical akinesia, is the presumed underlying mechanism. Hyperkinesia of the basal segment leads to reduction of LVOT cross-sectional area, accelerated blood flow across the LVOT, systolic anterior motion (SAM) of anterior mitral leaflet, and ultimately leading to LVOT obstruction. Significant posteriorly directed MR may also

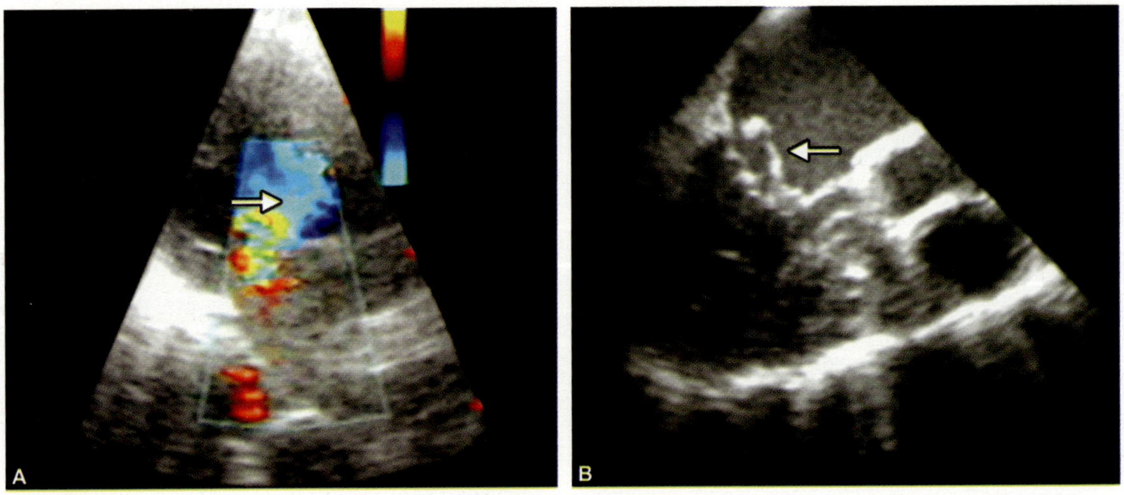

Figs. 6A and B: (A) Severe eccentric MR in inferior wall MI; (B) TEE showing ruptured papillary muscle in same patient.

lead to acute pulmonary edema. The incidence of dynamic LVOT obstruction after an acute MI is unknown. It is thought to be more common among women and in elderly patients having small LVOT area or basal septal hypertrophy due to chronic hypertension.[3,19]

Transthoracic echocardiography is the diagnostic modality of choice to assess LVOT obstruction, whereas TEE can be used for suboptimal acoustic windows. Common 2D echocardiography features include hypokinesia of anteroapical segments and hyperkinesia of basal segments and SAM of mitral valve. Color Doppler imaging will demonstrate turbulent flow across LVOT and posteriorly directed MR jet. CW Doppler of the LVOT from apical window will reveal dragger-shaped late peaking systolic jet where peak velocity corresponds to the degree of LVOT obstruction. The most important treatment strategy for these cases is intravenous fluid infusion, discontinuation of vasodilators or inotropes and administration of beta-blockers, alpha-agonists or both.

RIGHT VENTRICULAR INFARCTION

About half of acute inferior wall MIs are complicated by RV infarction. Significant hemodynamic compromise is relatively infrequent and long-term prognosis is usually favorable.[20] But according to the data of SHOCK Trial Registry, cardiogenic shock from RV infarction has similar risk of mortality when compared to those having cardiogenic shock from LV infarctions.[21]

Echocardiographic features of RV infarction have been noted in a few small studies. These include dilatation of RV cavity, variable degree of wall motion abnormalities in the RV free wall, systolic paradoxical ventricular septal motion, plethora of inferior vena cava, reduced RV ejection fraction, and reduced tricuspid annular plane systolic excursion.[22,23] Some studies have also demonstrated that the tissue Doppler systolic velocity (S') of the lateral tricuspid annulus is not only a sensitive and specific marker of RV involvement in an inferior wall MI, but also an independent predictor of cardiovascular outcome.[24,25] It is important to look carefully for other causes of RV enlargement and dysfunction, such as pulmonary hypertension and pulmonary embolism.

In patients who develop hypoxemia after an inferior wall MI, RV infarction and a clinically significant right to left shunt through a patent foramen ovale should be considered. This happens due to impaired RV compliance and elevated right atrial pressure in such cases. Color Doppler imaging or injection of agitated saline may help to establish the diagnosis. Alternatively, TEE may be the imaging test of choice having suboptimal acoustic window.

REFERENCES

1. Vaitcus PT, Barnathan ES. Embolic potential, prevention and management of mural thrombus complicating anterior myocardial infarction: a meta-analysis. J Am Coll Cardiol. 1993;22(4):1004-9.
2. Chiarella F, Santoro E, Domenicucci S, et al. Predischarge two-dimensional echocardiographic evaluation of left ventricular thrombosis after acute myocardial infarction in the GISSI-3 study. Am J Cardiol. 1998;81:822-7.
3. Oh JK, Seward JB, Tajik AJ (Eds). Coronary artery disease and acute myocardial infarction. The Echo Manual. 3. Philadelphia, Baltimore, New York, London, Buenos Aires, Hong Kong, Sydney, Tokyo: Lippincott Williams & Wilkins (a Wolters Kluwer business); 2006. pp. 154-74.
4. Visser CA, Kan G, Meltzer RS, et al. Embolic potential of left ventricular thrombus after myocardial infarction: a two-dimensional echocardiographic study of 119 patients. J Am Coll Cardiol. 1985;5:1276-80.
5. Mansencal N, Revault-d'Allonnes L, Pelage JP, et al. Usefulness of contrast echocardiography for assessment left

ventricular thrombus after acute myocardial infarction. Am J Cardiol. 2007;99:1667-70.

6. O'Gara PT, Kushner FG, Ascheim DD, et al. 2013 ACCF/AHA guideline for the management of ST-elevation myocardial infarction: a report of the ACCF/AHA Task Force on Practice Guideline. J Am Coll Cardiol. 2013;61:e78-140.
7. Hochman JS, Buller CE, Sleeper LA, et al. Cardiogenic shock complicating acute myocardial infarction—etiologies, management and outcome: a report from the SHOCK Trial Registry. J Am Coll Cardiol. 2000;36(3 suppl A):1063-70.
8. Helmcke F, Mahan EF 3rd, Nanda NC, et al. Two-dimensional echocardiography and Doppler color flow mapping in the diagnosis and prognosis of ventricular septal rupture. Circulation. 1990;81:1775-83.
9. López-Sendón J, González A, López de Sá E, et al. Diagnosis of subacute ventricular wall rupture after acute myocardial infarction: sensitivity and specificity of clinical, hemodynamic and echocardiographic criteria. J Am Coll Cardiol. 1992;19:1145-53.
10. Lehmann KG, Francis CK, Dodge HT. Mitral regurgitation in early myocardial infarction. Incidence, clinical detection, and prognostic implications. TIMI Study Group. Ann Intern Med. 1992;117:10-7.
11. Picard MH, Davidoff R, Sleeper LA, et al. Echocardiographic predictors of survival and response to early revascularization in cardiogenic shock. Circulation. 2003;107:279-84.
12. Stout KK, Verrier ED. Acute valvular regurgitation. Circulation. 2009;119:3232-41.
13. Sia YT, O'Meara E, Ducharme A. Role of echocardiography in acute myocardial infarction. Curr Heart Fail Rep. 2008;5:189-96.
14. Antman EA, Morrow DA. ST-segment elevation myocardial infarction: management. In: Bonow RO, Mann DL, Zipes DP, Libby P (Eds). Braunwald's Heart Disease: A Textbook of Cardiovascular Medicine, 9th edition. Philadelphia: Elsevier; 2012. pp. 1111-7.
15. Armstrong WF, Marcovitz PA. Dynamic left ventricular outflow tract obstruction as a complication of acute myocardial infarction. Am Heart J. 1996;131:827-30.
16. Bartunek J, Vanderheyden M, de Bruyne B. Dynamic left ventricular outflow tract obstruction after anterior myocardial infarction. A potential mechanism of myocardial rupture. Eur Heart J. 1995;16:1439-42.
17. Haley JH, Sinak LJ, Tajik AJ, et al. Dynamic left ventricular outflow tract obstruction in acute coronary syndromes: an important cause of new systolic murmur and cardiogenic shock. Mayo Clin Prac. 1999;74:901-6.
18. Joffe II, Riley MF, Katz SE, et al. Acquired dynamic left ventricular outflow tract obstruction complicating acute anterior myocardial infarction: serial echocardiographic and clinical examination. J Am Soc Echocardiogr. 1997;10: 717-21.
19. Matyal R, Warraich HJ, Karthik S, et al. Anterior myocardial infarction with dynamic left ventricular outflow tract obstruction. Ann Thorac Surg. 2011;91:e39-40.
20. Kinch JW, Ryan TJ. Right ventricular infarction. N Engl J Med. 1994;330:1211-7.
21. Jacobs AK, Leopold JA, Bates E, et al. Cardiogenic shock caused by right ventricular infarction: a report from the SHOCK Registry. J Am Coll Cardiol. 2003;41:1273-9.
22. D 'Arey B, Nanda NC. Two-dimensional echocardiographic features of right ventricular infarction. Circulation. 1982;65:167-73.
23. Goldberger JJ, Himelman RB, Wolfe CL, et al. Right ventricular infarction: recognition and assessment of its hemodynamic significance by two-dimensional echocardiography. J Am Soc Echocardiogr. 1991;4:140-6.
24. Dokainish H, Abbey H, Gin K, et al. Usefulness of tissue Doppler imaging in the diagnosis and prognosis of acute right ventricular infarction with inferior wall acute left ventricular infarction. Am J Cardiol. 2005;95:1039-42.
25. Kakouros N, Kakouros S, Lekakis J, et al. Tissue Doppler imaging of the tricuspid annulus and myocardial performance indexing the evaluation of right ventricular involvement in the acute and late phase of a first inferior myocardial infarction. Echocardiography. 2011;28:311-9.

28

CHAPTER

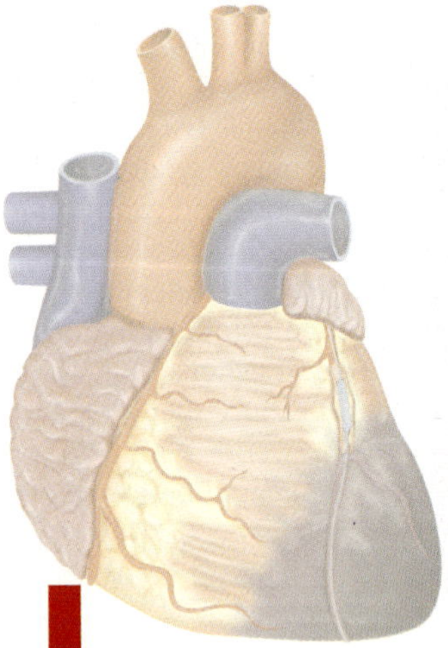

Coronary Artery Disease and Advances in Intravascular Ultrasound Imaging

Satyavan Sharma, Nikhil Raut

INTRODUCTION

Intravascular ultrasound (IVUS) is used in cardiac catheterization laboratory as a diagnostic modality, which provides cross-sectional imaging of coronary arteries. Bom and colleagues[1] developed the first ultrasound system nearly four decades ago. Over the years, IVUS has become an established imaging technology to provide insights into atherosclerosis, plaque morphology and practical guidance for percutaneous coronary intervention (PCI). Optical coherence tomography (OCT) is an alternate emerging coronary imaging technology.

This topic will be discussed under the following sub-headings:

- Basics of IVUS
- Normal vessel morphology and measurements
- Differences between OCT and IVUS
- Imaging of coronary atherosclerosis
- Clinical uses of IVUS:
  - Assessment of ischemia producing lesions
  - Left main coronary artery (LMCA)-PCI
  - Non-LMCA-PCI
  - Stent thrombosis (ST)
  - To prevent contrast-induced nephropathy
  - Chronic total occlusions (CTO)
- Lessons from the trials
- Guidelines.

BASICS OF INTRAVASCULAR ULTRASOUND

The IVUS imaging systems utilize reflected sound waves to image the vessel wall in a two-dimensional format analogs to a histological cross-section. The IVUS equipment consists of a catheter incorporating a miniaturized transducer and a console to reconstruct and display the images. IVUS catheters have the ability to display blood flow in color to facilitate distinction between lumen and wall boundaries. The current generation catheters range from 2.6 to 3.2 French in size and can be introduced through conventional 6 French guide catheters. IVUS transducer converts electrical energy into acoustical energy through piezoelectric crystalline material that expands and contracts to produce sound waves when electrically excited.[2] Several properties such as resolution, depth of penetration, and attenuation of the acoustic are dependent on the geometry and frequency of the transducer. The higher the frequency, better the axial resolution but lower the depth of penetration. For coronary imaging ultrasound, frequencies are centered at 20–40 MHz. IVUS uses an electronically generated scale with measurements performed using direct planimetry. There are two types of IVUS transducer systems. The rotational mechanical IVUS probes rotate a single piezoelectrical transducer at 1800 rpm and operate at frequencies between 30 MHz and 45 MHz whereas the electronically switched phased array systems operate at a central frequency of 20 MHz. Higher ultrasound frequencies are associated with better image resolution, but increasing the frequency beyond 45 MHz has been limited due to decreased tissue penetration.[2] With both systems, still frames and video images can be digitally achieved on local storage memory or a remote server using digital imaging and communications in medicine.

There are five companies that make IVUS equipment: (1) Boston Scientific, (2) Volcano, (3) Terumo, (4) Infraredx, and (5) ACIST. All five manufacture an IVUS catheter containing a rotating-transducer within a short-monorail imaging sheath to create cross-sectional IVUS images. All commercially available IVUS technologies produce equally valid diagnostic information, especially in the setting of PCI.[3] Newer applications like virtual histology (VH) and radiofrequency (RF)-IVUS allow to characterize plaque morphology and quantification of different components. It can also accurately quantify large lipid pool and visualize the entire vessel wall even in presence of large plaque burden. The most recent advance is the development of a single image catheter that permits simultaneous imaging with both IVUS (including RF analysis) and OCT during a single pull back.

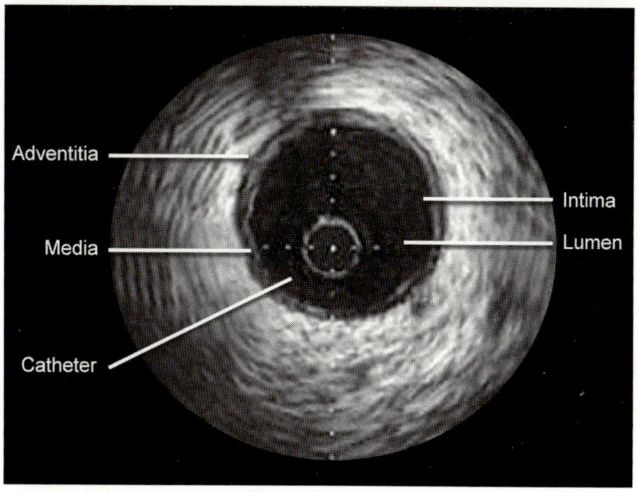

Fig. 1: Intravascular ultrasound image showing the trilaminar appearance of normal coronary arterial wall cross-section.

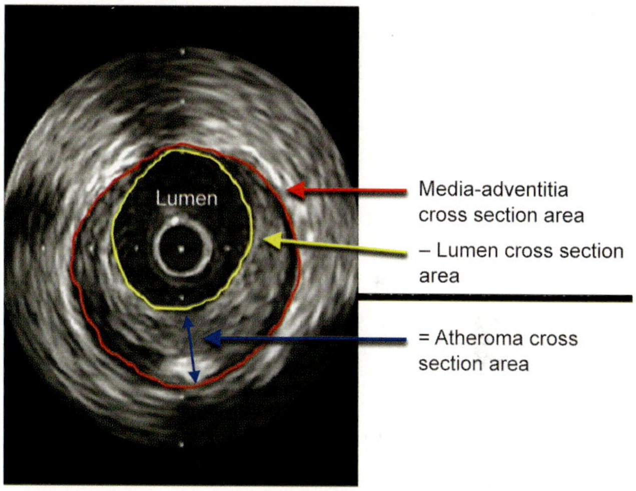

Fig. 2: Basic intravascular ultrasound measurements showing lesion severity.

NORMAL VESSEL MORPHOLOGY AND MEASUREMENTS

The interpretation of IVUS images is possible as the layers of a diseased arterial wall can be identified separately. In coronary vessel, the media of the vessel is characterized by a dark band compared with intima and adventitia. There are certain artifacts common during image acquisition. Qualitative and quantitative IVUS analysis are usually performed according to the American College of Cardiology Clinical Expert Consensus Document on standard for acquisition, measurement, and reporting of IVUS studies.[2] A motorized pullback device is used to image the entire vessel. Lumen cross-sectional area (CSA) is quantified by planimetry of the leading edge of the blood-intimal acoustic interface. The outer vessel border external elastic membrane (EEM)-CSA is detected as the interface between media and adventitia. Atheroma-CSA is calculated as the difference between EEM-CSA and lumen-CSA. Figure 1 delineates the cross-sectional image. Basic IVUS measurements for assessing lesion severity are shown in Figure 2.

DIFFERENCES BETWEEN IVUS AND OCT

Intravascular ultrasound uses ultrasound whereas OCT uses infrared. There are several key differences between IVUS and OCT (Table 1). The IVUS has useful applications even in the era of OCT. Because of shallower penetration, OCT may not be able to visualize the whole vessel structure including external elastic lamina, especially in presence of heavily lipid rich plaque burden. IVUS is superior in assessment of vascular remodeling and atheroma regression in atherosclerosis progression or regression trials. An Achilles heel of OCT is aortic ostia lesion, which cannot be visualized properly due to requirement of blood clearance. IVUS provides better information of this location. Many interventional cardiologists prefer IVUS guidance during PCI of ostia, left main and bifurcations. Another useful feature of IVUS that is lacking with OCT is full-thickness visibility of the vessel wall, which enables measurement of vessel size and achievement of large stent areas with low-risk of vessel perforation.

IMAGING OF CORONARY ATHEROSCLEROSIS

Atherosclerosis is the main cause of coronary artery disease (CAD) and continues to be a major health burden around

TABLE 1: Differences between intravascular ultrasound (IVUS) and optical coherence tomography (OCT).

	IVUS	*OCT*
Wave source	Ultrasound (10–40 MHz)	Near-infrared light
Acquisition speed	0.5 mm/s	25 mm/s
Axial resolution (µm)	100–150 µm	10–20 µm
Lateral resolution	200 µm	20 µm
Penetration depth (mm)	4–8 mm	2 mm
Minimum guide catheter size	5 French (Fr)	5 French (6 Fr preferable)
Aorto-ostial lesion visualization	+	–
Blood clearance	Not required	Contrast 10–15 mL

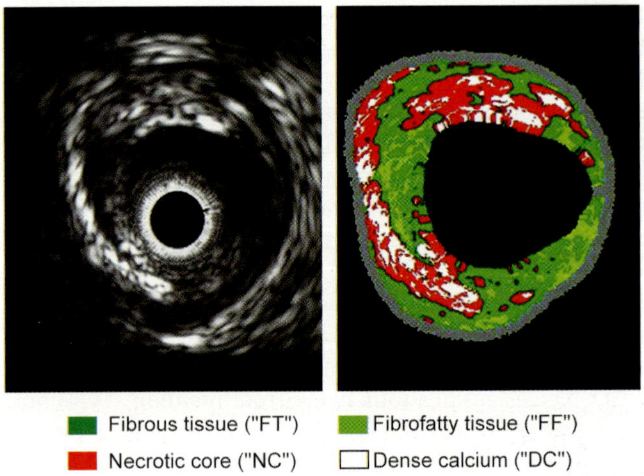

Fig. 3: Composition of atheroma plaque on intravascular ultrasound.

the globe. The process begins with accumulation of low-density lipoprotein (LDL) particles, cell death and formation of complex atherosclerotic plaques. At early stages of atheroma formation, there is remodeling of the vessel wall, which prevents plaques from encroaching on the lumen. Coronary angiography (CAG) fails to appreciate these changes. The intravascular imaging has played a key role in understanding the pathophysiology of CAD and various therapeutic and research applications. CAG depicts arteries as a planar silhouette of the contrast-filled lumen. A major limitation of CAG is that it fails to accurately determine anatomy, as it produces a two-dimensional representation of a three-dimensional coronary lumen. In addition, diffuse reference vessel disease, lesion foreshortening, angulations, calcification, eccentricity, vessel overlap, and streaming of contrast can complicate angiographic assessment of lesion severity. Table 2 summarizes other limitations of CAG. Angiographic assessment of atherosclerosis is often inadequate due to diffuse nature of the disease process as shown by pathological studies. IVUS, on the other hand, can outline the VH and assess the extent and severity. By gray scale IVUS on the basis of tissue echogenicity atheroma has been classified in four categories (Fig. 3):

1. Soft plaque (lesion echogenicity less than the surrounding adventitia)
2. Fibrous plaque (intermediate echogenicity between soft (echolucent) atheroma and highly echogenic calcified plaques)
3. Calcified plaque (echogenicity higher than the adventitia with acoustic shadowing)
4. Mixed plaques (no single acoustic subtype represents more than 80% of the plaque).

TABLE 2: Limitations of coronary angiography.

- Intra- and interobserver variability
- Under or over-estimation of lesion severity
- Discrepancy between angiographic severity and postmortem histology
- Luminogram (does not provide information on vessel wall)
- Does not quantify atheroma volume
- Not suitable for plaque characterization
- Inability to identify vulnerable plaques

Intravascular ultrasound accurately detects calcification as bright echoes. VH has a predictive accuracy of 96.7% for detection of dense calcification. The presence and distribution of calcification helps in selection of interventional device and predicting risk of the procedure.

Intravascular Ultrasound in Detection of Vulnerable Plaque

Acute coronary syndrome (ACS) is often the first manifestation of CAD and is caused by plaque rupture with or without thrombus. Plaque rupture occurs at the site of significant plaque accumulation but is often not highly stenotic by CAG due to positive vascular remodeling. IVUS played a significant role in understanding of vulnerable plaque. The frequency and distribution of ruptured plaques and their natural evolution has been studied.[4] Thrombus is usually recognized as an echolucent intraluminal mass with a layered or pedunculated appearance. Clinically, this target of vulnerable plaque imaging has so far remained illusive. The key to finding vulnerable plaques is detecting the composition of plaques in addition to their morphology.

Unstable plaques are characterized by presence of heterogeneous lipid-rich necrotic core covered by a thin fibrous cap (50–100 μm) that is weakened by inflammation (thin-capped fibroatheroma). These lesions frequently feature microcalcifications, increased microvascular density, and outward remodeling of the vessel.

Intravascular Ultrasound in Atherosclerosis Progression/Regression Trials

Intravascular ultrasound has been utilized as an imaging technique for a serial study of coronary atherosclerosis owing to its ability to provide accurate measurements, excellent resolution, reproducibility, and ability to detect even angiographically silent CAD. Several trials of antiatherosclerotic drugs have investigated the change of plaque geometry and composition. The effect of several therapeutic agents, e.g. statins, recombinant-apo A-1 Milano, nonstatin lipid modifying agents, antihypertensive and antidiabetic drugs and proprotein convertase subtilisin/kexin type-2 inhibitors on atheroma volume have been studied by IVUS.[5] Two large scale pharmaceutical intervention trials with serial volumetric IVUS reported the effects of statin therapy on coronary plaque progression-regression.[6,7] The Reversal of Atherosclerosis with Aggressive Lipid Lowering trial concluded that 80 mg atorvastatin treatment to a mean low-density lipoprotein (LDL) level of 78 mg/dL stopped progression of plaque volume.[6] Similarly, the ASTEROID study demonstrated that very high-intensity statin therapy with rosuvastatin to a mean LDL cholesterol level of 60.8 mg/dL resulted in significant reduction of atheroma volume.[7]

IVUS in Documentation of Coronary Vessel Remodeling

Arterial remodeling was described by Glagov et al.[8] and refers to characteristic changes of arterial size during plaque progression-regression. Coronary remodeling refers to a continuous process involving the changes in the vessel size measured by the EEM-CSA. Expansive (positive) remodeling is defined as an outward increase in EEM and is associated with inflammation, soft plaques, and plaque vulnerability in pathological studies and with ACS in clinical reports. Negative remodeling occurs when the EEM decreases in size (shrinkage of the vessel) and is seen in fibrocalcific plaques. Trials studying plaque size (progression-regression) showed useful insights into the serial remodeling behavior during pharmacological intervention. The data showed that apart from reduction in plaque size (regression), a shift of the remodeling pattern toward negative remodeling may be considered as a sign of plaque stabilization.

CLINICAL USES OF INTRAVASCULAR ULTRASOUND

Assessment of Ischemia Producing Lesions

In the current era, IVUS is not utilized for assessment of lesion severity. IVUS studies have shown a relatively high negative predictive value (72–96%) but a low-positive predictive value (39–73%). It may be useful to defer an intervention in selected situations based on minimal lumen area size, IVUS should not be used to justify an intervention.[9] Three randomized clinical trials, DEFER,[10] FAME[11] and FAME-2,[12] established fractional flow reserve as the gold standard to assess the significance of a non-LMCA lesion.

Left Main Coronary Artery–Percutaneous Coronary Intervention

For years, coronary artery bypass grafting has been the standard revascularization modality for LMCA disease owing to a large area of jeopardized myocardium and association with high mortality and morbidity.[13] Over the years, remarkable advances in stents, adjuvant technology and better medical treatment has led to improved PCI outcomes for unprotected LMCA disease. Two large trials EXCEL[14] and NOBLE[15] using second generation drug-eluting stents (DES) have demonstrated how much PCI has improved for LMCA treatment. In these two trials, IVUS-guided PCI was performed in more than 70% cases. The technique provided more reliable information than angiography on lesion characteristic, e.g. lumen size, plaque characterization and distribution. For distal LMCA bifurcation lesions, IVUS helps to decide stenting strategy and achieve large stent diameters. The best IVUS criteria of minimal stent area predicting angiographic restenosis were 5 mm for the left circumflex artery ostium, 6.3 mm for the left anterior descending ostium, 7.2 mm for the polygon of confluence, and 8.2 mm from the proximal LMCA above the polygon of confluence (so called 5-6-7-8 rule of criteria). Andell et al.[16] used data from the nationwide Swedish coronary angiography and angioplasty registry to determine the clinical impact of IVUS guidance for LMCA-PCI. In a multivariable adjusted model, compared with angiography alone, IVUS was associated with 37% reduction of primary composite end point (death, restenosis or definite ST) and 39% reduction of all-cause mortality. Based on Swedish registry and other data, IVUS is a valuable adjunctive tool for LMCA-PCI for preintervention lesion assessment and postinterventional stent optimization. However, a true clinical effect of IVUS guidance for LMCA-PCI can be only confirmed or refuted through randomized clinical trials. Figure 4 demonstrates mechanism of in-stent restenosis in distal left main due to unapposed stent.

Non-left Main Coronary Artery–Percutaneous Coronary Intervention

It is widely appreciated that IVUS and OCT are equivalent (and superior to angiography) in guiding and optimizing PCI procedures. Both modalities can identify features of optimal stent implantation as well as mechanisms of stent failure. Inadequate stent expansion, apposition, dissection, and thrombus can all be visualized with IVUS. Table 3 lists the information provided by IVUS whereas Table 4 shows advantages and limitations of the technique.

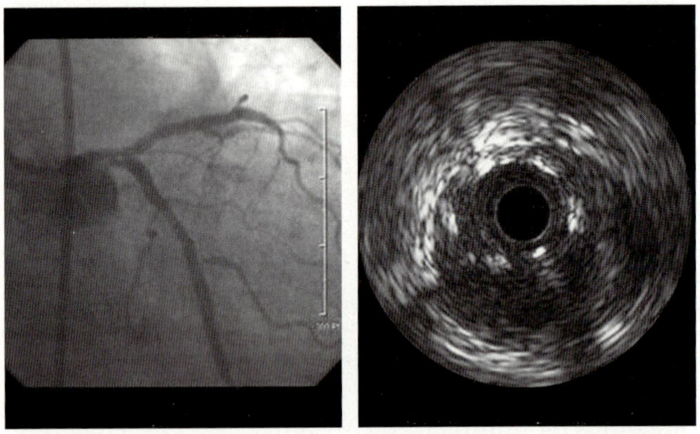

Fig. 4: Intravascular ultrasound demonstrating mechanism of in-stent restenosis. The in-stent restenosis at distal left main due to neointima developed from unapposed stent to vessel wall.

TABLE 3: Utility of intravascular ultrasound in percutaneous coronary intervention

- To identify superficial calcium and decide prestent lesion modification strategy
- Find reference lumen dimensions and lesion length for appropriate stent sizing
- Optimize stent deployment
- Study mechanism of stent failure

TABLE 4: Advantages and limitations of intravascular ultrasound for percutaneous coronary interventions.

Advantages:
- Clinical experience of three decades
- Extensive research data on procedural and clinical outcomes
- Imaging possible in most patients without predilation
- Allows true vessel stent sizing
- Better guidance for ostial, chronic total occlusions lesions
- Can minimize contrast use

Limitations
- Interpretation and low-resolution issues
- Limited tissue characterization
- Detection of thrombus difficult

Stent Thrombosis

Depending on the time since stent placement, ST is classified as early (0-30 days—post-procedure), late (more than 30 days), and very late (more than 12 months). The early ST can be acute (less than 24 hours) and subacute (1-3 days) events. IVUS has been utilized to understand the mechanism of ST. There are studies to suggest that increased utilization of IVUS at the time of initial stent implantation facilitates better stent deployment and reduces the chances of ST. IVUS has identified high prevalence of under expansion in early ST.[17] The other predictors of early ST identifies on IVUS include inflow or outflow tract disease (significant dissections, edge plaque burden, edge stenosis, and geographical miss). A higher incidence of malapposition is seen in very late ST. An optimal procedure result is important to minimize the risk of ST. Proper stent expansion and apposition over the full-length of the stent should be ascertained, and residual dissections should be avoided: A strong trend toward reduced ST after IVUS-guided stent implantation has been documented. Figure 5 shows visualization of ST on IVUS.

To Prevent Contrast-Induced Nephropathy

Intravascular ultrasound guided minimum or no contrast PCI has potentials to reduce contrast dose and prevent resultant acute kidney injury. PCI can be safely performed without contrast using IVUS and physiological guidance with high procedural success and without complications in patients with advanced renal failure.[18]

Chronic Total Occlusions

Percutaneous coronary intervention for CTO is a complex procedure and is associated with lower procedural success

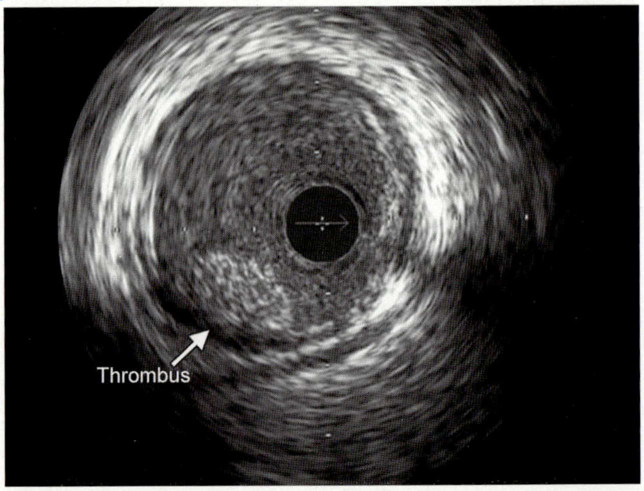

Fig. 5: Intravascular ultrasound demonstrating stent thrombosis.

rate, increased restenosis, and reocclusion compared with non-CTO procedures. IVUS provides valuable information in assessing the anatomy of the lesion. The technical challenges in CTO-PCI include passage of a guidewire and balloon catheter. Effective wiring strategies include antegrade wire escalation, parallel wiring, dissection and reentry, and the retrograde transcollateral approach. Angiography is able to provide only a two-dimensional image of contrast-filled lumen, which fails to assess the accurate anatomy. IVUS with its ability to provide cross-sectional images of the coronary artery provides elaborate information in this difficult subset. IVUS can be useful to classify anatomical structures better than on angiography. CTO recanalization with a guidewire is the crucial and most challenging step. IVUS can guide the precise location of guidewire(s) within the vessel (i.e. true lumen versus subintima), determine the entry point and evaluate penetration of the proximal cap. During PCI procedures, final diameter of opened vessel, stent expansion, apposition and edge dissection are better assessed by IVUS. Imaging can also determine the cause of stent failure, including in-stent restenosis and ST. The current available data suggest that the use of IVUS is beneficial for recanalizing CTO lesions and can improve long-term results.[19]

LESSONS FROM THE TRIALS

Coronary angiography (CAG) is the standard imaging modality for intraprocedural guidance of PCI. However, angiography has known limitations in assessing vessel size, plaque burden, calcium, eccentricity and lesion expansion. Intracoronary imaging techniques can overcome some limitations of CAG. A network meta-analysis[20] of 17,882 patients treated with either bare metal stents or DES from 17 randomized trials and registries showed that IVUS significantly reduced all-cause mortality (the primary outcome) compared with angiography alone. Benefits of IVUS guidance were also statistically significant for myocardial infarction, ST and repeat revascularization. There were no efficacy difference between the IVUS and the OCT imaging-related complications were rare, did not differ between two methods. In the present network meta-analysis, CAG guidance was rated as the worst of the three strategies.

GUIDELINES

The latest guidelines, which are currently available from European Society of Cardiology,[21] assign IVUS use a class II recommendation (Table 5). The trial results discussed above are quite compelling and call for wider clinical

TABLE 5: Recommendations* for intravascular ultrasound (IVUS) use in clinical practice.

Recommendations	*Class*	*Level*
IVUS in selected patients to optimize stent implantation	IIa	B
IVUS to assess severity and optimize treatment of unprotected left main lesions	IIa	B
IVUS to assess mechanism of stent failure	IIa	C

*Adapted from European Society of Cardiology guidelines.[21]

application of IVUS. It is quite likely that newer versions of the guidelines will upgrade the class of recommendation of imaging techniques.

CONCLUSION

Intravascular ultrasound provides high quality, tomographic imaging of the lumen, atheroma and vessel wall compared with CAG. It helps in practical guidance for PCI in optimizing stent diameter, length and vessel wall apposition. IVUS has become an important part of DES studies, representing an effective way to understand the mechanisms, effects and complications of stent technology. Newer applications like VH and RF-IVUS can accurately help in determining plaque composition and deciding appropriate PCI plan based on presence of calcium. Development of high definition IVUS, hybrid IVUS-OCT imaging or integration of novel techniques including IVUS and near-infrared spectroscopy has great potential to improve our current ability to identify plaques at high-risk of rupture.

REFERENCES

1. Bom N, Lancee CT, Honkoop J, et al. Ultrasonic viewer for cross-sectional analyses of moving cardiac structures. Biomed Eng. 1971;6:500-3.
2. Mintz GS, Nissen SE, Anderson WD, et al. American College of Cardiology Clinical Expert Consensus Document on Standards for Acquisition, Measurement and Reporting of Intravascular Ultrasound Studies (IVUS). A report of the American College of Cardiology Task Force on Clinical Expert Consensus Documents. J Am Coll Cardiol. 2001;37:1478-92.
3. Mintz GS. IVUS in PCI guidance. Expert analysis. JACC. 2006.
4. Suh WM, Seto AH, Margey RJ, et al. Intravascular detection of the vulnerable plaque. Circ Cardiovasc Imaging. 2011;4:169-78.
5. Hartmann M, Huisman J, Böse D, et al. Serial intravascular ultrasound assessment of changes in coronary atherosclerotic plaque dimensions and composition: An update. Eur J Echocardiogr. 2011;12:313-21.
6. Nissen SE, Tuzcu EM, Schoenhagen P, et al. Effect of intensive compared with moderate lipid-lowering therapy on progression of coronary atherosclerosis: a randomized controlled trial. JAMA. 2004;291:1071-80.

7. Nissen SE, Nicholls SJ, Sipahi I, et al. Effect of very high-intensity statin therapy on regression of coronary atherosclerosis: the ASTEROID trial. JAMA. 2006;295:1556-65.
8. Glagov S, Weisenberg E, Zarins C, et al. Compensatory enlargement of human atherosclerotic coronary arteries. N Engl J Med. 1987;316:371-5.
9. Raber L, Mintz GS, Koskinas KC, et al. Clinical use of intracoronary imaging. Part 1: guidance and optimization of coronary interventions. An expert consensus document of the European Association of Percutaneous Cardiovascular Interventions: Endorsed by the Chinese Society of Cardiology. Eur Heart J. 2018.
10. Zimmermann FM, Ferrara A, Johnson NP, et al. Deferral vs. performance of percutaneous coronary intervention of functionally non-significant coronary stenosis: 15-year follow-up of the DEFER trial. Eur Heart J. 2015;36:3182-8.
11. Van Nunen LX, Zimmermann FM, Tonino PA, et al. Fractional flow reserve versus angiography for guidance of PCI in patients with DES multivessel coronary artery disease (FAME): 5-year follow-up of a randomised controlled trial. Lancet. 2015;386:1853-60.
12. De Bruyne B, Pijls NH, Kalesan B, et al. Fractional flow reserve-guided PCI versus medical therapy in stable coronary disease. N Engl J Med. 2012;367:991-1001.
13. Park DW, Park SJ. Intravascular ultrasound-guided percutaneous coronary intervention for left main disease: does procedural fine tuning make a relevant clinical benefit? Circ Cardiovasc Interv. 2017;10(5). pii: e005293.
14. Gershlick AH, Kandzari DE, Banning A, et al. Outcomes after left main percutaneous coronary intervention versus coronary artery bypass grafting according to lesion site: results from the excel trial. JACC Cardiovasc Interv. 2018;11:1224-33.
15. Makikallio T, Holm NR, Lindsay M, et al. Percutaneous coronary angioplasty versus coronary artery bypass grafting in treatment of unprotected left main stenosis (NOBLE): a prospective, randomised, open-label, non-inferiority trial. Lancet. 2016;388:2743-52.
16. Andell P, Karlsson S, Mohammad MA, et al. Intravascular ultrasound guidance is associated with better outcome in patients undergoing unprotected left main coronary artery stenting compared with angiography guidance alone. Circ Cardiovasc Interv. 2017;10(5).
17. Claessen BE, Henriques JP, Jaffer FA, et al. Stent thrombosis: a clinical perspective. JACC Cardiovasc Interv. 2014;7:1081-92.
18. Ali ZA, Karimi Galougahi K, Nazif T, et al. Imaging- and physiology-guided percutaneous coronary intervention without contrast administration in advanced renal failure: a feasibility, safety, and outcome study. Eur Heart J. 2016;37:3090-5.
19. Galassi AR, Sumitsuji S, Boukhris M, et al. Utility of intravascular ultrasound in percutaneous revascularization of chronic total occlusions: an overview. JACC Cardiovasc Interv. 2016;9:1979-91.
20. Buccheri S, Franchina G, Romano S, et al. Clinical outcomes following intravascular imaging-guided versus coronary angiography-guided percutaneous coronary intervention with stent implantation: a systematic review and Bayesian network meta-analysis of 31 studies and 17,882 patients. JACC Cardiovasc Interv. 2017;10:2488-98.
21. Windecker S, Kolh P, Alfonso F, et al. 2014 ESC/EACTS Guidelines on myocardial revascularization: The Task Force on Myocardial Revascularization of the European Society of Cardiology (ESC) and the European Association for Cardio-Thoracic Surgery (EACTS) developed with the special contribution of the European Association of Percutaneous Cardiovascular Interventions (EAPCI). Eur Heart J. 2014;35:2541-619.

29

CHAPTER

Vulnerable Plaque Imaging in Acute Coronary Syndrome: When to Intervene?

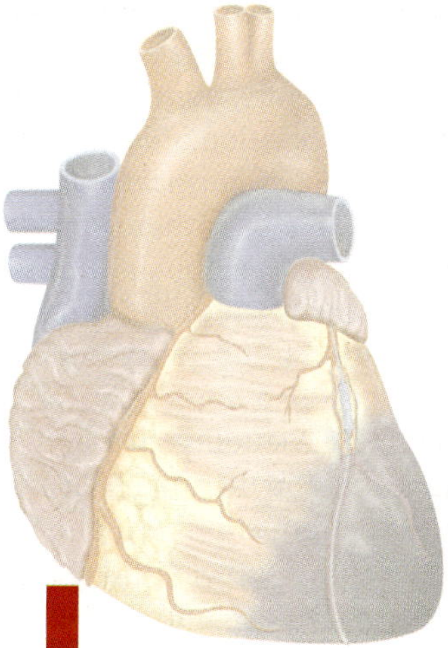

Sundeep Mishra

INTRODUCTION

Atherosclerosis, the most common form of vascular disease throughout the globe, accounts for approximately 30% of the total mortality.[1,2] The hallmark lesion of atherosclerosis is the atherosclerotic plaque. In spite of the indolent disease progression, its course is often punctuated by episodes of acute vascular thrombosis, superimposed on either plaque erosion or rupture. These episodes of thrombosis account for almost all cases of acute coronary syndromes (ACS) which include unstable angina, myocardial infarction (MI), and sudden cardiac death (SCD).[3] Approximately, 40% of cases of vascular thrombosis leading to SCD are caused by lesions less than 50% diameter stenosis.[4] The composition and vulnerability of the plaque are crucial determinants for the development of thrombosis, with soft and lipid-rich plaques being more dangerous than fibrous and collagen-rich plaques.[5] Clinical risk indices such as the Framingham criteria underestimate the 10-year probability of death due to a vascular event in young individuals.[6] Noninvasive imaging modalities such as stress single-photon emission-computed tomography (SPECT) or stress echocardiography provide an estimate of the significance of coronary stenosis and only allow the identification of severely stenosed lesions. However, most of the acute vascular events have been demonstrated to be due to either rupture or erosion of hemodynamically insignificant plaques. These plaques significantly outnumber the flow-limiting critically stenosed lesions. This accounts for the poor predictive value of noninvasive stress testing for the prediction of acute vascular events.[7] The term "vulnerable plaque" is used to describe lesions with a high probability of rupture and causing a coronary event. The intervention of this plaque before its destabilization may reduce the mortality caused by coronary artery disease (CAD). Coronary angiography has a low-predictive value in the detection of vulnerable plaque since most of these lesions do not show critical stenosis. Advanced techniques such as computed tomography coronary angiography (CTCA), intravascular ultrasound (IVUS), optical coherence tomography (OCT), and near-infrared spectroscopy (NIRS) guide the diagnosis and management of these plaques and play an important role in the prevention of CAD.[8]

DIAGNOSTIC CRITERIA AND PROGNOSTIC IMPLICATIONS

The vulnerable plaque hypothesis was proposed to explain the unpredictable nature of atherosclerosis. Vulnerable plaques have been defined as those plaques, which are prone to become culprit plaques, causing acute vascular events or death, irrespective of the shape, form or percentage stenosis. Hence, all erosion-prone, rupture-prone, hemorrhaging, calcified plaques and significantly stenosed plaques should be considered vulnerable. Plaque rupture, the most common form of plaque destabilization, accounts for almost two-thirds of all fatal MIs and SCDs. Hence, occasionally, the term vulnerable plaque has been loosely used to denote this specific subgroup of rupture-prone coronary plaques.[9] Atherosclerotic plaques consist of intimal thickening of medium and large-sized arteries. Oxidation of low-density lipoprotein (LDL) particles in these plaques leads to the expression of leukocyte adhesion molecules. This induces the infiltration of lymphocytes and macrophages, which convert into foam cells after taking up oxidized LDL particles via their scavenger receptors. Foam cell disintegration, loss of smooth muscle cells (SMCs), and production of matrix metalloproteinases by inflammatory cells lead to the formation of lipid-rich cores and rupture-prone plaques.[10,11] Mature plaques consist of soft, atheromatous gruel and hard fibrous tissue. The fibrous tissue consists of more than 70% of an average plaque. The atheromatous component is dangerous because it predisposes the plaque to rupture. Several studies have demonstrated that more severely stenosed plaques have a higher tendency to get occluded. However, the less obstructive plaques give rise to a higher total number of coronary occlusions due to their much higher number.[4,12,13]

Several studies have demonstrated that most vulnerable plaques are thin-cap fibroatheromas (TCFAs), which consist of a large eccentric necrotic core (25% of the plaque area) and a thin fibrous cap (<65 μm), with extensive lymphocyte and macrophage infiltration with a paucity of SMCs. The large Providing Regional Observations to Study Predictors of Events in the Coronary Tree (PROSPECT) trial showed that major adverse cardiac events (MACE) after percutaneous coronary interventions (PCI) could be attributed equally to recurrence at the site of culprit lesion and non-culprit lesions, which, though angiographically mild, were shown to be TCFAs by IVUS.[14] In addition, vulnerable plaques also show intraplaque hemorrhage, endothelial denudation, neoangiogenesis, and positive remodeling. ACS is usually secondary to rupture of such plaques, which exposes the blood to the thrombogenic material, thereby causing vascular thrombosis. Some culprit lesions also have calcified nodules, which have disruptive effects on plaque integrity.[15,16] A third of all vascular events are secondary to plaque erosion. Eroded plaques are more difficult to image than TCFAs because they have less severe stenosis, fewer calcifications, less extensive inflammation and angiogenesis and more negative remodeling. Several factors affect the vulnerability of a plaque. Plaque rupture commonly occurs at the thinnest point of the cap. This is commonly the junction of the plaque with native disease-free vessel, also called the shoulder region of the plaque. The vulnerability of the plaque also depends on the size of the necrotic core, the thickness of the fibrous cap, inflammation, and cap fatigue.[17]

THERAPEUTIC IMPLICATIONS

Current guidelines recommend immediate revascularization of the culprit lesion and staged revascularization of hemodynamically significant nonculprit lesions, with the goal of attaining complete revascularization in patients who present with ACS. Several studies have shown a reduced risk of MACE after revascularization of residual CAD after the treatment of culprit lesion.[18] Currently, there is limited evidence in the favor of intervention of vulnerable plaques not causing a significant reduction in coronary blood flow. There are several ongoing trials of catheter-based interventions of vulnerable plaques. Various systemic therapies have been tried to address these vulnerable plaques. Statins have demonstrated a mortality benefit in patients with CAD. Statins have also demonstrated a plaque stabilizing effect. Several CTCA studies have shown a reduction in plaque volume with statin therapy.[19] Several IVUS studies have demonstrated a reduction in high-risk plaque features and OCT studies have shown an increase in cap thickness with the introduction of statin therapy.[20] Additionally, high-intensity statins are better compared to low-intensity statins.[21] Another IVUS study showed superiority of combined ezetimibe with statin compared to statin alone in the regression of high-risk plaque features.[22] Studies have shown that proprotein convertase subtilisin/kexin type 9 (PCSK9) inhibitor alone or combined with statins is more effective than statin alone in reducing LDL levels.[23] In an IVUS study, PCSK9 inhibitor, evolocumab combined with statins was tested against statins alone. The PCSK9 inhibitor arm showed a greater regression of atheroma volume and greater plaque regression compared to statins alone.[24] Several anti-inflammatory drugs including methotrexate, canakimumab, and colchicine have demonstrated a benefit in small studies.[25-27] However, the role of these agents in human atherosclerosis remains to be established.

DISCUSSION

Coronary angiography is the preferred diagnostic test to depict significant coronary stenosis. However, angiography has several limitations. It provides data on the vascular lumen and not the vessel wall. Hazy angiographic sites can represent a thrombus, dissection or an irregular plaque. Additionally, diffuse atherosclerotic plaques can often be reported as normal with angiogram.[28] Several novel modalities have emerged that can identify vulnerable plaques in patients undergoing coronary angiography, radiofrequency (RF)-IVUS (RF-IVUS), OCT, and NIRS. RF-IVUS provides greater diagnostic accuracy compared to gray-scale IVUS. OCT provides better axial resolution, albeit at the cost of reduced penetration. NIRS analyzes the chemical composition of atherosclerotic plaque. All three modalities generate high quality cross-sectional images that depict high-risk coronary lesions. So how should these imaging tools be used to detect vulnerable plaque?

INTRAVASCULAR ULTRASOUND

Intravascular ultrasound is the one of the earliest and most widely adopted modality for the assessment of the nature of atherosclerotic plaques. It consists of a catheter with a piezoelectric catheter mounted at its distal end, which is connected to a computerized ultrasound apparatus. It provides gray-scale images perpendicular to the long axis of the vessel. It works on the principles of ultrasound generation, signal reception, data processing, and generation of a gray-scale image. It provides a resolution of 150 µm at a frame rate of 10–30 per second.[29] The anatomical characteristics of a plaque can be assessed with IVUS (Fig. 1). It assesses the features associated with vulnerable plaques: eccentric pattern, necrotic echolucent core, positive remodeling, the presence of thrombi, calcification, and neoangiogenesis. Serial imaging can demonstrate healing and stabilization of plaques following medical management with statins.[30] There are several limitations of IVUS. Due to the limited spatial resolution, IVUS cannot detect TCFAs and cap thickness. Gray-scale IVUS cannot detect the plaque composition due to image distortion during acquisition.[31]

Intravascular Ultrasound: Radiofrequency Analysis

Radiofrequency-IVUS overcomes some of the inherent limitations of gray-scale IVUS. Virtual histology (VH) IVUS, the most commonly used RF-IVUS, displays the plaque composition as a color-coded map superimposed on a gray-scale image. Plaque components are usually classified as fibrous, fibrofatty, calcific or necrotic. Vulnerable plaque is defined by VH as a focal lesion with a necrotic core (≥10% of plaque area) in direct contact with the lumen and atheroma volume more than 40%. It has a predictive accuracy of 88% for the detection of necrotic cores.[32] IVUS is the only imaging modality with a proven ability to predict major adverse cardiovascular events (MACE), as confirmed in the PROSPECT trial. The results implicated that RF-IVUS can predict MACE before their occurrence. The presence of TCFAs as assessed by RF-IVUS correlates well with the risk of MACE.[14] However, the specificity of RF-IVUS for the prediction of vascular events is low. RF-IVUS has several limitations. The low resolution precludes the assessment of cap thickness, which is one of the most important defining criteria for TCFAs. Also, it is unable to distinguish thrombi from other plaque components.[33] Hence, a combined assessment using RF-IVUS and OCT is generally more fruitful.[34]

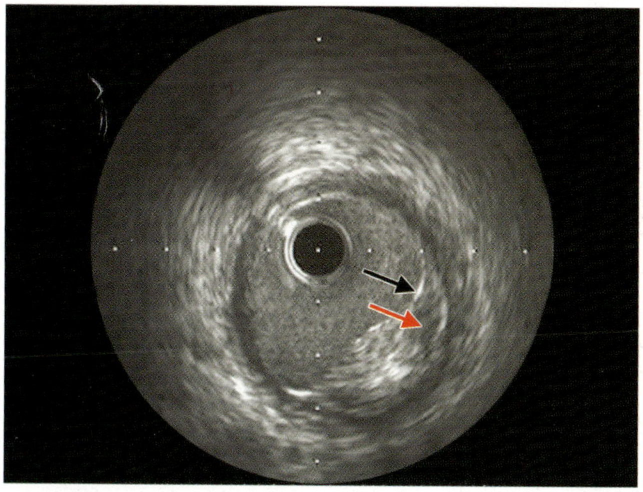

Fig. 1: Gray-scale intravascular ultrasound image of a patient who presented with crescendo angina, abnormal CT angiogram and an inconclusive coronary angiogram shows an eccentric echolucent plaque from 3 O'clock to 7 O'clock position with a thin cap of calcium (black arrow) overlying the echolucent necrotic core (red arrow).

PALPOGRAPHY

Palpography or intravascular elastography measures the strain in response to a pulsating force of blood pressure. It has been validated both ex-vivo and in-vivo. A good correlation has been found between TCFAs and high regional strain. It has a sensitivity of 100% and specificity of 80% for detection of fatty plaques in animal models.[35] Palpography is a research tool and may play an important role in the detection of vulnerable plaques in future.

OPTICAL COHERENCE TOMOGRAPHY

This works on a principle similar to IVUS but it uses infrared light with a wavelength of 1.3 µm instead of ultrasound waves. Since light has a smaller wavelength than ultrasound, OCT offers ten times higher resolution (10–20 µm) compared to IVUS (100–250 µm) (Table 1). Thus, OCT can visualize fibrous caps, collagen content, neovessels, thrombi and ruptures (Figs. 2A and B).[36] OCT is more accurate than IVUS for the identification of plaque rupture, erosions, and thrombi. Owing to its high resolution, OCT is the only available method to detect eroded plaques. It can measure the cap thickness and truly detect TCFAs.[37] Its sensitivity for the detection of TCFAs is 90% and specificity is 79% as compared to histology.[38] It can also be used to follow-up the thickness of the fibrous cap in patients on statin therapy. The imaging features of vulnerable plaque by OCT include: wide lipid arc more than 90°, necrotic lipid pools, superficial microcalcifications, and cap thickness less than 65 µm.[38] Micro-OCT offers higher axial and lateral resolution in the order of 1–2 µm, thus allowing molecular events such as

TABLE 1: Comparison of invasive imaging modalities.

	Coronary angiography	*Optical coherence tomography*	*Intravascular ultrasound*
Resolution	+	+++	+
Quantification	++	++	++
Imaging depth	–	+	++
Tissue characterization			
Intraluminal	+	++	+
Intramural	–	+	++
Thrombus	+	+++	–
Calcification	+	+++	++
Plaque characterization	+	++	+
Cap thickness estimation	–	+++	–

–: poor; +: good; +++; excellent.

leukocyte adhesion, diapedesis, fibrin strand formation, extracellular matrix (ECM) production, microcalcifications, cholesterol crystal formation to be visualized. Macrophage infiltration can also be recognized with OCT as bright spots with a high signal attenuation behind it.[39] There are some inherent limitations to the use of OCT. The high scattering of light prevents imaging at greater depths (>2 mm). Hence, the estimation of remodeling and necrotic core size remain inadequate. Since light is attenuated by blood, OCT needs the use of saline flushes to obtain good quality images.[40] This can be problematic in patients with renal dysfunction and left ventricular dysfunction, who are predisposed to develop pulmonary edema.

NEAR INFRARED SPECTROSCOPY

Near infrared spectroscopy allows for chemical characterization of plaque composition. It can be used to assess the lipid and protein content in atherosclerotic plaques. Studies have demonstrated that large lipid content correlated with TCFAs. Larger lipid cores can differentiate between culprit and nonculprit lesions in ACS.[41] The "Chemogram" generated by NIRS displays the lipid content at the site of interrogation. In vitro, NIRS offers a sensitivity of around 77–90% and specificity of 89–93% in detecting lipid-rich cores.[42] However, NIRS by itself cannot provide an idea about the lumen and plaque depth. Hence, it is commonly used along with IVUS as a single catheter. When combined with IVUS, it gives an idea about the plaque structure and composition and compares favorably with OCT.[43] Another limitation is the lower penetration of NIRS. Hence, information is obtained only from a depth of 1 mm or less.[44]

OTHER INVASIVE MODALITIES

Several other modalities have been tested to detect vulnerable plaques and study the components. Intravascular pulsed field gradient magnetic resonance imaging (MRI) has been studied in vivo and has demonstrated high sensitivity for the detection of lipid, fibrous, and calcified components: angioscopy, thermography, shear stress

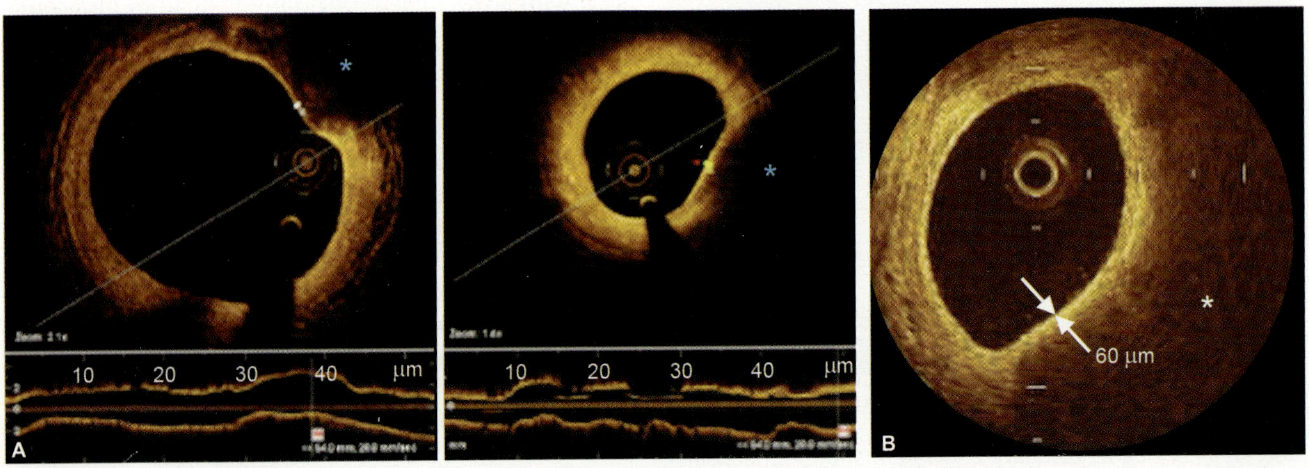

Figs. 2A and B: Optical coherence tomography features of a thin-cap fibroatheromas (TCFA). (A) Shows a lipid rich plaque (asterisk) and a thin cap. (B) Shows a cap with a thickness of 60 μm suggestive of TCFA.

imaging are the other methods studied for the detection of vulnerable plaques. However, these methods have remained research tools with poor accuracy.

NONINVASIVE TECHNIQUES

Multidetector Computed Tomography

Technical improvements in imaging have considerably improved the temporal and spatial resolution of multidetector computed tomography (MDCT).[46] MDCT with iodinated contrast has significant advantages. It can visualize the entire coronary circulation and can image the vessel wall along with the lumen.[47] The diagnostic accuracy of MDCT for detecting significant CAD exceeds 90%. MDCT detects some features of vulnerable plaque: positive remodeling (remodeling index ≥1.1), spotty calcifications (<3 mm), and lower plaque density (<30 HU).[48] The combined presence of these three features in a patient with ACS has a positive-predictive value of 90% in the identification of an unstable plaque.[49] These imaging criteria have been validated against VH-IVUS and histology in ACS patients. The presence of napkin-ring sign (necrotic core with low attenuation surrounded by ring of high attenuation) also has an excellent accuracy for the detection of TCFAs.[50] Thus, MDCT remains a first-line noninvasive modality for the detection of unstable plaques.[49] Its accuracy is noninferior to IVUS and has a negative-predictive value approaching 100%.[51] Coronary artery calcium score (CACS) is another method to detect coronary calcium without the need of iodinated dye. It is an attractive option for detection and monitoring of vulnerable plaques. It provides incremental information over conventional risk stratification.

Magnetic Resonance Imaging

Magnetic resonance imaging exposes the tissues to a strong magnetic field and evaluates their response. It provides information about the characteristics of the tissue, such as its water, lipid or fibrous content. It has an excellent ability to detect the soft tissue component of plaques and in detecting neoangiogenesis. T2-weighted images provide data about the lipid and fibrotic components of a plaque and can also measure the cap thickness, detect cap ruptures and hemorrhages.[52] However, MRI is best suited for the imaging of large arteries such as carotid vessels. Coronary arteries are difficult to image due to their constant motion. Targeted molecular imaging can be used along with MRI for the detection of plaque hemorrhages and neoangiogenesis.[53] However, further refinements are required before it can be used for human coronary vessels.

Nuclear Imaging

Positron emission tomography (PET) has been used more frequently than SPECT for detection of atherosclerosis due to the better spatial resolution and lower artifact rates.[54] ^{18}F-labeled fluorodeoxyglucose (FDG) remains the most widely used tracer. Areas with high FDG uptake correlate with areas of macrophage infiltration. FDG-PET signal is highly reproducible and has direct implications for treatment. However, its utility in coronary atherosclerosis is limited due to intense tracer uptake in the adjacent myocardium. An additional limitation of PET is the exposure to radiation, which limits follow-up studies.

LIMITATIONS

There are several limitations to the concept of vulnerable plaques and imaging methods. The vulnerable plaque hypothesis has predominantly focused on the plaque rupture leading to coronary thrombosis. A review of the literature reveals that more than 70% of fatal thrombi are due to plaque rupture.[55] However, OCT studies have shown a lower rate of plaque rupture in nonfatal ACS and non-ST-segment-elevation-MI.[56] Another limitation is that not all plaque ruptures and thrombosis are associated with a clinical event. Subclinical plaque ruptures are reported in 20% patients with ACS.[57] An important limitation of the concept is the poor positive predictive value of vulnerable plaques.[58] Also, studies have shown that plaque morphology may change during follow-up and may regress to stable lesions.[59] Additionally, the occurrence of clinical events heavily depends on blood and myocardial features; thus, the significance of treating rupture-prone plaques becomes unclear.

GUIDELINES

Numerous vulnerable plaques usually coexist in patients at risk for cardiovascular events. Additionally, vulnerable plaques may regress to a stable plaque with drug therapy. These factors argue the local treatment of vulnerable plaques and favor the implementation of systemic atherosclerosis treatment approaches. Exceptions to the above include nonculprit destabilized plaque detected during an acute event and presence of accelerated plaque progression with increasing stenosis. Hence, lipid-lowering treatment with statins and other drugs is warranted for most vulnerable plaques and local intervention reserved for a select few vulnerable plaques.[1]

CONCLUSION

Newer advances in imaging techniques have greatly improved the potential for identification of vulnerable coronary plaques. Although several studies have been published, more evidence is needed to establish the prognostic value of the various invasive and noninvasive plaque characteristics. Novel applications of invasive imaging modalities such as IVUS, OCT, and NIRS have paved the way for the evaluation of therapeutic agents specifically targeted at reducing plaque vulnerability. Reliable noninvasive modalities are necessary for the detection of vulnerable plaques in low-risk populations. Large studies of local treatment of these plaques are underway and will further guide the management of such high-risk plaques.

REFERENCES

1. Stefanadis C, Antoniou C-K, Tsiachris D, et al. Coronary atherosclerotic vulnerable plaque: Current perspectives. J Am Heart Assoc. 2017;6(3):e005543.
2. Members WG, Lloyd-Jones D, Adams RJ, et al. Executive summary: heart disease and stroke statistics—2010 update: A report from the American Heart Association. Circulation. 2010;121(7):948-54.
3. DeWood MA, Spores J, Notske R, et al. Prevalence of total coronary occlusion during the early hours of transmural myocardial infarction. N Engl J Med. 1980;303(16):897-902.
4. Ambrose JA, Tannenbaum MA, Alexopoulos D, et al. Angiographic progression of coronary artery disease and the development of myocardial infarction. J Am Coll Cardiol. 1988;12(1):56-62.
5. Fernández-Ortiz A, Badimon J, Falk E, et al. Characterization of the relative thrombogenicity of atherosclerotic plaque components: implications for consequences of plaque rupture. J Am Coll Cardiol. 1994;23:1562-9.
6. Kalantzi K, Korantzopoulos P, Tzimas P, et al. The relative value of metabolic syndrome and cardiovascular risk score estimates in premature acute coronary syndromes. Am Heart J. 2008;155(3):534-40.
7. Falk E, Shah PK, Fuster V. Coronary plaque disruption. Circulation. 1995;92(3):657-71.
8. Horváth M, Hájek P, Štěchovský C, et al. Vulnerable plaque imaging and acute coronary syndrome. Cor Vasa. 2014;56(4):e362-8.
9. Muller JE, Abela GS, Nesto RW, et al. Triggers, acute risk factors and vulnerable plaques: the lexicon of a new frontier. J Am Coll Cardiol. 1994;23(3):809-13.
10. Falk E. Pathogenesis of atherosclerosis. J Am Coll Cardiol. 2006;47(8 Supplement):C7-12.
11. Skålén K, Gustafsson M, Rydberg EK, et al. Subendothelial retention of atherogenic lipoproteins in early atherosclerosis. Nature. 2002;417(6890):750-4.
12. Alderman EL, Corley SD, Fisher LD, et al. Five-year angiographic follow-up of factors associated with progression of coronary artery disease in the Coronary Artery Surgery Study (CASS). CASS Participating Investigators and Staff. J Am Coll Cardiol. 1993;22(4):1141-54.
13. Nobuyoshi M, Tanaka M, Nosaka H, et al. Progression of coronary atherosclerosis: is coronary spasm related to progression? J Am Coll Cardiol. 1991;18(4):904-10.
14. Stone GW, Maehara A, Lansky AJ, et al. A prospective, natural-history study of coronary atherosclerosis. N Engl J Med. 2011;364(3):226-35.
15. Stone GW. In search of vulnerable plaque. Circ Cardiovasc Imaging. 2012;5(4):428-30.
16. Muller JE, Tofler GH, Stone PH. Circadian variation and triggers of onset of acute cardiovascular disease. Circulation. 1989;79(4):733-43.
17. Richardson PD, Davies MJ, Born GV. Influence of plaque configuration and stress distribution on fissuring of coronary atherosclerotic plaques. Lancet Lond Engl. 1989;2(8669):941-4.
18. Wald DS, Morris JK, Wald NJ, et al. Randomized trial of preventive angioplasty in myocardial infarction. N Engl J Med. 2013;369(12):1115-23.
19. Zeb I, Li D, Nasir K, et al. Effect of statin treatment on coronary plaque progression: a serial coronary CT angiography study. Atherosclerosis. 2013;231(2):198-204.
20. Kataoka Y, Puri R, Hammadah M, et al. Frequency-domain optical coherence tomographic analysis of plaque microstructures at nonculprit narrowings in patients receiving potent statin therapy. Am J Cardiol. 2014;114(4):549-54.
21. Nicholls SJ, Ballantyne CM, Barter PJ, et al. Effect of two intensive statin regimens on progression of coronary disease. N Engl J Med. 2011;365(22):2078-87.
22. Tsujita K, Sugiyama S, Sumida H, et al. Impact of dual lipid-lowering strategy with ezetimibe and atorvastatin on coronary plaque regression in patients with percutaneous coronary intervention: the Multicenter Randomized Controlled PRECISE-IVUS Trial. J Am Coll Cardiol. 2015;66(5):495-507.
23. Robinson JG, Nedergaard BS, Rogers, et al. Effect of evolocumab or ezetimibe added to moderate- or high-intensity statin therapy on LDL-C lowering in patients with hypercholesterolemia: the LAPLACE-2 randomized clinical trial. JAMA. 2014;311(18):1870-82.
24. Nicholls SJ, Puri R, Anderson T, et al. Effect of evolocumab on progression of coronary disease in statin-treated patients: the GLAGOV Randomized Clinical Trial. JAMA. 2016;316(22):2373-84.
25. Ridker PM, Howard CP, Walter V, et al. Effects of interleukin-1β inhibition with canakinumab on hemoglobin A1c, lipids, C-reactive protein, interleukin-6, and fibrinogen: a phase IIb randomized, placebo-controlled trial. Circulation. 2012;126(23):2739-48.
26. Micha R, Imamura F, Wyler von Ballmoos M, et al. Systematic review and meta-analysis of methotrexate use and risk of cardiovascular disease. Am J Cardiol. 2011;108(9):1362-70.

27. Nidorf SM, Eikelboom JW, Budgeon CA, et al. Low-dose colchicine for secondary prevention of cardiovascular disease. J Am Coll Cardiol. 2013;61:404-10.
28. Mintz GS, Painter JA, Pichard AD, et al. Atherosclerosis in angiographically "normal" coronary artery reference segments: an intravascular ultrasound study with clinical correlations. J Am Coll Cardiol. 1995;25(7):1479-85.
29. DeMaria AN, Narula J, Mahmud E, et al. Imaging vulnerable plaque by ultrasound. J Am Coll Cardiol. 2006;47(8 Supplement):C32-9.
30. Rioufol G, Gilard M, Finet G, et al. Evolution of spontaneous atherosclerotic plaque rupture with medical therapy: long-term follow-up with intravascular ultrasound. Circulation. 2004;110(18):2875-80.
31. Yamagishi M, Terashima M, Awano K, et al. Morphology of vulnerable coronary plaque: insights from follow-up of patients examined by intravascular ultrasound before an acute coronary syndrome. J Am Coll Cardiol. 2000;35(1):106-11.
32. Nasu K, Tsuchikane E, Katoh O, et al. Accuracy of in vivo coronary plaque morphology assessment: a validation study of in vivo virtual histology compared with in vitro histopathology. J Am Coll Cardiol. 2006;47(12):2405-12.
33. Surmely J-F, Nasu K, Fujita H, et al. Coronary plaque composition of culprit/target lesions according to the clinical presentation: a virtual histology intravascular ultrasound analysis. Eur Heart J. 2006;27(24):2939-44.
34. Sawada T, Shite J, Garcia-Garcia HM, et al. Feasibility of combined use of intravascular ultrasound radiofrequency data analysis and optical coherence tomography for detecting thin-cap fibroatheroma. Eur Heart J. 2008;29(9):1136-46.
35. Korte CL de, Sierevogel MJ, Mastik F, et al. Identification of atherosclerotic plaque components with intravascular ultrasound elastography in vivo: a Yucatan Pig Study. Circulation. 2002;105(14):1627-30.
36. Raffel OC, Tearney GJ, Gauthier DD, et al. Relationship between a systemic inflammatory marker, plaque inflammation, and plaque characteristics determined by intravascular optical coherence tomography. Arterioscler Thromb Vasc Biol. 2007;27(8):1820-7.
37. Kume T, Akasaka T, Kawamoto T, et al. Measurement of the thickness of the fibrous cap by optical coherence tomography. Am Heart J. 2006;152(4):755.
38. Kume T, Okura H, Yamada R, et al. Frequency and spatial distribution of thin-cap fibroatheroma assessed by 3-vessel intravascular ultrasound and optical coherence tomography: an ex vivo validation and an initial in vivo feasibility study. Circ J Off J Jpn Circ Soc. 2009;73(6):1086-91.
39. Tearney GJ, Regar E, Akasaka T, et al. Consensus standards for acquisition, measurement, and reporting of intravascular optical coherence tomography studies: a report from the International Working Group for intravascular optical coherence tomography standardization and validation. J Am Coll Cardiol. 2012;59(12):1058-72.
40. Brezinski M, Saunders K, Jesser C, et al. Index matching to improve optical coherence tomography imaging through blood. Circulation. 2001;103:1999-2003.
41. Madder RD, Puri R, Muller JE, et al. Confirmation of the intracoronary near-infrared spectroscopy threshold of lipid-rich plaques that underlie ST-segment-elevation myocardial infarction significance. Arterioscler Thromb Vasc Biol. 2016;36(5):1010-5.
42. Moreno PR, Lodder RA, Purushothaman KR, et al. Detection of lipid pool, thin fibrous cap, and inflammatory cells in human aortic atherosclerotic plaques by near-infrared spectroscopy. Circulation. 2002;105(8):923-7.
43. Roleder T, Kovacic JC, Ali Z, et al. Combined NIRS and IVUS imaging detects vulnerable plaque using a single catheter system: a head-to-head comparison with OCT. Euro Intervention. 2014;10(3):303-11.
44. Waxman S, Dixon SR, L'Allier P, et al. In vivo validation of a catheter-based near-infrared spectroscopy system for detection of lipid core coronary plaques: initial results of the SPECTACL study. JACC Cardiovasc Imaging. 2009;2(7):858-68.
45. Schneiderman J, Wilensky RL, Weiss A, et al. Diagnosis of thin-cap fibroatheromas by a self-contained intravascular magnetic resonance imaging probe in ex vivo human aortas and in situ coronary arteries. J Am Coll Cardiol. 2005;45(12):1961-9.
46. Cordeiro MAS, Lima JAC. Atherosclerotic plaque characterization by multidetector row computed tomography angiography. J Am Coll Cardiol. 2006;47(8 Supplement):C40-7.
47. Rodriguez-Granillo GA, Carrascosa P, Bruining N, et al. Defining the non-vulnerable and vulnerable patients with computed tomography coronary angiography: evaluation of atherosclerotic plaque burden and composition. Eur Heart J Cardiovasc Imaging. 2016;17(5):481-91.
48. Leber AW, Knez A, Becker A, et al. Accuracy of multidetector spiral computed tomography in identifying and differentiating the composition of coronary atherosclerotic plaques: a comparative study with intracoronary ultrasound. J Am Coll Cardiol. 2004;43(7):1241-7.
49. Motoyama S, Kondo T, Sarai M, et al. Multislice Computed Tomographic Characteristics of Coronary Lesions in Acute Coronary Syndromes. J Am Coll Cardiol. 2007;50(4):319-26.
50. Maurovich-Horvat P, Schlett CL, Alkadhi H, et al. The napkin-ring sign indicates advanced atherosclerotic lesions in coronary CT angiography. JACC Cardiovasc Imaging. 2012;5(12):1243-52.
51. Andreini D, Pontone G, Mushtaq S, et al. A long-term prognostic value of coronary CT angiography in suspected coronary artery disease. JACC Cardiovasc Imaging. 2012;5(7):690-701.
52. Chu B, Kampschulte A, Ferguson MS, et al. Hemorrhage in the atherosclerotic carotid plaque: a high-resolution MRI study. Stroke. 2004;35(5):1079-84.
53. Korosoglou G, Weiss RG, Kedziorek DA, et al. Noninvasive detection of macrophage-rich atherosclerotic plaque in hyperlipidemic rabbits using "positive contrast" magnetic resonance imaging. J Am Coll Cardiol. 2008;52(6):483-91.

54. Davies JR, Rudd JHF, Weissberg PL, et al. Radionuclide imaging for the detection of inflammation in vulnerable plaques. J Am Coll Cardiol. 2006;47(8 Supplement):C57-68.
55. Falk E, Nakano M, Bentzon JF, et al. Update on acute coronary syndromes: the pathologists' view. Eur Heart J. 2013;34:719-28.
56. Jia H, Abtahian F, Aguirre AD, et al. In vivo diagnosis of plaque erosion and calcified nodule in patients with acute coronary syndrome by intravascular optical coherence tomography. J Am Coll Cardiol. 2013;62(19):1748-58.
57. Arbab-Zadeh A, Fuster V. The myth of the "vulnerable plaque": transitioning from a focus on individual lesions to atherosclerotic disease burden for coronary artery disease risk assessment. J Am Coll Cardiol. 2015;65:846-55.
58. Cheng JM, Garcia-Garcia HM, de Boer SPM, et al. In vivo detection of high-risk coronary plaques by radiofrequency intravascular ultrasound and cardiovascular outcome: results of the ATHEROREMO-IVUS study. Eur Heart J. 2014;35(10):639-47.
59. Kubo T, Maehara A, Mintz GS, et al. The dynamic nature of coronary artery lesion morphology assessed by serial virtual histology intravascular ultrasound tissue characterization. J Am Coll Cardiol. 2010;55(15):1590-7.

30

CHAPTER

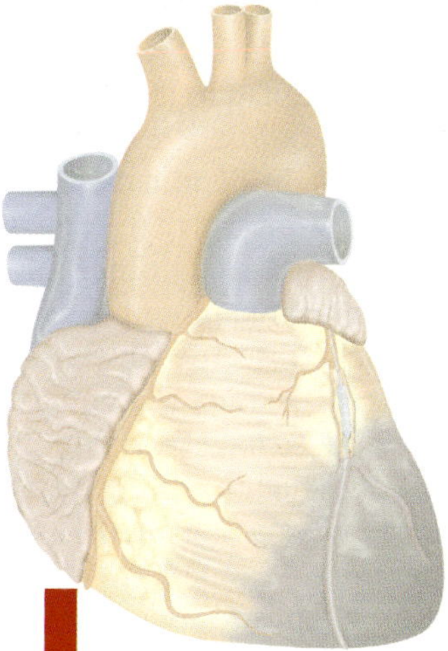

ST-elevation Myocardial Infarction and Advances in Optical Coherence Tomography

Raghav Bansal, Viveka Kumar

INTRODUCTION

Advent of intracoronary imaging has been an important development in the sphere of percutaneous coronary intervention (PCI) over the last 2 decades. The characterization of atherosclerotic plaque gives a better understanding of its pathophysiology and may help in treatment guidance. Developed in 1980s, intravascular ultrasound (IVUS) is currently the most commonly employed intracoronary imaging technique employed during angiography. In comparison to IVUS, optical coherence tomography (OCT) is relatively a newer technique being first put to use in human studies in 2008. Newer generation OCT provides quickly acquired uniquely detailed images of the vessel wall and reveals critical information regarding stability of the plaque in terms of thickness of fibrous cap, size of the necrotic core, and the presence of macrophages. Prior to stent implantation, OCT can be used to judge the lesion severity, stability of the plaque, and the diameter and the length of the lesion (thus, the exact size of the stent required). Poststent implantation, OCT allows for accurate assessment of adequate stent expansion and placement, and also ruling out complications such as dissection at the stent edge, which might not be visible on the coronary angiography. This may be transformed into better optimization of the stent implantation at the time of procedure leading to better future outcomes and lesser rates of stent restenosis. ST-elevation myocardial infarction (STEMI) is the manifestation of transmural ischemia cause by acute thrombotic occlusion of a coronary vessel. The underlying atherosclerotic mechanism of thrombotic occlusion may be associated with plaque rupture (most common), plaque erosion, or a calcific nodule rarely. However, in the standard contemporary practice, STEMI is treated with primary angioplasty and stenting in all of the cases irrespective of the underlying mechanism of the event. This is the case due to inability of fluoroscopic techniques to accurately identify the mechanism of thrombotic occlusion. OCT imaging allows differentiation of plaque rupture from an intact fibrous cap and thus, specific management of each which may lead to improved outcomes.

PRINCIPLES AND TECHNIQUE OF OPTICAL COHERENCE TOMOGRAPHY IMAGE ACQUISITION AND INTERPRETATION

Optical coherence tomography imaging is analogous to IVUS imaging with light from near-infrared spectrum being used as an energy source in contrast to ultrasound waves. A monorail OCT catheter with the energy source mounted over it, is introduced in the vessel lumen over a guidewire and the vessel is scanned in a spiral manner. Spiral scanning occurs by the virtue of motorized catheter pullback (2–3 mm/s) and rotation of the OCT device over the longitudinal axis of the catheter. The light emitted by the OCT device penetrates the tissue to a depth of 2–3 mm and the reflected light is captured by the OCT device followed by signal transmission back to the console for image generation. Latest generation OCT systems use Fourier-domain interferometry for image generation.

This means that each specific image point is calculated by the time taken by the light beam to penetrate, get reflected, and reach back to the device. The brightness of the point is determined by the intensity of the reflected light. Thus, OCT pullback creates a cylindrical dataset of the vessel wall coaxial to the OCT catheter. This dataset can be used to create any number of axial and longitudinal image slices. A lumenogram can also be generated with minimal lumen areas of each cross-section being taken into consideration along the length of the data acquisition (Fig. 1).

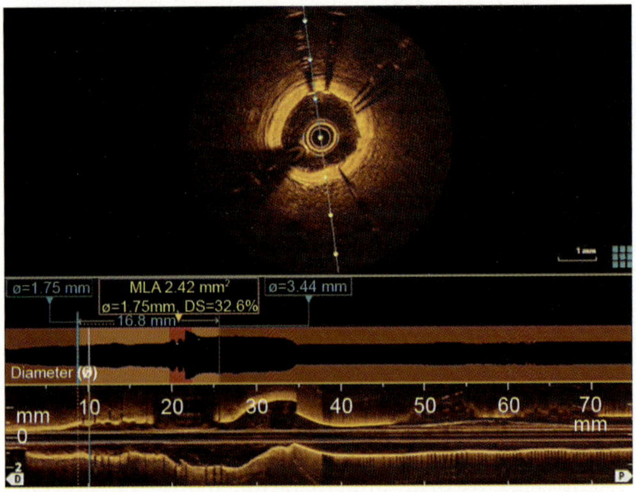

Fig. 1: Representation of optical coherence tomography (OCT) image acquisition. Axial section is seen in the upper part of the image. Longitudinal section (along the axis marked by a dotted line in the axial image) is seen in the lower part of the image. A lumenogram (two-dimensional longitudinal representation based on cross-sectional area rather than being in a single plane) is seen in the middle part of the section.

In a cross-sectional image, OCT clearly identifies three layers of the blood vessel, namely—(1) tunica intima, (2) tunica media, and (3) tunica adventitia (Fig. 2). In a vessel affected by atherosclerosis and plaque deposition, the differentiation of intimal layer may be lost. However, the fibrous cap along the lumen is accurately identified and its thickness can also be measured. A fibrous cap of thickness less than 65 µm is usually considered as a vulnerable plaque when associated with a significant amount of lipid burden. The nature of the plaque can be discerned by closely looking at the image characteristics. Two important image characteristics should be carefully looked for: (1) brightness and (2) shadowing. Fibrous plaque is highly reflective and casts a bright image, but still it allows significant amount of light to pass through and does not cast a shadow. A fatty plaque (lipid laden) instead absorbs light and appears dark. Due to its low transmittance of light, it causes a significant shadow. Whereas, a calcific plaque appears dark and well defined due to low reflectance. However, in contrast to a lipid-rich plaque, it does not cast any shadow. An algorithm for plaque morphology characterization is presented in Flowchart 1. The stent and the guidewire in the vessel lumen are highly reflective and also cast a significant shadow due to low transmittance of light. Red blood cells inside the vessel lumen also cast significant shadowing. Hence, the vessel needs to be cleared during image acquisition, which is achieved with contrast administration in the vessel at 3–4 mL/s during automated catheter pullback. This can be done preferably with a motorized injector or also with a hand injection. OCT also allows for identification of red and white thrombus in STEMI. The surface of red thrombus facing the catheter appears bright while it causes a significant shadow. In contrast, the white thrombus appears as a bright

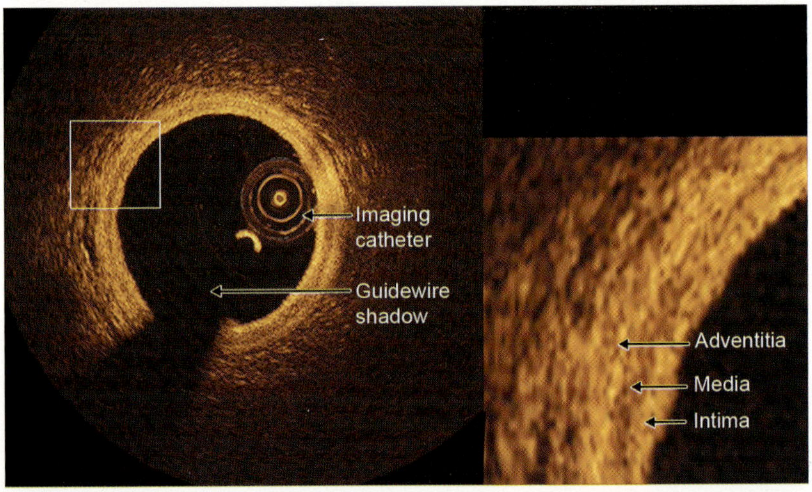

Fig. 2: Optical coherence tomography (OCT) image demonstrating cross-section of a normal epicardial coronary artery. Inset shows magnified image with differentiation of the three layers of the blood vessel namely—(1) tunica intima, (2) tunica media, and (3) tunica adventitia.

Flowchart 1: Algorithm for classification of plaque morphology on optical coherence tomography (OCT) imaging.

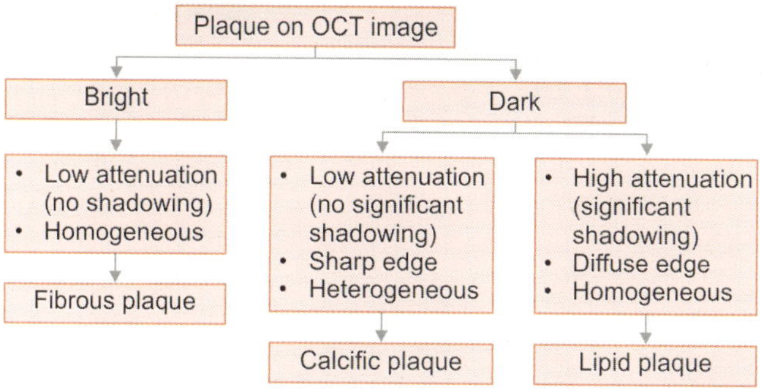

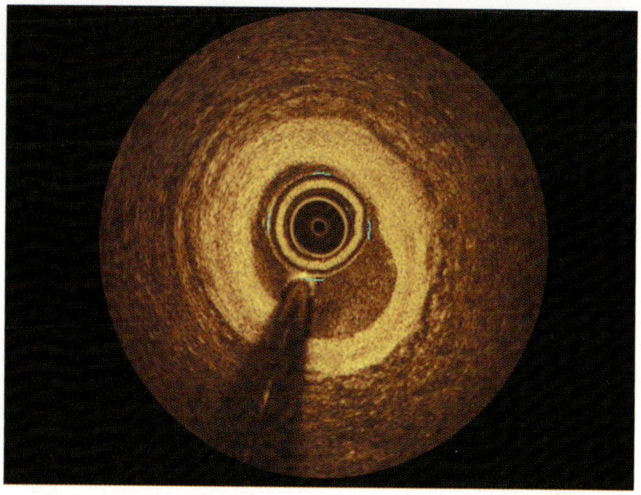

Fig. 3: Cross-sectional OCT image of a fibrous plaque (7 O'clock to 3 O'clock position). An arc of calcium is also seen from 3 O'clock to 5 O'clock position). Not made of saturation artifact due to highly reflective guidewire on the lumen at 6 O'clock to 7 O'clock positions. Incomplete clearance of blood vessel leading to presence of few RBCs in the lumen is also visualized. (OCT: optical coherence tomography; RBCs: red blood cells)

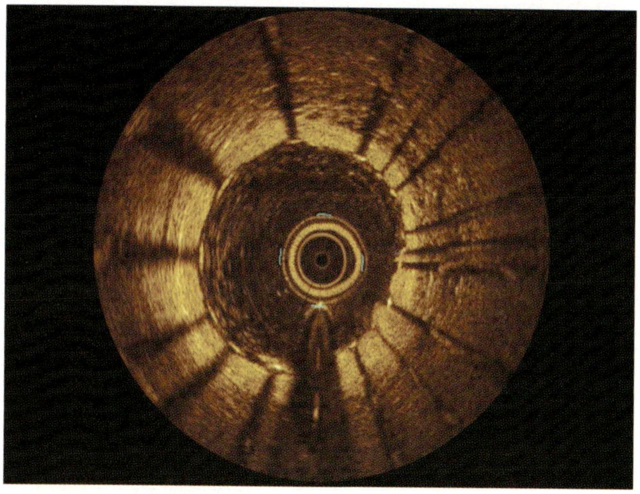

Fig. 4: Poststenting optical coherence tomography (OCT) demonstrating well-apposed stent struts. Note the presence of saturation artifacts due to highly reflective stent struts.

homogeneous mass inside the lumen without significant shadowing. Importantly for the current discussion, OCT allows imaging of the underlying culprit plaque in an acute coronary syndrome. A plaque rupture can be identified by presence of flaps that protrude in the lumen caused by tears in the fibrous cap. The communication between the plaque and vessel lumen causes the contents of the plaque to empty into vessel lumen and promote thrombus formation. The plaque may thus appear dark after a plaque rupture. Kubo et al. characterized plaque erosion on OCT with loss of endothelial lining and intimal tears without rupture of the entire thickness of the fibrous cap.[1] However, loss of endothelial lining is difficult to define and plaque erosion is identified with the presence of irregular thrombus deposition along the vessel wall in the absence of evidence of plaque rupture.[2] OCT is much more accurate than IVUS or any other imaging modality at detecting plaque erosion.[1] Figures 3 to 6 present examples of OCT images depicting morphology of plaque, stent apposition, red and white thrombus, and plaque erosion.

In comparison to IVUS, the main advantage of OCT is the exceptional quality of images due to its higher resolution. OCT gives an axial resolution of 10 μm and a lateral resolution of 20 μm, whereas the resolution of IVUS images is to the tune of 150–250 μm. However, OCT has limited depth of penetration (2–3 mm) as compared to IVUS (up to 10 mm) which makes IVUS the imaging modality of choice in larger vessels such as left main coronary artery.

IMPLICATIONS AND EVIDENCE FOR USE OF OCT IMAGING IN STEMI

Traditionally, the mechanism of STEMI was considered to be atherosclerotic plaque rupture followed by thrombotic occlusion of the vessel in all of the cases. However, with the advent of intracoronary imaging, it was increasingly recognized that plaque erosion with an intact fibrous cap is another important mechanism, which is the underlying mechanism in a sizeable proportion of STEMI cases. Although, plaque rupture remains the most common cause of thrombotic occlusion in STEMI, plaque erosion is definitely not an uncommon cause. In autopsy studies, plaque erosion constitutes up to 40% of the fatal cases with coronary thrombi.[3,4] In a combined OCT and IVUS study

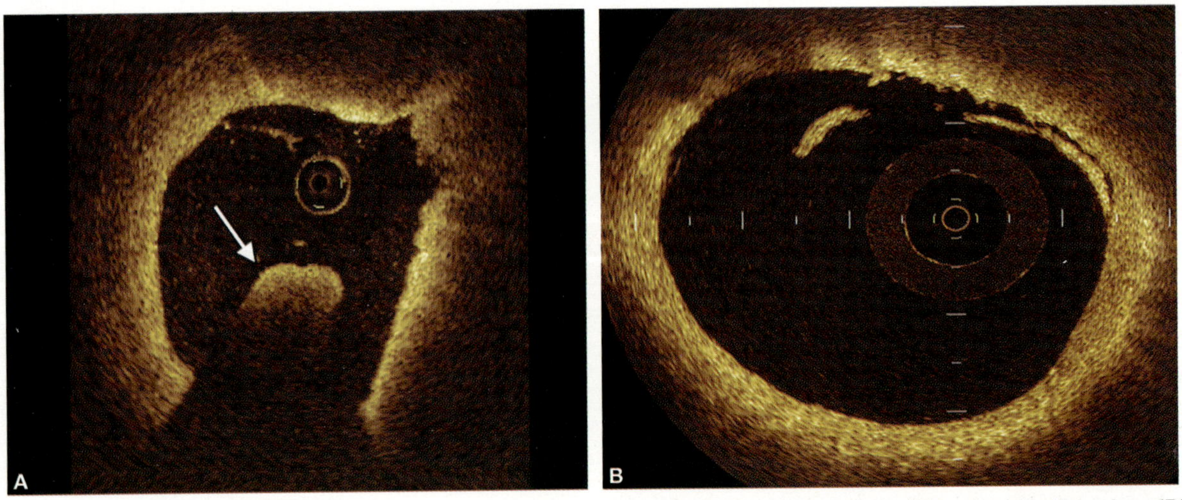

Figs. 5A and B: Optical coherence tomography (OCT) images demonstrating red thrombus (A) and white thrombus (B). Red thrombus is seen as an echogenic surface with significant shadowing. Whereas, white thrombus appears echogenic and heterogeneous but does not cause any significant shadowing.

of 112 STEMI, patients undergoing primary PCI within 12 hours by Higuma et al., plaque rupture, plaque erosion, and calcific nodule were found in 64.3%, 26.8%, and 8.0%, respectively.[5] Similar incidence has been reported from another interesting study called OCTAVIA trial in which OCT was performed on culprit lesions during acute events and on follow-up.[6] In another study of 126 patients, plaque erosion rate of 31% and a higher calcific nodule rate of 7.9% were noted.[7] Thus, plaque erosion seems to be the culprit in at least one-fourth of all cases of STEMI. Plaque erosion seems to be more common in younger population especially premenopausal women who are smokers.[7] Plaque erosion is also commonly seen in cases of non-ST-elevation acute coronary syndromes (ACSs).[7] Another interesting observation is the presence of less severe diameter culprit stenosis in plaque erosion as compared to plaque rupture.[7] Calcific nodules are characterized by significant luminal irregularity cause by a highly calcific and lipid-deficient matrix. Calcific nodules comprised 2–5% of cases in a series of sudden cardiac deaths, and were specifically more common in the mid-right coronary artery.[8] However, calcific nodules were found to be innocent bystanders with minimal added risk of ACS at up to 3 years follow-up in a prospective IVUS-based study of plaque morphology (PROSPECT trial).[9] Thus, plaque rupture and plaque erosion are the two most important mechanisms of acute myocardial infarction (MI) comprising most of the cases (Flowchart 2).

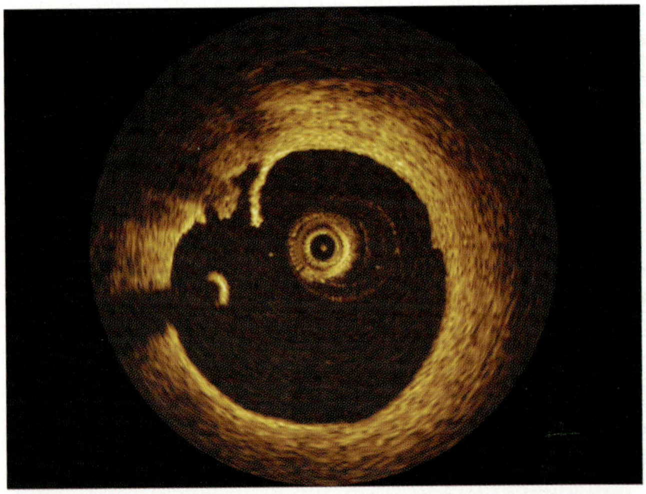

Fig. 6: High-resolution of optical coherence tomography (OCT) image allows visualization of small intimal tears and sometimes plaque erosions. A small thrombus is visualized at the site of the denuded endothelium.

Small observational studies have suggested impact of the morphology of culprit plaque on clinical outcomes. A study comprising of 72 patients demonstrated greater myocardial damage and poorer functional recovery among patients with MI cause by acute plaque rupture as compared to plaque erosion. In this study, the baseline wall motion score index (WMSI) on echocardiography at baseline was similar in both the groups. However, at 1 month of follow-up, the improvement in WMSI was significantly more pronounced in the plaque erosion group as compared to the plaque rupture group.[10] Another IVUS study also demonstrated larger infarct size in patients with acute MI associated with plaque rupture.[11] Thus, current evidence suggests better prognosis in patients with plaque erosion as compared to plaque rupture. OCT imaging can come handy during planning and optimization of PCI in general. In the ILUMIEN 1 trial, OCT led to a change in the management strategy in 57% of the cases with prestenting OCT imaging and 27% of the cases with poststenting OCT imaging.[12] In the recent DOCTORS trial, use of OCT imaging in non-ST elevation, ACS patients led to improved post-PCI fractional flow reserve (FFR) values and thus, a better functional result.[13] OCT imaging also helps to identify problems associated with stent structure (stent fracture) and implantation (malapposition and underexpansion) in cases with in-stent restenosis (ISR). This may reveal important information for decision making regarding need of a stent implantation versus a drug eluting balloon angioplasty for treatment of ISR. However, in both DOCTORS trial and ILUMIEN 3 trial, radiation dose, fluoroscopy time, and contrast dose were higher with the use of OCT imaging.[13,14] And the amount of benefit which OCT may confer in terms of reduced adverse clinical outcomes on long-term follow-up still remains uncertain. There remains a huge void requiring large scale and long-term studies to clarify the question of benefit conferred by OCT imaging during PCI. OCT imaging may be of a specific use in primary PCI during an STEMI situation.[15] Currently, all patients with STEMI situation are treated in a similar way irrespective of the plaque morphology. However, as discussed previously, patients with plaque erosion have milder degree of stenosis and possibly may do well only with thrombectomy without the need of a coronary stent. The hypothesis appears particularly appealing and was tested by Prati et al. in a small study of 31 patients with STEMI with plaque erosions.[15] 12 of the 31 patients were treated with thrombectomy only without any stent and the other 19 patients were treated in conventional manner with placement of a drug-eluting stent (Flowchart 3). At 2 years of follow-up, no patient in the thrombectomy alone group required repeat revascularization, thus confirming the feasibility of the strategy. Another study randomized 201 patients with STEMI to either primary PCI alone or OCT-guided primary PCI, and followed-up at 9 months with OCT imaging.[16] OCT guidance led to optimization of stent in 29% of the cases after primary PCI. The in-stent area stenosis was lower in the OCT-guided primary PCI at 9 months follow-up. However, to assert that these benefits translate into actual clinical benefits, larger trials with longer follow-up are needed.

Pitfalls of Optical Coherence Tomography Imaging

There are a number of technical limitations associated with OCT imaging. Imaging artifacts may be seen in up to one-third of the cases. The major limitation is the requirement of a blood-free field, necessitating a contrast flush. Even

Flowchart 2: Three major atherosclerotic pathophysiologic mechanisms of ST-elevation myocardial infarction (STEMI).

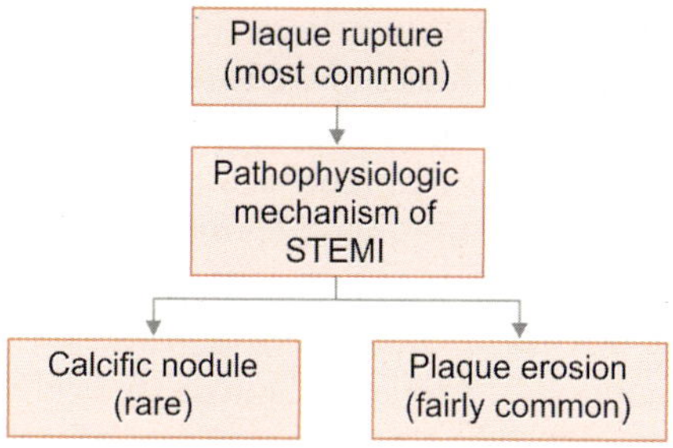

Flowchart 3: Proposed algorithm of OCT-guided treatment in STEMI patients as per study by Prati et al.[15]

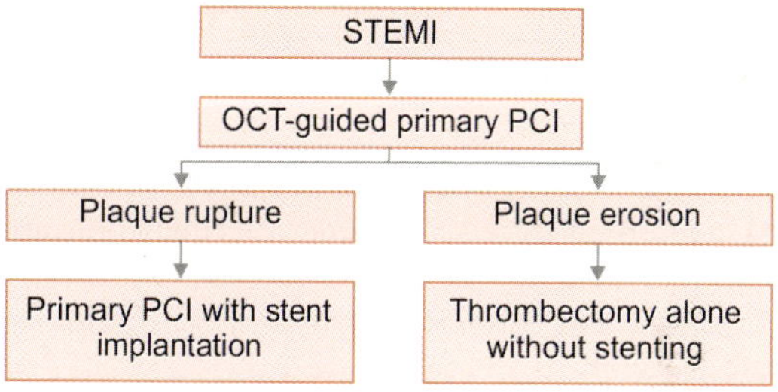

(OCT: optical coherence tomography; PCI: percutaneous coronary intervention; STEMI: ST-elevation myocardial infarction)

if there is small amount of blood left due to inadequate flush, red blood cells cast a significant shadow impairing image analysis and interpretation. Rotational artifacts and sew-up artifacts may also be noted due to abnormal rotation of the OCT probe or the OCT catheter inside the blood vessel. Another important limitation is the limited depth of penetration rendering it unusable in large vessels such as left main coronary artery and saphenous venous grafts. Differentiation of a calcific plaque from a lipid-rich plaque may be slightly more difficult as compared to IVUS due to similar hypoechoic pattern of both the plaques on OCT. Analysis of OCT imaging is time-consuming and leads to significant increment in procedural times in a busy catheterization laboratory. The time taken may be prohibitive for pre-PCI use during primary PCI in STEMI situation. Lastly, OCT imaging has significant costs involved and the benefits need to be significant for justifying its incorporation during PCI.

CONCLUSION

Optical coherence tomography imaging is an important tool in the interventional cardiologist's armamentarium. It gives excellent quality high-resolution images of the coronary vessels and the atherosclerotic plaques. It has allowed development of new insights regarding pathophysiology of atherosclerosis which leads to STEMI. Besides plaque rupture, plaque erosion has been recognized as an important and common mechanism of STEMI. Small clinical trials suggest utility of OCT imaging in identifying plaque erosion, which may be treated with thrombectomy alone without the implantation of a coronary stent. Also, OCT imaging allows optimization of stent implantation, which may improve outcomes. However, at present, routine use of OCT imaging during primary PCI cannot be recommended due to lack of adequate evidence. Also, increased procedural time, increased procedural cost, and increased contrast dose are significant issues that need to be addressed before routine uptake of OCT imaging in interventional practice.

REFERENCES

1. Kubo T, Imanishi T, Takarada S, et al. Assessment of culprit lesion morphology in acute myocardial infarction: ability of optical coherence tomography compared with intravascular ultrasound and coronary angioscopy. J Am Coll Cardiol. 2007;50:933-9.
2. Tearney GJ, Regar E, Akasaka T, et al. Consensus standards for acquisition, measurement, and reporting of intravascular optical coherence tomography studies: a report from the International Working Group for Intravascular Optical Coherence Tomography Standardization and Validation. J Am Coll Cardiol. 2012;59:1058-72..
3. van der Wal AC, Becker AE, van der Loos CM, et al. Site of initial rupture or erosion of thrombosed coronary atherosclerotic plaques is characterized by an inflammatory process irrespective of the dominant plaque morphology. Circulation. 1994;89:36-44.
4. Virmani R, Kolodgie FD, Burke AP, et al. Lessons from sudden coronary death. A comprehensive morphological classification scheme for atherosclerotic lesions. Arterioscler Thromb Vasc Biol. 2000;20:1262-75.
5. Higuma T, Soeda T, Abe N, et al. A Combined Optical Coherence Tomography and Intravascular Ultrasound Study on Plaque Rupture, Plaque Erosion, and Calcified Nodule in Patients with ST-Segment Elevation Myocardial Infarction: Incidence, Morphologic Characteristics, and Outcomes after Percutaneous Coronary Intervention. JACC Cardiovasc Interv. 2015;8:1166-77.
6. Saia F, Komukai K, Capodanno D, et al. Eroded versus ruptured plaques at the culprit site of STEMI: in vivo pathophysiological features and response to primary PCI. JACC Cardiovasc Imaging. 2015;8:566-75.
7. Jia H, Abtahian F, Aguirre AD, et al. In vivo diagnosis of plaque erosion and calcified nodule in patients with acute coronary syndrome by intravascular optical coherence tomography. J Am Coll Cardiol. 2013;62:1748-58.
8. Virmani R, Kolodgie FD, Burke AP, et al. Lessons from sudden coronary death: A comprehensive morphological classification scheme for atherosclerotic lesions. Arterioscler Thromb Vasc Biol. 2000;20:1262-75.
9. Xu Y, Mintz GS, Tam A, et al. Prevalence, distribution, predictors, and outcomes of patients with calcified nodules in native coronary arteries a 3-vessel intravascular ultrasound analysis from Providing Regional Observations to Study Predictors of Events in the Coronary Tree (PROSPECT). Circulation. 2012;126:537-45..
10. Tanaka A, Shimada K, Namba M, et al. Ruptured plaque is associated with larger infarct size following successful percutaneous coronary intervention in ST segment elevation acute myocardial infarction. Coron Artery Dis. 2009;20:260-6.
11. Kusama I, Hibi K, Kosuge M, et al. Impact of plaque rupture on infarct size in ST-segment elevation anterior acute myocardial infarction. J Am Coll Cardiol. 2007;50:1230-7.
12. Wijns W, Shite J, Jones MR, et al. Optical coherence tomography imaging during percutaneous coronary intervention impacts physician decision-making: ILUMIEN I study. Eur Heart J. 2015;36:3346-55.
13. Meneveau N, Souteyrand G, Motreff P, et al. Optical coherence tomography to optimize results of percutaneous coronary intervention in patients with non-ST-elevation acute coronary syndrome: Results of the multicenter, randomized DOCTORS (does optical coherence tomography optimize results of stenting). Circulation. 2016;134:906-17.
14. Ali ZA, Maehara A, Généreux P, et al. Optical coherence tomography compared with intravascular ultrasound and with angiography to guide coronary stent implantation (ILUMIEN III: OPTIMIZE PCI): a randomised controlled trial. Lancet. 2016;388:2618-28.
15. Prati F, Uemura S, Souteyrand G, et al. OCT-based diagnosis and management of STEMI associated with intact fibrous cap. JACC Cardiovasc Imaging. 2013;6:283-7.
16. Kala P, Cervinka P, Jakl M, et al. OCT guidance during stent implantation in primary PCI: A randomized multicenter study with nine months of optical coherence tomography follow-up. Int J Cardiol. 2018;250:98-103.

31

CHAPTER

Role of OCT in the Subset of CAD Postpercutaneous Coronary Intervention and Postcoronary Artery Bypass Graft

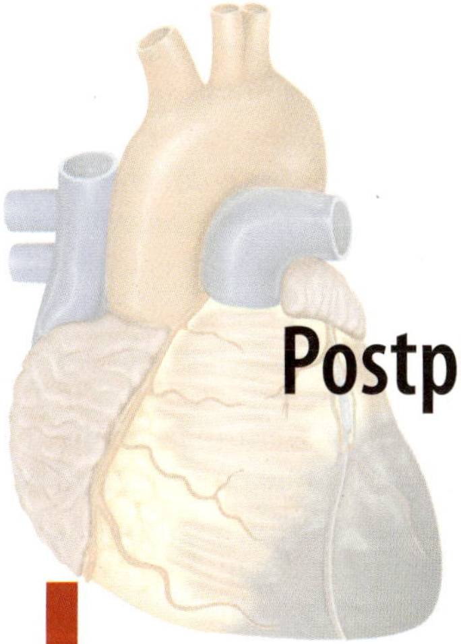

Binoy John

INTRODUCTION

Optical coherence tomography (OCT) is an optical analog of intravascular ultrasound (IVUS) which uses near-infrared light with a wavelength of about 1,300 nm for image acquisition. Over the past decades, IVUS and OCT have progressively evolved with respect to technical performance with higher resolution imaging and in procedural aspects with faster pullback, automatic vessel-lumen and plaque burden detection, measurements, and co-registration with angiography.[1] OCT can be used to visualize coronary arteries with 10 times greater resolution of 10–15 µm in comparison to IVUS, which has a resolution of only 100–150 µm.[2,3] This high-resolution of OCT helps to distinguish the intima, media, and adventitia of the coronary arteries and also to differentiate the internal and external elastic laminae clearly, which is otherwise not possible with IVUS. Based on the polarization properties, OCT can also differentiate tissue characteristics of plaques as being fibrotic, calcific, or lipid rich and even identify thin cap fibroatheroma (TCFA).[4] OCT has emerged as an important tool in the assessment of coronary artery disease (CAD) before revascularization in the optimization of percutaneous coronary interventions (PCIs) and also in the assessment and follow-up of CAD after revascularization. In the prePCI assessment of CAD, OCT gives detailed information on the severity of stenosis, length of stenosis, plaque composition, presence and extent of calcium, plaque rupture, presence of thrombus, and other anatomic characteristics, thereby aiding in the planning of PCI. It also provides precise information regarding the stent diameter and length to be used, thus aiding in a more scientific performance of PCI. Immediately post-PCI, OCT helps in the assessment of stent apposition and sizing of balloon for postdilatation, assessment of side-branch occlusion, and management strategies for side-branch angioplasty. OCT also helps to detect procedural complications or adverse sequelae like the presence of edge dissections, differentiation between thrombus and tissue prolapse, thus assisting in the optimization of PCI, providing better acute, subacute, and long-term results. In the post-PCI scenario, OCT can be used in the assessment of CAD especially pertaining to stent follow-up and features like stent strut endothelialization, neointimal coverage, in-stent restenosis (ISR), and the assessment of stent failure. OCT has been validated for use in assessment of strut coverage with an accuracy resembling that of histology.[5] OCT is also useful in the post-PCI assessment of etiology of stent thrombosis and thus, directing further strategies in the treatment and effective prevention of stent thrombosis. In the post-PCI scenario, in addition to assessment of native CAD in a manner similar to its pre-PCI assessment, OCT can also be used in the assessment of patency of side branches and side-branch stents. Similarly, OCT can be used to identify degeneration of coronary artery bypass grafts and provide insight into mechanisms of graft failure.

ROLE OF OPTICAL COHERENCE TOMOGRAPHY IN THE POSTPERCUTANEOUS CORONARY INTERVENTION SUBSET

Following PCI and stenting, stents variably get covered by endothelium, depending on the type of stent used, whether it is a bare metal stent (BMS) or a drug-eluting stent (DES). Even among DES, the endothelialization is variable depending on whether the stents are first or second or third generation or whether they are bioresorbable stents. OCT has shed immense light and provided a lot of insight and information on the patterns and mechanisms of endothelialization, ISR, and stent failure.

Restenosis is defined as a reduction in lumen diameter at the site of stenosis after PCI, either with or without stent implantation. It is a progressive phenomenon that starts soon after barotrauma associated with PCI. The three key mechanisms associated with restenosis include: (1) elastic recoil, (2) vascular remodeling, and (3) neointimal hyperplasia (NIH). In the absence of a stent, elastic recoil of the vessel at the site of the lesion and vascular remodeling are the predominant mechanisms, with the contribution of NIH to restenosis being limited. The internal and external elastic laminae of the coronary arteries contain elastin fibers which causes elastic recoil after balloon overstretch. Elastic recoil can result in up to 40% loss of luminal area, which can occur in a few seconds to minutes after balloon deflation.[6] Vascular remodeling is a more complex phenomenon, which consists of a medial and adventitial response to the barotrauma. The first two mechanisms for restenosis have been done away with, with the usage of stents. However, with the usage of stents, the mechanisms associated with ISR are different from restenosis after mere balloon angioplasty. ISR is characterized by excessive tissue proliferation stimulated by the presence of stent struts called NIH and a newly occurring atherosclerotic process in the neointima called neoatherosclerosis (NA).[7] NIH is characterized by vascular smooth muscle proliferation or migration and activation caused by vessel injury following mechanical stretch, rupture of internal elastic lamina, and medial dissection. ISR is a nonspecific inflammatory response to this injury and the persistent insult exercised by the foreign metal struts of the stent. The chronic wall stress due to stent strut protrusion into the tunica intima stimulates inflammatory processes and causes the migration of smooth muscle cells from tunica media and myofibroblasts from tunica adventitia to the tunica intima. In addition, the endothelial denudation leads to the exposure to circulating mitogens causing tissue proliferation. The vascular smooth cells, endothelial cells, platelets, and inflammatory cells also release mitogens and cytokines, which further enhances NIH. The myointimal barotrauma causes the atherosclerotic process also to change from its natural evolution of atherosclerotic plaque to a more aggressive local response at the site of injury. However, the NA occurring postPCI in response to myointimal barotrauma is different in that it is more focal and aggressive than the atherosclerosis associated with native CAD and is one of the reasons for late stent failure over time from stent thrombosis and acute coronary syndromes. Recent research based on histologic and intravascular imaging studies have indicated that NA within the neointimal region of the stented segment after coronary stent implantation is one of the mechanisms for late and very late stent thrombosis.[8] NA is characterized by the presence of clusters of lipid-laden foamy macrophages with or without necrotic core formation and or calcification within the neointimal tissue of stented segments.[8] Though histology can confirm diagnosis of NA, obtaining samples are difficult. So, OCT has now emerged as a tool in the characterization of various types of intimal tissue and the detection of morphological characteristics of NA such as macrophage infiltration, lipid accumulation, in-stent calcification, and neointimal rupture.[8] On OCT, OCT-defined NA is mainly confined to lipidic or calcific neointima. Lipidic neointima is seen as diffusely bordered, signal-poor regions with overlying signal-rich bands. Calcific neointima shows well delineated signal-poor regions with sharp borders.[9,10] NA was first described in BMS and later described in DES. One of the mechanisms for NA is the incomplete regeneration of endothelium, which results in an excessive uptake of the lipids circulating in the blood which causes an accelerated atherosclerosis of the new neointima. NA is, therefore, more common with DES than BMS due to the incomplete endothelialization associated with the drug in DES. In an OCT study of DES at 9 months and 2 years by Kim et al.,[11] it was shown that age after stent was a major predictor of NA. Lipid-laden neointima (27.6% vs 14.5%, $p = 0.009$) and thin cap neoatheroma (13.2% vs 3.9%, $p = 0.007$) were more common at 2 years than at 9 months post-DES implantation. Patients with NA had higher chances of symptoms or need for repeat revascularization. OCT defined rupture of lipidic neointima was observed in patients with very late stent thrombosis.[12] ISR has been considered as an enemy of the interventional cardiologist and is an independent predictor for mortality.[13] Diffuse restenosis has been shown to be associated with higher incidence of events at 1 year.[14] Thus, OCT with its superior axial resolution serves in the better visualization and understanding of the endothelialization patterns of the stent struts, NIH, NA, ISR, and mechanisms of late stent failure.

Optical coherence tomography also helps in quantitative and qualitative assessment of the artery, stenosis, and restenotic tissue. Restenotic tissue area is defined as stent area minus lumen area. Restenotic tissue burden is defined as mean restenotic tissue area/mean stent area × 100. Most of the quantitative information is now automatically derived with newer softwares. Qualitatively, restenotic tissue can be categorized as homogeneous, heterogeneous, layered, and NA. Restenotic tissue is described as homogeneous when the tissue has uniform optical properties and does not show focal variations in the backscattering pattern. It is described as heterogeneous, when the tissue has focally changing optical properties and shows various backscattering patterns. The restenotic tissue is described as layered when the tissue contains concentric layers of different optical properties. The restenotic tissue is described to have high backscatter when majority of the tissues appeared bright and it is described to have low backscatter when majority of the tissues appeared dark or black. OCT also aids in the detection of microvessels in the restenotic tissue, which appears within the arterial wall as well-delineated low backscattering structures less than 200 µm in diameter. OCT also helps to characterize the arterial lumen shape as being regular with sharp well-delineated smooth and circular borders, or irregular with tissue protrusions from the arterial wall into the lumen. A study of 24 patients with ISR by Gonzalo et al.[15] with OCT characterized restenotic tissue based on the earlier optical properties of backscatter, presence or absence of microvessels, and lumen shape. The morphology of ISR using OCT can also reveal macrophage infiltration, necrotic core, in-stent calcification, and neoatherosclerotic plaque rupture. OCT can also help in understanding the histologic pattern and composition of stent NIH, as has been shown in many studies.[16] The heterogeneous composition of NIH can be understood from the variations in light attenuation and intensity of backscattering. Fibrotic tissue appears as homogeneous signal, which is mostly seen in BMS restenosis, whereas heterogeneous signals are associated with early intimal changes due to fibrin accumulation and proteoglycans or from NA.[10,16,17] OCT, thus, helps in visualization of stent endothelialization, strut coverage, and the thickness of neointima (Fig. 1) and also the type of NIH (Fig. 2) and NA and also other factors inducing restenosis like chronic underexpansion of stent struts which occur in 18–40% cases and stent fracture which occurs in less than 5% of cases.[18,19] Three-dimensional OCT can, however, help in identifying stent fracture better than two-dimensional OCT.

Thus, OCT characterization of neointima after stent implantation can help to derive important information regarding possible mechanisms of stent failure and thus, aid in targeted preventive therapy.

Optical coherence tomography can also be used in the post-PCI scenario in the evaluation of cases of stent thrombosis and their possible underlying mechanisms. Delayed coverage of stent struts or failure of stent coverage by neointima or regenerated endothelium are the usual causes.[20] Stent thrombosis can occur due to several mechanisms such as incomplete stent apposition (ISA), incomplete strut coverage by endothelium, and stent strut fracture. OCT with its high-resolution gives pristine information in this regard and can precisely assess and

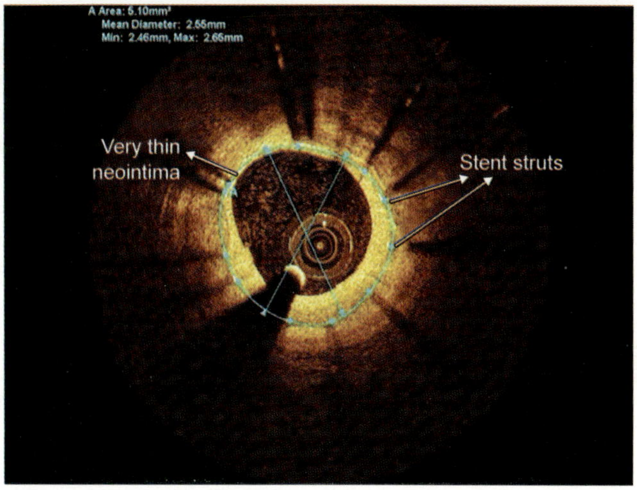

Fig. 1: Optical coherence tomography (OCT) showing completely endothelialized stent struts (homogeneous tissue with high backscatter).

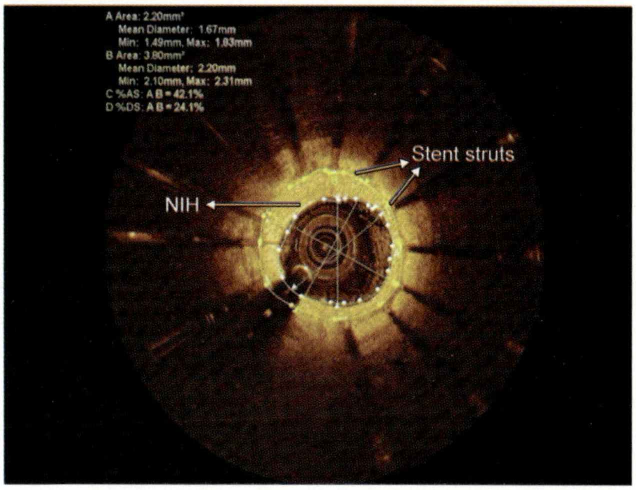

Fig. 2: Optical coherence tomography (OCT) showing completely endothelialized stent struts with eccentric neointimal hyperplasia (homogeneous restenotic tissue with high backscatter).

quantify stent coverage, ISA, and NIH.[21] Studies of pathology of stent thrombosis have shown that incomplete coverage of stent struts is one of the important mechanisms.[22,23] DES significantly suppress NIH and so have delayed neointimal coverage in contrast to BMS.[24] The stents may be covered with thin neointima less than 100 µm in thickness which is beyond the resolution of IVUS but can be picked up by OCT. In this regard, the first-generation stents were found to have uncovered struts even 5 years after index procedure.[25] Among second-generation stents, however, in a review of 33 studies by Papayannis et al.,[26] it was seen that sirolimus-eluting stents were found to have the highest frequency of uncovered and malapposed stent struts in contrast to paclitaxel-eluting struts and zotarolimus-eluting stents. The second-generation DES demonstrated more favorable vascular healing, better neointimal coverage, and less ISA than the first-generation DES. Impaired neointimal coverage was seen to be more commonly associated with ISA and nonapposed side-branch struts in contrast to well-apposed struts with the risk of delayed coverage being more common with ISA than nonapposed side-branch struts. OCT, especially three-dimensional OCT is useful in the post-PCI assessment of ostial restenosis of side branches and side-branch stent struts following bifurcation angioplasty, which may be usually overestimated by the oculostenotic reflex when using conventional angiography.

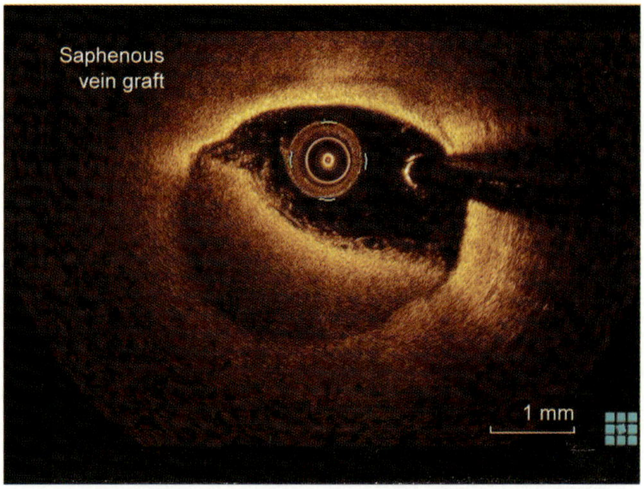

Fig. 3: OCT showing post-CABG surgery status of saphenous vein graft (without external and internal elastic laminae). (CABG: coronary artery bypass graft; OCT: optical coherence tomography)

ROLE OF OPTICAL COHERENCE TOMOGRAPHY IN POSTCORONARY ARTERY BYPASS GRAFT SURGERY SUBSET

Although, there is evidence on the superiority of arterial conduits over saphenous vein grafts (SVGS) in coronary artery bypass graft (CABG) surgery, SVGs continue to be used in large numbers. Serial angiographic studies have shown that approximately 10% of the SVGs get occluded in the first 1 year following CABG surgery and there is a continuous attrition of these grafts which accelerate as the graft ages and only 40% of the grafts are patent by 10 years. There is limited information available on the OCT characteristics of CABGs. In this scenario, OCT with its higher axial resolution, serves as an important tool in the better visualization of the graft vessel walls in contrast to angioscopy.[27,28] OCT is a validated method in the assessment of SVGs.[29] OCT differentiation of veins from arteries is by the absence of the elastic laminae in the veins (Fig. 3). OCT can also show the entire vein grafts and the distinct components of the anastomotic site including the midanastomotic segment and the "toe" segment of the graft, which connects to the native coronary artery. OCT has been used in many trials assessing the features of SVGs in various scenarios and subsets with a lot of information being drawn in comparison to native coronary arteries.

In a study by Keith et al.[30] using OCT and IVUS in 42 asymptomatic patients, 3 years after CABG surgery, it was seen that all grafts imaged had variable fibrocellular neointima but no stenotic disease. OCT, but not IVUS, showed findings of thin-cap fibroatheroma in 6 out of 16 SVGs and adherent thrombus in 4 out of 16 SVGs. The OCT findings suggest that these may be important markers of SVGs prone for future occlusion. Also, ACS occurring in patients with prior CABG surgery has been shown to occur in lesions located in SVGs in 70–80% of the cases. Pathological, angioscopic, and IVUS studies[31] have shown that lesions in SVGs are similar to as occur in native coronary arteries and in patients with ACS, SVGs may have features of rupture too. In a study by Davlouros et al.[32] using OCT to evaluate 28 SVGs with an average graft age of 14.6 years in ACS. It was seen that the grafts showed culprit lesions with fibrofatty composition, relatively thin fibrous cap, plaque rupture, and thrombus which correlated with the clinical spectrum of ACS suggesting that similar mechanisms with native vessel atherosclerosis may be involved in SVG-related ACS also. An OCT cutoff point of 65 µm was used to distinguish a TCFA. Calcifications within plaques were identified by the presence of well-delineated, low-backscattering heterogeneous regions. Plaque rupture was defined as a cavity communicating with the lumen with an overlying residual fibrous cap fragment. Red thrombi were defined as high-backscattering protrusions with signal free shadowing and white thrombi as signal rich, low-backscattering billowing projections protruding into the lumen. Most lesions in the SVG were complex (96.4%) with ulceration and thrombi. Calcification was seen in 32.1% and thrombi were seen with increasing frequency across the ACS spectrum moving from unstable angina to ST-elevation myocardial infarction (STEMI). TCFA were seen in 100% cases of STEMI and 53% cases of non-STEMI and 20% cases of unstable angina.

However, there are some OCT features, which were distinctive to SVGs. The atherosclerotic plaques are larger with aneurysmal dilatations which are frequent with intraluminal friable tissue compared with those in native coronaries.[33] This may, however, be related to the larger size of the SVGs. SVGs also have more of degenerated fragmented atheroma or friable plaque which corresponds to the loose fibroatheromatous debris lining on the internal surface of the vessel and is rarely found in native coronary arterial atherosclerosis. OCT showed circumferential signal-free zones inside the walls of the SVGs and over those, a distinct high-signal layer of tissue loosely attached and/or in discontinuity with the vein wall, correlating with areas of degenerated SVGs on angiography, which represent friable tissue. There is evidence that the presence of friable tissue or the age of the graft (age ≥ 3 years) correlates with the risk of distal embolization and periprocedural mortality during PCI.[34] The study had a 17.9% incidence of distal embolization with thrombolysis in myocardial infarction flow grade less than 3 during procedures in five grafts all of which had evidence of degeneration. Thus, this OCT study documented that severe graft degeneration, aneurysmal dilatation, and plaque friability with specific plaque characteristics such as tissue fragmentation are rare in native coronary arteries and are unique to SVGs.[32] Another interesting study, the venous external support trial (VEST) analyzed the effect of a novel external stent and its impact on intimal hyperplasia a year later by IVUS.[35] Later in a substudy of VEST, by Mario et al.,[36] OCT was used in 24 patients to assess SVG morphology and anatomy at 12 months after CABG surgery. In VEST at the time of CABG surgery, an expandable external stent made of braided cobalt-chromium-nickel-molybdenum-iron fibers, was placed to one of the SVGs with each patient having an unstented graft, which served as the control group. IVUS and OCT done for both the stented and unstented grafts showed that the lumen of the stented graft was more homogeneous in contrast to the unstented graft. The smaller lumen eccentricity index seen in stented grafts indicates a tendency for these vessels to be more circular and uniform, which may have an influence on blood flow patterns within the SVGs. Clinically, the VEST suggested that placement of an external stent could improve luminal flow patterns and hemodynamic parameters in the SVGs by reducing oscillatory shear stress.[37] Also, adherent thrombus was seen in 13% of unstented grafts which were not all picked up by IVUS. This study thus shows that OCT is advantageous for showing luminal characters of SVGs which were otherwise unappreciable by IVUS as seen in other studies.[30] The OCT findings also suggest that these early changes that occur in SVGs may be responsible for accelerated vein graft failure and that the placement of external stents can result in a more homogeneous and less eccentric lumen without thrombus formation and thus, possible better long-term patency rates. However, larger and longer follow-up studies will be required to further these inferences on SVGs.

Optical coherence tomography evaluation of left internal mammary arteries also has been done. In a study by Porto et al.,[38] an OCT evaluation of the morphological features of the left internal thoracic artery (LITA) and nonharvested right internal thoracic artery and endothelium dependent and independent vasoreactivity in response to selective infusion of acetylcholine and isosorbide dinitrate, respectively were done in 10 patients who were 10 years postCABG surgery. It was seen that LITA grafts showed intimal thickening, increased intima/media ratio, and maintained endothelium-derived vasodilatation, changes which were likely to be an adaptive response to the different flow dynamics typical of coronary circulation.

CONCLUSION

Thus, in the post-PCI subset, OCT with its superior spatial resolution serves as an excellent tool and helps us to have a better visual understanding of the pathophysiology and mechanisms associated with CAD, pertaining to quantification of plaques and their composition, mechanisms of stent failure, ISR, stent apposition and characterization of tissue in scenarios of NIH, NA, and evaluation of stent thrombosis. OCT also gives us an insight into the mechanisms of possible graft failure after CABG surgery and thus, help to improvise and develop newer techniques and technology to prevent or treat existing problems associated with early graft failure and thus, provide long-term patency rates.

REFERENCES

1. Raber L, Mintz GS, Koskinas KC, et al. Clinical use of intracoronary imaging. Part 1: guidance and optimization of coronary interventions. An expert consensus document of the European Association of Percutaneous Cardiovascular Interventions. Eur Heart J. 2018;39:3281-300..
2. Brezinski ME, Tearney GJ, Bouma BE, et al. Imaging of the coronary artery microstructure (in vitro) with optical coherence tomography. Am J Cardiol. 1996;77:92-103.
3. Jang IK, Bouma BE, Kang DH, et al. Visualization of coronary atherosclerotic plaques in patients using optical coherence tomography: comparison with intravascular ultrasound. J Am Coll Cardiol. 2002;39:604-9.
4. Terashima M, Kaneda H, Suzuki T. The role of optical coherence tomography in coronary intervention. Korean J Intern Med. 2012;27:1-12.
5. Murata A, Wallace-Bradley D, Tellez A, et al. Accuracy of optical coherence tomography in the evaluation of neointimal coverage after stent implantation. J Am Coll Cardiol Img. 2010;3:76-84.
6. Cortese B, Andolina G, Piraino D, et al. Understanding and managing in-stent restenosis: a review of clinical data, from pathogenesis to treatment. J Thorac Dis. 2016;8:1150-62.
7. Eeckhout E, Serruys PW, Wijns W, et al. Percutaneous Interventional Cardiovascular Medicine: the PCR-EAPCI Textbook. Europe: PCR Publications; 2012. pp. 785-826.

8. Hong SJ, Lee SY, Hong MK. Clinical implication of optical coherence tomography-based neoatherosclerosis. J Korean Med Sci. 2017;32:1056-61.
9. Tearney GJ, Regar E, Akasaka T, et al. Consensus standards for acquisition, measurement and reporting of intravascular optical coherence tomography studies: a report from the International Working Group for Intravascular Optical coherence tomography standardization and validation. J Am Coll Cardiol. 2012;59:1058-72.
10. Prati F, Regar E, Mintz GS, et al. Expert review document on methodology, terminology and clinical applications of optical coherence tomography: physical principles, methodology of image acquisition and clinical application for assessment of coronary arteries and atherosclerosis. Eur Heart J. 2010;31:401-15.
11. Kim JS, Hong MK, Shin DH, et al. Quantitative and qualitative changes in DES-related neointimal tissue based on serial OCT. JACC Cardiovasc Imaging. 2012;5:1147-55.
12. Ko YG, Kim DM, Cho JM, et al. Optical tomography findings of very late stent thrombosis after drug eluting stent implantation. Int J Cardiovasc Imaging. 2012;28:715-23.
13. Cassese S, Byrne RA, Schulz S, et al. Prognostic role of restenosis in 10,004 patients undergoing routine control angiography after coronary stenting. Eur Heart J. 2015;36:94-109.
14. Mehran R, Dangas G, Abizaid AS, et al. Angiographic patterns of in-stent restenosis: classification and implications of long term outcome. Circulation. 1999;100:1872-8.
15. Gonzalo N, Serruys PW, Okamura T, et al. Optical coherence tomography patterns of stent restenosis. Am Heart J. 2009;158:284-93.
16. Nakano M, Vorpahi M, Otsuka F, et al. Ex vivo assessment of vascular response to coronary stents by optical frequency domain imaging. JACC Cardiovasc Imaging. 2012;5:71-82.
17. Templin C, Meyer M, Muller MF, et al. Coronary optical frequency domain imaging (OFDI) for in vivo evaluation of stent healing: comparison with light and electron microscopy. Eur Heart J. 2010;31:1792-801.
18. Kang SJ, Ahn JM, Song H, et al. Comprehensive intravascular ultrasound assessment of stent area and its impact on restenosis and adverse cardiac events in 403 patients with unprotected left main disease. Circ Cardiovasc Interv. 2011;4:562-9.
19. Goto K, Zhao Z, Matsumura M, et al. Mechanisms and patterns of intravascular ultrasound in-stent restenosis among bare metal and first and second generation drug eluting stents. Am J Cardiol. 2015;116:1351-7.
20. Zivelongi C, Ghione M, Kilickesmez K, et al. Intracoronary optical coherence tomography: a review of clinical applications. J Cardiovasc Med. 2014;15:543-53.
21. Cook S, Ladich E, Nakazawa G, et al. Correlation of intravascular ultrasound findings with histopathological analysis of thrombus aspirates in patients with very late drug-eluting stent thrombosis. Circulation. 2009;120:391-9.
22. Finn AV, Joner M, Nakazawa G, et al. Pathological correlates of late drug eluting stent thrombosis: strut coverage as a marker of endothelialization. Circulation. 2007;115:2435-41.
23. Virmani R, Guagliumi G, Farb A, et al. Localized hypersensitivity and late coronary thrombosis secondary toa sirolimus eluting stent: should we be cautious? Circulation. 2004;109:701-5.
24. Chen BX, Ma FY, Luo W, et al. Neointimal coverage of bare metal and sirolimus eluting stents evaluated with optical coherence tomography. Heart. 2008;94:566-70.
25. Takano M, Yamamoto M, Inami S, et al. Long-term follow up evaluation after sirolimus eluting stent implantation by optical coherence tomography: do uncovered struts persist? J Am Coll Cardiol. 2008;51:968-9.
26. Papayannis AC, Cipher D, Banerjee S, et al. Optical coherence tomography evaluation of drug eluting stents: a systematic review. Catheter Cardiovasc Interv. 2013;81:481-7.
27. Kubo T, Imanishi T, Takarada S, et al. Assessment of culprit lesion morphology in acute myocardial infarction: ability of optical coherence tomography compared with intravascular ultrasound and coronary angioscopy. J Am Coll Cardiol. 2007;50:933-9.
28. Regar E, van Soest G, Bruining N, et al. Optical coherence tomography in patients with acute coronary syndrome. EuroIntervention. 2010;6 Suppl G:G154-60.
29. Ben-Gal Y, Taggart DP, Williams MR, et al. Expandable external support device to improve saphenous vein graft patency after CABG. J Cardiothoracic Surg. 2013;8:122.
30. Adlam D, Antoniades C, Lee R, et al. OCT characteristics of Saphenous Vein Graft Atherosclerosis. JACC Cardiovasc Imaging. 2011;4:807-9.
31. Pregowski J, Tyczynski P, Mintz GS, et al. Incidence and clinical correlates of ruptured plaques in saphenous vein grafts: an intravascular ultrasound study. J Am Coll Cardiol. 2005;45:1974-9.
32. Davlouros P, Damelou A, Karantalis V, et al. Evaluation of culprit saphenous vein graft lesions with optical coherence tomography in patients with acute coronary syndromes. J Am Coll Cardiol Interv. 2011;4:683-93.
33. Jang IK, Tearney GJ, MacNeill B, et al. In vivo characterization of coronary atherosclerotic plaque by use of optical coherence tomography. Circulation. 2005;111:1551-5.
34. Liu MW, Douglas JS, Lembo NJ, et al. Angiographic predictors of a rise in serum creatinine kinase (distal embolization) after balloon angioplasty of saphenous vein coronary artery bypass grafts. Am J Cardiol. 1993;72:514-7.
35. Taggart DP, Ben-Gal Y, Lees B, et al. A randomized trial of external stenting for saphenous vein grafts in coronary artery bypass grafting. Ann Thorac Surg. 2015;99:2039-45.
36. Webb CM, Orion E, Taggart DP, et al. OCT imaging of aorto-coronary vein graft pathology modified by external stenting: 1-year post-surgery. Eur Heart J Cardiovasc Imag. 2016;17:1290-5.
37. Meirson T, Orion E, Di Mario C, et al. Flow patterns in externally stented saphenous vein grafts as related to the development of intimal hyperplasia. J Thorac Cardiovasc Surg. 2015;150:871-9.
38. Porto I, Gaudino M, De Maria GL, et al. Long-term morophofunctional remodeling of internal thoracic artery grafts. A frequency-domain optical coherence tomography study. Circ Cardiovasc Interv. 2013;6:269-76.

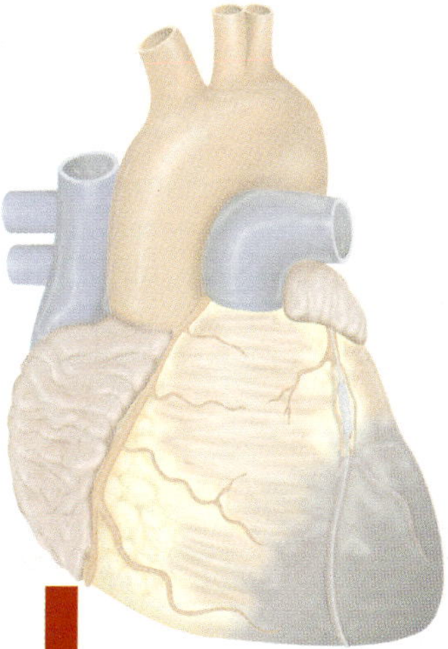

32

CHAPTER

Acute Coronary Syndrome: Bifurcation Lesion, Imaging, and Intervention Advances

Ravi Prakash, Viveka Kumar, Sunil Aggarwal

INTRODUCTION

Coronary bifurcation lesions comprise approximately 10–20% of percutaneous coronary interventions (PCIs).[1] Due to complexity of anatomy involved and the dynamic changes that occur during PCI, procedural and clinical outcomes associated with coronary bifurcation treatment are unfortunately suboptimal. Bifurcation lesions have been associated with lower rates of procedural success, higher restenosis rates, and adverse events compared with the treatment of relatively simpler, nonbifurcation lesions. Imaging has immense role to play in the management of bifurcation lesions. It may help in deciding the type and extend of the lesion, as well as kind of technique to be used for managing it. It is also useful in evaluation of postprocedural result, especially in left main bifurcation, where it is of utmost importance.

DEFINITION AND CLASSIFICATION

Analysis of bifurcation lesions involves assessment of lesion morphology in three important anatomic segments: (1) Proximal main branch (MB); (2) Distal MB; and (3) Side branch (SB). The carina is the point at which the proximal MB bifurcates into the distal MB and SB. The European Bifurcation Club defines a bifurcation lesion as a significant stenosis (i.e. > 50%) in a coronary artery adjacent to and/or involving the origin of an SB that is clinically significant.[2] Numerous classification schemes are available to characterize coronary bifurcation lesions. The simplest and most widely used is Medina classification.[3] The Medina classification assesses plaque burden based on the presence ("1") or absence ("0") of stenosis in the proximal MB, distal MB, and SB. A "true" bifurcation lesion involves significant stenosis in both the MB and the SB (i.e. Medina 1,1,1; 1,0,1; or 0,1,1), whereas all other lesion types would be classified as "nontrue". Here, we must understand that angiography has its limitations in its ability to appropriately classify bifurcation lesions, and adjunctive modalities such as intravascular ultrasound (IVUS) may be necessary to determine a lesion's true classification.

INDICATIONS OF PERCUTANEOUS CORONARY INTERVENTION

The indications for PCI of coronary bifurcation lesions follow the same general principles for revascularization of nonbifurcation lesions. The decision to pursue PCI or coronary artery bypass grafting (CABG) should be based on the present guidelines for nonbifurcation lesions, patient's preference, and the complexity and severity of coronary artery disease (CAD).

GENERAL APPROACH

Percutaneous coronary intervention of bifurcation lesions is undeniably and technically challenging. Each lesion can vary incredibly based on a number of anatomic characteristics, including bifurcation site, plaque location, plaque burden and morphology, bifurcation angle between the MB and SB, and vessel diameter. To complicate matters, bifurcation anatomy is dynamic and changes during PCI due to plaque or carina shift, bifurcation angle change, vessel spasm, and/or coronary dissection. The most important steps in PCI of coronary bifurcation are selection of appropriate treatment strategy and proper optimization of results of the intervention. The current prevailing opinion regarding the management is one of the "simpler is better" approaches; with provisional single stent strategy is the default strategy to go for in a suitable bifurcation lesion.

Treatment of bifurcation lesions with bare metal stents (BMSs) has yielded suboptimal results. Thus, drug-eluting stents (DESs) should be used for the treatment of bifurcation lesions.

One-stent versus Two-stent Approach

An important clinical decision is to determine a priori if a lesion will be approached using a one-stent (i.e. provisional) or two-stent approach. In a one-stent approach, the MB is stented and the SB is stented provisionally only if clinical symptoms and/or angiographic (e.g. < TIMI 3 flow) or adjunctive features [e.g. fractional flow reserve (FFR) < 0.80] warrant intervention. Whereas, a two-stent approach involves elective stenting of both the MB and SB. SB stenting should be considered: (1) When there is significant SB flow impairment (thrombolysis in myocardial infarction flow grade < 3); (2) In the presence of a major SB dissection; (3) When the SB is diseased and large enough to lead to significant residual ischemia; or (4) When future access toward the SB may be important.[4] Available data suggest that provisional SB stenting compared with elective SB stenting is the preferred approach due to equivalent clinical outcomes in both approaches and shorter procedural time and less contrast with the provisional approach. However, the generalizability of the clinical data to all bifurcation lesions is not appropriate. The heterogeneity and complexity of bifurcation lesions may warrant a one-stent or two-stent approach. No two bifurcations are alike, thus the therapeutic strategy should be determined in a lesion-specific manner. It is also important to remember that SB stenting is required in up to 30% of nonleft main and 50% of left-main bifurcation lesions.[5] The decision to perform elective SB stenting as part of a two-stent approach should be determined based on certain lesion characteristics.

TRUE BIFURCATION LESION

Typically, the two-stent approach has been reserved for lesions that have significant stenosis in both the MB and SB (i.e. Medina 1,1,1; 1,0,1; or 0,1,1), since the presence of two stents (versus just one stent in the bifurcation lesion) increases the risk of stent thrombosis. The SB length will also help to determine if a two-stent approach is needed (Fig. 1).

Bifurcation Angle

The bifurcation angle is determined by the internal angle between the MB and SB. Higher bifurcation angles are associated with increased rates of adverse events and SB closure. Importantly, the bifurcation angle should be assessed both before and after MB stenting, as the angle can change after treatment necessitating SB stenting. One-stent approaches are favored for bifurcation angles that are Y-shaped (<70°), whereas the two-stent approach should be considered for T-shaped (70–90°) or reverse-shaped (>90°).

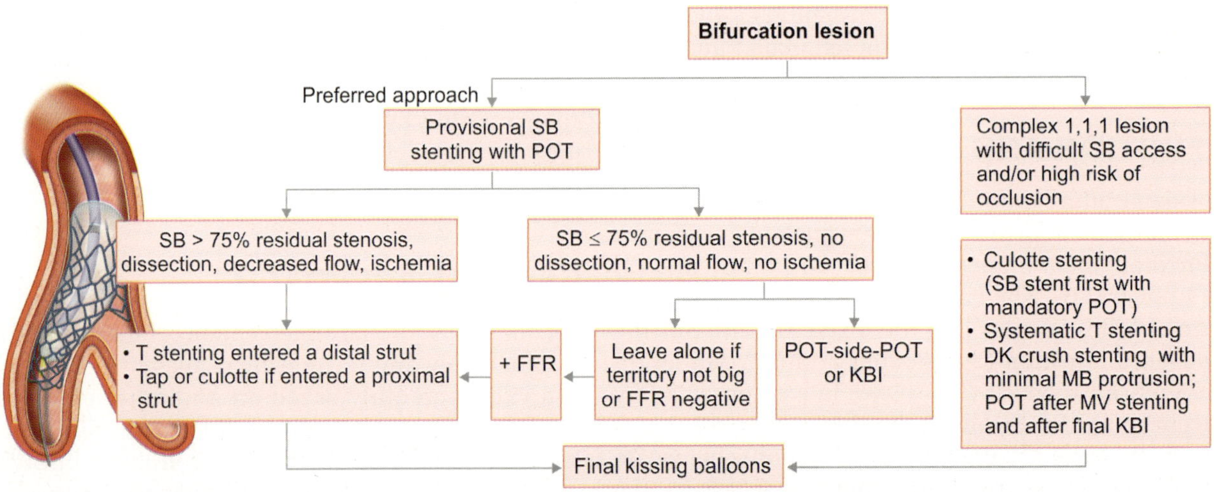

Fig. 1: Treatment algorithm for bifurcation lesion. (FFR: fractional flow reserve; SB: side branch)

Flowchart 1: Treatment algorithm for left main (LM) bifurcation lesion.

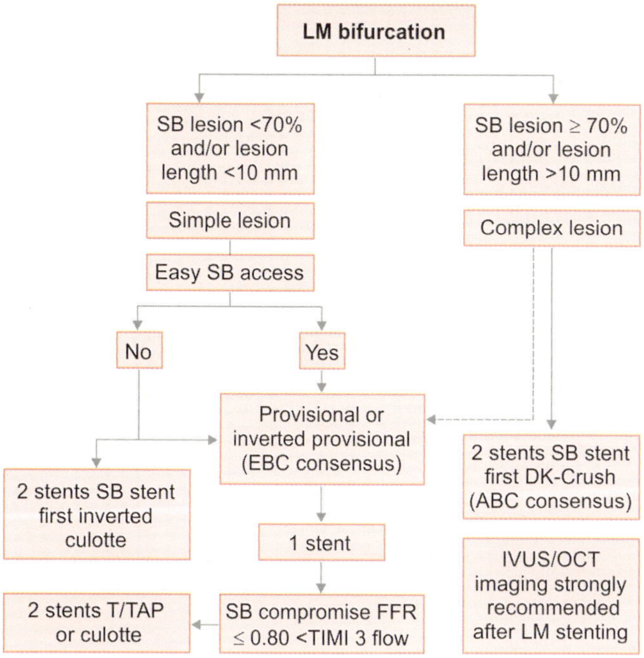

(FFR: fractional flow reserve; SB: side branch)

Side Branch Lesion Length

Isolated ostial or short SB lesions are less likely to occlude compared with long SB lesions. The two-stent technique is generally preferred for SB lesions more than or equal to 10 mm, whereas provisional SB stenting is typically reserved for focal lesions (≤5 mm). If an SB lesion is between 5 mm and 10 mm, clinical judgment should be used to select the most appropriate stenting strategy (Flowchart 1).

DEDICATED BIFURCATION STENTS

Dedicated bifurcation stents are designed to overcome limitations associated with conventional stents, such as SB protection and access, wire crossing through stent struts, multiple strut layering, ostial SB scaffolding gaps, and stent deformation and/or disruption. They are categorized into dedicated MB devices, which primarily provide access into the SB and only some coverage of the SB ostium, dedicated SB devices that are intended for primary SB treatment, dedicated MB plus SB devices that offer significant stent coverage of both branches but minimal coverage of the carina, and the MB stent with SB access port device that are designed primarily for MB stenting preserving access to the SB. Examples of dedicated stents are BIOSS stent, Stentys device, AXXESS stent, SLK view stent, and Tryton stent. However, going by available data, their superiority over the provisional strategy has yet to be demonstrated.

IMAGING

Alternative and/or Additional Procedures to Consider

It is very important to recognize that angiography is very limited in its ability to characterize bifurcation lesions. The use of adjunctive techniques such as intravascular ultrasound (IVUS), FFR, or optical coherence tomography (OCT) is often necessary for tailoring the appropriate PCI strategy for a given bifurcation lesion. IVUS and OCT can provide essential information for the assessment and treatment of BIF. They provide a better insight into plaque configuration and can diminish the unnecessary use of a two-stent procedure by identifying the extent of disease. This may play a role in improving outcomes and allowing selection of an appropriate stenting strategy. Before stenting, imaging may aid in vessel sizing and identify calcifications that may need rotational atherectomy. After stenting, both modalities can be used to evaluate stent expansion, edge dissection, or stent malapposition. OCT is also useful tool to aid recrossing into the jailed SB (distal strut), and achieve distal MB rewiring and favorable stent positioning against the SB ostium. Imaging should be mandatory for LM stenting, and as a minimum should be performed at the completion of the procedure to assess stent apposition and deployment (Flowchart 2).

Intravascular Ultrasound

Intravascular ultrasound can optimize the result following PCI and has the potential to reduce adverse cardiac events. Both IVUS (image resolution: 100–150 μ) and CT (resolution: 300–500 μ) lack the imaging resolution to fully appreciate the complex architecture of the bifurcation compared with OCT (OCT; image resolution: 10–20 μ). Fusion of CT and IVUS in obtaining three-dimensional (3D) reconstructions of human coronary bifurcation have successfully been undertaken to allow for wall shear stress analyses. This system, however, lacks the resolution obtainable with OCT. Several observational studies have shown that IVUS is associated with a reduction in adverse cardiac events. IVUS has many important uses in treatment of bifurcation lesions. Prior to PCI, IVUS can be used to assess plaque distribution and appropriately characterize the lesion ("IVUS Medina"), evaluate the extent of SB disease (especially for ostial lesions), appropriately size the vessel diameters of the MB and SB, and recognition of the IVUS "eyebrow" sign: a presenting marker for SB compromise. The information that IVUS provides when

Flowchart 2: Bifurcation lesion assessment through IVUS and FF.

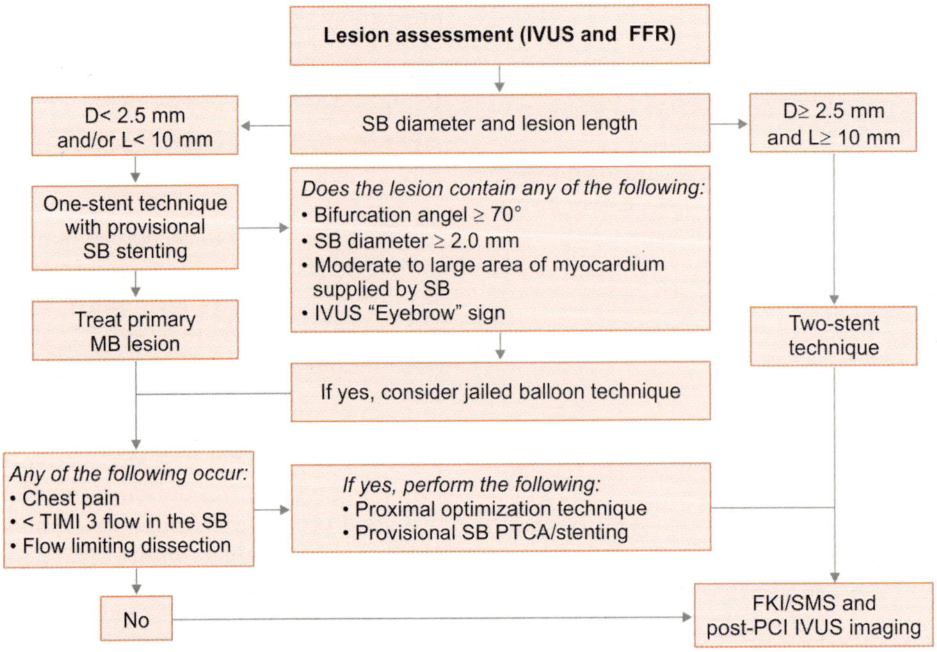

(FF: fractional flow; PCI: percutaneous coronary intervention; IVUS: intravascular ultrasound)

used prior to PCI allows for selection of stent size and length, type of stent, and the stenting technique. After PCI, IVUS can be used to assess for SB compromise, stent deformation of the MB, plaque shift in the MB or SB, proximal or distal edge dissection, stent malapposition, underexpansion, and stent lesion coverage including gaps.[6]

Fractional Flow Reserve

An fractional flow reserve (FFR) has the ability to assess the hemodynamic significance of a lesion. Given the importance of selecting the appropriate stenting technique for treatment of a bifurcation lesion, FFR can determine the ischemic potential of a given lesion and is most helpful for evaluating SB ostial disease. An FFR value less than 0.75 is the best cutoff value for determining if a lesion is hemodynamically significant; however, we should use the cutoff value of 0.80 as established in the FFR versus Angiography for Multivessel Evaluation (FAME) trial to improve the specificity of FFR and determine if a lesion should be treated. Another use of an FFR during treatment of bifurcation lesions is to assess the significance of a jailed SB following MB stenting. One study found that only 27% of jailed SB had an FFR value less than 0.75 and a jailed SB with an FFR more than 0.75 that did not undergo further treatment had very low rates of adverse clinical events. Thus, an FFR should be used to assess the significance of a jailed SB following MB stenting.[7]

Optical Coherence Tomography

Similar to IVUS, optical coherence tomography (OCT) can be used to optimize treatment of bifurcation lesions, both pre- and postprocedure. Compared to IVUS, OCT has a higher resolution, faster acquisition time, and smaller catheter size. It is limited by its tissue penetration, for which IVUS is superior. It can be particularly useful for evaluating lumen diameter, stent apposition and expansion, and lesion coverage. Current-generation Fourier domain optical coherence tomography (FDOCT) allows rapid pullback speeds and has allowed visualization of the coronary bifurcation with two-dimensional (2D) images in great detail. One of the major limitations of this technology, however, has been the lack of 3D images. Trying to mentally reconstruct a complex 3D structure from 2D images is difficult; 2D imaging may not allow a full appreciation of the anatomic features of the bifurcation and the effects of PCI. A limitation of OCT of the LM is the image interference with blood in a field that should be bloodless and filled only with contrast. Power injection of 20 mL of contrast over 5 s and a pressure of 500 psi can improve image quality.[8] Both IVUS and OCT can identify the preprocedure "spiky" carina or "eyebrow" sign at the origin of the SB that is a predictor of carinal shift and restenosis after LM stenting in a single-stent strategy. [8] 3D FDOCT reconstructions may have a clinical application in addition to tissue characterization.

Tissue characterization with 3D FDOCT imaging or fusion imaging of 2D FDOCT and IVUS virtual histology has the potential to aid in the identification of clinically useful areas of interest such as fibrocalcific plaque, lipid pools, and vulnerable plaque. Study utilizing longitudinal high-resolution IVUS has suggested that the effects of carina shift may be limited by the presence of fibrocalcific plaque at the carina, presumably because of resistance to expansion—using 3D FDOCT. This concept appears easier to appreciate; tissue characterization of intravascular imaging may ultimately aid in identifying these areas.

BIFURCATION LESIONS: TIPS AND TRICKS

- Use a 7-Fr or 8-Fr guide catheter, if possible.
- Pretreatment of IVUS and FFR is strongly encouraged.
- One-stent approach with provisional SB stenting will suffice for most lesions.
- Two-stent strategy should be used in lesions that are true bifurcation lesions with high bifurcation angles and/or long SB lesions (≥10 mm).
- If SB recrossing through MB stent struts is difficult, consider use of a second buddy wire, GuideLiner, or a low-profile 1.25 mm balloon.
- FKI should be performed in all cases.
- Post-treatment IVUS or OCT should be used to optimize the results.

CONCLUSION

Coronary artery bifurcation lesions pose a particular challenge in the field of interventional cardiology. Bifurcation interventions are associated with a higher rate of short- and long-term complications, with restenosis at the ostium of the side branch remaining the biggest problem. Currently, stenting the main branch with provisional side branch, stenting is the default approach in the majority of cases. IVUS should be employed at least in the more complex cases. These measures, if systematically applied, may further enhance the outcomes of bifurcation PCI, which nevertheless have already been substantially improved approximating those of nonbifurcation PCI. Expansion of the use of IVUS as well the introduction of new imaging modalities, such as OCT in the field of bifurcation PCI to guide optimal stent positioning and expansion apposition is warranted.

FINANCIAL AND COMPETING INTERESTS DISCLOSURE

The author has no relevant affiliations or financial involvement with any organization or entity with a financial interest in or financial conflict with the subject matter or materials discussed in the manuscript. No writing assistance was utilized in the production of this manuscript.

REFERENCES

1. Latib A, Colombo A. Bifurcation disease: what do we know, what should we do?. JACC Cardiovasc Interv. 2008;1:218-26.
2. Stankovic, G, Darremont O, Ferenc M. Percutaneous coronary intervention for bifurcation lesions: 2008 consensus document from the fourth meeting of the European Bifurcation Club. EuroIntervention. 2009;5:39-49.
3. Medina A, Suarez de Lezo J, Pan M. A new classification of coronary bifurcations lesions. Rev Esp Cardiol. 2006;59:183.
4. Latib A, Moussa I, Sheiban I, et al. When are two stents needed? Which technique is the best? How to perform? EuroIntervention. 2010;1:J81-7.
5. Katritsis DG, Siontis GC, Ioannidis JP. Double versus single stenting for coronary bifurcation lesions: a meta-analysis. Circ Cardiovasc Interv. 2009;2:409-15.
6. Rogacka R, Latib A, Colombo A. A IVUS-guided stent implantation to improve outcomes: a promise waiting to be fulfilled. Curr Cardiol Rev. 2009;5:78-86.
7. Koo BK, De Bruyne B. FFR in bifurcation stenting: what have we learned? EuroIntervention. 2010;1:J94-8.
8. Bezerra HG, Costa MA, Guagliumi G, et al. Intracoronary optical coherence tomography: a comprehensive review of clinical and research applications. JACC Cardiovasc Interv. 2009;2:1035-46.

33

CHAPTER

Quantitative Assessment of Myocardial Blood Flow and Fractional Flow Reserve and their Clinical Applications

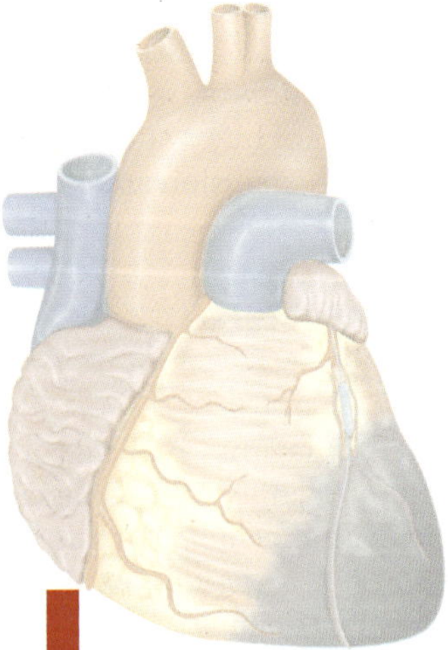

Ashwani Sood, Tinu T Lukose, Bhagwant R Mittal

INTRODUCTION

Presence of symptomatic or asymptomatic myocardial ischemia is an important risk factor in the clinical outcome of the patients with coronary artery disease (CAD). Early assessment and treatment of CAD will significantly reduce the morbidity and mortality even in asymptomatic patients who are at risk of developing CAD.[1] Various treatment strategies like medical therapy and percutaneous coronary intervention (PCI) depend upon the patients' clinical, biochemical and functional profile. The significance of functional assessment of coronary stenosis before percutaneous coronary intervention has been proven by various studies.[2-4] In this era of escalating medical costs, it is highly important to have accurate tests to support the clinical judgement, which may alter the patient management significantly. The tests with quantifiable parameters are preferable for providing both the diagnostic and prognostic functions.[5] Currently, a vast array of noninvasive and invasive imaging methods are used for the assessment of cardiac function and evaluation of epicardial coronary arteries, including computed tomography coronary angiography (CTCA), positron emission tomography (PET) and single-photon emission computed tomography (SPECT) myocardial perfusion imaging (MPI), functional cardiac MRI (CMR) and invasive coronary angiography.[6] This chapter aims to briefly review the quantification of the myocardial blood flow (MBF) and measurement of fractional flow reserve (FFR) using different methods. In addition, the various clinical implications, these parameters can bring into the diagnosis and management of CAD will also be discussed.

CORONARY PHYSIOLOGY

The myocardial blood flow is a tightly regulated process at various levels viz the epicardial coronary vessels, the resistance vessels, and the endothelium. The endothelium plays an important role in maintaining the coronary blood flow and thereby the myocardial perfusion in the normal coronary vasculature. Sympathetic stimulation leads to the release of endothelium-derived nitric oxide, which dilates the coronary arteries with maintenance of increased blood flow during stress/sympathetic activation. This coronary autoregulation helps to preserve the blood flow in atherosclerotic vessels by dilating and reducing the resistance of the distal vessels. An already maximally dilated vessel cannot further dilate in response to sympathetic stimulation, thereby leading to endothelial dysfunction. Studies have shown that coronary vessels can maintain resting blood flow in stenoses of up to 80% of the luminal diameter. Whereas, during maximal hyperemia in periods of stress, blood flow abnormalities start in stenoses greater than 40%.[7] Since endothelial dysfunction sets in early in the pathogenesis of CAD, functional evaluation of coronary vasculature in patients with significant CAD risk factors is of utmost importance.

Quantification of Myocardial Blood Flow and Myocardial Flow Reserve

Understanding of the coronary physiology has proved the need for functional evaluation of the coronary vessel and/or stenosis apart from the various anatomic imaging methods. The physiologic assessment of the coronary vasculature has been a major concern before planning therapy for a patient with CAD. The research in this field from the late 20th century onwards tried to develop various quantitative parameters for functional assessment of the coronary vasculature. Parameters like quantitative estimation of myocardial blood flow and flow reserve, fractional flow reserve, etc., are some among them. In conjunction with the anatomic imaging, noninvasive assessment of myocardial perfusion has gained popularity recently. Myocardial perfusion imaging using SPECT or PET tracers, CMR, CTCA, and myocardial contrast echocardiography are some among them.[8,9] Each one of them has its own weaknesses and strengths. The quantification of myocardial blood flow along with the perfusion imaging helps to provide the additional information during the imaging studies. This gives an objective parameter, which is usually more reproducible at different clinical settings and may also help in assessment of the physiologic significance of the stenosis. The measurement of coronary blood flow has varied over years from invasive methods such as intracoronary thermodilution, intracoronary Doppler wire (CFR), intracoronary pressure wire (FFR), TIMI frame counts or myocardial perfusion grade (blush) methods to noninvasive imaging modalities like PET, cardiac MR, Doppler echocardiography, contrast echocardiography and cardiac CT perfusion techniques, which can accurately measure the myocardial blood flow in terms of mL/min/g of myocardium.[10,11] Recent advances in the SPECT technology with cadmium-zinc-telluride (CZT) semiconductor detectors, MBF and myocardial flow reserve (MFR) can also be measured using SPECT tracers. Though, they underestimate the MBF at high flow rate.[12] A brief review of MBF quantification by currently used noninvasive methods are described below.

Myocardial Blood Flow using Multidetector CT

Dynamic perfusion CT scans can provide the myocardial blood flow along with anatomic evaluation of coronary stenosis. The 320-row multidetector CT (MDCT) can image the cardiac region within a single R-R interval compared to 64-slice CT. Thus, the advent of 320 rows MDCT has made it possible to acquire the dynamic studies in very less time and less radiation doses compared to the conventional 64 or 128 slices CT. Iodinated contrast is used as perfusion agent for stress and rest protocols, and time attenuation curve is obtained during the dynamic perfusion imaging. By measuring the inflow rate of iodinated contrast, absolute MBF is calculated from the relation between extraction fraction of the contrast agent and MBF.[13]

Myocardial Blood Flow Quantification by CMR

With ECG gating and breath holding, dynamic perfusion cardiac MRI is obtained in three planes in rest and stress (with intravenous adenosine infusion at 140 µg/kg/min). Perfusion sequence is started concurrently with Gd-DTPA administration (0.03 mmol/kg) at the rate of 4.0 mL/sec. In stress perfusion imaging, adenosine is infused for 3 minutes after which Gd-DTPA is administered and perfusion sequence is started. After completing both stress and rest imaging protocols, a total of 0.1 mmol/kg Gd-DTPA is administered for LGE (late gadolinium enhancement). Using a single-tissue compartment model and the Renkin-Crone equation, quantitative MBF values are calculated from the time-intensity curve data, which is converted into the myocardial gadolinium concentration.[14]

Positron Emission Tomography Quantification of MBF

Even though, various methods have been tried and tested in different backgrounds, PET assessment of MBF stands out because of its simplicity and noninvasive nature. PET quantification of absolute MBF involves an intravenous injection of the positron emitting perfusion radiotracer followed by dynamic acquisition of the tracer extraction and retention in left ventricular myocardium. PET estimation of MBF with ^{15}O-H_2O can be considered the gold standard for MBFestimation.[15] The added advantage of this technique is the measurement of the MFR, which is the ratio between the blood flow during stress and rest. The nomenclature of MBF and MFR is preferred now over previously used term CFR, as this technique measures blood flow through myocardial tissue, not in the epicardial coronary arteries. Physiologic reference ranges for the rest and stress MBF vary for tracers used (^{82}Rb may be having slightly higher values than ^{13}N-NH_3). Resting MBF measured with PET using different tracers is in range of 0.4–1.2 mL/g/min. The ideal perfusion PET tracer for quantifying MBF should have 100% extraction from vascular bed to myocardium and 100% retention without having washout from myocytes. This results in the linear relationship within MBF and measured tracer activity over varied range of blood flow. Several commonly used/promising radiotracers currently available for PET MPI are listed in Table 1. Each tracer has specific extraction/retention rates in the myocardium at varying coronary blood flow rates.[15] O-water has theoretically near perfect extraction with increasing coronary perfusion with negligible retention,[15] but the poor spatial resolution and short half-life reduces its utility as a PET perfusion tracer for myocardial blood flow quantification in clinical settings. ^{82}Rb is commonly tracer being used in clinical scenario but has poorer resolution and less extraction/retention at high flow rate. $^{13}NH_3$ has slightly higher resolution compared to the ^{15}O-water but has reduced extraction/retention fractions at high flow rates.[16] ^{18}F-flurpiridaz, a newer ^{18}F labeled perfusion tracer has shown high first pass extraction fraction even in high flow rates (~94% extraction). Higher tracer extraction enables for detection of smaller perfusion defects and

TABLE 1: Commonly used/promising radiotracers currently available for PET MPI.

Radiotracer	$T_{1/2}$	*Production*	*Extraction fraction**
^{82}Rb	76 sec	^{82}Sr– ^{82}Rb generator	~60%
^{15}O- water	2 min	Cyclotron	~95%
$^{13}NH_3$	10 min	Cyclotron	~80%
^{18}F- Flurpiridaz	110 min	Cyclotron	~94%

* Listed extraction fractions are for baseline MBF (1 mL/g/min)
(PET: positron emission tomography; MPI: myocardial perfusion imaging)

^{18}F-flurpiridaz cardiac PET has shown significant difference in the magnitude of reversible perfusion defects than SPECT MPI in phase III clinical trials.[17-20] Typical protocol is rest imaging followed by stress imaging on the same day. Maximal hypermedia is induced with coronary vasodilators for estimating stress MBF and MFR. Following intravenous injection of the tracer, recommended list mode dynamic image acquisition of the radiotracer flow through the central circulatory system and the tracer extraction and retention within the myocardium is obtained. Various tracer kinetic models have been developed (1–3 compartments), which will take into account the decay of tracer used, spill over of activity from LV myocardium, etc. to calculate the MBF in mL/g/min of myocardial tissue.[21] MFR is obtained by calculating the ratio of hyperemic flow during cardiac stress and resting myocardial blood flow (Figs. 1A and B).

Clinical Implications of Assessing MBF and MFR

Myocardial perfusion imaging (MPI) is one of the most frequently performed tests for assessment of CAD with its established clinical usefulness. However, its performance is limited because of two inherent drawbacks. The stress/rest myocardial perfusion imaging studies are assessed relatively, i.e. the myocardial region with the highest activity is considered normal, and rest of the myocardium is assessed compared to this region. Therefore, that in a global reduction in myocardial perfusion, flow limiting effects may go unnoticed in conventional MPI by SPECT and PET. Commonly used technetium labelled perfusion tracers and thallium have demonstrated low first pass extraction fraction at high flow rates, limiting the accuracy of MPI to estimate the tracer uptake during peak stress. SPECT MPI underestimates the disease and has limited sensitivity for multivessel disease.[22] It has been shown that prognosis is poor in high clinical risk subgroups with normal MPI. Measuring the regional and global MBF along with MFR may help to detect these lesions, because there will be reduction in the absolute MBF and hence MFR, corresponding to the vessels involved. Stress MBF and MFR in addition to MPI have shown improved diagnostic accuracy for CAD diagnosis, prognostic assessment and treatment guidance. MFR improves the risk assessment and provides incremental stratification beyond clinical risk factors, LV systolic function, extent and severity of myocardial ischemia and scar. It has been

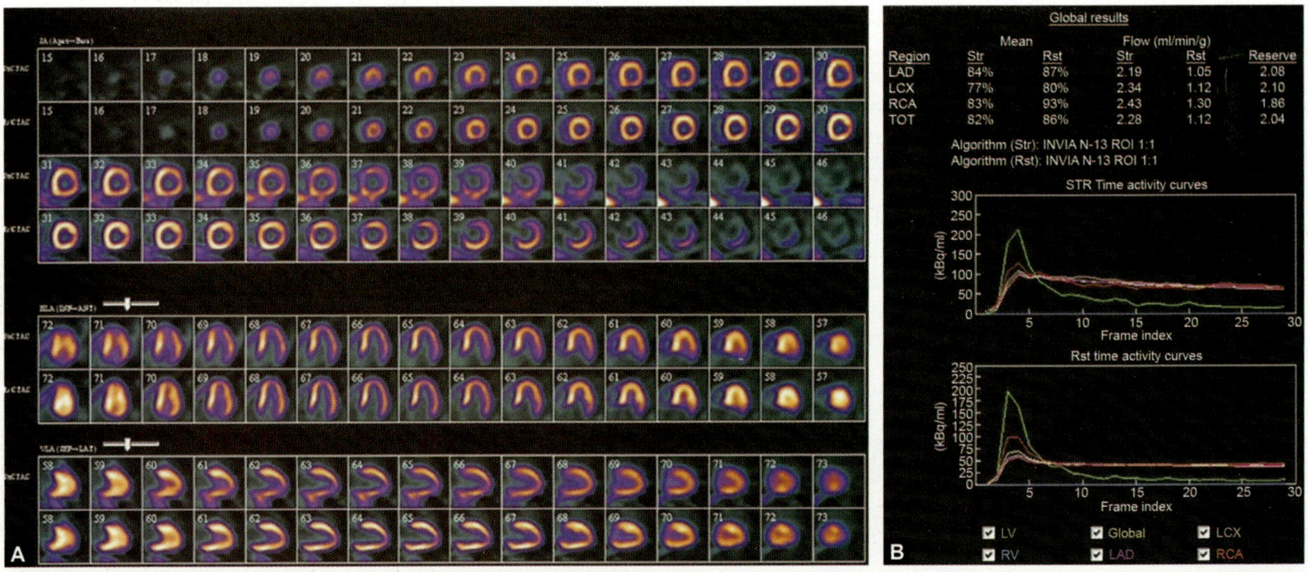

Figs. 1A and B: A 59-year-old long standing diabetic male patient underwent rest-stress $^{13}N\text{-}NH_3$ study using adenosine infusion, shows normal perfusion in stress and rest images with normal left ventricular ejection fraction (A). The global and regional MBF and MFR are also within normal limits except slight reduction of MFR in right coronary artery, though stress MBF in that territory is normal (B).

shown that impaired flow reserve is associated with 5.6 folds increased risk of cardiac death and MFR assessment led to risk reclassification in around 25% patients with nearly half of intermediate risk patients are reclassified. Preserved MFR (>2.0) has very high negative predictive value, though impaired MFR (<1.5) has modest positive predictive value for high risk CAD, i.e. left main or 3-vessels disease. Additional PET quantification of blood flow is preferable than conventional MPI in specific populations such as diabetes mellitus, chronic kidney disease, patients of cardiomyopathy and heart failure in addition to women and obese patients. It has been shown in various studies that impaired MFR is associated with increased rates of major cardiac events and cardiac deaths and preserved MFR has excellent NPV for excluding severe multivessel disease.[23-25] In a study by Ziadi et al. in 120 patients, comparing those without and with severe 3-vessel CAD, showed that MFR is globally reduced in patients with severe obstructive 3-vessel CAD.[26] In a study by Herzog et al. 229 patients were studied for long-term prognostication of CAD with PET MPI using $^{13}NH_3$. MBF and flow reserve were measured in all patients and were followed up for about 5.4 years for MACE, nonfatal MI, late revascularization, or hospitalization due to cardiac causes. The study concluded that the perfusion findings and flow reserve were strong outcome predictors and CFR was an independent predictor of adverse cardiac outcomes in patients with normal perfusion and abnormal flow reserve, providing a "warranty period" of three years if both flow reserve and perfusion are normal.[27] Farhad et al. in a prospective study of 324 patients concluded that myocardial perfusion findings with ^{82}Rb PET/CT were strong predictors of adverse cardiac events with median follow-up for 624 days. The study also found out that quantifying MBF had an added value of further risk stratification in patients with normal and abnormal perfusion.[28] PET MPI with measurement of regional or global MBF and/or MFR help in improving the accuracy of CAD and its severity is characterized. Global MFR less than 1.5 is a consistently high risk feature, but not always due to multivessel epicardial CAD and may be due to microvascular disease, diffuse disease or cardiomyopathy whereas regional stress MBF less than 1.5 or MFR less than 1.5 can indicate flow limiting disease in that territory.[20,29] According to the joint position paper of SNMMI Cardiovascular Council and ASNC (American Society of Nuclear Cardiology) on clinical quantification of MBF using PET, global hyperaemic MBF values of 2 mL/g/min and MFR values of 2 or more have a high negative predictive value for high risk angiographic CAD. Also, ASNC imaging guidelines/SNMMI procedure standard for PET nuclear cardiology procedures has given a possible list of indications in which MBF quantification is useful:[30]

- Patients suspicious of having myocardial ischemia
- For more specific physiological assessment of the coronary lesions
- If multivessel CAD is suspected
- To assess suspected microvascular dysfunction.

It is important to integrate the rest MBF, stress MBF and MFR parameters into the patients' reports.

Limitations of MBF Measurements

Although, measurement of MBF and MFR can add on to the diagnostic and prognostic utility of CAD, large-scale studies are not yet there which give optimal cut-off values. The cut-off values are also possibly different for different tracers due to their differences in myocardial extraction. Availability of tracers and hybrid PET/CT systems are also a main concern currently. Furthermore, potential sources of errors including detector saturation, patient motion and misregistration of CT and PET emission images while measuring the absolute blood flow and flow reserveneed to be better addressed.[18]

Assessment of Fraction Flow Reserve

Fractional flow reserve (FFR) gives a quantitative measure of the physiological significance of a coronary stenosis. It is simply the ratio between the maximal flow across a stenosis in an epicardial coronary vessel to the normal maximal flow in the artery in a hypothetical setting. It is derived as the ratio of mean distal coronary artery pressure to aortic pressure during maximal vasodilatation.[31,32] FFR is historically measured during invasive coronary angiography. However, the newer techniques also allow the measurement of FFR during CTCA. Various studies have proposed values of FFR ranging from 0.75 to 0.8 to be taken as a cut-off for deciding the intervention needed for the patients.[31-34] Studies have shown that FFR can be taken as an independent biomarker because of its relationship to the outcome and also as a reference for deciding treatment options in coronary artery diseases as revascularization alters the course of the disease.[2,4,33-35]

Measurement of FFR Using Angiography and CCTA

During coronary catheterization, pressure monitoring guidewire is advanced through the coronary catheter and is positioned distal to the stenosis under consideration. Adenosine is then infused intravenously (140 µg/kg/min) to induce maximal coronary blood flow. At steady-state hyperemia, the distal intracoronary pressure is measured using the pressure monitoring guidewire. FFR is then calculated as a ratio between mean distal intracoronary pressure across the stenosis and the mean arterial pressure measured by coronary catheter (Figs. 2A and B). FFR can also be measured by noninvasive coronary computed tomographic angiography (CCTA) with use of beta-blockers to control heart rate and scan is done immediately after giving sublingual nitroglycerine for coronary vasodilatation. 80–100 cc of contrast is then given intravenously during acquisition, followed by saline flush. FFR is then calculated from the CTA data using specific software such as HeartFlow™. Studies have shown that FFR measured by CT provides higher diagnostic accuracy and differentiates hemodynamically significant CAD.[36,37]

Clinical Implications of Assessing FFR

Multiple studies have shown the significance of measuring FFR for characterizing coronary culprit lesions. In patients with coronary stenosis without ischemia, FFR could identify those patients who would benefit from percutaneous transluminal coronary angioplasty (PTCA). The IRIS-FFR prospective registry included 5,846 patients who underwent

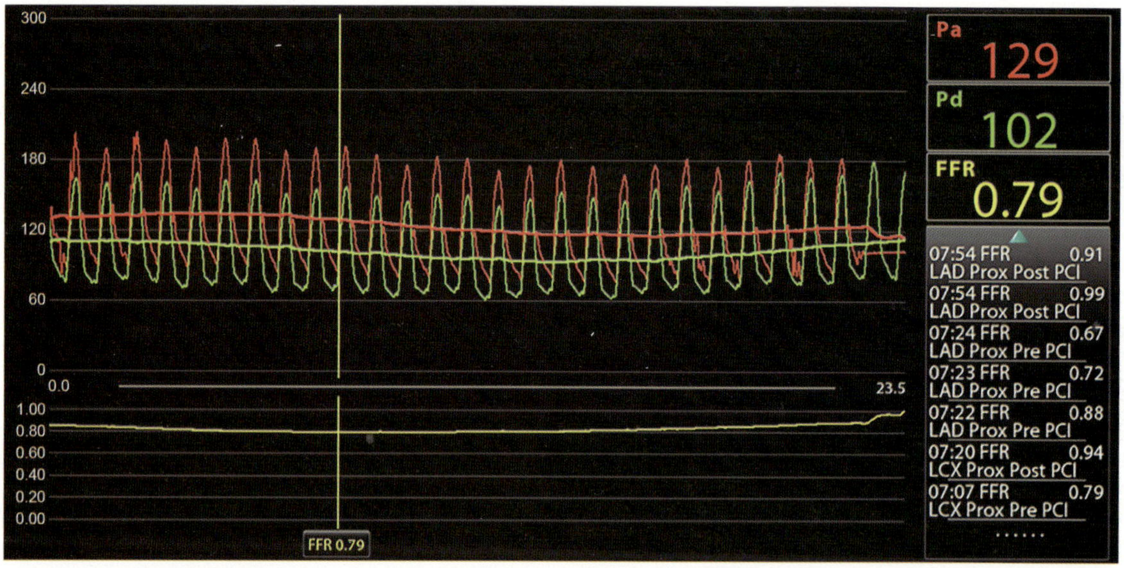

Fig. 2A: Fractional flow reserve (FFR) testing performed by the pressure wire technique in the proximal left circumflex coronary artery. After 200 µg of adenosine given intracoronary in the left circulation, the pressure distal to the stenosis (Pd) has fallen as compared to proximal (Pa) to stenosis. The fall in the pressure is significant (0.79).
(*Courtesy:* Dr Parag Barward, Department of Cardiology, PGIMER, Chandigarh, India).

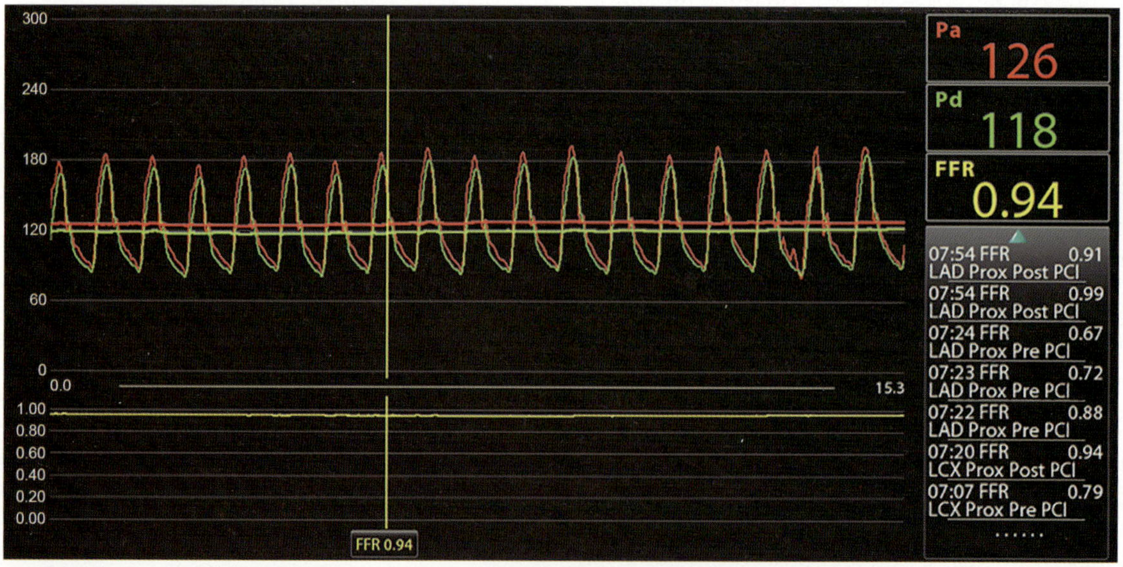

Fig. 2B: Fractional flow reserve (FFR) testing performed by the pressure wire technique in the proximal left circumflex coronary artery after stenting of the stenosis segment with a drug eluting stent. After 200 µg of adenosine given intracoronary in the left circulation, the pressure distal to the stenosis (Pd) has fallen nonsignificantly (Pd/Pa= 0.94).
(*Courtesy:* Dr Parag Barward, Department of Cardiology, PGIMER, Chandigarh, India).

FFR measurement for at least one coronary lesion. The study followed up patients for a median period of 1.9 years and end point was any major adverse cardiac event (MACE). The study showed that FFR values were linearly associated with the cardiac lesions, which were not revascularized. The study also concluded that revascularization of lesions with low FFR has better outcomes compared to medical therapy alone.[37] FFR more than 0.8 has very high predictive value for ruling out ischemia, whereas value less than 0.75 was associated with ischemia.[32] There were significantly reduced cardiac adverse events when decision of percutaneous coronary intervention was based on FFR values in addition to angiography as well FFR-guided PCI with medical treatment than medical treatment alone resulted in lesser urgent revascularization in FAME and FAME-2 trials.[2,4] It has been showed that PCI based on FFR is also economically better in the long run compared to medical therapy alone, other than having a good long-term outcome.[3]

Limitations of Fractional Flow Reserve

Measurement of FFR with catheterization of coronary arteries has shown to measure lower FFR when measured using pressure monitoring microcatheters. However, ACIST FFR study has shown that the diagnostic impact with these subtle decrease in FFR is minimal.[38] The estimation of FFR requires invasive coronary angiography which itself has got its own complications and contraindications. However, noninvasive CCTA can also measure FFR accurately, but this requires specific software for calculation of FFR. The values of FFR have not been validated well in patients with unstable angina, acute MI or microvascular dysfunction.[39]

CONCLUSION

The usefulness of absolute measurement of MBF and physiological impact of coronary stenosis in terms of FFR provide the better insight of coronary lesions and subclinical CAD. These may help in early intervention and treatment, which might change the clinical outcome in this subgroup of patients. Even though not widely implemented in the current management protocols of patients with high and intermediate risk of CAD, measurement of myocardial flow reserve has a special place in guiding the clinicians in management of these patients. Quantification of MBF and MFR has added substantial value, and quantification must be done carefully as there is still a learning curve. The newer generation noninvasive imaging modalities have made it easier for the physicians in determining the underlying pathological changes associated with coronary artery diseases.

REFERENCES

1. Greenland P, Alpert JS, Beller GA, et al. 2010 ACCF/AHA guideline for assessment of cardiovascular risk in asymptomatic adults: A report of the American College of Cardiology Foundation/American Heart Association Task Force on Practice Guidelines. J Am Coll Cardiol. 2010 14;56(25):e50-103.
2. Tonino PA, De Bruyne B, Pijls NHJ, et al. Fractional Flow Reserve versus Angiography for Guiding Percutaneous Coronary Intervention. N Engl J Med. 2009;360(3):213-24.
3. Fearon WF, Nishi T, De Bruyne B, et al. Clinical Outcomes and Cost-Effectiveness of Fractional Flow Reserve-Guided Percutaneous Coronary Intervention in Patients With Stable Coronary Artery Disease: Three-Year Follow-Up of the FAME 2 Trial (Fractional Flow Reserve Versus Angiography for Multivessel Evaluation). Circulation. 2018;30;137(5):480-7.
4. De Bruyne B, Pijls NHJ, Kalesan B, et al. Fractional flow reserve-guided PCI versus medical therapy in stable coronary disease. N Engl J Med. 2012;367:991-1001.
5. Bajaj NS, Singh S, Farag A, et al. The prognostic value of non-perfusion variables obtained during vasodilator stress myocardial perfusion imaging. J Nucl Cardiol. 2016; 23(3):390-413.
6. Hage FG, AlJaroudi WA. Review of cardiovascular imaging in the journal of nuclear cardiology in 2016: Part 2 of 2-myocardial perfusion imaging. J Nucl Cardiol. 2017; 6;24(4):1190-9.
7. Uren NG, Melin JA, De Bruyne B, et al. Relation between myocardial blood flow and the severity of coronary-artery Stenosis. N Engl J Med. 1994;330(25):1782-8.
8. Salerno M, Beller GA. Noninvasive assessment of myocardial perfusion. Circ Cardiovasc Imaging. 2009;2(5):412-24.
9. Jung J-H, Yoon YE. Advanced noninvasive cardiac imaging using cardiac magnetic resonance imaging in the diagnosis and evaluation of coronary artery disease. Ann Nucl Cardiol. 2017;3(1):143-9.
10. Marcus ML, Wilson RF, White CW. Methods of measurement of myocardial blood flow in patients: a critical review. Circulation. 1987;76(2):245-54.
11. Schelbert HR. Anatomy and physiology of coronary blood flow. Vol. 17, Journal of Nuclear Cardiology. 2010. pp. 545-54.
12. Nkoulou R, Fuchs TA, Pazhenkottil AP, et al. Absolute Myocardial Blood Flow and Flow Reserve Assessed by Gated SPECT with Cadmium-Zinc-Telluride Detectors Using 99mTc-Tetrofosmin: Head-to-Head Comparison with 13N-Ammonia PET. J Nucl Med. 2016; 57(12):1887-92.
13. Kikuchi Y, Oyama-Manabe N, Naya M, et al. Quantification of myocardial blood flow using dynamic 320-row multi-detector CT as compared with 15O-H2O PET. Eur Radiol. 2014;24(7):1547-56.
14. Tomiyama Y, Manabe O, Oyama-Manabe N, et al. Quantification of myocardial blood flow with dynamic perfusion 3.0 Tesla MRI: Validation with 15O-water PET. J Magn Reson Imaging. 2015; 42(3):754-62.

15. Williams MC, Mirsadraee S, Dweck MR, et al. Computed tomography myocardial perfusion vs 15O-water positron emission tomography and fractional flow reserve. Eur Radiol. 2017;27(3):1114-24.
16. Ziadi MC. Myocardial flow reserve (MFR) with positron emission tomography (PET)/computed tomography (CT): clinical impact in diagnosis and prognosis. Cardiovasc Diagn Ther. 2017;7(2):206-18.
17. Maddahi J, Packard RR. Cardiac PET perfusion tracers: Current status and future directions. Semin Nucl Med. 2014; 44(5):333-43.
18. Nakazato R, Heo R, Leipsic J, et al. CFR and FFR assessment with PET and CTA: Strengths and limitations. Curr Cardiol Rep. 2014;16(5):484.
19. Nakazato R, Berman D, Alexanderson E, et al. Myocardial perfusion imaging with PET. Imaging Med. 2013;5(1):35-46.
20. Murthy VL, Bateman TM, Beanlands RS, et al. Clinical quantification of myocardial blood flow using pet: joint position paper of the SNMMI Cardiovascular Council and the ASNC. J Nucl Med. 2018;59(2):273-93.
21. Schindler TH, Quercioli A, Valenta I, et al. Quantitative assessment of myocardial blood flow—Clinical and research applications. Semin Nucl Med. 2014;44(4):274-93.
22. Lima RS, Watson DD, Goode AR, et al. Incremental value of combined perfusion and function over perfusion alone by gated SPECT myocardial perfusion imaging for detection of severe three-vessel coronary artery disease. J Am Coll Cardiol. 2003;42(1):64-70.
23. Murthy VL, Naya M, Foster CR, et al. Coronary vascular dysfunction and prognosis in patients with chronic kidney disease. JACC Cardiovasc Imaging. 2012; 5:1025-34.
24. Shah NR, Charytan DM, Murthy VL, et al. Prognostic value of coronary flow reserve in patients with dialysis-dependent ESRD. J Am Soc Nephrol. 2016;27:1823-9.
25. Naya M, Murthy VL, Foster CR, et al. Prognostic interplay of coronary artery calcification and underlying vascular dysfunction in patients with suspected coronary artery disease. J Am Coll Cardiol. 2013;61:2098-106.
26. Ziadi MC, DeKemp RA, Williams K, et al. Does quantification of myocardial flow reserve using rubidium-82 positron emission tomography facilitate detection of multivessel coronary artery disease? J Nucl Cardiol. 2012;19(4):670-80.
27. Herzog BA, Husmann L, Valenta I, et al. Long-term prognostic value of 13N-Ammonia myocardial perfusion positron emission tomography. Added value of coronary flow reserve. J Am Coll Cardiol. 2009;54(2):150-6.
28. Farhad H, Dunet V, Bachelard K, et al. Added prognostic value of myocardial blood flow quantitation in rubidium-82 positron emission tomography imaging. Eur Heart J Cardiovasc Imaging. 2013;14(12):1203-10.
29. Murthy VL, Carli MF Di. Non-invasive quantification of coronary vascular dysfunction for diagnosis and management of coronary artery disease. J Nucl Cardiol. 2012;19(5):1060-72.
30. Dilsizian V, Bacharach SL, Beanlands RS, et al. ASNC imaging guidelines/SNMMI procedure standard for positron emission tomography (PET) nuclear cardiology procedures. J Nucl Cardiol. 2016;23(5):1187-226.
31. Pijls NH, Fearon WF, Tonino PA, et al. Fractional flow reserve versus angiography for guiding percutaneous coronary intervention in patients with multivessel coronary artery disease: 2-Year follow-up of the FAME (fractional flow reserve versus angiography for multivessel evaluation) study. J Am Coll Cardiol. 2010;56(3):177-84.
32. Pijls NH, de Bruyne B, Peels K, et al. Measurement of Fractional Flow Reserve to Assess the Functional Severity of Coronary-Artery Stenoses. N Engl J Med. 1996;27;334(26):1703-8.
33. Johnson NP, Tóth GG, Lai D, et al. Prognostic Value of Fractional Flow Reserve Linking Physiologic Severity to Clinical Outcomes. J Am Coll Cardiol. 2014;64(16):1641-54.
34. Ahn JM, Park DW, Shin ES, et al. Fractional Flow Reserve and Cardiac Events in Coronary Artery Disease: Data From a Prospective IRIS-FFR Registry (Interventional Cardiology Research Incooperation Society Fractional Flow Reserve). Circulation. 2017;6;135(23):2241-51.
35. Pijls NH, van Schaardenburgh P, Manoharan G, et al. Percutaneous coronary intervention of functionally nonsignificant stenosis: 5-year follow-up of the DEFER study. J Am Coll Cardiol. 2007;49:2105-11.
36. Koo BK, Erglis A, Doh JH, et al. Diagnosis of ischemia-causing coronary stenoses by noninvasive fractional flow reserve computed from coronary computed tomographic angiograms: Results from the prospective multicenter DISCOVER-FLOW (Diagnosis of Ischemia-Causing Stenoses Obtained Via Noninvasive Fractional Flow Reserve) study. J Am Coll Cardiol. 2011; 58(19):1989-97.
37. Nørgaard BL, Leipsic J, Gaur S, et al. Diagnostic performance of noninvasive fractional flow reserve derived from coronary computed tomography angiography in suspected coronary artery disease: the NXT trial (Analysis of Coronary Blood Flow Using CT Angiography: Next Steps). J Am Coll Cardiol. 2014;63(12):1145-55.
38. Fearon WF, Chambers JW, Seto AH, et al. ACIST-FFR Study (Assessment of Catheter-Based Interrogation and Standard Techniques for Fractional Flow Reserve Measurement). Circ Cardiovasc Interv. 2017;10(12).
39. Kern MJ. Coronary physiology revisited: Practical insights from the cardiac catheterization laboratory. Circulation. 2000;101(11):1344-51.

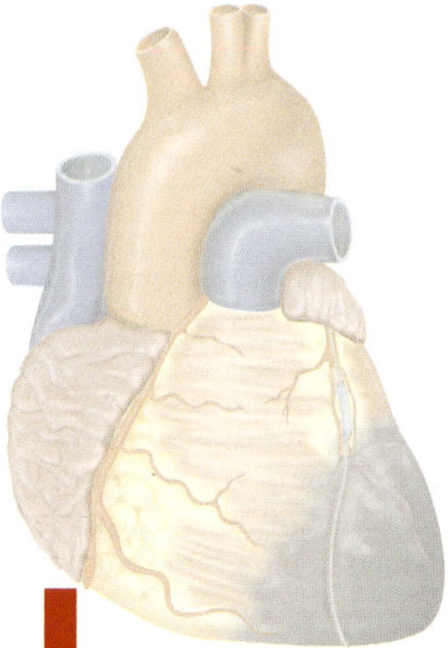

CHAPTER 34

ACS Coronary Intervention and Imaging: Recent Advances—Optical Coherence Tomography

Rony Mathew, Jo Joseph, Jabir A, Jimmy George

INTRODUCTION

Optical coherence tomography (OCT) has emerged as a powerful coronary intravascular imaging modality in the recent years due to their high resolution enabling visualization of vessel wall and related structures in great detail. The introduction of frequency domain (FD-OCT) has simplified the procedure and this has enabled its use in different clinical scenario both complex and simple. Even though, there was an initial inertia in its use in acute coronary syndromes, of late this modality is gaining importance in this difficult scenario as it is helpful in determining the mechanism of plaque disruption, thrombus burden and to guide percutaneous interventions (PCI). OCT is of particular importance in evaluating the cause of stent failure (Stent thrombosis and In-sent restenosis). This review will focus on the role of intracoronary imaging with OCT in acute coronary syndromes and its potential clinical uses.

LIMITATIONS OF CORONARY ANGIOGRAM

Coronary angiography provides a real-time “luminogram” of the coronary anatomy and remains the most widely used invasive imaging technique for diagnosing coronary artery disease and guiding PCI. However, angiography has a number of inherent limitations, including those arising from its two-dimensional projection of a three-dimensional coronary tree, as well as limitations in assessing the vessel wall, plaque composition, and extent and distribution of atherosclerosis.[1] Angiography is also associated with a high inter observer variability in the analysis of the degree of stenosis even among experienced operators. Though QCA has improved the diagnostic accuracy, its widespread clinical utility is limited. Additionally, coronary angiography cannot determine the morphology of the culprit lesion, or the status of the fibrous cap. Therefore, in every day practice, patients presenting with an ACS frequently end up with their culprit lesion stented regardless of the underlying mechanism for plaque disruption.[2] Failing to identify the underlying pathology not only meant adopting a “one size fits all” strategy, but also deprives us from understanding the natural history of different types of plaques, and prevents testing targeted therapeutic approaches for different plaque morphologies. So an intravascular imaging modality with sufficient resolution to visualize plaques, demonstrate its composition, identify vulnerable plaques and its natural history would definitely provide an ideal solution for both research and clinical practice.[3]

TECHNICAL CONSIDERATIONS

Optical coherence tomography is an imaging technique that can deliver three dimensional images from an optical scattering medium (like the arterial wall). It is real time and is able to assess and display tissue microstructure and provides close correlation with pathology. OCT basically delivers near infrared light to the wall of coronary artery through small diameter optical fibers, the light that illuminates the vessel is absorbed and reflected by structures to different degree, with an axial resolution of 2–15 μm. Different tissue types have different optic characteristics and the ability of OCT to create tomographic cross-sectional images of a vessel is based on optical interference of this near infrared light. Light is emitted and collected back from the tip of a small diameter optical fiber that rotates rapidly inside a transparent sheath and for longitudinal scanning of the vessel, a drive motor unit on the table pulls back the fibers it rotates within the sheath. The collected light carries information about the depth resolved back scattering reflectivity of the tissue structure at the illuminated spot.[4,5] The delivered images have high resolution with axial and lateral resolution better with OCT (10–20 μm) than by IVUS (100–150 μm) but maximum tissue penetration depth is limited to 1–2 mm.[6] Intracoronary OCT is performed by introducing the imaging catheter (2.7 French) over a guide wire (0.014 inch) distally into the coronary artery using standard guide catheters (6F or larger). A motorized pullback is performed to scan the coronary artery segment. The pullback speed is typically 20 mm/sec with a frame rate of 100 frames per second or higher. Since blood scatters the OCT signal, FD-OCT uses a contrast flush of 3–4 mL/s for 2–3 seconds to clear the blood column and allow clear path for the light beam to be emitted. The normal coronary arteries are seen as a 3-layered structure on OCT (Figs. 1A and B). Due to its high resolution, OCT can differentiate the internal elastic laminae, external elastic laminae as well as intima, media and adventitia.[7] The internal elastic lamina appears as a signal-rich 20 mm thick band that lies inside the dark band of the media and the further signal-rich band of external elastic lamina.[5] Agreement between the histopathological and OCT findings was high and interobserver and intraobserver reliabilities were good. Intimal thickness measured by OCT also correlated well with histology.[8]

Limitations

Optical coherence tomography images are prone to artifacts. In one study, 30.9% of the images contained artifacts and this improved with operator experience.[9] The more common are the seam line artifacts, which cause apparent breaks in the lumen contour on cross-sectional images. Decentration artifacts are caused by eccentric positioning of the imaging catheter within the artery and lead to image attenuation in remote structures. Caliber artifacts are caused by an arterial diameter greater than the penetration limits of the OCT and are a particular problem in vein grafts and in the left main.[10] Flow artifacts are caused by a failure to clear blood from either the vessel or the imaging catheter by flushing.

OCT IN ACUTE CORONARY SYNDROMES

The final common event in acute coronary syndromes (ACS) is coronary thrombosis and the three major mechanisms responsible are plaque rupture, plaque erosions and calcified nodule.[11,12]

Plaque rupture (Figs. 2A and B) is defined by an area of fibrous cap disruption whereby the overlying thrombus is in continuity with the underlying necrotic core. Ruptured

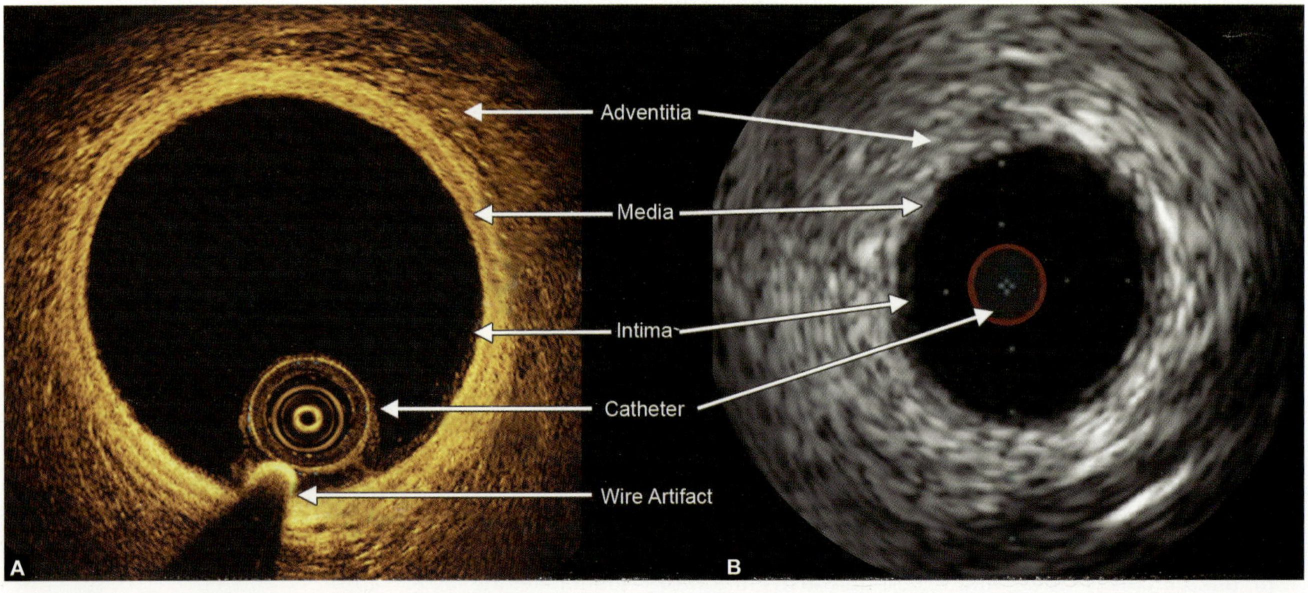

Figs. 1A and B: Normal artery: (A) Imaging with optical coherence tomography; and (B) Intravascular ultrasound.

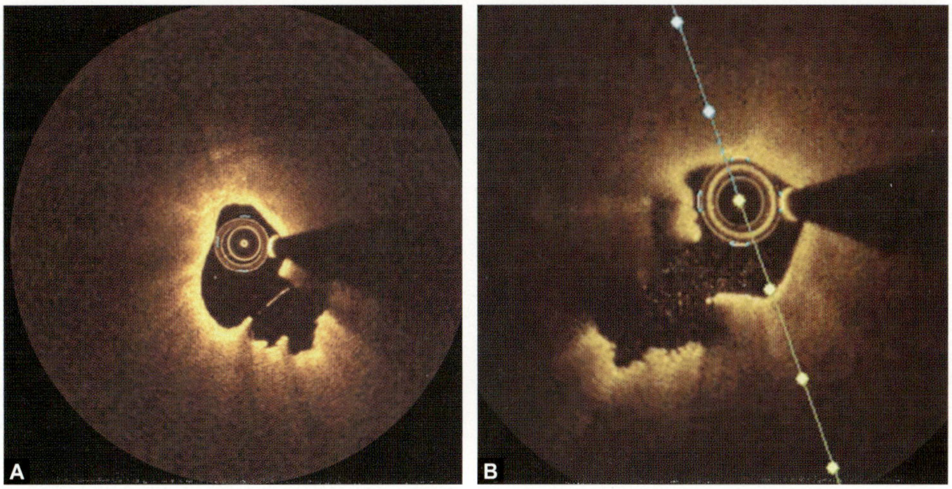

Figs. 2A and B: Plaque rupture (A) with empty cavity and (B) with thrombus in plaque cavity.

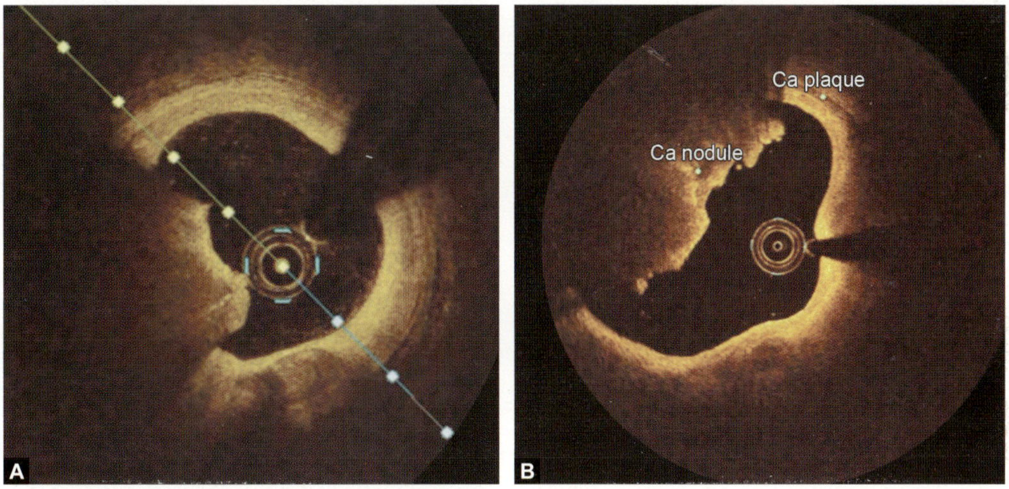

Figs. 3A and B: Calcific nodule without surface thrombus (A) and with thrombus (B).

lesions have large necrotic core and a disrupted fibrous cap infiltrated by macrophages and lymphocytes. The smooth muscle cell content within the fibrous cap at the rupture site is sparse. Plaque rupture is the most frequent cause of death in young men and older women.[13] Intraplaque hemorrhage is due to hemorrhage into plaque and occurs from cracks or fissures originating from the luminal surface.[14] The fissuring of the fibrous cap occurs at its thinnest portion, typically at the shoulder region, thereby allowing the entry of blood into the necrotic core may represent precursors or it may be a subtypes of plaque rupture.[15] Intraplaque hemorrhage is also proposed due to rupture of vasa vasorum, a common feature of advanced lesions with plaque rupture and luminal thrombi.

Calcified nodules (Figs. 3A and B) show highly calcified matrix causing substantial luminal irregularity with minimal or no lipid core.[16,17] They are also prone to rupture and were encountered in 2–5% of the sudden cardiac death cases and predominantly affects the mid-right coronary artery.[17] But the PROSPECT study suggested that calcific nodules were mostly "innocent bystanders" posing minimal added risk for ACS for up to 3 years of follow-up.[18] A calcified plaque will have a well-delineated low signal region with sharp borders, and a lipid rich plaque will show low signal region with diffuse borders.[19]

Plaque erosion (Fig. 4) is defined by absence of fibrous cap disruption and the presence of thrombus, or luminal surface irregularity in the absence of thrombus. In OCT erosion, there will be attenuation of underlying plaque by thrombus without superficial lipid or calcification immediately proximal or distal to the attached thrombus. OCT can differentiate between white and red thrombus due

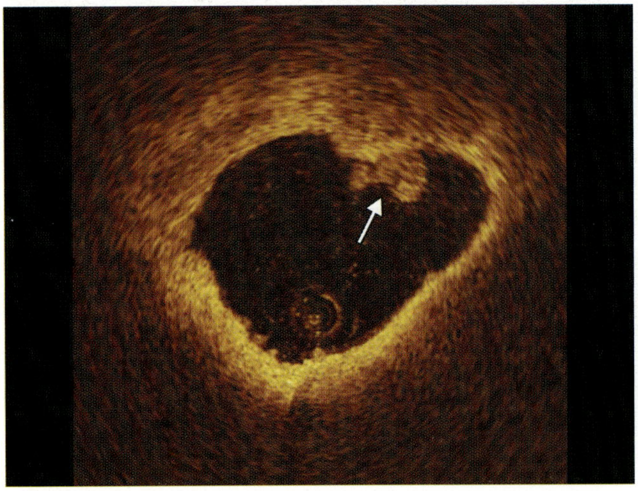

Fig. 4: Plaque erosion with irregular surface and thrombus (white arrow).

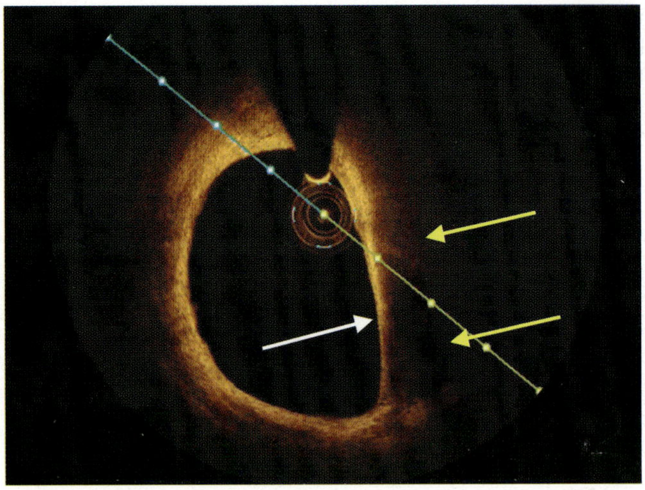

Fig. 5: Thin Cap Fibro Atheroma (TCFA) with Lipid core (yellow arrows) and thin cap less than 65 μm (white arrow).

to the high proportion of red blood cells in red thrombi, which cause greater attenuation of the OCT signal.[20] Definite OCT erosion was identified by the presence of attached thrombus overlying an intact visualized plaque. Probable OCT erosion was defined as either with luminal surface irregularity in the absence of thrombus, or attenuation of underlying plaque by the thrombus without superficial lipid or calcification immediately proximal or distal to the thrombus.[21] Plaque erosions are more common in young women and men less than 50 years of age and are associated with smoking, especially in premenopausal women.[13]

OCT and Vulnerable Plaques

Histological studies have identified the characteristics of "vulnerable" plaques that are implicated in the pathophysiology of ACS. These plaques which are prone to rupture have fibrous caps that are thinned out and rich in macrophages overlying a lipid pool.[22] In a study of hearts of 113 men who died suddenly, 41 had acute coronary thrombosis, and among them 95% had plaques with fibrous caps that have thickness less than 65 μm with an infiltrate of macrophages called thin cap fibro atheroma (TCFA)[23] (Fig. 5). OCT can identify TCFA and is defined as a lipid rich plaque with lipid arc within the plaque in more than 2 quadrants with a thin fibrous cap with thickness at the thinnest segment being less than 65 μm.[24] Because of its inherent high image resolution, OCT can identify these high-risk plaques, in vivo, however, there is still debate over the exact definition of a TCFA on OCT as the histological specimens of TCFA differ from OCT images, due to shrinkage of pathological specimens. Therefore, it is possible that the fibrous cap of a TCFA is thicker in vivo than on histology. The prevalence of TCFA was twice as high in those plaques with severe angiographic stenosis more than 70% compared with those with mild or moderate stenosis. TCFA in patients with severe lesions had greater plaque burden and more features of vulnerability, including microvessels, cholesterol crystal (Fig. 6), thinner fibrous cap, and higher vessel remodeling index. TCFAs are more common in patients with an acute or unstable clinical presentation than stable angina pectoris patients. A comparison of 26 acute ST-segment elevation myocardial infarction (STEMI) patients with 16 stable angina patients showed that STEMI patients had a higher proportion of OCT-TCFA in the culprit lesion (85% versus 13%, $p < 0.001$) and a thinner fibrous cap.[25] Patients with STEMI also had a higher prevalence of OCT-TCFA compared with patients with non ST-segment elevation ACS (78% versus 49%, $p = 0.008$).[26] Similar results have been shown in patients with

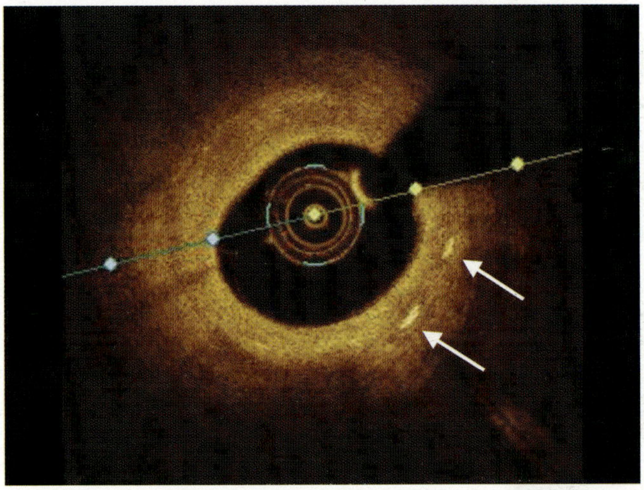

Fig. 6: Cholesterol crystals seen as signal rich with low attenuation (white arrows).

unstable angina compared to patients with stable angina (incidence of OCT-TCFA 81% versus 47%, p = 0.002).[27] Patients with ACS also have a higher proportion of OCT-TCFA than non ACS patients.[28] In patients with ACS, OCT-TCFAs are more commonly found in the proximal segments of the culprit vessel and plaque rupture of TCFA occurs more often away from the site of minimum lumen area in patients with STEMI and non-STEMI.[29] Studies have shown that TCFAs can transform into other plaque types and vice versa. There are studies that have shown TCFAs can undergo healing to stable lesions,[30] or remain unchanged.[31]

Macrophages and Neoangiogensis

The resolution of OCT may allow identification of macrophages (Fig. 7) within an atherosclerotic plaque. In ACS patients, a higher prevalence of macrophage infiltration in nonculprit plaques was found compared with non-ACS patients (82.4% vs. 37.9%, p= 0.001).[28] Plaques that exhibited an increase in luminal stenosis over time were more likely to have higher numbers of macrophages, TCFA, intimal laceration, and/or microchannels.[32] Plaque neovascularization and microchannel formation are known to be markers of plaque vulnerability and rupture as well as intraplaque hemorrhage, which can contribute to plaque progression.[33] In OCT images, this can be recognized as small black holes (microchannels) (Fig. 8). Patients with microchannels in the culprit lesion were more likely to have presented with unstable than stable angina, have a thinner fibrous cap, and have a trend toward a higher incidence of plaque rupture.[34] TCFA and microchannel findings in nonsignificant coronary plaque by optical coherence tomography correlate with subsequent progression of coronary atheromatous plaques.[32] Neo-angiogenesis is a predictor of luminal narrowing in clinical studies.[27]

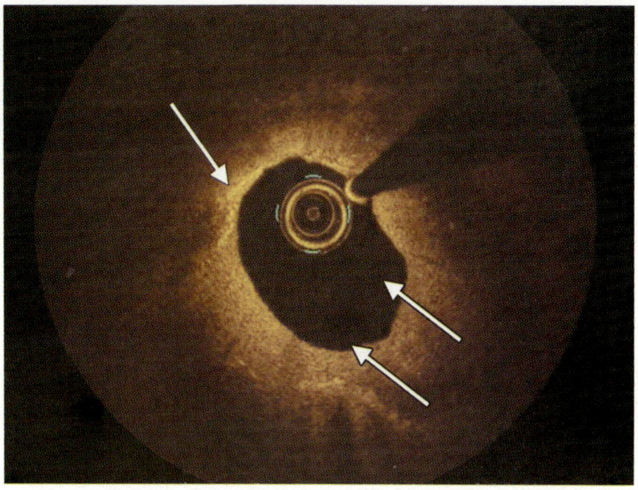

Fig. 7: Macrophages seen as signal rich with high attenuation (white arrows).

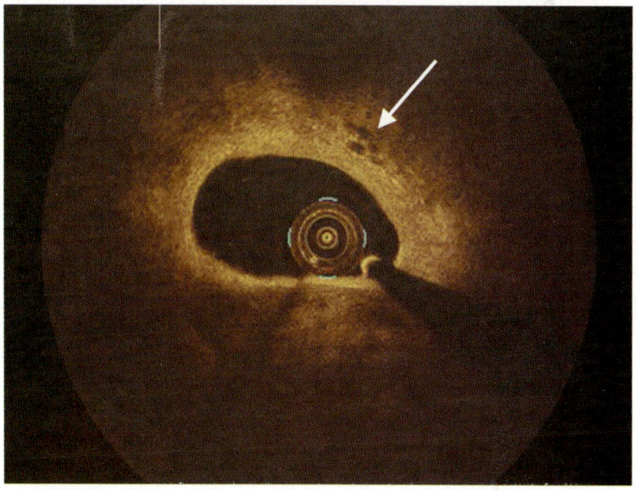

Fig. 8: Neovascularization seen as microchannels (arrow).

OCT in Coronary Physiology

Like IVUS, OCT has limited use in physiological assessment of coronary lesions. Minimal luminal area (MLA) on OCT correlates modestly with Fractional flow reserve (FFR) in vessels other than left main. OCT derived MLA thresholds are smaller than IVUS derived MLAs (median OCT-derived MLA 1.96 mm^2 vs. IVUS-derived MLA 2.8 mm^2).[35] OCT derived MLA thresholds have reasonably high positive predictive value (80–92%) but lower negative predictive value for physiological significance (66–89%). Thus a decision whether to perform PCI on the basis of OCT derived MLA alone can be erroneous in up to one third of cases and is not routinely recommended. Unlike IVUS, few studies have correlated clinical outcomes after OCT determined lesion severity versus FFR, particularly in the left main coronary artery.[36] Similarly, OCT determined lesion severity versus FFR in acute coronary syndrome is not well studied.

OCT IN ACUTE CORONARY SYNDROME: CLINICAL EVIDENCE AND IMPLICATIONS IN PRACTICE

In EROSION trial, a prospective study investigated the feasibility and safety of antithrombotic therapy without stenting in patients with ACS caused by plaque erosion with <70% luminal narrowing. The main findings of this study were that plaque erosion was a frequent (25.4%) underlying mechanism in patients with ACS, second only to plaque rupture (60.7%) and that thrombus volume significantly decreased (94.2%) in patients who were

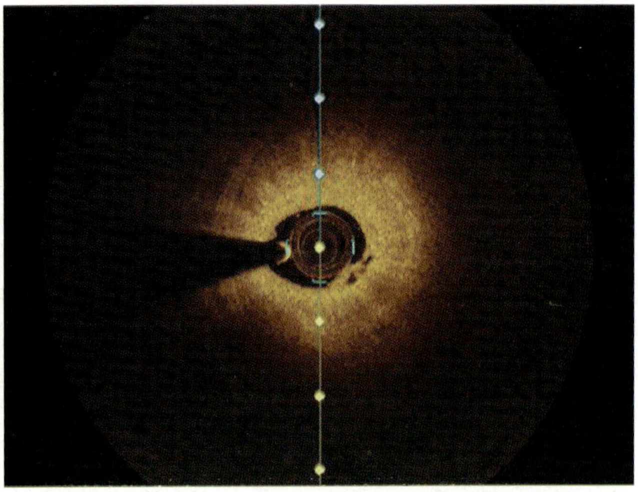

Fig. 9: Intact fibrous cap lesion with thrombus in STEMI patient.

treated with anti-thrombotic therapy at 1-month follow-up. All, but 2 patients treated with antithrombotic therapy without stent implantation remained asymptomatic. At 1 month, minimal lumen diameter increased and Diameter Stenosis decreased.[37] This was the first OCT based study to show the feasibility and safety of antithrombotic therapy without stenting in patients with ACS caused by plaque erosion.[37] TOTAL-OCT trial,[38] a prospective study of ST Elevation Myocardial Infarction (STEMI) patients treated with thrombectomy, has shown that mild residual stenosis were uncommon in intact fibrous cap (IFC) lesions and plaque rupture (PR) lesions. Lipid plaque was lower in IFC than in PR lesions but lipid composed the majority of plaques in both. Most STEMI patients have significant residual stenosis after thrombectomy, irrespective of the presence of plaque rupture or IFC at the culprit site. IFC stenosis in culprit lesions after thrombectomy is mainly composed of atherosclerotic plaque with a relatively minor contribution of thrombus, the quantity of which was not different between IFC and PR. The majority of IFC patients had postthrombectomy OCT lumen area stenosis >75% at the culprit lesion and mild stenosis were rare (Fig. 9). The mechanisms of coronary thrombosis in patients with IFC are not well known. In situ thrombus, formation may be stimulated by systemic exposures such as smoking or local factors such as shear stress. The presence of severe stenosis with small MLA may also be an important contributor. The smaller MLA could lead to occlusion with lower thrombus burden. In larger vessels, IFC lesions may be more likely to produce nonocclusive thrombi that do not present with ST-segment elevation, whereas plaque rupture lesions may be more thrombogenic and more likely to lead to vessel occlusion. This study has shown that both IFC and plaque rupture culprit lesions are advanced atherosclerotic lesions composed mainly of lipid-rich plaque, which may merit similar treatment strategies. The ability of OCT to determine the site of plaque rupture, thrombus burden and the longitudinal extent of the plaque as well as to measure the reference lumen, vessel diameter, and length of the lesion to be covered, specifies the potential utility of OCT to guide PCI in STEMI. Larger final minimum lumen diameter was obtained in patients who underwent OCT guided PCI because of the further dilatation of the sub- optimal stent results in the OCT arm.[39] Similarly, higher post-PCI-FFR values were achieved with OCT guided PCI in the DOCTORS randomized study, which included 240 patients with non STEMI.[40] In CLI-OPCI study, OCT predictors of stent-related events were under expansion, stent in flow and outflow disease, dissection at the distal stent edge >200 μm, intrastent plaque or thrombus protrusion.[41]

OCT in Stent Failure

With the current generation stents, though the incidence of stent thrombosis is low, the event can be catastrophic with mortality rates as high as 40%.[42] Important procedural risk factors for stent thrombosis include stent under-expansion and malapposition, edge dissection, and residual disease proximal or distal to the stent. Other mechanisms implicated in stent thrombosis include neo-atherosclerosis (with or without rupture), isolated uncovered struts, and evaginations related to late positive remodeling.[43,44] The treatment options in the patients presenting with stent thrombosis can be different depending upon the underlying mechanism with balloon dilatations for gross under expansion, restenting for neoatherosclerosis and thrombus aspiration followed by prolonged DAPT for those with isolated uncovered stent struts. OCT is able to identify the underlying mechanism in majority of cases and is therefore a perfect diagnostic tool in guiding therapy in such situations.[45] In the PESTO registry of 120 patients with definite stent thrombosis after metallic drug-eluting stent, OCT diagnosed an abnormality in 97% of cases. Malapposition (48%) and under expansion (26%) were associated with acute and subacute ST, whereas mal-apposition (31%) and Neo-atherogenesis (28%) were the prominent mechanisms associated with late ST and very late ST.[45] Similar findings were also observed in CLI-THRO registry and other prospective registries.[46,47] But among these factors, the role of malapposition remains unclear. Malapposition at the time of stent implantation is a common finding on OCT[48] and it is usually because of stent/vessel size mismatch and may not require correction if it is not associated with stent under expansion. Malapposition may persist (late persistent mal-apposition) or subsequently develop because of stent-related inflammation with positive vessel remodeling (late acquired malapposition). Malapposition regardless of the type was not shown to be of clinical consequence in a large OCT follow-up study.[49]

CONCLUSION

Optical coherence tomography is an exciting and powerful intravascular imaging modality, which can be used in both simple and complex coronary disease evaluation and management. Because of its high resolution, it can give vivid images and information about the in vivo pathology and disease process and help the clinician make better clinical decisions. However, we need large-scale prospective clinical studies to help the clinicians validate and utilize the multitude of information, and understand its impact on clinical outcomes and determine its cost effectiveness in various clinical scenarios including acute coronary syndromes. It will become the futuristic tool for performing a "perfect coronary angioplasty".

REFERENCES

1. Topol EJ, Nissen SE. Our preoccupation with coronary luminology. The dissociation between clinical and angiographic findings in ischemic heart disease. Circulation. 1995;92(8):2333-42.
2. Holmes DR, Lerman A, Moreno PR, et al. Diagnosis and management of STEMI arising from plaque erosion. JACC Cardiovasc Imaging. 2013;6(3):290-6.
3. Prati F, Uemura S, Souteyrand G, et al. OCT-based diagnosis and management of STEMI associated with intact fibrous cap. JACC Cardiovasc Imaging. 2013;6(3):283-7.
4. Tearney GJ, Waxman S, Shishkov M, et al. Three-dimensional coronary artery microscopy by intracoronary optical frequency domain imaging. JACC Cardiovasc Imaging. 2008;1(6):752-61.
5. Tearney GJ, Regar E, Akasaka T, et al. Consensus standards for acquisition, measurement, and reporting of intravascular optical coherence tomography studies: a report from the International Working Group for Intravascular Optical Coherence Tomography Standardization and Validation. J Am Coll Cardiol. 2012;59(12):1058-72
6. Prati F, Guagliumi G, Mintz GS, et al. Expert review document part 2: methodology, terminology and clinical applications of optical coherence tomography for the assessment of interventional procedures. Eur Heart J. 2012;33(20):2513-20.
7. Terashima M, Kaneda H, Suzuki T The role of Optical coherence tomography in coronary interventions. Korean J Intern Med. 2012;27(1):1-12.
8. Kume T, Akasaka T, Kawamoto T, et al. Assessment of coronary intima—media thickness by optical coherence tomography: comparison with intravascular ultrasound. Circ J. 2005;69(8):903-7.
9. Motreff P, Levesque S, Souteyrand G, et al. High-resolution coronary imaging by optical coherence tomography: feasibility, pitfalls and artifact analysis. Arch Cardiovasc Dis. 2010;103(4):215-26.
10. Moharram MA, Yeoh T, Lowe HC. Swings and roundabouts: intravascular optical coherence tomography (OCT) in the evaluation of the left main stem coronary artery. Int J Cardiol. 2011;148(2):243-4.
11. Crea F, Liuzzo G. Pathogenesis of acute coronary syndromes. J Am Coll Cardiol. 2013;61(1):1-11.
12. Libby P. Mechanisms of acute coronary syndromes and their implications for therapy. N Engl J Med. 2013;368(21):2004-13.
13. Virmani R, Kolodgie FD, Burke AP, et al. Lessons from sudden coronary death: a comparative morphological classification scheme for atherosclerotic lesions. Arterioscler Thromb Vasc Biol. 2000;20(5):1262-75.
14. Constantinides P. Plaque fissuring in human coronary thrombosis. J Atheroscler Res. 1966; 6:1-17.
15. Davies MJ, Thomas AC. Plaque fissuring: the cause of acute myocardial infarction, sudden ischemic death, and crescendo angina. Br Heart J. 1985;53(4):363-73.
16. Alfonso F, Virmani R. New morphological insights on coronary plaque rupture: Bridging the gap from anatomy to clinical presentation? JACC Cardiovasc Interv. 2011;4(1):83-6.
17. Virmani R, Kolodgie FD, Burke AP, et al. Lessons from sudden coronary death: A comprehensive morphological classification scheme for atherosclerotic lesions. Arterioscler Thromb Vasc Biol. 2000;20(5):1262-75.
18. Xu Y1, Mintz GS, Tam A, et al. Prevalence, distribution, predictors, and outcomes of patients with calcified nodules in native coronary arteries: a 3-vessel intravascular ultrasound analysis from Providing Regional Observations to Study Predictors of Events in the Coronary Tree (PROSPECT). Circulation. 2012;126(5):537-45.
19. Yabushita H, Bouma BE, Houser SL, et al. Characterization of human atherosclerosis by optical coherence tomography. Circulation. 2002;106(13):1640-5.
20. Kume T, Akasaka T, Kawamoto T, et al. Assessment of coronary arterial thrombus by optical coherence tomography. Am J Cardiol. 2006;97(12):1713-7.
21. Jia H, Abtahian F, Aguirre AD, et al. In vivo diagnosis of plaque erosion and calcified nodule in patients with acute coronary syndrome by intravascular optical coherence tomography. J Am Coll Cardiol. 2013;62(19):1748-58.
22. Farb A, Burke AP, Tang AL, et al. Coronary plaque erosion without rupture into a lipid core: A frequent cause of coronary thrombosis in sudden coronary death. Circulation. 1996;93(7):1354-63.
23. Burke AP, Farb A, Malcom GT, et al. Coronary risk factors and plaque morphology in men with coronary disease who died suddenly. N Engl J Med. 1997;336(18):1276-82.
24. Mitsuyasu T, Hideaki K, Takahiko S. The role of Optical coherence tomography in coronary interventions. Korean J Intern Med. 2012; 27(1): 1-12.
25. Kubo T, Imanishi T, Kashiwagi M, et al. Multiple coronary lesion instability in patients withacute myocardial infarction as determined byoptical coherence tomography. Am J Cardiol. 2010;105(3):318-22.

26. Ino Y, Kubo T, Tanaka A, et al. Difference of culprit lesion morphologies between ST-segment elevation myocardial infarction and non-ST segment elevation acute coronary syndrome: an optical coherence tomography study. JACC Cardiovasc Interv. 2011;4(1):76-82.
27. Tian J, Hou J, Xing L, et al. Significance of intraplaque neovascularization for vulnerability: optic coherence tomography study. Heart. 2012;98(20):1504-9.
28. Kato K, Yonetsu T, Kim SJ, et al. Nonculprit plaques in patients with acute coronary syndromes have more vulnerable features compared with those with nonacute coronary syndromes: a 3-vessel optical coherence tomography study. Circ Cardiovasc Imaging. 2012;5(4):433-40.
29. Toutouzas K, Karanasos A, Riga M, et al. Optical coherence tomography assessment of the spatial distribution of culprit ruptured plaques and thin-cap fibroatheromas in acute coronary syndrome. Euro Intervention. 2012;8(4):477-85.
30. Zhao Z, Witzenbichler B, Mintz GS, et al. Dynamic nature of nonculprit coronary artery lesion morphology in STEMI: a serial IVUS analysis from the HORIZONS-AMI trial. JACC Cardiovasc Imaging. 2013;6(1):86-95.
31. Diletti R, Garcia-Garcia HM, Gomez-Lara J, et al. Assessment of coronary atherosclerosis progression and regression at bifurcations using combined IVUS and OCT. JACC Cardiovasc Imaging. 2011;4(7):774-80.
32. Uemura S, Ishigami K, Soeda T, et al. Thin-cap fibroatheroma and microchannel findings in optical coherence tomography correlate with subsequent progression of coronary atheromatous plaques. Eur Heart J. 2012;33(1):78-85.
33. Moreno PR, Falk E, Palacios IF, et al. Macrophage infiltration in acute coronary syndromes: Implications for plaque rupture. Circulation. 1994;90(2):775-8.
34. Kitabata H, Tanaka A, Kubo T, et al. Relation of microchannel structure identified by optical coherence tomography to plaque vulnerability in patients with coronary artery disease. Am J Cardiol. 2010;105(12):1673-8.
35. D'Ascenzo F, Barbero U, Cerrato E, et al. Accuracy of intravascular ultrasound and optical coherence tomography in identifying functionally significant coronary stenosis according to vessel diameter: a meta-analysis of 2,581 patients and 2,807 lesions. Am Heart J. 2015;169(5):663-73.
36. Mintz GS. Clinical utility of intravascular imaging and physiology in coronary artery disease. J Am Coll Cardiol. 2014;64(2):207-22.
37. Haibo Jia, Jiannan Dai, Jingbo Hou, et al. Effective anti-thrombotic therapy without stenting: intravascular optical coherence tomography-based management in plaque erosion (the EROSION study). Eur Heart J. 2017;14;38(11):792-800.
38. Kajander OA, Pinilla-Echeverri N, Jolly SS, et al. Culprit plaque morphology in STEMI: an optical coherence tomography study: insights from the TOTAL-OCT substudy. Euro Intervention. 2016;12(6):716-23.
39. Sheth TN, Kajander OA, Lavi S, et al. Optical coherence tomography-guided percutaneous coronary intervention in ST-segment-elevation myocardial infarction: a prospective propensity matched cohort of the Thrombectomy Versus Percutaneous Coronary Intervention Alone trial. Circ Cardiovasc Interv. 2016;9(4):e003414.
40. Meneveau N, Souteyrand G, Motreff P, et al. Optical coherence tomography to optimize results of percutaneous coronary intervention in patients with non-ST-elevation acute coronary syndrome: results of the multicenter, randomized DOCTORS study (Does Optical Coherence Tomography Optimize Results of Stenting). Circulation. 2016;134(13):906-17.
41. Prati F, Romagnoli E, Gatto L, et al. Clinical impact of suboptimal stenting and residual intrastent plaque/thrombus protrusion in patients with acute coronary syndrome: the CLI-OPCI ACS substudy (Centro per la Lotta ControL'Infarto—Optimization of Percutaneous Coronary Intervention in Acute Coronary Syndrome). Circ Cardiovasc Interv. 2016;9(12):pii:e003726.
42. Schulz S, Schuster T, Mehilli J et al. Stent thrombosis after drug-eluting stent implantation: Incidence, timing, and relation to discontinuation of clopidogrel therapy over a 4-year period. Eur Heart J. 2009;30(22):2714-21.
43. van Werkum JW, Heestermans AA, Zomer AC, et al. Predictors of coronary stent thrombosis. The Dutch stent thrombosis registry. J Am Coll Cardiol. 2009;53(16):1399-409.
44. Kang S, Mintz GS, Akasaka T, et al. Optical coherence tomographic analysis of in-stent neoatherosclerosis after drug-eluting stent implantation. Circulation. 2011;123(25):2954-63.
45. Souteyrand G, Amabile N, Mangin L, et al. Mechanisms of stent thrombosis analyzed by optical coherence tomography: Insights from the national PESTO French registry. Eur Heart J. 2016;37(15):1208-16.
46. Prati F, Kodama T, Romagnoli E, et al. Suboptimal stent deployment is associated with subacute stent thrombosis: optical coherence tomography insights from a multicenter matched study. From the CLI Foundation Investigators: the CLI-THRO study. Am Heart J. 2015;169(2):249-56.
47. Taniwaki M, Radu MD, Zaugg S, et al. Mechanisms of very late drug-eluting stent thrombosis assessed by optical coherence tomography. Circulation. 2016;133(7):650-60.
48. Ali ZA, Maehara A, Genereux P, et al. Optical coherence tomography compared with intravascular ultrasound and with angiography to guide coronary stent implantation (ILUMIEN III: OPTIMIZE PCI): a randomized controlled trial. Lancet. 2016;388(10060):2618-28.
49. Im E, Kim BK, Ko YG, et al. Incidences, predictors, and clinical outcomes of acute and late stent malapposition detected by optical coherence tomography after drug-eluting stent implantation. Circ Cardiovasc Interv. 2014;7(1):88-96.

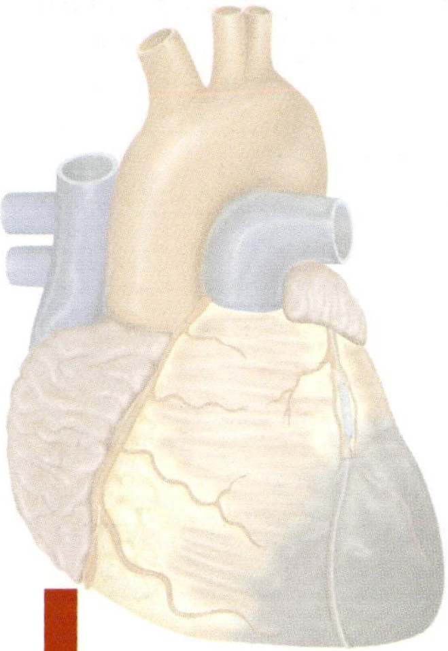

35

CHAPTER

Advances in CT Coronary Angiography in Evaluation of CAD

Harsh Mahajan, Suman Singhal, Puneet Sethi

INTRODUCTION

Computed tomography coronary angiography (CTCA) has been widely used in the diagnosis of coronary artery disease (CAD), which is the leading cause of death in men and women. Over the past few decades, computed tomography (CT) has undergone rapid breathtaking technological advancements *from single* slice to multislice CT (MSCT), which started from 4-slice systems in 1998 to the latest 256-slice and 320-slice CT systems. With wide array/volume scanners, smaller detector size, high pitch helical mode, faster gantry rotation speed, improved spatial and temporal resolutions of the 64- and post 64 MSCT scanners, coronary artery imaging has become a feasible, accurate and reliable noninvasive test significantly obviating the need of invasive coronary angiography in low to intermediate risk group population. It helps in detecting coronary calcium deposits, assessment of degree of coronary luminal stenosis, evaluation of stents, coronary artery grafts and in prediction of disease outcomes.[1-3] In this chapter Advances in CTCA in evaluation of CAD, recent guidelines, its role in new emerging areas like plaque characterization, CT-FFR, transluminal attenuation gradient and myocardial perfusion have been discussed. Further, recently introduced standardized reporting and data system in coronary artery disease CAD-RADS has been discussed.

The biggest challenges in cardiac CT today are coronary motion, calcium blooming, high heart rates, plaque characterization, and functional evaluation of coronary disease.

HEART RATE

The main limitation of 64-slice CT angiography is that patient's heart rate must be controlled with use of beta-blockers or calcium channel blockers to ensure optimal image quality for diagnostic purposes. This has been overcome to a greater extent with the development of dual-source CT as the temporal resolution has been significantly improved from 165 to 83 ms compared to single-source 64-slice CT.[4,5] Studies performed with dual-source CT coronary angiography have demonstrated high diagnostic accuracy for diagnosis of CAD, and most importantly the image quality is independent of heart rate[6] (Fig. 1). Further, technical developments and expansion of multislice CT systems from a 64-slice to 256- and 320-slice system have allowed acquisition of whole-heart coverage in one gantry rotation with extended z-axis coverage.[7,8] Despite these advantages, the temporal resolution (135 and 175 ms) of 256- and 320-slice CT is inferior to that of dual-source CT (83 ms).[9]

CALCIFICATIONS

The diagnostic value of CTCA is widely known to be hampered by the heavy calcification in the coronary artery tree. According to several meta-analyses,[10] high-density calcification produces blooming and beam hardening artifacts, which leads to overestimation of the degree of coronary stenosis. Specifically, calcium scores >400 were found to significantly reduce the diagnostic specificity. Stolzmann et al.[11] stated in their study that CTCA had

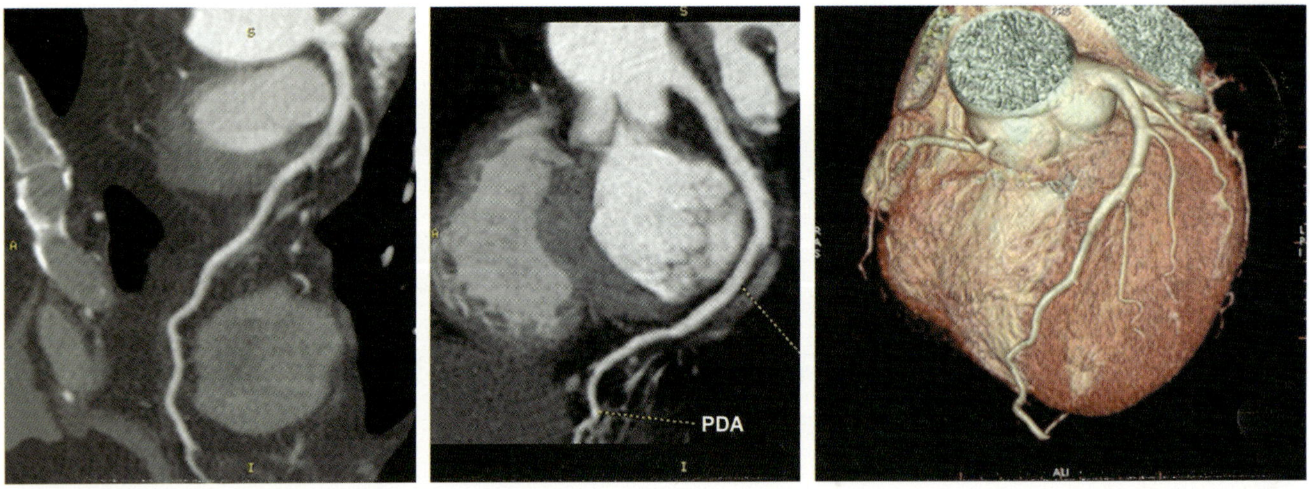

Fig. 1: Dual source-CT (DSCT) coronary angiography in a chronic obstructive pulmonary disease (COPD) patient with a heart rate of 90 bpm and no beta-blocker. Good quality curved multiplanar reformatted and volume rendered images show normal coronary arteries.

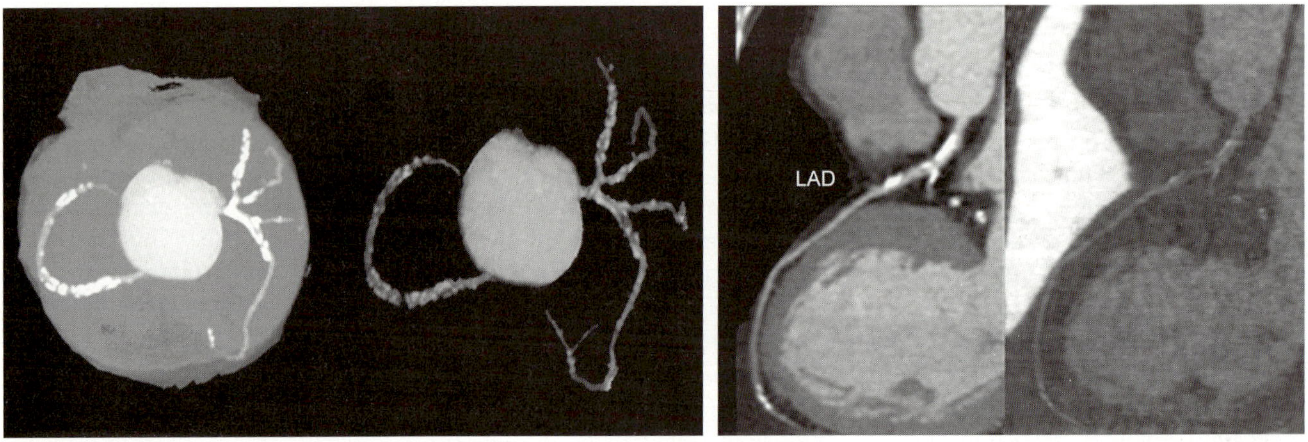

Fig. 2: Dual energy CT angiography in a patient with a history of chest pain and calcium score of 2,192. There is vessel visualization after calcium suppression in material density paired images (coronary tree and LAD) showing no significant luminal narrowing.

high diagnostic accuracy despite the presence of heavy calcifications with sensitivity and specificity being 99% and 99% in patients with median coronary artery calcium (CAC) score less than 316, and 98% and 99% in patients with median CAC score more than 316. Dual energy CT with Gem stone technology using material density and monochromatic imaging can better separate iodine and calcified plaque at different single keV energies enhancing both the visual and quantitative assessment of calcified plaque in the coronary vessels. It provides significant calcium suppression thus overcoming the beam hardening artifact (Fig. 2). Despite these promising results, further studies on 256- and 320-slice CT are needed to evaluate the diagnostic performance of CTCA in patients with high coronary calcium score.

CORONARY MOTION ARTIFACTS

Stair-step motion artifact occurs especially in patients with high heart rates, heart rate variability, and in the presence of irregular or ectopic heartbeats such as premature ventricular contractions and atrial fibrillation during image acquisition. It can be best recognized in a sagittal or coronal view. Therefore, beta-blockers or calcium channel blockers are used to lower the heart rate prior to the scan. Reduction of this artifact is achieved by reconstructing the dataset at different phases of the cardiac cycle.[12] Dual energy CT helps in cardiac motion correction by detecting vessel path and tracking coronary artery centre lines along with 3D phase reconstructions. It corrects the stair-step artifact and reconstructs the vessel within the same heart cycle (Fig. 3).

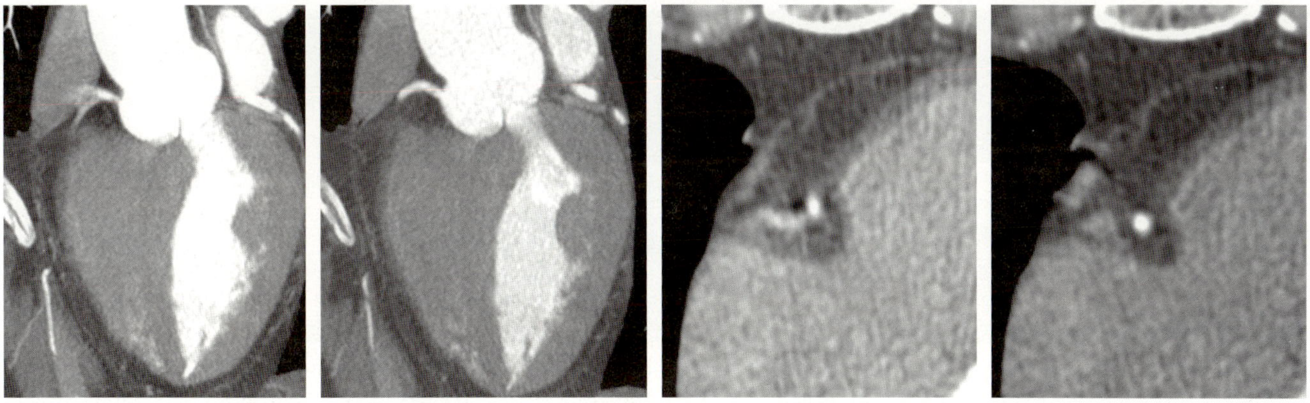

Fig. 3: Dual source CT curved multiplanar reformatted images and axial images; with and without snapshot freeze (cardiac motion correction sequence) showing improved visualization of right coronary artery (RCA).

PLAQUE CHARACTERIZATION

Classification of plaques by cardiac CT based on composition has important clinical implications, as increasing numbers of mixed plaques are associated with adverse major cardiac events.[13] Min et al. in their multicenter trial showed patients with mixed plaque composition more often demonstrated obstructive coronary stenosis at both per-segment and per-patient assessments when compared to those with noncalcified and calcified plaques, while calcified plaques rarely resulted in obstructive stenosis. Dual energy CT has potential for improved plaque differentiation, as there are algorithms that aim to differentiate between contrast opacified lumen of the vessel and hard plaques based on the spectral properties of iodine and calcium. Based on these monochromatic spectral images, color-coding is done (e.g. hard plaque algorithm) and HU spectral curves are obtained which give plaque material composition of different plaques (Fig. 4).

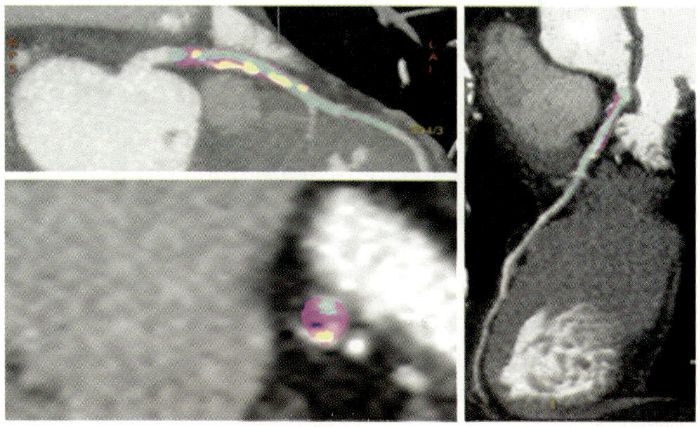

Fig. 4: DECT (Gem stone spectral imaging technology) images with color coding showing plaque composition. Lumen—green, lipid plaque—pink and calcified plaque—yellow.

VULNERABLE PLAQUE IDENTIFICATION WITH CTCA

Computed tomography coronary angiography with newer technological advancements and improved submillimeter, spatial resolution is able to assess plaque characteristics including identification of the "vulnerable plaque". Features associated with plaque vulnerability are positive remodeling, presence of spotty calcifications, and lower plaque density. In patients with acute coronary syndrome (ACS), the combined presence of these three features allows identification of the unstable lesion with a PPV, an NPV, and an accuracy of 95%, 60%, and 70%, respectively.[14] Motoyama and colleagues targeted positive remodeling (PR) (defined as diameter of plaque 10% larger than reference vessel) and low attenuation plaque (LAP) (less than 30 HU) as potential predictors of ACS (Figs. 5A to C). Patients with both factors had a 22.2% chance of developing ACS vs. 3.7% for only one of the above and 0.5% chance if a plaque had none of the above features. PR and/or LAP independently predicted acute coronary events HR 22.8 (95% CI, 6.9–75.2; P<0.001.[15] The Napkin ring sign describes an LAP surrounded by a rim of higher attenuation and helps in prediction of ACS. Important limitation of CT is that its spatial resolution does not permit measurement of fibrous cap thickness, preventing its use for the identification of thin cap fibroatheroma (TCFA).[16] The thin-cap (<65 μm) fibroatheroma (TCFA) has close resemblance to ruptured plaque but lacks luminal thrombosis and is, therefore, regarded as the most likely precursor lesion to plaque rupture.

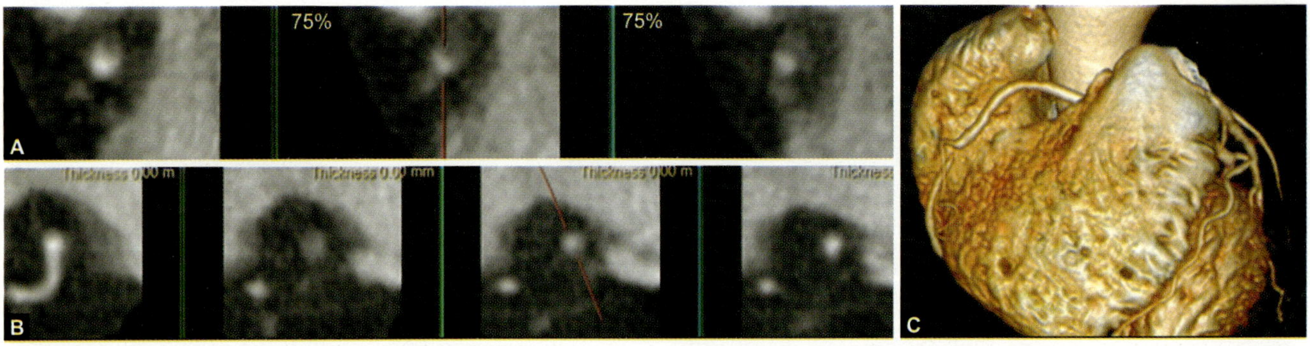

Figs. 5A to C: (A) Axial sections revealing eccentric low attenuation plaque (LAP) and positive remodeling (PR). (B and C) Axial sections and volume rendered images revealing significant focal luminal stenosis in RCA by concentric low attenuation plaque.

EVALUATION OF MYOCARDIAL PERFUSION

Myocardial perfusion imaging (CT-MPI) provides functional evaluation with hemodynamic assessment of obstructive coronary artery lesions. CT assessment of myocardial perfusion is based on the distribution of iodinated contrast material during its first pass through the myocardium. Because the contrast material's distribution is determined by the arterial blood supply, myocardial perfusion defects can be identified as hypoattenuating areas containing reduced amounts of contrast material.[17] Two different approaches are available for CT-MPI: static or dynamic, static CT myocardial perfusion imaging can further be categorized into single- and dual-energy techniques. Static myocardial perfusion evaluation at rest is generally performed using CTCA image sets already obtained for the morphologic assessment of the coronary arteries, thus, no additional acquisition time or radiation is necessary. If assessment of myocardial perfusion at stress is desired, an additional acquisition during pharmacologic stress is obtained. Ko et al.[18] determined the accuracy of dual-energy CT for the diagnosis of reversible ischemia identified by cardiac MRI with a sensitivity of 89% and a specificity of 78%. Ko et al.[19] also found the incremental diagnostic value of combined coronary CTA and CT perfusion compared with coronary CTA alone with a marked increase in sensitivity (91.8–93.5%), specificity (67.7–85.5%), PPV (73.6–88.3%), and NPV (87.5–91.4%).

Dynamic CT-MPI provides a quantitative estimation of myocardial time-attenuation curves and other parameters such as myocardial blood flow (MBF). Cutoff points between 75 and 78 mL/100 mL/min have been proposed as the optimal threshold values for the discrimination between significant and nonsignificant lesions.[20] The core limitation of dynamic CT-MPI is a significantly increased radiation dose compared with static CT-MPI, as well as the need for longer breath-holding that warrants the use of further motion correction algorithms.[21,22] A recently published multicenter study (CORE320—Coronary Artery Evaluation using 320-row Multidetector Computed Tomography Angiography and Myocardial Perfusion) has revealed that the overall performance of CT-MPI in the diagnosis of obstructive CAD was higher than that of SPECT (Figs. 6A to C).[23]

CT Functional Flow Reserve

Fractional flow reserve-computed tomography (FFR-CT) is a novel technology that enables determination of the functional significance of lesions noninvasively, using sophisticated computer algorithms based on computational fluid dynamics applied to coronary CTA. It is computed from commonly acquired coronary CT angiography scans without any modification of cardiac CT protocols, additional image acquisition, or administration of medications.

The CT FFR technology is based on three key principles. The first is that coronary supply meets myocardial demand at rest (total resting coronary flow is relative to ventricular mass). The second is that resistance of the microcirculation at rest is inversely but not linearly proportional to the size of the feeding vessel. The third principle is that microcirculation reacts predictably to maximal hyperemic conditions in patients with normal coronary flow. On the basis of these principles, a lumped parameter model representing the resistance to flow during simulated hyperemia is applied to each coronary branch of the segmented coronary CTA model.[24] The CT FFR was modeled for conditions of adenosine-induced hyperemia; an FFRCT ≤0.80 was considered to be diagnostic of lesion-specific ischemia.[25]

CT FFR was compared to invasive FFR and had a per-vessel accuracy of 84.3%, sensitivity of 87.9%, and specificity of 82.2% in the discover FLOW trial.[25] The DEFACTO trial revealed that FFR CT better discriminates coronary stenosis

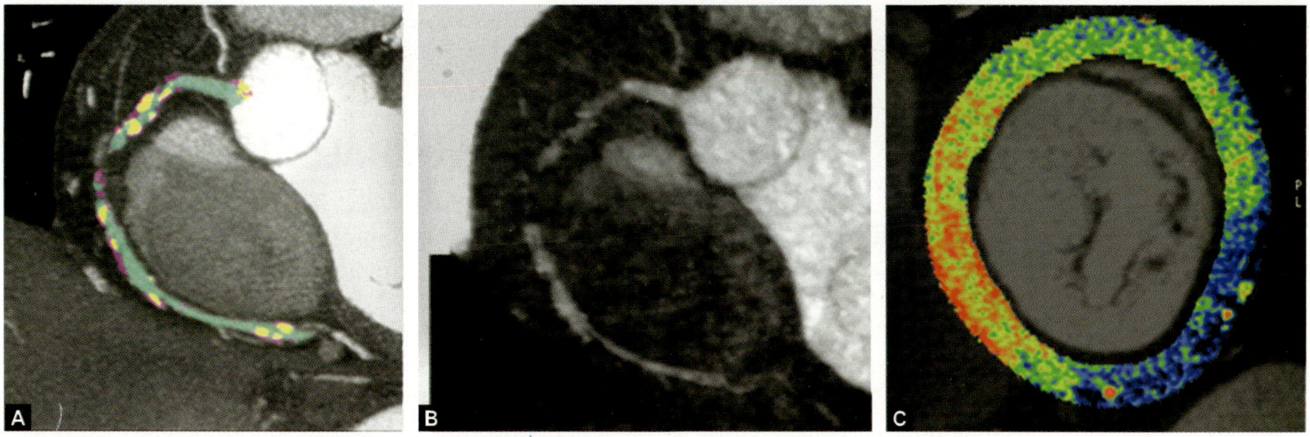

Figs. 6A to C: (A and B) CT coronary angiography in a patient with chest pain. Curved multiplanar reformatted image with plaque differentiation, curved multiplanar reformatted image show significant luminal stenosis in mid right coronary artery (RCA). (C) Myocardial perfusion image with color overlay showing semi-quantitative assessment of myocardial perfusion consistent with ischemia.

with ischemia AUC 0.81 (95% CI, 0.75–0.86; $P < 0.0001$) compared with CT alone AUC 0.68 (0.62–0.74).[26] Integrating CTMPI with CT FFR and reserving CT MPI for intermediate CTA FFR results, also improves diagnostic performance while omitting nearly one-half of the population from CT MPI examinations.[27]

Transluminal Attenuation Gradient

Transluminal attenuation gradient is a recently introduced image postprocessing method that provides functional assessment of CAD. Transluminal attenuation gradient is defined as the contrast opacification gradient along the length of a coronary artery.[28] It has been found that coronary CTA augmented with transluminal attenuation gradient has incremental diagnostic value in detecting hemodynamically significant CAD.[29] Both FFRCT and assessment of transluminal attenuation gradient are based on the conventional coronary CTA dataset and thus avoid additional radiation or contrast material exposure.[29]

RECENT GUIDELINES AND REPORTING SYSTEM IN EVALUATION OF CORONARY ARTERY DISEASE

Calcium Scoring

The calcium scoring is done using mean Agatston score and is routinely performed as an initial part of the entire cardiac CT examination. Prior 2010 ACC/AHA guidelines[30] on risk stratification of asymptomatic adults were more favorable for use of coronary artery calcium score offering a IIA recommendation for intermediate group patients, however, the recent 2013 ACC/AHA guidelines[31] give a IIB recommendation when a risk based treatment decision is uncertain.

Coronary Artery Disease-Reporting and Data System (CAD-RADS)

It is an expert consensus document of the Society of Cardiovascular Computed Tomography (SCCT), the American College of Radiology (ACR) and the North American Society for Cardiovascular Imaging (NASCI), Endorsed by the American College of Cardiology.[32] The main goal of CAD-RADS is to standardize reporting of coronary CTA results and to facilitate communication of test results to referring physicians along with suggestions for subsequent patient management. The suggested CAD-RADS classification is applied on a per-patient basis and represents the highest-grade coronary artery lesion documented by coronary CTA. It ranges from CAD-RADS 0 (Zero) for the complete absence of stenosis and plaque to CAD-RADS 5 for the presence of at least one totally occluded coronary artery and should always be interpreted in conjunction with the impression found in the report (Fig. 7). Specific recommendations are provided for further management of patients with stable or acute chest pain based on the CAD-RADS classification (Tables 1 and 2).

Radiation Dose

Radiation dose has always been a major concern with cardiac CT and a number of techniques have been introduced to reduce the radiation dose in cardiac CT imaging without compromising image quality. These

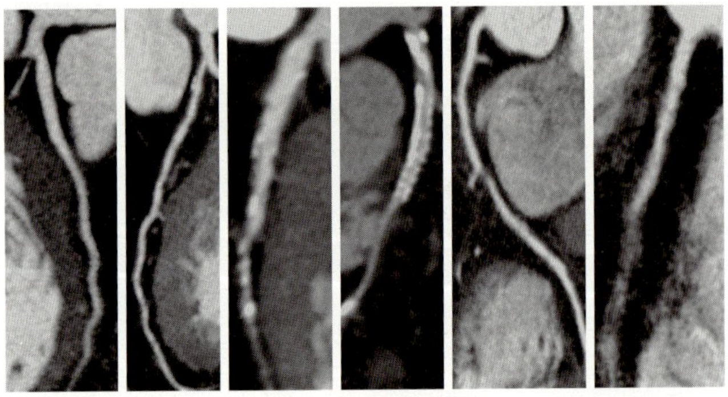

Fig. 7

dose-reduction techniques include ECG-controlled tube current modulation, lower X-ray tube voltage, high pitch, prospective ECG-triggered scanning, and reconstruction algorithms.[33,34] Of these dose-saving strategies, prospective ECG-triggering is the most effective approach in terms of dose reduction and high diagnostic accuracy when compared to conventional retrospective ECG-gated protocol (67-68). High pitch protocol is another strategy, which is only achievable with the second generation of dual-source CT scanners with dose lower than 1 mSv reported. Using many of the technologies and strategies discussed above, it is possible to lower the dose to <5 mSv, where doses of <1 mSv have been reported in the literature.[35]

CONTINUING CHALLENGES

The main challenge in cardiac CT is that there is a strong demand on high temporal resolution which translates into the time required to acquire cardiac images in a very short duration. Currently, a temporal resolution of 75 ms is achieved with the recent models of dual-source CT scanners, and this demonstrates a significant improvement in cardiac imaging. However, the temporal resolution of these models is still significantly inferior to that of invasive coronary angiography, which is 10 ms. The temporal resolution of 256–320 slice CT is inferior to that of dual source CT. The spatial resolution of current multislice CT scanners is excellent, which ranges from 0.3 mm to 0.5 mm, and this is close to the spatial resolution of invasive coronary angiography, which is between 0.1 and 0.2 mm. Despite this achievement, cardiac CT is unable to measure fibrous cap thickness, preventing its use for the identification of thin cap fibroatheroma (TCFA) which is a precursor of plaque rupture.

TABLE 1: CAD-RADS reporting and data system for patients presenting with stable chest pain.

Degree of maximal	*Coronary stenosis*	*Interpretation*	*Further cardiac investigation*	*Management*
CAD-RADS 0	0% (No plaque or stenosis)	Document absence of CAD*	None	Reassurance. Consider nonatherosclerotic causes of chest pain
CAD-RADS 1**	1–24%—minimal stenosis or plaque with no stenosis	Minimal nonobstructive CAD	None	Consider nonatherosclerotic causes of chest pain Consider preventive therapy and risk factor modification
CAD-RADS 2	25–49%—mild stenosis	Mild nonobstructive CAD	None	Consider nonatherosclerotic causes of chest pain Consider preventive therapy and risk factor modification, particularly for patients with nonobstructive plaque in multiple segments
CAD-RADS 3	50–69%—stenosis	Moderate stenosis	Consider functional assessment	Consider symptom-guided anti-ischemic and preventive pharmacotherapy as well as risk factor modification per guideline-directed care*** Other treatments should be considered per guideline-directed care***
CAD-RADS 4	A: 70–99%—stenosis or B: Left main > 50% or 3-vessel obstructive (≥70%) disease	Severe stenosis	A: Consider ICA**** or functional assessment. B: ICA is recommended	Consider symptom-guided anti-ischemic and preventive pharmacotherapy as well as risk factor modification per guideline-directed care*** Other treatments (including options of revascularization) should be considered per guideline-directed care***

Contd...

Contd...

Degree of maximal	*Coronary stenosis*	*Interpretation*	*Further cardiac investigation*	*Management*
CAD-RADS 5	100% (Total occlusion)	Total coronary occlusion	Consider ICA and/or Viability assessment	Consider symptom-guided anti-ischemic and preventive pharmacotherapy as well as risk factors modification per guideline-directed care*** Other treatments (including options of revascularization) should be considered per guideline-directed care***
CAD-RADS N	Non-diagnostic study	Obstructive CAD cannot be excluded	Additional or alternative evaluation may be needed	

The CAD-RADS classification should be applied on a per-patient basis for the clinically most relevant (usually highest-grade) stenosis. All vessels greater than 1.5 mm in diameter should be graded for stenosis severity. CAD-RADS will not apply for smaller vessels (<1.5 mm in diameter). MODIFIERS: If more than one modifier is present, the symbol "/" (slash) should follow each modifier in the following order: First: modifier N (non-diagnostic). Second: modifier S (stent). Third: modifier G (graft). Fourth: modifier V (vulnerability).

*CAD—coronary artery disease.

**CAD-RADS 1—this category should also include the presence of plaque with positive remodeling and no evidence of stenosis.

***Guideline-directed care per ACC Stable Ischemic Heart Disease Guidelines (Fihn et al. JACC 2012).

****ICA—invasive coronary angiography

TABLE 2: CAD-RADS reporting and data system for patients presenting with acute chest pain, negative first troponin, negative or non-diagnostic electrocardiogram and low to intermediate risk (TIMI Risk Score < 4) (Emergency Department or Hospital Setting).

Degree of Maximal	*Coronary Stenosis*	*Interpretation*	*Further Cardiac Investigation*	*Management*
CAD-RADS 0	0%	Document absence of CAD*	None	No further evaluation of ACS is required. Consider other etiologies
CAD-RADS 1**	1–24%	Minimal nonobstructive CAD	None	Consider evaluation of non-ACS etiology, if normal troponin and no ECG changes. Consider referral for outpatient follow-up for preventive therapy and risk factor modification
CAD-RADS 2	25–49%	Mild nonobstructive CAD	None	Consider evaluation of non-ACS etiology, if normal troponin and no ECG changes. Consider referral for outpatient follow-up for preventive therapy and risk factor modification. If clinical suspicion of ACS is high or if high-risk plaque features are noted, consider hospital admission with cardiology consultation
CAD-RADS 3	50–69%	Moderate stenosis	Consider functional assessment	Consider hospital admission with cardiology consultation, functional testing and/or ICA**** for evaluation and management. Recommendation for anti-ischemic and preventive management should be considered as well as risk factor modification. Other treatments should be considered if presence of hemodynamically significant lesion
CAD-RADS 4	A: 70–99% or B: Left main >50% or 3-vessel obstructive	Severe stenosis	A: Consider ICA*** or functional assessment. B: ICA is recommended	Consider hospital admission with cardiology consultation. Further evaluation with ICA and revascularization as appropriate. Recommendation for anti-ischemic and preventive management should be considered as well as risk factor modification

Contd...

Contd...

Degree of Maximal	*Coronary Stenosis*	*Interpretation*	*Further Cardiac Investigation*	*Management*
CAD-RADS 5	100% (Total occlusion)	Total coronary occlusion	Consider ICA and/or Viability assessment	Consider expedited ICA on a timely basis and revascularization if appropriate if acute occlusion***** Recommendation for anti-ischemic and preventive management should be considered as well as risk factor modifications
CAD-RADS N	Nondiagnostic study	Obstructive CAD cannot be excluded	Additional or alternative evaluation may be needed	Additional or alternative evaluation for ACS is needed

The CAD-RADS classification should be applied on a per-patient basis for the clinically most relevant (usually highest-grade) stenosis. All vessels greater than 1.5 mm in diameter should be graded for stenosis severity. CAD-RADS will not apply for smaller vessels (<1.5 mm in diameter). MODIFIERS: If more than one modifier is present, the symbol "/" (slash) should follow each modifier in the following order: First: modifier N (non-diagnostic). Second: modifier S (stent). Third: modifier G (graft). Fourth: modifier V (vulnerability).

*ACS—acute coronary syndrome.

**CAD-RADS 1—this category should also include the presence of plaque with positive remodeling and no evidence of stenosis.

***CAD-RADS—modifier 2/V can be used to indicate vulnerable/ high-risk plaque.

****ICA—invasive coronary angiography.

*****Unless the total coronary occlusion can be identified as chronic (through CT and clinical characteristics or patient history).

CONCLUSION

Computed tomography coronary angiography represents the most rapidly developing imaging modality in cardiac imaging. It has been increasingly used in the diagnosis of CAD due to improved spatial and temporal resolution with high diagnostic value. Dual energy CT allows tissue characterization, calcium suppression, assessment of myocardial perfusion and plaque differentiation. With further technological advancements, functional evaluation of coronary artery disease is possible with CT FFR, myocardial perfusion, transluminal attenuation gradient and assessment of atherosclerotic plaque characteristics. Detection of features of plaque vulnerability is possible with CTCA. The main disadvantage of cardiac CT imaging is radiation dose and various dose saving strategies have been introduced to reduce the effective radiation dose. CTCA provides an attractive alternative to invasive coronary angiography in routine clinical practice. CT coronary angiography with further developments in CT technology will continue to play an important role in the diagnostic evaluation of CAD and prediction of major adverse cardiac events.

REFERENCES

1. Nieman K, Oudkerk M, Rensing BJ, et al. Coronary angiography with multi-slice computed tomography. Lancet. 2001;357:599-603.
2. Achenbach S, Gieslar T, Ropers D, et al. Detection of coronary artery stenosis by contrast-enhanced, retrospectively electrocardiographically-gated multislice computed tomography. Circulation. 2001;103:2535-8.
3. Sun Z, Jiang W. Diagnostic value of multislice CT angiography in coronary artery disease: A meta-analysis. Eur J Radiol. 2006;60:279-86.
4. Johnson TR, Nikolaou K, Busch S, et al. Diagnostic accuracy of dual-source computed tomography in the diagnosis of coronary artery disease. Invest Radiol. 2007;42:684-91.
5. Alkadhi H, Stolzmann P, Scheffel H, et al. Radiation dose of cardiac dual-source CT: the effect of tailoring the protocol to patient-specific parameters. Eur J Radiol. 2008;68:385-91
6. Ropers U, Ropers D, Pflederer T, et al. Influence of heart rate on the diagnostic accuracy of dual-source computed tomography coronary angiography. J Am Coll Cardiol. 2007;50:2393-8.
7. Chao SP, Law WY, Kuo CJ, et al. The diagnostic accuracy of 256-row computed tomographic angiography compared with invasive coronary angiography in patients with suspected coronary artery disease. Eur Heart J. 2010;31:1916-23.
8. Rybicki FJ, Otero HJ, Steigner ML, et al. Initial evaluation of coronary images from 320-detector row computed tomography. Int J Cardiovasc Imaging. 2008;24:535-46.
9. Sun Z. Cardiac CT imaging in coronary artery disease: Current status and future directions. Quant Imaging Med Surg. 2012;2(2):98-105.
10. Sun Z, Lin CH, Davidson R, et al. Diagnostic value of 64-slice CT angiography in coronary artery disease: a systematic review. Eur J Radiol. 2008;67:78-84.
11. Stolzmann P, Scheffel H, Leschka S, et al. Influence of calcifications on diagnostic accuracy of coronary CT angiography using prospective ECG triggering. AJR Am J Roentgenol. 2008;191:1684-9.
12. Barrett JF, Keat N. Artifacts in CT: recognition and avoidance. Radiographics. 2004;24:1679-91.

13. Pundziute G, Schuijf JD, Jukema JW, et al. Head-to-head comparison of coronary plaque evaluation between multislice computed tomography and intravascular ultrasound radiofrequency data analysis. JACC Cardiovasc Interv. 2008;1:176-82.
14. Motoyama S, Kondo T, Sarai M, et al. Multislice computed tomographic characteristics of coronary lesions in acute coronary syndromes. J Am Coll Cardiol. 2007;50:319-26.
15. Motoyama S, Sarai M, Harigaya H, et al. Computed tomographic angiography characteristics of atherosclerotic plaques subsequently resulting in acute coronary syndrome. J Am Coll Cardiol. 2009;54:49-57.
16. Tomey M, Narula J, Kovacic J. Advances in the understanding of plaque composition and treatment options. J Am Coll Cardiol. 2014;63(16):1604-16.
17. George RT, Silva C, Cordeiro MA, et al. Multidetector computed tomography myocardial per-fusion imaging during adenosine stress. J Am Coll Cardiol. 2006; 48:153-60.
18. Ko SM, Choi JW, Song MG, et al. Myocardial perfusion imaging using adenosine-induced stress dual-energy computed tomography of the heart: comparison with cardiac magnetic resonance imaging and conventional coronary angiography. Eur Radiol. 2011;21:26-35.
19. Ko SM, Choi JW, Hwang HK, et al. Diagnostic performance of combined noninvasive anatomic and functional assessment with dual-source CT and adenosine-induced stress dual-energy CT for detection of significant coronary stenosis. AJR Am J Roentgenol. 2012;198:512-20.
20. Rossi A, Dharampal A, Wragg A, et al. Diagnostic performance of hyperemic myocardial blood flow index obtained by dynamic computed tomography: does it predict functionally significant coronary lesions? Eur Heart J Cardiovascular Imaging. 2014;15:85-94.
21. Mahnken AH, Klotz E, Pietsch H, et al. Quantitative whole heart stress perfusion CT imaging as noninvasive assessment of hemodynamics in coronary artery stenosis: preliminary animal experience. Invest Radiol. 2010;45:298-305.
22. Rossi A, Merkus D, Klotz E, et al. Stress myocardial perfusion: imaging with multidetector CT. Radiology. 2014;270:25-46.
23. George RT, Mehra VC, Chen MY, et al. Myocardial CT perfusion imaging and SPECT for the diagnosis of coronary artery disease: a head-to-head comparison from the CORE320 multicenter diagnostic performance study. Radiology. 2014;272:407-16.
24. Gonçalves Pde A, Rodríguez-Granillo GA, Spitzer E, et al. Functional Evaluation of Coronary Disease by CT Angiography. JACC: Cardiovascular Imaging. 2015; 8(11):1322-35.
25. Koo BK, Erglis A, Doh JH, et al. Diagnosis of ischemia-causing coronary stenoses by noninvasive fractional flow reserve computed from coronary computed tomographic angiograms. Results from the prospective multicenter DISCOVER-FLOW (Diagnosis of Ischemia-Causing Stenoses Obtained Via Noninvasive Fractional Flow Reserve) study. J Am Coll Cardiol. 2011;58:1989-97.
26. Min JK, Leipsic J, Pencina MJ, et al. Diagnostic accuracy of fractional flow reserve from anatomic CT angiography. JAMA. 2012;308:1237-45.
27. Coenen A, Rossi A, Lubbers MM, et al. Integrating CT Myocardial Perfusion and CT-FFR in the Work-Up of Coronary Artery Disease. JACC Cardiovasc Imaging. 2017;10(7):760-70.
28. Stuijfzand WJ, Danad I, Raijmakers PG, et al. Additional value of transluminal attenuation gradient in CT angiography to predict hemodynamic significance of coronary artery stenosis. JACC Cardiovasc Imaging. 2014;7:374-86
29. Wong DT, Ko BS, Cameron JD, et al. Transluminal attenuation gradient in coronary computed tomography angiography is a novel noninvasive approach to the identification of functionally significant coronary artery stenosis: a comparison with fractional flow reserve. J Am Coll Cardiol. 2013;61:1271-9.
30. Greenland P, Alpert JS, Beller GA et al. 2010 ACCF/AHA guideline for assessment of cardiovascular risk in asymptomatic adults: a report of the American College of Cardiology Foundation/American Heart Association Task Force on Practice Guidelines. J Am Coll Cardiol. 2010;56:e50-e103.
31. Goff DC Jr, Lloyd-Jones DM, Bennett G, et al. 2013 ACC/AHA guideline on the assessment of cardiovascular risk: a report of the American College of Cardiology/American Heart Association Task Force on Practice Guidelines. Circulation. 2014;129(25 Suppl 2):S49-73 .
32. Cury R, AbBara S, Achenbach S, et al. Coronary Artery Disease-Reporting and Data System. JACC Imaging. 2016;9(9):1099-113.
33. Sabarudin A, Sun Z, Ng KH. A systematic review of radiation dose ssociated with different generations of multidetector CT coronary angiography. J Med Imaging Radiat Oncol. 2012;56:5-17.
34. Sun Z, Ng KH. Multislice CT angiography in cardiac imaging. Part III: radiation risk and dose reduction. Singapore Med J. 2010;51:374-80.
35. Lell M, Marvan M, Schepis T, et al. Prospectively ECG-triggered high-pitch spiral acquisition for coronary CT angiography using dual source CT: technique and initial experience. Eur Radiol. 2009;19:2576-83.

36

CHAPTER

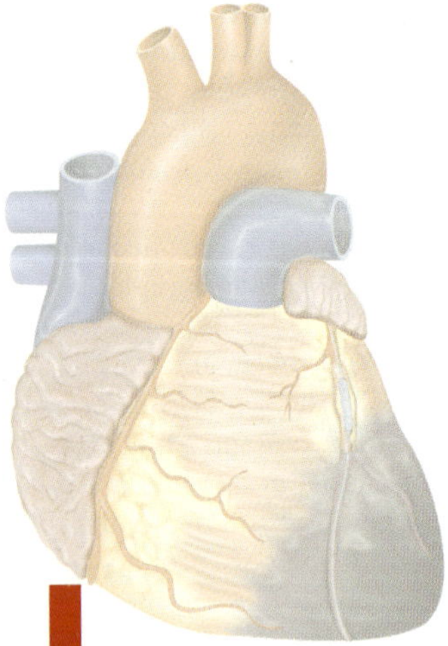

TNK Effect and Outcome Evaluation in STEMI by Echocardiography

SS Iyengar, Rajiv Ananthakrishna, Nagaraja Moorthy

INTRODUCTION

ST-elevation myocardial infarction (STEMI) is a product of profound myocardial ischemia that goes on to produce cardiac structural and functional alterations. Early recognition, prompt institution of reperfusion therapy with adjunctive and conjunctive measures, close watch for complications and a regular follow-up form the components of management. Primary percutaneous intervention (PCI) is the preferred form of reperfusion therapy, but fibrinolytic therapy is frequently used where primary PCI cannot be carried out within a stipulated time. Tenecteplase is a preferred fibrinolytic agent since it is conveniently administered as a single bolus and has established its efficacy and safety as evidenced by clinical trials and registries of fibrinolytic therapy and pharmacoinvasive strategy.[1-3] Diagnosis and management of STEMI could be quite challenging. Cardiac imaging is of great assistance and echocardiography is one of the simple and easily available imaging modalities. Echocardiography provides essential information (and sometimes unexpected findings) and is reported to be the second most frequently performed diagnostic procedure. [4] Echocardiography, after the initial development by Edler and Hertz in 1954 has evolved from one-dimensional (M mode) modality to 3D complex instrument with added features such as color Doppler, tissue Doppler, strain imaging, and contrast echocardiography. Echocardiography is essentially a noninvasive procedure, portable, simple to perform with low risk, could be used for serial studies and the information is obtained quickly. As one recalls "ischemic cascade" (Fig. 1),[5,6] myocardial diastolic and systolic abnormalities could be detected by echocardiography much before electrocardiography (ECG) changes and symptoms appear.

DIAGNOSIS OF STEMI

Decreased systolic thickening, regional wall motion abnormalities (delayed contractility of a segment, akinesia, dyskinesia) and reduced left ventricular ejection fraction (LVEF) indicate myocardial ischemia in a given clinical context. LVEF continues to remain as one of the

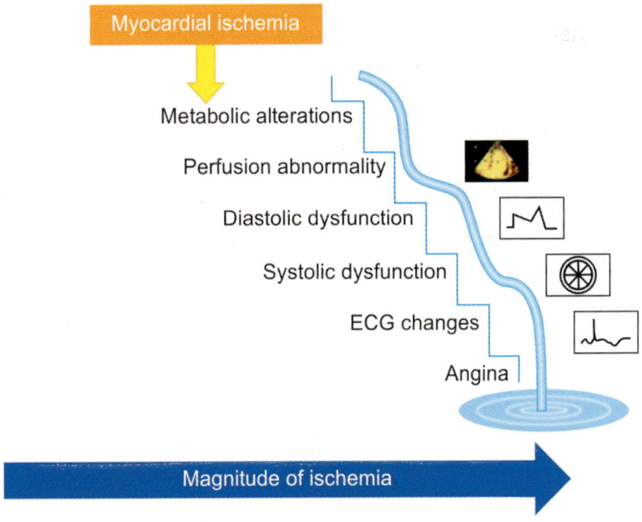

Fig. 1: Ischemic cascade.

Source: Maznyczka A, Sen S, Cook C, et al. The ischaemic constellation: an alternative to the ischaemic cascade—implications for the validation of new ischaemic tests. Open Heart 2015;2:e000178.

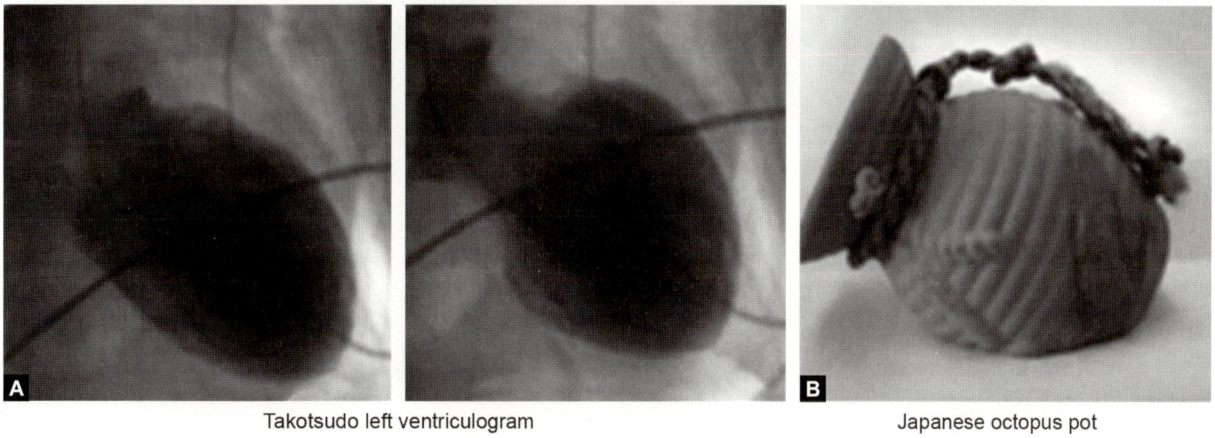

Figs. 2A and B: Left ventriculogram of a patient with stress cardiomyopathy showing typical apical ballooning (A), resembling takotsubo, i.e. a Japanese octopus pot (B).

important measurements with the greatest prognostic and clinical significance during and after MI.[7] Injection of an IV contrast agent may be tried to better delineate the endocardial borders for assessing LV function. Very proximal coronary artery lesions can be identified by examining the ostia of the coronary arteries with transesophageal echocardiogram (TEE). With history, clinical examination and ECG findings suggesting RV infarction, echocardiographic findings of RV dysfunction and infarction will substantiate the diagnosis. Other nonischemic cardiac causes of chest pain such as pericarditis, aortic or coronary aneurysm or dissection, myocarditis, cardiac contusion, and ruptured mitral chordae can be diagnosed by echocardiography. Takotsubo cardiomyopathy could be suspected by the classical picture of "apical ballooning" and confirmed once normal coronaries are seen on coronary angiogram (Figs. 2A and B). A careful analysis of the history, clinical examination findings, and ECG along with echocardiogram will help in the differential diagnoses and guide appropriate therapy.

Echocardiography After STEMI

Once the diagnosis of STEMI is established, concurrently and simultaneously with the institution of appropriate therapeutic measures, echocardiographic assessment for prognostication and complications should be carried out. Acute (first 48 hours) and subacute phase (3–7 days) of post-MI period is said to be the domain of echocardiography when it comes to cardiac imaging.[8] LV function, intracavitary thrombus and other complications are assessed.

Left Ventricular Ejection Fraction

Left ventricular systolic function is a key determinant of outcome after ST-segment elevation myocardial infarction (STEMI). LVEF, a measure of LV systolic function is a predictor of overall morbidity and mortality after STEMI and has been used as a surrogate endpoint in many major clinical studies. A left ventricular ejection fraction (LVEF) of 35% or less places, the patient at high risk for sudden cardiac death and is an indication for an implantable cardioverter-defibrillator (ICD) for primary prevention in selected patients with intraventricular conduction delay and heart failure 40 days after acute MI, or 3 months after coronary artery bypass graft (CABG) or percutaneous revascularization. After reperfusion, stunned or hibernating myocardium may recover function after sometime and hence the wait.[9] LVEF though used frequently and liked by many has several limitations. The estimation of ejection fraction is generally based on geometric assumptions. LVEF is both preload and afterload-dependent, and thus can change substantially based on loading conditions, and is not highly reproducible.[10]

LV Function as Assessed by LVEF After Tenecteplase

In a study,[11] 9 STEMI patients who were taken up for PPCI were noticed to have massive thrombus burden. These patients were administered low dose intracoronary thrombolysis via 6F-angioplasty guiding catheter. Intracoronary tenecteplase (TNK) administered was one-fifth of the systemic dose while remaining 4/5th was given through intravenous (IV) route and patients were maintained on heparin infusion. There was prompt and early ST resolution. There was improvement in thrombolysis in myocardial infarction (TIMI) flow and myocardial blush grade postlysis in all patients. Majority had recanalized infarct-related coronary artery thus obviating the need for stenting. Check coronary angiogram (CAG) was done after

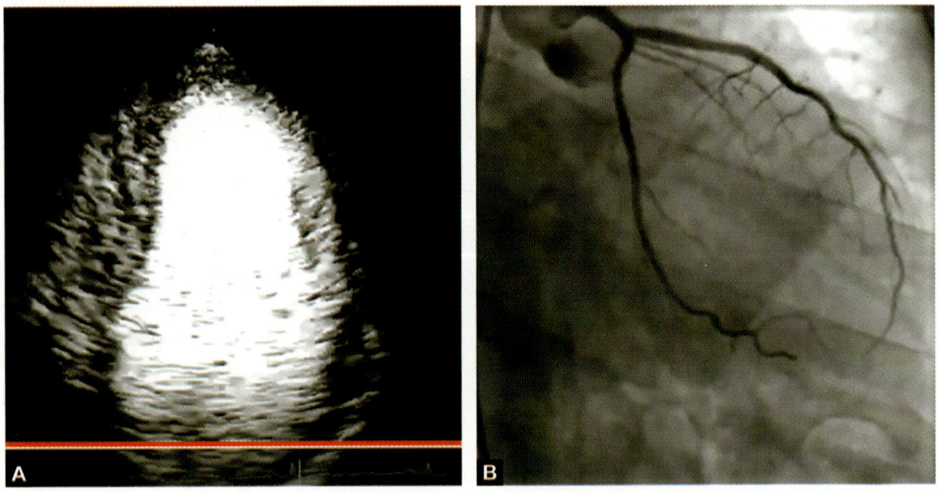

Figs. 3A and B: Myocardial contrast echocardiogram. (A) A 34-year-old male with acute anterior wall myocardial infarction (thrombolysed, window period of 3 hours). (B) Myocardial contrast echocardiography (A) showing good contrast opacification at the apical myocardium, correlating with a viable myocardium in a patent left anterior descending artery (coronary angiogram: B).

4 hour. All patients were followed up for a month for mortality, ventricular function, TIMI major or minor bleeding and stroke. There was no inhospital or 1 month mortality or bleeding events. At one month, majority had improvement of left ventricular function with no adverse events. In a substudy of the NORwegian study on DIstrict treatment of STEMI,[12] patients with STEMI of less than 6 hours of duration and more than 90 minutes of expected transfer delays to primary PCI were treated with tenecteplase, and randomized to early or late invasive strategy (N = 266). Left ventricular volumes and ejection fraction were assessed 3 months after the index infarction. In these patients treated with thrombolysis, no difference in left ventricular function after 3 months was found between patients treated with early versus late invasive strategy.

Echocardiographic Wall Motion Score Index[13]

Wall motion score index (WMSI) may be a better measure than LVEF (as measured by echocardiography) in predicting cardiac events such as rehospitalization for heart failure and mortality. On resting echocardiography, WMSI higher than 1.7 that persists after treatment of MI suggests a substantial (>20%) perfusion defect and increased risk for complications.

Other Tests

More refined techniques, including IV echocardiographic contrast enhancement to examine myocardial perfusion (Figs. 3A and B), low-dose dobutamine echocardiography, or regional strain analysis, may be useful in demonstrating whether segments that are still akinetic after reperfusion remain viable but hibernating. Global longitudinal strain has been reported to be a robust measure of LV function and noninferior to LVEF in prognostication. In a prospective historical prospective study, 576 patients underwent echocardiography within 24 hours after reperfusion therapy for STEMI and were followed up for 24 months. The end point was the composite of death, hospitalization with reinfarction, congestive heart failure, or stroke. The study concluded that global longitudinal strain (GLS) and WMSI were comparable and both were superior for early risk assessment compared with volume-based parameters such as LVEF and end-systolic volume (ESV).[14]

Diastolic Function

This factor is receiving more attention now in post-MI management of patients. E wave deceleration time less than 150 msec predicts poor prognosis, if associated with impaired pump function.[15] Another measure of LV filling pressure is E/e' (peak transmitral E wave velocity divided by peak early diastolic tissue velocity at the base of LV) and it has been shown by several studies that E/e' more than 15 early after infarction is a strong predictor of mortality and heart failure. [16] Left atrial size (>32 mL/m^2) and elevated pulmonary arterial systolic pressure which reflect elevated left atrial pressure are also independent predictors of poor prognosis.[17,18]

Right Ventricular Function

Right ventricle is no more an orphan or a forgotten chamber. RV infarction is a serious complication of inferior wall MI, and easily diagnosed on surface ECG. Fractional area shortening of RV (<32% one year after STEMI) and tricuspid annular systolic excursion (TAPSE) 14 mm or less confer a higher risk for mortality and heart failure.[19]

No Reflow Phenomenon

Flow in epicardial coronary arteries does not necessarily mean reperfusion at tissue level, and microvascular reflow may not be detected by coronary angiogram. Contrast echocardiography, either by intravenous or intracoronary injection can identify myocardial perfusion defects. These segmental perfusion defects strongly predict infarct remodeling and adverse prognosis.[20]

COMPLICATIONS OF STEMI

Mechanical Complications[21]

These are left ventricular free wall rupture (leading to tamponade or pseudoaneurysm), ischemic ventricular septal defect, and papillary muscle rupture. These are quite dramatic and catastrophic. These complications have decreased due to improved myocardial reperfusion strategies. Echocardiography is the diagnostic test of choice. Any sudden deterioration in clinical status of postMI patient should prompt one to immediately resort to echocardiography.

Ventricular free wall rupture: It is more common with left ventricle and is seen in about 1% of STEMI patients. Factors that increase the risk of rupture include reperfusion with a fibrinolytic agent rather than PCI, older age, female gender, hypertension, single-vessel disease without collateral circulation, and an anterior or first MI.[22] It exhibits a bimodal peak in first 24 hours and 3–5 days and may occur anytime up to 14 days post-MI. Usually, there is pericardial effusion with layered high acoustic echoes within the pericardial cavity. One may be able to visualize the tear directly and signs of tamponade would be present (Figs. 4A and B).

Ischemic ventricular septal defect: Those with an anterior wall MI tend to be apical in location. Those with inferior infarctions are associated with perforation of the basal septum and have a poorer outcome than those in an anterior location. It is seen in 1–3% of patients who do not receive any reperfusion therapy, 0.2–0.34% who receive fibrinolytic therapy and in 3.9% of patients who are in cardiogenic shock. Echocardiography shows left to right shunt on color flow Doppler echocardiography through the rupture and RV overload. It carries a mortality of 40–75%[22] (Figs. 5A and B).

Papillary Muscle Rupture

This occurs in about 1% of STEMI population. Posteromedial papillary muscle is more commonly affected because of its singular blood supply. Echocardiographic findings are hypercontractile LV, torn papillary muscle or chordae, flail mitral leaflet and severe mitral regurgitation. Color flow Doppler imaging is helpful in differentiating acute MR from VSD in the setting of STEMI (Fig. 6).[23]

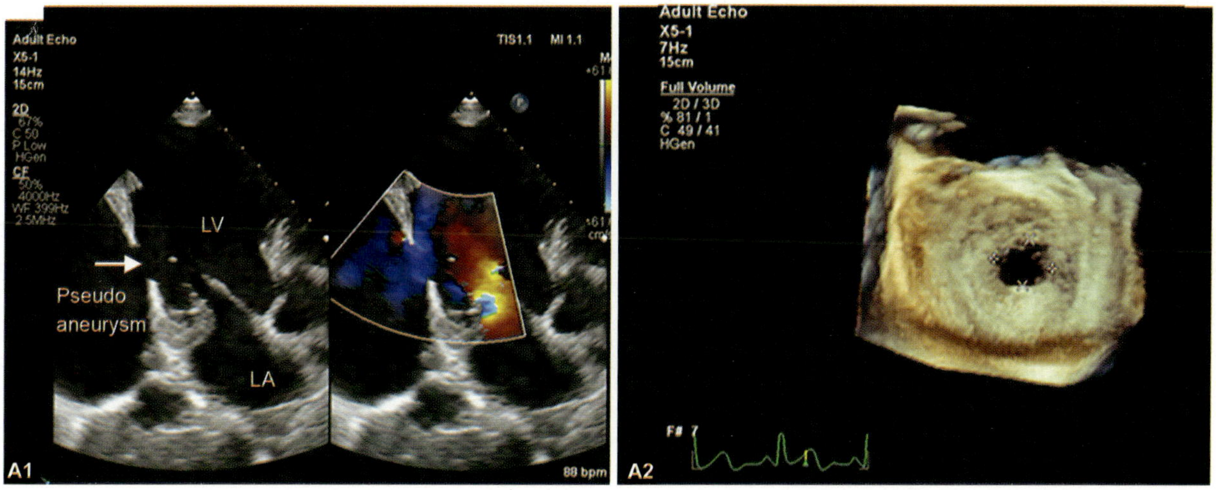

Fig. 4A: LV free wall rupture and pseudoaneurysm. A 67-year-old female with acute lateral and posterior wall myocardial infarction (thrombolysed, window period of 10 hours). Two-dimensional echocardiography on day 3 highlighting a contained free wall rupture of the left ventricle (arrow, A1). Three-dimensional echocardiography demonstrating the neck of the aneurysm (2.7 × 2.0 cm) (A2). (LA: left atrium, LV: left ventricle).

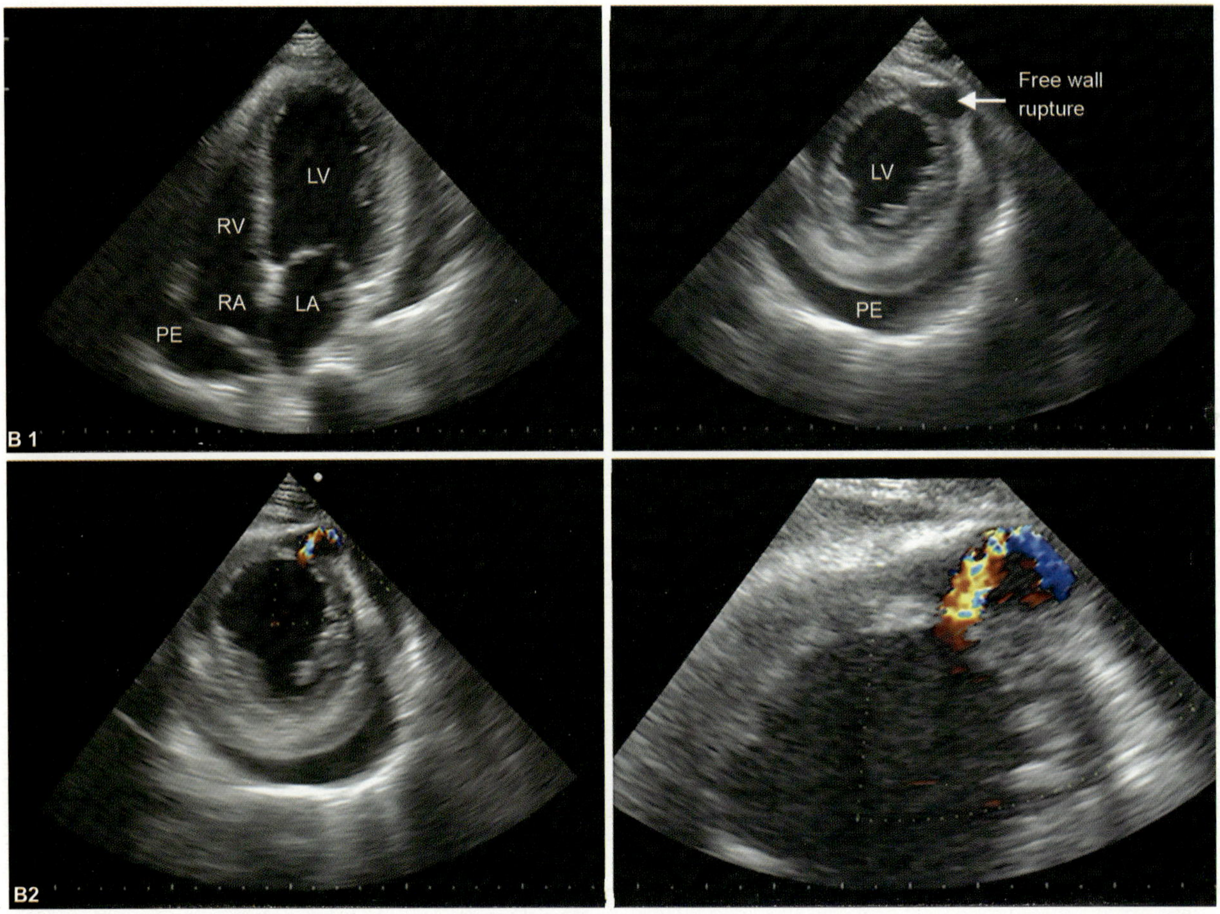

Fig. 4B: Free wall rupture and pericardial effusion. A 61-year-old male with anterior wall myocardial infarction (thrombolysed with streptokinase, window period of 9 hours). Two-dimensional echocardiography on day 2 showing pericardial effusion (B1). There is evidence of free wall rupture (arrow) in the short axis view at the apical level. Color flow evidence of free wall rupture is highlighted in the B2. (LA: left atrium, LV: left ventricle, PE: pericardial effusion RA: right atrium, RV: right ventricle).

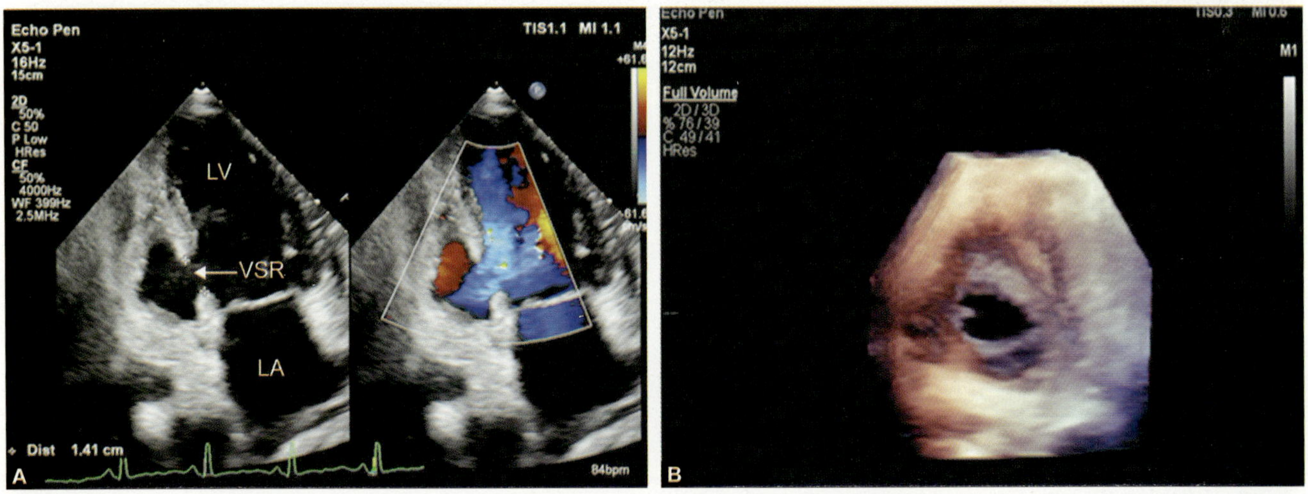

Figs. 5A and B: Ventricular septal rupture. A 69-year-old male with acute inferior wall myocardial infarction (thrombolysed, window period of 8 hours). (A) Two-dimensional echocardiography on day 2 showing ventricular septal rupture (basal septal segment). (B) Enface view of the defect from the right ventricular side on three-dimensional echocardiography. (LA: left atrium, LV: left ventricle, VSR: ventricular septal rupture).

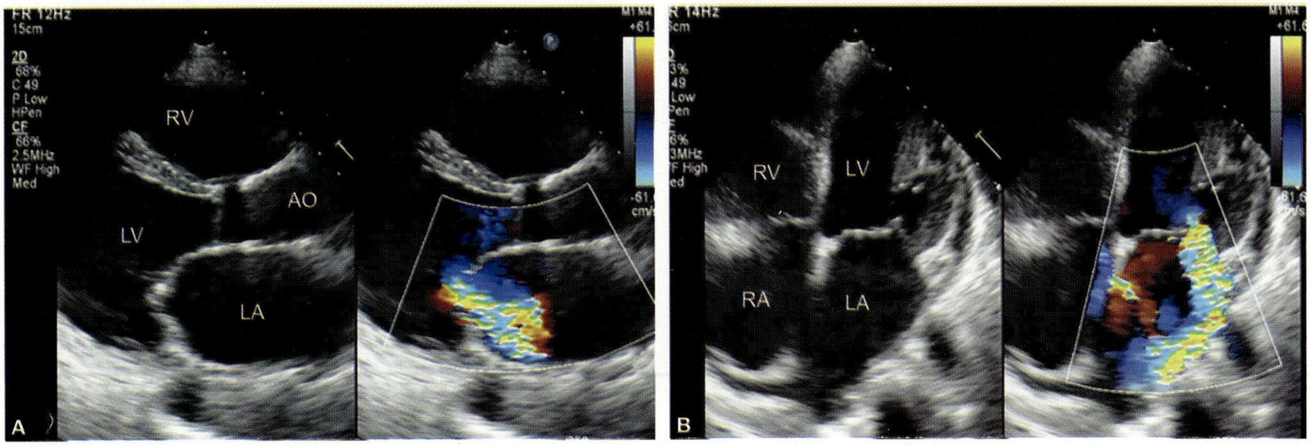

Fig. 6: Acute MR. A 51-year-old female with acute inferior wall myocardial infarction (thrombolysed, window period of 8 hours). Patient was in cardiogenic shock following thrombolysis. Two-dimensional echocardiography revealing severe mitral regurgitation (parasternal long axis view: A and apical 4C view: B).

Pseudoaneurysm

This is due to incomplete rupture of the myocardium and the wall does not have the myocardial element, unlike true aneurysm. The wall is composed of organized hematoma and pericardium. It has a narrow base and carries a high risk of rupture (*see* Fig. 4).

LV Thrombus (Fig. 7)

Inflammation and stasis are prothrombotic and lead to clot formation in STEMI. The incidence of LV thrombi has decreased from 20% to 5% as a result of aggressive management of STEMI and use of antithrombotics.[24] Formation of mural thrombi within 48 to 72 hours spells poor prognosis for the patient. Anticoagulation for 3–6 months with an oral vitamin K antagonist is reasonable for patients with demonstrable mural thrombi on echocardiogram.

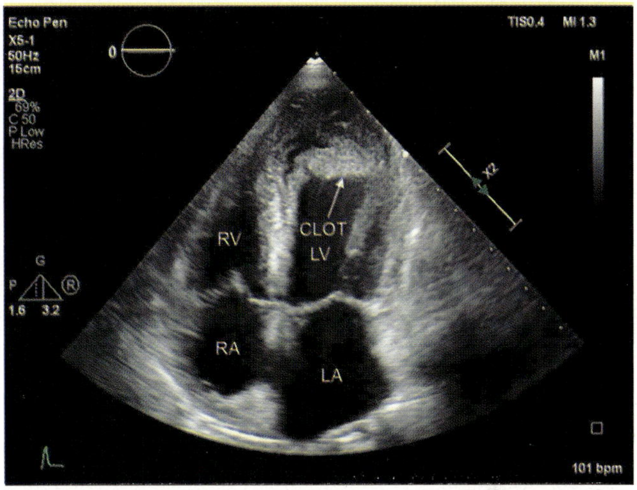

Fig. 7: LV thrombus. A 72-year-old male with acute anterior wall myocardial infarction (thrombolysed, window period of 9 hours). Patient had an episode of transient ischemic attack on day 4. Apical 4C view illustrating thrombus at the left ventricular apex. (LA: left atrium, LV: left ventricle, RA: right atrium, RV: right ventricle)

CONCLUSION

ST-elevation myocardial infarction (STEMI) is an acute coronary event, requires prompt recognition and rapid institution of therapy, including restoration of myocardial reperfusion. PCI is the reperfusion treatment of choice, and when it cannot be done within the time frame recommended, pharmacoinvasive strategy should be undertaken utilizing a fibrin specific bolus fibrinolytic agent. An echocardiogram should be performed in every patient immediately to substantiate diagnosis to assess regional and global, left and right ventricular function, and to recognize complications. A detailed study should be carried out subsequently as a follow-up and for risk stratification.

REFERENCES

1. The Assessment of the Safety and Efficacy of a New Thrombolytic Regimen (ASSENT)-3 Investigators. Efficacy and safety of tenecteplase in combination with enoxaparin, abciximab, or unfractionated heparin: the ASSENT-3 randomized trial in acute myocardial infarction. Lancet. 2001;358:605-13.
2. Armstrong PW, Gershlick AH, Goldstein P, et al. Fibrinolysis or Primary PCI in ST-segment Elevation Myocardial Infarction. N Engl J Med. 2013;368:1379-87.
3. Iyengar SS, Nair T, Hiremath JS, et al. Pharmacologic Reperfusion Therapy with Indigenous Tenecteplase in 15,222

patients with ST Elevation Myocardial Infarction—The Indian Registry. Indian Heart J. 2013;65(4):436-41.

4. Cheitlin MD, Alpert JS, Armstrong WF, et al. ACC/AHA Guidelines for the Clinical Application of Echocardiography: Executive Summary A Report of the American College of Cardiology/American Heart Association Task Force on Practice Guidelines (Committee on Clinical Application of Echocardiography). Circulation. 1997;95(6):1686-744.
5. Detry JMR. The pathophysiology of myocardial ischemia. Eur Heart J. 1996:17:48-52
6. Maznyczka A, Sen S, Cook C, et al. The ischaemic constellation: an alternative to the ischaemic cascade—implications for the validation of new ischaemic tests. Open Heart. 2015;2:e000178.
7. Mollema SA, Nucifora G, Bax JJ. Prognostic value of echocardiography after acute myocardial infarction. Heart. 2009;95:1732-45.
8. Flachskampf FA, Schmid M, Rost C, et al. Cardiac imaging after myocardial infarction. Eur Heart J. 2011;32:272-83.
9. Kusumoto FM, Calkins H, Boehmer J, et al. HRS/ACC/AHA expert consensus statement on the use of implantable cardioverter-defibrillator therapy in patients who are not included or not well represented in clinical trials. Circulation. 2014;130(1):94-125.
10. M Cikes, SD Solomon. Beyond ejection fraction: an integrative approach for assessment of cardiac structure and function in heart failure. Eur Heart J. 2016;37(21):1642-50.
11. Jayagopal PB, Sarjun Basha KM. Intracoronary tenecteplase in STEMI with massive thrombus. Indian Heart J. 2018;70(3):446-49.
12. Mistry N, Bøhmer E, Hoffmann P, et al. Left ventricular function in acute myocardial infarction treated with thrombolysis followed by early versus late invasive strategy. Am. 2010;160(1):73-9.
13. Thune JJ, Køber L, Pfeffer MA, et al. Comparison of Regional Versus Global Assessment of Left Ventricular Function in Patients with Left Ventricular Dysfunction, Heart Failure, or Both After Myocardial Infarction: The Valsartan in Acute Myocardial Infarction Echocardiographic Study. J Am Soc Echocardiogr. 2006;19:1462-5.
14. Munk K, Andersen NH, Terkelsen CJ, et al. Global Left Ventricular Longitudinal Systolic Strain for Early Risk Assessment in Patients with Acute Myocardial Infarction Treated with Primary Percutaneous Intervention. J Am Soc Echocardiogr. 2012;25:644-51.
15. Meta-Analysis Research Group in Echocardiography (MeRGE). AMI Collaborators Møller JE, Whalley GA, et al. Independent prognostic importance of a restrictive left ventricular filling pattern after myocardial infarction: an individual patient: meta-analysis research group in echocardiography acute myocardial infarction. Circulation. 2008;117:2591-8.
16. Kruszewski K, Scott AE, Barclay JL, et al. Non-invasive assessment of left ventricular filling pressure after acute myocardial infarction a prospective study of the relative prognostic utility of clinical assessment, echocardiography, and B-type natriuretic peptide. Am Heart J. 2010;159:47-54.
17. Møller JE, Hillis GS, Oh JK, et al. Left atrial volume: a powerful predictor of survival after acute myocardial infarction. Circulation. 2003;107:2207-12.
18. Møller JE, Hillis GS, Oh JK, et al. Prognostic importance of secondary pulmonary hypertension after acute myocardial infarction. Am J Cardiol. 2005; 96:199-203.
19. Engstrom AE, Vis MM, Bouma BJ, et al. Right ventricular dysfunction is an independent predictor for mortality in ST-elevation myocardial infarction patients presenting with cardiogenic shock on admission. Eur J Heart Fail. 2010;12:276-82.
20. Hayat SA, Senior R. Myocardial contrast echocardiography in ST elevation myocardial infarction: ready for prime time? Eur Heart J. 2008;29:299-314.
21. Bohula EA, MaorrowDA. ST Elevation Myocardial Infarction. In: Braunwald's Heart Disease: A Textbook of Cardiovascular Medicine, 11th edition. New York: Elsevier; 2018.
22. ER Bates. Reperfusion therapy reduces the risk of myocardial rupture complicating ST-elevation myocardial infarction. J Am Heart Assoc. 2014;3(5):e001368.
23. O'Gara PT, Kushner FG, Ascheim DD, et al. 2013 ACCF/AHA guideline for the management of ST-elevation myocardial infarction: a report of the American College of Cardiology Foundation/American Heart Association Task Force on Practice Guidelines. Circulation. 2013;127(4):e362-425.
24. Delewi R, Zijlstra F, Piek JJ. Left ventricular thrombus formation after acute myocardial infarction. Heart. 2012;98(23):1743-9.

37

CHAPTER

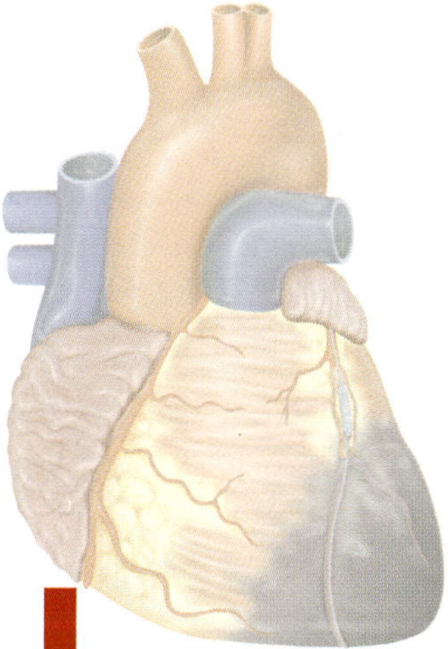

Prognosis and Risk Outcome by Echocardiography in AMI Patients Post-thrombolysis

Rohit Tandon, Harshit Gupta, Mohammed Nazir, Devinder Mahal, Bishav Mohan

INTRODUCTION

Fibrinolytic therapy and primary percutaneous coronary intervention (PPCI) are the two exclusively used modalities of reperfusion therapies in acute STEMI (ST-elevation myocardial infarction). PPCI although has been proven superior but is not available universally. Patency rates of the infarct-related artery[1-5] are 48–60% with fibrinolytic agents. Ongoing chest pain, lack of more than 50% ST-segment resolution and the absence of reperfusion arrhythmias at 60–90 minutes after fibrinolytics administration are considered as treatment failure indicating thrombolysis in myocardial infarction (TIMI) flow less than 3 in infarct-related artery.[6] Coronary artery patency is restored within 90 minutes in around 75% of people with acute STEMI after fibrinolysis, but complete reperfusion with normal flow in the infarct-related coronary artery is observed in only 50%.[7-9]; residual narrowing may predispose the vessel to reocclusion in around 18–32% of people within 3 months[10,11] resulting in recurrent ischemia. In post-thrombolysis patients, guidelines suggest early angiography to assess the patency of the infarct-related artery, extent of disease in other coronary arteries so as to consider the need for myocardial revascularization rather than watchful waiting or predischarge ischemia-guided strategy which may pose patients to risk of reinfarction (Gracias, CARESS AMI, WEST trials) but the recommended approach is not still universally available and acceptable. Although there has been advances in imaging modalities [viz. cardiac computed tomography (CT), magnetic resonance imaging (MRI), positron emission tomography (PET)] in acute myocardial infarction (AMI) patients to assess postinfarct remodeling, risk for subsequent ischemia; but echocardiography still holds promise in guiding management in these patients especially with improvement in advanced echocardiography techniques like speckle tracking and 3D echocardiography due to its widespread availability and large experience. The extent of myocardial necrosis following AMI is directly related to: (1) The total duration of coronary artery occlusion; (2) The extent of myocardium supplied by the infarct-related artery; and (3) The quality of collateral circulation. Myocardial dysfunction after reperfusion may also occur either as a result of stunning or no-reflow state despite restoration of epicardial coronary patency due to lack of perfusion at microvascular level also. In the immediate reperfusion period coronary hyperemia may occur which results in underestimation of myocardial necrosis (Flowchart 1).

ASSESSMENT OF LEFT VENTRICULAR VOLUMES AND EJECTION FRACTION

Left ventricular ejection fraction (LVEF) has a well-established short-term and long-term prognostic value. Its estimation should be done from 3rd day and re-evaluated at 14th day so as to overcome the effects of myocardial stunning as shown in PREDICT study. Patients who show improvement have 1.2% mortality risk while those who do not carry mortality risk of 5.6%. LVEF mortality curve after AMI exhibits a typical hyperbolic increasing with

Flowchart 1: Risk stratification in acute myocardial infarction (MI).

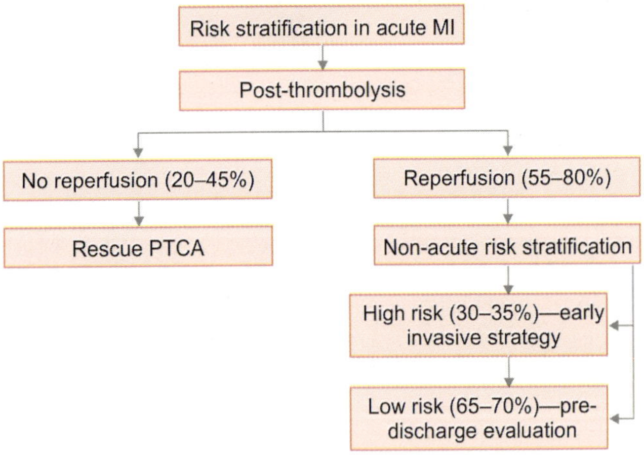

(PTCA: percutaneous transluminal coronary angioplasty)

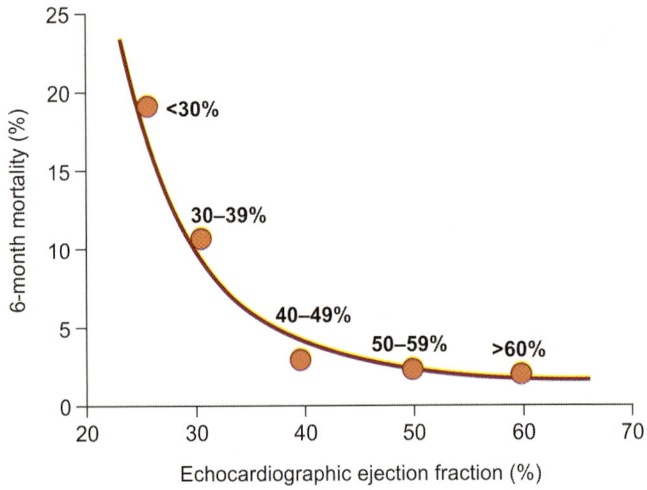

Fig. 1: Hyperbolic inverse relation between left ventricle ejection fraction (LVEF) and 6-month all-cause mortality after acute myocardial infarction (AMI).

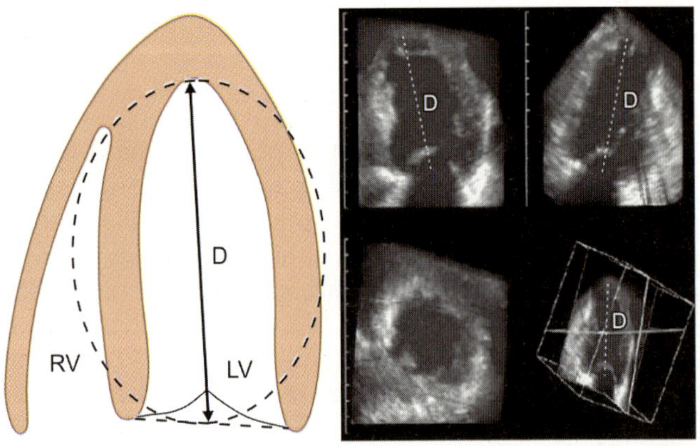

Fig. 2: Three-dimensional sphericity index.

an upturn in mortality occurring at values less than 40%. In 417 patients with AMI, an LVEF less than 40% was an independent predictor of the combined endpoint of death, congestive heart failure (HF), and recurrent AMI at 30 days after AMI [odds ratio (OR) 3.82]. Also patients with LVEF less than 30% and LVEF between more than 30% and less than 40% had an increased risk for sudden cardiac death (SCD) [hazard ratio (HR) = 5.99 and 3.37, respectively] and all-cause mortality (HR = 3.85 and HR= 2.06, respectively) compared to those with LVEF more than 40%. Thus after thrombolytic reperfusion EF dictates further management strategy. If patient has sustained a large MI (EF <35%) viability assessment is priority before revascularization while patients with EF more than 40% restoring patency of culprit vessel gains priority. Decisions based on EF should be individualized as EF being a volumetric-based determination suffers from large interobserver and test-retest variability (Fig. 1).

Usefulness of 3D Echocardiography for Assessing Post-MI Adverse LV Remodeling

Three-dimensional echocardiography may prove more useful in assessment of adverse remodeling on follow-up due to its inherent advantages over 2D datasets. Mannaerts et al. and Li et al. in two separate small studies on AMI after 6 months follow-up have suggested 3D sphericity index and 3D conic index as better marker of remodeling than 2D LV volumes assessment (Fig. 2).

Evaluation of Myocardial Wall Motion Abnormalities

Accuracy of the qualitative assessment of wall motion is influenced by image quality, imaging plane, experience of the observer.[12-15] Thickening is preferred for regional systolic function evaluation because of the counter-clockwise rotation of the LV around its long axis during systole. Normal LV wall motion score index of 1 increase as wall motion abnormalities increase in severity. There is a good correlation between the wall motion score index and functional LV impairment. An index of 1.1–1.6 represents small infarct while index more than 2.0 predicts occurrence of complications. In 144 patients with a first AMI treated with thrombolytic therapy, a predischarge resting wall motion score index (WMSI) more than 1.50 was superior to LVEF less than 40% to identify patients who had post-AMI cardiac death, unstable angina, nonfatal reinfarction, and HF.[16] In 767 AMI patients, WMSI was an independent predictor of death and HF hospitalization, whereas LVEF was not. WMSI, unlike EF which is a marker of global LV functions, represents regional LV functions therefore it reflects mild wall motion abnormalities because it is not affected by compensatory hyperkinesia of remote segments.[17]

Remodeling Assessment in Acute Phase: Infarct Expansion and Remodeling

Cardiac imaging in the acute (0–48 hours) and subacute (Day 3–7) phase is targeted to assessment of segmental and overall left ventricular systolic function, intracavitary thrombus formation, and mechanical complications. In acute phase, left ventricle undergoes rapid morphological changes influenced by extent and reversibility of ischemia, myocardial edema, passive myocardial stretch depending on loading conditions, and use of reperfusion therapy. Within seconds of ischemia the infarcted area bulges and extends, if not revascularized in time it leads to infarct expansion in ensuing hours. Left ventricle acutely responds by hyperkinesia of remote myocardial areas and further dilates over the course of days and weeks, thus recruiting preload reserve. This process is compounded by ventricular dilatation and apical tethering of papillary muscles termed as "infarct remodeling." Postinfarction remodeling of left ventricle infarct remodeling is defined as an increase in end-diastolic left ventricular volume by 20% at 6 months after MI compared with baseline. This progressive increase in left ventricular volumes after indicates worse prognosis seen in approximately 30% of patients although EF remains the same due to parallel increase in both end-systolic and end-diastolic volume. Factors associated with postinfarction remodeling are infarct size, anterior location, late or unsuccessful reperfusion therapy both at the epicardial vessel level and at the microvasculature level, gender as higher incidence and more aggressive course in men, possibly due to a higher rate of myocyte apoptosis in the peri-infarction zone. Assessment of LV function in this early stage of MI could overestimate the extent of irreversible infarct area because of myocardial stunning. Myocardial contrast echocardiography (MCE) assesses the infarct area through the absence/reduction of tissue-level perfusion providing better prognostic information in patients with impaired LVEF. In a study by Lepper et al. the *size of persistent MCE perfusion defect after revascularization for AMI had a high predictive value for LV remodeling during a 4-week follow-up period.*

Contrast defect index (CDI): This was calculated as the sum of the contrast scores (1 = homogeneous opacification; 2 = heterogeneous opacification; 3 = minimal/absent contrast opacification) of all LV interpretable segments divided by the number of LV segments analyzed. At multivariable analysis, elevated CDI, as a marker of lower residual myocardial viability, was a predictor of the composite endpoint of cardiac death and nonfatal AMI and of cardiac death, whereas LVEF and end-systolic volume (ESV) did not achieve statistical significance. The optimal *cut-off of CDI was 1.86* for the composite endpoint of cardiac death and nonfatal AMI (sensitivity, 62%; specificity, 84%) and for cardiac death (sensitivity, 87%; specificity, 84%) in a study by Dwivedi et al. Sakuma et al. evaluated 50 patients of AMI post-thrombolytic therapy day 2 and concluded presence of reduced perfusion on myocardial contrast echocardiography as predictive of major cardiac events (death, nonfatal MI, or admission for heart failure) during a mean follow-up of 22 months (event rate 28% in patients with reduced perfusion versus 4% in those with preserved perfusion, $p < 0.05$). Therefore, resting myocardial contrast echocardiography should be routinely employed in this setting; to quantify stunned versus infarcted myocardium using CDI and to demonstrate microvascular integrity postreperfusion (Figs. 3A and B).

Other 2D and M-mode parameters helpful in post-MI acute risk stratification are LV mass, mitral annular plane systolic excursion (MAPSE), tricuspid annular plane systolic excursion (TAPSE) and left atrial volume index (LAVI), and LA distensibility. MAPSE less than 8 mm, TAPSE less than

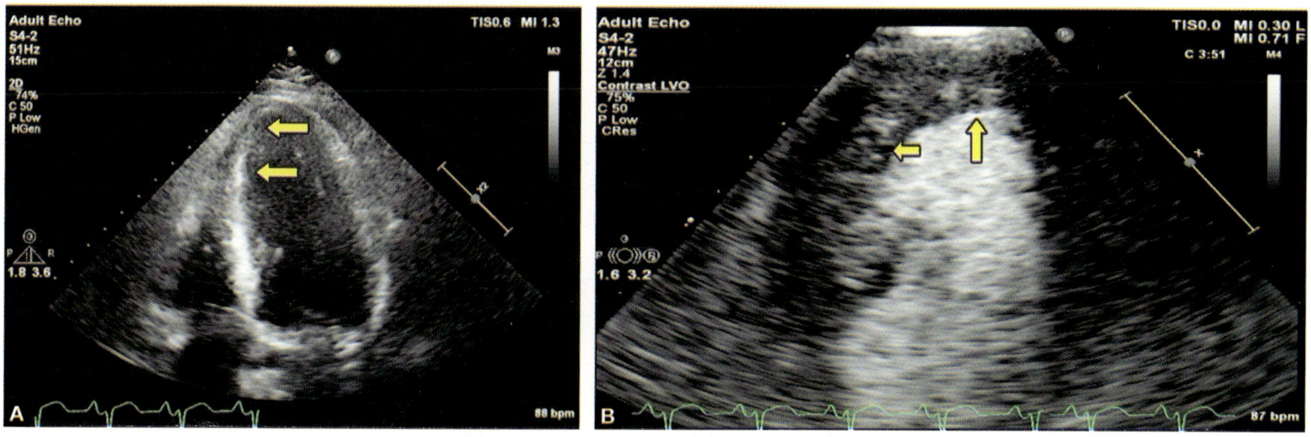

Figs. 3A and B: Yellow arrows showing difference in delineation between the contrast uptake in fibrotic scarred myocardium (A) and viable myocardium (B).

15 mm, LAVI more than 32 mL/m^2, LA distensibility less than or equal to 60%, LV mass increases 10 g/m^2 or 0.1 unit increase in relative wall thickness (RWT) was independently associated with all-cause mortality, cardiovascular (CV) death, and HF hospitalization on follow up in patients with large AMI in various studies.

Doppler Flow Patterns of Remodeling

In postinfarction patients with LVEF less than 35%, a mitral deceleration time less than 120 ms, deceleration time of the diastolic component of the pulmonary venous flow less than 160 ms, systolic fraction of the pulmonary venous flow smaller than 45%, TEI index more than 0.6, E/Vp by color M-mode more than 2 denotes pulmonary capillary wedge pressure (PCWP) more than 20 mm Hg and the reversibility of these parameters at pre discharge is associated with a more favorable late outcome, whereas its persistence was the most powerful independent predictor of late mortality and adverse LV remodeling. In patients with EF more than 40% PCWP more than 20 mm of Hg can be reliably predicted by E/e' value derived from Nageuh formula. Recently regional diastolic strain rate has been proposed as a further marker of elevated LV filling pressure. In a study of 1,048 post-AMI patients with mildly impaired LV systolic functions the ratio of transmitral E velocity to global diastolic strain rate (E/e'sr at cut-off value >1.25) was superior to E/e' ratio and in predicting all-cause mortality, HF hospitalization, stroke, and new onset AF (Figs. 4A and B).

Detecting No-reflow

Microvascular obstruction may be detected by coronary angiography as "no-reflow" after a technically successful coronary intervention by lack of brisk coronary flow despite an open vessel with no or minor residual obstruction. However, microvascular "no-reflow" may also go undetected by coronary angiography. Absence of reperfusion at the tissue level, shown as nonopacification of the corresponding segmental myocardium, is a strong predictor of later infarct remodeling. Contrast echocardiography can identify and semiquantify myocardial perfusion.

GUIDANCE OF REVASCULARIZATION STRATEGIES AND PROGNOSTIC STRATIFICATION

The extent of coronary disease and the presence of inducible ischemia in territories other than the infarcted one is one of the crucial clinical questions after MI. Low-dose dobutamine echocardiography or adenosine/dipyridamole stress echocardiography ± MCE helps in detecting inducible ischemia, both in "remote" myocardial territories and in the periphery of the infarcted area.

Prediction of Functional Recovery after Acute Myocardial Infarction

Extent and severity of perfusion defects after acute MI have been shown to correlate (inversely) with the likelihood of functional recovery at follow-up. Patients with large perfusion defects (indicating nonviable tissue) seem to have a low likelihood of functional recovery after acute MI, whereas dysfunctional regions with preserved perfusion (indicating viable myocardium) frequently exhibit improvement of function during follow-up. Candidates for pre discharge evaluation are those who did not undergo revascularization or those who underwent partial revascularization provided that they had stable electrocardiography (ECG) and no episode of HF or angina at least 72 hours before testing. To detect residual ischemia from stunned segments mainly two responses

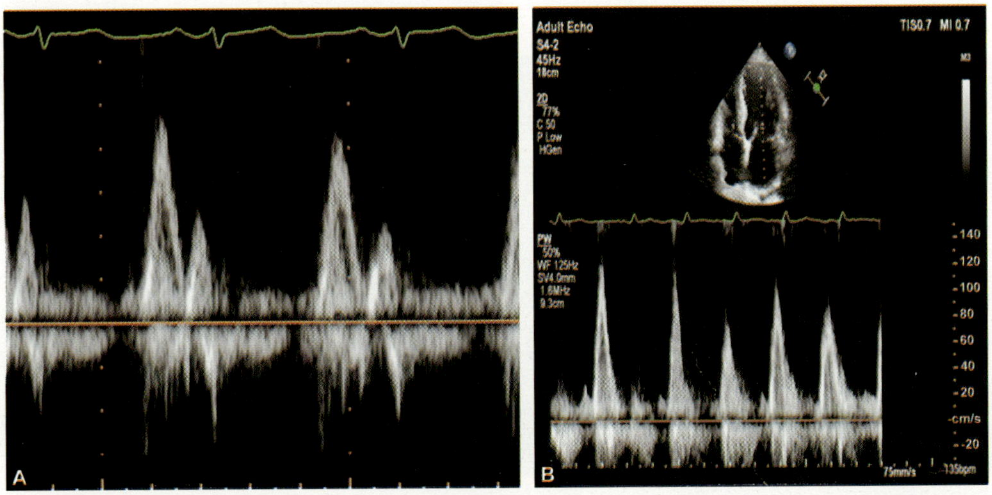

Figs. 4A and B: Examples of restrictive filling pattern in post-thrombolysis patients.

are yielded one is that of sustained improvement (100% specific) signifying absence of residual stenosis and other is biphasic response (80% sensitive and specific) for residual stenosis requiring revascularization. In recent years many studies using MCE and speckle-tracking imaging (STE) have established cut off values to distinguish viable segments longitudinal strain (LS) less than –14.92% and LS rate less than –1.30/sec at low dose of dobutamine predicted LV regional recovery with 86% sensitivity and 87% specificity. SE also identifies AMI patients at increased risk of subsequent adverse events. In a large-scale multicenter prospective study, 755 in-hospital patients underwent pharmacological SE with either dipyridamole or dobutamine and an exercise ECG 10 days from AMI. At multivariate analysis, peak stress WMSI was an independent predictor of all-cause mortality; WMSI difference between rest and peak stress was the most important predictor of the composite endpoint of death, nonfatal AMI, and rehospitalization for unstable angina. The viability-guided angioplasty after acute myocardial infarction trial demonstrated that in patients with sub-AMI, not treated by primary or rescue PCI, the detection of myocardial viability at low-dose dobutamine identified a subgroup to be referred to viability-guided PCI of infarct-related coronary artery. Picano et al. studied the value of dipyridamole stress echocardiography in predicting reinfarction in 1,080 patients assessed early (10 ± 5 days) after uncomplicated AMI with follow-up of 1 year. The results of stress echocardiography were positive for ischemia in 475 patients (44%). During follow-up, reinfarction occurred in 30 patients with positive and 20 with negative results (6.3% vs. 3.3%, p = 0.01). Bansal et al. (2010) reported that increment in longitudinal strain (optimal cutoff - 3.0, for sensitivity and specificity 0.70) and increasing of strain rate (optimal cutoff: - 0.24, for sensitivity: 0.77 and specificity: 0.68) with dobutamine stimulation were also good predictors of recovery.

USEFULNESS OF SPECKLE TRACKING ECHOCARDIOGRAPHY

Conventional parameters as discussed above have proven their long-term predictive implications in AMI patients in large studies albeit in large infarcts or EF less than or equal to 35% but there is limited data on patients with EF more than or equal to 40% to predict LV adverse remodeling. Strain imaging helps to risk stratify these patient subgroups as it is able to detect subtle changes in patients with small infarcts and relatively preserved or mildly impaired systolic functions. Global longitudinal strain (GLS) assessment (cut off <–14%) has led to identification of adverse remodeling post discharge and risk of heart failure during hospital stay in as much as one-third of the patients. Ersbøll et al.[18] found that impaired systolic GLS but not reduced LVEF (<40%) is a powerful independent predictor of a composite endpoint of all-cause of mortality and HF hospitalization and cardiac death. A systolic GLS less than or equal to 14% was associated with a three-fold increase in risk for the combined endpoint of all-cause mortality and HF hospitalization (HR = 3.21). In a study of 576 AMI patients treated by primary PCI, systolic GLS, and WMSI were independently associated with the composite endpoint of all-cause mortality, reinfarction, hospitalization, HF, or stroke within 1 year, whereas LVEF and ESV did not enter the model. 47 patients with systolic GLS less than or equal to 10% experienced more adverse events than patients with systolic GLS less than or equal to 15% (HR = 4.6). In a recent study of 100 patients with successfully reperfused first AMI, 3D STE determined global area strain discriminated transmural from nontransmural extent of scar and predicted microvascular obstruction. In patients who have large infarcts with EF after 6 weeks less than or equal to 35% recommendations for implantable cardioverter defibrillator (ICD) implantation apply but trial failed to show incremental benefit based on this recommendation. Calculation of mechanical dispersion using strain analysis (>50 ms) may help to select optimally patients at high risk for ventricular arrhythmias. In another study of Ersbøll et al.[18] on 988 AMI patients, systolic GLS (HR = 1.24), and mechanical dispersion [SD of average time from ECG-derived peak R to peak systolic LS (HR = 10 m = 1.15)] were both associated with risk of ventricular arrhythmias and SCD after AMI at multivariate analysis. There is also good comparison of STE with other techniques single-photon emission computed tomography (SPECT), contrast-enhanced cardiovascular magnetic resonance (ceCMR) as shown by Martin et al. (2013).[19] The peak longitudinal systolic strain optimal cutoff –5.3% identified segments with delayed enhancement more than 75% on ceCMR (sensitivity = 83.1%, specificity = 84.6%). Roes SD et al. in 2009[20] found that a regional longitudinal strain cutoff value of –4.5% distinguished nontransmural from transmural infarction with high sensitivity and specificity (81.2% and 81.6%, respectively) global circumferential strain (GCS) although has been used to predict adverse LV remodeling but results at present are inconsistent probably because of small sample size of studies. Despite complete revascularization of the infarcted area, LV remodeling may escalate overtime due to lack of microcirculation and tissue perfusion. VALIANT (The VALsartan In Acute myocardial iNfarcTion) echo substudy had proven that besides viable segments adjacent to infarcted segments, GCS is strongly predictive of adverse LV remodeling due to complex interdependence on ventricular shape, deformation, and infarct size as integrity of circumferential fibers prevents LV dilatation (Figs. 5A and B, Table 1).

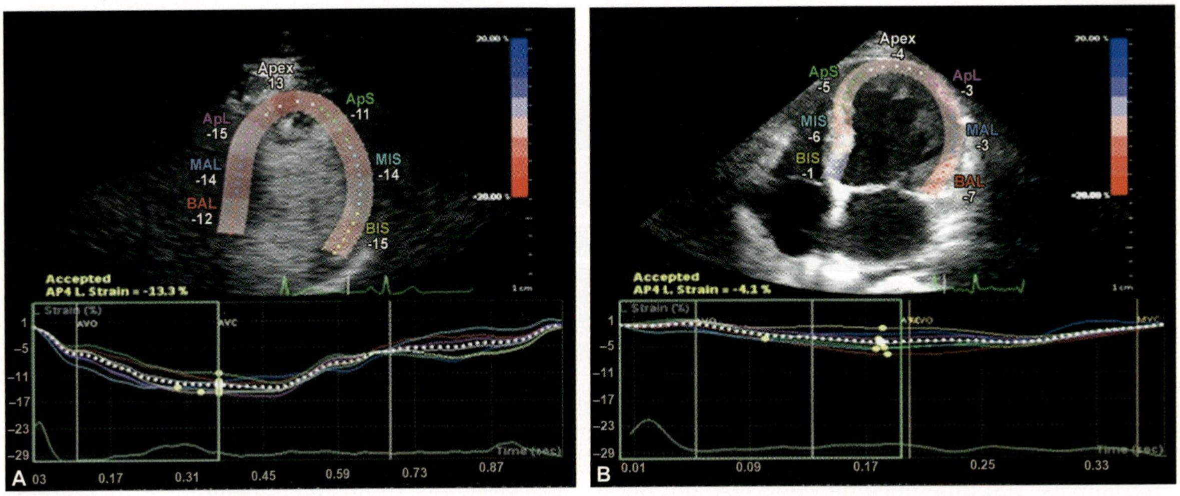

Figs. 5A and B: Left ventricular global longitudinal strain (GLS) values in small (−13.5%) and large infarct (−4.5%).

TABLE 1

First author	*Patient characteristics*	*Strain derivation*	*Strain cutoff*	*Sensitivity*	*Specificity*
Zaliaduonyte-Peksiene et al.	141 first STEMI	GLS	NA	NA	NA
Zaliaduonyte-Peksiene et al.	82 first STEMI	GLS	≥ −11.6%	78%	73%
Park et al.	50 first anterior STEMI	GLS	≥ −10.2%	90.9%	85.7%
Joyce et al.	1,041 first STEMI	GLS	≥ −15%		
D'Andrea et al.	70 first NSTEMI	GLS	≥ −12%	84.8%	87.8%
Zito et al.	46 STEMI	GCS	Associated, not predicted	NA	NA
Hung et al.	380 post-MI patients with evidence of LV dysfunction	GCSr	OR: 1.3	NA	NA
Spinelli et al.	75 post-MI patients	Torsion for RR	≥ −1.34°/cm	88%	80%
Nucifora et al.	120 first STEMI	Torsion	≥ −1.44°/cm	95%	77%
Li et al.	61 NSTEMI	Area	≤32%	86.1%	68%
Bochenek et al.	66 first STEMI	GLS	≤−12.5%	69%	79%
Lacalzada et al.	97 first STEMI	GLS	≤−12.5%	85.2%	86.27%
Altiok et al.	55 first STEMI 38 frist NSTEMI	GLS	≤−12.8%	81.8%	80.5%
Liszka et al.	39 frist STEMI 24 NSTEMI	GLS	>−9.98%	80.3%	64.7%
Cong et al.	127 first STEMI	GLS	>−10.85%	89.7%	91.7%

(GCS: global circumferential strain; GLS: global longitudinal strain; LV: left ventricular; MI: myocardial infarction; NSTEMI: non-ST-elevation myocardial infarction; RR: reverse remodeling; STEMI: ST-elevation myocardial infarction).

RECOMMENDATIONS

- Perform a limited emergency study as quickly as possible in every patient as long as reperfusion therapy is not delayed. Assess regional and global left and right ventricular functions, exclude other causes of chest pain, e.g. Type A aortic dissection, identify mechanical complications impending rupture, papillary muscle rupture, and right ventricular infarction.
- Identify signs of increased left ventricular filling pressures restrictive mitral inflow pattern, E/e' ratio, LA size, and pulmonary artery (PA) systolic pressures.
- If large akinetic or dyskinetic left ventricular regions are present exclude thrombi, also see for acute

Flowchart 2: Diagnosis of acute myocardial infarction (MI).

Diagnosed acute MI	
Estimate EF, WMSI, ESV, LAVI preferably 3D	Exclude mechanical complications, acute infarct expansion and remodelling

↓

Advanced techniques	
Myocardial contrast for CDI, actual infarct size, EDWT	STE for GLS, mechanical dyssynchrony

↓

Doppler hemodynamics	
Look for RF pattern, E/E' for filling pressures	Pre-discharge low dose DSE to identify high-risk subset

(CDI: contrast defect index; DSE: dobutamine stress echocardiography; EDWT: end-diastolic wall thickness; EF: ejection fraction; ESV: end-systolic volume; GLS: global longitudinal strain; LAVI: left atrial volume index; WMSI: wall motion score index)

ischemic remodeling in apical segments.[2] Myocardial contrast echocardiogram is very helpful in accurate categorization of stunned and scar segments estimate CDI (≥1.86), and exclude no reflow.[3] GLS, GCS should be estimated in patients with small infarcts or baseline EF more than or equal to 40% and in patients with EF less than or equal to 35% for mechanical dispersion.

- A stress test preferably using MCE should be performed after the acute phase of MI once the patient is stable usually after 4 days for identification of inducible ischemia typically in a patient who did not undergo coronary angiography or who has intermediate coronary nonculprit lesions on the acute coronary angiogram, or identification of viable myocardium typically in a patient with impaired global left ventricular systolic function suitable coronary anatomy amenable to revascularization (Flowchart 2).

REFERENCES

1. Martin GV, Sheehan FH, Stadius M, et al. Intravenous streptokinase for acute myocardial infarction. Effects on global and regional systolic function. Circulation. 1988;78:258-66.
2. The GUSTO Angiographic Investigators. The effects of tissue plasminogen activator, streptokinase, or both on coronary-artery patency, ventricular function, and survival after acute myocardial infarction. N Engl J Med. 1993;329:1615-22.
3. Antithrombotic Trialists' Collaboration. Collaborative meta-analysis of randomised trials of antiplatelet therapy for prevention of death, myocardial infarction, and stroke in high risk patients. BMJ. 2002;324:71-86.
4. AIMS Trial Study Group. Effect of intravenous APSAC on mortality after acute myocardial infarction: preliminary report of a placebo-controlled clinical trial. Lancet. 1988;1:545-9.
5. Cannon C, McCabe C, Gibson C, et al. TNK-tissue plasminogen activator in acute myocardial infarction. Results of Thrombolysis in Myocardial Infarction (TIMI) 10A dose ranging trial. Circulation. 1997;95:351-6.
6. Sutton AG, Campbell PG, Price DJ, et al. Failure of thrombolysis by streptokinase: detection with a simple electrocardiographic method. Heart. 2000;84:14956.
7. de Lemos JA, Braunwald E. ST-segment resolution as a tool for assessing the efficacy of reperfusion therapy. J Am Coll Cardiol. 2001;38(5):1283-94.
8. Goldman LE, Eisenberg MJ. Identification and management of patients with failed thrombolysis after acute myocardial infarction. Ann Intern Med. 2000;132(7):556-65.
9. The GUSTO Investigators. An international randomized trial comparing four thrombolytic strategies for acute myocardial infarction. N Engl J Med. 1993;329(10):673-82.
10. Gurewich V. Coronary rethrombosis after successful thrombolysis. Circulation. 1993;87(5):1759-61.
11. Verheugt FW, Meijer A, Lagrand WK, et al. Reocclusion: The flip side of coronary thrombolysis. J Am Coll Cardiol. 1996;27(4):766-73.
12. Bhatnagar SK, Al-Yusuf AR. Significance of early two-dimensional echocardiography after acute myocardial infarction. Int J Cardiol. 1984;5:575-84.
13. Loh IK, Charuzi Y, Beeder C, et al. Early diagnosis of nontransmural myocardial infarction by two-dimensional echocardiography. Am Heart J. 1982;104:963-8.
14. Deutsch HJ, Curtius JM, Leischik R, et al. Reproducibility of assessment of left-ventricular function using intraoperative transesophageal echocardiography. Thorac Cardiovasc Surg. 1993;41:54-8.
15. Otto CM, Stratton JR, Maynard C, et al. Echocardiographic evaluation of segmental wall motion early and late after thrombolytic therapy in acute myocardial infarction: the Western Washington Tissue Plasminogen Activator Emergency Room Trial. Am J Cardiol. 1990;65:132-8.
16. Carluccio E, Tommasi S, Bentivoglio M, et al. Usefulness of the severity and extent of wall motion abnormalities as prognostic markers of an adverse outcome after a first myocardial infarction treated with thrombolytic therapy. Am J Cardiol. 2000;85:411-5.
17. Møller JE, Hillis GS, Oh JK, et al. Wall motion score index and ejection fraction for risk stratification after acute myocardial infarction. Am Heart J. 2006;415:419-25.
18. Ersbøll M, Valeur N, Mogensen UM, et al. Prediction of all-cause mortality and heart failure admissions from global left ventricular longitudinal strain in patients with acute myocardial infarction and preserved left ventricular ejection fraction. J Am Coll Cardiol. 2013;61:2365-73.
19. Martin H, Tomas S, Milan K, et al. Speckle tracking echocardiography derived systolic longitudinal strain is better than rest single photon emission tomography perfusion imaging for nonviable myocardium identification. Biomed Pap Med Fac Univ. 2013;157:12-21.
20. Roes SD, Mollema SA, Lamb HJ, et al. Validation of echocardiographic two-dimensional speckle tracking longitudinal strain imaging for viability assessment in patients with chronic ischemic left ventricular dysfunction and comparison with contrast-enhanced magnetic resonance imaging. Am J Cardiol. 2009;104:312-7.

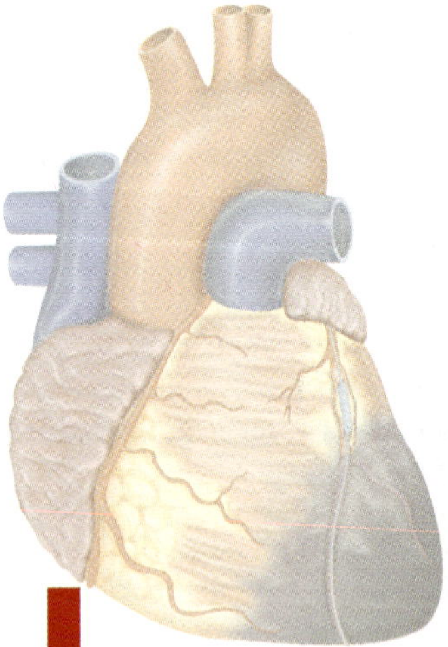

38

CHAPTER

TNK Effect and Outcome Evaluation in STEMI by Coronary Angiography

KN Srinivasan, I Sathyamurthy

INTRODUCTION

Tenecteplase (TNK-tPA) is a variant of the native tissue-type plasminogen activator (tPA) molecule that has a longer half-life, slower plasma clearance, 14-fold greater fibrin specificity than alteplase (accelerated tPA), and 80-fold greater resistance to inhibition by plasminogen activator inhibitor type 1. Its half-life of approximately 18 minutes allows single-bolus administration.

Success of thrombolysis is assessed clinically by relief of angina, biochemically by early raise in cardiac enzymes, electrocardiographically by resolution of ST segment elevation more than 50% at 90 minutes after initiation of thrombolysis, appearance of new reperfusion arrhythmias like accelerated idioventricular rhythm (AIVR) and angiographically by Thrombolysis In Myocardial Infarction (TIMI) flow, corrected TIMI frame count, and myocardial blush score in the culprit artery at 90-minute coronary angiogram. Visual quantification of epicardial flow was proposed by the TIMI investigators.[1] There are four grades. When there is no perfusion, it is grade 0. When contrast penetrates the thrombus with no distal perfusion, it is grade 1. When there is partial perfusion with slow entry of dye into the distal coronary bed of culprit artery compared to other arteries, it is grade 2. Complete normal flow into the distal bed is marked as grade 3. Initially, grade 2 and grade 3 TIMI flows were considered as successful reperfusion. But soon, it was realized that, it is not so. Hence, the TIMI flow grading was standardized by corrected TIMI frame count (CTFC). CTFC[2] is the number of cine frames required for contrast to first reach standardized distal coronary landmarks in the culprit artery and is measured by use of a frame counter on a cine viewer. Faster flow (lesser CTFC) was correlated to better clinical outcomes. CTFC has been shown to stratify patients with TIMI 3 flow into low- and high-risk groups.

The importance of myocardial perfusion was highlighted by Gibson,[3] who proposed myocardial blushing as an index of microvascular circulation. TIMI myocardial perfusion (TMP) grading is an easy method, wherein angiographically, dye passing into and out of myocardium is assessed in mid-diastole and is adjusted for the heart rate of the patient (Box 1).[3] Ideal view for assessing myocardial blush for right coronary artery (RCA) is left anterior oblique (LAO) with cranial tilt and for the left anterior descending (LAD) is right anterior oblique (RAO) with cranial tilt and for LCx is RAO with caudal tilt. By quantifying this blush, TMP is categorized into 4 grades (0 to 3). In TMP grade 3, there is the normal diffuse ground glass appearance of myocardial blush. At the end of the washout phase, dye is only mildly persistent or cleared. The washout phase is the time after the end of dye injection during which dye would normally be expected to clear from the epicardial vessels during opacification of the myocardium, followed by clearing from the myocardium. In TMP grade 2, dye enters the myocardium, but accumulates and exits more slowly, so that at the end of the washout phase dye in the myocardium is strongly persistent; however, dye totally clears by the next injection. In TMP grade 1, the dye does not leave the myocardium and there is a stain on the next injection. In TMP grade 0, dye does not enter the myocardium and there is minimal or no blush apparent during the injection and washout phases. It is found to be a better and independent predictor of mortality after adjusting for the age, TIMI flow, and infarct location. When TMP grading is used along with TIMI flow grading, it gives additional risk stratification into low- and high-risk groups.

Tenecteplase has undergone one phase-I, three phase-II, and one large phase-III trials. TNK-tPA in the treatment of ST-elevation myocardial infarction (STEMI) was studied for the first time in TIMI-10A trial.[4] It is a phase I trial, wherein 113 patients with STEMI received single bolus dose of TNK-tPA over 5–10 seconds and the dose ranged from 5 mg to 50 mg (eight ascending doses). Efficacy and safety of TNK-tPA was assessed by TIMI grade 3 flow at 90 minutes, TIMI frame counting, bleeding complications, coagulation parameters, and allergic reactions. TIMI grade 3 flow at 90 minutes[1] was greatest in 30 mg and 50 mg dosages (59% and 64%), respectively (Fig. 1). Serious bleeding occurred in 6.2% of the patients. There was no stroke or intracerebral hemorrhage observed. Pharmacokinetic property TNK-tPA like slow plasma clearance was also confirmed in this trial.

Weight-adjusted TNK-tPA doses were analyzed and found to have more percentage of TIMI 3 grade flow with 0.5 mg/kg TNK-tPA dose[3] (62–63%; Fig. 2), below which, significantly fewer patients achieved TIMI grade 3 flow. Similarly with more than 0.55 mg/kg TNK-tPA dose, there was increase in the risk of serious bleeding and intracranial hemorrhage (ICH), irrespective of the heparin dosage. This trail concluded that TNK-tPA at a dose of 0.5 mg/kg has similar efficacy and safety compared to accelerated tPA arm. TNK-tPA was observed to have a prolonged half-life and to be highly fibrin specific compared to tPA, features that explains its efficacy when administered as a 5–10 seconds single bolus.

Thrombolysis in myocardial Infarction-10B (TIMI-10B) is a phase II trial,[5] wherein 886 patients were randomized

BOX 1: Definitions of TIMI myocardial perfusion (TMP) grades.[3]

- *TMP Grade 0*: Failure of dye to enter the microvasculature. Either minimal or no ground-glass appearance ("blush") or opacification of the myocardium in the distribution of the culprit artery, indicating lack of tissue-level perfusion
- *TMP Grade 1*: Dye slowly enters but fails to exit the microvasculature. There is the ground-glass appearance ("blush") or opacification of the myocardium in the distribution of the culprit lesion that fails to clear from the microvasculature, and dye staining is present on the next injection (30 seconds between injections)
- *TMP Grade 2*: Delayed entry and exit of dye from the microvasculature. There is the ground-glass appearance ("blush") or opacification of the myocardium in the distribution of the culprit lesion that is strongly persistent at the end of the washout phase (i.e. dye is strongly persistent after three cardiac cycles of the washout phase and either does not or only minimally diminishes in intensity during washout)
- *TMP Grade 3*: Normal entry and exit of dye from the microvasculature. There is the ground-glass appearance ("blush") or opacification of the myocardium in the distribution of the culprit lesion that clears normally and is either gone or only mildly/moderately persistent at the end of the washout phase (i.e. dye is gone or is mildly/moderately persistent after three cardiac cycles of the washout phase and noticeably diminishes in intensity during the washout phase), similar to that in an uninvolved artery. Blush that is of only mild intensity throughout the washout phase but fades minimally is also classified as grade 3

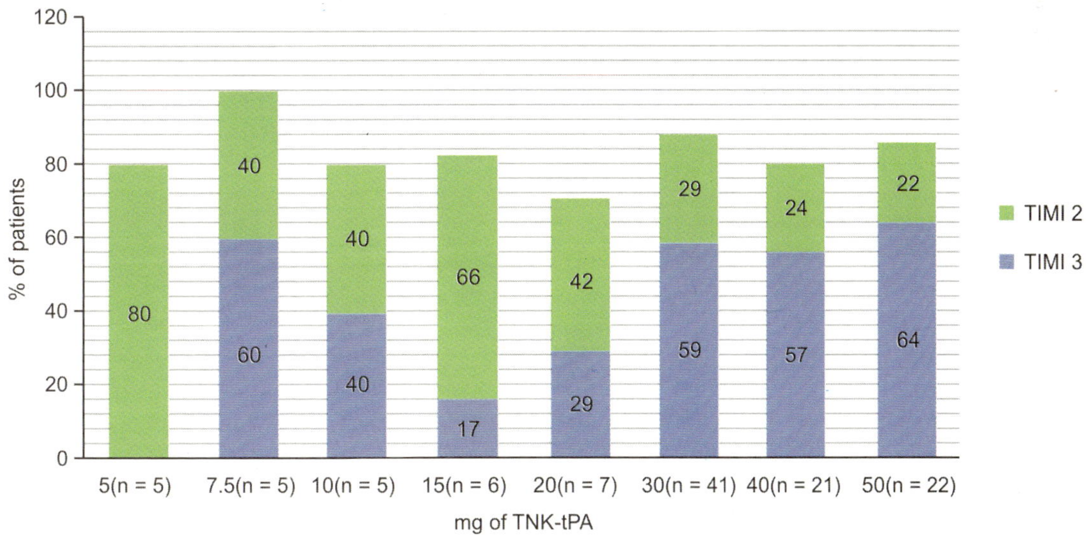

Fig. 1: TIMI 10A Trial. Culprit vessel patency rates with ascending doses of TNK-tPA.[4] (TIMI: Thrombolysis In Myocardial Infarction; TNK-tPA: tenecteplase)

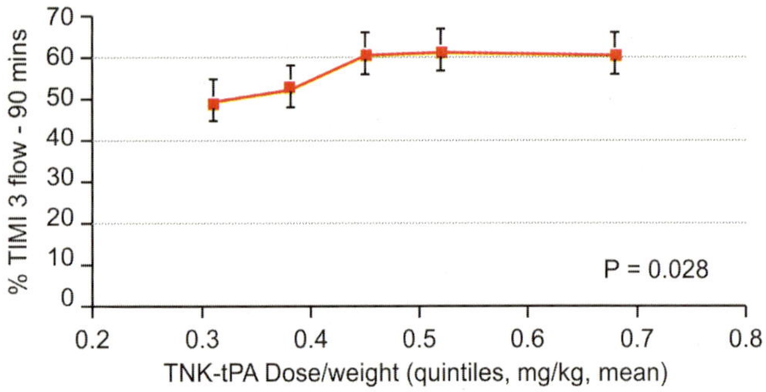

Fig. 2: TIMI flow grade at 90 minutes among TNK-tPA–treated patients, with dose expressed in mg TNK-tPA per patient body weight.[3] (TIMI: Thrombolysis In Myocardial Infarction; TNK-tPA: tenecteplase)

to receive 30 mg or 50 mg of TNK-tPA or 100 mg accelerated tPA. Angiograms were performed 90 minutes after thrombolytic administration. The primary endpoint of this trail was TIMI grade 3 flow at 90 minutes. Secondary endpoints were TIMI grade 3 at 60 and 75 minutes, TIMI grade 2 and 3 flow, TIMI frame counting, pharmacokinetic profiling, coagulation parameters, reinfarction, and serious bleeding. TIMI 3 flow at 90 minute was 54% with 30 mg TNK-tPA, 63% with 40 mg TNK-tPA, 66% with 50 mg TNK-tPA as against 63% with r-tPA (Table 1).[5] There was increased risk of ICH noted with higher dose of TNK-tPA. In view of excess ICH, 50 mg of TNK-tPA was replaced with 40 mg TNK-tPA and heparin doses were reduced. After downgrading the dosage of TNK-tPA and heparin, incidence of ICH and serious bleeding was lower in all treatment groups.

Out of 886 patients from TIMI-10B trail, 762 patients had both TMP and 30-day mortality data available for analysis. Coronary angiogram performed at 90 minutes following thrombolysis, showed more patients in the 40 mg TNK-tPA group to have less than 28 CTFC (40.8%) as against the other groups (30 mg TNK-tPA, 50 mg TNK-tPA) (p = 0.04; Table 2).[5] Mortality increases in a stepwise fashion with decreasing TMP grades. Patients with TMP grade 0 had higher 30-day mortality rate (6.2%) than patients with TMP grade 1 (5.1%), TMP grade 2 (4.4%), or TMP grade 3 (2.0%; Fig. 3).[3]

Mortality in patients with epicardial TIMI grade 3 flow (3.5%) was significantly lower than mortality in patients with TIMI flow 0 to 2 (6.8%; p = 0.04). Among patients with epicardial TIMI grade 3 flow, mortality increased as myocardial perfusion decreased from 0.73% for TMP grade 3 to 2.9% for TMP grade 2 to 5.0% for TMP grades 0/1 (p = 0.03 for TMP grade 3 vs grades 0 through 2; 3-way p = 0.066 Fig. 4).[3] Likewise, among patients with epicardial TIMI grades 0 through 2 flow, mortality tended to be lower in the TMP grade 3 group (4.7%; Fig. 4).[3] Lowest mortality was observed in patients who had grade 3 flow in both their epicardial artery and their myocardium (successful reperfusion). The 30-day mortality rate was 0.73% in this group. Highest mortality occurred in patients who had an occluded epicardial artery and no angiographically

TABLE 1: TIMI-10B trail–culprit artery patency rates at 90 minutes postlysis.[5]

	Accelerated rtPA <100 mg (n = 311)	*TNK-tPA 30 mg (n = 302)*	*TNK-tPA 40 mg (n = 148)*	*TNK-tPA 50 mg (n = 76)*
TIMI Grade 3 flow	63%	54%	63%	66%
TIMI Grade 2/3 flow	82%	77%	79%	88%
95% CI (TIMI 2/3 flow)	(77%, 86%)	(72%, 81%)	(72%, 85%)	(79%, 94%)

(CI: confidence interval; tPA: tissue-type plasminogen activator; TIMI: Thrombolysis In Myocardial Infarction; TNK-tPA: tenecteplase)

TABLE 2: Angiographic results: TIMI frame count from TIMI-10B trail.[5]

	TNK-tPA 30 mg,%	*TNK-tPA 40 mg,%*	*TNK-tPA 50 mg,%*	*Accelerated rtPA mg%*
90-minute angiogram No. of patients	297	147	74	306
Median	>38[1]	>32	33.5	33.5
25th, 75th percentiles	25, 100	22, 78	21, 46	23, 58
CTFC <40%	53.5[2]	62.6	66.2	60.8
CTFC <28%	31.0[3]	40.8	36.5	36.9

- CTFC indicates corrected TIMI frame count.
- 1 p = 0.065 vs. tPA, p = 0.07 vs. 40 mg TNK-tPA, p = 0.05 vs. 50 mg TNK-tPA
- 2 p = 0.07 vs. tPA and vs. 40 mg TNK-tPA, P = 0.05 vs. 50 mg TNK-tPA;
- 3 p = 0.04 vs. 40 mg TNK-tPA.

(TIMI: Thrombolysis In Myocardial Infarction; TNK-tPA: tenecteplase) apparent flow in myocardium (grade 0 or 1 for both TIMI and TMP grades) (failed lysis). The 30-day mortality rate was 10.9% in this group. Intermediate mortality was seen in patients who did not fall into either of the previous two groups (incomplete perfusion). Three-way p value between groups was less than 0.001 (Fig. 5).[3]

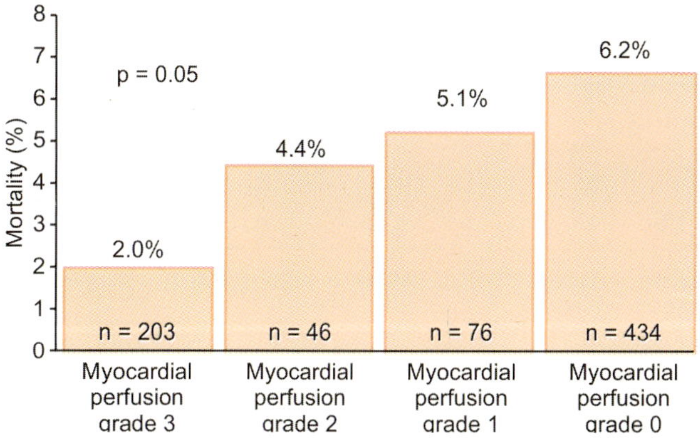

Fig. 3: Relationship between myocardial perfusion grade and mortality.[3]

CONCLUSION

Impaired myocardial perfusion by TMP grading is correlated to higher risk of mortality following thrombolysis and is found to be independent of TIMI flow in the epicardial coronary arteries. When both TMP grading and TIMI flow grading combined in a given patient, it gives additional prognostic information to the conventional epicardial TIMI flow grades and TIMI frame counts. Except 30 mg TNK-tPA group, the other two TNK-tPA groups had comparable TIMI grade 3 patency rate at 90 minutes to those of accelerated tPA group in TIMI-10B trail. While choosing a thrombolytic agent, one should consider age of the patient, timing of thrombolytic treatment, cost effectiveness, risk of bleeding including ICH and risk of mortality. Both TNK-tPA and tPA are comparable in all subgroup analyses with reference to their efficacy and risk of bleeding, except patients presenting late (>4 hours from the onset of symptoms), in whom the mortality rate was 7.0% with TNK-tPA and 9.2% with accelerated tPA. Among the available agents, TNK-tPA has the advantage of single bolus injection that makes it convenient for prehospital thrombolysis.

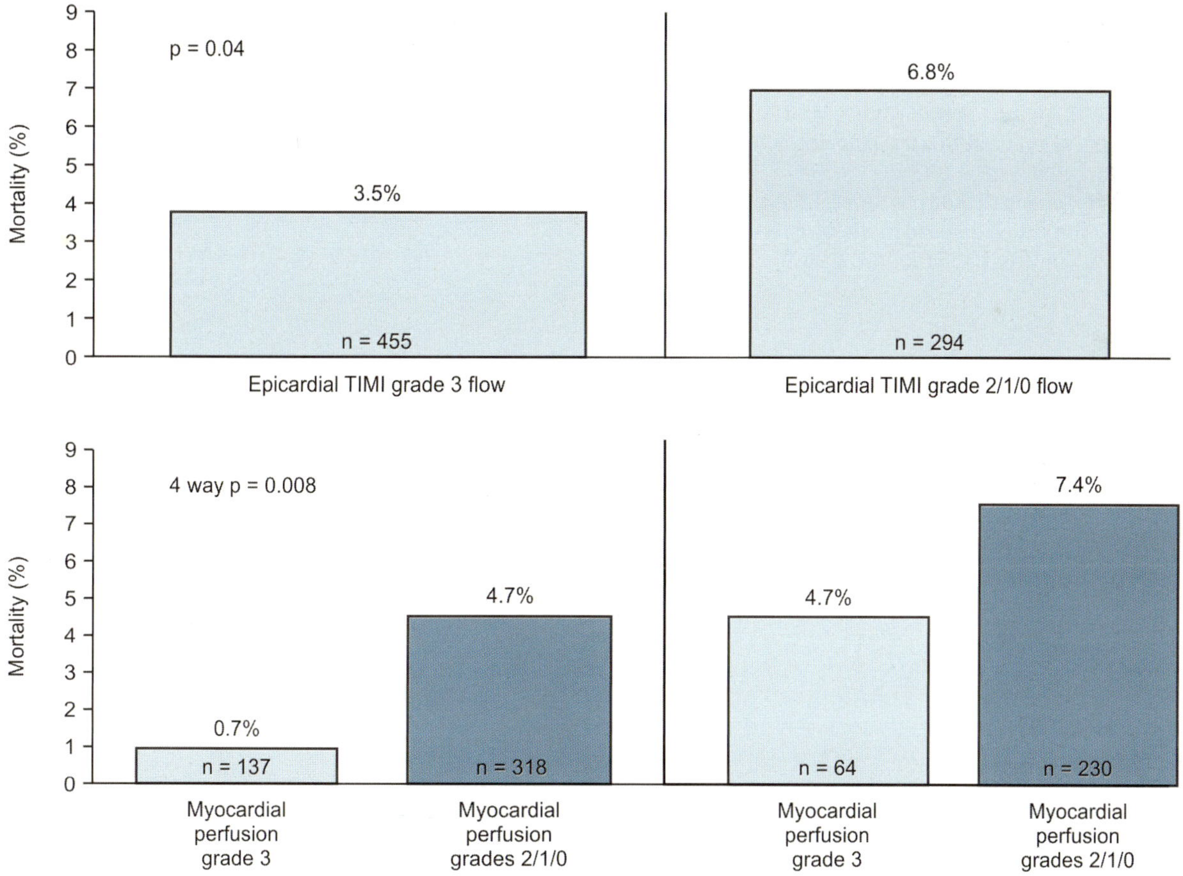

Fig. 4: Relationship of both TIMI epicardial flow grade and TMP grade to 30-day mortality.[3] (TMP: TIMI myocardial perfusion; TIMI: Thrombolysis In Myocardial Infarction)

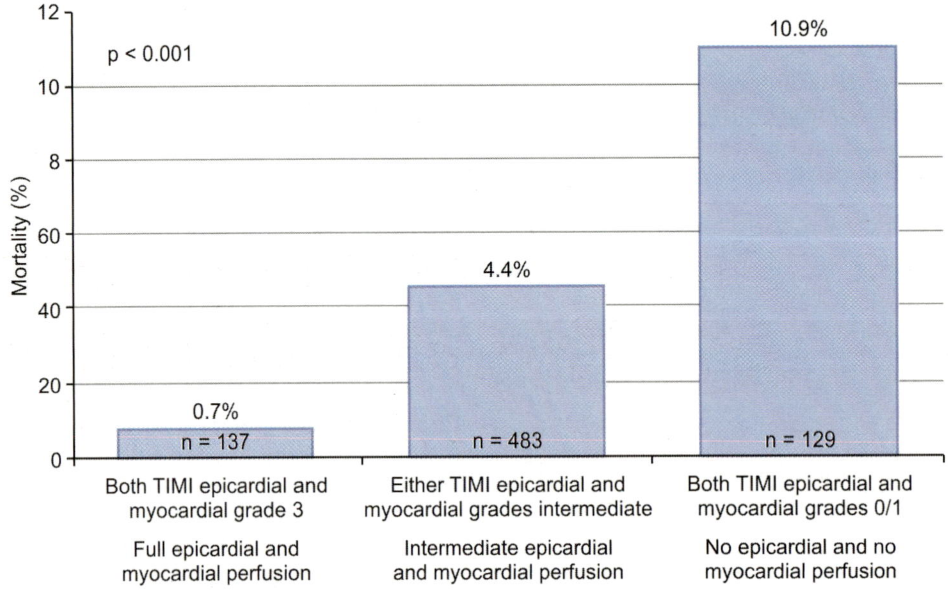

Fig. 5: Relationship between mortality and combined epicardial flow and myocardial perfusion.[3]

REFERENCES

1. The TIMI study group. The Thrombolysis in Myocardial Infarction (TIMI) trial. Phase I findings. N Engl J Med. 1985;312(14):932-6.
2. Gibson CM, Cannon CP, Daley WL, et al. TIMI frame count: a quantitative method of assessing coronary artery flow. Circulation. 1996;93:879-88.
3. Gibson CM, Cannon CP, Murphy SA, et al. Relationship of TIMI myocardial perfusion grade to mortality after administration of thrombolytic drugs. Circulation. 2000;101:125-30.
4. Cannon CP, McCabe CH, Gibson CM, et al. TNK-tissue plasminogen activator in acute myocardial infarction. Results of the Thrombolysis in Myocardial Infarction (TIMI)-10A dose-ranging trial. Circulation. 1997;95:351-6.
5. Cannon CP, Gibson CM, McCabe CH, et al. TNK-tissue plasminogen activator compared with front-loaded alteplase in acute myocardial infarction: results of the TIMI 10B trial. Thrombolysis in Myocardial Infarction (TIMI)-10B investigators. Circulation. 1998;98:2805-14.

39

CHAPTER

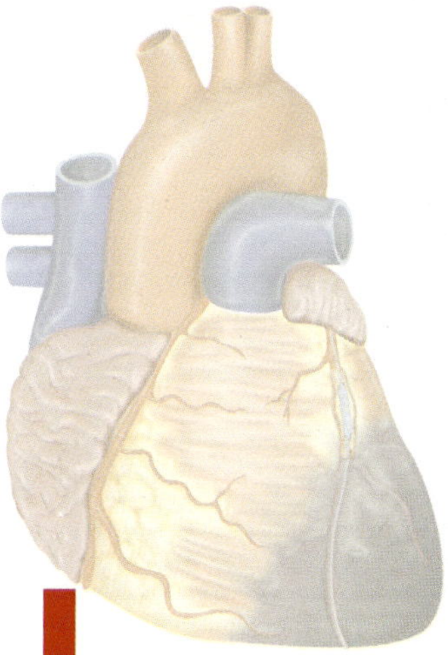

Thrombolytic Therapy Effect/Outcome Evaluation by Intravascular Ultrasound

K Venugopal

INTRODUCTION

Thrombolytic therapy is one of the major therapeutic advances that revolutionized the management of STEMI (ST-segment elevation myocardial infarction), the other being primary percutaneous coronary intervention (PCI).[1] Following thrombolysis, patients require further evaluation including coronary angiography to plan optimal management of the condition (pharmacoinvasive therapy). Following unsuccessful thrombolysis, urgent coronary angiography is needed to rescue percutaneous coronary angioplasty (Rescue PCI). Role of intravascular ultrasound (IVUS) in these situations is for optimization of the procedures, identification of causes for No Reflow phenomenon and assessment of noninfarct-related vessels.

PATHOPHYSIOLOGY OF ST-SEGMENT ELEVATION MYOCARDIAL INFARCTION

Mechanisms of acute myocardial infarction are spontaneous rupture of a vulnerable plaque, plaque erosion, calcific nodules, spontaneous coronary dissection, and subsequent thrombus formation resulting in complete occlusion of the culprit vessel and STEMI.[2] Though the basic pathophysiology of STEMI and non-STEMI (NSTEMI) is similar, clinical manifestations differ. Plaque rupture is seen in more than 76% in men and 55% in women and in older patients.[3] Plaque erosion is seen more in women than men and occurs in around 30%.[4] Calcific nodule is seen in around 2–7%. Occlusion, reperfusion, and reocclusion characterizes NSTEMI.

THROMBOLYTIC THERAPY IN ACUTE MYOCARDIAL INFARCTION

The thrombolytic action of streptokinase was discovered by Dr. Tillet in 1933.[5] Streptokinase was first used intravenously by Fletcher in 1958 for the treatment of myocardial infarction but the routine use of intravenous thrombolytic therapy gained momentum after the publication of major trials—GISSI (Gruppo Italiano per lo Studio della Streptochinasi nell' Infarcto Miocardio) and ISIS-2 (Second International Study of Infarct Survival).[6-8] The landmark study of DeWood in 1980 showed that 87% of patients presenting with acute myocardial infarction (AMI) within 4 hours had total coronary occlusion and this led to the mega trials which established the use of this form of treatment in AMI. It was recognized that while thrombolysis was beneficial in patients presenting with STEMI, its use in NSTEMI was associated with poorer outcomes and considered inappropriate. The success of initial agents like streptokinase and urokinase led to the development of newer more effective, more rapidly acting and more fibrin-specific agents like alteplase (t-PA), reteplase, and tenecteplase. Compared to primary angioplasty, thrombolysis is more easily available, can be administered even in settings with minimal facilities and is cheaper but the major problems are lesser rates of reperfusion, more bleeding problems, and need for angioplasty in settings of failed thrombolysis (Rescue PCI). Around 30% patients who present with STEMI are ineligible to receive the treatment due to absolute and relative contraindications. In developing countries like India thrombolysis still remains the more commonly performed revascularization strategy. Attempts at prehospital thrombolysis have shown similar benefits to primary PCI. In an ideal setting, the administration of thrombolytic therapy should be done with a Door-to-Needle time of 20–30 minutes as per the new guidelines [The American College of Cardiology/American Heart Asso- ciation, European Society of Cardiology (ACC/AHA, ESC)].

MARKERS OF SUCCESSFUL REPERFUSION AFTER THROMBOLYSIS

Relief of pain, ST-segment resolution more than 50%, occurrence of reperfusion arrhythmias, earlier release of biomarkers like troponin, myoglobin, and creatine kinase are some of the indices of successful reperfusion. Disadvantage of thrombolysis is an increased incidence of hemorrhagic complications especially intracerebral bleed.[9] Current guidelines indicate routine coronary angiography within 24–48 hours (Pharmacoinvasive therapy). Patients who undergo unsuccessful thrombolysis need urgent coronary angiography and revascularization with angioplasty.

INTRAVASCULAR ULTRASOUND FINDINGS IN AMI

Preprocedural Intravascular Ultrasound Findings

- *Plaque erosions and rupture:* The main mechanisms in STEMI are plaque rupture and erosions. Multiple plaque ruptures are suggested by the presence of smooth lumen between ruptured plaques with cavities. Hong et al. reported the presence of ruptured plaques in 46% patients with STEMI compared to 29% patients with NSTEMI. They also reported that multiple plaque ruptures tended to be more present in STEMI compared to NSTEMI (19% vs. 13%).[10] Positive remodeling and soft plaques were more associated with plaque rupture (Figs. 1 and 2).[11]
- *Thrombus:* Occlusive thrombus is seen in around 34% patients with STEMI and 21% patients with NSTEMI.[12] Compared to optical coherence tomography (OCT), detection of thrombus is less definite with IVUS due to its low-resolution rate. The points for detection of thrombus include speckled plaque, hypoechoic mass, detached mass, and evacuated plaque cavity (Fig. 3).
- *Positive remodeling*: The diagnosis of positive remodeling is by assessing the remodeling index. The lesion site external elastic membrane cross sectional area is compared to the average of the distal and proximal reference sites. When the index is more than 1.05 it is said to be positive remodeling while an index of less than 0.95 is negative remodeling (Figs. 4 and 5).[13]

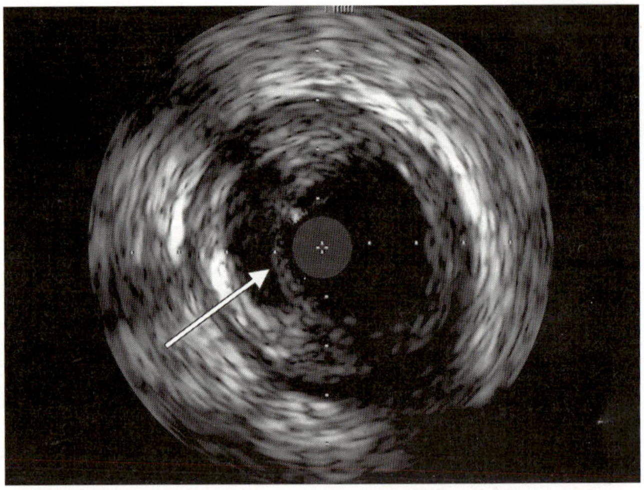

Fig. 1: Anterior wall MI, postlysis. Ulcerated plaque in LAD (arrow). (LAD: left anterior descending; MI: myocardial infarction)
Courtesy: Dr K Venugopal, Dr Deepak Davidson.

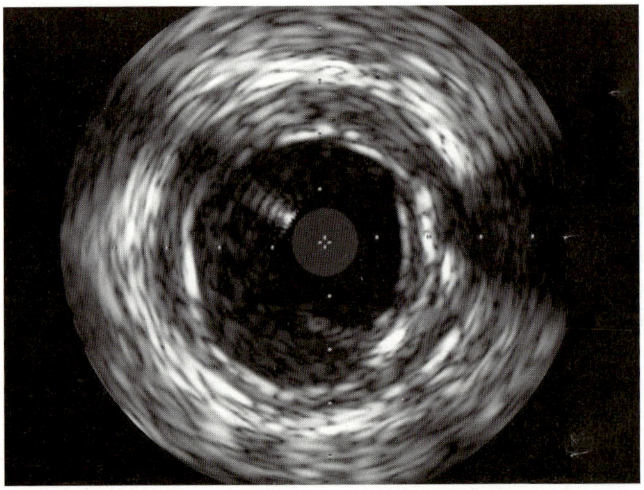

Fig. 2: Poststenting of the patient in Figure 1.
Courtesy: Dr K Venugopal, Dr Deepak Davidson.

- *Thin cap fibroatheroma (TCFA)*: The most common lesion which predisposes to plaque rupture, thrombus formation, and subsequent events is the TCFA. Attenuated plaque is a hypoechoic plaque without calcification or fibrosis.[14] Attenuated plaque was seen in 39.6% STEMI and 17.6% NSTEMI.[15] Elderly patients were more likely to have predominantly calcified lesions, longer lesions with less-positive remodeling.[16]

No Reflow Phenomenon

Distal embolization of the thrombus with subsequent microcirculatory loss characterizes No Reflow phenomenon. Following PCI occurrence of periprocedural myocardial infarction is associated with No Reflow. IVUS can identify

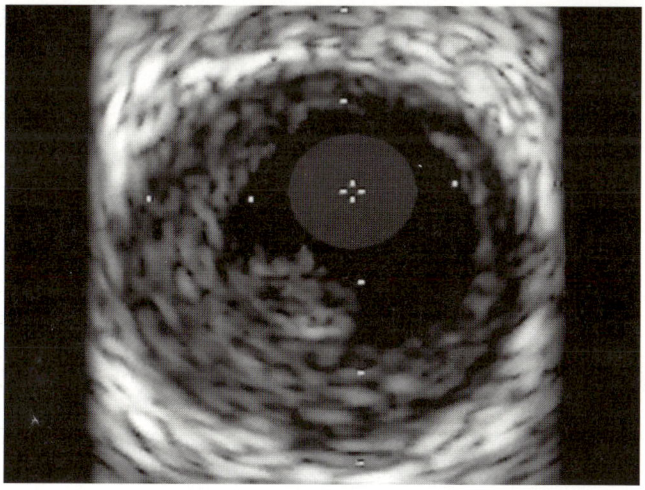

Fig. 3: Hazy lesion in left anterior descending on intravascular ultrasound.
Courtesy: Dr K Venugopal, Dr Deepak Davidson.

lesions likely to develop No Reflow. Plaque rupture, positive remodeling, tissue prolapse, and thrombus were associated with No Reflow.

Left Main Coronary Artery Lesions

Post-thrombolysis, a significant number of patients have multi vessel disease or involvement of the left main coronary artery (LMCA). IVUS can assess the luminal characteristics in LMCA disease and also the wall characteristics. It is superior to OCT in the visualization of ostium in LMCA disease. Minimal lumen area for significant LMCA stenosis is 6 mm^2,[16] but in Asian population values of 4.5–4.8 has been proposed. IVUS is also useful in plaque distribution and plaque characteristics especially calcium. IVUS will be useful in assessing the vascular bed preparation especially with rotablation. Stent sizing is another important aspect of IVUS use in LMCA stenting. Poststenting IVUS should also be done to see if the stent is well opposed to the lumen.

Nonculprit Vessel Angioplasty

Following primary PCI of the culprit vessel, the treatment of the nonculprit vessels with significant lesions is currently a debated topic. While the treatment of nonculprit vessels in cardiogenic shock is noncontroversial, the same approach in hemodynamically stable patients is still a matter of controversy. Use of IVUS in these situations is greatly helpful (Fig. 6).

CONCLUSION

Thrombolysis is a major revascularization strategy in STEMI especially in developing countries where immediate access to primary interventional therapy may not be available.

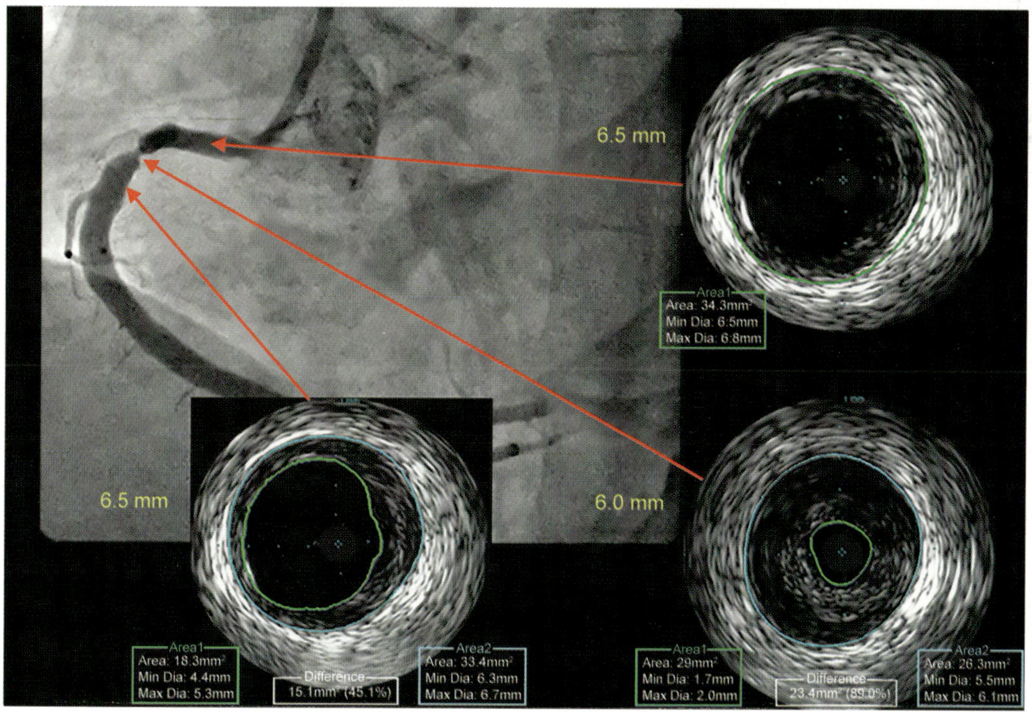

Fig. 4: Negative remodeling on intravascular ultrasound (IVUS) study.
Courtesy: Dr K Venugopal, Dr Deepak Davidson.

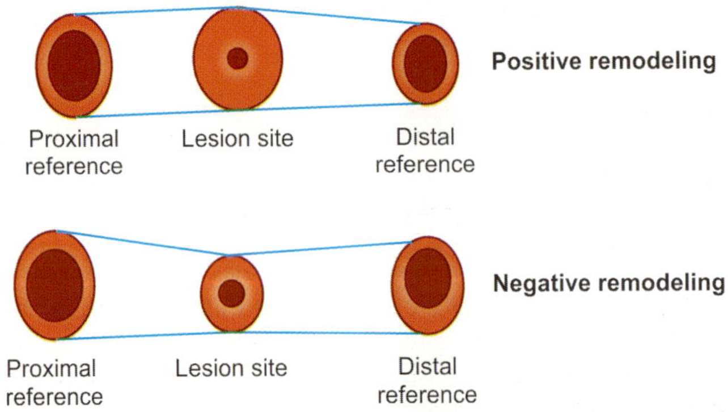

Fig. 5: Positive and negative remodeling.

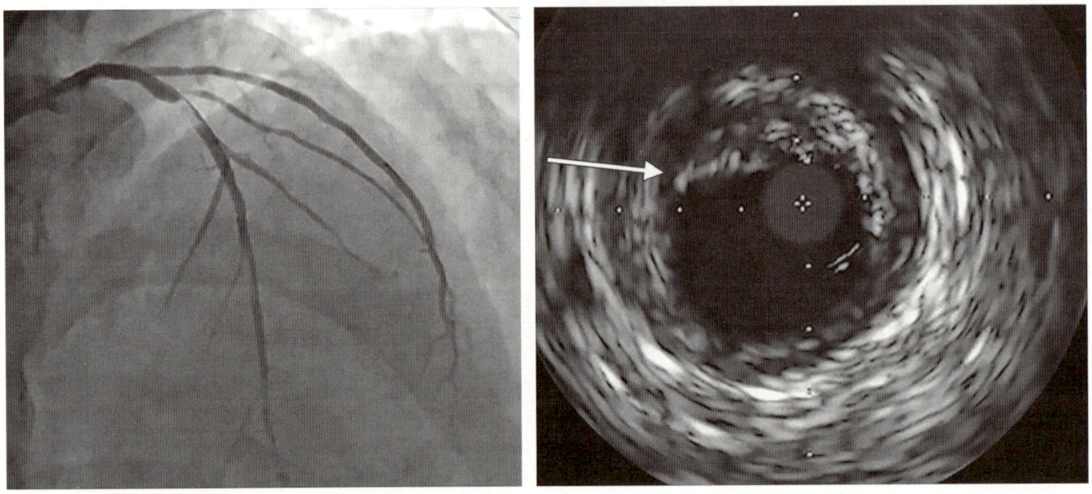

Fig. 6: Anterior wall MI thrombolyzed. Hazy lesion in LMCA on angiogram. IVUS study showing undermined ulcer in LMCA. (IVUS: intravascular ultrasound; LMCA: left main coronary artery; MI: myocardial infarction).
Courtesy: Dr K Venugopal, Dr Deepak Davidson.

Following thrombolysis patients should ideally undergo coronary angiography within 3–24 hours or up to 48 hours. IVUS use in these situations is extremely valuable in the characteristics of plaque rupture, erosion, and predicting probability of No Reflow phenomenon and positive remodeling. The role of IVUS in left main lesions is now accepted for better procedural outcomes. IVUS thus remains an integral part of post-MI revascularization strategies after thrombolysis.

REFERENCES

1. Fibrinolytic Therapy Trialists (FTT) Collaborative group. Indications for fibrinolytic therapy in suspected AMI: Collaborative overview of early mortality and major morbidity results from all randomized trials of more than 1000 patients. Lancet. 1994;343:311-22.
2. Virmani R, Burke AP, Farb A, et al. Pathology of the vulnerable plaque. J Am Coll Cardiol. 2006;47(8):C13-8.
3. Falk E, Nakano M, Benton JF, et al. Update on acute coronary syndromes: The pathologists view. Eur Heart J. 2013;34:719.
4. Jia H, Abtahian F, Aguirre AD, et al. In vivo diagnosis of plaque erosion and calcified nodules in patients with acute coronary syndrome by intravascular optical coherence tomography. J Am Coll Cardiol. 2013;62:1748.
5. Tillet WS, Garner RL. Fibrinolytic activity of Streptococci. J Exp Med. 1933;58:485-502.
6. Fletcher AP, Alkajaersign N, Smyrniotis FE, et al. The treatment of patients suffering from early myocardial infarction with massive and prolonged streptokinase therapy. Trans Assoc Am Physicians. 1958;71:287-96.
7. Gruppo Italiano per lo Studio della Streptochinasi nell' Infarcto Miocardico (GISSI). Effectiveness of intravenous thrombolytic treatment in acute myocardial infarction. Lancet. 1986;1:397-402.
8. ISIS-2 (Second International Study of Infarct Survival) Collaborative Group. Randomized trial of intravenous streptokinase, oral aspirin both or neither among 17187 cases of suspected acute myocardial infarction. Lancet. 1988;332(8607):349-60.
9. De Jaegere PP, Arnold AA, Balk AH, et al. Intracranial hemorrhage in association with trombolytic therapy: Incidence and clinical predictive factors. J Am Coll Cardiol. 1992;19(2):289-94.

10. Hong YJ, Jeong MH, Choi YH, et al. Differences in intravascular ultrasound findings in culprit lesions in infarct-related arteries between ST-segment elevation myocardial infarction and non-ST-segment elevation myocardial infarction. J Cardiol. 2010;56:15-22.
11. Kusama I, Hibi K, Kosuge M, et al. Impact of plaque rupture on infarct size in ST-segment elevation anterior acute myocardial infarction. J Am Coll Cardiol. 2007;50: 1230-7.
12. Hong YJ, Jeong MH, Choi YH, et al. Differences in intravascular ultrasound findings in culprit lesions in infarct-related arteries between ST-segment elevation myocardial infarction and non-ST-segment elevation myocardial infarction. J Cardiol. 2010;56:15-22.
13. Nakamura M, Nishikawa H, Mukai S, et al. Impact of coronary artery remodeling on clinical presentation of coronary artery disease: An intravascular ultrasound study. J Am Coll Cardiol. 2001;37:63-9.
14. Endo M, Hibi K, Shimizu T, et al. Impact of ultrasound attenuation and plaque rupture as detected by intravascular ultrasound on the incidence of no-reflow phenomenon after percutaneous coronary intervention in ST-segment elevation myocardial infarction. JACC Cardiovasc Interv. 2010;3:540-9.
15. Lee SY, Mintz GS, Kim SY, et al. Attenuated plaques detected by intravascular ultrasound; clinical angiographic and morphologic features and post percutaneous coronary intervention complications in patients with acute coronary syndromes. JACC Cardiovasc Interv. 2009;2(1):65-72.
16. Jasti V, Ivan E, Yalamanchili V, et al. Correlations between fractional flow reserve and intravascular ultrasound in patients with an ambiguous left main coronary artery stenosis. Circulation. 2004;110:2831-6.

40

CHAPTER

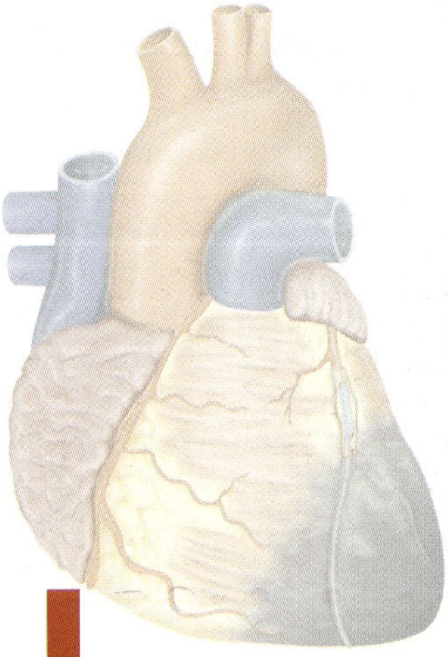

Role of Myocardial Perfusion Imaging in Patients of Chronic Stable Angina

E Prabhu, S Santhosh

INTRODUCTION

Indian scriptures quote that our hearts are suffused with "*kshamã (forbearance).*" The scriptures also extolled that forbearance as sacrifice, truth, nonviolence, compassion, righteousness, the truth, the vedas and that which confers happiness and heavenly bliss, possibly because we think through our hearts. In our country, where healthcare expenses are predominantly met "out of pocket" by each family, chronic heart disease—especially the coronary artery disease (CAD) is causing a remarkably high financial burden on them. In growing economies like India and South-East Asia, there is a rising trend of cardiovascular morbidity and mortality, while in developed countries in the west—especially the USA, there is a steady decline in cardiovascular deaths in recent years, possibly because of their robust action plans.[1,2] In India, the data studied in ICMR depicts that between 1998 and 2004, there is 9.19% increase in the burden of ischemic heart diseases in India and the number of death due to ischemic heart disease has also progressively increased.[3] Multiple, small, clinical, and subclinical myocardial events occurring over a long time as a consequence of CADs, generate a sequence of events over a period of time to manifest as diverse clinical manifestations summed up as chronic cardiac ischemia. Such prolonged and repetitive ischemic events lead to three common chronic ischemic manifestations: "precondition," "stunning," and "hibernation."[4,5] Off late, several studies have demonstrated that CAD is the commonest cause of chronic heart failure. The main trick lies in differentiating between the viable and nonviable myocardium before planning and justifying any cardiac intervention. Several cardiologists prefer to do some kind of intervention in a patient with chronic CAD because of the general perception that their intervention will possibly improve the left ventricular (LV) dysfunction to some definite extent. stress-rest myocardial perfusion study has helped in identification of patients with inducible ischemia and enhanced survival in patients undergoing early revascularization instead of optimal medical therapy. Overt clinical evidence of CAD without obvious ischemia or with minimal ischemia, was found to be benefitted by medical management.[6]

BACKGROUND

Nuclear cardiology helps in understanding chronic ischemia in a majority of asymptomatic patients. Stress-rest myocardial perfusion imaging (MPI) has long been established as a modality to objectively establish the extent of ischemia in obstructive CAD. In chronic ischemia, the various data collected to definitely convince us to about its ability to risk stratify the patients with angina. Although clinical trials have convinced us the importance of invasive coronary angiography to understand the level of luminal obstruction and its functional significance, MPI has added value to this by including information about the myocardial blood flow and tissue perfusion to understand the clinical significance of the luminal obstruction. In recent times, we are adopting newer strategies for performing better MPI with conventional cardiac single photon emission computed tomography (SPECT) like elimination of ^{201}Thallium and dual isotope imaging protocols (^{201}Tl - ^{99m}Tc) so as to keep radiation exposure to less than 9 mSv, use of newer count-density softwares with conventional gamma cameras, adopting stress first/stress only imaging protocols and modification of imaging hardwares by incorporating focused collimators and solid state detectors.[7]

DIAGNOSTIC CRITERIA

Exercise testing has conventionally been well established for about 3 decades in our country, with the availability of appropriate facilities and protocols as specified in the Joint Commission International (JCI) or National Accreditation Board for Hospitals & Healthcare Providers (NABH) standards like appropriate equipment like the treadmill test (TMT) or the Bicycle ergometer, devices for continuous monitoring of electrocardiography (ECG) and blood pressure, availability of emergency drugs and protocols, informed consent, trained personnel, standardized patient preparation, etc. There are specific recommendations for performing MPI in specific patients like in women, older patients, and asymptomatic patients or like those requiring cardiopulmonary exercise stressing for undergoing heart surgeries.[8-10] Absolute contraindications for exercise stress test MPI include—those with high risk of unstable angina, heart failure, hypertension [systolic blood pressure (SBP) > 200 mm Hg and diastolic blood pressure (DBP) > 110 mm Hg at rest], cardiac arrhythmias, aortic stenosis, pulmonary hypertension pulmonary embolism, acute myocardial infarction (MI), myocarditis, and other severe medical illness. Already known patient with significant left main disease, asymptomatic aortic stenosis, physical/mental impairment for performing physical stress, and conduction abnormalities including tachy and brady arrhythmias, left bundle branch block (LBBB), and Wolff-Parkinson-White (WPW) syndrome. In patients who cannot be motivated to perform adequate stress and reach targeted heart rates and those with musculoskeletal disease and peripheral vascular disease exercise testing has its own inherent limitations and are recommended for pharmacological stress testing. Patients for stress MPI are required to avoid caffeine-containing drinks for minimum 12 hours before test, BP medications like beta-blockers or calcium channel blockers can be withheld, if possible and have a very light breakfast - like fruits and cereals. Nothing should be eaten at least 3–4 hours before study. Stress test should be terminated when patient develops chest pain, shortness of breath, fatigue, ST depression less than 2 mm or elevation more than 1 mm from baseline, drop in SBP more than 10 mm Hg despite increasing workload, sustained arrhythmias, SBP more than 230 mm Hg and DBP more than 130 mm Hg, achievement of about 85% of targeted heart rate are the common indications of terminating stress without achievement of maximum age adjusted targeted heart rate. The inability to monitor the ECG and patients with implantable defibrillators are also to be closely monitored for rapid loss in heart rate.

In India, pharmacological vasodilator agents are also administered like the adenosine and dipyridamole. Adenosine's analogue regadenoson is not available in several centers and they cause selective stimulation of A_{2A} receptors. This causes 3–4-fold increase myocardial blood flow. Adenosine, in addition also activates A_1, A_{2B}, and A3 receptors, producing unpleasant atrioventricular (AV) blocks, peripheral vasodilation, and severe bronchospasm. These effects are not seen in regadenoson. Adenosine infusion is administered at the rate of 140 microgram per Kg body weight is administered over standard 6 minutes IV infusion. ^{99m}Tc-methoxyisobutylisonitrile (MIBI) (tracer) is injected at 3 minutes and the infusion is continued for rest 3 minutes. For as shorter duration of study, injection of tracer is given 2 minutes following adenosine infusion and the infusion is continued 2 minutes further following tracer injection. Patients commonly may experience flushing, chest discomfort, giddiness, nausea, dyspnea, and symptomatic hypotension. Rarely AV block, ST segment changes from baseline level, headaches, atrial fibrillations, headaches, stroke, and seizures have been reported. As the half-life of adenosine is less than 10 seconds, most of the above adverse effects resolve spontaneously, rarely requiring aminophylline infusion.

Adenosine causes modest BP changes—may decrease BP by 10 to 20 mm Hg, and pulse/heart rate may increase to about 10–20 per minute. Adenosine stress MPI is commonly indicated in inability of the patient to perform physical stress—like amputation of the lower limb and other musculoskeletal constraints, pulmonary, peripheral vascular or mental disorders, cardiac medications like beta blockers, nitrates and calcium antagonists, baseline ECG abnormalities, like the LBBB, WPW syndrome, ventricular pacing device implanted, and clinically stable but high-risk patient for acute myocardial infarction. It is not administered in patients with history of bronchospasm, nonfunctioning of ventricular pacing in patients with II or III degree heart block, patient with pleuropericardial diseases, severe aortic stenosis, cerebral vascular diseases, stroke or in patients with SBP less than 90 mm Hg, known hypersensitivity to adenosine, recent study with adenosine vasodilation or in unstable angina and acute coronary syndromes. Patients who are ambulant can be subjected to adenosine infusion in combination with low-level physical stress in a TMT (work load up to 1.7 METS, 0% gradient). This had significant decrease in the adverse effects of adenosine-like prevention of sudden drop in BP and improved the image quality with low background level. Conduction abnormalities like the LBBB, WPW syndrome, and patients with pacemaker implantation are the contraindications for low-level stress–adenosine study. Adenosine infusion is stopped immediately upon noticing rapid drop in BP (SBP <80 mm Hg), patient becomes symptomatic with development of AV block, shock, severe chest pain, and pallor with ST segment variation more than 2 mm or patient's request because of his discomfort. In case of development of wheeze or bronchospasm or hemodynamic changes; dobutamine infusion for stress study causes direct dose dependent b_1 and b_2 stimulation, causing increase in BP, heart rate, and cardiac contractility. Regional myocardial blood flow is enhanced in dobutamine, similar to exercise testing. Normal ventricle will have similar, dose-related increase in blood flow which is supplied by normal coronaries, whereas, in ischemia, the blood flow changes are very minimal in ischemic myocardium. Dobutamine is infused at 5–10 µg/kg/min, which in increased at intervals of 3 minutes to 20, 30, and 40 µg/kg/min. Once peak heart rate is achieved, radioactivity is injected and peak heart rate maintained for 1 more minute. The plasma half-life of dobutamine is 2 minutes and its onset of action is about 1–2 minutes, while it may require up to 10 minutes to obtain peak effect.

Hemodynamic effect of dobutamine may vary, causing increase in about 45 beats per minute, heart rate and BP may increase to about 30 mm Hg. Headache, palpitations, chest pain, breathlessness, and arrhythmias can happen with dobutamine infusion. ST segment changes occur if ischemia happens and all adverse effects can be reversed by IV administration of short-acting beta blocker (esmolol 0.5 mg/kg over 1 minute). Uncontrolled hypertension (SBP >200 mm Hg, DBP >110 mm Hg), unstable angina, arrhythmias, prior history of ventricular tachyarrhythmias and dobutamine hypersensitivity are contraindications for dobutamine stress test. Early termination of dobutamine infusion is indicated if more than 85% increase in heart rate, severe hypertension, severe hypotension, signs of poor perfusion, or technical constraints.

In chronic ischemia and pharmacological stress MPI studies are useful in patients with hypersensitive airway disease, chronic obstructive pulmonary disease (COPD), LBBB, WPW syndromes, and chronic kidney disease (CKD).

Tracers for Myocardial Perfusion Imaging

^{99m}Tc sestamibi and ^{99m}Tc tetrofosmin are commonly used agents for MPI. They are lipophilic, cationic, physical half-life of 6 hours, produces gamma photons of 140 keV energy, taken-up by the mitochondria depending upon the blood flow and transmembrane energy potentials. Excretion of these tracers is mainly through the hepatobiliary tract. 201-Thallium (^{201}Tl) which is an analogue of potassium and its physical half-life is 73.1 days. It decays by emitting predominantly X-rays with 68 and 80 keV energy. It has a very high first-pass myocardial extraction, active transport into the membrane and rapid clearance, excretion mainly through the kidneys. The effective radiation delivered by Thallium is higher than other tracers and hence, following ALARA (As Low As Reasonably Achievable) principle, Thallium is scarcely used routinely in India as well as elsewhere the world for MPI. In order to keep radiation dose minimal, several institutions have begun to adopt Stress Only Protocol for chronic ischemia imaging, although, many are comfortable with single day stress-rest protocol or rest-stress protocol with ^{99m}Tc-based tracers or 2-day protocol in higher number of studies for time management.[11]

Prognostic and Therapeutic Implications

Hachamovich et al.[6] in their study have clearly demonstrated that presence of substantial volume of myocardium with inducible ischemia in patients have demonstrated with MPI, have demonstrated to have enhanced survival for undergoing revascularization procedure when compared with those with optimal medical therapy. In patients who do not have inducible ischemia, as demonstrated by MPI, without prior CAD, without prior revascularization procedure, have found to be benefitted more by optimal medical therapy than revascularization procedure. In patients with a large, prior MI, the therapeutic benefit of revascularization was blunted as demonstrated by the MPI. These findings concur with the current level of understanding of the value of ischemia testing with MPI in chronic stable angina. The exact cut-off value beyond which, demonstration of reversible ischemia will be recommended for optimum medical therapy is not understood clearly. In the presence of extensive MI and absence of reversible ischemia by MPI, the survival benefit is not obvious as seen in several studies. However, even in the presence of extensive reversible ischemia, without prior history of MI, there is definite benefit for early revascularization procedures than optimal medical therapy alone, as demonstrated by MPI. Detailed studies performed on diabetic patients with multi-vessel CAD and dysfunctional myocardium have been found to be extensively benefitted in determining the best possible treatment strategy with the guidance of MPI. Several diabetic patients also have other comorbidities like hypertension, obesity, hyperlipidemias, diabetic kidney diseases, etc., there is greater incidences of CAD and mortality associated with it. As a consequence, they might already be on long-term medications like statins, antiplatelet agents, angiotensin-converting enzyme-angiotensin-receptor blockers (ACE-ARBs) etc., which modify the morbidity and mortality rates in them. In the nuclear substudy of the COURAGE (The Clinical Outcomes Utilizing Revascularization and Aggressive Drug Evaluation) report, it was found to have better survival rate of patients who have undergone revascularization for moderate to severe ischemia than with optimal medical therapy,[12] although, in another separate study there was no significant relationship between the extent of ischemia, ischemia severity, MI, and consequent death.[13]

Therefore, ISCHEMIA (International Study of Comparative Health Effectiveness with Medical and Invasive Approaches) trial[14] was commenced to understand whether the routine cardiac catheterization and revascularization in patients with severe ischemia will improve prognosis or derive some clinical benefit in an invasive approach of management. Patient with equal to or more than 10% ischemic myocardium demonstrated by nuclear stress test were included for the study, in addition to those who demonstrated 3/16 segments with stress induced hypo or akinesis in echocardiography or cardiac MRI. In ECG-TMT without imaging, patients who had typical angina during test, absence of ST depression of 1 mm or more and elevation of 2 mm or more in any specific vascular territory is accepted for this study. It was decided to enroll 10,000 participants, taking into account for screen failures and ensure an appropriate sample size to provide 90% power to obtain a 15% reduction in MI or cardiovascular (CV) death (primary composite end point) within 4 years—20% in conservative strategy group and 17% in invasive strategy group. Thus, this study is expected to address the gaps in our scientific understanding on the management strategy for patients with moderate to severe ischemic heart disease.

DISCUSSIONS

Following chronic ischemia, a complex and dynamic remodeling process happens in the left ventricle, including hypertrophy, apoptosis, proteolysis, and fibrosis. As a consequence, the geometry of ventricle is altered, causing progressive stress on the walls of the ventricle—stretching and dilating it, decreasing its contraction and causing heart failure. There is expansion of the infarct size and recruitment of border-zone viable myocardium into the scar tissue, thereby further altering its geometry and decreasing its contractile efficiency.[15] Therefore, there is an urgent need for a highly integrated, interdisciplinary method for understanding the distribution of the viable myocardium and its role in improving the contractile efficiency of an already jeopardized left ventricle. The sensitivity and specificity of measuring the cardiac biomarkers, including the troponin I, the troponin T, and the brain natriuretic peptide (BNP) is debatable as they may also be present in individuals without a chronic ischemia and may be vary in levels from individual to individual. Newer approaches like gene characterization, study of RNA, proteins, peptides, and metabolites as possible biomarkers to noninvasively understand chronic ischemia is still an evolving science. MRI is more extensively available and its real strength lies in imaging the inherent tissue contrast. It easily measures the ventricular volumes, mass, and contractile function and with gadolinium containing extracellular T1 shortening contrast agents, tissue characterization is possible. Myocardial edema can easily be imaged with T2-weighted imaging. The gadolinium-contrast agents are not distributed in cellular spaces and help to image the extracellular and vascular compartments. Therefore, in the event of acute MI where the cellular integrity is lost and in myocardial fibrosis, there is augmentation of interstitial compartment and higher concentration of the gadolinium contrast. Because of the higher spatial resolution of an MRI, the transmural extent of an infarction or distribution of tracer can be easily seen and its pathology quantified.

The stress myocardial perfusion images demonstrate that the salutary effects of revascularization are not mechanistically linked to the extent of viable myocardium. It only brings out the jeopardized myocardium that is identified as inducible ischemia on stress perfusion imaging. In MPI, high-risk features with annual mortality rate greater than 3% is seen as severe resting LV dysfunction [ejection fraction (EF) <35%]; Severe exercise LV dysfunction (EF < 35%), stress-induced large perfusion defect, particularly in the left anterior descending artery (LAD) territory, stress-induced moderate sized multiple perfusion defects, large-fixed perfusion defect with dilated LV, and/or increased lung uptake; stress-induced moderate-sized multiple perfusion defects with dilated LV and a low heart rate.[16] The nuclear substudy of BARI-2D (Bypass Angioplasty Revascularization Investigation 2 Diabetes) follow-up SPECT was performed after 1 year in 1,505 patients showed that those who had been treated with intervention has lesser incidence of ischemia.[17] Abnormal myocardial perfusion predicted subsequent infarction, significant association with scaring, and death. In the nuclear substudy of COURAGE, which is widely quoted, 314 patients who had stress test at baseline and follow-up stress test again at 6–18 months, stress-induced ischemic myocardium was reduced by more than 5% in patients treated by revascularization than medical therapy alone. Additional analysis based on the outcomes at the time of follow-up studies reveals more than 5% reduction of event rates, regardless of randomization. Thus, as on date, the best evidence based on use of stress SPECT test identification of patients with chronic CAD, in an observational study on 10,627 patients with no prior CAD reveal that they are more likely to benefited from intervention than optimal medical therapy alone.[18] The WOMEN (What is the Optimal Method for ischemia Evaluation in WomeN) study randomized women with good functional capacity and normal resting ECG to ECG testing alone or ECG plus SPECT. The results showed no difference in outcomes.[19] In a subsequent larger subgroup analysis as ECG alone have higher false-positive rates, 2,235 patient study by Cerci et al. shows incremental benefits of stress SPECT MPI over other clinical variables and LV dysfunction.[20] In many elderly patients, there are lot of comorbidities or physical deconditioning that make them incapable of performing stress ECG. Stress SPECT MPI is found to be safe, noninvasive, and effective with now cardiac event rates in normal studies in comparison to similar studies in younger population.[21] With increasing incidence of diabetes in our population, there is definitive data available on the importance of stress SPECT MPI has an incremental prognostic value over stress ECG alone for the assessment of cardiac death and nonfatal MI.[22] Similarly, hypertension and CKD is also in the raise in recent times. The progressively increasing incidence of CKD, measured as raising estimated glomerular filtration rate (eGFR) in our clinical practice has found to have 10–20-fold increase in cardiac death. With advanced CKD, CAD is not manifested as obvious chest pain. Before planning for renal transplantation in them, stress SPECT MPI is found to detect and risk-stratify patients with CAD in them. Hakeem et al. found that on patients with eGFR less than 60, there is substantial increase in cardiac death in patients with abnormal stress SPECT MPI results.[23] The annual rates of all-cause mortality for cardiac death and nonfatal MI were significantly higher in them. With CKD and diabetes, the all-cause mortality was still higher with abnormal stress SPECT MPI values (Summed Stress Score >8) especially in those undergoing renal transplantation.

In studies conducted on patients with CAD and normal or slightly reduced LV systolic function, there is inadequate evidence suggesting the decision on the method of treatment adopted has an important role based on stress MPI SPECT results. The ongoing ISCHEMIA study results could possibly reveal the best possible treatment strategy in normal patients with EF less than 35%. Studies based on Surgical Treatment for IsChemic Heart Failure (STICH) trial although did not have a serial testing data for patients undergoing coronary artery bypass graft (CABG) or optimal medical therapy as it was not mandated by the study design, CABG definitely reduced the rate of sudden cardiac death and fatal MI as followed up with stress SPECT MPI studies.[24]

LIMITATIONS

The process of atherosclerotic CAD itself is a dynamic process, with the patient's comorbidities like diabetes and hypertension taking several medications including statins, ACE-ARBs, and antiplatelet agents. Once severe LV dysfunction and ventricular remodeling sets-in, the occurrence of inducible ischemia has limited role in understanding the LV functional abnormalities because of the distorted geometry of the ventricle. The revascularization procedure, including surgical intervention may not be mechanistically related to the process of inducible ischemia on stress testing in patients with normal or mildly reduced LV systolic function. Subsequent analysis of the STICH trial showed definite evidence of reduction of fatal MIs and sudden cardiac deaths, with improved quality of life in patients as it protected the jeopardized myocardium. However, it could not prevent subsequent atherosclerotic occlusion of artery might precipitate lethal arrhythmias that may not be associated with previous arterial occlusion. The introduction of appropriate use criteria[25] has not only refined our understanding on the patient selection, but also on the variables that could affect the patient outcomes whether optimal medical therapy or surgical intervention is beneficial in stable CAD, with due emphasis on shared decision making and patient preferences (Table 1, Flowchart 1).

TABLE 1: Depicting the common image interpretations, artefacts, and their possible explanations in stress SPECT MPI in chronic ischemia evaluation.

Common interpretations of myocardial perfusion SPECT artefacts commonly seen while imaging chronic ischemia		
S. No.	*Image description terms*	*Most probable explanation*
1	Apical defect	Physiological thinning possibly due to attenuation correction and elliptical orbit of the SPECT detector.
2	Basal septal defect	Physiological membranous tissue in the atrioventricular valve plane.
3	Fixed/reversible anterior and/or lateral wall defect	Attenuation of the left breast tissue or lateral chest wall fat.
4	Fixed inferior or inferolateral defect	Attenuation of the left hemidiaphragm (common in men)
5	Diffusely reduced myocardial uptake	Normalization to noncardiac maximal activity

Contd...

Contd...

Common interpretations of myocardial perfusion SPECT artefacts commonly seen while imaging chronic ischemia		
S. No.	*Image description terms*	*Most probable explanation*
6	Fixed/reversible defects confined to the septum	LBBB causes asynchronous relaxation of the septum, resulting in shortened diastolic perfusion period in this region.
7	Fixed inferobasal defect	Depth dependent attenuation in obese patients
8	Anteroseptal or inferobasal linear defects.	Attenuation at the insertion points of the free wall of the RV (11 and 7 o'clock defects).
9	Opposed defects in the contralateral walls	Technical errors in image acquisition like flood field nonuniformity, errors in center of rotation, camera head tilt in multi-head detectors, immediate postexercise acquisition, patient motions (> 2 pixels)
10	Apical "Hot Spots" and basal defects	Truncation or localized apical hypertrophy
11	Anterior defect and normal or increased inferior uptake	Scatter from subdiaphragmatic tracer accumulation artificially increases inferior wall count density, exaggerated attenuation correction by the equipment
12	Inferior defect and increased anterior uptake	Intense subdiaphragmatic activity, adjacent to the inferior wall which is removed together with the count density of the inferior wall by ramp filtering.
13	Loss of details and contrast resolution	Increased detector to patient distance and decreased critical frequency of processing filter
14	Excessive Noise	Decreased count density and increased critical frequency of processing filter
15	Decrease in lateral to septal wall tracer activity	Left ventricular hypertrophy
16	Hotspots in the anterolateral and inferolateral walls	Hypertension with hypertrophy of papillary muscles.

(LBBB: left bundle branch block; MPI: myocardial perfusion imaging; RV: right ventricle; SPECT: single photon emission computed tomography)

Flowchart 1: Depicting the strategy for evaluation of chronic ischemia with stress SPECT myocardial perfusion imaging.

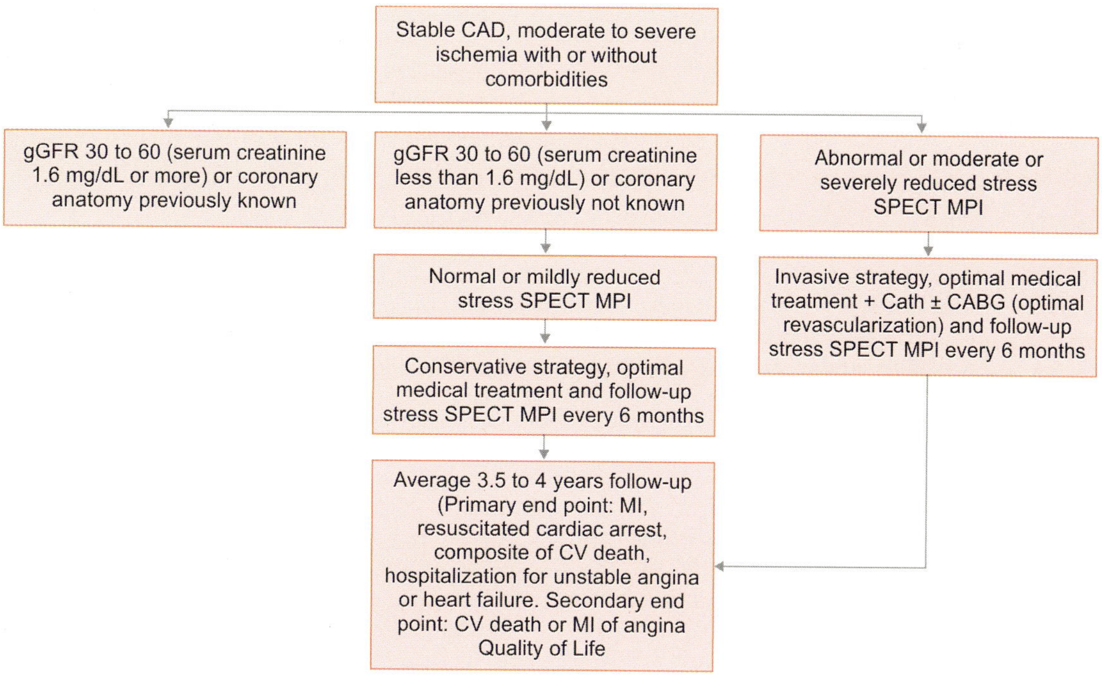

(CABG: coronary artery bypass graft; CAD: coronary artery disease; CV: cardiovascular; eGFR: estimated glomerular filtration rate; MI: myocardial infarction; MPI: myocardial perfusion imaging; RV: right ventricle; SPECT: single photon emission computed tomography)

CONCLUSION

Myocardial perfusion imaging is an important component for evaluation of chronic ischemic heart disease which determines the strategy for its comprehensive management, either interventions or optimal medical management. This is an established procedure for several years in which the standard method is either exercise or pharmacological stress-rest MPI for detection and risk stratification of the CAD. Patients selection criteria and the test procedure are being further refined periodically by appropriateness criteria considering the current technological development and predominantly balancing carefully the clinical benefits and radiation risks to the patient. Current practices like use of stress only imaging and predominant use of technetium-based radiopharmaceuticals help to reduce radiation exposure of the patient to a large extent. As only tracer quantities (picogam/nanogram) medications are administered, it is safe for the kidneys even in advanced CKD and in heart failure. Current innovations in instrumentation, like fusion imaging with CT/MRI, newer and better cameras, computers and softwares have revolutionized the field of SPECT MPI by providing functional as well as anatomical data. Considering the overall cost-containment in the management of chronic CAD, inappropriate imaging methods are decreased especially in screening of an asymptomatic individual for possible CAD. Finally, until the ISCHEMIA trial provides a definitive evidence on the use of stress SPECT MPI as a strategy for selecting the patient for undergoing revascularization, current clinical management of chronic stable angina shall continue to prevail mainly on individual judgment and experience instead of evidence based.

REFERENCES

1. Prabhakaran D, Singh K, Roth GK, et al. Cardiovascular diseases in India compared to the United States. J Am Coll Cardiol. 2018;72(1):79-85.
2. Public Health England. (2018). Action plan for cardiovascular disease prevention 2017–2018. [online] Available from https://assets.publishing.service.gov.uk/government/uploads/system/uploads/attachment_data/file/648190/cardiovascular_disease_prevention_action_plan_2017_to_2018.pdf [Accessed October 2018].
3. Upadhyay RP. An overview of the burden of noncommunicable diseases in India. Iran J Public Health. 2012;41(3):1-8.
4. Depre C, Vatner SF. Cardio-protection in stunned and hibernating myocardium. Heart Fail Rev. 2007;12:307-17.
5. Heusch G, Schulz R, Rahimtoola SH. Myocardial hibernation: A delicate balance. Am J Physiol Heart Circ Physiol. 2005;288:H984-H999.
6. Hachamovich R, Rozanski A, Shaw LJ, et al. Impact of ischaemia and scar on the therapeutic benefit derived from myocardial revascularization versus medical therapy among patients under-going stress-rest myocardial perfusion scintigraphy. Eur Heart J. 2011;32:1012-24.
7. DePeuy EG. Editorial: Myocardial perfusion SPECT just keeps getting better and better. J Nucl Cardiol. 2017;24:605-10.
8. Mieres JH, Gulati M, Bairey Merz N, et al. Role of non-invasive testing in the clinical evaluation of women with suspected ischemic heart disease: A consensus statement from the American Heart Association. Circulation. 2014;130:350-79.
9. Balady GJ, Arena R, Sietsema K, et al. Clinician's guide to cardiopulmonary exercise testing in adults: A scientific statement from the American Heart Association. Circulation. 2010;122:191-225.
10. Fleisher LA, Fleischmann KE, Auerbach AD, et al. 2014 ACC/AHA guideline on perioperative cardiovascular evaluation and management of patients undergoing noncardiac surgery: Executive summary: A report of the American College of Cardiology/American Heart Association task force on practice guidelines. J Nucl Cardiol. 2015;22:162-215.
11. Henzlova MJ, Duvall WL, Einstein AJ, et al. ASNC imaging guidelines for SPECT nuclear cardiology procedures: Stress, protocols, and tracers. J Nucl Cardiol. 2016;23(3):606-39. (Available at https://www.asnc.org/files/Guidelines%20and%20Quality/ASNC%20SPECT%20ProtocolsTracers%20Guidelines2016.pdf).
12. Shaw LJ, Berman DS, Maron DJ, et al. Optimal medical therapy with or without percutaneous coronary intervention to reduce ischemic burden: Results from the Clinical Outcomes Utilizing Revascularization and Aggressive Drug Evaluation (COURAGE) trial nuclear substudy. Circulation. 2008;117:1283-91.
13. Shaw LJ, Weintraub WS, Maron DJ, et al. Baseline stress myocardial perfusion imaging results and outcomes in patients with stable ischemic heart disease randomized to optimal medical therapy with or without percutaneous coronary intervention. Am Heart J. 2012;164:243-50.
14. Maron DJ, Hochman JS, O'Brein SM, et al. International Study of Comparative Health Effectiveness with Medical and Invasive Approaches (ISCHEMIA) trial: Rationale and design. Am Heart J. 2018;201:124-35.
15. White HD, Norris RM, Brown MA, et al. Left ventricular end-systolic volume as the major determinant of survival after recovery from myocardial infarction. Circulation. 1987;76:44-51.
16. Gibbons RJ, Miler TD. Should extensive myocardial ischemia prompt revascularization to improve outcomes in chronic coronary heart disease? Eur Heart J. 2015;36:2281-7.
17. Shaw L, Cerqueira M, Brooks M. Impact of left ventricular function and the extent of ischemia and scar by stress myocardial perfusion imaging on prognosis and therapeutic risk reduction in diabetic patients with coronary artery disease: Results from the Bypass Angioplasty Revascularization Investigation 2 Diabetes (BARI 2D) trial. J Nucl Cardiol. 2012;19:658-69.
18. Hachamovitch R, Hayes S, Friedman J, et al. Comparison of the short-term survival benefit associated with revascularization compared with medical therapy in patients with no prior

coronary artery disease undergoing stress myocardial perfusion single photon emission computed tomography. Circulation. 2003;107:2900-6.

19. Mieres JH, Shaw LJ, Hendel RC, et al. The WOMEN study: What is the Optimal Method for ischemia Evaluation in WomeN? A multi-center, prospective, randomized study to establish the optimal method for detection of coronary artery disease (CAD) risk in women at an intermediate-high pretest likelihood of CAD: study design. J Nucl Cardiol. 2009;16:105-12.
20. Cerci MS, Cerci JJ, Cerci RJ, et al. Myocardial perfusion imaging is a strong predictor of death in women. J Am Coll Cardiol Imaging. 2011;4: 880-8.
21. Hachamovitch R, Kang X, Amanullah AM, et al. Prognostic implications of myocardial perfusion single-photon emission computed tomography in the elderly. Circulation. 2009;120:2197-2206.
22. Zellweger MJ, Hachamovitch R, Kang X, et al. Prognostic relevance of symptoms versus objective evidence of coronary artery disease in diabetic patients. Eur Heart J. 2004;25: 543-50.
23. Hakeem A, Bhatti S, Dillie KS, et al. Predictive value of myocardial perfusion single-photon emission computed tomography and the impact of renal function on cardiac death. Circulation. 2008;118:2540-9.
24. Panza JA, Holly TA, Asch FM, et al. Inducible myocardial ischemia and outcomes in patients with coronary artery disease and left ventricular dysfunction. J Am Coll Cardiol. 2013;61:1860-70.
25. Patel MR, Calhoon JH, Dehmer GJ, et al. ACC/AATS/AHA/ASE/ASNC/SCAI/SCCT/STS 2017 appropriate use criteria for coronary revascularization in patients with stable ischemic heart disease. J Nucl Cardiol. 2017;24(5): 175962.

41

CHAPTER

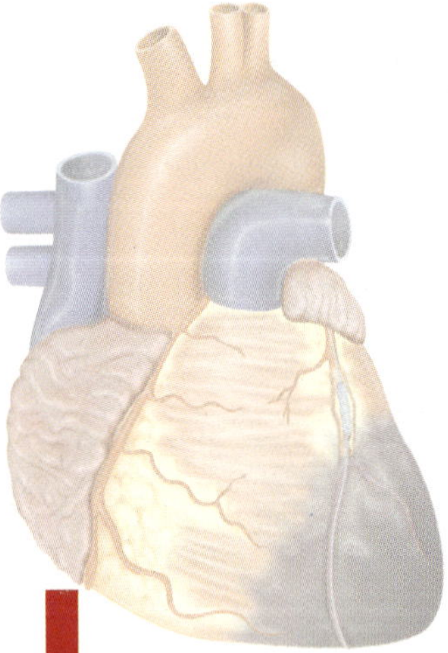

STEMI Intervention: Femoral versus Radial by Conventional Coronary Angiography

Brian Pinto, Neeraj A Desai, Ankeet Dedhia

INTRODUCTION

Percutaneous coronary intervention (PCI) is an integral part of treatment for ischemic heart disease. Coupled with evidence-based pharmacological strategies, the use of PCI in appropriate patients reduces morbidity and mortality across the spectrum of risk.[1] Continual evolution of antithrombotic therapy and device technology has resulted in the application of PCI to a wider population of patients.[2] Procedural success rates are high and ischemic complications relatively rare,[3] thus, attention has turned to periprocedural bleeding complications.[4] Transradial intervention (TRI) approach for PCI has emerged as an alternative to transfemoral intervention (TFI) in many settings and serves as a default access strategy for operators experienced in this technique. The radial artery (RA) is the preferred approach arm, compared with the brachial artery because, in most patients, the hand can remain perfused in the case of RA occlusion via the ulnar artery and a patent palmar vascular arch. This is not the circumstance with brachial access; the brachial artery serves as an end blood supply to the forearm and hand via the radial and ulnar arteries and its occlusion can be devastating. In addition, vascular compression and hemostasis are more consistent in the radial distribution and wrist compared with the upper arm post-PCI. TRI can be used successfully in many complex coronary lesion subsets, including left main disease, bifurcations, multivessel disease, chronic total occlusion, thrombotic, and calcified lesions.[5-15] The efficacy of TRI seems comparable to TFI when used by experienced operators. The learning curve includes proper patient selection, radial access assessment, trouble shooting arm vessel anomalies,[16] guide catheter selection and engagement, augmentation of guide support, and adjunctive device selection. With TRI-specific experience, the operator can effectively utilize this approach in most patients if desired, and maintain the femoral approach as a crossover technique as needed. In this setting, efficacy appears comparable between TRI and TFI. Although vascular complications exist with both approaches, the mechanism of the complications often differs between the radial and femoral routes. TRI in the appropriate settings seems to reduce major and minor bleeding.[17-23]

BLEEDING AND ADVERSE EVENTS IN MYOCARDIAL INFARCTION

Periprocedural blood loss, as defined by thrombolysis in myocardial infarction (TIMI) and GUSTO (Global Use of Strategies to Open coronary arteries) criteria, as well as blood transfusion are associated with higher rates of death and recurrent ischemia in the short-term and long-term in patients with acute myocardial infarction (AMI) and acute coronary syndrome.[24,25] Elderly patients, women, and patients with very high or very low body surface area have higher rates of vascular adverse events post-PCI as well.[26-28] It is noteworthy that patients with myocardial infarction are at the highest risk for bleeding for multiple reasons, but particularly related to anticoagulant/antiplatelet/thrombolytic status and the emergent nature of their procedures. It is also troublesome that bleeding complications in this patient subset are much more likely to be associated with repeat ischemia as well as short-term and long-term adverse cardiac events, including mortality. Major and minor bleeding, which can be particularly life-threatening in the clinical setting of AMI or acute coronary syndrome are lower with TRI. Bleeding events do still occur and remain associated with poorer outcome and therefore cannot be trivialized even with TRI approach,[29] but TRI appears to have a different vascular adverse event profile compared with TFI in terms of the nature and frequency of events. Radial artery occlusion (RAO) is found in ~5% of cases during the post-TRI follow-up period,[30] and a much higher percentage of patients may experience long-standing impairment of RA vasomotor tone of uncertain significance.

It is not currently clear if newer coated sheath designs, improved compression techniques, and increased operator experience have contributed to a reduction in RAO over time. In addition, RA access with inadequate compression technique is prone to pseudoaneursym formation, as is the femoral artery (FA), but with much lower apparent frequency.[31] Finally, a critical ischemic limb complication involving a dominant hand may be a catastrophic life event for a patient, though these complications in the lower extremity can be equally serious and impairing. It is unclear if systematic utilization of TRI for myocardial infarction can compress morbidity and mortality in this clinical patient subset by virtue of reduction in vascular complications, but preliminary data are encouraging.

Why Radial Better?

Numerous studies have shown the superiority of radial access over femoral access regarding the access site complications. Day by day, the radial access site is becoming more preferable and its range of applications is also increasing. Recent studies show a trend toward improvement in outcomes of death and myocardial infarction, whereas previously, the data only supported decreased bleeding, early ambulation, and improved patient satisfaction. These data will continue to increase the number of operators choosing this approach as their default. The biggest reason behind the superiority is its ease of access and relatively small diameter of artery which makes it very easy to achieve hemostasis and can be attained immediately after the PCI procedures.

The RIVAL (RadIal vs. femorAL) study, a multicenter, multinational randomized study evaluated 7,021 patients with an acute coronary syndrome from 152 hospitals in 32 countries randomized to undergo PCI from either RA or FA.[32] A significant reduction in the rates of major vascular access complications from 3.7% to 1.4% with the use of RA compared with FA was observed but no substantial differences in overall rates of bleeding or in mortality were found.

RIFLE-STEACS (Radial versus Femoral Randomized Investigation in ST-Elevation Acute Coronary Syndrome) study, a multicenter, randomized, parallel-group study enrolling 1,001 patients with acute ST elevation acute coronary syndrome (ACS) from 2009 to 2011 also showed significant decrease in access site bleeding (TRI 2.6 % vs. TFI 6.8%, p = 0.002). The cardiac death for the same reason also showed significantly decrease with radial access.[33]

In RIFLE-STEACS, the radial approach was associated with a 36% relative reduction in the primary outcome (13.6% vs. 21%; p = 0.003). Importantly, cardiac death was also reduced with the radial approach compared with the femoral approach (5.3% vs. 9.2%; p = 0.020). The difference was attributed by the researchers to the reduction of bleeding (7.8% vs. 12.2%; p = 0.026), and particularly access site bleeding, because no difference in nonaccess site bleeding was observed between the two groups.[33]

Two studies further address the issue of RA versus FA for primary PCI (PPCI) for STEMI (ST-elevation myocardial infarction). First, Bernat et al.[34] present the results of the STEMI-RADIAL trial (ST-Elevation Myocardial Infarction Treated by RADIAL or Femoral Approach), a multicenter (n ¼ 4) randomized trial of PPCI for STEMI. The study was designed to evaluate only PPCI for STEMI, and excluded patients with thrombolysis or cardiogenic shock who were included in the STEMI subgroup of RIVAL and in RIFLE-STEACS. The primary endpoint was the cumulative incidence of major bleeding and access site complications at 30 days, with a second primary endpoint of net adverse clinical events (NACE) defined as a composite of death, myocardial infarction, stroke, and major bleeding/vascular complications. The primary endpoint occurred in 1.4% of RA (n = 348) and 7.2% of FA (n = 359; p = 0.001). NACE occurred in 4.6% of RA and 11.0% of FA (p = 0.028), although mortality rates were similar (2.3% vs. 3.6%, respectively; p = 0.31). The authors concluded that "in patients with STEMI undergoing PPCI by operators experienced in both access sites, the radial approach was associated with significantly lower incidence of major bleeding and access site complications and superior net clinical benefit. These findings support the use of the radial approach in PPCI as first choice after proper training."

The results of the RADIAL-STEMI trial and the RIVAL substudy complement the observations made from the STEMI subgroup of RIVAL and RIFLE-STEACS trials. Each of the studies used slightly different endpoints so it is difficult to precisely compare results, but some reasonable generalizations can be made about these studies. The reduction in access site complications with RA compared with FA was directionally similar in all studies. Interestingly, overall bleeding was not reduced in these studies, largely because nonaccess site bleeding was not different for the RA and FA groups, and accounted for at least 50% of overall major bleeding. Mortality was lower in the RA versus FA groups in the STEMI subgroup of RIVAL and in RIFLE-STEACS trials, but not in the RADIAL-STEMI trial. As the authors of the RADIAL-STEMI trial concluded, the results from these studies make a strong argument for considering a paradigm shift to RA rather than FA for PPCI of STEMI. The RA approach was introduced several decades ago but received little uptake because of issues including spasm, variations in the pathway from the wrist to the ascending aorta, limitations in catheter sizes, as well as less than optimal equipment tailored specifically for the radial approach. However, improvements in technology, and in technique, have dramatically overcome many of these limitations. Yet several concerns persist among interventionalists, particularly with regard to PCI performed from the RA, that continue to limit wider utilization of this approach, including concern that RA takes longer and is associated with higher radiation exposure than FA cases; the RA will make adherence to a 90-minute door-to-balloon time (DTB) metric problematic; and that it may limit interventional options in complex cases.

The perception that RA has a "steep learning curve," takes longer to perform, and is associated with higher radiation exposure have been addressed by multiple studies as well as by a post-hoc analysis of the RIVAL trial.[32] In the RIVAL trial, overall fluoroscopy times were slightly longer for radial than femoral 9.3 minutes [95% confidence interval (CI): 5.8–15.0 minutes] versus 8.0 minutes (95% CI: 4.5 to 13.0 minutes; $p < 0.01$) but these differences were substantially mitigated by high-volume operators and centers. In the RADIAL-STEMI trial, DTBs were very low and similar in both RA and FA groups, 32 ± 11 minutes and 31 ± 11 minutes, respectively ($p = 0.31$).[34] There also has been concern among interventionalists that the radial approach may limit their options in complex cases, and that the urgent need for revascularization in a STEMI case requires the most flexible approach be taken (i.e. FA). However, techniques have evolved that allow complex PCI, for example use of a sheathless guide technique, and sequential two-stent strategies among others, as well as treatment of graft patients via the left RA. Finally, patients with shock complicating a STEMI are problematic. If support devices are expected to be required, a FA approach is needed for the support device, with PPCI performed from RA or FA on the basis of the operators' experience and comfort level. Ultimately, these technical considerations do not appear to be issues among high-volume RA operators at high-volume center.

CONCLUSION

The studies reviewed above are helping shape the evidence base surrounding the relative benefits of RA versus FA for PPCI for STEMI. What should we take away from these studies? First, in experienced centers with experienced operators, procedures performed from the RA can be performed in the same length of time, using the same amount of radiation and contrast, as the same procedures performed from the FA. Second, access site complications are consistently lower with RA than FA, as would be expected. Third, PPCI for STEMI can be performed via RA with DTBs clinically equivalent to those performed from FA after adequate experience and training. Finally, mortality is the same or possibly lower with RA versus FA for PPCI for STEMI. Based on these considerations is it time for a paradigm shift to a preferred RA approach for PPCI for STEMI? Based on these new studies the answer appears to be yes. Moreover, this transition from preferred FA to preferred RA for PPCI for STEMI represents a natural evolution of strategies aimed at improving safety of coronary interventions. To reap the full benefit of the radial approach, however, a concerted effort by both interventional centers and operators to achieve proficiency in performing PCI from the RA will be needed.

REFERENCES

1. Patel MR, Dehmer GJ, Hirshfeld JW, et al. ACCF/SCAI/STS/AATS/AHA/ASNC 2009 appropriateness criteria for coronary revascularization: A report of the American College of Cardiology Foundation Appropriateness Criteria Task Force, Society for Cardiovascular Angiography and Interventions, Society of Thoracic Surgeons, American Association for Thoracic Surgery, American Heart Association, and the American Society of Nuclear Cardiology. Circulation. 2009;119:1330-52.
2. Batchelor WB, Anstrom KJ, Muhlbaier LH, et al. Contemporary outcome trends in the elderly undergoing percutaneous coronary interventions: Results in 7,472 octogenarians. National Cardiovascular Network Collaboration. J Am Coll Cardiol. 2000;36:723-30.
3. Singh M, Rihal CS, Gersh BJ, et al. Twenty-five-year trends in in-hospital and long-term outcome after percutaneous coronary intervention: A single-institution experience. Circulation. 2007;115:2835-41.
4. Doyle BJ, Rihal CS, Gastineau DA, et al. Bleeding, blood transfusion, and increased mortality after percutaneous coronary intervention: implications for contemporary practice. J Am Coll Cardiol. 2009;53:2019-27.
5. Cheng CI, Wu CJ, Fang CY, et al. Feasibility and safety of transradial stenting for unprotected left main coronary artery stenoses. Circ J. 2007;71:855-61.
6. Hsueh SK, Hsieh YK, Wu CJ, et al. Immediate results of percutaneous coronary intervention for unprotected

left main coronary artery stenoses: Transradial versus transfemoral approach. Chang Gung Med J. 2008;31:190-200.

7. Jabara R, Gadesam R, Pendyala L, et al. Ambulatory discharge after transradial coronary intervention: preliminary US single-center experience (Same-day TransRadial Intervention and Discharge Evaluation, the STRIDE Study). Am Heart J. 2008;156:1141-6.
8. Louvard Y, Krol M, Pezzano M, et al. Feasibility of routine transradial coronary angiography: a single operator's experience. J Invasive Cardiol. 1999;11:543-8.
9. Ranjan A, Patel TM, Shah SC, et al. Transradial primary angioplasty and stenting in Indian patients with acute myocardial infarction: acute results and 6-month follow-up. Indian Heart J 2005;57:681-7.
10. Rathore S, Hakeem A, Pauriah M, et al. A comparison of the transradial and the transfemoral approach in chronic total occlusion percutaneous coronary intervention. Catheter Cardiovasc Interv. 2009;73:883-7.
11. Saghir T, Jan DM, Masood T, et al. Transradial diagnostic and percutaneous coronary intervention. J Coll Physicians Surg Pak. 2003;13:242-7.
12. Sharma GL, Loubeyre C, Morice MC. Safety and feasibility of the radial approach for primary angioplasty in acute myocardial infarction during pregnancy. J Invasive Cardiol. 2002;14:359-62.
13. Yang YJ, Xu B, Chen JL, et al. Comparison of immediate and follow-up results between transradial and transfemoral approach for percutaneous coronary intervention in true bifurcational lesions. Chin Med J (Engl). 2007;120:539-44.
14. Ziakas A, Klinke P, Mildenberger R, et al. A comparison of the radial and the femoral approach in vein graft PCI. A retrospective study. Int J Cardiovasc Intervent. 2005;7:93-6.
15. Ziakas A, Klinke P, Mildenberger R, et al. Comparison of the radial and femoral approaches in left main PCI: a retrospective study. J Invasive Cardiol. 2004;16:129-32.
16. Yokoyama N, Takeshita S, Ochiai M, et al. Anatomic variations of the radial artery in patients undergoing transradial coronary intervention. Catheter Cardiovasc Interv. 2000;49:357-62.
17. Cruden NL, Teh CH, Starkey IR, et al. Reduced vascular complications and length of stay with transradial rescue angioplasty for acute myocardial infarction. Catheter Cardiovasc Interv. 2007;70:670-5.
18. De Carlo M, Borelli G, Gistri R, et al. Effectiveness of the transradial approach to reduce bleedings in patients undergoing urgent coronary angioplasty with GPIIb/IIIa inhibitors for acute coronary syndromes. Catheter Cardiovasc Interv. 2009;74:408-15.
19. Eichhofer J, Horlick E, Ivanov J, et al. Decreased complication rates using the transradial compared to the transfemoral approach in percutaneous coronary intervention in the era of routine stenting and glycoprotein platelet IIb/IIIa inhibitor use: a large single-center experience. Am Heart J 2008;156:864-70.
20. Hamon M, Sabatier R, Zhao Q, et al. Mini-invasive strategy in acute coronary syndromes: direct coronary stenting using 5 Fr guiding catheters and transradial approach. Catheter Cardiovasc Interv. 2002;55:340-3.
21. Lo TS, Hall IR, Jaumdally R, et al. Transradial rescue angioplasty for failed thrombolysis in acute myocardial infarction: reperfusion with reduced vascular risk. Heart. 2006;92:1153-4.
22. Mann T, Cubeddu G, Bowen J, et al. Stenting in acute coronary syndromes: a comparison of radial versus femoral access sites. J Am Coll Cardiol. 1998;32:572-6.
23. Philippe F, Larrazet F, Meziane T, et al. Comparison of transradial vs. transfemoral approach in the treatment of acute myocardial infarction with primary angioplasty and abciximab. Catheter Cardiovasc Interv. 2004;61:67-73.
24. Stone GW, Witzenbichler B, Guagliumi G, et al. Bivalirudin during primary PCI in acute myocardial infarction. N Engl J Med. 2008;358:2218-30.
25. White HD, Ohman EM, Lincoff AM, et al. Safety and efficacy of bivalirudin with and without glycoprotein IIb/IIIa inhibitors in patients with acute coronary syndromes undergoing percutaneous coronary intervention 1-year results from the ACUITY (Acute Catheterization and Urgent Intervention Triage strategy) trial. J Am Coll Cardiol. 2008;52:807-14.
26. Floyd KC, Jayne JE, Kaplan AV, et al. Age-based differences of percutaneous coronary intervention in the drug-eluting stent era. J Interv Cardiol. 2006;19:381-7.
27. Thompson CA, Kaplan AV, Friedman BJ, et al. Gender-based differences of percutaneous coronary intervention in the drug-eluting stent era. Catheter Cardiovasc Interv. 2006;67:25-31.
28. Thompson CA, Kaplan AV, Jayne JE, et al. Impact and temporal trends of percutaneous coronary intervention in the drug-eluting stent versus bare metal stent eras. Am J Cardiol. 2005;96:668-72.
29. Bertrand OF, Larose E, Rodes-Cabau J, et al. Incidence, predictors, and clinical impact of bleeding after transradial coronary stenting and maximal antiplatelet therapy. Am Heart J. 2009;157:164-9.
30. Sakai H, Ikeda S, Harada T, et al. Limitations of successive transradial approach in the same arm: the Japanese experience. Catheter Cardiovasc Interv. 2001;54:204-8.
31. Rao SV, Ou FS, Wang TY, et al. Trends in the prevalence and outcomes of radial and femoral approaches to percutaneous coronary intervention: a report from the National Cardiovascular Data Registry. J Am Coll Cardiol Interv. 2008;1:379-86.
32. Jolly SS, Yusuf S, Cairns J, et al. Radial versus femoral access for coronary angiography and intervention in patients with acute coronary syndromes (RIVAL): a randomised, parallel group, multicentre trial. The Lancet. 2011;377(9775):1409-20.
33. Romagnoli E, Biondi-Zoccai G, Sciahbasi A, et al. Radial versus femoral randomized investigation in ST-segment elevation acute coronary syndrome: The RIFLE-STEACS (Radial Versus Femoral Randomized Investigation in ST-Elevation Acute Coronary Syndrome) study. J Am Coll Cardiol. 2012;60(24):2481-9.
34. Bernat I, Horak D, Stasek J, et al. ST-segment elevation myocardial infarction treated by radial or femoral approach in a multicenter randomized clinical trial: The STEMI-RADIAL trial. J Am Coll Cardiol. 2014;63(10):964-72.

42

CHAPTER

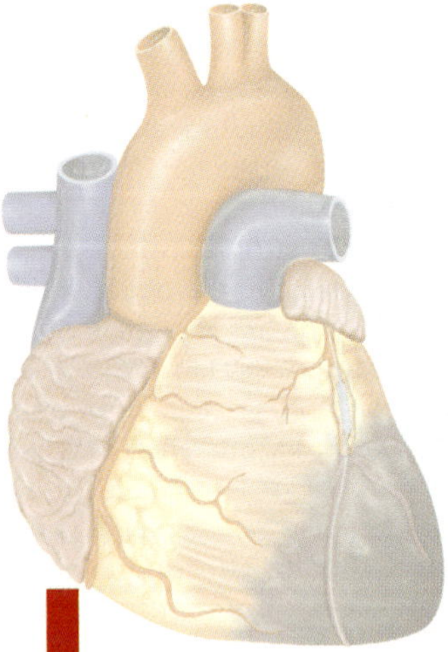

ARBs, ACEIs Effect and Outcome Evaluation in STEMI by Echocardiography

PB Jayagopal, SKM Sarjun Basha

INTRODUCTION

Activation of renin-angiotensin-aldosterone system (RAAS) occurs actively in the process of left ventricular (LV) remodeling. LV remodeling includes changes in ventricular structure, volume, and shape after an acute myocardial infarction (AMI). The process develops in two phases: an early phase with expansion limited to the infarct zone and a late remodeling phase, when the entire left ventricle undergoes progressive dilatation. LV remodeling eventually results in chamber dilatation and sphericity. Initially, ventricular dilatation maintains adequate cardiac output but progressive dilatation may lead to dysfunction and heart failure. Angiotensin converting enzyme (ACE) inhibitors have been shown to attenuate LV enlargement thus reducing mortality after myocardial infarction (MI). Angiotensin receptor blockers (ARB) are another means of inhibiting RAAS that is associated with favorable effects on LV structure and function.

PARAMETERS FOR ASSESSING LEFT VENTRICULAR REMODELING BY ECHOCARDIOGRAPHY

- Left ventricular ejection fraction (LVEF) is the most common metric of cardiac performance in clinical practice, but is influenced by many factors.[1] LVEF estimated by biplane Simpson's method is considered to be the most accurate and the gold standard. Mid myocardial fractional shortening and myocardial performance index are other measures of LV systolic function.
- *LV volume*: End-diastolic volume (EDV) and end-systolic volume (ESV) are calculated using Simpson's method
- LV mass is determined by linear method and 2D method (the area length method and the truncated ellipsoid method)
- Wall motion score index (WMSI) which is obtained by dividing the LV into 16 segments model, and the score for each segment is graded according to the following system: normal-1, hypokinesia-2, akinesia-3, dyskinesia-4. The total WMS is obtained by adding the score of each segment. The WMSI is calculated by dividing the total wall motion score by 16.
- Strain and strain rate.

Longitudinal strain (LS) that is predominantly governed by the subendocardial region is most vulnerable and sensitive to the presence of myocardial disease. While mid myocardial and epicardial region contribute more to LV circumferential (CS) and radial strain (RS), they are relatively preserved or compensated to maintain the LV systolic function in the initial process. A strain value of –15% has 83% sensitivity and 93% specificity at the global level and 76% sensitivity 95% specificity at the territorial level to identify infarction. Global LS, global CS, and global RS represent the global LV contractility and perhaps do not reflect the severity of the infarct area in a cohort with preserved EF. *Injury LS* defined as the average of segmental longitudinal strain more than –15% was a significant predictor of LV remodeling especially in patients with preserved ejection fraction after AMI.[2]

- *Left atrial volume index (LAVI)*: It is the LA volume calculated by biplane area length or Simpsons method and indexed to body surface area. Left atrial enlargement becomes a powerful predictor of long-term outcome. Moreover left atrial dilatation has been shown to predict both all-cause and cardiovascular mortality.[3] Deterioration of diastolic dysfunction is associated with a rise in LV end-diastolic pressure. As *LAVI* is influenced by LV filling pressure, it may be a powerful predictor for the development of LV remodeling.
- Ischemic mitral regurgitation (IMR) can be evaluated semiquantitatively from the area of regurgitant jet by color Doppler or by PISA (proximal isovelocity surface *area*) method.

Two-dimensional echocardiography (ECHO) is a well-established means of assessing LV remodeling. White et al.[4] demonstrated that within groups with varying degrees of post-MI LV dysfunction (defined by LVEF), analysis of LV ESV further risk-stratified patients, thus supporting that it is a more powerful index. Kober et al.[5] established the accuracy of echocardiographic LV volumes using the Simpson's method compared with *in vitro* canine measurements. Subsequently, harmonic imaging and contrast echocardiography have improved 2D echocardiographic image quality. However, estimates of LV volumes derived from 2D images are subject to variability and error caused by inaccuracies in identifying endocardial border, geometric assumptions, beat-to-beat variation in LV volume and function, and selection of imaging plane. LVEF determined by conventional echocardiography and the WMSI has been reported as useful predictor for LV remodeling and clinical outcomes.[6]

Real-time 3D echocardiography has superior accuracy in quantifying ventricular volume, mass, and ejection fraction. It can be performed rapidly, avoids the geometric assumption and problems of image plane position that are associated with 2D ECHO.

EVIDENCE OF ACE AND ARB EFFECTS ON LV REMODELING IN STEMI BY ECHOCARDIOGRAPHY

Measures of LV remodeling have been used extensively to gauge the effect of drug on cardiac structure and function. ACE inhibitors and ARBs have been shown to attenuate left ventricular enlargement thus reducing mortality after myocardial infarction.[7]

The Survival And Ventricular Enlargement (SAVE) trial[8] was a landmark trial which enrolled patients with left ventricular dysfunction (ejection fraction less than 40%) after AMI treated with captropril vs placebo. *Echocardiographic substudy* of the SAVE trial[9] demonstrated reduction of ventricular enlargement after 12 months and was associated with a significant reduction in morbidity and mortality. *SOLVD (Studies of Left Ventricular Dysfunction) trial*[10] in patients with acute myocardial infarction with ejection fraction less than 35% randomized to enalapril or placebo showed improved survival in patient receiving the ACE inhibitor. An *echocardiographic substudy of the SOLVD trial*[11] showed a trend toward reduction in left ventricular EDV in enalapril group compared to placebo. In echo substudy of Gruppo Italiano per lo Studio della sopravvivenza nell' Infarto Miocardico (GISSI3) trial[12] comparing lisinopril vs placebo in AMI showed improved outcomes with reduction in LV volumes and LV enlargement. In the perindopril and remodeling in elderly with AMI *(PREAMI) trial*[13] in elderly postmyocardial infarction patients (at least 65 years) with EF at least 40% comparing perindopril versus placebo showed significant reduction in composite end points of death, admissions to hospital. The *echocardiographic substudy* showed daily dose of 8 mg of perindopril was associated with prevention of progressive left ventricular dilatation.[14]

Similarly ARBs are associated with favorable effects on LV structure and function. Echocadiographic data from the *Valsartan heart failure trial (Val - HeFT)* showed changes in LV end-diastolic dimension index and LVEF over a period of time were independent predictors of patient outcome.[15] The Valsartan in Acute Myocardial Infarction (VALIANT) trial enrolled high-risk MI patients with evidence of reduced left ventricular systolic function and randomized them to captopril, valsartan or both. *VALIANT Echo study*[16] showed similar changes in cardiac volume, ejection fraction, and infarct segment length between baseline and 20 months after MI between captopril, valsartan, combination of captopril plus valsartan. Baseline LVEF, EDV, and ESV were each independent predictors of the primary combined end point of death or heart failure hospitalization. The Optimal Trial in Myocardial Infarction with Angiotensin II Antagonist Losartan (*OPTIMAAL*) compared losartan with captopril. The Echo substudy[17] demonstrated a small but significant decrease in WMSI in patients receiving captopril. The noninferiority of losartan compared with captopril could not be shown. Hence, the role of ARBs in STEMI has at best been as an alternative to ACEI.

Ischemic mitral regurgitation occurs as a consequence of global or regional LV remodeling despite a structurally normal valve, which cause the leaflet tethering by displacement of papillary muscles.[18,19] IMR has been identified as an independent predictor of heart failure (HF) and reduced long-term survival.[20,21] Recent study demonstrated that the use of RAAS inhibitors was associated with better long-term prognosis in patients with MI and significant (> moderate) IMR.[22]

CONCLUSION

Left ventricular remodeling after MI has been identified as a predictor of adverse outcome and as a relevant therapeutic target. Echocardiography is a reliable and noninvasive means to study the process of LV remodeling and dysfunction after MI. RAAS inhibition with ACE inhibitor or ARB in the setting of AMI represents an established strategy to reduce cardiovascular mortality and morbidity.

REFERENCES

1. Konstam MA, Udelson JE, Anand IS, et al. Ventricular remodeling in heart failure: Acredible surrogate endpoint. J Card Fail. 2003;9:350-3.
2. Hsiao JF, Chung CM, Chu CM, et al. Two-dimensional speckle tracking echocardiography predicts left ventricular remodeling after acute myocardial infarction in patients with preserved ejection fraction. PLoS One. 2016:11(12):e0168109.
3. Tsang TS, Barnes ME, Gersh BJ, et al. Left atrial volume as a morphophysiologic expression of left ventricular diastolic dysfunction and relation to cardiovascular risk burden. Am J Cardiol. 2002;90(12):1284-9.
4. White HD, Norris RM, Brown MA, et al. Left ventricular end-systolic volume as the major determinant of survival after recovery from myocardial infarction. Circulation. 1987;76:44-51.
5. Kober L, Torp-Pedersen C, Carlsen J, et al. An echocardiographic method for selecting high risk patients shortly after acute myocardial infarction, for inclusion in multi-centre studies (as used in the TRACE study). TRAndolapril Cardiac Evaluation. Eur Heart J. 1994;15:1616-20.
6. Moller JE, Hillis GS, Oh JK, et al. Wall motion score index and ejection fraction for risk stratification after acute myocardial infarction. Am Heart J. 2006;151(2):419-25.
7. Yoon HJ, Jeong MH, Bae JH, et al. Dyslipidemia, low left ventricular ejection fraction and high wall motion score index are predictors of progressive left ventricular dilatation after acute myocardial infarction. Korean Circ J. 2011;41(3):124-9.
8. Pfeffer MA, Braunwald E, Moye LA, et al. Effect of captopril on mortality and morbidity in patients with left ventricular dysfunction after myocardial infarction. Results of the survival and ventricular enlargement trial. The SAVE Investigators. N Engl J Med. 1992;327:669-77.
9. St. John Sutton M, Pfeffer MA, Plappert T, et al. Quantitative two-dimensional echocardiographic measurements are major predictors of adverse cardiovascular events after acute myocardial infarction. The protective effects of captopril. Circulation. 1994;89:68-75.
10. Pouleur H. Results of the treatment trial of the studies of left ventricular dysfunction (SOLVD). The SOLVD Investigators. Am J Cardiol. 1992;70:135C-136C.
11. Greenberg B, Quinones MA, Koilpillai C, et al. Effects of long-term enalapril therapy on cardiac structure and function in patients with left ventricular dysfunction. Results of the SOLVD echocardiography substudy. Circulation. 1995;91:2573-81.
12. Temporelli PL, Giannuzzi P, Nicolosi GL, et al. Doppler derived mitral deceleration time as a strong prognostic marker of left ventricular remodeling and survival after acute myocardial infarction: Results of the GISSI-3 echo substudy. J Am Coll Cardiol. 2004;43:1646-53.
13. Ferrari R. Effects of angiotensin-converting enzyme inhibition with perindopril on left ventricular remodeling and clinical outcome: Results of the randomized Perindopril and Remodeling in Elderly with Acute Myocardial Infarction (PREAMI) Study. Arch Intern Med. 2006;166:659-66.
14. Nicolosi GL, Golcea S, Ceconi C, et al. Effects of perindopril on cardiac remodelling and prognostic value of pre-discharge quantitative echocardiographic parameters in elderly patients after acute myocardial infarction: The PREAMI echo sub-study. Eur Heart J. 2009;30:1656-65.
15. Wong M, Staszewsky L, Latini R, et al. Severity of left ventricular remodeling defines outcomes and response to therapy in heart failure: Valsartan heart failure trial (Val-HeFT) echocardiographic data. J Am Coll Cardiol. 2004;43:2022-7.
16. Solomon SD, Skali H, Anavekar NS, et al. Changes in ventricular size and function in patients treated with valsartan, captopril, or both after myocardial infarction. Circulation. 2005;111:3411-9.
17. Moller JE, Dahlstrom U, Gotzsche O, et al. Effects of losartan and captopril on left ventricular systolic and diastolic function after acute myocardial infarction: Results of the Optimal Trial in Myocardial Infarction with Angiotensin II Antagonist Losartan (OPTIMAAL) echocardiographic substudy. Am Heart J. 2004;147:494-501.
18. Otsuji Y, Handschumacher MD, Liel-Cohen N, et al. Mechanism of ischemic mitral regurgitation with segmental left ventricular dysfunction: Three-dimensional echocardiographic studies in models of acute and chronic progressive regurgitation. J Am Coll Cardiol. 2001;37:641-8.
19. Kumanohoso T, Otsuji Y, Yoshifuku S, et al. Mechanism of higher incidence of ischemic mitral regurgitation in patients with inferior myocardial infarction: Quantitative analysis of left ventricular and mitral valve geometry in 103 patients with prior myocardial infarction. J Thorac Cardiovasc Surg. 2003;125:135-43.
20. Aronson D, Goldsher N, Zukermann R, et al. Ischemic mitral regurgitation and risk of heart failure after myocardial infarction. Arch Intern Med. 2006;166:2362-8.
21. Amigoni M, Meris A, Thune JJ, et al. Mitral regurgitation in myocardial infarction complicated by heart failure, left ventricular dysfunction, or both: Prognostic significance and relation to ventricular size and function. Eur Heart J. 2007;28:326-33.
22. Okura H, Kataoka T, Yoshida K. Renin-angiotensin system inhibitors in patients with myocardial infarction and secondary mitral regurgitation. Heart. 2016;102:694-700.

43

CHAPTER

Beta Blockers Effect and Outcome Evaluation in STEMI by Echocardiography

Arnab Banerjee, Debabrata Roy

INTRODUCTION

Beta blockers have been the cornerstone of the medical therapy after acute myocardial infarction (AMI) for decades. They impart an immediate benefit of reducing the infarct size, decreasing the incidence of ventricular arrhythmias, and in the long-term, prevent adaptive ventricular remodeling, heart failure, and sudden cardiac death. But most of the trials that have proven the beneficial effects of beta blockers are from the pre-reperfusion era. Effects of these drugs on survival and quality of life are less well defined in the post-reperfusion era, with the advent of improvised reperfusion strategies along with antiplatelets, statins, angiotensin-converting enzyme inhibitors (ACEIs) and angiotensin-receptor blockers (ARBs). Recently, questions have been asked about whether treating patients with beta blockers after an AMIs holds any rationale at all; provided the change in dynamics of the patient profile of present times compared to that of a patient from the seventies or early eighties.[1] All these questions are pertinent because the beta blockers have a considerable amount of side effects (viz. bradycardia, hypotension, bronchospasm, fatigue, reduced libido, depression, new onset diabetes mellitus, and additional burden of an extra medication),[2] and are frequently very poorly tolerated by patients. We try to find answers to some of these questions in our review article as well as shed light on some of the emerging fields in the horizon of the beta blocker spectrum in the subsequent paragraphs.

BACKGROUND

In patients presenting with an AMI, sympathetic activation occurs in response to pain, anxiety, and the acute reduction in cardiac output, initially aimed as a compensatory mechanism to increase cardiac output. However, sympathetic activation leads to a number of negative consequences:

- It increases demand, which in the setting of diminished blood flow leads to infarct expansion.
- It decreases ventricular fibrillation threshold, resulting in increased propensity for sudden cardiac death.

Sympathetic activation over the long-run results in ventricular remodeling and heart failure (HF).

Beta blockers, by their antiadrenergic action, reduces this sympathetic drive and the ensuing neurohormonal imbalance and thereby ameliorate all the negative impacts of the neurohormonal spurt that occurs after AMI.[3,4] They have been shown to reduce the deterioration of left ventricular (LV) function and progression to higher stages of heart failure, and by this they have also been shown to reduce the incidence of malignant ventricular and supraventricular tachycardias after MI and sudden cardiac death.[5] Reduction in the use of other antiarrhythmic medications, incidence of chest pain syndrome[6] and early and late reinfarctions have also been shown.[7] However in patients with compromised LV function, they have also been shown to reduce blood pressure further and increase the incidence of mortality and cardiovascular morbidity and hospitalization, thereby preventing the use of beta blockers in the subgroup of patients who may have needed those drugs the most to put a stop to the harmful mechanism of neurohormonal imbalance and ventricular remodeling, thus leading to a further worsening of heart failure. Again, in most of the studies, that have defined the benefits of beta blockers after an MI, there has never been a clear cut consensus about the duration of use of beta blockers, the dose of beta blockers that provides optimal benefit without increasing the risk of side effects, and the effectiveness of intravenous or oral beta blockers in reducing the magnitude of infarct size and improvement of other echocardiographic parameters.

Diagnostic Modalities of the Left Ventricular Function Postmyocardial Infarction

Various parameters have been used to measure the infarct size. These include quantitative assessment of cardiac biomarkers (troponin I and T, CK-MB mass, etc.), 2D echocardiography to measure LV ejection fraction and WMSI (wall motion score index) and contrast enhanced magnetic resonance imaging (MRI). Although the measurement of cardiac biomarkers is widely available, the predictability of the infarct size from the levels of the same is quite modest. In recent years however, the contrast enhanced MRI can quantify the size of the infarct tissue quite accurately and is being hailed as the new gold standard in LV infarct size estimation. However, the nonavailability of this test at the bedside is a concern. In contrast, 2D echocardiographic measurements are quite accurate and at the same time readily available at the bedside and are comparatively easy to obtain, and hence is arguably the favorite among cardiologists to measure the infarct size after an MI.

Methods of Measurement of Infarct Size and Left Ventricular Dysfunction after Acute Myocardial Infarction by Echocardiography

As already told earlier, LV ejection fraction (LVEF) and WMSI are by far the most commonly used techniques to assess the LV structure and function after an AMI. The reasons being easy availability and bedside assessment; however, these methods of echocardiographic assessments are largely affected by the technical acumen of the person performing the procedure, hence predisposing to interobserver bias. Novel echocardiographic imaging techniques such as speckle-tracking strain imaging provide sound information on the function of the myocardial tissue, over and above that provided by LVEF and WMSI to predict LV functional recovery and clinical outcome after an acute MI. LV global longitudinal strain (LVGLS) assessment after STEMI (ST-elevation myocardial infarction) has also demonstrated considerable accuracy in the assessment of LV function compared to LVEF.

An interesting study was published by Joyce et al. in 2014.[8] In STEMI, patients treated with primary PCI, baseline LVGLS was measured with 2-dimensional speckle-tracking echocardiography. At first baseline apical 4-, 2-, and 3-chamber views were stored and then they were processed offline using commercially available speckle-tracking analysis software. The end systolic frame was defined as the view obtained after the closure of the aortic valve. The LV endocardial border was then traced at the end of systole in all the three views, and the region of interest created automatically was adjusted manually to the thickness of the entire myocardium. Segments were rejected if the quality of tracking was found to be poor after assessment of quality. LVGLS was provided by the software as the average value of peak systolic longitudinal strain of the three apical views, using a 17-segment model in a bull's eye plot. Patients were divided into two groups according to the median value. All these patients were treated according to the institutional MISSION! protocol as per recent guidelines. The independent relationship between GLS groups and LV end-diastolic volume at 3 and 6 months (adjusted for clinical and echocardiographic variables) was measured. The final study population comprised of 1,041 patients (60 +/– 12 years; 76% men). Median LVGLS was –15.0%. Patients with baseline LVGLS more than –15.0% exhibited greater LV dilatation at 3 and 6 months compared with patients with GLS less than or equal to –15.0% (LV end-diastolic volume 123 +/– 44 mL versus 106 +/– 36 mL and 121 +/– 43 versus 102 +/– 34 mL, respectively; $p < 0.001$). This association retained the same statistical significance after adjustment for various relevant demographic, clinical, and echocardiographic characteristics. Further, net reclassification improvement index demonstrated significant incremental value of LVGLS for prediction of LV end-diastolic volume increase ($p = 0.04$). From this study it was evident that LVGLS can readily be used as a marker of LV function after STEMI, albeit with greater accuracy and interobserver variations which plague conventional echocardiographic techniques.

Another study by Grayburn et al. published in 2005 found that three echocardiographic variables: LV end-diastolic volume index, mitral deceleration time, and the vena contracta width of MR predicted the combined end point of death (events-75), heart failure hospitalization (events-97), and transplant (events-9) quite accurately in patients with heart failure.[9] Optimal cut-off points for these variables were 120 mL/m^2, 150 ms, and 0.4 cm, respectively. However, the patients in this study with heart failure were not exclusively due to myocardial infarction, but due to all causes of heart failure. The point that we are trying to make by citing this study is that these three parameters can well be used to predict the mortality and morbidity of patients with myocardial infarction resulting in heart failure, and can be used as measureable parameters in future studies to compare response to different classes of therapies (Table 1).

ROLE OF BETA BLOCKERS AFTER AN ACUTE MYOCARDIAL INFARCTION IN THE POSTREPERFUSION ERA: ARE BETA BLOCKERS OVER-RATED?

In a recent study, data from patients enrolled between 2000 and 2007 in the Global Registry of Acute Coronary Events (GRACE) were used to extrapolate outcomes in three

TABLE 1: Effect of beta blockers.

Trial or meta-analysis	*Principal study*	*Patient population = n*	*Results*
Goteborg trial	Effect of metoprolol on survival during early phase of AMI	1,395	16% decrease in index infarctions, 36% reduction in mortality, 35% reduction in late MI, decrease in VF in the metoprolol treated group at 90 days. Benefit maintained at 1 year
MIAMI (Metoprolol in AMI) trial	IV metoprolol within 24 hours of symptom onset versus placebo, f/b oral treatment for 15 days	5,778	• No statistical difference in mortality • 29% decrease in mortality in high-risk patients in retrospective analysis (p = 0.033) • Nonsignificant decrease in VF and reinfarction
Comprehensive analysis by Yusuf et al.	Mortality and morbidity rates in RCTs of beta blockers after AMI		• Nonsignificant benefit in mortality • No effect on ventricular arrhythmias or infarct size • Significant reductions in cardiac enzyme release, chest pain and development of full AMI in cases of threatened MI
ISIS-1(First International Study of Infarct Survival)	Immediate IV atenolol, f/b oral administration for 7 days versus placebo	16,027	• 15% relative risk reduction in vascular mortality, benefit limited to administration during days 0–1 • Significant lower overall vascular mortality at 1 year (35% versus 25% in controls) • Significant increase in use of inotropes • Nonsignificant increases in complete heart block, nonfatal reinfarctions and cardiac arrests, and no effect on the magnitude of cardiac enzyme release
TIMI-II-B (Thrombolysis in myocardial infarction) study	Effects of immediate versus deferred BB therapy (IV metoprolol f/b oral versus oral metoprolol from D6) in patients receiving IV recombinant tissue-type plasminogen activator	1,434	• Immediate beta blockade produced no improvement in LVEF, nor reduced mortality • Lower incidence of reinfarction (2.7% versus 5.1%, p = 0.02) and recurrent chest pain (18.8% versus 24.1%, p < 0.02) at 6 days versus deferred therapy, but no difference at one year (8.6% versus 9.6%, p = 0.44) • Mean discharge LVEF in both groups was 50% and was unchanged at 1 year
GUSTO-I trial (Pfisterer et al.)	30-day mortality of fibrinolytic-treated patients with ST-elevation MI who received any atenolol (IV, oral or both) or no atenolol		• Use of atenolol was associated with decreased mortality, stroke, shock, and arrhythmias • Increased recurrent ischemia and reinfarction • IV atenolol was contraindicated
Meta-analysis by Freemantle et al. (1999)	82 RCTs analyzed	29,260	• Small and nonsignificant reduction in the odds of death (0.4 deaths in 100 patients) in beta blocker treated patients

Contd...

Contd...

Trial or meta-analysis	*Principal study*	*Patient population = n*	*Results*
COMMIT study	Early IV metoprolol followed by oral metoprolol or placebo within 24 hours of suspected AMI onset. Treatment was up to discharge or 4 weeks in the hospital	45,852	• Early BB therapy had no effect on the primary composite outcome of death, reinfarction or cardiac arrest • Reduction in the risks of reinfarction by 18%, ventricular fibrillation by 17%, and death due to arrhythmia by 22% • 29% increase in death due to cardiogenic shock and a 12% increase in development of CHF
Meta-analysis by Al-Reesi et al.	Eighteen studies assessing the 6 weeks mortality in patients getting beta blockers within 72 hours of index event	74,643	• No survival benefit from acute intervention with BB at 6 weeks • A subgroup analysis after exclusion of high-risk patients (Killip class III and IV) showed small but significant absolute risk reduction of 0.4% in short-term mortality
Norwegian Timolol trial	Effect of timolol administered 7–28 days after AMI, and followed patients for 12–33 months conducted mainly on low risk, clinically stable patients	1,884	• 39.4% reduction in mortality, a 44.6% reduction in sudden death, and a 28.4% reduction in reinfarction rates • Mortality curves showed divergence up to 30 months after which they become parallel • Pedersen et al. reported similar divergence of the curves of the same group of patients on follow-up upto 6 years, in older and high-risk patients
BHAT (American beta blocker heart attack) trial	Randomized patients 5–21 days after acute MI to propranolol, or placebo with a mean follow-up of 27 months	3,837	• Total mortality was reduced by 25%, sudden death by 28% and arteriosclerotic heart disease by 27% • Survival curves diverged for the first year, then became parallel • Recommended propanolol use for at least 3 years
Stockholm Metoprolol study	Oral metoprolol versus placebo for 3 years	301	Significant reduction in cardiac death in patients with a large infarct (32% versus 12.5%), and a significant decrease in sudden death (59%) and nonfatal reinfarction rates (45%) in the metoprolol group
Meta-analysis by Kernis et al. (2004)	Outcome of patients treated with or without BBs in the PAMI-2, PAMI No SOS, Stent PAMI and Air PAMI trials	2,442	• Lower 6 months mortality and Major Adverse Cardiac Events (MACE), with the benefit seen in patients with decreased LVEF (<50%) and multivessel coronary artery disease • Beneficial effect was NOT seen in patients with LVEF>50% and single-vessel CAD

(AMI: acute myocardial infarction; BB: beta blocketer; CAD: coronary artery disease; CHF: congestive heart failure; COMMIT: CLOpidogrel and Metoprolol in Myocardial Infarction Trial; GUSTO-I: Global Use of Strategies to Open Occluded Coronary Arteries; LVEF: left ventricular ejection fraction; MI: myocardial infarction; PAMI: primary angioplasty in myocardial infarction; RCT: randomized controlled trial; VF: ventricular fibrillation)

cohorts of patients admitted with STEMI, based on the use of beta blockers after an MI—early intravenous (+/– oral; 1st 24 hours), only early oral, or delayed (after the 1st 24 hours). Around 13,110 patients were evaluated. Twenty-one percent received early IV beta blockers, 65% received only early oral beta blockers, and the rest 14% received delayed oral beta blockers. Early beta blocker were less likely to be used in older patients, patients with moderate to severe LV dysfunction, and in those presenting with inferior myocardial infarction or Killip class II or III heart failure. IV and delayed beta blocker use were associated with higher rates of cardiogenic shock, sustained ventricular fibrillation or tachycardia, and acute cardiac failure. In hospital mortality was increased with IV beta-blocker use (propensity score adjusted odds ratio, 1.41; 95% confidence interval, 1.03–1.92) but significantly reduced with delayed beta blocker administration (propensity adjusted odds ratio, 0.44; 95% confidence interval, 0.26–0.74). They concluded that oral beta blockers were associated with a decreased risk of cardiogenic shock, ventricular arrhythmia, and acute heart failure.[10]

In spite of the multitude of studies involving the beta blockers, few questions remain unanswered. In the prereperfusion era, the modus operandi was usually to continue beta blockers in a patient after an AMI. But in the reperfusion era, this question becomes very pertinent and has been vexing the cardiologists from times immemorial. How long shall the beta blockers be continued after an index event? Are they at all necessary? Very few studies have dared to tread on these gray areas, and in this age of relentless litigation, these questions become even more evident.

In a study published recently by Jin Joo Park et al., they tried to answer the question about the efficacy of beta blockers up to 3 years after a myocardial infarction.[11] They enrolled all the patients presenting with AMI at Seoul National University Bundang Hospital, between June 2003 and February 2015. The primary end-point was 5-year all-cause mortality, depending on whether the patient was getting beta blockers at discharge, 1 year after AMI, and 3 years after AMI. Of 2,592 patients enrolled in the study, 72%, 69%, 63%, and 60% of the patients were receiving beta blockers at discharge and at 1, 3, and 5 years after AMI, respectively. Patients on beta-blocker therapy had more favorable clinical features, such as younger age (62 versus 65 years; $p < 0.001$). They received one or the other form of reperfusion therapy more frequently (92% versus 80%; $p < 0.001$) than those who were not on any beta blockers. Univariate analysis revealed a lower 5-year all-cause mortality for patients treated with beta blockers at all points. However, beta blockers were not associated with reduced mortality at 3 years of therapy compared to 1 year therapy in the Cox model after statistical adjustment. The authors concluded that the beneficial effect of beta blocker therapy after AMI may be limited until up to 1 year after AMI and whether late beta blocker therapy beyond that period offers any benefit remains to be seen with further randomized clinical trials.

Few of the newer studies in the postreperfusion era have questioned the role of beta blockers after an AMI in the present scenario. The Clopidogrel and Metoprolol in Myocardial Infarction Trial (COMMIT) (n = 45,852 patients, metoprolol versus placebo within 24 hours, 4-week follow-up) revealed that beta blockers had no effect on total mortality, and a reduction of reinfarction and ventricular fibrillation that they commanded was counterbalanced by increased risk of cardiogenic shock.[12] It was also found that the beta blockers had no role in altering the eventuality of cardiovascular events in patients with stable coronary artery disease.

In the largest study till date, based on the data available in Reduction of Atherothrombosis for Continued Health (REACH) registry, 44,708 patients from general practice were included in the period between 2003 and 2004.[13] Thirty-one percent of these patients have suffered an AMI, and they were distributed over a geographical kaleidoscope of 44 countries. No difference in cardiovascular mortality between patients with and without beta blockers was found after a follow-up period of 3.6 years, when propensity score matching was used after adjusting and eliminating factors which may skew the study with bias.

In another study from northern France, CORonariens stables en region NORd-Pas-de-Calais (the CORONOR study) 4,184 patients were enrolled, 2,612 (62%) of whom had suffered infarctions.[14] The follow-up period was 2 years, and a statistically significant reduction in cardiovascular mortality was seen.

A meta-analysis of randomized, controlled studies reviewed 102,003 patients from 60 studies, 12 of which were published in the postreperfusion era (1991–2013).[15] Beta blockers were found to have no effect on mortality, whereas the 1 month incidence of reinfarction and angina were decreased with a reciprocal increase in heart failure and cardiogenic shock. The other 48 studies were published during the prereperfusion era (1966 – 1999), where it was found that beta blockers were inversely correlated with mortality, infarction, and angina.

In yet another recent meta-analysis, 10 observational studies of treatment with beta blockers after percutaneous coronary intervention (PCI)-treated infarction were reviewed.[16] Around 2,168 patients enrolled in this study had been given beta blockers and 15,705 did not receive any beta blockers after the index incident. The primary endpoint was total mortality. In adjusted analyses, mortality was reduced, but the beneficial effect was only seen in study populations with a reduced ejection fraction and those who were not on any other medicinal treatment or were using them irregularly. No effect was observed on cardiac mortality, reinfarction or hospitalizations for heart failure. The authors concluded that there is now no evidence for routine beta blocker therapy for sufferers of myocardial infarction, and that new studies are necessary for further clarification.

CONCLUSION

Most of the studies that involved the beta blockers primarily assessed the mortality and survival benefits of the patients post an AMI. Few of the studies have conclusively shown that beta blockers do comprehensively improve cardiac systolic function post-MI, or more precisely prevent further deterioration of LV function and dilatation of the heart after the index coronary event over a prolonged period of time. In all these trials, the beta blockers have been used along with the standard protocols of care and management as prevalent during the time of conduction of the trials. Keeping in mind the ever evolving field of echocardiography, and the improvement in echocardiographic parameters like LVGLS, there is a scope of immense research in this field, specially the correlation between the effect of beta blockers, ACEIs, ARBs with echocardiographic parameters of the heart post an AMI.

REFERENCES

1. Tidsskriftet. (2016). Is the evidence base for post-myocardial infarction beta-blockers outdated? [online] Available from: https://tidsskriftet.no/en/2016/04/evidence-base-post-myocardial-infarction-beta-blockers-outdated [Accessed October 2018].
2. Kezerashvili A, Marzo K, De Leon J. Beta blocker use after acute myocardial infarction in the patient with normal systolic function: when is it "ok" to discontinue? Curr Cardiol Rev. 2012;8:77-84.
3. Lange R, Kloner RA, Braunwald E. First ultra-short-acting beta adrenergic blocking agent: its effect on size and segmental wall dynamics of reperfused myocardial infarcts in dogs. Am J Cardiol. 1983;51(10):1759-67.
4. Mueller HS, Ayres SM. Propranolol decreases sympathetic nervous activity reflected by plasma catecholamines during evolution of myocardial infarction in man. J Clin Invest. 1980;65(2):338-46.
5. Norris RM, Barnaby PF, Brown MA, et al. Prevention of ventricular fibrillation during acute myocardial infarction by intravenous propranolol. Lancet. 1984;2(8408):883-6.
6. Ramsdale DR, Faragher EB, Bennett DH, et al. Ischemic pain relief in patients with acute myocardial infarction by intravenous atenolol. Am Heart J. 1982;103(4 Pt 1):459-67.
7. Waagstein F, Hjalmarson AC, Wasir HS. Apex cardiogram and systolic time intervals in acute myocardial infarction and effects of practolol. Br Heart J. 1974;36(11):1109-21.
8. Joyce E, Hoogslag GE, Leong DP, et al. Association between left ventricular global longitudinal strain and adverse left ventricular dilatation after ST-segment elevation myocardial infarction. Circ Cardiovasc Imaging. 2014;7:74-81.
9. Grayburn PA, Appleton CP, DeMaria AN, et al. Echocardiographic predictors of morbidity and mortality in patients with advanced heart failure: the Beta-blocker Evaluation of Survival Trial (BEST). J Am Coll Cardiol. 2005;45:1064-71.
10. Park KL, Goldberg RJ, Anderson FA, et al. Beta-blocker use in ST-segment elevation myocardial infarction in the reperfusion era (GRACE). Am J Med. 2014;127:503-11.
11. Par JJ, Kim SH, Kang SH, et al. Effect of beta blockers beyond 3 years after acute myocardial infarction. J Am Heart Assoc. 2018;7:e007567.
12. COMMIT (CLOpidogrel and Metoprolol in Myocardial Infarction Trial) collaborative group. Early intravenous then oral metoprolol in 45,852 patients with acute myocardial infarction: randomized placebo-controlled trial. Lancet. 2005;366:1622-32.
13. Bangalore S, Steg G, Deedwania P, et al. β-Blocker use and clinical outcomes in stable outpatients with and without coronary artery disease. JAMA. 2012;308:1340-9.
14. Bauters C, Lemesle G, Meurice T, et al. Prognostic impact of β-blocker use in patients with stable coronary artery disease. Heart. 2014;100:1757-61.
15. Bangalore S, Makani H, Radford M, et al. Clinical outcomes with β-blockers for myocardial infarction: a meta-analysis of randomized trials. Am J Med. 2014;127:939-53.
16. Huang B-T, Huang FY, Zuo Z-L, et al. Meta-analysis of relation between oral β-blocker therapy and outcome in patients with acute myocardial infarction who underwent percutaneous coronary intervention. Am J Cardiol. 2015;115:1529-38.

44

CHAPTER

Post-PCI Effect and Evaluation in STEMI by Echocardiography

Ankush Sachdeva, Sameer Shrivastava

INTRODUCTION

An early echocardiogram is needed in every patient with ST-elevation myocardial infarction (STEMI) and it has now become a mandate and part of routine protocol to screen every such patient prior to shifting the patient to cath lab. The purpose is to look for regional and global function for both left and right ventricle and to rule out mechanical complications due to STEMI. Echocardiography has a definitive role in deciding revascularization strategies and follow-up postpercutaneous coronary intervention (PCI) using exercise or pharmacological stress testing. Echocardiography helps in managing heart failure in post-STEMI patients, aids to recognize persistent or inducible ischemia, myocardial viability, and need for anticoagulation.

LEFT VENTRICLE FUNCTION AND STRUCTURE

Left ventricle (LV) undergoes changes in acute-phase STEMI depending upon the extent and severity of underlying ischemia. This change is influenced by many factors like presence of edema, use of thrombolytic therapy, loading conditions, and passive myocardial stretch. The bulge in infracted segment further increases overtime as surrounding endocardial area gets involved; the process is termed as infarct expansion. After an acute myocardial infarction, a wide variety of abnormalities can be detected on echocardiography which can suggest decreased blood flow to the involved territory. The ischemic cascade consists of diminished perfusion which can be picked up early using contrast echo.[1] The development of diastolic dysfunction is earliest evidence in favor of STEMI. Use of tissue Doppler and strain rate imaging can pick lesser degree of ischemia early in STEMI. Regional wall motion abnormality occurs before electrocardiographic (ECG) changes develop. Chronic ischemia can show scar and aneurysm formation on echo in long run.[2,3] Impaired contractility of affected segments produces regional wall motion abnormalities on echo. The left ventricle is divided into 17 segments and segmental function is in relation to perfusion territories of three coronary arteries which help to identify infarct-related artery as shown in Figure 1.

The left ventricular dysfunction on echo can be graded as follows:

- *Normokinetic*: Normal contractility and preserved wall thickness
- *Hypokinetic*: Reduced longitudinal shortening or wall thickening

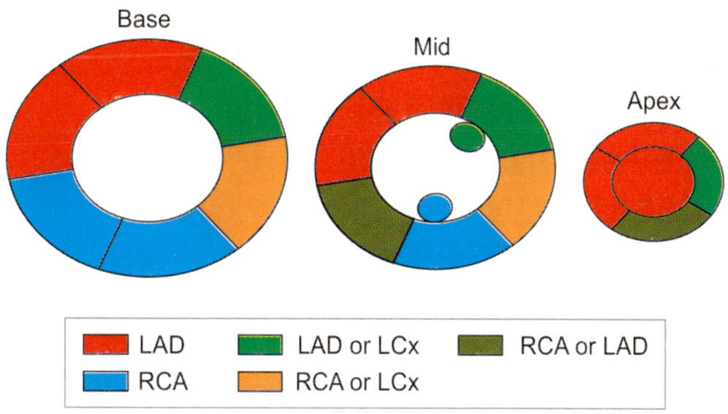

Fig. 1: Representative image of 17 segment model with coronary territory on short axis on echo at base, papillary muscle level, and apex.

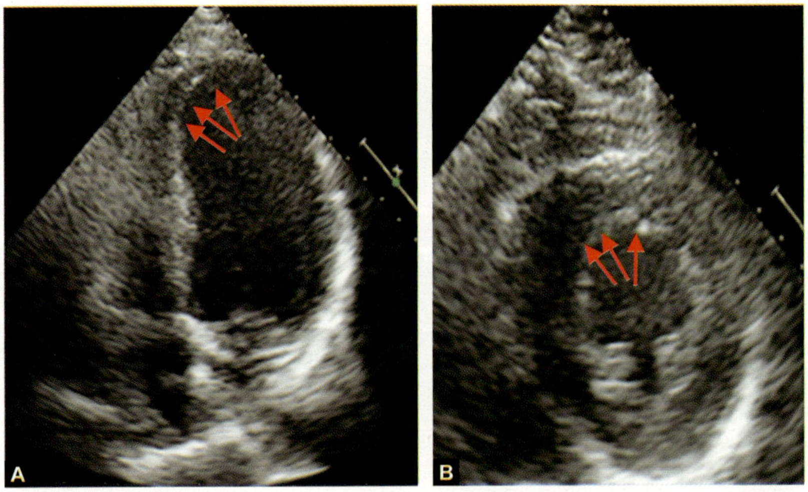

Figs. 2A and B: Regional wall motion abnormality (RWMA) in left anterior descending (LAD) territory in a patient with ongoing chest discomfort in apical four-chamber view and short axis, respectively.

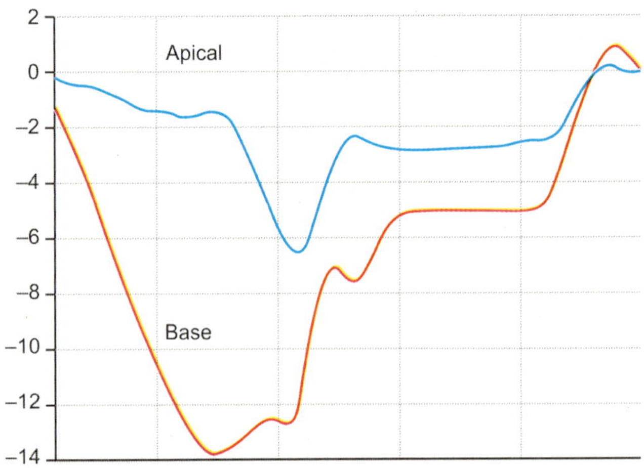

Fig. 3: Decreased strain in distal interventricular septum compared to base in a patient with anteroseptal myocardial infarction (MI).

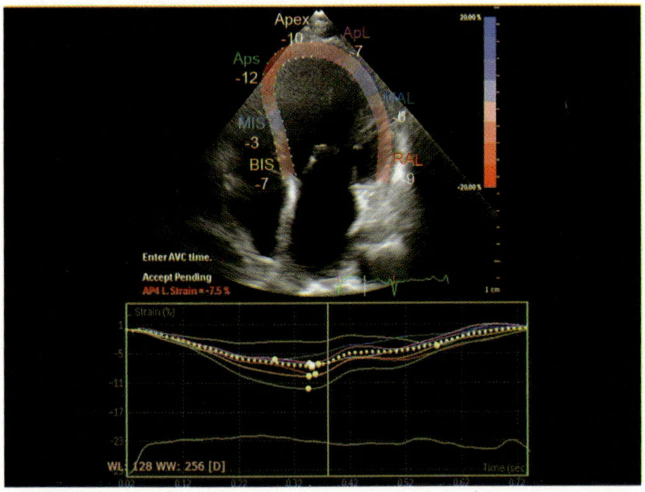

Fig. 4: Figure showing decreased global longitudinal strain in post-PCI patient with history of STEMI. (PCI: percutaneous coronary intervention; STEMI: ST-elevation myocardial infarction).

- *Akinetic*: No deformation
- *Dyskinetic*: Outward segment motion in systole (Figs. 2 to 4).

COMPLICATIONS OF ST-ELEVATION MYOCARDIAL INFARCTION DIAGNOSED ON ECHOCARDIOGRAPHY

Acute Thrombus Formation

Approximately 5% of patients with acute myocardial infarction (AMI) may develop left ventricular thrombus. They are located in akinetic or dyskinetic segments and appear as homogeneous echogenic mass. The more the mobile portions or protruding filaments, the more are the chances of embolic phenomenon due the thrombus. Clot formation in LV may be seen within 24 hours of AMI, some develop at 2 weeks after an event and late thrombus formation after AMI is seen with worsening of systolic function of the LV (Fig. 5).[4]

Right Ventricular Infarction

Right ventricular myocardial infarction (RVMI) should be considered in a patient with inferior wall MI. Clinically hypotension with jugular vein distension and clear lung fields and ECG help to clinch the diagnosis. Echo can show

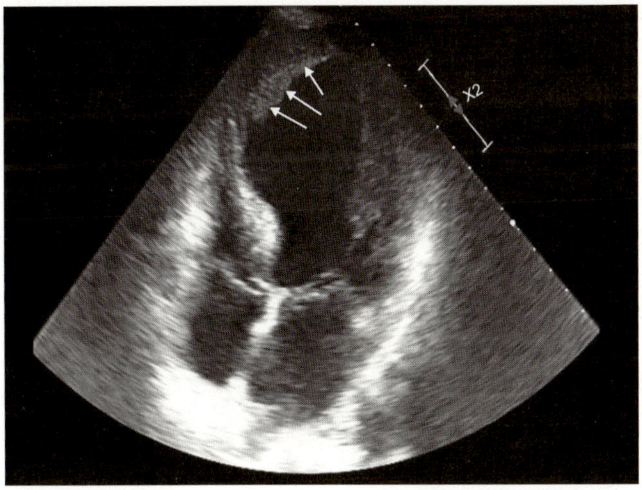

Fig. 5: Soft left ventricular (LV) apical thrombus in a case of acute anterior wall myocardial infarction.

a RV dilatation with depressed RV systolic function with tricuspid regurgitation (Fig. 6).

Acute Mitral Regurgitation (Functional versus Papillary Muscle Rupture)

Acute mitral regurgitation is seen either due to rupture of mitral apparatus which includes the chordae tendinae, the papillary muscles, or a muscle head. There may be impaired coaptation due to papillary muscle ischemia, LV remodeling, and dilatation. The posteromedial papillary muscle is more likely to rupture as it is supplied only by right coronary artery (RCA) in comparison to anterolateral papillary muscle with receives dual blood supply both from left anterior descending (LAD) and left circumflex (LCx) . The rupture leads to sudden volume overload to left ventricle and left atrium which is transmitted to lungs leading to acute pulmonary edema (Fig. 7).[5]

Ventricular Septal Defects

Ventricular septal rupture (VSR) incidence has decreased from 0.5–3% to 0.2–0.3% with reperfusion treatment. Clinically, it is diagnosed by a new onset holodiastolic murmur. Echocardiography can define its location and size, the right ventricular systolic pressures (RVSP). Abnormal communication between right and the left ventricle will lead to oxygenated blood to flow from left into right ventricle and mixing with deoxygenated blood (Fig. 8).

Free Wall Rupture/Pseudoaneurysm

True aneurysms on echocardiography appear as echogenic area of thinned and scarred myocardium and due to stagnant blood flow, clot formation may be seen within these aneurysms. Pseudo or false aneurysms develop after AMI when ventricular free wall rupture is contained by local pericardial adhesions. Pseudoaneurysms are characterized by a narrow neck communicating into left ventricle with tendency to expand and rupture (Fig. 9).[6]

STRESS TEST POSTPERCUTANEOUS CORONARY INTERVENTION

The need for a stress test is determined by a cardiologist. Routine stress testing after coronary intervention has not shown to be beneficial and hence is not indicated.[7-15] A treadmill test (TMT) is done for patients who have undergone PCI when their symptoms and signs have

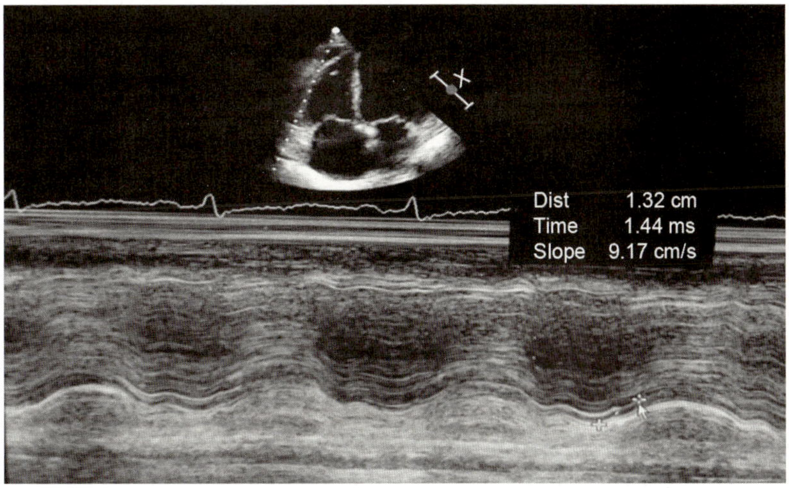

Fig. 6: Right ventricular dilatation and decreased tricuspid annular plane systolic excursion (TAPSE) in a patient with inferior and right ventricular myocardial infarction (RVMI).

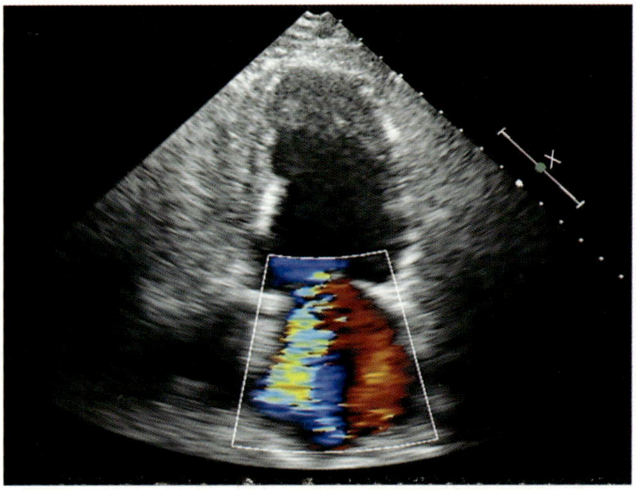

Fig. 7: Apical four-chamber view showing mitral regurgitation a case of acute inferior wall myocardial infarction due to papillary muscle dysfunction.

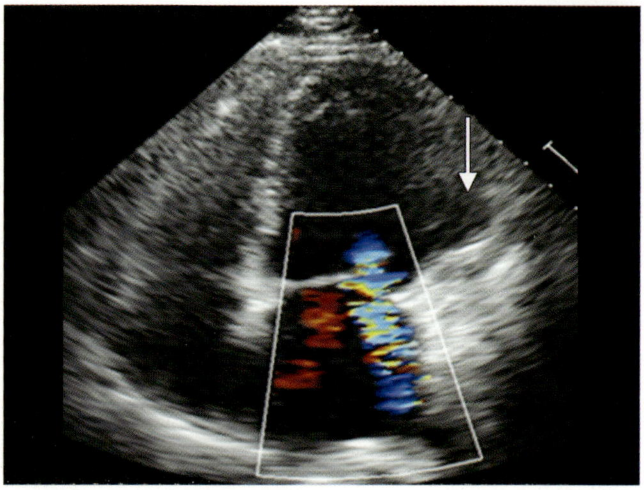

Fig. 9: Aneurysm formation in basal lateral wall (arrow) and mitral regurgitation in a patient with inferior wall myocardial infarction.

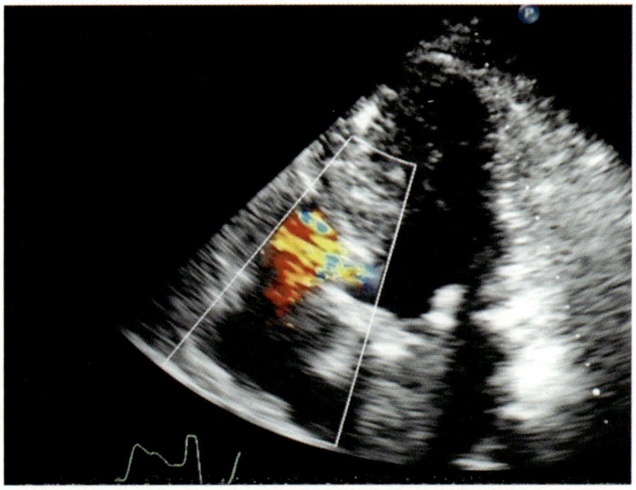

Fig. 8: Ventricular septal rupture (VSR) in basal septum in a patient with acute inferior wall myocardial infarction.

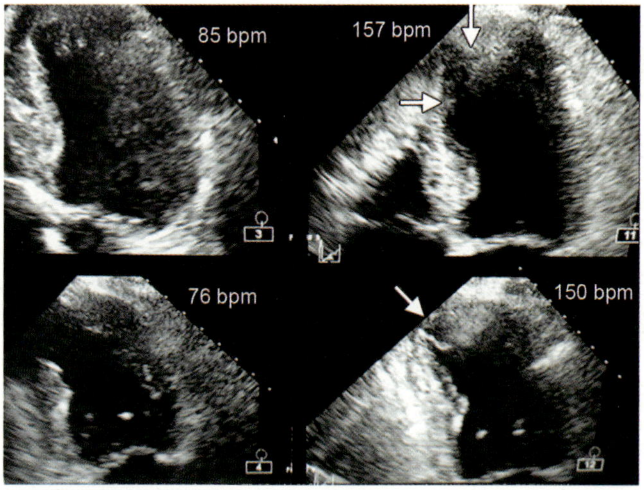

Fig. 10: An exercise stress echo test which is positive for reversible myocardial ischemia in left anterior descending (LAD) territory.

changed or if there is a clinical suspicion that their coronary artery disease (CAD) has become worse. Patients who cannot tolerate physical stress of an adequate intensity should have an imaging study under pharmacologically-induced stress using stress echocardiography, stress magnetic resonance imaging (MRI), or single-photon emission computed tomography (SPECT).[15] Patients with known CAD who develop symptoms again despite treatment and for whom the site of ischemia, the functional quantification of stenosis, or cardiac viability are important questions should undergo an imaging study under physical or pharmacologically induced stress rather than a TMT. An imaging modality should be chosen that is locally available and can be carried out with ease; the adverse effects of ionizing radiation, contrast media, and pharmacological stressors have to be taken into account. The high-risk patients for stress testing include chronic CAD patients or patients with severe left ventricular dysfunction, underlying multivessel disease, patients with diabetes, silent MI, and those who have survived cardiac arrest in the past (Fig. 10).

Diastolic Function

Diastolic function is of prime importance for prognosis and management after STEMI. Restrictive mitral inflow pattern where peak E-wave velocity is more than double on peak

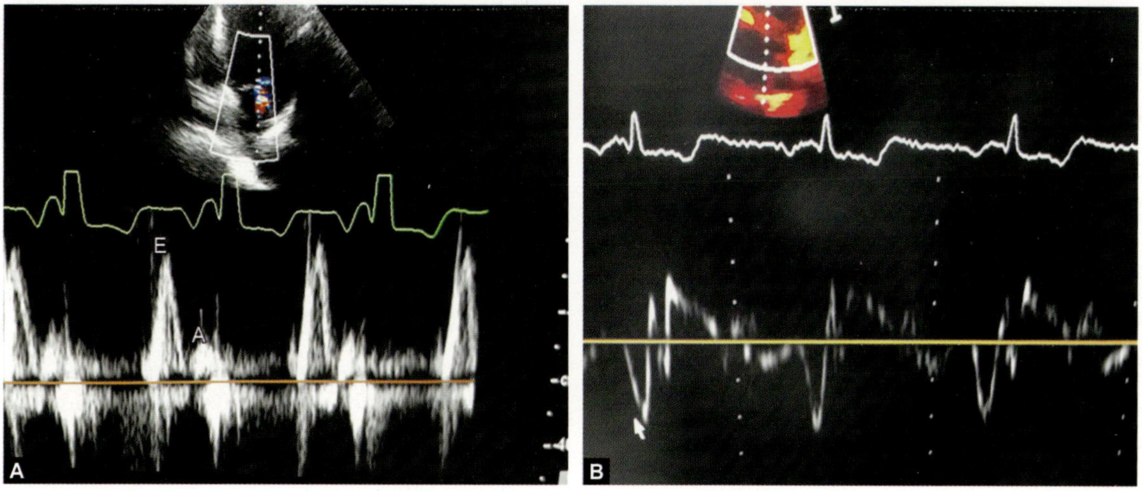

Figs. 11A and B: Restrictive mitral inflow pattern in a post-ST-elevation myocardial infarction (STEMI) patient with severe left ventricle (LV) systolic dysfunction.

A-wave velocity is suggestive of impaired prognosis and when associated with low LVEF has shown to have worse prognosis in large meta-analysis. E/e' ratio when 15 or more is suggestive of increased LV filling pressures and is a predictor of heart failure and mortality (Figs. 11A and B).[16-19]

Other important parameters on echo which suggest adverse prognosis are increased left atria (LA) size (32 mL/m^2) and elevated systolic pulmonary artery pressures measured on echo using tricuspid regurgitation (TR) velocity.[20-22]

MYOCARDIAL VIABILITY

Myocardial stunning is reversible if perfusion is restored early post-MI. If there is a delay and myocardial ischemia persists the cardiomyocytes may remain viable and can potentially recover once perfusion is restored and this phenomenon is termed as hibernation. Hibernating myocardium is studied using low-dose dobutamine stress echo. Echo deformation imaging using tissue Doppler or speckle tracking at rest has been studied for predicting recovery of contractile function.[23-27] In post-PCI cases, the amount of LV dysfunction and the timing of revascularization determine the functional recovery of the myocardium.

CONCLUSION

Echocardiography is accurate for diagnosis of STEMI and the territory involved. It provides prognostic information in patients with STEMI. It can track recovery of function after intervention and identify all mechanical complications of AMI and advanced imaging techniques such as contrast echo, tissue Doppler and strain rate imaging and stress testing have a vital role to play in thorough evaluation and follow-up of patient with myocardial infarction.

REFERENCES

1. Czitrom D, Karila-Cohen D, Brochet E, et al. Acute assessment of microvascular perfusion patterns by myocardial contrast echocardiography during myocardial infarction: relation to timing and extent of functional recovery. Heart. 1999;81:12-6.
2. Neskovic AN, Bolognese L, Picard MH. Echocardiography in acute myocardial infarction. Emerg Echocardiogr. 2005;129-46.
3. Ioannidis JPA, Salem D, Chew PW, et al. Accuracy of imaging technologies in the diagnosis of acute cardiac ischemia in the emergency department: a meta-analysis. Ann Emerg Med. 2001;37:471-7.
4. Jugdutt BI, Sivaram CA. Prospective two-dimensional echocardiographic evaluation of LV thrombus and embolism after acute myocardial infarction. J Am Coll Cardiol. 1989;13:554-64.
5. Kishon Y, Iqbal A, Oh JK, et al. Evolution of echocardiographic modalities in detection of post myocardial infarction ventricular septal defect and papillary muscle rupture: study of 62 patients. Am Heart J. 1993;126:667-75.
6. Lopez-Sendon J, Gonzalez A, Lopez de Sa E, et al. Diagnosis of subacute ventricular wall rupture after acute myocardial infarction: Sensitivity and specificity of clinical, hemodynamic and echocardiographic criteria. J Am Coll Cardiol. 1992;19:1145-53.
7. Levine GN, Bates ER, Blankenship JC, et al. ACCF/AHA/ SCAI guideline for percutaneous coronary intervention: a report of the American College of Cardiology Foundation/American Heart Association Task Force on Practice Guidelines and the Society for Cardiovascular Angiography and Interventions. Circulation. 2011;124:e574-651.
8. Wijns W, Kolh P, Danchin N, et al. Guidelines on myocardial revascularization. Eur Heart J. 2010;31:2501-55.

9. Scanlon PJ, Faxon DP, Audet AM, et al. ACC/AHA guidelines for coronary angiography: Executive summary and recommendations. A report of the American College of Cardiology/American Heart Association Task Force on Practice Guidelines (Committee on Coronary Angiography) developed in collaboration with the Society for Cardiac Angiography and Interventions. Circulation. 1999;99:2345-57.
10. Hamm CW, Bassand JP, Agewall S, et al. ESC guidelines for the management of acute coronary syndromes in patients presenting without persistent ST-segment elevation: The task force for the management of acute coronary syndromes (ACS) in patients pre-stenting without persistent ST-segment elevation of the European Society of Cardiology (ESC). Eur Heart J. 2011;32:2999-3054.
11. Wright RS, Anderson JL, Adams CD, et al. 2011 ACCF/AHA focused update of the guidelines for the management of patients with unstable angina/non-ST-elevation myocardial infarction (updating the 2007 guideline): a report of the American College of Cardiology Foundation/American Heart Association Task Force on Practice Guidelines developed in collaboration with the American College of Emergency Physicians, Society for Cardiovascular Angiography and Interventions, and Society of Thoracic Surgeons. J Am Coll Cardiol. 2011;57:1920-59.
12. George JC, Dangas GD. 2009 Focused updates to guidelines in ST-elevation myocardial infarction and percutaneous coronary intervention: Application to interventional cardiology. JACC Cardiovasc Interv. 2010;3:256-8.
13. Smith SC, Feldman TE, Hirshfeld JW, et al. ACC/AHA/SCAI 2005 guideline update for percutaneous coronary intervention: a report of the American College of Cardiology/American Heart Association Task Force on Practice Guidelines (ACC/AHA/SCAI Writing Committee to Update 2001 Guidelines for Percutaneous Coronary Intervention). Circulation. 2006;113:e166-286.
14. Cheitlin MD, Armstrong WF, Aurigemma GP, et al. ACC/AHA/ASE 2003 guideline update for the clinical application of echocardiography: summary article: a report of the American College of Cardiology/American Heart Association Task Force on Practice Guidelines (ACC/AHA/ASE Committee to Update the 1997 Guidelines for the Clinical Application of Echocardiography). Circulation. 2003;108:1146-62.
15. Klocke FJ, Baird MG, Lorell BH, et al. ACC/AHA/ASNC guidelines for the clinical use of cardiac radionuclide imaging—executive summary: a report of the American College of Cardiology/American Heart Association Task Force on Practice Guidelines (ACC/AHA/ASNC Committee to Revise the 1995 Guidelines for the Clinical Use of Cardiac Radionuclide Imaging). Circulation. 2003;108:1404-18.
16. Yamamoto K, Nishimura RA, Chaliki HP, et al. Determination of left ventricular filling pressure by Doppler echocardiography in patients with coronary artery disease: Critical role in left ventricular systolic function. J Am Coll Cardiol. 1997;30:1819-26.
17. Meta-analysis Research Group in Echocardiography (MeRGE) AMI Collaborators. Independent prognostic importance of a restrictive left ventricular filling pattern after myocardial infarction: An individual patient meta-analysis: Meta-analysis research group in echocardiography acute myocardial infarction. Circulation. 2008;117:2591-8.
18. Cerisano G, Pucci PD, Valenti R, et al. Comparison of the usefulness of Doppler-derived deceleration time versus plasma brain natriuretic peptide to predict left ventricular remodeling after mechanical revascularization in patients with ST-elevation acute myocardial infarction and left ventricular systolic dysfunction. Am J Cardiol. 2005;95:930-4.
19. Hillis GS, Moller JE, Pellikka PA, et al. Noninvasive estimation of left ventricular filling pressure by E/e' is a powerful predictor of survival after acute myocardial infarction. J Am Coll Cardiol. 2004;43:360-7.
20. Kruszewski K, Scott AE, Barclay JL, et al. Noninvasive assessment of left ventricular filling pressure after acute myocardial infarction a prospective study of the relative prognostic utility of clinical assessment, echocardiography, and B-type natriuretic peptide. Am Heart J. 2010;159:47-54.
21. Møller JE, Hillis GS, Oh JK, et al. Left atrial volume: A powerful predictor of survival after acute myocardial infarction. Circulation. 2003;107:2207-12.
22. Møller JE, Hillis GS, Oh JK, et al. Prognostic importance of secondary pulmonary hypertension after acute myocardial infarction. Am J Cardiol. 2005;96:199-203.
23. Rahimtoola SH, Dilsizian V, Kramer CM, et al. Chronic ischemic left ventricular dysfunction: from pathophysiology to imaging and its integration into clinical practice. JACC Cardiovasc Imaging. 2008;1:536-55.
24. Carluccio E, Biagioli P, Alunni G, et al. Effect of revascularizing viable myocardium on left ventricular diastolic function in patients with ischaemic cardiomyopathy. Eur Heart J. 2009;30:1501-9.
25. Kim RJ, Wu E, Rafael A, et al. The use of contrast-enhanced magnetic resonance imaging to identify reversible myocardial dysfunction. N Engl J Med. 2000;343:1445-53.
26. Ichikawa Y, Sakuma H, Suzawa N, et al. Late gadolinium-enhanced magnetic resonance imaging in acute and chronic myocardial infarction. Improved prediction of regional myocardial contraction in the chronic state by measuring thickness of nonenhanced myocardium. J Am Coll Cardiol. 2005;45:901-9.
27. Knuesel PR, Nanz D, Wyss C, et al. Characterization of dysfunctional myocardium by positron emission tomography and magnetic resonance: relation to functional outcome after revascularization. Circulation. 2003;108:1095-1100.

45

CHAPTER

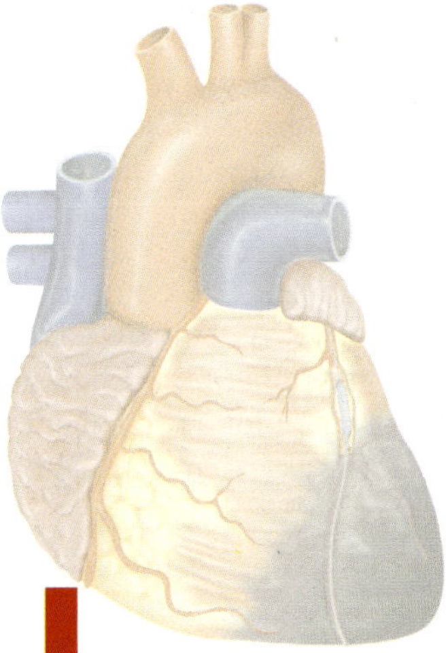

Coronary Artery Disease Evaluation by Coronary Doppler Imaging

Anjaneyulu V Anne

INTRODUCTION

Though several new cardiac imaging techniques have emerged, invasive coronary angiography remains the gold standard in evaluating coronary arteries for measuring anatomic severity of the stenotic lesion and assisting in intracoronary interventions. Transthoracic echocardiography (TTE) evaluation of coronary artery disease (CAD) was mostly limited to assessment of regional and global myocardial function. Several workers[1-3] have attempted to image the coronary arteries by echocardiography. With improvements in ultrasound machines and introduction of harmonic imaging and high-frequency transducers, direct visualization of long segments of all three coronary arteries is now possible. Though the entire artery cannot be reconstructed, multiple segments can be visualized, flow velocity can be measured, thus enabling us to obtain useful anatomic and physiologic information. Careful evaluation of coronary flows can be translated into a wide variety of clinical applications (Box 1).

TECHNICAL CONSIDERATIONS

A high-quality ultrasound machine gives good quality imaging for coronaries. 5.0 MHz or 3.5 MHz narrow-band sector transducers in second harmonic mode are used for B-mode examination and color Doppler mapping and spectral Doppler coronary flow velocity assessment are performed at 2.5 MHz or 2 MHz. After obtaining good quality B-mode image, coronary segments should be searched, using color flow with or without use of harmonics. Sample size of color Doppler should be at minimum, velocity range should be set with a low Nyquist limit (15–20 cm/s), and filters should be decreased. Some ultrasound systems provide special color maps for coronary artery evaluation including second or third harmonics of B-mode and color, low Nyquist limit, special gain for B-mode and Doppler mode, etc.

SEGMENTAL EVALUATION OF CORONARY ARTERIES

Standard parasternal short- and long-axis views from second or third intercostal space or low parasternal long- or short-axis views from fourth or fifth intercostals space should be used. Coronary arteries appear as linear

BOX 1: Clinical applications.

- Identification of coronary stenosis in the LM, LAD, and PDA
- Measurement of coronary flow velocity at rest and after stress
- Diagnosis of reperfusion in LAD after acute anterior myocardial infarction
- Identification of chronic occluded LAD and RCA
- Assessment of endothelial function
- Measurement of coronary flow reserve noninvasively
- Detection of restenosis after percutaneous interventions in the LM, LAD, and RCA
- Differentiating ischemic from nonischemic cardiomyopathy
- Assessment of coronary bypass graft patency.

(LAD: left anterior descending; LM: left main; PDA: posterior descending artery; RCA: right coronary artery) intramyocardial color segments of approximately 0.5–2.5 cm in length and 2–4 mm in diameter. Initially after obtaining a short segment, step-by-step movement of the transducer along the course of the vessel will bring longer segments into view.

Left Main and Left Anterior Descending Artery

With the patient in left lateral decubitus position, parasternal short-axis view of the great vessels is obtained. In the plane immediately below the pulmonary trunk, left main (LM) and proximal left anterior descending (LAD) can be visualized by B-mode. Consecutive clockwise and cranial rotation of the transducer helps to locate these segments. The LM has approximately 1–3 cm length and is usually visualized along its entire course bifurcation of the vessel into the LAD and circumflex (Cx) (Fig. 1A) delineates the distal LM. The apical view is used for visualizing the distal LAD and its flow velocity measurements.

Left Circumflex Artery

The circumflex is visualized in parasternal short-axis view in a plane immediately below the pulmonary trunk just below the left atrial appendage. The normal antegrade flow in proximal Cx appears as blue linear color signal.

Right Coronary Artery

Proximal right coronary artery (RCA) can be easily visualized in parasternal short-axis plane. Middle and distal RCA segments need color Doppler assistance for their visualization. Distal RCA can be assessed using apical window.

Normal Flow Velocities

Coronary flow is biphasic, predominantly diastolic. Normal flow velocity spectrum consists of two forward flow components: smaller, dome-like systolic, and bigger diastolic (Fig. 1C). The maximal flow velocities in

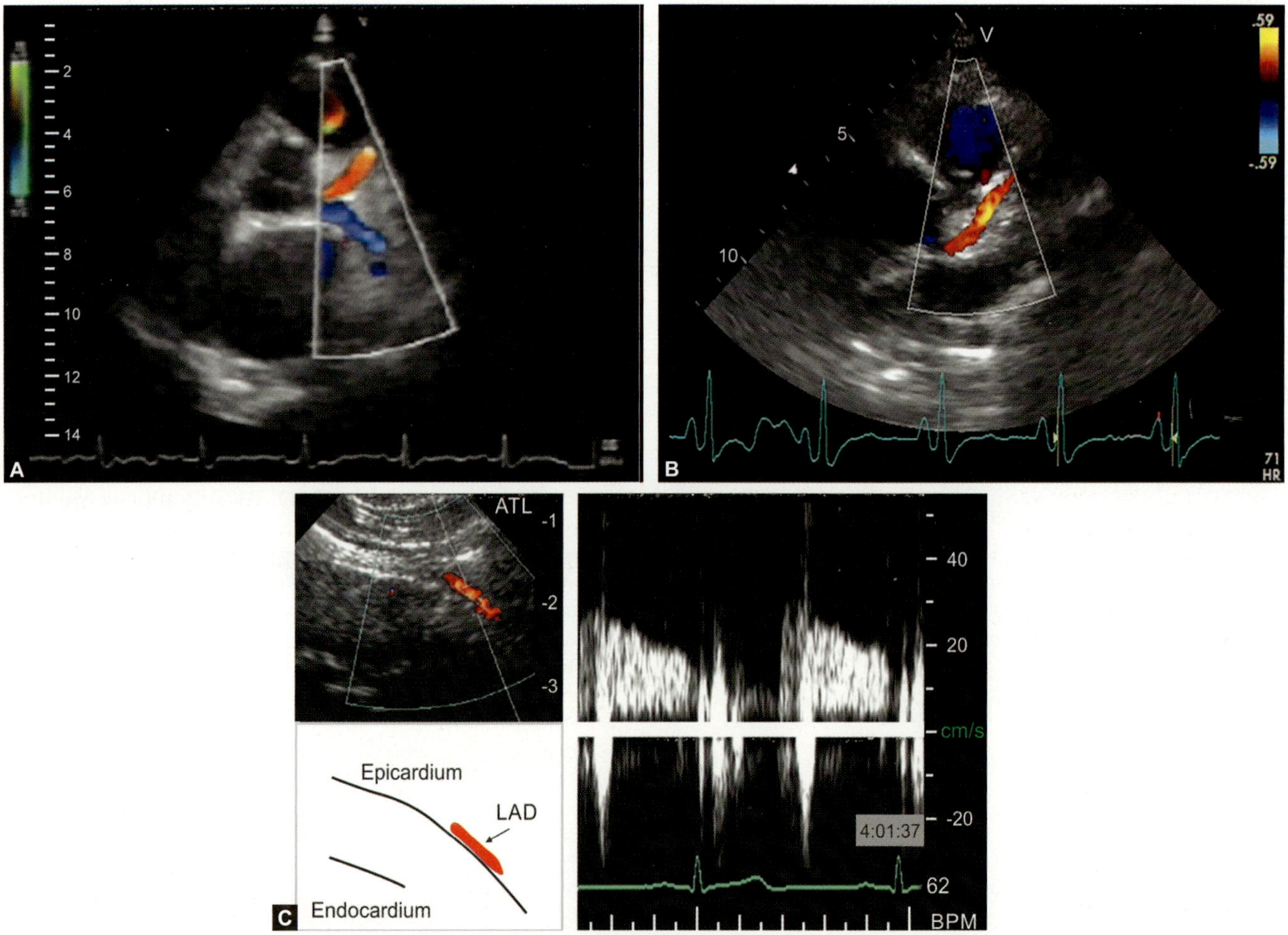

Figs. 1A to C: Normal coronary flows. (A) Short left main coronary artery dividing into LAD, and Cx—both of them showing laminar flows; (B) Laminar flow in LM continuing into proximal LAD; and (C) Normal Doppler flow velocity in distal LAD (0.3 m/s). (Cx: circumflex; LAD: left anterior descending).

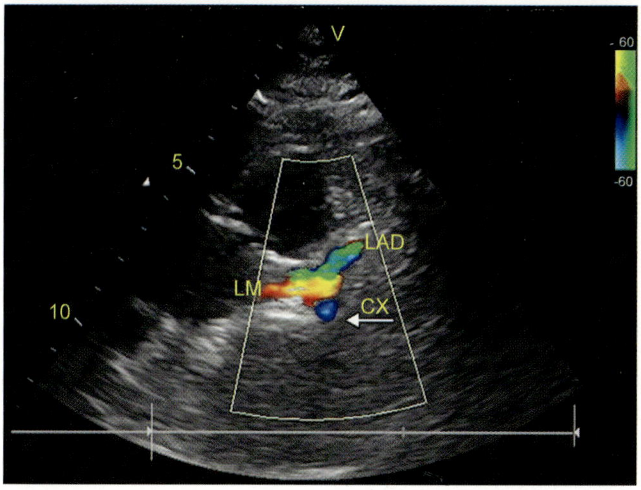

Fig. 2: Mosaic flow in proximal left anterior descending (LAD).

nonstenosed proximal parts of LAD, Cx, and RCA is in the range of 0.7 m/s. Control subjects with normal coronary angiograms and normal LV function had a peak diastolic velocity in the distal LAD in the range of 21.2 ± 7.9 cm/s. The velocity increases at the site of stenosis. The proportion of maximal flow *in* diastole velocities to systole change distal to a significant stenosis. Flow velocities vary considerably depending on many factors: heart rate, blood pressure, thickness of myocardium, hyperdynamic circulatory states—hyperthyroidism, anemia, and renal failure, etc.

The color Doppler pattern in the normal coronary artery is uniformly consistent with laminar flow (Fig. 1B). At the site of stenosis, focal flow acceleration and turbulence may be detected as aliasing zone (Fig. 2). The Doppler velocity should be measured at the point of focal aliasing. Krznowski[2] et al. and Saraste[3] et al. showed that a local peak diastolic flow velocity more than 2.0 m/s could be used as a sign of diameter reduction of more than 50% for all three main coronary arteries. Since LM and proximal LAD segment are almost horizontal and exceed the 60° angle, one can rely on mosaic flow to determine significant stenosis in these segments. A local maximal flow velocity more than 1.5 m/s is also a reasonably accurate sign of stenosis (Anjaneyulu et al., 2008).[4] Hozumi et al.[5] have observed localized aliasing by color flow mapping in 100% of patients with LAD restenosis of more than 50% after coronary angioplasty and 56% of patients without restenosis. The ratio of stenotic to prestenotic velocities of more than 2.0 has been used by most workers, as this allows exclusion or minimization of hemodynamic influence.

Artifacts and other Sources of Errors

Most of the artifacts are due to the heart movement and make the examination difficult—especially for RCA and Cx. Flow in the adjacent pericardial sac can create a strong signal which may be confused with flow within a coronary artery. This can be resolved by timing—pericardial flow signal is systolic while coronary flow is predominantly diastolic. Some large branches of coronary arteries—the ramus, diagonal, and marginal branches can be confused with principal coronary arteries, mostly the LAD and Cx.

FEASIBILITY OF VISUALIZING CORONARY ARTERIES BY TRANSTHORACIC ECHOCARDIOGRAPHY

Feasibility of visualizing coronary arteries with the addition of harmonics, newer transducers, and contrast agents has been reported to be as high as 100% for distal LAD and 33–97% for posterior descending artery (PDA). Imaging of entire Cx and mid-RCA has been possible with a low rate. Only skilled operators can be expected to achieve a 90% success rate in visualizing the coronary arteries. TTE with both the use of peak diastolic flow velocity more than 2.0 m/s and stenotic to prestenotic peak velocity ratio more than 2.0 revealed 48% of all LAD stenoses, 30% of all Cx stenoses, and 14% of all RCA stenosis (Table 1).

TABLE 1: Diagnostic accuracy of Doppler TEE in the detection of more than 50% stenosis in main coronary arteries (Boshchenko et al., 2008).

Coronary artery	*Coronary angiography*				*Transthoracic echocardiography*			
	Stenosis	*Stenosis*	*False positive*	*False negative*	*Sensitivity*	*Specificity*	*Positive predictive value*	*Negative predictive value*
LMCA (n = 100)	1	0	0	1	-	100	-	97
LAD (n = 300)	55	39	8	24	56	96	79	89
Cx (n = 300)	28	6	4	26	7	94	33	70
RCA (n = 300)	47	21	9	35	26	93	57	78

(Cx: circumflex; LAD: left anterior descending; LMCA: left main coronary artery; RCA: right coronary artery; TTE: transthoracic echocardiography)

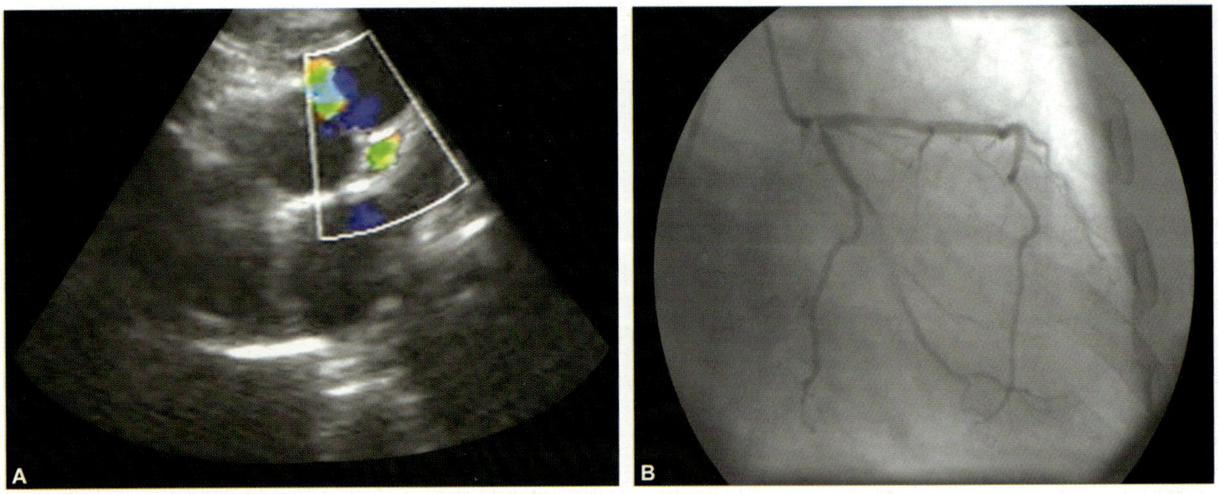

Figs. 3A and B: LM stenosis. (A) Mosaic flow in left main coronary artery; and (B) Coronary angiography showing severe left main stenosis in the same patient.

Left Main Coronary Artery Stenosis

Anjaneyulu et al.[4] studied a total of 1,456 patients with CAD of which 801 patients (55%) had adequate coronary flow assessment by TTE. Using the criteria of either color aliasing (Figs. 3A and B) or a peak diastolic flow velocity of more than 1.5 m/s, LM stenosis of more than 50% could be diagnosed with a sensitivity of 85% and specificity of 88%. In view of this high degree of specificity and sensitivity, LM flows should be assessed by TTE in patients with rest angina, familial hypercholesterolemia, Takayasu disease (aorto-arteritis). LM flow evaluation is also useful in patients who undergo LM stenting—to assess stent patency. Prior knowledge of LM stenosis will enable the angiographer to take precautions, while engaging the LM ostium during coronary angiography and also to counsel the relatives about the need for an urgent intervention.

Detection of Total Coronary Occlusion: Coronary Collaterals

Absence of coronary flow on color Doppler map is not a reliable sign of total occlusion. At present, TTE is not a suitable method to diagnose acute coronary occlusions. However, chronic total occlusions (CTOs) can be picked up by identifying coronary collaterals. Watanabe et al.[6] proposed the reversal of coronary flow in epicardial collateral vessels to be the main ultrasound sign of CTO. It has been established that retrograde flow in distal LAD is a good marker of total LAD occlusion with 88% sensitivity and 100% specificity (Hirata et al.)[7] and retrograde flow in PDA is a good marker of RCA occlusion with 67% sensitivity and 100% specificity (Otsuka et al.).[8] Identifying intramyocardial collaterals in the interventricular septum (Figs. 4A and B) have increased the sensitivity in the CTO detection from 88% to 96% for the LAD and from 67% to 80% for the RCA (Otsuka et al., Saraste et al.).[8] Identifying collateral flow in interventricular septum is a vital clue to diagnose anomalous left coronary artery origin from pulmonary artery (ALCAPA) (Fig. 4C).[9]

Detection of Recanalized Left Anterior Descending after Thrombolysis by Transthoracic Echocardiography

Anjaneyulu et al.[10] have attempted to show reperfusion after thrombolysis in LAD in 12 patients of acute anterior wall myocardial infarction. Color flow imaging in proximal, mid, and distal LAD segments was done every 15 minutes for 6 hours after initiating thrombolysis. In seven patients, flow could be demonstrated in LAD within 15 minutes to 6 hours after initiating thrombolysis. Also, a focal area of color turbulence could be shown in these patients in LAD after the reappearance of flow (Figs. 5A and B), which correlated with the site of significant stenosis on coronary angiography.

CORONARY STENT ASSESSMENT

Maxted et al.[11] attempted to locate stents in proximal and mid-LAD, using criteria such as—increased echogenicity, stented lumen with relatively straight edges, and a diameter approximately equal to the deployed stent. Stents were determined in 10 of 13 cases. Direct assessment of stent flow is possible in LM and proximal LAD segments. Any turbulence with increased flow velocities more than 1.5 m/s would suggest restenosis (Fig. 6). Indirect assessment of LAD

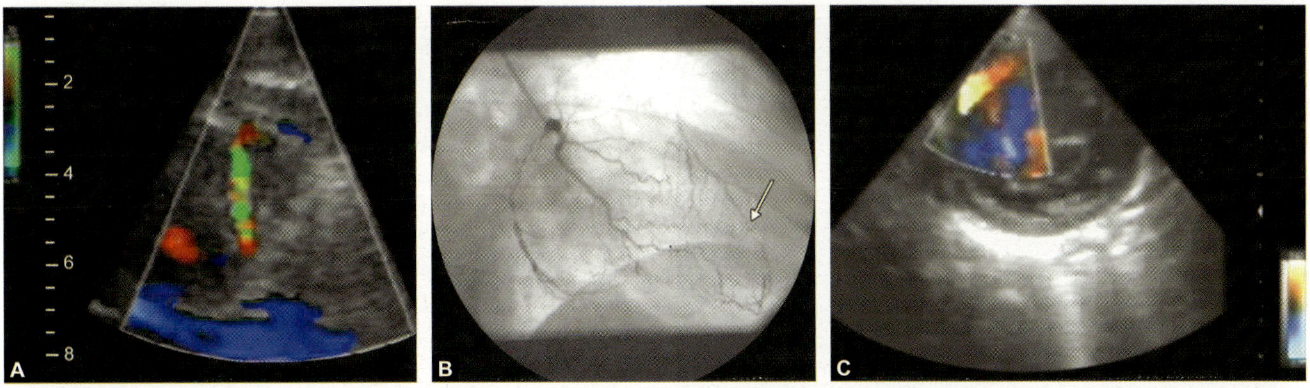

Figs. 4A to C: Coronary collaterals by TTE. (A) Mosaic collateral flow in distal inter ventricular septum directed from base to apex of left ventricle (RCA → LAD collaterals); (B) RCA injection in the same patient showing LAD opacification through collaterals at the apex; and (C) Continuous flow in interventricular septum directed anteriorly in a case of ALCAPA. (ALCAPA: anomalous left coronary artery origin from pulmonary artery; LAD: left anterior descending; RCA: right coronary artery; TTE: transthoracic echocardiography).

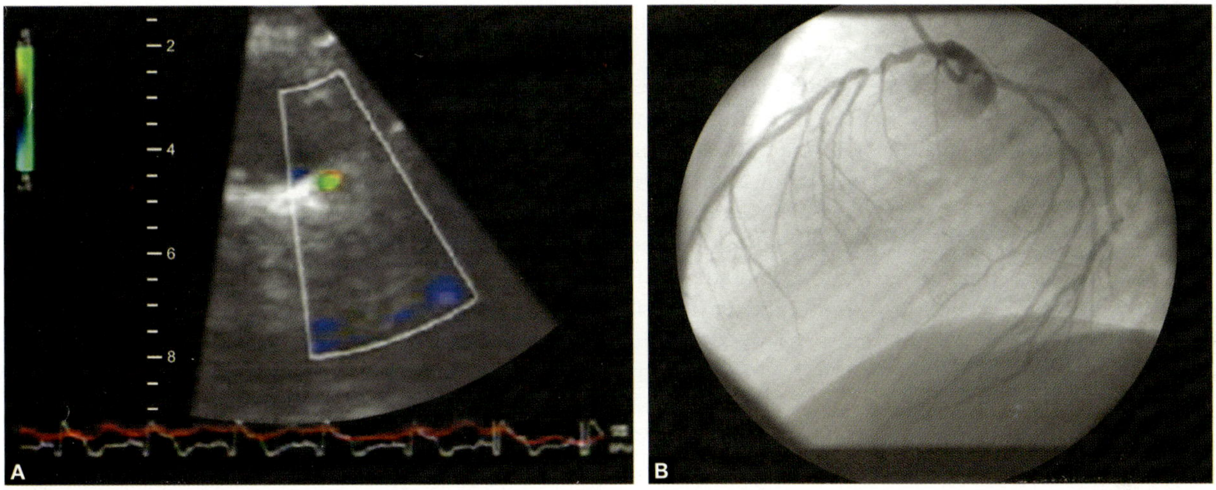

Figs. 5A and B: Recanalized left anterior descending (LAD) flow 20 minutes after thrombolysis. (A) Focal area of mosaic flow in mid-LAD; and (B) Coronary angiogram in the same patient showing severe stenosis (90%) in mid-LAD.

and RCA stents can be done by evaluating coronary flow reserve (CFR). A CFR value of less than 2 after intravenous adenosine in distal LAD would suggest significant in-stent restenosis in proximal or mid-LAD. Similar finding in PDA would suggest in-stent restenosis in RCA.

ISCHEMIC CARDIOMYOPATHY

When a diagnosis of dilated cardiomyopathy is made by TTE, the presence of mosaic flow pattern in proximal coronary arteries (LM, LAD, or Cx) is a strong pointer to ischemia as the cause for myocardial dysfunction (Figs. 7A and B). It is worthwhile to interrogate the proximal coronary segments by TTE to diagnose ischemic cardiomyopathy in which myocardial dysfunction can be improved with revascularization.

Noninvasive Assessment of Coronary Flow Reserve by Transthoracic Echocardiography

It has been demonstrated that CFR measurements provide lot of additional information on the function of coronary artery and assist in the decision making process of coronary interventions. CFR is defined as the ability of coronary blood flow volume to increase under maximal coronary hyperemia when compared with flow volume at rest. Intracoronary Doppler with adenosine or papaverine infusion remains to be the reference standard for the assessment of CFR. Hozumi et al.[12] performed the first validation of TTE comparing CFR in the LAD with simultaneous intracoronary Doppler guidewire assessment. TTE reflected invasive measurement of coronary flow velocity and CFR accurately, and the

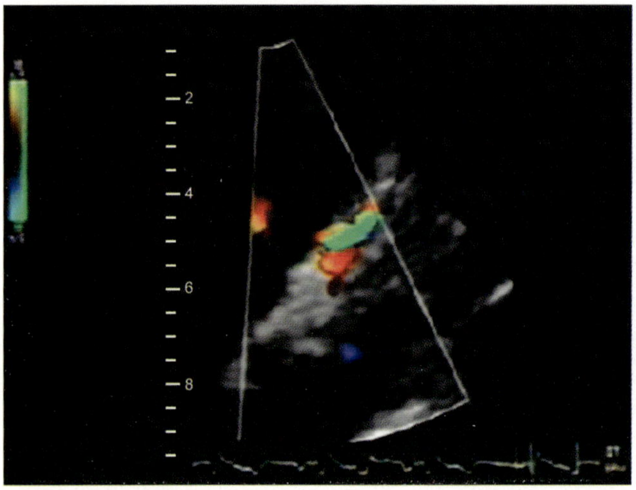

Fig. 6: Stent in mid left anterior descending (LAD) showing mosaic flow.

agreement between the two methods was 0.98 for diastolic peak velocity and 0.97 for CFR.

Coronary flow reserve assessment may be performed at the bedside within a few minutes. Echocontrast agent administration can enhance the coronary color flow signals. Adenosine should be infused intravenously at the rate of 140 μg/kg/min for 2 minutes. Coronary flow velocities are measured in distal LAD before and immediately after the cessation of adenosine infusion. The cut-off value for CFR is generally accepted to be 2.0 for predicting significant LAD stenosis, for decision making regarding intervention, after intracoronary intervention for assessing in-stent restenosis. In one study,[13] CFR with a cut-off value less than 2.0 was a significantly better predictor (90% sensitivity, 96% specificity) of LAD stenosis than multidetector computed tomography (80% sensitivity, 93% specificity). Unlike intracoronary Doppler studies with the guidewire or guiding catheter which may influence the coronary flow dynamics, TTE, being a noninvasive technique is devoid of this effect and can more accurately reflect the changes in coronary flow. A transthoracic CFR in the LAD less than 2.0 provided data consistent with those obtained by single photon emission computed tomography for physiologic estimation of stenosis severity with 94% sensitivity and 100% specificity (Hirate).[14] TTE can be used as a possible substitute of the invasive method for clinical measurement of CFR.

Coronary Flow Reserve and Prognosis in Coronary Artery Disease

Coronary flow reserve is able to detect the absence of microvascular reperfusion in the presence of a patent epicardial coronary artery. Ueno et al.[15] reported that CFR measured in open infarct-related LAD on day 1 after successful primary angioplasty was a good predictor of recovery of LV function at discharge. In the study of Meimoun et al.,[16] a cut-off CFR value of 1.7 was an independent predictor of both LV function recovery at 3-month follow-up, and in-hospital adverse cardiac events including death, recurrent myocardial infarction (MI), and acute heart failure.

In patients undergoing dobutamine stress echocardiography (DSE), CFR evaluation gives additional useful information. Even when DSE is negative, CFR assessment can detect moderate coronary stenoses inducing no wall motion abnormalities during stress test. Also in patients on anti-ischemic therapy with negative DSE result, CFR can be useful for the detection of severe stenosis.

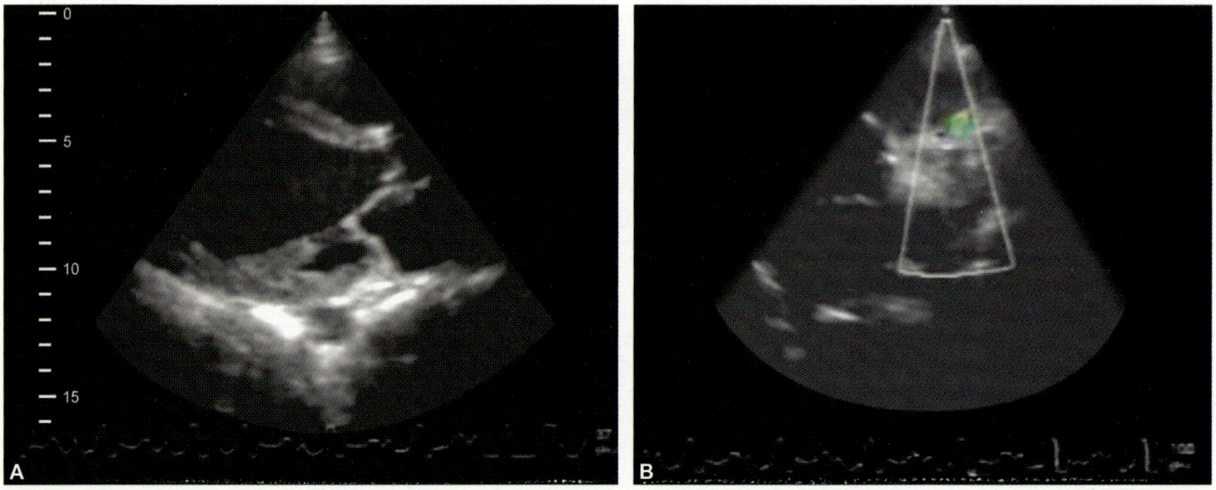

Figs. 7A and B: Proximal coronary flows in a case of dilated cardiomyopathy. (A) Parasternal long-axis view showing dilated left ventricle with severe left ventricular (LV) dysfunction; and (B) Mosaic flow in proximal left anterior descending (LAD) in the same patient.

Coronary Flow Reserve and Coronary Microvascular Disease

Coronary flow reserve can identify severe microvascular disease. Coronary microvascular dysfunction does not normally induce wall motion abnormalities but has been linked to adverse outcomes. In a prospective study in 394 patients with angiographically normal coronary arteries and preserved regional and global LV function at baseline and during stress, CFR less than 2.0 adds incremental value to the prognostic stratification.[17]

Coronary Flow Reserve and Coronary Bypass Graft Patency

In a large study,[18] using CFR assessment in distal LAD and PDA, the identification rate for patency of mammary grafts was 100%, for saphenous vein grafts to LAD 91%, and for vein grafts to RCA was 96%.

CONCLUSION

TTE with the help of harmonic imaging, contrast agents, and high frequency transducers can be used for the diagnosis of coronary stenosis as a noninvasive, inexpensive, non-X-ray, and high-time resolution technique. Doppler TTE assessment of coronary flows in CAD patients can provide lot of useful functional information with a wide range of clinical applications—including detection of coronary stenosis in LM, proximal coronary arteries, identifying CTO of major coronary arteries, and measurement of CFR noninvasively. However, due to limited visualization of coronary arteries, TTE cannot be accepted as an alternative to coronary angiography.

REFERENCES

1. Krzanowski M, Bodzon W, Dimitrow PP. Imaging of all three coronary arteries by transthoracic echocardiography: an illustrated guide. Cardiovasc Ultrasound. 2003;1:16.
2. Krzanowski M, Bodzon W, Brzostek T, et al. Value of transthoracic echocardiography for the detection of high-grade coronary artery stenosis prospective evaluation in 50 consecutive patients scheduled for coronary angiography. J Am Soc Echocardiogr. 2000;13:109-19.
3. Saraste M, Vesalainen RK, Yitalo A, et al. Transthoracic Doppler echocardiography as a noninvasive tool to assess coronary artery stenosis: a comparison with quantitative coronary angiography. J Am Soc Echocardiogr. 2005;18:679-85.
4. Anjaneyulu A, Raghu K, Chandramukhi S, et al. Evaluation of left main coronary artery stenosis by transthoracic echocardiography. J Am Soc Echocardiogr. 2008;21:855-60.
5. Hozumi T, Yoshida K, Akasaka T, et al. Value of acceleration flow and the prestenotic to stenotic coronary flow velocity ratio by transthoracic color Doppler echocardiography in noninvasive diagnosis of restenosis after percutaneous transluminal coronary angiography. J Am Coll Cardiol. 2000;35:164-8.
6. Watanabe N, Akasaka T, Yamaura Y, et al. Noninvasive detection of total occlusion of the left anterior descending coronary artery with transthoracic Doppler echocardiography. J Am Coll Cardiol. 2001;38:1328-32.
7. Hirata K, Watanbe H, Hozumi T, et al. Simple detection of occluded coronary artery suing retrograde flow in septal branch and left anterior descending coronary artery by transthoracic Doppler echocardiography at rest. J Am Soc Echocardiogr. 2004;17:108-13.
8. Otsuka R, Watanabe H, Hirata K, et al. A novel technique to detect total occlusion in the right coronary artery using retrograde flow by transthoracic Doppler echocardiography. J Am Soc Echocardiogr. 2005;18:704-9.
9. Anjaneyulu A, Christopher J, Raju P, et al. Coronary collaterals by transthoracic echocardiography in coronary artery disease. J Am Soc Echocardiogr. 2004;17:466-9.
10. Anjaneyulu A, Raghavaraju P, Raghu K, et al. Demonstration of recanalized left coronary artery after thrombolysis by transthoracic echocardiography. J Am Soc Echocardiogr. 2005;18:686-92.
11. Maxted WC Jr, Swanson ST, Huntley M, et al. Location of stents in the left anterior descending coronary artery using three dimensionally acquired two dimensionally displayed transthoracic echocardiography. Am J Cardiol. 1998;82:1434-6.
12. Hozumi T, Yoshida K, Akasaka T, et al. Noninvasive assessment coronary flow and coronary flow velocity reserve in the left anterior descending coronary artery by Doppler echocardiography. Comparison with invasive technique. J Am Coll Cardiol. 1998;32:1251-9.
13. Pizzuto F, Voci P, Bartlmucci F, et al. Usefulness of coronary flow reserve measured by echocardiography to improve the identification of significant left anterior descending coronary artery stenosis assessed by multidetector computed tomography. Am J Cardiol. 2003;92:1320-4.
14. Hirata K, Watanabe H, Otsuka R, et al. Noninvasive diagnosis of restenosis by transthoracic Doppler echocardiography after percutaneous coronary intervention: Comparison with exercise TI-SPECT. J Am Soc Echocardiogr. 2006;19:165-71.
15. Ueno Y, Nakamura Y, Kinnoshita M, et al. Can coronary flow velocity reserve determined by transthorcic Doppler echocardiography predict the recovery regional left ventricular function in patients with acute myocardial infarction? Heart. 2002;88:137-41.
16. Melmoun P, Malaquin D, Benali T, et al. Noninvasive coronary flow reserve after successful primary angioplasty for acute anterior myocardial infarction is an independent predictor of left ventricular recovery and in-hospital cardiac events. J Am Soc Echocardiogr. 2009;22:1071-9.
17. Sicari R, Rigo F, Cortigiani L, et al. Additive prognostic value of coronary flow reserve in patients with chest pain syndrome and normal or near-normal coronary artery. Am J Cardiol. 2009;103:626-31.
18. Chirillo F, Bruni A, Balestra G, et al. Assessment of internal mammary artery and saphenous vein graft patency and flow reserve using transthoracic Doppler echocardiography. Heart. 2001;86:424-31.

46

CHAPTER

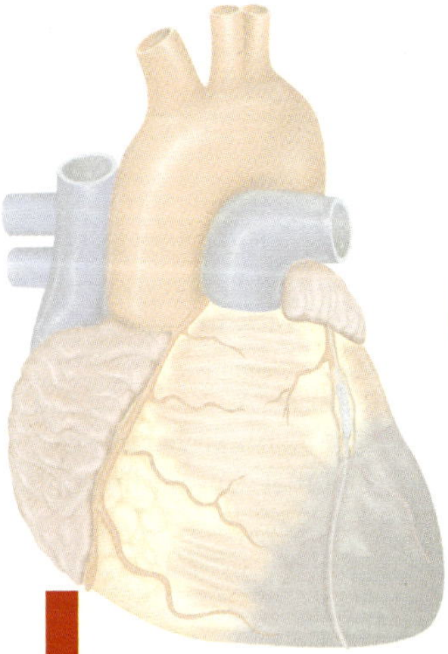

Dobutamine Stress Echocardiography in Assessment of Myocardial Viability

CK Ponde, Pranav A Oza

INTRODUCTION

Presence of viable myocardium has been considered as a prerequisite for any tangible benefit from revascularization either by angioplasty or coronary artery bypass surgery.[1] Various methods are available for the assessment of viable myocardium, viz. low-dose dobutamine stress echocardiography (LD-DSE), positron emission tomography (PET), radionuclide imaging, and cardiac magnetic resonance imaging (MRI) with late gadolinium enhancement (LGE).[2] Concept of viable myocardium translating into demonstrable patient benefit has been questioned in view of recent trials. We will discuss specifically LD-DSE in this review. Viable myocardium is defined as segment of myocardium with contractile dysfunction at rest which has potential of significant recovery after revascularization.[3] Viable myocardium occurs in several clinical settings, viz. patients with acute coronary syndrome, chronic coronary artery disease (CAD), and patients with heart failure. Revascularization in patients with viable myocardium offers substantial benefit which translates into patient's symptomatic improvement, improvements in cardiac function measurements, and survival.[4]

CHARACTERISTICS OF VIABLE MYOCARDIUM[5]

- Has the ability to generate high energy phosphates [creatine phosphate (PCr) and adenosine triphosphate (ATP)],
- Has an intact sarcolemma in order to maintain ionic/electrochemical gradients, and
- Has sufficient perfusion, both for the delivery of substrates and O_2 and for the adequate washout of potentially noxious metabolites.

As a result of coronary blood flow reduction, acute and chronic adaptations of the myocardium prevent irreversible myocardial damage.

Stunned myocardium is a type of viable myocardium that occurs after brief and intense ischemia and has ability to recover its function. The term hibernating myocardium means viable myocardium in regions which are insufficiently perfused at rest and recover function after reestablishing adequate coronary blood flow. Hibernating and stunned myocardium have a positive inotropic reserve, which is in contrast to irreversibly damaged myocardium, i.e. necrosis or scar.[6]

MYOCARDIAL STUNNING

In 1973, Chatterjee et al. reported improved myocardial wall motion abnormalities following revascularization in the CAD patients in the absence of myocardial scar.

A year later, Horn et al. (1974) concluded that myocardial wall motion abnormalities improved by inotropic stimulation with epinephrine infusion in patients with CAD and left ventricular (LV) asynergy.

Heyndrickx et al. in the mid-1970s showed that brief periods of coronary occlusion in dogs result in prolonged depression of myocardial function in the ischemic zone with recovery of function on restoration of blood flow.

In 1982, Braunwald et al. described the ischemic process after brief coronary occlusion as "hit, run, and stun": myocardial ischemia acutely affects myocardial function (hit); after reestablishing myocardial perfusion (run) the myocardial function is impaired for a prolonged period. This prolonged, postischemic ventricular dysfunction is called "stunned myocardium."

The myocardial stunning is prolonged, fully reversible myocardial dysfunction that persists even after restoration of coronary blood flow. Main feature being a normal perfusion with a depressed myocardial function. In absence of recurrent ischemia, the function normalizes in 1 week. The duration and severity of ischemia determines the duration of postischemic dysfunction.

Cellular mechanisms involve free radical-mediated myocardial injury and reduced myofilament calcium sensitivity.[7]

HIBERNATING MYOCARDIUM

It is persistent depression of myocardial function in the presence of CAD, with improvement of function postrevascularization, first coined by Diamond and colleagues in 1978, and later defined by Rahimtoola et al. in 1985.

The term hibernating myocardium means viable myocardium in regions which are insufficiently perfused at rest and recover function after reestablishing adequate coronary blood flow. Another hypothesis is repetitive ischemia causing recurrent episodes of myocardial dysfunction eventually resulting in sustained depression of myocardial function (Flowchart 1).[8]

Flowchart 1: Types of myocardium.

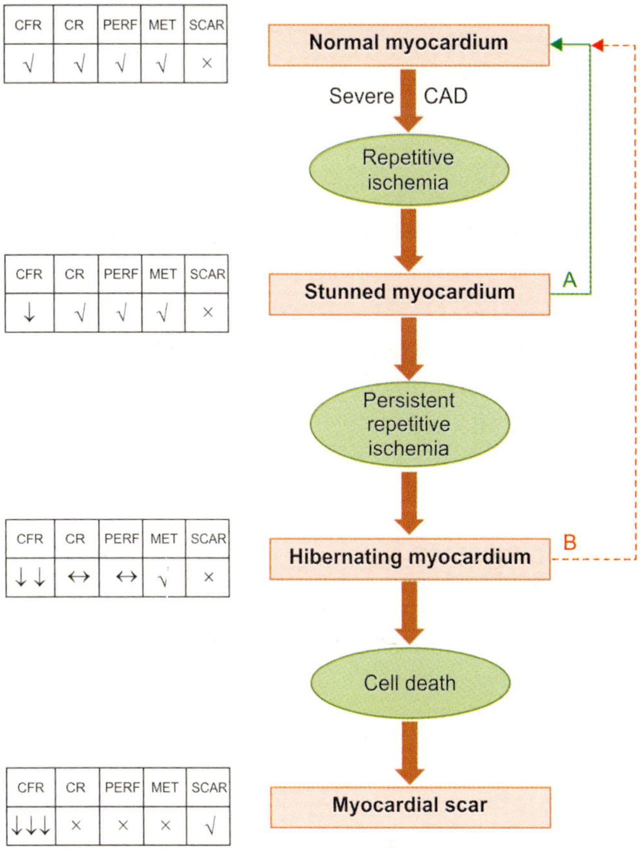

NONINVASIVE METHODS OF VIABILITY ASSESSMENT[9]

- *Single photon emission computed tomography*:
  - Depends on presence of intact cell membrane.
  - Thallium-201 and Technetium Tc99m–labeled tracers are the commonly used radionuclides.
- *Positron Emission Tomography*:
  - Uses fluorodeoxyglucose (FDG) which is transported into the cell by the same sarcolemmal carrier as glucose, where it is phosphorylated to FDG-6-phosphate by the enzyme, hexokinase.
- *Magnetic resonance*:
  - Uses gadolinium diethylenetriamine penta-acetic acid (DTPA) which is excluded by healthy cells
- *Echocardiography*:
  - Echocardiography is the most easily available, low cost, reproducible modality and has high sensitivity and specificity for assessment of myocardial viability.
  - End-diastolic wall thickness (EDWT):[10]
    - End-diastolic wall thickness shows the presence of sufficient mass of recruitable myocytes to produce effective systolic thickening.
    - End-diastolic wall thickness less than 5.5 mm in previous myocardial infarction (MI) is suggestive of myocardial necrosis.
    - Decreased diastolic wall thickness (<5 mm) is highly accurate in identifying resting regional left ventricular dysfunction that is unlikely to improve after revascularization.
    - The sensitivity and specificity of the end-diastolic thickness for the diagnosis of myocardial viability is 72% and 89%, respectively.
    - In akinetic segments (but with EDT preserved), 44% of segments are found viable in PET.
  - Viable myocardium on echo is identified as areas of myocardium with near normal thickness and contractile dysfunction, viz. hypokinesia, akinesia, or mere absence of systolic thickening or areas of myocardium with grossly reduced regional strain values despite normal thickness (Fig. 1).

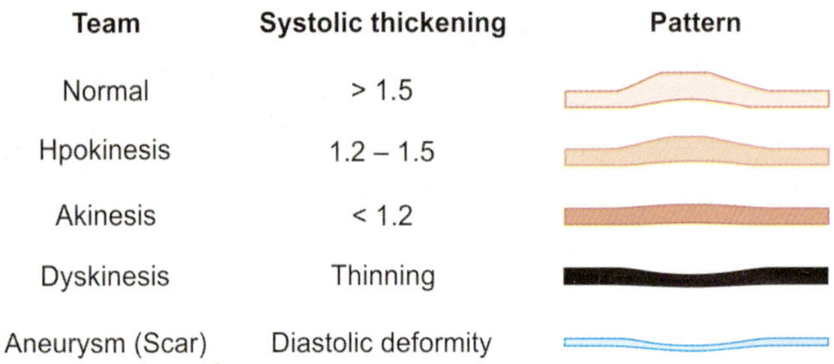

Fig. 1: Wall motion abnormalities.

- Nonviable myocardium is identified as myocardial segments with severe thinning and/or scarring with akinesia or dyskinesia.
- In echocardiography, both chronic ischemic (hibernation) and postischemic (stunning) left ventricular dysfunction appear as severe wall motion abnormalities at rest.
- Addition of dobutamine infusion helps in assessment of contractile reserve.
- Stress echocardiography aims at detecting a stimulated positive inotropic response in segmental wall motion.
- The positive inotropic response leads to an improvement in impaired regional wall motion.

LOW-DOSE DOBUTAMINE STRESS ECHOCARDIOGRAPHY

This chapter focuses on low-dose dobutamine echocardiography. DSE is the most widely available and most studied test to evaluate for presence of viable myocardium. Most widely used criterion for assessment of viable myocardium is contractile reserve. Usually low-dose dobutamine is used by infusion of 5–10 mcg/kg/min which increases contractility in dysfunctional but viable myocardium while nonviable myocardium does not show this contractile reserve.

Mechanism of Dobutamine[11]

It is a synthetic catecholamine that causes increase in heart rate, wall stress, contractility, and cardiac work, predominantly through beta-adrenergic stimulation in a dose-dependent manner. There is some alpha-2-adrenergic stimulation, and afterload is reduced by peripheral artery dilation. These effects, along with dobutamine's half-life of about 2 minutes, make it useful for cardiac stress testing. Dobutamine has a similar effect on heart rate as exercise, but there is typically less of an increase in blood pressure.

In akinetic segments, wall motion and systolic thickening may improve without steep rise in myocardial oxygen demand. The visually seen improvement in systolic function depends on the quantity of surviving myocytes and intact contractile apparatus in myocytes and the recruitable coronary vasodilator reserve. Dobutamine induced contractile response if highly specific predictor of viability. A positive dobutamine response is useful to rule in viability although negative response cannot rule out viability. This means that if very small segments of myocardium have viability these may not show a distinct improvement in wall motion on dobutamine challenge.

Method of Performing Dobutamine Stress Echocardiography

Patient should be fasting for 2–3 hours, with chest shaving and secure left arm intravenous access. Antianginals and beta blockers may be stopped 24 hours prior to test if considered necessary by the physician. Requirements are 12-lead electrocardiography (ECG) monitoring, an automated blood pressure cuff, an infusion pump for dobutamine, and a pulse oximetry. A typical protocol requires four standard echocardiography views: (1) parasternal long axis, (2) parastenal short axis, (3) apical four-chamber, and (4) apical two-chamber.

The dobutamine infusion is started at a low dose (5–10 μg/kg/min). At approximately 2.5-minute intervals, the infusion is increased by 10 μg/kg/min increments until a maximum dose of 40 μg/kg/min is reached. Intravenous (IV) administration of atropine 0.5–2 mg can supplement the stress test if 85% of the maximal predicted heart rate [(220 – age) × (0.85)] is not achieved. Atropine increases the sensitivity of dobutamine echocardiography in patients receiving beta blockers and in those with single-vessel disease.

The DSE test is terminated under following endpoints:

- When the target heart rate is achieved
- If angina or its clinical equivalent occurs
- After significant hemodynamic compromise or arrhythmia
- When significant ECG changes occur (which, when present, can improve the positive predictive power), or
- If diagnostic wall motion abnormalities are observed.

Standard DSE images are obtained at rest, with low-dose (5 μg/kg/min) and peak-dose dobutamine, and after several minutes of recovery when heart rate has largely normalized.

Patients are closely monitored until they are asymptomatic and stable. The development of hyperdynamic ventricular wall motion is considered normal. Abnormal responses include the development of new regional wall motion abnormalities (hypokinesis, akinesis, or dyskinesis) or a worsening of a baseline wall motion abnormality.

If the dobutamine effect needs to be antagonized clinically, an IV beta blocker can be administered (e.g. metoprolol 5 mg IV).

Indicators of Viability on Dobutamine Stress Echocardiography

For wall motion analysis, the 16 segment model for LV myocardial segmentation is used as recommended by the American Society of Echocardiography (ASE).

At low dose (5–10 μg/kg/min) dobutamine augments contractility without any increase in myocardial oxygen demand. With increase in doses, there is increase in heart rate (HR) and myocardial oxygen demand as a result of which the hibernating segment will improve in contractility at low dose but worsen at high doses. In contrast a stunned myocardium or nonischemic, tethered segment will show sustained improvement in contractility at both low and peak doses. When there is no change in contractility even at low doses it indicates nonviable myocardium.

Four different types of responses to LD-DSE:[12]

1. *Biphasic*: Improvement in contractility at low dose and akinesia at higher dose suggesting viable and ischemic myocardium. Most specific and most accurate for myocardial viability and functional recovery after revascularization (specificity 89% and sensitivity 74%).
2. *Sustained*: Continued improvement in contractility with increasing doses. Indicates viable, stunned, remodeled, myopathic tethered segment, or subendocardial infract without ischemia. This response is highly sensitive but has lower specificity to predict improvement after revascularization. However, in practice both biphasic and sustained responses are reported as presence of viability to improve sensitivity.
3. *Deterioration*: Hypokinetic segments becoming akinetic to dyskinetic with dobutamine. These are segments with critical resting low myocardial blood flow.
4. *No response*: Segments continue to be akinetic. These are nonviable scarred segments and are unlikely to improve with revascularization (Table 1).

Side Effects

Palpitations, nausea, headache, chills, urinary urgency, and anxiety and are usually well tolerated, without the need for test termination.

The most common cardiovascular side effects are angina, hypotension, and cardiac arrhythmias. Severe, symptomatic hypotension necessitating test termination occurs only rarely. Frequent premature atrial or ventricular contractions occur in about 10% of patients and supraventricular or ventricular tachycardias each occur in about 4% of patients.

Ventricular tachycardias are usually nonsustained and more frequently encountered in patients with a history of ventricular arrhythmias or baseline wall-motion abnormalities. On the basis of combined diagnostic and safety reports on dobutamine stress echocardiography, it is estimated that ventricular fibrillation or MI occurs in 1 of 2,000 studies.

Inadequate images occur in about 5% of patients and may preclude interpretation of DSE results.

TABLE 1: Stress echocardiography in four equations.

Rest + Stress = Diagnosis		
Rest	*Stress*	*Diagnosis*
Normokinesis	Normo or hyperkinesis	Normal
Normokinesis	Hypokinesis, akinesis, or dyskinesis	Ischemia
Akinesis	Hypokinesis or normokinesis	Viability
Akinesis or dyskinesis	Akinesis or dyskinesis	Necrosis

Sensitivity and Specificity of Dobutamine Stress Echocardiography for Myocardial Viability[13]

Low-dose dobutamine stress echocardiography shows average sensitivity of 75–80% and a specificity of 80–85% for the prediction of functional recovery either early after infarction or in case of severe LV dysfunction.

Diagnostic accuracy improves significantly when dobutamine response is combined with presence of diastolic wall thickness of more than or equal to 6 mm (sensitivity 88% and specificity 77%). The highest sensitivity for detection of viability is noted when improvement at low-dose dobutamine echocardiography is considered; highest specificity is achieved when a biphasic response occurs.

Global LV functional recovery postrevascularization depends on the number of segments showing viability on LD-DSE. Improvement in left ventricular ejection fraction (LVEF) of 5–6% is predicted if there are 2–5 viable segments and improvement in LVEF of more than 10% is predicted if there are six or more viable segments detected on DSE.

TABLE 2: Comparison of various modalities for viability assessment.

Modality	Sensitivity	Specificity
Low-dose dobutamine echocardiography	79%	78%
Tl-201 reinjection	87%	50%
Positron emission tomography (PET)	92%	63%
Late gadolinium enhancement	84%	63%

Strengths and Limitations of Dobutamine Stress Echocardiography

- *Strengths*:
  - Higher specificity
  - Viability and ischemia assessed
  - MR can be detected
  - Good spatial resolution
  - Widely available
  - Lower cost
  - Predictive of clinical outcomes.
- *Limitations*:
  - Poor window in 30%
  - Lower sensitivity
  - Viable regions with absent flow reserve will not show thickening.
    - Reductions in blood flow that lead to hibernation likely do so across a significant range of flows, with a corresponding spectrum of metabolic reserve. Those regions with greater metabolic reserve will likely retain the ability to respond to an inotropic stimulus while those regions with profoundly reduced flow—just on the threshold of viability—will have no ability to respond. Such regions will therefore appear to be nonviable on a dobutamine-echocardiography challenge.
  - Reliance on visual assessment (Table 2).

NEWER MODALITIES FOR DETECTION OF VIABILITY

With LD-DSE, the improvement in systolic and early diastolic strain rate values of akinetic segments has been proposed as markers of viability. Increase in systolic strain rate more than 0.23 or increase in early diastolic strain rate more than 0.8 predicted viability with sensitivity of 83% and specificity 84%, respectively. Strain rate increment of more than 0.25/s predicted functional recovery after revascularization with sensitivity 80% and specificity 75%. In a study comparing Doppler tissue velocity imaging (TVI) and strain imaging by speckle tracking echocardiography (STE) only TVI-based longitudinal strain and strain ratio (SR) on LD-DSE showed incremental value over wall motion analysis in detecting postrevascularization recovery. STE identified viability only in left anterior descending (LAD) territory but TVI strain and SR identified viability in both LAD and left circumflex artery/right coronary artery (LCx/RCA) territories.

In a study by park et al. SR measurement was better method than velocity-time integral (VTI) for identification of viable myocardium in patients with ST-elevation myocardial infarctions (STEMIs) who underwent percutaneous coronary intervention (PCI). Patients with functional recovery from anterior wall STEMI showed better diastolic function SR and more isovolumic contraction.

ALGORITHMS FOR MYOCARDIAL VIABILITY ASSESSMENT

First step is to accurately measure EDWT of akinetic segment on echocardiography. A preserved segment with EDWT more than 5–6 mm suggest more than 50% probability of recovery while a thinned out segment with EDWT of less than 5 mm indicates less than 5% probability of recovery. In presence of EDWT more than 5–6 mm either LD-DSE or SPECT imaging is sufficient to establish viability. In EDWT less than 5 mm further tests are required if LD-DSE is negative or equivocal, like combination of LD-DSE and LGE MRI or LD-DSE and FDG PET.

REFERENCES

1. Vanonerschelde JL, Pasquet A, Gerber B, et al. Pathophysiology of myocardial hibernation: Implications for the use of dobutamine echocardiography to identify myocardial viability. Heart. 1999;82(Suppl 3):1111-7.
2. Partington SL, Kwong RY, Dorbala S. Multimodality imaging in the assessment of myocardial viability. Heart Fail Rev. 2011;16(4):381-95.
3. Biessaux YG, Piérard LA. Viable myocardium. Definition and identification. Rev Med Liege. 1997;52(9):589-92.
4. Bhat A, Gan GCH, Tan TC, et al. Myocardial viability: From proof of concept to clinical practice. Cardiol Res Pract. 2016;2016:1020818.
5. Heusch G, Schulz R. Characterization of hibernating and stunned myocardium. Eur Heart J. 1997;18(Supplement D):D102-10.
6. Ferrari R, Ferrari F, Benigno M, et al. Hibernating myocardium: Its pathophysiology and clinical role. In: Cohen MV, Gelpi RJ, Downey JM (Eds). Myocardial Ischemia and Reperfusion. Molecular and Cellular Biochemistry (An International Journal for Chemical Biology in Health and Disease). Boston, MA: Springer; 1998.
7. Rahimtoola SH, Canna GL, Ferrari R. Hibernating myocardium: Another piece of the puzzle falls into place. J Am Coll Cardiol. 2006;47(5):978-80.

8. Rahimtoola SH. The hibernating myocardium. Am Heart J. 1989;117(1):211-21.
9. Elfigih IA, Henein MY. Non-invasive imaging in detecting myocardial viability: Myocardial function versus perfusion. Int J Cardiol Heart Vasc. 2014;5:51-6.
10. Cwajg JM, Cwajg E, Nagueh SF, et al. End-diastolic wall thickness as a predictor of recovery of function in myocardial hibernation: Relation to rest-redistribution Tl-201 tomography and dobutamine stress echocardiography. J Am Coll Cardiol. 2000;35(5):1152-61.
11. Ruffolo RR. The mechanism of action of dobutamine. Ann Intern Med. 1984;100:313-4.
12. Elhendy A, Cornel JH, Roelandt JR, et al. Relation between contractile response of akinetic segments during dobutamine stress echocardiography and myocardial ischemia assessed by simultaneous thallium-201 single-photon emission computed tomography. Am J Cardiol. 1996;77(11):955-9.
13. Geleijnse ML, Krenning BJ, van Dalen BM, et al. Factors affecting sensitivity and specificity of diagnostic testing: Dobutamine stress echocardiography. J Am Soc Echocardiogr. 2009;22(11):1199-208.

47

CHAPTER

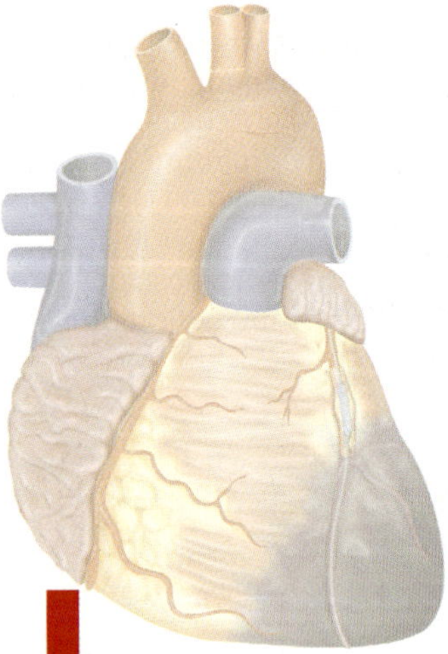

Assessment of Myocardial Viability: Advantages and Pitfalls of Various Modalities

Mythri Shankar

INTRODUCTION

Ischemic heart disease/coronary heart disease is leading cause of a morbidity and mortality. Left ventricular (LV) function and myocardial viability is by far the most important parameter in determining prognosis and making decisions toward medical or invasive options in managing ischemic coronary artery disease (CAD). Reserving invasive and expensive and revascularization procedures to select patient groups who show evidence of viable myocardial tissue will have a much higher chance of benefiting from such interventions compared to those who exhibit nonviable myocardium. Functional abnormalities [LV dysfunction, left ventricular ejection fraction (LVEF), and reservoir-wave approach (RWA)] can arise from multiple case scenarios like infarction, necrosis, hibernation, and stunning. It becomes very important to distinguish between these, particularly to further stratify patients with salvageable myocardium. Several recent studies have been done to confer prognosis of interventional/revascularization versus medical management and to determine an optimal strategy. The assessment of myocardial viability is the sole determining factor while deferring interventional/revascularization procedures in patients with coronary heart disease who have reduced LVEF.

DIAGNOSTIC CRITERION

Key Concepts

Myocardial viability refers to the state of dysfunctional myocardium, which has intact glucose at cellular level and in which restoration of coronary blood flow (following revascularization) will improve myocardial performance and LVEF, and therefore, better prognosis.

Myocardial stunning refers to the myocardium, which has undergone significant reversible injury due to ischemia (e.g. coronary spasm, postmyocardial infarction, or postcardiopulmonary bypass secondary to "cardiac off time" status postsuccessful postinfarct revascularization).

Myocardial hibernation refers to the sustained depressed functional state of myocardium, which is reversible.

Identifying such conditions is of significant clinical importance as it represent potentially salvageable myocardium which will result in improved contrafunctional upon cardiac revascularization if such conditions are less untreated they have the potential to progress into cardiac failure.

A meta-analysis of several trials (the STICH trial, The HEART trial, PARR-2 trial, and Ottawa-FIVE substudy) revealed a significant association between revascularization and improvement in mortality utilizing viability testing in patients with known ischemic cardiomyopathy. This finding was shared irrespective of imaging modality chosen. Primary limitations of these studies, however, included lack of standardization and adherence to optimal medical therapy during this period, with outcome reviews having been retrospective in nature.

PROGNOSTIC AND THERAPEUTIC IMPLICATIONS

Viability assessment helps mainly to:

- Identify those patients who might benefit most from revascularization

- Choose the most appropriate revascularization approach
- Avoid unnecessary procedures and risk in those patients with minimal or absent viability.

Recent European Guidelines on heart failure do not clearly recommend revascularization as a specific intervention in patients with chronic ischemic LV dysfunction unless they suffer from angina. Coronary artery bypass surgery in patients with severe LV systolic dysfunction is associated with higher periprocedural complications and mortality (approximately 3% stroke, approximately 5% death within 30 days postsurgery). Furthermore, recent studies provide evidence that percutaneous coronary interventions (PCIs) can be used safely to achieve complete revascularization in patients with severe CAD (Table 1). There is compelling evidence that revascularization of dysfunctional but viable myocardium may lead to reverse LV remodeling and confer prognostic benefits in patients with postischemic heart failure.[1] Several imaging modalities have become available in assessment of myocardial viability and the merits and limitations of each has been listed in the discussion here.[1]

Electrocardiography

The pathologic Q waves have traditional shown to have poor correlation with viability. The sensitivity is low at 41–65% and specificity 69–70% when compared to other imaging modalities. ST segment elevation during stress increases in the sensitivity to 82% and specificity 200%. Normalization of abnormal T waves during exercise has poor sensitivity and conflicting reports in the literature.

Echocardiography

Echocardiography is an important parameter to assess LV morphology and viability. Severe dilatation of LV and high end-systolic volume indices more than 130 mL are associated with poor functional recovery and reduced 3 years survival rates. End-diastolic wall thickness less than 5–6 mm indicates lack of contractile reserve. End-diastolic wall thickness greater than 5 mm has a sensitivity of 100% and specificity of 28% in predicting contractile function improvement in patients with LVEF of less than 50%.

Stress Echo (Dobutamine)

Out of the four classic responses, biphasic response has the greatest predicative capability with sensitivity and specificity is modestly high at 71–97% and 63–95%, respectively.[2] Diagnostic accuracy of dobutamine-echocardiography is reduced with increasing severity of regional and global LV dysfunction. It is not currently possible to detect transmural variations. This technique underestimates the extent of viability: 39% of all recovering LV segments failed to exhibit inotropic contractile reserve. It fails to identify 45% of the segments that ultimately regain function. Hibernating myocardium with more than 17% fibrosis failed to exhibit contractile reserve when challenged with low-dose dobutamine.[3,4]

It is relatively less expensive diagnostic test performed consistently worse than perfusion single-photon emission computed tomography (SPECT) in predicting hard clinical outcomes—spatial resolution wise,

TABLE 1: Indications for diagnostic testing in patients with suspected CAD and stable symptoms.

	Aymptomatic		*Symptomatic*						
			Probability of significant disease						
			Low (<15%)		*Intermediate (15–85%)*		*High (>85%)*		
	Class	*Level*	*Class*	*Level*	*Class*	*Level*	*Class*	*Level*	*Ref*
Anatomical detection of CAD									
Invasive angiography	III	A	III	A	IIb	A	I	A	50–52.54
CT angiography	III	B	III	C	IIa	A	III	B	57–62
Functional test									
Stress echo	III	A	III	A	I	A	III	A	63–65
Nuclear imaing	III	A	III	A	I	A	III	A	60.66–70
Stress MRI	III	B	III	C	I	A	III	B	71–75
PET perfusion	III	B	III	C	I	A	III	B	67,69,70,76,77
Combined or hybrid imaging test									
	III	C	III	C	IIa	B	III	B	78–83

Echo Contrast (Myocardial Contrast Echocardiography)

This has relatively higher sensitivity (78–90%). However, low specificity (51–72%), in demonstrating myocardial contractile recovery postrevascularization relative to dobutamine stress echocardiography (DSE; which on average has a relatively high specificity but lower sensitivity). A combination of the two modalities seems to be optimal in echocardiographic assessment of myocardial viability (sensitivity 96% and specificity 63%).

Echocardiography (Doppler Imaging Strain Analysis)

It allows more complete assessment of wall motion overcoming the challenge of 2D echo; ease of procedure and widespread availability as well as its noninvasive qualities; an ability to monitor functional response to accurate uptitration of inotropic therapy; sensitivity of 83% and specificity of 84% in discerning viable myocardium as determined by 18-fludeoxyglucose (^{18}FDG); additionally, radial strain more than 9.5% was associated with a sensitivity of 83.9% and specificity of 81.4%, whereas a change in longitudinal strain more than 14.6% provided a sensitivity of 86.7% and specificity of 90.2% in detection of viable myocardium using strain imaging with adenosine stress.

There is high operator dependency with resultant inter- and intraobserver variability. Patients with comorbidities such as obesity, chronic obstructive airflow limitation, and thoracic chest wall abnormalities limit the acoustic window and thus impair LV views. Assessment relies heavily on subjective visual interpretation of wall motion abnormalities.

Single Photon Emission Computed Tomography (Myocardial Perfusion/Stress Thallium/Gated SPECT)

Single photon emission computed tomography (SPECT) utilizes radionuclides to assess myocardium perfusion and function. Tracer-like sestamibi, tetrofosmin, thallium, which reflux uptake sodium, potassium ATPa system; percent uptake threshold on the distinction between salvageable and infarcted myocardium with a recommended threshold of 60%.

%WT and ejection fraction (EF)% estimates are obtainable by gated-SPECT which are useful in patients with nondiagnostic echocardiograms (e.g. due to severe pulmonary obstructive disease or extreme obesity). Attenuation correction (inferior wall artifacts, etc.) is now possible. It is of sensitivity (64–72%) and specificity (45–88%). Primary limitations include cost, ionizing radiation exposure, low spatial resolution, and attenuation artifacts. These artifacts can be removed via integration of multislice CT and SPECT.

Positron Emission Tomography

Gold-standard noninvasive test having passed the test of time; myocardial perfusion imaging with $^{13}NH_3$, $H_2{}^{15}O$, and ^{82}Rb extremely short half-lives permit repeat measurements, degree of improvement in exercise capacity could be predicted by the extent of viable myocardium identified by positron emission tomography (PET) perfusion/metabolism testing, but not with dobutamine echocardiography.

The FDG has the highest sensitivity[5] since PET requires the least amount of viable myocardium (25.8%) in comparison with DSE (35.9%), and SPECT (38.7%). "PET viable" is based on the established threshold of more than 50% FDG uptake compared with remote myocardium or as "magnetic resonance imaging (MRI) viable" when late gadolinium enhancement (LGE) transmurality of less than or equal to 50% was present. Spatial resolution is limited approximately 6 mm tall width of half maximum (FWHM) with specificity (88% and 73%, respectively) better spatial resolution and superior average sensitivity and as little as 7% of the myocardium as mismatch may be needed to yield an outcome benefit from revascularization. It is possible to evaluate cardiac magnetic resonance (CMR), a highly sensitive method to detect scarred myocardium. PET-FDG data also can be analyzed using a quantitative approach that, however, requires longer dynamic acquisitions. A threshold value for the metabolic rate of glucose of 0.25 mol/g/min allows the best prediction of improvement in functional class of at least 1 grade after revascularization.[6,7]

N-13 ammonia ($^{13}NH_3$)/FDG-PET is classified as class I level of evidence B for the prediction of the improvement in regional and global LV function. The ability to predict improvement in heart failure symptoms after revascularization is less well established and is classified as IIa level of evidence B for PET. Relatively high cost and poor availability of PET, regarding how substrate is utilized (i.e. oxidative metabolism versus anaerobic glycolysis), the ability to resume and maintain oxidative metabolism is an important predictor of subsequent functional recovery. It shows superior predictive value in direct relation to blood.

Variability of FDG uptake is the primary limitation. Other factors, including cardiac output, sympathetic activity, heart failure status, and degree of ischemia, impact FDG uptake and, thus, scan quality. PET scanners are not easily available due to the required infrastructure and cost involved.

Magnetic Resonance Imaging

Magnetic resonance imaging (MRI) has excellent spatial imaging at 3 T, has an ability to discern transmural variations in viability, and provision of accurate quantification of nonviable, infarcted or necrotic tissue with a sensitivity of 83% and specificity of 88%. No other modality can depict subendocardial infarct high-spatial resolution (2–2.8 mm voxels) with high image contrast quantify the transmural extent of infarct. The minimum amount of myocardium that can be imaged is 1 g with a spatial resolution of 2 mm. The transmural extent of infarction correlates with the likelihood of functional recovery of functional myocardium after revascularization. Limitations cost, poor availability, and prolonged study periods are requiring patient immobility and breath holding.

Poor spatial resolution at conventional field-strengths: at 1.5 T, the average voxel size interrogated by 31 P magnetic resonance spectroscopic imaging (MRSI) is on the order of 25 cm^3. This is problematic, as neighboring liver or skeletal muscle from the chest wall may contaminate the myocardial HEP peaks. There are no differences between reversibly damaged and normal myocardium, in terms of either T1- or T2-based signal intensity. Cine MR images are generally of much better quality with a sensitivity and specificity of dobutamine-induced systolic wall-thickening, as determined by cine MRI were 88% and 87%, respectively before and 4–6 months postrevascularization revealed a sensitivity and specificity of 89% and 94%, respectively, for functional improvement. In general, myocardial scar or fibrosis involving more than 50% of myocardial wall thickness at cardiac MR imaging is unlikely to recover contractile function following coronary revascularization. Distinguishing acute versus chronic infarction may be difficult with these MR imaging methods. Cost, availability, and trained personnel are the other limiting factors.

CONCLUSION

Of the several modalities available for evaluation of myocardial viability, PET remains the gold standard. MRI is an option when evaluation of small-sized infarcts with morphologic detailing is required. The available literature and data is based on relatively small sample size, with no additional correction algorithms and no angiographic correlation and stress imaging with MRI also not performed.

REFERENCES

1. Bhat A, Gan GC, Tan TC, et al. Myocardial viability: From proof of concept to clinical practice. Cardiol Res Pract. 2016;2016:10.
2. Thornhill RE, Prato FS, Wisenberg G. The assessment of myocardial viability: a review of current diagnostic imaging approaches. J Cardiovasc Magn Reson. 2002;4(3):381-410.
3. Camici PG, Prasad SK, Rimoldi OE. Stunning, hibernation, and assessment of myocardial viability. Circulation. 2008;117:103-14.
4. Vogel-Claussen J, Rochitte CE, Wu KC, et al. Delayed enhancement MR imaging: utility in myocardial assessment. Radiographics. 2006;26:795-810.
5. Ghosh N, Rimoldi OE, Beanlands RS, et al. Assessment of myocardial ischemia and viability: role of positron emission tomography. Eur Heart J. 2010;31(24):2984-95.
6. Rischpler C, Langwieser N, Souvatzoglou M, et al. PET/MRI early after myocardial infarction: evaluation of viability with late gadolinium enhancement transmurality vs. 18F-FDG uptake. Eur Heart J. Cardiovasc Imaging. 2015;16(6):661-9.
7. Lee VS, Resnick D, Tiu SS, et al. MR imaging evaluation of myocardial viability in the setting of equivocal SPECT results with 99mTc sestamibi1. Radiology. 2004;230:191-7.

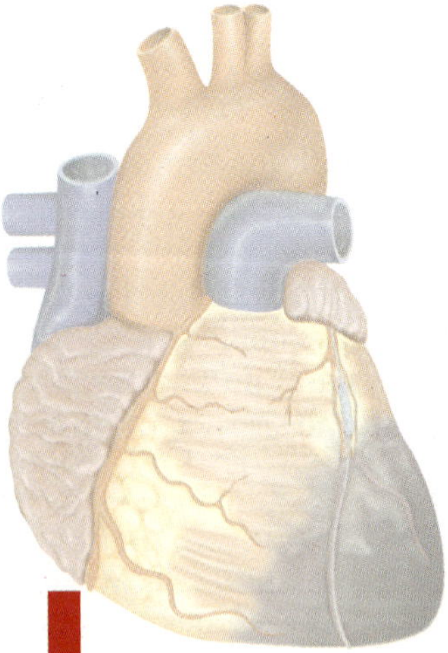

48

CHAPTER

Small Vessel Coronary Artery Disease

Sayeed Raheem, Upendra Kaul

INTRODUCTION

Annually 500,000 patients are diagnosed with angina in the United States.[1] In patients with angina who undergo coronary angiography, no or nonobstructive coronary artery disease (CAD) is a common finding. Even in patients with obstructive CAD who undergo revascularization, percutaneous coronary intervention (PCI) or coronary artery bypass graft (CABG), still continue with angina. Microvascular dysfunction can explain this angina. Coronary microvascular dysfunction (CMVD) is common in patients with angina with both obstructive and nonobstructive epicardial CAD.[2] Main attention has been focused on epicardial CAD. The term cardiac syndrome X was coined by Harvey Kemp in 1973, in patients with angina and ischemic electrocardiographic changes in the absence of epicardial obstructive CAD.[3,4] Angina with normal coronary arteries, microvascular angina, cardiac syndrome X, all these terms are used interchangeably for chest pain associated with CMVD. Because of lack of a standard definition, there is some impetus to abandon the term syndrome X.[5]

PREVALENCE AND RISK FACTORS

Angina patients undergoing coronary angiography (CAG), a significant proportion, mainly women show normal epicardial coronary arteries. In 25,000 patients in coronary artery surgery study (CASS) registry, patients of angina who underwent CAG, 39% women and 11% men had normal epicardial coronary arteries.[6] In the American College of Cardiology—National Cardiovascular Data Registry (NCDR) and Women's Ischaemic Syndrome Evaluation (WISE) study women had more nonobstructive CAD.[7,8] Chest pain and normal coronaries are more commonly seen in blacks as compared to whites. Blacks had more nonobstructive CAD as compared to other ethnicities (59% black, 53% Hispanic, 50% white, 47% Asian, and 45% native American) as observed in NCDR registry.[7] Cardiac syndrome X is seen more in estrogen-deficient females and after hysterectomy.[9] Hyperlipidemia, hypertension, and insulin resistance are known risk factors for microvascular CAD.[10] In last decade, microvascular CAD is validated as a cause of myocardial ischemia and has been associated with many diseases. In 20–30% of individuals who undergo CABG still continue with angina, which can be explained because of microvascular disease.[11] In patients with microvascular dysfunction, coronary flow reserve (CFR) is abnormal. False-positives stress tests in which ischemia is diagnosed may be because of microvascular CAD, as coronary angiography show normal epicardial coronary arteries.[5] Various diseases linked to microvascular CAD are Takotsubo cardiomyopathy,[12] heart failure with preserved ejection fraction,[13] various chronic inflammatory diseases, e.g. rheumatoid arthritis and systemic lupus erythematous. Oxidative stress and inflammation may lead to endothelial dysfunction, vasomotion abnormalities of coronary microcirculation, and finally increased risk of premature CAD.[14]

PATHOPHYSIOLOGY OF CORONARY MICROVASCULAR DYSFUNCTION

Resistance vessels which include both prearterioles (100–500 μm in diameter vessels) and arterioles (<100 μm) are responsible for abnormal flow in coronary arteries. Among various theories explaining the pathophysiology of microvascular CAD, structural abnormalities leading to increased vessel resistance due to smooth muscle hypertrophy as seen in left ventricular hypertrophy secondary to hypertension or hypertrophic cardiomyopathy, is one of mechanism for coronary microvascular disease.[15] Risk factors are shared by both epicardial and microvascular CAD.[5] Most commonly proposed mechanism of microvascular CAD is reduced nitric oxide production which leads to impaired endothelium-dependent vasodilatation in patients of stable microvascular angina. Reduced coronary blood flow (CBF) to acetylcholine has proved endothelium-independent mechanism of microvascular CAD. Both mechanisms can be tested with adenosine and acetylcholine (ACh).[5] ACh binds to muscarinic receptors (M3) on vascular smooth muscle cells endothelial (M3) receptors. By binding to M3 receptors on smooth muscle cells, it causes intracellular calcium release and vasoconstriction, and by acting on endothelial M3 receptors, it causes calcium release which activates endothelial nitric oxide synthase (NOS) leading to nitric oxide release (via calmodulin-dependent pathway). Nitric oxide by activating soluble guanylate cyclase, converts guanosine triphosphate (GTP) into guanosine monophosphate (GMP). GMP activates protein kinases, which induce cascade of intracellular events which leads to decrease intracellular calcium and vasodilatation. On vascular smooth cells, adenosine activates adenylate cyclase by binding on receptors A2a, which in turn increase cyclic adenosine monophosphate level (cAMP) and cAMP-dependent activates protein kinase. The latter results in potassium channel opening, resulting in a hyperpolarization of vascular smooth muscle cells, inhibits the entry of calcium and also activates inducible NOS (iNOS or NOS2), thus producing vasodilation.[16-18] While there is a reduction in the endothelium-dependent vasodilation due to changes in CBF, this does not seem sufficient to fully account for CMVD in these patients. The potential direct vasoconstrictor effects of ACh are not highly specific for the assessment of endothelial function, and in some studies, the metabolic pathway of NO did not seem to be affected.[19] Basal microvascular constriction was suggested by slow flow coronaries finally, in some typical patients of cardiac syndrome X. In some patients, ACh-induced angina was associated with a reduction of CBF in the absence of epicardial vasoconstriction (Flowchart 1).[5]

TESTS FOR SMALL VESSEL CORONARY ARTERY DISEASE

Noninvasive testing with multiple imaging modalities can be used to quantitatively assess myocardial perfusion and to determine absolute myocardial blood flow (MBF). Various imaging techniques have emerged to determine small vessel CAD, such as, positron emission tomography (PET), single-photon emission tomography (SPECT), and computed tomography (CT), magnetic resonance imaging (MRI), myocardial contrast echocardiography (MCE). PET is most commonly used tool, other techniques have emerged also with great promise for determination of small vessel CAD.[5] CBF is defined as blood flow during maximum hyperemia divided by baseline coronary blood flow, both in epicardiac and small vessel disease. Majority of research publications consider CFR of less than two abnormal to result into ischemia; however, normal value greatly depends on technique used for estimation. Adenosine, regadenoson, and dipyridamole, are frequently used agents to achieve hyperemia via endothelium-independent vasodilatation.[20] Unlike the previously mentioned vasodilators, dobutamine raises coronary flow by increasing cardiac workload via beta adrenergic receptor activation, mimicking exercise-induced physiological changes.[20] Coronary flow augmentation have been reported to be underperformed by exercise and dobutamine as compared to adenosine.

Cold Pressor Testing

Patient's hand or foot is immersed in ice cold water which leads to increase in heart rate and blood pressure, flow-mediated prearteriolar coronary vasodilatation occurs and which can be detected by dynamic imaging. Abnormal coronary microvascular pathology associated with many diseases show impaired cold pressor testing (CPT).[21-25] Endothelial function assessment can be performed with CPT.[20] Fraction of myocardium volume occupied by blood is intramyocardial blood volume (IMBV). SPECT can be used to estimate IMBV at equilibrium, as the tracer concentration in the myocardium over the tracer concentration in the blood pool.[26]

Myocardial Contrast Echocardiography

Intravascular gas-filled microbubbles are employed to estimate IMBV.[27,28] IMBV can be also estimated noninvasively from first pass perfusion cardiovascular magnetic resonance (CMR)[29] and by fast volumetric CT acquisition.[30]

Computed Tomography Imaging

Additional novel diagnostic markers can help in differentiating CAD and small vessel CAD in CT imaging. Transluminal attenuation gradient (TAG), defined as the linear regression

Flowchart 1: Proposed algorithm for the diagnosis of microvascular angina.

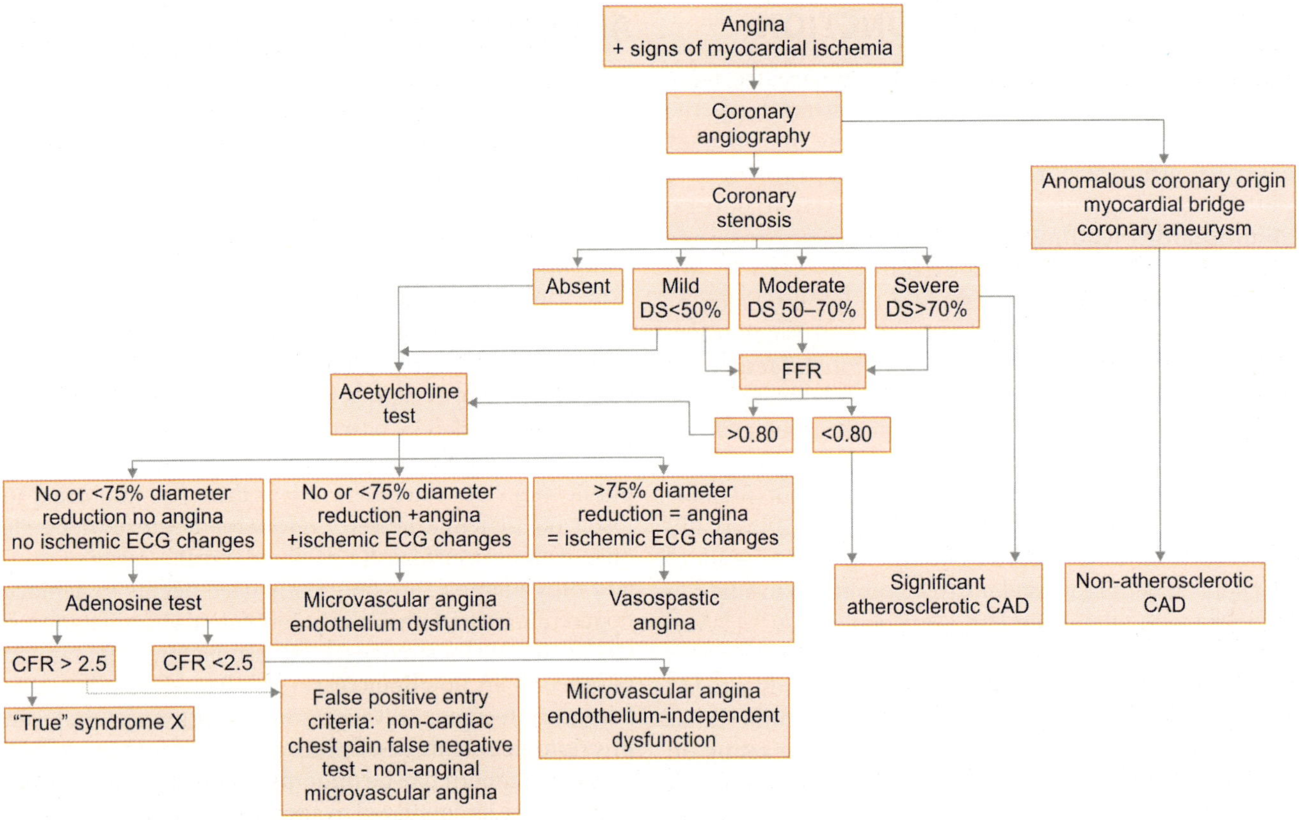

(CAD: coronary artery disease; CFR: coronary flow reserve; DS: diameter stenosis; ECG: electrocardiography; FFR: fractional flow reserve)
Source: Reprinted with permission from Elsevier by Radico F, Cicchitti V, Zimarino M, et al. Angina pectoris and myocardial ischemia in the absence of obstructive coronary artery disease: practical considerations for diagnostic tests. JACC Cardiovasc Interv. 2014;7:453-63.

coefficient between luminal contrast attenuation (measured in Hounsfield units) and axial distance on coronary CT angiography images, is a novel CT marker used for the evaluation of the degree of coronary stenosis.[31] It is particularly useful in the assessment of calcified stenotic lesions. The application of computational fluid dynamics to contrast CT angiography can also provide a unique opportunity for noninvasive estimation of fractional flow reserve (FFR).[32] As TAG and CT-FFR are markers of epicardial stenosis, it is reasonable to assume, that they are not affected by alterations in the microcirculation. Historically invasive coronary angiography was done for estimation of invasive CFR. Since, with almost 3 decades of experience, for the assessment of noninvasive CFR, PET became an alternative gold standard noninvasive imaging modality. CFR of less than 2.5 is most frequently used cutoff value based on study by Bergmann et al. in 11 healthy volunteers with PET.[33]

Positron Emission Tomography

With almost 3 decades of experience, the most studied noninvasive imaging modality for MBF quantification is PET using ^{15}O-water, ^{13}N-ammonia, and ^{82}Rubidium (^{82}Rb) for blood flow quantification. ^{82}Rb can be produced at the scanner by a portable generator; there is no need for an on-site cyclotron.[34] Newer ^{18}F labeled myocardial perfusion radiotracers (^{18}F-flurpiridaz), shows favorable characteristics for dynamic PET imaging.[35,36] ^{18}F-flurpiridaz was demonstrated to be superior to SPECT for diagnosing CAD, especially in women, obese, and CAD.[37] PET offers enhanced image quality when compared to SPECT and PET tracers usually permit lower radiation exposure than SPECT perfusion tracers. Because of high-cost associated with PET imaging has limited clinical application, due to the requirement of either onsite cyclotrons or expensive generators. However, the availability of Food and Drug Administration (FDA)-approved automated software packages for kinetic modeling and quantitative analysis of flow has made routine assessment of MBF and CFR feasible in the everyday clinical setting.[38] PET is considered one of the most reliable methods to evaluate microvascular dysfunction. PET uses a flow tracer that allows the determination of total regional MBF at rest and after a vasodilator challenge.[5] PET also has the advantage of assessing all three coronary distributions, thus allowing a more accurate assessment of microvascular dysfunction, as coronary microvascular dysfunction (CMD) has been shown to have a heterogeneous distribution over the three vessels.[39]

Computed Tomography Imaging

Computed tomography is relatively cost effective and has better spatial resolution. CT provides better anatomic and functional assessment of both the myocardium and coronary circulation. CT provides both luminal and extraluminal structural information about the epicardial coronary arteries information about the coronary microcirculation. CT scan with sufficient spatial resolution is enabled to differentiate between the endocardium and the epicardium, and the attenuation difference between these two layers, (when assessed during rest and stress conditions) can provide unique and sufficient information about the microcirculation. The decreased endocardial over epicardial contrast ratios and associated CT attenuation values has been associated with microvascular abnormalities.[40] Linear spatial variations in iodine concentration along the vessel (transluminal attenuation gradient) can also be calculated with CT perfusion imaging.[31] The new CT scanners operating at lower kVp, and the application of newer acquisition protocols and advanced reconstruction have the potential to reduce the radiation exposure.[41]

Magnetic Resonance Imaging

Magnetic resonance imaging (especially 3 T and more) because of high resolution is an excellent tool for estimation of MBF. MRI quantifies IMBV accurately using first pass perfusion. The main advantage of MRI is lack of ionizing radiation, detailed cardiovascular assessment of structure and mechanical function, and transmural MBF charecterization.[42]

The MRI is most reliable test for evaluation of microvascular dysfunction. Gadolinium enhances better visualization of subendocardial region of heart and stress agent (adenosine) is used to increase the CBF. Changes in gadolinium enhancement are correlated with an abnormal coronary flow and microvascular dysfunction. The main disadvantage of MRI is being expensive, time consuming, challenging in patients with devices, and limited by motion artifact.[43-46]

Myocardial Contrast Echocardiography

In MCE, most widely used contrast agents are microbubbles with shell containing lipid, albumin, or biopolymer which are filled with perfluoropropane.[47] MCE has been validated for quantification of flow in preclinical studies against microspheres, and it provides a good correlation with PET-derived MBF in humans.[48] In post-PCI patients flow limiting microvascular obstruction (no reflow phenomena) has been detected with extensive use of MCE.[49] The major advantage of MCE is lack of ionizing radiation and major disadvantage is operator dependence.

Transthoracic Doppler Echocardiography

Transthoracic Doppler echocardiography (TTDE) can measure distal left anterior descending (LAD) artery CBF velocity, which is a surrogate for CBF. CFR is measured as the ratio of peak CBF velocity after vasodilator and CBF velocity at rest.[50] CFR velocity measurements have been found to be highly reproducible.[51] CFR measured by this way show excellent correlation with CFR as measured with PET or invasively.[52] TTDE is cheap as compared to other noninvasive techniques. The main disadvantage is that TTDE is limited to LAD artery.[53] A ratio less than 2.0 (normal 2.5–5.0) is used as a marker of microvascular dysfunction.[5]

TREATMENT OF SMALL VESSEL CORONARY ARTERY DISEASE

There is limited guidance for making diagnosis of small vessel CAD by standard guidelines. In acute coronary syndrome patients if coronary angiogram is normal or show nonobstructed epicardial CAD, the American College of Cardiology/American Heart Association (ACC/AHA) guidelines recommend to consider invasive CFR if small or microvascular CAD is suspected (Class IIb indication, level of evidence: B).[54] The European Society of Cardiology (ESC) recommends noninvasive imaging modalities for CFR quantification by transthoracic Doppler echocardiography in LAD, PET for the diagnosis of microvascular angina and without consensus in regards to the use of MCE or MRI for quantification of MBF.[55] Data collected for medical management of small vessel CAD have been extrapolated from many meta-analysis, all utilizing same definition for small vessel CAD. The diagnosis of small vessel CAD was defined as CFR less than 2.5 by using cardiac MRI, PET, and invasive coronary Doppler. Cases with epicardial CAD (>50%) were excluded.[56] It can be assumed that angina is secondary to small vessel CAD when CFR is impaired on invasive or noninvasive quantification of MBF in patients with chest pain and nonobstructive CAD, so appropriate treatment strategies can be implemented. Evidence is less for effective treatment strategies of primary small or microvascular CAD. Besides controlling risk factors, traditional antianginal therapies [beta-blockers, nitrates, and CCBs (calcium channel blockers)] nontraditional drugs (nicorandil, aminophylline, and ivabradine) for angina management have been proposed for treatment of small vessel CAD.[57] Lifestyle modifications are very important. Patients must be encouraged to participate in weight loss programs, to do regular exercise and stop smoking.[58,59] Apart from lifestyle modifications, hypertension and diabetes should be controlled as per recommendations and focus on other parameters of control in CAD.[59] Microvascular CAD has been classified as with normal coronary arteries, obstructive CAD, and with myocardial diseases. Thus, treatment may also vary depending on the type of small vessel CAD. Studies have not assessed whether treating small vessel CAD results in any long-term prognostic benefits.[56]Long-acting nitrates are not recommended, they have no effect on microvessels as they do in epicardial vessels and thus not recommended.[60] Sildenafil, quinapril, enalapril, atenolol, estrogens, and transcutaneous electrical nerve stimulation (TENS) application, studies on these agents demonstrated benefits in their respective endpoints.[61] Angiotensin-converting enzyme (ACE) inhibitors, estrogens, TENS, and NO modulators were the drug classes that met strict inclusion criteria in studies and demonstrated benefits in their respective endpoints.

Mechanisms of these Drugs and their Benefits

Sildenafil acts by inhibiting breakdown of cGMP and thus, leads to smooth muscle relaxation. Guanylate cyclase activation by NO leads to increased cyclic guanosine monophosphate (cGMP). Improvement in CFR was shown by a small study on sildenafil but did not assess symptoms. NO activates guanylate cyclase and increases cGMP.[62] ACE inhibitors may directly modulate coronary microvascular tone.[63] Quinapril showed improvement in angina and CFR in a small placebo controlled trial.[64] As estrogen deficiency is associated with small vessel CAD, administration of ethinyl-estradiol showed an improvement in anginal symptoms in a small study.[65] The existing studies of beta-blockers included patients with signs and symptoms of ischemia, but not with a definitive diagnosis of CMD. Myocardial oxygen consumption is reduced and diastolic filling time is increased by beta blockers. Atenolol has shown to decrease the number of angina episodes[66] and improve the ischemic threshold.[67] Although well studied in obstructive epicardial CAD and in CMD in patients with structural heart disease, there is no currently published study that met our inclusion criteria in patients with microvascular angina.[63] CCBs, which are considered as a reasonable first-line drugs for microvascular angina, in one of the study of intracoronary diltiazem did not show improvement in CFR in microvessel angina. CCBs had predominant vasodilatory effect on the epicardial artery.[68] Despite this patients with abnormal CFR had improved symptoms, decrease nitrate usage, and improved exercise tolerance after being treated with nifedipine or verapamil.[69] Among statins data show improvement in CFR with the use of fluvastatin and even greater improvement when combined with diltiazem.[70] Addition of atorvastatin also shows improvement in CFR as shown in two pilot studies.[71] The utility of ranolazine for microvascular CAD has been conflicting. In patients with low CFR ranolazine use improved this, in women with no CAD and symptoms of angina were also improved with use of ranolazine.[72] Another study showed some improvement in symptoms but no effect on coronary microvascular function.[73]

PROGNOSIS OF MICROVASCULAR CORONARY ARTERY DISEASE

Small vessel CAD is associated with worse cardiovascular outcomes (stroke, MI, death, and worsening angina) as shown consistently in various prognostic studies. Patients with severe endothelial dysfunction (with intracoronary ACh testing) found to have 14% cardiac events on follow-up compared with no events in patients with moderate to severe endothelial dysfunction.[74] In a study by Schachinger et al., 30% patients with microvascular coronary artery dysfunction develop obstructive CAD at 10-year follow-up.[75] Both endothelial-dependent and endothelial-independent mechanisms of microvascular CAD predict adverse prognosis. Endothelial-dependent dysfunction is an independent risk factor for cardiac events regardless of the severity of a patient's CAD.[76,77] Endothelial-independent mechanism characterized by reduced CFR was also significantly associated with adverse cardiovascular events at 5-year mean follow-up which was demonstrated in 189 women in Women's Ischemia Syndrome Evaluation (WISE) study.[54] Reduced benefit was seen with revascularization inpatients with abnormal CFR.[78] Another study showed 5%, 10%, and 18% adverse cardiovascular events respectively in mild, moderate, and severe microvascular CAD.[79] Diabetics without known CAD but abnormal CFR and nondiabetics with CAD have similar yearly event rate (2.8% vs 2%) as studied by Murthy et al.[80]

CONCLUSION

Small vessel disease, which cannot be detected by invasive CAG, results in microvascular angina. It is an important entity, which needs an emphasis for practicing physicians. It has a scientific basis and therapeutic solutions. The prognosis of this entity is related to its pathophysiology. The entity has several subsets and should not be labeled as one entity.

REFERENCES

1. Phelps CE, Buysman EK, Gomez Rey G. Costs and clinical outcomes associated with use of ranolazine for treatment of angina. Clin Ther. 2012;34:1395-407.e4.
2. Corcoran D, Young R, Adlam D. Coronary microvascular dysfunction in patients with stable coronary artery disease: the CE-MARC 2 coronary physiology substudy. Int J Cardiol. 2018;266:7-14.
3. Kemp HG. Left ventricular function in patients with the anginal syndrome and normal coronary arteriograms. Am J Cardiol. 1973;32:375-6.
4. Camici PG, Crea F. Coronary microvascular dysfunction. N Engl J Med. 2007;356:830-40.
5. Alrifai A, Kabach M, Nieves J, et al. Microvascular coronary artery sisease: review article. USC. 2018;12:41-5.
6. Davis KB, Chaitman B, Ryan T, et al. Comparison of 15-year survival for men and women after initial medical or surgical treatment for coronary artery disease: a CASS registry study. Coronary Artery Surgery Study. J Am Coll Cardiol. 1995;25:1000-9.
7. Shaw LJ, Shaw RE, Merz CN, et al. Impact of ethnicity and gender differences on angiographic coronary artery disease prevalence and in-hospital mortality in the American College of Cardiology-National Cardiovascular Data Registry. Circulation. 2008;117:1787-801.
8. Shaw LJ, Merz CN, Pepine CJ, et al. The economic burden of angina in women with suspected ischemic heart disease: results from the National Institutes of Health-National Heart, Lung, and Blood Institute--sponsored Women's Ischemia Syndrome Evaluation. Circulation. 2006;114:894-904.
9. Rosano GM, Collins P, Kaski JC, et al. Syndrome X in women is associated with oestrogen deficiency. Eur Heart J. 1995;16:610-4.
10. Jadhav ST, Ferrell WR, Petrie JR, et al. Microvascular function, metabolic syndrome, and novel risk factor status in women with cardiac syndrome X. Am J Cardiol. 2006;97:1727-31.
11. Abbate A, Biondi-Zoccai GG, Agostoni P, et al. Recurrent angina after coronary revascularization: a clinical challenge. Eur Heart J. 2007;28:1057-65.
12. Galiuto L, De Caterina AR, Porfidia A, et al. Reversible coronary microvascular dysfunction: a common pathogenetic mechanism in apical ballooning or Tako-Tsubo syndrome. Eur Heart J. 2010;31:1319-27.
13. Tschöpe C, Van Linthout S. New insights in (inter)cellular mechanisms by heart failure with preserved ejection fraction. Curr Heart Fail Rep. 2014;11:436-44.
14. Faccini A, Kaski JC, Camici PG. Coronary microvascular dysfunction in chronic inflammatory rheumatoid diseases. Eur Heart J. 2016;37:1799-806.
15. Opherk D, Zebe H, Weihe E, et al. Reduced coronary dilatory capacity and ultrastructural changes of the myocardium in patients with angina pectoris but normal coronary arteriograms. Circulation. 1981;63:817-25.
16. Motz W, Vogt M, Rabenau O, et al. Evidence of endothelial dysfunction in coronary resistance vessels in patients with angina pectoris and normal coronary angiograms. Am J Cardiol. 1991;68:996-1003.
17. Chauhan A, Mullins PA, Taylor G, et al. Both endothelium-dependent and endothelium-independent function is impaired in patients with angina pectoris and normal coronary angiograms. Eur Heart J. 1997;18:60-8.
18. Bøttcher M, Botker HE, Sonne H, et al. Endothelium-dependent and -independent perfusion reserve and the effect of l-arginine on myocardial perfusion in patients with syndrome X. Circulation. 1999;99:1795-801.
19. Desideri G, Gaspardone A, Gentile M, et al. Endothelial activation in patients with cardiac syndrome X. Circulation. 2000;102:2359-64.
20. Salerno M, Beller GA. Noninvasive assessment of myocardial perfusion. Circ Cardiovasc Imaging. 2009;2:412-24.
21. Morita K, Tsukamoto T, Naya M, et al. Smoking cessation normalizes coronary endothelial vasomotor response assessed with ^{15}O-water and PET in healthy young smokers. J Nucl Med. 2006;47:1914-20.
22. Schindler TH, Cardenas J, Prior JO, et al. Relationship between increasing body weight, insulin resistance, inflammation, adipocytokine leptin, and coronary circulatory function. J Am Coll Cardiol. 2006;47:1188-95.
23. Quercioli A, Montecucco F, Pataky Z, et al. Improvement in coronary circulatory function in morbidly obese individuals after gastric bypass-induced weight loss: relation to alterations in endocannabinoids and adipocytokines. Eur Heart J. 2013;34:2063-73.
24. Alexanderson E, Ochoa JM, Calleja R, et al. Endothelial dysfunction in systemic lupus erythematosus: evaluation with 13N-ammonia PET. J Nucl Med. 2010;51:1927-31.
25. Prior JO, Quinones MJ, Hernandez-Pampaloni M, et al. Coronary circulatory dysfunction in insulin resistance, impaired glucose tolerance, and type 2 diabetes mellitus. Circulation. 2005;111:2291-8.
26. Jayaweera AR, Edwards N, Glasheen WP, et al. In vivo myocardial kinetics of air-filled albumin microbubbles during myocardial contrast echocardiography: comparison with radiolabeled red blood cells. Circ Res. 1994;74:1157-65.
27. Wei K, Jayaweera AR, Firoozan S, et al. Quantification of myocardial blood flow with ultrasound-induced destruction of microbubbles administered as a constant venous infusion. Circulation. 1998;97:473-83.
28. Wu CC, Feldman MD, Mills JD, et al. Myocardial contrast echocardiography can be used to quantify intramyocardial blood volume: new insights into structural mechanisms of coronary autoregulation. Circulation. 1997;96:1004-11.
29. McCommis KS, Zhang H, Goldstein TA, et al. Myocardial blood volume is associated with myocardial oxygen consumption: an experimental study with cardiac magnetic resonance in a canine model. JACC Cardiovasc Imaging. 2009;2:1313-20.
30. Mohlenkamp S, Beighley PE, Pfeifer EA, et al. Intramyocardial blood volume, perfusion and transit time in response to embolization of different sized microvessels. Cardiovasc Res. 2003;57:843-52.
31. Choi JH, Min JK, Labounty TM, et al. Intracoronary transluminal attenuation gradient in coronary CT angiography for determining coronary artery stenosis. JACC Cardiovasc Imaging. 2011;4:1149-57.

32. Koo BK, Erglis A, Doh JH, et al. Diagnosis of ischemia-causing coronary stenoses by noninvasive fractional flow reserve computed from coronary computed tomographic angiograms Results from the prospective multicenter DISCOVER-FLOW (Diagnosis of Ischemia-Causing Stenoses Obtained Via Noninvasive Fractional Flow Reserve) study. J Am Coll Cardiol. 2011;58:1989-97.
33. Bergmann SR, Herrero P, Markham J, et al. Noninvasive quantitation of myocardial blood flow in human subjects with oxygen-15-labeled water and positron emission tomography. J Am Coll Cardiol. 1989;14:639-52.
34. El Fakhri G, Kardan A, Sitek A, et al. Reproducibility and accuracy of quantitative myocardial blood flow assessment with (82)Rb PET: comparison with (13)N-ammonia PET. J Nucl Med. 2009;50:1062-71.
35. Huisman MC, Higuchi T, Reder S, et al. Initial characterization of an 18F-labeled myocardial perfusion tracer. J Nucl Med. 2008;49:630-6.
36. Nekolla SG, Reder S, Saraste A, et al. Evaluation of the novel myocardial perfusion positron-emission tomography tracer 18F-BMS-747158-02: comparison to 13N-ammonia and validation with microspheres in a pig model. Circulation. 2009;119:2333-42.
37. Maddahi J, Flurpiridaz F. 18 MPI: Recent clinical trial data. Eur Heart J Cardiovasc Imaging. 2015:16.
38. Nesterov SV, Deshayes E, Sciagra R, et al. Quantification of myocardial blood flow in absolute terms using (82)Rb PET imaging: the RUBY-10 Study.JACC Cardiovasc Imaging. 2014;7:1119-27.
39. Marroquin OC, Holubkov R, Edmundowicz D, et al. Heterogeneity of microvascular dysfunction in women with chest pain not attributable to coronary artery disease: Implications for clinical practice. Am Heart J. 2003;145(4):628-35.
40. Kuhl JT, George RT, Mehra VC, et al. Endocardial-epicardial distribution of myocardial perfusion reserve assessed by multidetector computed tomography in symptomatic patients without significant coronary artery disease: insights from the CORE320 multicentre study. Eur Heart J Cardiovasc Imaging. 2016;17:779-87.
41. Danad I, Raijmakers PG, Appelman YE, et al. Hybrid imaging using quantitative H215O PET and CT-based coronary angiography for the detection of coronary artery disease. J Nucl Med. 2013;54:55-63.
42. Liu A, Wijesurendra RS, Francis JM, et al. Adenosine stress and rest T1 mapping can differentiate between ischemic, infarcted, remote, and normal myocardium without the need for gadolinium contrast agents. JACC Cardiovasc Imaging. 2016;9:27-36.
43. Frans S. Noninvasive assessment of coronary microvascular dysfunction. Heart Metab. 2008;40:15-9.
44. Lanza GA, Crea F. Primary coronary microvascular dysfunction: clinical presentation, pathophysiology, and management. Circulation. 2010;121:2317-25.
45. Lanza GA, Camici PG, Galiuto L, et al. Methods to investigate coronary microvascular function in clinical practice. J Cardiovasc Med (Hagerstown). 2013;14:1-18.
46. Panting JR, Gatehouse PD, Yang GZ, et al. Abnormal subendocardial perfusion in cardiac syndrome X detected by cardiovascular magnetic resonance imaging. N Engl J Med. 2002;346:1948-53.
47. Wei K, Jayaweera AR, Firoozan S, et al. Quantification of myocardial blood flow with ultrasound-induced destruction of microbubbles administered as a constant venous infusion. Circulation. 1998;97:473-83.
48. Vogel R, Indermuhle A, Reinhardt J, et al. The quantification of absolute myocardial perfusion in humans by contrast echocardiography: algorithm and validation. J Am Coll Cardiol. 2005;45:754-62.
49. Feher A, Chen SY, Bagi Z, et al. Prevention and treatment of no-reflow phenomenon by targeting the coronary microcirculation. Rev Cardiovasc Med. 2014;15:38-51.
50. Dimitrow PP. Transthoracic Doppler echocardiography: Noninvasive diagnostic window for coronary flow reserve assessment. Cardiovasc Ultrasound. 2003;1:4.
51. Saraste M, Koskenvuo J, Knuuti J, et al. Coronary flow reserve: Measurement with transthoracic Doppler echocardiography is reproducible and comparable with positron emission tomography. Clin Physiol. 2001;21:114-22.
52. Caiati C, Montaldo C, Zedda N, et al. Validation of a new noninvasive method (contrast enhanced transthoracic second harmonic echo Doppler) for the evaluation of coronary flow reserve: comparison with intracoronary Doppler flow wire. J Am Coll Cardiol. 1999;34:1193-200.
53. Chen C, Wei J, AlBadri A, et al. Epidemiology, pathogenesis, prognosis, diagnosis, risk factors and therapy. Circ J. 2017;81:3-11.
54. Amsterdam EA, Wenger NK, Brindis RG, et al. 2014 AHA/ACC guideline for the management of patients with non-ST-elevation acute coronary syndromes: a report of the American College of Cardiology/American Heart Association Task Force on Practice Guidelines. Circulation. 2014;130: e344-426.
55. Montalescot G, Sechtem U, Achenbach S, et al. 2013 ESC guidelines on the management of stable coronary artery disease: the task force on the management of stable coronary artery disease of the European Society of Cardiology. Eur Heart J. 2013;34(38):2949-3003.
56. Löffler AI, Bourque JM. Coronary microvascular dysfunction, microvascular angina, and management. Curr Cardiol Rep. 2016;18:1.
57. Crea F, Camici PG, Bairey Merz CN. Coronary microvascular dysfunction: An update. Eur Heart J. 2014;35:1101-11.
58. Pepine CJ, Ferdinand KC, Shaw LJ, et al. Emergence of nonobstructive coronary artery disease: a woman's problem and need for change in definition on angiography. J Am Coll Cardiol. 2015;66:1918-33.
59. Chen C, Wei J, AlBadri A, et al. Coronary microvascular dysfunction: epidemiology, pathogenesis, prognosis, diagnosis, risk factors and therapy. Circ J. 2016;81:3-11.
60. Russo G, Di Franco A, Lamendola P, et al. Lack of effect of nitrates on exercise stress test results in patients with microvascular angina. Cardiovasc Drugs Ther. 2013;27: 229-34.

61. Marinescu MA, Löffler AI, Ouellette M, et al. Coronary microvascular dysfunction, microvascular angina, and treatment strategies. JACC Cardiovasc Imaging. 2015;8:210-20.
62. Denardo SJ, Wen X, Handberg EM, et al. Effect of phosphodiesterase type 5 inhibition on microvascular coronary dysfunction in women: a women's ischemia syndrome evaluation (WISE) ancillary study. Clin Cardiol. 2011;34:483-7.
63. Marinescu MA, Loffler AI, Ouellette M, et al. Coronary microvascular dysfunction, microvascular angina, and treatment strategies. JACC Cardiovasc Imaging. 2015;8:210-20.
64. Pauly DF, Johnson BD, Anderson RD, et al. In women with symptoms of cardiac ischemia, nonobstructive coronary arteries, and microvascular dysfunction, angiotensin-converting enzyme inhibition is associated with improved microvascular function: a double-blind randomized study from the national heart, lung and blood institute women's ischemia syndrome evaluation (WISE). Am Heart J. 2011;162:678-84.
65. Merz CNB, Olson MB, McClure C, et al. A randomized controlled trial of low-dose hormone therapy on myocardial ischemia in postmenopausal women with no obstructive coronary artery disease: results from the national institutes of health/national heart, lung, and blood institute–sponsored women's ischemia syndrome evaluation (WISE). Am Heart J. 2010;(159):987.
66. Lanza GA, Colonna G, Pasceri V, et al. Atenolol versus amlodipine versus isosorbide-5-mononitrate on anginal symptoms in syndrome X. Am J Cardiol. 1999;84:854-6.
67. Leonardo F, Fragasso G, Rossetti E, et al. Comparison of trimetazidine with atenolol in patients with syndrome X: effects on diastolic function and exercise tolerance. Cardiologia. 1999;44:1065-9.
68. Sutsch G, Oechslin E, Mayer I, et al. Effect of diltiazem on coronary flow reserve in patients with microvascular angina. Int J Cardiol. 1995;52:135-43.
69. Cannon RO 3rd, Watson RM, Rosing DR, et al. Efficacy of calcium channel blocker therapy for angina pectoris resulting from small-vessel coronary artery disease and abnormal vasodilator reserve. Am J Cardiol. 1985;56:242-6.
70. Zhang X, Li Q, Zhao J, et al. Effects of combination of statin and calcium channel blocker in patients with cardiac syndrome X. Coron Artery Dis. 2014;25:40-4.
71. Eshtehardi P, McDaniel MC, Dhawan SS, et al. Effect of the interaction between atorvastatin and selective serotonin reuptake inhibitors on the blood redox equilibrium. Exp Ther Med. 2016;12:3440-4.
72. Mehta PK, Goykhman P, Thomson LE, et al. Ranolazine improves angina in women with evidence of myocardial ischemia but no obstructive coronary artery disease. JACC Cardiovasc Imaging. 2011;4:514-22.
73. Villano A, Di Franco A, Nerla R, et al. Effects of ivabradine and ranolazine in patients with microvascular angina pectoris. Am J Cardiol. 2013;112:8-13.
74. Suwaidi JA, Hamasaki S, Higano ST, et al. Long-term follow-up of patients with mild coronary artery disease and endothelial dysfunction. Circulation. 2000;101:948-54.
75. Schachinger V, Britten MB, Zeiher AM. Prognostic impact of coronary vasodilator dysfunction on adverse long-term outcome of coronary heart disease. Circulation. 2000;101:1899-906.
76. Halcox JP, Schenke WH, Zalos G, et al. Prognostic value of coronary vascular endothelial dysfunction. Circulation. 2002;106:653-8.
77. Von Mering GO, Arant CB, Wessel TR, et al. Abnormal coronary vasomotion as a prognostic indicator of cardiovascular events in women: results from the National Heart, Lung, and Blood Institute sponsored Women's Ischemia Syndrome Evaluation (WISE). Circulation. 2004;109:722-5.
78. Murthy VL, Naya M, Foster CR, et al. Improved cardiac risk assessment with noninvasive measures of coronary flow reserve. Circulation. 2011;124:2215-24.
79. Britten MB, Zeiher AM, Schachinger V. Microvascular dysfunction in angiographically normal or mildly diseased coronary arteries predicts adverse cardiovascular long-term outcome. Coron Artery Dis. 2004;15:259-64.
80. Murthy VL, Naya M, Foster CR, et al. Association between coronary vascular dysfunction and cardiac mortality in patients with and without diabetes mellitus. Circulation. 2012;126:1858-68.

SECTION 5

Advances in Echocardiography: Clinical Implications

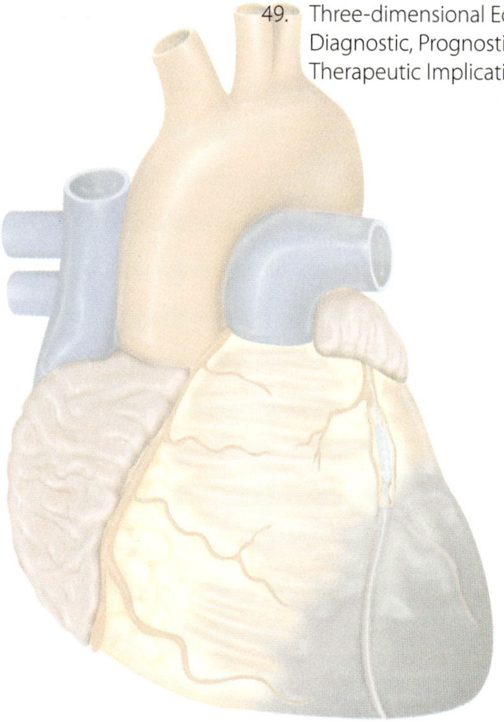

49

CHAPTER

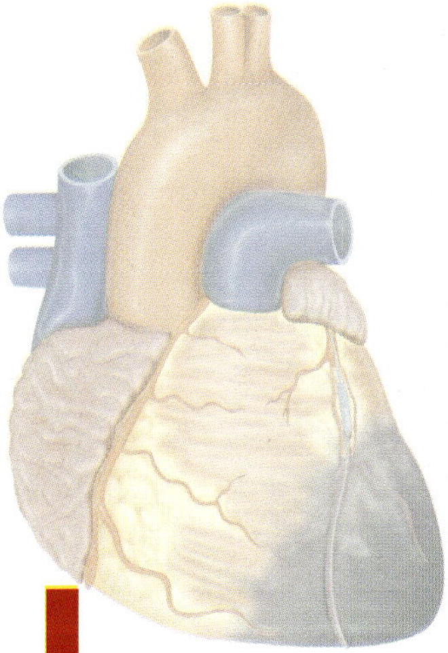

Three-dimensional Echocardiography: Diagnostic, Prognostic, and Therapeutic Implications

Aiman M Smer, Navin C Nanda, Ahmed Y Salama, Raziye E Akdogan, Hanan Fadala, HK Chopra

INTRODUCTION

Three-dimensional (3D) echocardiography is currently one of the main evolving advances in the field of cardiovascular ultrasound. The technology is based on matrix array transducers which consist of 3,000 piezoelectric crystals each of which emits an ultrasound beam resulting in 3D image acquisition of a large section of the heart.[1] These images can be acquired in real-time with limited elevation depth in Z-axis or in full volume mode utilizing several beats with elevation depth and lateral size decided by the operator keeping in mind that increases in the size of the acquired data set result in lower frame rates and hence lower image resolution. 3D zoom view lets the examiner focus on a smaller area of particular interest while 3D color Doppler acquisition provides color Doppler images useful to assess intracardiac shunts and valvular and paravalvular regurgitation. The 3D technology has been incorporated in both transthoracic and transesophageal transducers and more recent advances have resulted in faster dataset acquisition and improved image quality. The unique ability of 3D echocardiography to visualize the heart structures from 3D perspective has improved the diagnostic accuracy and clinical decision-making process.

DIAGNOSTIC CRITERION

Three-dimensional echocardiography is a powerful imaging modality and in several clinical conditions is considered superior to two-dimensional (2D) echocardiography (Table 1). Transthoracic 3D echocardiography has clearly improved the accuracy of chamber quantification. It

TABLE 1: Advantages and disadvantages of three-dimensional echocardiography.

Advantages	Disadvantages
1. Views normal and pathological cardiac structures in 3D providing comprehensive evaluation. 2. Provides assessment of third dimension (depth) of any structure. 3. Accurate assessment of size of any structure/masses/defects. Often underestimated by 2DTTE/multiplane 2DTEE 4. Obtains reliable enface views. 3D cropping plane can be positioned exactly parallel to any orifice or defect (stenotic, regurgitant or shunt) in short-axis to obtain accurately its area facilitating quantification of severity. Cannot ensure parallel orientation with 2D echo.	1. 3D echo not used as a stand-alone technique. However, complements 2D echo in many clinical scenarios. 2. 3D echo image resolution is inferior to 2D echo with lower frame rates, hence best quality 2D images required for 3D acquisition. 3. Needs additional training. May take considerable time and effort to change mind set to adapt to 3D images 4. Takes additional time to acquire, crop and interpret 3D echo data sets.

Contd...

Contd...

Advantages	Disadvantages
5. Facilitates systematic assessment of any cardiac structure or cavity by sequential cropping. Minimizes missing any abnormality.	5. Artifacts occur due to arrhythmia or patient/transducer movement during 3D acquisition (single beat acquisition obviates this).
6. Since 3D data sets contain multiple structures, their relationship can be accurately delineated	6. 3D echo systems more expensive than 2D equipment.
7. Morphology of a structure or mass can be studied by taking sections and viewing them enface.	
8. Volume of any structure or lesion can be measured to provide superior assessment of size. 2D echo provides only linear dimensions.	
9. Volume of any cardiac cavity (LV, RV, LA and RA) can be measured without making geometrical assumption of shape (as done by 2D echo).	

(2D echo: two-dimensional echocardiography; 3D echo: three-dimensional echocardiography; 2DTEE: two-dimensional transesophageal echocardiography; 2DTTE: two-dimensional transthoracic echocardiography; LA: left atrium; LV: left ventricle; RA: right atrium; RV: right ventricle)

Source: Reproduced with permission from Nanda NC, Karakus G, Degirmencioglu A. Manual of Echocardiography, 1st edition. New Delhi: Jaypee Brothers Medical Publishers (P) Ltd; 2016.

BOX 1: Major clinical applications of three-dimensional echocardiography in clinical practice.

- Valvular stenosis orifice planimetry for assessment of severity (MS, AS, TS, and PS).
- Native and prosthetic valvular regurgitation site determination and vena contracta planimetry to quantify severity (MR, AR, TR and PR).
- Assessment of individual prosthetic valve leaflet motion, thrombus (usually protruding from prosthesis) and pannus (usually does not protrude from prosthesis).
- Valvular prolapse (MV, AV, TV, and PV). Assessment of individual MV scallop/segment prolapse and chordae rupture.
- Aortic dissection and aneurysm. Differentiation from artifact as dissection flap appears sheet-like on 3D echo and not linear.
- Global LV/RV volumes and function. LV mass. Regional function. Diagnosis and assessment of LV/RV noncompaction/thrombus.
- Characterization of valvular masses. Vegetations and abscesses. Assessment of extent of valvular destruction.
- Characterization of cardiac masses and tumor mimics. Thrombus in LV, RV, RA, LA, and LAA (individual lobes can be examined). Differentiation of thrombus, myxoma, hemangioma, lipoma/fibroma, and malignancy.
- Differentiation of bicuspid from tricuspid AV.
- Enface planimetry of congenital and acquired defects (ASP, PFO, ASD, VSD, VSR, PDA, aorto-pulmonary window, fistulas, and complex defects).
- Planimetry of other obstructive lesions (sub/supravalvular stenosis, hypertrophic cardiomyopathy, atrial membranes, etc.).

(AR: aortic regurgitation; AS: aortic stenosis; ASD: atrial septal defect; ASP: atrial septal pouch; AV: aortic valve; LA: left atrium; LAA: left atrial appendage; LV: left ventricle; MR: mitral regurgitation; MS: mitral stenosis; MV: mitral valve; PDA: patent ductus arteriosus; PFO: patent foramen ovale; PR: pulmonary regurgitation; PS: pulmonary stenosis; PV: ulmonary valve; RA: right atrium; RV: right ventricle; TR: tricuspid regurgitation; TS: tricuspid stenosis; TV: tricuspid valve; VSD: ventricular septal defect; VSR: ventricular septal rupture)

Source: Reproduced with permission from Nanda NC, Karakus G, Degirmencioglu A. Manual of Echocardiography, 1st edition, New Delhi: Jaypee Brothers Medical Publishers (P) Ltd; 2016.

provides accurate measurements of left ventricular mass, volumes, wall motion, and ejection fraction without making assumptions regarding the geometric shape of the left ventricle inherent in 2D technology. Also, 3D echo helps eliminate apical foreshortening which is common with 2D echo and reduces its accuracy in the assessment of left ventricular function. When compared to a different imaging modality such as cardiac magnetic resonance (CMR), these 3D measurements show a good correlation and have much better intra- and interobserver variability than 2D echocardiography.[2] In patients with heart valves disease, 3D echocardiography offers valuable diagnostic information as well as provides real-time guidance for surgical and percutaneous valve repair procedures. 3D echocardiography is more accurate than 2D mitral and aortic valve area planimetry measurements and has strong correlation with invasive hemodynamic measurements of mitral valve area.[3] Moreover, 3D echocardiography offers the ability to accurately measure the effective orifice area of both stenotic and regurgitant valve lesions from multiple orthogonal 2D angles in a multiplanar reconstruction tool (Box 1 and Figures 1 to 14).[4]

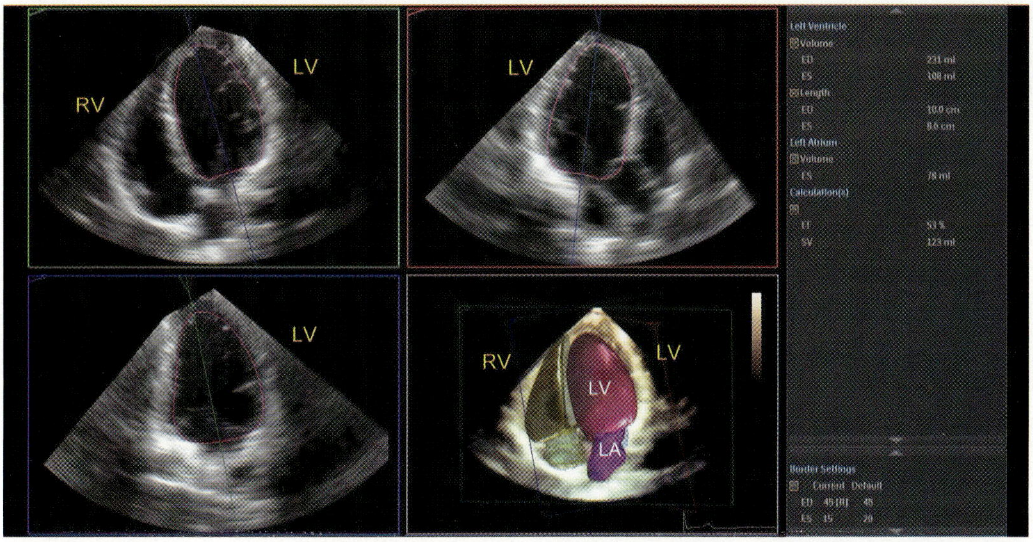

Fig. 1: An example of transthoracic three-dimensional heart-model dataset with surface reconstruction display of all four cardiac chambers, left atrium volume, left ventricle volumes, and ejection fraction. (LV: left ventricle; RV: right ventricle).

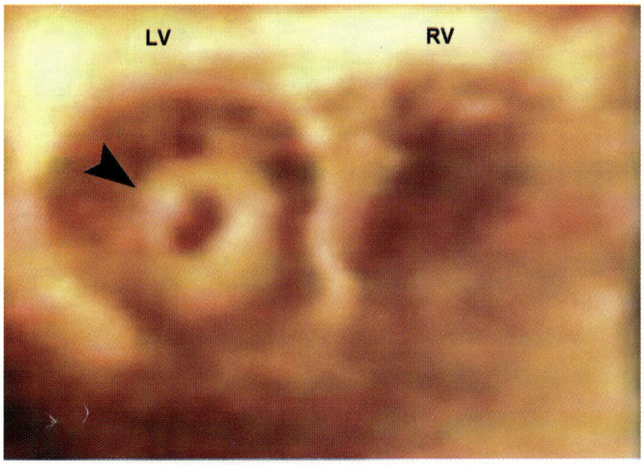

Fig. 2A: Live/real-time three-dimensional transthoracic echocardiography in mitral stenosis. Arrow head points to the tip of the MV orifice. (LV: left ventricle; MV: mitral valve; RV: right ventricle).
Source: Reproduced with permission from Singh V, Nanda NC, Agrawal G, et al. Live three-dimensional echocardiographic assessment of mitral stenosis. Echocardiography. 2003;20:743-50.

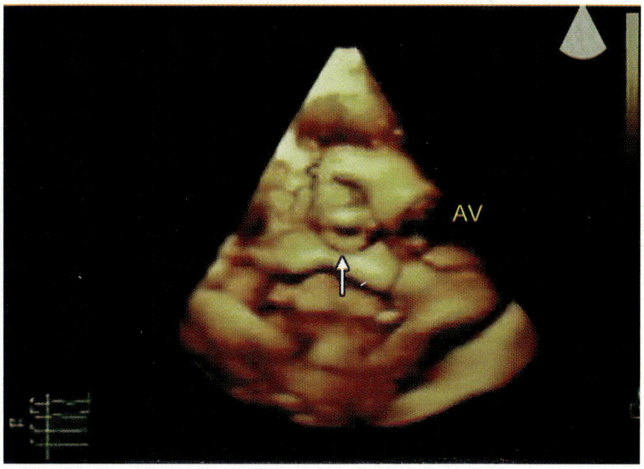

Fig. 2B: Live/real-time three-dimensional transthoracic echocardiography. Arrow points to severe bicuspid AV stenosis. (AV: aortic valve).
Source: Reproduced with permission from Nanda NC, Karakus G, Degirmencioglu A. Manual of Echocardiography, 2nd edition. New Delhi: Jaypee Brothers Medical Publishers (P) Ltd; 2018.

PROGNOSTIC IMPLICATIONS

Several echocardiographic parameters, such as left ventricular ejection fraction and left atrium volume index, have been shown to provide prognostic implications. Also, 3D longitudinal strain has been showing to be an independent predictor of segmental and global left ventricular improvement after myocardial infarction.[5] 3D echocardiography measurements of left atrial size and volume are more accurate and reproducible than 2D measurements, when compared to CMR imaging, and has a strong correlation with cardiovascular outcomes.[6]

THERAPEUTIC IMPLICATIONS INCLUDING MEDICAL, MECHANICAL, AND SURGICAL

Three-dimensional echocardiography could provide additive value in the management of patients with

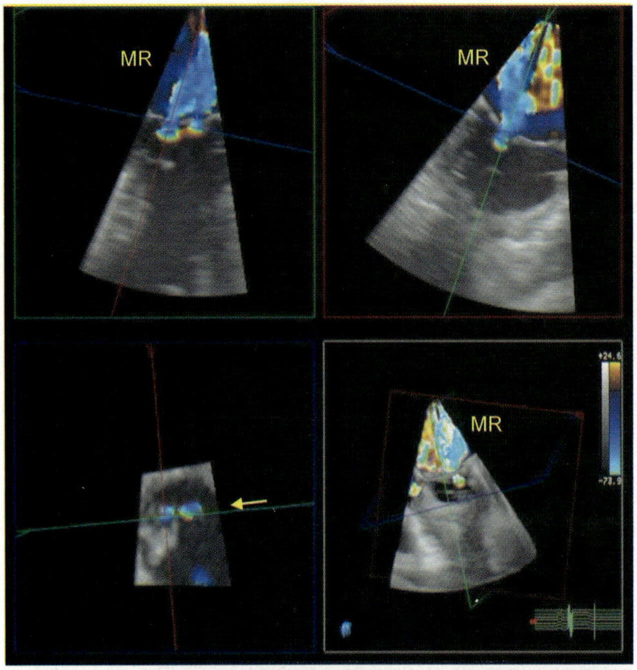

Fig. 3: Measurement of vena contracta dimensions and area from three-dimensional transesophageal color Doppler images of mitral regurgitation using the multiplanar reconstruction (MPR) technique. Arrow points to the vena contracta. (MR: mitral regurgitation).

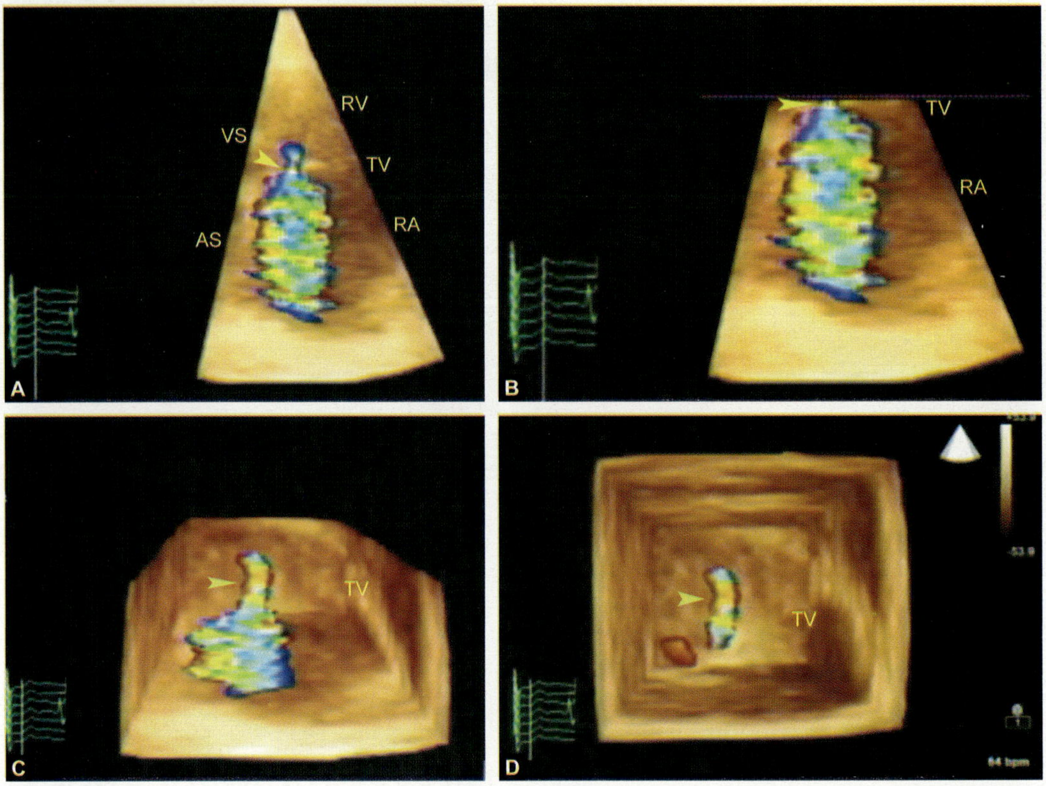

Figs. 4A to D: Live/real-time three-dimensional transthoracic echocardiographic assessment of tricuspid regurgitation vena contracta. (A) The three-dimensional data set was first cropped posteroanteriorly to detect the tricuspid regurgitation jet, flow acceleration (PISA) and the vena contracta (arrow head); (B) The cropping plane was then moved from the top toward the bottom and placed at the level of the vena contracta making sure it is parallel to it; and (C and D) The dataset was tilted to view the vena contracta enface. The size of the vena contracta can then be measured by planimetry. (AS: atrial septum; RA: right atrium; TV: tricuspid valve; VS: ventricular septum).

Source: Reproduced with permission from Velayudhan DE, Brown TM, Nanda NC, et al. Quantification of tricuspid regurgitation by live three-dimensional transthoracic echocardiographic measurements of vena contracta area. Echocardiography. 2006;23:793-800.

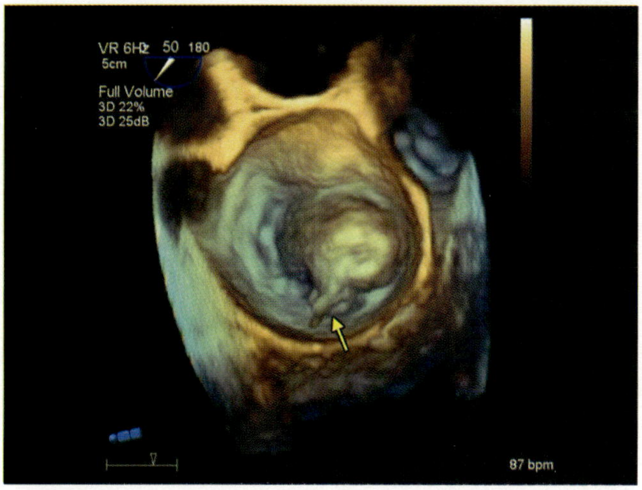

Fig. 5: Transesophageal 3D zoom imaging of the mitral valve in enface view from the left atrial side. Arrow points to a flail A2 scallop with a ruptured chord.

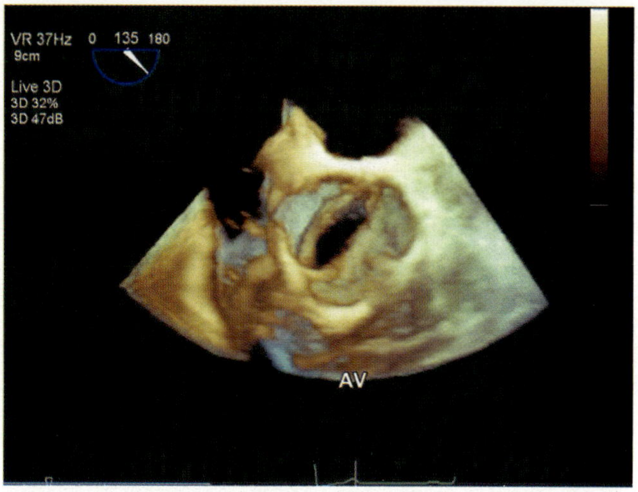

Fig. 7: Live three-dimensional transesophageal echocardiogram showing enface view of a bicuspid aortic valve with fusion of the right and left coronary cusps.

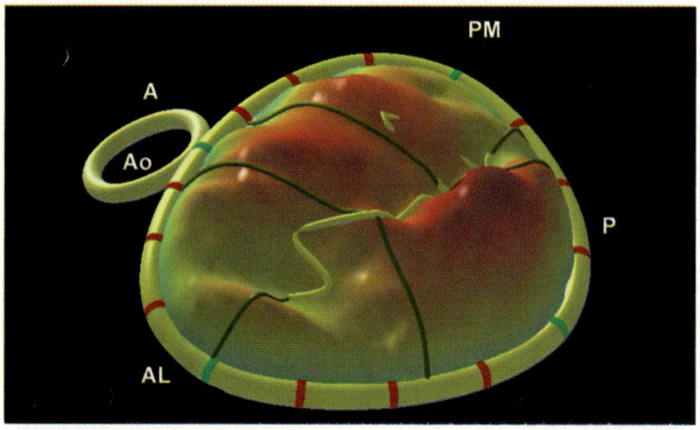

Fig. 6: An image of mitral valve obtained from a patient with Barlow's disease. 3D mitral valve quantification analysis demonstrates a saddle-shaped mitral annulus and bileaflet prolapse. (A: aortic valve; Ao: aorta; AL: anterolateral; PM: posteromedial; P: posterior).

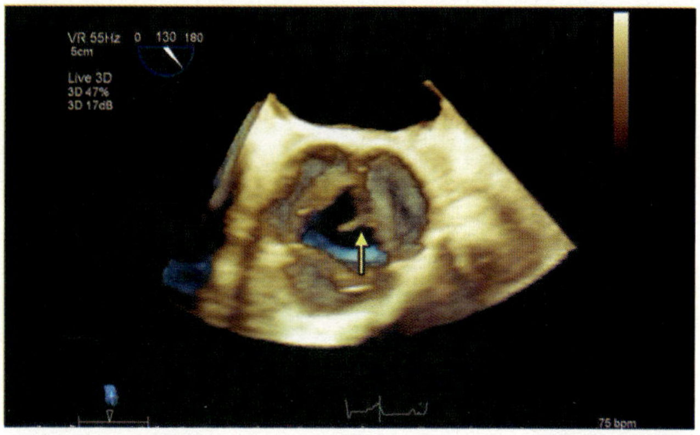

Fig. 8: Live three-dimensional transesophageal mid-esophageal short-axis view of the aortic valve. Arrow points to a linear mobile echodensity at the tip of the left coronary cusp consistent with a Lambl's excrescence.

cardiac conditions. For example, transesophageal 3D echocardiography allows direct visualization of the mitral valve leaflets from the left atrial side in "en face" perspective, also known as "the surgeon's view". This unique advantage of 3D echocardiography provides unprecedented views of the mitral valve apparatus and allows for accurate diagnosis of individual leaflet or scallop pathology in patients with organic mitral regurgitation. The use of 3D echocardiography has been shown to improve the diagnostic accuracy and the decision making process in patients undergoing mitral valve repair.[7] In patients with pacemakers presenting with significant tricuspid regurgitation, 3D echocardiography has a useful role in determining whether pacemaker or defibrillator leads interfere with tricuspid valve function.[8] The benefit of 3D echocardiography is invaluable in the assessment of patients with malfunctioning prosthetic valves. Transesophageal 3D echocardiography can be very instrumental in the evaluation of prosthesis degeneration, suture dehiscence, and paravalvular regurgitation. 3D color Doppler echocardiography is most helpful in not only pinpointing the location of the paravalvular leak but also determining the size of the regurgitation vena contracta.[9] When closing paravalvular mitral regurgitation in the cardiac catheterization laboratory, 3D echocardiography is routinely used for accurate device deployment and 3D color Doppler supplements 2D color Doppler imaging to evaluate for residual leak postdevice deployment. Moreover, 3D transesophageal echocardiography is crucial for successful MitraClip procedure firstly to puncture the atrial septum at the optimal site by visualizing it en face and then

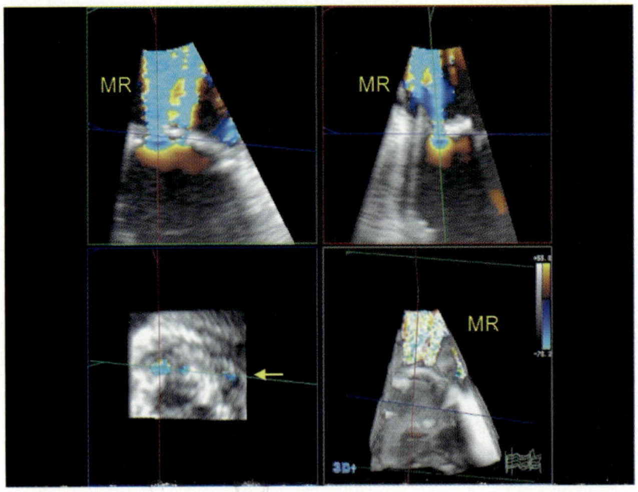

Fig. 9: Three-dimensional transesophageal color Doppler enface view of a mitral valve prosthesis showing the location of three separate paravalvular leaks (arrow). Quantitative assessment of leakage size using three-dimensional analysis software and multiplanar reconstruction (MPR) mode. (MR: mitral regurgitation).

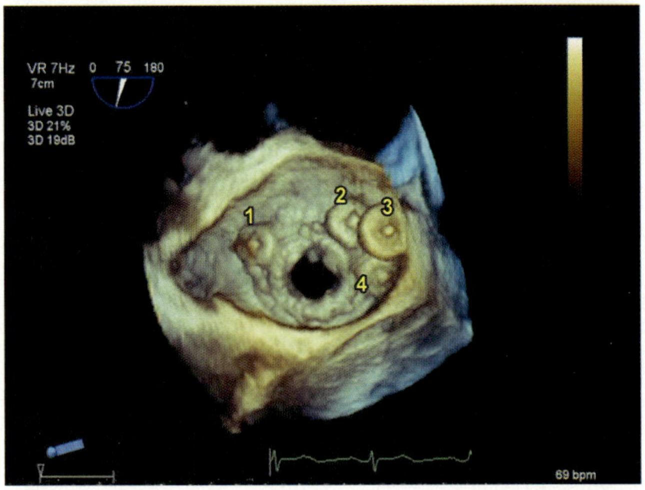

Fig. 11: Live/three-dimensional transesophageal echocardiography enface view of the mitral valve. #1, #2, #3, and #4 represent four Amplatzer occluder devices implanted around the bioprosthetic mitral valve ring for severe paravalvular leaks.

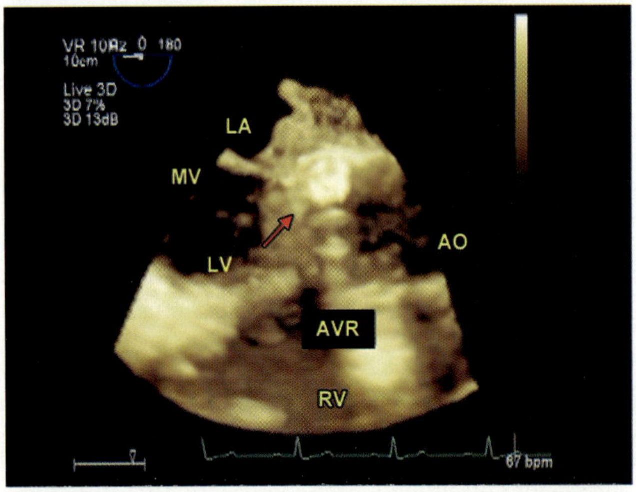

Fig. 10: Live/real-time three-dimensional transesophageal echocardiography. Arrow points to vascular Amplatzer plug used to close paravalvular aortic regurgitation (AR) in this patient with aortic valve (AV) prosthesis. (AVR: aortic valve replacement; LA: left atrium; MV: mitral valve).

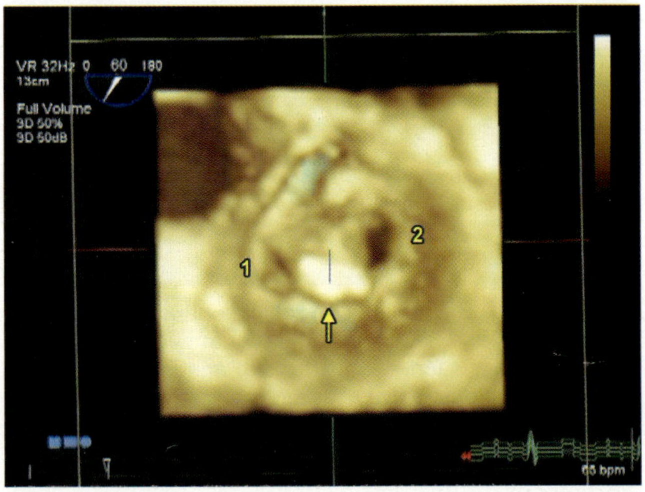

Fig. 12: Live/real-time three-dimensional transesophageal echocardiography. Arrow points to Mitraclip #1 and #2 represent the two mitral orifices resulting from mitraclip device placement.
Source: Reproduced with permission from Nanda NC, Karakus G, Degirmencioglu A. Manual of Echocardiography, 2nd edition, New Delhi: Jaypee Brothers Medical Publishers (P) Ltd; 2018.

to position the device successfully converting the single mitral orifice into two orifices with a resultant decrease in mitral regurgitation severity.[4] 3D echocardiography measurements are more accurate than 2D transesophageal echocardiography in the assessment of the left atrial appendage ostium dimensions and circumference as well as depth in patients who would benefit from left atrial appendage occlusion with the Watchman or some other device. In this procedure also, 3D echo is useful in guiding trans-septal puncture and assessing the appendage before, during and following device placement. Importantly, 3D echocardiography is an essential diagnostic modality in the evaluation and management of patients with congenital heart disease.[10] Overall, there are three main important clinical applications of 3D echocardiography in these patients: (1) en face viewing and assessment of size of

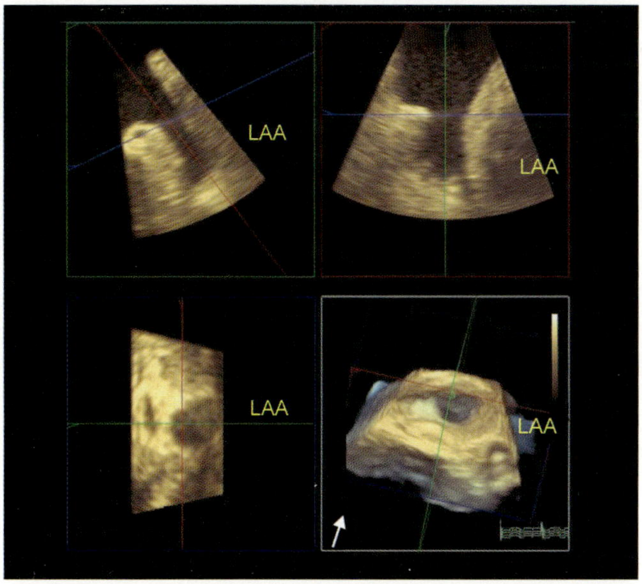

Fig. 13: Three-dimensional transesophageal zoom image of left atrial appendage viewed in multiplanar reconstruction (MPR) mode for accurate measurement of orifice size and depth prior to Watchman procedure (arrow). (LAA: left atrial appendage).

congenital heart defects together with the surrounding structures, (2) cardiac chambers visualization in 3D and quantitative evaluation of their size and function, and (3) guidance of percutaneous cardiac interventions. Moreover, 3D echocardiography is useful in evaluation of intracardiac masses, which improve the diagnostic accuracy and delineate treatment options in cases of cardiac thrombi, vegetations, and tumors. In one study, live transesophageal 3D echocardiography identified cardiac thrombi in up to 78% of cases compared to only 33% via conventional 2D echocardiography.[11]

DISCUSSION

Three-dimensional echocardiography has become a powerful diagnostic tool in the field of cardiology. The clinical use of 3D echocardiography will continue to evolve and provide more accurate assessments of cardiac chamber characteristics, better in-depth understanding of cardiac anatomy, and real-time guidance for percutaneous cardiac procedures. The ongoing improvements in 3D technology will probably overcome current limitations and further enhance the clinical applications of 3D echocardiography.

LIMITATION

For now, it is important to realize that 3D echocardiography does not completely replace 2D imaging for most clinical indications and remains a supplementary technique. The quality of 3D echo is lower as compared to 2D imaging and hence an attempt needs to be made in all patients to acquire the best quality 2D images for 3D acquisition. With further advances in technology, one would expect increased frame rates and improved spatial resolution which will further enhance its utility in clinical practice.

GUIDELINES

Both the American Society of Echocardiography and the European Association of Echocardiography guidelines recommend routine use of 3D echocardiography in: (1) left

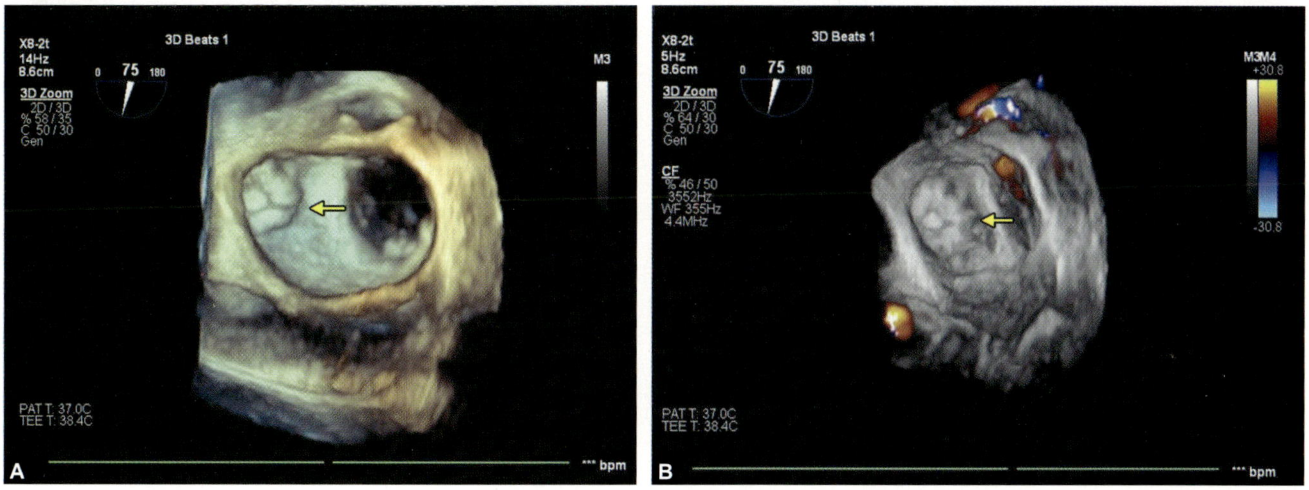

Figs. 14A and B: (A) Live/real-time three-dimensional transesophageal image shows a well-seated Watchman device (arrow) within the left atrial appendage; and (B) Three-dimensional color Doppler image shows appropriate device placement (arrow) with no peridevice leak.

ventricular volumes and ejection fraction, (2) assessment of valvular heart disease, and (3) guidance for transcatheter procedures.[12]

CONCLUSION

Three-dimensional echocardiography is a safe, valuable, and noninvasive diagnostic tool. Both transthoracic and transesophageal 3D echocardiography provide not only impressive images of cardiac structures but also can view them using planes not available with 2D imaging. En face views using 3D echocardiography provide valuable information in many cardiac disease entities. This advantage has further improved the diagnostic accuracy of echocardiography. Future directions and advancements of 3D echocardiography would be expected to provide accurate, efficient, and fast measurements of cardiac chamber function, stenotic areas, various types of cardiac defects, and volumes of masses thus, contributing to time-saving and cost-saving strategies in the management of cardiac patients.

REFERENCES

1. Wang XF, Deng YB, Nanda NC, et al. Live three-dimensional echocardiography: Imaging principles and clinical application. Echocardiography. 2003;20(7):593-604.
2. Nikitin NP, Constantin C, Loh PH, et al. New generation 3-dimensional echocardiography for left ventricular volumetric and functional measurements: Comparison with cardiac magnetic resonance. Eur J Echocardiogr. 2006;7(5):365-72.
3. Singh V, Nanda NC, Agrawal G, et al. Live three-dimensional echocardiographic assessment of mitral stenosis. Echocardiography. 2003;20(8):743-50.
4. Nanda N, Karakus G, Degirmencioglu A. Manual of Echocardiography, 2nd edition. New Delhi: Jaypee Brothers Medical Publishers (P) Ltd; 2018.
5. Abate E, Hoogslag GE, Antoni ML, et al. Value of three-dimensional speckle-tracking longitudinal strain for predicting improvement of left ventricular function after acute myocardial infarction. Am J Cardiol. 2012;110(7):961-7.
6. Pritchett AM, Jacobsen SJ, Mahoney DW, et al. Left atrial volume as an index of left atrial size: A population-based study. J Am Coll Cardiol. 2003;41(6):1036-43.
7. Ben Zekry S, Nagueh SF, Little SH, et al. Comparative accuracy of two- and three-dimensional transthoracic and transesophageal echocardiography in identifying mitral valve pathology in patients undergoing mitral valve repair: Initial observations. J Am Soc Echocardiogr. 2011;24(10):1079-85.
8. Nucifora G, Badano LP, Allocca G, et al. Severe tricuspid regurgitation due to entrapment of the anterior leaflet of the valve by a permanent pacemaker lead: Role of real time three-dimensional echocardiography. Echocardiography. 2007;24(6):649-52.
9. Alli OO, Hsiung MC, Guvenc T, et al. Incremental value of three-dimensional transesophageal echocardiography over the two-dimensional technique in percutaneous closure of aortic paraprosthetic regurgitation. Echocardiography. 2014;31(9):1154-8.
10. Simpson J, Lopez L, Acar P, et al. Three-dimensional echocardiography in congenital heart disease: An expert consensus document from the European Association of Cardiovascular Imaging and the American Society of Echocardiography. J Am Soc Echocardiogr. 2017;30(1):1-27.
11. Anwar AM, Nosir YF, Ajam A, et al. Central role of real-time three-dimensional echocardiography in the assessment of intracardiac thrombi. Int J Cardiovasc Imaging. 2010;26(5):519-26.
12. Lang RM, Badano LP, Tsang W, et al. EAE/ASE recommendations for image acquisition and display using three-dimensional echocardiography. Eur Heart J Cardiovasc Imaging. 2012;13(1):1-46.

50

CHAPTER

TEE: Overview, Diagnostic, Prognostic and Therapeutic Implications

Kaustubh Mahamine, CK Ponde

INTRODUCTION

Echocardiography is the most commonly used imaging modality for cardiac assessment. Transthoracic echocardiography (TTE) is widely available and provides quick, low cost, and clinically relevant information regarding cardiac structure and function. TTE is inadequate in certain clinical conditions where transesophageal echocardiography (TEE) provides incremental diagnostic and prognostic information that helps in clinical decision making. TEE is performed by inserting a small ultrasound transducer via a flexible probe into patients esophagus. Images of heart thus obtained are from posterior position permitting use of higher frequency transducer. Images thus obtained have higher spatial resolution and superior image quality. TEE being semi-invasive is used as an adjunctive investigation to TTE (Box 1 outlines advantages and disadvantages of TEE).

Frazin et al.[1] in 1976 were first to report use of TEE using modified rigid endoscopic probe with single M-mode crystal. Current generation probes use phased array technology to steer at an angle of 180° thereby providing a 360° panoramic image of heart. Adult TEE probes operate at 3.5–7 MHz and pediatric probes at 7–10 MHz. All modalities like M-mode, color flow Doppler, color M-mode, and real-time 3D imaging are possible with multiplanar probes. Integration of 3D TEE with fluoroscopy[2] now is used in many advanced cardiac catheterization labs worldwide to aid various therapeutic procedures like trans-septal puncture, left atrial appendage closure, pulmonary vein isolation, and even transcatheter aortic valve replacement (TAVR).

INDICATIONS

Most common indications of TEE are to investigate cryptogenic stroke or source of embolism, to rule out left atrial appendage (LAA) clot prior to cardioversion of atrial fibrillation and prosthetic valve endocarditis. Indications are discussed in details in subsequent sections. Though TEE usually follows an initial TTE certain situations demand initial evaluation by TEE (Box 2).

CONTRAINDICATIONS

In contrast to TTE, transesophageal imaging has the disadvantage of being semi-invasive. Detail history should be taken to rule out contraindications (Box 3) to TEE.

BOX 1: Advantages and disadvantages of TEE.

Advantages:
- Higher resolution
- Superior imaging of mitral and aortic valve, left atrium, pulmonary veins, aortic arch
- No ribs shadowing-continuous acoustic window

Disadvantages:
- Semi-invasive, requires sedation
- Risk associated with probe intubation
- May not visualize left ventricular (LV) apex and right sided structures
- Blind acoustic spot where trachea is interposed between heart and esophagus

BOX 2: Indications of TEE as the first modality of imaging.

- Suspected acute aortic pathology (i.e. dissection, trans-section, intramural hematoma)
- Suspected prosthetic valve dysfunction (thrombus, pannus ingrowth, vegetation, or regurgitation)
- Suspected complications of endocarditis (e.g. fistula, abscess)
- Evaluation for left atrial/LAA thrombus in a patient with atrial fibrillation/atrial flutter to facilitate clinical decision making regarding anticoagulation, cardioversion, or ablation
- Evaluation of source of embolism in a young (<50 years) patient

(TEE: transesophageal echocardiography; LAA: left atrial appendage)

BOX 3: Contraindications of TEE.

Absolute contraindications:
- Perforated viscus
- Esophageal stricture
- Esophageal tumor
- Esophageal perforation/laceration
- Esophageal diverticulum
- Active upper gastrointestinal (GI) bleed

Relative contraindications:
- Altered mental status or an uncooperative patient
- History of radiation to neck or mediastinum
- History of GI surgery
- Recent upper GI bleed
- History of Barrett's esophagus
- Esophageal varices
- Active esophagitis
- Active peptic ulcer disease
- Symptomatic hiatal hernia
- Tenuous cardiorespiratory status (consider endotracheal intubation prior to TEE for airway protection)
- Surgical interposition of the esophagus
- History of odynophagia or dysphagia (consider screening endoscopy and/or barium swallow prior to TEE)
- Cervical spine arthritis with reduced range of motion
- Severe thrombocytopenia (less than 50k), elevated international normalized ratio (greater than 3), or prolonged partial thromboplastin time (>150 seconds)
- Obstructive sleep apnea/airway compromise (consider sedation by anesthesia)

PATIENT PREPARATION

- Obtain informed consent. Patient should be counseled and procedure should be explained in detail to ensure full cooperation.
- Patient should be fasting for 6 hours. Clear fluids can be allowed 3 hours prior to procedure.
- Metoclopramide may be indicated in patients with delayed gastric emptying.
- Venous access is obtained with 20G catheter. Left hand is preferred due to high incidence of left superior vena cava (LSVC) (4.3%) in patients referred for cardiac evaluation.[3] Intravenous access is required for administering medication as well as contrast injection.
- Sedation and Anesthesia
  Patients undergoing TEE belong to either of the three groups mentioned below. Level of sedation differs for different patients.
  - Outpatients or ambulatory awake inpatients.
  - Ventilated patients in intensive care units.
  - Patients in operating rooms under general anesthesia.

Conscious Sedation

Awake patients should be given sedation enough to allay procedure related anxiety. Intravenous midazolam in small doses of 1–2 mg is preferred for its fast onset (1–2 minutes) and short half-life of 15–30 minutes. Diazepam and lorazepam are longer acting agents. Prior assessment of airway is warranted before administration of sedation. The echocardiography lab should be equipped with emergency intubation tray and crash cart. Vital parameters such as heart rate, blood pressure, and arterial oxygen saturation should be monitored. Opioids (e.g. Fentanyl) can be used as adjuncts to benzodiazepine with intention to reduce the probe-related discomfort. Reversal agents, flumazenil (0.2 mg every 10 minutes till reversal) for benzodiazepines and Naloxone (0.4 mg) for opioids can be used in case of toxicity.

Anesthesia

Oropharynx anesthesia can be achieved by topical application of local anesthesia (lignocaine, benzocaine, or cetacaine) in form of spray, gel or viscous gargles. Spray is preferred as drug can be directed towards posterior pharyngeal wall (*see* Fig. 4). Topical anesthesia should be applied until patient reports loss of sensation.

PROCEDURE

Transesophageal Echocardiography Probe

The TEE probe has been described in Figures 1 to 3.

Probe Insertion Techniques

Patient is turned in lateral position to allow drainage of oral secretions. Block bite (Fig. 4) is placed in patients mouth. Water soluble jelly is applied over the probe. Probe is introduced in pharynx in an anteflexed position and patient is encouraged to swallow. Swallowing of air should be avoided. Probe is advanced into esophagus, synchronized with the deglutition movements of patient to avoid trauma.

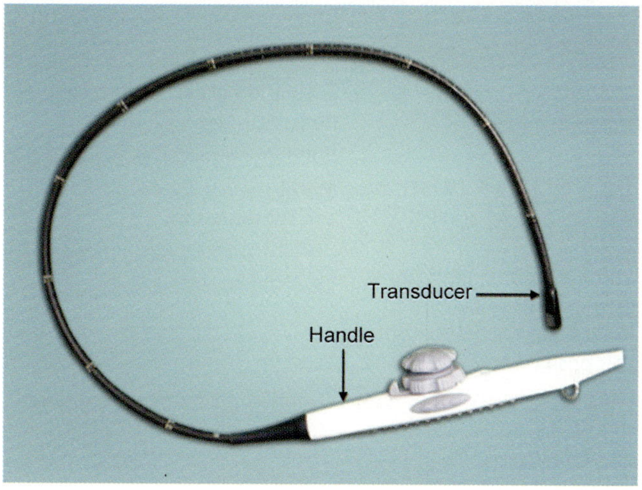

Fig. 1: TEE probe.

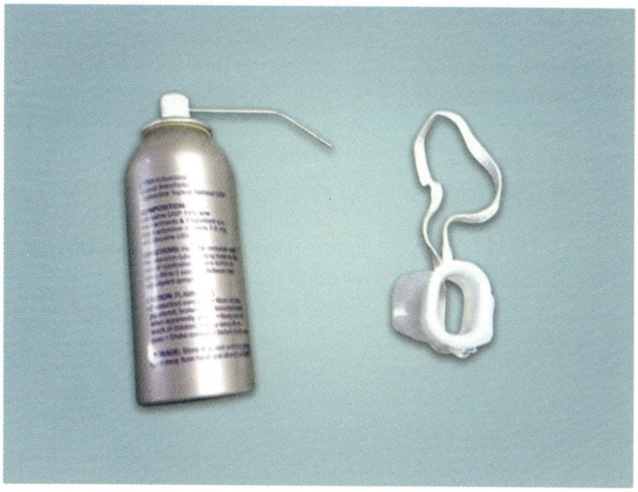

Fig. 4: Lignocaine spray and bite guard.

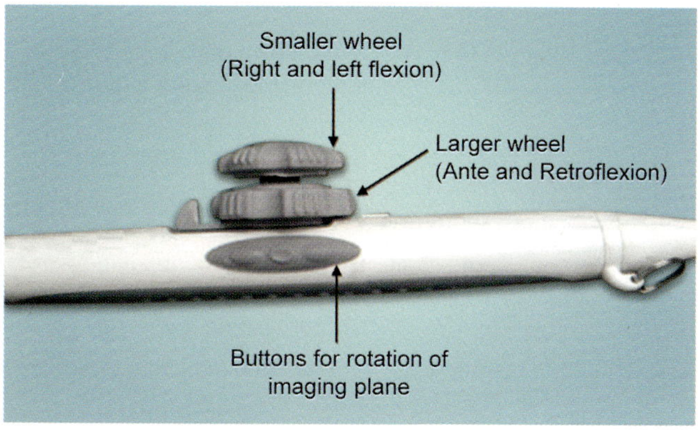

Fig. 2: TEE probe handle.

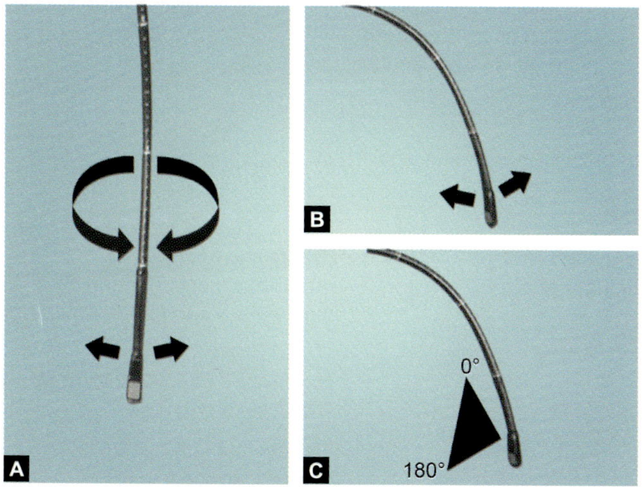

Figs. 3A to C: Movements of the TEE probe: (A) Right and left flexion and manual rotation; (B) Ante- and retroflexion; (C) Rotation of transducer.

Probe has markers to guide level of intubation, e.g. a midesophageal view is 33 cm from incisors. Image should guide the movement of the probe.

Manipulation of the Probe

A TEE probe has two control wheels and two buttons over the handle. Smaller wheel is used for right or left flexion. Larger wheel causes anteflexion and retroflexion. Pressing the buttons causes rotation of imaging plane from 0° to 180°. Apart from these, probe can be manually rotated clockwise and anticlockwise. Standard terminology used to define movements of TEE probe are as follows (Figs. 3A to C):

- Advancing—pushing probe distally
- Withdrawing—pulling of probe proximally
- Anteflexion—rotating larger wheel clockwise
- Retroflexion—rotating larger wheel anticlockwise
- Right flexion—rotating smaller wheel clockwise
- Left flexion—rotating smaller wheel anticlockwise
- Turn to right—manual clockwise rotation of probe
- Turn to left—manual counterclockwise rotation of probe.

Transesophageal Echocardiography Views

American Society of Echocardiography (ASE) and Society of Cardiovascular Anesthesiologists (SCA) have proposed 28 views as a part of comprehensive TEE examination.[4] Though a comprehensive TEE examination is advised it may not be feasible given patient's clinical condition and time constraints. Hence, it is wise to perform a transthoracic echo study prior and determine "what to look for" in TEE exam. Nevertheless, whenever situation permits a comprehensive TEE should be performed. Standard TEE views are subsequently described in this section (Table 1 and Fig. 5).

TABLE 1: Comprehensive TEE views.

	View	*Sequential probe position*	*Structures viewed*	*Clinical application*
1.	ME five-chamber view	• 30 cm from incisors • 10° rotation of transducer	RA, LA, LV, RV, AV, LVOT, MV (A2-A1 and P1-P2) and TV	Evaluation of aortic, mitral and tricuspid valve structure and regurgitation
2.	ME four-chamber view	30–35 cm until MV seen clearly, 20° angle to remove AV and LVOT from image and max tricuspid annulus is seen. Retroflexion may be necessary	RA, LA, IAS, RV, LV, IVS, TV (STL and PTL), MV (A3–A2 and P2P1) Most comprehensive view. All major structures can be viewed with slight manipulation of probe from this position.	Mitral, tricuspid valve structure and regurgitation.
3.	ME mitral commissural view	Further rotate transducer angle to 50°–70°	• MV (P3-A3A2A1-P1) • Anterolateral and posteromedial papillary muscles and their chordae • Coronary sinus • Turning probe to right and left shows prosthetic valve sewing rings	Commissural mitral regurgitation jets, paravalvar leaks
4.	ME two-chamber view	80°–100° from ME commissural view	LA, LAA, LV and MV (P3-A3A2A1)	Mitral valvar pathology, LAA clot, inferior and anterior regional wall motion
5.	ME LAX view (like three-chamber view)	120°–140° rotation	LA, LV, AV, LVOT, aortic root, proximal aorta, CS, MV (P2-A2), RVOT and membranous septum	Inferolateral and anteroseptal wall motion, AR
6.	ME AV LAX	• Withdraw probe while maintaining 120°–140° • Turn probe right	LVOT, AV, aortic root and proximal aorta	Evaluation of AV, obtaining dimensions of the annulus and sinotubular junction
7.	ME ascending aorta LAX view	Withdraw probe, rotation of transducer to 90°–110°	Proximal aorta, right pulmonary artery	Evaluation of proximal ascending aorta
8.	ME ascending aorta SAX view	Transducer rotation to 0°–30°	Ascending aorta, SVC, MPA, MPA bifurcation (turn to right), LMCA, LMCA bifurcation	Evaluation of proximal aorta and MPA
9.	ME right pulmonary vein view	Advance probe in 0° and turn to right	Right inferior pulmonary vein (at 90° to insonation beam) and right superior pulmonary vein (parallel to insonation beam), SVC and ascending aorta	PV flow assessment
10.	ME AV SAX view	Reposition probe to center aorta in image, advance the probe and rotate transducer to 25°–45°	AV morphology, LMCA and RCA, IAS	AV evaluation, detection of PFO and ASD
11.	ME RV inflow-outflow view	Advance probe slightly rotating transducer to 50–70° and turn probe to right till RVOT and PV appear	TV, RV (on left of display), RVOT (on the right of display), PV and MPA	RV size and function, TV morphology and function, PV morphology and function
12.	ME modified bicaval view	In same position probe is turned to right until TV is centered in image	LA, RA, IAS, IVC, and TV	Eccentric TR directed toward IAS visualized in this view
13.	ME bicaval view	Transducer rotated to 90°–110° and probe turned to right	LA, RA, IAS, IVC, SVC	PFO detection, IVC and SVC rim measurement in OS–ASD for determining feasibility of device closure, detection of sinus venosus ASD

Contd...

Contd...

	View	*Sequential probe position*	*Structures viewed*	*Clinical application*
14.	ME right and left pulmonary vein view	Transducer angle 90°–110° turning probe further right images right pulmonary veins and turning probe left past LA images left pulmonary veins	Pulmonary veins	Left superior pulmonary vein flow can be assessed
15.	ME LA appendage view	From left pulmonary vein view turn probe to right with advancement will open LAA	LAA	Pulsed-wave Doppler to assess LAA velocity, detection of LAA clot or spontaneous echo contrast
16.	TG basal SAX view	Transducer angle 0°–20° probe is advanced into stomach, then anteflexed	Short-axis "Fish mouth" view of MV	MV morphology, commissures, to assess feasibility of PTMC. Regurgitant orifice
17.	TG midpapillary SAX view	Transducer turned back to neutral position and advanced further into stomach maintaining same 0°–20° transducer angle	LV	LV size, volume, and regional function
18.	TG apical SAX view	Further advance probe with same angle	LV apex and RV apex (rotate probe to right)	Regional wall motion, apical thrombi
19.	TG RV basal view	Return to TG Basal SAX view and turn probe to right	RV, TV	TV morphology and regurgitant orifice
20.	TG RV inflow/ outflow view	Maximal right flexion	ATL and PTL, right and left cusp of PV	TV and PV morphology
21.	Deep TG five-chamber view	Probe advanced deep anteflexed and left flexed	LVOT, AV, MV	Doppler assessment of AV and MV as Doppler beam is in alignment with LVOT and AV
22.	TG two-chamber view	Probe returned to midpapillary TG view, transducer angle rotated to 90°–110°	Anterior and inferior walls of LV, papillary muscles, chordae and MV	Regional wall motion
23.	TG RV inflow view	Turn probe to right	RV free wall, papillary muscles and chordae of TV	TV evaluation
24.	TG LAX view	Turn to left, rotate transducer to 120°–140°	Anterior septum and inferolateral wall of LV, LVOT, and AV	Regional wall motion, Doppler assessment of AV
25.	Descending aorta LAX view	Return transducer to 0°–10° and turn probe to left and withdraw till diaphragm	Descending aorta	Aortic dissection, aortic aneurysm, atherosclerotic plaques
26.	Descending aorta SAX view	From TG LAX view return transducer to 90°–100° and turn probe to left and withdraw	Descending aorta	Aortic dissection, aortic aneurysm, atherosclerotic plaques
27.	UE aortic arch view	Withdraw probe till left subclavian artery is imaged, then turn probe to right	Aortic arch and branches	Aortic dissection, aortic aneurysm, atherosclerotic plaques
28.	UE aortic arch SAX view	Rotate transducer to 70°–90°	Aortic arch and branches	Aortic dissection, aortic aneurysm, atherosclerotic plaques

(AR: aortic regurgitation; ASD: atrial septal defect; ATL: anterior leaflet; AV: aortic valve; CS: coronary sinus; IAS: interatrial septum; IVS: interventricular septum; LA: left atrium; LAA: left atrial appendage; LAX: long axis; LMCA: left main coronary artery; LV, left ventricle; LVOT: left ventricular outflow tract; ME: midesophageal; MPA: main pulmonary artery; MV, mitral valve; PFO: patent foramen ovale; PTL: posterior leaflet; PV: pulmonary vein; RA: right atrium; RV: right ventricle; RCA: right coronary artery; RVOT: right ventricular outflow tract; SAX: short axis; STL: septal tricuspid leaflet; SVC: superior vena cava; TG: transgastric; TV: tricuspid valve; UE: upper esophageal)

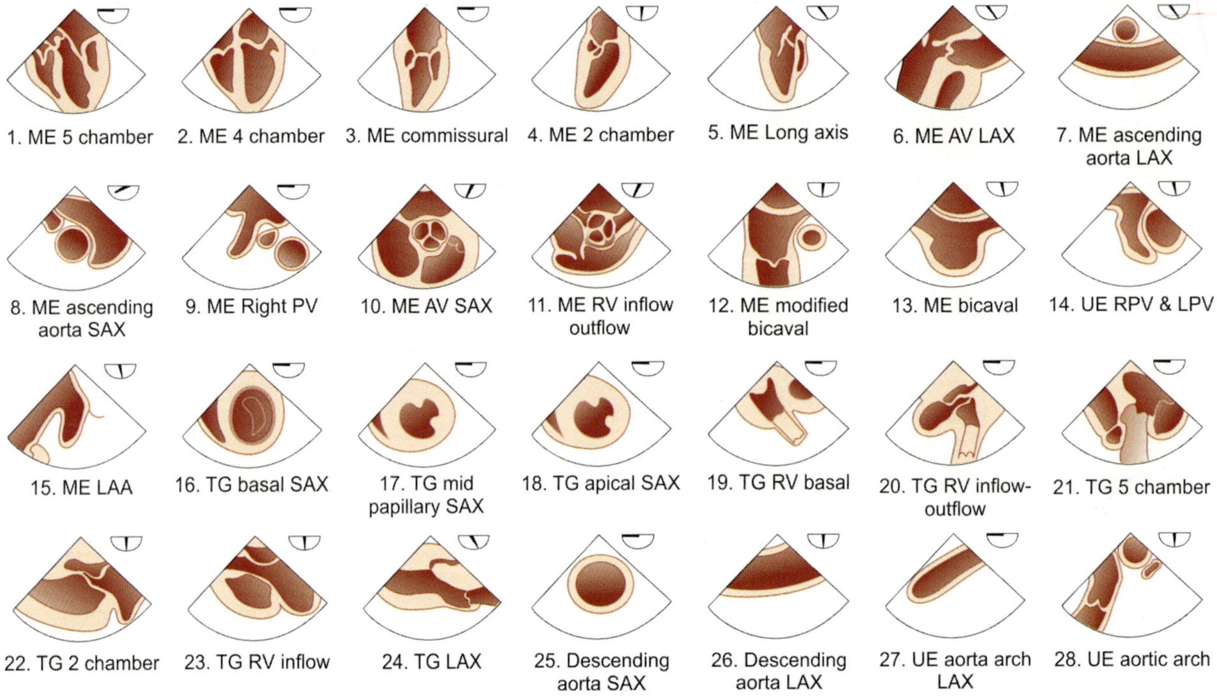

Fig. 5: Comprehensive TEE examination views. (ME: midesophageal; LAX: long axis; SAX; short axis; PV: pulmonary vein; AV: aortic vein; TG: transgastric; UE: upper esophageal; LAA: left atrial appendage).

Probe manipulation to obtain most common transducer position and angle are mentioned but image-guided fine tuning may be required to get a good quality image.

Three-dimensional TEE

Real-time 3D images can be obtained with currently available TEE probes. 3D TEE is widely used for valvar evaluation and during percutaneous cardiac procedures. Normal or pathological structures can be viewed from different perspectives and enables better understanding of cardiac anatomy.

Specific Indications of TEE

Apart from indications mentioned in Table 2, TEE is mainly indicated in cases where TTE is either inadequate or inconclusive. In general clinical applications of TEE can be classified as given below (Box 4).

BOX 4: Clinical applications of TEE[5]

Evaluation of:
- Native valve
- Prosthetic valve function/dysfunction
- Cardiac masses
- ICU patient with hemodynamic instability
- Congenital heart disease
- Cardioversion in atrial fibrillation

Detection of:
- Aortic dissection
- Complications of endocarditis
- Potential etiologies of stroke

Adjunct to:
- Percutaneous cardiac interventional procedures
- Cardiac surgical procedures

Native Valve Evaluation

Mitral Valve

Mitral valve and left atrium lie in the far field of all imaging planes of TTE. Hence, TEE is a crucial investigation modality to assess mitral valve disease in following scenarios:

- To assess the severity and cause of mitral regurgitation[6] especially in presence of eccentric regurgitant jet, Mitral valve prolapse, chordal rupture, secondary MR and papillary muscle dysfunction.
- To measure Mitral annulus for mitral valve repair.[7] Mitral annulus is measured in LAX view.
- To evaluate submitral apparatus, Mitral commissures, mitral regurgitation and LA clot in mitral stenosis to assess feasibility of percutaneous balloon mitral commissurotomy (Figs. 6 and 7)
- To detect vegetations (Fig. 8).

Aortic Valve

Transesophageal echocardiography (TEE) evaluation of aortic valve (AV) usually involves morphologic assessment. Hemodynamic assessment of aortic valve stenosis is best accomplished by TTE as it is difficult to align the aortic jet

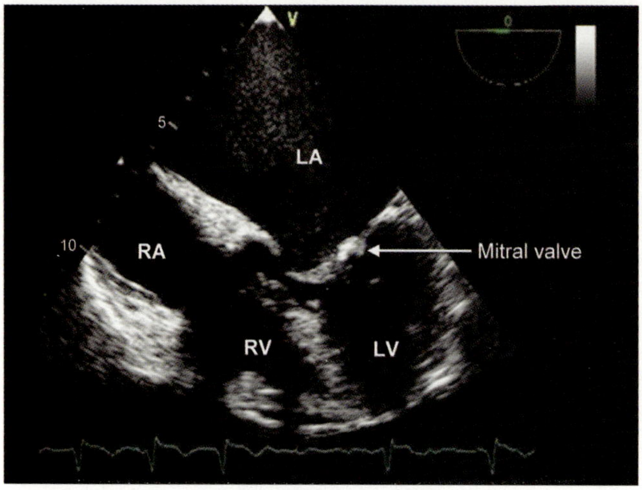

Fig. 6: Midesophageal 4-chamber view showing thickened, calcific and immobile mitral valve in a patient of rheumatic mitral stenosis.

to ultrasound beam in TEE. Measurement of aortic annulus by 3D TEE is comparable to computed tomography.[8] Aortic valve and LV outflow tract morphology is best seen in midesophageal LAX and SAX views of aortic valve (Figs. 9 and 10). TEE is more sensitive than TTE to detect aortic valve vegetations.

Tricuspid Valve

Tricuspid valve (TV) lies in far field of TEE probe, hence, TEE may not be of much use to diagnose tricuspid valve disease yet vegetation in right sided endocarditis particularly on septal leaflet are best seen on TEE. Turning the probe to right from midesophageal four-chamber view brings in TV in image. Transgastric view of TV may give better images of vena contracta for complex TR jets.

Pulmonary Valve

Plane of pulmonary valve is oblique to the plane of AV. PV also lies in the far field of the transducer hence difficult to image. Turning the probe left from midesophageal ascending aorta LAX and SAX views brings PV in the view. Transgastric view of PV is used for Doppler assessment of PV flow.

Prosthetic Valve

Reverberation and artifacts arising from mechanical valves prohibit adequate morphological assessment of prosthetic valves by TTE. The posterior position of TEE provides good quality images of paraprosthetic mitral and tricuspid anatomy. A combination of multiple views including both esophageal and transgastric views is essential for complete assessment of prosthetic aortic valves. TEE is a better investigation to diagnose paravalvular leaks. Thrombus, vegetation, and pannus are visualized better using TEE than other imaging techniques. Thrombi are generally larger with softer echo density and reduced video intensity when compared to pannus (Figs. 11 and 12).[9] In addition to its diagnostic utility, TEE can be used to monitor the effectiveness of thrombolytic therapy when treating valve thrombosis.

Infective Endocarditis

Transesophageal echocardiography (TEE) offers better images to detect vegetation with a sensitivity of 82–100% for

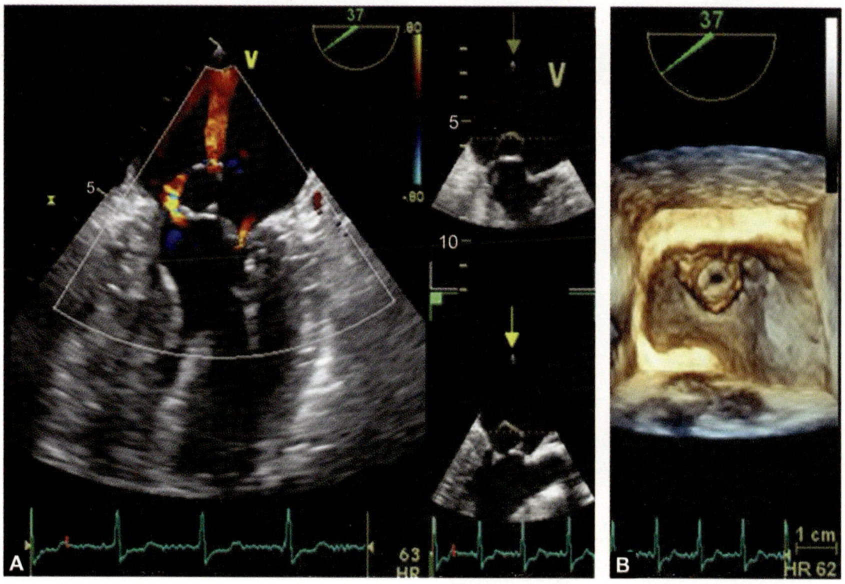

Figs. 7A and B: (A) Communicating aneurysm of AML with color flow showing flow across aneurysm into left atrium (LA). (B) 3D enface view of mitral valve showing opening of aneurysm into the LA.

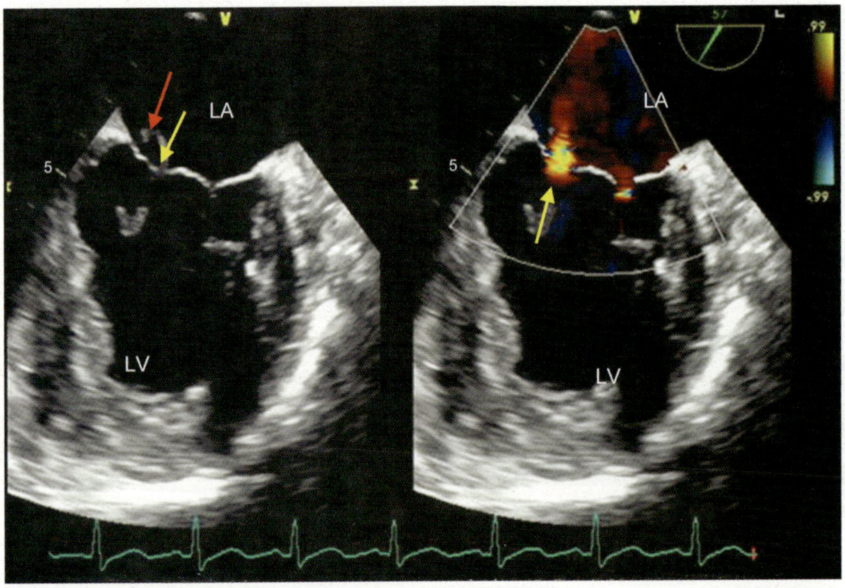

Fig. 8: Midesophageal commissural view. Left: Anterior mitral leaflet vegetation (red arrow) with perforation (yellow arrow). Right: Color Doppler showing regurgitant flow through perforated segment.

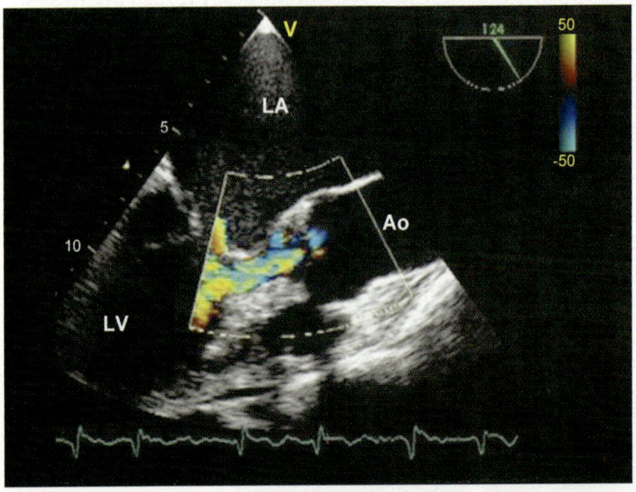

Fig. 9: Midesophageal 3-chamber view with color Doppler across aortic valve showing aortic regurgitation.

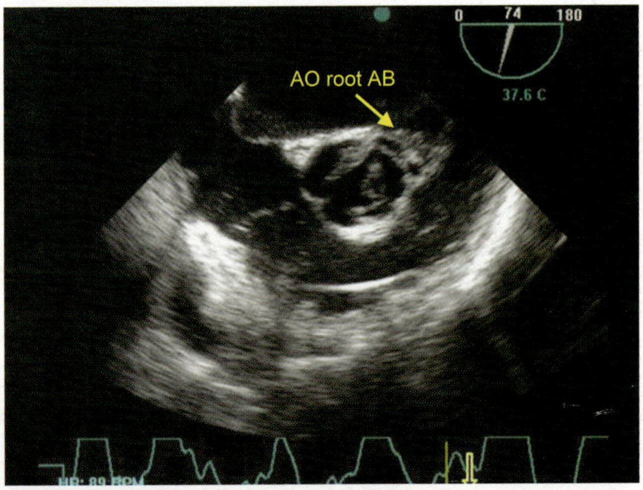

Fig. 10: ME AV SAX showing aortic abscess (arrow). (AV: aortic valve; ME: midesophageal; SAX: short axis).

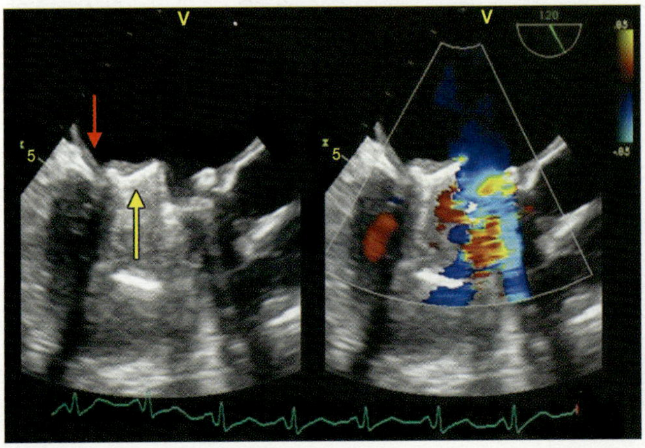

Fig. 11: Midesophageal 3-chamber view showing bileaflet mechanical valve pannus (red arrow) with stuck disc (yellow arrow).

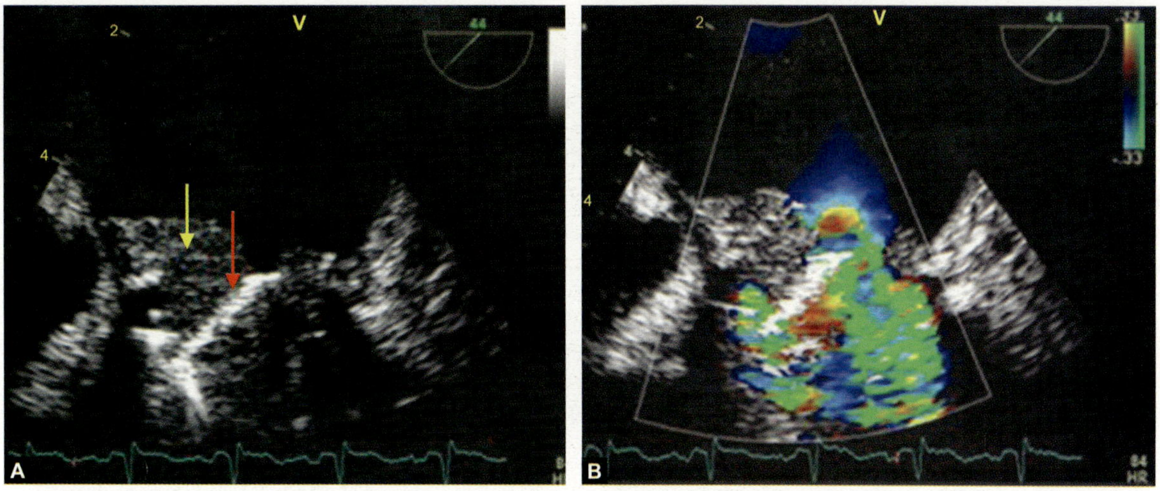

Figs. 12A and B: Midesophageal (ME) commissural view. (A) Mechanical valve thrombus (yellow arrow) with stuck leaflet (red arrow). (B) Color Doppler showing flow from the mobile leaflet.

native valves and 77–94% for prosthetic valves, specificity of 88–100%. TEE is preferred over TTE as initial tool for diagnosing infective endocarditis (IE) in patients with difficult window, with prosthetic valves or those who are a high risk of developing complications (including those with staphylococci bacteremia, systemic to pulmonary shunts, cyanotic congenital diseases, and prior IE). TEE is helpful in diagnosing complications of IE such as paravalvular extension, perforation of valve (Figs. 8 and 13), and abscess. Indications of surgical intervention based on echocardiography criteria are given in Box 5.

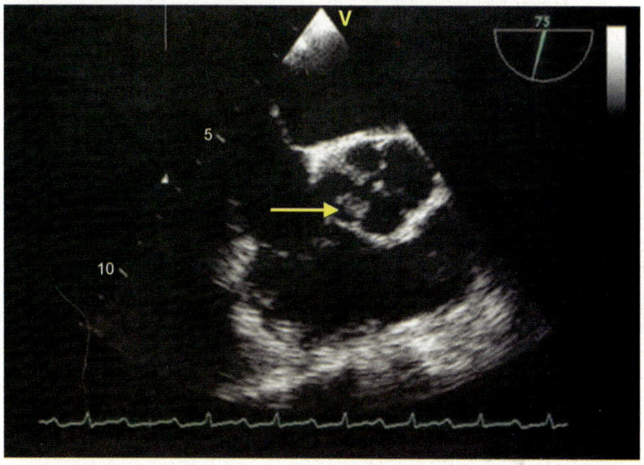

Fig. 13: ME SV SAX view showing aortic valve vegetation. (ME: midesophageal; SAX: short axis; SV: sinus venosus)

Cardiac Masses

TEE offers better images than TTE to delineate cardiac masses and provide clues regarding etiology. Cardiac masses are often accidentally discovered during a TTE performed for some other reason or during evaluation of embolic stroke. TEE gives a fair idea about size, morphology, hemodynamic effects, point of attachment, homogeneity, vascularity, and calcification. Cardiac magnetic resonance imaging (MRI) adds incremental information and is superior to TEE for detection of tissue characteristics. Cardiac masses in order of common to rare occurrence are mentioned in the Table 2.

Assessment in Atrial Fibrillation Prior to Cardioversion

Atrial fibrillation (AF) carries a risk of thrombus formation in the left atrium more commonly in the left atrial appendage (Fig. 14). This predisposes the patient with AF for thromboembolism. Stroke Prevention in Atrial Fibrillation (SPAF) trial confirmed the usefulness of TEE for predicting

BOX 5: Echocardiographic indications for surgical intervention in IE.

Vegetation

- Persistent vegetation after systemic embolization
- Anterior mitral leaflet mobile vegetation >1 cm size
- Increase in size of vegetation despite appropriate antimicrobial therapy

Valve related

- Acute valvular regurgitation with signs of LV failure
- Valve perforation or rupture
- Paravalvular extension
- Valve dehiscence, rupture or fistula
- New onset heart block
- Myocardial abscess

(IE: infective endocarditis; LV: left ventricular)

TABLE 2: Cardiac masses.[10]

Cardiac mass	*TEE characteristics*
Thrombus	Density different than surrounding tissue, does not enhance with contrast. Limitation of TEE is the difficulty to view some regions such as the left ventricular apex, distal ascending aorta, and proximal aortic arch
Vegetation	Independent mobility, associated valvar regurgitation predisposing valvar pathology
Primary benign cardiac tumors (85%)	
Myxoma (common in adults)	Site- LA side of IAS (75–80%), RA (15–20%) Heterogeneous mobile mass either Polypoid (larger with smooth surface and lucencies and cystic within due to hemorrhages and necrosis) or Papillary (smaller with multiple villi)
Papillary fibroelastoma	Found on endocardial surface, smaller with frond-like projections with independent mobility
Rhabdomyoma (common in children)	Homogeneous lobulated mass embedded in myocardium often brighter than surrounding tissue, serial examination may show spontaneous resolution.
Others (lipoma, fibroma, hemangioma, teratoma)	
Primary malignant cardiac tumors (15%)	Broad-based heterogeneous masses. Associated with pericardial effusion.
Sarcomas (most common)	
Primary cardiac lymphoma (rare)	Infiltrating nodules with restrictive physiology. Pericardial effusion often present
Mesothelioma	Thick pericardial nodules with effusion.
Secondary tumors	
Direct invasion (breast, lung, lymphoma, esophagus)	Local invasion from adjacent primary site.
Hematogenous spread (malignant melanoma)	Pericardium frequently involved with nodular metastasis
Vascular extension (renal cell carcinoma)	Tumor may be seen in IVC

(LA: left atrium; IAS: interatrial septum; IVC: inferior vena cava; RA: right atrium)

thromboembolism as the rate of stroke was increased over threefold when TEE evidence of dense spontaneous echo contrast was present, increased by threefold for reduced (<20 cm/second) left atrial appendage peak ejection velocity and for left atrial appendage thrombus.[11] According to one study sensitivity and specificity of TEE to detect LAA thrombus is 93–100% and 99–100%.[12] Midesophageal two-chamber view and midesophageal LA appendage view are useful (*see* Table 1). It is imperative to rule out LA thrombus before embarking on cardioversion in treatment of acute AF. TEE rules out majority of LA clots. Even in patients with chronic AF and inadequate anticoagulation (<3 weeks) can undergo cardioversion, if TEE demonstrates absence of LA clot.

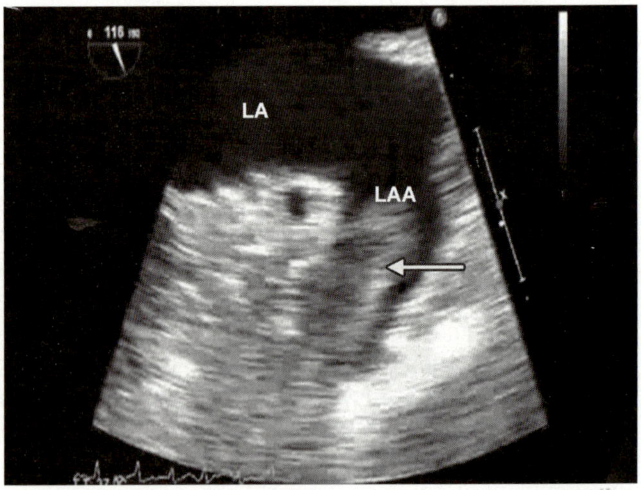

Fig. 14: ME LAA view, showing LAA clot (arrow). (ME: midesophageal; LAA: left atrial appendage)

Aortic Dissection

TEE is a rapid and reliable tool for the diagnosis of aortic dissection, allowing differentiation of dissection from intramural hematoma and penetrating aortic ulcers. TEE has sensitivity of 98% and specificity of 95% to detect aortic dissection[13] which is comparable to MRI and computed tomography; however, the aortic arch and distal descending thoracic aorta may be poorly visualized by TEE. Advantage of TEE over other imaging modalities is that it can be performed bedside in a critically ill patient.

Congenital Heart Diseases

Need for general anesthesia in pediatric population for TEE makes it less used investigation in this age group. TEE is widely used in perioperative period, though. In adult congenital diseases, TEE should be used whenever TTE is insufficient. Table 3 mentions a few common indications

TABLE 3: Use of TEE for evaluation of congenital heart disease.

	Primary lesions	*Associated lesions*
ASD (Figure 15 showing sinus venosus defect)	Location, size and number, and suitability for device closure (rims) ME four-chamber, ME AV SAX, and ME bicaval	*Partial anomalous pulmonary venous drainage (right upper and/or right middle, with sinus venosus defect):* ME right pulmonary vein view *Inlet ventricular septal defect (primum ASD):* ME four-chamber *Cleft mitral valve:* TG basal SAX Subaortic obstruction (AV septal defects)
Ventricular septal defect	*Location, size, number:* ME 5-chamber, ME four-chamber, ME three-chamber, ME AV SAX, TG basal SAX, deep TG five-chamber view	*AV prolapse (supracristal defects):* ME three-chamber and ME AV SAX *Double-chamber RV:* ME AV SAX and ME RV inflow-outflow
LVOT obstruction	*Site of obstruction:* Subvalvular versus valvular versus *supravalvular (discrete vs dynamic):* ME AV LAX , deep TG five-chamber view and TG LAX	*Ascending aortopathy:* ME AV LAX, ME ascending aorta LAX, ME ascending aorta SAX,
Right heart: Ebstein anomaly	Morphology of leaflets, and suitability for repair (mobility of anterior leaflet, chordal attachments to right ventricular outflow tract,): ME four-chamber, ME RV inflow outflow, TG RV inflow-outflow	*Interatrial shunt:* *Noncompaction of left ventricle:* ME four chamber and ME two chamber, TG two chamber

(ASD: atrial septal defect; AV: aortic valve; LAX: long axis; LVOT: left ventricular outflow tract; ME: midesophageal; RV: right ventricle; SAX: short axis; TG: transgastric)

Apart from above-mentioned indications TEE is frequently used to assess the functional status after various cardiac surgeries such as atrial switch surgeries, Fontan operation, etc.

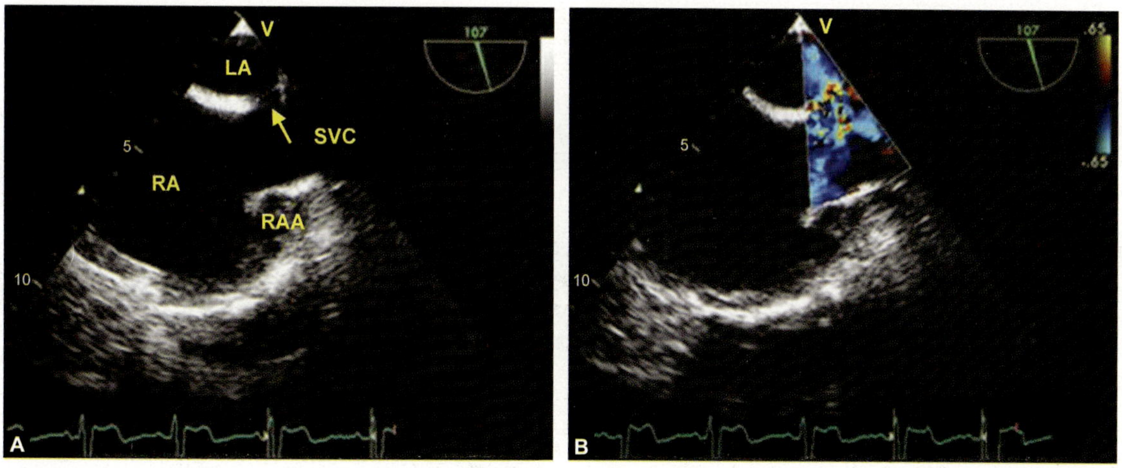

Figs. 15A and B: ME bicaval view. (A) 7 mm SVC type sinus venosus atrial septal defect (arrow). (B) Right to left shunt across the defect. (SVC: superior vena cava)

where TEE offers incremental diagnostic and therapeutic advantage over TTE.

TEE AS AN ADJUNCT TO THERAPEUTIC INVASIVE PROCEDURES

Adjunct to Percutaneous Procedures

Traditionally fluoroscopy and angiography guidance has been used to guide various percutaneous cardiac procedures. TEE is used during these procedures help to delineate

Percutaneous paravalvular leak closure: Percutaneous closure of paravalvular leak is a safe and feasible alternative to high-risk redo surgery. 3D TEE is an important tool used to define anatomy, defect sizing, and procedure guidance. TEE helps in improving procedure success and reducing both fluoroscopy and procedure time.[14]

Percutaneous Balloon Mitral Commissurotomy (PBMC)

TEE plays a crucial adjunctive role in identifying patients feasible for PBMC, aids in transseptal puncture and guides in balloon inflation during the procedure. Another major advantage of TEE during PBMC is that it can rapidly and accurately diagnose complications such as acute MR, cardiac rupture, and residual atrial septal defect.[15]

Transeptal Puncture

Transeptal puncture is the major step in many percutaneous procedures namely PBMC, LAA closure, paravalvular leak closure, AF ablation, etc. and can lead to catastrophic complications. TEE is not *per se* required for trans-septal puncture but if used improves safety and outcome of procedure and reduces the procedure time. TEE can directly visualize puncture needle and fossa ovalis.

Pulmonary Vein Isolation

Online TEE performed during pulmonary vein isolation helps in trans-septal puncture, guiding ablation balloon catheter in each of the pulmonary veins, and documenting its occlusion by balloon.[16]

Patent Foramen Ovale (PFO) and Atrial Septal Defect (ASD) Closure

TEE offers the advantage of visualizing the interatrial septum in real time, thus guiding device closure of PFO/ASD. TEE has a vital role in determining the size of occlusion device and directly visualizing the adequacy of rims around the defect. TEE also clearly differentiates Eustachian valve and Chiari network from rims preventing wrong deployment of closure device.

If the device is seen impinging on any nearby structure or has embolized, it can be immediately detected and device can be retrieved and redeployed.[17]

Left Atrial Appendage (LAA) Closure

Prior to LAA closure TEE is required to rule out LA thrombus and active endocarditis. TEE also gives the morphology and measurements of LAA to determine the size of LAA closure device and helps to decide proper site of its deployment.[18]

Transcatheter Aortic Valve Replacement (TAVR)

TAVR is nowadays preferred alternative to Surgical Aortic valve replacement (SAVR) especially in patients with high and prohibitive surgical risk. Indication for TAVR is now expanded to include intermediate risk patients as well. Percutaneous aortic valve is deployed under guidance of fluoroscopy and TEE. Role of TEE at various stages of TAVR is mentioned in the following text.

- *Annulus sizing:* Aortic annulus is measured in multiple views namely ME AV LAX and ME AV SAX. TEE gives fairly accurate annulus measurement but CT is better modality for this purpose.
- *Guidewire placement:* Crossing the aortic valve is facilitated by TEE in ME AV LAX view.
- *Balloon valvoplasty:* TEE is essential to place the balloon across aortic valve to ensure universal dilatation and assessment of regurgitation postvalvoplasty.
- *Valve replacement and assessment:* Valve is deployed under fluoroscopic and TEE guidance. Postdeployment TEE is used to assess paravalvular leaks if any.

Other procedures such as percutaneous mitral valve repair, pulmonary valvoplasty and replacement, ruptured sinus of valsalva closure, etc. are done under TEE guidance.

Perioperative TEE

Perioperative TEE is routinely employed during cardiovascular surgery in many centers. Major uses of intraoperative TEE are as follows:

- *Coronary artery bypass grafting (CABG):* TEE is frequently employed to monitor biventricular function, to detect air, and confirm success of de-airing techniques. The rare complication of bronchopulmonary fistula can be promptly diagnosed on TEE.[19]
- *Valvar surgeries:* TEE is used for measurement of annulus, to detect paravalvar leaks, and confirm prosthetic valve function during valve replacement surgery. Assessment of severity of valvar regurgitation should not be done under anesthesia, though.[20]
- *Noncardiac surgery in a cardiac patient:* TEE offers the advantage of continuous monitoring of cardiac status and volume loading condition during noncardiac surgery in a patient with LV dysfunction or valvulopathy.
- *Neurosurgery:* TEE is used to detect air embolism during neurosurgeries done in sitting position.

TEE IN CRITICAL CARE

A TTE study in a critically ill patient is limited by difficult echo window because of multiple tubes, dressing, wounds, patient position, and mainly mechanical ventilation. These disadvantages are negated by TEE. Usual indications of TEE in these patients are assessment of ventricular function (especially in patients with unexplained hypotension), valvulopathies, suspicion of aortic dissection or rupture of the aorta, localization of an embolic cardiac focus, mechanical complications of myocardial infarction, postoperative complications of cardiovascular surgery, and diagnosis of IE in the intensive care unit.[21]

TEE DURING CARDIOPULMONARY RESUSCITATION

Cardiopulmonary resuscitation (CPR) mandates continuous high quality chest compressions while intermittently looking for signs of spontaneous circulation and performing a rapid evaluation to find reversible causes of cardiac arrest. TEE is

TABLE 4: TEE during cardiopulmonary resuscitation.

View	*Findings*
ME four-chamber, ME LAX, and TG SAX	Organized cardiac activity versus cardiac standstill
ME four-chamber, ME LAX, TG SAX	LV systolic function, mitral valve function
ME four-chamber, TG SAX	Increased RV : LV ratio, septal fluttering
ME four-chamber, TG SAX, ME LAX	Under filled ventricles
ME four-chamber, TG SAX	Pericardial effusion

(LAX: long axis; LV: left ventricle; ME: midesophageal; RV: right ventricle; SAX: short axis; TG: transgastric)

being frequently used during CPR as it provides continuous imaging without interrupting CPR thus obviating need to check pulse and simultaneously allowing diagnostic evaluation. Recently Advanced Cardiac Life Support (ACLS) and European Resuscitation Council have endorsed use of TEE during CPR.[22,23] As few as three views are sufficient for diagnostic and therapeutic purpose (Table 4).[24]

CONCLUSION

Technological advances over last decade have permitted to reduce the size of probe. Also physicians are becoming more familiar with TEE. All these factors have led to widespread use of TEE. Instant bedside hemodynamic assessment has made TEE an indispensable tool in intensive care units and emergency rooms. 3D TEE provides added advantage over TTE during various percutaneous procedures such as mitral valve repair, transcatheter aortic valve repair, balloon mitral valvoplasty, LAA closure, etc. TEE is deployed in operation theaters for continuous hemodynamic monitoring during cardiac procedures such as mitral valve replacement, CABG, etc. In future more cardiac surgeries will be replaced by percutaneous procedures and will require high resolution real-time 3D imaging for guidance. TEE has become quintessential in determining success and outcome of this procedure. Cardiac physicians and anesthesiologists should continually develop skills and expertise required to perform diagnostic and periprocedure TEE.

REFERENCES

1. Frazin L, Talano JV, Stephanides L, et al. Esophageal echocardiography. Circulation. 1976;54(1):102-8.
2. Jain A, Gutierrez L, Stanton D. 3D TEE registration with X-ray fluoroscopy for interventional cardiac applications BT—functional imaging and modeling of the heart. In: Ayache N, Delingette H, Sermesant M (Eds). Functional imaging and modeling of the heart. Berlin, Heidelberg: Springer; 2009. pp. 321-9.
3. Winter FS. Persistent left superior vena cava: Survey of world literature and report of thirty additional cases. Angiology. 1954;5:90-132.
4. Hahn RT, Abraham T, Adams MS, et al. Guidelines for performing a comprehensive transesophageal echocardiographic examination: Recommendations from the American Society of Echocardiography and the Society of Cardiovascular Anesthesiologists. J Am Soc Echocardiogr. 2013;26(9):921-64.
5. Peterson GE, Brickner ME, Reimold SC. Transesophageal echocardiography. Circulation. 2003;107(19):2398-402.
6. Stewart WJ, Currie PJ, Salcedo EE, et al. Evaluation of mitral leaflet motion by echocardiography and jet direction by Doppler color flow mapping to determine the mechanisms of mitral regurgitation. J Am Coll Cardiol. 1992;2:1353-61.
7. Foster GP, Dunn AK, Abraham S, et al. Accurate measurement of mitral annular dimensions by echocardiography: Importance of correctly aligned imaging planes and anatomic landmarks. J Am Soc Echocardiogr. 2009;22:458-63.
8. Messika-Zeitoun D, Serfaty JM, Brochet E, et al. Multimodal assessment of the aortic annulus diameter: Implications for transcatheter aortic valve implantation. J Am Coll Cardiol. 2010;55:186-94.
9. Barbetseas J, Nagueh SF, Pitsavos C, et al. Differentiating thrombus from pannus formation in obstructed mechanical prosthetic valves: An evaluation of clinical transthoracic and transesophageal echocardiographic parameters. J Am Coll Cardiol. 1998;32:1410-7.
10. Mankad R, Herrmann J. Cardiac tumors: Echo assessment. Echo Res Pract. 2016;3(4):R65-77.
11. Transesophageal echocardiographic correlates of thromboembolism in high-risk patients with nonvalvular atrial fibrillation. The Stroke Prevention in Atrial Fibrillation Investigators Committee on Echocardiography. Ann Intern Med. 1998;128(8):639-47.
12. Manning WJ, Weintraub RM, Waksmonski CA, et al. Accuracy of transesophageal echocardiography for identifying left atrial thrombi: A prospective, intraoperative study. Ann Intern Med. 1995;123(11):817-22.
13. Evangelista A, Flachskampf FA, Erbel R, et al. Echocardiography in aortic diseases: EAE recommendations for clinical practice. Eur J Echocardiogr. 2010;11(8):645-58.
14. Gafoor S, Franke J, Bertog S, et al. A quick guide to paravalvular leak closure. Interv Cardiol Rev. 2015;10(2):112-7.
15. Goldstein SA, Campbell AN. Mitral stenosis: Evaluation and guidance of valvuloplasty by transesophageal echocardiography. Cardiol Clin. 1993;11(3):409-25.
16. Kenneth KE, Curtis H, James M. Transesophageal echocardiography during pulmonary vein cryoballoon ablation for atrial fibrillation. Echocardiography. 2014;32(2):281-90.
17. Bartel T, Müller S. Contemporary echocardiographic guiding tools for device closure of interatrial communications. Cardiovasc Diagn Ther. 2013;3(1):38-46.
18. Wunderlich NC, Beigel R, Swaans MJ, et al. Percutaneous interventions for left atrial appendage exclusion. JACC Cardiovasc Imaging. 2015;8(4):47288.

19. Hsaad AH, Bleich S, Nanda NC, et al. Transesophageal echocardiographic diagnosis of bronchopulmonary vein fistula complicating mitral valve replacement. Echocardiography. 2013;30(7):850-2.
20. Shapira Y, Vaturi M, Weisenberg DE, et al. Impact of intraoperative transesophageal echocardiography in patients undergoing valve replacement. Ann Thorac Surg. 2004;78(2):574-9.
21. Cobo-Molinos J, Cobo-Molinos A. Indications and use of transesophageal echocardiography in intensive care patients: Systematic review. J Med Diagn Meth. 2017;6:1-3.
22. Link MS, Berkow LC, Kudenchuk PJ, et al. Part 7: Adult advanced cardiovascular life support. Circulation. 20153;132(18 suppl 2):S444-64.
23. Soar J, Nolan JP, Böttiger BW, et al. European Resuscitation Council guidelines for resuscitation 2015. Resuscitation. 2015;95:100-47.
24. Fair J, Mallin M, Mallemat H, et al. Transesophageal echocardiography: Guidelines for point-of-care applications in cardiac arrest and resuscitation. Ann Emerg Med. 2018;71(2):201-7.

SECTION 6

Emergency Imaging in Chest Pain

51

CHAPTER

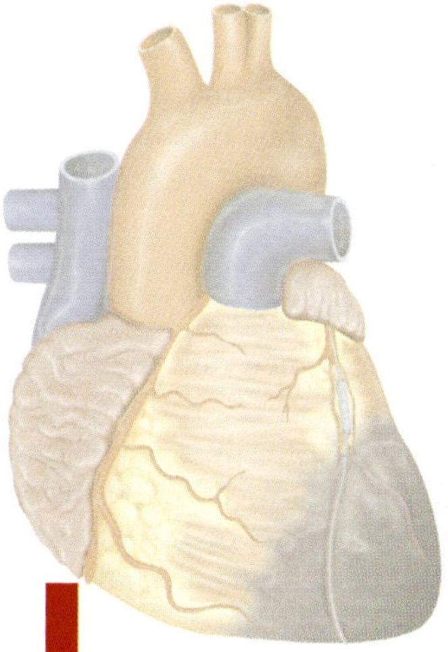

Emergency Imaging in Chest Pain: Echocardiographic Evaluation

BP Singh, Ravi Vishnu Prasad

INTRODUCTION

Chest pain is one of the most frequent reasons for patient visits in emergency departments (EDs). Acute chest pain is a common diagnostic dilemma in the emergency department and its impact on the health care system is substantial. Emergency physicians and cardiologists are commonly required to decide whether to admit a patient with acute chest pain based on clinical judgment and a rough estimation of risk. Optimal triage requires a quick noninvasive test that is cost effective and is readily available to identify all patients with acute coronary syndrome (ACS). Moreover, a triage test should also be able to accurately identify patients in whom significant coronary artery disease can be excluded and who can thus safely be discharged.

CAUSES OF CHEST PAIN ENCOUNTERED IN EMERGENCY

Possible causes of chest pain are numerous and diverse, but importantly, several conditions, such as ACS, pulmonary embolism (PE), aortic dissection (AD), tension pneumothorax, and pericardial tamponade require urgent management and, in some cases, may be life-threatening. Echocardiography can help to distinguish between cardiac versus noncardiac etiologies of chest pain (Box 1). Therefore, a challenge for clinicians in EDs is rapid identification of those patients with chest pain who require urgent management and those with more benign entities who do not require admission.

Acute Coronary Syndrome

At one end of the spectrum are patients with abnormal electrocardiography (ECG) and thus definite ACS who require immediate invasive diagnostic procedures and possibly coronary intervention. At the other end of the spectrum are patients with atypical and noncardiac chest discomfort and normal ECG who can be sent home safely. In between these two extremes

BOX 1: Role of echocardiography in emergency room.

- Acute coronary syndrome
- Assessment of chest trauma
- Pulmonary embolism.
- *Evaluation of thoracic aorta*:
  - Acute aortic syndromes (aortic dissection, intramural hematoma, penetrating ulcer)
  - Aortic aneurysm.
- *Identification of pericardial effusion*:
  - Pericardial effusion versus pleural effusion
  - Identify pericardial tamponade.
- *Evaluation of valvular heart disease*:
  - Acute valvular dysfunction
  - Prosthetic valve dysfunction.
- Detection of etiology of shock
- Evaluation of volume status including hypovolemia (IVC diameter, RV/LV size).

(IVC: inferior vena cava; LV: left ventricular; RV: right ventricular) are numerous patients with atypical presentation of ischemic chest pain and normal or nondiagnostic ECG who might have ACS. Cardiac imaging may play an important role in triaging and directing clinical management of these patients. Echocardiography is a noninvasive, portable, and relatively inexpensive bedside imaging technique that is available in most hospitals. In these patients, echocardiography gives additional information on:

- Left ventricular (LV) systolic function
- Size of infarcted area
- Presence of LV thrombus
- *Mechanical complications of myocardial infarction (MI)*: Papillary muscle rupture, ventricular septal rupture, or free wall rupture
- Pericardial effusion/tamponade
- Left ventricular pseudoaneurysm.

It can assess both left ventricular systolic function and regional wall motion analysis (WMA) and, therefore, provides valuable diagnostic as well as prognostic information (Fig. 1). Because of the close relationship between wall motion and myocardial blood flow (MBF), echocardiography is a very useful tool in patients with suspected ACS. Development of WMAs is preceded by considerable reductions in MBF.

Rest Echocardiography

When echocardiography is performed soon after a patient arrives at the emergency department or during a chest pain episode, WMAs are detected in up to 90% of the cases. However, chest pain has subsided in most patients at the time of evaluation and the resting echocardiogram may be completely normal. Rest echocardiography is associated with high specificity but unsatisfactory sensitivity for adverse events within 30 days, including MI, revascularization, or unstable angina.

Contrast-enhanced Echocardiography

Microbubble contrast agents enhance delineation of endocardial borders, which facilitates wall motion assessment (Figs. 2A and B). Imaging using these agents also provides important information about myocardial perfusion and viability. In a prospective analysis of 114 patients with cardiac chest pain and no clinical manifestations of acute myocardial infarction (AMI), Kang et al. found that the addition of contrast material improved the sensitivity of echocardiography from 49% (43/87) to 77% (67/87), whereas specificity was similar, 78% (74/95) versus 73% (69/95), for the detection of ACS at the index visit. Patients presenting with mechanical complications of an untreated MI are typically in florid heart failure at the time of presentation. Transthoracic echocardiography (TTE) or transesophageal echocardiography (TEE) demonstrating papillary muscle rupture or ventricular septal rupture can lead to life-saving emergency surgery. Free wall rupture is rare in the emergency room and is typically rapidly fatal unless recognized immediately. In stable patients, assessment of longitudinal strain has been shown to be

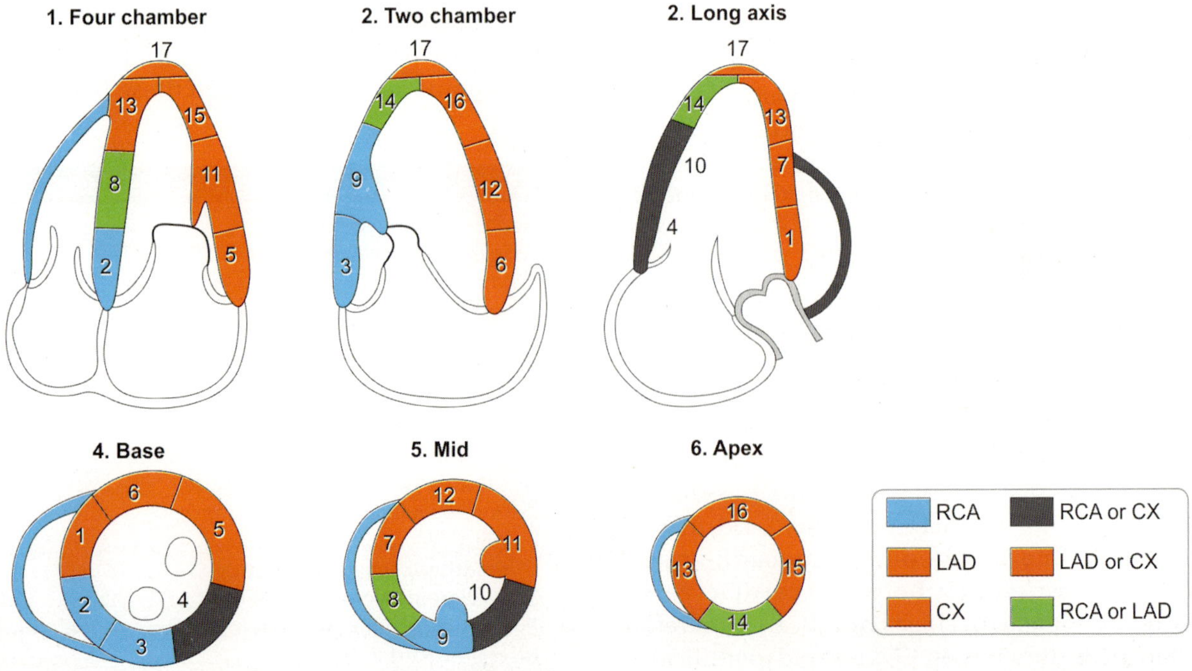

Fig. 1: Left ventricular segmentation in apical (1, 2, 3) and short-axis (4, 5, 6) views according to typical coronary artery distribution.

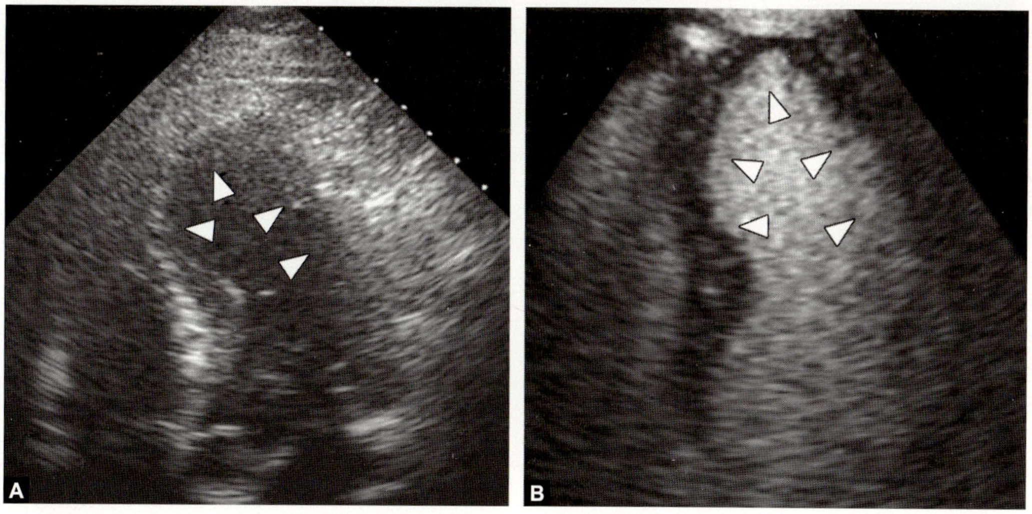

Figs. 2A and B: A 67-year-old man suspected to have myocardial ischemia who was referred for echocardiography. (A and B) Microbubble contrast agents were used to enhance delineation of endocardial borders. Arrowheads in A indicate endocardial borders on unenhanced echocardiography, and arrowheads in B indicate improved delineation of endocardial borders by using contrast agents.

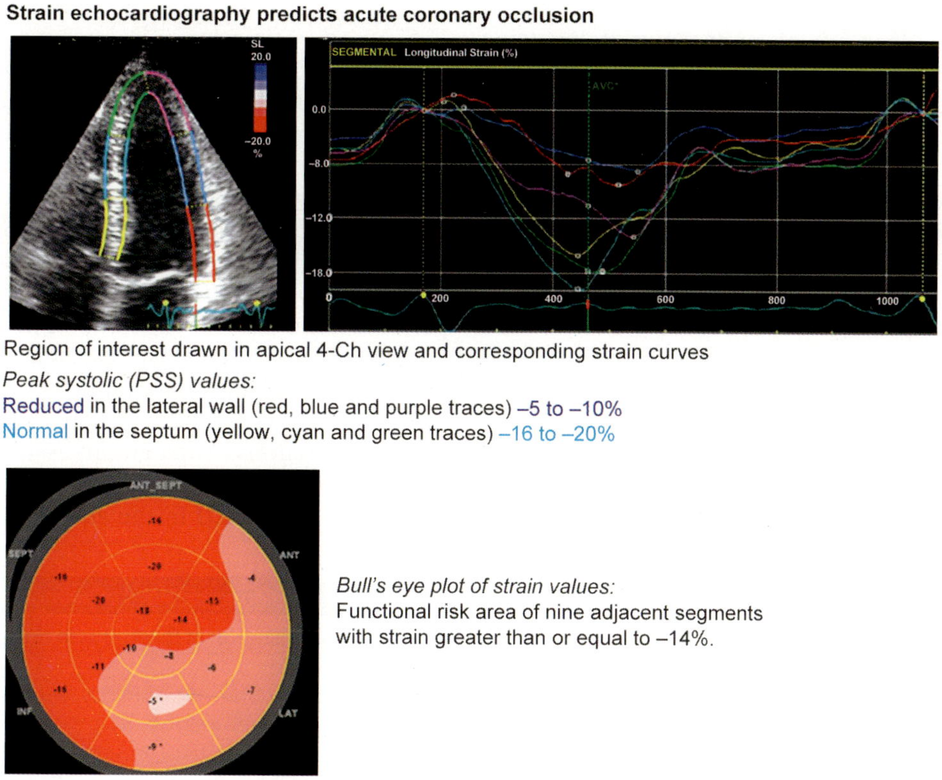

Fig. 3: Strain echo in acute coronary syndrome.

Source: Eek C, Grenne B, Brunvand H, et al. Strain echocardiography predicts acute coronary occlusion in patients with non-ST-segment elevation acute coronary syndrome. Eur J Echocardiogra. 2010;11:501-8.

reasonably accurate for the diagnosis of significant coronary artery disease in patients presenting with chest pain to the emergency room. Such patients typically show reduced global longitudinal strain, reduced peak segmental strain in a coronary distribution, abnormal postsystolic strain index, and postsystolic shortening in the affected segment (Fig. 3).

Trauma

Blunt injuries to the chest wall may be the result of assault, road traffic accidents, or falls/fallen objects. From a cardiac perspective, such injuries compress the anterior-posterior dimension of the thorax and internal structures, resulting in myocardial contusion, hemopericardium, hemothorax, right ventricular free wall and/or right atrial rupture, traumatic injury to the valves, or partial/complete aortic transection. Myocardial contusion is the most common result of blunt injuries to the chest wall and occurs as a direct pressure on the myocardium caused by either sudden deceleration forces that directly affect the chest or indirectly due to shear stress or increased intrathoracic pressure. Although technically a histological diagnosis, myocardial contusion is usually diagnosed based on a history of blunt chest trauma or deceleration injury combined with the characteristic echo findings of regional wall motion abnormalities, valvular involvement, focal wall rupture, or pericardial effusion. ECG may show ST depression or arrhythmias, and cardiac biomarkers are typically mildly elevated. Penetrating injuries to the chest may be the result of assault or trauma and can lead a wide variety of cardiac injuries, including hemopericardium and/or tamponade. Aortic transection is a classic example of traumatic injury to the great vessels, and result from a sudden deceleration injury such as a road traffic accident (e.g. an unrestrained driver whose chest hits the steering wheel after a head-on collision) or fall from a height. The aorta is torn or transected at the aortic isthmus. Most patients die immediately by exsanguination into the thorax immediately at the site of the accident.

Chest X-ray typically shows a widened mediastinum and hemothorax. TTE from the parasternal window can be helpful, but due to limited windows TEE is often required. Blood around the aortic arch in a trauma patient is characteristic. A large flap in the distal aortic arch is also common, and can be distinguished from a dissection flap by its thickness (equal to the thickness of the normal aortic wall) and its vertical alignment with the aorta in the long-axis view, unlike dissection flaps, which usually run parallel to the long axis of the aorta.

Pulmonary Embolism

The diagnosis of PE is made using a combination of clinical findings, D-dimer testing, computed tomography (CT) angiography of the pulmonary arteries, compression venous sonography, lung scintigraphy (i.e. V/Q scan), and/or echocardiography. PE is classified as either "high-risk PE" in patients who present with suspected or confirmed PE in the presence of shock or persistent arterial hypotension, or as "not high-risk PE" in their absence.

Echo can be useful in the suspected high-risk group, where echo can exclude other causes of hypotension or shock such as right ventricular (RV) MI, pericardial tamponade, AD, hypovolemia, acute valvular dysfunction, and LV dysfunction. An important indication for echo in the hypotensive patient with suspected PE is when immediate CT angiography is not available. In such patients, the presence of RV dilation or dysfunction on echo is sufficient evidence to start reperfusion therapy.

Apart from the presence of a mobile thrombus in the RV or a saddle embolus in the main pulmonary artery, there are no echo signs that are 100% sensitive or specific for PE. *McConnell's sign* (depressed RV free wall contractility compared to apex) has fair positive predictive value of 67%. Unfortunately, other common findings such as RV dilation and global RV dysfunction are not specific to PE. Since a normal TTE has a negative predictive value of only 40–50%, a normal study does not exclude PE. Important differential diagnoses for PE include RVMI (dilated RV with dyskinesia of the inferior and posterior left ventricle walls) and pericardial tamponade. Common echocardiographic findings in PE are listed in Box 2.

Acute Aortic Syndrome

Aortic dissection, intramural hematoma, and penetrating atherosclerotic ulcer comprise the acute aortic syndromes. Due to their high morbidity and mortality, rapid diagnosis and treatment is required. AD accounts for 80–90% of acute aortic syndromes. AD is defined as acute if less than 2 weeks in duration; acute AD has the highest mortality, regardless of location (type A or B). Acute type A AD is a true surgical emergency due to very high mortality: 1–3% per hour after presentation and approximately 36–72% within 48 hours of diagnosis. Diagnosis of AD is typically made by computed tomography or echocardiography. MRI is usually reserved for follow-up of uncomplicated type B dissections. Angiography is seldom used today. The role of echocardiography in patients with suspected acute or subacute AD in the emergency room is to: (1)

BOX 2: Echocardiographic signs of pulmonary embolism.

- Direct visualization of thrombus in right heart/pulmonary artery
- Right ventricular hypokinesis with hyperdynamic RV apex (McConnell's sign)
- Right ventricular (RV) enlargement, decrease in left ventricular (LV) size, RV/LV end diastolic dimension ratio > 0.7
- Interventricular septal shift (D sign)
- Increased pulmonary artery diameter
- Dilation of IVC with loss of respiratory variation
- Increased velocity of TR jet (<3.9 msec)
- Shortened pulmonary ejection acceleration time (PAT < 60 msec).

(IVC: inferior vena cava; TR: tricuspid regurgitation)

BOX 3: Echocardiography features of aortic dissection.

- *Mobile dissection (intimal flap) within*:
  - Aortic root (PLAX, A2C)
  - Sinotubular junction-ascending aorta (high PLAX)
  - Aortic arch
  - Descending thoracic aorta (PLAX, A2C)
  - Proximal abdominal aorta
  - Aortic root dissections.
- Acute aortic insufficiency
- Wall motion abnormality
- Pericardial effusion or tamponade
- Differential color Doppler flow patterns within true and false lumen
- Pulse wave Doppler examination of flow/exit sites and within true and false lumen.

(PLAX: parasternal long axis; A2C: apical two-chamber)

distinguish between a type A versus type B dissection; and (2) evaluate life-threatening complications of type A dissection such as acute aortic regurgitation, regional wall motion abnormalities in a coronary territory (suggesting coronary artery dissection), large pleural effusions, and pericardial effusion suggestive of hemopericardium. Other findings, such as aortic aneurysm may further guide management. The common echocardiographic features of AD are described in Box 3.

Standard TTE windows for assessment of AD include the parasternal long axis (PLAX), high PLAX, apical four-chamber, apical two-chamber, suprasternal notch, and subxiphoid views. Use of nonstandard windows, such as the right parasternal border view of the ascending aorta (with the patient turned to a right lateral decubitus), may assist in diagnosing a type A AD. Long-axis views of the intrarenal abdominal aorta can also be performed for evaluation of an abdominal aortic aneurysm. However, TTE does not evaluate the entire thoracic or abdominal aorta, and a negative TTE does not rule out AD. Overall sensitivity of TTE for diagnosis of AD is 59–83% and specificity is 63–93%.

When TTE is nondiagnostic or suspicion for dissection is high, TEE should be performed. The sensitivity and specificity of TEE for AD is 99% and 89%, respectively. TEE can sometimes be limited by difficulty in visualizing the superior ascending aorta and proximal arch due to the shadowing from the main stem bronchus. Care should be taken to avoid reverberation or mirror image artifacts which can simulate a type A dissection.

Pericardial Tamponade

Patients presenting with hemodynamic instability postpenetrating injury or blunt force chest trauma should be evaluated for myocardial contusion or pericardial effusion/tamponade. Even a small amount of pericardial fluid accumulating rapidly within the pericardium is sufficient to cause tamponade (Figs. 4A and B). Typical echocardiographic features of cardiac tamponade are listed in Box 4.

Acute Valvular Regurgitation

Patients with acute valvular regurgitation typically present in heart failure, including florid pulmonary edema. Acute mitral regurgitation can be the result of penetrating of blunt chest wall trauma, myocardial infarction, or endocarditis with secondary leaflet, chord, or papillary muscle involvement. In addition to determining the severity of regurgitation, the echo should determine the mechanism of mitral regurgitation and the feasibility of repair.

Acute severe aortic regurgitation is most commonly seen in blunt trauma, type A AD, and infective endocarditis. On physical examination, the pulse pressure may be normal as compared to chronic aortic regurgitation. Echo may show premature closure of mitral valve, diastolic fluttering of anterior mitral leaflet, and diastolic mitral regurgitation.

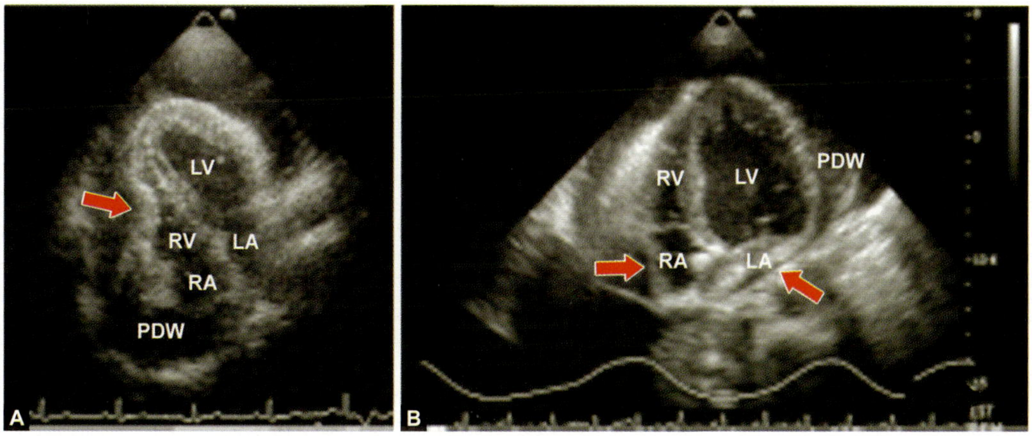

Figs. 4A and B: Right ventricle (RV) collapse (A) in early diastole (end of T-wave) in a patient with cardiac tamponade. (B) Collapse of both atria in another patient with signs of tamponade.

BOX 4: Echocardiographic features of pericardial tamponade.

- Pericardial effusion
- Right atrial systolic inversion (sensitivity 50–100%; specificity 33–100%)
- RV diastolic collapse (sensitivity 48–100%; specificity 72–100%)
- Respirophasic variation of right to left volume
- *Exaggerated respirovariation on Doppler of transvalvular flow*:
  - >40% increase in the transtricuspid valve flow
  - >25% decrease in transmitral flow in inspiration
- Inferior vena cava (IVC) plethoric with the loss of respirophasic variation.

TABLE 1: Major advantages and disadvantages of imaging techniques for the detection of acute coronary syndrome.

Imaging technique	*Major advantages*	*Major disadvantages*
Echocardiography	Readily accessible Portable Safe Less expensive than MPI and CTA Allows assessment of many nonischemic causes of acute chest pain	Poor sensitivity Operator and reader dependent Poor thoracic window in at least 10% of patients
Radionuclide MPI	High sensitivity and high specificity	Logistic barrier Radiation exposure Expensive
Coronary CTA	High sensitivity and high specificity Identification of noncoronary conditions fast	Radiation exposure

(CTA: computed tomography angiography; MPI: myocardial perfusion imaging)

Focused versus Comprehensive Echo

A focused echo examination is targeted toward specific clinical question such as ruling out pericardial tamponade and AD in road traffic accident. Focused echo is the most appropriate in serious or critically ill patients in whom information is required quickly. TTE is adequate in most cases but sometimes TEE may be in nondiagnostic cases. Comprehensive echo in emergency room are typically done when a complex but stable patient requiring comprehensive evaluation prior to treatment decision or discharging home from emergency room, and when information from focused echo and clinical scenario is discordant.

LIMITATIONS

There are some key concerns regarding the use of echocardiography in the ED. Evaluation of remains a subjective and difficult skill to master. Interpreters should therefore be experienced readers. Second, a considerable number of patients have a poor thoracic imaging window resulting in indeterminate findings. Discriminating between existing WMAs and newly developed WMAs is difficult, and both conditions may even coexist in the same patient. The images should be stored for later reviewing and as a document to provide evidence of findings (Table 1).

CONCLUSION

Echocardiography (Echo) with other imaging techniques is of paramount importance for early diagnosis, timely intervention and may help in improving the vascular inflicted mortality and morbidity benefits.

BIBLIOGRAPHY

1. Amuthan V, Parashar KS, Nanda CN. Textbook of Echocardiography. Indian Academy of Echocardiography. New Delhi: Jaypee Brothers Medical Publishers (P) Ltd; 2018.
2. Christenson J, Innes G, McKnight D, et al. Safety and efficiency of emergency department assessment of chest discomfort. CMAJ. 2004;170:1803-7.
3. Dedic A, Genders TS, Nieman K, et al. Imaging strategies for acute chest pain in the emergency department. AJR Am J Roentgenol. 2013;200(1):W26-38.
4. Fruergaard P, Launbjerg J, Hesse B, et al. The diagnoses of patients admitted with acute chest pain but without myocardial infarction. Eur Heart J. 1996;17:1028-34.
5. Gibler WB, Runyon JP, Levy RC, et al. A rapid diagnostic and treatment center for patients with chest pain in the emergency department. Ann Emerg Med. 1995;25:1-8.
6. Gomez MA, Anderson JL, Karagounis LA, et al. An emergency department-based protocol for rapidly ruling out myocardial ischemia reduces hospital time and expense: Results of a randomized study (ROMIO). J Am Coll Cardiol. 1996;28:25-33.
7. Kang DH, Kang SJ, Song JM, et al. Efficacy of myocardial contrast echocardiography in the diagnosis and risk stratification of acute coronary syndrome. Am J Cardiol. 2005;96:1498-502.
8. Lee TH, Rouan GW, Weisberg MC, et al. Clinical characteristics and natural history of patients with acute myocardial infarction sent home from the emergency room. Am J Cardiol. 1987;60:219-24.
9. McCarthy BD, Beshansky JR, D'Agostino RB, et al. Missed diagnoses of acute myocardial infarction in the emergency department: Results from a multicenter study. Ann Emerg Med. 1993;22:579-82.
10. Peels CH, Visser CA, Funke Kupper AJ, et al. Usefulness of two-dimensional echocardiography for immediate detection of myocardial ischemia in the emergency room. Am J Cardiol. 1990;65:687-91.
11. Tatum JL, Jesse RL, Kontos MC, et al. Comprehensive strategy for the evaluation and triage of the chest pain patient. Ann Emerg Med. 1997;29:116-25.

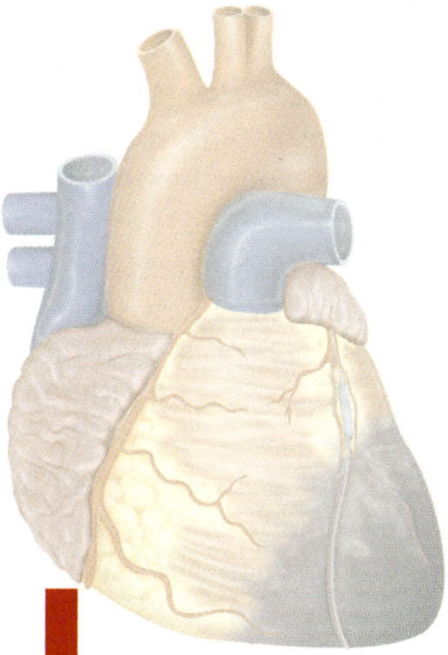

52

CHAPTER

Chest Pain: Emergency Echocardiographic Evaluation

Debika Chatterjee

INTRODUCTION

Chest pain is one of the most common complaints that brings a patient to the hospital and needs immediate attention. In an emergency setting, echocardiography is of great value for evaluation of such patients with chest pain. Emergency echocardiographic evaluation of chest pain is a comprehensive and focused study that can quickly rule in or rule out cardiac versus noncardiac etiology of chest pain, identify critical abnormalities which may affect the management of the patient and support the need for additional testing, imaging, procedures or urgent admission of the patients with high-clinical risk and discharge of the patients with low-clinical risk. It should be distinguished from the traditional full echocardiography where a detailed study is done. This is often challenging as the possible causes of chest pain are numerous and diverse, and the decisions must be taken quickly. Moreover, the quality of the echocardiographic images may be suboptimal due to abnormal chest wall configuration, obesity, pulmonary emphysema, or improper position of the patient. Standard echocardiographic views may not be always available. Inaccurate interpretation in these situations may lead to a potentially dangerous conclusion. Ideally, therefore, an expert who is competent enough to perform and interpret echocardiography independently even in the presence of limited echo windows and has the capacity to fully integrate echocardiographic information into clinical decision-making should perform the study. Inexperienced operators without supervision should not attempt to do it.

Two-dimensional (2D) and color Doppler study are the cornerstones for emergency evaluation of chest pain. Tissue-Doppler imaging, speckle tracking for myocardial deformation, and three-dimensional echocardiography and stress echocardiography have limited role.[1] Transthoracic echo (TTE) is the initial diagnostic modality of choice to start with, but transesophageal echocardiography (TEE) should also be performed, whenever the information from TTE is inadequate, nondiagnostic or does not fit into the clinical scenario. Views in TTE should be focused and goal-directed including parasternal long axis (LAX), parasternal short axis (SAX), apical four, three, two chambers, subcostal, and suprasternal views. In an emergency situation, the echocardiographer may have to obtain and interpret the nonstandardized views of the heart, as the pathological finding may not be seen in standard imaging planes. Similarly, TEE also to be done using goal-directed views such as midesophageal (ME) four and five chamber, ME bicaval, ME RV inflow-outflow, transgastric (TG) midpapillary SAX, and TG midpapillary LAX views.

The initial critical findings of the echocardiography should be communicated immediately to the treating physician so that the urgent treatment can be initiated. A detailed report may be given later. Though differential diagnosis of chest pain includes numerous cardiac and noncardiac diseases but importantly, few of these conditions, such as acute coronary syndrome (ACS), acute pulmonary embolism, and acute aortic dissection may be life-threatening and require urgent identification and management. Echocardiography can identify these catastrophic conditions. Echo also can provide clues to rule out less important causes of chest pain like pericarditis or musculoskeletal pain, esophagitis, etc.

Acute coronary syndromes are caused by a sudden occlusion of a coronary artery. The sequence of events after coronary occlusion, the so-called ischemic cascade, provides the theoretical basis of using echocardiography in patients presenting with chest pain. After acute coronary occlusion, regional wall motion abnormalities (RWMAs) appear almost instantaneously and appear before electrocardiography (ECG) changes and chest pain. Thus, TTE detection of RWMA using different precordial views is more sensitive method to pick up evidence of ischemia as compared to ECG changes. Early emergency echocardiography in the patients presenting with chest pain due to ACS may facilitate early diagnosis and management in those patients with clinical suspicion of myocardial infarction (MI) but a nondiagnostic ECG. It may diagnose unstable angina, if performed during chest pain. A new onset RWMA is a very strong indicator of chest pain being due to ongoing myocardial ischemia and provides a quick and specific marker of ongoing myocardial necrosis. New-onset RWMA predicts increased likelihood of MI with positive predictive accuracy of 50%, while absence of RWMA predicts that the patient is likely to have MI with negative predictive value (NPV) of 95%.[2] In a study involving 260 patients presenting with chest pain, echocardiography was done within 4 hours of presentation and compared with ECG. New-onset RWMA and LV dysfunction predicted cardiac events with 91% sensitivity, while sensitivity of ECG was found to be only 40%. In multivariate analysis, only male gender and positive echocardiographic study predicted cardiac events.[3] Echocardiography has the sensitivity of 90–95% (NPV 95%) for MI diagnosis. In a study of 169 patients presenting to the emergency room (ER) with chest pain, out of those 88 patients who had no RWMA, only two patients has raised cardiac enzymes, while out of those 87 patients who had RWMAs, 31% were ultimately determined to have an MI.[4] Other than detection of RWMA, TTE also helps to assess the size of infarcted area, left ventricular (LV) systolic function, to rule out presence of LV thrombus and mechanical complications of acute myocardial infarction (AMI) such as ventricular septal defect (VSD), papillary muscle (PM) rupture, pericardial effusion/tamponade. Detection of PM rupture or VSD by TTE or TEE can save the life of the patients by doing emergency surgery on them. Free wall rupture is rapidly fatal can also be identified by TTE (Figs. 1A and B).

Although speckle tracking is not done routinely for emergency echocardiographic evaluation of chest pain, it can be done in a stable patient with chest pain as assessment of longitudinal strain has been shown to be reasonably accurate for the diagnosis of significant coronary artery disease. These patients show reduced global longitudinal strain, reduced peak segmental strain in a coronary distribution, abnormal postsystolic strain index, and postsystolic shortening in the affected segments.[5]

Common echocardiographic features of MI are listed in Box 1.

Chest pain may be due to *aortic dissection (AD)*, which should be diagnosed as early as possible and should be managed aggressively as an extraordinary high mortality is associated with type A acute AD. About 40% of acute AD patients die immediately and survivors carry an added mortality of 1–3%/h after presentation and approximately 36–72% within 48 hours of diagnosis.[6] So, key to success in treating acute AD is prompt diagnosis where echocardiography plays a great role. Demonstration of the presence of an intimal flap that divides the aorta into true and the false lumen forms the basis of echocardiographic diagnosis of the AD. However, TTE often faces a major challenge in demonstrating the intimal flap in aorta, as

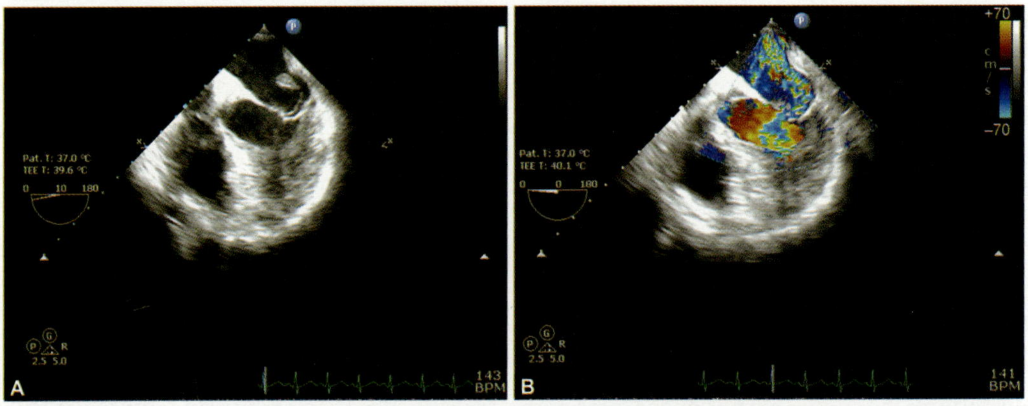

Figs. 1A and B: The images are showing postmyocardial infarction (MI) papillary muscle rupture with severe eccentric wall hugging jet of mitral regurgitation in transesophageal echo.

BOX 1: Echocardiographic features of myocardial infarction.

- RWMA
- LV systolic function
- Size of the infarcted area
- LV thrombus
- VSD, PM rupture, and free wall rupture
- Pseudoaneurysm.

(LV: left ventricular; PM: papillary muscle; RWMA: regional wall motion abnormality; VSD: ventricular septal defect)

linear reverberation artifacts are common in aortic root and ascending aorta especially when they are dilated. The low NPV of TTE does not permit to rule out the diagnosis of AD. Regardless of the visualization of a dissection flap, TTE is useful in almost all cases of suspected AD for demonstrating the presence of a bicuspid aortic valve (particularly in a young patient with chest pain), aortic regurgitation, a dilated aortic root, associated pericardial effusion, or RWMA due to involvement of origin of coronary artery is suggestive of acute type A AD, whereas their absence is reassuring (but cannot definitely exclude the diagnosis). The presence of a pericardial effusion with an ascending aortic dissection is a sign of poor prognosis. Therefore, despite its relatively poor diagnostic accuracy, emergency TTE is an extremely valuable clinical tool in assessing acute aortic dissection, identifying its related complications. Most importantly, it has a vital role in identifying patients at high risk and directing their referral to the relevant cardiothoracic surgical department promptly. Standard transthoracic windows for evaluation for AD are standard parasternal long axis (PLAX) and high PLAX, parasternal short axis (PSAX) at the level of aorta, apical four-chamber (AP4ch), apical five-chamber (AP5ch), apical three-chamber (AP3ch), suprasternal, and subcostal views. Nonstandard off-axis views are also to be used to look for dissection flap. Overall sensitivity of TTE for diagnosis of AD is 59–83% and specificity is 63–93%. The sensitivity and specificity of TTE for type A AD is 78–97% and 86–97%, respectively.[7]

If the high clinical suspicion of AD exists despite of initial negative imaging by TTE, then consideration should be given to TEE. TEE is a highly accurate imaging modality for AD with sensitivity and specificity of 99% and 89%, respectively. The most recent comparative study with nonhelical computed tomography (CT), magnetic resonance imaging (MRI), and TEE shows high equal sensitivity of all with CT having better specificity. Scrupulous attention must be paid while doing TEE in suspected cases of acute AD. TEE should be done by an expert in intensive care unit under continuous monitoring of blood pressure (BP), heart rate, and oxygen saturation. BP is to be maintained low as high BP may cause further propagation of dissection. Careful conscious intravenous sedation is to be given to the patient so that the TEE probe

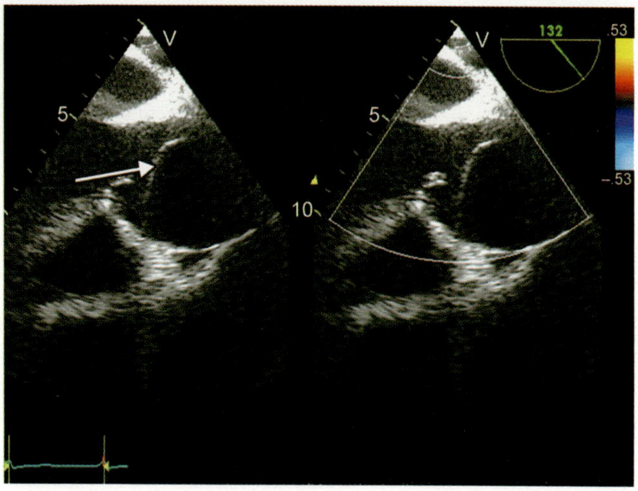

Fig. 2: Intimal flap in aortic root in transesophageal echo (arrow).

BOX 2: Echocardiographic features of aortic dissection.

- Mobile dissection flap in aorta
- Demonstration of true and false lumen
- Demonstration of entry point from true to false lumen
- Dilated aortic root
- Aortic regurgitation
- Demonstration of involvement of coronary arteries by the dissection and RWMA
- Pericardial effusion/tamponade.

(RWMA: regional wall motion abnormality)

can be introduced with maximal patient cooperation and minimal agitation. With the help of TEE it is possible to demonstrate the intimal flap, true and false lumen, entry tear from true to false lumen, involvement of coronary arteries, mechanism and severity of aortic regurgitation, and presence of pericardial effusion. However, it is often difficult to comment on the involvement of first and second branch of arch by TEE because of interposition of bronchus in between this part of aorta and esophagus resulting in a blind spot (Fig. 2).

Echocardiographic features of AD are listed in Box 2.

Acute pulmonary embolism (PE) is a condition where the patient may come with chest pain. PE is an important cause of morbidity and mortality but is often underdiagnosed. Because of limited specificity, echocardiography is not suitable as routine imaging modality to diagnose PE and should not be used as standalone imaging technique. However, occasionally a free-floating thrombus transiting through the right heart can be visualized in echocardiography which is a very useful information to diagnose PE especially when the patient is too unstable to transport for CT pulmonary angiography

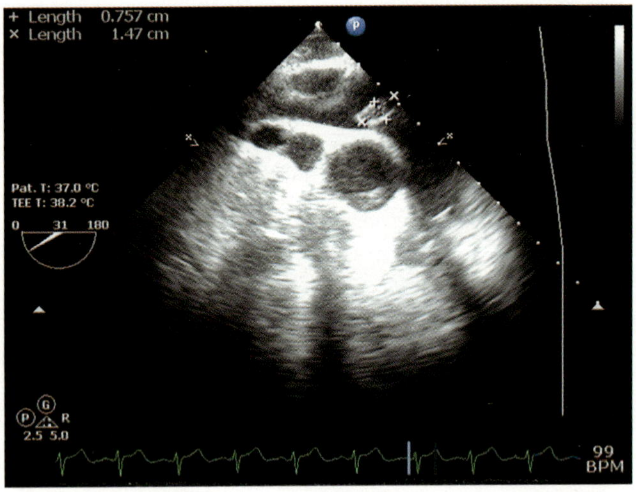

Fig. 3: A thrombus in pulmonary artery in transesophageal echo in a case of acute pulmonary embolism.

or when immediate CT is not available. PE causes acute right ventricular (RV) dysfunction due to abrupt increase of pulmonary artery pressure. As this happens, a distinct pattern of RV wall motion abnormality can be detected in apical RV-focused or RV-modified views of TTE, called the McConnell sign consisting of akinesia of RV mid-free wall but normal motion at the apex. These findings are both sensitive and specific for PE.[8,9] Moreover, RV dysfunction is also a good predictor of increased mortality.[10,11] When CT is not available, presence of RV dilatation or dysfunction on echo is sufficient evidence to start reperfusion therapy.[12] TEE can be done in suspected cases of PE. With TEE, it is possible to visualize the right-sided cardiac structures more clearly especially the main pulmonary artery (MPA), a significant portion of the right pulmonary artery (RPA), and a portion of left pulmonary artery (LPA). RPA can be followed until it branches to the right lobar pulmonary arteries. However, interposition of the left main bronchus interferes with the ultrasound beam in the middle portion of LPA. So, thromboembolism is more difficult to detect in LPA. TEE can visualize thrombi in the central pulmonary arteries (MPA, RPA, and proximal portion of LPA) with high specificity (>90%). Important differential diagnosis for PE is right ventricular MI where there is RV dilatation with akenesia of RV-free wall and pericardial tamponade (Fig. 3).[13]

Common echocardiographic features of PE are listed in Box 3.

BOX 3: Echocardiographic features of pulmonary embolism.

Two-dimensional features:
- Direct visualization of thrombus in right heart/pulmonary artery
- McConnell sign (akinesia of RV mid-free wall, normal motion at apex)
- Right ventricular dilatation
- Decrease in left ventricular size
- RV/LV end diastolic dimension ratio > 0.7
- Flattening of the IVS
- Interventricular septal shift (D sign)
- Dilated inferior vena cava with loss of respiratory variation.

Doppler features:
- Increased velocity of tricuspid regurgitation jet (<3.9 ms)
- Shortened pulmonary acceleration time (PAT < 60 ms).

(LV: left ventricular; IVS: interventricular septum; RV: right ventricular)

CONCLUSION

Emergency echocardiographic evaluation of chest pain is a focused, goal-directed echocardiography to evaluate, diagnose, and manage the patient. Making a correct diagnosis of a patient with chest pain is a challenge for the physician, as decision has to be taken quickly for risk stratification, for further investigation, and for hospital admission. Echocardiography can be easily performed at bedside, which makes it a very useful adjunct in evaluating patients with chest pain and thus, resulting in lower morbidity and mortality rates. Early identification of patients with unstable angina may significantly reduce the risk of MI. Emergency echocardiographic evaluation of chest pain should be very systematic, thorough and is to done under the assumption that any patient with chest pain could potentially be having a critical cardiovascular risk as, a successful management depends on timely diagnosis and appropriate management of the patient including surgical intervention.

REFERENCES

1. Neskovic AN, Hagendorff A, Lancellotti P, et al. Emergency echocardiography: The European Association of Cardiovascular Imaging recommendations. Eur Heart J Cardiovasc Imaging. 2013;14:1-11.
2. Oh JK, Gibbons RJ, Christian TF, et al. Correlation of regional wall motion abnormalities detected by two-dimensional echocardiography with perfusion defect determined by technetium 99m sestamibi. Am Heart J. 1996;131:32-7.
3. Kontos MC, Arrowood JA, Paulsen WH, et al. Early echocardiography can predict cardiac events in emergency department patients with chest pain. Ann Emer Med. 1998;31;550-7.
4. Sabia P, Afrookteh A, Touchstone DA, et al. Value of regional wall motion abnormality in diagnosis of acute myocardial infarction. Circulation. 1991;84:I85-92.
5. Geyer H, Caracciola G, Abe H, et al. Assessment of myocardial mechanics using speckle tracking echocardiography fundamentals and clinical application. J Am Soc Echocardiogr. 2010;23:351-69.

6. Balgia R, Nienaber CA, Eduardo B, et al. The role of imaging in aortic dissection and related syndromes. J Am Coll Cardiol Imaging. 2014;7:406-24.
7. Evangelista A, Flachskamp F, Raimund E, et al. Echocardiography in aortic disease: EAE recommendations for clinical practice. Euro J Echo. 2010;11:645-58.
8. Goldhaber SZ. Echocardiography in the management of pulmonary embolism. Ann Intern Med. 2002;136:691-700.
9. McConnell MV, Solomon SD, Rayan ME, et al. Regional right ventricular dysfunction detected by echocardiography in acute pulmonary embolism. Am J Cardiol. 1996;78:469-73.
10. Ribeiro A, Lindmaker P, Juhlin-Dannfelt A, et al. Echocardiography Doppler in pulmonary embolism: Right ventricular dysfunction as a predictor of mortality rate. Am Heart J. 1997;134:479-87.
11. Kucher N, Luder CM, Dornhofer T, et al. Novel management strategy for patients with suspected pulmonary embolism. Eur Heart J. 2003;4:366-76.
12. Grifoni S, Olivotto I, Cecchini P, et al. Short-term clinical outcome of patients with acute pulmonary embolism, normal blood pressure, and echocardiographic right ventricular dysfunction. Circulation. 2000;101:2817-22.
13. Ginghina C, Caloianu GA, Serban M. Right ventricular myocardial infarction and pulmonary embolism differential diagnosis: A challenge for clinicians. J Med Life. 2010;3:242-53.

53

CHAPTER

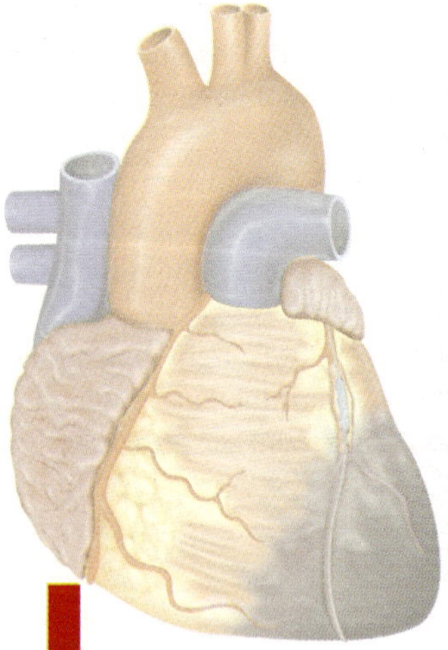

Imaging in Chest Pain: Computed Tomography Coronary Angiography Evaluation

Nidhi Goyal, Parveen Gulati, Arif Mirza, Aishwarya Gulati

INTRODUCTION

Early triage of patients presenting with acute chest pain to the emergency department brings a big challenge for early accurate diagnosis and is important for both prognosis and treatment. Patients at high risk for adverse outcomes are greatly benefited by early treatment with revascularization and low-risk patients may be discharged without a long-term risk of myocardial ischemia.[1] Patients presenting with acute chest pain are initially clinically evaluated for acute coronary syndrome (ACS). ACS describes the clinical manifestations of acute myocardial ischemia secondary to coronary artery disease (CAD) and includes unstable angina, non-ST elevation myocardial ischemia (NSTEMI), and ST elevation myocardial ischemia (STEMI). Of all the patients presenting with acute chest pain to the emergency,[2] only 25% have a confirmed diagnosis of acute chest syndrome at the time of discharge, with failure rate in diagnosis of up to 2–5%.[3,4] There are more chances of missing the diagnosis of ACS in younger patients, and such patients tend to have an atypical presentation with nondiagnostic ECG readings.[5] Age, gender, and clinical presentation are well-delineated parameters that can be used to define patients with possible ACS. The traditional cardiac risk factors like family history of coronary disease, hypertension, hypercholesterolemia, and other clinical parameters may be prognostic factors, but have limited value in the evaluation of acute chest pain. A quick and noninvasive examination with multidetector computed tomography (MDCT) for the presence and extent of CAD substantially improves the diagnosis and clinical care as well as outcome of patients who present to the emergency department with acute chest pain.

RISK STRATIFICATION

The initial workup of these patients includes a detailed clinical history, electrocardiography (ECG) evaluation, and cardiac biomarker values. Patients with a high probability of acute myocardial infarction or a proven acute myocardial infarction are benefited from immediate intervention (i.e. catheter angiography). A large number of patients, approximately 55–85% of patients with chest pain, do not have ACS and will be categorized as having an intermediate or low risk of ACS.[6,7]

Electrocardiography results and cardiac biomarker values enable early risk stratification but do not identify which patients can be discharged safely without a period of observation.[3,8,9] Risk-stratification algorithms, which combine clinical and ECG findings, have also not been considered accurate enough to identify low-risk patients and may have a 30-day risk for a major adverse cardiac event (MACE) of less than 1%.[7] Early utilization of cardiac CT angiography (CTA) through a quick and noninvasive examination with MDCT in patients with a low to intermediate risk of ACS should provide an efficient, safe, reliable, and cost-effective strategy for further risk stratification. The selection of patients for CTA is based on the pretest probability of ACS. The widely used Thrombolysis In Myocardial Infarction (TIMI) risk score determines the probability of ACS,[10] which is based on the patient's demography, past history of CAD, initial ECG results, and measurements of cardiac biomarkers and applies one point to each of the following risk factors:

- Age greater than 65 years
- Known CAD (documented previous coronary artery stenosis >50%)
- Severe angina (more than two episodes of chest pain in the preceding 24 hours)
- ST segment changes (persistent depression or transient elevation) on admission ECG
- Elevated serum markers of myocardial ischemia (troponins)
- Use of aspirin in the 7 days before presentation
- Three or more conventional risk factors for CAD (family history, diabetes mellitus, hypertension, hypercholesterolemia, smoking).

Patients with TIMI score of 5–7 are considered at high risk and usually are referred for urgent coronary invasive angiography and intervention.[11] Patients at intermediate risk (TIMI score 3–4) and low risk (TIMI score 0–2) are admitted for observation and undergo serial ECG and cardiac biomarker testing and are candidates for CT coronary angiography evaluation. The patients with low to intermediate risk of ACS are typically identified using clinical judgment and thorough clinical evaluation, and guided by initial risk assessment data from clinical history. Following this protocol, cardiac CTA can be ordered for approximately 60–70% of patients with suspected ACS.[7] The American College of Cardiology and the American College of Radiology, in collaboration with other societies, are trying to create protocols and criteria for the imaging of patients presenting with chest pain (Rybicki F, written communication, 2015). Patients with non-ST elevation ACS, on the basis of initial ECG results, and cardiac enzyme markers, will be benefited from cardiac CTA even in the setting of negative or equivocal ECG or troponin results.

CLINICAL ROLE OF COMPUTED TOMOGRAPHY ANGIOGRAPHY

Multidetector CT is now easily available and is widely used to for noninvasive assessment of CAD, with high accuracy and good image quality. With the advent of 64 and above detector row MDCT, ECG-gated scanning provides a quick, cost-effective, noninvasive technology for coronary artery evaluation, as well as additional information about cardiac morphology and adjacent thoracic structures simultaneously. A normal CT coronary angiogram confidently excludes significant CAD as a cause of acute chest pain. It can provide invaluable information about cardiac morphology, thoracic aorta, cardiac valves, and thoracic aorta. Advancements in evaluation of plaque morphology and myocardial perfusion will make it a comprehensive noninvasive cardiac assessment tool in near future. Many studies have proven the safety and efficacy of cardiac CTA for the triage of patients presenting with chest pain who have a low to intermediate risk of ACS, and for allowing safe and rapid discharge when possible.[12-14] Recent studies concluded that in low to intermediate risk patients CTA used in triage is less costly and more conclusive than decisions based on either stress ECG and stress echocardiography.[15] Authors of another recent study suggested that compared to other strategies, CTA is safe and incurs the lowest cost, and decreases the length of hospital stay leading to early discharge of patients.[16] Cardiac CTA has a high sensitivity (86–100%) and a high negative predictive value (93–100%), although the positive predictive value, with invasive coronary angiography as a gold standard, is still limited (50–90%).[12-14] Various studies evaluated the early use of cardiac CTA in low- to intermediate-risk ACS patients presenting with acute chest pain and established that cardiac CTA, reduces the time of diagnosis, facilitates discharge, and may lower costs compared with the usual protocol in appropriately selected patients.[10,17,18] Various causes of acute noncardiac chest pain are broad and include aortic dissection, pulmonary embolism (PE), tension pneumothorax, pericardial tamponade, and mediastinitis, all of which may also be depicted on cardiac CTA done for coronary artery evaluation. Based on its high negative predictive value, easy availability and short diagnostic time, CTA has been proved to be cost effective for evaluating patients presenting with acute chest pain with suspected ACS.

RADIATION EXPOSURE AND RISKS

Radiation exposure remains the main concern with CT. However, the recent advancements in technology and reconstruction algorithms have made it possible a CTA with an effective dose as low as 1 mSv. The effective radiation dose in older cardiac CT is 6.7–7.6 mSv in men and 8.1–9.2 mSv in women.[19] By comparison mean effective radiation dose with conventional angiography ranges from 3 to 6 mSv.[20,21] With the use of prospective gated axial scanning technique, the effective radiation dose is approximately 2–6 mSv, with mean 4 mSv, and is reduced by about 70–80% compared to that of retrospective gated imaging and is also lower than catheter coronary angiography.[22-24]

CORONARY ANATOMY

A comprehensive knowledge and understanding of the coronary artery anatomy is a prerequisite for the interpretation of CT coronary angiography and for the correct diagnosis of chest pain related to CAD (Figs. 1 to 3). According to the AHA (American Heart Association) system

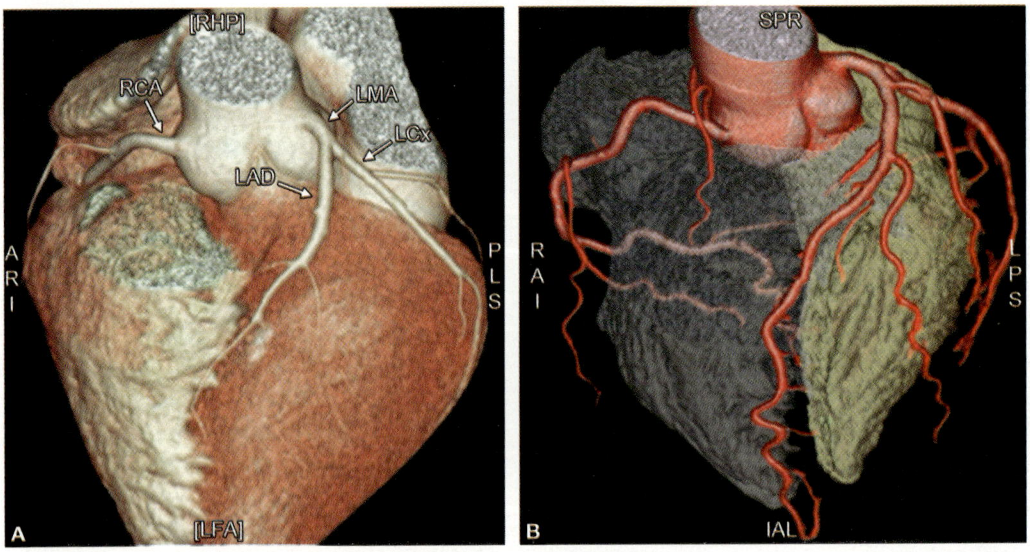

Figs. 1A and B: Volume rendering (VR) images showing—(A) entire heart in a single view with visualization of origin and course of coronary arteries. (B) VR images showing different color coding of chambers and coronary arteries. (LAD: left anterior descending; LCx: left circumflex artery; LMA: left main artery; RCA: right coronary artery)

of classification, the coronary artery tree is divided into 17 segments.[25,26] Four main arteries and their branches are evaluated, i.e. the left coronary artery (LCA), the left anterior descending (LAD), the left circumflex artery (LCx), the right coronary artery (RCA). The average diameter of coronary arteries varies, ranging from 5 mm (LCA in males) to 2 mm [posterior descending artery (PDA) in females].[27] The LAD courses anterolaterally into the atrioventricular (AV) groove, down to the apex, and supplies the majority of left ventricle. The major branches of the LAD are septal perforating arteries and diagonal branches. Septal perforating arteries course medially and supply the interventricular septal and AV bundle. Diagonal branches, which course laterally, supply the left ventricular free wall.[28] LAD is divided into proximal middle and distal parts according to the origin of diagonal branches. The LCx courses in the left AV groove and gives off obtuse marginal branches and supplies the left ventricular free wall.[28] LCx is divided into proximal and distal segments based on the origin of obtuse marginal arteries. LCX may also give rise to posterolateral branch and posterior descending artery in cases of left dominant circulation. In approximately 15% of patients, a thin branch, the ramus intermedius (RI), is seen arising at the division of LCA, resulting in trifurcation (Fig. 4).[29] The RCA arises from the anterior aspect of the right coronary sinus and courses into right AV groove toward the posterior interventricular septum where the AV groove transects the interventricular septum (IVS) perpendicularly. In majority of the patients (50–60%), the first branch of the RCA is the conus artery unless the conus is arising directly from the right coronary sinus and supplies the right ventricular outflow track.[30] The origin of the sinoatrial branch is variable with about 58% of the cases arising from RCA and 42% arising from LCx (Fig. 5).[31] Few other branches called acute marginal branches arise from RCA and supply the free wall of right ventricle. The RCA is divided into proximal, middle, and distal segments for which the landmark is based on the origin of the acute marginal (AM). The proximal and middle segments are the two halves before the origin of the AM and distal RCA is from AM origin up to the origin of PDA. PDA and posterior left ventricular (PLV)/posterolateral branch supply the diaphragmatic wall of the left ventricle. The origin of the PDA and posterolateral branch decides the dominance. When PDA and posterolateral branches arise from RCA, it is a right dominant circulation, which is the case in 70%. In 10% cases, it is a left dominant circulation and in the remaining 10%, it is a codominant circulation.[28]

MULTIDETECTOR COMPUTED TOMOGRAPHY TECHNIQUE AND PROTOCOLS

Continuously beating heart makes it mandatory to perform coronary CTA on a multislice CT. Minimum 64 slice is required for coronary evaluation, however the advent of 256 and 512 slice CT has made the evaluation easier and more accurate.

Patient Evaluation and Preparation

Patients who require CT coronary angiography are thoroughly evaluated by radiologist or anesthesiologist or trained CT technicians for any possible severe allergic reactions to an iodinated contrast media. Creatinine level

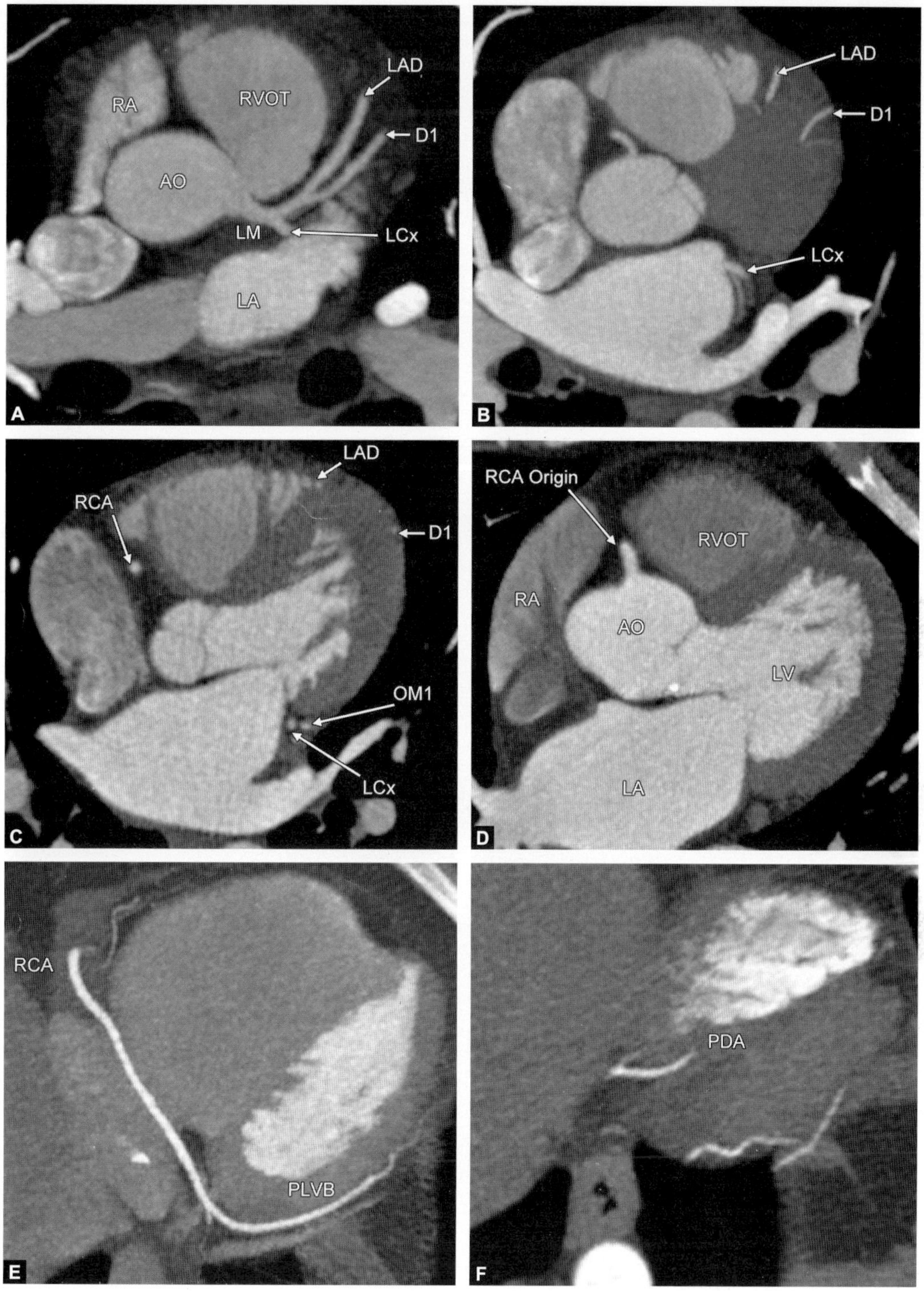

Figs. 2A to F: Axial images showing normal anatomy of coronary arteries. (A to D) Show normal LAD artery coursing in the interventricular groove toward LV apex with septal and diagonal branches. LCX and RCA coursing in the left and right atrioventricular groove respectively. LCx giving off obtuse marginal branches. (E and F) PDA and PLV are arising from RCA in a right dominant circulation. (LAD: left anterior descending; LCx: left circumflex artery; PDA: posterior descending artery; PLV: posterior left ventricle; RCA: right coronary artery; LA: left artery; LV: left ventricle; LVOT: left ventricular outflow tract; AO: Aorta; LM: left main artery; PA: pulmonary artery; RA: right artery).

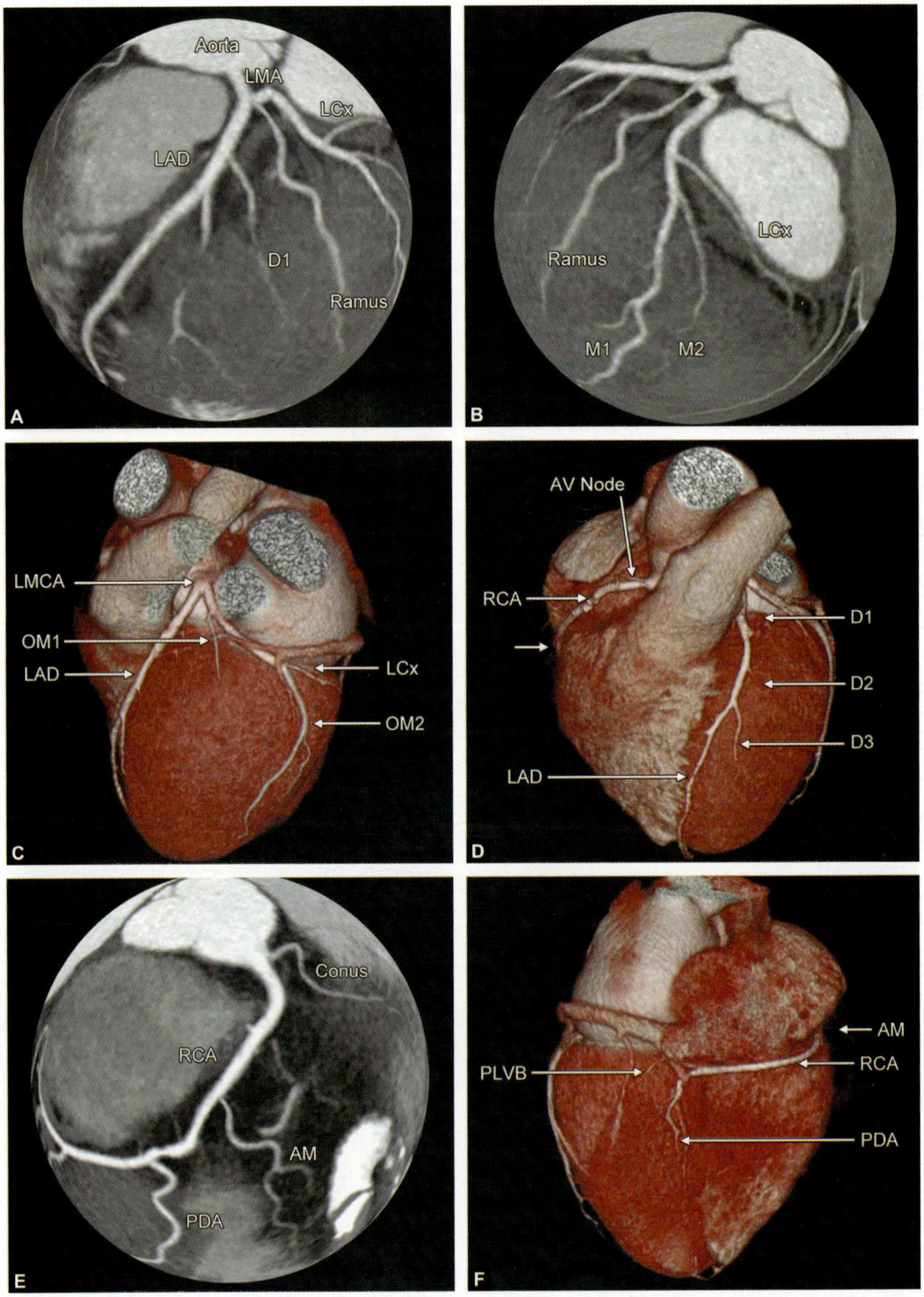

Figs. 3A to F: Volume rendering (VR) and global views showing normal anatomy of coronary arteries. Conus and acute marginal (AM) arteries are also seen arising from right coronary artery (RCA). (LAD: left anterior descending; LCx: left circumflex artery; LMA: left main artery; LMCA: left main coronary artery; PDA: posterior descending artery; PLV: posterior left ventricle)

more than 1.5 mg/dL is also considered a relative contraindication for administration of contrast media in these times.[32] The pulse and blood pressure are evaluated. Normal sinus rhythm is a preferable as the presence of arrhythmias will be a challenge for ECG-gated coronary imaging, therefore, patients having arrhythmias, e.g. atrial fibrillations are exempted. However, now, this is no longer an absolute contraindication and beta-blockers may be

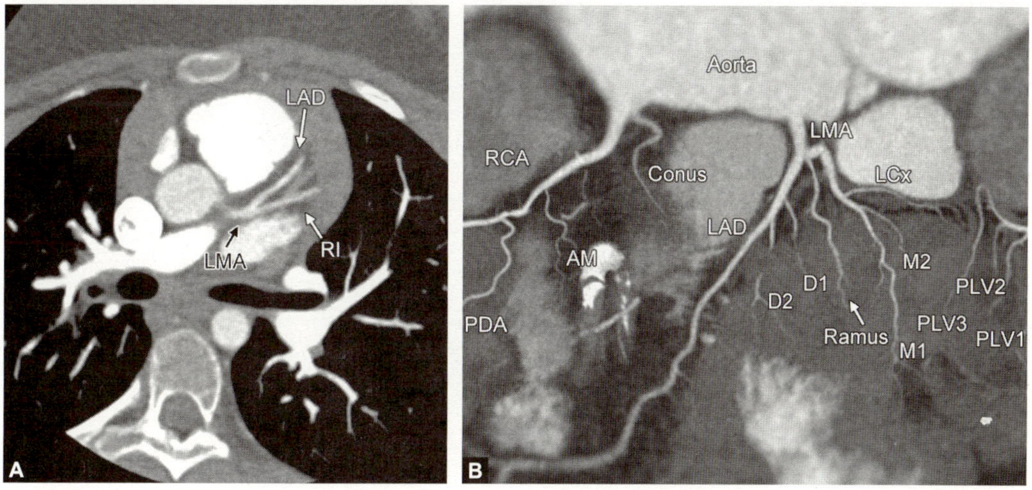

Figs. 4A and B: Axial images showing Ramus intermedius (RM) arising between LAD and LCx arteries resulting from trifurcation of LMA (left main artery). (LAD: left anterior descending; LCx: left circumflex artery).

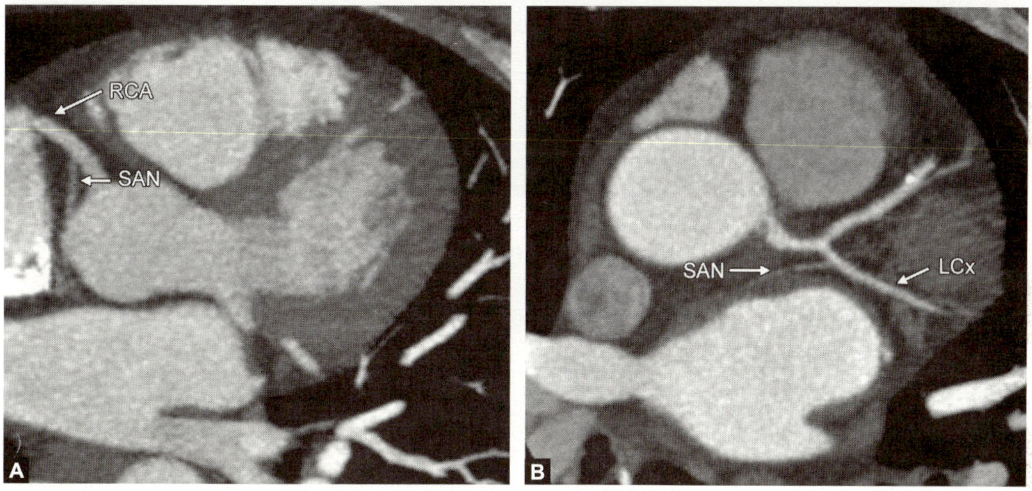

Figs. 5A and B: Axial images showing sinoatrial nodal branch (SAN) arising from RCA in (A) and from LCX in (B). (LCx: left circumflex artery; RCA: right coronary artery).

used to reduce ectopy. The most quiescent phase of the cardiac cycle is the diastolic phase, hence, a heart rate of 70 beats or less per minute is necessary for data acquisition in an adequate timed diastolic phase to ensure diagnostic image quality. Patients with heart rate higher than 70 beats per minute receive intravenous/oral beta blockers for regularizing and achieving the required heart rate. IV metoprolol with a dose of 5 mg is usually administered within the CT suite, and the effect occurs typically in 5–10 minutes and additional doses may be given up to four doses. Oral administration of drug with an initial dose of 50–100 mg is performed at least 1 hour before imaging and up to 200 mg of dose can be given to achieve required heart rate.[33] In patients with contraindications to beta blockers, like congestive heart failure, asthma and bradycardia, calcium channel blockers can be considered as an alternative with diltiazem as the preferred drug with IV bolus up to 0.25 mg/kg.[34] Constant monitoring with a cardiac resuscitation trained person is necessary.

PROTOCOLS

Scanogram is obtained as a starting point to precisely localize the position of the heart and limit the area of exposure. This is followed by unenhanced and angiographic phases. The image volume should include the area 1–2 cm below the carina to the bottom of heart. The ECG of the patient is recorded during scanning for synchronization of heart motion to data acquisition (Fig. 6).

Plain/unenhanced scan is acquired for the evaluation of calcium score and other thoracic structures, and is

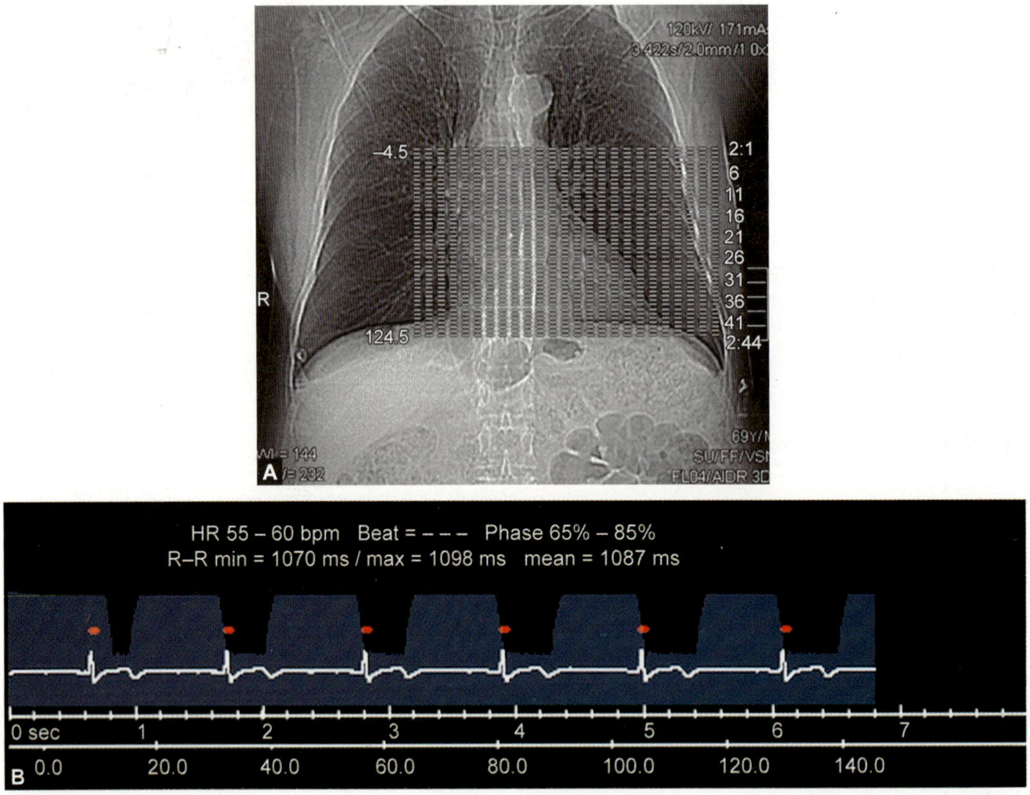

Figs. 6A and B: Scanogram is obtained to plan area of scanning: (A) Below the carina to base of heart (between the dashed lines); (B) Electrocardiogram (ECG) is continuously monitored and the scan data is obtained; Information about the heart cycle is used to reconstruct the data: Retrospective gating.

obtained using a high-pitch helical scan or prospectively triggered acquisition. Contrast-enhanced angiographic phase is acquired using weight-based IV injection of nonionic iodinated contrast material (generally 60–120 mL) followed by 20–40 mL of saline at a rate of 4–5 mL/s. A rightly timed and optimized contrast injection leads to maximal opacification of the left heart and coronary arteries and mild opacification of the right heart and superior vena cava while using a minimal contrast dose. Contrast bolus transmit time, which is the contrast material arrival time in the heart, is crucial for accurate and adequate opacification of coronary arteries. This time varies, depending upon the patient's blood circulation time and ranges from 8 seconds to 40 seconds.[35] The scanning time factors in contrast bolus transmit time through test bolus tracking/automated bolus tracking in administration of contrast.

IMAGE ACQUISITION

Retrospective ECG-gated helical CT is the prevailing technique, acquiring data throughout the cardiac cycle with simultaneous ECG monitoring over multiple heartbeats (Fig. 6).

The major advantage of retrospective coronary imaging is functional evaluation of the heart in addition to coronary artery analysis. The major disadvantage is increased radiation dose, which has led to the use of prospective ECG-triggering/step and shoot method.[36] This technique has a lower radiation dose as the data is acquired for short periods and not throughout the entire cardiac cycle with disadvantage that functional assessment of the heart is not possible. High-pitch helical acquisition with prospective ECG-synchronization is a newer method that enables diagnostic imaging at a potentially even lower dose,[37] available with dual source scanners.

Reconstruction Methods and Postprocessing of the Data

Multiplanar reformation is used to generate cross-sectional images of coronary arteries, such as short axis and long axis views (Fig. 7).

Curved multiplanar imaging allows the visualization of the entire coronary artery in a single image. The centerline of the vessel is followed and image plane is adjusted accordingly to place the entire vessel in a single plane from ostium to the end.

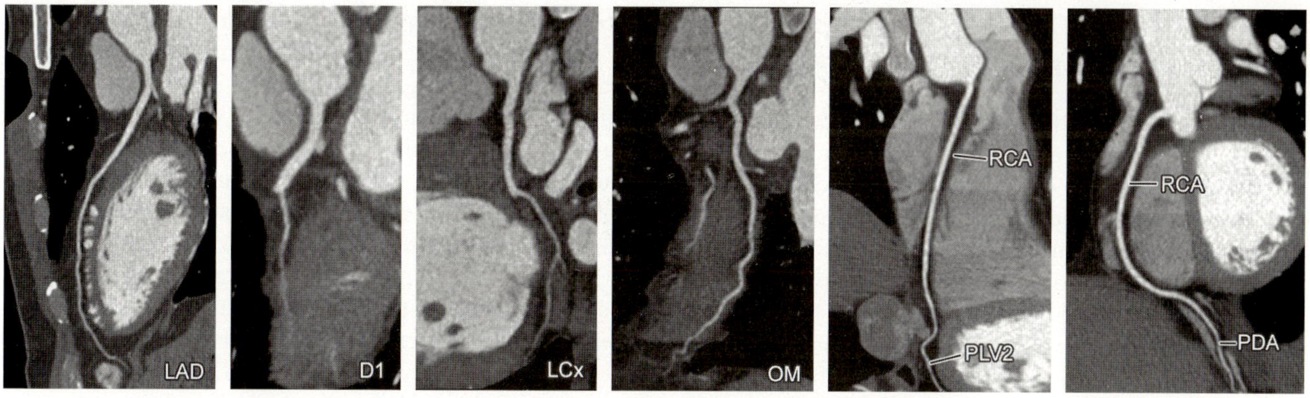

Fig. 7: Maximum intensity projections (MIP) showing all coronary arteries. (LAD: left anterior desending: LCx: left circumflex artery; PDA: posterior descending artery; PLV: posterior left ventricle; RCA: right coronary artery)

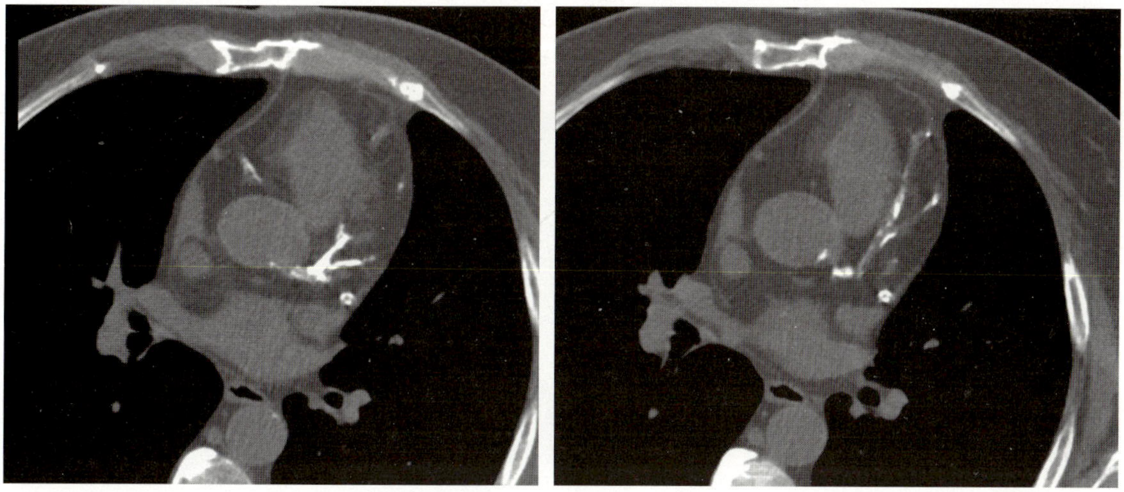

Fig. 8: Dense calcified plaques in LMA, LAD and LCx in calcium scoring scan, limiting the evaluation of vessel lumen. Calcium score was near 700. (LAD: left anterior descending; LCx: left circumflex artery; LMA; left main artery).

Maximum intensity projection (MIP) stacks multiple axial section images together and allows visualization of longer lengths of coronary vessel lumen and accurate detection of intraluminal lesions/disease.

Volume rendering (VR) involves reconstruction of the entire volume of image data. The acquired data is summed up pixel by pixel to obtain a single composite image. Single composite image can be evaluated in multiple planes as required and most helpful in coronary artery anomalies and for surgical planning (*see* Fig. 1).[38,39]

Calcium Scoring

Patients who present with acute chest syndrome are very likely to have calcifications in their coronary arteries. There have been multiple retrospective studies for predicting cardiac events in patients having coronary calcium and an increased risk of death.[40-42] Prospective studies have also confirmed these results and demonstrated that coronary calcium scoring provides additional prognostic information in addition to clinical and laboratory tests.[43]

In patients having CAD, there is also a high burden of noncalcified plaques, therefore it is necessary to evaluate and monitor patients experiencing coronary event even in absence of calcium along coronary vessels.[44,45]

Nonetheless, patients with a high burden of calcium are likely to be greatly benefited from coronary imaging. Calcified plaques can be a deterrent to the evaluation of CT coronary angiography as coronary disease can be overestimated due to blooming artifacts from the calcium component. An indeterminate coronary CT evaluation is much more likely in patients with extensive calcium burden, with scores typically ranging from more than 400 to 1000, depending upon the MDCT hardware, and postprocessing techniques used (Fig. 8).

CORONARY ARTERY DISEASE: COMPUTED TOMOGRAPHY FINDINGS

It is recommended to assess the raw data as well as processed data for complete and accurate evaluation. Mild to moderate stenosis of coronary artery with calcified, noncalcified, and mixed plaque is evaluated in axial images and using other postprocessing parameters. Information about the presence and extent of CAD is evaluated through arterial luminal opacification. (Figs. 9 to 14) The presence, amount, and composition of noncalcified coronary atherosclerotic plaque and the resultant luminal narrowing is assessed on CTA. CT clearly allows identification of calcified, noncalcified, and mixed plaques with high sensitivity (92%) and specificity (88%) and also enables further stratification of noncalcified plaques as either fibrous or lipid rich.[46-48] The quantification of lumen narrowing of coronary stents by neointimal hyperplasia with MDCT is limited due to beam-hardening artifacts caused by metallic stents (Figs. 15 and 16). However, despite these limitations, single-center studies using 64-slice MDCT have shown reasonable diagnostic performances for in-stent restenosis detection. Recent pooled analyses reported an overall sensitivity of in-stent restenosis detection of 84% with un-assessable stents in up to 13% of cases.[49-52]

A variety of postoperative complications may manifest as dyspnea and chest pain, thereby mimicking recurrent angina secondary to graft occlusion. Chest pain is common after coronary artery bypass graft (CABG) surgery and can have a variety of etiologies including, but not limited to, recurrent angina secondary to graft occlusion, sternal infection, and pleural or pericardial effusion. In this setting, MDCT can offer a rapid, convenient, and noninvasive means of discerning the correct underlying diagnosis

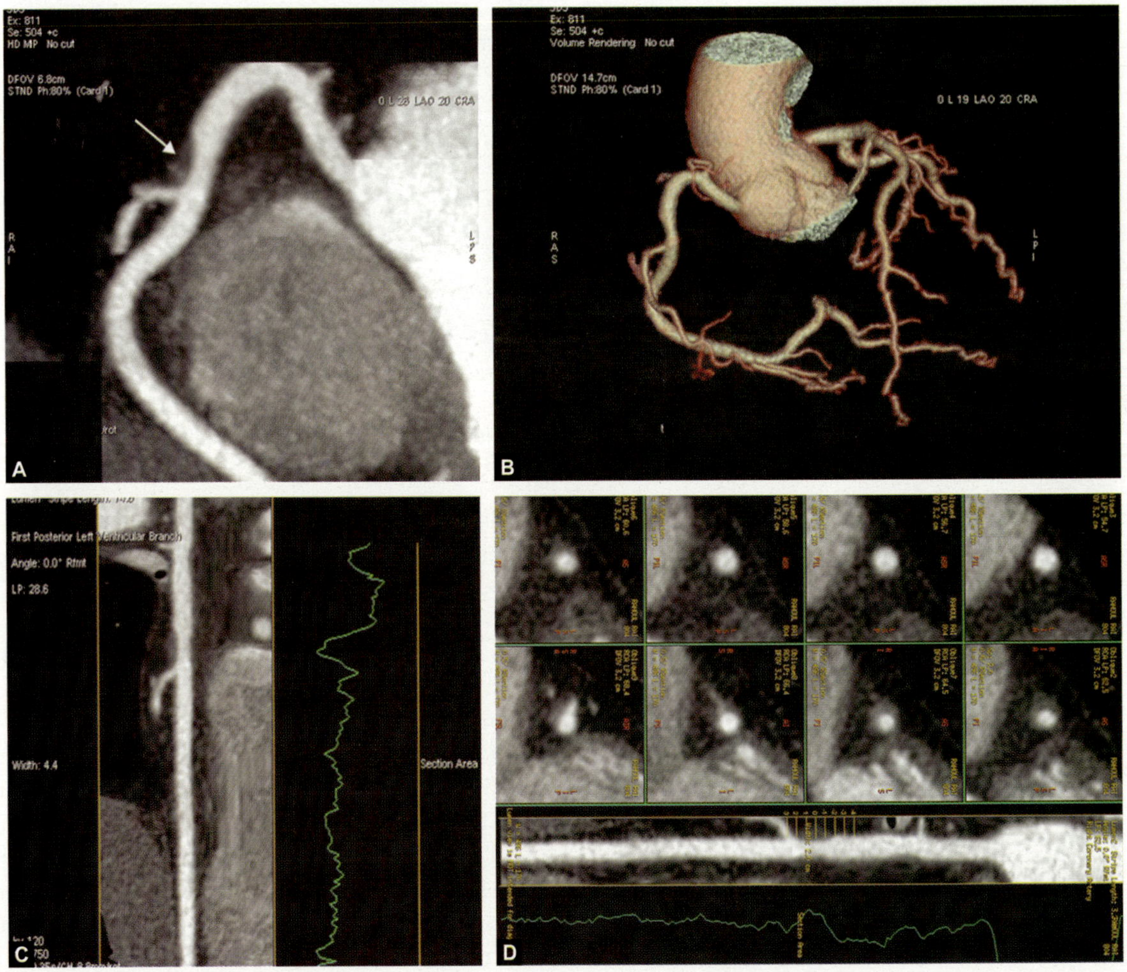

Figs. 9A to D: (A) MPR and (B) VR images showing single vessel disease with predominantly soft plaque (arrow) in proximal RCA causing mild to moderate stenosis with about 30% luminal narrowing. (C and D) Straightened lumen curved MPR and corresponding axial sequences in same case showing predominantly soft plaque in proximal RCA with mild to moderate luminal narrowing in cross sectional images. (MPR: multiplanar reconstruction; RCA: right coronary artery; VR: volume rendering).

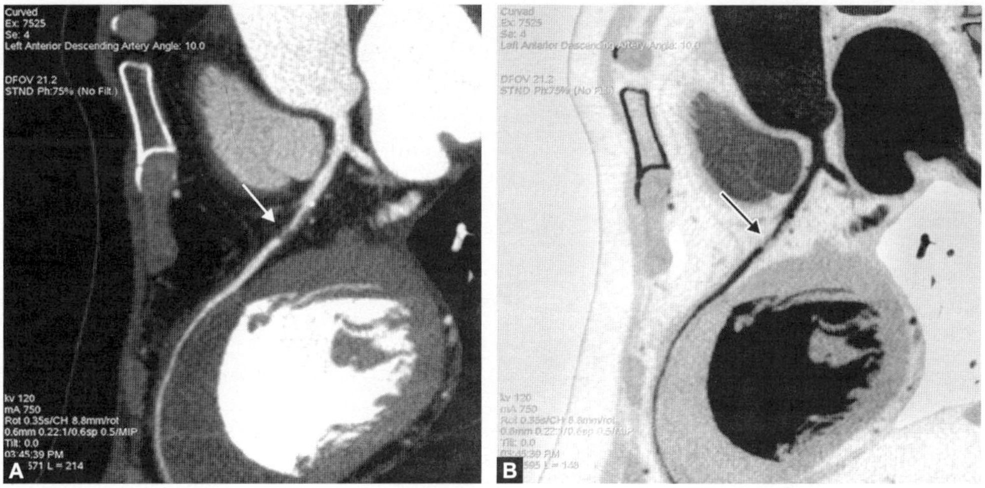

Figs. 10A and B: MPR images showing diseased proximal LAD secondary to mixed soft and calcified plaque causing short segment of severe narrowing (arrows) in a patient complaining of acute chest pain. (LAD: left anterior descending; MPR: multiplanar reconstruction)

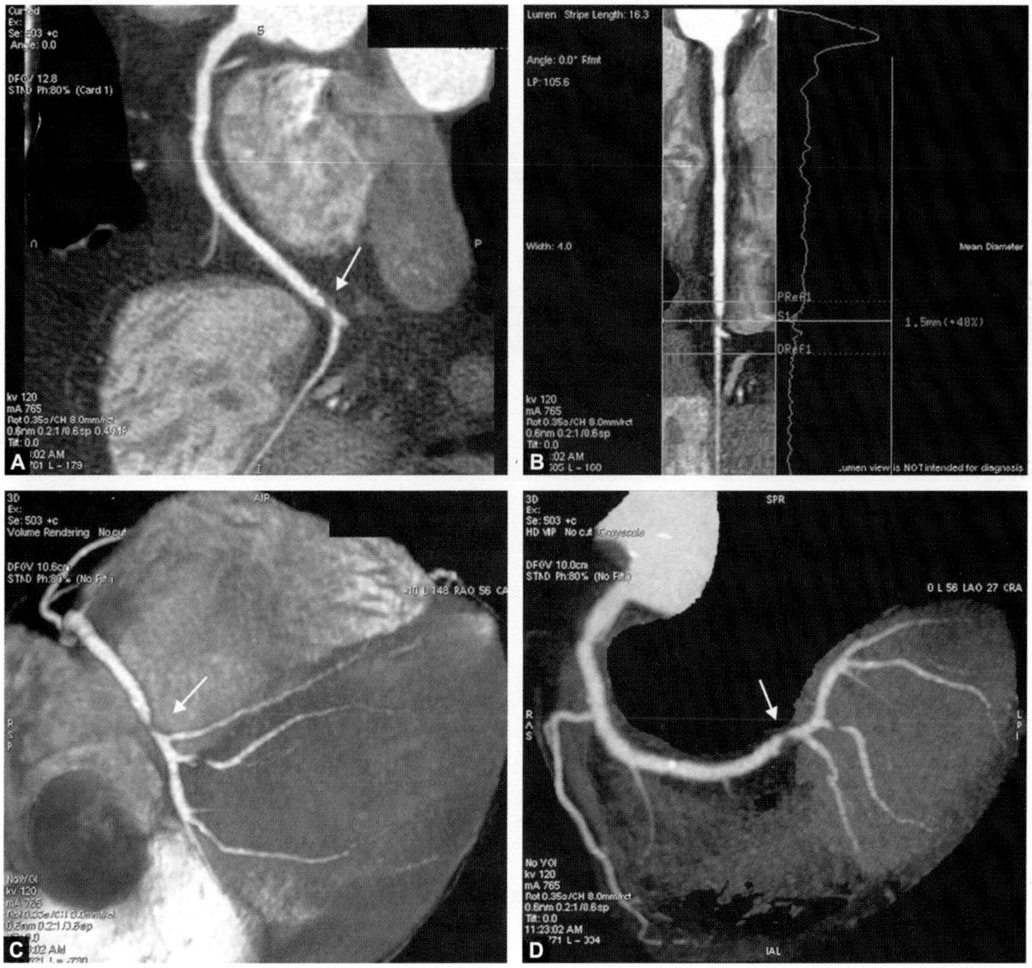

Figs. 11A to D: Patient presented to emergency with acute chest pain with normal ECG. (A and B) MPR and MIP images showing single vessel disease with focal area of severe narrowing (arrow) in distal RCA. (C and D) VR images showing focal area of severe narrowing (arrow) in distal RCA just proximal to origin of PDA and PLV. (ECG: echocardiography; PDA: posterior descending artery; PLV: posterior left ventricle; MIP: maximum intensity projections; MPR: multiplanar reconstruction; RCA: right coronary artery; VR: volume rendering)

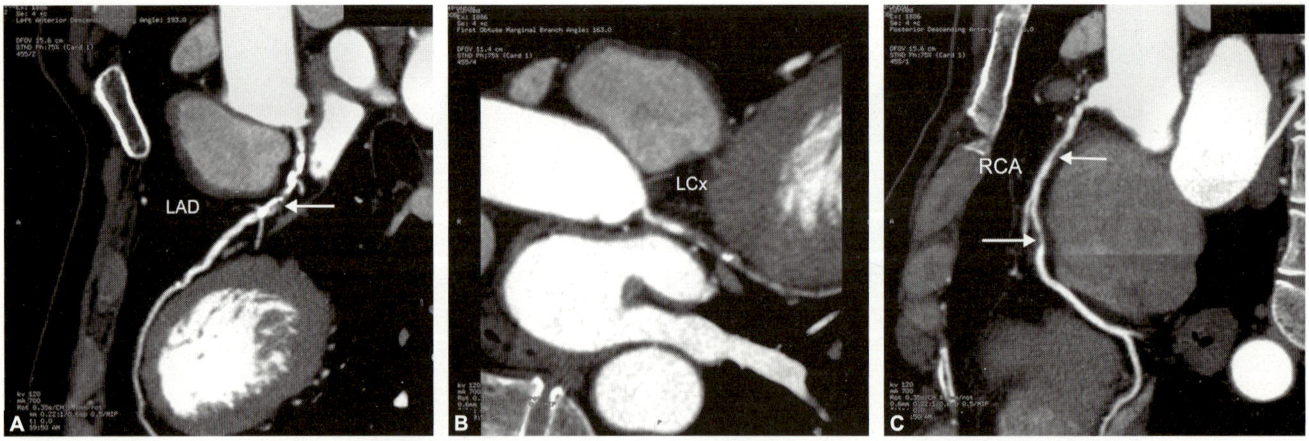

Figs. 12A to C: MPR images showing triple vessel disease with mixed soft and calcified plaques in all three vessels causing irregular outline of the lumen and area of severe narrowing (arrows) in proximal LAD, LCX and distal RCA. Patient had history of unstable angina, with multiple risk factors but with no acute changes in ECG or biochemical markers. (ECG: echocardiography; LAD: left anterior descending; LCX: left circumflex artery; MPR: multiplanar reconstruction; RCA: right coronary artery)

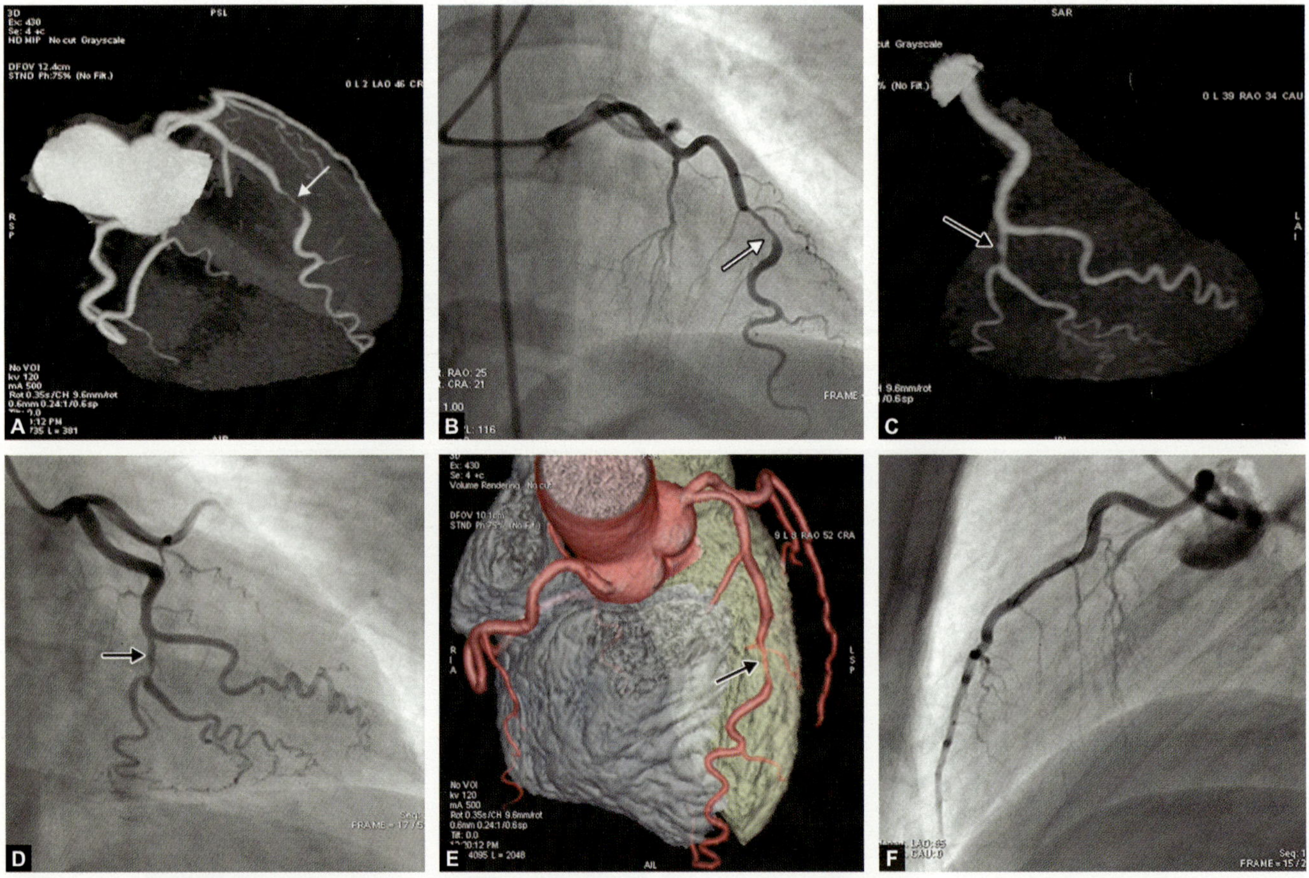

Figs. 13A to F: (A and B) CTA images in various projections showing short segment diseased LAD mid segment (white arrows). (C and D) Corresponding catheter images showing short segment luminal narrowing (black arrows) in LAD in similar views, confirming the findings. (E) Catheter angiography showing the successful post angioplasty stenting of LAD (arrow). (F) VR image with color coding of ventricles and coronary vessels with diseased LAD. (CTA: computed tomography angiography; LAD: left anterior descending; VR: volume rendering).

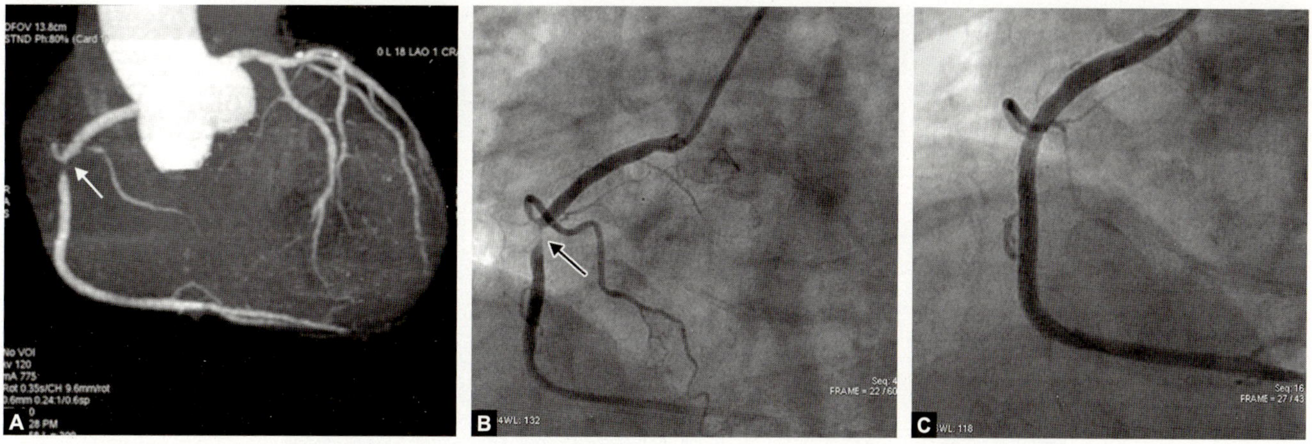

Figs. 14A to C: (A) CTA VR image showing short segment severe narrowing of RCA (white arrow). (B) Corresponding catheter images confirming area of narrowing in RCA (black arrow. (C) Catheter angiography showing the post angioplasty stenting of RCA. (CTA: computed tomography angiography; RCA: right coronary artery; VR: volume rendering).

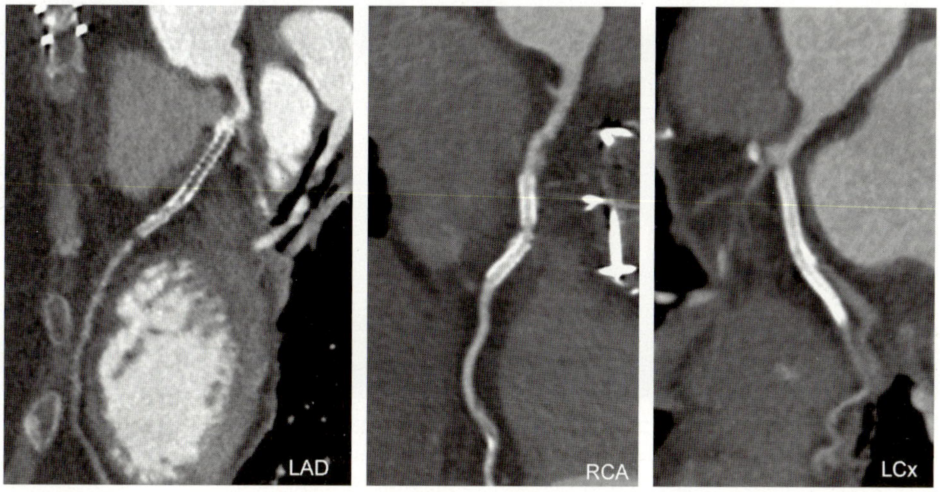

Fig. 15: Past history of stenting in all three vessels, presented to emergency with acute chest pain. MIP CT angiography images reveal complete thrombosis of stent in LAD, with opacification of distal LAD likely from collaterals. There are patent stents seen in LCx and RCA with normal opacification of distal vessels. (LAD: left anterior descending; LCx: left circumflex artery; MIP: maximum intensity projections; RCA: right coronary artery).

(Figs. 16–18). Assessment of procedural complications can also be assessed or confirmed using CT coronary angiography (Fig. 19). Anomalous origin of coronary arteries like RCA from LMA can predispose the patients to myocardial ischemia and arrhythmias (Figs. 20 to 22) can be well evaluated with CT and should always be looked for and commented upon.

Computed Tomography Perfusion Imaging

Evaluation of morphology without functional assessment is the major limitation of traditional CTA, therefore what level of coronary stenosis will lead to myocardial ischemia cannot be predicted. Inducible ischemia associated with coronary disease is predictive of risk of coronary event and hence the benefit from revascularization compared to medical treatment and is a part of entire coronary evaluation.[53,54]

The CTA needs to provide both anatomical and functional information about CAD for a comprehensive evaluation of coronary disease.

Several studies have been done to perform CT perfusion to evaluate myocardial status. First pass dynamic evaluation of myocardial perfusion is likely the most accurate technique, however dynamic evaluation needs multiple phases of scanning resulting in increased radiation dose. To reduce radiation burden, studies have been published using single arterial phase scanning for myocardial perfusion based on myocardial blood pool enhancement as a part of CTA, followed by a delayed phase low dose

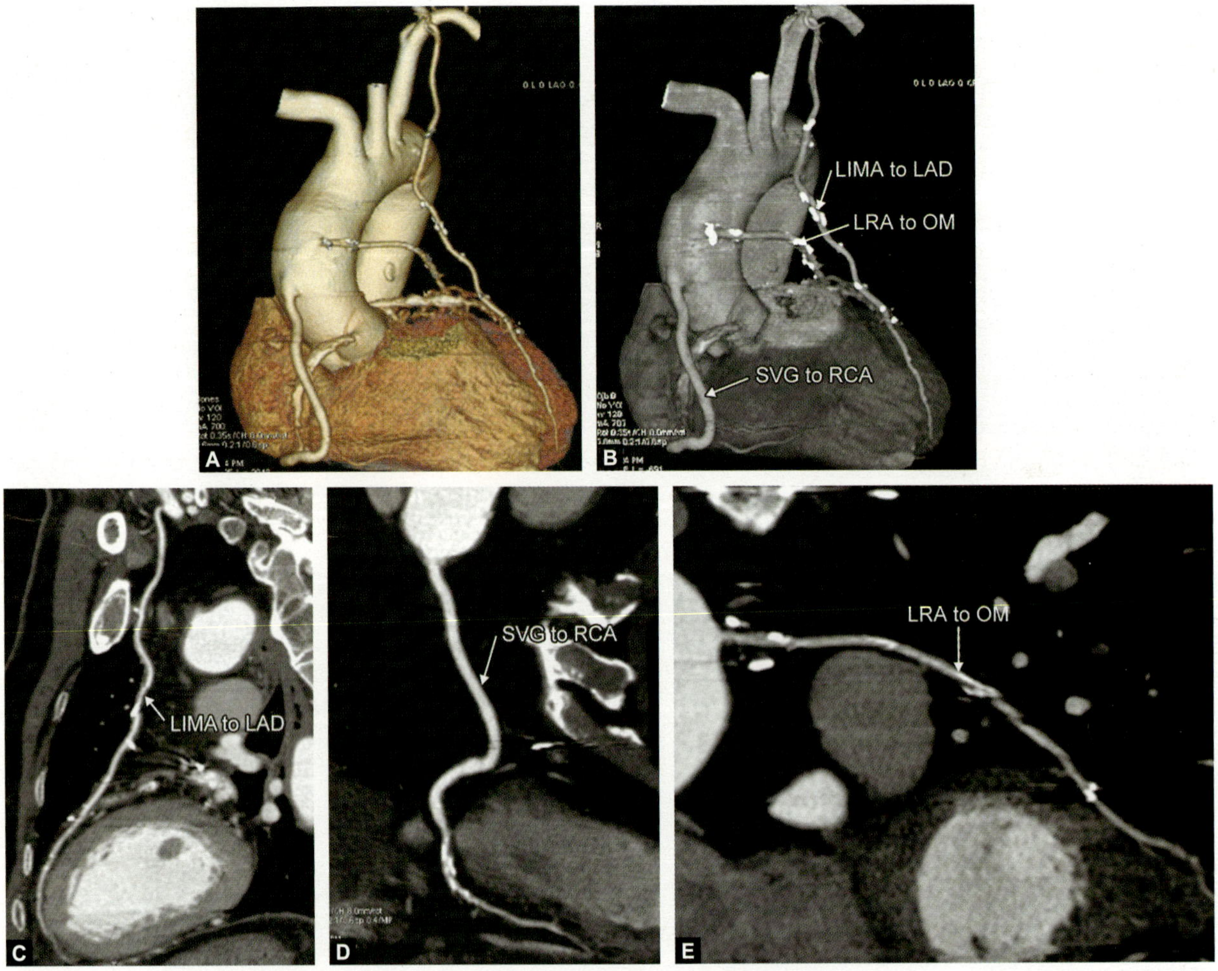

Figs. 16A to E: Patient underwent bypass graft cardiac surgery a year back and now presented with mild chest pain. (A and B) CTA VR images, (C to E) MIP images showing patent arterial, venous, and radial grafts with well visualized proximal and distal anastomosis. Negative predictive value of CTA helps to confidently rule out cardiac cause of chest pain. (CTA: computed tomography angiography; MIP: maximum intensity projections; VR: volume rendering).

scan to evaluate myocardial enhancement indicative of myocardial ischemia.[55,56] Various other techniques, including dobutamine stress study, are used for myocardial perfusion with the limitation of compromised image quality due to tachycardia induced by dobutamine. Using adenosine as vasodilator for CT stress imaging for measuring transmural perfusion (subendocardial attenuation density/ subepicardial attenuation density) to detect myocardial perfusion has proven to have a sensitivity/specificity of 86%/92% on a per-patient analysis.[57] Dual source CT scanner using relatively high kVp for coronary imaging and a low kVp for "iodine perfusion map" displayed as a color overlay on high resolution CTA provides excellent quality diagnostic correlation with SPECT imaging (sensitivity 91%; specificity 92%).[58]

TRIPLE RULE OUT

Triple-rule-out (TRO) CT angiography provides a quick and cost-effective evaluation of the coronary arteries along with aorta and pulmonary arteries and simultaneous visualization of adjacent intrathoracic structures in patients with acute chest pain in same sitting. TRO CT is most appropriate in the setting of low to intermediate risk for ACS in patients with acute chest syndrome where symptoms are not specific for CAD and may also be attributed to other acute pathologic conditions of the aorta or pulmonary arteries. Newer CT scanners with 64 or more detector rows allow rapid ECG-gated imaging to provide high-quality images in patients with a heart rate of up to 80 beats per minute. Injection of iodinated contrast material ranges from 80 mL to 120 mL and is tailored to provide

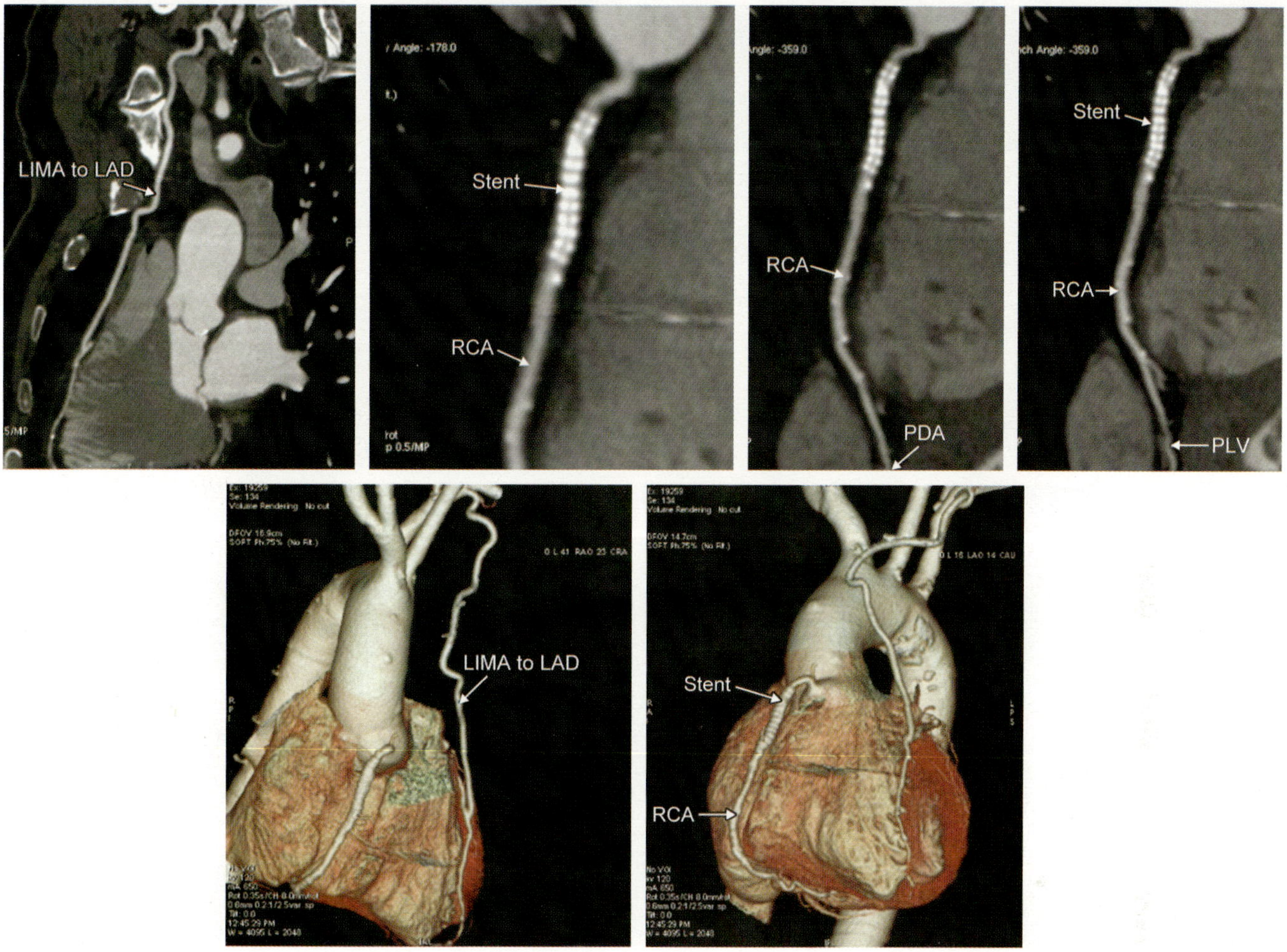

Fig. 17: Patient came after two years of bypass surgery with chest pain and CTA was done which showed one patent LIMA–LAD graft and a patent stent in native RCA and normal contrast opacification of the vessels and branches. VR images showing patent graft and stent. (CTA: computed tomography angiography; LAD: left anterior descending; LIMA: left internal mammary artery; RCA: right coronary artery; VR: volume rendering).

simultaneous high levels of arterial enhancement in the coronary arteries and aorta (300 HU) and in the pulmonary arteries (200 HU). Limiting the study to incorporate the aortic arch down through the heart decreases radiation exposure. Other methods like choosing the right scanning parameters, including prospective ECG tube current modulation and prospective ECG gating with the "step-and-shoot" technique, are utilized to reduce radiation exposure (optimally, 5–9 mSv).[32] When performed with appropriate attention to timing and technique, TRO CT provides coronary image quality equal to that of dedicated coronary CT angiography and pulmonary arterial images that are free of motion artifact related to cardiac pulsation. In an appropriately selected emergency department patient population, TRO CT can safely eliminate the need for further diagnostic testing in over 75% of patients (Fig. 23).[32]

NOVEL IMAGING TECHNIQUE

With continuing developments in technology and intense scientific and clinical evaluations, CT coronary angiography has come out of the realms of research and has established a definitive role in evaluation of coronary arteries and sounds promising to replace catheter angiography. There are still many more advancements under research, which are gradually becoming a part of all routine coronary angiographic examinations, to overcome shortcomings in the present scenario. Even with applications like ECG controlled tube current modulation and low-tube voltage, standard coronary CT with a retrospective ECG-gated helical scan with a tube voltage of 120 kVp on CT scanners with 64 or more detectors there are various limitations as listed:

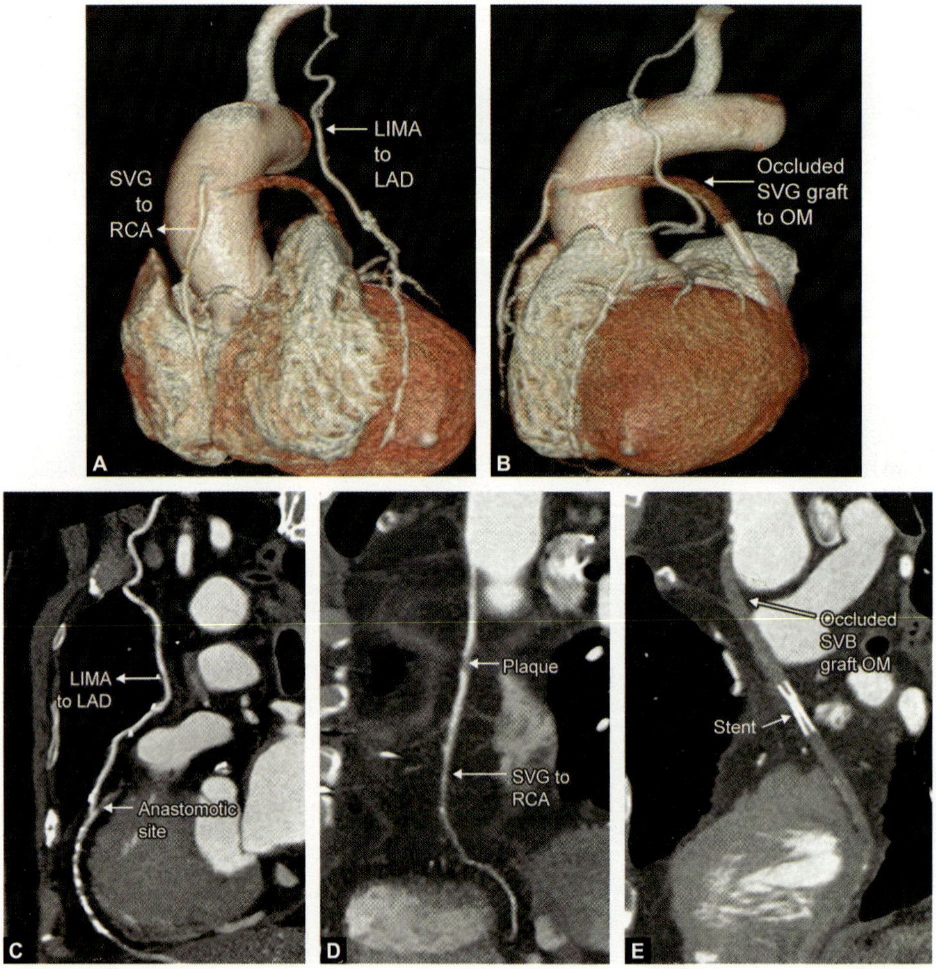

Figs. 18A to E: Follow-up case of cardiac surgery: Post-CABG status with stenting done in venous SVG graft. (A and B) CTA VR images reveal patent LIMA-LAD graft and blocked SVG-OM graft. (C to E) MIP images showing patent LIMA-LAD graft. SVG-OM graft is completely occluded with blocked stent in situ. There is soft tissue plaque seen in SVG-RCA graft with sever narrowing: Cause of clinical presentation of chest pain. (CABG: coronary artery bypass graft; CTA: computed tomography angiography; LAD: left anterior descending; LIMA: left internal mammary artery; OM: obtuse marginal; RCA: right coronary artery; SVG: saphenous vein graft; VR: volume rendering).

- Exposure to nephrotoxic contrast medium
- Stair-step artifacts, due to varying/higher heart rate or inability to hold breath
- Irregular heart rate and arrhythmias
- Beam-hardening artifacts, due to excessive calcification
- Coronary plaque characterization
- Limited information for the functional assessment of coronary stenosis
- Radiation dose.

There are many new techniques proposed and gradually being widely used to overcome these shortcomings. Detailed discussion of these techniques is beyond the scope of this chapter, however an introduction and brief summary is shared.

- *Variable heart rate:* Beat to beat variable delay algorithm always picks same percentage delay in diastole and cardiac delay algorithm dynamically integrates changes.
- *To overcome high and variable heart rates, and breathing artifacts:* Adaptive multicycle reconstruction uses the patient's recorded ECG information to reconstruct data using the optimal number of cardiac cycles. With lower heart rates fewer cycles are necessary to produce a good image. Higher heart rate multicycle reconstruction is used for producing good cardiac images, as it uses a smaller data set from multiple cycles. It combines a portion of projections from one heart cycle with the portion of projections from another to make full 180°.
- *Irregular heart rate and arrhythmias:* ECG editing helps in automatic detection of abnormal beats and

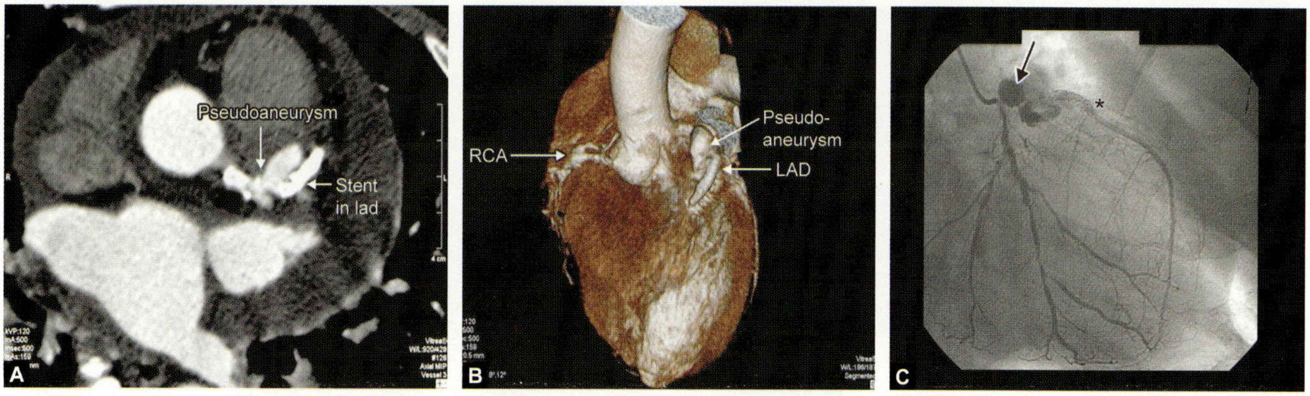

Figs. 19A to C: (A) A 50-year-old male underwent LAD stenting for single vessel disease in LAD. One day post procedural patient presented with severe chest pain. ECG was unremarkable and patient was referred for CTA to evaluate the stent status and to look for in-stent restenosis. CTA revealed pseudoaneurysm in proximal LAD likely a rare complication of procedure. (B) VR images showing the out pouching in proximal LAD. Patient was immediately taken for catheter angiography and (C) images revealed extravasation of contrast (black arrow) at the proximal end of stent (*) in LAD. (CTA: computed tomography angiography; LAD: left anterior descending; VR: volume rendering).

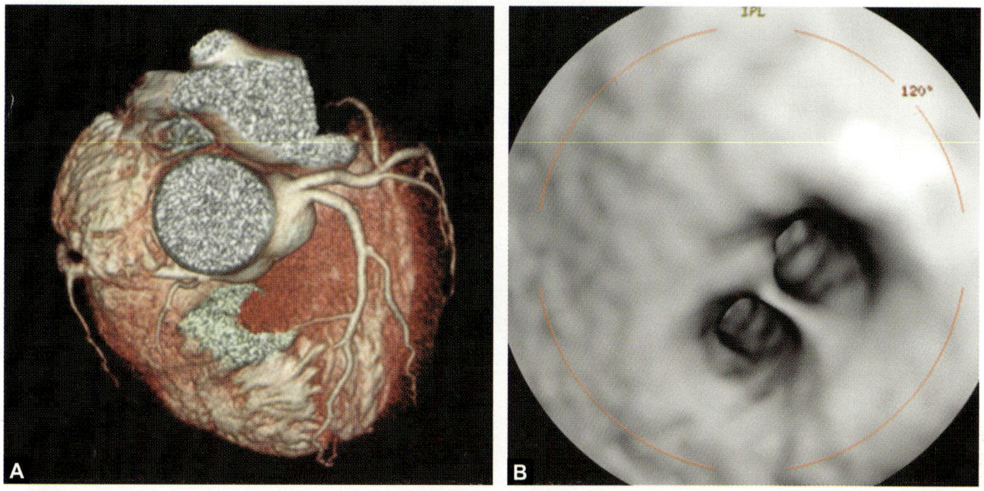

Figs. 20A and B: VR and endovascular views showing separate and origins of LAD and LCx from aorta with absent left main artery. (LAD: left anterior descending; LCx: left circumflex artery; VR: volume rendering).

their deletions. System recreates image data sets using raw data, abnormal beats are then excluded and data regenerated using the edited data sets devoid of artifacts.

- *Dose modulation tools:* Low mAs used during non-diagnostic part of the cycle, step and shoot prospective triggering, a wide coverage with advanced MDCT detectors, accurate synchronization of the X-ray with rate-responsive technology, real-time monitoring of the ECG signal irregularities, and arrhythmia rejection via advanced algorithms, precise prospective identification of the quiet physiological phase with the beat-to-beat algorithm and 3D cone-beam reconstruction algorithms for thin-slice imaging are other methods of dose modulation.
- Functional evaluation of heart through cardiac CT is done using retrospective gating and software automatically calculates ventricular stroke volume, ventricular ejection fraction, ventricular cardiac output, left ventricular wall muscle mass, and end systolic and diastolic ventricular volume (Fig. 24).
- Advances in CTA image processing software is manifold and includes:
  - Automatic cardiac segmentation
  - Automatic vessel tracking and extraction
  - Vessel measurements tools
  - Stent planning software
  - Plaque analysis software
  - *True View:* Conventional catheter projections

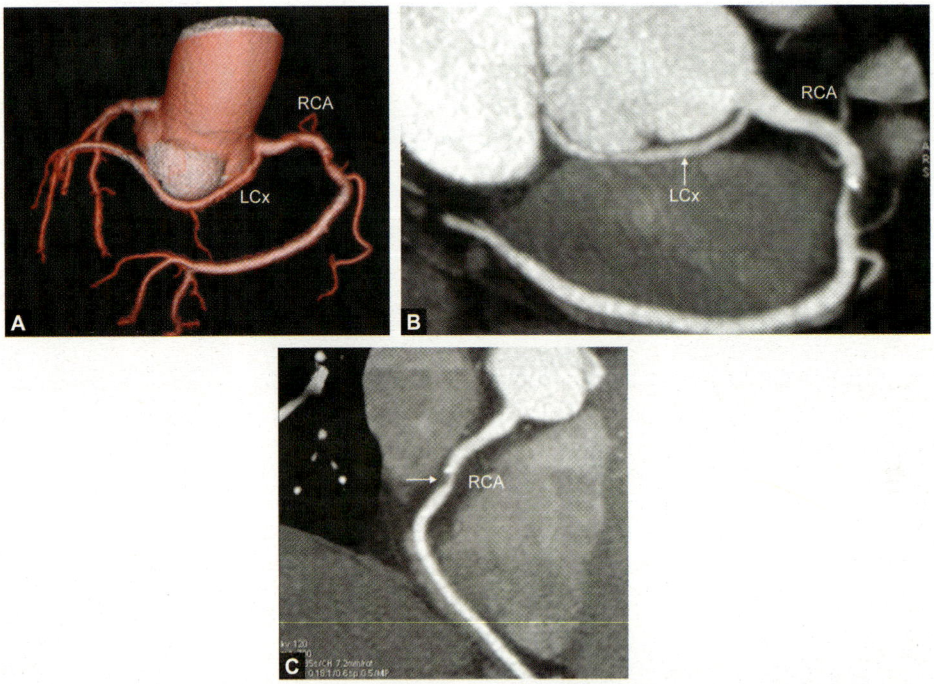

Figs. 21A to C: (A) VR and (B and C) curved MIP images: LCx arising from RCA and traversing posterior to aorta to enter left atrioventricular groove. Mixed plaque (white arrow) in (C) is seen in RCA. (LCx: left circumflex artery; MIP: maximum intensity projections; RCA: right coronary artery; VR: volume rendering).

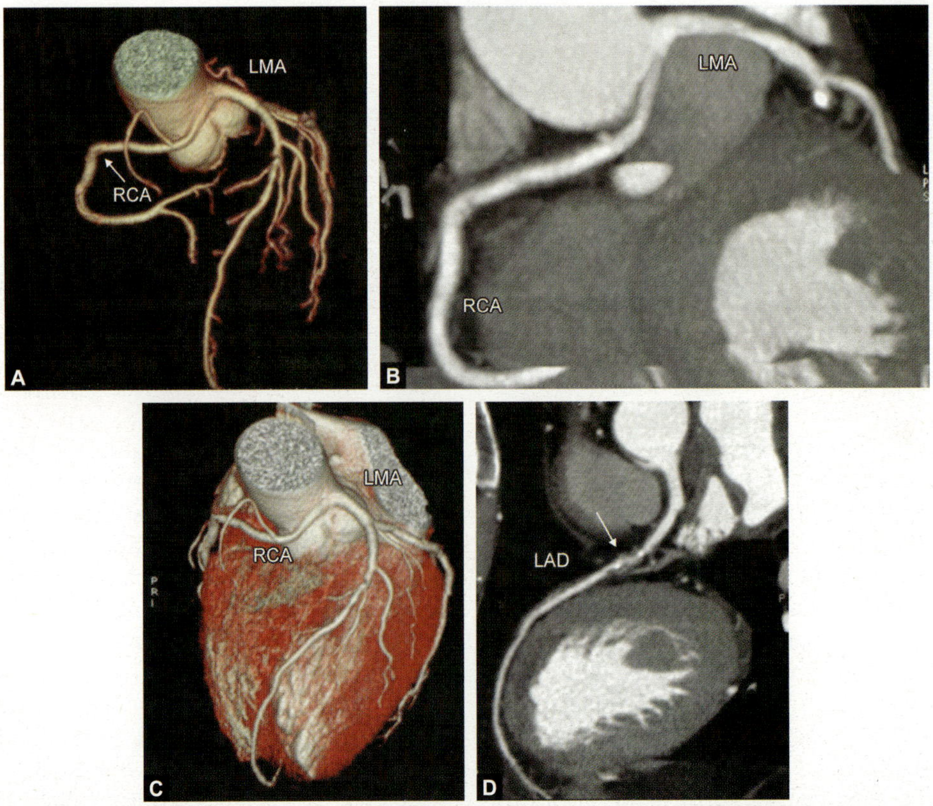

Figs. 22A to D: (A and B) VR and (C and D) curved MIP images: RCA arising from LMA. Mixed plaque (white arrow) in (D) is seen in LAD is causing significant luminal narrowing: Cause for acute chest pain. (LAD: left anterior descending; LMA: left main artery; MIP: maximum intensity projections; RCA: right coronary artery; VR: volume rendering).

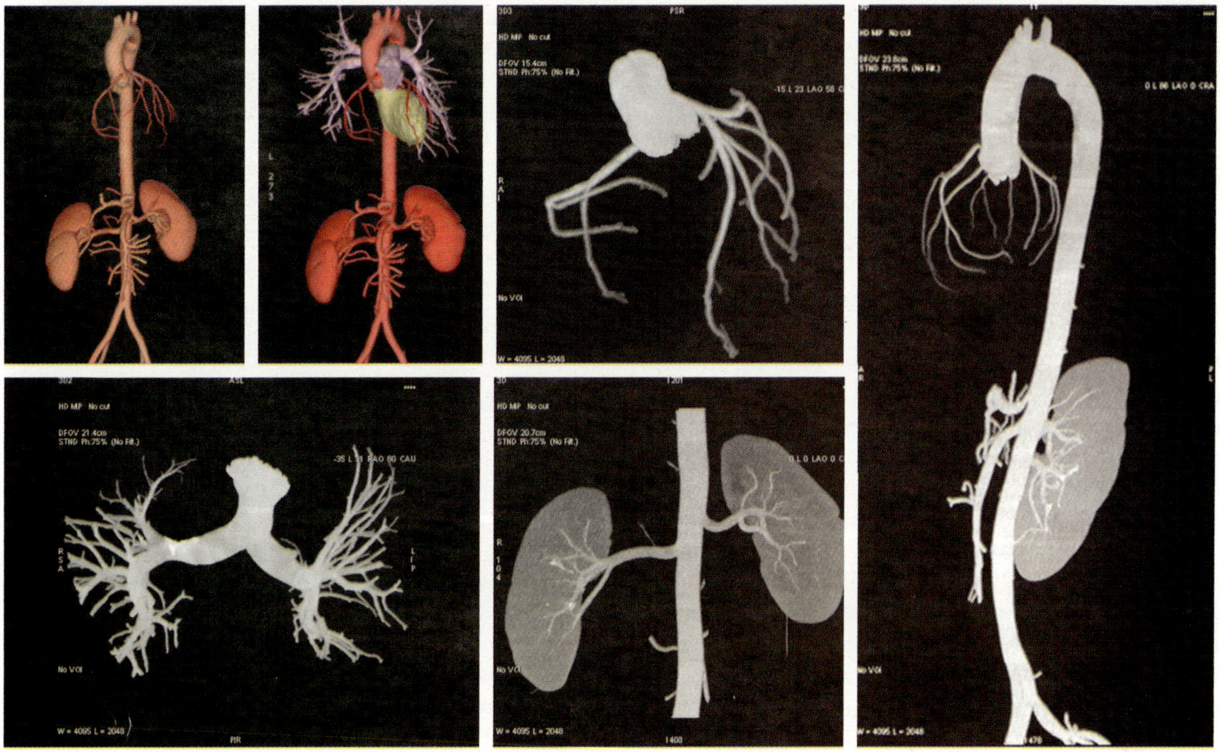

Fig. 23: Triple rule out.

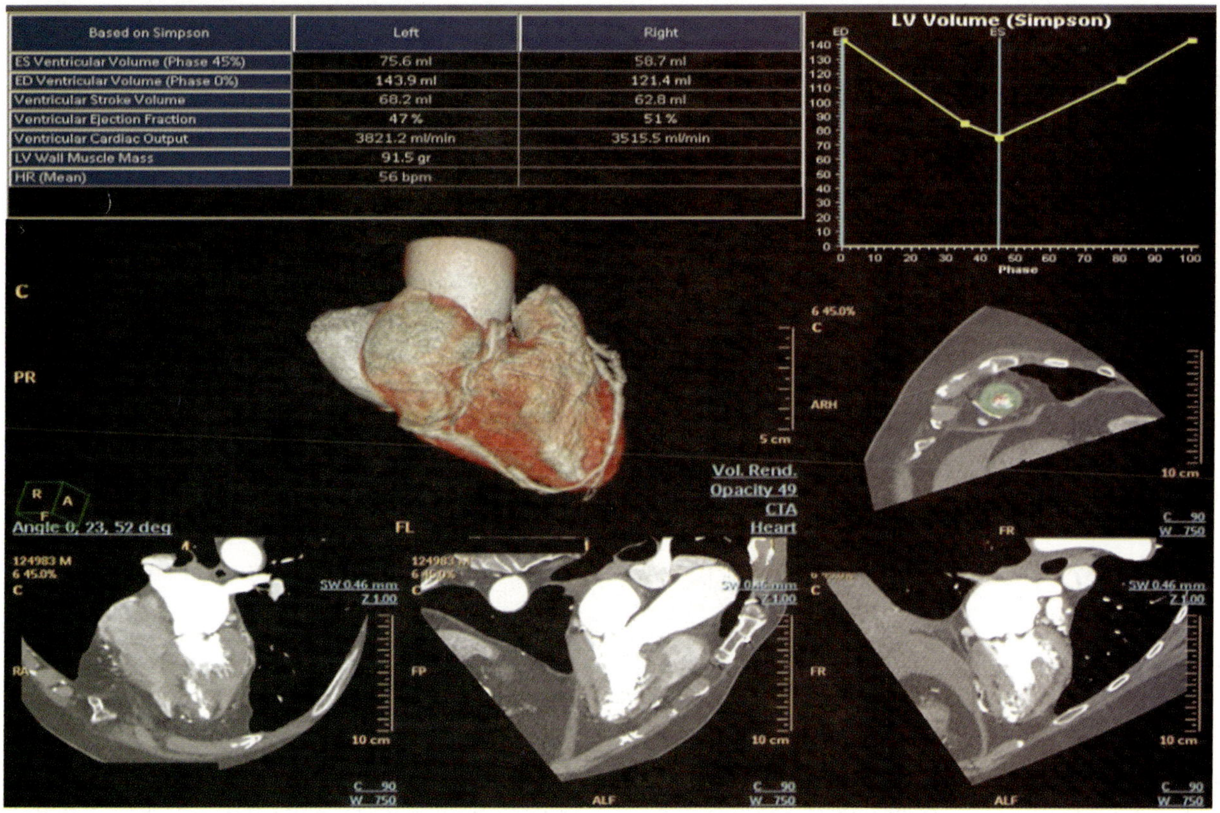

Fig. 24: Functional evaluation in cardiac computed tomography.

  - Functional analysis
  - Dual energy applications.
- Single-source dual-energy CT with fast tube voltage switching to reduce beam hardening.

CONCLUSION

Advances in CT technology over the past few years have resulted in marked improvements in image quality along with reduction in effective radiation dose.

The current triage of emergency department patients with acute chest pain is ineffective, leading to many unnecessary hospital admissions and discharges. Fast and noninvasive detection of the presence and extent of CAD with MDCT, which provides information that cannot be obtained with the standard clinical evaluation, may help to take more definitive diagnosis and substantially improves the clinical care of such patients. The major indication for cardiac CT is CTA for evaluation of CAD in symptomatic patients with low to intermediate risk of CAD. High-risk symptomatic patients should be triaged directly to cardiac catheterization. CTA is useful in these patients to follow-up on positive stress tests in order to avoid catheterization of patients with false-positive stress test results. While 64-section and above multidetector CT allows triple rule out with simultaneous evaluation of coronary arteries, aorta, and pulmonary arteries in a single scan. Upcoming advances are been gradually adapted in day to day practice to overcome the present limitations of radiation exposure, irregular heart rate. New techniques and software are been introduced for better image quality and functional assessment.

REFERENCES

1. Prina LD, Decker WW, Weaver AL, et al. Outcome of patients with a final diagnosis of chest pain of undetermined origin admitted under the suspicion of acute coronary syndrome: a report from the Rochester Epidemiology Project. Ann Emerg Med. 2004;43:59-67.
2. Pope JH, Selker HP. Acute coronary syndromes in the emergency department: diagnostic characteristics, tests, and challenges. Cardiol Clin. 2005;23(4):423-51, v-vi.
3. Pope JH, Aufderheide TP, Ruthazer R, et al. Missed diagnoses of acute cardiac ischemia in the emergency department. N Engl J Med. 2000;342(16):1163-70.
4. Christenson J, Innes G, McKnight D, et al. Safety and efficiency of emergency department assessment of chest discomfort. CMAJ. 2004;170(12):1803-7.
5. Rusnak RA, Stair TO, Hansen K, et al. Litigation against the emergency physician: common features in cases of missed myocardial infarction. Ann Emerg Med. 1989;18(10):1029-34.
6. Anaya P, Moliterno DJ. CT angiography for emergency decision making in acute coronary syndromes: applying future vision now. Curr Cardiol Rep. 2012;14:537-9.
7. Hollander JE, Chang AM, Shofer FS, et al. One-year outcomes following coronary computerized tomographic angiography for evaluation of emergency department patients with potential acute coronary syndrome. Acad Emerg Med. 2009;16:693-8.
8. Kontos MC, Jesse RL. Evaluation of the emergency department chest pain patient. Am J Cardiol. 2000;85:32B-39B.
9. Tatum JL, Jesse RL, Kontos MC, et al. Comprehensive strategy for the evaluation and triage of the chest pain patient. Ann Emerg Med. 1997;29:116-25.
10. Cury RC, Feuchtner GM, Batlle JC, et al. Triage of patients presenting with chest pain to the emergency department: implementation of coronary CT angiography in a large urban health care system. AJR. 2013;200:57-65.
11. Braunwald E, Antman EM, Beasley JW, et al. ACC/AHA guideline update for the management of patients with unstable angina and non-ST-segment elevation myocardial infarction-2002: Summary article: A report of the American College of Cardiology/American Heart Association Task Force on Practice Guidelines (Committee on the Management of Patients With Unstable Angina). Circulation. 2002;106:1893-900.
12. Rubinshtein R, Halon DA, Gaspar T, et al. Usefulness of 64-slice cardiac computed tomographic angiography for diagnosing acute coronary syndromes and predicting clinical outcome in emergency department patients with chest pain of uncertain origin. Circulation. 2007;115:1762-8.
13. Beigel R, Oieru D, Goitein O, et al. Usefulness of routine use of multidetector coronary computed tomography in the 'fast track' evaluation of patients with acute chest pain. Am J Cardiol. 2009;103:1481-6.
14. Fazel P, Peterman MA, Schussler JM. Three-year outcomes and cost analysis in patients receiving 64-slice computed tomographic coronary angiography for chest pain. Am J Cardiol. 2009;104:498-500.
15. Khare RK, Courtney DM, Powell ES, et al. Sixty-four-slice computed tomography of the coronary arteries: cost-effectiveness analysis of patients presenting to the emergency department with low-risk chest pain. Acad Emerg Med. 2008;15(7):623-32.
16. Chang AM, Shofer FS, Weiner MG, et al. Actual financial comparison of four strategies to evaluate patients with potential acute coronary syndromes. Acad Emerg Med. 2008;15(7):649-55.
17. Hoffmann U, Truong QA, Schoenfeld DA, et al. Coronary CT angiography versus standard evaluation in acute chest pain. N Engl J Med. 2012;367:299-308.
18. Litt HI, Gatsonis C, Snyder B, et al. CT angiography for safe discharge of patients with possible acute coronary syndromes. N Engl J Med. 2012;366:1393-403.
19. Morin RL, Gerber TC, McCollough CH. Radiation dose in computed tomography of the heart. Circulation. 2003;107:917-22.
20. Mahesh M. Cardiac imaging: Technical advances in MDCT compared with conventional x-ray angiography. In: Boulton E, ed. US Cardiology 2006: the Authoritative Review of the Clinical and Scientific Issues Relating to Cardiology

with Perspectives on the Future. London, England: Touch Briefings (http://www.touchcardiology.com); 2006. pp. 115-9.
21. Hunold P, Vogt FM, Schmermund A, et al. Radiation exposure during cardiac CT: effective doses at multi-detector row CT and electron-beam CT. Radiology. 2003;226:145-52.
22. Earls JP, Berman EL, Urban BA, et al. Prospectively gated transverse coronary CT angiography versus retrospectively gated helical technique: improved image quality and reduced radiation dose. Radiology. 2008;246(3):742-53.
23. Herzog BA, Husmann L, Burkhard N, et al. Accuracy of low-dose computed tomography coronary angiography using prospective electrocardiogram-triggering: first clinical experience. Eur Heart J. 2008;29(24):3037-42.
24. Sun Z, Ng KH. Prospective versus retrospective ECG-gated multislice CT coronary angiography: a systematic review of radiation dose and diagnostic accuracy. Eur J Radiol. 2012;81(2):e94-e100.
25. Austen WG, Edwards JE, Frye RL, et al. A reporting system on patients evaluated for coronary artery disease. Report of the ad hoc Committee for Grading of Coronary Artery Disease, Council on Cardiovascular Surgery, American Heart Association. Circulation. 1975;51:5-40.
26. Wallentin L, Lagerqvist B, Husted S, et al. Outcome at 1 year after an invasive compared with a non-invasive strategy in unstable coronary-artery disease: the FRISC II invasive randomised trial. FRISC II Investigators. Fast Revascularisation during Instability in Coronary Artery Disease. Lancet. 2000;356:9-16.
27. Yang F, Minutello RM, Bhagan S, et al. The impact of gender on vessel size in patients with angiographically normal coronary arteries. J Interv Cardiol. 2006;19(4):340-4.
28. Malouf JF, Edwards WD, Tajik AJ, et al. Functional anatomy of the heart. In: Fuster V, Alexander RW, O'Rourke RA, et al. (Eds). Hurst's The Heart, 11th edition. New York, NY: McGraw-Hill; 2005. pp. 45-82.
29. Hoffmann U, Pena AJ, Cury RC, et al. Cardiac CT in emergency department patients with acute chest pain. Radio Graphics. 2006;26(4):963-80.
30. Stankovic I, Jesic M. Morphometric characteristics of the conus coronary artery. McGill J Med. 2004;8:2-6
31. DiDio LJ, Lopes AC, Caetano AC, et al. Variations of the origin of the artery of the sinoatrial node in normal human hearts. Surg Radiol Anat. 1995;17(1):19-26.
32. Halpern EJ. Triple-rule-out CT angiography for evaluation of acute chest pain and possible acute coronary syndrome. Radiology. 2009;252(2):332-45.
33. Abbara S, Arbab-Zadeh A, Callister TQ, et al. SCCT guidelines for performance of coronary computed tomographic angiography: a report of the Society of Cardiovascular Computed Tomography Guidelines Committee. J Cardiovasc Comput Tomogr. 2009;3:190-204.
34. Halpern EJ. Clinical Cardiac CT: Anatomy and Function. New York, NY: Thieme; 2008. pp. 272.
35. Fleischmann D, Kamaya A. Optimal vascular and parenchymal contrast enhancement: the current state of the art. Radiol Clin North Am. 2009;47:13-26.
36. Lee AM, Engel LC, Shah B, et al. Coronary computed tomography angiography during arrhythmia: radiation dose reduction with prospectively ECG-triggered axial and retrospectively ECG-gated helical 128-slice dual-source CT. J Cardiovasc Comput Tomogr. 2012;6:172.e2-183.e2.
37. Srichai MB, Lim RP, Donnino R, et al. Low-dose, prospective triggered high-pitch spiral coronary computed tomography angiography: comparison with retrospective spiral technique. Acad Radiol. 2012;19:554-61.
38. Achenbach S, Ropers D, Regenfus M, et al. Diagnostic value of 2 and 3-dimensional image reconstruction techniques for the detection of coronary artery stenoses by contrast-enhanced electronbeam CT. J Am Coll Cardiol. 2000;36:44-50.
39. Ropers D, Moshage W, Daniel WG, et al. Visualization of coronary artery anomalies and their anatomic course by contrast-enhanced electron beam tomography and three-dimensional reconstruction. Am J Cardiol. 2001;87:193-7.
40. Kondos GT, Hoff JA, Sevrukov A, et al. Electron-beam tomography coronary artery calcium and cardiac events: a 37-month follow-up of 5635 initially asymptomatic low- to intermediate-risk adults. Circulation. 2003;107:2571-6.
41. Shaw LJ, Raggi P, Schisterman E, et al. Prognostic value of cardiac risk factors and coronary artery calcium screening for all-cause mortality. Radiology. 2003;228:826-33.
42. Budoff MJ, Shaw LJ, Liu ST, et al. Long-term prognosis associated with coronary calcification: observations from a registry of 25, 253 patients. J Am Coll Cardiol. 2007;49:1860-70.
43. Greenland P, LaBree L, Azen SP, et al. Coronary artery calcium score combined with Framingham score for risk prediction in asymptomatic individuals. JAMA. 2004;291:210-5.
44. Marwan M, Ropers D, Pflederer T, et al. Clinical characteristics of patients with obstructive coronary lesions in the absence of coronary calcification: an evaluation by coronary CT angiography. Heart. 2009;95:1056-960.
45. Gottlieb I, Miller JM, Arbab-Zadeh A, et al. The absence of coronary calcification does not exclude obstructive coronary artery disease or the need for revascularization in patients referred for conventional coronary angiography. J Am Coll Cardiol. 2010;55:627-34.
46. McLaughlin VV, Balogh T, Rich S. Utility of electron beam computed tomography to stratify patients presenting to the emergency room with chest pain. Am J Cardiol. 1999;84:327-8.
47. Leber AW, Knez A, Becker A, et al. Accuracy of multidetector spiral computed tomography in identifying and differentiating the composition of coronary atherosclerotic plaques: a comparative study with intracoronary ultrasound. J Am Coll Cardiol. 2004;43:1241-7.
48. Achenbach S, Moselewski F, Ropers D, et al. Detection of calcified and noncalcified coronary atherosclerotic plaque by contrast-enhanced, submillimeter multidetector spiral computed tomography: a segment-based comparison with intravascular ultrasound. Circulation. 2004;109:14-17.
49. Rixe J, Achenbach S, Ropers D, et al. Assessment of coronary artery stent restenosis by 64-slice multi-detector computed tomography. Eur Heart J. 2006;27(21):2567-72.
50. Ehara M, Kawai M, Surmely JF, et al. Diagnostic accuracy of coronary in-stent restenosis using 64-slice computed

tomography: comparison with invasive coronary angiography. J Am Coll Cardiol. 2007;49(9):951-9.
51. Andreini D, Pontone G, Bartorelli AL, et al. Comparison of feasibility and diagnostic accuracy of 64-slice multidetector computed tomographic coronary angiography versus invasive coronary angiography versus intravascular ultrasound for evaluation of in-stent restenosis. Am J Cardiol. 2009;103(10):1349-58.
52. Hamon M, Champ-Rigot L, Morello R, et al. Diagnostic accuracy of in-stent coronary restenosis detection with multislice spiral computed tomography: a meta-analysis. Eur Radiol. 2008;18(2):217-25.
53. Hachamovitch R, Hayes SW, Friedman JD, et al. Comparison of the short-term survival benefit associated with revascularization compared with medical therapy in patients with no prior coronary artery disease undergoing stress myocardial perfusion single photon emission computed tomography. Circulation. 2003;107(23):2900-7.
54. Hachamovitch R, Kang X, Amanullah AM, et al. Prognostic implications of myocardial perfusion single-photon emission computed tomography in the elderly. Circulation. 2009;120(22):2197-206.
55. Ko SM, Seo JB, Hong MK, et al. Myocardial enhancement pattern in patients with acute myocardial infarction on two-phase contrast-enhanced ECG-gated multidetector-row computed tomography. Clin Radiol. 2006;61(5):417-22.
56. Kopp AF, Heuschmid M, Reimann A, et al. Evaluation of cardiac function and myocardial viability with 16- and 64-slice multidetector computed tomography. Eur Radiol. 2005;4:D15-D20.
57. George RT, Arbab-Zadeh A, Miller JM, et al. Adenosine stress 64- and 256-row detector computed tomography angiography and perfusion imaging: a pilot study evaluating the transmural extent of perfusion abnormalities to predict atherosclerosis causing myocardial ischemia. Circ Cardiovasc Imaging. 2009;2(3):174-82.
58. Ruzsics B, Lee H, Zwerner PL, et al. Dual-energy CT of the heart for diagnosing coronary artery stenosis and myocardial ischemia-initial experience. Eur Radiol. 2008;18(11): 2414-24.

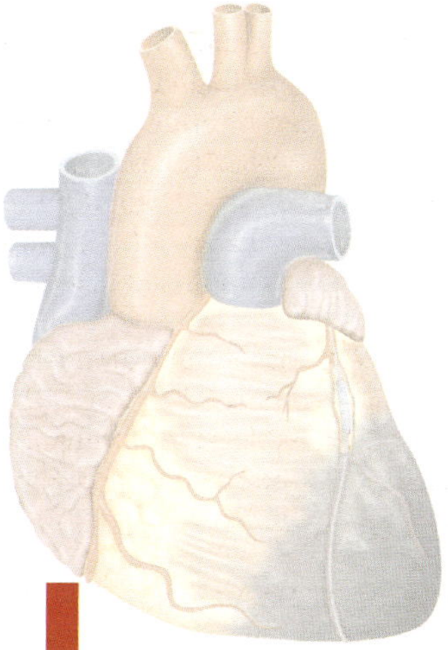

54

CHAPTER

Radionuclide Imaging in Patients with Acute Chest Pain

Uma Ravishankar, Arjun Ravishankar

INTRODUCTION

Chest pain and related symptoms are the second leading cause of emergency department (ED) visits in the United States, accounting for 5.3% of the 137 million ED visits in 2015.[1] Between 2006 and 2014, ED visits for nonspecific chest pain increased by nearly 26%.[2] Patients with confirmed acute coronary syndrome (ACS), and those with very low risk of ACS are easily triaged; the former going for coronary angiography with or without primary PCI, and the latter being discharged from the ED. The low- to intermediate-risk groups who have no clear evidence of ACS, i.e. abnormal electrocardiography (ECG) findings or positive cardiac biomarkers, represent a diagnostic dilemma and require further workup to determine whether the etiology of the chest pain is cardiac. No currently used diagnostic procedure meets all the criteria for an "ideal" marker of acute myocardial infarction (AMI), and therefore an unmet need exists for a test that is both highly sensitive and specific for acute infarction and provides early information following the onset of chest pain to help make appropriate therapeutic decisions.

ACUTE REST MYOCARDIAL PERFUSION IMAGING

Rationale for Acute Rest Myocardial Perfusion Imaging

In the ischemic cascade, myocardial perfusion heterogeneity occurs before the development of left ventricular dysfunction, ECG changes, chest pain, and myocardial necrosis. Therefore, nuclear imaging can identify areas of myocardial ischemia and infarction long before biochemical markers of myocardial necrosis appear in serum (Fig. 1).

Tracers Used for Myocardial Perfusion Imaging

Thallium 201 Chloride

Tl^{201} is cyclotron produced with a half-life of 73 hours. It is transported across the myocardial cell membrane via the Na-K ATPase pump. More than 85% of Tl^{201} is extracted by the myocardial cell on first pass through the coronary capillary circulation. Extraction is proportional to relative regional perfusion over a wide range of flow rates. Thallium 201 can only be extracted. After uptake, it undergoes redistribution, which is a continual dynamic exchange of Tl^{201} between myocardial cell and vascular blood pool. There are certain drawbacks of thallium Tl 201 especially while using it in the ED.

- Relatively high-radiation dosimetry because of its long biological and physical half-life, thus limiting the maximum administrate dose to 3.5–4 mci.
- The low-administrated dose results in a poor count rate with poor quality images.
- The low photo energy emission (69–83 KUV) compared to technetium Tc99m (140 KUV) makes it poorly suited for modern day gamma cameras.
- Redistribution issue—as the patient has to be imaged immediately after injection and that may not be possible in the emergency setting.

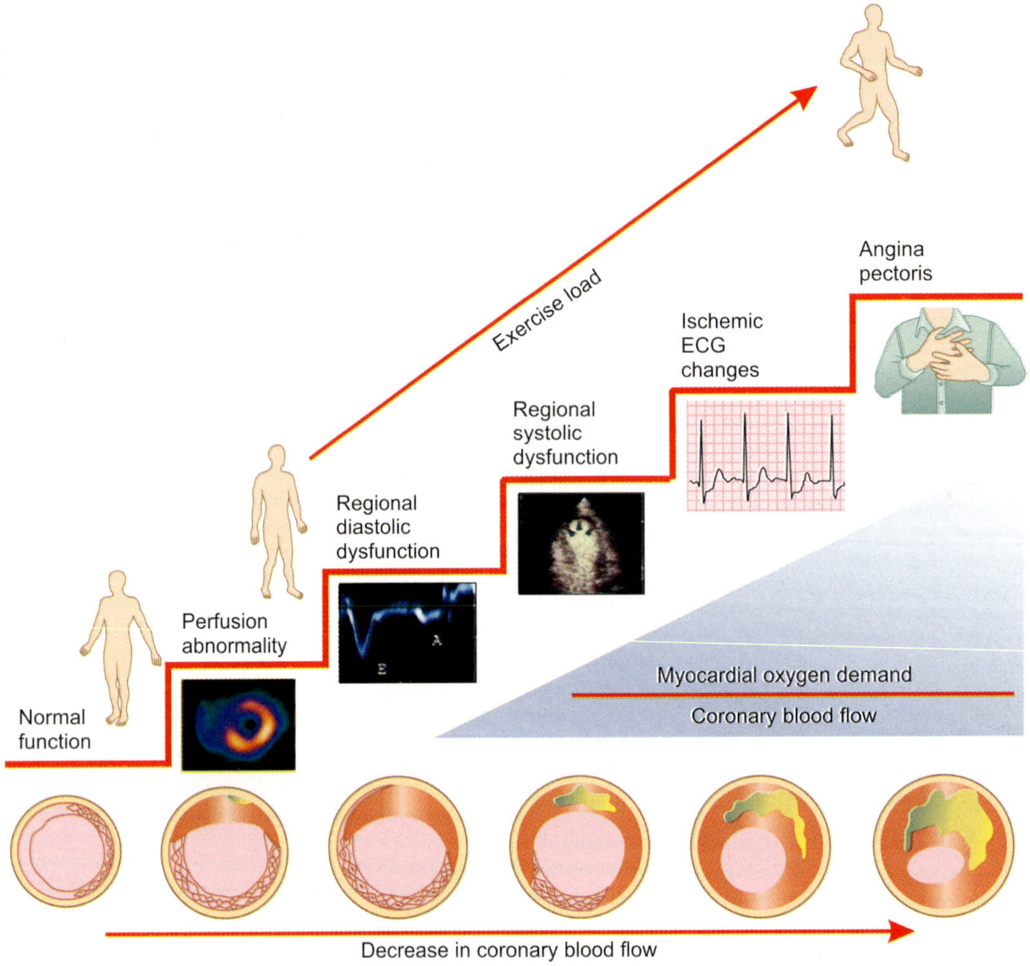

Fig. 1: Ischemic cascade: Perfusion abnormality occurs much earlier in the ischemic cascade.
Source: Gaemperli O, Lüscher TF, Bax JJ. Viewpoint: What should the future design of clinical imaging studies be? Eur Heart J. 2013;34(31):2432-5.

Tc99m Perfusion Agents (Sestamibi and Tetrofosmin)

Tc99m has a half-life of 6 hours and energy of 140 keV. Technetium with its higher energy profile and less attenuation also has advantage of higher quality images compared with thallium. Tc perfusion agents are lipophilic cation that localizes and are retained within mitochondria. Unlike the redistribution of thallium, the clearance half time from the myocardium is long, and for practical purposes, they remain fixed within myocardium. This allows for an imaging window of several hours after administration. Imaging usually begins 45–60 minutes after tracer administration. This property allows patient stabilization without loss of sensitivity and helps technetium agent to be the preferred agents for acute rest myocardial perfusion imaging (ARMPI).

Positron Emission Tomography Tracers

Positron emission tomography tracers are biologically active allowing for assessment of perfusion, myocardial viability, angiogenesis, etc. Naturally occurring biological molecules can be radioactively labeled and administered to the patient. Clinical cardiac PET tracers include ^{13}N-ammonia, ^{15}O-water, and ^{82}rubidium for myocardial perfusion and ^{18}F-fluorodeoxyglucose (^{18}FDG) for cardiomyocyte metabolism and viability. The radioactive tracer decays, emitting a positron which travels in the tissue for a short distance before interacting with an electron, causing an annihilation event producing two 511 keV photons moving in opposite directions. The PET system detects these photons and, therefore, the localization of the annihilation event. Correction for attenuation is a standard practice in PET imaging to improve accuracy and quantify concentrations of radioactive tracers. A meta-analysis showed that sensitivity and specificity to detect obstructive cardiovascular disease (CVD)-induced ischemia with PET imaging was 84–92%, while 81–85% was achieved using single-photon emission computed tomography (SPECT), demonstrating the higher diagnostic value of PET.[3]

Timing of Injection and Image Acquisition

The preferred agent for ARMPI is Tc99m-based myocardial perfusion agents. The timing of injection in relation to symptoms is important in the successful use of ARMPI. Wackers et al. demonstrated when the imaging was performed within 6 hours of pain in AMI, the incidence of a perfusion abnormality was 84% but decreased to 19% at 12–18 hours after the onset of pain.[4] Acquisition can be done up to 6 hours postinjection as the tracer will get retained in the myocardial mitochondria with no redistribution. The patient injected in the ER can be managed for his symptoms and stabilized and then shifted to nuclear medicine for imaging.

Patterns

A normal perfusion scan is defined by uniform myocardial uptake and normal regional wall thickening (Figs. 2A and B). A normal myocardial perfusion scan rules out an acute on going cardiac problem. Various studies have demonstrated a negative predictive value (NPV) of 99–100%. An abnormal scan is defined as an area of decreased myocardial tracer uptake or a regional area of decreased myocardial thickening (Figs. 3A and B). Equivocal scans can be regarded as abnormal. Perfusion defect seen in the scan can be due to acute ischemia, unstable angina (UA), and old infarct. A detailed history of previous myocardial infarction is essential.

DISCUSSION

Various studies and trials have established that MPI is an excellent tool in ruling out ACS in the ED setting. While initial studies showed that MPI has a high sensitivity and NPV for diagnosis of MI, the first randomized trial Emergency Room Assessment of Sestamibi for Evaluating Chest Pain (ERASE) was reported in 2002 which confirmed the ability to safely discharge a patient after negative acute MPI. Around 2,475 patients were randomized to routine care or ED MPI, in which patients were injected with Tc99m sestamibi in the ED and then underwent acute imaging. All patients, whether admitted or discharged, underwent subsequent marker analysis and further diagnostic evaluation with either stress testing or coronary angiography. There was no difference between the two groups, in the percentage of ACS patients with MI (97% vs 96%) or unstable angina (83% vs 81%) who were admitted. However, there was a significantly lower admission rate and a higher rate of direct discharge from the ED in the MPI arm of the study compared to the standardized care arm. A meta-analysis by Romero et al. in 2015 compared noninvasive imaging modalities in the assessment of acute chest pain in the ED.[5] Thirteen of the 37 studies in the meta-analysis used SPECT, and enrolled a total of 2,752 patients. They found weighted mean sensitivity, specificity, positive predictive value (PPV), NPV, and overall accuracy for SPECT were 85% [confidence interval (CI): 82–88%], 86% (CI: 85–87%), 57% (CI: 54–61%), 95% (CI: 95–96%), and 88% (CI: 86–%), respectively.

COMPARISON OF MYOCARDIAL PERFUSION IMAGING WITH CARDIAC BIOMARKERS

Cardiac biomarkers, including creatine kinase muscle-brain (CKMB) and cardiac troponins (cTn), have long assisted in the diagnosis of MI. In 2000, the guidelines for diagnosis of MI were changed, suggesting cTn as the preferred biomarker.[6] However, the use of troponin early at presentation for a reliable diagnosis of ACS is hampered by its low sensitivity. A study of 1,047 patients found sensitivity of first troponin sample of just 40%.[7] Similarly, Kontos et al. found that sensitivity of MPI (92%) and serial cTnI measurements (90%) were comparable, but were significantly higher than sensitivity of initial cTnI (39%).[8] A prospective study of 75 patients compared acute rest MPI and cardiac biomarkers, and found that MPI had a much better sensitivity and equal specificity for diagnosis of MI compared to serum biomarkers.[9] In the same study, abnormal acute MPI was a predictor of symptomatic coronary artery disease (CAD), but not serum cardiac biomarkers.

COMPARISON OF MYOCARDIAL PERFUSION IMAGING WITH ECHOCARDIOGRAPHY

Transthoracic echocardiography (TTE) has the advantages of being readily accessible, portable, noninvasive, and fast and it may detect significant findings that are misdiagnosed or not detected on initial clinical evaluation, including myocardial ischemia, acute aortic dissection, pulmonary embolism, significant valvular heart disease, and pericardial pathologies. The presence of regional wall motion abnormalities (RWMAs) can be visualized echocardiographically within seconds of a coronary artery occlusion and even prior to the onset of ECG changes or symptoms. Chest pain in the absence of RWMAs is very unlikely from active myocardial ischemia: however, the presence of RWMAs does not establish the diagnosis of ischemia. There are numerous reasons for RWMAs, including a prior myocardial infraction, focal myocarditis, prior surgery, right ventricular volume overload, left bundle branch block, Wolff-Parkinson-White syndrome and ventricular pre-excitation, and cardiomyopathy.

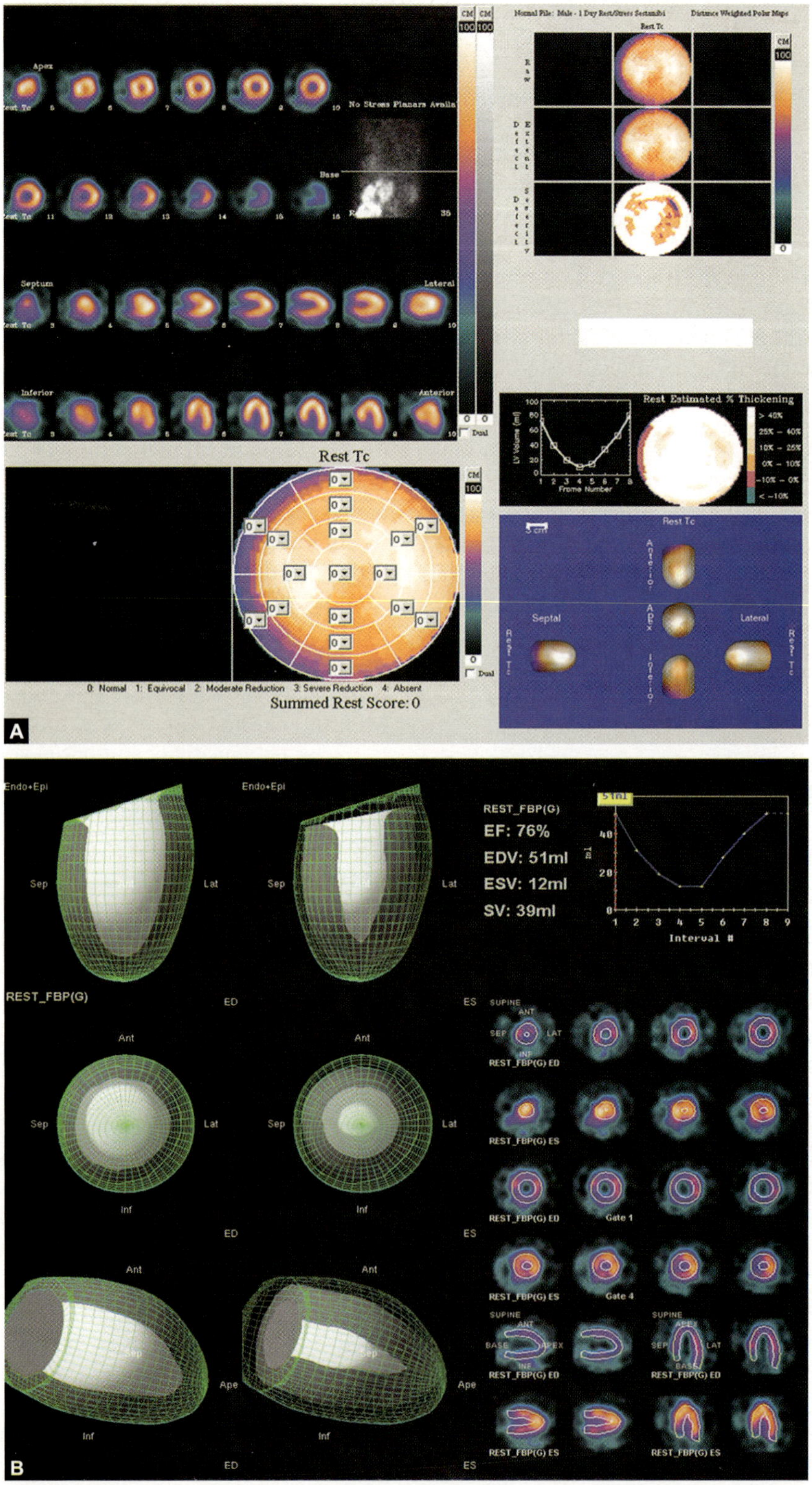

Figs. 2A and B: (A) Tc99m sestamibi single-photon emission computed tomography (SPECT) resting images showing normal perfusion to all segments of myocardium; and (B) Gated SPECT quantification—normal ejection fraction (EF), wall motion, and wall thickening.

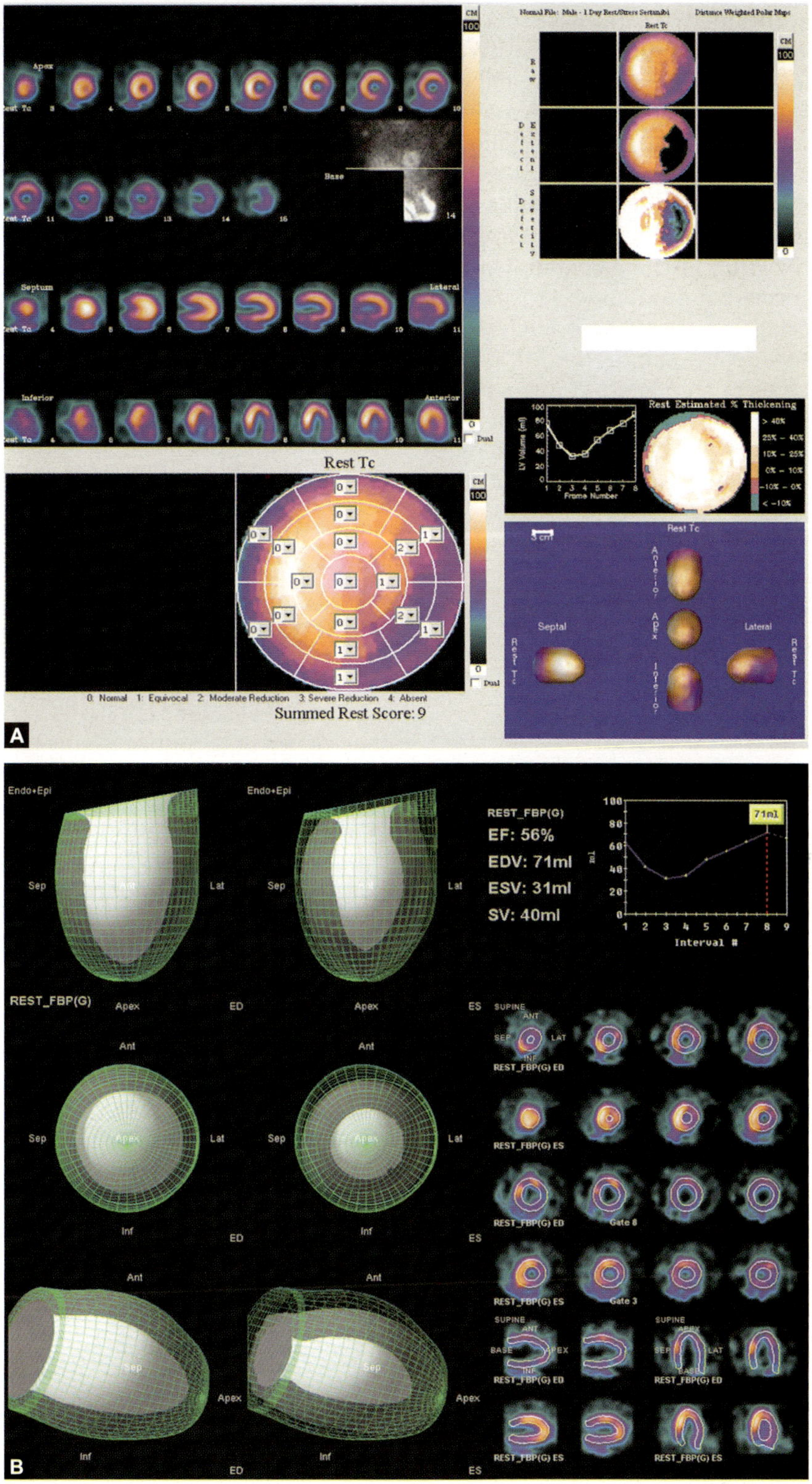

Figs. 3A and B: Tc99m sestamibi resting single-photon emission computed tomography (SPECT) images showing perfusion defect in lateral wall of myocardium. Gated SPECT quantification—Adequate ejection fraction (EF), impaired wall motion, and wall thickening in lateral wall.

Different studies have reported varied results about stress echocardiography for diagnosing ACS with sensitivities ranging from 24%[10] to 92%.[11] Stress echo has been compared to exercise ECG and shown to be better in risk stratifying and more cost effective.[12] A study that compared echo and MPI performed both investigations in 185 patients found a high concordance (89%) between the two techniques, and both identified patients at high risk who required admission and those who could be safely discharged from the ED.[13] There is a lack of information from large, prospective, randomized clinical trials comparing both nuclear and echo for the diagnosis of chest pain in the ED setting. However, a meta-analysis of coronary CT angiography, stress echocardiography, and SPECT MPI used for chest pain evaluation in the ED showed no significant difference between stress echocardiography and SPECT MPI in all of the studied parameters (sensitivity, specificity, PPV, NPV, and overall accuracy).[5]

COMPARISON OF MYOCARDIAL PERFUSION IMAGING WITH CORONARY COMPUTED TOMOGRAPHY ANGIOGRAPHY

The use of coronary CT angiography (CCTA) is rapidly expanding and recommendations for the use of this imaging test are included in several relevant guidelines. The ACC foundation "appropriate use criteria for cardiac computed tomography" have endorsed CCTA as an appropriate test in the context of acute chest pain with normal or nondiagnostic ECG, and normal or equivocal biomarkers in the groups determined pretest to have low or intermediate likelihood of an ACS.[14] High-quality CTCA is feasible with multidetector CT scanners acquiring more than or equal to 64 slices, and these scanners are now widely available, including in many emergency departments. In the ROMICAT 1 trial (Rule Out Myocardial Infarction using Computer Assisted Tomography), the diagnostic accuracy of 64-slice CCTA in 368 acute chest pain ED patient with low to intermediate risk for ACS with negative initial troponin, normal or nonischemic ECG, and no prior history of CAD revealed sensitivity and specificity for detection of ACS using the criterion of presence of any plaque were 100% and 54% and using the criterion of presence of coronary stenosis were 77% and 87%.[15] In a similar study, looking at the 15-month follow-up, the value of 64-slice CCTA for diagnosing ACS and predicting outcomes showed that the sensitivity and specificity for diagnosis of ACS were 100% and 92%, sensitivity and specificity for predicting major adverse cardiovascular events (death, myocardial infarction, or revascularization) were 92% and 76%.[16] Results of the PROSPECT trial (Prospective Randomized Outcome trial comparing radionuclide Stress myocardial Perfusion imaging and ECG-gated CCTA) which compared coronary CTA to stress MPI in the care of ED patients with acute chest pain, were reported in 2015. The two groups, CCTA and MPI, did not differ in the primary outcome which was cardiac catheterization within 1 year. Most other outcomes (incidence of death, nonfatal cardiovascular events, rehospitalization, emergency department visit, and outpatient cardiology visits) also did not differ; however, the CCTA arm had less radiation exposure (24 vs 29 mSv) than the MPI arm.[17] However, there are limitations to using CT angiography. The diagnostic value of CCTA is hampered by calcification in the coronary arteries. High-density calcification produces blooming artifacts, which leads to overestimation of the degree of coronary stenosis, thus resulting in low PPV.[18] Other limitations are inability to receive beta blockers (obstructive lung disease, heart block), arrhythmia, contrast-related issues (allergy, renal insufficiency, metformin use), etc.

PROGNOSTIC IMPLICATIONS

Hilton et al. used SPECT MPI to evaluate 150 patients with typical anginal chest pain. In the 87 patients with a normal scan, no adverse cardiac events (cardiac death, nonfatal MI, readmission) were present on 90 days of follow-up.[19] Tatum et al., in a study of 1,187 patients complaining of chest pain in the ED, risk stratified the patients, and performed immediate resting MPI on those with moderate-high probability of UA. Within 30 days of the ED encounter, 2.1% of patients with normal MPI findings underwent revascularization, compared to 30% of those with abnormal MPI. On 1 year follow-up, only 0.9% of patients with normal MPI underwent revascularization, and none had an MI or died of cardiac causes.[20] In a Danish study, 272 patients with acute nonspecific chest pain who were discharged after evaluation for ACS underwent adenosine stress SPECT MPI and were followed up for a median of 3.7 years. They found that perfusion deficits predicted the primary outcome (cardiac death, ACS, or revascularization; hazard ratio—7.54) as well as the secondary outcome (all cause death, composite measure of cardiac death, ACS, revascularization, and stroke; hazard ratio—2.93). In the same study, clinical cardiac risk classification could not differentiate between patients with and without perfusion deficits.[21]

LIMITATIONS

Acute RMPI has some limitations when used to assess chest pain patients. Acute MI, acute ischemia, and prior MI all-cause perfusion defects, and differentiation are not possible based on the images alone. Sensitivity for identifying necrosis is imperfect for MPI, since at least 3–5% of the left ventricle must be ischemic for a defect to be visible.

GUIDELINES

The 2014 American Heart Association/American College of Cardiology (AHA/ACC) revision of their 2007 guidelines for the management of non–ST-segment elevation acute coronary syndromes (NSTE-ACS) includes the following recommendations for management of patients with suspected ACS:[22]

- For patients with suspected ACS who have normal serial ECGs and cardiac troponin levels, it is reasonable to obtain a treadmill ECG (level of evidence: A), stress myocardial perfusion imaging, or stress echocardiography before discharge or within 72 hours after discharge. (level of evidence: B)
- In patients with suspected ACS but a normal ECG, normal cardiac troponin levels, and no history of CAD, it is reasonable to initially perform (without serial ECGs and troponins) CCTA to assess the coronary artery anatomy (level of evidence: A) or rest myocardial perfusion imaging with a technetium-99m radiopharmaceutical to exclude myocardial ischemia. (level of evidence: B)

In 2015, various American societies released a joint "Appropriate Utilization of Cardiovascular Imaging in Emergency Department Patients With Chest Pain" document in which resting SPECT MPI was "appropriate" for patients with equivocal initial troponin or single troponin elevation without additional evidence of ACS and "may be appropriate" for patients whose ischemic symptoms resolved hours before testing or who had normal/nonischemic initial ECG and normal initial troponin. In the same document, stress/rest SPECT was deemed "appropriate" in patients with serial ECG and troponins negative/borderline for ACS.[23] The UKs National Institute for Health and Care Excellence (NICE) in their 2016 update of guidelines for chest pain of recent onset recommends the use of SPECT MPI as one of the modalities for diagnosis of myocardial ischemia if CCTA has shown CAD of uncertain functional significance or is nondiagnostic.[24]

CONCLUSION

Triaging of patients presenting with chest pain remains a significant issue, with ECG being the primary tool, but lacking the sensitivity to rule out ongoing ischemia. MPI using SPECT is a sensitive tool with a high NPV to rule out perfusion abnormalities in patients with chest pain in the ED, and it has been shown to be useful, safe, and cost effective for this purpose.

REFERENCES

1. Centers for Disease Control and Prevention. (2015). 2015 NHAMCS Emergency Department summary tables. [online]. Available from https://www.cdc.gov/nchs/data/nhamcs/web_tables/2015_ed_web_tables.pdf. [Accessed October, 2018].
2. Moore BJ, Stocks C, Owens PL. (2014). Trends in Emergency Department Visits, 2006–2014. [online]. Available from https://www.hcup-us.ahrq.gov/reports/statbriefs/sb227-Emergency-Department-Visit-Trends.pdf. [Accessed October, 2018].
3. Jaarsma C, Leiner T, Bekkers SC, et al. Diagnostic performance of noninvasive myocardial perfusion imaging using single-photon emission computed tomography, cardiac magnetic resonance, and positron emission tomography imaging for the detection of obstructive coronary artery disease. J Am Coll Cardiol. 2012;59(19):1719-28.
4. Wackers FJ, Lie KI, Liem KL, et al. Potential value of thallium-201 scintigraphy as a means of selecting patients for the coronary care unit. Br Heart J. 1979;41(1):111-7.
5. Romero J, Husain SA, Holmes AA, et al. Non-invasive assessment of low risk acute chest pain in the emergency department: A comparative meta-analysis of prospective studies. Int J Cardiol. 2015;187:565-80.
6. Myocardial infarction redefined—a consensus document of The Joint European Society of Cardiology/American College of Cardiology Committee for the redefinition of myocardial infarction. Eur Heart J. 2000;21(18):1502-13.
7. Polanczyk CA, Lee TH, Cook EF, et al. Cardiac troponin I as a predictor of major cardiac events in emergency department patients with acute chest pain. J Am Coll Cardiol. 1998;32(1):8-14.
8. Kontos MC, Jesse RL, Anderson FP, Schmidt KL, Ornato JP, Tatum JL. Comparison of myocardial perfusion imaging and cardiac troponin I in patients admitted to the emergency department with chest pain. Circulation. 1999;99(16):2073-8.
9. Duca MD, Giri S, Wu AH, et al. Comparison of acute rest myocardial perfusion imaging and serum markers of myocardial injury in patients with chest pain syndromes. J Nucl Cardiol. 1999;6(6):570-6.
10. Iglesiasgarriz I, Rodriguez M, Garciaporrero E, et al. Emergency nontraumatic chest pain: Use of stress echocardiography to detect significant coronary artery stenosis. J Am Soc Echocardiogr. 2005;18(11):1181-6.
11. Tsutsui JM, Xie F, O'Leary EL, et al. Diagnostic accuracy and prognostic value of dobutamine stress myocardial contrast echocardiography in patients with suspected acute coronary syndromes. echocardiography. 2005;22(6):487-95.
12. Jeetley P, Burden L, Stoykova B, et al. Clinical and economic impact of stress echocardiography compared with exercise electrocardiography in patients with suspected acute coronary syndrome but negative troponin: A prospective randomized controlled study. Eur Heart J. 2006;28(2):204-11.
13. Kontos MC, Arrowood JA, Jesse RL, et al. Comparison between 2-dimensional echocardiography and myocardial perfusion imaging in the emergency department in patients with possible myocardial ischemia. Am Heart J. 1998;136(4 Pt 1):724-33.
14. Taylor AJ, Cerqueira M, Hodgson JM, et al. ACCF/SCCT/ACR/AHA/ASE/ASNC/NASCI/SCAI/SCMR 2010 appropriate use criteria for cardiac computed tomography. J Am Coll Cardiol. 2010;56(22):1864-94.

15. Hoffmann U, Bamberg F, Chae CU, et al. Coronary computed tomography angiography for early triage of patients with acute chest pain. J Am Coll Cardiol. 2009;53(18):1642-50.
16. Rubinshtein R, Halon DA, Gaspar T, et al. Usefulness of 64-slice cardiac computed tomographic angiography for diagnosing acute coronary syndromes and predicting clinical outcome in emergency department patients with chest pain of uncertain origin. Circulation. 2007;115(13):1762-8.
17. Levsky JM, Spevack DM, Travin MI, et al. Coronary computed tomography angiography versus radionuclide myocardial perfusion imaging in patients with chest pain admitted to telemetry. Ann Intern Med. 2015;163(3):174.
18. Sun Z, Choo GH, Ng KH. Coronary CT angiography: Current status and continuing challenges. Br J Radiol. 2012;85(1013):495-510.
19. Hilton T, Fulmer H, Abuan T, et al. Ninety-day follow-up of patients in the emergency department with chest pain who undergo initial single-photon emission computed tomographic perfusion scintigraphy with technetium 99m-labeled sestamibi. J Nucl Cardiol. 1996;3(4):308-11.
20. Tatum JL, Jesse RL, Kontos MC, et al. Comprehensive strategy for the evaluation and triage of the chest pain patient. Ann Emerg Med. 1997;29(1):116-25.
21. Stochkendahl MJ, Mickley H, Vach W, et al. Clinical characteristics, myocardial perfusion deficits, and clinical outcomes of patients with non-specific chest pain hospitalized for suspected acute coronary syndrome: A 4-year prospective cohort study. Int J Cardiol. 2015;182(3):126-31.
22. Amsterdam EA, Wenger NK, Brindis RG, et al. 2014 AHA/ACC guideline for the management of patients with non-ST-elevation acute coronary syndromes. J Am Coll Cardiol. 2014;64(24):e139-228.
23. Rybicki FJ, Udelson JE, Peacock WF, et al. 2015 ACR/ACC/AHA/AATS/ACEP/ASNC/NASCI/SAEM/SCCT/SCMR/SCPC/SNMMI/STR/STS appropriate utilization of cardiovascular imaging in emergency department patients with chest pain. J Am Coll Radiol. 2016;13(2):e1-29.
24. NICE. (2010). Guidance and guidelines. Chest pain of recent onset: assessment and diagnosis. [online] Available from https://www.nice.org.uk/guidance/cg95/chapter/Recommendations. [Accessed October, 2018].

55

CHAPTER

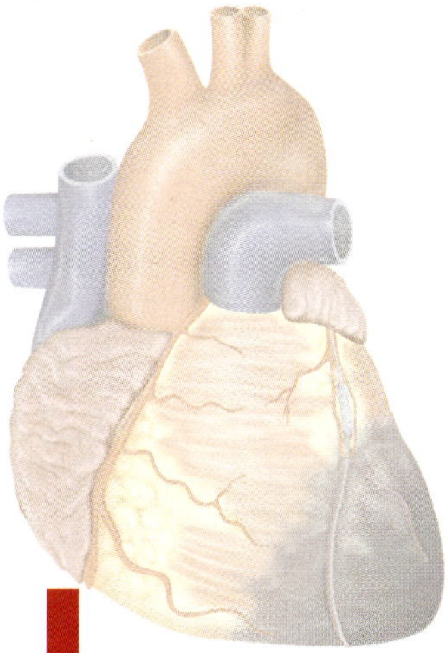

Cardiovascular Imaging in Emergency Department in Patients of Chest Pain

Satyendra Tewari, Roopali Khanna, Nikunj Kotecha

INTRODUCTION

Acute chest pain is the most common cause of cardiac emergency department. It is important to differentiate life-threatening causes of chest pain (acute aortic dissection, pulmonary embolism, and acute coronary syndrome) from more benign conditions (like costochondritis, gastric reflux disease). Though in majority of cases diagnosis can be reached by proper history and physical examination but in few cases diagnostic imaging becomes essential to exclude or diagnose life-threatening causes. Although acute chest pain raises the probability of acute coronary syndrome (ACS) but only 10–15% patients with acute chest pain had ACS.[1] The diagnosis of ACS is missed in 2% cases which increased the risk of short-term mortality and it is also essential to differentiate between ACS and other life-threatening cardiac and noncardiac conditions. Cardiac imaging is useful and complementary to clinical history, physical examination, electrocardiography (ECG), and cardiac biomarkers. Cardiac imaging is helpful for identification of ACS which reduces the rate of misdiagnosis of ACS and also helpful for identifying life-threatening non-ACS cardiac conditions. Imaging modality can evaluate anatomy or myocardial function or myocardial perfusion. Cardiovascular imaging which is useful in chest pain evaluation are echocardiography, treadmill test, computed tomography (CT) coronary angiography, cardiac magnetic resonance (CMR) imaging (MRI), cardiac nuclear imaging, and coronary angiography. But it is inappropriate to do all imaging modalities in a patient and proper selection of case is must because it will add to the cost with increase radiation exposure. This article will review the utility and feasibility of available cardiovascular imaging modalities and how it helps in early diagnosis and treatment. Patients with classical history of ischemic chest pain, ischemic ECG changes, and raised cardiac biomarkers should be directly referred to cardiologist and treated according to the evidence-based guidelines. Among various noninvasive imaging, echocardiography is the most important imaging modality in acute setting because it is rapid, real-time imaging, and portable; so transthoracic echocardiography (TTE) is often used as first-line imaging for emergency evaluation of chest pain.

DIAGNOSTIC CRITERIA

For diagnosis of ACS, echocardiography is helpful in diagnosis of myocardial ischemia or infarction in patients who are presented with acute chest pain. Severe ischemia or infarction can produce regional wall motion abnormality which can be detected as early as within seconds of ischemia and even before ECG and biomarker changes. However, regional wall motion abnormalities (RWMA) can also present because of previous myocardial infarction, myocarditis, and left bundle branch block. Similarly absence of RWMA cannot rule ACS. In a study of 280 patients with suspected ACS, the role of echocardiography in patients with equivocal ECG, echocardiography demonstrated a sensitivity of 71%, specificity of 91%, and a negative predictive value of 73% for diagnosing ACS.[2] Detection of other causes of acute chest pain, echocardiography also excludes conditions like acute aortic dissection, pulmonary embolism, and pericardial effusion. Detection of complication of acute myocardial infarction, echocardiography is very useful for detection various complication of acute myocardial infarction such as acute severe mitral regurgitation, free wall rupture.

PROGNOSTIC IMPLICATION

Left ventricular ejection fraction (LVEF) is considered as the most important prognostic parameter in case of patients who had ACS who presented with acute chest pain. Other parameters which are detected by echocardiography which had prognostic implication are detection of various complications of acute myocardial infarction and decreased in global longitudinal strain.

LIMITATION

It cannot possible to differentiate that RWMA is due to acute ischemia or previous infarction. When the patients were asymptomatic, use of these tests decreases sensitivity of echocardiography to detect ACS.

CONTRAST ECHOCARDIOGRAPHY

Diagnostic Criteria

Use of contrast agent improve the endocardial border detection, hence improve the detection of RWMA and real-time contrast echocardiography is helpful by identifying myocardial perfusion. In multicenter study comparing myocardial contrast echocardiography versus single-photon emission computed tomography (SPECT) found that contrast echocardiography improves the detection of ACS over and above symptoms, ECG and biomarkers and equivalent to SPECT for risk stratification.[3]

Prognostic Implication

Contrast echocardiography apart from providing information regarding wall motion abnormality it also helpful in detecting myocardial perfusion hence provides prognostic information above routine echocardiography. In study of multivariate logistic regression analysis, in which myocardial contrast echocardiography, Thrombolysis In Myocardial Infarction (TIMI) risk score, abnormal ECG, and troponin T levels were compared in 100 patients, myocardial contrast echocardiography was the strongest predictor of ACS, and it correlated the measured perfusion defect size with the ejection fraction at the 4-week follow-up.[4]

Limitation

Contrast perfusion imaging requires expertise hence its role in routine practice is limited.

STRESS ECHOCARDIOGRAPHY

Diagnostic Implication

It can be performed with exercise or dobutamine or with vasodilator. It is recommended in patients without recurrence of chest pain, normal ECG findings, negative troponin, and low risk score. The sensitivity and specificity of stress echocardiography for significant CAD is approximately 88% and specificity is 83% as compare to nuclear imaging.[5] Another important use of stress echocardiography is to assess viability of myocardium. A biphasic response in which improvement in wall thickening occurs at low dose and then deteriorates at high dose which is the most specific sign of viability.

Prognostic Implication

In patients with suspected ACS normal stress echocardiography implies excellent prognosis in which coronary angiography can be safely avoided.

Strain Imaging

This novel imaging provides additional information over RWMA. Ischemic segment tends to stretch as intraventricular pressure rises steeply during isovolumetric contraction phase. Strain imaging can identify this process in patients with suspected ACS.

COMPUTED TOMOGRAPHY CORONARY ANGIOGRAPHY

Diagnostic Criteria

High-quality coronary angiography can be performed with use of 64-slice CT system.[6] In patients presented with acute chest pain CT coronary angiography provide reliable coronary artery visualization, detection, and to rule out CAD. CT coronary angiography indicated in patients presented with acute chest pain with low pretest probability of CAD such as normal or diagnostic ECG, negative biomarker as a rule out test. In multicenter trial which include patients with low-risk ACS, CT coronary angiography has sensitivity of 95–99%, specificity of 64–83%, and negative predictive value of 97–99% and positive predictive value is 64–86% because CT coronary angiography overestimate coronary artery stenosis at site of calcification. CT coronary angiography is safe and effective investigation to rule out CAD in patients presenting acute chest pain.

Prognostic Indication

Ruling out significant coronary artery disease in patients present with acute chest pain has good prognostic value.

CT coronary angiography allow visualization of coronary atherosclerotic plaque, positive remodeling, and low CT attenuation in plaque area are consider to be high-risk features but their value in patients presenting with acute chest pain is not known.

Limitation

CT coronary angiography is not much useful in patients with arrhythmia, obesity, and those who cannot hold breath.

NUCLEAR IMAGING

Diagnostic Indication

Radionuclide imaging is very well-established imaging modality for evaluation of myocardial ischemia and viability of myocardium. Myocardial perfusion imaging includes stress test and rest test with use of radiouptake tracer labeled with thallium 201 or technetium 99m. Rest perfusion imaging becomes abnormal as soon as myocardial blood flow is disturbed. Rest imaging is helpful for detection of myocardial scar and stress test helpful for identifying inducible ischemia. Stress test can be done either via exercise or pharmacological stress. Rest imaging has sensitivity of 90% and specificity of 80% for detection of acute myocardial infarction. Nuclear imaging has very high negative predictive value which is reported as more than 99% means normal rest myocardial perfusion imaging in patients presented with acute chest pain rule out ACS.

Prognostic Indication

Patients with normal rest imaging had very low (<1%) event rate as compared to abnormal rest imaging which has 10–30% event rate at 30 days.[7] Although rest myocardial perfusion imaging appear to be ideal investigation for evaluation of chest pain but it is infrequently used because most of the patients become chest pain free hence according to guideline the stress test become the investigation of choice.

Ischemic Memory Imaging

Many patients who are asymptomatic, this novel approach can be useful. During ischemia myocardium utilizes glucose instead of free fatty acid and this metabolism persists for approximately 30 hours despite ischemia has resolved. This decreased metabolism can be visualized by using I-123 β-iodophenyl-pentadecanoic acid (BMIPP) imaging. This often known as ischemic memory imaging. ^{18}F-fluorodeoxyglucose (^{18}FDG) is glucose analog tracer used in positron emission tomography (PET) scan. It is accumulated in both normal and ischemic myocardium but in fasting condition it is accumulate in ischemic myocardium, hence FDG PET imaging is usually done in fasting state.

CARDIAC MAGNETIC RESONANCE

Diagnostic Indication

In recent years, CMR has undergone tremendous technological advancement and it can be utilized for diagnosis and management of patients with ACS who are clinically stable. CMR provides both structural and functional information in patients with ACS such as RWMA, late-gadolinium enhancement for scar, myocardial perfusion imaging both rest and stress, myocardial edema, and microvascular obstruction. T2-weighted imaging is able to differentiate acute versus chronic myocardial infarction. A study published in 2004 showed that CMR was feasible and safe in 72 patients with recent non-ST-segment elevation ACS. CMR within 3 days of the event had 96% sensitivity and 83% specificity for significant CAD (stenosis ≥70%) defined by invasive angiography.[8] Although it is difficult to do CMR in emergency basis because it is not easily available at everywhere but study had shown that cine, late gadolinium, and T2-weighted edema imaging can be done within 30 minutes in low-risk patients. Myocardial edema develops before ischemic necrosis or even troponin release. The edema can persist even when ECG changes and myocardial dysfunction have resolved and can persist up to 1 month. A study in which myocardial edema-sensitive T2-weighted imaging (T2W-imaging) was added to the CMR showed increased specificity, positive predictive value, and overall accuracy (96%, 85%, and 93%, respectively) compared with the conventional CMR protocol while sensitivity remained at 85%.[9] In addition, in this study, edema-sensitive T2W-imaging accurately identified all patients with acute MI, often before cardiac biomarkers were elevated. CMR has good safety profile. CMR stress test is done with dobutamine. The negative dobutamine stress test had good negative predicated value.[10] CMR also helpful in identifying condition like aortic dissection and myocarditis.

CORONARY ANGIOGRAPHY

Conventional coronary angiography is gold standard test in evaluation of patients with acute chest pain. It is accurately differentiate between ischemic versus nonischemic cause of chest pain. It also helpful to identify other than atherosclerotic cause of chest pain such as coronary artery dissection, coronary artery spasm, coronary aneurysm, and coronary arteritis. It is imaging modality of choice when other modalities are not available or technically not feasible or there are discrepancies between test result and patients clinic symptoms.

DISCUSSION

For evaluation of acute chest pain, use of imaging modalities depends upon whether patients who are hemodynamically stable or not, symptoms are present or not, patients can be able to exercise or not, ECG is interpretable or not, biomarker is positive or not and TIMI risk score which include age, risk factors of CAD, known case of CAD, use of aspirin in last 7 days, severe angina, ECG changes, and positive biomarker. In case of patients who is able to exercise and ECG is interpretable exercise stress testing without imaging is indicated. In case of patients who are able to exercise and ECG is not interpretable due to left bundle branch block or ventricular paced rhythm, and low or high TIMI risk score and biomarker is equivocal or borderline either radionuclide perfusion imaging or echocardiography is preferable. According to the American College of Cardiology Foundation (ACCF) "appropriate use criteria for echocardiography," published in 2011 and "appropriate use criteria for nuclear imaging," published in 2009, the role of 2D-TTE or radionuclide imaging in suspected ACS as "appropriate".[11,12] According to appropriate use criteria for CMR imaging published in 2006, patients who has intermediate pretest probability of CAD and ECG is not interpretable and patients or unable to exercise use of CMR is appropriate.[13] In case of patients who are not able to exercise then pharmacological stress test with imaging is indicated.

GUIDELINES

ACCF/ASNC/ACR/AHA/ASE/SCCT/SCMR/SNM 2009 Appropriate Use Criteria for Cardiac Radionuclide Imaging

The ACCF/ASNC/ACR/AHA/ASE/SCCT/SCMR/SNM 2009 appropriate use criteria for cardiac radionuclide imaging are given in Table 1.

ACCF/ACR/SCCT/SCMR/ASNC/NASCI/SCAI/SIR 2006 Appropriateness Criteria for Cardiac Computed Tomography and Cardiac Magnetic Resonance Imaging

The ACCF/ACR/SCCT/SCMR/ASNC/NASCI/SCAI/SIR 2006 appropriateness criteria for cardiac computed tomography and cardiac magnetic resonance imaging are described in Table 2.

TABLE 1: Detection of coronary artery disease (CAD): Symptomatic.

Indication		*Appropriate use score (1- 9)*
	Evaluation of ischemic equivalent (non-acute)	
1.	• Low pretest probability of CAD • ECG interpretable AND able to exercise	I (3)
2.	• Low pretest probability of CAD • ECG uninterpretable OR unable to exercise	A (7)
3.	• Intermediate pretest probability of CAD • ECG interpretable AND able to exercise	A (7)
4.	• Intermediate pretest probability of CAD • ECG uninterpretable OR unable to exercise	A (9)
5.	• High pretest probability of CAD • Regardless of ECG Interpretability and ability to exercise	A (8)
	Acute chest pain	
6.	• Possible ACS • ECG—no ischemic changes or with LBBB or electronically ventricular paced rhythm • Low-risk TIMI score • Peak troponin: Borderline, equivocal, minimally elevated	A (8)
7.	• Possible ACS • ECG—no ischemic changes or with LBBB or electronically ventricular paced rhythm • High-risk TIMI score • Peak troponin: Borderline, equivocal, minimally elevated	A (7)

Contd...

Contd...

Indication		*Appropriate use score (1- 9)*
8.	• Possible ACS • ECG—no ischemic changes or with LBBB or electronically ventricular paced rhythm • Low-risk TIMI score • Negative peak troponin levels	A (8)
9.	• Possible ACS • ECG—no ischemic changes or with LBBB or electronically ventricular paced rhythm • High-risk TIM I score • Negative peak troponin levels	A (8)
10.	• Definite ACS*	I(1)
	Acute chest pain (Rest imaging only)	
11.	• Possible ACS • ECG—no ischemic changes or with LBBB or electronically ventricular paced rhythm • Initial troponin negative • Recent or ongoing chest pain	A (7)

*See definition of ACS in Appendix A (based on ACC/ AHA Guidelines for the Management of Patients With ST-Elevation Myocardial Infarction).
(A: appropriate; I: inappropriate; ACS: acute coronary syndrome; AMI: acute myocardial infarction; CAD: coronary artery disease; ECG: electrocardiography)

TABLE 2: Appropriateness criteria for cardiac computed tomography and cardiac magnetic resonance imaging.

Indication		*Appropriateness criteria (median score)*
	Evaluation of chest pain syndrome (Use of vasodilator perfusion CMR or dobutamine stress function CMR}	
1.	• Low pretest probability of CAD • ECG interpretable AND able to exercise	I (2)
2.	• Intermediate pretest probability of CAD • ECG interpretable AND able to exercise	U (4)
3.	• Intermediate pretest probability of CAD • ECG uninterpretable OR unable to exercise	A (7)
4.	• High pretest probability of CAD	U (5)
	Evaluation of chest pain syndrome (Use of MR coronary angiography)	
5.	• Intermediate pretest probability of CAD • ECG interpretable AND able to exercise	I (2)
6.	• Intermediate pretest probability of CAD • ECG uninterpretable OR unable to exercise	I (2)
7.	• High pretest probability of CAD	I (1)
	Evaluation of Intracardiac structures (Use of MR coronary angiography)	
8.	Evaluation of suspected coronary anomalies	A (8)
	Acute chest pain (Use of vasodilator perfusion CMR or dobutamine stress function CMR)	
9.	• Intermediate pretest probability of CAD • No ECG changes and serial cardiac enzymes negative	U (6)
10.	• High pretest probability of CAD • ECG—ST-segment elevation and/or positive cardiac enzymes	I (1)

(A: appropriate; I: Inappropriate; U: uncertain; CAD: coronary artery disease; CMR: cardiac magnetic resonance; ECG: electrocardiography)

TABLE 3: Detection of coronary artery disease (CAD) in symptomatic patients without known heart disease.*

Indication		*Appropriate use score (1–9)*		
Nonacute symptoms possibly representing an ischemic equivalent				
	Pretest probability of CAD	Low	Intermediate	High
1.	• ECG interpretable AND • Able to exercise	U (5)	A (7)	I (3)
2.	• ECG uninterpretable OR • Unable to exercise	A (7)	A (8)	U (4)
Acute symptoms with suspicion of ACS (Urgent presention)				
3.	Definite MI	I (1)		
4.	Persistent ECG ST-segment elevation following exclusion ol MI	U (6)		
5.	Acute chest pain of uncertain cause (differential diagnosis Includes pulmonary embolism, aortic dissection, and ACS ["triple rule out·])	U (6)		
	Pretest probability of CAD	Low	Intermediate	High
6.	Normal ECG and cardiac biomarkers	A (7)	A (7)	U (4)
7.	ECG uninterpretable	A (7)	A (7)	U (4)
8.	• Nondiagnostic ECG OR • Equivocal cardiac biomarkers	A (7)	A (7)	U (4)

*All indications are for GTA unless otherwise noted.

(A: appropriate; I: inappropriate; U: uncertain; ACS: acute coronary syndrome; CAD: coronary artery disease; ECG: electrocardiography; MI: myocardial infarction)

ACCF/SCCT/ACR/AHA/ASE/ASNC/NASCI/SCAI/SCMR2010 Appropriate Use Criteria for Cardiac Computed Tomography

The ACCF/SCCT/ACR/AHA/ASE/ASNC/NASCI/SCAI/SCMR2010 appropriate use criteria for cardiac computed tomography are illustrated in Table 3.

CONCLUSION

There are various imaging modalities available to assess the patients in emergency department who are presenting with acute chest pain. Subjecting the patients to all modalities is inappropriate and depending upon probability of CAD, specific imaging modality can be done. It is essential to diagnose the patient presenting with acute chest pain and to rule out life-threatening complications in which the above mentioned imaging modalities are helpful in managing the CAD patients.

REFERENCES

1. Yiadom MY. Acute Coronary Syndrome Clinical Presentations and Diagnostic Approaches in the Emergency Department. Emerg Med Clin North Am. 2011;29:689-97.
2. Di Pasquale P, Cannizzaro S, Scalzo S, et al. Sensitivity, specificity and predictive value of the echocardiography and troponin-T test combination in patients with non-ST elevation acute coronary syndromes. Int J Cardiovasc Imaging. 2004;20:37-46.
3. Kaul S, Senior R, Firschke C, et al. Incremental value of cardiac imaging in patients presenting to the emergency department with chest pain and without ST-segment elevation: a multicenter study. Am Heart J. 2004;148:129-36.
4. Korosoglou G, Labadze N, Hansen A, et al. Usefulness of real-time myocardial perfusion imaging in the evaluation of patients with first time chest pain. Am J Cardiol. 2004;94:1225-31.
5. Fisch SD, Garlin JM, Abrams J, et al. 2012 ACCF/AHA/ACP/AATS/PCNA/SCAI/STS guideline for the diagnosis and management of patients with stable ischemic heart disease force on practice guidelines, and the American College of Physicians, American Association for Thoracic Surgery, Preventive Cardiovascular Nurses Association, Society for Cardiovascular Angiography and Interventions, and Society of Thoracic Surgeons: A report of the American College of Cardiology Foundation/American Heart Association Task. J Am Coll Cardiol. 2012;60:e34-44.
6. Meijboom WB, Meijs MF, Schuijf JD, et al. Diagnostic accuracy of 64-slice computed tomography coronary angiography: a prospective, multicenter, multivendor study. J Am Coll Cardiol. 2008;52:2135-44.
7. Wackers FJ. Chest pain in the emergency department: role of cardiac imaging. Heart. 2009;95:1023-30.
8. Kwong RY, Schussheim AE, Rekhraj S, et al. Detecting acute coronary syndrome in the emergency department with cardiac magnetic resonance imaging. Circulation. 2003;107:531-7.

9. Cury RC, Shash K, Nagurney JT, et al. Cardiac magnetic resonance with T2-weighted imaging improves detection of patients with acute coronary syndrome in the emergency department. Circulation. 2008;118:837-44.
10. Ingkanisorn WP, Kwong RY, Bohme NS, et al. Prognosis of negative adenosine stress magnetic resonance in patients presenting to an emergency department with chest pain. J Am Coll Cardiol. 2006;47:1427-32.
11. Douglas PS, Garcia MJ, Haines DE, et al. ACCF/ASE/AHA/ASNC/HFSA/HRS/SCAI/SCCM/SCCT/SCMR 2011 Appropriate Use Criteria for Echocardiography. A Report of the American College of Cardiology Foundation Appropriate Use Criteria Task Force, American Society of Echocardiography, American Heart Association, American Society of Nuclear Cardiology, Heart Failure Society of America, Heart Rhythm Society, Society for Cardiovascular Angiography and Interventions, Society of Critical Care Medicine, Society of Cardiovascular Computed Tomography, and Society for Cardiovascular Magnetic Resonance Endorsed by the American College of Chest Physicians. J Am Coll Cardiol. 2011;57:1126-66.
12. Taylor AJ, Cerqueira M, Hodgson JM, et al. ACCF/SCCT/ACR/AHA/ASE/ASNC/NASCI/SCAI/SCMR 2010 appropriate use criteria for cardiac computed tomography. A report of the American College of Cardiology Foundation Appropriate Use Criteria Task Force, the Society of Cardiovascular Computed Tomography, the American College of Radiology, the American Heart Association, the American Society of Echocardiography, the American Society of Nuclear Cardiology, the North American Society for Cardiovascular Imaging, the Society for Cardiovascular Angiography and Interventions, and the Society for Cardiovascular Magnetic Resonance. J Am Coll Cardiol. 2010;56(22):1864-94.
13. Hendel RC, Patel MR, Kramer CM, et al. ACCF/ACR/SCCT/SCMR/ASNC/NASCI/SCAI/SIR 2006 appropriateness criteria for cardiac computed tomography and cardiac magnetic resonance imaging: A report of the American College of Cardiology Foundation Quality Strategic Directions Committee Appropriateness Criteria Working Group, American College of Radiology, Society of Cardiovascular Computed Tomography, Society for Cardiovascular Magnetic Resonance, American Society of Nuclear Cardiology, North American Society for Cardiac Imaging, Society for Cardiovascular Angiography and Interventions, and Society of Interventional Radiology. J Am Coll Cardiol. 2006;48:1475-97.

SECTION 7

Valvular Heart Disease

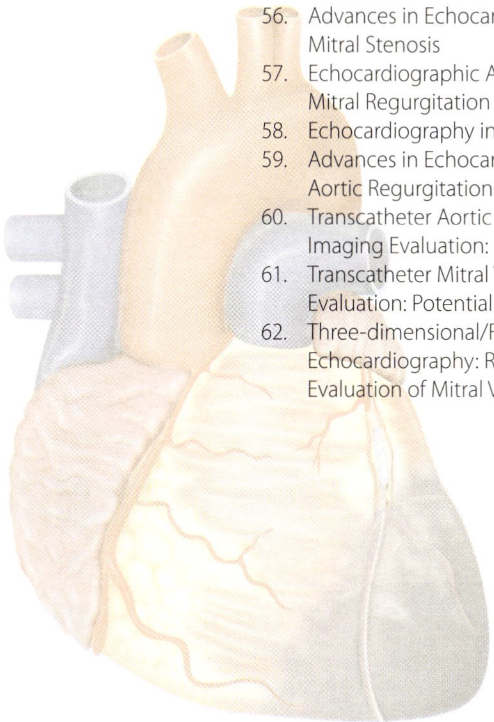

56

CHAPTER

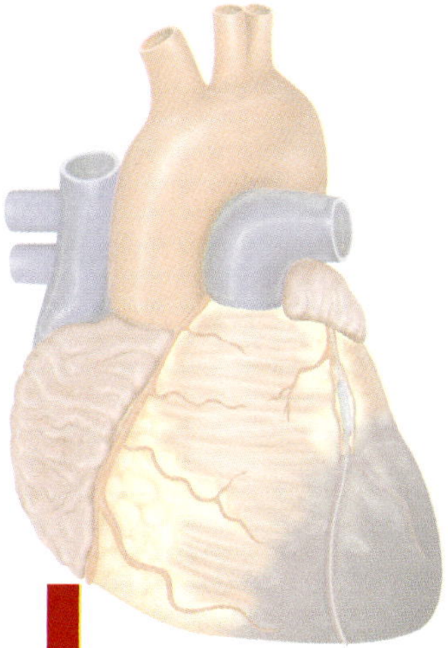

Advances in Echocardiographic Evaluation of Mitral Stenosis

Rakesh Gupta, N Chidambaram, SKD Bhardwaj, Sunil Mangla

INTRODUCTION

The American Heart Association/American College of Cardiology guidelines for the management of patients with valvular heart disease[1] state that transthoracic and transesophageal echocardiography are the imaging modality of choice for the assessment of patients with valvular heart disease. Many partially invasive therapies, such as percutaneous or transcatheter interventions, have been introduced for the treatment of structural heart disease. Many of these procedures require extensive multimodality imaging guidance including echocardiography and has lead to increased interest in advances in echocardiography. Various recent advancements in echocardiography are of particular relevance to valvular diseases and in this chapter, we will discuss the application of these new technologies to diagnose, manage, and prognosticate mitral stenosis (MS).

REAL-TIME THREE-DIMENSIONAL TRANSESOPHAGEAL ECHOCARDIOGRAPHY

Real-time transthoracic and transesophageal three-dimensional (3D) echocardiography may be useful in enhancing the objective assessment of mitral valve morphology, especially to visualize the narrowest orifice of mitral valve for planimetry. It is also more accurate than 2D techniques in identifying specific mitral valve pathology in the setting of complex disease but the diagnosis can be made more rapidly. Real-time 3D (RT3D) echo improves the accuracy and reproducibility of planimetry measurements of mitral valve area (MVA) in the setting of rheumatic disease by ensuring on-axis imaging of the short-axis view.[2-5] Subvalvular fusion is better appreciated by 3D echocardiography. 3D estimation of MVA correlates better with catheter-derived values. The advantage of 3D echocardiography is that mitral valve morphology is assessed in its entirety from single-imaging plane. Real-time 3D echo scoring system for MS objectively assess mitral valve morphology (Figs. 1A and B).[6] Each scallop of both leaflets is given a score taking into account, thickness, mobility, and calcification. Subvalvular apparatus is divided into three segments: (1) proximal, (2) middle, and (3) distal third and given score based on thickness and separation (Fig. 2). All the score points are summed to calculate total RT3DE score ranging from 0 to 31 points (Fig. 3). Score more than 14 indicates severe mitral valve involvement (Table 1).

STRAIN IMAGING

Left ventricular (LV) deformation is reduced in patients with severe MS and is related to hemodynamic severity of MS.[7] Balloon mitral valvuloplasty (BMV) results in rapid improvements in LV deformation, which is correlated with serial improvement in LV diastolic loading. Hence, suggesting that reduced diastolic filling rather than an irreversible myocardial structural abnormality contributes predominantly to reduced LV mechanical performance in patients with MS (Figs. 4A and B).

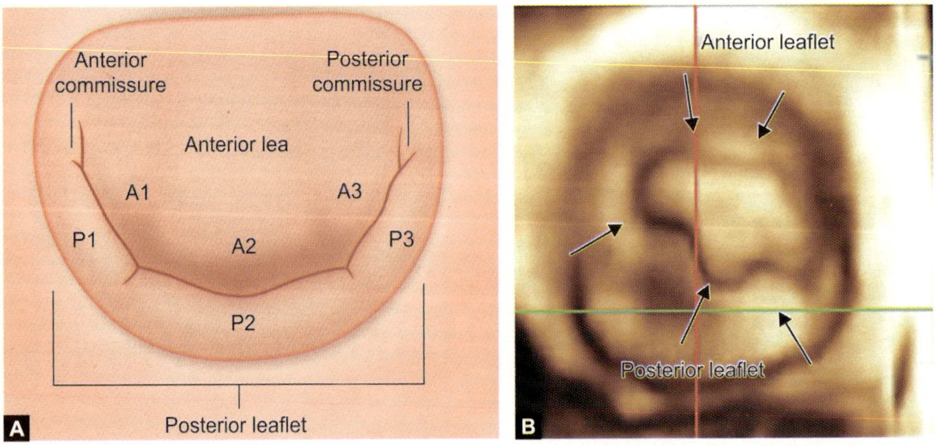

Figs. 1A and B: (A) Schematic diagram showing the three scallops of each leaflet (A1, A2, A3, P1, P2, and P3); and (B) Real-time three-dimensional echocardiography en face view of the mitral valve (MV) as seen from the ventricular aspect.

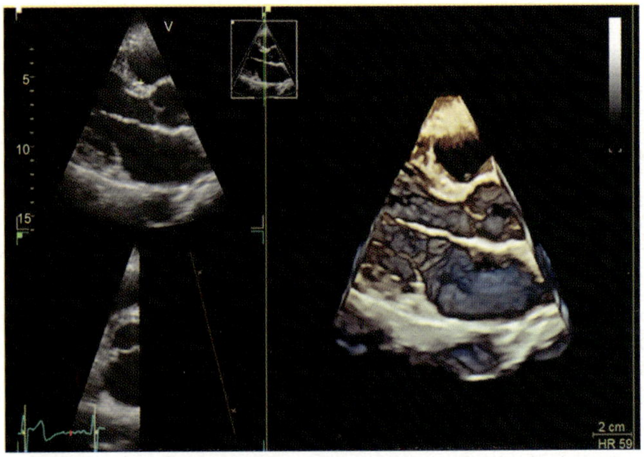

Fig. 2: Image of three-dimensional (3D) echo of normal mitral valve and mitral stenosis valve.

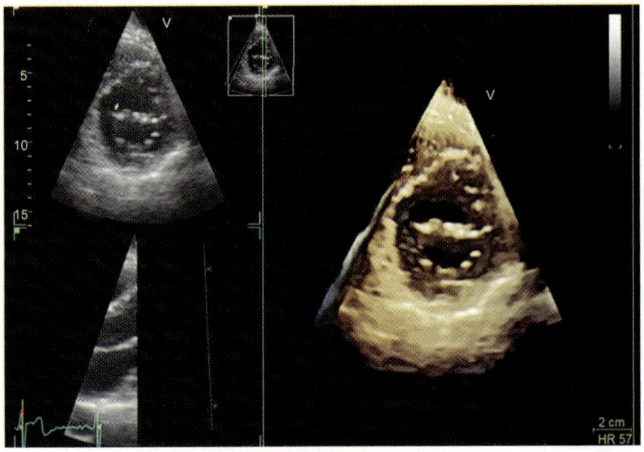

Fig. 3: Image of three-dimensional (3D) echo of normal mitral valve with commissure.

TABLE 1: Real-time three-dimensional echocardiography (RT3DE) score of mitral valve (MV).

	Anterior leaflet			*Posterior leaflet*		
	A1	*A2*	*A3*	*P1*	*P2*	*P3*
Thickness (0-6) (0 = normal, 1 = thickened)*	0–1	0–1	0–1	0–1	0–1	0–1
Mobility (0-6) (0 = normal, 1 = limited)*	0–1	0–1	0–1	0–1	0–1	0–1
Calcification (0-10) (0 = no, 1-2 = calcified)†	0–2	0–1	0–2	0–2	0–1	0–2
	Subvalvular apparatus†					
	Proximal third		Middle third		Distal third	
Thickness (0-3) (0 = normal, 1 = thickened)	0–1		0–1		0–1	
Separation (0-6) (0 = normal, 1 = partial, 2 = no)	0–1, 2		0, 1, 2		0, 1, 2	

*Normal = 0, mild = 1 to 2, moderate = 3 to 4, severe ≥ 5.
†Normal = 0, mild = 1 to 2, moderate = 3 to 5, severe ≥ 6.

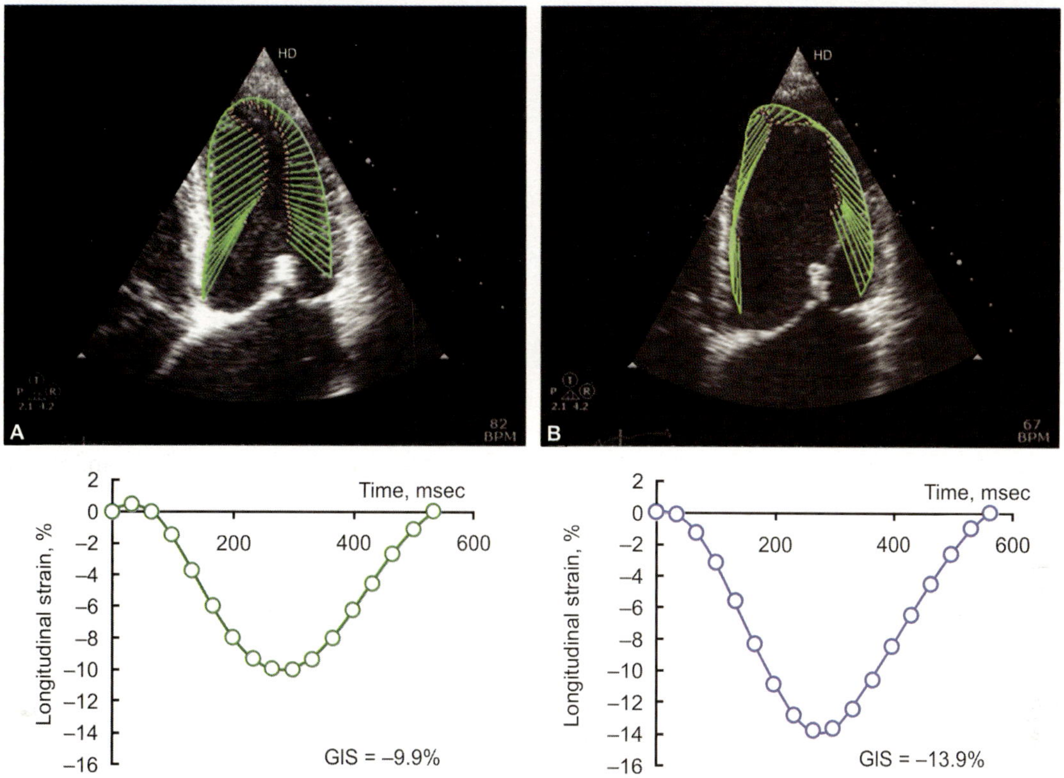

Figs. 4A and B: GLS measured from the apical four-chamber view in a patient with MS. (A) Baseline; and (B) After BMV. (BMV: balloon mitral valvuloplasty; GLS: global longitudinal strain; MS: mitral stenosis).

CONCLUSION

Real-time three-dimensional transesophageal echocardiography and strain imaging are of tremendous clinical relavance in evaluation of mitral stenosis including diagnostic, prognostic and therapeutic implications.

REFERENCES

1. Nishimura RA, Otto C. 2014 ACC/AHA valve guidelines: Earlier intervention for chronic mitral regurgitation. Heart. 2014;100(12):905-7.
2. Zamorano J, Cordeiro P, Sugeng L, et al. Real-time three-dimensional echocardiography for rheumatic mitral valve stenosis evaluation: An accurate and novel approach. J Am Coll Cardiol. 2004;43(11):2091-6.
3. Schlosshan D, Aggarwal G, Mathur G, et al. Real-time 3D transesophageal echocardiography for the evaluation of rheumatic mitral stenosis. JACC Cardiovasc Imaging. 2011;4(6):580-8.
4. Min SY, Song JM, Kim YJ, et al. Discrepancy between mitral valve areas measured by two-dimensional planimetry and three-dimensional transesophageal echocardiography in patients with mitral stenosis. Heart. 2013;99(4):253-8.
5. Wunderlich NC, Beigel R, Siegel RJ. Management of mitral stenosis using 2D and 3D echo-Doppler imaging. JACC Cardiovasc Imaging. 2013;6(11):1191-205.
6. Anwar AM, Attia WM, Nosir YF, et al. Validation of a new score for the assessment of mitral stenosis using real-time three-dimensional echocardiography. J Am Soc Echocardiogr. 2010;23:13-22.
7. Sengupta SP, Amaki M, Bansal M, et al. Effect of percutaneous balloon mitral valvotomy on left ventricular deformation in patients suffering from isolated severe mitral stenosis: A speckle-tracking strain echocardiographic study. J Am Soc Echocardiogr. 2014;27:639-47.

57

CHAPTER

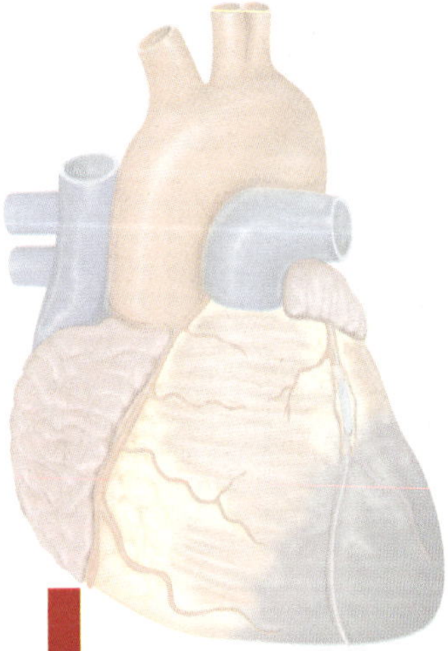

Echocardiographic Advances in the Diagnosis of Mitral Regurgitation

Rakesh Gupta, N Chidabaram, SKD Bhardwaj, Sunil Mangla

INTRODUCTION

Amongst imaging modality of choice for the assessment of valvular heart disease, echocardiography plays a significant role. Echocardiographic advancements have made a particular impact on the assessment and management of patients with valvular heart disease. Newer advancements, such as three-dimensional echocardiography, strain imaging, intracardiac echocardiography, and fusion imaging in this patient population is immensely helpful in diagnosis, prognosis, and therapeutics (Fig. 1).

THREE-DIMENSIONAL ECHOCARDIOGRAPHY

The echocardiographic advancement that has had the most impact on the diagnosis of valvular heart disease is real time three-dimensional (RT3D) echocardiography. The advantages of three-dimensional (3D) imaging over two-dimensional (2D) imaging have been well described in the most recent societal guidelines: "Recommendations for cardiac chamber quantification by echocardiography in adults" update[2] and "Recommendations for image acquisition and display using 3D echocardiography."[1] These guidelines review the significant data supporting the improved accuracy and reproducibility of 3D imaging for ventricular volumes and mass, as well as valvular morphology, and function. Initially introduced in the year 2000, the continued improvement of 3D technology has led to its widespread availability and its growing utility, particularly for valvular heart disease (Figs. 2 and 3).

Valve morphology RT3D transesophageal echocardiography (TEE) has significantly changed the assessment of valvular pathology and has revolutionized patient selection not only for surgical repair but also for newer transcatheter procedures like transcatheter aortic valve replacement (TAVR) and Mitraclip.

RT3D TEE is not only more accurate than 2D techniques in identifying specific mitral valve pathology in the setting of complex disease but the diagnosis can be made more rapidly, which is of particular use in the intraoperative evaluation of patients undergoing mitral valve repair. RT3D has also been integral to our understanding of the dynamic nature of the mitral valve complex in normal patients, as well as in primary and secondary mitral valve disease.[2-6]

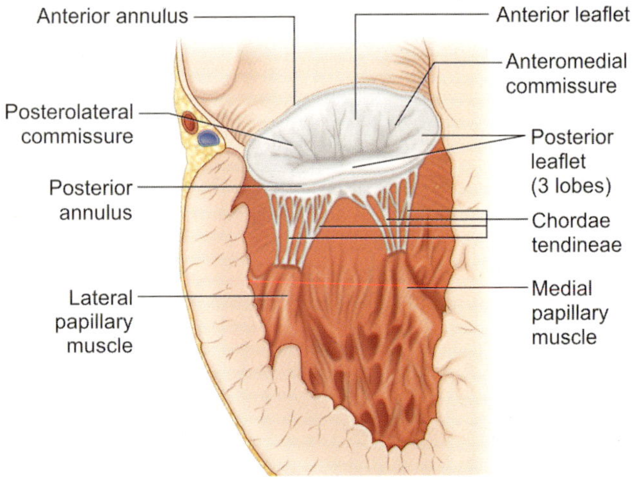

Fig. 1: Mitral valve diagram.

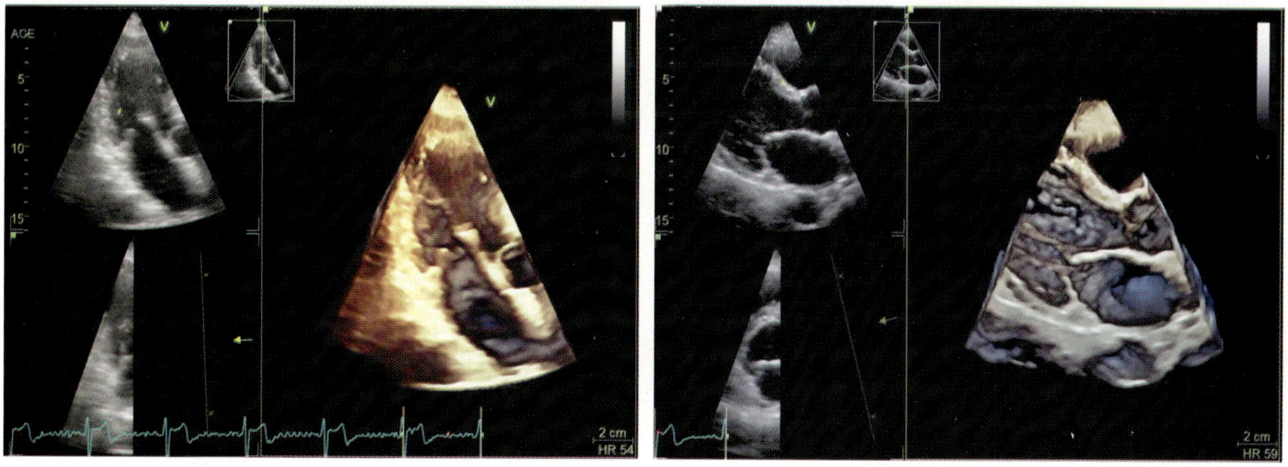

Figs. 2 and 3: Three-dimensional image of mitral valve.

Recent RT3D TEE studies have shown a coupling of mitral and aortic valve dynamic anatomy. Mitral valve diseases may affect normal mitral-aortic coupling and aortic valve function; different patterns of abnormal mitral-aortic coupling are associated with different Carpentier types of mitral regurgitation.[7] Conversely, changes in aortic morphology may affect mitral valve function, particularly in the setting of aortic stenosis and calcification of the aortic-mitral fibrous continuity.[8] RT3D TEE has shown changes in mitral valve morphology following surgical aortic valve replacement[9] as well as TAVR.[10] Notably, a decrease of tenting area predicted those patients whose mitral regurgitation improved following TAVR.

Quantification of valvular function three-dimensional color Doppler may overcome the limitations of 2D and standard Doppler measurements for quantifying regurgitation.[1,11,12] Studies have shown the feasibility of measuring the 3D vena contracta (narrowest portion of the regurgitant jet) on RT3D echocardiography to assess the severity of regurgitation for native regurgitant valve disease[11,13-15]as well as following surgical[16] or transcatheter interventions (Fig. 4).[17]

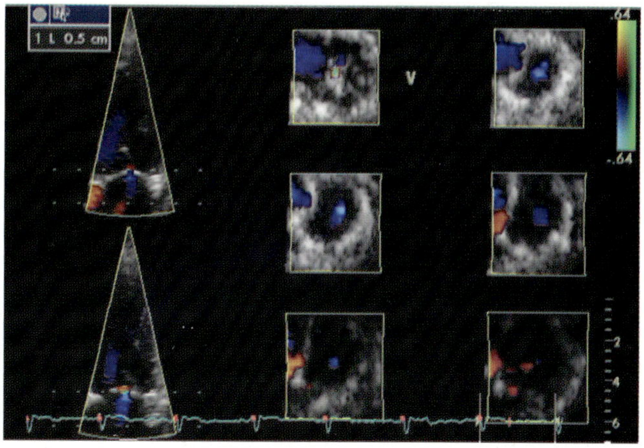

Fig. 4: Three-dimensional vena contracta. Figure shows vena contracta more than 0.4 cm, suggestive of severe mitral regurgitation.

Calculation of regurgitant volume in native valvular disease using the proximal isovelocity surface area (PISA) method[18] has known technical limitations, primarily the geometric assumptions of PISA shape required to calculate effective regurgitant orifice area. Multiple studies have validated the use of single-beat RT3D echocardiographic color Doppler imaging allowing the direct measurement of PISA without geometric assumptions for aortic, mitral, and tricuspid regurgitation assessment (Fig. 5).[19-22]

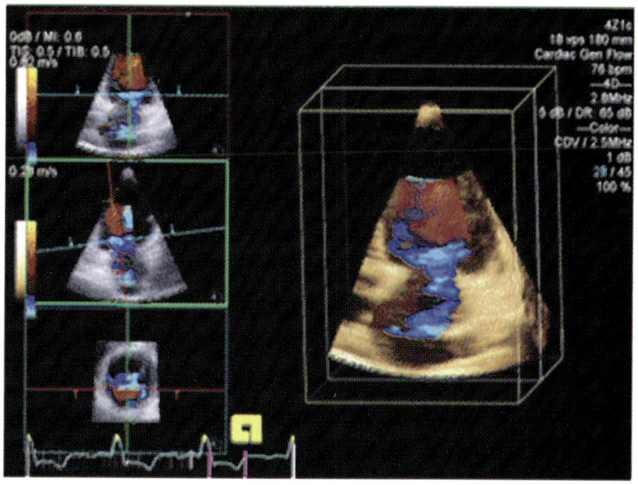

Fig. 5: Three-dimensional (3D) proximal isovelocity surface area (PISA).

Newer methods of determining relative flows within the heart make use of the velocity and direction of flow information which can be derived from color Doppler. Off-line and recently introduced online software has been

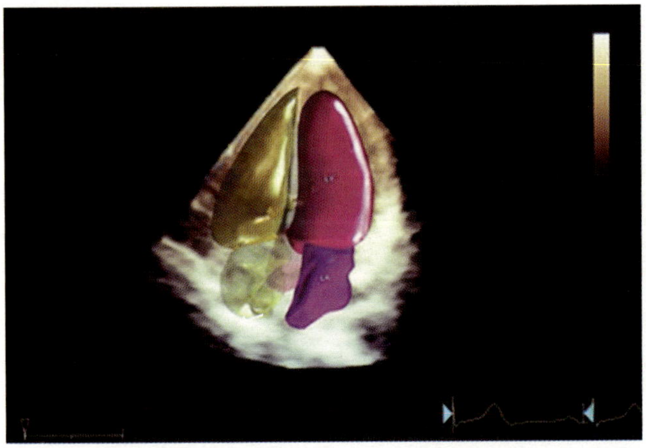

Fig. 6: Heart model for regurgitant volume.

developed which uses 2D color Doppler images to determine the velocity, flow rate, and flow volume in any given region of the heart.[23] Extension of this technology to 3D color Doppler volume sets is now possible and allows rapid, accurate, and reproducible quantitation of relative stroke volumes.[24,25] Thavendiranathan et al.[25] used the velocity information encoded in the volume color Doppler data, targeting the appropriate region of interest by using the simultaneous 3D imaging of the mitral annulus and left ventricular outflow tract. Color Doppler velocity is multiplied by a known area of this cross-section (a voxel area), and the resulting spatially averaged flow rates are used to generate flow-time curves that resemble those obtained by magnetic resonance imaging. The temporal integration of the flow-time curve generates the stroke volume. There was excellent correlation between the automated measured mitral inflow and aortic stroke volumes, and magnetic resonance imaging stroke volume ($r = 0.91$, 95% confidence interval [CI], 0.83–0.95, and $r = 0.93$, 95% CI, 0.87–0.96, respectively, $P < 0.001$) and very low interobserver variability. Automation of the measurement process allowed calculations of mitral inflow and aortic stroke volumes to be performed very rapidly. This methodology will likely become the standard for measurement of regurgitant volumes in the future (Fig. 6).

Three-dimensional TEE may also improve procedural success and shorten procedure time for the MitraClip™ device (Abbott Vascular Structural Heart, Menlo Park, CA).[26-28] Altiok et al.[27] performed a structured analysis to compare information and guidance capability provided by RT3D TEE compared to 2D TEE and found 3D TEE advantageous in 9 of 11 steps of the percutaneous mitral repair procedure, including optimizing trans-septal puncture site, guidance of the clip delivery system, precise positioning of the clip delivery system simultaneously in anterior-posterior, and lateral-medial direction, valvular regurgitation jet position, adjustment and visualization of the clip position relative to the valvular orifice, and assessment of remaining regurgitant jets.[27] Following MitraClip, assessment of residual regurgitation could also be assessed by 3D color Doppler43. A more than 50% reduction in regurgitant volume using the product of vena contracta areas defined by direct planimetry of RT3D color Doppler and velocity time integral using continuous-wave Doppler was associated with greater left atrial and ventricular remodeling (Fig. 7).

Strain imaging: Recent American Society of Echocardiography Chamber Quantification guidelines strongly recommend routine assessment of ventricular systolic function by quantification of ventricular volumes and calculation of ejection fraction (EF).[29] Cardiac mechanics, however, can now be assessed with the use of both tissue Doppler and speckle tracking for the measurement of myocardial displacement.[30] The measurement of myocardial deformation or "strain" is the fractional change in the length of a myocardial segment (expressed as a percentage of the baseline length). Strain rate is the rate of change in strain. The deformation of the myocardium is directional: lengthening would be represented by positive strain, and shortening by negative strain. Systolic strain can be measured along the anatomic coordinates of the cardiac chambers: longitudinal (negative strain), radial (positive strain), and circumferential (negative strain). The strengths and weaknesses of strain measurement have been well described;[30] however, the recent standardization of strain Digital Imaging and Communications in Medicine (DICOM) format will reduce inter-vendor variability which, along with improved software analysis and automation packages, will likely increase the clinical acceptability and use of this powerful technique (Fig. 8).

Chronic mitral regurgitation is associated with complex left ventricular adaptive remodeling, eccentric hypertrophy, and, eventually, reduced EF. Current guidelines recommend intervening on severe, asymptomatic mitral regurgitation in the setting of reduced EF because of a high incidence of persistent or worsening dysfunction.[31] In chronic severe degenerative mitral regurgitation, numerous studies have shown that a reduced baseline global longitudinal strain (GLS) signifies a maladaptive preload-related change that is associated with a reduction in left ventricular EF immediately after mitral valve repair.[32-34] A GLS cutoff of >-19.9% was a strong independent predictor of long-term left ventricular dysfunction and may become an appropriate indication for intervention in the setting of normal EF.[33]

INTRACARDIAC ECHOCARDIOGRAPHY

Although TEE imaging is well established and provides exceptional images, particularly for intra-procedural guidance, it most commonly requires general anesthesia

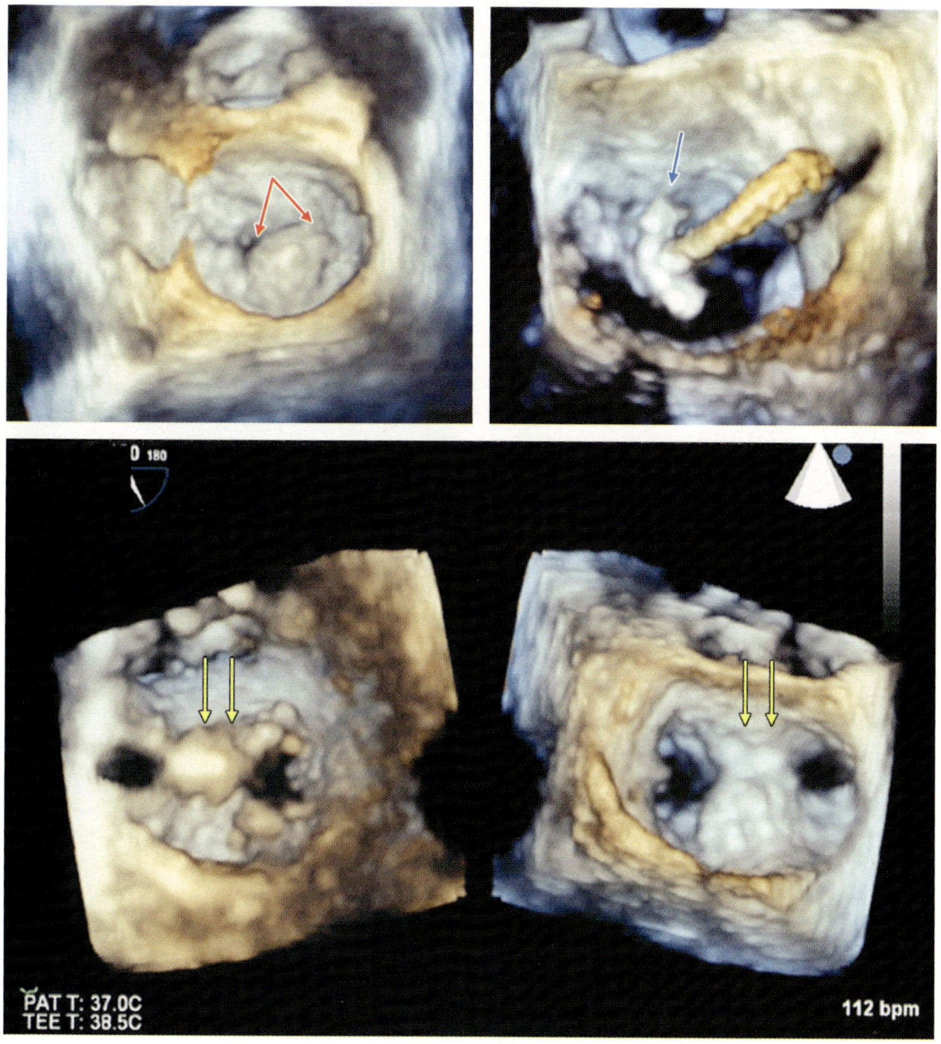

Fig. 7: Position of wire for puncture and Mitraclip.

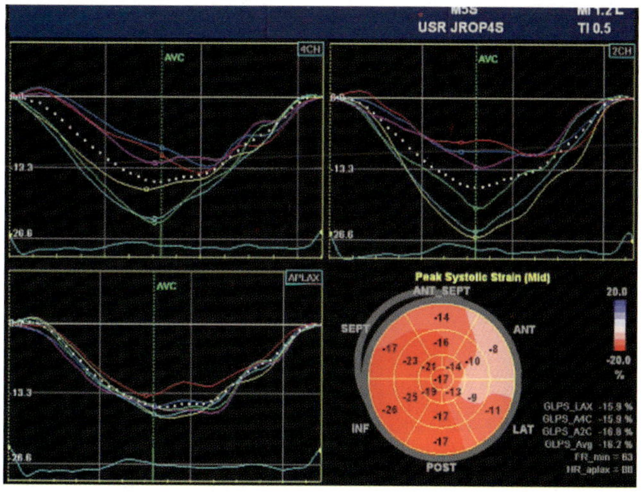

Fig. 8: Strain image in 4c view.

and may be associated with intermittent obstruction of fluoroscopic viewing.[35] With the current move toward conscious sedation for structural heart disease interventions, intra-cardiac echocardiography (ICE) may be an acceptable alternative in some patients with no other adequate intra-procedural imaging options. Evidence that ICE guidance can improve safety and outcome of interventional procedures is still lacking; however, ICE imaging for paravalvular leak closure has been reported to be feasible and advantageous.[36,37] A reduction in contrast use has also been reported with 2D ICE when used in TAVR.[38] The recently introduced AcuNav® V catheter (Siemens Inc. Mountain View, USA) represents the only commercially available RT3D ICE system. The 10F catheter carries a matrix transducer providing a 22° × 90° real-time volume image. This small volume represents the main limitation, particularly in near field applications, such as structural heart disease interventions (Fig. 9).

FUSION IMAGING

Combining images from two or more different imaging techniques, or fusion imaging, has been accomplished most recently with real-time echocardiography and fluoroscopy.[39-41] This technology, which co-registers the TEE probe position with the intervention table and the angulation of the fluoroscopy C-arm, allows for relatively accurate placement of the TEE image onto the fluoroscopic image. This integration eliminates the need for two different image display monitors and the mental integration of two very different imaging datasets by the operator of structural heart disease interventions.

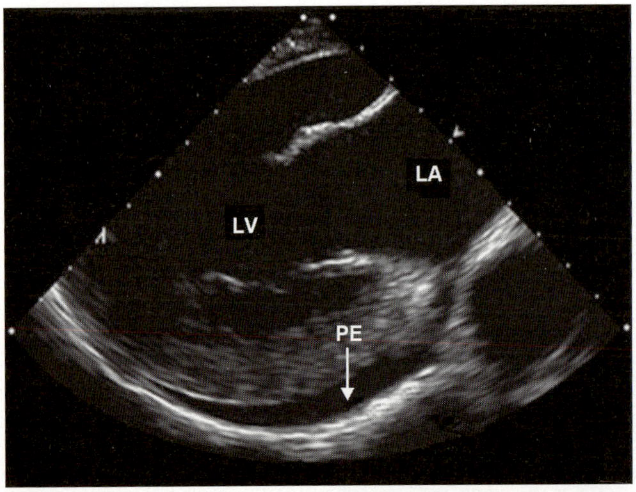

Fig. 9: Intra-cardiac echocardiography (ICE): Transventricular long-axis view of the left ventricular (LV) and the left atrium (LA) in patient with pericardial effusion. (PE: Pericardial effusion)

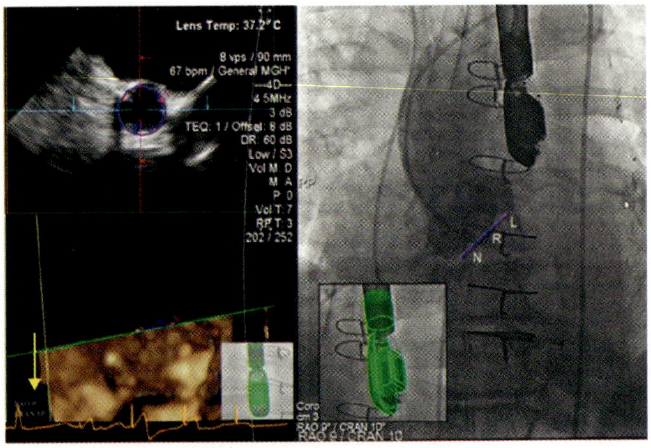

Fig. 10: Fusion imaging.

The ability to define targets on echocardiographic images (whether 2D or 3D), and coregister these targets onto the fluoroscopic images, should improve guidance of structural heart disease interventions. This technology has been shown to be safe and feasible for the transcatheter mitral repair procedure with the MitraClip™ device (Abbott Vascular Structural Heart, Menlo Park, CA) and shows a trend toward reduction of fluoroscopy and procedure time (Fig. 10).[42]

CONCLUSION

Echocardiography is the primary imaging modality for the diagnosis and management of patients with valvular heart disease. Improvement in surgical outcomes and advances in interventional techniques require further refinements in echocardiographic imaging. Three-dimensional echocardiography, strain imaging, intracardiac echocardiography, and fusion imaging have significant application in advancing our understanding of pathophysiology and anatomy, as well as the diagnosis and management of patients with valvular heart disease.

REFERENCES

1. Lang RM, Badano LP, Tsang W, et al. EAE/ASE recommendations for image acquisition and display using three-dimensional echocardiography. J Am Soc Echocardiogr. 2012;25(1):3-46.
2. Levine RA, Handschumacher MD, Sanfilippo AJ, et al. Three-dimensional echocardiographic reconstruction of the mitral valve, with implications for the diagnosis of mitral valve prolapse. Circulation. 1989;80(3):589-98.
3. Topilsky Y, Vaturi O, Watanabe N, et al. Real-time 3-dimensional dynamics of functional mitral regurgitation: a prospective quantitative and mechanistic study. J Am Heart Assoc. 2013;2(3):e000039.

4. Grewal J, Suri R, Mankad S, et al. Mitral annular dynamics in myxomatous valve disease: New insights with real-time 3-dimensional echocardiography. Circulation. 2010;121(12):1423-31.
5. Watanabe N, Ogasawara Y, Yamaura Y, et al. Mitral annulus flattens in ischemic mitral regurgitation: Geometric differences between inferior and anterior myocardial infarction: A real-time 3-dimensional echocardiographic study. Circulation. 2005;112(9 Suppl):I458-62.
6. Zeng X, Nunes MCP, Dent J, et al. Asymmetric versus symmetric tethering patterns in ischemic mitral regurgitation: Geometric differences from three-dimensional transesophageal echocardiography. J Am Soc Echocardiogr. 2014;27(4):367-75.
7. Looi JL, Lee AP, Fang F, et al. Abnormal mitral-aortic intervalvular coupling in mitral valve diseases: A study using real-time three-dimensional transesophageal echocardiography. Clin Res Cardiol. 2015;104(10):831-42.
8. Tsang W, Meineri M, Hahn RT, et al. A three-dimensional echocardiographic study on aortic-mitral coupling in transcatheter aortic valve replacement. Eur Heart J Cardiovasc Imaging. 2013;14(10):950-6.
9. Mahmood F, Warraich HJ, Gorman JH, 3rd, et al. Changes in mitral annular geometry after aortic valve replacement: A three-dimensional transesophageal echocardiographic study. J Heart Valve Dis. 2012;21(6):696-701.
10. Shibayama K, Harada K, Berdejo J, et al. Effect of transcatheter aortic valve replacement on the mitral valve apparatus and mitral regurgitation: Real-time three-dimensional transesophageal echocardiography study. Circ Cardiovasc Imaging. 2014;7(2):344-51.
11. Perez de Isla L, Zamorano J, Fernandez-Golfin C, et al. 3D color-Doppler echocardiography and chronic aortic regurgitation: A novel approach for severity assessment. Int J Cardiol. 2013;166(3):640-5.
12. Gonçalves A, Almeria C, Marcos-Alberca P, et al. Three-dimensional echocardiography in paravalvular aortic regurgitation assessment after transcatheter aortic valve implantation. J Am Soc Echocardiogr. 2012;25(1):47-55.
13. Mori Y, Shiota T, Jones M, et al. Three-dimensional reconstruction of the color Doppler-imaged vena contracta for quantifying aortic regurgitation: studies in a chronic animal model. Circulation. 1999;99(12):1611-7.
14. Fang L, Hsiung MC, Miller AP, et al. Assessment of aortic regurgitation by live three-dimensional transthoracic echocardiographic measurements of vena contracta area: Usefulness and validation. Echocardiography. 2005;22(9):775-81.
15. Chen TE, Kwon SH, Enriquez-Sarano M, et al. Three-dimensional color Doppler echocardiographic quantification of tricuspid regurgitation orifice area: Comparison with conventional two-dimensional measures. J Am Soc Echocardiogr. 2013;26(10):1143-52.
16. Franco E, Almería C, de Agustín JA, et al. Three-dimensional color Doppler transesophageal echocardiography for mitral paravalvular leak quantification and evaluation of percutaneous closure success. J Am Soc Echocardiogr. 2014;27(11):1153-63.
17. Altiok E, Hamada S, Brehmer K, et al. Analysis of procedural effects of percutaneous edge-to-edge mitral valve repair by 2D and 3D echocardiography. Circ Cardiovasc Imaging. 2012;5(6):748-55.
18. Zoghbi WA, Enriquez-Sarano M, Foster E, et al. Recommendations for evaluation of the severity of native valvular regurgitation with two-dimensional and Doppler echocardiography. J Am Soc Echocardiogr. 2003;16(7):777-802.
19. Pirat B, Little SH, Igo SR, et al. Direct measurement of proximal isovelocity surface area by real-time three-dimensional color Doppler for quantitation of aortic regurgitant volume: An in vitro validation. J Am Soc Echocardiogr. 2009;22(3):306-13.
20. Little SH, Igo SR, Pirat B, et al. In vitro validation of real-time three-dimensional color Doppler echocardiography for direct measurement of proximal isovelocity surface area in mitral regurgitation. Am J Cardiol. 2007;99(10):1440-7.
21. de Agustín JA, Marcos-Alberca P, Fernandez-Golfin C, et al. Direct measurement of proximal isovelocity surface area by single-beat three-dimensional color Doppler echocardiography in mitral regurgitation: A validation study. J Am Soc Echocardiogr. 2012;25(8):815-23.
22. de Agustín JA, Viliani D, Vieira C, et al. Proximal isovelocity surface area by single-beat three-dimensional color Doppler echocardiography applied for tricuspid regurgitation quantification. J Am Soc Echocardiogr. 2013;26(9):1063-72.
23. Li C, Zhang J, Li X, et al. Quantification of chronic aortic regurgitation by vector flow mapping: a novel echocardiographic method. Eur J Echocardiogr. 2010;11(2):119-24.
24. Little SH, Igo SR, McCulloch M, et al. Three-dimensional ultrasound imaging model of mitral valve regurgitation: design and evaluation. Ultrasound Med Biol. 2008;34(4):647-54.
25. Thavendiranathan P, Liu S, Datta S, et al. Automated quantification of mitral inflow and aortic outflow stroke volumes by three-dimensional real-time volume color-flow Doppler transthoracic echocardiography: Comparison with pulsed-wave Doppler and cardiac magnetic resonance imaging. J Am Soc Echocardiogr. 2012;25(1):56-65.
26. Biner S, Perk G, Kar S, et al. Utility of combined two-dimensional and three-dimensional transesophageal imaging for catheter-based mitral valve clip repair of mitral regurgitation. J Am Soc Echocardiogr. 2011;24(6):611-7
27. Altiok E, Becker M, Hamada S, et al. Optimized guidance of percutaneous edge-to edge repair of the mitral valve using real-time 3-D transesophageal echocardiography. Clin Res Cardiol. 2011;100(8):675-81.
28. Guarracino F, Baldassarri R, Ferro B, et al. Transesophageal echocardiography during MitraClip® procedure. Anesth Analg. 2014;118(6):1188-96.
29. Lang RM, Badano LP, Mor-Avi V, et al. Recommendations for cardiac chamber quantification by echocardiography in adults: An update from the American Society of Echocardiography and the European Association of

Cardiovascular Imaging. J Am Soc Echocardiogr. 2015;28(1):1-39.e14.

30. Mor-Avi V, Lang RM, Badano LP, et al. Current and evolving echocardiographic techniques for the quantitative evaluation of cardiac mechanics: ASE/EAE consensus statement on methodology and indications endorsed by the Japanese Society of Echocardiography. J Am Soc Echocardiogr. 2011;24(3):277-313.
31. Nishimura RA, Otto CM, Bonow RO, et al. 2014 AHA/ACC guideline for the management of patients with valvular heart disease: Executive summary: A report of the American College of Cardiology/American Heart Association Task Force on Practice Guidelines. J Am Coll Cardiol. 2014;63(22):2438-88.
32. de Isla LP, de Agustin A, Rodrigo JL, et al. Chronic mitral regurgitation: A pilot study to assess preoperative left ventricular contractile function using speckle-tracking echocardiography. J Am Soc Echocardiogr. 2009;22(7):831-8.
33. Witkowski TG, Thomas JD, Debonnaire PJMR, et al. Global longitudinal strain predicts left ventricular dysfunction after mitral valve repair. Eur Heart J Cardiovasc Imaging. 2013;14(1):69-76.
34. Pandis D, Sengupta PP, Castillo JG, et al. Assessment of longitudinal myocardial mechanics in patients with degenerative mitral valve regurgitation predicts postoperative worsening of left ventricular systolic function. J Am Soc Echocardiogr. 2014;27(6):627-38.
35. Smith LA, Monaghan MJ. Monitoring of procedures: Peri-interventional echo assessment for transcatheter aortic valve implantation. Eur Heart J Cardiovasc Imaging. 2013;14(9):840-50.
36. Rihal CS, Sorajja P, Booker JD, et al. Principles of percutaneous paravalvular leak closure. JACC Cardiovasc Interv. 2012;5(2):121-30.
37. Osman F, Steeds R: Use of intra-cardiac ultrasound in the diagnosis of prosthetic valve malfunction. Eur J Echocardiogr. 2007;8(5):392-4.
38. Bartel T, Bonaros N, Edlinger M, et al. Intracardiac echo and reduced radiocontrast requirements during TAVR. JACC Cardiovasc Imaging. 2014;7(3):319-20.
39. Corti R, Biaggi P, Gaemperli O, et al. Integrated x-ray and echocardiography imaging for structural heart interventions. EuroIntervention. 2013;9(7):863-9.
40. Gao G, Penney G, Ma Y, et al. Registration of 3D trans-esophageal echocardiography to X-ray fluoroscopy using image-based probe tracking. Med Image Anal. 2012;16(1):38-49.
41. Kaiser M, John M, Heimann T, et al. 2D/3D registration of TEE probe from two non-orthogonal C-arm directions. Med Image Comput Comput Assist Interv. 2014;17(Pt 1):283-90.
42. Quaife RA, Salcedo EE, Carroll JD. Procedural guidance using advance imaging techniques for percutaneous edge-to-edge mitral valve repair. Curr Cardiol Rep. 2014;16(2):452.

58

CHAPTER

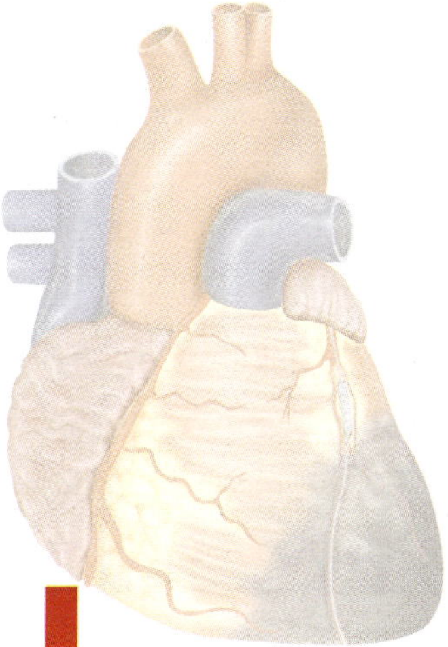

Echocardiography in Aortic Stenosis

R Alagesan, Satish Govind

INTRODUCTION

Echocardiography is the first imaging test done in the diagnosis of aortic stenosis (AS) when AS is first suspected. It provides for not only detection but to also assess the severity and anatomical characteristics of the valve. It can also provide findings on left ventricular (LV) function, coexisting valvular diseases, LV outflow tract abnormalities (LVOT), pulmonary hypertension (PH), and diseases of aorta. Just like any other echocardiogram, before starting the procedure, it is important to review patient's clinical status, findings, and related tests and record the body surface area (BSA). A comprehensive assessment of AS made by echocardiography can provide information from which diagnostic, prognostic, therapeutic, and surgical decisions are made.[1] Cardiac catheterization is necessary only for the diagnosis of coronary artery disease and rarely for the hemodynamic assessment of AS. AS may be valvular, subvalvular, supravalvular, or at multiples level. Transthoracic echocardiography (TTE) from different windows and views (Figs. 1 to 3) is useful to diagnose the pathology and anatomy. In patients with poor transthoracic

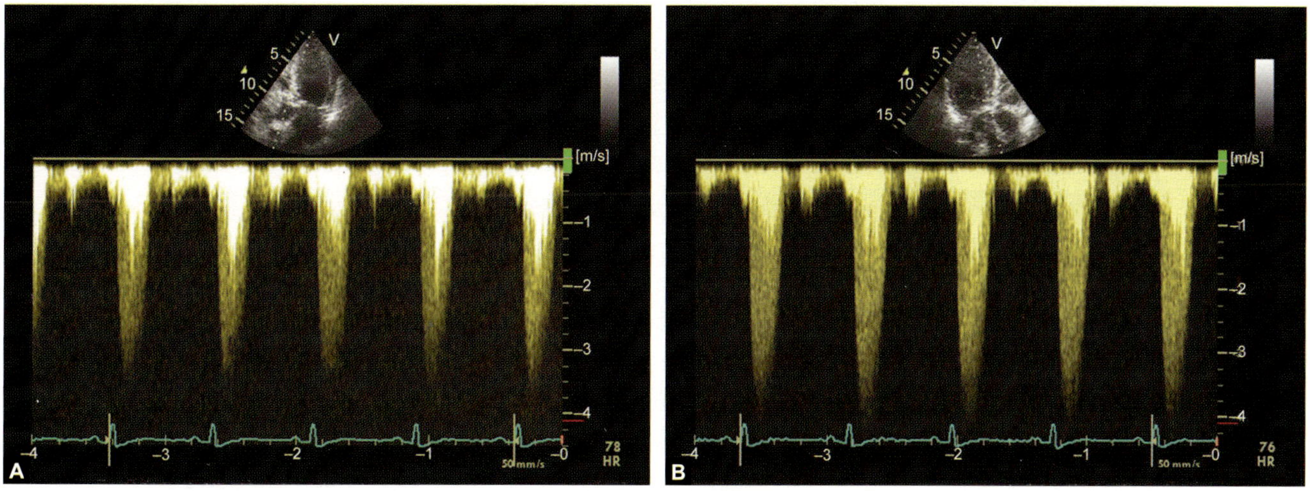

Figs. 1A and B: Importance of recording Doppler from different views in aortic stenosis. (A) Lower velocity when recorded from apical five-chamber view, but when it is more optimally aligned with color flow in apical three-chamber view, it shows increased velocity as seen in (B). Figure B is the preferred Doppler tracing to be measured.

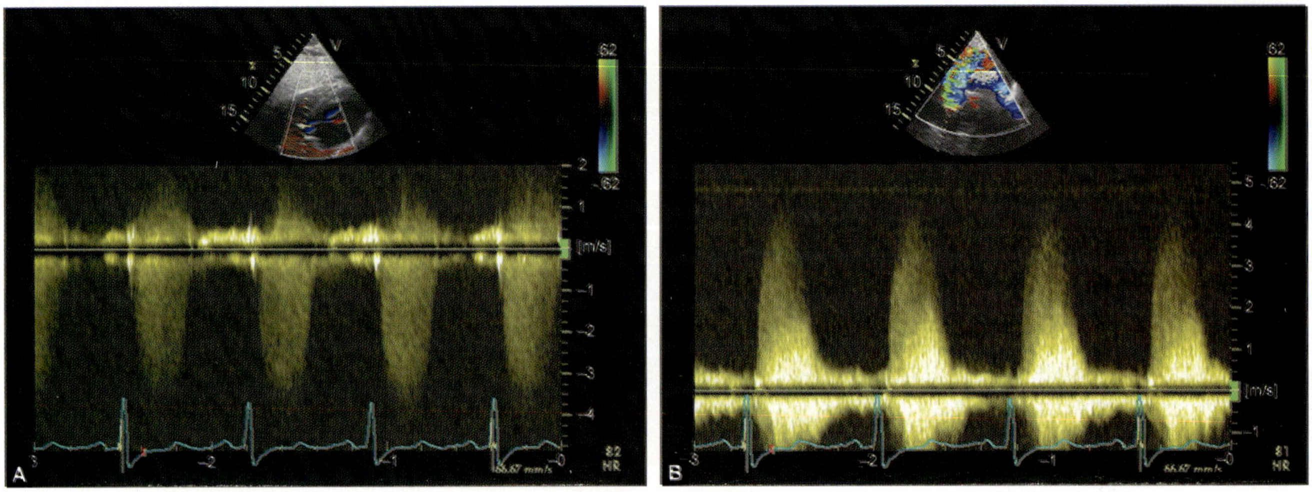

Figs. 2A and B: Other views from which Doppler recording should be attempted in aortic stenosis are shown. The view which displays the highest Doppler recording should be reported: (A) Subcostal view, (B) Suprasternal view.

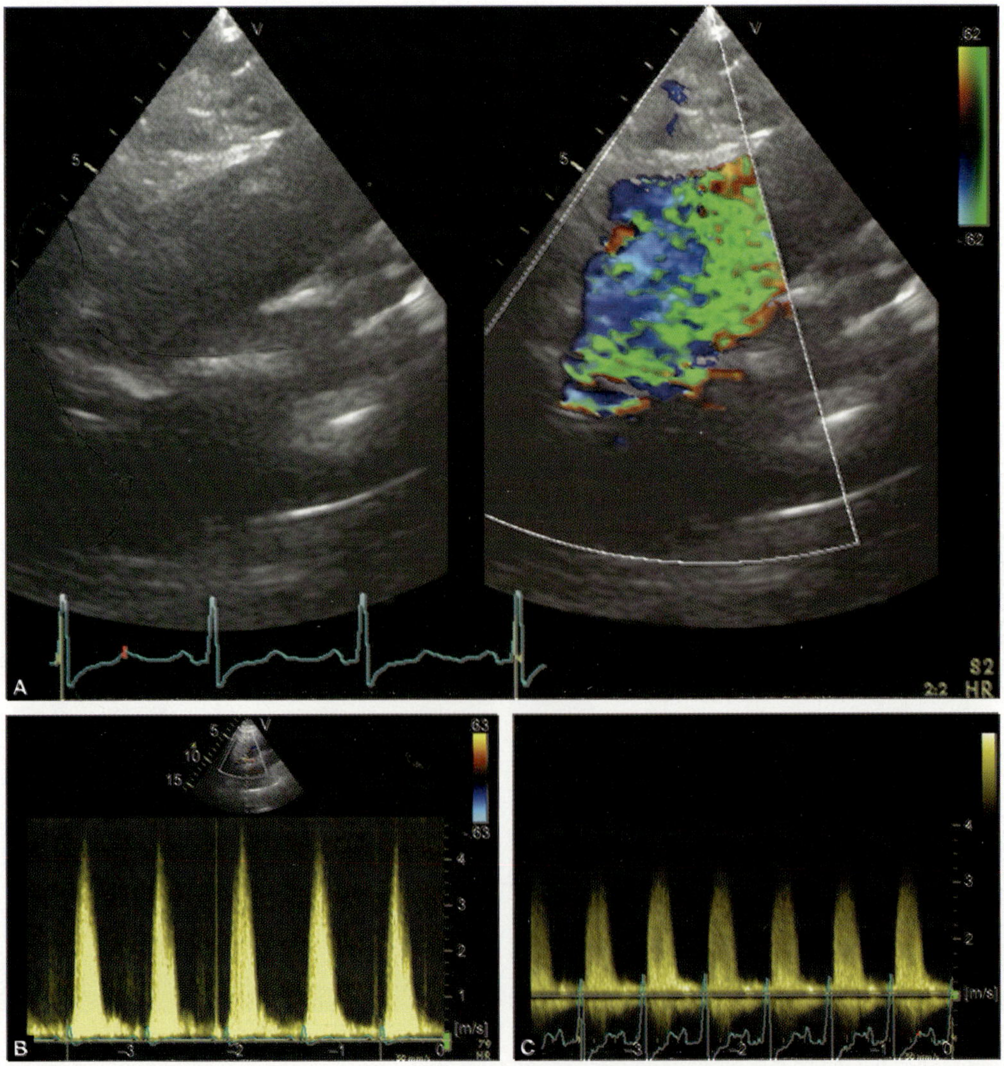

Figs. 3A to C: Right parasternal view (A) as shown, provides incremental information and should be done in all patients in aortic stenosis whenever possible. (B) Doppler obtained from adult matrix transducer. (C) Doppler obtained from nonimaging Pedoff transducer. The view which displays the highest Doppler recording should be reported.

windows transesophageal echocardiography (TEE) can be done. Three-dimensional echocardiography (3DE) can give incremental information about the diagnosis and severity of AS. The most important part of the echocardiographic examination is the Doppler echocardiography for the diagnosis and assessment of severity of AS along with two-dimensional echocardiography (2DE) for LV function, aorta, shunts, and LV mass.[2] Dobutamine stress echocardiography (DSE) can be useful in patients with low-flow low-gradient AS with reduced LV ejection fraction (LVEF). Exercise stress echocardiography (ESE) is useful to unmask the symptoms in patients with asymptomatic severe AS. Speckle-tracking echocardiography (STE) strain is useful as a predictor of adverse events. Echocardiography is also useful during balloon aortic valvuloplasty and during aortic valve replacements (AVR), by either surgical or by transcatheter approach.

TYPES

Valvular

Congenital

Bicuspid aortic valve (BAV) is the most common congenital abnormality of the heart occurring in 1–2% of normal population. In most of the cases, it does not produce any stenosis or regurgitation and goes unrecognized. But in certain percentage of patients it is associated with stenosis, regurgitation, or both. It is also associated with increased risk of infective endocarditis. The most common form of BAV is due to fusion of the right and left coronary cusps with a large anterior cusp and a small posterior cusp with commissure between the cusps. There may be a raphe in the region of fused commissure of right and left coronary cusps and both the coronary arteries arise from the anterior sinus. The next common type is the fusion of the right and noncoronary cusps resulting in a large right and small left cusp.[3] The raphe is in the region of the fused commissure of right and noncoronary cusps and the right coronary artery arises from the large right sided sinus and the left coronary from the smaller left sinus. Sometimes the raphe may be incomplete or completely absent. Fusion of the noncoronary cusp and left coronary cusp is rare. Unicuspid aortic valve has got usually an eccentric orifice, the common type being the unicommissural, unicuspid aortic valve. These valves are stenotic at birth and produce severe stenosis. Quadricuspid aortic valve usually produces aortic regurgitation (AR) than stenosis.

Calcific

Normal tricuspid aortic valve is thin and semitransparent, but as age advances there is some thickening of the valve because of the high-pressure gradient to which it is subjected to. Apart from this there are pathological changes of the valve including fibrosis, thickening, and calcification similar to atherosclerosis. The changes are more marked in patients with diabetes mellitus, systemic hypertension (HTN), dyslipidemia, and smoking, the same risk factors which produces atherosclerosis in the large and small arteries. These changes happen after the 5th and 6th decade of life where calcific aortic valve disease is more common after the 6th decade. Aortic valve commissural fusion and calcification starts from near the aorta and spreads slowly toward the center of the valve and hence the stenosis does not become severe till later in life. When the calcification is severe and involves the entire commissures, it is invariably associated with significant AS.

Rheumatic

Rheumatic heart disease (RHD) is multivalvular, where mitral valve is more commonly affected followed by the aortic valve. Usually, the mitral valve disease is dominant with insignificant to hemodynamically significant disease of the aortic valve.[4] Predominant aortic valve disease with mild involvement of the mitral valve is less commonly encountered. AS is a slow process where the main pathology is thickening and fusion of the commissure resulting in stenosis. Invariably, it is associated with varying degrees of AR and calcification of aortic valve which occurs in adult life.

Subvalvular

Fixed

Congenital fixed stenosis may be due to a membrane extending from the interventricular septum and getting attached to the base of anterior mitral leaflet (AML). The membrane may not be present at birth or early childhood and may develop later in life-producing subaortic stenosis. The jet of subaortic stenosis can strike the aortic valve producing structural damage of the aortic valve leading to AR. For this reason, the subaortic stenosis should be operated early, even if the stenosis is not severe. Sometimes the subaortic obstruction may be fibromuscular appcaring as a ridge and rarely may affect the entire LVOT producing a tunnel type of subaortic stenosis. Congenital subaortic stenosis may be associated with other defects, especially ventricular septal defect and patent ductus arteriosus.

Dynamic

Dynamic subaortic stenosis or obstruction occurs typically in patients with hypertrophic obstructive cardiomyopathy (HOCM). This is genetically inherited where there is marked thickening of LV muscle and occasionally right ventricular (RV) muscle with the characteristic pathological

TABLE 1: Severity of aortic stenosis.

Severity	*Peak velocity (m/s)*	*Mean gradient (mm of Hg)*	*Aortic valve area (cm²)*	*Aortic valve area-indexed (cm²)*
Mild	2.6–2.9	<20	>1.5	>0.85
Moderate	3.0–4.0	20–40	1.0–1.5	0.60–0.85
Severe	>4.0	>40	<1.0	<0.60
Very severe/critical	>5		<0.7	

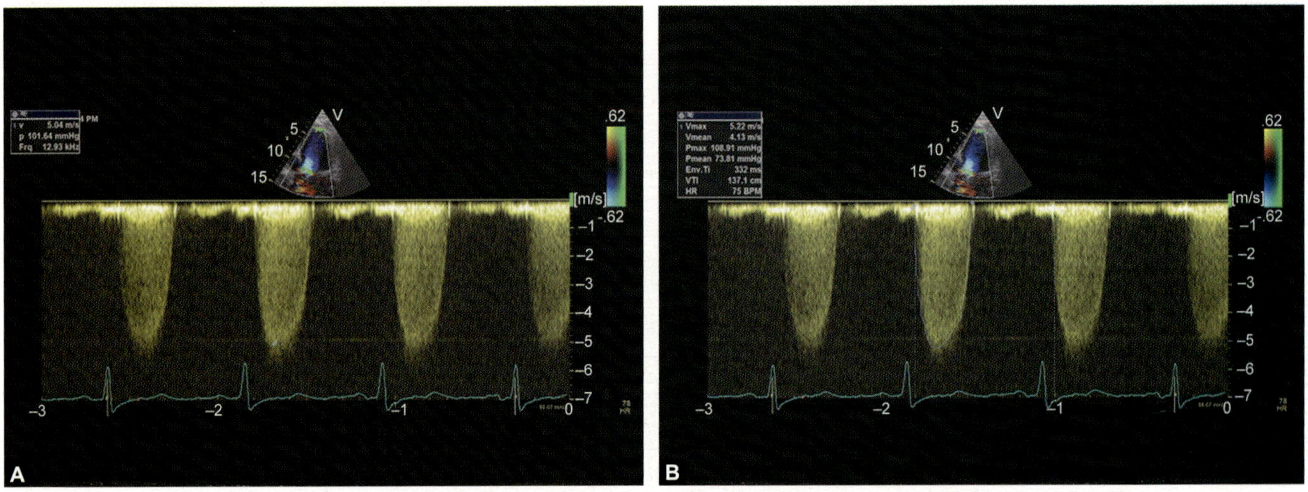

Figs. 4A and B: Velocity and gradient measurements in assessment of aortic stenosis severity.

pattern of myocardial fiber disarray. In patients with LVOT obstruction, there is systolic anterior motion of the mitral valve producing varying degree of obstruction. Because of the abnormal movement of AML,[5] there is posteriorly directed mitral regurgitation (MR), the severity of which is proportional to the severity obstruction. Dynamic subaortic obstruction may also occur following acute anterior myocardial infarction and also after mitral valve repair surgery.

Supravalvular

Supravalvular AS is rare. It may form part of the William's syndrome in which the patients also present with elfin facies, mental retardation, and pulmonary artery stenosis also. The common type is the hour-glass type where there is narrowing of the aorta above the aortic sinuses resulting in stenosis. Rarely, there may be diaphragm-like membrane with normally sized aorta and very rarely the entire ascending aorta and brachiocephalic vessels may be hypoplastic. The increased pressure inside the aortic sinuses produces dilatation of the sinuses and thickening of aortic valve. The coronary arteries may be dilated, and rarely there may be coronary ostial stenosis.

ASSESSMENT OF SEVERITY

The recommendations of the American Society of Echocardiography for the diagnosis and assessment of severity in AS is described in Table 1 (Figs. 4 and 5).

Peak Velocity

Peak velocity should be obtained by keeping the continuous wave Doppler (CWD) beam parallel to the AS color Doppler jet. This is possible when the aortic valve is not calcified, and the opening of the aortic cusps can be clearly visualized. Most of the times the highest velocity is recorded from the apical five-chamber view or apical long axis views (Fig. 6). In addition to these views, the velocity should be obtained from high parasternal long axis view, suprasternal long axis view and right parasternal view.[6] The highest AS velocity is measured and reported and the view from which the highest velocity is obtained should be mentioned in the report. This helps when serial studies are performed for comparison.

The brightest point at the tip of the Doppler velocity wave form should be used for calculating the gradients. The faint linear strands near the tip should be discarded, as these are artifacts. The gain setting should not be too high and only the high velocity signals should be recorded

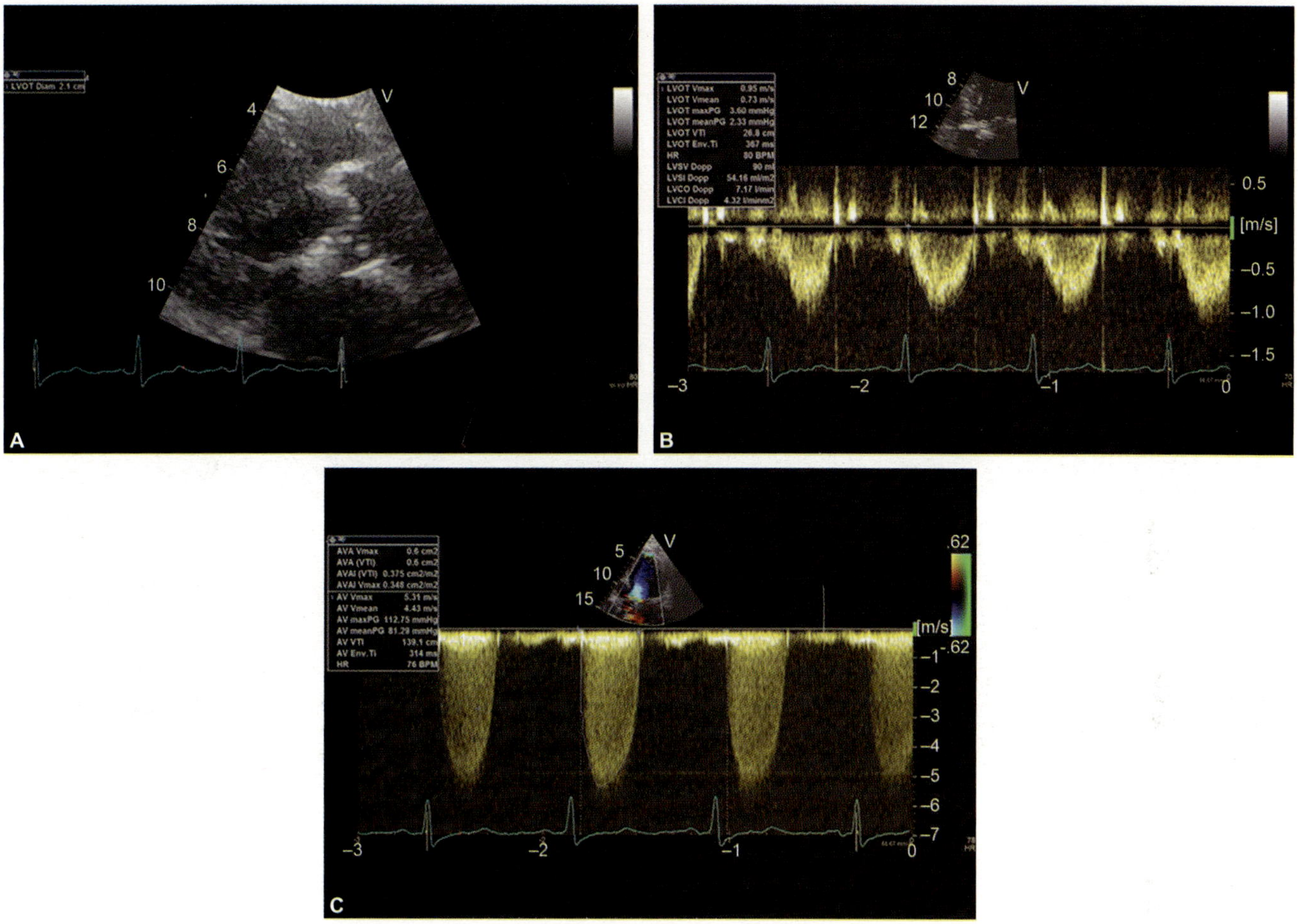

Figs. 5A to C: Aortic valve area calculation by continuity equation. (A) Left ventricular outflow tract measurement, (B) Left ventricular outflow tract velocity time integral measurement, and (C) Aortic valve stenosis tracing.

by suppressing the low velocity. The velocity wave form should not be colorized, and the measurements should be done from the grey scale images. It is better to average three consecutive beats when the patient is in sinus rhythm and at least five beats when the patients is in atrial fibrillation, while the beat following ventricular premature beats should be avoided. The shape of CWD velocity wave from is useful in the diagnosis of the type and level of AS. Fixed AS has a triangular appearance whereas dynamic LVOT obstruction in HOCM has a curvilinear appearance with late peaking.[7] The shape of the AS velocity is triangular in mild AS where the peak is reached early and the peak is delayed in severe AS where the peak is reached in the mid systole and apex is rounded.

Mean Gradient

The peak of the aortic pressure occurs later than the LV peak pressure in systole; hence, the gradient is underestimated in invasive studies. If the mean gradient (MG) is measured it correlates well between cardiac catheterization and Doppler. The MG is calculated by averaging the gradients obtained at equal intervals throughout systole. The MG and velocity time integral (VTI) are measured automatically by the computer once the AS wave form is traced.

The Bernoulli equation considers the convective acceleration, flow acceleration, and viscous friction. But in clinical settings the effect of flow acceleration and viscous friction is negligible, and it can be simplified by considering only the convective acceleration.[8] So, the modified Bernoulli equation derived gradient across a stenosis is calculated by the formula $4V^2$ where V is the peak velocity distal to the stenosis. There is another longer formula which considers the proximal velocity also, the gradient across a stenosis is equal to $4(V_2^2 - V_1^2)$ where, V_2 is the velocity distal to the stenosis and V1 is the velocity proximal to the stenosis. When the distal velocity is high, and the proximal velocity is less than 1 m/s the shorter formula can be used for calculating the peak gradient (PG). When the proximal velocity is more than 1 m/s as it happens in certain patients

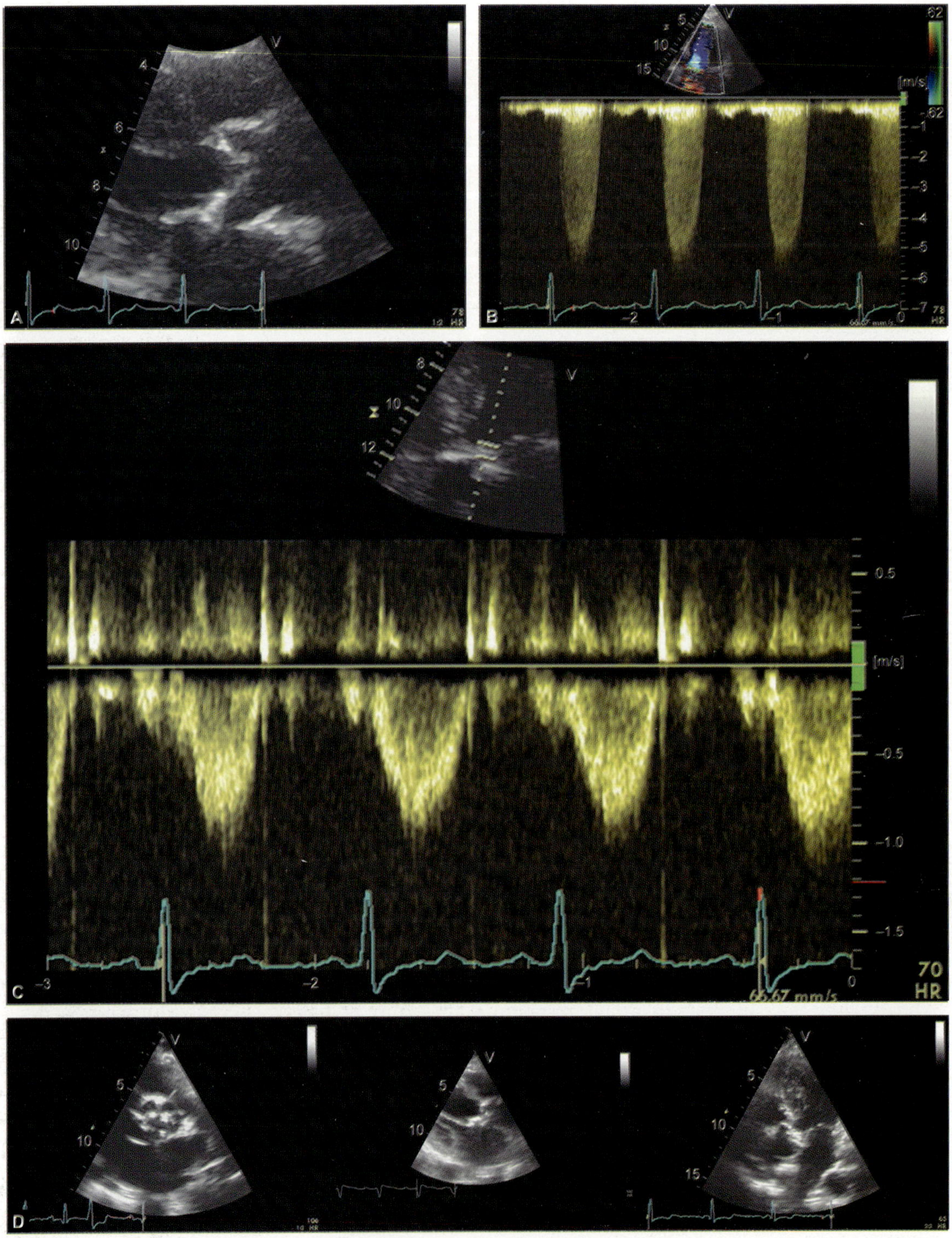

Figs. 6A to D: Techniques for proper measurement. (A) Image to be zoomed when aortic annulus and left ventricular outflow tract is to be measured. (B) Color flow to be properly aligned with cursor for accurate measurement of Doppler. (C) Doppler sampling of left ventricular outflow tract. (D) Calcified aortic stenosis seen in different views. Calcification can cause measurement errors.

with AS and AR, in renal failure, hyperthyroidism and anemia the longer formula should be used. When the AS is mild, and the peak velocity is below 3 m/s the longer formula should be used. This avoids overestimation of the PG. Calculation of the MG will be overestimated in these situations and one cannot apply any correction for the higher proximal velocity. In these clinical situations, the PGs should be given more importance to decide about the severity. However, the calculated valve orifice area will not be affected by the increased proximal velocity.

Valve Area

The valve area in AS is calculated from continuity equation in the absence of significant valvular regurgitation or shunts. By applying this for AS, the flow across the left LVOT is equal to the flow across the stenosed aortic valve. The flow across the LVOT is calculated by measuring the LVOT diameter and VTI of LVOT velocity. The aortic valve stenosis VTI is measured from the highest AS velocity. The LV, LVOT, and aortic valve are imaged in parasternal long axis view. The LVOT and aortic valve are imaged in zoom mode and three cardiac cycles are stored.[9] The LVOT diameter is measured in mid-systole from the inner edge of interventricular septum to the base of the AML. Accurate measurement of the LVOT is of paramount importance since any error will be accentuated when used in the formula.

Usually, the LVOT velocity is obtained 5–10 mm below the aortic valve and the LVOT measurements should be done at this level. Sometimes the pulsed Doppler (PWD) sample volume has to be moved further down to avoid the flow acceleration and the LVOT measurement should be done at the same level from the where the LVOT velocity is recorded. The problem in moving the sample volume further down in the LVOT is the shape of the LVOT becomes elliptical and the LVOT area is underestimated. The LVOT velocity is recorded using PWD by keeping the sample volume 5–10 mm below the aortic valve in apical five-chamber view or apical long axis view and color Doppler can be used to guide the positioning to avoid flow acceleration which happens in the LVOT. When the sampling volume is kept in the middle of LVOT, the velocity is recorded without any late peaking where the closing click of aortic valve may be recorded but not the opening click. In older patients the long axis of the LV and the LVOT are at an angle and in these patients the flow acceleration may start further below the aortic valve, and in these patient's sample volume has to be moved further below the 5–10 mm level and the LVOT diameters also should be measured at this level. Despite taking all care, if the LVOT is elliptical the resultant value may still not reflect the true valve area

The aortic valve area to a certain extent is dependent on the volume flow across the stenosed valve and when the LV function is normal the flow across the AS is normal and the valve area calculation is accurate. When there is LV dysfunction, the reduced flow is not able to open the thickened calcified aortic valve and the measurement of the area may not be accurate. The same finding has been observed in patients with severe MR where the thickened and calcified aortic valve opening is much more affected by the flow across the valve. So, in patients with severe LV dysfunction, DSE should be done to differentiate severe AS with LV dysfunction from mild AS with LV dysfunction due to low output.

In simplified continuity equation instead of using the VTI from LVOT and AS, velocity alone is used. This assumes that the ratio of the velocities is equal to the ratio of the VTI. The VTI is a more physiological measurement which represents the flow across the area.

Aortic Valve Planimetry

In certain patients with AS the PG, MG and valve area do not correlate with each other even after careful attention to the technical accuracy of obtaining these data. In these patients planimetry of the anatomical area of the AS will be useful to assess the severity. It will be difficult to go through the narrowest region of AS by transthoracic 2DE, but TEE, especially 3DE can be used to visualize the AS.[10] The orifice can be visualized, and the area can be planimetered even in patients with significant calcification after adjustment of the gain settings. 3DE by using TTE or TEE also can be used to visualize the AS from aortic side and measure the anatomical area (Figs. 7 and 8).

Ideally the aortic valve area either by planimetry or by continuity equation has to be indexed to the BSA of patients. A value of 0.6 cm^2/m^2 BSA is considered severe.

Dimensionless Index

Another simplified method is to remove the LVOT diameter and area from the calculation and expressing the severity of the AS as ratio of LVOT VTI to AS VTI. The normal aortic valve area is 3–4 cm^2, and in severe stenosis when the area is narrowed to 25% of normal, between 0.75 and 1.0 cm^2, a dimensionless index of 0.25 or less will indicate severe AS. The dimensionless index being a ratio need not be normalized to the BSA. But this can be helpful in those cases where the LVOT diameter cannot be measured accurately.

SPECIAL SITUATIONS

Low-flow low-gradient AS with reduced left ventricular ejection fraction: When MG indicate mild or moderate AS and the valve area is below 1.0 cm^2 the first thing to do is to review and confirm that the measurements are correct. The next step is to assess LV function and measure the stoke volume (SV) index by Doppler and confirm the same with biplane 2DE or 3DE.[11] When LVEF is less than 40% with reduced SV index then these patients are having low flow low gradient AS with reduced LVEF. In these patients DSE is done to differentiate from pseudo-AS. In those with reduced

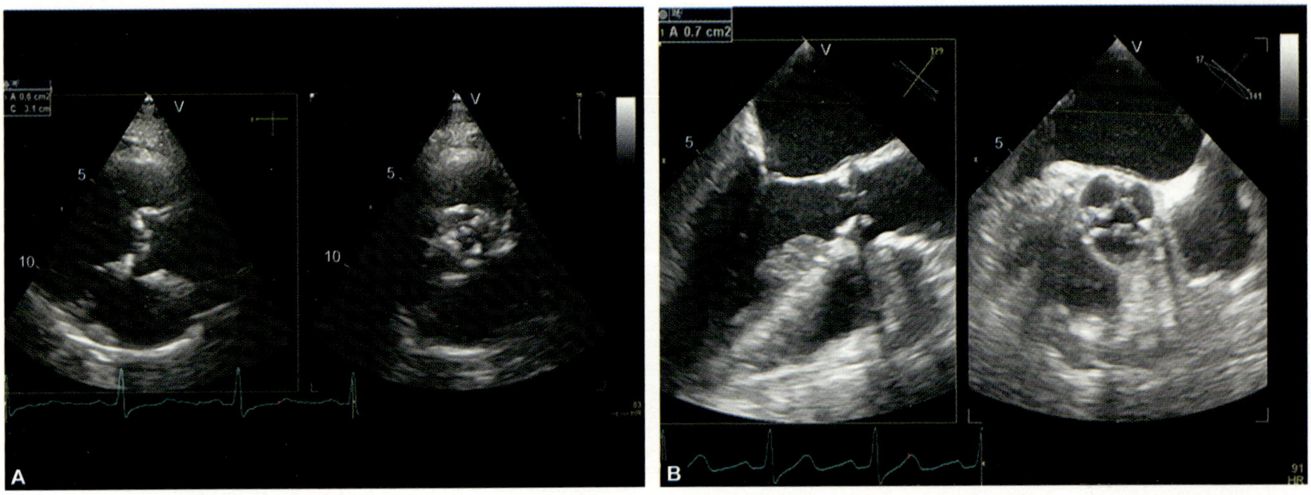

Figs. 7A and B: Planimetry of aortic valve area using bi-plane or X-plane method. (A) Transthoracic approach. (B) Transesophageal approach.

LVEF but MG more than 40 mm Hg, LVEF is reduced due to increase in afterload which will improve after AVR and DSE is not necessary.

Paradoxical low-flow low-gradient AS with preserved left ventricular ejection fraction: When the LV volume is small due to marked LV hypertrophy (LVH), significant mitral stenosis (MS), MR, tricuspid regurgitation, impaired diastolic filling, and increased ejection time of LV with preserved LVEF, then these patients have reduced SV index of less than 35 mm/m^2 BSA resulting in low flow, low gradient severe AS with preserved LVEF. In a small group of patients when the area is less than 1.0 cm^2 it may correspond to moderate AS when the BSA is less than 1.5 m^2. In these groups of patient's, velocity and area represents moderate AS which can be confirmed by dimensionless index and indexed aortic valve area.

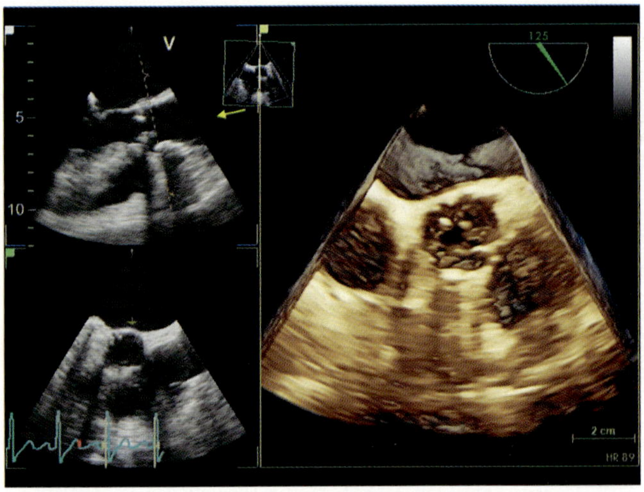

Fisg. 8A and B: Three-dimensional echocardiography of the aortic valve by transesophageal echocardiography.

SPECIAL PROCEDURES

Transesophageal Echocardiography

The important indication for TEE is suboptimal TTE study. The LV, LVOT, aortic valve, annulus, aortic sinuses, and the ascending aorta can be clearly visualized in TEE. Color Doppler flow imaging can be done to visualize the AS or AR jets. Measurement of the maximum velocity and gradient will require deep transgastric view. The LV contraction can be assessed in midesophageal and transgastric view and any regional wall motion abnormalities present can be detected.[12] The LVOT diameter can be accurately measured and with 3DE the aortic valve area and LVOT short axis can be obtained in the orthogonal plane and the area can be measured by planimetry. The anatomical AS area can be measured by the TEE by getting the 50-degree short axis section across the tip of the aortic valve. Again, this measurement can be done more reliably using the biplane section or from 3DE. The aortic sinuses, sinus tubular junction, and the ascending aorta are better visualized with TEE.

Stress Echocardiography

Patients with AS develop LVH as the AS severity increases. Because of increased afterload at one point, LV starts to develop systolic dysfunction. When there is significant LV systolic dysfunction with LVEF below 40%, the SV decreases, and the gradient across the AS decreases as also the calculated valve area and this condition is called low-flow low-gradient AS with reduced ejection fraction.

In contrast, there is a group of patients with is thickened calcified aortic valve with only mild stenosis where the LV systolic dysfunction is not related to AS.[13] In these patients also, the flow and gradient are low and because the reduced blood flow is not able to open the thickened aortic valve, the calculated aortic valve area may be reduced. These patients must be differentiated from true severe AS with LV dysfunction.

Dobutamine: In DSE, dobutamine is given intravenously which improves the contractility of the LV so that it generates more pressure and increases the flow across the aortic valve. In patients with true anatomically severe AS the LVOT velocity and AS velocity increases equally and so the effective valve area remains the same. In patients with mild AS and LV dysfunction due to myocardial diseases the LVOT velocity increases but there is no proportional increase in AS velocity and the calculated valve area increases significantly.

DSE is indicated in patients with MG below 40 mm Hg with LVEF below 40%. The aim is to increase the LV contractility and increase the SV by at least 25%. The protocol for DSE is to start with 2.5–5.0 μg/kg/min and increase by 5 μg/kg/mm every 3–5 minutes upto a maximum of 10–20 μg/kg/min. The initial action of dobutamine is ionotropic and the heart rate should not increase by more than 10–20 beats/min.[14] At each stage the LVOT VTI and AS velocity and the valve area are calculated. Apart from this, if dobutamine does not show improvement in LV contractility, these patients have low LV contractile reserve and the operative mortality for AVR is higher and prognosis is poorer. The test should be stopped when symptoms occur, when heart rate increases more than 10–20 bpm/min compared to baseline or increases beyond 100 bpm/min or when blood pressure falls.

Exercise: ESE in patients with AS can be done in asymptomatic patients with AS. It is not indicated in symptomatic patients with severe AS and for the diagnosis of associated coronary atherosclerotic heart disease in AS. ESE is primarily done to assess the exercise capacity in patients with AS and to unmask symptoms. The test should be done under careful supervision by a trained physician and the test should be stopped once there are symptoms or there is fall in systolic blood pressure.

Speckle-tracking Echocardiography

Left ventricular ejection fraction is not a sensitive marker of LV systolic function, especially when it comes to detecting subclinical dysfunction. In AS, there is increased mechanical stress on the LV because of the high afterload created by the stenotic valve. This causes subendocardial fibrosis which is not detected by traditional LVEF measurement of LV systolic function. This alters LV contractility and will have an adverse outcome and hence needs to be identified at an early stage before it starts to cause a significant decline in LV systolic function which is conventionally assessed by LVEF.[15] A more sensitive and accurate method is required to detect patients with subclinical dysfunction and identify those who can be sent for surgery for AVR before there is a decline in LV systolic function to improve their outcome. Global longitudinal strain (GLS) by 2D STE is one such parameter which has shown to be effective in such a scenario. Impaired GLS less than 12% is a predictor of adverse outcomes and also a marker of lack of improvement of LV systolic dysfunction (Fig. 9).

SPECIAL CONSIDERATIONS

Aortic Regurgitation

Aortic stenosis frequently coexists with AR to a varying severity (Figs. 10A and B). When AR is moderate or severe, then the SV is increased which in turn increases the AS gradient. When the AS is moderate and AR is also moderate the AS gradient is increased and will be in severe AS range. Anatomically, the AS is moderate but hemodynamically it is a severe stenosis due to AR and these patients tend to have more symptoms. Clinical decision making requires accurate quantification of both AS and AR and correlate with symptoms.

Mitral Valve Disease

Mitral stenosis: MS may be associated with AS in patients with RHD (Figs. 11A and B). Rarely congenital MS may be associated with bicuspid AS. In older patients calcific AS may be associated with MS due to severe mitral annular

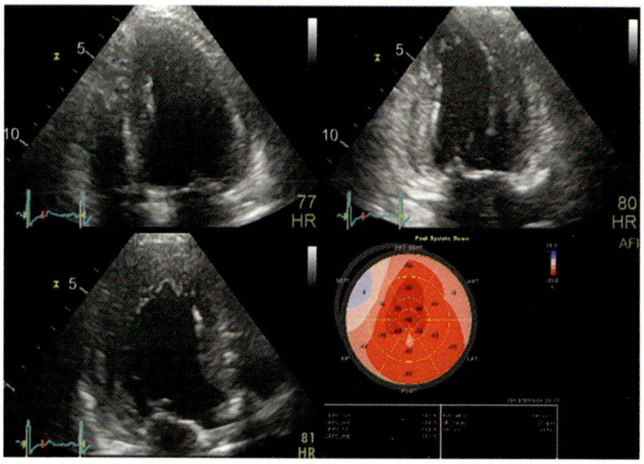

Fig. 9: Speckle-tracking echocardiography showing Bull's eye view with segmental and longitudinal strain.

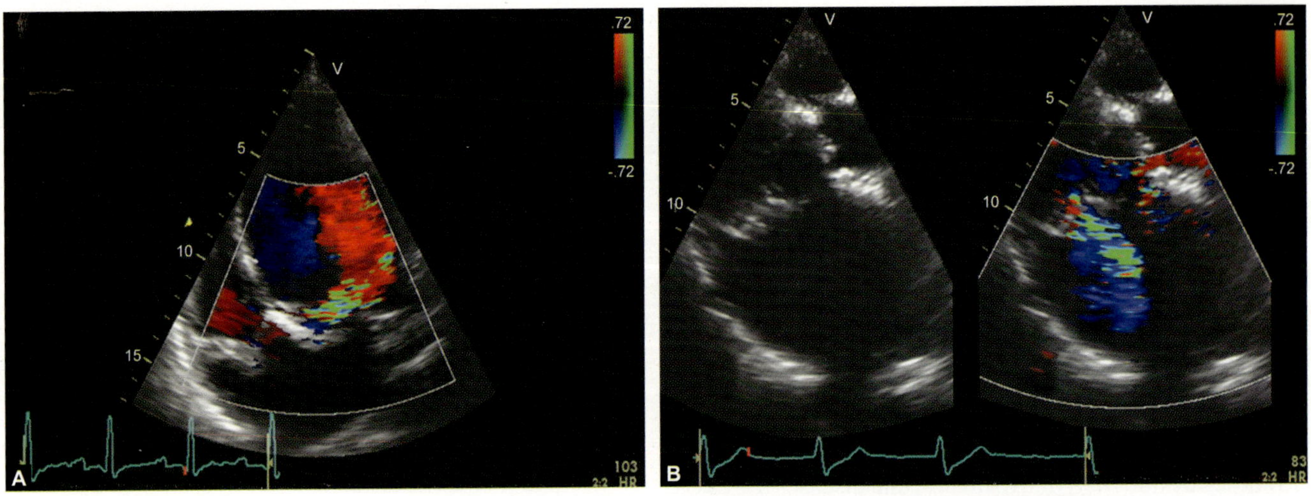

Figs. 10A and B: (A) Aortic stenosis with aortic regurgitation, and (B) mitral regurgitation.

calcification. LV filling may be reduced due to MS and this may reduce the SV and AS gradient resulting in low-flow low-gradient AS with preserved LVEF.

Mitral regurgitation: Primary disease of mitral valve may be present in patients with AS. Sometimes due to the pressure over load the mitral valve may start leaking and significant secondary MR may occur. One of the technical problems is not to mistake the MR jet for the AS jet. The MR jet has longer duration and the shape is rounded. MR when significant can decrease the SV and produce low-flow low-gradient AS with preserved LVEF. There is also the question in patients undergoing AVR whether the mitral valve will require replacement or repair. When the mitral valve is structurally normal, MR should be assessed before and after AVR intraoperatively and the decision to repair or replace the mitral valve should be considered when there is significant MR persisting after AVR.

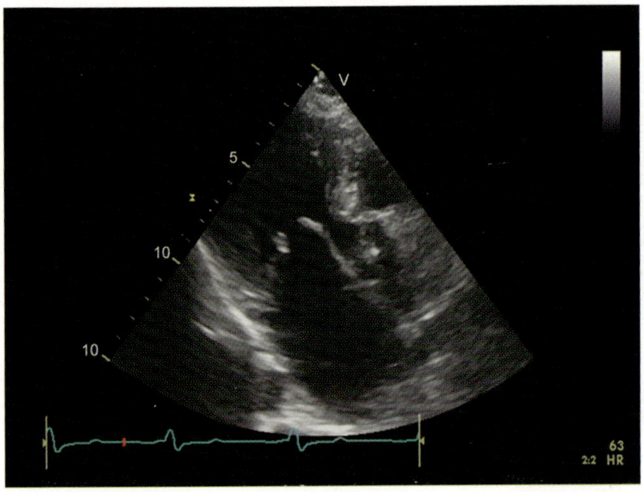

Fig. 11: Aortic stenosis with mitral stenosis seen in rheumatic heart disease.

Systemic Hypertension

Hypertension is frequently associated with calcific AS. Patients with AS and HTN tend to have marked LVH, decreased LV volume and SV and the gradient may be lower with severe AS, but the valve area will be decreased. It is a good practice to measure and report the blood pressure at the time of echocardiography, in patients with HTN the gradient and valve area should be reassessed after control of blood pressure. The measurement of the Z_{VA} which is the valvuloarterial impedance should be considered when the both AS and HTN coexist. In valvuloarterial impedance, it is the total load imposed on the LV due to combined effect of AS and increased systolic blood pressure when divided by the SV index which gives the "impedance" or the resistance to the blood flow. Even though the concept is attractive, there are no longitudinal prospective studies.

High Output States

Often causes of increased SV and increased AS velocity and gradient in the presence of mild or moderate AS are anemia, hyperthyroidism, volume overload in patients on hemodialysis and arteriovenous fistula. In these patients the SV should be carefully measured which will be high and the AS velocity is also high resulting in aortic valve area more than 1.0 cm^2. The LVOT-VTI is increased, the AS velocity and VTI are increased with aortic valve orifice area of more than 1.0 cm^2. Careful attention to anatomy and CWD waveform will help to avoid under or overestimation of AS severity.

Ascending Aorta

In patients with BAV, the aorta may be dilated due to aortopathy resulting in dilatation of aortic sinuses and

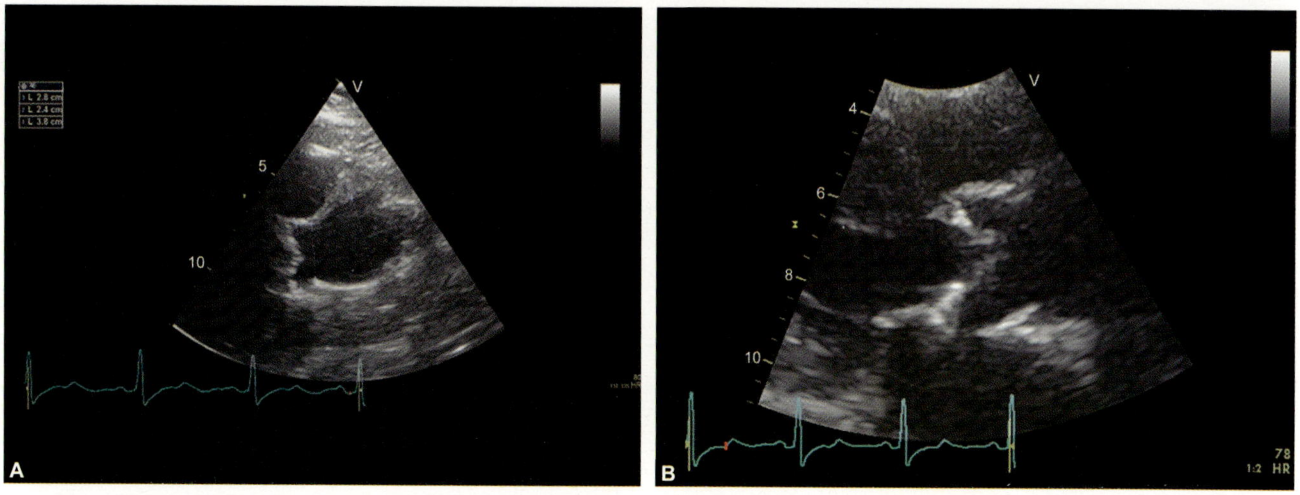

Figs. 12A and B: (A) Measurement of ascending aorta, sinotubular junction, and aortic sinus, and (B) Aortic annulus.

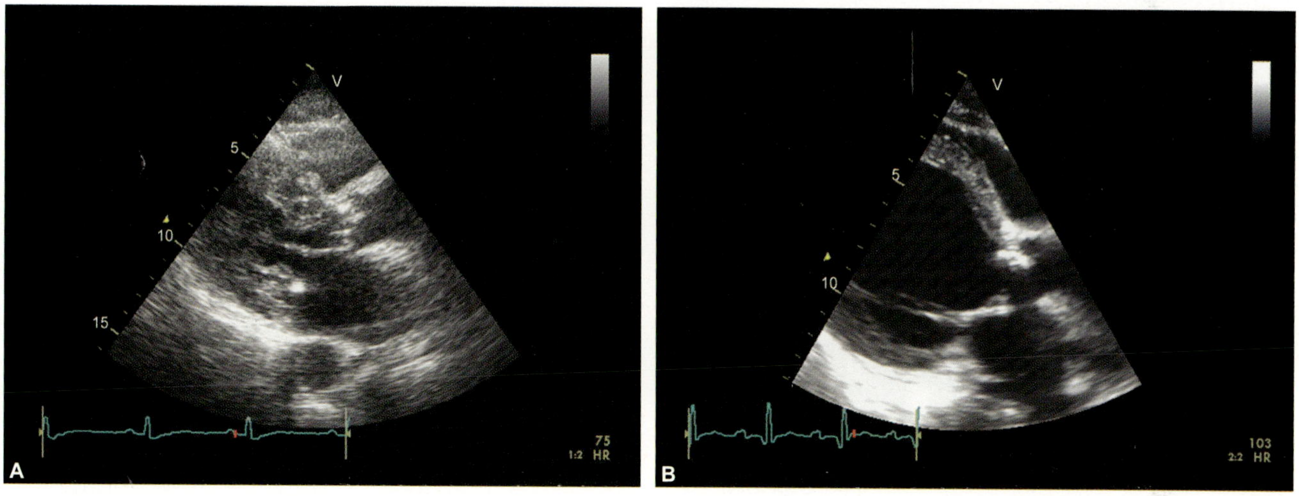

Figs. 13A and B: (A) Left ventricular (LV) hypertrophy and small LV cavity associated with low-flow low-gradient aortic stenosis with preserved LV ejection fraction, and (B) Dilated LV cavity with LV dysfunction associated with low-flow low-gradient aortic stenosis with reduced LV ejection fraction.

ascending aorta (Figs. 12A and B). The aortic sinuses and ascending aorta may show significant atherosclerotic plaques in patients with calcific AS. Aorta should be assessed with TTE and TEE and in certain cases computerized tomography scan or cardiac magnetic resonance imaging may be required.

Left Ventricular Hypertrophy

Left ventricular hypertrophy occurs frequently in patients with significant AS. LVH is more marked when AS is associated with HTN resulting in a small LV cavity (Figs. 13A and B). This may produce the low-flow low-gradient AS with preserved LVEF especially in women since they have smaller LV size. The LVH is marked and asymmetric in patients with hypertrophic cardiomyopathy, and hence different when compared to AS patients.

Left Ventricular Function

Left ventricular function is maintained till the late stages of AS. Once LV function starts decreasing the patients becomes symptomatic with a downhill course. On the other hand, AVR in patients with early symptoms improves LV function, reduces LVH, apart from improving symptoms and survival. The LV volumes, LVEF can be measured by 2DE and 3DE.

Left Atrium

Left atrium may be dilated due to LVH and patients with grade 2 and grade 3 diastolic dysfunctions have much more dilatation of LA. E/e′ can be used to assess the elevation in LV filling pressure. In advanced cases, there is PH and the right atrial pressure is increased with hepatic venous congestion.

REFERENCES

1. Sathyamurthy I, Jayanthi K. Asymptomatic severe aortic stenosis with normal left ventricular function: a review. Indian Heart J. 2016;68(4):576-80.
2. Nishimura RA, Otto CM, Bonow RO, et al. 2014 AHA/ACC guideline for the management of patients with valvular heart disease: Executive summary: A report of the American College of Cardiology/American Heart Association Task Force on Practice Guidelines. Circulation. 2014;129(23):2440-92.
3. Baumgartner H, Hung J, Bermejo J, et al. American Society of Echocardiography; European Association of Echocardiography. Echocardiographic assessment of valve stenosis: EAE/ASE recommendations for clinical practice. J Am Soc Echocardiogr. 2009;22(1):1-23.
4. Rajani R, Hancock J, Chambers JB. The art of assessing aortic stenosis. Heart. 2012;98(Suppl 4):iv14-22.
5. Pandian NG, Ramamurthi A, Applebaum S. Role of echocardiography in aortic stenosis. Prog Cardiovasc Dis. 2014;57(1):47-54.
6. Everett RJ, Newby DE, Jabbour A, et al. The role of imaging in aortic valve disease. Curr Cardiovasc Imaging Rep. 2016;9:21.
7. Badiani S, van Zalen J, Treibel TA, et al. Aortic stenosis: a left ventricular disease: Insights from advanced imaging. Curr Cardiol Rep. 2016;18(8):80.
8. Clavel MA, Magne J, Pibarot P. Low-gradient aortic stenosis. Eur Heart J. 2016;37(34):2645-57.
9. Izumi C. Asymptomatic severe aortic stenosis: Challenges in diagnosis and management. Heart. 2016;102(15):1168-76.
10. Rashedi N, Otto CM. Aortic stenosis: Changing disease concepts. J Cardiovasc Ultrasound. 2015;23(2):59-69.
11. Garbi M, Chambers J, Vannan MA, et al. Valve stress echocardiography: A practical guide for referral, procedure, reporting, and clinical implementation of results from the HAVEC group. JACC Cardiovasc Imaging. 2015;8(6):724-36.
12. Saikrishnan N, Kumar G, Sawaya FJ, et al. Accurate assessment of aortic stenosis: A review of diagnostic modalities and hemodynamics. Circulation. 2014;129(2):244-53.
13. Heuvelman HJ, van Geldorp MW, Eijkemans MJ, et al. Progression of aortic valve stenosis in adults: A systematic review. J Heart Valve Dis. 2012;21(4):454-62.
14. Pibarot P, Dumesnil JG. Improving assessment of aortic stenosis. J Am Coll Cardiol. 2012;60(3):169-80.
15. Ozkan A, Kapadia S, Tuzcu M, et al. Assessment of left ventricular function in aortic stenosis. Nat Rev Cardiol. 2011;8(9):494-501.

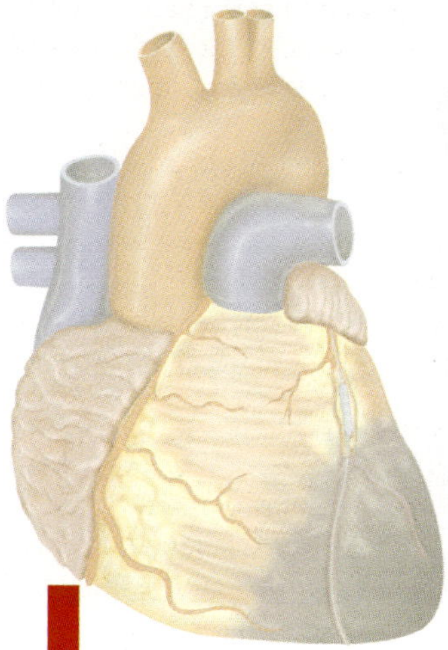

59

CHAPTER

Advances in Echocardiographic Evaluation of Aortic Regurgitation

Simmi Manocha, Kumar Hrishikesh, Prateek Bajaj

INTRODUCTION

Aortic valve disease is the most common form of heart valve disease in developed countries.[1] Imaging remains pivotal to the diagnosis and risk stratification of patients with both aortic stenosis (AS) and aortic regurgitation (AR) and has traditionally been performed with echocardiography. Indeed, echocardiography remains the cornerstone of aortic valve imaging in patients of AR, as it is cheap, widely available, and provides critical information concerning valve hemodynamic and ventricular function and helps in deciding medical/surgical management of disease. Nowadays advancement in various echocardiographic techniques and availability of advance machines ensures more precise and detailed evaluation of AR.

ASSESSMENT OF AORTIC REGURGITATION

Assessment of AR includes study of jet direction and its quantification. It should also include information about anatomy and functioning of aortic cusps, aortic root, ascending aorta, left ventricular (LV) dimensions, and systolic function of LV. Assessment of severity of AR is more nuanced than AS, requiring the integration of different visual, semi-quantitative, and quantitative parameters as recommended by clinical guidelines.[2,3]

DIAGNOSIS

Study of Valve Morphology

Traditional modalities M-mode and 2D-Echo provide good assessment of aortic valve anatomy, whether it is tricuspid (normal), bicuspid, monocuspid or quadricuspid. Cusp pathology is also very important to diagnose the etiology of AR, whether cusps are retracted (rheumatic), calcified (senile), perforated, or prolapsed (myxomatous) and noncoapting. With above information, we can utilize Carpentier classification of AR (Table 1).[4] However, modalities like 3D-Echo and TEE allow more precise examination of aortic cusps morphology, which is important for deciding surgical intervention.

Aortic Root and Ascending Aorta Dimensions

Though computed tomography (CT) aortogram is the gold standard for measuring ascending aorta and aortic root dimension, but 2D-Echo and transesophageal echocardiography (TEE) also provides good alternative. Measuring aortic root and ascending aorta is important for functional (Carpentier's) classification of AR (Table 1) and deciding need of replacement of aortic root/ascending aorta with/without aortic valve replacement (i.e. Bentall procedure). Normally patient with severe AR with aortic

TABLE 1: Carpentier's classification.[5]

Dysfunction	Echo finding
I. Enlargement of the aortic root with normal cusps	Dilatation of any component of aortic root (Annulus, sinus of valsalva, sinotubular junction)
IIa. Cusp prolapse with eccentric AR jet (cusp flail) partial/whole cusp prolapse	Complete eversion of a cusp/ cusp prolapse into the LVOT in long-axis views
IIb. Free edge fenestration with eccentric AR jet	Presence of an eccentric AR jet without definite evidence of cusp prolapse
III. Poor cusp quality or quantity	Thickened and rigid valves with reduced motion, tissue destruction (endocarditis), large calcification spots/ extensive calcification of all cusps interfering with cusps motion

(LVOT: left ventricular outflow tract; AR; aortic regurgitation)

root diameter more than or equal to 55 mm, more than or equal to 50 mm for bicuspid aortic valve, and more than or equal to 45 mm for myxomatous aortic valve, patient needs aortic root replacement (Bentall procedure).

Quantification of Aortic Regurgitation Jet

Quantification of AR jet can be done by various methods, which can be broadly divided into qualitative, semiquantitative, and quantitative methods.

Qualitative methods include:

- *AR jet width ratio to left ventricular outflow tract (LVOT) diameter* (>65% makes it severe)[6]
- *Continuous wave (CW) signal of AR jet*: Although CW AR Doppler jet density is a poor marker of severity, the rate of deceleration (pressure half-time, PHT) is a useful adjunct. A value of <250 ms is considered severe with measurements critically dependent on obtaining an aligned Doppler signal. PHT is best used in addition to other parameters as it is affected by LV compliance, blood pressure, and usually reduced in acute AR of any severity.
- *Diastolic flow reversal in proximal descending thoracic aorta* is measured by color M-mode and CW Doppler. Holodiastolic flow reversal in the descending aorta, especially when associated with an end-diastolic velocity of more than 20 cm/s, is specific but not sensitive for severe AR.[7]

Various *semiquantitative-quantitative methods include:*

- *Measuring vena contracta (VC) width*: Apical five-chamber view (for central jet) or parasternal long-axis view (PLAX)/apical three-chamber view (for eccentric jet) are preferred. Optimize color gain/scale. Reduce the color sector size and imaging depth to maximize frame rate. Expand the selected zone (Zoom). Use the cine loop to find the best frame for measurement. Measure the smallest VC (immediately distal to the regurgitant orifice, perpendicular to the direction of the jet).

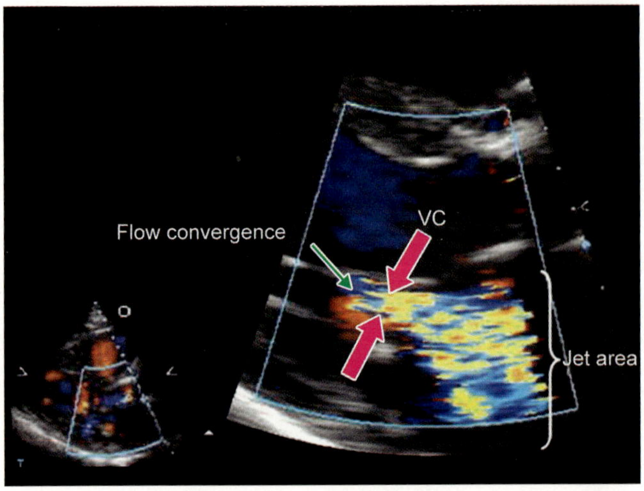

Fig. 1: Flow convergence.[8]

- *Calculation of effective orifice area (EROA) and regurgitant volume (RVol) by proximal isovelocity surface area (PISA) (Flow convergence method):* Apical five-chamber view (for central jet) or PLAX/apical three-chamber view (for eccentric jet) are preferred. Optimize color gain/scale of AR jet. Zoom the image of the regurgitant aortic valve. Increase the Nyquist limit in apical views/decrease or increase in PLAX. With the cine mode select the best PISA. Display the color off and on to visualize the AR orifice. Measure the PISA radius at diastole using the first aliasing and along the direction of the ultrasound beam. Measure AR peak velocity and time–velocity interval (TVI) (CW). Calculate flow rate, EROA, regurgitant volume of AR (Figs. 1 and 2).
- *Calculation of RVol and regurgitant fraction (RF) by Doppler volumetric method:* Flow across the mitral valve is measured by measuring the mitral inflow velocity–time integral (VTI) by placing the pulsed wave (PW) sample volume at the mitral annulus (apical four-chamber view) and mitral annulus diameter (d) at the maximal opening of the mitral valve (2–3 frames after the end systole) (Fig. 3 and Table 2).

  Mitral Inflow $= 0.785 \times$ *Mitral Inflow VTI* $\times d^2$

  Flow across the aortic valve is measured by calculating the LVOT VTI by placing the PW sample volume 5 mm below the aortic cusps (apical five-chamber view) and measuring the LVOT diameter (D) (parasternal long axis view).

  Aortic outflow $= 0.785 \times$ *LVOT VTI* $\times D^2$

  Regurgitant volume (RVol) = Mitral inflow – Aortic outflow

  Regurgitant fraction (RF) = (RVol/Aortic outflow) × 100

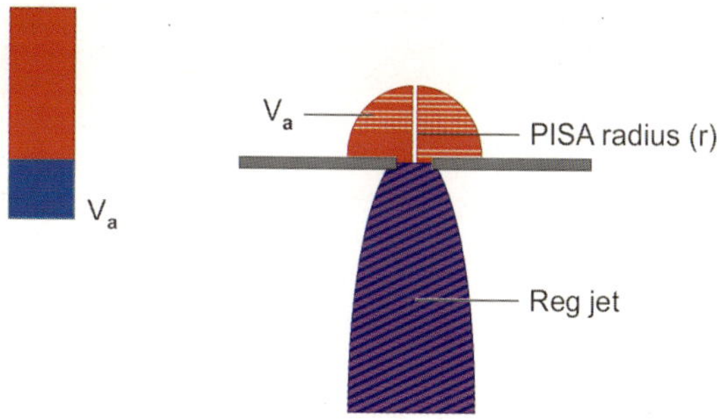

$$\text{Reg flow} = 2\pi r^2 \times V_a$$
$$\text{EROA} = \text{Reg flow} / \text{Pk } V_{Reg}$$

Fig. 2: Flow convergence method.[8]

Grading of Aortic Regurgitation

On the basis of above qualitative and quantitative methods, AR is divided into mild, moderate, and severe grades as tabulated in Table 3.

KEY POINTS

- Wherever possible, the measurement of vena contracta width is recommended to quantity AR. VC of more than or equal to 0.6 cm indicates severe AR
- PISA method is highly recommended to quantity the severity of AR. It can be used both in central and eccentric jet of AR. An ERDA more than or equal to 0.3 cm^2 and RVol more than or equal to 60 mL indicates severe AR
- Measurement of diastolic flow reversal for proximal DTA is recommended, when assessable. It is the strongest addition parameter to evaluate AR severity (end-diastolic velocity more than 20 cm/s, is specific marker of severe AR)

Assessment of Left Ventricular Dimension and Systolic Function

Exact quantification of LV dimension is important in knowing the chronicity of AR, deciding time of surgery, deciding prognosis of AR. Asymptomatic patient with severe

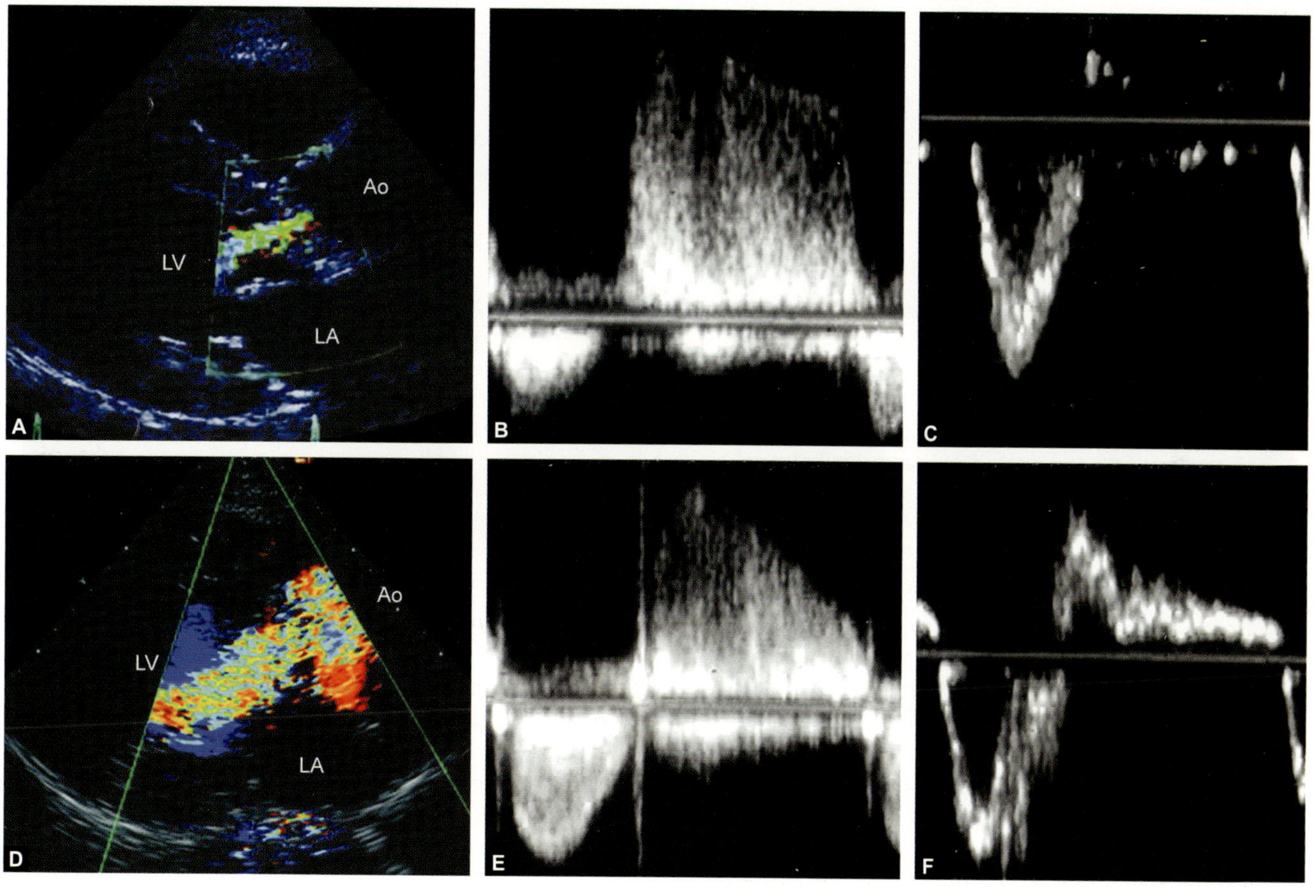

Figs. 3A to F: Echo Doppler evaluation of aortic regurgitation (AR): Panels A, B, C—mild AR; panels D, E, F—severe AR. (A) Narrow color Doppler jet in mild AR (parasternal long-axis view). (B) Continuous wave (CW) Doppler tracing in mild AR (slow velocity-decay). (C) Pulsed wave (PW) Doppler tracing from the descending aorta (suprasternal approach) in mild AR (minimal diastolic flow reversal). (D) Broad color Doppler jet and large convergence zone in severe AR (parasternal long-axis view). (E) CW Doppler tracing in severe AR (steep diastolic velocity decay). (F) PW Doppler tracing from the descending aorta (suprasternal approach) in severe AR (holodiastolic flow reversal). (Ao: aorta; LA: left atrium; LV: left ventricle)[8]

TABLE 2: Echocardiographic parameters used to quantify aortic regurgitation severity, their advantages, and limitations.[5]

Parameters	*Usefulness/Advantages*	*Limitations*
• Valve morphology • Color flow AR jet width and area	• Flail valve (if visualized), is specific for significant AR • Ease of use • Evaluates the spatial orientation of AR jet • Quick screen for AR	• Other abnormalities are non-specific of significant AR • Influenced by technical and hemodynamic factors • Inaccurate for eccentric jet • Expands unpredictably below the orifice • Not valid for multiple jets
• VC width	• Relatively quick and easy. • Relatively independent of hemodynamics and instrumentation factors • Not affected by other valve leak • Can be used in eccentric jet	• Small values; small measurement errors lead to large % error • Intermediate values need confirmation • Affected by systolic charges in regurgitant flow
• PISA method	• Can be used in eccentric jet • *Quantitative:* Estimate lesion severity (EROA) and volume overload (RVol)	• *PISA shape affected:* – by the aliasing velocity – in the case of noncircular orifice – by systolic changes in regurgitant flow – by adjacent structures (flow constrainment) • PISA radius is more a hemiellipse • Interobserver variability • Not valid for multiple jets • Feasibility limited by aortic valve calcifications
• Doppler volumetric method (PW)	• *Quantitative:* Estimate lesion severity (ERO) and volume overload (RVol) • Valid in multiple jets	• Time consuming • *Requires multiple measurements:* Source of errors • Not applicable in the case of significant MR (use the pulmonic site)
• CW AR jet profile	• Simple	• Qualitative, complementary finding • Complete signal difficult to obtain in eccentric jet
• Pressure half time	• Simple	• Affected by LV compliance, blood pressure, acuity of AR
• Diastolic flow reversal in descending aorta	• End-diastolic velocity of >20 cm/s is specific for chronic significant AR	• Affected by sample volume location and acuity of AR • Affected by aortic compliance • Brief velocity reversal is normal • Cut-off validated for distal aortic arch

(AR: aortic regurgitation; CW: continuous-wave; EROA: effective regurgitant orifice area; LV: left ventricle; PISA: proximal isovelocity surface area; PW: pulse wave; RVol: regurgitant volume; VC: vena contracta)

AR with LV end-systolic diameter (LVESD) more than 50 mm is a class-I indication for aortic valve surgery (Table 4).[7-10] Similarly exact estimation of LV systolic function (LVEF) is needed for deciding time of surgery and prognosticating it. Asymptomatic patient with severe AR with LVEF less than 50% is a class-I indication of aortic valve surgery.

Precise 2D-Echo is sufficient for LV dimension measurement, but use of contrast agent is done for better endocardial visualization (when endocardium is less than 80% visualized) and *3D-Echo modality* is better method for LV dimension and LV volume measurement. Similarly biplane summation method (Simpson's) is adequate for LVEF measurement, but in borderline LVEF cases (i.e. LVEF: 50–55%), use of *tissue Doppler imaging (TDI) and 2D and 3D speckle-tracking method (Longitudinal and radial strain imaging)* are more sensitive methods. A tissue Doppler peak systolic velocity of medial annulus less than 9.5 cm/s, indicates poor exercise response. Similarly, average global longitudinal strain value less than 16 indicates early systolic dysfunction of LV with borderline normal LVEF.

Exercise echocardiography (stress echo) is another modality useful in predicting outcome in patient in severe AR, who is appropriately asymptomatic at rest. It also indicates absence of contractile reserve of LV. In case of

TABLE 3: Grading the severity of aortic regurgitation[5]

Parameters	*Mild*	*Moderate*	*Severe*
Qualitative:			
Aortic valve morphology	Normal/Abnormal	Normal/Abnormal	Abnormal/flail/large coaptation defect
Color flow AR jet width	Small in central jets (<25% of LVOT)	Intermediate (25%–65% of LVOT)	Large in central jet (>65% of LVOT diameter), variable in eccentric jets
CW signal of AR jet*	Incomplete/faint	Dense	Dense
Diastolic flow reversal in descending thoracic aorta	Brief, early diastolic flow reversal	Intermediate	Holodiastolic flow reversal (end-diastolic velocity >20 cm/s)
Semiquantitative:			
VC width (mm)	<3	3–6	>6
Pressure half time (ms) †	>500	250–500	<250
Quantitative (PISA):			
EROA‡ (cm^2)	<0.1	0.1–0.29	≥0.3
R Vol§ (mL)	<30	30–59	≥60
RF & LV Size‖	<30%	30–49%	≥50%

(AR: aortic regurgitation; CW: continuous-wave; LA: left atrium; EROA: effective regurgitant orifice area; LV: left ventricle; RVol: regurgitant volume; RF: regurgitant fraction; VC: vena contracta)

*At Nyquist limit of 50–60 cm/s.

†Pressure half-time (PHT) is shortened with increasing LV diastolic pressure, vasodilator therapy and in patients with a dilated compliant aorta or lengthened in chronic AR.

‡ EROA = Flow/Max AR jet velocity,

§R Vol = EROA X (VTI of AR jet CW).

‖Unless for other reasons, the LV size is usually normal in patients with mild AR. In acute severe AR, the LV size is often normal. In chronic AR, the LV is classically dilated. Accepted cut-off values for nonsignificant LV enlargement are LV end-diastolic diameter <56 mm, LV end-diastolic volume <82 mL/m^2, LV end-systolic diameter <40 mm, LV end-systolic volume <30 mL/m^2.

decrease in LVEF by 5% at exercise, is useful in predicting time of surgery and prognosticating patients with severe AR with borderline LVEF (50–55%) or borderline LVESD (~50 mm).

MANAGEMENT OF AORTIC REGURGITATION

Medical Therapy

Medical therapy can provide symptomatic improvement in individuals with chronic severe AR, in whom surgery is not feasible. In these patients medical therapy with use of angiotensin-converting enzyme (ACE) inhibitors/ angiotensin-receptor blockers (ARBs) and beta-blockers is reasonable.[13,14] Treatment of hypertension [systolic blood pressure (SBP) >140 mm Hg] is recommended in patients with chronic severe AR preferably with dihydropyridine calcium channel blockers (CCBs) or ACE or ARBs.[15] Diuretics are used for symptoms if patient is in heart failure. In asymptomatic patients with severe AR careful follow-up of symptomatic status and LV size and LV function is mandatory.

TABLE 4: The European Society of Cardiology/ European Association for Cardio-Thoracic Surgery (ESC/EACTS) Guidelines 2017.

Indications for surgery	*Class*	*Level*
Severe aortic regurgitation		
Surgery is indicated in symptomatic patients[9-12]	I	B
Surgery is indicated in asymptomatic patients with resting LVEF≤50%[9,10]	I	B
Surgery is indicated in patients undergoing CABG or surgery of the ascending aorta or of another valve	I	C
Heart team discussion is recommended in selected patients in whom aortic valve repair may be a feasible alternative to valve replacement	I	C
Surgery should be considered in asymptomatic patients with resting ejection fraction > 50% with severe LV dilatation: LVEDD > 70 mm or LVESD > 50 (or LVESD > 25 mm/m^2 BSA in patients with small body size)[9,11]	IIa	B

(CABG: coronary artery bypass grafting; LVEF: left ventricular ejection fraction; LVEDD: left ventricular end-diastolic diameter; LVESD: left ventricular end-systolic diameter)

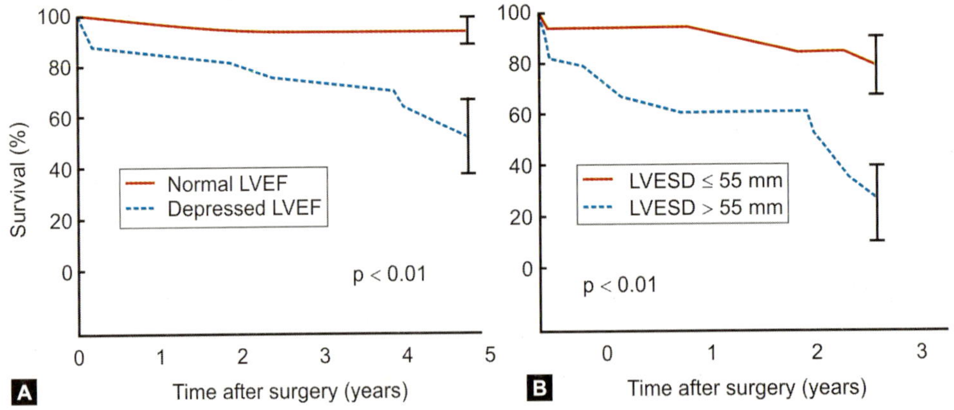

Figs. 4A and B: Prognosis of aortic regurgitation (AR) patient after surgery on left ventricular ejection fraction (LVEF) and LV end systolic diameter (LVESD) indices.[16,17]

Surgical Management

Surgical management includes aortic valve replacement (AVR) with or without aortic root replacement (i.e. Bentall procedure). Normally patient with severe AR with aortic root diameter more than 55 mm, more than 50 mm for bicuspid aortic valve and more than or equal to 45 mm for myxomatous aortic valve, patient needs aortic root replacement (Bentall procedure).

Though conservative approach of the surgical management is open heart surgery for AVR, but newer modality of surgery is transcatheter aortic valve replacement (TAVR).

Indications for surgery in (A) severe aortic regurgitation and (B) aortic root disease (irrespective of the severity of aortic regurgitation).

The strongest indication for valve surgery is presence of symptoms (spontaneous or on exercise testing) and/or the documentation of LVEF less than 50% and/or LV systolic diameter more than 50 mm.

Prognosis of AR patient after surgery on LVEF and LVESD indices: Low LVEF and LVESD, adversely affect postsurgery survival time of AR patients as depicted in Figures 4A and B.

Transcatheter Aortic Valve Replacement in Aortic Regurgitation

The use of TAVR for pure AR presents several potential challenges, as these devices are specifically designed for stenotic aortic valves.

A registry study done[18] in 2017 showed a relatively high procedural success rate and relatively low rate of cardiovascular death in selected patients undergoing TAVR for severe native AR. Newer devices had significantly higher success rates, with markedly lower rates of significant AR and need for second valve implantation. These improvements likely represent improved valve design and procedural techniques and much of the differences was driven by changes between the *older CoreValve device and the newer Evolut R device.* Based on results of limited data it may be reasonable to consider TAVR for pure AR on a case-to-case basis when patients are not candidates for surgical AVR and more long-term follow-up and further randomized control trials (RCTs) are required to determine the appropriate role of TAVR in this population.

CONCLUSION

Although various newer modalities of echocardiography are now available for more accurate diagnosis and quantification of AR, which help us in timely diagnosis and early start of medical/surgical management of the patient; but further research (RCTs) are needed for effective newer modality of treatment, i.e. TAVR. Extensive utility of newer modalities like strain imaging, 3D-Echo, and advanced TEE, will help us further for precise diagnosis and quantification of AR.

REFERENCES

1. Nkomo VT, Gardin JM, Skelton TN, et al. Burden of valvular heart diseases: A population-based study. Lancet. 2006;368:1005-11.
2. Joint task force on the management of valvular heart disease of the European Society of Cardiology (ESC), European Association for Cardio-Thoracic Surgery (EACTS), Vahanian A, et al. Guidelines on the management of valvular heart disease (version 2012). Eur Heart J. 2012;33(19):2451-96.
3. Nishimura RA, Otto CM, Bonow RO, et al. 2014 AHA/ACC guideline for the management Of patients with valvular heart disease: executive summary: A report of the American

College of Cardiology/American Heart Association Task Force on Practice Guidelines. Circulation. 2014;129(33):2440-92.

4. El Khoury G, Glineur D, Rubay J, et al. Functional classification of aortic root/valve abnormalities and their correlation with etiologies and surgical procedures. Curr Opin Cordial. 2005;20:115-21.
5. Recommendations for the valvular regurgitation: Part 1: Aortic regurgitation (Native Valve Disease).
6. Perry GJ, Helmcke F, Nanda NC, et al. Evaluation of aortic insufficiency by Doppler color flow mapping. JACC. 1987;9:952-9.
7. Tribouilloy C, Avinée P, Shen WF, et al. End diastolic flow velocity just beneath the aortic isthmus assessed by pulsed Doppler echocardiography: A new predictor of the aortic regurgitant fraction. Br Heart J. 1991;65:37-40.
8. American Society of Echocardiography: recommendations for evaluation of the severity of native valvular regurgitation with two-dimensional and Doppler echocardiography: A report from the American Society of Echocardiography's Nomenclature and Standards Committee and The Task Force on Valvular Regurgitation, developed in conjunction with the American College of Cardiology Echocardiography Committee, The Cardiac Imaging Committee, Council on Clinical Cardiology, The American Heart Association, and the European Society of Cardiology Working Group on Echocardiography.
9. Chaliki HP, Mohty D, Avierinos JF, et al. Outcomes after AVR in patients with severe AR & reduced LV function. Circulation. 2002;106:2687-93.
10. Tomos P, Sambola A, Permanyer-Miralda G, et al. Long-term outcome of surgically treated AR: influence of guideline adherence towards early surgery. J AM Coll Cardiol. 2017;69:1372-82.
11. Dujrdin KS, Enriquez-Sarano M, Schaff HV, et al. Mortality and morbidity of AR in clinical practice. a long-term follow-up study. Circulation. 1999:99:1851-7.
12. Klodas-E, Enrique-Sarano M, Tajik AJ, et al. Optimizing timing of surgical correction in patients with AR: Role of symptoms. J AM Coll Cardiol. 1997:30;746-52.
13. Zendaoui A, Lachance D, Roussel E, et al. Usefulness of Carvidelol in treatment of chronic AR. Circ Heart Fail. 2011;4:207-13.
14. Elder DH, Wei L, Szwejkowski BR, et al. The impact of reinin angiotensin-aldosterone system blockade on heart failure outcomes & mortality In patients having AR. A large population cohort study. J AM Coll Cardiol. 2011;58:2084-91.
15. Nishimura RA, Otto CM, Bonow RO, et al. 2014 AHA/ACC guideline for the management of patients with valvular heart disease. Circulation. 2014;129(23):e521-643.
16. Bonow RO, Picone AL, McIntosh CL, et al. Survival and functional results after valve replacement for aortic regurgitation from 1976 to 1983: Impact of preoperative left ventricular function. Circulation. 1985;72:1244-56.
17. Bonow RO, Rosing DR, Kent KM, et al. Timing of operation for chronic aortic regurgitation. Am J Cardiol. 1982;50:325-36.
18. Yoon SH, Schmidt T, Bleiziffer S, et al. Transcatheter aortic valve replacement in pure native aortic valve regurgitation. J Am Coll Cardiol. 2017;70:2752-63.

60

CHAPTER

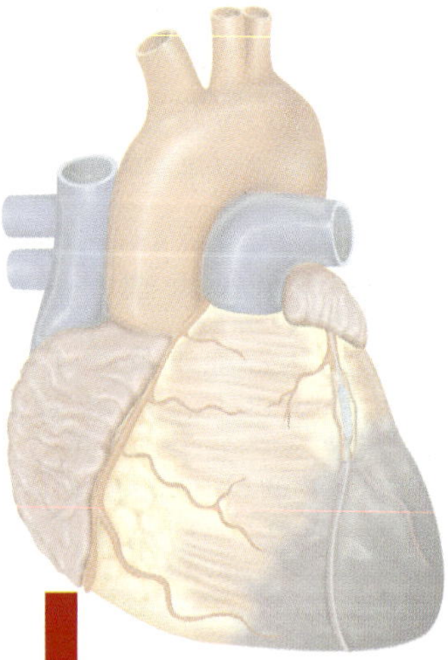

Transcatheter Aortic Valve Replacement Imaging Evaluation: Status 2018

R Keshava, Satish Govind

INTRODUCTION

Aortic stenosis (AS) was first described by French physician Lazare Rivière in 1663.[1] Major causes of valvular AS include rheumatic heart disease (RHD), degenerative calcific stenosis, and bicuspid aortic valve. Bicuspid and degenerative calcific AS is common in western world and rheumatic AS common in the developing world. It is estimated that around 2% of the population above the age of 65 years have AS.[2] The treatment of AS has evolved from balloon aortic valvotomy to valve repair or valve replacement.

The population at risk for AS is growing.[3] The elderly population will be more than double between now and the year 2050.[4] AS is also more likely to affect men than women, 80% of adults with symptomatic AS being male.[5] Patients may live with AS for many years during a latent, asymptomatic period even before symptoms of the disease develop and present. However, once patients begin experiencing symptoms, it is urgent they receive some form of interventional treatment.

AORTIC VALVE REPLACEMENT

Open-Heart Surgery

Surgical aortic valve replacement (SAVR) through open-heart surgery is a more invasive approach for treating severe AS. It has been performed over decades on patients who need valve replacement using either a mechanical or tissue valve. Aortic valve replacement can also be performed through minimal incision valve surgery (MIVS). During MIVS, the surgeon replaces the diseased valve through a smaller incision; however, cardiopulmonary bypass is still used. MIVS is an option for some patients who are candidates for surgery.

Transcatheter Approach

For patients suffering from severe AS unless determined to be at low surgical risk for traditional open-heart surgery, transcatheter aortic valve replacement (TAVR) may be another treatment option. TAVR is a less invasive procedure that does not require open-heart surgery. During the TAVR procedure, a bioprosthetic valve is inserted over a diseased native aortic valve. The TAVR procedure can be performed through multiple approaches (transfemoral, transapical, or transaortic). This procedure was approved in Europe in 2007 and in United States of America in 2011. With increasing clinical experience, outcomes of TAVR have continuously improved since the time it was first introduced. Early randomized controlled trials demonstrated that it is a therapeutic option in patients who are inoperable.[5] Later, it was found to be an effective treatment option in patients at high risk for surgery. Prospective randomized data from the PARTNER-B (Placement of Aortic Transcatheter Valve) cohort have demonstrated that it is superior to medical therapy in inoperable patients up to 5 years after valve implantation[6] Reardon et al. have compared the 2-year outcome of TAVR versus SAVR in patients at high risk which showed that TAVR has lower mortality.[7]

New data from randomized intermediate-risk patients in PARTNER-2 trial have again demonstrated no difference in 1-year mortality between TAVR and SAVR, with the lowest mortality observed in transfemoral TAVR patients.[8] It has been observed in TAVR that major bleeding complications were reduced and need for permanent pacemaker was less, but it showed higher risks of vascular access complications, paravalvular leak, and conduction blocks when compared to SAVR. Apart from these promising outcomes in native aortic valve disease, TAVR has also been identified as a treatment option in patients with tissue valve failure, who potentially may need redo-SAVR.[9] An important issue to consider is that the present studies on TAVR outcomes have focused on patients with mean age of 80 years, while there are scant data available for outcomes in younger patients. Hence, existing data on TAVR do not truly represent the general cohort of AS and also do not apply in multivalvar disease (especially in RHD) as also coexisting significant coronary artery disease (CAD), bicuspid or unicuspid aortic valves, and small aortic annulus. In such scenarios, it has to be seen how the outcomes of TAVR would vary with such a wide variety of AS patients.

TYPES OF VALVES

Over time TAVR has undergone major advancements, transforming a complex intervention into a safe and acceptable procedure. The newest generation of valves has been designed so as to facilitate easy deployment, capable of being repositioned and also have retrieval capability.[10] They can be categorized as balloon-expandable and self-expanding according to the type of deployment. A TAVR valve is usually made by suturing three leaflets (porcine or bovine pericardium) with a skirt and a self-expanding frame made of nitinol.

EVOLUT R, the CoreValve (Medtronic) is made from porcine pericardial tissue; it has three leaflets mounted inside a self-expandable nitinol frame.[11] It is designed such that it allows for self-expansion and exclusion of the native calcified valve and is supported by a stent. It has the capacity of recapturability and repositionability along with other improvements in its design.

SAPIEN 3 heart valve (Edwards Lifesciences) is the most recent in the Sapien series of valves. It has a cobalt-chromium frame, three bovine pericardial leaflets, with an inflow portion skirt and an outer sealing skirt to minimize paravalvular leaks.[12]

PORTICO valve (St. Jude Medical) is a self-expanding stent, made of bovine leaflets and a porcine pericardial sealing cuff. The larger area and annular positioning allow for a convenient implantation with respect to coronary ostia. The large area of the device minimizes paravalvular leak as it adjusts and adapts around the calcific nodules present at the annulus.

ACURATE NEO (Symetis) is a valve with flaps composed of porcine pericardium sewn into a stent made of self-expanding nitinol, covered both outside and inside by a porcine pericardial skirt. The valve has three arches for stabilization along with an axial alignment to the aortic annulus and a crown at the top with a bottom that can fully align on the native valve.[13]

JENAVALVE (JenaValve Technology GmbH) is a porcine valve mounted on a self-expanding nitinol stent.[14] It is available as either a stentless (Elan valve, Vascutek Ltd.) or stented (Aspire valve, Vascutek Ltd.) for surgical bioprosthesis. The porcine root leaflets are connected to the flexible stent to reduce leaflet stress during diastole. The special feature of this prosthesis is that it relies on active clip fixation to the native aortic leaflets, which provides for secure anchorage even when there are no calcifications. It is the only valve to have a CE Mark approval for noncalcified aortic regurgitation (AR).[15]

ALLEGRA (NVT AG) is a self-expandable valve with a nitinol stent frame and bovine pericardium (annular skirt and leaflets). The annular portion of the frame has a sealing skirt above which the leaflets are sewn where this forms the functional portion and is positioned supra-annular.

LOTUS (Boston Scientific Corporation) valve consists of a trileaflet bovine pericardial valve supported on a nitinol frame. This frame is covered with an adaptive seal at the inflow segment that adapts to the uneven surface of the aortic root and limits paravalvular leak.[16] This is the only latest generation valve that is recapturable and repositionable even after the valve has been completely deployed.[17] However, it has a high rate of conduction disturbances needing pacemaker implantation, which has led to further changes in the newer generation Lotus Edge valve.[18]

The evolution of TAVR over the last decade has made this into a routine and widely used intervention with complication rates progressively declining. This is because of better valve design along with cumulative experience of operators and mounting data, which has led to standardization of the procedure. But despite such improvements, there still exists complications that can affect procedural outcomes.[19]

IMAGING

An ideal center for TAVR (and also those doing complex aortic valve surgeries) should have extended imaging diagnostic facilities, such as three-dimensional (3D) echocardiography, transesophageal echocardiography (TEE), stress echocardiography, computerized tomography

(CT) scan, magnetic resonance imaging (MRI), and also positron emission tomography (PET)-CT apart from an advanced catheterization laboratory. Role of two-dimensional (2D) echocardiography in TEE is limited due to its inability to provide crucial imaging planes and views when compared to 3D TEE.

Vascular Access Site Imaging

Transfemoral route is the preferred approach in TAVR. Despite the reduced size of delivery systems and sheaths sizes of present day, vascular complications are seen in about 16% of all transfemoral procedures.[20] The complications are divided as bleeding complications, dissections, and vascular occlusions after removal of the sheath.

There are several well-defined risk factors for access related or vascular complications including sheath to artery ratio, circumferential calcification, and severe tortuosity. It is important to bear these factors in mind during the preinterventional workup in order to choose an adequate access strategy. Arterial Doppler could be done to delineate the access site and calculate sheath to artery ratio and areas of calcification. A groin shoot with contrast also helps to determine the tortuosity, branches, and stenosis before beginning the procedure.[21] But, presently, a preprocedural CT scan is widely advocated to examine aorta and peripheral arterial/femoral vessels since it provides comprehensive information about the vasculature for vascular access planning. Minimum specifications for a CT scanner required for vascular imaging are at least 64 detectors, a minimum spatial resolution of 0.6 mm, and a workstation, which can offer 3D reconstruction.

Vascular complications are less seen in transapical approach in comparison to a transvascular route. It is suggested that TEE should routinely be performed just before and after a transapical procedure. In the case of worsening of patient's condition or an unstable patient, intraprocedural TEE helps to detect complications, such as an apical tear or rupture which has led to cardiac tamponade.[22]

Cardiac Imaging

Transthoracic echocardiography (TTE) is presently the imaging modality of choice when diagnosing significant AS, in periprocedural TAVR guidance and at follow-up for assessing valve gradients, the severity of AR and left ventricular (LV) function. TEE is used to better assess the location and severity of paravalvular leaks. It can also detect complications, such as impingement of coronary ostia [(by detecting new regional wall motion abnormalities (RWMA)], dislodgment and migration of device, new or increasing pericardial effusion, aortic dissection, and mitral regurgitation (MR).[23,24]

Angiography is used if there is any suspicion of coronary involvement post TAVR and to also identify iliofemoral access site complications. Newer imaging techniques, such as 3D rotational angiography and C-arm CT, appear promising for improving the success and safety of TAVR procedures.[25,26] The role of multidimensional CT (MDCT) in follow-up imaging is still yet to be established.

Patient Selection

Patient selection is very important for TAVR. The 2014 American College of Cardiology valvular heart disease guidelines give a class I recommendation for heart team evaluation of patient for TAVR, where one of the most important roles of this multidisciplinary team is patient selection. Imaging forms an integral part to assess and identify patients who are likely to benefit from TAVR. Patients with asymmetrical or severe calcifications, unfavorable aortic root morphology, LV thrombus, bicuspid valves, severe CAD, severe primary mitral valve disease, severe tricuspid regurgitation (TR), ascending aorta aneurysm, hypertrophic obstructive cardiomyopathy requiring myomectomy, and low-set coronary ostia may benefit from SAVR, and these patients are identified with multi-imaging modalities.

Society of Thoracic Surgeons score as a risk assessment model utilizes multiple parameters, including clinical and laboratory parameters.[27] Imaging parameters include valve status, LV function, peripheral arteriopathy, and coronary anatomy.[28] EuroSCORE (ES) (European System for Cardiac Operative Risk Evaluation) is a risk model, which allows the calculation of the risk of death after a heart operation and needs 17 parameters of information about the patient.[29] Three of these parameters require imaging—extracardiac arteriopathy, LV function, and pulmonary hypertension (PH). Patients are scored as low, intermediate, and high risk for TAVR, ES < 10% low, ES between 10% and 20% intermediate, and ES > 20% high.

Transcatheter aortic valve replacement as a valve-in-valve (VIV) procedure is a treatment option for bioprosthetic valve failure, where redo surgery has increased morbidity. Though TAVR VIV has not been compared to SAVR, it has shown good results in high-risk older patients. Large bioprostheses show good hemodynamic improvements, while small prostheses result in increased transvalvular gradients which may lead to patient prosthesis mismatch.

Preprocedural

Annulus sizing: Proper sizing of the aortic annulus plays a critical role prior in device implantation. Unintentional undersizing of aortic annulus leads to paravalvular leak, while unintentional oversizing may cause bundle branch block, complete heart block (due to adjacent compression of the device), or annular rupture. The aortic annulus shape is frequently underestimated in the sagittal plane when measured in the parasternal long-axis view by 2D echocardiography. This method is not accurate; hence, it should not be used. The annulus most of the times is more oval than circular and becomes more elliptical with increasing severity of AS. As it constantly changes shape and size throughout the cardiac cycle, measurement is even more of a challenge. 3D TEE, which is superior to 2D TEE, measures (annulus size) in midsystole when the annulus is at its maximal size and when it is more likely to be circular (since it correlates more with TAVR devices which are circular). On the other hand, measurement by MDCT (annulus area) is made during diastole, though an optimal image at any point in the cardiac cycle is acceptable. MDCT when compared to TEE oversizes to some extent, though this has not caused any major errors in choosing the right device.

There is an interesting debate whether the annulus should be assessed by either area or perimeter measurements.[30] Though both of them have good correlation, it is thought that perimeter measurement would be superior, since area is more likely to underestimate due to the elliptical nature of the annulus in a severely stenotic valve. MDCT is presently the preferred approach to assess aortic annulus since 3D TEE tends to undersize by about 9–12%. TEE in TAVR for the sole purpose of annulus sizing is considered unnecessary though it can be an alternative in patients who have contraindications for contrast used in MDCT.[31] But it should be kept in mind that TEE is invaluable in clinical indications, such as assessment of ventricular function, valvular function, intracardiac pressures, etc. TEE can provide accurate and reliable information in the hands of a skilled and experienced operator. Attempts to study MRI in the assessment of aortic annulus size, aorta, and femoral vasculature for vascular access have shown good results, but no incremental value when compared to cardiac CT. It is inferior to cardiac CT in the measurement of internal diameters of vessel walls and in the detection of calcification.[32]

Low-gradient AS: The different types of low-gradient AS with its diagnostic challenges and adverse outcomes have drawn attention to this unique subgroup and its association with TAVR. Studies are underway to look at this special population with and without LV dysfunction where randomized studies are investigating medical therapy versus TAVR. Stress echocardiography is the preferred test in diagnosing patients with low flow, low-gradient AS with LV dysfunction.[33] It is only when there is a contraindication to stress echocardiography that MDCT has a role to play where it has focused on the aortic valve calcium burden and severity of AS. A recent study called TOPAS-TAVI (True Or Pseudo severe AS-Transcatheter Aortic Valve Implant) sought to look at outcomes and improvement in LV ejection fraction (LVEF) following TAVR in low-gradient AS. It showed good procedural outcomes, with low 30-day mortality, but one third of patients died at 2-year follow-up due to showing poor long-term outcomes.[34] Dobutamine stress echocardiography does not have the predictive capability to demonstrate LVEF improvement or adverse events, post TAVR. TAVR should be the preferred choice of treatment, especially for those having minimal or no LV contractile reserve.

Coronary arteries: 3D TEE not only assesses the annulus but can also visualize and delineate the coronary arteries and measure length of left coronary cusp to evaluate potential problem of coronary ostial obstruction when the device is deployed. The wide use of MDCT in various scenarios of TAVR has tempted investigators to look at its utility as an alternative to routine coronary angiography. Existing studies show mixed results varying from good sensitivity and specificity to a limited one, where only the left main stem, proximal or midlevel segments are better imaged. Extensive calcification seen in most TAVR patients is a limiting factor to visualize them. Once the technology of fractional flow reserve by CT improves, then probably MDCT can be considered a serious alternative to conventional coronary angiogram (CAG). At present, MDCT for coronary arteries is mainly useful in patients who have undergone coronary artery bypass grafts.

Periprocedural

With increasing operator experience over the years, the actual procedure of TAVR is now done under conscious sedation; in which, fluoroscopic imaging plays a prominent role. A minimalist approach has been adopted in recent years where there is more use of TTE than TEE. This has been shown to reduce procedural costs without affecting procedural success and outcome. On the other hand, studies show that the use of TEE in procedural guidance has shown lower mortality, reduced fluoroscopy time, reduced acute kidney injury, and decreased complications in randomized controlled trials. However, the use of TEE has gradually come down, and its present-day use is mainly restricted to detection of cardiac tamponade, RWMA, aortic dissection, and valvular regurgitation assessment. TTE is the preferred choice periprocedurally, and TEE is used only when needed or when TTE is providing limited images.

Hybrid or fusion imaging is another technique, which has been explored where fluoroscopy when combined with echocardiography has enabled operators to implant the device with more ease and success. Cardiac CT-fluoroscopy is another type of fusion imaging, a promising technique which has been investigated in some centers and found to be feasible. It is a complex piece of equipment having many technical layers, which poses formidable challenges when it is being used. At present, it is still a research tool, with potential to develop into a handy clinical application later.

Postprocedural

Data accumulated since the time TAVR first started has also provided new insights about certain echocardiographic parameters. More severe the diastolic dysfunction prior to TAVR and lack of reverse remodeling post TAVR is associated with increased 1-year mortality. Apart from this, other reasons for adverse prognosis in a patient scheduled for TAVR are significant PH, LV systolic dysfunction, and primary MR. Tricuspid annular diameter assessed at the time of patient selection can provide insights about worsening of TR post TAVR, which has been shown to be associated with increased 1-year mortality.

Imaging of TAVR valve in terms of its long-term durability and function is an area, which has scant data. Generally, the risk of structural valve degeneration is low in elderly patients in SAVR at 10 years, and as a natural corollary, it would be expected that the same should hold good for TAVR where such data is not available. But, with the present wide variety of designs that are now available for TAVR, obtaining data to predict its long-term outcome would be an extremely difficult exercise. At present, a good number of young patients are undergoing TAVR for whom there is no outcome data, and it is this group that needs particular attention where imaging should be focused to detect signs of early degeneration, valve dysfunction, etc. and to see its progress.

Just like any other device, the threat of infective endocarditis (IE) is ever present. Vegetations when present can be seen mainly on the leaflets and to a lesser extent on the stent frame, or both. Complications, such as abscesses, are seen more often than fistulas. Satellite lesions have been reported on the mitral valve with a small percentage showing secondary involvement.[35] TEE plays a leading role in the detection and diagnosis of IE, supported by CT, MRI, and PET as supportive imaging modalities. TEE detection of vegetations can be difficult in TAVR since different varieties of implants, type of implantation, remnants of the native valve, lack of sewing ring, significant calcification, and related artifacts can confound imaging. High transvalvular aortic gradients and atypical thickening of leaflets are frequently seen in IE and should arouse strong suspicion of IE. Cardiac CT can be helpful to delineate the prosthetic valve, perivalvular area, and periannular complications. PET-CT can also be used to look for active areas of IE, which has moderate sensitivity and specificity. A heart team approach combined with multimodality imaging can be quite effective in the diagnosis of IE in TAVR.

Coronary artery disease is a progressive disease, and this can be a challenge when imaging needs to be done in post TAVR patients to assess CAD. With the recent approach of TAVR implantation in younger patients, the onset of CAD at a later stage can pose challenges if and when CAG is considered. Difficulty in coronary ostial engagement has been encountered particularly in patients where the device has been implanted extending above the ostia and in self-expanding valves.[36] In situations where coronary status needs to be evaluated and difficulties in CAG are anticipated, a heart team approach is required, and decision can be taken if cardiac CT angiography would be a better option. If conventional CAG is necessary, a different approach may be planned with a slight change in technique and use of smaller catheters.

Strain by cardiac MRI in TAVR and SAVR patients has been another area that has been investigated, and it has been reported that rotational mechanics of LV decline 6 months after the procedure, while strain and strain rate remained unchanged.[37]

Recent data in low-risk patients undergoing TAVR shows that it is safe. Complications were reported to be low in accordance with the previous data of high-risk patients. Imaging of these patients showed no new RWMA or paravalvular leaks.

CONCLUSION

Since the early recommendations of TAVR, much has changed in terms of indications, technique, the types of devices implanted, and the role of imaging.[38,39] Multimodality imaging is increasingly being used, and it plays a central role in patient selection, procedural guidance, and postprocedural monitoring. 3D when compared to 2D TEE should be used whenever available. Use of TEE intraprocedurally for guidance has decreased with a minimalist approach being followed during implantation by choosing TTE imaging. MDCT plays an important role at many stages of TAVR and is increasingly being preferred for accurate measurements and structural information, while echocardiography is essential as a provider of functional information.

REFERENCES

1. Saura D, de la Morena-Valenzuela G. Historical note on the attribution of the first description of aortic stenosis in the modern era. Int J Cardiol. 2014;172(1):229-30.

2. Leopold JA. Cellular mechanisms of aortic valve calcification. Circ Cardiovasc Interv. 2012;5(4):605-14.
3. Cribier A, Eltchaninoff H, Bash A, et al. Percutaneous transcatheter implantation of an aortic valve prosthesis for calcific aortic stenosis: first human case description. Circulation. 2002;106(24):3006-8.
4. Leon MB, Smith CR, Mack M, et al. Transcatheter aortic-valve implantation for aortic stenosis in patients who cannot undergo surgery. N Engl J Med. 2010;363(17):1597-607.
5. Smith CR, Leon MB, Mack MJ, et al. Transcatheter versus surgical aortic-valve replacement in high-risk patients. N Engl J Med. 2011;364(23):2187-98.
6. Kapadia SR, Leon MB, Makkar RR, et al. 5-Year outcomes of transcatheter aortic valve replacement compared with standard treatment for patients with inoperable aortic stenosis: a randomized controlled trial. Lancet. 2015;385(9986):2485-91.
7. Reardon MJ, Adams DH, Kleiman NS. 2-Year outcomes in patients undergoing surgical or self-expanding transcatheter aortic valve replacement. J Am Coll Cardiol. 2015;66(2):113-21.
8. Leon MB, Smith CR, Mack MJ, et al. Transcatheter or surgical aortic-valve replacement in intermediate-risk patients. N Engl J Med. 2016;374(17):1609-20.
9. Webb JG, Wood DA, Ye J, et al. Transcatheter valve-in-valve implantation for failed bioprosthetic heart valves. Circulation. 2010;121(16):1848-57.
10. Van G L, Tchetche D, Latib A, et al. TAVI with current CE-marked devices: strategies for optimal sizing and valve delivery. EuroIntervention. 2016;12Y:Y22-7.
11. Manoharan G, Walton AS, Brecker SJ, et al. Treatment of symptomatic severe aortic stenosis with a novel resheathable supra-annular self-expanding transcatheter aortic valve system. JACC Cardiovasc Interv. 2015;8:1359-67.
12. Kodali S, Thourani VH, White J, et al. Early clinical and echocardiographic outcomes after SAPIEN 3 transcatheter aortic valve replacement in inoperable, high-risk and intermediate-risk patients with aortic stenosis. Eur Heart J. 2016;37:2252-62.
13. Kempfert J, Holzhey D, Hofmann S, et al. First registry results from the newly approved ACURATE TA TAVI system. Eur J Cardiothorac Surg. 2015;48:137-41.
14. Nijenhuis VJ, Swaans MJ, Michiels V, et al. First experience with JenaValve™: a single-centre cohort. Neth Heart J. 2015;23:35-41.
15. Reuthebuch O, Koechlin L, Kaufmann BA, et al. Transapical transcatheter aortic valve implantation using the JenaValve: a one-year follow-up. Thorac Cardiovasc Surg. 2015;63:493-500.
16. Meredith IT, Worthley SG, Whitbourn RJ, et al. Transfemoral aortic valve replacement with the repositionable Lotus valve system in high surgical risk patients: the REPRISE I study. EuroIntervention. 2014;9(11):1264-70.
17. Dumonteil N, Meredith I, Blackman D, et al. Need for permanent pacemaker following implantation of the repositionable LOTUS valve for the transcatheter aortic valve replacement in 250 patients: results from the REPRISE II trial extended cohort. EuroIntervention. 2017;13(7):796-803.
18. Rampat R, Khawaja MZ, Byrne J, et al. Transcatheter aortic valve replacement using the repositionable LOTUS valve: United Kingdom experience. JACC Cardiovasc Interv. 2016;9(4):367-72.
19. Kappetein AP, Head SJ, Genereux P, et al. Updated standardized endpoint definitions for transcatheter aortic valve implantation: the Valve Academic Research Consortium-2 consensus document. Euro Heart J. 2012;33(19):2403-18.
20. Genereux P, Head SJ, Van Mieghem NM, et al. Clinical outcomes after transcatheter aortic valve replacement using valve academic research consortium definitions: a weighted meta-analysis of 3,519 patients from 16 studies. J Am Coll Cardiol. 2012;59(25):2317-26.
21. Sharma A, Arbab-Zadeh A, Dubey D, et al. Access site bleeding after transcatheter aortic valve implantation. J Thromb Thrombolysis. 2013;35(4):463-8.
22. Rezq A, Basavarajaiah S, Latib A, et al. Incidence, management, and outcomes of cardiac tamponade during transcatheter aortic valve implantation: a single-center study. JACC Cardiovasc Intervent. 2012;5(12):1264-72.
23. Stewart WJ. Imaging the future of transcatheter aortic valve replacement. JACC Cardiovasc Imaging. 2008;1(1):25-8.
24. Moss RR, Ivens E, Pasupati S, et al. Role echocardiography in percutaneous aortic valve implantation. JACC Cardiovasc Imaging. 2008;1(1):15-24.
25. Krishnaswamy A, Tuzcu EM, Kapadia SR. Three dimensional computed tomography in cardiac catheterization laboratory. Catheter Cardiovasc Interv. 2011;77(6):860-5.
26. Schwartz JG, Neubauer AM, Fagan TE, et al. Potential role of 3D rotational angiography and C arm CT for valvular repair and implantation. Int J Cardiovasc Imaging. 2011;27(8):1205-22.
27. Dewey TM, Brown D, Ryan WH, et al. Reliability of risk algorithms in predicting early and late operative outcomes in high-risk patients undergoing aortic valve replacement. J Thorac Cardiovasc Surg. 2008;135(1):180-7.
28. van Mieghem NM, Head SJ, van der Boon RM, et al. The SURTAVI model: proposal for a pragmatic risk stratification for patients with severe aortic stenosis. EuroIntervention. 2012;8(2):258-66.
29. Chin CW, Pawade TA, Newby DE, et al. Risk stratification in patients with aortic stenosis using novel imaging approaches. Circ Cardiovasc Imaging. 2015;8(8):e003421.
30. Bleakley C, Monaghan MJ. The pivotal role of imaging in TAVR procedures. Curr Cardiol Rep. 2018;20(2):9.
31. Hahn RT, Nicoara A, Kapadia S, et al. Echocardiographic imaging for transcatheter aortic valve replacement. Am Soc Echocardiogr. 2018;31(4):405-33.
32. Naqvi TZ. Echocardiography in transcatheter aortic valve implantation—Part 1—Transthoracic echocardiography. Echocardiography. 2018;35(7):1005-19.
33. Ribeiro HB, Lerakis S, Gilard M, et al. Transcatheter aortic valve replacement in patients with low-flow, low-gradient aortic stenosis: the TOPAS-TAVI Registry. J Am Coll Cardiol. 2018;71(12):1297-308.

34. Généreux P. Low-flow, low-gradient aortic stenosis: TAVR in, dobutamine stress echocardiography out?. J Am Coll Cardiol. 2018;71(12):1309-12.
35. Salaun E, Sportouch L, Barral PA, et al. Diagnosis of infective endocarditis after TAVR: value of a multimodality imaging approach. JACC Cardiovasc Imaging. 2018;11(1): 143-6.
36. Yudi MB, Sharma SK, Tang GHL, et al. Coronary angiography and percutaneous coronary intervention after transcatheter aortic valve replacement. J Am Coll Cardiol. 2018;71(12): 1360-78.
37. Mayr A, Klug G, Reinstadler SJ, et al. Is MRI equivalent to CT in the guidance of TAVR? A pilot study. Eur Radiol. 2018.
38. Thonghong T, De Backer O, Søndergaard L. Comprehensive update on the new indications for transcatheter aortic valve replacement in the latest 2017 European guidelines for the management of valvular heart disease. Open Heart. 2018;5(1):e000753.
39. Musa TA, Uddin A, Swoboda PP, et al. Cardiovascular magnetic resonance evaluation of symptomatic severe aortic stenosis: association of circumferential myocardial strain and mortality. J Cardiovasc Magn Reson. 2017;19(1):13.

61

CHAPTER

Transcatheter Mitral Valve Interventions Imaging Evaluation: Potentials and Tips

S Venkatesh, Satish Govind

INTRODUCTION

Mitral regurgitation (MR) is the most common valvular lesion found either in isolation or in combination with mitral stenosis (MS), aortic or tricuspid valve disease. Isolated MR is seen in around 25% of all patients of valvular lesions in India with rheumatic and myxomatous etiologies accounting for roughly 40% each.[1] Moderate and severe MR can lead to significant symptoms related to left ventricular (LV) dysfunction, heart failure, and pulmonary hypertension. While medical management may be useful in treating heart failure or cardiac rhythm abnormalities associated with chronic MR, nearly 90% of patients will have either undergone surgery or have died by 10 years after being diagnosed to have chronic organic MR.[2] Therefore, eventually surgical intervention may be required in a significant proportion of these patients having mitral valve (MV) disease. MV replacement or MV repair by open heart surgery are the dominant surgical treatment options for patients with chronic MR. However, significant number of these patients may not actually undergo open heart surgery because of perioperative risk and patient comorbidities. Mirabel et al. reported that surgery was denied in 49% of patients with severe symptomatic MR. Impaired left ventricular ejection fraction (LVEF), older age, and comorbidities were the most striking characteristics of patients who were denied surgery.[3] Similarly, the EURO Heart Survey showed that nearly 50% of patients admitted with symptomatic severe MR were not referred for MV surgery, due to older age, comorbidities, and LV dysfunction. Only 15% of octogenarians undergo surgery for MR as compared to 60% in patients less than 70 years of age. In octogenarians, mortality and morbidity following MV surgery is also considerably high.[4] Under these circumstances, a less invasive transcatheter mitral valve repair (TMVR) or replacement (TMVRep) become attractive options for such patients.

MITRAL REGURGITATION

Outcomes of patients with chronic MR depend on several factors, of which etiology, severity of MR, and LV function are quite important.[5] Progression of mild MR to severe MR and its rate of progression is unpredictable and varies between patients.[6] MR result from the structural abnormalities of the MV apparatus (primary MR) or from distortion of MV geometry due to regional or global LV dysfunction leading to papillary muscle distortion or dilatation of MV annulus (secondary MR). In secondary MR, the structural components of MV are normal. The distinction is important because surgical correction of MR in primary MR is curative, whereas it may not make a substantial difference in the outcomes of secondary MR unless the underlying cause is addressed. Understandably, the indications for MR surgery in secondary MR are less well-defined. However, percutaneous techniques for repair or replacement have been developed for both primary and secondary MR.

Timing of Interventional Therapies for Mitral Regurgitation

Mild and Moderate Mitral Regurgitation

Patients with mild or moderate MR (seen as having mitral regurgitant fraction of <50%, or a regurgitant volume of <60 mL, or a regurgitant orifice area of <0.4 cm^2) remain asymptomatic and with preserved LV function for prolonged periods of time. Therefore, at this time, surgery or transcatheter interventions are not indicated.

Severe Mitral Regurgitation

Asymptomatic patients with severe MR and normal LV function have a very good short-term prognosis and most guidelines recommend expectant treatment for these patients unless they become symptomatic or develop LV dysfunction. However, since valve repairs carry low mortality in expert hands or at experienced centers, it is suggested that the option of valve repair as against replacement must be offered to such patients.[7]

SYMPTOMATIC PATIENTS WITH NORMAL LEFT VENTRICULAR FUNCTION

Even though LV function has a very important role in determining the prognosis of patients with MR, the onset of symptoms also have a major impact on outcomes in patients with normal LV function.[8] Therefore, MR surgery, especially MV repair, should be performed as soon as symptoms develop.

TRANSCATHETER MITRAL VALVE REPAIR TECHNIQUES

Chiam and Ruiz elegantly classified the technologies of percutaneous MV procedures based on the part of the MV anatomy that is targeted. Currently available devices target the (a) leaflets, (b) annulus, (c) chordae, and (d) LV. The coronary sinus reshaping devices that may result in unequal tension on the left atrium (LA) or MV annulus or causing functional MS are currently not viewed favorably.[9] Therefore, currently available TMVR devices can be classified either as leaflet or chordae targeted (Table 1).

TABLE 1: Transcatheter devices for mitral valve repair.

Target: leaflet	*Company*
Edge-to-edge repair	
MitraClip	Evalve, United States of America
PASCAL	Edwards
MitraFlex	Transcardiac Therapeutics, United States of America
Leaflet ablation	
ThermoCool ablation electrode	Biosense Webster, United States of America
Target: Chordae	
V-Chordal Adjustable system	Valtech Cardio, Israel

Leaflet Techniques

For degenerative MR, Alfieri and colleagues described a simple, yet innovative surgical edge-to-edge stitch technique commonly known as the Alfieri stitch. This repair that often produced a double-barreled MV orifice, was designed to reduce the MV orifice size or improve coaptation and thus, restore MV competence.[10] Percutaneous edge-to-edge MV repair has emerged into a successful technique from this surgical concept. The MitraClip and the PASCAL systems have been developed using this technique.

MitraClip

MitraClip is the most common percutaneous technology in TMVR therapies with the largest clinical experience so far. The device was developed by Evalve, which has been acquired by Abbott. First use of MitraClip in animals was described in 2003.[11] The first-in-man implant was done in 2003, in a patient with MV prolapse. At 2 years follow-up, patient had showed only mild MR.[12] Following the encouraging results, human use was adapted and the device is now on an approved list of regulatory agencies around the world. The procedure is performed where the MR jet guides the positioning of the clip. The rapid success of the system is attributable to an elegant delivery system, excellent visibility under echocardiographic guidance and the ability to reposition or retrieve the device. The MitraClip implantation procedure is performed under general anesthesia with transesophageal echocardiography (TEE) and fluoroscopic guidance. The steps of implantation are described in through a sequence of standardized steps that have been described by the Endovascular Valve Edge-to-Edge Repair Study (EVEREST) investigators.[13] The MitraClip consists of a triaxial delivery system. The steerable guide catheter is 24F at the hub and tapers to 22F. The implantable clip is composed of cobalt or chromium and has two arms and two "grippers" for grasping the leaflets. The clip arms and grippers are polyester covered to promote tissue healing. The implant is performed under general anesthesia and guided by TEE and fluoroscopy. Septal puncture is performed in the mid-superioposterior aspect of the fossa ovalis and heparin is administered.

The clip delivery system is advanced via the guide catheter into the LA, perpendicular to the annular plane. The clip is centered over the MR jet, above the regurgitant orifice under TEE guidance. The clip arms are opened to 180° and advanced into the LV below the line of coaptation. The clip is partially closed to get a "V" shape. Mitral leaflets are grasped by gentle retraction of the clip toward the left atrium. The grippers of the device are dropped to secure the leaflets and the clip is closed to approximately 60° and leaflet insertion is confirmed by TEE. Then the clip is closed, the MR is quantified and if satisfactory, the clip is released. If the result is unsatisfactory, the clip can be opened, the leaflets released, and device repositioned. Sometimes, a second clip or even a third clip can be used to improve the result. The EVEREST II trial was a prospective randomized multicenter controlled trial which randomized patients with moderate to severe MR to MitraClip ($n = 184$) and mitral valve surgery ($n = 95$) in a 2:1 fashion. The study enrolled 279 patients at 37 sites between September 2005 and November 2008. The primary composite endpoint for efficacy was freedom from death, from surgery for mitral-valve dysfunction, and from grade 3+ or 4+ MR at 12 months. The primary safety endpoint was a composite of major adverse events within 30 days.[14] At 12 months, the rates of the primary endpoint for efficacy were 55% in the percutaneous-repair group and 73% in the surgery group ($p = 0.007$). Mortality and freedom from grade 3+ or 4+ MR were similar in either group, though the need for surgery for MV dysfunction was much more frequent in the percutaneous repair group. Major adverse events occurred in 15% of patients in the percutaneous-repair group and 48% of patients in the surgery group at 30 days ($p < 0.001$). The investigators concluded that percutaneous repair was less effective at reducing MR than conventional surgery, but it was associated with better safety with similar improvements in clinical outcomes. Several registries have since then evaluated MitraClip of which ACCESS-EU[15] are most prominent. Over 50,000 patients have been treated worldwide using MitraCLip. Most of these included patients with symptomatic secondary or functional MR with LV dysfunction. The number of primary or degenerative MR cases included is less. Most patients have to confirm to the so-called EVEREST criteria to have a successful outcome with MitraClip. When there is deviation from these criteria, the results have been less satisfactory.[16]

PASCAL Repair System

PASCAL-TMV repair system is another novel edge-to-edge leaflet repair system developed by Edwards Lifesciences. In the first-in-man study,[17] results were shown in 23 patients with symptomatic, severe degenerative, functional or combined MR. In their series of 23 patients, following a heart team approach, most were deemed not suitable for MitraClip procedure. The procedure was successful in 22 patients (96%), there were no procedural deaths. Postprocedural MR was zero or one in 17 patients and 22 patients showed MR of grade 2+ or less. In six patients, a second device was implanted. Two patients suffered from procedural complications, three patients died during the 30-day follow-up and reduction in the New York Heart Association class to less than and equal to grade II was seen in 95% of cases. Similar to MitraClip device, the PASCAL system also requires transseptal puncture under TEE guidance. The PASCAL system consists of a steerable guide sheath (22F), a steerable catheter, and an implant catheter with the implant preattached at the distal end. The implant consists of a 10-mm spacer, which acts as a filler in the regurgitation orifice. The spacer is attached to two paddles with 25 mm width in grasping position and clasps of 10 mm lengths. Compared to the MitraClip device, the spacer width is more and the paddles longer. The operator can grasp the anterior and posterior leaflet independently unlike MitraClip. These differences appear to allow to treat patients with more complex MV anatomy (both secondary and primary MR) compared to MitraClip.

Chordal Techniques

Babic Device

The *Babic device* purports to create artificial chords by creating two continuous guiding tracks from the LV apical puncture through the mitral leaflets. Eventually, the chords are anchored at the LV apex with a loop lock to prevent sliding. After the leaflets are punctured, the wires are snared in the LA and then exteriorized via the transseptal catheter and femoral vein. A polymer loop is apposed onto the venously exteriorized guiding tracks via docking adapters and is anchored onto the atrial leaflet surface by retracting the guiding tracks from the epicardial end. An elastic polymer tube is interposed between the leaflet and the free myocardial wall and secured to the epicardial surface by an adjustable knot. According to the inventors, the Babic device is ideally suited for flail or prolapsed MV without annular dilatation. A series of 11 patients was presented in transcatheter cardiovascular therapeutics 2015 wherein the procedural success was seen in 10 patients and there was no procedural mortality.

MitraFlex

The *MitraFlex* device utilizes a thoracoscopic, transapical approach to place two anchors: one, in the inner LV myocardium and another on the leaflet and then connects the two with a synthetic chord; the device can also be used to perform a concomitant edge-to-edge repair. Several other techniques and devices for transcatheter mitral repair targeting different parts of the MV apparatus have been described (*see* Table 1). Most of these have completed animal studies and are in the preclinical stage of development. Some have crossed the first-in-man implantation stage. None of them, other than MitraClip device, have been approved for clinical use.

TRANSCATHETER MITRAL VALVE REPLACEMENT TECHNIQUES

Transcatheter MV replacement carries a major disadvantage that only a limited number of patients are eligible for the therapy due to morphological issues pertaining to the MV itself. Moreover, a significant proportion of patients undergoing TMVR also need a combination of percutaneous procedures (leaflet repair plus annuloplasty) for better procedural outcomes. TMVRep can potentially overcome these two problems.

However, compared to transcatheter aortic valve replacement (TAVR), TMVRep (Table 2) is more difficult due to:

- Larger MV annulus size
- D-shaped MV annulus as against more uniform one for the aortic valve
- Presence of subvalvular apparatus unlike the aortic valve
- Interaction of the transcatheter MV with the LV outflow tract (LVOT)
- Large devices, requiring large delivery systems.

Ideal TMVRep device should be:

- Flexible delivery system, because both transseptal and transaortic-retrograde implantation routes are sinuous.
- D-shaped to confirm to the MV annulus, fitting well enough to prevent paravalvular leaks.
- Consist of the complex MV apparatus: Leaflets, chordae, and papillary muscle.

TABLE 2: The differences between transcatheter aortic and mitral valve replacement.

	Transcatheter aortic valve replacement	*Transcatheter mitral valve replacement*
Annulus size	Smaller	Larger
Shape of annulus	Circular or oval	D-shaped
Subvalvular apparatus	Absent	Present, complex
Impinging on adjacent structures	Coronary arteries	Left ventricular outflow
Device size/ delivery system	Smaller	Larger
Septal puncture	Not necessary	Essential
Transaortic delivery	Most often	Sometimes

- Should not perforate the LA or coronary sinus.
- Should not impinge unduly on the LVOT causing obstruction.
- Other attributes of durability, low thrombogenicity, tenacity to withstand high LV forces, and movements of the mitral ring as in any other prosthetic valve.

Bioprosthetic Valves

Current cardiac surgical practice has increasingly shifted to bioprosthetic rather than mechanical valves for valve replacement surgery in order to avoid the need for lifelong oral anticoagulation and its attendant hemorrhagic or thromboembolic risk. Even in patients aged less than 60 years, some of the newer tissue valves have an excellent durability and complication free survival. Bourguignon et al. reported 25-year follow-up of 450 Carpentier-Edwards PERIMOUNT valve and showed that the expected valve durability was 16.6 years for the entire cohort, 11.4, 16.6, and 19.4 years for patients aged less than 60, 60-70, and more than 70 years, respectively.[18] Despite this, bioprosthetic valves eventually fail in most cases. In such cases, repeat open heart surgery and surgical replacement carry very high-risk. Transcatheter valve replacement is a less invasive and a less risky alternative. A good amount of data is available documenting the procedure and outcomes of transcatheter valve-in-valve procedures in patients with failed bioprosthetic aortic valves.[19] For these type of cases, dedicated TMVRep devices are not available. Taking advantage of the near-circular shape of the previous bioprosthetic valve or surgical annuloplasty ring, investigators have used transcatheter aortic devices for this purpose. The most commonly studied device has been the Edwards Sapien XT device. Other aortic transcatheter valves such as Melody (Medtronic), Sapien 3 (Edwards), Inovare (Braile), and Lotus (Boston) have also been used for treating failed surgical valves and rings. At EuroPCR 2015, data from the Valve-in-Valve International Data (VIVID) registry was presented pertaining to 437 transcatheter mitral [349 patients with MV-in-valve and 88 with valve-in-ring (VIR)] implantations in patients with failed bioprosthetic valves. Patients were high risk or surgery with average Society of Thoracic Surgeons score of 12.9. 45% of failed bioprosthetic valves showed MR, 23% showed MS, and the rest had a combination of both. The median time from the first surgery to the transcatheter procedure was 9 years. The valve-in-valve (VIV) or VIR was performed via transapical route in 79% of cases, via direct left atrial puncture in 2.5% and via transseptal route in the rest. The median postprocedure follow-up was for 408 days. Transcatheter procedure in a patient with prior surgical valve less than 25 mm size predicted an elevated postprocedure gradient [adjusted odds ratio (OR) 3.7]. In the VIV group, the mean postprocedural valve area was 1.99 cm^2 and in the VIR group, it was 2.33 cm^2. Potentially, catastrophic LVOT obstruction was seen in 2.6% of VIV procedures and in 8% of VIR procedures. Compared to the mitral VIR, the VIV intervention had better procedural and subsequent outcomes. Postprocedurally, moderate-to-severe MR was seen in only 2.6% of patients undergoing mitral VIV, as against 14.8% undergoing mitral VIR. The VIVID registry also documented that the 30-day primary composite endpoint in the mitral VIV group was 11.2%, which was encouraging considering that the patients belonged to a very high-risk cohort. Compared to this, 28.4% patients in the VIR group had a composite adverse event endpoint at 30 days. These data suggest that transcatheter MV replacement procedure is more reasonable in patients with failed bioprosthetic valve rather than failed surgical rings.

Native Mitral Valve

Intuitively, it should appear that TMV replacement may offer several advantages over TMV repair. The most prevalent technique of transcatheter repair, i.e. MitraClip is theoretically designed to reduce the severity of MR. A well-designed transcatheter MV should potentially eliminate MR with an acceptable forward gradient. This optimism stems from the experience of surgically treating MR with surgical valves. The greatest challenge, however, has been that the MV including the mitral apparatus is a complex anatomical structure and considerable variations exist in individual valve size and shape. The morphological basis of MR or MS differs from patient to patient. These factors render the one design or few sizes fit all concept of transcatheter aortic valves inapplicable in transcatheter MV design. Also, patients with severe MV disease, especially MR who are not surgical candidates, are sicker and have multiple comorbidities and consequently are at high-risk and therefore, recruiting these patients for evaluation of transcatheter devices is not easy.

Problems of TMV replacement in native MV:

- Unlike VIV or VIR native MV does not afford a scaffold support
- Left ventricular outflow tract obstruction from the protrusion of the device into LVOT
- Left ventricular outflow tract obstruction due to displacement of the anterior mitral leaflet into the LVOT.

Transcatheter mitral valve replacements indications:

- Previous surgical bioprosthetic valves or annuloplasty rings
- Native valves
- Severe mitral annular calcification (MAC).

Currently, patients with primary MR who are denied open heart MV replacement due to high surgical risk are potential candidates for TMV repair or replacement. Prior to admitting such patients to percutaneous MV replacement, a suitability for MitraClip procedure should be assessed. This is because TMV repair with MitraClip is shown to have a similar symptom relief and survival compared to surgery (despite more residual MR) in high-risk candidates and has been approved for use in high-risk primary MR patients. Secondary MR patients who are anatomically unsuitable for MitraClip, can be recruited into TMV replacement with one or the other devices.

IMAGING

Preprocedural

It is important to plan the TMV procedure meticulously since it involves a lot of complexity and precision at the time of implantation. Success of TMVR depends on an experienced heart valve team. A close association between the cardiac imagers and the interventionalists is crucial to a good outcome of the procedure. Multimodality imaging plays a crucial role to characterize MR, assess the MV apparatus and adjacent anatomy (like LVOT), identify at-risk patients, evaluate for likely complications, appropriate device selection, measure LVEF, and to determine other important measurements that are necessary during implantation.[20]

Echocardiography [both transthoracic TTE and trans-esophageal echocardiography (TEE)] is the first-line imaging modality. With availability of three-dimensional (3D) echocardiography, this takes on an invaluable role especially when there is a limitation in the use of contrast in cardiac computerized tomography (CCT). TTE is economical and provides first-hand information about the pathology, anatomy, and Doppler hemodynamics. When speckle tracking echocardiography and 3D-TEE are applied, it makes the study comprehensive. 3D-TEE can provide for accurate MV annulus sizing, area and vena contract a measurement. A complete echocardiography should consider systemic blood pressure, heart rate, sedation, and presence of associated diseases like anemia, etc. when flow dynamics is being assessed. The many uses of echocardiography are:

- Identify valve pathology (prolapse, stenosis, and calcification) and anatomy (leaflets, chordae, and papillary muscles)
- Evaluating severity of the regurgitant or stenotic lesion
- Doppler hemodynamics
- Extent of MAC
- Size of MV annulus

- Aortomitral assessment
- Left ventricular and right ventricular function
- Pulmonary hypertension
- Left ventricular, LV, and LVOT size
- Evaluation of LA appendage and interatrial septum
- Assessment of aortic valve and aortic pathology
- Associated pericardial or cardiac disease.

Echocardiography provides for excellent imaging quality of mitral leaflets. It starts with examination of mobility, thickness, length and calcification and extent of prolapse, presence of flail segments, clefts, and those at risk of LVOT obstruction by the anterior mitral leaflet. Present day software allows for quantitative evaluation of annulus and leaflet which provides multiple measurements. Valve hemodynamics should be done in a detailed manner and if required stress echocardiography should be considered. 3D-TEE can provide incremental information about leaflets and annular dynamics. Severe MV annulus calcification is a technical challenge for TMVRep, imaging guides the operator to understand the extent of calcification and plan the procedure properly. Calcification can be a source of paravalvular leak where assessment of calcification is made mainly from the parasternal short axis by echocardiography. When there is minimal or no anterior MV annular calcification but presence of severe posterior calcification, this can lead to anterior displacement of the implanted valve, which in turn may lead to LVOT obstruction. Predictors of LVOT obstruction are: increased aortomitral angle, anterior mitral leaflet length, interventricular septal thickness, and the potential increase of neo-LVOT area. If the valve is undersized, this may lead to migration, paravalvular leak, or embolization. The assessment of LV and LA is also of grave importance where it is important to look for chamber enlargement, annular dilatation, wall motion abnormalities, leaflet tethering, chordal apparatus, and abnormal papillary muscles. Design of the valve devices and the implantation techniques are not favorable for optimal LVOT flow dynamics, hence the LVOT has to be imaged and assessed carefully to avoid significant obstruction after the device is implanted. An interesting concept of a neo-LVOT that is formed postprocedure has been put forward by Blanke et al.[21] This is a potentially dangerous complication following TMVRep. The original native LVOT bordered by the interventricular basal septum and the aortomitral curtain continues to be the same. But, there is elongation of the LVOT created posteriorly due to the displacement of the anterior mitral leaflet or by the presence of a bioprosthetic vale or due the struts of the newly implanted device and this is called as the neo-LVOT. Reduced LVOT area can either be due to a preexisting small LVOT or it can be due to the newly implanted device.

Cardiac Computerized Tomography

Despite the many advantages of echocardiography, CCT scan is the imaging modality that is used to make critical decisions. The 3D volumetric datasets in CCT provides for detailed and comprehensive images of the MV anatomy and geometry, especially when echocardiographic images are not adequate. An appropriate selection of a device is made after reviewing such images. Additionally, images of the thoracic cage and pelvic anatomy are easily obtained by CT which may be helpful if either a transapical or transfemoral approach is chosen. Despite CCT being the preferred imaging modality, many of these measurements are not standardized since they have not been validated in the required manner. Measurements for patient selection and for choosing an appropriate device are likely to get more accepted as increasing experience and evidence accumulates over period of time. Presence of MAC and small LVOT should be identified and examined carefully for good procedural outcome. CCT is the investigation of choice when LVOT is being assessed. CCT preprocedural planning can provide advance information to the cardiac imager to optimize imaging when doing periprocedural echocardiography to guide septal puncture, proper aligning of the device and catheter during deployment and can ensure proper positioning of the device thus, limiting or avoiding paravalvular leak and LVOT obstruction.[22]

The various anatomical structures of MV and LV that are evaluated by CCT are shown here:

- *Annulus of MV*: For annular height, shape, extent of calcification, annular trajectory, intercommissural + septal/lateral + trigone distance, perimeter measurement by 3D, and also projected perimeter and area.
- *Leaflets of MV*: Length, mobility, and calcification.
- *Papillary muscles*: Interpapillary muscle heads distance and projected distance to the MV annulus.
- *LVOT*: Aortomitral angle and cross-sectional area of neo-LVOT.
- *LV*: Long axis width and diameter and LV apex location for best intercostal space + distance from midline for transapical approach.
- *Interventricular septum*: Thickness.
- *LA*: Short-axis and long-axis diameter, height and LA appendage ostium to MV annulus distance.

Presently, preprocedural multimodality imaging is the preferred approach to plan for TMV procedures to ensure a good procedural outcome. Cardiac magnetic resonance imaging (CMRI) has been shown to have utility but is used in a limited way due to prolonged imaging time, operator expertise, and its availability. It is useful in identifying valve morphology and flow dynamics, especially when CCT due to its low temporal resolution cannot be relied upon giving accurate information about mobility of leaflets, structural information of MV, LV and LA, and Doppler hemodynamics. It has limitations in imaging leaflet and annular calcification.

Three-dimensional printing has also been investigated and has been shown to be useful when looking into it as a bridge between CCT and echocardiography images. CCT and CMRI digital images are the ones presently being used to create a 3D print, while 3D print from echocardiography is still an evolving technique. The value of an actual 3D print provides the interventionalist to better understand the anatomy and gives a unique perspective when guiding catheter and the device.

Periprocedural

Procedures are usually performed in a hybrid laboratory supported by high-end echocardiography equipment. Availability of fusion imaging (echocardiography and fluoroscopy) can be an added advantage. Once patient is sedated and intubated, TEE is done to document baseline measurements and images for future comparisons, select good imaging planes, review structural abnormalities (wall motion abnormalities, etc.), assess severity of valve dysfunction, presence or absence of pericardial effusion, and also to look for LA or LA appendage thrombus. Good communication system should be there between the cardiac imager and the interventionalist for a successful outcome of the procedure. Guidance for septal puncture is provided in transfemoral approach by using the bicaval and short-axis views (biplane image from 3D-TEE is faster and better) while the LV apex is identified when a transapical approach is selected. Sometimes, a hybrid method is adopted by way of an arteriovenous or a venous-arterial rail creation. Imaging is also crucial to identify a proper landing site for the device (neither too far into the LV, which will cause LVOT obstruction, nor too much into LA where it may lead to embolization). Presence of calcification or a previous device makes for easier identification of the landing site before deployment.

Procedural evaluation involves assessing for successful outcome in terms of the technique adopted, looking at stability or inappropriate fixation of the valve, observing for complications like valve dislocation and embolization, assessing MR in terms of its severity, measuring mitral transvalvular gradients, determining LVOT obstruction, monitoring of LVEF, detection of new wall motion abnormality, to observe for device or leaflet malfunction, to decide about the need for a second valve, to assess its relation to a previous aortic valve implant, and also anticipate the likelihood or requirement for open-heart surgery. Small LVOTs are usually at risk of life-threatening obstruction. A thickened basal septum and displaced anterior mitral leaflet will result in a neo-LVOT, which may result in obstruction to flow across LVOT. The risk of paravalvular leak is low, whereas the MV mean gradient is not affected and has been found to be around less than 3 mm Hg. There is always the rare possibility of valve thrombosis that one should be aware of. Devastating complications like MV annular rupture, severe LVOT obstruction, cardiac tamponade and valve dislodgement, and other life-threatening complications are higher in TMVRep.

In the event of significant LVOT obstruction, septal ablation even in a normal-sized interventricular septum may be helpful to reduce the flow obstruction. In such scenarios, an alternative unique approach has been advocated which involves periprocedural laceration of the anterior mitral leaflet for improved flow dynamics. These methods are heavily dependent on imaging.

Postprocedural

This entails imaging for flow dynamics across the device and the LVOT, for paravalvular leak, new pericardial effusion or wall motion abnormality, valve migration, and to observe for stability of the valve. Expansion of the device can cause myocardial perforation and compression of the left circumflex artery, while pulmonary vein perforation can happen in the event of a rail approach that was selected.

Follow-up imaging starts with a predischarge TTE to document baseline measurements and flow dynamics and this can be repeated at 1, 6, and 12 months and, thereafter every 12 months if the course is uneventful. Parameters to be observed are LVEF, iatrogenic atrial septal shunts, abnormal leaflet motion, presence of thrombus on the valve, right ventricular function, presence of pulmonary hypertension, and valve degeneration in addition to parameters mentioned earlier.

ONGOING TRIALS ON TRANSCATHETHER MITRAL VALVE REPLACEMENT

Trials recruiting for TMV replacement are: MITRAL, SITRAL, PRELUDE, RELIEF, TIARA II, early feasibility study of CardiAQ TMVI system, early feasibility study of TIARA valve, Tendyne MV system and NHLBI DIR LAMPOON study. At present both nitinol-based self-expanding valves as well as balloon expandable valves are available for TMVRep. For primary MR, the self-expanding valves are more appropriate compared to the balloon expandable valves. The latter are likely to be appropriate for patients with more uniform annuluses as in MS secondary to annular calcium or in failed bioprostheses and failed surgical annuloplasty rings.

CardiAQ Device (Edwards Lifesciences)

It was the first device to be used for transcatheter MV replacement. CardiAQ device consists of a self-expanding nitinol frame, which houses a trileaflet of bovine pericardial tissue valve. The device is covered with a membrane to minimize paravalvular leak. The frame contains two opposing sets of LV anchors thus, allowing annular attachment without radial force. The frame is designed to preserve patient's subvalvular apparatus. A first-generation device was used in the first-in-human transfemoral CardiAQ case. The procedure was done under general anesthesia and required cardiopulmonary bypass (CPB) for a short duration. Though the procedure was successfully done, the patient died 68 hours later due to systemic inflammatory response syndrome, possibly because of the CPB. A second-generation device, which was designed to improve load distribution with optimized flow properties in the LA and lesser potential for paravalvular leak received the United States of America Food and Drug Administration (FDA) approval in 2015. However, as on February 2017, Edwards Lifesciences announced that it had paused enrollment for the clinical trials of CardiAQ device.

Intrepid Device (Medtronic)

This valve has a self-expandable double-stent design with a nitinol outer stent for fixation and sealing and an inner stent containing a trileaflet bovine pericardium valve with an effective orifice area of 24 mm^2. Currently, the valve is available for transapical implantation while the transvenous, transseptal device is expected to be ready for clinical trials. A pilot study involving 50 patients demonstrated procedural success in 48 patients with a median deployment time of 14 minutes. Thirty-day mortality was 14%, there were no disabling strokes or repeat interventions. At last follow-up (median 173 days), there was mild or no residual MR in all patients who received implants and nearly 80% patients showed improvement in functional class.[23] Currently, recruitment is on for the large multicenter APOLLO trial involving 1,380 patients comparing the study device to conventional MV surgery. The study is expected to complete in 2025 (Source: ClinicalTrials.gov).

Tendyne Valve (Abbott Vascular)

It is also a self-expanding nitinol valve with a double-frame design. The circular inner frame has a trileaflet porcine pericardial valve. The outer frame is D-shaped to fit into the MV annulus and has a cuff to seal the annulus. The valve is delivered transapically. This is the only fully retrievable and repositionable valve used for TMVRep. A feasibility study, which included 30 patients, was reported. Procedural success was seen in 28 patients, with 27 patients having no residual MR. Based on high procedural success and low complication rates, an expanded clinical trial is ongoing.[24] In May 2018, experience of first 100 patients in a global study with favorable 30-day outcomes was presented during late-breaking trials session at the EuroPCR in Paris. To date this is the largest experience in TMVRep that is published or presented, and the trial is intending to enroll 350 patients.

FORTIS Device (Edwards Lifesciences)

The FORTIS transcatheter heart valve system consists of a nitinol stent frame including two paddles and a valve with three leaflets of bovine pericardial tissue-sutured inside. The device is deployed transapically using a 40 F catheter. Early device implantation was associated with paravalvular leak.[25] In May 2015, Edwards halted enrolment of patients for trials involving this device because of "thrombus" issues as per the company website.

TIARA Device (NeoVasc)

Tiara valve consists of a nitinol self-expanding frame and bovine pericardial trileaflet valve. The frame has an asymmetric shape to fit the D-shaped MV annulus. The atrial part of the valve fits the atrial aspect of the MV. Ventricular anchoring structures secure the valve into the fibrous trigones and the posterior shelf of the annulus. The 32-F delivery system is designed to enter the LV apex without a delivery sheath. The early feasibility study in man, aiming to study 30 patients in total, is expected to complete implantation in the last patient by end of 2018 (Source: ClinicalTrials.gov). The manufacturer provided data in September 2017 about the 34 patients who have undergone TMVRep with Tiara device and reported an all-cause mortality of 12%. Currently, implantation of the device is being performed under three parallel investigational programs: (1) an FDA Early Feasibility trial, TIARA-I, (2) a European pivotal CE Mark trial, TIARA-II, and (3) compassionate use or special access treatment across multiple centers. The TIARA-II study, which is the primary focus of the Tiara program, is a 115 patient, nonrandomized, prospective clinical study evaluating Tiara's safety and performance.

The other valves or devices, which are undergoing evaluation for TMV replacement, are listed in Table 3. A detailed technical analysis of these devices is also available.[26]

TABLE 3: Valves or devices, which are undergoing evaluation for transcatheter mitral valve replacement.

Device name	Company	Country
Cardiovalve	Valtech/Edwards	Israel/United States of America
Double-crowned mitral valve	Zhejiang University and Vaudois University Hospital	China/Switzerland
Endovalve	Micro Interventional Devices	United States of America
Gorman	University of Pennsylvania	United States of America
HighLife	HighLife Medical	France/United States of America
Medtronic TMV	Medtronic	United States of America
MitralSeal	Avalon Medical	United States of America
MitrAssist	MitrAssist Medical	Israel
MiVAR	Trinity College Dublin	Ireland
NaviGate	Navigate Vardiac Structures	United States of America

TRANSCATHETER MITRAL VALVE REPLACEMENT IN NATIVE MITRAL VALVE DISEASE DUE TO SEVERE MITRAL ANNULAR CALCIFICATION

Patients with MAC with severe valvular dysfunction who are high risk for surgical valve replacement theoretically present with a unique problem-solving opportunity. Unlike other forms of primary MR, these patients have a natural skirt of calcium, and when the annulus is stenotic, they have a more regular annular shape. Investigators have exploited these two factors and have attempted to perform TMVRep in these patients with balloon-expandable stents. For the purpose, the valves used for TAVR appears to be highly suitable. In fact, a large majority of patients who have undergone TMVRep for this indication have received the Edwards Sapien-XT and Sapien 3 valves. In some cases, the Lotus Edge valve (Boston Scientific) and Direct Flow (Direct Flow Medical) have been used but both these valves have since been withdrawn.

The TMVRep in MAC global registry collects the safety and efficacy data on TMVRep in patients with severe MAC. The experience in the first 64 patients was published in 2016.[27] 95% of valves used were Sapien, Sapien-XT or Sapien 3 and 5% were Innovare Braille valves. Access was transatrial in 15.6%, transapical in 43.8% and transseptal in 40.6%. Technical success was achieved in 46 (72%) patients, primarily due to the need for a second valve in 11 (17.2%). Six patients (9.3%) had LVOT obstruction with hemodynamic compromise. Mean mitral gradient postprocedure was 4 ± 2.2 mm Hg, paravalvular regurgitation was mild or absent in all. 30-day all-cause mortality was 29.7% with cardiovascular mortality being 12.5%. The report concluded that TMVRep with balloon-expandable valves in patients with severe MAC is feasible but may be associated with significant adverse events and therefore, recommended reserving this strategy as an alternative for selected high-risk patients with limited treatment options. A subsequent analysis presented at the EuroPCR 2016 which included 104 patients demonstrated that the procedural success as well as 30-day mortality was better in progressive tertiles of patients thus, pointing to a steep learning curve for the procedure. In 2017, further data from 116 patients showed an all-cause mortality of 25% at 30 days and 55% at 1 year. LVOT obstruction by the device and mitral reintervention were major determinants of cardiovascular mortality, which stood at 25% at 1 year.

CONCLUSION

Transcatheter MV interventions purport to fill the felt gap in the unmet need of patients with severe MR who are denied open heart surgery. At present, a limited proportion of these patients are candidates for undergoing transcatheter MV repair using MitraClip procedure, the only one approved in this situation. The major drawbacks of TMV repair are applicability in few patients, low predictability of MR reduction, and recurrence of MR. Transcatheter MV replacement theoretically has many advantages: it is perhaps applicable to a larger proportion of patients with primary MR. Unlike TMV repair, MR reduction may be more predictable, and the replacement procedure may be technically simpler, once an ideal valve that fits most anatomies is designed. At this time, however, the ideal TMVRep device is yet to evolve. Unlike TAVR, which rapidly gained acceptability due to device successes, the progress in TMV replacement has been slow. While a number of trials are recruiting patients for clinical trials with various devices, the procedural success, serious complication rates and outcomes are far from ideal. In addition, the implant procedure including requirement of transapical access and extracorporeal circulation continues to be daunting and presents a steep learning curve for the physician. Moreover, the large body of evidence from surgical field, which clearly shows the superiority or MV repair over MV replacement, should also be considered. In summary, currently TMV repair with leaflet repair technology, specifically MitraCLip procedure appears to be the only credible procedure likely to be available to patients commercially. These procedures are complex and require a lot of technical skills from all members of the team involved. It is a rapidly growing field which requires multimodality imaging for a successful outcome.

REFERENCES

1. Manjunath CN, Srinivas P, Ravindranath KS, et al. Incidence and patterns of valvular heart disease in a tertiary care high-volume cardiac center: a single center experience. Indian Heart J. 2014;66:320-6.
2. Enriquez-Sarano M, Sundt TM. Early surgery is recommended for mitral regurgitation. Circulation. 2010;121:804-12.
3. Mirabel M, Lung B, Baron G, et al. What are the characteristics of patients with severe, symptomatic, mitral regurgitation who are denied surgery? Eur Heart J. 2007;28:1358-65.
4. Iung B, Baron G, Butchart EG, et al. A prospective survey of patients with valvular heart disease in Europe: the Euro Heart Survey on Valvular Heart Disease. Eur Heart J. 2003;24:1231-43.
5. Benjamin MM, Smith RL, Grayburn PA. Ischemic and functional mitral regurgitation in heart failure: natural history and treatment. Curr Cardiol Reports. 2014;16:517) (Delling FN, Vasan RS. Epidemiology and Pathophysiology of Mitral Valve Prolapse. New insights into disease progression, genetics and molecular basis. Circulation. 2014;129:2158-70.
6. Enriquez-Sarano M, Basmadjian AJ Rossi A, et al. Progression of mitral regurgitation: a prospective Doppler echocardiographic study. J AM Coll Cardiol. 1999;34:1137-44.
7. Nishimura RA, Otto CM, Bonow RO, et al. 2014 AHA/ACC Guideline for the management of patients with valvular heart disease: executive summary. Circulation. 2014;129:2440-92.
8. Tribouilloy CM, Enriquez-Sarano M, Schaff HV, et al. Impact of preoperative symptoms on survival after surgical correction of organic mitral regurgitation: rationale for optimizing surgical indications. Circulation. 1999;99:400-5.
9. Chiam PT, Ruiz CE. Percutaneous transcatheter mitral valve repair: a classification of the technology. J Am Coll Cardiol Cardiovasc Interv. 2011;4:1-13.
10. Fucci C, Sandrelli L, Pardini A, et al. Improved results using this surgical technique has led to. Eur J Cardiothorac Surg. 1995;9:621-6.
11. St Goar FG, Fann JI, Komtebedde J, et al. Endovascular edge-to-edge mitral valve repair: short-term results in a porcine model. Circulation. 2003;108:1990-3.
12. Condado JA, Acquatella H, Rodriguez L, et al. Percutaneous edge-to-edge mitral valve repair: two-year follow-up in the first human case. Catheter Cardiovasc Interv. 2006;67:323-5.
13. Feldman T, Kar S, Rinaldi M. Percutaneous mitral repair with the MitraClip System. Safety and midterm durability in the initial EVEREST (Endovascular Valve Edge-to-Edge REpair Study) cohort. J Am Coll Cardiol. 2009;54:686-94.
14. Feldman T, Foster E, Glower DD, et al. Percutaneous repair of surgery for mitral regurgitation. N Engl J Med. 2011;364: 1395-406.
15. Maisano F, Franzen O, Baldus S, et al. Percutaneous mitral valve interventions in the real world: early and 1-year results from the ACCESS-EU, a prospective, multicenter, nonrandomized post-approval study of the MitraClip therapy in Europe. J Am Coll Cardiol. 2013;62:1052-61.
16. Lesevic H, Karl M, Braun D, et al. Long-term outcomes after mitraclip implantation according to the presence or absence of EVEREST inclusion criteria. Am J Cardiol. 2017;119:1255-61.
17. Praz F, Spargias K, Chrissoheris M, et al. Compassionate use of the PASCAL transcatheter mitral valve repair system for patients with severe mitral regurgitation: a multicentre, prospective, observational, first-in-man study. Lancet. 2017;390:773-80.
18. Bourguignon T, Bouquiaux-Stablo A, Loardi C, et al. Very late outcomes for mitral valve replacement with the Carpentier-Edwards pericardial bioprosthesis: 25-year follow-up of 450 implantations. J Thorac Cardiovasc Surg. 2014;148: 2004-11.
19. Dvir D, Webb JG, Bleiziffer S, et al. Transcatheter aortic valve implantation in failed bioprosthetic surgical valves. JAMA. 2014;312:162-70.
20. Regueiro A, Granada JF, Dagenais F, et al. Transcatheter mitral valve replacement: insights from early clinical experience and future challenges. J Am Coll Cardiol. 2017;69(17):2175-92.
21. Blanke P, Naoum C, Dvir D, et al. Predicting LVOT obstruction in transcatheter mitral valve implantation: concept of the neo-LVOT. JACC Cardiovasc Imaging. 2017;10(4):482-5.
22. Mackensen GB, Lee JC, Wang DD, et al. Role of echocardiography in transcatheter mitral valve replacement in native mitral valves and mitral rings. J Am Soc Echocardiogr. 2018;31(4):475-90.
23. Bapat V, Rajagopal V, Meduri C, et al. Early experience with new transcatheter mitral valve replacement. J Am Coll Cardiol. 2018;71:12-21.
24. Muller DW, Farivar RS, Jansz P, et al. Transcatheter mitral valve replacement for patients with symptomatic mitral regurgitation: a global feasibility trial. J Am Coll Cardiology. 2017;69:381-91.
25. Abdul-Jawad Altisent O, Dumont E, Dagenais F, et al. Transcatheter mitral valve implantation with the FORTIS device: insights into the evaluation of device success. JACC Cardiovasc Interv. 2015;8(7):994-5.
26. Preston-Maher GL, Torii R, Burriesci G. A technical review of minimally invasive mitral valve replacements. Cardiovasc Eng Technol. 2015;6:174-84.
27. Guerrero M, Dvir D, Himbert D et al. Transcatheter mitral valve replacement in native mitral valve disease with severe mitral annular calcification: results from the first multicenter global registry. JACC Cardiovasc Interv. 2016; 9:1361-71

62

CHAPTER

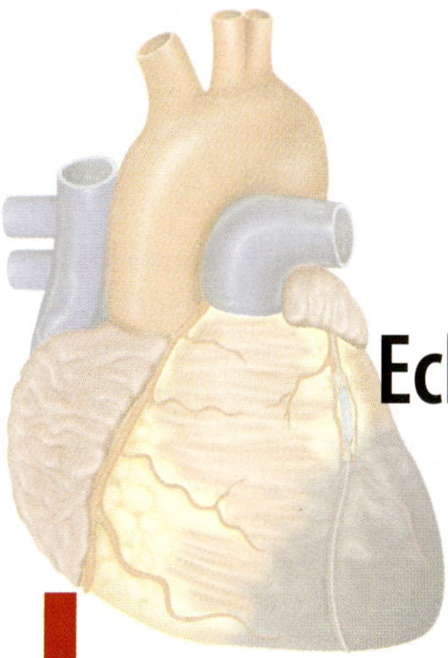

Three-dimensional/Four-dimensional Echocardiography: Recent Advances in the Evaluation of Mitral Valve

V Amuthan, RVA Ananth, AB Gopalamurugan

INTRODUCTION

Echocardiography, since its inception from the days of Elder, has revolutionized the management of cardiac patients. From the days of single crystal probe to M-mode, two-dimensional (2D), color flow mapping, the advancement has reached the stage of three-dimensional (3D) echocardiogram with the added fourth dimension of time (four-dimensional echocardiography—the real-time 3D echocardiography). The cumbersome big mechanical probes are now replaced with smaller matrix probes with more than 3,000 elements, which can acquire images from a single cardiac cycle.[1-3] The introduction of the first phased-array real-time volumetric 3D imaging system (Duke University, Durham, North Carolina) enabled transthoracic real-time acquisition of 3D echocardiographic data sets.[4,5]

ADVANCES IN THE TRANSDUCER TECHNOLOGY

A breakthrough in the area of transthoracic real-time 3D echocardiography was achieved with the so-called Live 3D (Sonos 7500, Philips, Andover, Massachusetts) and Csound technology-derived probes [4Vc Probes, General Electric (GE)]. In addition to transthoracic real-time acquisition, simultaneous presentation of perspective images became possible; the spatial and temporal image resolution was considerably improved. The technological advances have made it possible for the 3D echocardiography from a single crystal A-mode to 2D B-mode with 2D phased array transducer to the 3D matrix array transducers with Csound technology (Fig. 1). The 3D matrix array transducer acquires a pyramidal cone of data set. The transducers are of the same size as that of 2D phased array transducers. The Csound technology utilizes the replacement of the hardware beam former with software beam former (Fig. 2). The advantages of this technology are that confocal imaging is now available without the loss of frame rate and without the line artifacts usually present as a result of multiline acquisition and/or multifocal stitching. Adaptive contrast enhancement is the second feature enabled by the Csound architecture.

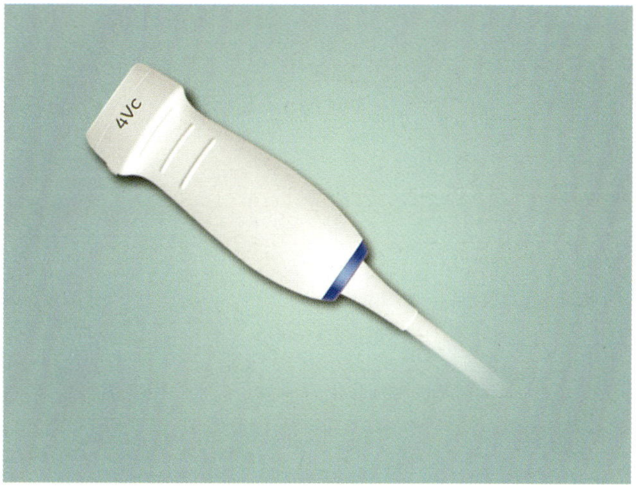

Fig. 1

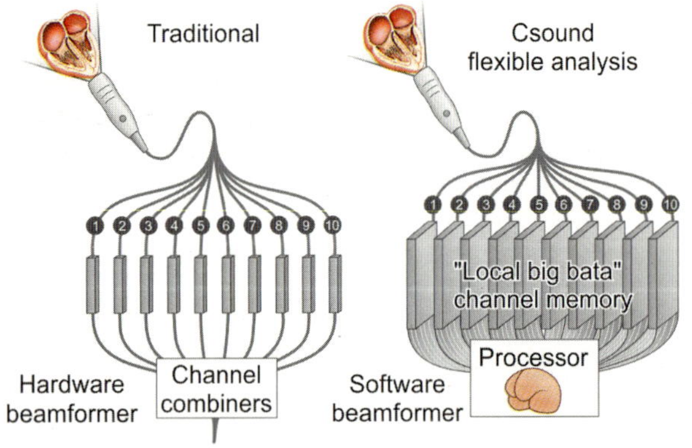

Fig. 2

THE PROCEDURE OF THREE-DIMENSIONAL ECHOCARDIOGRAPHY FOR MITRAL VALVE

The performance of the 3D echocardiogram has the same methodology of standard 2D echocardiography.[6-8] The image data set is essentially acquired from the same parasternal and apical windows. More commonly the apical window is chosen.[9-13] One standard requirement for the acquisition of 3D echocardiography is the connection of standard electrocardiography. Another important factor to be kept in mind is the acquisition of optimized 2D images. These images can be viewed in different formats.[14-23] The advantages and disadvantages of the different formats are given in Table 1.

MULTIPLANE VIEW

Simultaneously orthogonally two opposite planes of 2D echocardiograms can be viewed in biplane. Mitral valve (MV) can be acquired from parasternal long axis or from the apical window (Fig. 3). MV can also be seen in triplane view with the slices of 60° apart.

- *Zoom view:* Zoomed views are used frequently to study MV in both transthoracic and transesophageal views. The MV can be selected in four-chamber plane; the elevation plane is adjusted and can be zoomed in (Figs. 4 and 5).
- *Narrow angle:* A narrow angle slice of data set is acquired in real time, usually 60° in azimuthal plane (x-axis) and 30° in the elevation plane (z-axis). The elevation plane angle can be increased.
- *Full volume:* A full-volume acquisition usually consists of cone of data set: 90° in the azimuthal plane (x-axis) and 90° in the elevation plane (z-axis). In the initial versions of the equipment, five cardiac cycles were used for this feature. In more recent equipment the number of cardiac cycles can be selected from a single beat to up to 6 beats. However, during the selection of multibeats for analysis, the stich artifacts are to be avoided. The full-volume images can be viewed as volume-rendered image or surface-rendered image. Surface rendering is a visualization technique that shows the surfaces of structures or organs in a solid appearance.
- *Tomographic slices:* After acquiring the images in the full volume, 3–12 tomographic slices of the images can be made (In GE systems). The top and bottom levels of

TABLE 1: Advantages and disadvantages of various modes in 3D echocardiography.

	Live	*Zoom*	*Full volume*
Dimensions	60° × 30° × depth of 2D image	20° × 20° × variable height to 90° × 90°	90° × 90° × depth of 2D image
Real time	Yes	Yes	• Single beat—Yes • Multibeat—depends on vendor
Frame rate	20–30 Hz	5–10 Hz	• 20–40 Hz (4 beats) • 40–50 Hz (7 beats)
Temporal resolution	Good	Lowest	
Spatial resolution	Mild	Highest	Lowest
Cardiac structure	Any 2D image	• Cardiac valves • Interatrial septum • Left atrial appendage	• Mitral valve • Aortic valve • Left ventricle
Clinical application	To guide interventional procedures	Examine anatomy	• LV function • Color Doppler

(2D: two-dimensional; 3D: three-dimensional; LV: Left ventricular)

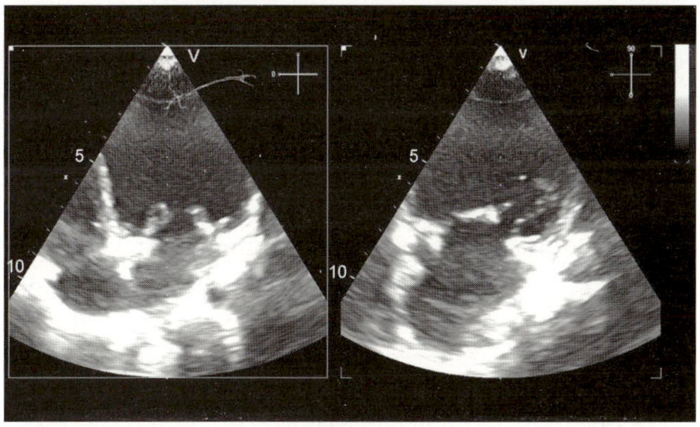

Fig. 3

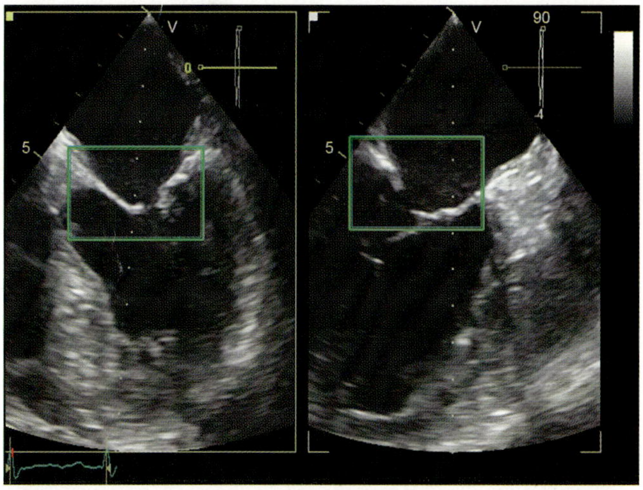

Fig. 4

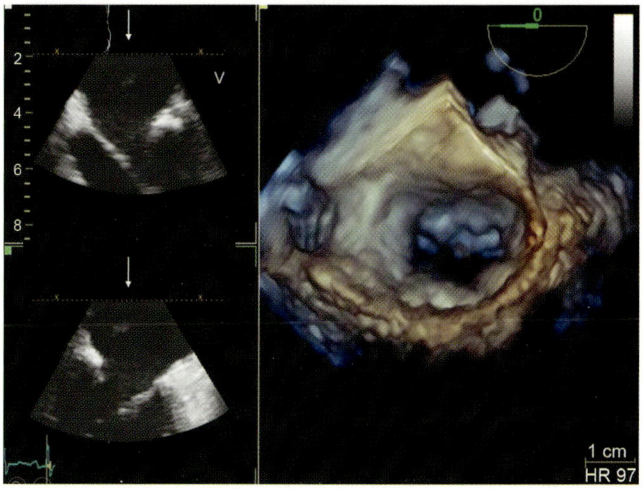

Fig. 5

cuts can be adjusted. The *iScan* (Philips systems) can be used to have the options of serial short-axis sections at apical, mid-left ventricular (LV), and MV level. The tomographic slices offer the advantages of views similar to Radionuclide studies.

- *Three-dimensional color full volume:* In this mode, the color flow mapping can be done within the three dimensionally acquired image. The advantages of the 3D color full-volume acquisition are the ease of identification of the area of vena contractae in regurgitant lesions and to identify the site of regurgitation in differentiation of valvular and paravalvular leaks.[24-26]

TOOLS FOR THREE-DIMENSIONAL ECHOCARDIOGRAPHY—CROPPING

Cropping is an important tool in 3D echocardiography. The machine after acquisition of the image displays it as an autocropped image in the coronal plane. To view the full pyramid, the image can be rotated through 90°, and the crop box can be moved in coronal plane. By cropping, the unwanted elements in the images can be removed. Oblique crop boxes are also available, which can be used for oblique cropping. In more modern machines the cropping has been simplified. In both GE and Philips systems, Click 2 Crop is used. Any two points can be clicked, and a rectangular area in between them can be cropped. We can even select the direction to view the cropped images. In Philips system a rectangular box can be used, which is called iCrop.

3D TRANSESOPHAGEAL ECHOCARDIOGRAPHY

A typical 3D transesophageal echocardiography (TEE) probe is similar to 2D TEE probe and consists of an ultrasound transducer, mounted at the tip of a flexible endoscope. The handle of the probe has two knobs that flex the tip anteroposteriorly or laterally. By advancing, withdrawing, rotating, or flexing the probe, it can be optimally positioned in the patient. The core of the modern transesophageal real-time 3D echocardiography system is a newly designed transducer with approximately 3,000 elements in contrast to the 2D TEE probe systems with 64 elements. Initially, biplane imaging is done to optimize the image size in azimuthal, axial, and elevation planes by adjusting the elevation plane width. The 3D zoom mode, which displays a smaller, magnified pyramidal volume, is commonly used to image MV and different cardiac structures, including other native valves, fossa ovalis, and the left atrial appendage.

SAFETY CONSIDERATIONS AND THE PROCEDURE OF THREE-DIMENSIONAL TRANSESOPHAGEAL ECHOCARDIOGRAPHY

The TEE probe is inserted after a light sedation in anxious patients and bite guard should always be used. Proper local anesthesia with Xylocaine spray and application of Xylocaine jelly are used to lubricate at the tip of the transducer for up to 20 cm. The torque of the rotating probe is limited to a low level by means of a mechanical system. This should prevent injury to the epithelium, even if the protective sheath should break. Moreover, the sheath is filled with nontoxic oil in case there is a leak. There is slight warming of the probe of about 2°C due to the rotation. Heating to more than 41°C is prevented by sensors. The probe is rotated by a flexible drive shaft. The ultrasonic signals are supplied via a rotating coupling from an electronic unit, consisting of the transmitter/receiver and digitizer module. The probe could be introduced without sedation in 2 min. The examination generally lasts for a total of about 10 min. The procedure is generally safe and, in sick patients, may require SPO_2 monitoring. The TEE probe is passed into the stomach at 35–40 cm, and the transgastric views are obtained. The scope is slowly withdrawn to 30–35 cm for lower esophageal and midesophageal views, then to upper esophageal cuts, and finally is rotated backward to view the descending aorta. Generally, a scheme very similar to 2D TEE is followed. However, there are very important differences which are the awesome multiplane imaging for sizing the image, the 3D zoom mode, and in addition, specialized software is available for quantification, which will be described later.

THREE-DIMENSIONAL EVALUATION OF MITRAL VALVE

The MV is a complex structure ideally suited for examination by 3D echocardiography as mental makeup of the valve by 2D echocardiography is difficult. Three dimensionally, it consists of atrioventricular junction or the mitral annulus, anterior and posterior mitral leaflets with commissures in medial and lateral aspects, chordae tendinae, anterolateral, and posteromedial papillary muscles, and the ventricular myocardial attachments.[27] The anterior leaflet comprises roughly the two-thirds of the valve area, is about twofold longer than the posterior leaflet (PL), and is somewhat triangular. The PL is more elongated and rectangular. The anterior leaflet is attached to the septum and fibrous annulus of the heart, and it is relatively nondistensible. Although the anterior leaflet accounts for the two-thirds of the MV area, its attachment to the mitral annulus accounts for only approximately one-third of the mitral annular circumference. The anterior mitral leaflet spans the distance between the two fibrous trigones and is in direct continuity with the noncoronary cusp of aortic valve. The posterior MV leaflet is attached to the posterior two-thirds of the mitral annulus, which runs along the free wall of the left ventricle and is primarily muscular with little fibrous tissue (explaining its tendency to distend and elongate).[27]

STEPS INVOLVED IN THREE-DIMENSIONAL ACQUISITION OF MITRAL VALVE

- Mitral valve can be viewed from long-axis view, short-axis view, or apical window, transthoracically, and at midesophageal level, transesophagically. Whatever view is used, the aorta is rotated in the *z* axis and kept in 12-o'clock position.
- *Multiplane view:* Generally examination of MV is started in long-axis window with biplane mode. In the long axis, by placing the cursor across the tip of the MV, short-axis view of the MV is displayed on the right hand side. Thus, from exactly the tip of MV, the MV area can be calculated accurately by planimetry (Fig. 6). Similarly from apical window, biplane and triplane modes are used. This will be especially helpful in 3D TEE from midesophageal location to identify the mitral scallops (Fig. 7).

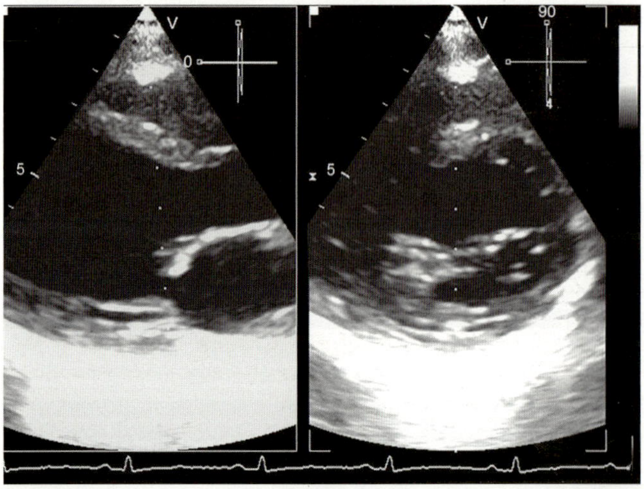

Fig. 6

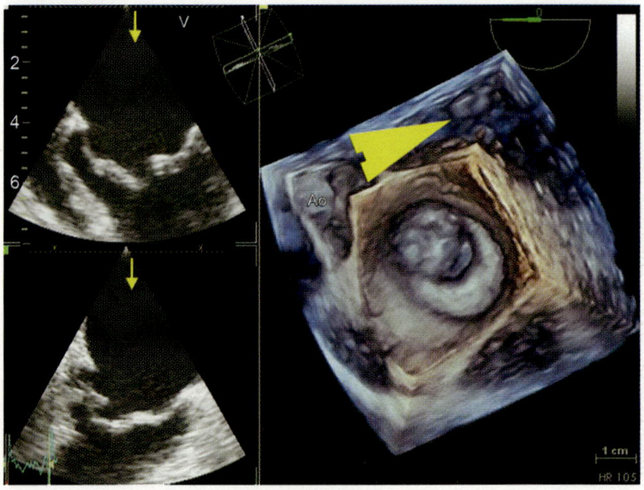

Fig. 7

- *Zoom view*: From the biplane view zoom, acquisition window is applied, and the elevation plane width is adjusted and clicked. Both from transthoracic echocardiogram and TEE, the 3D data set is rotated to bring the aorta to 12 o'clock position (Fig. 8). Unlike, 2D echocardiography, where viewing of MV is only possible from LV side only, in 3D echocardiography, viewing from both LV side and left atrial (LA) side (Surgeons' view) is possible. By selecting the dual layout format, simultaneous viewing of MV from both LA and LV side is possible. The surgeons' view is the preferred view to obtain the anterior and posterior mitral leaflets and the several indentations dividing them into segments or scallops. The anterior leaflet has three scallops: A1—anterolateral, A2—middle, and A3—posteromedial. Similarly, the PL has three scallops: P1—anterolateral, P2—middle, and P3—posteromedial. The anterior and PLs are fused for 3–8 mm medially and laterally at the trigones and usually form distinct commissures (anterolateral and posteromedial). The LA appendage is also seen at 9 o'clock position in this view. This is also the best view for mitral interventions in the cardiac catheterization laboratory.
- *Full volume*: Before selecting full volume, the image is acquired in narrow angle view. Here the gain setting and the elevation plane width can be adjusted. After full-volume acquisition, from the apical window, either Click 2 Crop or iCrop can be used to crop the MV and view. After the acquisition of MV in full thickness from parasternal long-axis view, the image can be rotated 90° counterclockwise, to view the MV and the entire subvalvular apparatus (Fig. 8).

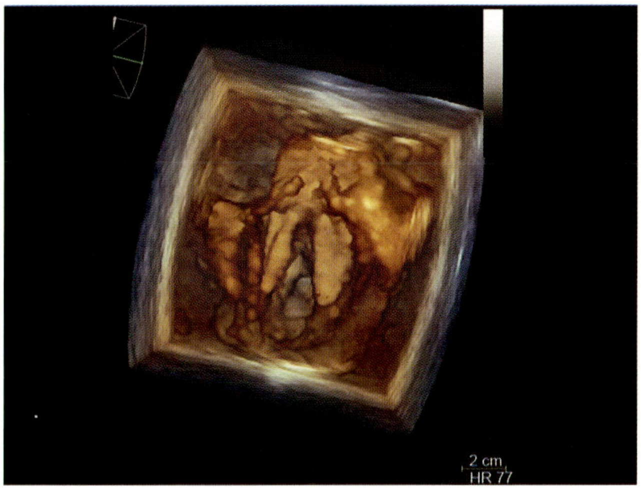

Fig. 8

THREE-DIMENSIONAL EVALUATION OF MITRAL STENOSIS

The severity of mitral stenosis is assessed mainly by the estimation of the MV area. At present, the available 2D echocardiographic and Doppler techniques have their well-known limitations. The advent of 3D echocardiography has refined the assessment of MV area to such an extent that today it is considered a gold standard. When compared to traditional 2D and Doppler measurements, such as 2D planimetry, pressure halftime, and flow convergence, 3D echocardiography best agreed with mitral orifice area calculations derived using the Gorlin formula during cardiac catheterization.[28,29] In addition, Anwar et al. have introduced the new 3D echocardiographic indices and scoring system which further improves the diagnosis of mitral stenosis and helps in the assessment of the morphology of the MV for the success of balloon mitral valvuloplasty compared to the 2D-based Wilkinson criteria.[30] In this method, thickness, mobility, and calcification for each MV scallop are assessed qualitatively and scored as follows: normal thickness and mobility are scored as 0 and abnormal thickness or restricted mobility as 1. An absence of calcification is scored as 0, calcification in middle scallop (A2 or P2) is scored as 1, and calcification of the commissural scallops of both leaflets (A1, A3, P1, and P3) is scored as 2. Scoring of the subvalvular apparatus includes chordal thickness and distance of separation between the chordae which are as follows: Normal thickness is scored as 0 and abnormal thickness as 1, normal chordal separation (distance in between >5 mm) is scored as 0, partial separation (distance in between <5 mm) as 1, and the absence of separation is scored as 2 (Table 2).

STEPS INVOLVED IN THREE-DIMENSIONAL EVALUATION FOR MITRAL VALVE AREA

- The zoomed images of MV are acquired as enumerated above (Figure 9 shows transthoracic image viewed from left ventricle, and Figure 10 shows transesophageal image viewed from left atrium).
- The middiastolic image with maximal opening of MV is selected. Now, the translational line can be moved to place exactly across the tip of the mitral leaflets as shown on the four-chamber or two-chamber views depicted on the left hand side.
- The planimetry can be directly done from this using the crop plane area planimetry tool.
- Alternatively, Flexi Slice can be selected, and the central points of the cursor can be aligned to the center of the mitral leaflets (Fig. 11), and planimetry can be done.

TABLE 2: Anwar 3D echocardiographic scoring of mitral stenosis.

	Anterior leaflet			*Posterior leaflet*		
	A1	*A2*	*A3*	*P1*	*P2*	*P3*
Thickness (0–6) (0 = normal, 1 = thickened)*	0–1	0–1	0–1	0–1	0–1	0–1
Mobility (0–6) (0 = normal, 1 = limited)*	0–1	0–1	0–1	0–1	0–1	0–1
Calcification (0–10) (0 = normal, 1–2 = calcified)†	0–2	0–1	0–2	0–2	0–1	0–2
	Subvalvular apparatus					
	Proximal third	*Middle third*			*Distal third*	
Thickness (0–3) (0 = normal, 1 = thickened)	0–1	0–1			0–1	
Separation (0–6) (0 = normal, 1 = partial, 2 = no)	0, 1, 2	0, 1, 2			0, 1, 2	

(3D: Three-dimensional)

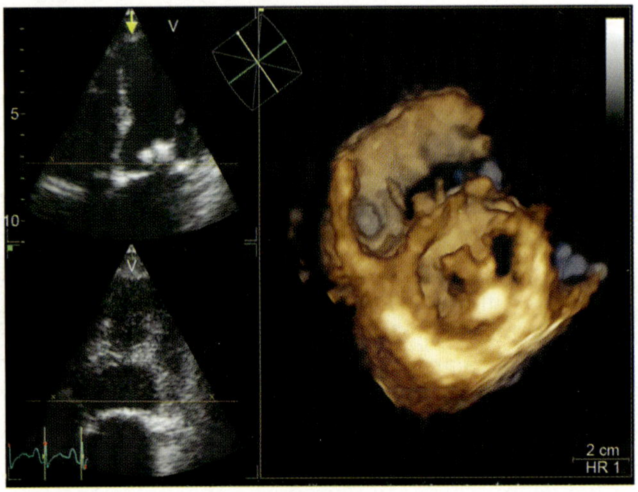

Fig. 9

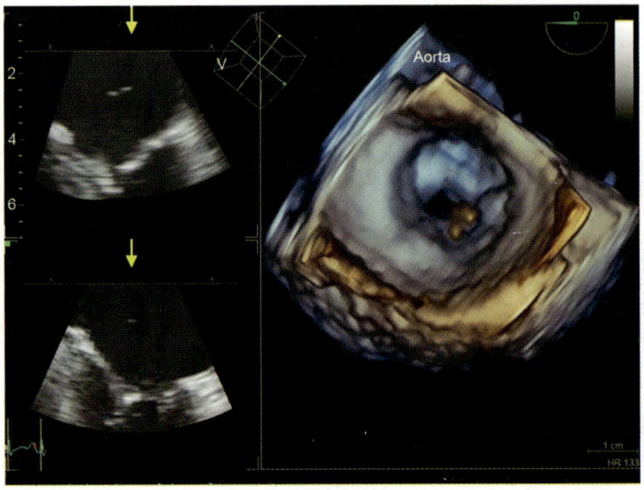

Fig. 10

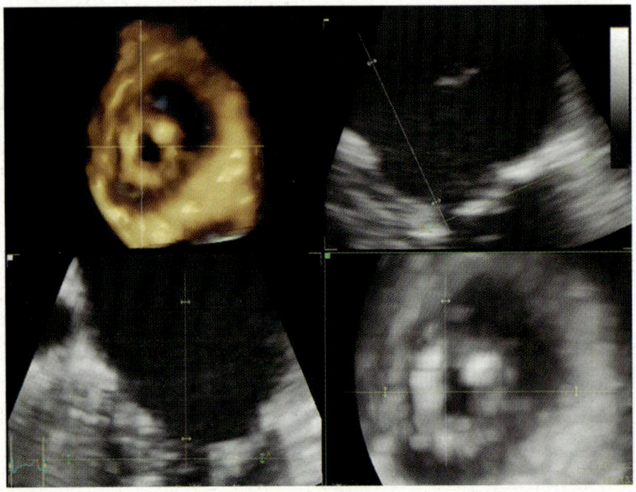

Fig. 11

THREE-DIMENSIONAL EVALUATION OF MITRAL REGURGITATION

Three-dimensional echocardiography has led to improved insight into the complex geometry of the saddle-shaped MV, the mechanisms of functional and ischemic mitral regurgitation (MR), and the abnormalities in MV prolapse, and infective endocarditis. Carpenter has classified the mitral valvular lesions according to the disease, valvular lesions, and the type of valvular dysfunction, which are called Carpenter's triad. The Carpenters' classification of valvular dysfunction is further summarized in Table 3.[31] The 3D echocardiogram is ideally suited for the analysis of this kind and also helps to guide surgical repair.[32,33] The classification of mitral dysfunction is based on the position of the leaflet margins with respect to the mitral annulus plane:

TABLE 3: Carpenters, classification of mitral valvular dysfunction.

- *Type I* dysfunction implies normal leaflet motion with isolated annular dilation, leading to poor leaflet coaptation
- *Type II* dysfunction is defined by excess motion of the margin of a leaflet segment above the annular plane and is the most common type of dysfunction in degenerative MV disease
- *Type III* restricted motion of the leaflet margin, which can be further subdivided
- *Type IIIa*: Restriction of motion in both systole and diastole (usually due to fibrosis of the subvalvular apparatus)
- *Type IIIb*: Restriction of motion only in systole (which usually results from ventricular remodeling with papillary displacement and leaflet tethering)

(MV: mitral valve)

- Type I dysfunction, normal leaflet motion with severe annular dilatation (central regurgitant jet) or perforation of one of the leaflets (Figure 12A shows a patient with severe annular dilatation and B shows the central jet)
- Type II dysfunction, excessive leaflet motion generally secondary to pathologic elongation or rupture of the chordae tendinae (in which case, regurgitant jet is directed to the opposite side of the affected leaflet) (Figure 13 shows A2, A3, and P3 Prolapse)
- Type III dysfunction, restricted leaflet motion due to the retraction of the subvalvular apparatus
  - IIIa: Rheumatic disease or inflammatory processes [Figure 14A shows thick MV in a patient with rheumatic MR biplane view, (B) shows the 3D evaluation in the same patient, (C) shows Flexi Slice evaluation, (D) shows the thick subvalvular apparatus, and (E) shows the transesophageal 3D of the thick mitral leaflets].
  - IIIb: Papillary muscle displacement (ischemic remodeling or dilated cardiomyopathy) causing apical displacement (tethering) of the valve. The MV tenting area is measured as the area enclosed between the annular line and MV leaflets (Fig. 15). The coaptation distance is defined as the distance between the annular line and the leaflet's coaptation point. The PL angle is the angle in between annular line and the coaptation point of the PL length.[32]

STEPS IN FOUR-DIMENSIONAL COLOR FLOW EVALUATION OF MITRAL REGURGITATION

- Four-dimensional color flow imaging is the most common way to assess MR severity. The general assumption is that as the severity of the MR increases, the size and the extent of the jet into the LA also increase. Theoretically, larger color jets that extend deep into the left atrium represent more MR than smaller thin jets that appear just beyond the mitral leaflets. Initially, triplane view can be selected and to view MR severity in three-chamber, four-chamber, and two-chamber planes (Fig. 16A). Subsequently the full-volume color flow can be acquired (Fig. 16B). The 12-segment analysis can be done at this point, and color flow can be quantified (Fig. 16C). However, the relationship between jet size and MR severity presents a large range of variability because, in addition to regurgitation severity, the color flow display depends on many technical and hemodynamic factors. For a similar severity, patients with increased LA pressure or with eccentric jets that hug the LA wall or in whom the LA is enlarged may exhibit smaller jet

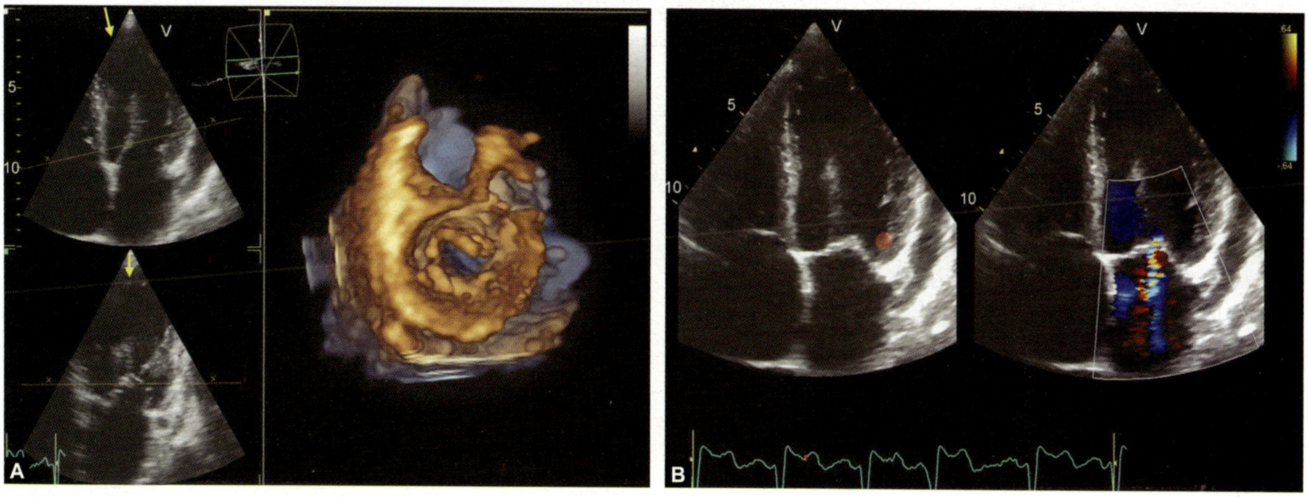

Figs. 12A and B

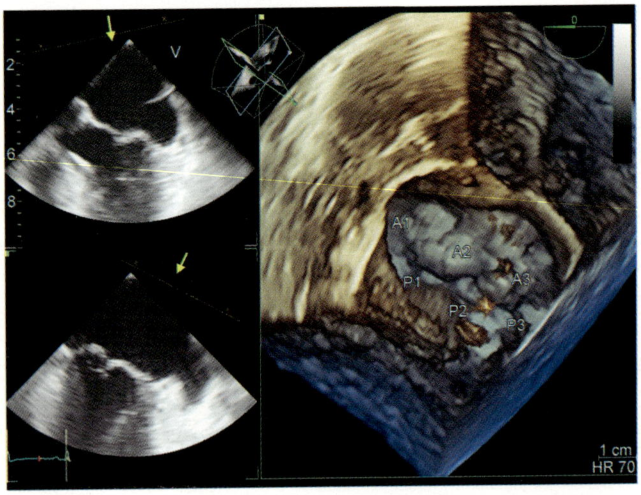

Fig. 13

area than those with normal LA pressure and size or with central jets.

- *Four-dimensional assessment of vena contracta width and anatomic regurgitant orifice area*: By moving the translation line to the narrowest portion of the flow convergence, the assessment of the vena contracta in the biplane view is possible (Fig. 17A). In addition, by looking from 3D echocardiographic perspective, the anatomic regurgitant orifice area can be planimetered (Fig. 17B). Direct measurement of MR anatomic regurgitant orifice area correlates well with effective regurgitant orifice area by proximal convergence method and vena contracta area. Agreement between methods is better for patients with a circular regurgitation orifice area than in patients with a noncircular regurgitation orifice area.[34]

THREE-DIMENSIONAL EVALUATION OF MITRAL VALVE BY TOMTEC SOFTWARE

- The data set is oriented with left atrium above left ventricle.
- The frame of interest is selected for the end-diastolic and the end-systolic frame.
- The MV annulus is marked in the midsystole, and the mitral annulus position is set in upper and lower long-axis view. This is followed by the marking of the LV outflow tract (LVOT) in the middle of LVOT. The end of coaptation of MV is marked (Fig. 18A) (Media 11A).
- The calculated 3D MV is checked and edited (Fig. 18B).
- The various parameters of MV coaptation are displayed.

THREE-DIMENSIONAL EVALUATION OF MITRAL VALVE BY ECHOPAC

- The images are acquired from TEE in zoomed view of MV with a frame rate of ≥12/s, and images are aligned in 3D short-axis view, midcommissural view, and long-axis view (Fig. 19A).
- The end-diastolic and end-systolic frames are set, and landmark points in the annulus, coaptation point, and the aorta are marked.
- The reference frames are chosen for scallops and commissures, and the adjustments are made (Fig. 19B).
- The results and the various parameters of leaflets and commissures are displayed (Fig. 19C).

THREE-DIMENSIONAL EVALUATION OF PROSTHETIC MITRAL VALVE

Prosthetic valve evaluation by echocardiography is the gold standard, and the recent guidelines by American Society of Echocardiography and European Association of Cardiovascular Imaging have upheld this.[35] The 3D echocardiography plays a major role in the evaluation of structure and function of all the bioprosthetic and mechanical valve types:

- *Caged ball (Starr–Edwards valve) (Fig. 20):* This valve is no more used for implantation now.
- *Single-disc tilting valve (Chitra valve) (Fig. 21):* This is the commonest valve implanted in India.
- Bileaflet valve (St. Judes) (Fig. 22).

By the unquestionable clarity, the 3D echocardiography remains the best method to evaluate the prosthetic valve obstruction, regurgitation, and paravalvular regurgitation.[36]

THREE-DIMENSIONAL ECHOCARDIOGRAPHY DURING MITRAL VALVE INTERVENTIONS

Balloon mitral valvuloplasty: Intraprocedural imaging techniques are continuously evolving as there are mitral interventional advances. Since 1984, when Kenji Inoue introduced the Inoue Balloon, this technique has become the procedure of choice for mitral stenosis. At present, 3D echocardiography is used during various steps of balloon mitral valvuloplasty, such as septal puncture and placement of the Inoue balloon across the MV and dilatation.[37-39] Figure 23 shows the 3D TEE-guided placement of the Inoue balloon across the MV.

Edge-to-edge repair of MV regurgitation: Percutaneous edge-to-edge repair of MV regurgitation using MitraClip system mimics the surgical mitral repair introduced by Otavio Alfieri in the year 1991. The EVEREST I (Endovascular Valve Edge-to-Edge Repair Study) showed the safety and efficacy of the MitraClip system (Evalve Inc., Menlo Park, California). The mortality was low, and the severity of the MR was reduced remarkably.[39,40] TEE showing biplane 2D and color flow image with MitraClip in situ, having been optimally "clipped" to the mitral leaflets (Fig. 24).

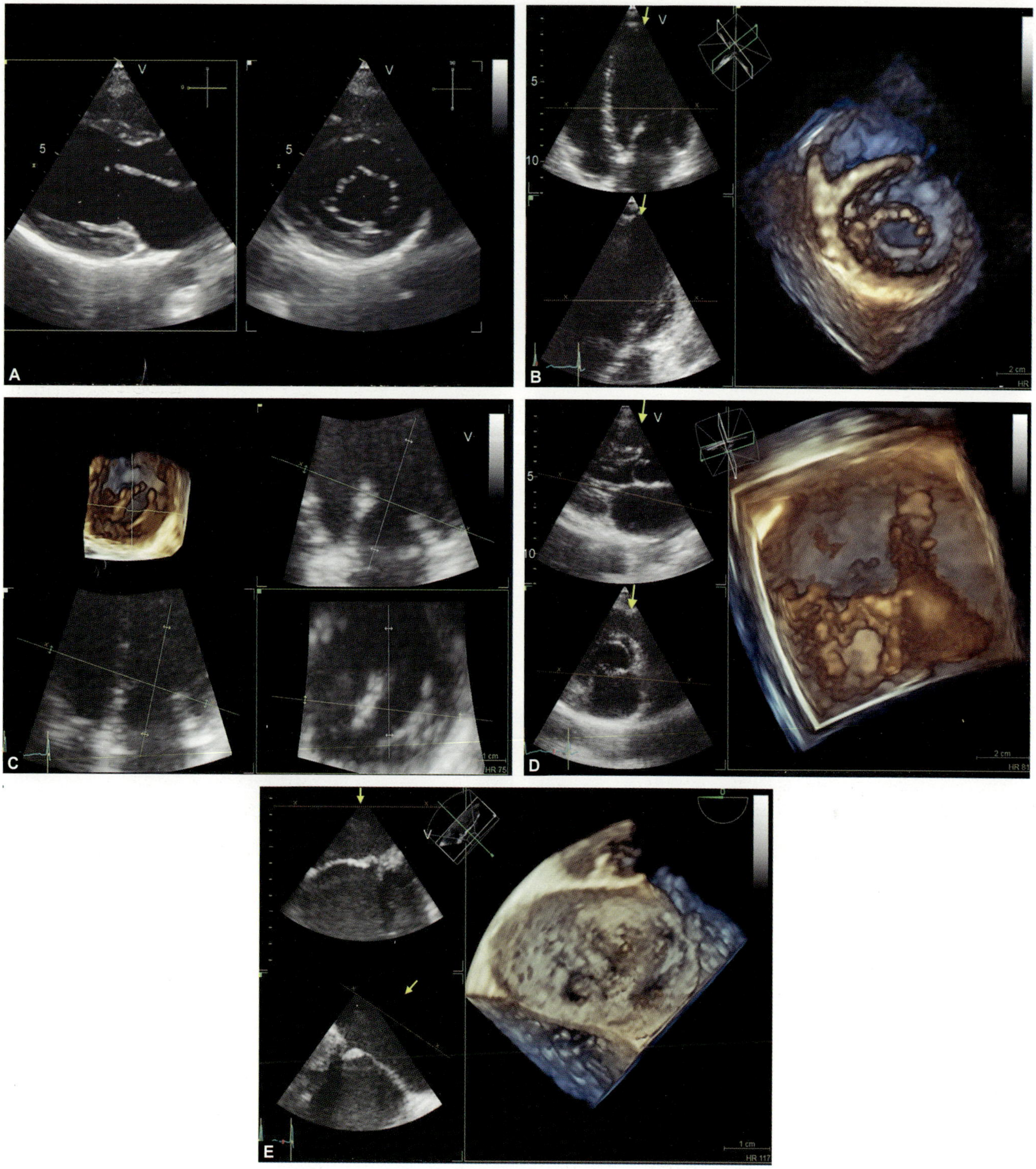

Figs. 14A to E

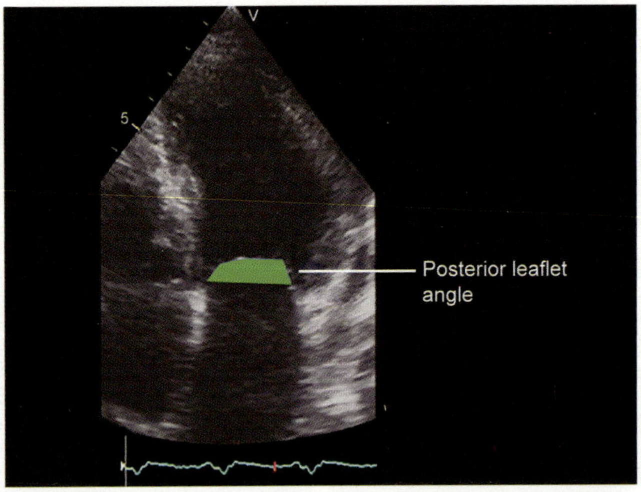

Fig. 15

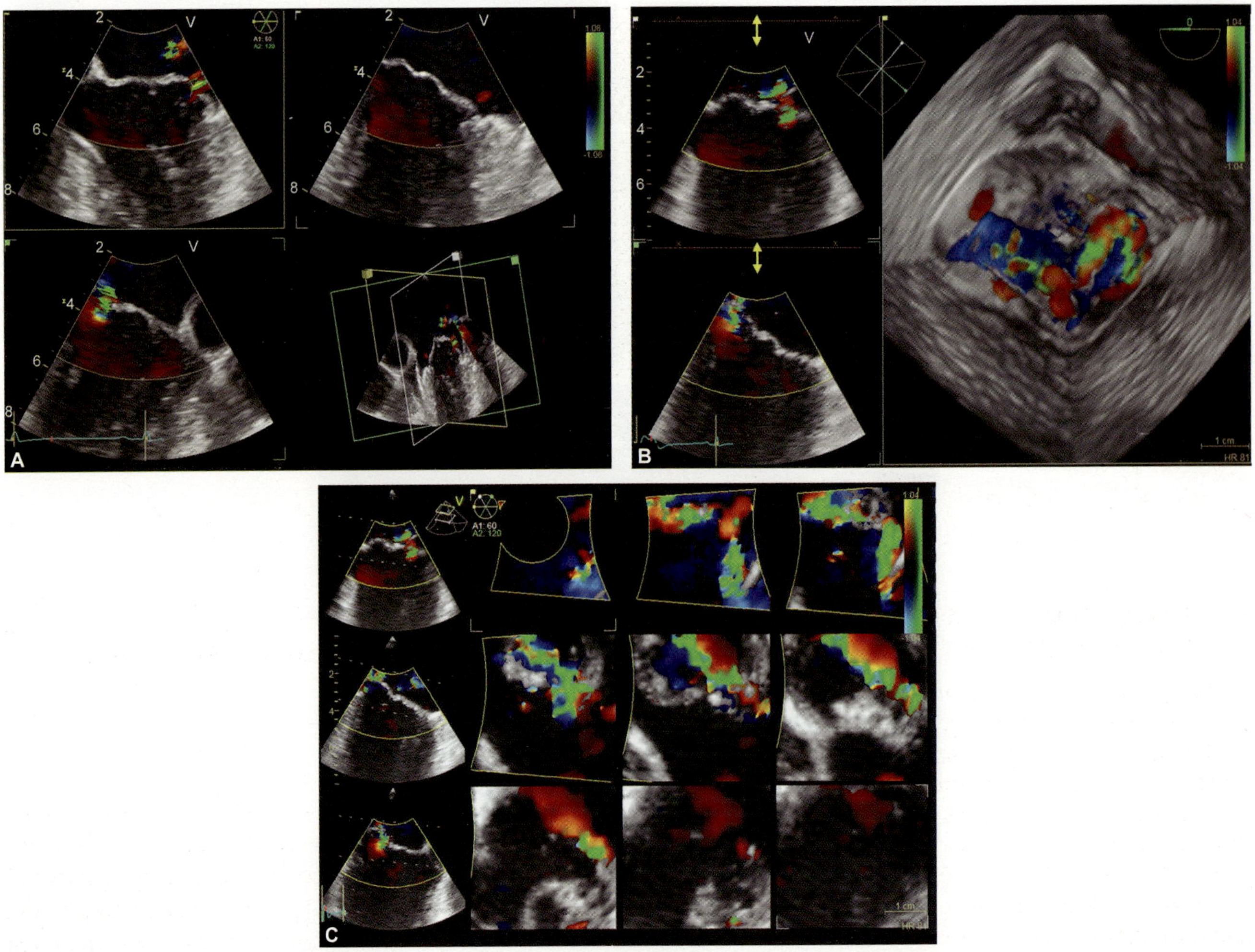

Figs. 16A to C

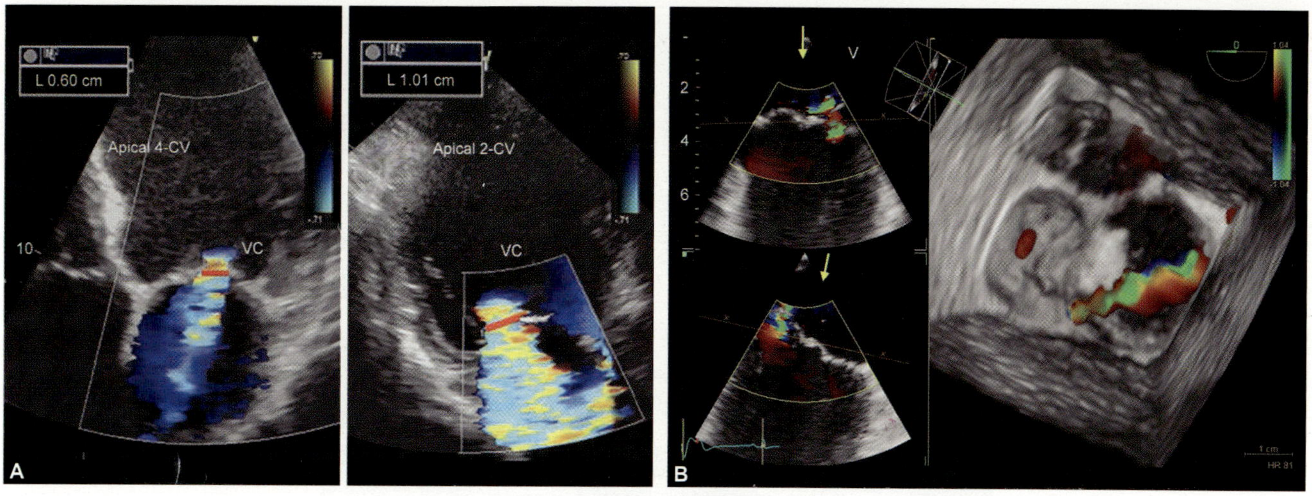

Figs. 17A and B

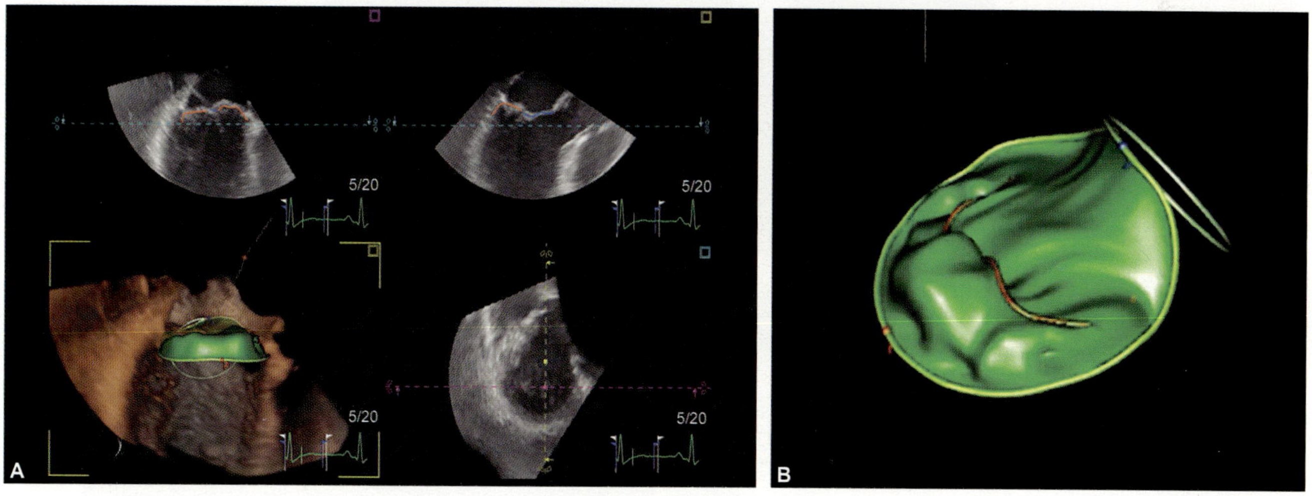

Figs. 18A and B

TEE showing 3D image of the MV from the LA side with MitraClip in place (Fig. 25).

Percutaneous MV replacement: World's first percutaneous MV replacement was done and reported by Gopalamurugan et al. in a 75-year-old man with previous coronary artery bypass grafting surgery and implantation of St. Jude porcine valve in mitral position and bioprosthetic valve dysfunction.[41] A valve in valve implantation using 26 mm Sapien XT valve (Edwards Lifesciences) was deployed successfully. Figure 26 shows the 3D echocardiography demonstrating the success of the procedure. Transcutaneous MV replacement for native MV has emerged as an exciting new development in structural heart disease intervention.[42]

CONCLUSION

The ever-increasing use and the literature on 3D echocardiography is a proof of the acceptance of this technique in the real world. However, with more and more development of techniques and transducer technology, special and temporal resolution of the 3D data sets is increased, and there is single-beat acquisition possible to avoid the stitch

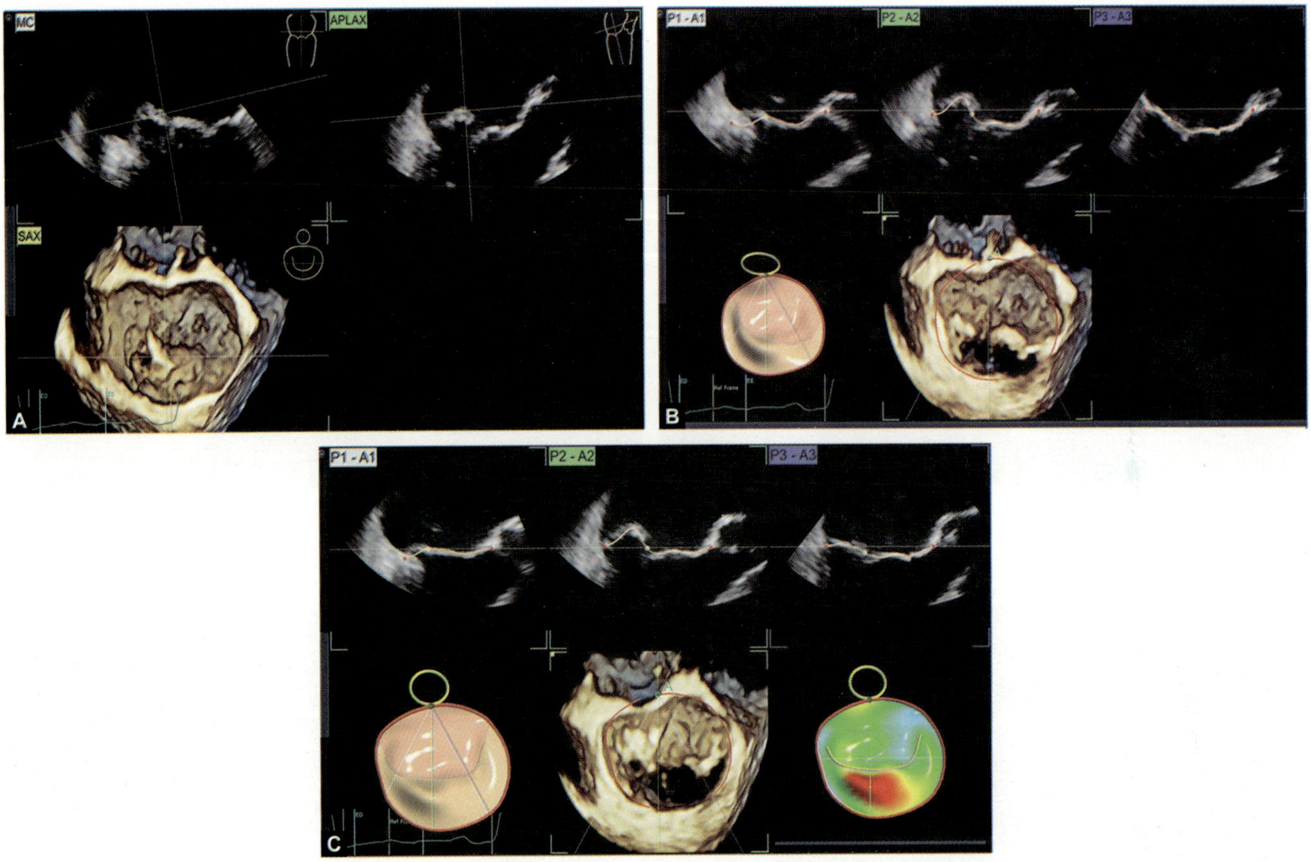

Figs. 19A to C

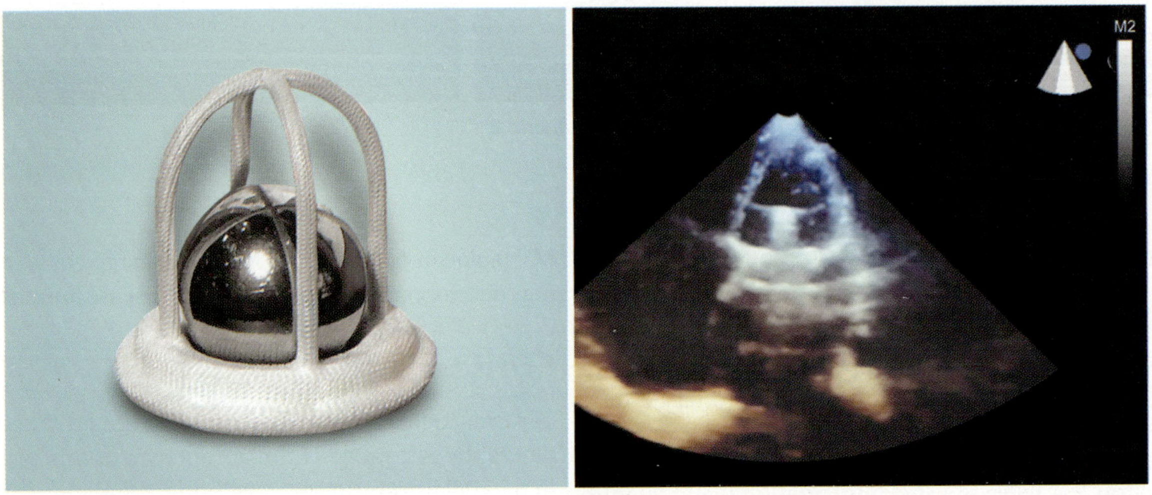

Fig. 20

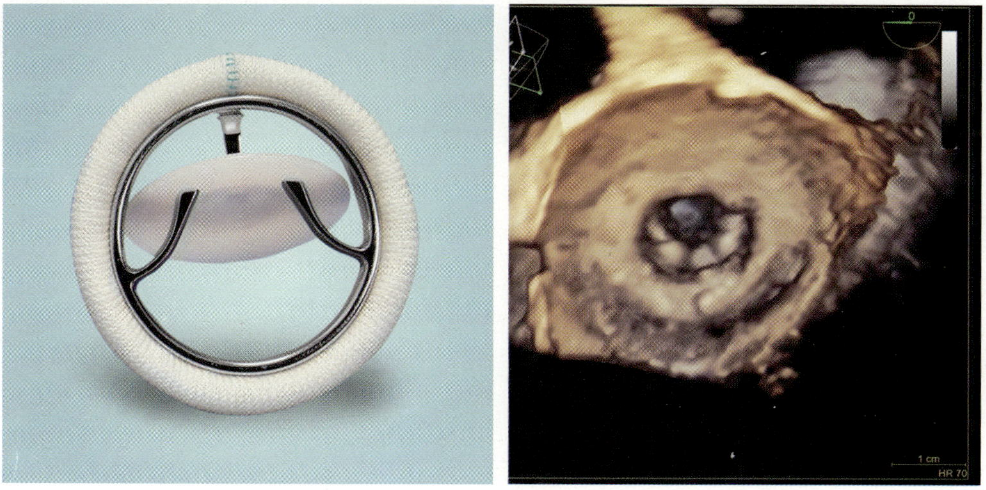

Fig. 21

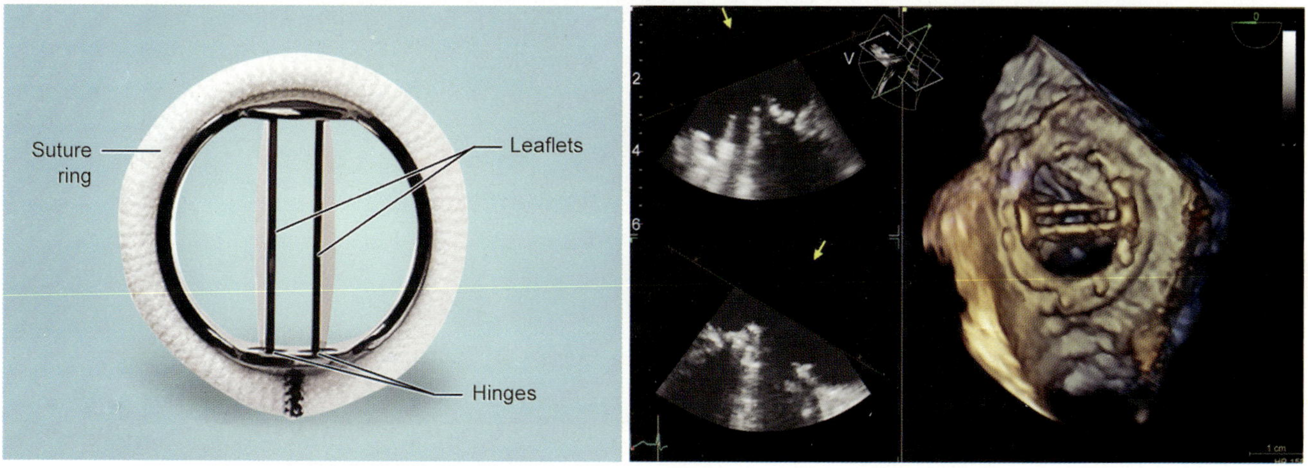

Fig. 22

artifact. At present the following are the areas where 3D echocardiography has demonstrated the usefulness.[43] Major advantages of 3D echocardiography compared to traditional 2D echocardiography are as follows: (1) LV function assessment—improved accuracy of evaluation of LV chamber volumes (by eliminating the need for geometric modeling as well as a reduction in errors caused by foreshortened views); principal reasons for requesting an echocardiogram in clinical practice include the assessment of LV chamber size and systolic function. (2) Realistic visualization of cardiac valves and congenital abnormalities. Volume-rendered 3D displays of transthoracic or transesophageal images enable improved evaluation of the anatomy of the heart valves and their supporting structures. Accordingly, 3D imaging is particularly helpful to the cardiac surgeon or interventional cardiologist to provide the most detailed anatomic and functional information.

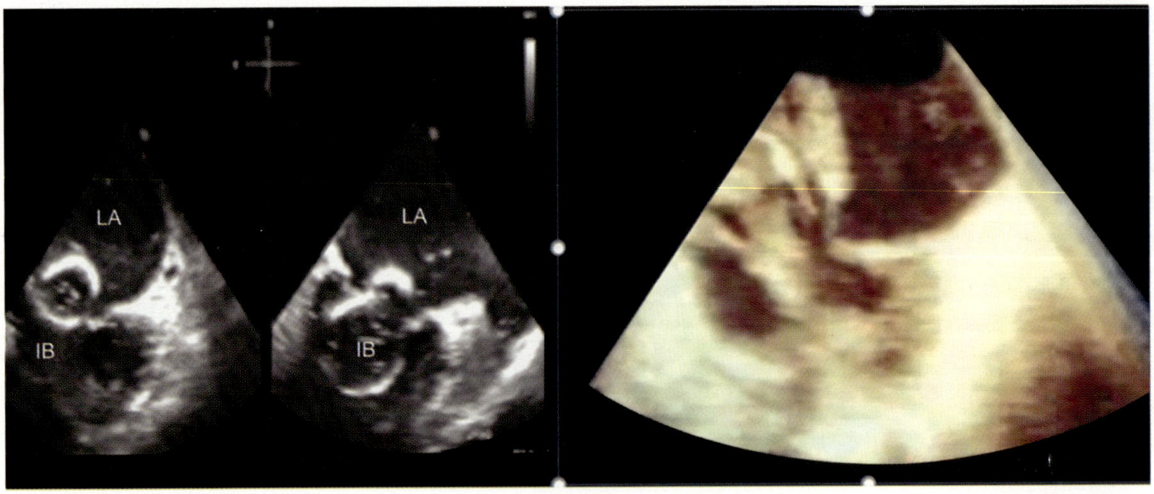

Fig. 23

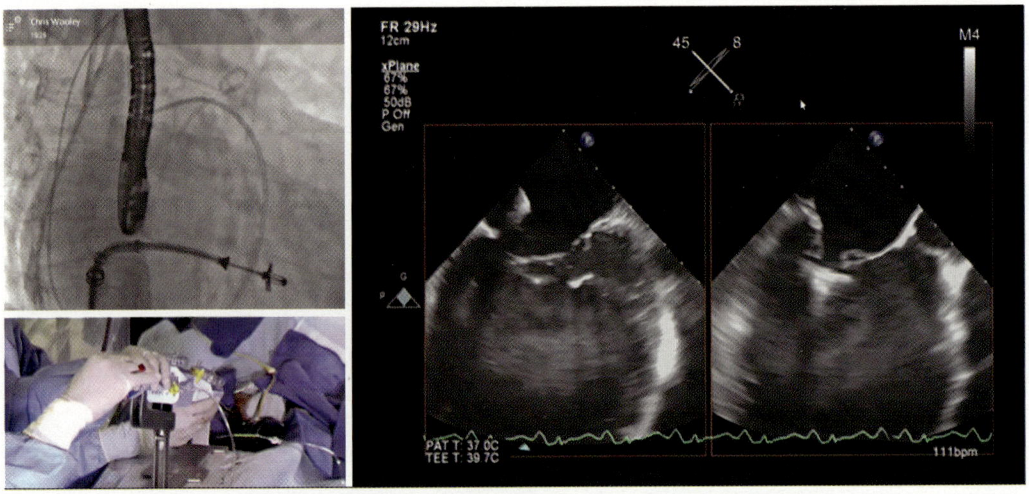

Fig. 24

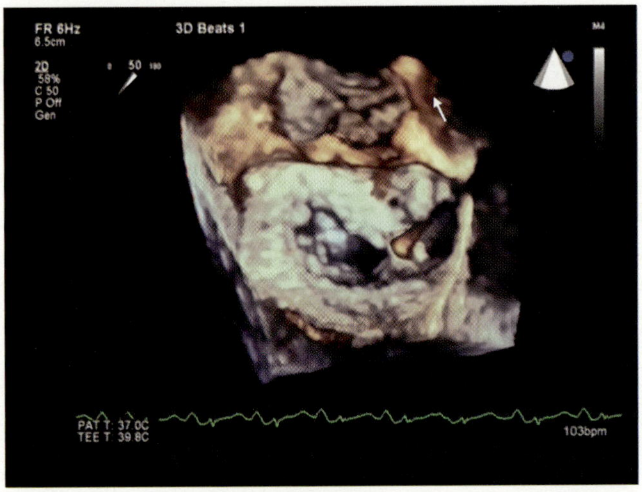

Fig. 25

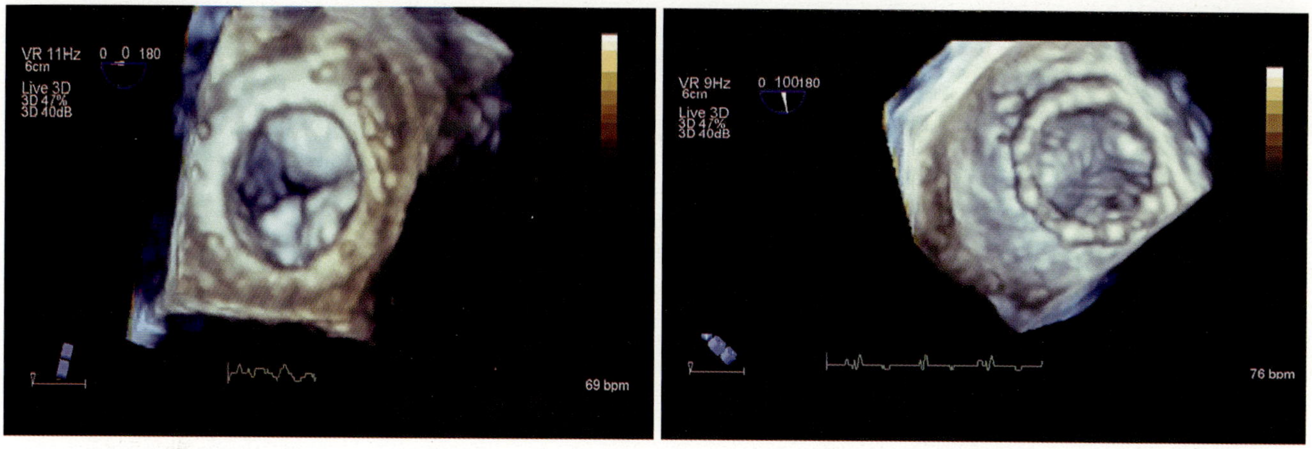

Fig. 26

REFERENCES

1. Hung J, Lang R, Flachskampf F, et al. 3D echocardiography: a review of the current status and future directions. J Am Soc Echocardiogr. 2007;20(3):213-33.
2. Lang RM, Badano LP, Tsang W, et al. EAE/ASE recommendations for image acquisition and display using three-dimensional echocardiography. J Am Soc Echocardiogr. 2012;25:3-46.
3. Amuthan V. Manual of 3D echocardiography. JP Brothers; 2013.
4. Handke M, Heinrichs G, Moser U, et al. Transesophageal real-time three-dimensional echocardiography. Methods and initial in vitro and human in vivo studies. J Am Coll Cardiol. 2006;48:2070-6.
5. Sugeng L, Shernan SK, Salgo IS, et al. Live 3-dimensional transesophageal echocardiography initial experience using the fully-sampled matrix array probe. Am Coll Cardiol. 2008;52:446-9.
6. Mor-Avi V, Sugeng L, Lang RM. Real-time 3-dimensional echocardiography. an integral component of the routine echocardiographic examination in adult patients? Circulation. 2009;119:314-29.
7. Bhan A, Kapetanakis S, Monaghan MJ. Three-dimensional echocardiography. Heart. 2010;96:153-63.
8. Johri AM, Passeri JJ, Picard MH. Three-dimensional echocardiography: approaches and clinical utility. Heart. 2010;96:390-7.
9. Faletra FF, Ho SY, Auricchio PA. Anatomy of right atrial structures by real-time 3D transesophageal echocardiography. JACC Cardiovasc Imaging. 2010;3(3):966-75.
10. Pearlman AS. Echocardiography 2020: opportunities and challenges. J Am Soc Echocardiogr. 2010;23(8):898-900.
11. Latcu DG, Rinaldi JP, Saoudi N. Real-time three-dimensional transoesophageal echocardiography for diagnosis of left atrial appendage thrombus. Eur J Echocardiogr. 2009;10: 711-2.
12. Szmigielski C, Rajpoot K, Grau V, et al. Real-time 3D fusion echocardiography. JACC Cardiovasc Imaging. 2010;3: 682-90.
13. Hilberath JN, Oakes DA, Shernan SK, et al. Safety of transesophageal echocardiography. J Am Soc Echocardiogr. 2010;23:1115-27.
14. Franke A, Rulands D, Breithardt OA, et al. Transthoracic high-resolution real-time three-dimensional echocardiography for the analysis of regional left-ventricular wall motion patterns in patients with cardiac resynchronization therapy. Eur Heart J. 2003;24(Abstr. Suppl.):396.
15. Kapetenakis S, Murray O, Rance K, et al. Contrast enhanced real-time three-dimensional echocardiography, is it feasible? Eur Heart J. 2003;24(Abstr. Suppl.):700.
16. Kühl HP, Rulands D, Schreckenberg M, et al. Assessment of left-ventricular volumes and function using high-resolution transthoracic real-time three-dimensional echocardiography: comparison of semi-automatic border detection with manual contour tracing. Eur Heart J. 2003;24(Suppl):352.
17. Marx G. The real deal: real-time 3-D echocardiography in congenital heart disease. Pediatr Cardiol Today. 2003;1(1): 9-11.
18. Shirali G. Live 3-D echo clarifies anatomy of recurrent subaortic stenosis and a shadow in the left atrium. RT Image. 2003;16(25).
19. Lang R, Sugeng L. A fantastic journey: 3D cardiac ultrasound goes live. Radiol Manage. 2002;24(6):18-22.
20. Ahmad M, Xie T, Chamoun AJ, et al. Images in cardiovascular medicine. Real-time three-dimensional echocardiography with real-time volume rendering in assessment of left ventricular apical thrombi. Circulation. 2002;106(13):e53.
21. Belohlavek M, Tanabe K, Jakrapanichakul D, et al. Rapid three-dimensional echocardiography: clinically feasible alternative for precise and accurate measurement of left ventricular volumes. Circulation. 2001;103(24):2882-4.

22. Qin JX, Shiota T, McCarthy PM, et al. Real-time three-dimensional echocardiographic study of left ventricular function after infarct exclusion surgery for ischemic cardiomyopathy. Circulation. 2000;102(19 Suppl. 3):III101-6.
23. Yao J, Cao QL, Masani N, et al. Three-dimensional echocardiographic estimation of infarct mass based on quantification of dysfunctional left ventricular mass. Circulation. 1997;96(5):1660-6.
24. Hung J, Guerrero JL, Handschumacher MD, et al. Reverse ventricular remodeling reduces ischemic mitral regurgitation: echo-guided device application in the beating heart. Circulation. 2002;106(20):2594-600.
25. Kwan J, Shiota T, Agler DA, et al. Real-time three-dimensional echocardiography study. Geometric differences of the mitral apparatus between ischemic and dilated cardiomyopathy with significant mitral regurgitation: real-time three-dimensional echocardiography study. Circulation. 2003;107(8):1135-40.
26. Buck T, Mucci RA, Guerrero JL, et al. The power-velocity integral at the vena contracta: a new method for direct quantification of regurgitant volume flow. Circulation. 2000;102(9):1053-61.
27. Salustri A, Becker AE, van Herwerden L, et al. Three-dimensional echocardiography of normal and pathologic mitral valve: a comparison with two-dimensional transesophageal echocardiography. J Am Coll Cardiol. 1996;27:1502-10.
28. Zamorano J, Cordeiro P, Sugeng L, et al. Real time three dimensional echocardiography for rheumatic mitral valve stenosis evaluation: an accurate and novel approach. J Am Coll Cardiol. 2004;43:2091.
29. Sugeng L, Weinert L, Lammertin G, et al. Accuracy of mitral valve area measurements using transthoracic rapid freehand 3-dimensional scanning: comparison with noninvasive and invasive methods. J Am Soc Echocardiogr. 2003;16:1292.
30. Anwar AM, Attia WM, Nosir YF, Soliman OI, Mosad MA, Othman M et al. Validation of a new score for the assessment of mitral stenosis using real-time three-dimensional echocardiography. J Am Soc Echocardiogr. 2010;23:13-22.
31. Carpentier A, Adams DH, Filsoufi F. Carpentier's reconstructive valve surgery. Maryland Heights, MO: Saunders-Elsevier; 2010.
32. Castillo JG, Solís J, González-Pinto A, et al. Surgical echocardiography of the mitral valve. Rev Esp Cardiol. 2011;64(12):1169-81.
33. Magne J, Pibarot P, Dagenais F, et al. Preoperative posterior leaflet angle accurately predicts outcome after restrictive mitral valve annuloplasty for ischemic mitral regurgitation. Circulation. 2007;115:782-91.
34. Altiok E, Hamada S, van Halla S, et al. Comparison of direct planimetry of mitral valve regurgitation orifice area by three-dimensional transesophageal echocardiography to effective regurgitant orifice area obtained by proximal flow convergence method and vena contracta area determined by color Doppler echocardiography. Am J Cardiol. 2011;107(3):452-8.
35. Lancellotti P, Pibarot P, Chambers J, et al. Recommendations for the imaging assessment of prosthetic heart valves: a report from the European Association of Cardiovascular Imaging endorsed by the Chinese Society of Echocardiography, the Inter-American Society of Echocardiography, and the Brazilian Department of Cardiovascular Imaging. Eur Heart J Cardiovasc Imaging. 2016;17:589-90.
36. Sordelli C, Severino S, Ascione L, et al. Echocardiographic assessment of heart valve prostheses. J Cardiovasc Echogr. 2014;24(4):103-13.
37. Eng MH, Salcedo EE, Quaife R, et al. Implementation of real time three-dimensional transesophageal echocardiography in percutaneous mitral balloon valvuloplasty and structural heart disease interventions. Echocardiography. 2009;26:958-66.
38. Navarro MA, Kim M, Salcedo EE. Real-time 3D echocardiography in percutaneous balloon mitral valvuloplasty. 2013.
39. Cavalcante JL, Rodriguez L, Kapadia S, et al. Role of echocardiography in percutaneous mitral valve interventions. JACC Cardiovasc Imaging. 2012;5:733-46.
40. Feldman T, Kar S, Rinaldi M, et al.; EVEREST Investigators. Percutaneous mitral repair with the MitraClip system: safety and midterm durability in the initial EVEREST (Endovascular Valve Edge-to-Edge REpair Study) cohort. J Am Coll Cardiol. 2009;54:686-94.
41. Gopalamurugan AB, Pantazis A, Schievano S, et al. Percutaneous transvenous mitral valve implantation. J Am Coll Cardiol. 2013;61(7).
42. Regueiro A, Granada JF, Dagenais F, et al. Transcatheter mitral valve replacement: insights from early clinical experience and future challenges. J Am Coll Cardiol. 2017;69:2175-92.
43. Avi VM, Lang RM. Three dimensional echocardiography. UpToDate; 2015. pp. 1-18.

63

CHAPTER

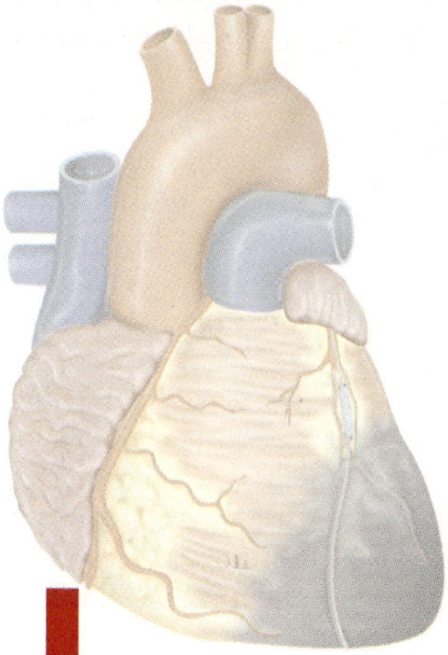

Mitral Clipping Evaluation by Echocardiography

Ahmed K Pasha, Rajesh Janardhanan

INTRODUCTION

Severity of mitral regurgitation (MR) is strongly associated not only with heart failure but also with death.[1] Surgical management is the gold standard for MR if indicated, however, numerous comorbidities in patients, especially elderly, precludes them from the intervention due to significant perioperative risk. For these patients with substantial risk, United States Food and Drug Administration (USFDA) approved MitraClip (Abbott, Menlo Park, CA) percutaneous intervention for mitral valve repair in October 2013.[2]

INDICATIONS

Mitral regurgitation can be primary or secondary (Table 1).[3] Percutaneous mitral valve repair has a recommendation of IIb for severe symptomatic patients with severe primary MR who have a high surgical risk due to accompanying comorbidities.[4] Percutaneous MitraClip entails "edge-to-edge coaptation" of valve leaflets, making it a double orifice valve (Fig. 1), which is similar to the Alfieri technique performed surgically.[5] EVEREST trial criteria for MitraClip procedure is stated in Box 1.[6]

ROLE OF ECHOCARDIOGRAPHY

Transesophageal echocardiogram (TEE) is an integral part of this procedure. It helps in patient selection, provides a roadmap during the procedure and very helpful in recognizing postprocedural complications. TEE has an appropriate use score of 9 for assessment of valvular heart disease, assessment and planning of this intervention.[7] Three-dimensional (3D) TEE views provide excellent details over two-dimensional (2D) TEE views.[8]

TABLE 1: Etiology of mitral regurgitation.

Organic/primary mitral regurgitation (MR)	*Secondary/functional MR*
• Leaflet abnormality • Chordae tendineae abnormality.	• Papillary muscle dysfunction • Annular dilatation • Left ventricular dysfunction.

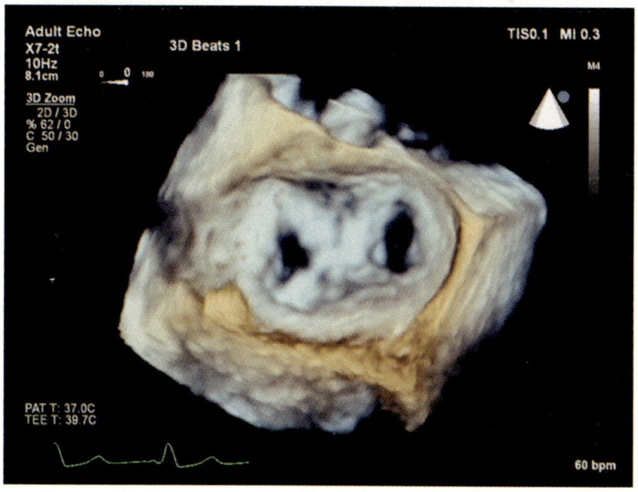

Fig. 1: "Surgeon's view" on 3D-TEE revealing a double orifice mitral valve in a patient who had two MitraClips deployed.

BOX 1: Inclusion and exclusion criteria for EVEREST study.[6]

Inclusion criteria:
- Candidate for mitral valve repair or replacement
- Moderate to severe (3+) or severe (4+) mitral valve regurgitation and symptomatic with LVEF > 25% and LVIDs ≤ 55 mm or asymptomatic with one or more additional criteria.
  - LVEF > 25–60%
  - LVIDs ≥ 40–55 mm
  - New onset atrial fibrillation
  - Pulmonary hypertension with pulmonary artery systolic pressure > 50 mm Hg at rest or > 60 mm Hg with exercise.

Exclusion criteria:
- Recent myocardial infarction
- Any interventional or surgical procedure within 30 days of the index procedure
- Mitral valve orifice area < 4 cm^2
- Renal insufficiency, endocarditis, and rheumatic heart disease
- Previous mediastinal surgery.

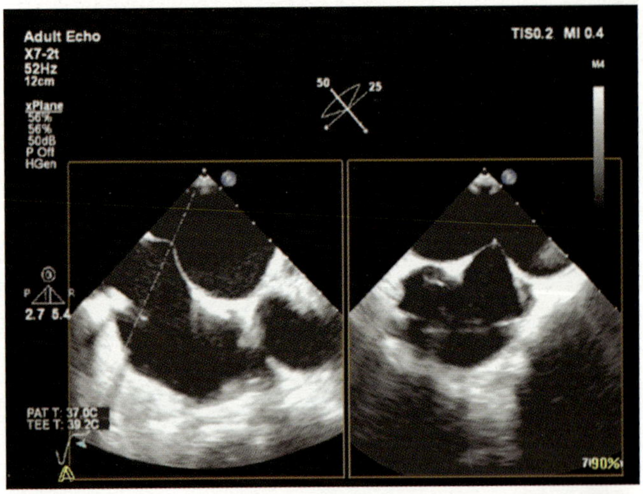

Fig. 2: Posterior and superior transseptal puncture site identified on biplane imaging on 3D-TEE. The panel on the left (basal short-axis view) indicates a posterior puncture and the panel on the right (bicaval view) indicates a superior puncture.

Patient Selection

Transthoracic echocardiogram (TTE) is a screening tool for evaluation of mitral valve but TEE holds an important place in the percutaneous mitral valve repair. TEE determines the qualitative and quantitative function of the mitral valvular regurgitation, its etiology; hence, it helps in recruitment of the right patient per EVEREST trial criteria stated in Box 1. Morphologic evaluation of the mitral valve leaflets is the corner stone of patient selection. The MR jet should ideally be at the level of A2/P2. For leaflet prolapse, coaptation depth less than 11 mm and coaptation length of at least 2 mm is required. For flail leaflets, flail gap should be less than 10 mm and flail width less than 15 mm. Also, TEE helps in assessing if there is enough leaflet tissue for the clip to grasp on.[9] Procedure yields good results in patients with favorable morphology. TEE also assesses if there is any left atrial (LA) thrombus present, which would necessitate delaying the procedure.[8]

TABLE 2: Various TEE views for intraprocedural guidance.

TEE view	*Structures visualized*
Bicaval view (Fig. 2)	During TSP and visualization of the septum after removal of CDS
Short-axis view (Fig. 2)	Puncture of the IAS
Long-axis view	When positioning the clip in the anteroposterior plane
Commissural view	For medial or lateral alignment
LV outflow tract view	Positioning the clip, moving the clip to the center of the valve, advancing the clip in the LV, grasping the leaflets, and to confirm grasping
3D enface view (surgeon's view) (Fig. 3)	Helps in alignment of the clip at the target area

(3D: three-dimensional; CDS: clip-delivery system; IAS: interatrial septal; LV: left ventricle; TEE: transesophageal echocardiography; TSP: transseptal puncture)

Intraprocedural Guidance

Two-dimensional and 3D-TEE views along with fluoroscopy are utilized in various steps of the procedure.[8]

Transseptal puncture (TSP) is the key step for procedural success. The ideal location of TSP is posterior and superior aspect of the interatrial septal (IAS) (Fig. 2) approximately 4-5 cm above the leaflet coaptation plane. This height above the plane will provide room for maneuverability of the MitraClip system.[10] Mid-esophageal aortic short-axis and four-chamber views are of paramount importance during this stage of the procedure. Continuous TEE is mandatory during this phase to guide the right trajectory of the needle. Important TEE views used during the procedure and their rationale is summarized in Table 2.[11] TEE guides the interventional cardiologist during the TSP, advancement and maneuvering the clip delivery system (CDS) in LA, adequate positioning of CDS above mitral valve, advancing the CDS into the left ventricle, grasping the leaflets, and comprehensive assessment of the valve after clip deployment. 3D TEE view from the roof of the left atrium (surgeon's view) helps in the alignment of the clip (Fig. 3) to the target area. Details of each stage are beyond the scope of this chapter.

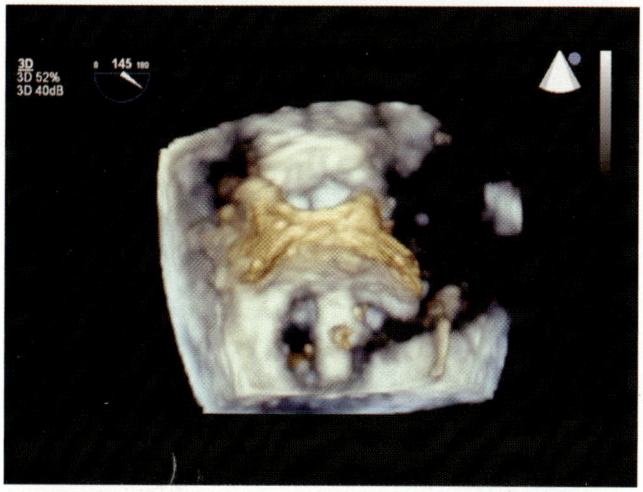

Fig. 3: "Surgeon's view" on 3D-TEE confirming the correct alignment of the MitraClip inside the left atrium.

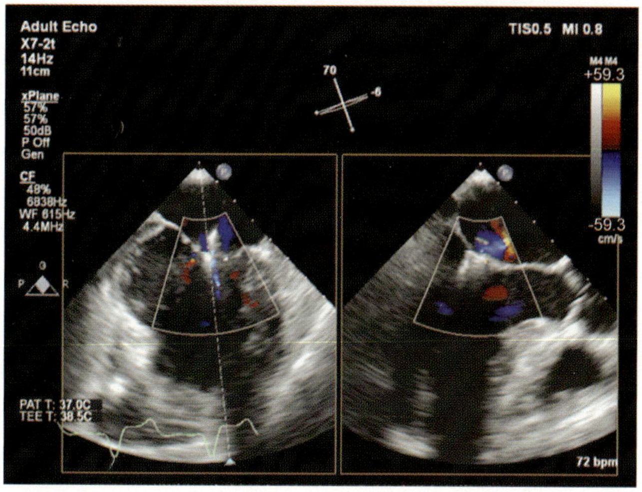

Fig. 4: Color Doppler biplane imaging on 3D-TEE performed to check for residual mitral regurgitation before final deployment of the MitraClip.

Valve Assessment after MitraClip Deployment

After leaflet grasping, but prior to final deployment of the clip, it is important to assess the residual MR (Fig. 4), amount of grasping tissue, transmitral gradient, and residual mitral valve area. Mean transmitral gradient less than 5 mm Hg and mitral valve area (MVA) more than 2 cm^2 is considered ideal.[2] Decreased survival is associated with transmitral valve gradient more than 5 mm Hg.[12] Decision is made if additional clips are required depending upon residual mitral valve regurgitation and transmitral gradients.

EVALUATION OF COMPLICATIONS

Complications compared to the open surgical repair are significantly less but can occur pertaining to the procedure, access site, and general anesthesia. TSP could lead to pericardial effusion and/or tamponade, aortic puncture due to malpositioning of the puncture needle. Patients are also at risk for thrombus formation, partial or complete clip detachment, entrapment of clip in the chordae tendineae, injury to chordae, gastrointestinal injury. Fortunately, all these complications could be detected during the procedure with the help of TEE. Device embolization is extremely rare.[11]

CONCLUSION

Percutaneous mitral valve repair has a promising future. Besides MitraClip, which is approved by FDA, numerous other percutaneous modalities are in various stages of development or approval for mitral valve repair. Leaflet ablation, direct and indirect annuloplasty, chordal implantation, and left ventricle remodeling are to name a few. Percutaneous mitral valve replacement technology is also being developed for a select group of nonsurgical patients.[13] All these modalities would require real-time imaging with TEE during the procedure. Real-time fusion of echocardiographic and fluoroscopy images have helped reduce the time required for TSP. This technology is safe and efficacious.[14] Intracardiac echocardiography has been utilized in patients where clear images via TEE cannot be obtained due to various reasons with promising results.[15] At the time of writing this book chapter, cardiovascular Outcomes for Assessment of the MitraClip Percutaneous Therapy for Heart Failure Patients with Functional MR (COAPT) trial is underway to assess the outcomes of nonsurgical candidates with functional mitral regurgitation and underlying cardiomyopathy. The trial results could add more to the select group of patient who could potentially benefit from this percutaneous mitral valve repair.[16]

REFERENCES

1. Bursi F, Enriquez-Sarano M, Nkomo VT, et al. Heart failure and death after myocardial infarction in the community: The emerging role of mitral regurgitation. Circulation. 2005;111(3):295-301.
2. Nyman CB, Mackensen GB, Jelacic S, et al. Transcatheter Mitral Valve Repair Using the Edge-to-Edge Clip. J Am Soc Echocardiogr. 2018;31(4):434-53.
3. Rogers JH, Franzen O. Percutaneous edge-to-edge MitraClip therapy in the management of mitral regurgitation. Eur Heart J. 2011;32(19):2350-7.

4. Nishimura RA, Otto CM, Bonow RO, et al. 2014 AHA/ACC Guideline for the Management of Patients With Valvular Heart Disease: executive summary: a report of the American College of Cardiology/American Heart Association Task Force on Practice Guidelines. Circulation. 2014;129(23):2440-92.
5. Alfieri O, Maisano F, De Bonis M, et al. The double-orifice technique in mitral valve repair: a simple solution for complex problems. J Thorac Cardiovasc Surg. 2001;122(4):674-81.
6. Feldman T, Kar S, Rinaldi M, et al. Percutaneous mitral repair with the MitraClip system: safety and midterm durability in the initial EVEREST (Endovascular Valve Edge-to-Edge REpair Study) cohort. J Am Coll Cardiol. 2009;54(8):686-94.
7. Douglas PS, Garcia MJ, Haines DE, et al. ACCF/ASE/AHA/ASNC/HFSA/HRS/SCAI/SCCM/SCCT/SCMR 2011 Appropriate Use Criteria for Echocardiography. A Report of the American College of Cardiology Foundation Appropriate Use Criteria Task Force, American Society of Echocardiography, American Heart Association, American Society of Nuclear Cardiology, Heart Failure Society of America, Heart Rhythm Society, Society for Cardiovascular Angiography and Interventions, Society of Critical Care Medicine, Society of Cardiovascular Computed Tomography, and Society for Cardiovascular Magnetic Resonance Endorsed by the American College of Chest Physicians. J Am Coll Cardiol. 2011;57(9):1126-66.
8. Altiok E, Becker M, Hamada S, et al. Real-time 3D TEE allows optimized guidance of percutaneous edge-to-edge repair of the mitral valve. JACC Cardiovasc Imaging. 2010;3(11):1196-8.
9. Yuksel UC, Kapadia SR, Tuzcu EM. Percutaneous mitral repair: patient selection, results, and future directions. Curr Cardiol Rep. 2011;13(2):100-6.
10. Singh GD, Smith TW, Rogers JH. Targeted Transseptal Access for MitraClip Percutaneous Mitral Valve Repair. Interv Cardiol Clin. 2016;5(1):55-69.
11. Alegria-Barrero E, Chan PH, Paulo M, et al. Edge-to-edge percutaneous repair of severe mitral regurgitation--state-of-the-art for Mitraclip(R) implantation. Circ J. 2012;76(4):801-8.
12. Neuss M, Schau T, Isotani A, et al. Elevated Mitral Valve Pressure Gradient After MitraClip Implantation Deteriorates Long-Term Outcome in Patients With Severe Mitral Regurgitation and Severe Heart Failure. JACC Cardiovasc Interv. 2017;10(9):931-9.
13. Chiam PT, Ruiz CE. Percutaneous transcatheter mitral valve repair: a classification of the technology. JACC Cardiovasc Interv. 2011;4(1):1-13.
14. Afzal S, Veulemans V, Balzer J, et al. Safety and efficacy of transseptal puncture guided by real-time fusion of echocardiography and fluoroscopy. Neth Heart J. 2017;25(2):131-6.
15. Saji M, Rossi AM, Ailawadi G, et al. Adjunctive intracardiac echocardiography imaging from the left ventricle to guide percutaneous mitral valve repair with the MitraClip in patients with failed prior surgical rings. Catheter Cardiovasc Interv. 2016;87(2):E75-82.
16. Stewart MH, Jenkins JS. The evolving role of percutaneous mitral valve repair. Ochsner J. 2016;16(3):270-6.

64

CHAPTER

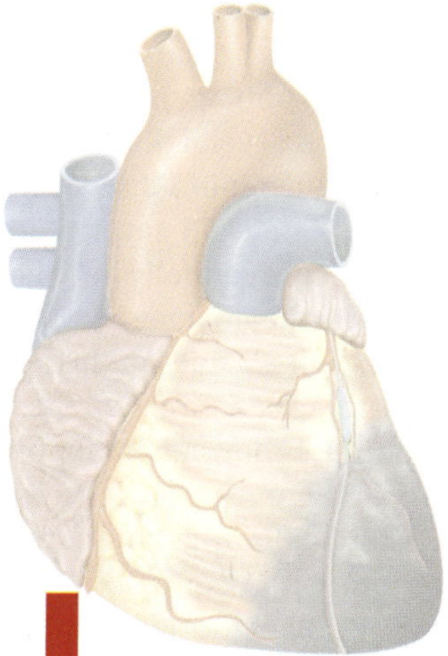

Evaluation of Tricuspid Valve Regurgitation and Stenosis: Advances in Echocardiography

Vinay Sharma, Sameer Shrivastava, HK Chopra

INTRODUCTION

Echocardiography is the mainstay to assess the severity of tricuspid valve disease in clinical practice. As with all valve lesions, the initial evaluation starts with an anatomical assessment of the valve by two-dimensional (2D) echocardiography, using the multiple windows such as parasternal right ventricular inflow, parasternal short-axis, apical four-chamber and subcostal four-chamber views to elucidate the suspected etiology (Box 1). The assessment of severity of tricuspid regurgitation (TR) is performed using color Doppler flow mapping, size of the jet, assessment of vena contracta width, and flow convergence calculations. The evaluation of tricuspid stenosis severity is primarily done using the hemodynamic information provided by continuous-wave Doppler.

ASSESSMENT OF SEVERITY OF TRICUSPID REGURGITATION

Role of Two-dimensional Echocardiography in Assessment of Tricuspid Valve Anatomy

Normal tricuspid valve function depends on the integrity and coordination of interactions among various components of the tricuspid valve complex. Tricuspid valve complex consists of three leaflet, named after their positions as the anterior, posterior, and septal leaflets, fibrous annulus, 2–3 papillary muscles, chordae tendinea and adjacent right atrial and right ventricular myocardium. The tricuspid valve (TV) leaflets (anterior, posterior and septal) are attached to a fibrous annulus and are of unequal size: the anterior leaflet is the largest leaflet; the septal leaflet is usually the second largest leaflet, while the posterior leaflet is the smallest of the three. The leaflets are supported by 2 or 3 papillary muscles: the anterior papillary muscle provides chordae to the anterior and posterior leaflets, and the medial papillary

BOX 1: Causes of tricuspid valve diseases.

- *Tricuspid regurgitation*
  - Primary causes (25%)
    - Rheumatic
    - Myxomatous
    - Ebstein anomaly
    - Endomyocardial fibrosis
    - Endocarditis
    - Carcinoid disease
    - Traumatic (blunt chest injury, laceration)
    - Iatrogenic (pacemaker/defibrillator lead, RV biopsy)
  - Secondary causes (75%)
    - Left heart disease (LV dysfunction or valve disease) resulting in pulmonary hypertension
    - Pulmonary hypertension (chronic lung disease, pulmonary thromboembolism, left to right shunt)
    - Any cause of RV dysfunction (myocardial disease, RV ischemia/infarction)
- *Tricuspid stenosis*
  - Rheumatic
  - Infective endocarditis
  - Carcinoid
  - Cardiac tumors

muscle provides chordae to the posterior and septal leaflets. The septal wall gives chordae to the anterior and septal leaflets (there is no formal septal papillary muscle as with the anterior and posterior papillary muscles).[1]

The normal tricuspid annulus is a saddle-shaped structure with the highest points in an anteroposterior orientation and the lowest points in a mediolateral orientation. In patients with functional tricuspid regurgitation, the annulus dilates and becomes more circular and planar. Normal TV diameter in adults is 28 ± 5 mm, as measured in the apical four-chamber view. Significant tricuspid annular dilatation is defined by a diastolic diameter more than 21 mm (>35 mm). The most common cause of TR is impaired valve coaptation caused by dilation of the right ventricle and/or of the tricuspid annulus which is often secondary to left heart failure from myocardial or valvular causes, right ventricular volume and pressure overload, and dilation of cardiac chambers. A variety of disease can also affect the TV complex directly and lead to valve incompetence: Infective endocarditis, congenital disease like Ebstein anomaly or atrioventricular canal, rheumatic fever, carcinoid syndrome, endomyocardial fibrosis, myxomatous degeneration of the TV, penetrating and nonpenetrating trauma, and iatrogenic damages during cardiac surgery, biopsies, and catheter placement in right heart chambers.[2,3]

Rheumatic TR is a consequence of deformity, shortening and retraction of one or more leaflets of the TV as well as shortening and fusion of the chordae tendinea and papillary muscles. Degenerative myxomatous disease can be diagnosed by real-time three-dimensional echocardiographic (RT-3DE) as bulging or protrusion of one or more segments of a single or multiple TV leaflets, with or without of chordal rupture. The carcinoid disease is characterized by the thickened leaflets with markedly restricted motion (frozen appearance of tricuspid valve). Ebstein's anomaly is a congenital defect of the TV, characterized by apical displacement of the septal or posterior leaflets into the right ventricle with a large sail-like anterior leaflet. Two-dimensional echocardiographic (2DE) can show the characteristic displacement of the septal leaflet and the redundant and elongated anterior leaflet. The excessive apical displacement of the valve, i.e. the displacement index more than 8 mm/m^2, is associated with the Ebstein's anomaly.

COLOR DOPPLER METHODS FOR EVALUATION OF TRICUSPID REGURGITATION

Jet area: It is the most commonly used parameter for assessing the severity of TR and the operator should append time in careful planning to visualize the largest jet area. Using jet area for initial assessment of TR severity is perfectly fine and that is how it should start, but one should remember that unless severe or clear cut mild (supported by appropriate valve morphology), using jet area as sole method to quantify TR has several pitfalls and is not recommended as the sole parameter of TR severity. Jet area markedly under or overestimate TR severity in eccentric jets. Color jets that are directed centrally into the rheumatoid arthritis (RA) generally appear larger because they entrain red blood cells (RBCs) on all sides of the jet. In contrast, eccentric jets tend to appear smaller than central jets of similar severity because they flatten out on RA wall and also cannot entrain RBC from sides of the jet. Eccentric jets in setting of structural abnormalities of the valve (e.g. prolapse, flail, or perforation), frequently in the leaflet or cusp opposite to the direction of the jet in setting of eccentric should alert to presence of significant TR unless proven otherwise. Jet area is also influenced by flow momentum, i.e. the TR jet may appear larger by increasing the driving pressure across the valve. Hence, patient with marked elevation of right ventricular systolic pressure may have a large jet area even with lesser degree of TR. The same regurgitant flow will produce larger or smaller jets depending on the size of the atrium, which has led to indexing for atrial area.

Vena contracta (VC): These pitfalls of jet area can be avoided by use of the VC, which is the narrowest portion of regurgitant jet, as a marker of severity of TR. VC is independent of flow characteristics and much less effected by driving pressure and is neither effected by pulse-repetition-frequency, as the flow at level of VC is characterized by high velocity laminar flow probe is manipulated in apical four-chamber till clear differentiation of the area of proximal flow acceleration, VC and the downstream expansion of the jet is seen. The area of VC is zoomed up and size of sector is reduced to smallest possible to achieve maximal temporal and lateral resolution. Color gain is kept just enough till background noise just disappeared. Nyquist velocity is kept at 50–60 cm/s. VC measured as the narrowest portion of the jet just downstream from the orifice.

Effective regurgitant orifice area (EROA): VC is basically a surrogate of EROA assuming it to be circular. However, "direct measurement of EROA" may be more useful as EROA may not be circular. Further, in multiple TR jets, where the respective widths of the VC are not additive, but their cross-sectional areas can be added. Since direct measurement of EROA in SAX under color flow imaging (CFI) is very fallacious, so it can be "calculated indirectly" by proximal isovelocity surface area (PISA) or flow convergence method. As blood approaches a regurgitant orifice, its velocity increases, forming concentric, roughly hemispheric shells of increasing velocity and decreasing surface area. These hemispheres can be visualized on CFI by shifting the baseline toward the direction of flow, or by lowering the Nyquist limit, or both. EROA is calculated as = 6.28 × R^2 × Va (aliasing velocity) divided by maximal velocity of jet by continuous wave.

Even PISA has its own pitfalls. It is usually easy to identify the aliasing line of the hemisphere. However, it can be difficult to judge the precise location of the orifice. Any error introduced is then squared. PISA is basically for mitral regurgitation and considerably less experience with using PISA to assess TR.

PULSED WAVE DOPPLER METHODS FOR EVALUATION OF TRICUSPID REGURGITATION

Assessment of TR severity based on color jet is at best a qualitative assessment, as the color jet, being a velocity map, do not reflect the absolute regurgitant volume (RV) at that point in time. Actual quantification may be an advantage in the case of eccentric or multiple regurgitant TR jets, where PISA is not as accurate and VC is not applicable in the latter situation. For actual quantification of RV, regurgitant fraction (RF) and EROA, we need to use pulsed wave Doppler based methods. Stroke volume (SV) is calculated at tricuspid and pulmonary valves. In the presence of regurgitation of one valve, without any intracardiac shunt, the flow through the affected valve is larger than through other competent valves (normally it is equal). The difference is the "regurgitant volume":

= TV flow – RVOT flow

= (.785 × tricuspid annulus diameter^2 × tricuspid VTI) – (.785 × RVOT annulus diameter^2 × LVOT-VTI)

Regurgitant volume divided by forward SV at the regurgitant valve is RF. It is a better way to assess severity as absolute RV, being dependent on hemodynamic variables and chamber size, can change overtime. In severe TR in a small RV may have ↓ RV but ↑ RF and EROA. There are no data regarding indexing these measurements to body surface area. RV divided by velocity-time integral (VTI) of regurgitant jet is EROA. Quantitative Doppler generates a mean EROA as its calculations are based on the regurgitant stroke volume and the VTI of the regurgitant flow signal.

Three-dimensional Echocardiographic Assessment of the Tricuspid Valve Anatomy

Two-dimensional echocardiographic assessment of the TV morphology is challenging due to difficulty in accessing retrosternal position of the valve. Retrosternal position together with nearly vertical (approximately 45° to the sagittal plane) position of the valve makes it impossible to simultaneously visualize all three leaflets in any one standard transthoracic echocardiography 2DE (TTE-2DE) views. Thus, the TV morphology has to be evaluated by a series TTE-2DE views from the standard parasternal right ventricular inflow view, parasternal short-axis, apical four-chamber and subcostal views. 3DE has the unique capability of obtaining a short-axis plane of the TV allowing simultaneous visualization of the all three leaflets. 3DE supplements 2DE with detailed images of the morphology of the valve including leaflets size and thickness, annulus shape and size and their anatomic relationships, allowing a more objective evaluation of TV anatomy and function. Matrix array 3DE transducer can acquire 3D images in both RT-3DE and in full-volume acquisition (i.e. four consecutive cardiac cycles merged together). The real-time zoom mode has several advantages over the full-volume acquisition, including higher resolution and absence of stitch artifacts. Full-volume acquisition covers a wider region, allowing delineation of relevant adjacent structures and their spatial relationships (e.g. leaflets, chordae and papillary muscles). There are three main approaches to be used with RT-3DE: parasternal, apical and subcostal. The parasternal long-axis position is modified to visualize right ventricular inflow, the overall gain control is set higher than normal, the TV is centered in the 3D volume, and the transducer is adjusted to simultaneously view all three leaflets and image is acquired. Acquisition of full-volume 3D dataset is best done from apical four-chamber view. After acquisition, cropping from the apex toward the base or from the atrial roof toward the apex will display the enface view of the TV from the ventricular and from atrial ("surgical view") side, respectively. RT-3DE can be useful for a better characterization of valve lesions in different primary valve diseases.

Rheumatic TR is a consequence of deformity, shortening and retraction of one or more leaflets of the TV as well as shortening and fusion of the chordae tendinea and papillary muscles. The diagnosis is established on the "enface" view of the TV is obtained by RT-3DE to visualize the commissural fusion. Assessment of TV apparatus deformities requires the full-volume data set which includes the entire valve apparatus, to examine the apparatus from multiple different perspectives. This is an important advantage of 3DE as 2DE cannot reliably detect morphological abnormalities of the valve apparatus involvement. Degenerative myxomatous disease can be diagnosed by RT-3DE as bulging or protrusion of one or more segments of a single or multiple TV leaflets, with or without of chordal rupture. The carcinoid disease is characterized by the thickened leaflets with markedly restricted motion. In patients with TV endocarditis, RT-3DE may show the stereoscopic morphology and attachments of vegetations, mobility of vegetations with blood flow, and possible complications such as leaflet prolapse or perforation. Ebstein's anomaly is characterized by deformed leaflets and the characteristic bubble-like aspect of septal and posterior leaflets as effect of tethering of the leaflet where the chordae are attached. The VC as measured by 3DE may be more accurate as not effected by the shape of the orifice. The area of the VC of the tricuspid regurgitant jet can be assessed by cropping the RT-3DE color Doppler data set with imaging planes exactly parallel to the TV orifice (Figs. 1A to D, Table 1).[4]

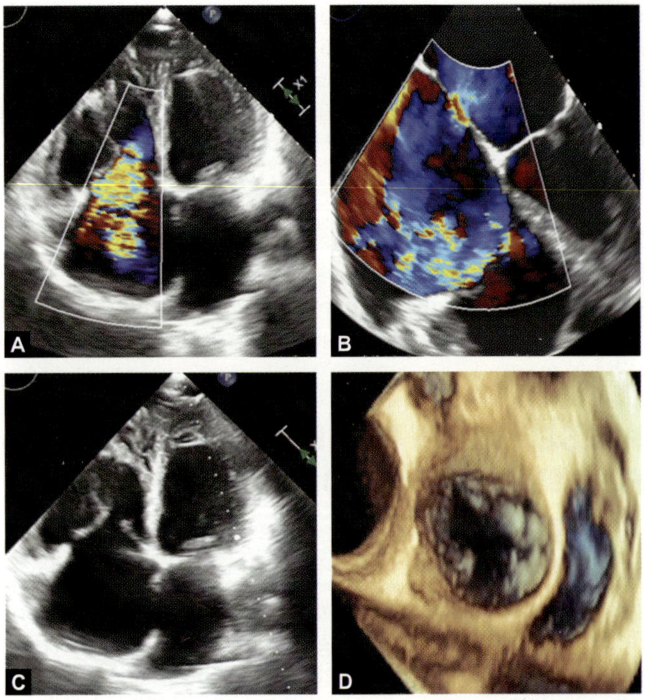

Figs. 1A to D: Images from a patient with severe rheumatic tricuspid regurgitation. Image A and B are 2D images from transthoracic and transesophageal echocardiography. Image C shows noncoapting thickened tricuspid leaflets and dilated RV and RA. Image D is enface view of tricuspid valve in 3D-TEE.

ASSESSMENT OF TRICUSPID STENOSIS

Two-dimensional Echocardiographic Assessment of the Tricuspid Valve Anatomy

Rheumatic, heart disease is the most common cause of tricuspid stenosis (TS). Rheumatic TS is often accompanied by mitral stenosis. Rheumatic TS is characterized by diastolic doming, valve thickening and/or calcification, restricted mobility, and right atrial enlargement. Other causes of TS include rare congenital malformations and mechanical obstruction by valvular or pacemaker endocarditis and benign or malignant tumors. Carcinoid syndrome can lead to TS, but tricuspid regurgitant is the predominant lesion in all of them. Echocardiographic appearance of carcinoid involvement of TV has been described a frozen appearance, characterized by severe immobility of the leaflets. Detection of valve obstruction by atrial tumors, metastatic lesions, or giant vegetations is a straightforward diagnosis. The normal valve area in adults is 4–6 cm^2. Unlike for mitral valve direct

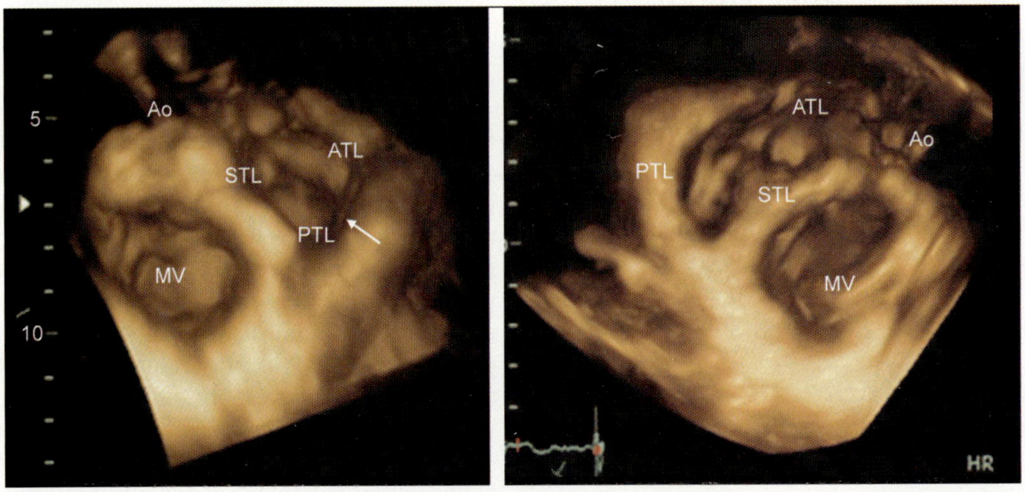

Figs. 2A and B: Normal tricuspid valve leaflets visualized by real-time three-dimensional echocardiography from atrial (A) and ventricular side (B). (ATL: anterior tricuspid leaflet; Ao: aorta; MV: mitral valve; PTL: posterior tricuspid leaflet; STL: septal tricuspid leaflet).

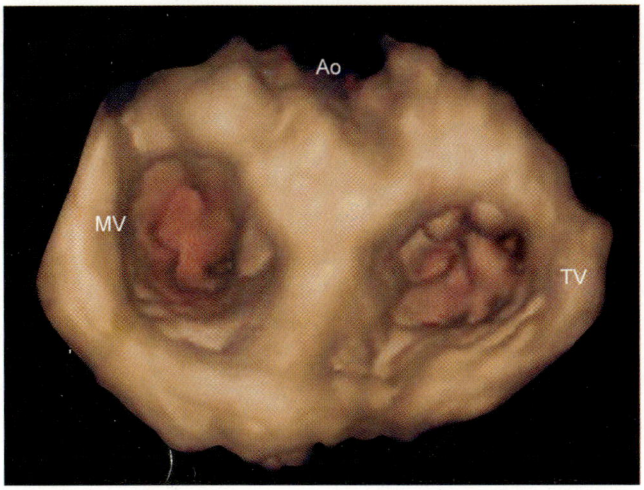

Fig. 3: Right atrial view of the tricuspid valve (TV) in a normal subject with a clear delineation of the tricuspid annulus and its spatial relationships with mitral valve (MV) and aorta (Ao). (B) Reconstructed tricuspid annulus viewed from profile and showing its saddle shape, with the highest points located in an anterior–posterior orientation and the lowest points in a mediolateral orientation. (C) Reconstructed tricuspid annulus viewed from the right atrium.

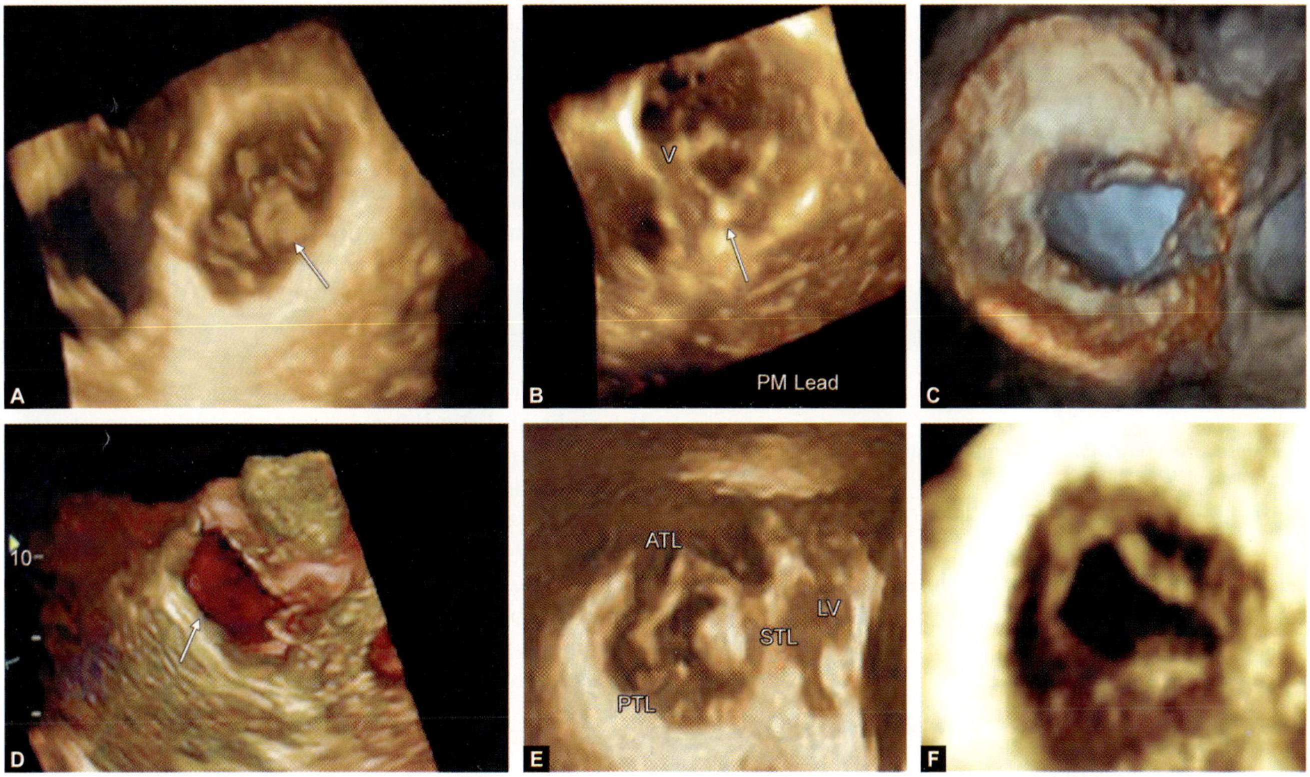

Figs. 4A to F: Three-dimensional assessment of the mechanism of regurgitation in various tricuspid valve disease. Anterior tricuspid leaflet prolapse with ruptured chordae (A, right atrial "surgical" view); pacemaker lead interference causing immobilization of the septal leaflet (B, right atrial view); carcinoid tricuspid valvulopathy with adhesion of the valve leaflets to right ventricular walls that prevent the valve to close during systole (C, right ventricular view. Courtesy by Andreas Hagendorff, Leipzig, Germany); nearly complete detachment of the posterior tricuspid leaflet during biopsy in a heart transplant patient (D, right ventricular view); functional tricuspid regurgitation, dilated annulus, and tenting of the three leaflets with loss of systolic coaptation (E, right ventricular view); rheumatic tricuspid valve steno-insufficiency (F, right ventricular view).

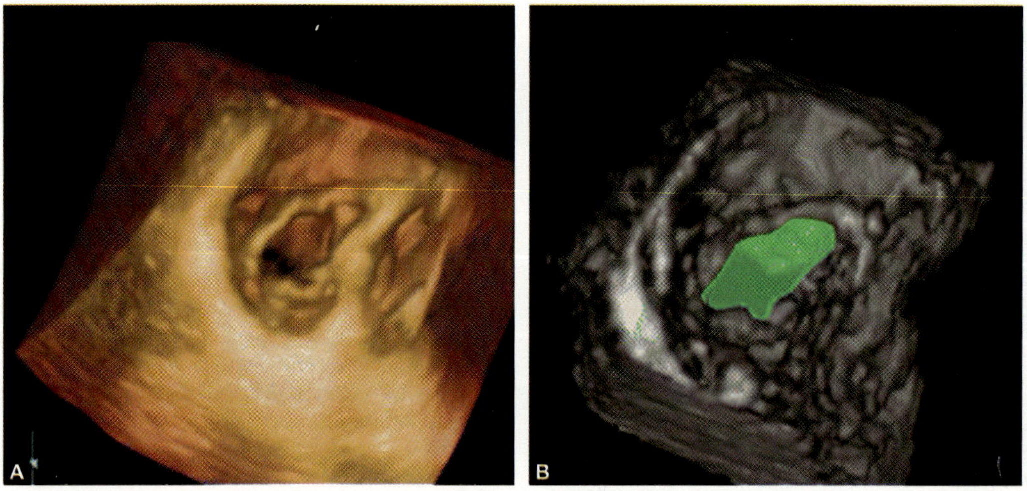

Figs. 5A and B: Rheumatic tricuspid valve stenosis seen from the right ventricle. (A) The deformed and thickened leaflets are clearly visualized as well as fused commissures and the stenotic orifice of the valve. (B) Stenotic tricuspid valve orifice can easily and accurately be planimetered to obtain an objective measure of stenosis severity.

TABLE 1: Findings indicative of hemodynamically significant tricuspid stenosis

Specific findings	
Mean pressure gradient	>5 mm Hg
Inflow time velocity integral	>60 cm
Pressure half-time	>190 millisecond
Valve area by continuity equation	<1 cm^2
Supportive findings	
Enlarged right atrium	
Dilated inferior vena cava	

Reproduced from: EAE/ASE Recommendations for Echocardiographic Assessment of Valve Stenosis

calculation of TV area is not possible on TTE as the TTE-2DE cannot provide an enface view the stenotic orifice.

Doppler Assessment of Severity of Tricuspid Stenosis

Doppler recordings of trans tricuspid flow velocity allow calculation of mean gradient and pressure half-time valve area as described for the mitral valve. The tricuspid inflow velocity is best recorded from the apical four-chamber view. All measurements taken must be averaged throughout the respiratory cycle or recorded at end-expiratory apnea. In patients with atrial fibrillation, measurements from a minimum of five cardiac cycles should be averaged. The transvalvular gradient is clinically more relevant for assessment of severity and decision-making than the actual stenotic valve area, which is difficult to measure. The pressure half-time method has been applied in a manner analogous to mitral stenosis (MS) but is not very accurate. Some authors have used the same constant of 220, while others have proposed a constant of 190 with valve area determined as: 190/T1/2.93. Although validation studies with TS are less than those with MS, valve area by the T1/2 method may be less accurate than in MS. This is probably due to differences in atrioventricular compliance between the right and the left side, and the influence of right ventricular relaxation, respiration, and TR on the pressure half-time. However, as a general rule, a longer T1/2 implies a greater TS severity with values frequently associated with significant (or critical) stenosis. In theory, the continuity equation can be used to calculate the effective valve area as SV divided by the tricuspid inflow VTI. However, as severity of TR increases, valve area is progressively underestimated by this method (Table 2).

3D Echocardiographic Assessment of the Stenotic Tricuspid Valve Anatomy

Three-dimensional echocardiography is the only echocardiographic method that can provide enface view of the valve allowing direct measurement of valve area and visualization of commissural fusion. However, the methodology is neither standardized nor sufficiently validated to be recommended as a method of choice.

TABLE 2: Echocardiographic and Doppler parameters used in grading TR severity.

Parameter	*Mild*	*Moderate*	*Severe*
Tricuspid valve	Usually normal	Normal or abnormal	Abnormal/flail leaflet/poor coaptation
RV/RA/IVC size	Normal	Normal or dilated	Usually dilated
Jet area-central jets (cm^2)	<5	5–10	>10
VC width (cm)	Not defined	Not defined, but <0.7	>0.7
PISA radius (cm)			
Jet density and contour	Soft and parabolic	Dense, variable contour	Dense, triangular with early peaking
Hepatic vein flow	Systolic dominance	Systolic blunting	Systolic reversal

RV: right ventricle; RA: right atrium; IVC: inferior vena cava; VC: vena contracta; PISA: proximal isovelocity surface area
Adopted from American Society of Echocardiography Recommendations for Evaluation of the Severity of Native Valvular Regurgitation with Two-dimensional and Doppler Echocardiography.

REFERENCES

1. Anwar AM, Geleijnse ML, Soliman OI, et al. Assessment of normal tricuspid valve anatomy in adults by real-time three-dimensional echocardiography. Int J Cardiovasc Imaging. 2007;23(6):717-24.
2. Ton-Nu TT, Levine RA, Handschumacher MD, et al. Geometric determinants of functional tricuspid regurgitation: insights from 3-dimensional echocardiography. Circulation. 2006;114(2):143-9.
3. Fukuda S, Saracino G, Matsumura Y, et al. Three-dimensional geometry of the tricuspid annulus in healthy subjects and in patients with functional tricuspid regurgitation: a real-time, 3-dimensional echocardiographic study. Circulation. 2006;114(1 Suppl):1492-8.
4. Shiina A, Seward JB, Edwards WD, et al. Two-dimensional echocardiographic spectrum of Ebstein's anomaly: detailed anatomic assessment. J Am Coll Cardiol. 1984;3(2 Pt 1): 356-70.

65

CHAPTER

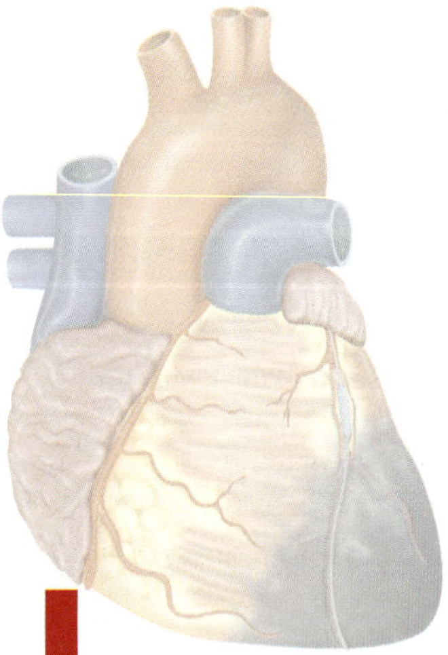

Advances in Echocardiographic Assessment of Pulmonary Regurgitation and Stenosis

Rohit Tandon, Rajiv Gupta

INTRODUCTION

Nanda and Raymond gave the first description of pulmonary valve (PV) anatomy using M-mode echocardiography in 1972.[1] Since then, there has been tremendous progress in understanding and interrogating PV anatomy using advanced three-dimensional (3D) echocardiography especially from interventionist point of view.

PULMONARY VALVE ANATOMY

Pulmonary valve is separated by the smooth myocardial right ventricular outflow tract (RVOT) and the pulmonary artery. It is the most anterior structure of the heart and lies directly beneath the sternum and anterolateral to the aortic valve. It is a semilunar valve with three distinct cusps, whose nomenclature reflects their relationship to the aortic valve; hence the anterior cusp lies most anterior to the aorta, the right cusp lies to the right of the aortic valve directly facing the right coronary cusp of the aortic valve, and the left cusp lies to the left of the aortic valve and is directly facing the left coronary cusp of the aortic valve while anterior cusp does not face any of the aortic cusp (Figs. 1A and B).

Unlike other cardiac valves, it is not connected to the fibrous skeleton of the heart and is mainly supported by valve sinuses. Mean pulmonary valve diameters in

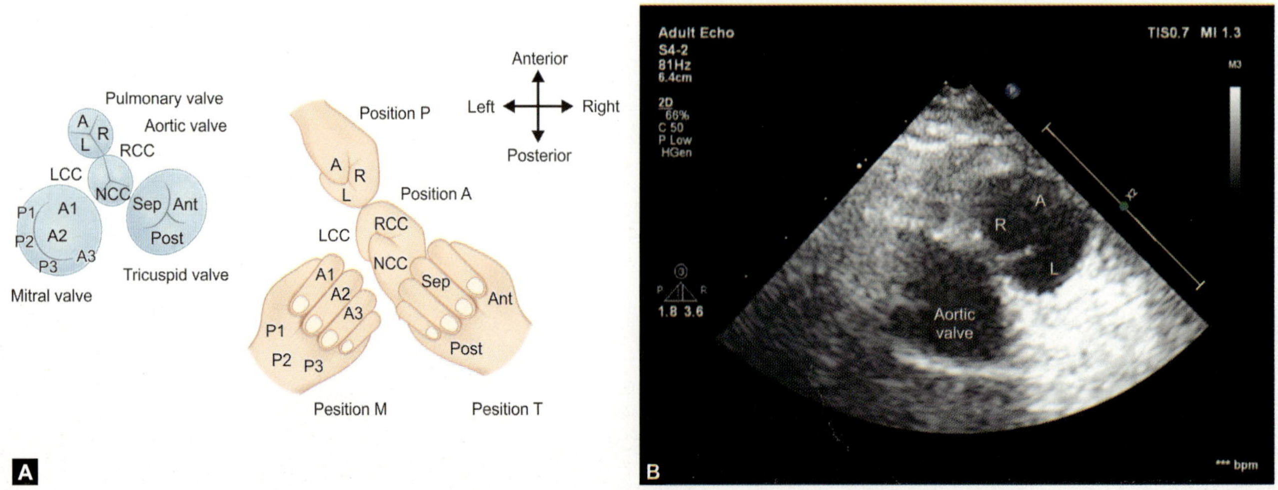

Figs. 1A and B

anatomical dissections measure approximately 23.9 ± 2.2 mm in women and 26.2 ± 2.3 mm in men.

ECHOCARDIOGRAPHY VIEWS FOR PULMONARY VALVE ASSESSMENT

Transthoracic echocardiogram (TTE) views include:

- Right ventricular outflow tract view in the parasternal long-axis view by tilting the probe caudally
- Right ventricular (RV) inflow-outflow in the parasternal short-axis view
- Right ventricular outflow tract view in subcostal view

Transthoracic echocardiogram views include:

- Midesophageal RV inflow-outflow view (45°)
- Upper esophageal aortic arch short-axis view (0° and 90°)
- Transgastric RVOT and pulmonary artery view (20°).

Additional views are:

- Transgastric RV inflow-outflow view (between 20° and 40°)
- Deep transgastric RV inflow-outflow (120–140°—gentle anteflexion) (Fig. 2).

LIMITATIONS OF TWO-DIMENSIONAL ASSESSMENT

Assessment of PV morphology using 2D-TTE is challenging as it cuts PV in its long-axis, so only two cusps can be visualized simultaneously. A short-axis view like that of aortic valve is not generally obtained by 2D-TTE, although in rare cases in which the orientation of the pulmonary artery is dilated, this could be possible. 3D-TTE is advantageous as it provides volumetric datasets that can then be cropped and reoriented to assess the zone of interest from any perspective.

CARDIAC IMAGING IN PULMONARY REGURGITATION

Although cardiac magnetic resonance is regarded as the gold standard for morphological assessment of PV, and right side morphology and function; echocardiography is the first line imaging modality and the most frequent used imaging modality for follow-up due to its universal availability, low cost, and acceptable sensitivity.

ECHOCARDIOGRAPHIC ASSESSMENT OF PULMONARY REGURGITATION

Goals of imaging are to evaluate valve cusp morphology (bicuspid, quadricuspid valves; hypoplasia, dysplasia, absence of PV) and motion (doming or prolapse) and RVOT morphology.

COMMON ETIOLOGIES OF PULMONIC REGURGITATION

Mild pulmonic regurgitation (PR) is found in 40-78% of patients with normal PV anatomy. Severe PR though is found in patients with significant structural right heart

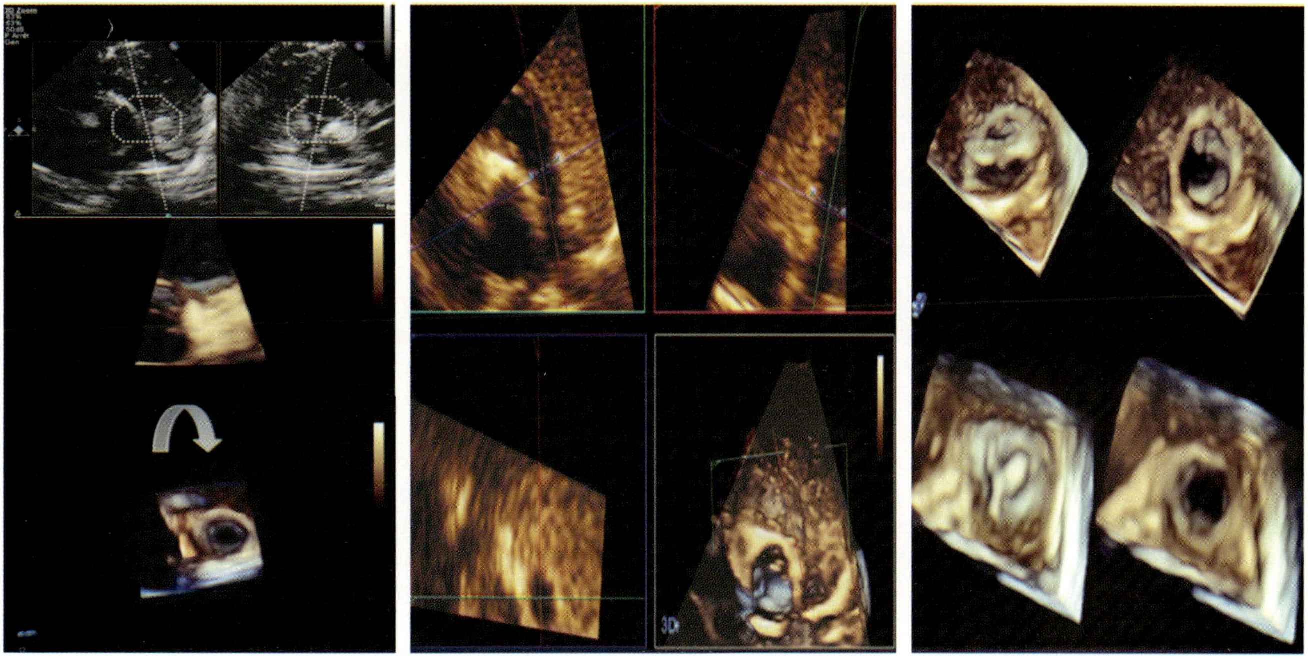

Fig. 2

disease such as congenital heart disease (approximately 20% have abnormality in RVOT or PV) or acquired valvular dysfunction (carcinoid, rheumatic and endocarditis). Severe PR can lead to RV dilation, dysfunction, right heart failure, arrhythmia, and cardiac death. The amount of regurgitation is influenced by several factors; size of the regurgitant orifice, right ventricle afterload, RV diastolic compliance, and the time in diastole. The low pressure system and low resistance of the right ventricle can allow pulmonary regurgitation to go undetected with little clinical significance for years until progressive RV dilation occurs. Thus, assessment of PR at "routine intervals" is warranted.

GOALS OF IMAGING

Assessment of PR should take into account the following determinants of its degree of severity: (1) size of regurgitant orifice, (2) hydraulic impedance or afterload, (3) the ventricular diastolic compliance, and (4) diastolic filling time significance of the regurgitant volume varies proportionally with the RV size and stroke volume, as such, in patients with a modest regurgitant volume and normally sized RV may have the same regurgitation fraction as a patient with a more severe regurgitant jet but with a proportionate increase in RV volume and stroke volume size and systolic and diastolic function of the RV must be included in the echocardiographic evaluation and are in fact also part of the criteria considered to formulate a potential surgical indication.

Color flow Doppler allows visualization of regurgitant jet origin, jet width [vena contracta (VC)], and the spatial orientation of jet area in the right ventricle. When regurgitation is more than mild, flow convergence into the regurgitant orifice an also be visualized using computational fluid dynamics (CFD). Maximization of the frame rate, reducing the color sector size and image depth and optimization of color or gain scale including a Nyquist limit of 50-60 s/min are essential for a correct evaluation. The CFD quantification of PR severity relies on three methods: (1) color jet assessment, (2) VC, and (3) flow convergence method.

Pathological PR has a longer duration, is usually holodiastolic, and has a wider flow jet than the common physiological functional PR which is usually small (<10 mm in length), spindle-shaped, and originates centrally from coaptation site. The color jet area depends mostly on the driving pressure between the pulmonary artery and the right ventricle, but in severe PR, equalization between diastolic pulmonary and RV pressures occurs rapidly, and the color jet can be brief and misleading. The color jet diameter width is estimated by the diameter of the jet in diastole immediately below the valve (RV outflow tract and pulmonary annulus). A jet width occupying more than 65% of RV outflow tract suggests severe PR (highly interobserver dependent) and presence of color flow reversal in branch pulmonary arteries is a specific sign of severe PR proximal jet width (VC) is probably the most widely used semiqualitative color Doppler method. This parameter is less dependent on driving pressures and is simple and more reproducible. The VC width of the PR is commonly expressed as a ratio relative to the PV annulus diameter. A ratio of more than 0.5 is correlated with severe PR measured by cardiac magnetic resonance (CMR). It is important to note that in severe PR with normal PA pressures (e.g. primary PR), the color jet can be difficult to detect as the PR jet velocities are low, laminar, and brief in duration due to rapid equilibration of pressures across the PV. In secondary PR with pulmonary hypertension, the jet is aliased, of high velocity, and usually holodiastolic. Effective regurgitant orifice area calculation by VC method (the narrowest portion of a jet that occurs at or just downstream from the orifice) is based on the assumption of a circular or elliptical regurgitant flow, which is available in only some cases. There are no available studies validating the use of proximal isovelocity surface area method for grading PR severity as both these methods are not applicable when free PR occurs (as with anastomosis between the pulmonary artery and the RV infundibulum) or when PR originates in the distal pulmonary arteries as with tetralogy of Fallot (TOF) patients.

Severe PR will have a dense jet that rapidly decelerates so that regurgitant flow ends around mid-diastole while mild-to-moderate PR flow persists throughout diastole; occasionally, a jet of mild PR will decelerate quickly, but its signal density is low. By contrast, velocity of flow is not proportional to severity of regurgitation. Higher velocities suggested by aliasing of the color Doppler signal or by high continuous wave (CV) Doppler peak velocity reflect higher pressure gradients between RVOT and pulmonary circulation.

Spectral Doppler

Spectral jet density is considered a qualitative visual method for grading PR severity. The duration of the jet is not yet specific but may be indicative of severe regurgitation when a rapid deceleration rate with early termination (mid-to-late diastole) occurs. Also, the pressure half-time less than 100 ms demonstrated high-sensitivity and specificity to identify hemodynamically significant PR in congenital population. The PR index (PRi) expressed as the ratio between the duration of PR and the total diastole (measured from the end of forward pulmonary flow to the beginning of the next forward pulmonary flow curve) has shown excellent sensitivity and sensibility in a single study compared with

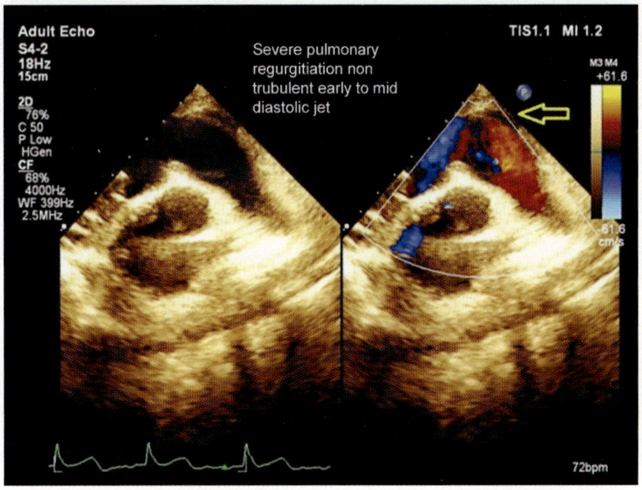

Parameter	*Mild*	*Moderate*	*Severe*
Pulmonic valve	Normal	Normal or abnormal	Abnormal and may not be visible
RV size	Normal	Normal or dilated	Dilated
Jet size, color Doppler	Thin (usually <10 mn in length) with a narrow origin	Intermediate	Broad origin; variable depth of penetration
Radio of PR jet width/pulmonary annulus			>0.7
Jet density and contour (CW)	Soft	Dense	Dense; early termination of diastolic flow
Deceleration time of the PR spectral Doppler signal			Short, <260 msec
Pressure half-time of PR jet			<100 sec
PR index		<0.77	<0.77
Diastolic flow reversal in the main or branch PAs (PW)			Prominent
Pulmonic systolic flow (VTI) compared to systemic flow (LVOTVTI) by PW	Silghtly	Intermediate	Greatly increased
RF	<20%	20–40%	>40%

Fig. 3

pulmonary regurgitant fraction on CMR for identifying significant PR in TOF asymptomatic patients.

The main limitations of these CW-based methods are the presence of elevated diastolic pulmonary pressures and RV restrictive physiology, defined as RV "unfillable" in late diastole, such that atrial contraction induces an anterograde forward flow due to rapid opening of PV could induce the early termination of the regurgitant jet. The peak velocity measured with CW Doppler at the beginning and end of diastole allow a direct measurement respectively of the mean and diastolic pulmonary pressure applying the Bernoulli equation shape of PR at CW Doppler (pandiastolic plateau, biphasic, peak and plateau, and early diastolic triangular types) may give some additional information regarding the severity of PR and the PA-RV pressure gradient including the RV diastolic properties (Figs. 3 and 4).

TIMING OF SURGERY

Overall, there is sufficient evidence that support the benefits of pulmonic valve replacement as shown by clinical improvement, ventricular remodeling with improved mechanics, lower degree of tricuspid regurgitation (TR), and improved RV functions has been well-demonstrated with proliferative vitreoretinopathy (PVR). Timing of surgery in patients with PR who require PVR is the main challenge in this surgical approach. The decision is influenced by the lack of consensus on clinical parameters that determine the best timing for PVR. The vast evidence of PVR is from clinical investigations inpatients with repaired TOF. Previous evidence in experimental models shows decreased right ventricle contractility as early as 3 months after the onset of PI and eventually producing clinical symptoms, and RV failure. This sequence of events can predispose

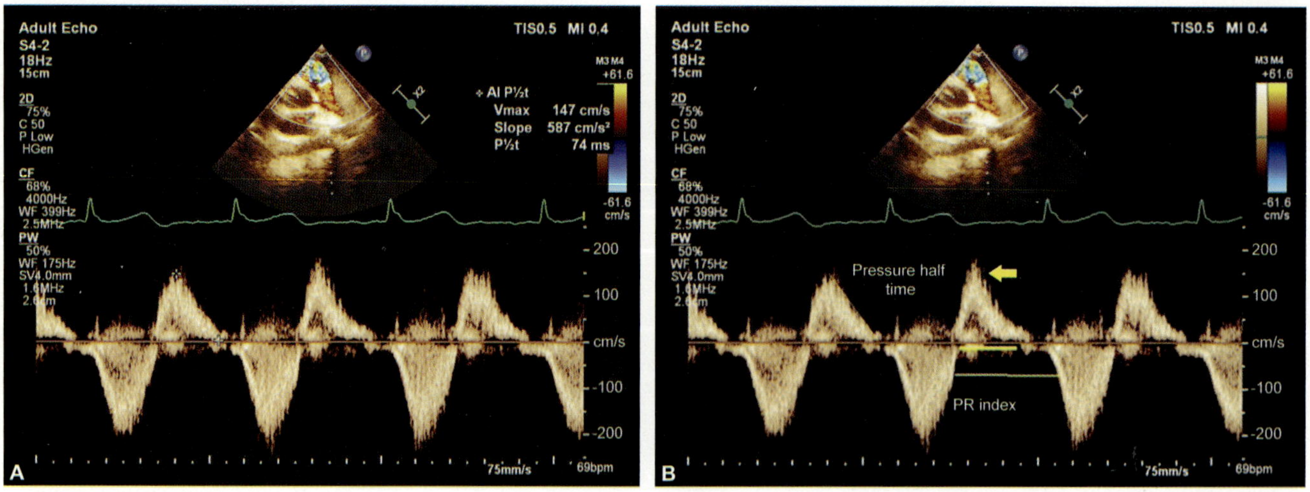

Figs. 4A and B

patients to ventricular arrhythmias. The decision to undergo PVR should be based on a risk/benefit ratio, taking into consideration the natural history and pathophysiology of each underlying condition leading to PR and the likelihood of valve failure following PVR.[2,3] Adult patients with corrected TOF who require PVR have, on average, low mortality and 5-year survival of over 92%. Unfortunately, a surgical decision for PVR based on clinical symptoms would delay recognition of the best surgical timing because the RV is markedly dilated and biventricular failure can be present at that time. Geva et al. found a mean RV end-diastolic volume of 201 ± 37 mL/m^2 when patients were more symptomatic. PVR is recommended in asymptomatic patients with previous TOF repair, if regurgitation fraction is more than 24% by CMR and if at least two of the following measurements are found:

- RV ejection fraction less than 45%
- Indexed end-diastolic volume more than 150 mL/m^2
- Indexed end-systolic volume more than 70 mL/m^2
- Right ventricular outflow tract aneurysm
- Clinical symptoms [heart failure, decreased functional capacity, syncope, and sustained ventricular tachycardia (VT)].

Valve failure is perhaps the most limiting factor on long-term PVR success. In general, PVR at earlier age is associated with higher valve failure and reoperation.[2-5]

ROLE OF ECHOCARDIOGRAPHY IN TRANSCATHETER VALVE REPLACEMENT FOR PULMONARY REGURGITATION

Percutaneous pulmonic valve implantation is obviously becoming the technique of choice for failed bioprosthetic PV and in cases of dysfunctional right ventricle-to pulmonary-artery conduits using Melody valve or Sapien valves.

The first prospective trial of percutaneous PVR in congenital heart disease patients with previous surgical intervention and RVOT conduit dysfunction has showed promising results with this approach. The implantation success rate was over 95% with low complication rate and short-term good outcomes. Finally, percutaneous PVR can be considered in high-risk patient population such as those hemodynamically unstable during pregnancy.

Dilated RVOT remains a limiting factor for the effective utilization of percutaneous valve implantation. A more recent hybrid approach for off-pump percutaneous PVR in patients with dilated RVOT has been described with potential decreased perioperative morbidity and mortality.

Severe RVOT obstruction with no or mild-pulmonary regurgitation, with either of the following:

- Symptoms related to RVOT obstruction (<65% of expected exercise tolerance) plus a peak CW Doppler velocity of more than 3.5 m/s
- No symptoms plus RVOT obstruction with peak CW Doppler velocity more than 4.0 m/s or RVOT obstruction with RV systolic pressure greater than two-thirds of systemic systolic pressure.

Severe pulmonary regurgitation and little or no RVOT obstruction, with RV end-diastolic volume index more than 150 cm/m^2 by cardiovascular magnetic resonance imaging Candidates for percutaneous pulmonic valve implantation (PPVI) must also meet the following two criteria:

1. Adequate RVOT conduit size to accommodate a covered stent. We do not have a lower size limitation. The upper size limitation is usually a diameter less than 29 mm. In selected cases, a slightly larger diameter may be successfully treated after prestenting to a smaller diameter to create a suitable "landing zone".

2. *Adequate body size*: There is no absolute lower age limit but an adequate body size (e.g. weight > 20 kg) is required to accommodate femoral placement of the introducer.

EXCLUSION CRITERIA (ADAPTED FROM THE EUROPEAN SOCIETY OF CARDIOLOGY 2010 GUIDELINES)

Risk of coronary compression by the expanded implant as determined by balloon testing, central vein occlusion or significant obstruction, active infection (such as endocarditis) or high-risk of infection (such as intravenous drug abuse), surgery is preferred when additional interventions are considered such as tricuspid annuloplasty, coronary artery bypass, or arrhythmia surgery.

Major society guidelines for the management of grown-up congenital heart disease include the following indications for surgical intervention or PPVI in patients with RV to pulmonary artery conduits:

- Intervention is recommended in symptomatic patients with RV systolic pressure more than 60 mm Hg (TR velocity > 3.5 m/s; may be lower in cases with reduced flow) and/or moderate-to-severe PR.[2-5] Intervention is suggested in asymptomatic patients with severe RVOT obstruction and/or severe pulmonary regurgitation when at least one of the following criteria is present:
    1. Decrease in exercise capacity on cardiopulmonary exercise testing
    2. Progressive RV dilation
    3. Progressive RV systolic dysfunction
    4. Progressive TR (at least moderate)
    5. Right ventricular systolic pressure more than 80 mm Hg (TR velocity > 4.3 m/s)
    6. Sustained atrial or ventricular arrhythmias.

PULMONARY VALVE STENOSIS

The PV may be dysplastic, thickened, and/or tethered causing restriction of the flow of blood from the right ventricle to the main and branch pulmonary arteries.

- *Domed*—42%
- *Tricuspid*—6%
- *Bicuspid*—10%
- *Unicommissural*—16%
- *Hypoplastic annulus*—6%
- *Dysplastic*—20%.

It may present as critical pulmonary stenosis in newborn when the ductal flow is critical to maintain adequate pulmonary perfusion or may present in three predominant forms:

1. Dome-type pulmonic valve stenosis, which is characterized by a narrow central opening with preserved valve motion. Three rudimentary raphes are generally present without clear-cut commissures. The pulmonary trunk may be dilated due to a medial abnormality and eccentric flow from the stenotic valve (poststenotic dilatation). Calcification of the valve is rare but is noted in some older patients.
2. Approximately, 20% of cases present with valve dysplasia, with thickened valve leaflets and relative immobility of the valve. Pulmonary artery dilation is not commonly associated with dysplastic valves. Dysplastic PVs are a common component of Noonan syndrome, occurring in up to half of patients.
3. More complex congenital heart disease, such as cases of tetralogy of Fallot or transposition of the great arteries, may be associated with an obstructive unicuspid or bicuspid PV.

Acquired RV outflow obstruction may occur after surgical reconstruction for congenital cardiac disorders such as TOF, pulmonary atresia, truncus arteriosus, double outlet right ventricle, or transposition of the great arteries with pulmonic stenosis. Reconstruction often entails the placement of a PV prosthesis, right ventricle-to-pulmonary artery homograft, or valved conduit, which degenerates overtime, manifesting as stenosis, regurgitation, or both.

Valvular pulmonic stenosis can also be classified by the presence or absence of associated stenosis in the subvalvar or supravalvar region. The subvalvar stenosis can be due to the muscle bundle proliferation in a pressure-overloaded right ventricle. The supravalvar stenosis is more commonly associated with a syndrome like Noonan, or as a part of a lesion complex like TOF (Figs. 5 and 6).

GOALS OF ECHOCARDIOGRAPHY EXAMINATION

- Pressure gradient across the PV—calculated using the Bernoulli's equation with the peak velocity of flow across the valve. This can underestimate the obstruction in the setting of high pulmonary vascular resistance or pulmonary hypertension.
- Right ventricular pressure—based on the TR velocity, or the orientation of the interventricular septum, or direction of shunting at an atrial septal communication or a patent ductus arteriosus, if present.
- Right ventricular systolic and diastolic dysfunction—using TAPSE or tissue Doppler imaging.
- Morphology of the PV—number of leaflets, dysplastic appearance, and doming of leaflets in systole. Also, presence of poststenotic dilation is typical for isolated valvular pulmonary stenosis.

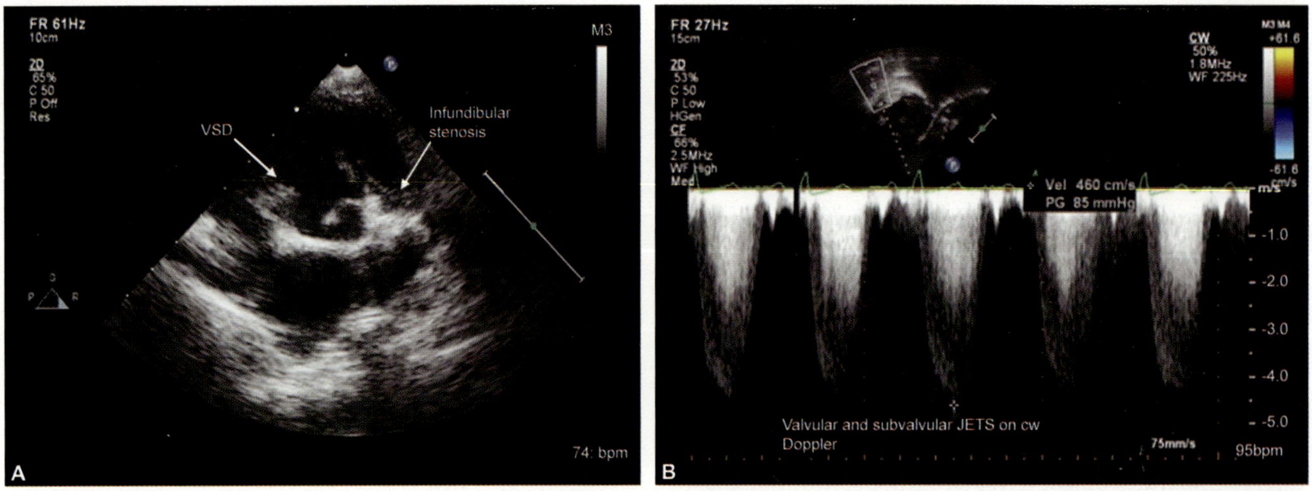

Figs. 5A and B

- Associated presence of subvalvar pulmonary stenosis—by using pulse wave Doppler and note the characteristic dagger-shaped infundibular stenosis jet pattern.
- Associated presence of supravalvar stenosis and see for difference in ostial size.

The severity of pulmonic stenosis is classified by major society guidelines using the following criteria:

- Mild pulmonic stenosis is identified by a peak Doppler gradient across the valve less than 36 mm Hg (equal to peak Doppler jet velocity < 3 m/s) or a peak Doppler gradient less than 30 mm Hg.
- Moderate stenosis is identified by a peak Doppler gradient of 36–64 mm Hg (peak jet velocity of 3–4 m/s) or peak Doppler gradient of 30–50 mm Hg.
- Severe pulmonic stenosis is identified by a peak Doppler gradient more than 64 mm Hg (peak jet velocity of > 4 m/s) or peak Doppler gradient more than 50–60 mm Hg or mean Doppler gradient more than 30–40 mm Hg.

INDICATIONS FOR INTERVENTION [2008 AMERICAN COLLEGE OF CARDIOLOGY/AMERICAN HEART ASSOCIATION (ACC/AHA)]: ADULT CONGENITAL HEART DISEASE RECOMMENDATIONS FOR INTERVENTION IN PATIENTS WITH PULMONIC STENOSIS

- For asymptomatic patients with a domed pulmonic valve and peak instantaneous Doppler gradient more than 60 mm Hg or a mean Doppler gradient more than 40 mm Hg (in association with < moderate pulmonic valve regurgitation), balloon valvotomy is recommended.

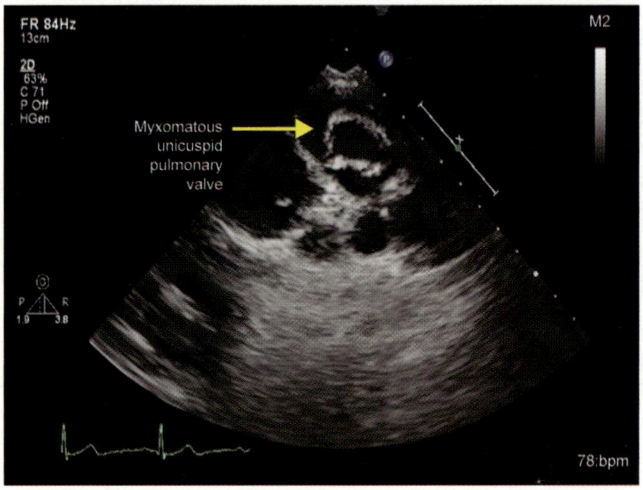

Fig. 6

- For symptomatic patients with a domed pulmonic valve and peak instantaneous Doppler gradient more than 50 mm Hg or a mean Doppler gradient more than 30 mm Hg (in association with < moderate pulmonic valve regurgitation), balloon valvotomy is recommended.
- Surgical therapy is recommended for patients with severe pulmonic stenosis and an associated hypoplastic pulmonary annulus, severe pulmonary regurgitation, subvalvular pulmonic stenosis, or supravalvular pulmonic stenosis. Surgery is also preferred for most dysplastic valves and when there is associated severe TR, the need for a surgical Maze procedure or other cardiac surgical procedure that warrants operative intervention.

Balloon valvotomy is less effective in patients with a dysplastic valve (with or without Noonan syndrome), so surgery is generally preferred. However, the 2008 ACC/AHA guidelines note that balloon valvotomy may be reasonable in patients with a dysplastic PV who are either asymptomatic with a peak Doppler gradient more than 60 mm Hg or mean Doppler gradient more than 40 mm Hg or symptomatic with a peak Doppler gradient more than 50 mm Hg or a mean Doppler gradient more than 30 mm Hg.

Procedural Considerations

Use of an oversized balloon (approximately 1.2–1.25 times), the measured pulmonary annulus aids in achieving a successful result (defined as a final-peak valvular gradient of < 20 mm Hg). Transient severe RVOT obstruction ("suicidal right ventricle") has been reported after the pulmonic valvular obstruction has been relieved.[6-9] This may be treated by volume expansion and beta-blocker therapy and tends to regress with time.

REFERENCES

1. Gramiak R, Nanda NC, Shah PM. Echocardiographic detection of the pulmonary valve. Radiology. 1972;102:153-7.
2. Shillcutt SK, Tavazzi G, Shapiro BP, et al. Pulmonic regurgitation in the adult cardiac surgical patient. J Cardiothorac Vasc Anesth. 2016;31:215-28.
3. Awad SM, Masood SA, Gonzalez I, et al. The use of intracardiac echocardiography during percutaneous pulmonary valve replacement. Pediatr Cardiol. 2015;36:76-83.
4. Chessa M, Butera G, Carminati M. Intracardiac echocardiography during percutaneous pulmonary valve replacement. Eur Heart J. 2008;29:2908.
5. Chowdhury SM, Hijazi ZM, Rhodes J, et al. Early echocardiographic changes after percutaneous implantation of the Edwards SAPIEN transcatheter heart valve in the pulmonary position. Echocardiography. 2013;30:786-93.
6. Silversides CK, Bradley T, Webb GD, et al. Canadian Consensus Conference on Adult Congenital Heart Disease 1996. Can J Cardiol. 1998;14:395-452.
7. Baumgartner H, Hung J, Bermejo J, et al. Echocardiographic assessment of valve stenosis: EAE/ASE recommendations for clinical practice. J Am Society Echocardiography. 2009;22:1-23.
8. Nishimura RA, Otto CM, Bonow RO, et al. 2014 AHA/ACC Guideline for the Management of Patients with Valvular Heart Disease: executive summary: a report of the American College of Cardiology/American Heart Association Task Force on Practice Guidelines. Circulation. 2014;129:2440-92.
9. Rao PS. Percutaneous balloon pulmonary valvuloplasty: State-of-the-art. Catheter Cardiovasc Interv. 2007;69:747-63.

66

CHAPTER

Echocardiographic Evaluation of the Prosthetic Valve

Ashok K Omar, Rahul Kumar, Mitu Minocha, Shailendra Bhadoriya

INTRODUCTION

Patients with significant valvular heart disease may undergo interventions like valvuloplasty, surgical repair and replacement. Prosthetic heart valves have been successfully used in heart valve replacement over the past 50 years.[1] More than 43 thousand aortic or mitral valve replacement operations (with or without coronary artery bypass were reported to the society of thoracic surgeons (STS). National adult cardiac database in 2015.[2] About 4 million prosthetic heart valve (PHV) replacement have been performed over the past 50 years.[3] Some of those valve designs are no more under use. After prosthetic valve replacement, prognosis depends on hemodynamics, durability, thrombogenicity and other complications like endocarditis. To reduce the morbidity and mortality of the patient, evaluation of prosthetic valve function at regular intervals is required to detect any early valvular dysfunction. Although physical examination and clinical features may indicate prosthetic valve dysfunction, diagnostic methods are needed to evaluate and assess the prosthetic valve function. Echocardiography with the Doppler is the method of choice for noninvasive evaluation of prosthetic valve. As per design, prosthetic valves are always obstructive in nature which corresponds to the type and the size of the prostheses. Prosthetic valves may also be associated with trivial or mild transprosthetic regurgitation as per its design which should be considered while prosthetic valve function assessment. A full transthoracic echocardiographic study requires multiple angulation of probes and use of off-axis views. On rare occasions intermittent obstructions are suspected and prolonged Doppler examination may be required. Quiet often transthoracic echo is not adequate and transesophageal echocardiography (TEE) is needed for evaluation of PHV related complications. The past six decades have witnessed significant advancement in patient's survival and functional outcomes following heart valve replacement surgery.[1]

Heart valve team have been formed to provide multidisciplinary assessment and treatment of complex patients including the use of transcatheter heart valve.

TYPES OF PROSTHETIC HEART VALVES

Ideal PHV should have:

- Optimal hemodynamics
- Nonobstructive in systole
- Competent in diastole
- Nonthrombogenecity
- Durability
- Ease of insertion
- Resistance of infection
- Low noise level.

None of the PHV available today, fulfills the above criteria.

Prosthetic valves are generally grouped as mechanical and biological (Fig. 1).

Most frequently implanted biological types are those made from animal tissues, Xenografts usually made from the pig aortic valve or bovine pericardium. Stentless xenograft valves were introduced in hope of improving hemodynamic function durability and complications.

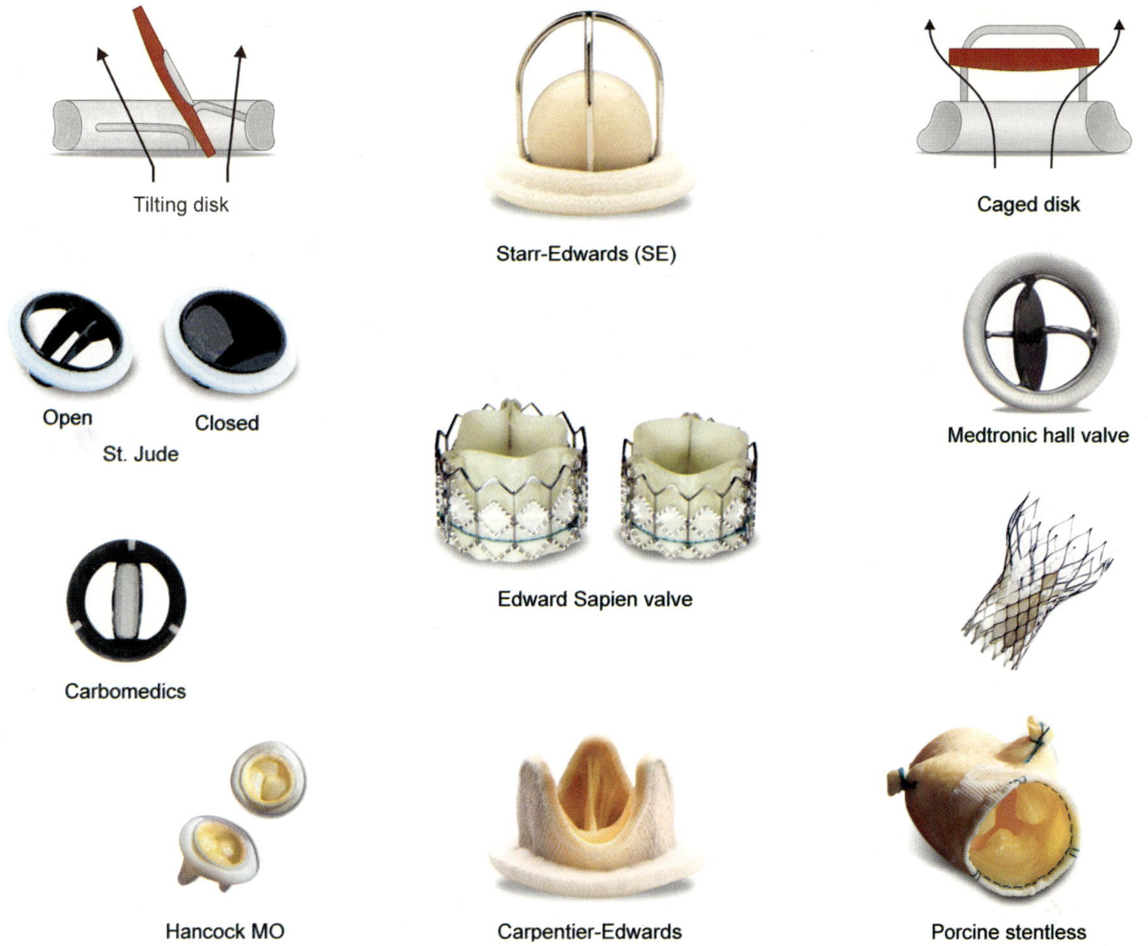

Fig. 1: Types of prosthetic valves.

Homografts (allografts) are stentless human valves. Homografts have long durability even in younger subjects and they resist infection and can be useful for patients with infective endocarditis. The Ross procedure involves auto transplanting the patient's pulmonary valve to the aortic position and replacing it with a homograft. It has a good durability, may grow in children and less likely to become infected than xenograft.[4] The three classes of mechanical valves are tilting disk, bileaflet and ball in cage which differ primarily in the type and function of occluder. Most frequently implanted mechanical valves is bileaflet mechanical valve but tilting disk valves are still used. Ball in cage valves though not used now will still require echocardiography (Table 1).

Transcatheter valves are essentially bioprosthetic mounted in aortic and pulmonary in particular position, percutaneous aortic valve implantation is an alternative to standard aortic valve replacement in patients with symptomatic aortic stenosis with moderate or high operative risk (Fig. 2).[5-7] Most frequently implanted biological valves are stented xenografts and most frequently implanted mechanical valves are bileaflet valves. Various valve types can differ also by their implantation position relative to the valve annulus, mainly in aortic valve.

- Intra-annular
- Partially supra-annular
- Wholly supra-annular.

TABLE 1: Types of prosthetic valves.

Biological			*Mechanical*
Stented	Stentless	Percutaneous	
Porcine xenograft	Porcine xenograft	Core	Bileaflet
Pericardial xenograft	Pericardial xenograft	Sapien	Single tilting disk
	Homograft (allograft)		Caged ball
	Autograft		

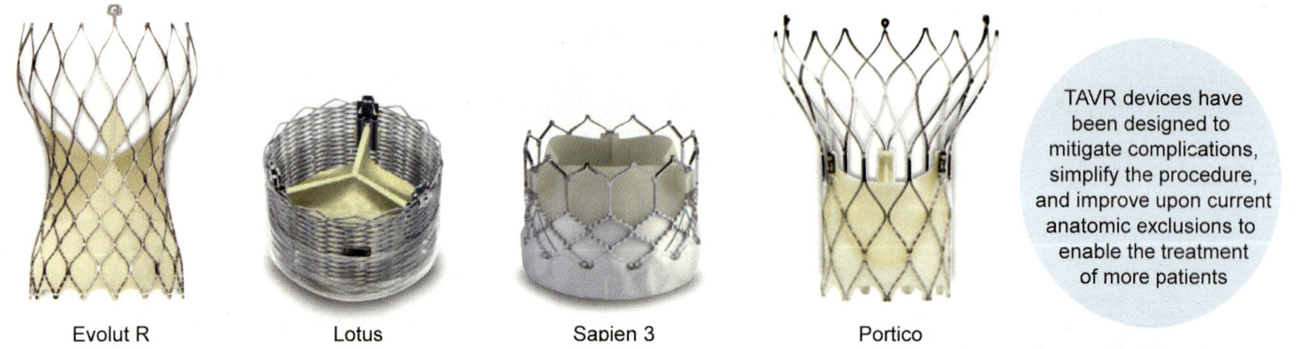

Frame	*Nitinol*	*Nitinol*	*Cobalt Chromium*	*Nitinol*	*Nitinol*
PVL management	Extended skirt	Adaptive seal	PET fabric skirt	Pericardial cuff	Pericardial skirt
Annular range	18–30 mm	20–27 mm	16–28 mm	19–27 mm	21–27 mm
Positioning	Recapturable	Recapturable	—	Recapturable	—
Caliber	14 Fr/16 equiv.	18 Fr	14 Fr/16 Fr	18 Fr/19 Fr	18 Fr

Fig. 2: TAVR—newer designs.

Suprannular position is designed to lift as much of the replacement valve above the annulus to maximize the orifice area, available for flow.[8]

ECHOCARDIOGRAPHY FOR PROSTHETIC HEART VALVES

Echocardiography is main stay for assessment of replacement of valves and is indicated immediately after surgery to confirm the normal function and baseline hemodynamic parameters for the individual valve.

It should be done between 3 week and 12 week after the surgery.

Routine echocardiography studies after this are not indicated for mechanical valves, since their risk of primary failure is effectively nil. Echocardiography should be performed for older biological valves annually after 5 years of implantation according to European Society of Cardiology and 10 years after surgery as per American Heart Association (Table 2). The bioprosthetic valve failure rate is 20% in aortic position and 40% for mitral position in 10 years. Frequency of follow-up, however, may need to be individualized due to various factors like valve design, age of implantation, patient prosthesis mismatch (PPM), etc.

In patients with abnormal symptoms or sign, echocardiography has to differentiate PHV dysfunction from left ventricular (LV) or right ventricular (RV) dysfunction or other valve dysfunction.

A complete echocardiography includes two-dimensional (2D) imaging of prosthetic valve, evaluation of valve leaflet/occluder morphology and mobility, measurement of transprosthetic gradients, effective valvular orifice area (EOA), degree of regurgitation, LV size and function and systolic pulmonary arterial pressure. It is extremely important to know:

- The type and size of the replacement valve
- The date of valve surgery
- Blood pressure and heart rate
- The patient's height, weight, and body surface area (BSA) to identify a possible PPM.

Goals for the 2D Echocardiography

- Determine the specific types of prosthesis
- Confirm the opening and closing motion of the prosthesis
- Confirm stability of the sewing ring
- Presence of leaflet calcification or any other abnormal echodensity
- Calculate valve gradients and effective orifice area

TABLE 2: Guideline indications for echocardiography for replacement heart valves.

- Immediately after surgery to confirm normal function
- *Routine late after implantation to detect structural degeneration*:
  - More than and equal to 5 years for biological mitral valves or biological aortic valves in patients aged less than 50[9]
  - More than and equal to 10 years for biological aortic valves in patients aged more than 50[10]
- If dysfunction is suspected based on a new murmur or symptom
- If there is clinical evidence of infective endocarditis
- Before and during pregnancy (every trimester)
- Before major noncardiac surgery

- To confirm normal blood flow patterns
- Detection of any transvalvular or paravalvular regurgitation.

Echocardiography on PHV is more demanding both to perform and interpret in comparison to assessment of native valves. Acoustic shadowing and artifacts created by prosthetic valves make echo study difficult. Transesophageal echo helps in overcoming some of these difficulties.

Qualitative Parameters

In bioprosthetic valve, the thickening of leaflets is earliest sign of degeneration. Bright echos on the cusps shows calcification. There may be flail cusps. Stentless homografts or autografts valves may be indistinguishable from the native valves. TEE allows more detailed assessment of cusp calcification, vegetations, thrombus, pannus, reduced disk or ball movements. Prosthetic valve stenosis is associated with abnormal morphology and mobility. There may be presence of thrombus in relation to PHV. Pannus formation is also important to recognize which is in growth and leads to progressive obstruction. Prosthetic valve dehiscence is characterized by rocking motion of entire prosthesis.

A normal functioning porcine aortic PHV leaflets opening resembles normal native valve. Unless historical information is available, sometimes they are mistaken as normal valves. When examined carefully, sewing ring is more echogenic and tend to obscure leaflets. In ball and cage valve protruding highly echo-dense cage in left ventricle is well seen. Ball movement can be seen forward and backward during real-time examination. Single leaflet tilting disk prosthetic valve is very well seen with the disk movement showing a major and minor opening. A bileaflet type (St. Jude) PHV seen as two hemidisks opening like two parallel line and move to close the PHV orifice during systole (Figs. 3A to F).

Significant shadowing occurs in left atrium due to these valve.

Assessment of leaflet or occluder movement can be difficult. However, through careful interrogation rapid movement of leading edge of disk or ball generally can be recorded. Motion is usually brisk and consistent with each beat. M-mode imaging is also useful to record a sharp closing and opening leaflets (Fig. 4).

Quantitative Parameters

Purpose of Doppler assessment across the prosthetic valve is to look for pattern of flow which is unique for each valve, quantitative assessment of the gradients and detection of abnormal regurgitation.

Basic principles of Doppler assessment are same as for native valves.

Following parameters are measured for the prosthetic valve assessment.[11]

- Transprosthetic velocity and pressure gradient
- Transprosthetic jet contour and acceleration time
- Doppler velocity index (DVI)
- Effective valvular orifice area (EOA)
- Pressure half-time.

Transprosthetic Velocity and Gradient

With the help of pulsed wave (PW), continuous wave (CW) and color Doppler and flow velocity through the prosthetic valve can be calculated, similarly as for the native valves. To minimize angulation between the Doppler beam and flow direction and to obtain the highest velocity, we should take multiple windows.[12] Fluid dynamics of mechanical valves may differ from that of native valves. Sometimes, we get an abnormally high jet velocity by CW Doppler through the smaller central orifice of bileaflet mechanical aortic or mitral prosthesis which leads us to overestimate the jet velocity and gradients. The flow is eccentric for monoleaflet valves and of three separate jets for bileaflet valves.[11]

Flow velocities are higher in normal functioning prosthetic valve and make them inherently stenotic. This is due to various reasons:

- Smaller sewing ring
- Growing age of the patient
- EOA is significantly small than area of sewing ring
- Occluder mechanism occupies central space
- Preservation process for leaflets in bioprosthesis makes them stiffer.

Both valve size and type determine the normal velocity and gradients of particular valve.

Pressure gradient (PG) is calculated by Bernoulli equation, $PG = 4 \times V_{pr}^2$, where V_{pr} is the peak transprosthetic jet flow velocity in m/s. Prosthetic valve stenosis is associated with increased transprosthetic peak-flow velocity and mean gradient, i.e. for aortic prostheses peak velocity more than and equal to 3 m/s, mean PG more than and equal to 20 mm Hg and for mitral prostheses peak velocity more than and equal to 1.9 m/s, as mean PG more than and equal to 6 mm Hg.[9-12] But, on increased velocity and gradient is not proof of prosthetic valve obstruction, it may also be because of PPM, high flow conditions (anemia) and prosthetic valve regurgitation, increased heart rate, localized central jet velocity in bileaflet valve.

Transprosthetic jet contour and acceleration is very helpful parameter to evaluate prosthetic valve function. For prosthetic valve in aortic position, the contour of the CW flow velocity is usually of triangular shape with early peaking of the velocity and shorter acceleration time (<80 ms). In conditions of prosthetic aortic valve stenosis, a more

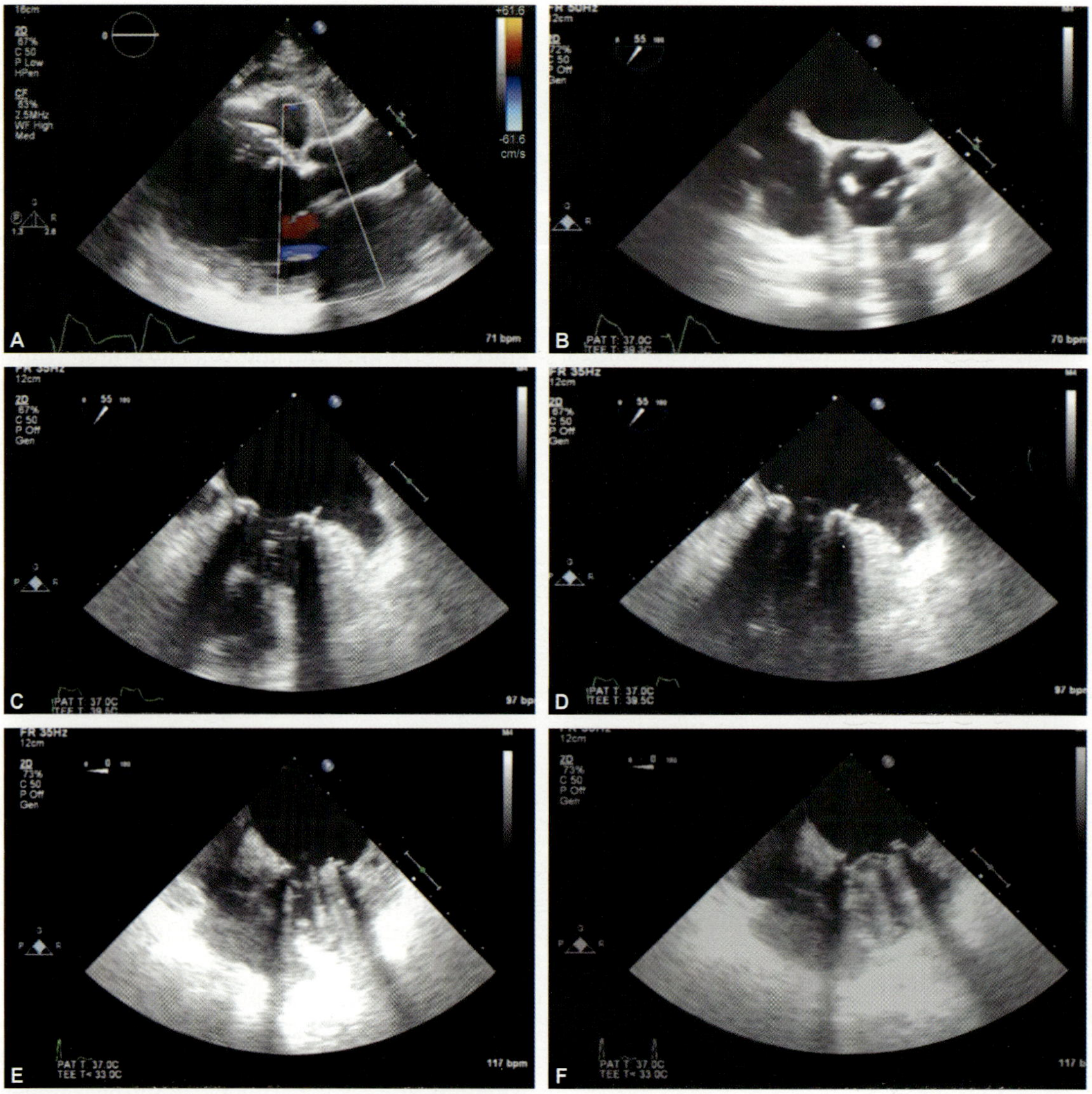

Figs. 3A to F: Various prosthetic valves. (A and B) Bioprosthetic PHV aortic position; (C and D) Starr-Edward PHV mitral position; (E and F) Bi Leaflet PHV mitral position.

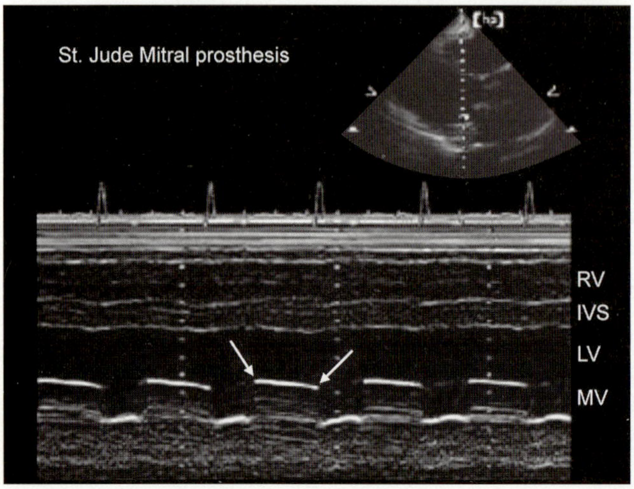

Fig. 4: M-mode echocardiogram of a St. Jude mitral prosthetic valve. M-mode echocardiography is ideal to record the brisk opening and closing of the disks (arrows).

Suggests Stenosis	
Peak velocity	>4 m/s
Mean gradient	>35 mm Hg
Doppler velocity index	<0.25
Effective orifice area	< 0.8 cm²
Contour of the jet	Rounded, symmetrical contour
Acceleration time	>100 ms

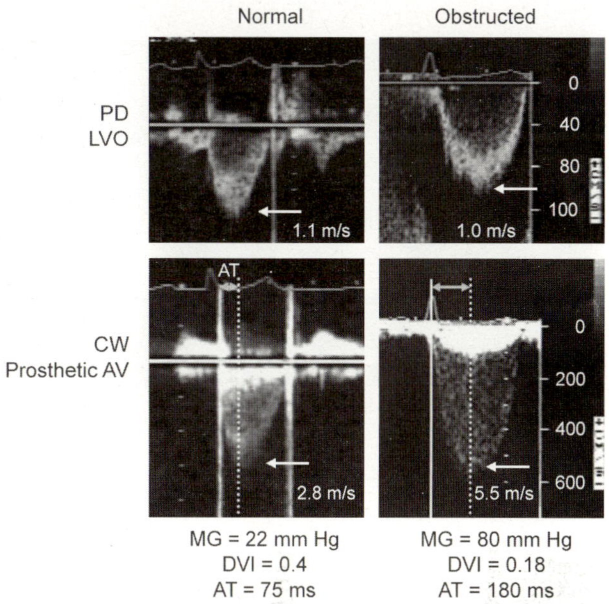

Fig. 5: Doppler parameters of prosthetic aortic valve function.

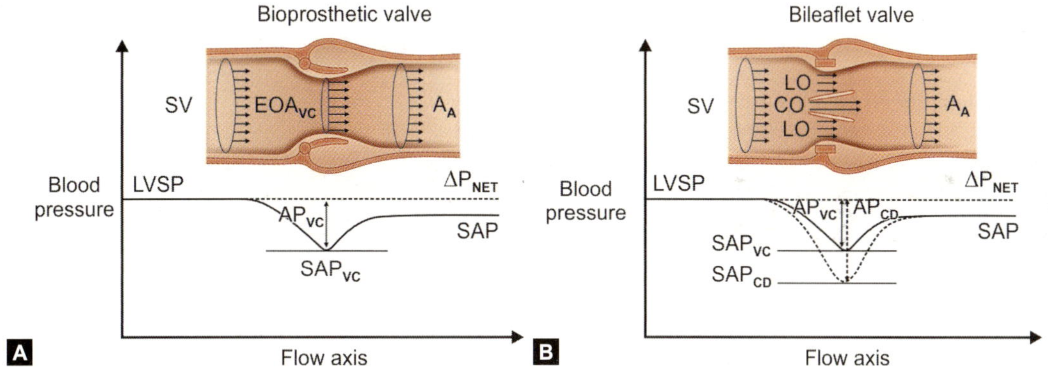

Figs. 6A and B: Evaluation of valve leaflets by CT, TEE, and fluoroscopy.

rounded velocity contour is observed, with the velocity peaking in mid ejection, longer acceleration time (Fig. 5).[13]

A bileaflet PHV has three orifice central orifice is small and produces highest velocity across the PHV and if this flow is sampled it will give erroneously high PG which is explained by pressure recovery phenomenon especially in aortic position. Pressure recovery phenomenon occurs when a portion of the kinetic energy released as blood across the valve is recovered in form of pressure downstream. Amount of energy recovered depends on how smoothly transition of flow occurs between valve and downstream conduit. Pressure Recovery is clinically relevant for bileaflet PHV in aortic position. Effect of pressure recovery is very high gradient but this is localized immediately distal to disks (Figs. 6A and B).

For prosthetic mitral valve, the condition is reversed. Initially the contour is parabolic with longer acceleration time with late peaking of velocity in mid-ejection. But, as severity increases contour becomes triangular with early peaking of the velocity and shorter acceleration time (Fig. 7).

Flow through Starr Edwards PHV comes through all around the ball instead of a well-defined orifice. Flow through bioprosthesis is usually triangular in shape.

Normal pressure gradients across the various mitral and aortic position are depicted in Tables 3 and 4.

Doppler Velocity Index

It is the ratio of velocity time integral (VTI) of left ventricular outflow tract (LVOT) and VTI of tranprosthetic flow (Fig. 8).

$$DVI_{PrAV} = VTI_{LVOT}/VTI_{PrAV}.$$

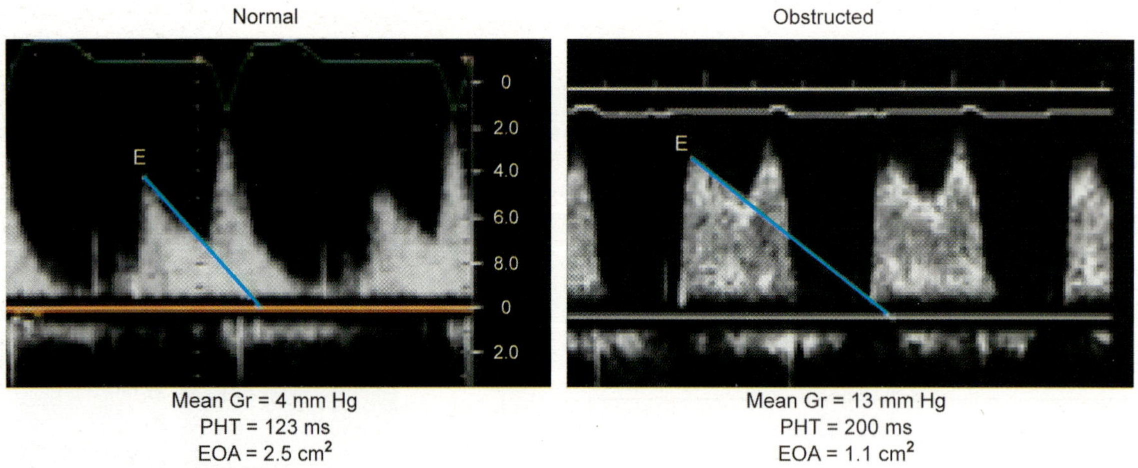

Suggests Significant Stenosis	
Peak velocity	≥ 2.5 m/s
Mean gradient	>10 mm Hg
EOA (continuity)	< 1 cm^2
Pressure half-time	>200 ms

Fig. 7: Doppler parameters of prosthetic mitral valve function.
Source: Zoghbi WA, Chambers JB, Dumesnil JG, et al. American Society of Echocardiography's Guidelines and Standards Committee; Task Force of Prosthetic Valves. J Am Soc Echocardiogr. 2009;22:975-1014.

TABLE 3: Normal gradients for PHV mitral position.

Mitral PHV: Normal mean PG						
	Mechanical			*Porcine*		
Valve type	Bileaflet (St. Jude)	Tilt-disk (BS)	Ball-cage (SE)	Ionescu-Shiley	Carpentier-Edwards	Hancock
Gradient	4 ± 1	3 ± 2	5 ± 2	3 ± 1	6 ± 2	4 ± 2

In place of VTI, absolute peak velocities also can be used. For prosthetic mitral valve, DVI is calculated by dividing VTI of transprosthetic flow by VTI of LVOT.

$$DVI_{Pr\,MV} = VTI_{PrMV}/VTI_{LVOT}$$

For prosthetic aortic valve DVI should be more than 0.3 while for the mitral valve prosthesis it should be less than 2.2.[14]

Pressure Half-Time

Pressure half-time (PHT) is defined as the duration in milliseconds between the maximum mitral PG and early diastole and the time point where PGs become half of the maximum. In case of normal valves and in mild stenosis rate of flow across mitral valve depends on atrial and ventricular compliance. For normally functioning prosthetic mitral valve, PHT remains less than 130 ms. Values more than 200 ms indicates prosthetic valve obstruction. PHT should not be obtained in conditions like 1° heart block and tachycardia because in these conditions E and A waves merge with each other and period of diastole becomes shorter.[8]

TABLE 4: Normal gradients for PHV aortic position.

Aortic PHV: Normal mean PG					
Size	*Bileaflet (St. Jude)*	*Tilt-disk (BS-MH)*	*Ball-cage (SE)*	*Porcine (Hancock CE)*	*Homograft*
19	20 (10–30)	21 ± 7		16 ± 2	
21	14 (10–30)	16		15 ± 6	
23	12 (10–30)	14 ± 5	24 ± 4	13 ± 6	7 ± 3
25	12 (5–30)	13 ± 3		11 ± 2	
27	11 (5–20)	10 ± 3		10 ± 1	
29	10 (5–15)	7 ± 6		12	
31	10 (5–15)	-		-	

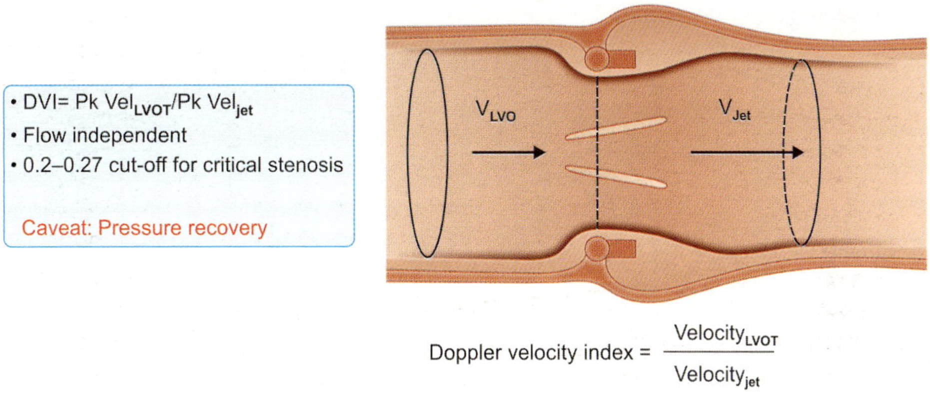

Fig. 8: Doppler velocity index.

Effective Orifice Area

The EOA of prosthetic aortic valve is calculated by continuity equation:

$$EOA_{prAV} = \text{Stroke volume}/VTI_{PrAV}$$

i.e. $EOA_{PrAV} = CSA_{LVOT} \times VTI_{LVOT}/VTI_{PrAV}$

Where CSA_{LVOT} is cross-sectional area (CSA) of LVOT which is derived by diameter measurement just beneath the prosthetic aortic valve in parasternal long-axis (PLAX) view.

VTI_{LVOT} is calculated in apical 5 chamber view using PW Doppler. It is VTI proximal to the leaflet. It is important to locate the PW Doppler sample volume adjacent to the prosthesis.

VTI_{PrAV} is calculated from the same signals that are used for measurement of prosthetic peak velocity and mean gradient using CW Doppler.[15,16]

For prosthetic mitral valve, EOA is calculated as

$EOA_{PrMV} = \text{Stroke volume}/VTI_{Pr\,MV} = CSA_{LVOT} \times VTI_{LVOT}/VTI_{PrMV}$

Where VTI_{PrMV} is calculated from the same signals that are used for measurement of prosthetic peak velocity and mean gradient using CW Doppler.

Patient Prosthetic Mismatch

When the EOA of normally functioning prosthetic valve is too small in relation to the body size of the patient to cause abnormally high postoperative gradients across the prosthetic valve, this condition is called prosthesis - patient mismatch.[11] It may result in abnormally high postoperative gradients, i.e. mean gradient more than 20 mm Hg.[17,18] It is not an intrinsic prosthetic valve dysfunction per se. The identification of patient prosthethic mismatch (PPM) and its differentiation from dysfunction is achieved by calculating the projected indexed EOA.

Patient prosthetic mismatch causes worse hemodynamics, slower and incomplete regression of left ventricular hypertrophy (LVH) or LV dysfunction, worse New York Heart Association (NYHA) class, exercise capacity and quality of life and more cardiac events and decreased survival (short-term and long-term) is associated with LV dysfunction.[19]

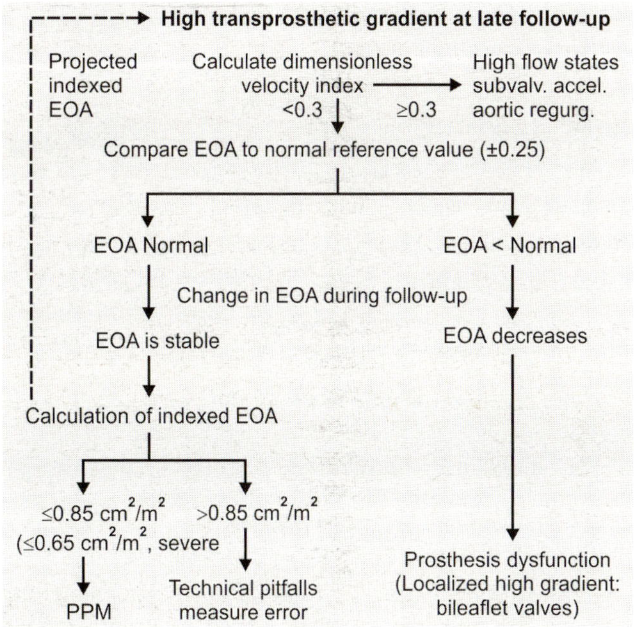

Fig. 9:

PPM can largely be avoided by the calculation of projected indexed EOA of the prosthesis to be implanted. If PPM is anticipated we should choose for alternative prosthesis or consider root enlargement surgery (Fig. 9 and Table 5).

Findings supportive of presence of PPM:

- PPM is present from the time early after surgery to anytime on subsequent echocardiography.
- Morphology and movement of valve leaflets are normal.
- Presence of lower measured indexed EOA.[20]

TABLE 5: Normal reference value of EOAs for the aortic prosthesis.

	Prosthetic valve size (mm)					
	19	21	23	25	27	29
Aortic stented bioprosthesis:						
Mosaic	1.1 ± 0.2	1.2 ± 0.3	1.4 ± 0.3	1.7 ± 0.4	1.8 ± 0.4	2.0 ± 0.4
Hancock II	—	1.2 ± 0.1	1.3 ± 0.2	1.5 ± 0.2	1.6 ± 0.2	1.6 ± 0.2
Carpentier-Edwards Perimount	1.1 ± 0.3	1.3 ± 0.4	1.50 ± 0.4	1.80 ± 0.4	2.1 ± 0.4	2.2 ± 0.4
Carpentier-Edwards Magna*	1.3 ± 0.3	1.7 ± 0.3	2.1 ± 0.4	2.3 ± 0.5	—	—
Biocor (Epic)*	—	1.3 ± 0.3	1.6 ± 0.3	1.8 ± 0.4	—	—
Metrofow*	1.1 ± 0.1	1.3 ± 0.1	1.5 ± 0.2	1.8 ± 0.2	—	—
Aortic stent less bioprosthesis:						
Medtronic freestyle	1.2 ± 0.2	1.4 ± 0.2	1.5 ± 0.3	2.0 ± 0.4	2.3 ± 0.5	—
St. Jude Medical Toronto SPV	—	1.3 ± 0.3	1.5 ± 0.5	1.7 ± 0.8	2.1 ± 0.7	2.7 ± 1.0
Aortic mechanical prosthesis:						
Medtronic-Hall	1.2 ± 0.2	1.3 ± 0.2	—	—	—	—
Medtronic advantage*	—	1.7 ± 0.2	2.2 ± 0.3	2.8 ± 0.6	3.3 ± 0.7	3.9 ± 0.7
St. Jude Medical standard	1.0 ± 0.2	1.4 ± 0.2	1.5 ± 0.5	2.1 ± 0.4	2.7 ± 0.6	3.2 ± 0.3
St. Jude Medical regent	1.6 ± 0.4	2.0 ± 0.7	2.2 ± 0.9	2.5 ± 0.9	3.6 ± 1.3	4.4 ± 0.6
MCRI on-X	1.5 ± 0.2	1.7 ± 0.4	2.0 ± 0.6	2.4 ± 0.8	3.2 ± 0.6	3.2 ± 0.6
Carbomedics standard	1.0 ± 0.4	1.5 ± 0.3	1.7 ± 0.3	2.0 ± 0.4	2.5 ± 0.4	2.6 ± 0.4

EOA is expressed as mean values available in the literature.
*These results are based on a limited number of patients and this should be interpreted with caution.

Caveats where we have to be careful during assessment of PPM:

- EOA indexed for body surface area (BSA) may overestimate the severity of PPM in obese (BMI >/30).[21.] So, we should take lower cut off points for indexed EOA for obese.[22]
  Because obese patient's cardiac output requirements are lower for same BSA as with nonobese. Thus, detrimental effects are lower for obese.[8]
- In conditions of low flow, PPM may be associated with normal or flow gradients, while it is associated with high gradient normally.
- PPM may be concomitantly present with prosthetic valve dysfunction. If stenosis is present indexed EOA is significantly low and valve leaflet movement/morphology, abnormal.

For prosthetic aortic valves EOA between 0.85 cm²/m² and 1.2 cm²/m². BSA indicates possible stenosis while between 0.60 cm²/m² and 0.85 cm²/m² and less than 0.60 cm²/m² indicates moderate and severe stenosis, respectively.

For prosthetic mitral valves EOA between 1.20 cm²/m² and 2.0 cm²/m². BSA indicates possible stenosis while between 0.9 cm²/m² and 1.2 cm²/m² and less than 0.9 cm²/m² indicates moderate and severe stenosis (PPM), respectively. (Table 6).[8]

Tables 7 and 8 show the various parameters for the prosthetic valve obstruction in aortic and mitral position.

Evaluation of Prosthetic Valve Regurgitation

It is very important to distinguish physiologic from pathologic regurgitation during the assessment of prosthetic valve regurgitation, as mechanical prostheses have a normal back flow leakage (physiological regurgitation), while

TABLE 6: Patient prosthetic mismatch.

Aortic PHV		
PPM	EOA	
Insignificant	>0.85 cm²/m²	*Effects:* • Reduced short and long time survival especially if with LV dysfunction • Less regression of LVH • Increased cardiac events • Less improvement of functional class
Moderate	>0.65–0.85 cm²/m²	
Severe	>0.65 cm²/m²	
Mitral PHV		
EOA should be more than 1.2–1.3 cm²/m² • Persistant PAH • ↓Longtime survival		

TABLE 7: Doppler parameters of prosthetic aortic valve (PrAV) function.

Doppler parameters of prosthetic aortic valve function (PrAV)			
Parameter	*Normal*	*Possible stenosis*	*Significant stenosis*
Peak velocity (m/s)	<3	3–4	>4
Mean gradient (mm Hg)	<20	20–35	>35
DVI	>0.30	0.29–0.25	<0.25
EOA	>1.2	1.2–0.8	<0.8
Contour of the jet velocity, through the PrAV	Triangular-early peaking	Triangular-to-intermediate	Rounded, symmetrical contour
AT (ms)	<80	80–100	>100

(DVI: Doppler velocity index; EOA: effective valvular orifice area)
Source: A report from the American Society of Echocardiography guidelines and standards committee and the task force on prosthetic valves.

TABLE 8: Doppler parameter of prosthetic mitral valve (PrMV) function.

Doppler parameter of prosthetic mitral valve (PrMV) function			
	Normal	*Possible stenosis*	*Significant stenosis*
Peak velocity (m/s)	<1.9	1.9–2.5	≥2.5
Mean gradient (mm Hg)	≤5	6–10	>10
VTI_{PrMV}/VTI_{LVO}	<2.2	2.2–2.5	>2.5
EOA (cm^2)	≥2.0	1–2	<1
PHT (ms)	<130	130–200	>200

(VTI: aortic valve area; EOA: effective orifice area; PHT: pressure half-time)

pathological regurgitant jets tend to be of high velocity, broad and highly aliased physiological regurgitation jets are of short duration, narrow and symmetric (Figs. 10A to E).[23]

Parameters of the Severity of Prosthetic Mitral Valve Regurgitation

During evaluation by transthoracic echocardiography (TTE), enlarged LV size and structural abnormality of prosthetic valve can be an earliest indication of prosthetic valve dysfunction and these lead us to think about prosthetic regurgitation.

Assessment of severity of magnetic resonance (MR) in prosthetic mitral valve is complex and difficult because of:

- Lack of single qualitative parameter that can be applied in all patients.
- Shadowing and artifacts created by prosthetic valve.[11]

Prosthetic MR evaluation by TTE is difficult because of acoustic shadowing of prosthesis decreases visibility of left atrial (LA) while TEE provides an excellent visualization of LA and MR jet but visualization of LV is largely limited by acoustic shadowing of metallic component of prosthetic valve. Minimal and large flow convergence defined as a flow convergence radius less than 0.4 and more than and equal to 0.9 cm for central jets, respectively. For eccentric jet, it may be higher.

If during systole, there is large flow convergence in LV side of prosthetic mitral valve, it denotes severe regurgitation, while no or minimal flow convergence indicates mild prosthetic MR.[8] Jet density and jet contour of regurgitation by CW Doppler signal is also helpful in grading severity of prosthetic regurgitation. Prosthetic mitral regurgitation can also be assessed by evaluating the retrograde systolic flow in pulmonary veins. Severe MR is associated with swirling motion of jet within the atrium and retrograde systolic flow in pulmonary veins that can be more accurately assessed by TEE.[11] Prosthetic MR is usually eccentric or multiple jets, thus the proximal isovelocity surface area cannot be used, instead we use volumetric method for quantification of prosthetic MR.[23,24] Quantitative parameter for assessment of prosthetic MR are vena contracta (VC), jet width, regurgitant volume, regurgitant fraction and effective regurgitant orifice area in cm^2, respectively. Their values and severity are given in Table 9. But, these quantitative parameters are less well-validated than in native MR.

After these, we evaluate the regurgitation jet by Doppler examination. We measure jet and calculate the percentage with respect to LA area. If jet area is less than 4 cm^2 as less than 20% of LA, it reflects mild regurgitation, while if jet area is more than 8 cm^2 or more than 40% of LA, it is indicative of severe LA (Figs. 11A to E).[24]

Thus, a combined approach of TTE plus TEE is applied. During TTE prosthetic mitral MR should be suspected if there is presence of:

- Flow convergence in LV side of prosthetic mitral valve during systole.
- Increased peak E-wave
- Mean gradient more than 6 mm Hg
- DVI more than 2.2
- Unexplained or new worsening of pulmonary hypertension.
- Dilated LV.

Vena Contracta

It is defined as the narrowest central flow region of a jet at or just downstream to the orifice of regurgitant valve. Its characteristics are high velocity, laminar flow, etc.

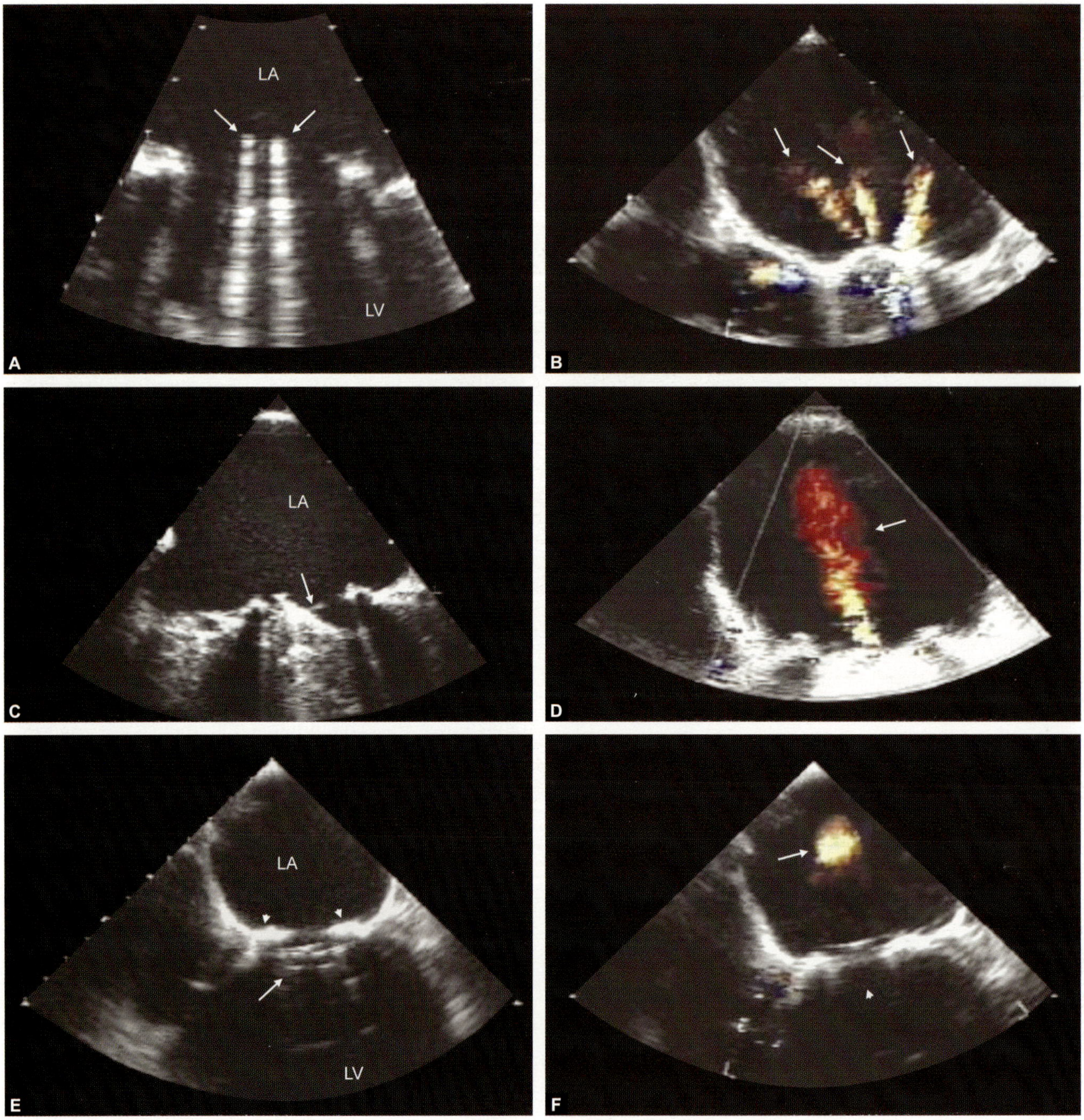

Figs. 10A to E: PHV regurgitation. (A and B) St. Jude mitral; (C and D) Medtronic hall mitral; (E and F) Starr-Edward mitral.

It is smaller than the anatomic regurgitant orifice. Width of the VC less than 3, 3–6 and more than 6 mm indicates respectively mild moderate and severe regurgitation.[11]

Regurgitant Volume and Regurgitant Fraction

Regurgitant volume (RV) is the amount of blood leaking back to the atrium by MV during systole. It is less than 30,

TABLE 9: Features of severe mitral prosthetic heart valve regurgitation.

- Increased mitral inflow peak velocity (≥2.5 m/s) and pressure half-time ≤ 150 m/s
- Dense mitral regurgitation-continuous-wave signal
- Regurgitant fraction ≥ 55%
- Effective regurgitant orifice ≥ 0.35 cm^2
- Systolic flow reversals in the pulmonary veins

Source: Oh JK, Seward JB, Tajik AJ. The Echo Manual, 3rd edition. Philadelphia: Lippincott Williams and Wilkins; 2006.

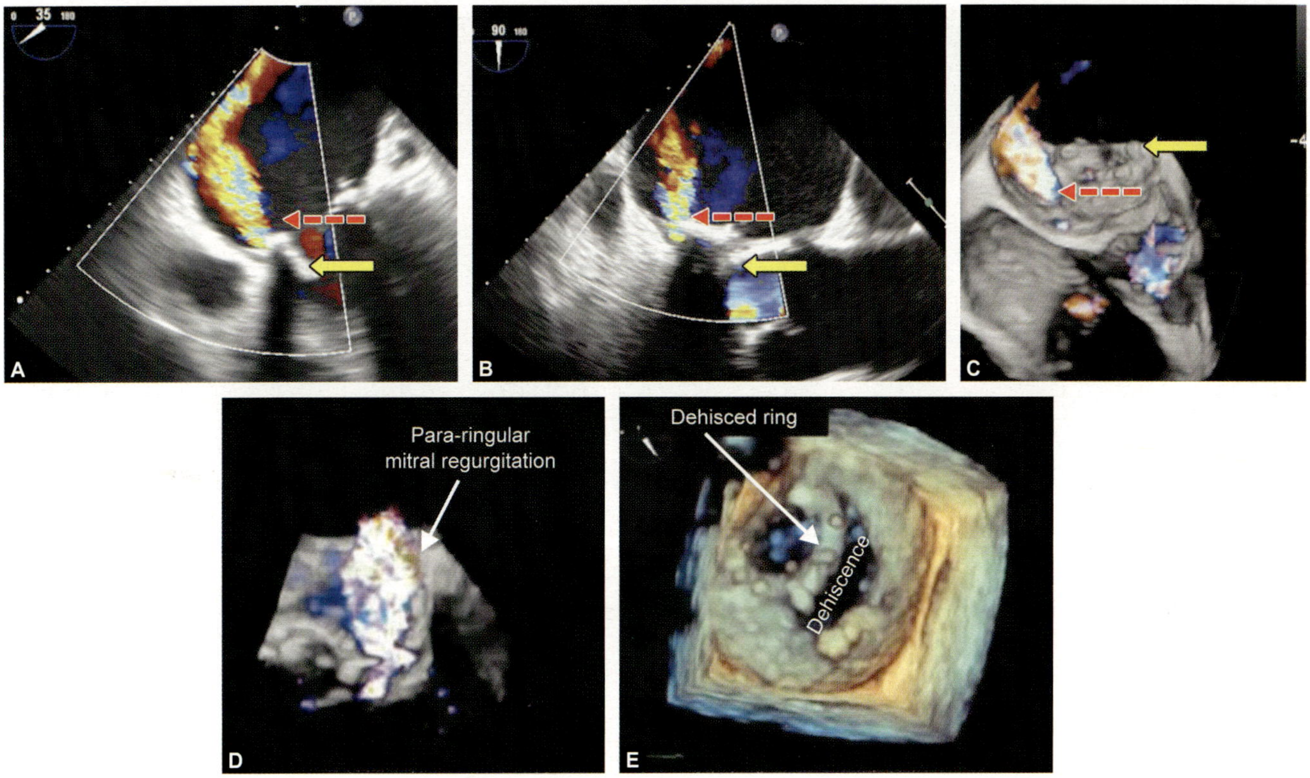

Figs. 11A to E: PHV mitral regurgitation.

30–59 and more than per 60 mL/beat for mild, moderate, and severe regurgitation, respectively.

Regurgitant fraction (RF) is the percentage of blood that regurgitates back through the mitral valve to the LA due to MR. RF less than 30, 30–49 and more than per 50% are indicative of mild moderate and severe regurgitation respectively.[11]

RV and RF are quantitative and advantageous in multiple jets and eccentric jets. These provide information about both lesion severity and volume overload status.

Limitation of RV and RF are cumbersome, needs more expertise and it is also less reliable in calcific MV and annulus.

Effective Regurgitation Orifice Area

It is calculated as the ratio of regurgitant volume or regurgitant jet velocity time integral. It is less than 0.20, 0.20–0.49 and more than and equal to 0.50 cm^2, respectively for mild moderate and severe regurgitation.[8] It brings addictive information to other quantitative indexes in the comprehensive assessment of valvular regurgitation.

Prosthetic Aortic Valve Regurgitation

Transthoracic echocardiography usually provide a good visualization of prosthetic aortic valve regurgitation either of transvalvular or paravalvular.[25]

But, the regurgitant jet may be occulted by acoustic shadowing, especially in noncoronary sinus region. On account of these difficulties, we can use TEE. It helps in identifying origin and mechanism of regurgitation (Figs. 12A and B).[20]

Assessment of Severity of Prosthetic Aortic Regurgitation

Although the estimation of the severity of prosthetic aortic valve regurgitation is done in a similar way as for the native valves,[23] but values of application of parameters such as width of regurgitant jet or VC, effective regurgitation orifice area (EROA), regurgitant volume are limited in the context of prosthetic valves.

Color Doppler Parameters

The ratio of regurgitant jet diameter to LVOT diameter from PLAX view and of jet area to LVOT area from parasternal short-axis (PSAX) view just below the prosthesis can be used to assess the severity of central jet. A ratio of jet D/LVOT D, less than 25%, more than 25% and more than 65 indicate mild, moderate and severe regurgitation, respectively.[11] But, we can over estimate regurgitation severity in case of eccentric or crescent-shaped jets and under estimate in case of jets impinging of LVOT wall and anterior mitral leaflets, by using this method.[26]

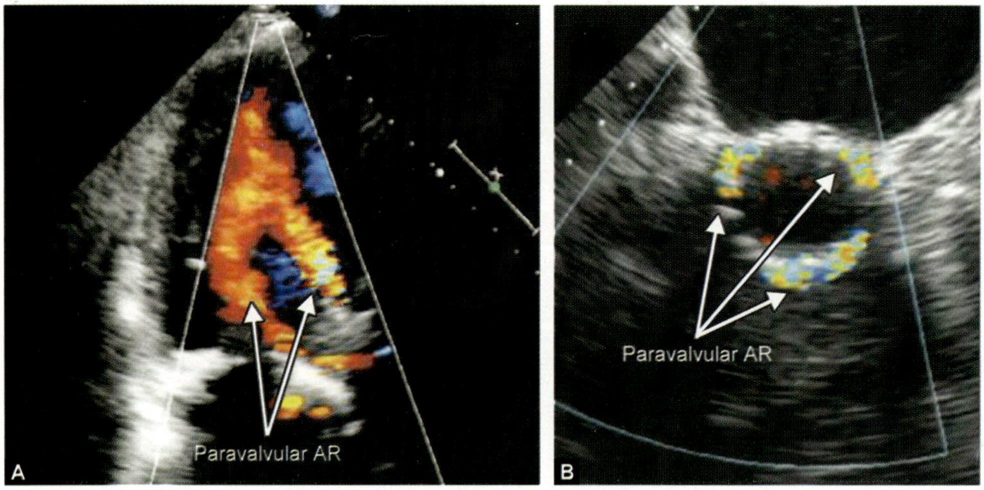

Figs. 12A and B: PHV aortic regurgitation.

It is very difficult to measure VC width in PLAX view, due to acoustic shadowing, unlike the native valve.[11] Using a Nyquist limit of 50–60 cm/s, a VC width of less than 3 mm indicate mild while width more than 6 mm indicate severe AR.[26]

For semi quantitative evaluation of paravalvular aortic regurgitation (AR), careful imaging of the neck of the jet in PSAX view at the level of prosthetic sewing ring or stent is required for defining circumferential extent.[26]

A jet occupying less than 10%, 10–20% and more than 20% of the sewing ring or stent circumference indicate mild, moderate, and severe regurgitation, respectively. If there is rocking movement of prosthesis, i.e. more than 40% circumference suggests dehiscence.[24]

In case of multiple jets, TEE may be helpful to identify the origin and estimate its circumferential extent.[11]

Quantitative assessment based on proximal isovelocity surface area (PISA) is difficult to apply to mechanical aortic prosthetic valve.[27] When assessable, usually in bioprosthesis with central regurgitant jet, imaging of the flow-convergence zone is done mainly in apical three or five-chamber or PLAX views. Regurgitant volume and EROA and RF are obtained from standard formulas. Regurgitant volume more than and equal to 60 mL, RF more than 50%.[26] An EROA more than and equal to 30 mm^2 indicates severe prosthetic AR (Table 10).

Spectral Doppler Parameters

These parameters are very useful in case of prosthetic valve regurgitation, as these are very less sensitive to position, shadowing and artifacts of prosthesis.[11] For eccentric jet, better signals are obtained from right parasternal window. The PHT of CW regurgitant jet signal is useful when PHT is less than 200 ms, suggestive of severe AR or more than 500 ms, indicating mild AR. Values 200–500 ms are less specific as these are influenced by other variable such as heart rate, LV compliance and pressures and acuteness of AR. In acute AR, PHT is shorter.[28]

TABLE 10: Features of severe aortic prosthetic heart valve regurgitation.

- Pressure half-time ≤ 250 ms
- Restrictive mitral inflow pattern (in acute aortic regurgitation)
- Holodiastolic reversal in the descending thoracic aorta
- Regurgitant fraction ≥ 55%
- *Color Doppler*: Proximal jet width/cross-sectional area; vena contracta > proximal isovelocity surface area; Beware of eccentric jets

For imaging diastolic flow reversal in descending aorta, we place sample volume just distal to the origin of left subclavian artery, PW Doppler is aligned along the major axis of aorta, Doppler filter is decreased to lowest setting and velocity scale is set to 60–80 cm/s. Reversal of flow is limited to early diastole and is brief in case of mild regurgitation. As the severity of regurgitation increases, duration, and velocity of diastolic flow reversal also increases. The presence of holodiastolic flow reversal indicates at least moderate AR when end-diastolic velocity is more than 20 m/s. it indicates severe AR.[29]

TRANSCUTANEOUS AORTIC VALVE REPLACEMENT

This minimally invasive surgical procedure repairs the valve without removing the old damaged valve. Two devices are most commonly used for transcutaneous aortic valve replacement (TAVR). Edwards Sapien valve, containing three pericardial leaflets, mounted within a balloon - expandable stent. Core valve revolving system, containing

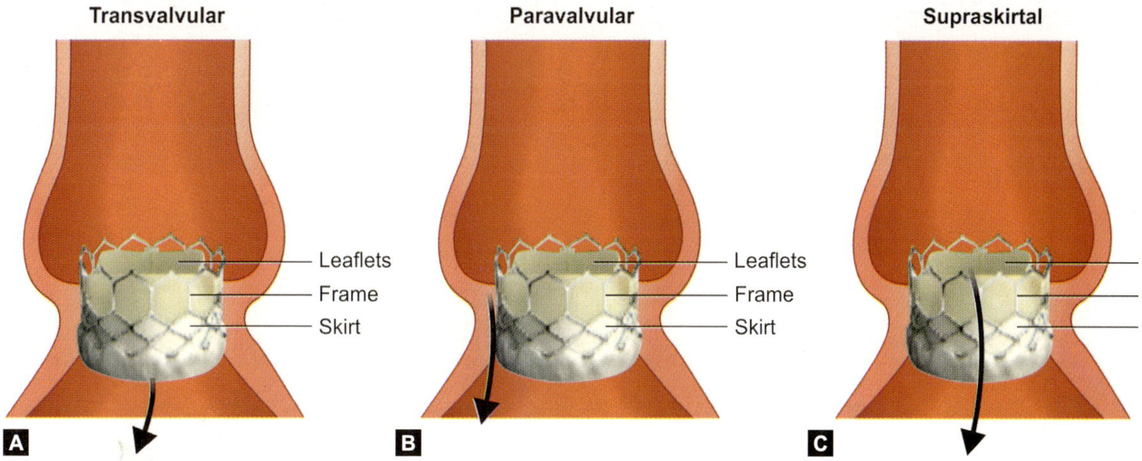

Figs. 13A to C: Mechanism of different forms of AR (TAVR).

three pericardial leaflets mounted in a self-expanding, nitinol frame.[11] We take either transfemoral or transapical approach for TAVR. AR is the MC drawback of TAVR which may be transvalvular or paravalvular or both occurring together. Recently, supraskirtal AR, a third form of AR associated with TAVR has been described.[30]

Mechanism of Different Forms of AR (Figs. 13A to C)

- Transvalvular AR: Due to leaflet destruction, restricted leaflet movement and over dilation of the valve
- Paravalvular AR: Due to incomplete opposition of the prosthesis to the aortic annulus
- Supraskirtal AR: Due to implantation of prosthesis in a position, too low in the aortic position.[31]

Three-dimensional Echocardiography

Three-dimensional (3D) echo, particularly 3D TEE is more suitable for PHVs and provide add on advantage after 2D echo. The 3D surgical "enface" view of the valve is much helpful for determining PHV function and extent of regurgitant jet.[32] It also allows for an accurate assessment of prosthetic valve disk and planimetric evaluation of prosthetic valve area. It is superior to 2D TEE in assessment of paravalvular leak (PVL), its localization and size and shape of PVL.[33] It also helps in overcoming the problems of poor window due to acoustic shadowing. Ventricular side of prosthetic mitral valve, which is difficult to visualize in 2D echo can be seen by 3D TEE.[34]

For improvement of communication, between the interventionist and the echocardiographer, different structures and PVL are seen by 3D echo should be depicted in a clockwise fashion from a surgeon's view.[11] Conventionally the mitral image, as viewed from the LA perspective is rotated to position the aortic valve at 12 o'clock (top of mitral ring), LA appendage at 9 o'clock, commissure between left and right coronary sinuses at 5 o'clock, commissure between noncoronary and left coronary sinuses at 8 o'clock and between right and noncoronary cusps are located, aortic PVL, more commonly.[35] The most common location of mitral PVL are near anterolateral commissure.[33]

Limitations of 3D Echo

- Due to their increased distance from the TEE probe anterior cardiac structures like aortic and posterior tricuspid leaflets and posterior cardiac structures are not well-visualized by 3D echo.
- Three-dimensional echo mode provides images of high spatial resolution at the expense of temporal resolution. This hampers ability to visualize fast moving structures like vegetations.
- Tissue dropout.[36]

However with improved resolution of 3D probes (TTE and TEE) and various acquisition modes, the small cardiac structures like thrombus and vegetations are well-visualized (Figs. 14A to E).

TRICUSPID PROSTHETIC VALVE

Tricuspid PHV lies in anterior position, so TTE is superior to TEE.[37] Views in TTE for prosthetic tricuspid valve:

- Parasternal (PSAX/PLAX of RV inflow)
- Apical four-chamber
- Subcostal views.

Multiple tilting or rotations are used.

Views in TEE for prosthetic tricuspid valve:

- Mid-esophageal four-chamber
- Modified bicaval views
- Mid-esophageal inflow outflow view and
- Transgastric RV inflow–outflow views

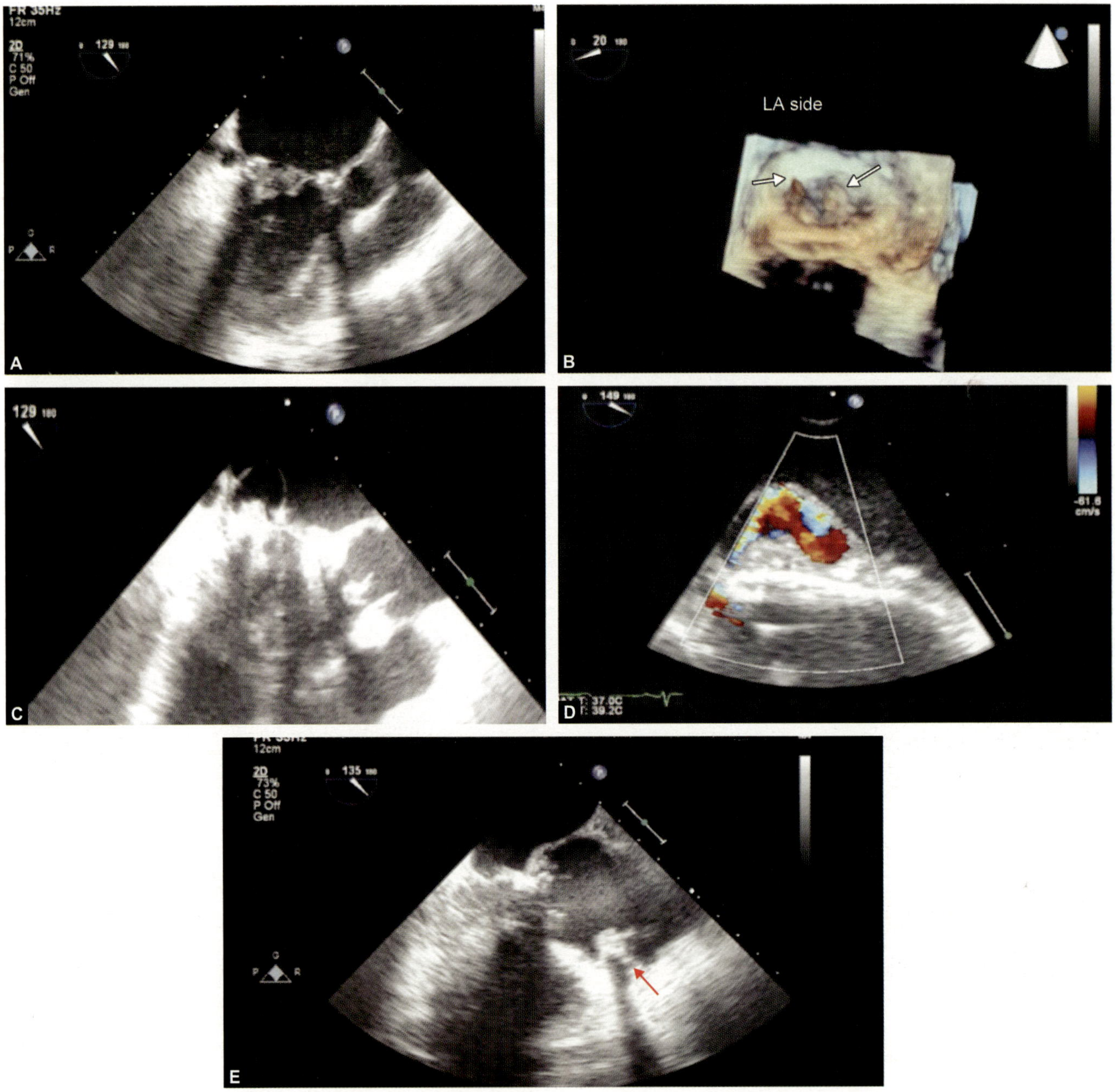

Figs. 14A to E: PHV endocarditis. (A and B) Bioprosthetic PHV vegetations; (C and D) paravalvular MR and abcess; (E) Aortic root vegetation

ACQUIRED TRICUSPID PHV OBSTRUCTION (FIGS. 15A TO D)

Doppler Assessment

Tricuspid inflow peak early diastolic velocity (E) is normally less than 2 m/s and gradient less than 6–9 mm Hg.[38] If these parameter are more than these reference values, it is suggestive of possible tricuspid prosthetic obstruction. Again a short PHT is indicative of normal tricuspid PHV, while prolonged PHT suggests possible stenosis. These parameters are influenced by respiration, heart rate, RA/RV size and compliance. DVI used to distinguish stenosis from regurgitation. In the absence of AR, DVI more than per 3.2 for tissue valve and more than and equal to 2 for mechanical valves suggests stenosis. EOA have to be calculated by continuity equation which is valid only in absence of AR. If AR is present, RVOT is assessed. There is no cutoff value of EOA for stenosis.[26]

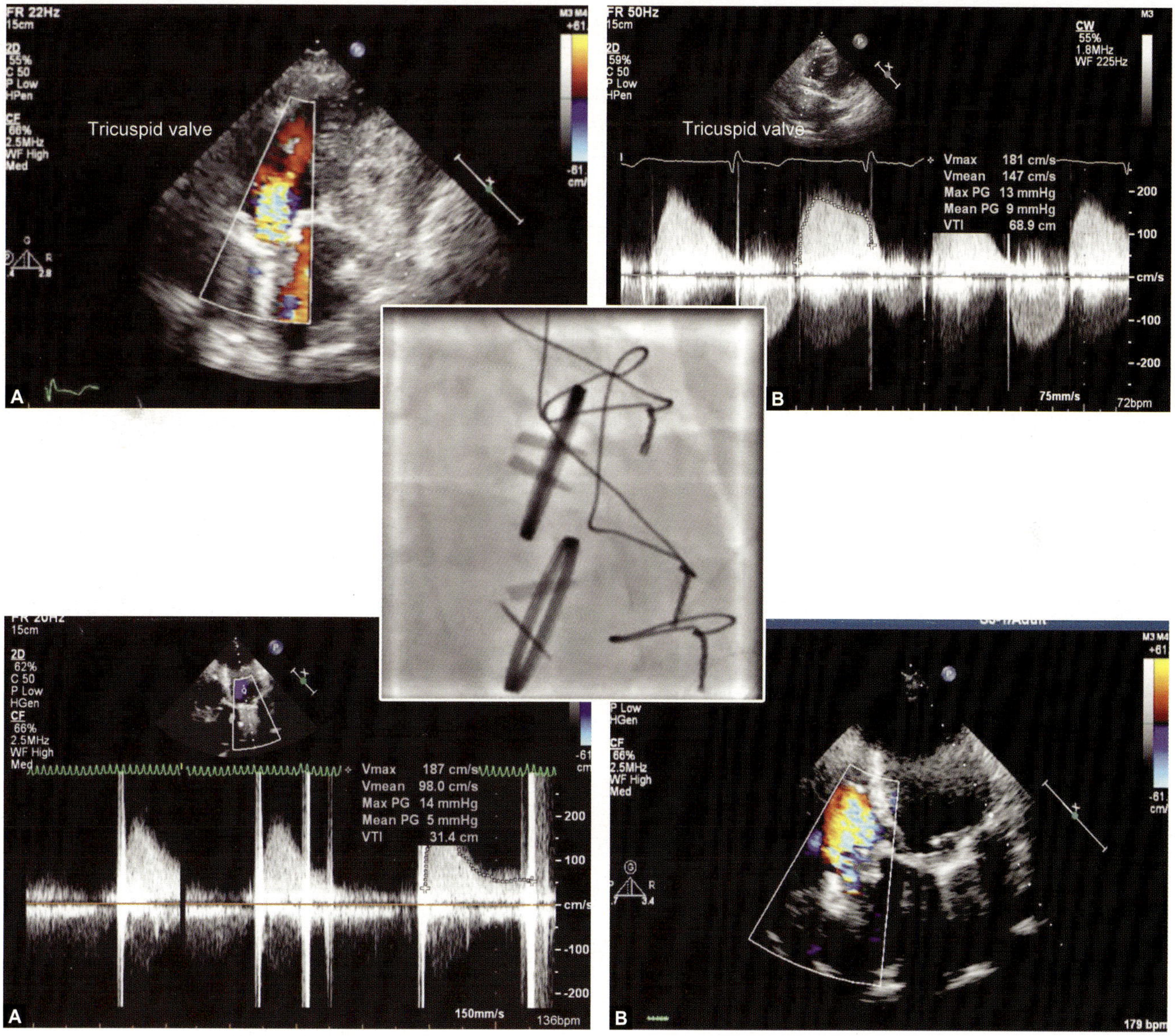

Figs. 15A to D: Tricuspid prosthetic valve obstruction.

Differential Diagnosis of High-Pressure Gradient across Tricuspid PHV

- Tachycardia
- PPM
- Hyperdynamic flow (fever, thyrotoxicosis, anemia, frequency, AV fistula)
- Regurgitation.

PROSTHETIC TRICUSPID REGURGITATION

Color flow imaging is useful for indicating the presence of tricuspid regurgitation (TR) but not useful for assessing severity. Generally,

- Large eccentric jet, swirling and reaching to the posterior wall indicates severe TR.
- Small thin central jets indicate mild TR.

Vena Contracta

In the apical four-chamber view, VC more than per 7 mm indicates severe TR while less than 6 mm may be mild or moderate TR. Acoustic shadowing and multiple jets create difficulty in assessing TR.

Spectral Doppler Parameters

In the absence of triangularis sterni (TS), increased peak E velocity more than per 1.9–2.1 cm/s suggests severe TR.

Presence of holosystolic reversed of flow by PW Doppler in hepatic vein also indicates significant TR.[39] In CW Doppler, TR signal of high density and truncated with of triangular contour and an early peaked velocity indicates severe TR.[26] Besides, these we should see the size of RA and RV and IVC with respiratory variation to assess chronic significant TR.

PULMONARY PROSTHETIC HEART VALVE

Pulmonary valve is located anteriorly and superiorly and views in TTE for pulmonary PHV.

- PSAX at the level of aortic valve
- RVOT view
- Subcostal view.

Views in TEE

High esophageal view at 50–90 was the level of short-axis view of aortic valve slight withdrawal of the probe from this position facilities viewing of pulmonic valve, mean pulmonary artery and its bifurcation.
Deep transgastric view in 120° imaging plane.

PULMONARY PHV OBSTRUCTION

Both CW and PW Doppler at the level of pulmonary valve are used to measure velocity and gradient. For bioprosthesis, transvalvular peak velocity more than 3.2 m/s and mean gradient more than per 20 mm Hg. For homografts more than 2.5 m/s and mean gradient more than and equal to 15 mm Hg are indicative of obstruction. Besides increased peak velocity, increased RV systolic pressure and newly impaired RV function also indicates stenosis in pulmonary PHV.

PULMONARY PHV REGURGITATION

Color Doppler Assessment

A diastolic jet in right ventricular outflow tract (RVOT) directed toward RV, indicate pulmonic regurgitation (PR). Color jet diameter is measured in diastole just below pulmonary valve (PV) in PSAX and subcostal view. A jet width more 50-65% of RVOT measured in the same frame indicates severe PR. Reversal of color Doppler flow in pulmonary arteries is a specific sign of significant PR.

A short PHT (<100 ms) and dense CW-PR jet indicates severe PR but these are not specific.[40]

Because PHT also depends on diastolic intrapulmonary pressure and diastolic properties of the RV, with shorter PHT when RV physiology is restrictive.

PW Doppler is used for regurgitant volume and regurgitant fraction assessment. RF less than 30% suggests mild while RF more than 50% is consistent with severe PR.

RV dilatation with flattening of interventricular septum (IVS) in diastole and paradoxical motion is also suggestive of severe PR. In mild or acute PR, it is absent.

OTHER IMAGING MODALITIES

Cine Fluoroscopy

Fluoroscopy, the first noninvasive technique used for the identification of type of prosthetic valve and evaluation of its function, is used mainly in case of abnormally raised gradients.[41] By this fluoroscopic examination. we can evaluate the mobility of valvular leaflets, valvular ring motion. Presence of rocking movement of the prosthetic valve ring indicates extensive valve dehiscence, impaired excursion of the moving parts indicates tissue in growth or thrombus.[8]

For fluoroscopy study, patient has to lie down in supine position. Three projections are used for viewing PHVs.

- *In situ projections*: In this, radiographic beam is projected posterior-anterior (0°) and lateral (90°) to evaluate orientation of the valve.
- *In profile projection*: Radiographic beam is projected parallel to both the valve ring plane and the tilting axis of disk. It helps in calculation of opening and closing angles.
- *Enface projection*: In this, radiographic beam is projected parallel to the valve outflow tract. It is used only for mitral valve prosthesis.

For aortic position, disk motion is better evaluated by cine fluoroscopy than echocardiography,[42] but it does not allow hemodynamic assessment and does not give information about the etiology of reduced disk movement.

For mechanical prosthetic valves, it is easily applied because of radiopaque ring and ball or disk occluder but it is of limited valve for tissue valves.[43]

For cine fluoroscopic examination, a short, i.e. 10 beats of each projection is taken and from these, some frames are selected for evaluation and measuring the disk motion. In fully open and closed positions, opening and closing angles are calculated, as the distance between the two leaflets are in respective positions.

For single disk prosthesis, opening angles is distance between the housing and the disk at fully opened position. For bileaflet disk prosthesis, opening angle is distance between the leaflets in fully opened position (Figs. 16A to D).[26]

Cardiac Computed Tomography

Till now, there is no definitive indication for CT in assessing PHVs dysfunction. It is not used routinely. Uses of cardiac CT in PHVs assessment:

- CT can be used as an alternative to fluoroscopy for mechanical PHV to measure opening angles.

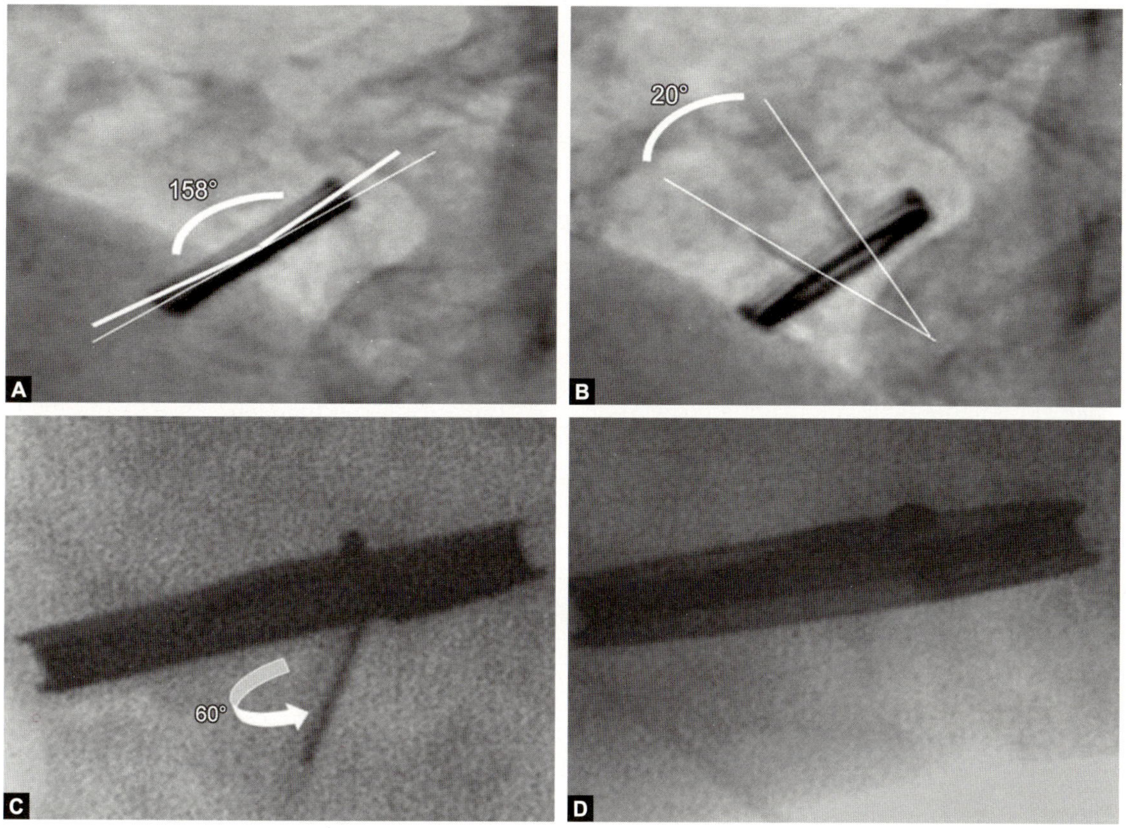

Fig. 16: Cinefluoroscopy. (A and B) Opening and closing angles bileaflet PHV; (C and D) Opening and closing angles single leaflet PHV.

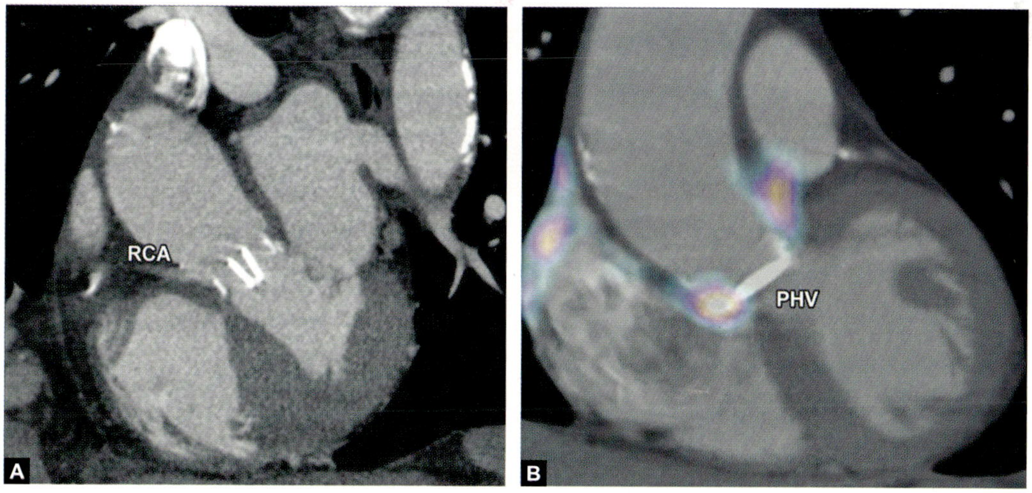

Figs. 17A and B: CT for prosthetic valve.

- CT can distinguish thrombus from pannus.
- Rocking movement of the valve ring on dynamic CT indicate ring dehiscence.
- It quantifies severity of stenosis in a bioprosthesis by planimetry.
- Paravalvular regurgitation and malcoaptation are also identified.
- Ventricular or atrial dilation or stasis, which are morphological consequences of obstructive or regurgitation valves are also identified.[26]
- Calcification on CT could aid in the detection of early primary failure of biologic replacement valves.
- It helps in imaging of pannus, vegetation and thrombus (Figs. 17A and B).[8]

Disadvantages of Cardiac CT

- In this, iodine contrast medium is used and there is need for ionizing radiation.
- It is unable to assess hemodynamics and flow pattern.
- Pledget material adjacent to the valve ring can be misinterpreted as regurgitation. But, this problem can be resolved by evaluating the density.[44]

Cardiovascular Magnetic Resonance

Cardiovascular magnetic resonance (CMR) also has some value for assessing the function of PHV, as a complementary method when TEE is undesirable and TTE is nondiagnostic. For assessment of cardiac chamber volumes and flow patterns, it is an excellent technique.[26]

Anatomy of PHV can be assessed by taking short-axis; two-, three- and four-chamber long-axis views with oblique long-axis view in the line of coaptation.[45]

Phase-contrast velocity mapping by CMR helps in obtaining blood flow patterns and velocity. Thus, it may be very helpful in assessing regurgitation.[46]

CMR with late gadolinium enhancement is widely used to assess cardiac fibrosis in cardiomyopathy.[47]

Nuclear Cardiology

In assessment of PHV, there is limited role of nuclear imaging. Further studies are needed to determine whether this technique may be used to identify the mineralization or degeneration of bioprosthetic valve. 18–FDP can help in PHV endocarditis and 18 F-sodium fluoride positron emission tomography (PET)/CT identify calcification.[48]

Cardiac Catheterization

It is used for measurement of flow patterns and PGs across the PHV. These parameter helps in calculating EOA by Gorlin formula. In case of mechanical valves, catheter should not be crossed across PHV, because it may cause complications like regurgitation.[49]

Catheterization of biological valves can be done easily but if the PHV is degenerated or calcified, it will be friable. Thus, it may cause prosthetic valve leaflet rupture leading to acute severe regurgitation.[8]

Measurement of transmitral gradient should be done by direct measurement of LA pressure instead of using pulmonary capillary wedge pressure (PCWP) because measurement of PCWP can overestimate gradients and underestimate EOA. For measurement of LA pressure, we use transseptal approach for invasive mitral prosthetic gradient.[50]

COMPLICATIONS OF PROSTHETIC VALVES

Early Complications

- Valvular dysfunction—due to technical challenges during surgery or early infection
- Paravalvular leak
- Early prosthetic thromboembolism
- Acute endocarditis.

Late Complications

- Late valvular dysfunction
- Thrombosis and thromboembolism
- Pannus formation
- Valve degeneration
- Annular abscess
- Endocarditis
- Dehiscence
- PPM
- Primary failure
- Hemolysis.

ENDOCARDITIS (*SEE* FIG. 14)

In a stable patient with PHV and fever first, we should exclude other common causes of fever. If we are unable to get a definite cause, we perform echo for endocarditis. On the other hand, if the patient is severely ill or there is medium or high clinical suspicion for endocarditis, we perform echocardiography.

Vegetations in PHVs tend to form in valve ring area, which may spread to involve other components of PHV and impair opening and closing movement of leaflets. Vegetations are identified as an irregularly shaped, freely mobile mass of low echogenicity on echocardiography.

Complications of Endocarditis

- *Abscess may lead to*:
  - Conduction system defect if it involves IVS.
  - Shunt between two chambers.
- Suture dehiscence and paravalvular regurgitation in all PHVs.
- Valve destruction in bioprosthetic valves.

Indications of TEE in Endocarditis

TEE is superior in detecting vegetations to TTE with higher sensitivity and specificity.

- It is used in detection of perivalvular abscess in posterior aortic root.[51]

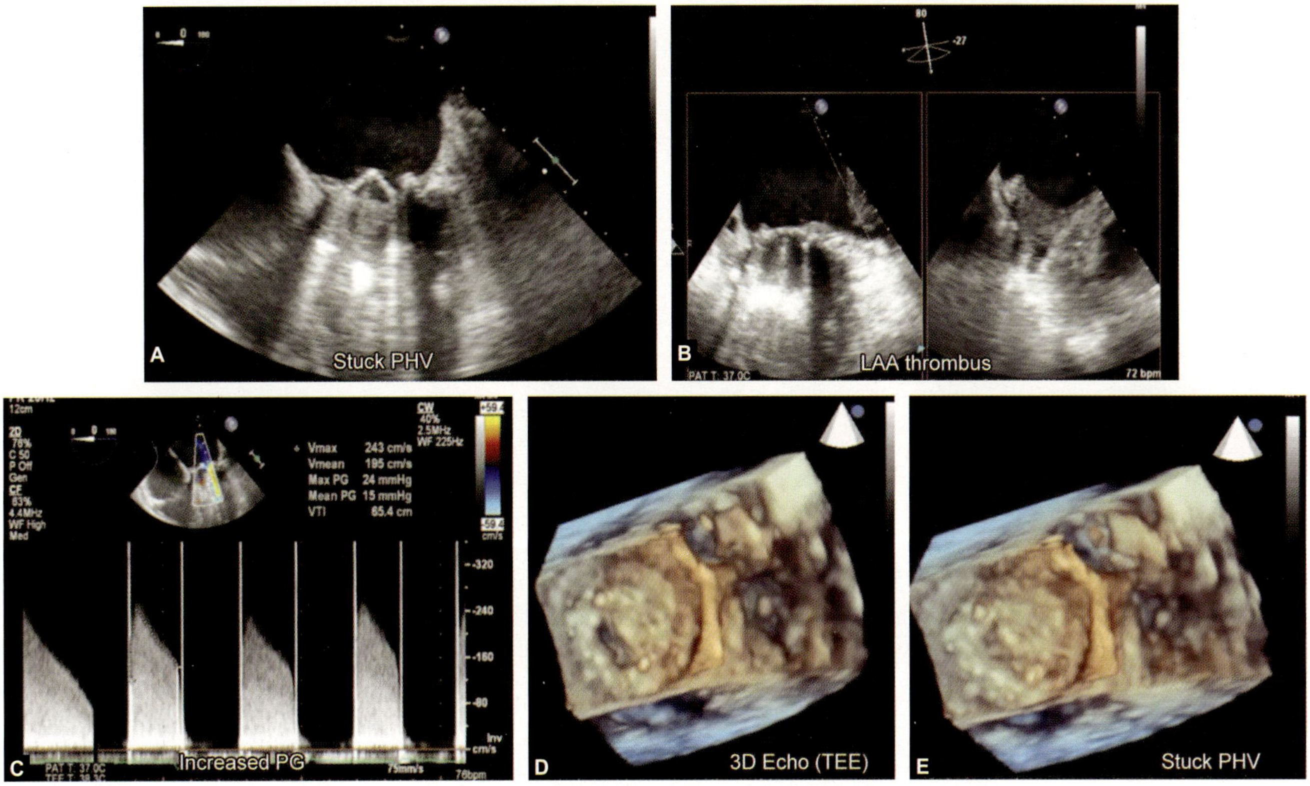

Figs. 18A to E: Bileaflet stuck PHV, with Thrombus + LAA Thrombus.

- If we are unable to find a significant lesion of endocarditis in TTE and clinical suspicion is high, we should use TEE for this.[52]
- If signs of infection persist or worsens despite adequate antimicrobial treatment, we should use TEE for complications like abscess or shunt.

A combined approach with TEE and TTE gives best diagnostic accuracy. Anterior structures are better seen by TTE and posterior structures by TEE.[47] Despite the combined approach some small percentage of cases can be missed.[53] A repeat study after 7–10 day should be recommended, in such circumstances.

PROSTHETIC VALVE THROMBUS AND PANNUS AND THEIR DIFFERENTIATION

Thrombus

Mainly mechanical valves are associated with thrombus formation. Bioprosthetic valves are less commonly associated with thrombosis. Usually, thrombosis is associated with obstruction, regurgitation and embolism, but sometimes it may be silent.[54] Thrombus formation leading to significant obstruction may be catastrophic. It is treated by redo operation or fibrinolytic therapy (treatment of choice for tricuspid valve thrombosis). TEE and Doppler echo is used to assess serially for success of thrombolytic therapy and improved hemodynamics or valve motion.[55] Sometimes, thrombus and pannus occur together and even after successful thrombolysis, residual pannus can lead to rethrombosis of the prosthesis (Figs. 18A to E).[8]

If on TEE, thrombus area is more than 0.85 cm^2, it confers a higher risk of embolism and death associated with thrombolysis.[56]

Pannus

After prosthetic valve implantation, a membrane of granulation tissue as a response to healing, forms which may cause obstruction. This granulation tissue is called pannus.

Per year, the incidence of prosthetic valve obstruction is 4%.

- Pure thrombus (75%)
- Pure pannus (10%)
- Combination of both (15%)

Difference between thrombus and pannus is described in the Table 11.

If we are going to perform thrombolytic therapy, it is important to differentiate between thrombus and pannus. TEE can be used to differentiate between the two (Figs. 19A to C).[56]

TABLE 11: Difference between thrombus and pannus.

Thrombus	Pannus
Occurs at any time after surgery	Occurs between 1 year and 5 years
If International-normalized ratio (INR) decreases, increased chance of thrombus formation	No relationship with INR
Involves both mitral and aortic valves equally	Involves more commonly to aortic valves
It is larger and soft	It is small dense
Thrombi in mitral position may extend from surgical ring to left atrial (LA) and LA appendage	Pannus is mainly limited to valves

STRESS ECHOCARDIOGRAPHY

Stress echocardiography is a valuable tool for the evaluation of PHVs hemodynamic function, especially when there is discordance between the patient's symptomatic status and the PHVs hemodynamics. If patients symptoms are mild or equivocal exercise stress echocardiography is preferred especially with supine ergometery. If symptoms are moderate to severe, use of low dose dodutamine (up to 20 µg/kg/min) stress echocardiography is recommended.

In aortic PHV, there is least increase in PG during stress especially in stent less porcine than stented PHV. Most increase is in PG during exercise is in mechanical PHV.

Increase of more than 15 mm Hg during stress echocardiography is abnormal.

In mitral PHV, increase of gradient more than 18 mm Hg is indicative of pannus or obstruction.

CONCLUSION

Physicians who take care of patients with a prosthetic valve should be familiar with the characteristics of normal and abnormally functioning prosthetic valves. Echocardiography with Doppler evaluation of PHV is mainstay for diagnosis and management of prosthetic valves. TEE is often necessary for the evaluation. Advent of 3D transthoracic and transesophageal echo, has made

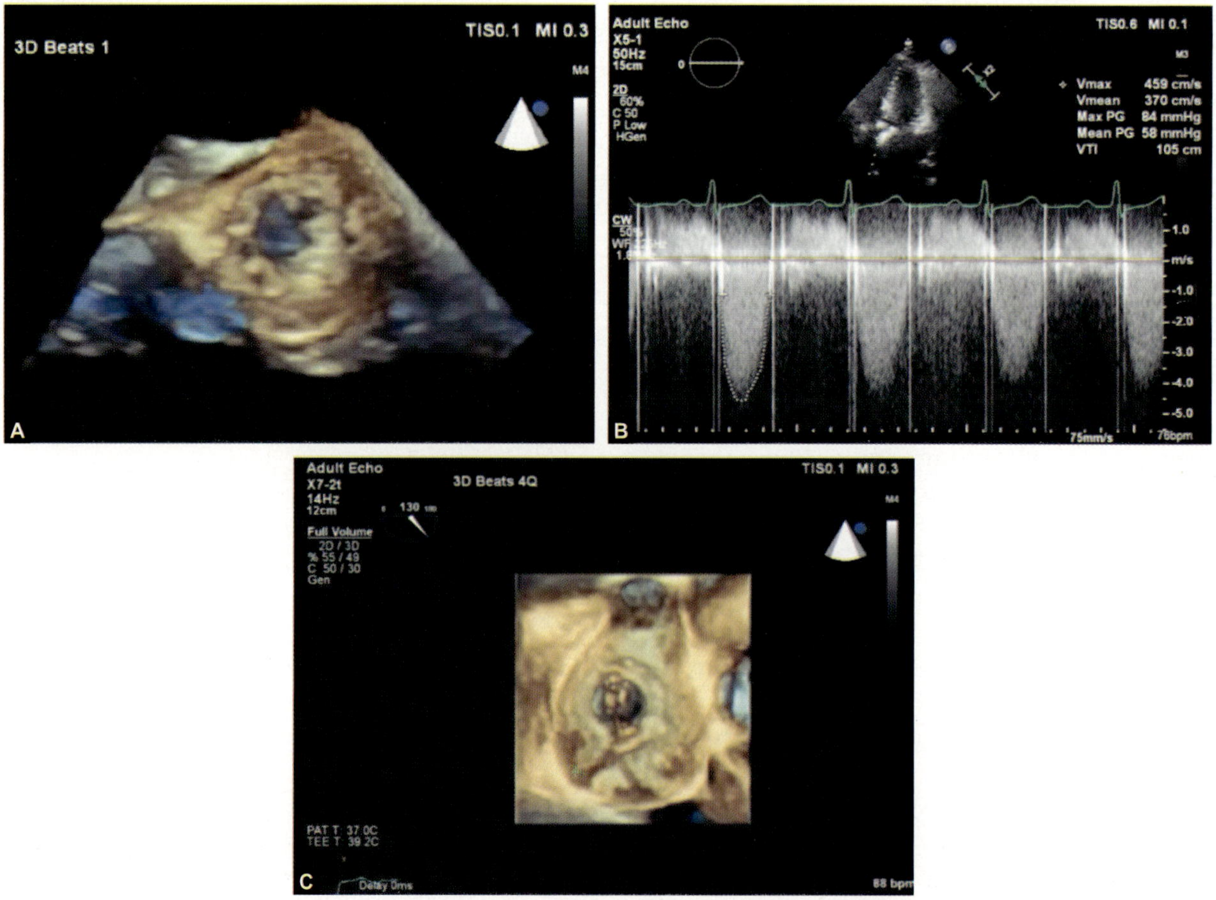

Fig. 19: Pannus—Aortic position

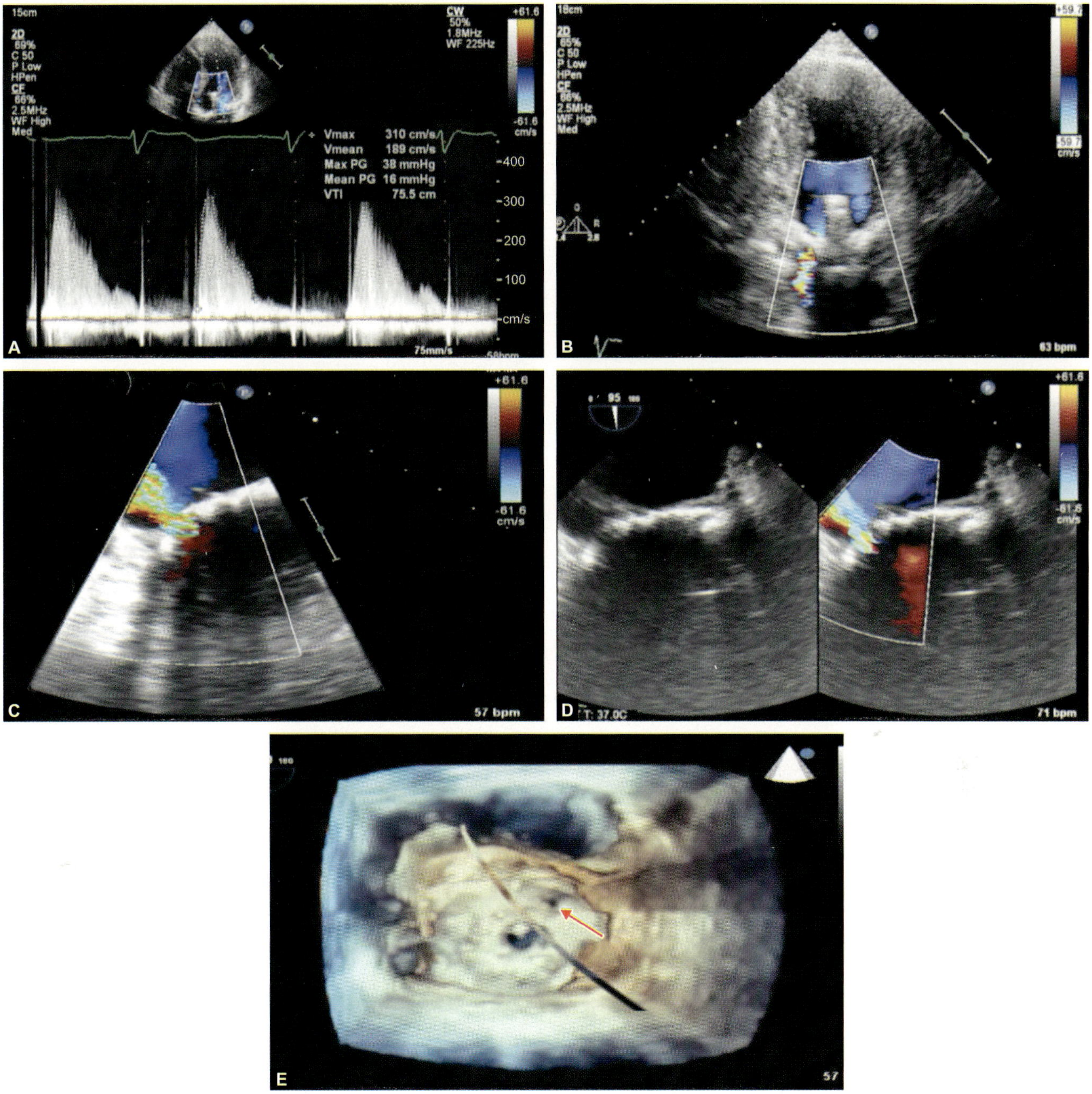

Figs. 20A to E: Paravalvular MR.

easy to recognize the complication related to PHV. Other imaging modalities like cine-fluoroscopy, CT scan, MRI are sometime helpful.

REFERENCES

1. Hermiller J, Samspon AJ, Utilization and mortality trends in transcatheter and surgical aortic valve replacement: the New York state experience – 2011 to 2012. JACC Cardiovasc Interv. 2016:9:586-8.
2. Society of Thoracic Surgeons. (2015) Executive report. [online] http://www.sts.org/sites/default/files/documents/2015Harvest4_Executive summary. pdf. [Accessed October, 2016].
3. Dunning J, Goa H, Chambers J, et al. Aortic valve surgery: marked increases in volume and significant decrease in mechanical valve use – an analysis of 41227 patients over 5 years from the Society for Cardiothoracic Surgery in Great Britain and Ireland National database J Thorac Cardiovasc Surg. 2011:142:776-82.

4. Chambers JB. Echocardiography of replacement of the heart valves. Echo Res Prac. 2016;32.
5. Cribier A, Eltchaninoff H, Tron C, et al. Early experience with percutaneous transcatheter implantation of heart valve prosthesis for the treatment of end-stage inoperable patients with calcific aoric stenosis. J Am Coll Cardiol. 2004;43:698-703.
6. Webb JG, Chandavimol M, Thrompson CR, et al. Percutaneous Aortic valve implantation retrograde from the femoral artery. Circulation. 2006;113:842-50.
7. Grube E, Schuler G, Buellesfeld L, et al. Percutaneous aortic valve replacement for severe aortic stenosis in high-risk patients using the second -and current third generation - expanding Core Valve prosthesis: Device success and 30-day clinical outcome. J Am Coll Cardiol. 2007:50:69-76.
8. Zoghbi WA, Chambers JB, Dumesnil JG, et al, Recommendation for evaluation of prosthetic valves with echocardiography and Doppler ultrasound. J.Echo. 2009:975-1006.
9. Vahanian A, Alfieri O, Andreotti F, et al. Guidelines on the management of valvular heart disease (version 2012). Eur Heart J. 2012;33:2451-96.
10. Nishimura RA, Otto CM, Bonow RO, et al.2014.2014 AHA/ACC guideline for the management of patients with valvular heart disease; a report of the American College of Cardiology/American Heart Association Task Force on Practice Guidelines. Circulation. 129:e521-e643.
11. Sordelli C, Severino S. Echocardiographic assessment of heart valve prosthesis. J Cardiovasc Echogr. 2014;24(4):103-13.
12. Vahanian A, Baumgartner H, Bax J, et al. Task Force on the Management of Valvular Heart Disease of the European Society of Cardiology. ESC Committee for Practice Guidelines. Guidelines on the management of valvular heart disease: The task force on the management of valvular heart disease of the European society of cardiology. Eur Heart J. 2007:28:230-68
13. Zoghbi WA, Chambers JB, Dumesnil JG et al. American Society of Echocardiography's Guidelines and Standards Committee; Task Force of Prosthetic Valves. J Am Soc Echocardiogr. 2009;22:975-1014.
14. Coppolino P, Coppolino F. L'ecocardiographianellavalutaz ionedelleprotesicardiache. Giornaleitaliano di Cardiologia pratica. 2012.
15. Pibarot P, Dumesnil JG. Hemodynamic and clinical impact of prosthesis-patient mismatch in the aortic valve position and its prevention. J Am Coll Crdiol. 2000;36:1131-41.
16. Rahimtoola SH. The problem of valve prosthesis-patient mismatch. Circulation. 1978;58:20-4.
17. Dumesnil JG, Honos GN, Beauchemin J, et al. Validation and application of mitral prosthetic valvular areas calculated by Doppler echocardiography. Am J Cardiol. 1990;65:1443-8.
18. Pibarot P, Dumesnil JG. Hemodynamic and clinical impact of prosthesis-patient mismatch in the aortic valve position and its prevention. J Am Coll Cardiol. 2000;36:1131-41.
19. Pibarot P, Weissman NJ, et al Incidence and sequelae of prosthesis -patient mismatch in transcatheter versus surgical valve replacement in high risk patients with severe aortic stenosis - APARTNER trial cohort A analysis. J Am Coll Cardiol. 2014;64:1323-34.
20. Vesey JM, Otto CM. Complication of prosthetic heart valves. Curr Cardiol Rep. 2004;6:106-11.
21. Mohty D, Dumesnil JG. Impact of prosthesis patient mismatch on long term survival after aortic valve replacement influence of age, obesity and left ventricular dysfunction J Am Coll Cardiol. 2009:53:39-47.
22. Kappetein AP, Head SJ. Updated standardized endpoint definitions for transcatheter aortic valve implantation the Valve Academic Research Consortium-2 consensus document. Eur J Cardiothorac Surg. 2012;42:545-60.
23. Zoghbi WA, Enriquez-Sarano M. American Society of Echocardiography. Recommendations for evaluation of the severity of native valvular regurgitation with two-dimensional and Doppler echocardiography. J Am Soc Echocardiogr. 2003;16:777-802.
24. Fernandes V, Olmos L. Peak early diastolic velocity rather than pressure half -time is the best index of mechanical prosthetic mitral valve function. Am J Cardiol. 2002;89:704-10.
25. Vitarelli A, Conde Y. Assessment of severity of mechanical prosthetic mitral regurgitation by transesophageal echocardiography. Heart. 2004;90:539-44.
26. Lancellotti P, Pibarot P, Chambers J, et al. Recommendations for the imaging assessment of Prosthetic heart valves. Eur Heart J Cardiovasc Imaging. 2016;17(6):589-90.
27. Pouleur AC, de Waroux JB. Accuracy of the flow convergence method for quantification of aortic regurgitation in patients with central versus eccentric jets. Am J Cardiol. 2008;102:475-80.
28. Samstad SO, Hegrenaes L. Half time of the diastolic aortoventricular pressure difference by continuous wave Doppler ultrasound a measure of AR? Br Heart J. 1989;61:336-43.
29. Tribouilloy C, Avinee P. End diastolic flow velocity just beneath the aortic isthmus assessed by pulsed Doppler echocardiography: a new predictor of the aortic regurgitant fraction. Br Heart J. 1991;65:37-40.
30. Gotzmann M, Korten M. Long term outcome of patients with moderate and severe prosthetic aortic valve regurgitation after transcatheter aortic valve implantation. Am J Cardiol. 2012;110:1500-6.
31. Anwar AM, Nosr YF. Real time three dimensional transthoracic echocardiography in daily practice: initial experience. Cardiovasc Ultrasound. 2012;10:14.
32. Anwar AM, Nosir YFl. Real time three dimensional transthoracic echocardiography: a novel approach for the assessment of prosthetic heart valves. Echocardiography. 2014;31:188-96.
33. Kronzon I, Sugeng L. Real time 3-dimensional transesophageal echocardiography in the evaluation of post-operative mitral annuloplastyring and prosthetic valve dehiscence. J Am Coll Cardiol. 2009;53:1543-7.
34. Singh P, Manda J. Live Real time 3 dimensional Transesophageal echocardiographic evaluation of mitral and aortic valve prosthetic paravalvular regurgitation. Echocardiography. 2009;26:980-7.
35. De Cicco G, Loruso R. Aortic valve periprosthetic leakage—anatomic observations and surgical results. Ann Thorac Surg. 2005;79:1480-5.

36. ZamoranoJL, Badano LP. EAE/ASE recommendations for the use of echocardiography in new transcatheter interventions for valvular heart disease. Eur Heart J. 2011;32:2189-214.
37. Blauwet LA, Burkhart HM, et al. Comprehensive echocardiographic assessment of mechanical tricuspid valve prosthesis based on early postimplantation echocardiographic studies. J Am Soc Echocardiogr. 2011;24:414-24.
38. Kobayashi Y, Nagata S Ohmori F, et al. Serial Doppler echocardiographic evaluation of bioprosthetic valves in the tricuspid position. J Am Coll Cardiol. 1996;27:1693-7.
39. Gonzalez A, Vilchez F, Zarauza L, et al. Assessment of tricuspid regurgitation by Doppler color flow imaging: angiographic correlation. Int J Cardiol. 1994;44:275-83.
40. Silversides CK, Veldtman GR, Crossin J, et al. Pressures Halftime predicts hemodynamically significant pulmonary regurgitation in adult patients with repaired tetralogy of Fallot. J Am Soc.Echocardiogr. 2003;16:1057-62.
41. CanclulliT, Lax J. Cinefluoroscopic assessment of mechanical disc prosthesis; its value as a complementary method to Echocardiography. J Heart Valve Dis. 2005;14:664-73.
42. Muratori M, Montorsi P. Dysfunction of bileaflet aortic prosthesis accuracy of echocardiography versus fluoroscopy. JACC Cardiovasc Imaging. 2013;6:196-205.
43. Castaneda-Zuniga W, Nicoloff D. In vivo radiographic appearance of the St. Jude valve prosthesis. Radiology. 1980;134:775-6.
44. Habets J, Meijer TS, Budde RP, et al. CT attenuation measurements are valuable to discriminate pledgets used in prosthetic heart valve implantation from paravalvular leakage. Br J Radiol 2012;85:e616-21.
45. Han Y, Peters DC. Cardiovascular magnetic resonance characterization of mitral valve prolapse. JACC Cardiovasc Imaging. 2008;1:294-303.
46. Pennekamp W, Geyhan N. Determination of flow profiles of different mechanical aortic valve prosthesis using phase-contrast MRI. J Cardiovasc Surg. 2011;52:277-84.
47. Clavel MA, Pibarot P. Assessment of low-flow, low gradient aortic stenosis:multiple modality imaging is the key to success. EuroIntervention. 2014;10(Suppl U):U52-60.
48. Dweck MR, Jones C. Assessment of valvular calcification and inflammation by positron emission tomography in patients with aortic stenosis. Circulation. 2012;125:76-86.
49. Palicov RE, Walsh WF. Retrograde crossing of aortic Bjork-Shiley prosthetic. Am J Cardiol. 1979;43:1062-4.
50. Dunn M. Is transseptal catheterization necessary? J Am Coll Cardiol. 1985;5:1393-4.
51. Mugge A. Echocardiographic detection of cardiac valve vegetations and prognostic implications. Infect Dis Clin North Am. 1993;7:877-98.
52. Lowry RW, Zoghbi WA. Clinical impact of transesophageal echocardiography in the diagnosis and management of infective endocarditis. Am J Cardiol. 1994;73:1089-91.
53. Bayer AS. Infective endocarditis. Clin Infect Dis. 1993;17:313-20.
54. Gueret P, Vignon P, Bensaid J, et al. Transesophageal echocardiography for the diagnosis and management of nonobstructive thrombosis of mechanical mitral valve prosthesis. Circulation. 1995;91:103-10.
55. Tong AT, Roudaut R, Girard SE, et al. Transesophageal echocardiography improves risk assessment of thrombolysis of prosthetic valve thrombosis: results of the international PRO-TEE registry. J Am Coll Cardiol. 2004;43:77-84.
56. Barbetseas J, Nagueh SF, Pitsavos C, et al. Differentiating thrombus from pannus formation in obstructed mechanical prosthetic valve:an evaluation of clinical, transthoracic and transesophageal echocardiographic parameters. J Am Coll Cardiol. 1998;32:1410-7.

67

CHAPTER

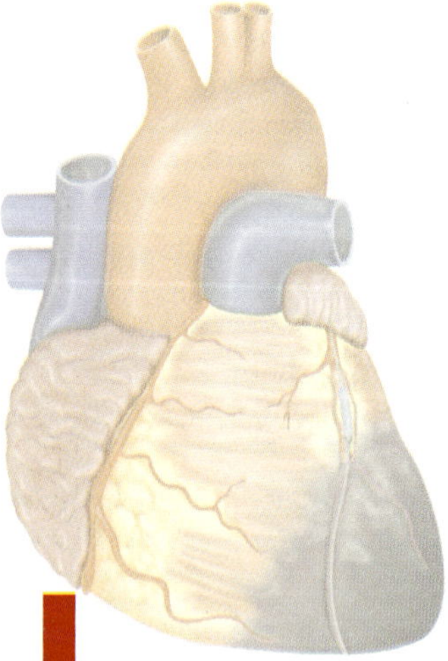

Magnetic Resonance Imaging in Valvular Heart Disease

Kartik Ganga, Arun Sharma, Gurpreet S Gulati

INTRODUCTION

Valvular heart disease (VHD) accounts for 10–20% of all cardiac surgeries in the developed world, where the most common cause is degenerative disease.[1] In the developing world, however, where 60% of the world's population lives, half of all cases of cardiovascular disease are rheumatic in etiology. The prevalence of rheumatic fever in India has declined significantly from a pandemic scale that was seen earlier. However, it continues to be a major public health concern. The prevalence of rheumatic heart disease among rural school children is reported to be 0.67/1,000 school children.[2] Calcific degeneration, myxomatous disease, and bicuspid aortic valve are the other common forms of VHD affecting our population.[3]

IMAGING MODALITIES

Valvular assessment is usually performed using echocardiography (ECHO) and when used in conjunction with angiography, a complete structural and functional assessment is usually possible. Transthoracic ECHO is, however, operator-dependant and can be restricted by poor acoustic windows. Transoesophageal ECHO has superior spatial and temporal resolution and can offer better evaluation of VHD. However, it is invasive, and some patients may not tolerate it. Angiography, being the "gold standard" investigation for VHD, is associated with a mortality of approximately 0.1%.[4] Advances in computed tomography (CT) have led to it being used in valvular assessment. Though CT can be used for structural assessment of the valves, it cannot be used be used for flow assessment or gradient calculations and is associated with radiation and use of potentially nephrotoxic contrast. Cardiac magnetic resonance imaging (CMRI), on the other hand, can provide the required information in a single investigation, that is noninvasive, safe, and without exposure to ionizing radiation. It has excellent spatial and temporal resolution for the purpose of valvular assessment. It can be used to assess both the stenotic and regurgitant lesions with a high degree of accuracy with complete evaluation of function and relevant vascular anatomy. In addition to assessment of the valve morphology and quantification of severity of dysfunction, it allows for accurate and early quantification of left ventricular (LV) function, thus helping in prognostication.

Goals of Valvular Imaging

The goals of any imaging modality for VHD are to offer the following information (Table 1).

- Etiology (structural or functional)
- Severity (qualitative and quantification)
- Ventricular function (estimation of ejection fractions and end-diastolic/systolic volumes)
- Associated abnormalities—such as presence of aortic coarctation in patients with bicuspid aortic valve

TABLE 1: CMRI assessment for valvular heart disease.

Etiology/Morphology	*Function*	*Additional information*
	Aortic regurgitation	
• Valve morphology, e.g. bicuspid valve/ degenerative/dysplastic • Aortic root dimensions	• Regurgitant jet visualization and quantification with phase contrast MRI • LV volume and systolic functional assessment • LV mass	*Assess for* • Marfans syndrome • Dissection • Infection • Vegetation • Abscess
	Aortic stenosis	
• Valve morphology presence of leaflet fibrosis • *Lesion location*: Supravalvar, valvar or subvalvar	• Aortic valve area by planimetry • Gradient quantification with phase contrast—MRI • LV volume and systolic functional assessment/LV mass	• Ascending aortic poststenotic dilatation • Aortic coarctation
	Mitral regurgitation	
• Mitral apparatus dysfunction—dysplastic, rheumatic, mitral valve prolapse, papillary muscle infarction • 2° dilatation of mitral annulus—LV dysfunction (DCM either ischemic or nonischemic)	• Direct quantification with phase contrast—MRI • Indirect quantification using LV inflow/outflow/aortic forward flow	*Assess for* • Vegetation • Abscess • Infarction • Cardiomyopathy
	Mitral stenosis	
• Valve leaflet morphology—dysplastic, thickened fused, or tethered • Valvar support evaluation—single papillary muscle, shortened chordae	• Mitral valvar area (planimetry) • Peak velocity, mean gradient using phase contrast—MRI • LV volumes, systolic function	• *Assess for* • 2° pathology— atrial thombi or myxoma • Supramitral membrane • Left atrial dilatation • Pulmonary hypertension
	Pulmonary valve assessment	
• The imaging assessment as under aortic regurgitation and stenosis apply for investigation of the pulmonary valve • In addition CMRI is the investigation of choice in post-tetralogy of Fallot repair to assess for – Regurgitant fraction – RV outflow tract anatomy to r/o aneurysm – Infundibular, muscular RV outflow tract obstruction – Main and branch pulmonary artery anatomy – RV/LV systolic function and diastolic/systolic volumes – Qp:Qs—To evaluate for residual VSD		
	Tricuspid valve assessment	
• The imaging assessment as under mitral regurgitation and stenosis apply for investigation of the tricuspid valve • In addition, CMRI is the investigation of choice in evaluation of Ebstein anomaly – Location and dilation of annulus (tricuspid:mitral ratio) – Degree of displacement of valve leaflets/regugitant fraction – Assessment of functional/atrialized right ventricle – Assessment of ventricular volumes and function		

(CMRI: cardiac magnetic resonance imaging; DCM: dilated cardiomyopathy; LV: left ventricular; MRI: magnetic resonance imaging; RV: right ventricular; VSD: ventricular septal defect)

CARDIAC MAGNETIC RESONANCE IMAGING TECHNIQUE

Cardiac magnetic resonance imaging sequences are broadly divided into two types (Table 2).

1. Bright blood—These are bright blood images which depict the high signal intensity of fast-flowing blood as bright areas, as opposed to relatively immobile structures, such as myocardium, depicted as dark areas. These sequences reflect the relatively high T2/T1 ratio of blood and are typically b-SSFP (balanced steady-state free precession) sequences. Cine sequences are an example of bright blood technique.
2. Dark blood—Here, the signal from blood alone is nulled (double inversion recovery) or signals from both blood and fat are nulled (triple inversion recovery). Routine

TABLE 2: Overview of CMRI sequences used for valvular heart disease assessment.

Cine SSFP imaging (non–contrast bright blood sequence)	Anatomical assessment	• Leaflet motion and morphology • Valve area • Atrial size • Assessment of other abnormalities
	Functional assessment	• Disease severity quantification (regurgitation or stenosis) • Ventricular size and function (volumes and mass) • Regional wall motion abnormalities
Native T1 mapping (non–contrast dark blood sequence)	• Assessment of extracellular volume and identification of early fibrosis	
Perfusion (post–contrast sequence contrast dark blood sequence)	• Assessment for myocardial ischemia/infarction	
Late gadolinium enhancement (post–contrast sequence contrast dark blood sequence)	• Myocardial tissue characterization for assessment of fibrosis and infarction	
Post–contrast T1 mapping (dark blood sequence)	• Along with native T1 mapping, helps quantify extracellular volumes and quantification of fibrosis	
Phase contrast (non–contrast sequence)	• Flow volume, peak systolic velocity, and direction of flow assessment • Calculation of regurgitation fractions	

(CMRI: cardiac magnetic resonance imaging; SSFP: steady-state free precession)

T1, T2, and postcontrast images are examples of these sequences.

Cardiac magnetic resonance imaging is performed either on a 1.5-T or a 3-T scanner using a standardized imaging protocol, with additional planes being acquired according to the specific clinical question. Initial localizer black-blood images are acquired in axial and coronal planes as contiguous sections, covering the thorax from the diaphragm to the thoracic inlet. Cine b-SSFP sequences are then acquired in short-axis, two- and four-chamber planes (Figs. 1A to F). Further planes are acquired for assessment of the specific valve under study. These are followed by acquisition of T1-weighted and T2-weighted images along both four-chamber and short-axis planes. T1- and T2-mapping sequences are acquired in the short-axis views to assess for fibrosis and edema, respectively. The patient is administered an intravenous injection of gadolinium-based contrast agent to assess enhancement of the myocardium. Late gadolinium enhancement images are acquired after 5 and 15 minutes of contrast injection in the short-axis, two- and four-chamber planes, using phase-sensitive inversion recovery sequence. The information gained from these sequences is summarized in Table 2.

Cine Sequences

These noncontrast sequences are the workhorse of CMRI and help in assessment of cardiac chamber function and valve motion assessment. Cardiac motion, depicted as beating heart images, are displayed as cine loops with high spatial (up to 1–2 mm) and temporal resolution (20–50 ms). They are useful for both functional as well as structural assessment.

- *Functional assessment using cine sequences*
  - Calculated using software, ventricular function can be calculated manually or by using semiautomated contour detection algorithms (Figs. 2A to D). The impact of valve lesion on the ventricles is best assessed by precise calculation of ventricular volumes, functions, and mass. Poor function and increased volumes are poor predictor of recovery. Right ventricular (RV) volumes are particularly well evaluated, being difficult to accurately assess by other methods, such as ECHO. Both in vivo and in vitro experiments have validated both the accuracy as well as reproducibility of these CMRI-based indices as opposed to ECHO, which is operator-dependent and subject to obtaining a good acoustic window.[5,6] In addition, LV myocardial mass has been demonstrated to be a more accurate measure of the effect of aortic stenosis than wall thickness.[7]
  - Cine sequences are also useful in identifying regional wall motion abnormalities.
  - Flow turbulence, depicted as a black jet (also known as "signal void"), alerts the examiner to the presence of regurgitant or stenotic lesions. The width of such jets can allude to the severity if the lesion as less severe leaks have narrower jets in general. In combination with phase-contrast (PC) imaging, disease severity in terms of stenosis assessment and regurgitation fraction can be obtained.

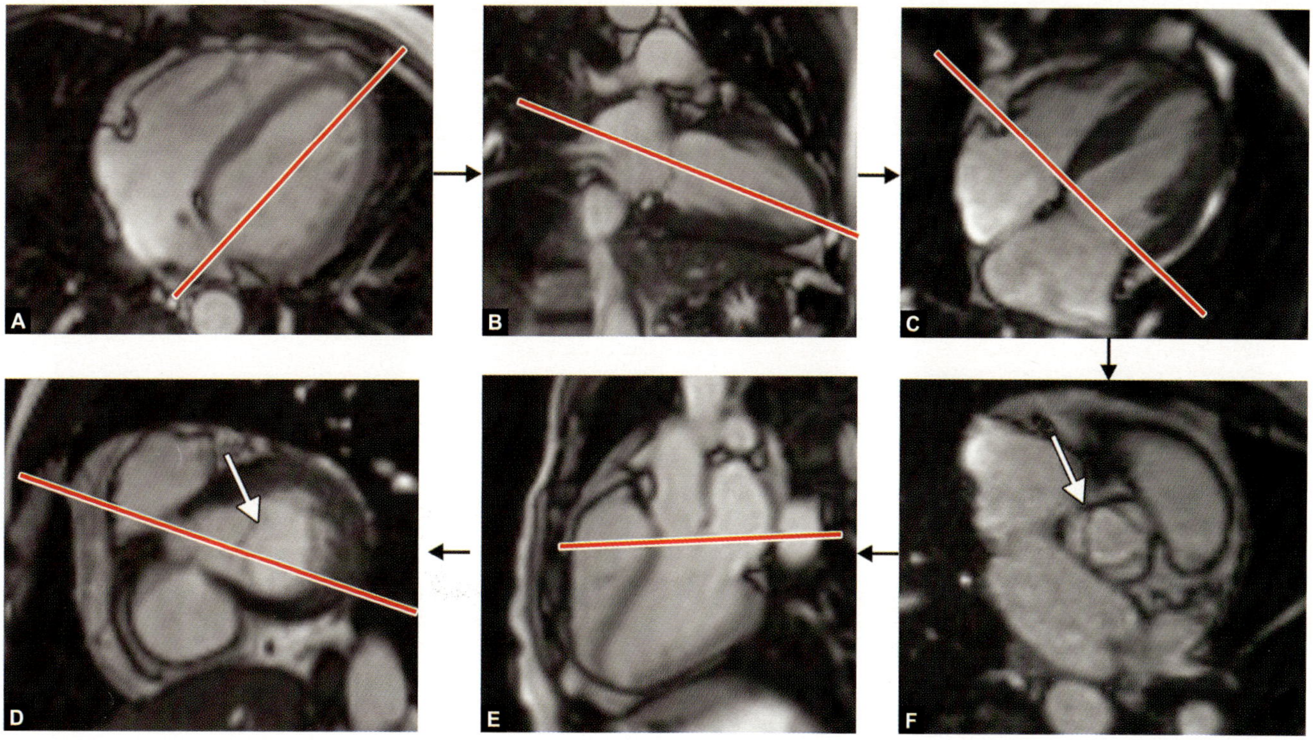

Figs. 1A to F: Imaging planes used in cardiac MRI. The figure demonstrates the order in which the planes are acquired. Arrows indicate the relationship between prescription and resultant image. (A) axial localizer image, (B) vertical long-axis view, (C) four-chamber view, (D) short-axis image; arrow depicts normal mitral valve leaflets with normal mitral valve area (E) three-chamber view (F) aortic annulus view; arrow shows normal tricuspid aortic valve leaflets with normal aortic valve area. (MRI: magnetic resonance image)

- *Anatomical assessment using cine sequences:*
  - Cine sequences enable assessment of all of the valvular components (papillary muscles, chordae tendineae, and leaflets). Abnormal valve morphology, such as bicuspid aortic valve, displaced valve leaflets as in Ebstein anomaly (Figs. 3A and B) aberrant papillary muscle anatomy (parachute mitral valve), increased leaflet thickness, presence of calcification, leaflet redundancy (in mitral valve prolapse (MVP)), and fusion of the leaflets are well assessed. Due to their exceptional temporal resolution, the cine images can also evaluate abnormal valve motion (Figs. 4A and B) and can be used for assessing valve area (Fig. 5).
  - Information about infective vegetation's, bland thrombi, or tumors attached to the valves, including site and mobility, can be effectively obtained by cine mitral regurgitation (MR). Additional anatomical findings that can be assessed on cine sequences are left atrial (LA) size and presence of LA thrombus. This is important if mitral valvuloplasty is being considered, both for risk estimation as well as prognostication.

Phase-contrast Imaging

This is a noncontrast sequence that helps in flow evaluation/gradient estimations by assessing velocity, volume, and direction of flow. It can quantitate gradients across stenosis and calculate regurgitant fractions. These sequences are based on the phase of moving protons in blood. After obtaining the images perpendicular to the vessel of interest, reactive oxygen intermediates (ROIs) are drawn over the vessel in each frame to obtain the peak systolic velocity (V_{max}). Using the simplified Bernoulli equation ($4 \times V^2_{max}$), the peak systolic velocity is calculated. PC has been shown to be accurate with an error of less than 5 m/s in studies when comparing it with flow phantoms.[8] These measurements being repeatable and consistent can also be used for follow-up and postoperative monitoring purposes. Flow volumes are then calculated using the velocity maps, after similar ROI placement. The velocity is multiplied by the area of the region of interest, to obtain the flow volume (cm^3/s) per cardiac cycle. The flow volume is plotted against the time to visualize flow and its relationship to the cardiac cycle. Using these curves, forward and regurgitant volumes can be evaluated (Figs. 6A to D). These flow

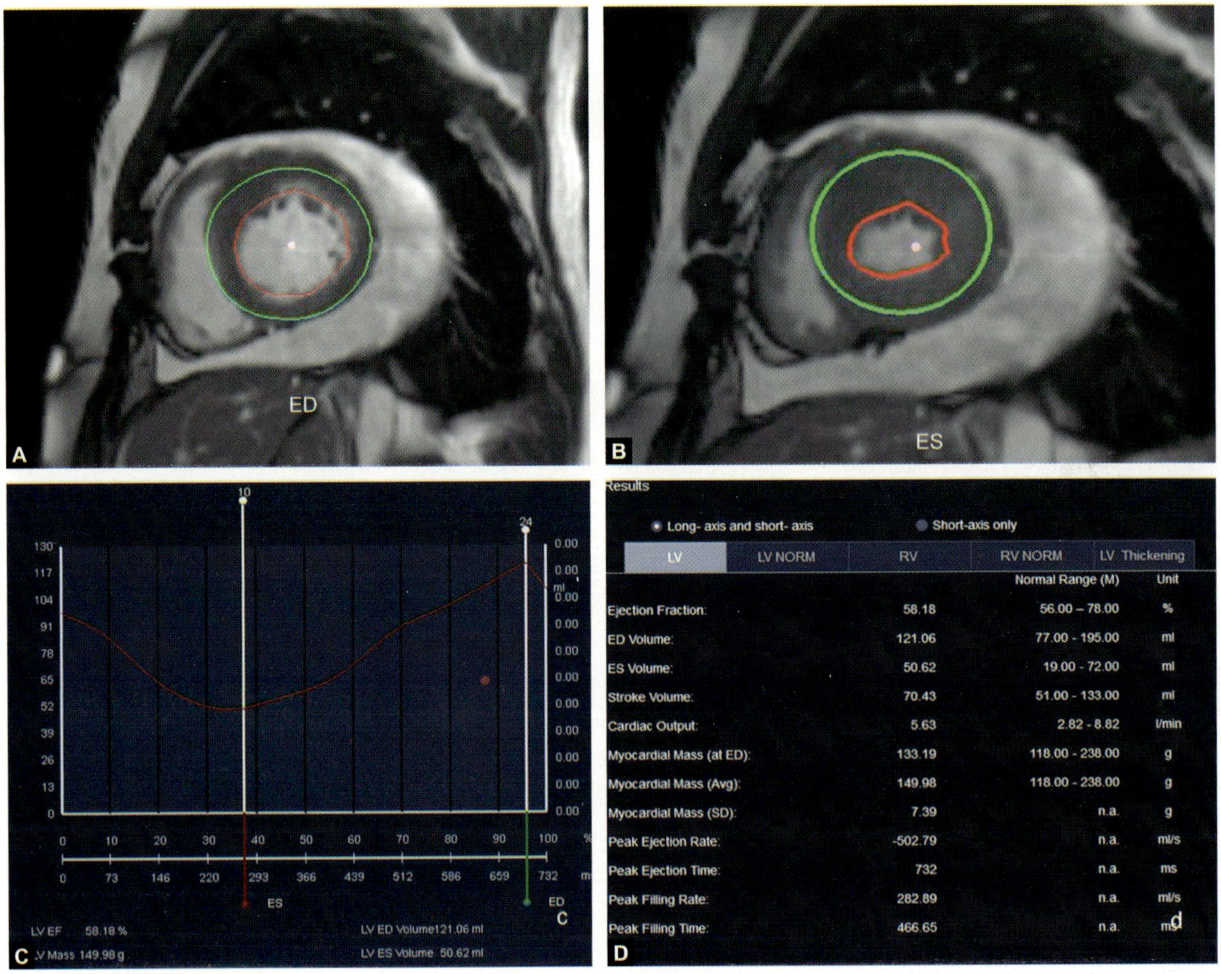

Figs. 2A to D: Functional assessment of the left ventricle using CMRI. (A and B) Semiautomated endocardial and epicardial contour detection in end-diastole and end-systole. (C and D) Graphical representation of volumetric change of the left ventricle throughout the cardiac cycle and results pane of the volumetric analysis. (CMRI: cardiac magnetic resonance imaging)

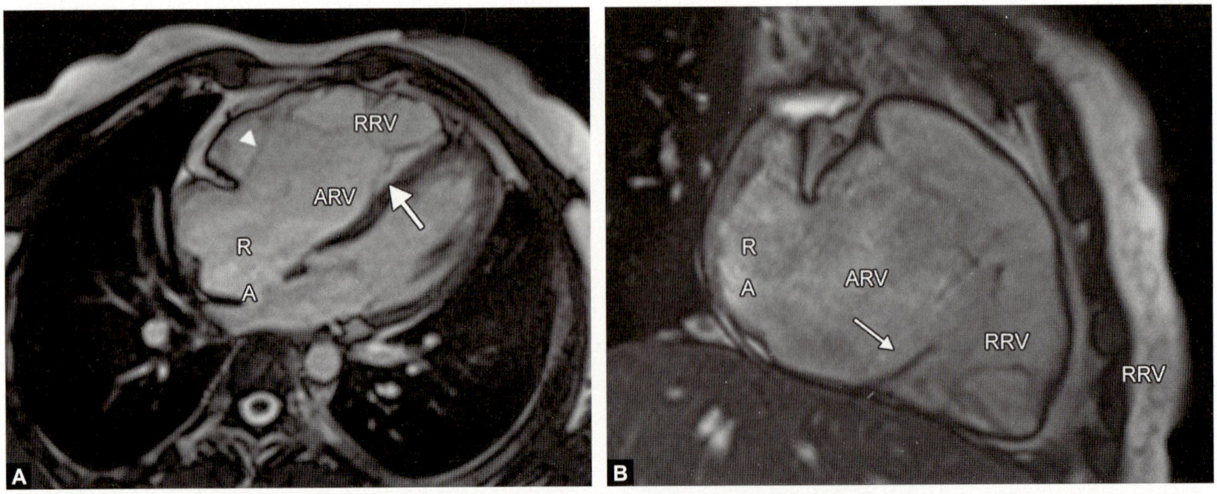

Figs. 3A and B: Four-chamber and vertical long-axis view bright-blood cine MR image showing displaced septal (arrow in A) and posterior leaflet (arrow in B) of the tricuspid valve. The anterior leaflet (arrowhead in A) of the tricuspid valve (though long and redundant), and its annulus are in their normal anatomical position. (MR: Magnetic resonance)

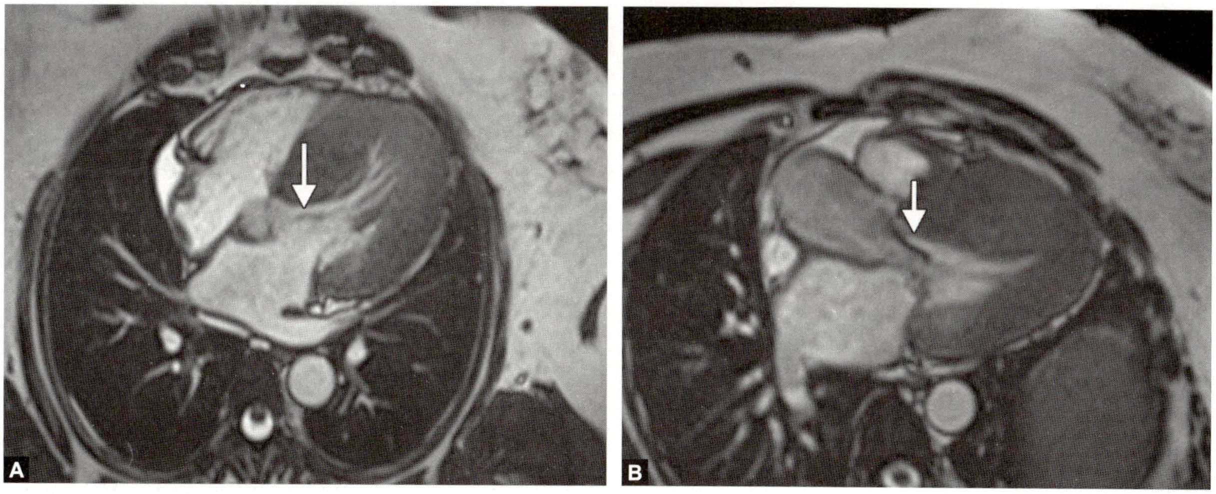

Figs. 4A and B: (A) Bright-blood cine MR image showing systolic anterior motion of the mitral leaflet causing narrowing of the outflow tract in systole in a case of hypertrophic cardiomyopathy. (B) Three-chamber view shows the dephasing jet in the outflow tract caused by an associated aortic regurgitation. (MR: magnetic resonance)

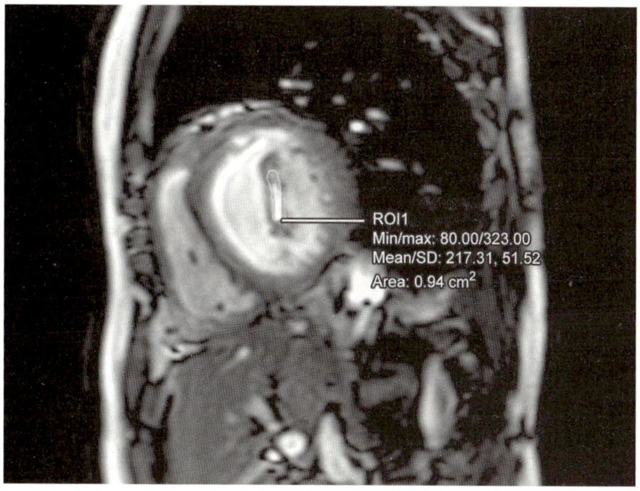

Fig. 5: Bright-blood cine MR image showing severe mitral stenosis. Planimetry showing a mitral valve area of less than 1 cm^2. Compare with Figure 1D where the mitral valve area is normal. (MR: magnetic resonance)

measurements are however dependent on presence of a homogenous magnetic field, ensuring that the image slice is perpendicular to the vessel and placed just proximal or distal to the valve annulus. The values thus obtained can be erroneous if strict protocols are not adhered to.[9] Velocity and gradient assessment by CMRI is especially useful in cases of angulated roots where correct assessment of the stenotic jet by ECHO can be difficult, since many stenotic jets are not parallel to the LV outflow tract.

Assessment of Valvular Stenosis

Valve areas are assessed primarily for the aortic and mitral valves. However, the same techniques can be employed for the tricuspid and pulmonary valves, if required. For mitral valve area assessment, besides planimetry, pressure halftime (PHT) method may be used.

- Anatomical—The mitral valve area can be determined by drawing a contour around the smallest valve orifice on a diastolic image obtained in a plane perpendicular to the direction of flow through the valve (Fig. 5).
- Pressure halftime method—Electrocardiography-gated short-axis sequences are obtained 1.5 cm above the mitral valve leaflets. Analogous to E and A waves as obtained by ECHO, similar information can be generated from the flow velocity curve.[10]

Pressure halftime is defined as the time in milliseconds between the maximum mitral gradient in early diastole and the time point where the gradient is half the maximum initial value. Mitral valve area is then calculated using a generic formula—[MVA = 220/PHT].

For aortic valve area measurement, two methods are available—(1) anatomical and (2) physiological area.

1. Anatomical valve area is the planimetered area of the aortic valve leaflets in its maximally open position. This can be done directly on cine SSFP images, and these values correlate well with area assessments on transoesophageal ECHO (Fig. 1F). This method however may be incorrect when assessing calcified valves where the calcification may cause erroneous area measurement due to artifacts.[11]

2. Physiological valve area is useful in presence of calcified valves where the area of the flow stream (seen as a dephasing jet) is calculated as it passes through the valve.[12] This is similar to vena contracta method[13] used in ECHO but is no longer preferred as it is an unreliable indicator of disease severity.

ASSESSMENT OF VALVULAR REGURGITATION

Multiple methods are used for the evaluation of disease severity using a combination of information obtained by of cine sequences and PC sequences.

- Visualization of a jet is often the first feature used to detect regurgitation. Evaluation of severity of regurgitation, based on jet length or area, is no longer performed as mentioned above.
- Phase-contrast sequences to directly sample MR/aortic regurgitation (AR)/pulmonary regurgitation (PR)/tricuspid regurgitation (TR) jet to obtain regurgitant volume. This is the easiest of the techniques to perform and is the most widely used sequence to calculate the regurgitant fractions (Figs. 6A to D).
- The stroke volumes of both the ventricles (calculated using cine sequences) are equal in the absence of disease. With regurgitation, the regurgitant volume is the difference in stroke volumes of the ventricles as long as only one valve is dysfunctional and no intracardiac shunting is present.
- Aortic regurgitant volume is the difference between total LV stroke volume and forward stroke volume in the aorta (calculated using PC sequences) in the absence of MR.
- Aortic regurgitant volume is the difference between forward stroke volume between aortic and mitral valve (calculated using PC sequences to sample flow at the respective valves) in the absence of MR.

Tricuspid and PR can also be quantified using the same methods.

Tissue Characterization

The ability of CMRI to perform tissue characterization is the most significant advantage of this modality compared to other cardiac imaging techniques. Many cardiac diseases are identified by the abnormal increase in extracellular space where contrast (gadolinium) accumulates. Lateral

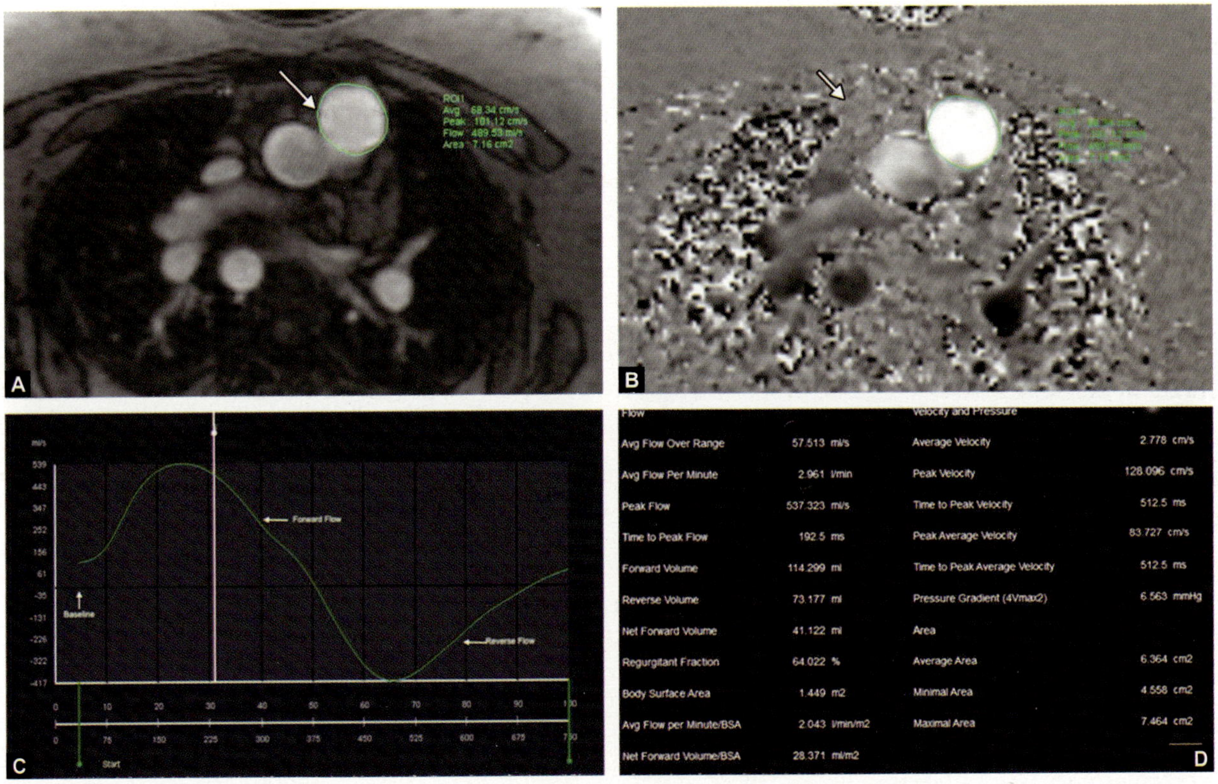

Figs. 6A and B: Phase contrast MRI in a postoperative case of tetralogy of Fallot showing calculation of pulmonary regurgitation fraction. (A and B) Magnitude and phase velocity image showing ROI placed on the main pulmonary artery. (C) Flow mapping curve from the ROI in the main pulmonary artery shows severe pulmonary regurgitation (represented as reverse flow) with a regurgitant fraction of 64%. (D) Results tab showing the various indices automatically obtained from the flow mapping curve. (MR: magnetic resonance imaging; ROI: reactive oxygen intermediate)

ganglionic eminence (LGE) is the gold standard for quantification of fibrosis in cardiomyopathies (both ischemic and nonischemic). LGE has been shown to adequately assess fibrosis that is known to occur in cases of volume or pressure overload to the ventricles. Especially in the case of aortic stenosis, where myocardial hypertrophy occurs, studies have shown that presence of fibrosis is an adverse prognostic marker for improvement after valve replacement. Other studies have shown that the presence of LGE, and its severity predicted the perioperative risk and all-cause mortality in patients with ankylosing spondylitis.[14,15] LGE can also assess for fibrosis of papillary muscles in cases of ischemia-related functional MR. The identification of this fibrosis either in the papillary muscles or the LV myocardium has been associated with increased risk of arrhythmias, as fibrotic tissue acts as a potent arrythmogenic substrate.[16] Papillary muscle fibrosis has also been theorized to be of predictive valve in stratifying clinical outcomes in patents with MVP.[17] Tissue characterization can now also be performed with newer pulse sequences, using various principles of MRI, to assess tissue composition which do not require contrast injection. T1 mapping, for example, can assess for the presence of myocardial fibrosis and T2 mapping can identify foci of myocardial edema/inflammation. These sequences help in identifying earlier subtle degrees of fibrosis as compared to LGE. The presence of altered native or postcontrast T1 values may help in earlier institution of treatment and prognostication.[18]

Cardiac Magnetic Resonance Imaging for Preoperative Assessment

Cardiac magnetic resonance imaging can be used for preoperative planning purposes as well as to help in prognostication. This is especially relevant in preprocedure planning for transcatheter aortic valve implantation (TAVI). Accurate anatomical assessment of the aortic annulus which is the key to TAVI is best done by three-dimensional (3D) imaging that is best performed by either CT or CMRI. CMRI with its high spatial resolution and its capability for 3D multiplanar reconstructions is an attractive alternative to the gold standard CT examination. Studies have demonstrated close agreement between measurements on CT and CMR and their ability to predict paravalvular leaks (PVL).[19] The prognostic valve of tissue characterization using LGE as well as T1 mapping as discussed earlier is of value in both the ischemic and nonischemic myocardial pathologies including VHDs.

Cardiac Magnetic Resonance Imaging for Postoperative Assessment

Cardiac magnetic resonance imaging can help in monitoring of response to valvular interventions. The presence of a PHV is not a contraindication for performing an MR scan at 1.5 T. This is because the force that the valve undergoes during every beat far exceeds the amount of force exerted by the magnet. However, for all devices, it is recommended that the practitioner review the most current literature on each device for MR safety (http://www.MRIsafety.com). The artifacts caused by the valve, however, may impede assessment of the surrounding structures. Leaflet motion of certain valves may be assessed (though suboptimal) by CMRI by careful slice selection and angulation; however, this information is readily and more accurately obtained by X-ray fluoroscopy.[20] The presence and quantification of PVL (as assessed using a combination of cine and PC sequences) associated with long-standing surgically placed aortic and mitral valves can be assessed by CMRI. Cine CME is also a highly sensitive examination for assessment of residual MR postpercutaneous or surgical mitral valve replacement.[21,22] CMRI is also the imaging method of choice in assessing the postoperative morphologic and functional changes that occur following repair of tetralogy of Fallot. The most common postoperative complications including recurrent or residual ventricular septal defect, PR, RV outflow tract aneurysm and dyskinesis, conduit failure, residual pulmonary artery stenosis, TR, and RV failure. All of these can be accurately assessed by CMRI. This is particularly important since CMRI-derived results for ventricular volumes and pulmonary regurgitant fraction are useful for decision-making regarding timing of pulmonary valve replacement (a detailed discussion on the same is beyond the scope of this discussion). Recently, CMRI has been used for assessing LV reverse remodeling following mitral valve interventions. CME assessment showed a strong correlation between postoperative LV remodeling and MR severity as opposed to ECHO which was not found to establish this correlation.[23] CMRI can also be an ideal and comprehensive technique to preoperatively and postoperatively assess and follow-up patients undergoing percutaneous balloon mitral valvuloplasty as LA chronic compliance changes makes immediate postprocedure assessment of multiple sclerosis unreliable.[24]

Limitations of Cardiac Magnetic Resonance Imaging

- Clinically unstable or uncooperative patients cannot be adequately imaged as it is a time-consuming examination.
- Irregular heart rates degrade the image quality of CMRI. Complex algorithms are used to reconstruct images using data that are acquired over multiple cardiac cycles. Irregular heart rates therefore lead to imprecise segmentation of data leading to excessive blurring of images leading to nondiagnostic studies. This disadvantage can be offset by using advanced CMRI

sequences that either are less dependent on heart rate or by using faster sequences that can acquire date over fewer cardiac cycles. Real-time cine CMRI belongs to the former category as it leads to acquisition of bright blood cardiac images at less than 1 s per slice without breath holding.[25] This faster acquisition is however associated with poorer spatial resolution as evidenced by blurrier images. Compressed sensing CMRI is another exciting new set of sequences that has the potential to accelerate MR scans beyond what is possible with any other method.[26] This method is, however, more complicated than the usually used Fourier transformation in conventional MR imaging, making it computationally heavy and thus time-consuming. With faster computers and processors available today, this limitation will likely be overcome, making these sequences the standard in CMRI.
- Inability to assess hemodynamic abnormalities directly. This is a limitation with all imaging modalities, including ECHO and CT. Although CMRI can calculate velocity and thereby gradient across a lesion, it is essentially an indirect estimation of the pressure within the chamber or vessel.

FUTURE DIRECTIONS

Time-resolved multidimensional (4D) velocity flow CMRI is a new sequence that helps to quantify MR more accurately than current two-dimensional (2D) PC-CMRI. Direct estimation of MR via 2D PC-CMRI is hampered due presence of multidirectional regurgitant patterns. Using 4D flow, velocity is measured in x-, y-, and z-vectors, effectively overcoming the limitations of the former. Excellent correlation has been obtained between 4D flow and 3D ECHO in assessment of MR.[27] Computational modeling by machine learning algorithms has been used to study stress–strain relationships by dividing the area of interest in multiple small finite elements and observing the relationships between them.[28] Computational modeling is being used to study geometric and functional alterations that occur postoperatively and can assess the stress distribution over valve leaflets. For example, this technique was used by researchers to simulate two different approaches to MVP repair which suggested the superiority and better durability of one surgery over the other, thus enabling the best surgical repair to be used.[29]

The possibility of real-time CMRI-guided TAVI is another exciting area of active research. Implantation of transcatheter aortic valves under real-time CMR guidance has been performed in animal models.[30] However, due to obvious logistic challenges, this remains firmly within the realms of research institutes.

CONCLUSION

Advances in CMRI technology allow for accurate and noninvasive evaluation of cardiac valves. The advantage of CMRI assessment of VHD is its reproducible assessment of ventricular volumes and function in patients with chronic AR, MR, and PR. CMRI also provides a measure of valve stenosis, regurgitant fraction and volume. Precise assessment of valve dysfunction and measures of ventricular function are also possible using CMRI. Its ability to perform both pre- and postoperative assessment noninvasively with no radiation concerns and possibility of multiple follow-up studies makes it a very attractive imaging modality for valvular assessment.

REFERENCES

1. Maganti K, Rigolin VH, Sarano ME, et al. Valvular heart disease: diagnosis and management. Mayo Clin Proc. 2010;85:483-500.
2. Ramakrishnan S, Juneja R. Rheumatic heart disease in India: 'Buried alive'. Natl Med J India. 2014;27:65-9.
3. Manjunath CN, Srinivas P, Ravindranath KS, et al. Incidence and patterns of valvular heart disease in a tertiary care high-volume cardiac center: a single center experience. Indian Heart J. 2014;66:320-6.
4. Davis K, Kennedy JW, Kemp HG, Jr., et al. Complications of coronary arteriography from the Collaborative Study of Coronary Artery Surgery (CASS). Circulation. 1979;59:1105-12.
5. Rehr RB, Malloy CR, Filipchuk NG, et al. Left ventricular volumes measured by MR imaging. Radiology. 1985;156:717-9.
6. Sechtem U, Pflugfelder PW, Gould RG, et al. Measurement of right and left ventricular volumes in healthy individuals with cine MR imaging. Radiology. 1987;163:697-702.
7. Debl K, Djavidani B, Buchner S, et al. Delayed hyperenhancement in magnetic resonance imaging of left ventricular hypertrophy caused by aortic stenosis and hypertrophic cardiomyopathy: visualisation of focal fibrosis. Heart. 2006;92:1447-51.
8. Mostbeck GH, Caputo GR, Higgins CB. MR measurement of blood flow in the cardiovascular system. AJR Am J Roentgenol. 1992;159:453-61.
9. Gatehouse PD, Rolf MP, Graves MJ, et al. Flow measurement by cardiovascular magnetic resonance: a multi-centre multi-vendor study of background phase offset errors that can compromise the accuracy of derived regurgitant or shunt flow measurements. J Cardiovasc Magn Reson. 2010;12:5.
10. Lin SJ, Brown PA, Watkins MP, et al. Quantification of stenotic mitral valve area with magnetic resonance imaging and comparison with Doppler ultrasound. J Am Coll Cardiol. 2004;44:133-7.
11. Schlosser T, Malyar N, Jochims M, et al. Quantification of aortic valve stenosis in MRI-comparison of steady-state free precession and fast low-angle shot sequences. Eur Radiol. 2007;17:1284-90.

12. Caruthers SD, Lin SJ, Brown P, et al. Practical value of cardiac magnetic resonance imaging for clinical quantification of aortic valve stenosis: comparison with echocardiography. Circulation. 2003;108:2236-43.
13. Little SH. The vena contracta area: conquering quantification with a 3D cut? JACC Cardiovasc Imaging. 2012;5:677-80.
14. Barone-Rochette G, Pierard S, De Meester de Ravenstein C, et al. Prognostic significance of LGE by CMR in aortic stenosis patients undergoing valve replacement. J Am Coll Cardiol. 2014;64:144-54.
15. Dweck MR, Joshi S, Murigu T, et al. Midwall fibrosis is an independent predictor of mortality in patients with aortic stenosis. J Am Coll Cardiol. 2011;58:1271-9.
16. Basso C, Perazzolo Marra M, Rizzo S, et al. Arrhythmic mitral valve prolapse and sudden cardiac death. Circulation. 2015;132:556-66.
17. Perazzolo Marra M, Basso C, De Lazzari M, et al. Morphofunctional abnormalities of mitral annulus and arrhythmic mitral valve prolapse. Circ Cardiovasc Imaging. 2016;9:e005030.
18. Bui AH, Roujol S, Foppa M, et al. Diffuse myocardial fibrosis in patients with mitral valve prolapse and ventricular arrhythmia. Heart. 2017;103:204-9.
19. Jabbour A, Ismail TF, Moat N, et al. Multimodality imaging in transcatheter aortic valve implantation and post-procedural aortic regurgitation: comparison among cardiovascular magnetic resonance, cardiac computed tomography, and echocardiography. J Am Coll Cardiol. 2011;58:2165-73.
20. Botnar R, Nagel E, Scheidegger MB, et al. Assessment of prosthetic aortic valve performance by magnetic resonance velocity imaging. MAGMA. 2000;10:18-26.
21. Thavendiranathan P, Phelan D, Thomas JD, et al. Quantitative assessment of mitral regurgitation: validation of new methods. J Am Coll Cardiol. 2012;60:1470-83.
22. Simprini LA, Afroz A, Cooper MA, et al. Routine cine-CMR for prosthesis-associated mitral regurgitation: a multicenter comparison to echocardiography. J Heart Valve Dis. 2014;23:575-82.
23. Uretsky S, Gillam L, Lang R, et al. Discordance between echocardiography and MRI in the assessment of mitral regurgitation severity: a prospective multicenter trial. J Am Coll Cardiol. 2015;65:1078-88.
24. Park JH, Han MC, Im JG, et al. Mitral stenosis: evaluation with MR imaging after percutaneous balloon valvuloplasty. Radiology. 1990;177:533-6.
25. Francone M, Dymarkowski S, Kalantzi M, et al. Real-time cine MRI of ventricular septal motion: a novel approach to assess ventricular coupling. J Magn Reson Imaging. 2005;21: 305-9.
26. Kido T, Kido T, Nakamura M, et al. Compressed sensing real-time cine cardiovascular magnetic resonance: accurate assessment of left ventricular function in a single-breath-hold. J Cardiovasc Magn Reson. 2016;18:50.
27. Marsan NA, Westenberg JJ, Ypenburg C, et al. Quantification of functional mitral regurgitation by real-time 3D echocardiography: comparison with 3D velocity-encoded cardiac magnetic resonance. JACC Cardiovasc Imaging. 2009;2:1245-52.
28. Wenk JF, Zhang Z, Cheng G, et al. First finite element model of the left ventricle with mitral valve: insights into ischemic mitral regurgitation. Ann Thorac Surg. 2010;89:1546-53.
29. Morgan AE, Pantoja JL, Grossi EA, et al. Neochord placement versus triangular resection in mitral valve repair: a finite element model. J Surg Res. 2016;206:98-105.
30. Horvath KA, Guttman M, Li M, et al. Beating heart aortic valve replacement using real-time MRI guidance. Innovations (Phila). 2007;2:51-5.

SECTION 8

Rheumatic Heart Disease

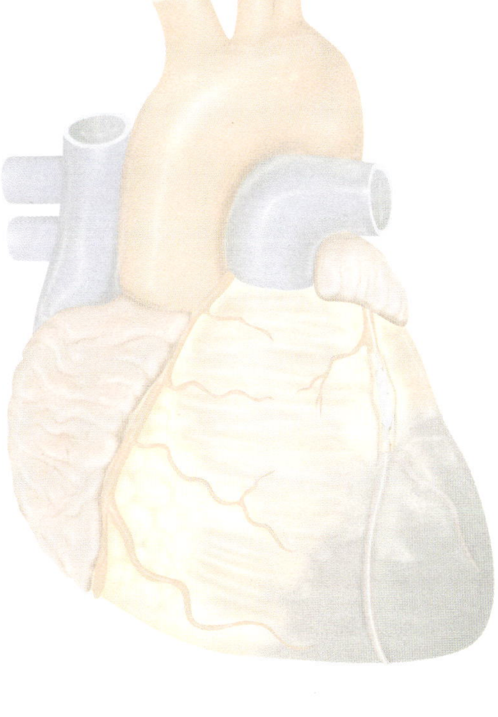

68

CHAPTER

Recent Advances in Echocardiographic Navigation in Acute Rheumatic Fever Evaluation

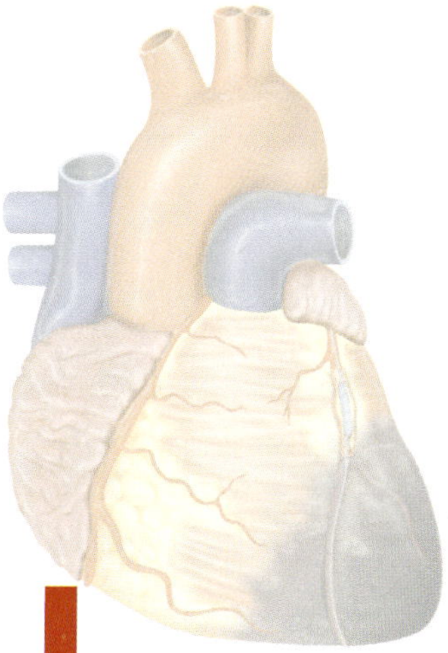

B Vijayalakshmi

INTRODUCTION

Acute rheumatic fever (ARF) and its long-term sequel rheumatic heart disease (RHD) is still a major burning problem in children, adolescents and young adults in emerging economies such as India. Globally, India contributes nearly 25–50% of newly diagnosed cases of ARF, hospitalizations, and deaths due to its sequel RHD.[1] According to World Health Organization bulletin of 1981, more than 50% of ARF/RHD detected in surveys and health checkup camps are unaware of their disease and more than 70% do not receive secondary prophylaxis regularly. This inappropriate secondary prophylaxis leads to repeated attacks of recrudescence of rheumatic activity and further damage to valves in juveniles. Unfortunately, "carditis" is the only presentation of ARF that causes death during acute stage or leads to permanent damage with long-term morbidity and mortality due to RHD and congestive heart failure. In the past, precise and early diagnosis of "carditis" in ARF was eluding the clinicians as no single pathognomonic test was available to detect carditis other than echocardiography. Hence, it is very important to know the recent advances in echocardiographic navigation in ARF.

DIAGNOSTIC CRITERION

The diagnostic accuracy for ARF has advanced tremendously since the pioneering work of Dr. T. Duckett Jones in the 1940s.[2] Since then the American Heart Association (AHA) has been a partner in revising, modifying, and publicizing "Jones Criteria" several times. In all the earlier criteria, a clinical diagnosis was principal, and echocardiography was not given any role in the diagnosis of carditis. Now that echocardiography has evolved over the past two decades and become widely available, there are several papers published documenting utility of echocardiography in early and precise diagnosis of carditis even in the absence of overt clinical findings ("subclinical carditis").[3,4] In the recently revised Jones criteria (2015), for the first time technology-driven echocardiography is included as major criteria in Jones criterion.[5] The serial changes made in original Jones criteria over the decades are shown in Table 1.[1] The revised Jones criteria are aimed at bringing more patients in the net of secondary prophylaxis. Echocardiography has also become a cornerstone in worldwide screening programs to evaluate the prevalence of RHD.

TWO-DIMENSIONAL ECHOCARDIOGRAPHY

Two-dimensional transthoracic echocardiography (TTE) can distinguish pathological mitral regurgitation (MR) from functional MR and can also distinguish rheumatic from nonrheumatic MR. TTE can detect mechanism of MR, e.g. valvulitis, valve prolapse, annulitis, ventricular enlargement, chordal rupture (rarely) causing valve regurgitation more precisely. All these cannot be detected by clinical examination. TTE can assess the severity of MR—mild, moderate, and severe—which has prognostic significance. Not only that, TTE can distinctly detect both clinical and subclinical carditis. It can also detect pericarditis with pericardial effusion. The various echocardiographic features

TABLE 1: Serial changes made in original Jones criteria over the decades and addition of echocardiography as a major criterion in 2015.

Symptoms	1944	1956	1965	1984	1992	2002	2015
Carditis	Major	Major	Major	Major	Major	Major	Major Subclinical
Polyarthritis	Major	Major	Major	Major	Major	Major	Major
Polyarthralgia	Major	Minor	Minor	Minor	Minor	Minor	Major
Chorea	Major	Major	Major	Major	Major	Major	Major
Subcutaneous nodules	Major	Major	Major	Major	Major	Major	Major
Erythema marginatum	Major	Major	Major	Major	Major	Major	Major
Echocardiography							Major

in ARF cases are given in Box 1.[5] The incidence of various features of carditis detected on echocardiography in our study is given in Table 2.[3]

BOX 1: Echocardiographic features of carditis in acute rheumatic fever.

Morphological findings on echo in mitral valve in acute carditis
- Annular dilation
- Chordal elongation
- Chordal rupture resulting in flail leaflet with severe mitral regurgitation
- Anterior (or less commonly posterior) leaflet tip prolapse
- Beading/nodularity of leaflet tips
- Leaflet thickening
- Chordal thickening
- Restricted leaflet motion
- Aortic valve changes in acute carditis
- Irregular or focal leaflet thickening
- Coaptation defect
- Restricted leaflet motion
- Leaflet prolapse

M-Mode Echocardiographic Features of Carditis in Acute Rheumatic Fever

- Left ventricle (LV) and left atrium (LA) are dilated. Hence, LA:abdominal obesity ratio is altered (Figs. 1A and B).
- The mitral/aortic/tricuspid valve leaflets are thickened >4 mm (normal ≤3 mm).
- Mild pericardial effusion may be seen.

Two-Dimensional Echo Features of Carditis in Acute Rheumatic Fever

- The thickened anterior mitral leaflet and posterior mitral leaflet >4 mm is best seen in the parasternal long-axis view (Fig. 2A). Hyperechogenicity of the submitral structures, such as chordae tendinae, due to inflammation, thickening, and elongation (Fig. 2B).
- Irregular thickening of mitral valve, aortic valve, tricuspid valve giving rise to beaded appearance, especially in parasternal short-axis view (Fig. 3A).

TABLE 2: Incidence of various features of carditis detected on echocardiography.

Sl. No.	Type of involvement	No. of cases	Percentage
1.	Mitral valvar thickness greater than 4 mm with reduced mobility	132	93.62
2.	Mitral regurgitation grades I–III	118	83.69
3.	Mitral valvar prolapse	80	56.74
4.	Rheumatic nodules (beaded appearance)	38	26.95
5.	Aortic regurgitation	31	21.99
6.	Tricuspid regurgitation	31	21.99
7.	Pancarditis	13	9.22
8.	Pericardial effusion	13	9.22
9.	Chordal tear	4	2.84

Doppler study is used to distinguish between physiological and pathological MR. Holosystolic jet with a well-defined, dense, high-velocity spectral envelope is seen in pathological MR (Fig. 4) and tricuspid regurgitation. The spectral is holodiastolic in aortic regurgitation. If the peak velocity is <3 m/s then it is functional, and >3 m/s means that it is pathological (Box 2).[5]

Color Doppler

Color Doppler echo can differentiate functional MR of nonrheumatic etiology. In functional MR, there is a central jet with normal valves and dilated LV with reduced ejection fraction (Fig. 5A). In MR of rheumatic etiology, there is a wall-hugging eccentric jet with reflux into pulmonary veins in severe MR (Fig. 5B).

Substantial color jet with mosaic pattern seen in two planes extending >1 cm beyond cooptation point color jet of MR passes over the posterior wall of LA, holosystolic jet with a well-defined, dense, high-velocity spectral envelope graded as trivial, grade I, II, III. Unless valve regurgitation is associated with other features, such as "thickened valves, beaded appearance, hyperechogenic submitral structures," with an echo score of >6 according to Vijaya's Echo score, it is not taken as significant pathological MR of rheumatic etiology.[4]

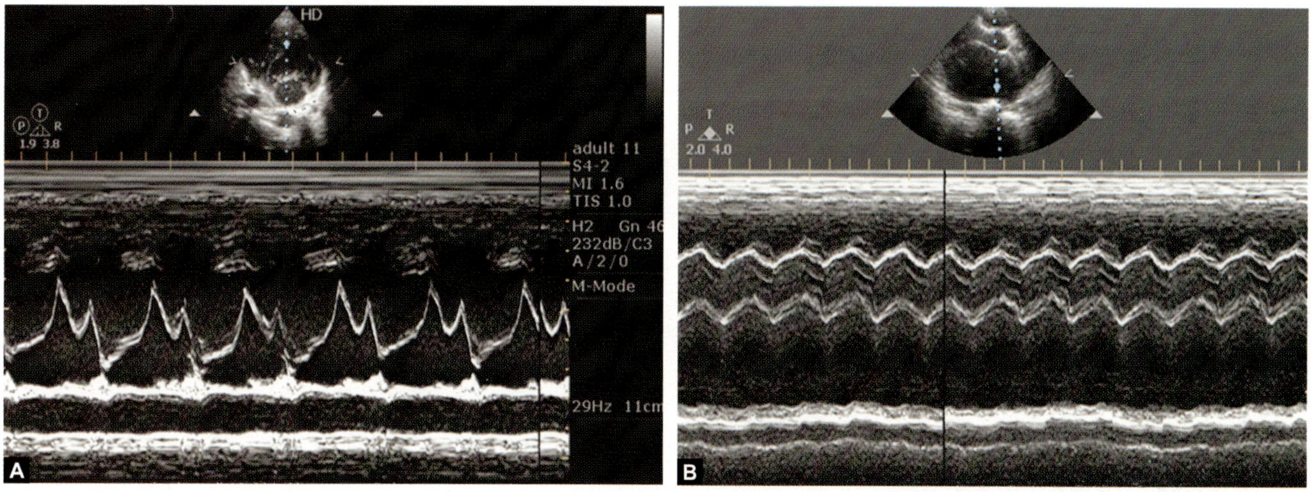

Figs. 1A and B: (A) M-mode echo shows thickened anterior mitral and posterior mitral leaflets with reduced excursion in a 12-year-old girl with ARF; (B) M-mode echo shows left atrium dilated and pericardial effusion in a 12-year-old girl with ARF with carditis. (ARF: acute rheumatic fever)

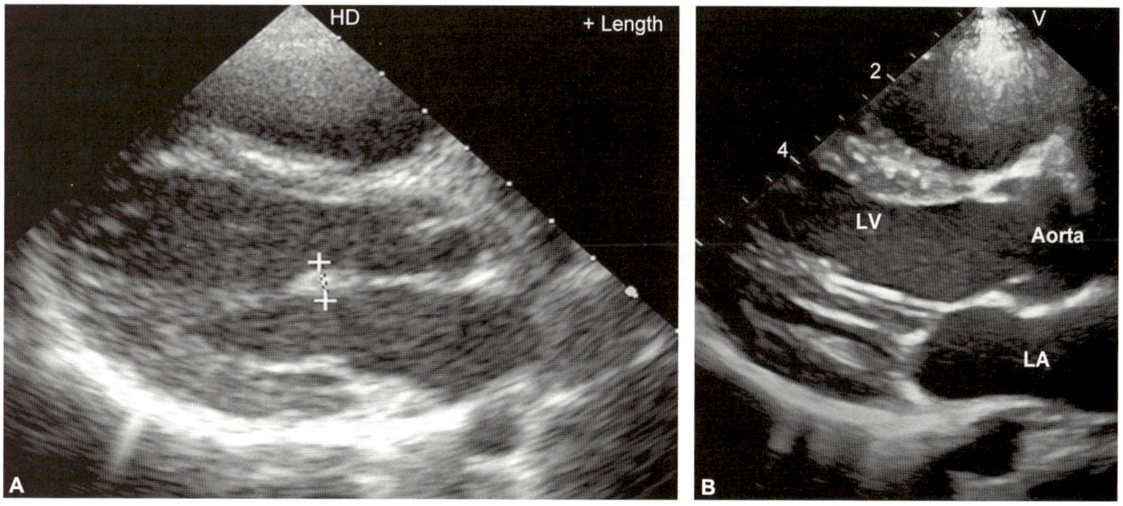

Figs. 2A and B: (A) Parasternal long-axis view shows thickened mitral valve (6 mm); (B) Modified three-chamber view shows thickened aortic valve and hyper echogenic submitral structures like chordae tendinae in a 6-year-old girl with ARF. (ARF: acute rheumatic fever)

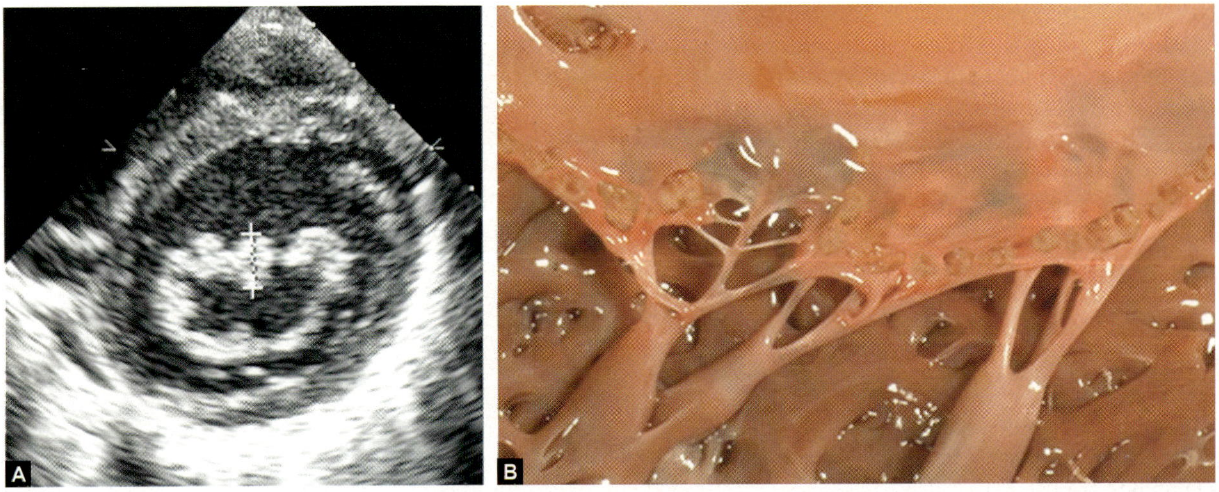

Figs. 3A and B: (A) Parasternal short-axis shows thickened beaded appearance of anterior mitral leaflet and posterior mitral leaflet in 12-year-old girl with ARF; (B) Autopsy specimen of mitral valve shows small thrombi form on the valve at the edge giving rise to a ridge or a row of small pink nodules seen on echocardiography as beaded appearance of the valve. (ARF: acute rheumatic fever)

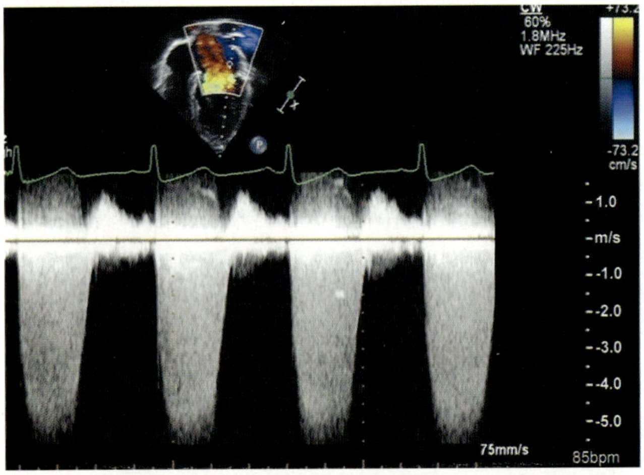

Fig. 4: Doppler study shows holosystolic jet with a well-defined, dense, high-velocity spectral envelope in a case of MR in an 8-year-old girl. (MR: mitral regurgitation)

BOX 2: Doppler findings in rheumatic valvulitis.

Pathological mitral regurgitation (all four criteria met)
- Seen in at least 2 views
- Jet length ≥2 cm in at least 1 view
- Peak velocity >3 m/s
- Pansystolic jet in at least 1 envelope

Pathological aortic regurgitation (all four criteria met)
- Seen in at least 2 views
- Jet length ≥1 cm in at least 1 view
- Peak velocity >3 m/s
- Pandiastolic jet in at least 1 envelope

APPLICATION OF VIJAYA'S ECHO CRITERIA

Our own study clearly showed that echocardiography can prevent both underdiagnosis and overdiagnosis.[3] Our two studies titled, "Role of echocardiography in diagnosing carditis in setting of acute rheumatic fever"[3] and "Efficacy of echocardiographic criteria for diagnosis of carditis in acute rheumatic fever,"[4] are quoted in the 2015 revised Jones criteria.[3] The echocardiographic score to be calculated according to Vijaya's criteria is given in Table 3.[4] Any patient getting <6 scores is unlikely to be ARF. Unless valve regurgitation is associated with other features, such as thickened valves, reduced mobility, beaded appearance, hyperechogenic submitral structures, and chordal tear, with an echo score of >6, it is not taken as significant and pathological (Figs. 6A and B).

PROGNOSTIC IMPLICATIONS

The presence of carditis is a reason for lifelong prophylaxis. Therefore, echo can bring more number of patients of ARF in the net of secondary prophylaxis in the developing countries. Doing echo at the time of discontinuing prophylaxis might make more sense because if valves have become normal, one can discontinue it safely. Patients with carditis are more likely to be detected during their first attacks of ARF. Detecting subclinical carditis will prevent from a more relaxed and inappropriate secondary prophylaxis. There is a significant prognostic implication

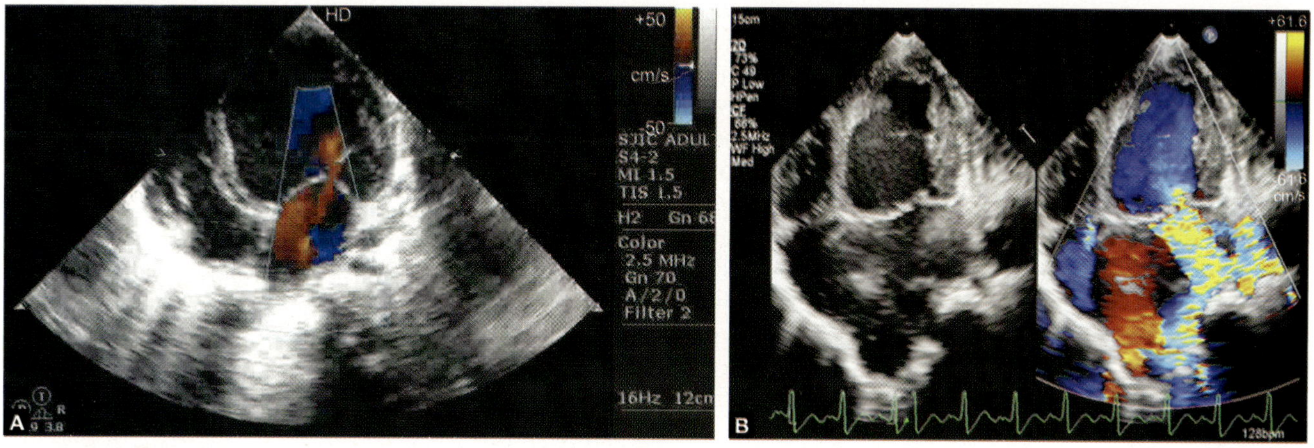

Figs. 5A and B: (A) Apical four-chamber view shows dilated left ventricle with central MR jet without any thickening of mitral valve in an 8-year-old boy with dilated cardiomyopathy. (B) Apical four-chamber view with color Doppler shows thickened mitral valve with mitral valve prolapse, exccentric wall hugging jet of MR with reflux into pulmonary viens in an 8-year-old girl with ARF. (ARF: acute rheumatic fever; MR: mitral regurgitation)

TABLE 3: Shows Vijaya's echo score.

Sl. No.	Echo feature	Score
1.	Thicknesses of mitral and aortic leaflets >4 mm	2
2.	Mitral, aortic, or tricuspid regurgitation	2
3.	Prolapse of mitral, aortic, or tricuspid valves	2
4.	Rheumatic nodules, giving beaded appearance	2
5.	Reduced mobility of leaflets	2
6.	Chordal tear	2
7.	Increased echogenicity of submitral structures	2
8.	Pericardial effusion	2
	Total score	16

of finding a normal heart or finding unrelated causes of murmurs in this population. Timely echocardiography can change epidemiological face of ARF.

THERAPEUTIC IMPLICATIONS

The focus in the current AHA guidelines is on epidemiological differences seen in high-risk and low-risk populations, so that more ARF patients are detected in time and receive secondary prophylaxis. Patients with carditis are more likely to be detected during their first attacks of ARF. There is a significant prognostic implication of finding a normal heart or finding unrelated causes of murmurs in this population. Timely echo can change epidemiological face of ARF.

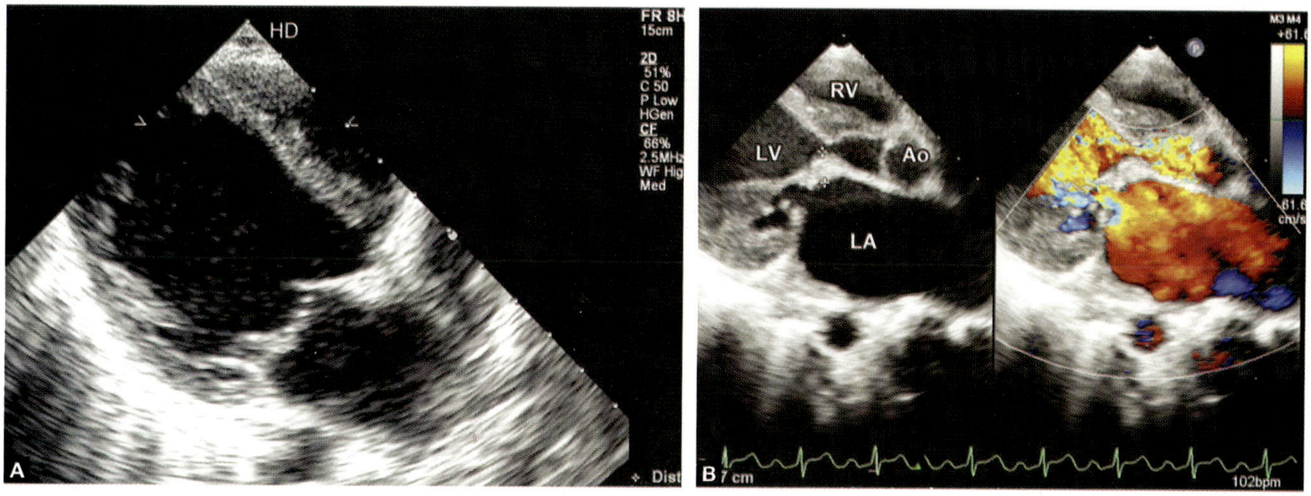

Figs. 6A and B: (A) Parasternal long-axis view in a 4-year-old patient with clinical diagnosis of mucopolysaccharidosis with MR shows myxomatous redundant mitral valve with prolapse of scallops. Echo score is 4; MVP, 2; and MR, 2. Hence, this MR is not of rheumatic etiology. (B) Parasternal long-axis view in a 10-year-old boy clinical diagnosis of MR and AR shows mitral and aortic valve thickening, 2; hyperechogenic submitral structures, 2; MR and AR, 2; beaded appearance, 2. The echo score is 8. Hence, this is of rheumatic etiology. (AR: aortic regurgitation; MR: mitral regurgitation; MVP: mitral valve prolapse)

Medical

Medical management includes mainly secondary prevention of ARF, because ARF is a recurrent disease with recurrence per infection of 40–60%. Permanent cardiac damage increases with every recurrence. For this medical management, echocardiography plays an important role in detecting the degree of valvulitis and valve regurgitation. If there is significant regurgitation of mechanical ventilation (MV) and/or atrioventricular then angiotensin-converting-enzyme inhibitors are given to preserve LV geometry and prevent LV failure.

Surgical

The medical treatment is not curative in some rare cases of chordal rupture and severe MR due to flail mitral valve (Fig. 7A). In such cases, mitral valve repair/replacement, mitral annuloplasty, mitral valve repair gives excellent results. For all this, the echocardiography plays a crucial role in management strategy and avoids complications due to abuse of steroids.

DISCUSSIONS

Pathogenesis of ARF and RHD is a complex maze of events that are immunologically intricate, pathologically significant, and clinically devastating for the patients.[1] Hence, precise early diagnosis and appropriate management of ARF is very important. Echo is useful in precise and early diagnosis of carditis in ARF. It is a key technique used to assess the valve damage, decide the management strategy, and monitor the progression of chronic RHD.

Despite the modification, revision, and re-revision of Jones criteria repeatedly, the "CARDITIS" in ARF is underdiagnosed, leading to nearly 50% of RHD patients detected in heart checkup camps are not aware and 70% of patients do not receive prophylaxis. Relying on traditional characteristic, auscultatory findings for diagnosis of carditis lead to either underdiagnosis or overdiagnosis. The accurate diagnosis of "CARDITIS" is very essential, as timely management can make the heart normal in 35–40% of cases and prevent recrudescence of rheumatic activity and further damage to the valves by adequate secondary prophylaxis. Subclinical carditis refers exclusively to the circumstance in which classic auscultatory findings of valvar dysfunction either are not present or are not recognized by the diagnosing clinician, but Doppler studies reveal pathological mitral or aortic regurgitation due to valvulitis.[5] Echocardiography is now recognized as an essential clinical compliment to the physical exam, electrocardiogram, and serum diagnostic studies. Up until this point, echocardiographic findings were not considered essential and had always been considered secondary to other clinical findings of carditis. More than 25 studies are available to substantiate subclinical carditis. A review of 23 articles showed the prevalence of subclinical carditis from 0% to 53%, emphasizing the high variability of the finding. This includes two of our large series from India. Pooled evidence puts the prevalence of subclinical carditis at 16.8% of ARF.[5] Importantly, newer evidence suggests that by adding subclinical carditis, identified by echocardiography, an additional 15–20% of patients with ARF can be identified who otherwise would have been missed.[6,7] The valve is slightly thickened and displays small vegetations—"verrucae" seen on echocardiography as

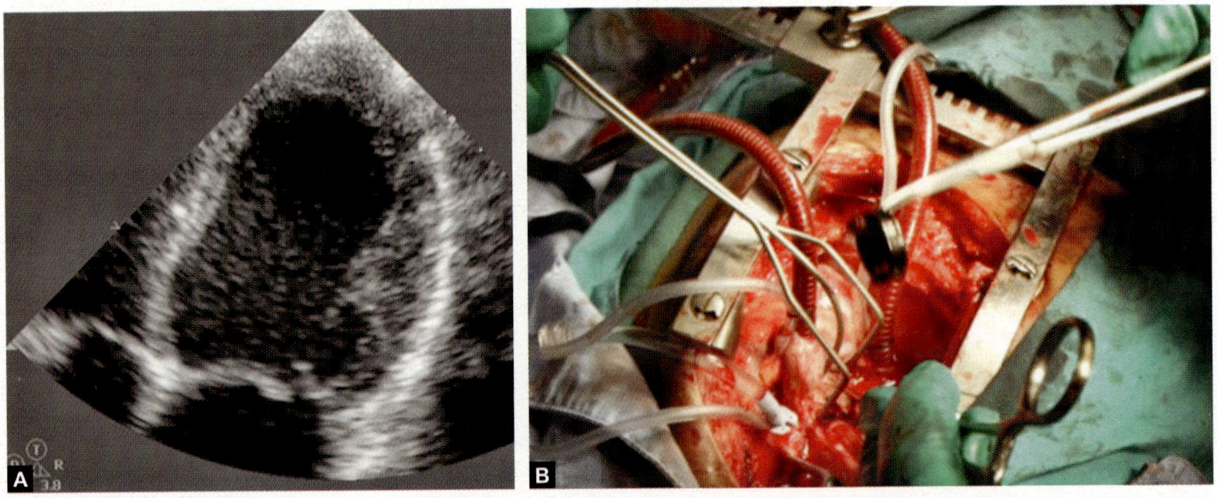

Figs. 7A and B: Echo shows chordal tear of both AML and PML with severe MR caused by flail MV underwent surgery after rheumatic activity subsided in a 14-year-old boy. (AML: anterior mitral leaflet; MR: mitral regurgitation; MV: mechanical ventilation; PML: posterior mitral leaflet)

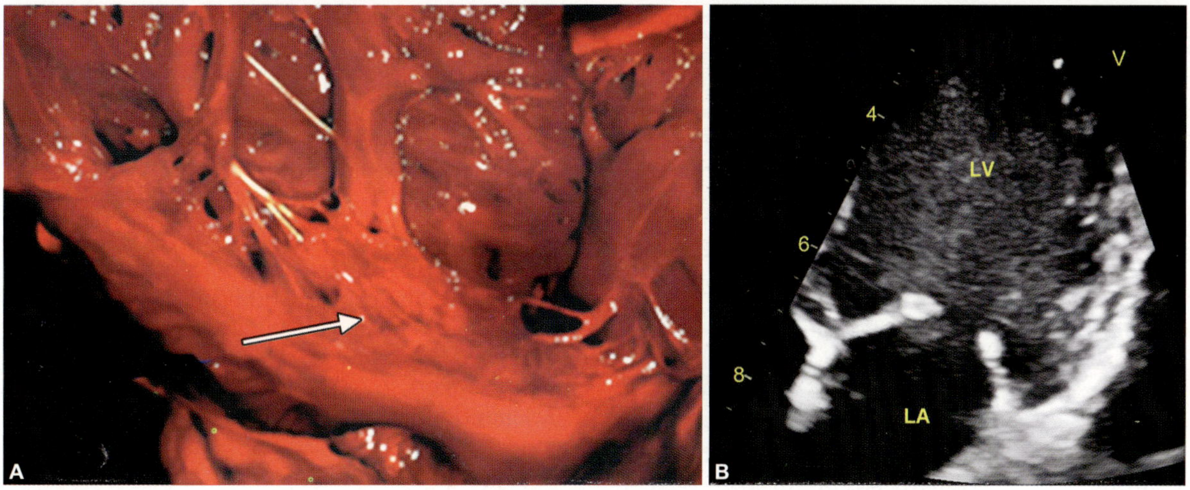

Figs. 8A and B: (A) Small verrucae on free edge of valve seen as nodule in autopsy case of ARF. (B) Apical two-chamber view shows thickened club-like nodule at the tip of AML and PML in a 9-year-old girl with ARF. (ARF: acute rheumatic fever; AML: anterior mitral leaflet; PML: posterior mitral leaflet)

thickened nodules. The nodules are seen just proximal to free edge of MV, where the cusps come into apposition, at the site of maximum natural trauma (*see* Fig. 3B). Nodules on body and tip of mitral leaflets do not have chaotic motion, such as vegetation, and may reduce in size or disappear on follow-up (Fig. 8B). The nodules on the valves may be equivalents of verrucae seen/at autopsy in patients who died of ARF.[8]

Limitation: There are no long-term double blind studies to show what happens to subclinical carditis with and without secondary prophylaxis.

GUIDELINES[5]

Technology-driven (ECHO) and also focus on epidemiological differences seen in high-risk and low-risk populations, so that more ARF patients are detected in time. In view of the heterogeneity in global disease burden, a single set of diagnostic criteria may no longer be sufficient for all population groups and in all geographic regions. The addition of echocardiography and Doppler to the armamentarium of tests in the diagnosis of ARF will lead to diagnosis of more cases. The introduction of especially subclinical carditis and polyarthralgia as major criteria in high-risk populations, such as in India, will bring more patients into the net of secondary prophylaxis.

Echocardiography with Doppler should be performed in all cases of confirmed and suspected ARF.

- Echocardiography with Doppler should be performed in all cases of confirmed and suspected ARF (Class I; Level of Evidence B).
- It is reasonable to consider performing serial echocardiography/Doppler studies in any patient with diagnosed or suspected ARF even if documented carditis is not present on diagnosis (Class IIa; Level of Evidence C).
- Echocardiography/Doppler testing should be performed (strictly fulfilling the findings) to assess whether carditis is present in the absence of auscultatory findings, particularly in moderate-to-high-risk populations and when ARF is considered likely (Class I; Level of Evidence B).
- Echocardiography/Doppler findings not consistent with carditis should exclude that diagnosis in patients with a heart murmur otherwise thought to indicate rheumatic carditis (Class I; Level of Evidence B).

Arthritis and Polyarthritis

At present, consideration that monoarthritis may be a part of the ARF spectrum should be limited to patients from moderate-to-high-risk populations (Class I; Level of Evidence C). The inclusion of polyarthralgia as a major manifestation is applicable only for moderate- or high-incidence populations and only after careful consideration and exclusion of other causes of arthralgia, such as autoimmune, viral, or reactive arthropathies (Class IIb; Level of Evidence C).[5]

Evidence of Preceding Streptococcal Infection[5]

- Increased or rising antistreptolysin O titer or other streptococcal antibodies (anti-deoxyribonuclease B) (Class I; Level of Evidence B). A rise in titer is better evidence than a single-titer result.

- A positive throat culture for group A β-hemolytic streptococci (Class I; Level of Evidence B).
- A positive rapid group A streptococcal carbohydrate antigen test in a child whose clinical presentation suggests a high pretest probability of streptococcal pharyngitis (Class I; Level of Evidence B).

What to do if Diagnosis is not Certain?

- Where there is genuine uncertainty, it is reasonable to consider offering 12 months of secondary prophylaxis followed by reevaluation to include a careful history and physical examination in addition to a repeat echocardiogram (Class IIa; Level of Evidence C).
- In a patient with recurrent symptoms (particularly involving the joints) who has been adherent to prophylaxis recommendations but lacks serological evidence of group A streptococcal infection and lacks echocardiographic evidence of valvulitis, it is reasonable to conclude that the recurrent symptoms are not likely related to ARF, and discontinuation of antibiotic prophylaxis may be appropriate (Class IIa; Level of Evidence C).[5]

CONCLUSION

The accurate diagnosis of "carditis" is very essential, as timely management can make the heart normal in 35–40% of cases and prevent recrudescence of rheumatic activity and further damage to the valves by adequate secondary prophylaxis. In this direction, echocardiography can navigate the evaluation of both clinical and subclinical carditis. Hence, it should be performed in all cases of confirmed and suspected ARF. To avoid morbidity, mortality, heavy expenditure on sophisticated treatment with balloon and valve replacement, in an early precise diagnosis of ARF, more patients are brought in the net of secondary prophylaxis. Echocardiography is a very simple, noninvasive, reproducible, and most useful investigation, which will certainly change the epidemiological face of RHD. Echocardiography as a major criterion for navigation of evaluation should be followed as per revised 2015 Jones criteria.

REFERENCES

1. World Health Organization. Rheumatic fever and rheumatic heart disease: report of a WHO expert consultation. Geneva, 29 Oct-1 Nov 2001. World Health Organ Tech Rep Ser. 2004;923:1-122.
2. Jones TD. Diagnosis of rheumatic fever. JAMA. 1944;126:481-4.
3. Vijayalakshmi IB, Mithravinda J, Deva AN. The role of echocardiography in diagnosing carditis in the setting of acute rheumatic fever. Cardiol Young. 2005;15:583-8.
4. Vijayalakshmi IB, Vishnuprabhu RO, Chitra N, et al. The efficacy of echocardiographic criterions for the diagnosis of carditis in acute rheumatic fever. Cardiol Young. 2008;18:586-92.
5. Gewitz MH, Baltimore RS, Tani LY, et al. Revision of the Jones criteria for the diagnosis of acute rheumatic fever in the era of Doppler echocardiography: a scientific statement from the American Heart Association Committee on Rheumatic Fever, Endocarditis, and Kawasaki Disease of the Council on Cardiovascular Disease in the Young. Circulation. 2015;131:1806-18.
6. Beg A, Sadiq M. Subclinical valvulitis in children with acute rheumatic fever. Pediatr Cardiol. 2008;29:619-23.
7. Caldas AM, Terreri MT, Moises VA, et al. What is the true frequency of carditis in acute rheumatic fever? A prospective clinical and Doppler blind study of 56 children with up to 60 months of follow-up evaluation. Pediatr Cardiol. 2008;29:1048-53.
8. Vasan RS, Shrivastava S, Vijayakumar M, et al. Echocardiographic evaluation of patients with acute rheumatic fever and rheumatic carditis. Circulation. 1996;94:73-82.

69

CHAPTER

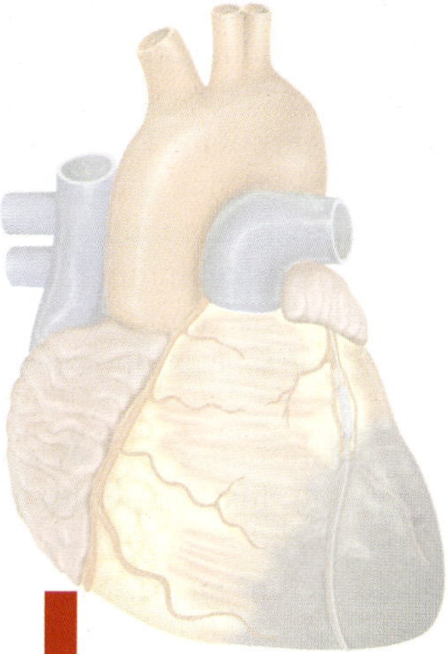

Balloon Valvotomy in Rheumatic Mitral Stenosis: Echocardiographic Evaluation

CN Manjunath, Ravi S Math

INTRODUCTION

Echocardiography has revolutionized the management and diagnosis of rheumatic mitral stenosis (MS). It has become fundamental to the diagnosis of MS, determines the etiology, quantifies the severity, detects concomitant valve involvement, assesses suitability for balloon mitral valvotomy (BMV), and enables serial follow-up. BMV is the procedure of choice for relieving MS. It is recommended for the following groups of patients[1]: (1) symptomatic patients (classes II–IV) with severe MS [mitral valve (MV) area (MVA) ≤ 1.5 cm^2] (class 1 indication) or asymptomatic patients with very severe MS (MVA ≤ 1.0 cm^2) (class 2a indication) with a favorable valve morphology in the absence of left atrial (LA) thrombus and moderate-to-severe mitral regurgitation (MR); (2) asymptomatic patients with severe MS (MVA ≤ 1.5 cm^2) with new-onset atrial fibrillation (AF) and suitable valve anatomy (class 2b indication); (3) symptomatic patients with MVA > 1.5 cm^2 and hemodynamically significant MS during exercise (mean MV gradient >15, pulmonary capillary wedge pressure >25 mm Hg, class 2b indication); and (4) severely symptomatic patients (New York Heart Association classes III–IV) with severe MS (MVA ≤ 1.5 cm^2) with suboptimal valve anatomy and high risk for surgery (class 2b indication). Absolute contraindications to BMV are bicommissural calcification, presence of LA/left atrial appendage (LAA) thrombus, and presence of MR of Grades 3–4 severity. The mechanical obstruction to the mitral inflow can be assessed by a two-dimensional (2D) or three-dimensional (3D) echocardiography (3DE), whereas the functional consequences of MS can be discerned by Doppler echocardiography. Despite the availability of 3DE, the backbone of a good echocardiographic evaluation of MS remains a thorough 2D scan and a careful Doppler assessment. This chapter will assess the role of echocardiography before, during, and after BMV that is relevant to day-to-day practice.

BEFORE BALLOON MITRAL VALVOTOMY

Historically, MS was first evaluated by M-mode echocardiography.[2] This showed thickened MV leaflets, reduced amplitude of E and A waves, and reduced EF slope (Fig. 1). Due to leaflet rigidity, the posterior mitral leaflet (PML) does not move posteriorly during diastole; rather, it parallels the motion of anterior mitral leaflet (AML). It is a semiquantitative method and has a limited role in the current era. The 2D echocardiography helps evaluate the morphology and severity of obstruction at the mitral valvular and subvalvular level. In addition, it enables assessment of the size and functions of cardiac chambers, presence of clot, pericardial effusion, and associated valvular abnormalities, all of which have a bearing on the management decisions related to MS. Each component of the MV apparatus should be assessed individually (Fig. 2). These consist of the AML and PML, medial and lateral commissures, and the submitral apparatus (the anteromedial and posterolateral papillary muscles and

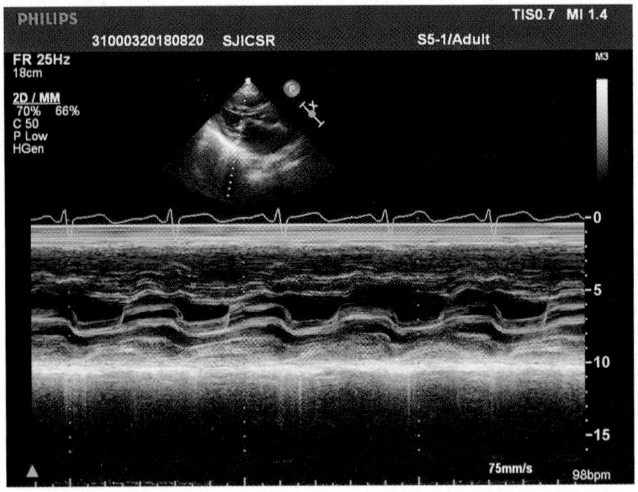

Fig. 1: M-mode echocardiography showing reduced EF slope, thickened leaflets, and anterior motion of posterior mitral leaflet.

the chordae tendineae connecting papillary muscles to the leaflet surfaces). The leaflets show doming, asymmetric thickening, nodularity, restricted movement, calcification, or prolapse. Typically, there is a hockey-stick appearance of the AML (Fig. 2A) and restricted mobility of the PML. Due to leaflet rigidity and thickening, the PML does not move posteriorly during diastole, rather it parallels the motion of AML. The thickening is usually uneven with thin hinge points in midportion and thickened base and tips. The leaflet morphology is best seen in parasternal long-axis and apical views.

The commissures are best seen in the parasternal short-axis view (Fig. 2B). They may be split, fused, thickened, partially, or fully calcified. To determine if an area is calcified, it is necessary to turn down the gain sufficiently to hide most of the other cardiac structure. If the area still remains bright, it is said to be calcified. Another indicator

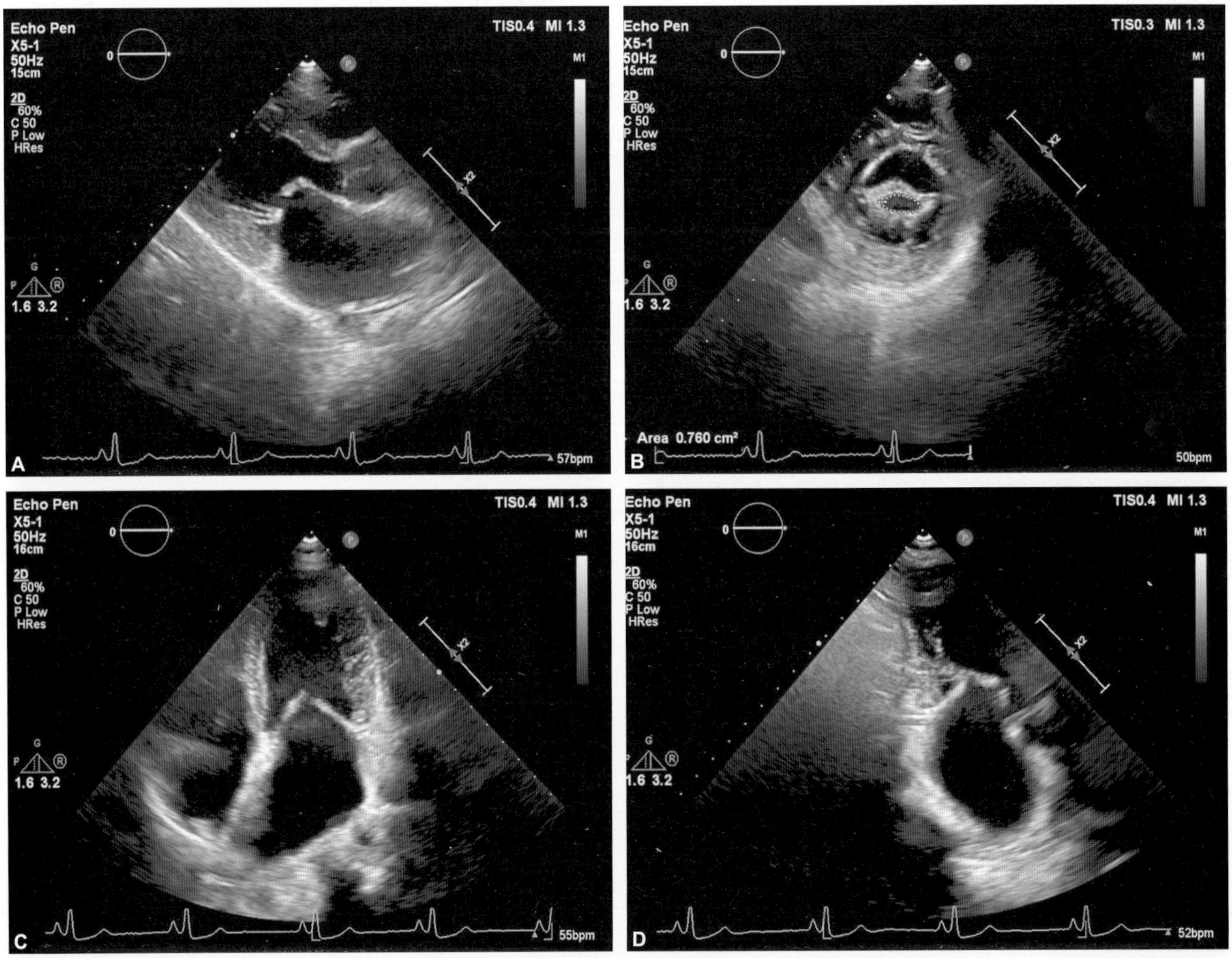

Figs. 2A to D: (A) Parasternal long-axis view showing hockey-stick appearance (doming) of anterior mitral leaflet. Posterior mitral leaflet is thickened, shortened with reduced mobility. (B) Parasternal short-axis view showing fused commissures giving "fish-mouth appearance." (C) Apical four-chamber view. (D) Apical two-chamber view showing anterior and posterior papillary muscles which are thickened and deformed.

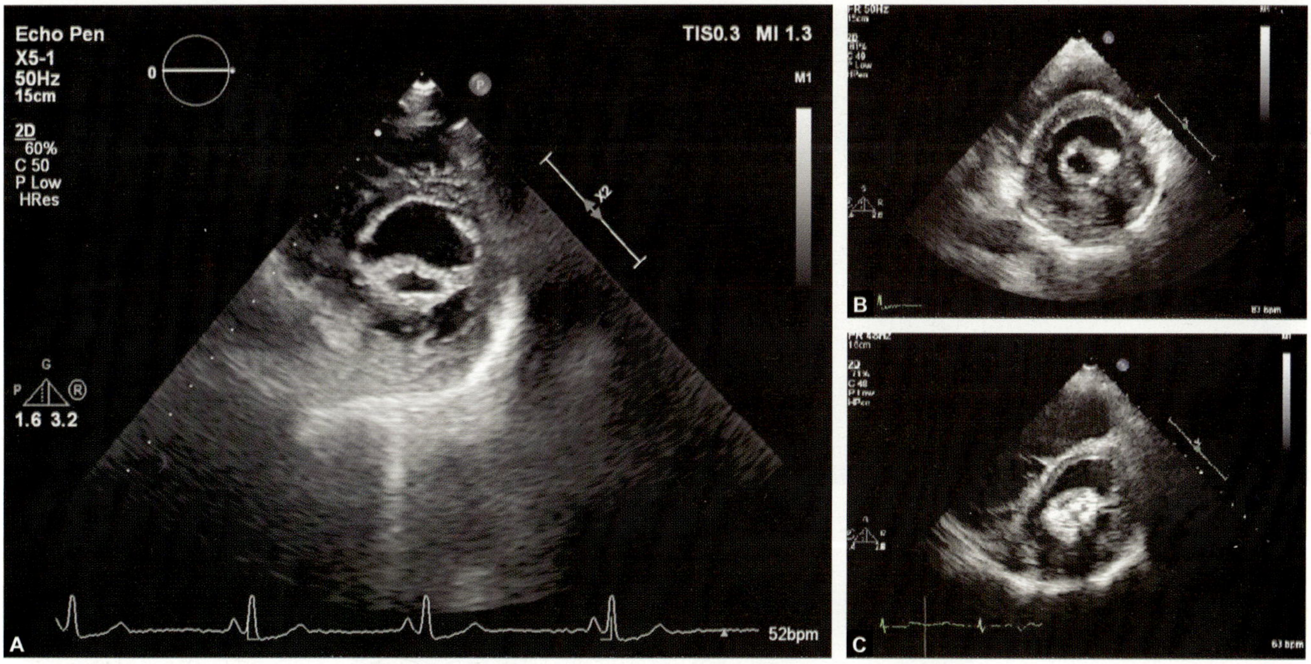

Figs. 3A to C: Parasternal short-axis view (A) medial and lateral commissures are fused and thickened. No calcification seen. (B) Lateral commissure calcified and fused. (C) Both medial and lateral commissures are fused and calcified.

of calcification is shadowing. Calcification of commissures is the most important factor in deciding BMV as the mechanism of BMV is splitting of commissures (Figs. 3A to C). Increasing commissural calcification leads to greater complications. Bilateral commissural calcification is a contraindication for BMV (Fig. 3C). However, patients with unilateral commissural calcification may still undergo BMV using a graded inflation technic. The subvalvular apparatus consists of the chordae tendinae and the two papillary muscles (Figs. 2D and 4A to C). The subvalvular apparatus thickens and retracts with advancing disease. At times, it may so happen that the narrowest portion of the MV is located in the subvalvular apparatus rather than at the tips of leaflets. The subvalvular apparatus is best evaluated in parasternal long-axis view where tilting and gently adjusting the probe anteriorly or posteriorly will bring into focus the anterolateral or the posteromedial papillary muscle, respectively. Another useful view is the apical two-chamber view (with a slight tilt, Fig. 2D). Lastly, the apical four-chamber view can be used to further delineate the subvalvular apparatus (Figs. 4A to C). Increasing degrees of subvalvular deformity leads to increasing complications and reduced success rates. As the MV is a complex 3D structure, it is important to utilize all possible views to inspect the valvular and subvalvular structures.

Assessment of Mitral Stenosis Severity

The normal MVA is 4–6 cm^2. A MV gradient is rare in patients with an MVA > 2 cm^2. In the past, MS was classified as mild, moderate, and severe using MVA cutoffs of >1.5 cm^2, 1–1.5 cm^2, and <1 cm^2, respectively (Table 1).[3] A new staging system has now been proposed similar to the heart failure staging system.[1] Patients are classified as being in Stages A to D ranging from at risk patients (Stage A) to progressive obstruction (Stage B), to severe asymptomatic (Stage C), and symptomatic MS (Stage D). The definition of "severe" MS has now been based on the severity at which symptoms occur and at a level when interventional treatment improves symptoms. Severe MS has now been defined as ≤1.5 cm^2 unlike previous guidelines where it was ≤1.0 cm^2. Patients with MVA ≤ 1.0 cm^2 are considered to have very severe MS (Table 2). This makes comparisons with historical cohorts problematic. For the sake of consistency, we will use the American College of Cardiology 2006 definitions of mild, moderate, and severe MS. It needs to be emphasized that the classification of MS as mild, moderate, and severe is based on theoretical thresholds of pulmonary edema at a certain cardiac output, heart rate, and MVA. The MV gradient is directly proportional to the square of mitral flow in diastole (cardiac output) and inversely proportional to the time in diastole (heart rate). Thus, even patients with mild MS

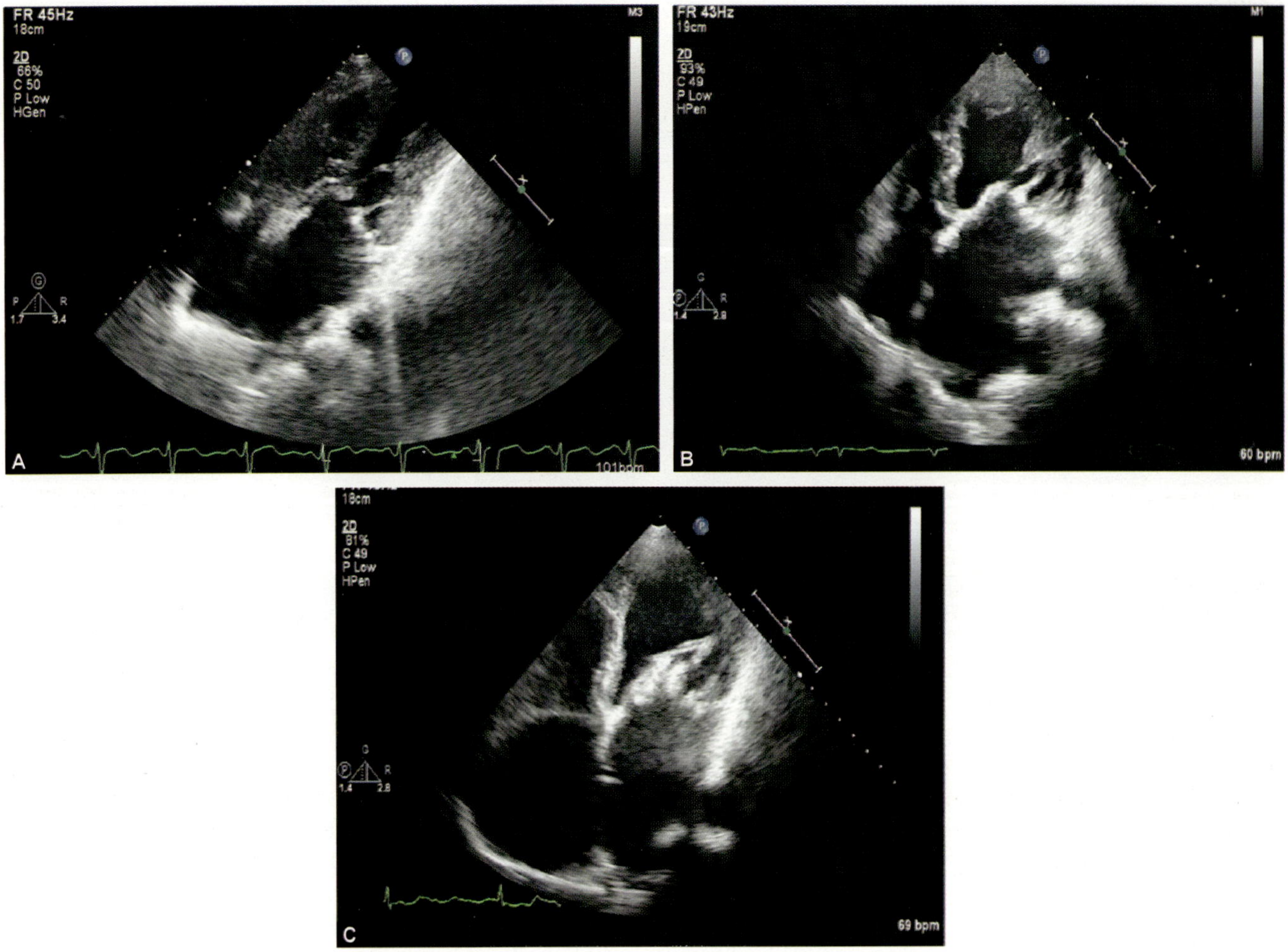

Figs. 4A to C: Apical four-chamber view showing—(A) mild, (B) moderate, and (C) severe degrees of subvalvular disease.

TABLE 1: Mitral stenosis severity as per ACC/AHA 2006 guidelines.[3]

Mild MS	MVA >1.5 cm^2, mean gradient <5 mm Hg*, PASP <30 mm Hg
Moderate MS	MVA 1–1.5 cm^2, mean gradient 5–10 mm Hg*, PASP 30–50 mm Hg
Severe MS	MVA <1.0 cm^2, mean gradient >10 mm Hg*, PASP >50 mm Hg

(ACC/AHA: American College of Cardiology/American Heart Association; MS: mitral stenosis; MVA: mitral valve area; PASP: pulmonary artery systolic pressure)
*Valve gradients are dependent upon transvalvular flow. The gradients suggested in this table assume a normal cardiac output and may not pertain to patients with abnormally high or low transvalvular flows. Criteria applicable when heart rate between 60 and 90 beats/min.
Source: Data from American College of Cardiology/American Heart Association 2006 Guidelines for the Management of Patients with Valvular Heart Disease.[5]

TABLE 2: Stages and severity of mitral stenosis.[1]

Stage	*Definition*	*Valve anatomy*	*Valve hemodynamics*	*Hemodynamic consequences*	*Symptoms*
A	At risk of MS	Mild diastolic valve doming	Normal transmitral flow velocity	None	None
B	Progressive MS	1. Rheumatic valve changes with commissural fusion and diastolic doming of the mitral valve leaflets 2. Planimetered MVA >1.5 cm^2	1. Increased transmitral flow velocities 2. MVA > 1.5 cm^2 3. Diastolic pressure half-time <150 ms	1. Mild-to-moderate LA enlargement 2. Normal pulmonary pressure at rest	None

Contd...

Contd...

Stage	*Definition*	*Valve anatomy*	*Valve hemodynamics*	*Hemodynamic consequences*	*Symptoms*
C	Asymptomatic severe MS	1. Rheumatic valve changes with commissural fusion and diastolic doming of the mitral valve leaflets 2. Planimetered MVA ≤ 1.5 cm^2 (MVA ≤ 1.0 cm^2 with very severe MS)	1. MVA ≤ 1.5 cm^2 (MVA ≤ 1.0 cm^2 with very severe MS) 2. Diastolic pressure half-time ≥150 ms (diastolic pressure half-time ≥220 ms with very severe MS)	1. Severe LA enlargement 2. Elevated PASP > 30 mm Hg	None
D	Symptomatic severe MS	1. Rheumatic valve changes with commissural fusion and diastolic doming of the mitral valve leaflets 2. Planimetered MVA ≤ 1.5 cm^2	1. MVA ≤ 1.5 cm^2 (MVA ≤ 1.0 cm^2 with very severe MS) 2. Diastolic pressure half-time ≥150 ms (diastolic pressure half-time ≥220 ms with very severe MS)	1. Severe LA enlargement 2. Elevated PASP > 30 mm Hg	1. Reduced exercise tolerance 2. Exertional dyspnea

(LA: left atrial; MS: mitral stenosis; MVA: mitral valve area; PASP: pulmonary artery systolic pressure)
Data from American College of Cardiology/American Heart Association 2014 Guidelines for the Management of Patients with Valvular Heart Disease.[1]

may develop pulmonary edema. Thus the management of MS (including the decision to perform BMV) should not be based solely on arbitrary cutoff values of MVA. Rather, it should be viewed as a disease spectrum taking into consideration the hemodynamic and symptomatic status of the individual patient.

Planimetry

The most accurate method to assess MVA is by planimetry by an experienced operator. This is done in the parasternal short-axis view (Fig. 5). The foundation for a good short-axis view is an optimal parasternal long-axis view wherein the maximum excursion of the mitral leaflets should be at the center of the screen. From this point, the transducer is rotated clockwise to obtain the short-axis view. The typical "fish mouth" appearance of the MV is seen. Certain important features need to be borne in mind. The cross section should be uninterrupted with no echocardiography dropouts. Second, it should be the most apical cross section. Lastly, the area should be measured in middiastole. This can be easily determined in the presence of electrocardiography gating but can also be deducible as the maximal outward excursion of the leaflets. Usually multiple estimations (at least three) should be done and averaged. This is especially important in AF and the cases of incomplete commissural fusion. Finally, the area seen within the commissures is also a part of the cross-sectional area and hence should be included in the measurement.

If the estimated MVA does not fit with the overall echocardiographic picture, multiple measurements of MVA should be taken. For example, moderate MS by MVA in the presence of severe pulmonary artery (PA) hypertension (PAH), controlled heart rates, and no other pathology identified. A useful semiquantitative method for estimating MS severity is the mitral leaflet separation (MLS) index.[4] This measures the distance between the tips of the mitral leaflets in diastole in parasternal long-axis and apical four-chamber view (Figs. 6A and B). While there is significant overlap, values of less than 0.8 cm and more than 1.2 cm can diagnose severe and nonsevere MS reliably.

Continuous Wave Doppler

Despite its shortcomings, continuous wave (CW) Doppler forms an essential part in the assessment of MS severity. It is easy and quickly reproducible. It not only provides the pressure gradient across the MV but also enables the estimation of MVA by the pressure halftime (PHT) method. The pressure gradient is measured using the simplified Bernoulli equation. It is done in the apical four-chamber view with the beam aligned to maximal turbulence (as assessed by color flow Doppler). The mean diastolic gradient (MDG) is the most important parameter that indicates the hemodynamic severity (Fig. 7A). The heart rate should always be reported. In the presence of AF, an average of 5 beats should be taken as MDG of <5 mm Hg, 5–10 mm Hg, and >10 mm Hg which indicates mild, moderate, and severe MS (for stable heart rates of 60–80 beats/min).[3] As the MDG is affected by other parameters, such as heart rate, cardiac output, and the presence of MR, it is only a useful complementary tool for assessing MS severity.

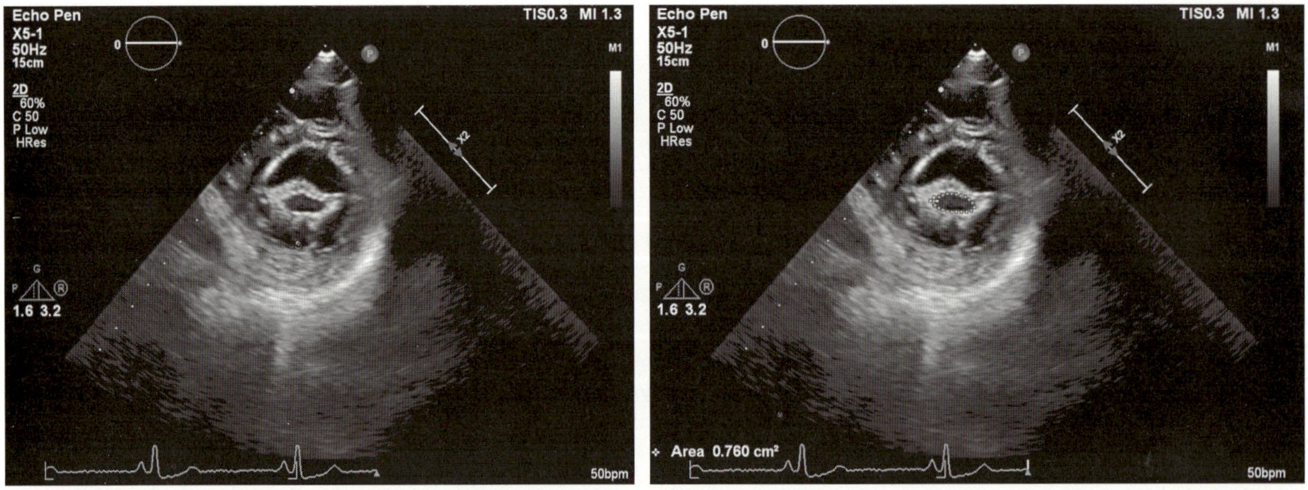

Fig. 5: Calculation of mitral valve area by planimetry. Mitral valve area of 0.76 cm^2.

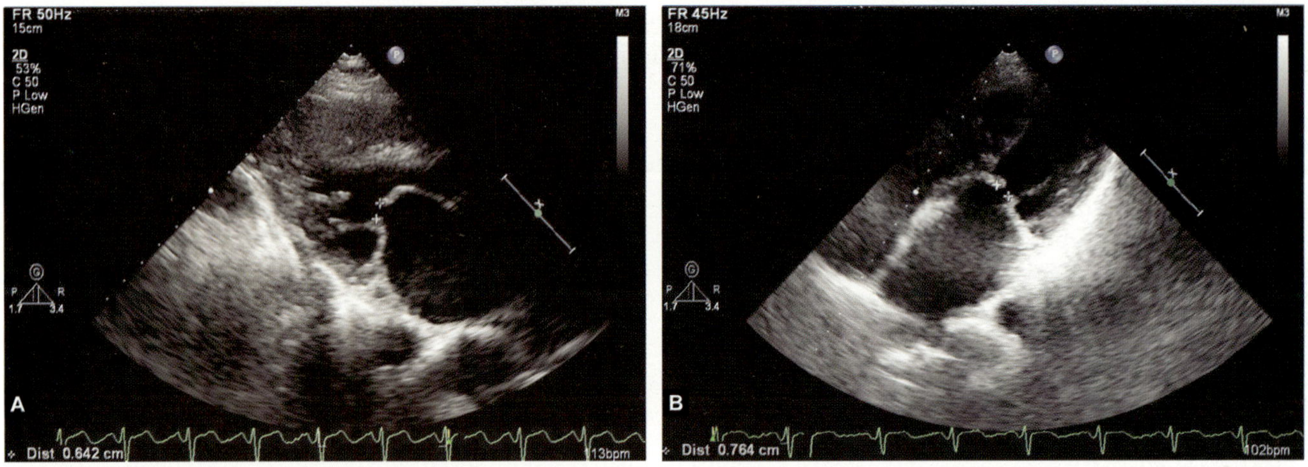

Figs. 6A and B: Mitral leaflet separation index. Average of the maximum distance between the leaflet tips in diastole in the parasternal long-axis (A) and apical four-chamber view (B). A value <0.8 cm denotes severe MS. (MS: mitral stenosis).

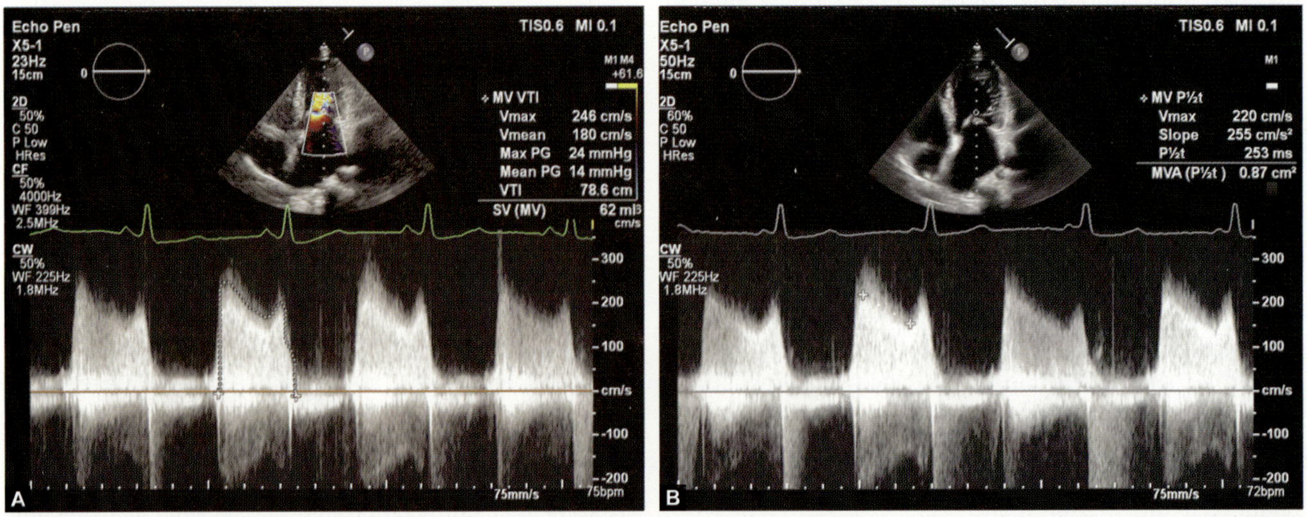

Figs. 7A and B: Continuous wave Doppler across mitral valve: (A) mean transmitral gradient of 14 mm Hg at heart rate of 75 beats/min, (B) calculation of MVA by pressure half-time method. The MVA is 0.87 cm^2 which is very close to MVA by planimetry as in Figure 4 (0.76 cm^2). (MVA: mitral valve area).

Pressure halftime is the time in milliseconds for the transmitral gradient to decrease by half of its original value in early diastole. It was developed by Hatle et al.[5] who provided the equation for empirical calculation of MVA from PHT. MVA (cm^2) = 220/T1/2 (ms) where T1/2 is the PHT on the deceleration slope of the E wave. The CW Doppler trace is used for this purpose (Fig. 7B). The gain and filter settings should be optimized to get a clear trace and the sweep speed increased to 75–100 mm/s. Sometimes, the deceleration slope is not even and has a rapid initial deceleration. In such cases the deceleration slope in the middiastole (instead of early diastole) should be employed. Very short cycles of AF should be avoided. An average of multiple cycles should be taken in AF. While the PHT method shows good accuracy to cardiac catheterization in estimation MVA, it is affected by LA compliance, initial LA diastolic pressure, as well as left ventricular (LV) diastolic function. It is unreliable immediately after percutaneous transvenous mitral commissurotomy (PTMC) where there is a sudden change in LA compliance. Other methods to assess MVA include the continuity equation and the proximal isovelocity surface area method. These are time consuming and not commonly used in routine clinical practice. They remain useful in experienced hands. The assessment of PA pressures (PAPs) and its effects on the right-sided cardiac chambers form a critical aspect of assessment of MS severity. While there is no strict correlation between MVA and PAH, generally PAPs increase with the increasing severity of MS and can be used to prognosticate as well as decide management in borderline cases. The commonest method to estimate PA systolic pressure is by calculating the maximum velocity (and thus gradient) of a regurgitant jet across the tricuspid valve (TV) and adding this gradient to presumed right atrial (RA) pressure (this is done by visualizing inferior vena cava). Most of the cases with MS have tricuspid regurgitation (TR), allowing estimation of PAPs. Multiple views of TR gradient should be used in addition to the standard four-chamber view, e.g. modified two-chamber apical view, tilted parasternal long-axis view, epigastric view, etc. The dense part of the spectral envelope should be used to calculate TR gradient. With the development of fixed PAH and right ventricular (RV) dysfunction, reduction in cardiac output may actually lower PAP. Development of PAH [pulmonary artery systolic pressure (PASP) > 30 mm Hg], at baseline or after exercise stress, implies significant MS that needs to be corrected while severe PAH (PASP > 50 mm Hg) due to MS should be addressed on a priority basis because of its impact on survival. With severe PAH, there is progressive dilatation of right atrium and ventricle, and flattening of the interventricular septum causing a D-shaped left ventricle. With severe RV dilatation, it is important to measure the (tricuspid annulus) TV annulus diameter in four-chamber apical view during diastole, in case the patient is destined for open heart surgery. A TV annulus of >40 mm or >21 mm/m^2 body surface area (BSA) is an indication for TV annuloplasty, even if TR is mild.

Color Doppler

Color Doppler echocardiography is essential for the assessment of coexistent MR which may be central or eccentric (Figs. 8A and B). Central MR is usually due to a fixed mitral orifice and regresses after successful PTMC. Thus patients, with central MR with a grade of ≤2/4 can undergo PTMC. Greater degrees of central MR warrant surgical intervention. Eccentric MR may be due to AML prolapse or severe subvalvular diseases, both of which increase the risk of severe MR during PTMC. Thus, an eccentric MR of Grade 2/4 severity should lead to surgical intervention if the patient is not high risk for surgery. Patients with mild eccentric MR (Grade 1/4) may undergo BMV if there are no other high-risk morphological parameters [e.g. severe small vessel disease (SVD), severe calcification]. An inappropriately enlarged LA is a clue to significant MR. Different views should be used to quantify the degree of MR and its origin. The assessment of MR should be done in at least apical four- and two-chamber views, parasternal long-axis view, and short-axis (commissural level). The quantification of MR is done as in other causes of MR. Color Doppler echocardiography also provides clues to the severity of MS and presence of subvalvular disease. A turbulent jet with a mosaic pattern suggests significant MS (Fig. 8C). However, this may not be so in the cases with poor antegrade flow (e.g. decreased cardiac output). On the other hand, a laminar flow across the MV indicates a successful PTMC. The presence of more than one antegrade jets suggests the presence of extensive SVD.

Evaluation of the Mitral Valve Apparatus for Suitability of Percutaneous Transvenous Mitral Commissurotomy

Balloon mitral valvotomy is the preferred modality for relieving MS. The selection of the optimal patient for BMV is based on echocardiography. As mentioned earlier, there are three absolute contraindications for BMV, namely the presence of LA/LAA thrombus, extensive bicommissural calcification, and severe MR, all of which are determined by echocardiography (Grades 3–4). The outcomes of BMV are determined by valve morphology. These outcomes include the short-term outcomes in terms of achieving the desirable increase in MVA and/or the development of severe MR and the long-term outcomes in terms of attrition of MVA, redo-interventions and survival. Various scores have been utilized

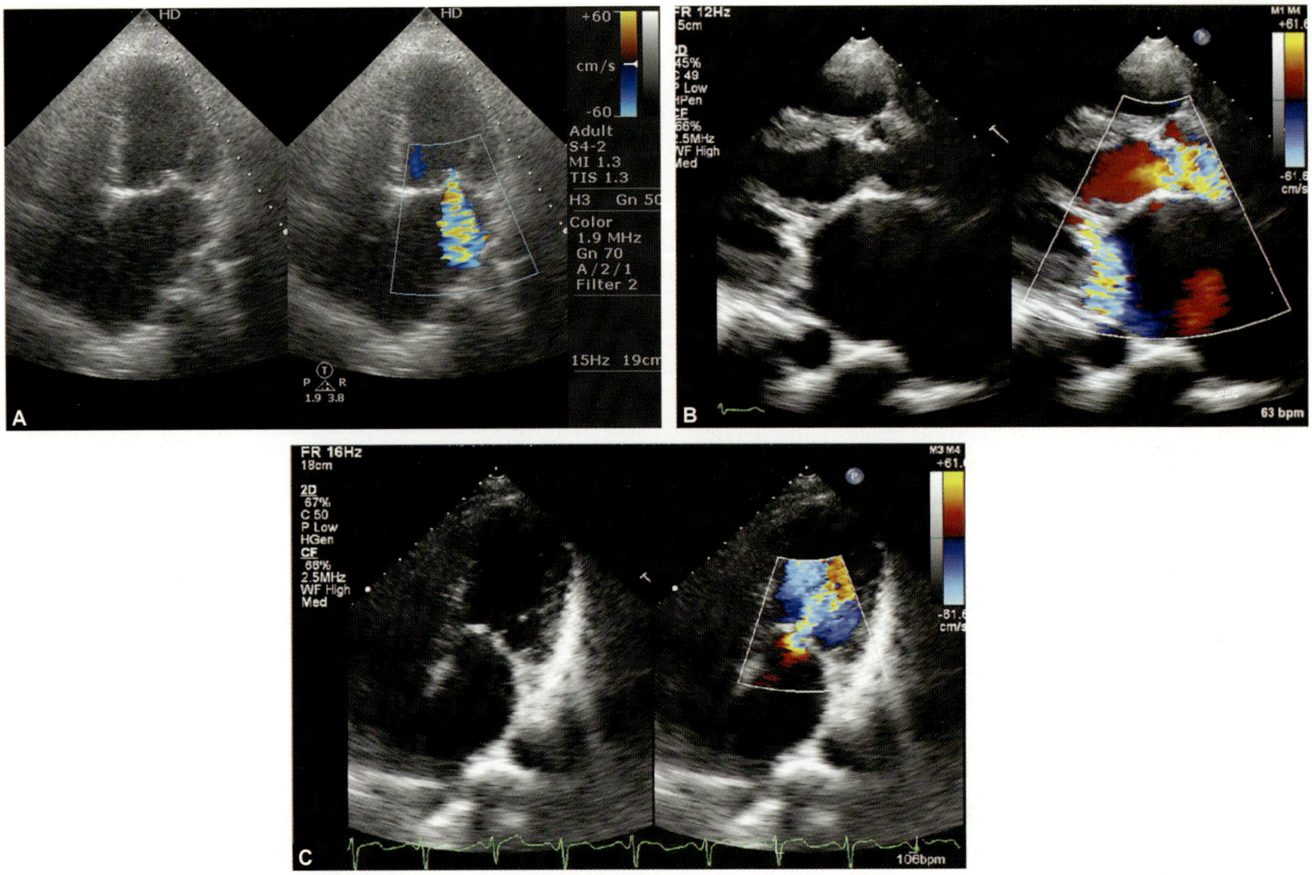

Figs. 8A to C: Color Doppler echocardiography. (A) Severe MS with moderate central MR. Patient underwent successful BMV. (B) Severe MS with moderate eccentric MR. Patient did not undergo BMV. (C) Severe MS showing turbulent jet with mosaic pattern. (BMV: balloon mitral valvotomy; MR: mitral regurgitation; MS: mitral stenosis).

to aid in the selection of the ideal patient. The multitude of scores is a testimony that no one echocardiographic score is perfect. Second, most echocardiographic scores use a combination of variables to determine outcomes. Some of the scores tend to predict procedural success better, whereas others predict the development of MR. Third, no particular value of an individual score is by itself a contraindication to BMV. Patients with a high (adverse) score can still achieve a good result but the success rates are less. In such a scenario, it is essential to assess other clinical characteristics. Those patients who are at a high surgical risk may be offered PTMC despite unfavorable anatomic characteristics (e.g. elderly, kyphoscoliosis, renal failure, cardiac failure, chronic obstructive airway disease, etc.). Finally, as the focus of BMV is on commissural splitting, most interventionalist believe that it is the commissural morphology that is most important. PTMC is a relative contraindication if the obstruction is subvalvular without any commissural fusion.

The oldest and the most commonly used score is the Massachusetts General Hospital score or the Wilkins score[6] (Table 3). It scores the four variables on a scale of 1–4 with the range of score being 4–16. No specific score is a complete contraindication for PTMC. A score <8 with no more than moderate MR is the best candidate for PTMC. This does not mean that those with a score of >8 are denied BMV. The latter may still undergo BMV with the understanding that success rates will be lower. The valve morphology becomes more adverse with increasing score. However, as it does not take into account commissural morphology and asymmetry of scarring, several studies have shown its poor ability to predict acute leaflet tear (and subsequent severe MR) and success following PTMC. Nunes et al.[7] developed a new score addressing the shortcomings of the Wilkins score incorporating commissural morphology and maximal leaflet displacement in diastole. They validated it in a separate patient population with good results. Baseline MVA ≤1 cm^2, maximum leaflet displacement, commissural area ratio, and subvalvular thickening were the only factors found significant. However, the overall calculation of score is lengthy and cumbersome. Lung and Cormier[8] devised a simpler score measuring the length of chordae of AML in

TABLE 3: Components and scoring of the Wilkins or the MGH score.[6]

Grade	*Mobility*	*Thickening*	*Calcification*	*Subvalvular disease*
1	Highly mobile with only leaflet tip restricted	Near normal thickness 4–5 mm	Single area of increased echo brightness	Minimal thickening just below the leaflets
2	Leaflet mid and base have normal mobility	Mid leaflet normal; considerable thickening of margins 5–8 mm	Scattered area of echo brightness confined to leaflet margins	Thickening of the chordal structures extending to one third of the chordal length
3	Valve moves forward in diastole, mainly from base	Thickening throughout the leaflet 5–8 mm	Brightness extending to midportion of the leaflet	Thickening of the chordal structures extending to distal one third of the chordal length
4	No or minimal forward movement of leaflet in diastole	Considerable thickening of the entire leaflet tissue >8–10 mm	Extensive brightness throughout the leaflet tissue	Extensive thickening and shortening of all chordae extending down to the papillary muscles

TABLE 4: Lung and Cormier risk score for commissurotomy.[8]

Grade	*Description*
1	Pliable noncalcific AML and mild subvalvular disease (thin chordae ≥10 mm long)
2	Pliable noncalcific AML and severe subvalvular disease (thickened chordae <10 mm long)
3	Calcification of mitral valve of any extent on fluoroscopy irrespective of SVD extent

(AML: anterior mitral leaflet: SVD: small vessel disease)

the parasternal long-axis view on echocardiography and assessing calcification on fluoroscopy (Table 4). Fluoroscopy was advised because of the difficulty of differentiating calcification with nodular fibrosis on echocardiography. Another method is to examine the calcium (Canaan score[9]) in each of the anterolateral and posteromedial commissures. The extent of commissural calcification is quantified by giving each half of the commissures a score of one. Commissural calcification can therefore range from Grade 0 (no calcification) to grade. Commissural calcium was defined by bright echocardiographic density with acoustic shadowing. Calcium was said to be present if the brightness was more as compared to that of adjacent aortic root. Increasing commissural calcium with this score identifies poor outcome after PTMC, especially among those with Wilkins' score ≤8.

Padial et al.[10] devised a score consisting of extent and unevenness of individual leaflet thickness and calcification, commissural calcium, and subvalvular disease to better predict development of acute MR after PTMC (total score 0–16). A score ≥10 had a good discriminatory value for this outcome. Bhalgat et al.[11] found that only subvalvular pathology, seen independently for each papillary muscle and summed into an easy score, was predictive of outcomes. In their study, none of the patients with extensive SVD had an acute favorable outcome (increase in valve area and no significant MR). However, the score was not independently validated.

A real-time transthoracic 3DE-based score has also been developed looking at determinants for individual leaflet (thickness, mobility, and calcification) and subvalvular apparatus (thickness and separation of proximal, middle, and distal third).[12] The score ranges from 0 to 31 with <8, 8–13, and ≥14 indicating mild, moderate, and severe MV involvement. But real-time transthoracic 3DE is not widely available and also with a poorer resolution, it's not clear whether it offers any advantage over a thoroughly conducted 2D echocardiogram.

To summarize, no individual score is superior to another in all respects. Each score is semiquantitative, and to some extent, subjective. While the Wilkin's score is more predictive of procedural success (in terms of acute gain in valve area), the Padial and Canaan score are more predictive of procedural severe MR. Thus, each scoring system should be considered complementary to one another. Each component of mitral apparatus should be examined and described in detail with the greatest importance being given to commissural morphology. It is extremely important to identify patients who are likely to have failed procedure (no increase in valve area and/or severe MR requiring surgery) so that they do not undergo a potentially harmful or unsuccessful procedure.

Transesophageal Echocardiography

Transesophageal echocardiography (TEE) has superior resolution as compared to transthoracic echocardiography (TTE). It can be used for the assessment of the MV if TTE images are suboptimal. It also helps evaluate the degree of MR accurately. However, its main role in MS is to rule out the presence of LAA thrombus. Usually, a parasternal short-axis view with anterior tilt is sufficient to visualize the LAA on TTE (Fig. 9A). Thus, in patients with sinus rhythm, a TEE is not routinely performed except in the presence of a prior embolic event, dense spontaneous echocardiographic contrast in LA, and suboptimal transthoracic imaging of LAA. On the other hand, all patients with AF should undergo a TEE prior to BMV (Fig. 9C).

Another important use of TEE is during the BMV procedure for guiding transseptal puncture (TSP). The presence of LA/LAA thrombus has traditionally been a contraindication to BMV. Some studies have shown that it is feasible to perform BMV in selected patients with LA/LAA appendage thrombus after 8–12 weeks of anticoagulation. The LA/LAA thrombus was classified into five types (Table 5; Fig. 9C).[13] Patients with thrombus types Ia, Ib, and IIa can successfully undergo BMV. In one study, 108 patients with LA thrombus types Ia, Ib, and IIa underwent BMV using a modified over the wire technique that virtually excluded the LA from the track of the septal dilator and balloon catheter exchanges. BMV was successfully performed in 98% of cases. Only one patient had a transient ischemic attack 6 hours after the procedure and recovered completely. It is to be noted that BMV was performed by experienced operators (>500 procedures) in this study.

Three-Dimensional Echocardiography

Real-time 3DE uses a phased, matrix array transducer probe to obtain full-volume images of the MV for real-time or offline analysis. It is to be done by transthoracic and transesophageal route. The acquired volume can then be rotated, steered, and sliced along all the three axes at any desired level. The smallest MV orifice can be measured using

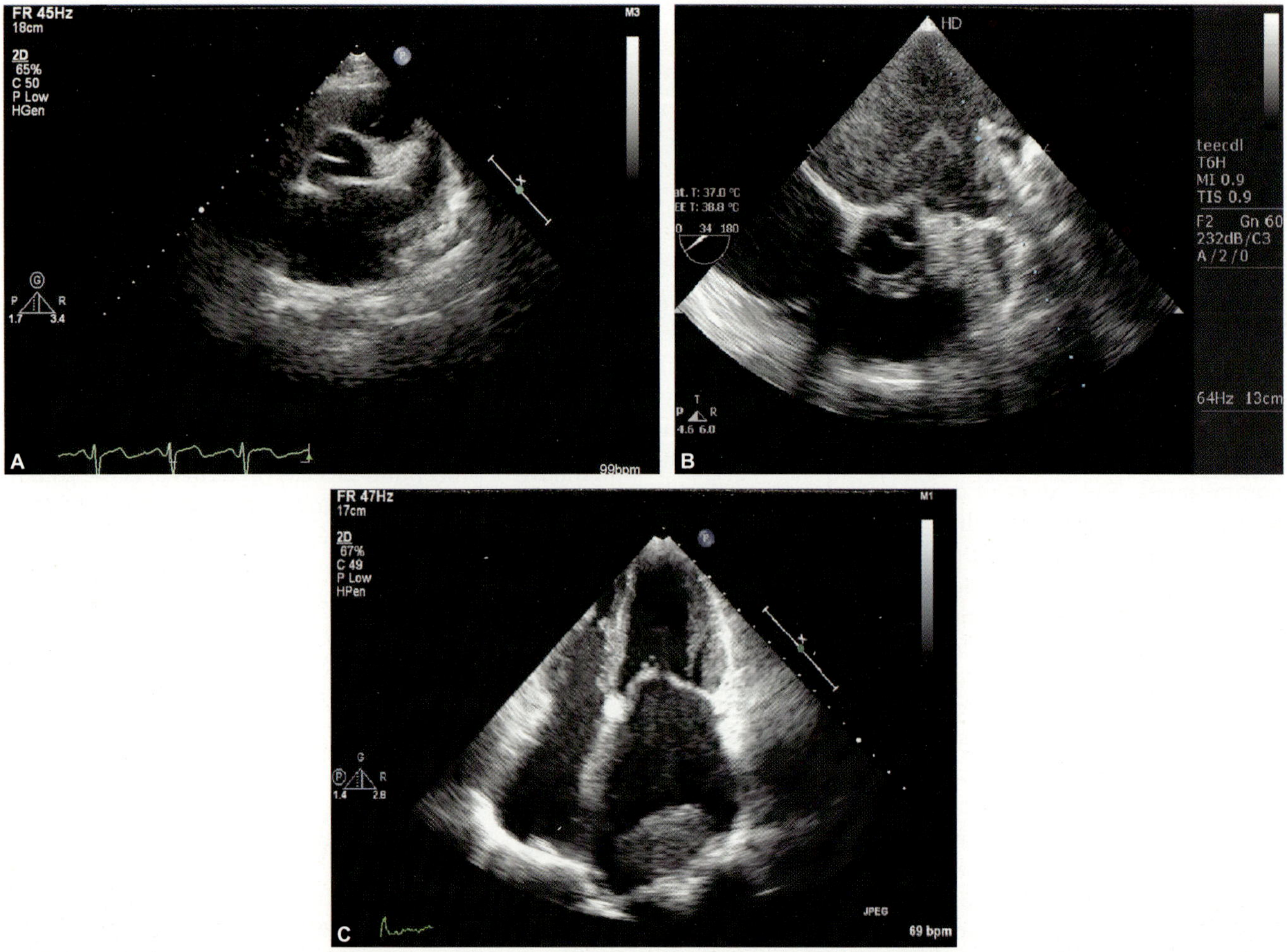

Figs. 9A to C: (A) Transthoracic parasternal short axis with an anterior tilt demonstrating left atrial appendage. (B) Transesophageal echocardiogram demonstrating LAA thrombus and spontaneous echocardiographic contrast in left atrium. (C) Large thrombus in left atrium. (LLA: left atrial appendage)

TABLE 5: LA/LAA clot classification.[13]

Type Ia	LA appendage clot confined to appendage
Type Ib	LA appendage clot protruding into LA cavity
Type IIa	LA roof clot limited to a plane above the plane of fossa ovalis
Type IIb	LA roof clot extending below the plane of fossa ovalis
Type III	Layered clot over the IAS
Type IV	Mobile clot which is attached to LA free wall or roof or IAS
Type V	Ball valve thrombus (free floating)

(IAS: interatrial septum; LA: Left atrium; LAA: left atrial appendage)

either atrial or ventricular view (Figs. 10A and B). Planimetry by 3DE has better reproducibility and intraobserver variability than 2D echocardiography[14] and has the closest agreement with invasive Gorlin-derived MVA. It has also been shown to better visualize the commissural opening, thus helping guide appropriate treatment, especially for restenosed valve which could be narrowed due to valve rigidity per se rather than commissural fusion. On the other hand, 3DE is not widely available in the developing countries (where the actual burden of MS lies); the acquisition may be suboptimal with uncontrolled ventricular rates and needs operator appearance, and the spatial resolution is still low.

ECHOCARDIOGRAPHY DURING BALLOON MITRAL VALVOTOMY

Echocardiography during BMV has now become indispensable and is mandatory. A complete invasive hemodynamic assessment before and after BMV is rarely performed in the present era. Most of this data is available through echocardiography, thereby reducing procedure time and radiation exposure. Immediately prior to the procedure, on the catheterization laboratory table, an abridged echocardiogram is performed noting the transmitral mean gradient, commissural status, the degree of MR, the presence of LA/LAA thrombus (occasional surprises have been noted), and preprocedural PASP. In addition, two more important aspects should be noted. First is the presence/absence of pericardial effusion at baseline (which may be due to congestive heart failure or rheumatic carditis). If this effusion is missed, the subsequent appearance of a pericardial effusion later in the procedure may be wrongly attributed to cardiac perforation leading to the procedure being abandoned. Sometimes, pericardial fat may be mistaken for pericardial effusion. The second aspect is the orientation and morphology of the interatrial septum (IAS). This aids in guiding TSP. The IAS may bulge toward the right atrium (with high LA pressures) or toward the left atrium (in the presence of severe PAH and/or TV disease causing RA volume overload). The curve of the Brockenbrough needle can be suitably adjusted depending on the IAS bulge (more acute angle for straight IAS and lesser angle for IAS bulging into RA). Usually, TSP is done under fluoroscopic guidance. However, in challenging cases, echocardiographic guidance (TTE or TEE) may be needed for TSP as in instances of thoracic deformities, severe bulging of the IAS, or an aneurysmal septum (Figs. 11A and B). Following TSP, a TTE is again performed to assess the site of septal puncture (appropriate, high, or low) and for the appearance of new pericardial effusion. Depending on the site of septal puncture and the size of LA, the curve of the J-shaped stylet can be increased or

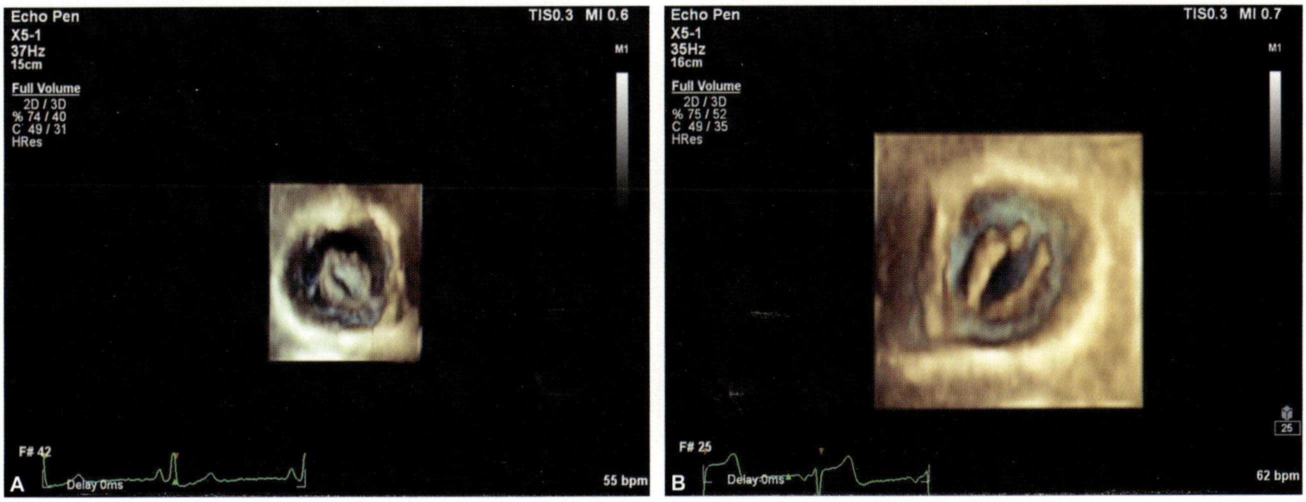

Figs. 10A and B: Three-dimensional echocardiography of mitral before (A) and after BMV (B) showing fused and split commissures, respectively. (BMV: Balloon mitral valvotomy).

decreased to aid LV entry (greater diameter for larger LA and vice versa, smaller curve for low puncture). If the stainless steel guidewire is not seen to traverse in the vicinity of the fossa ovalis, a consideration should be made for redoing the TSP as the TSP may have been through one of the gutters.

After each balloon inflation, TTE is performed to assess the success of BMV (commissural splitting) in terms of MVA and mean transmitral gradient and for the appearance of MR. Successful BMV has been defined as a postprocedure valve area >1.5 cm^2 (without >Grade 2 MR), in the absence of major complications that require emergency surgery.[1] Some studies have also utilized a 50% increase in the baseline area as a measure of success.[15] At least one commissure should be shown to be completely split for the procedure to be considered successful (Fig. 12A). Sometimes, it may be difficult to assess commissural splitting as the patient cannot be turned to the left lateral position. In such cases, apart from the reduction in transmitral gradient, certain other aspects may be useful to guide further balloon dilation. The presence of laminar flow across the MV on color Doppler (Figs. 13A and B), an MLS index of more than 1.2, and straightening of the AML (which is normally hockey-stick shaped Figs. 13A and B) are all indicative of a successful BMV. Grade 2/4 MR or increase in MR by one grade is an indication for the termination of BMV. Post-BMV MR requiring urgent surgical attention is usually due to leaflet tear or chordal rupture. However, as PTMC opens the valve by splitting commissures, a commissural MR (sometimes even severe) can often be seen (Figs. 14A to C). This however decreases with time due to the remodeling

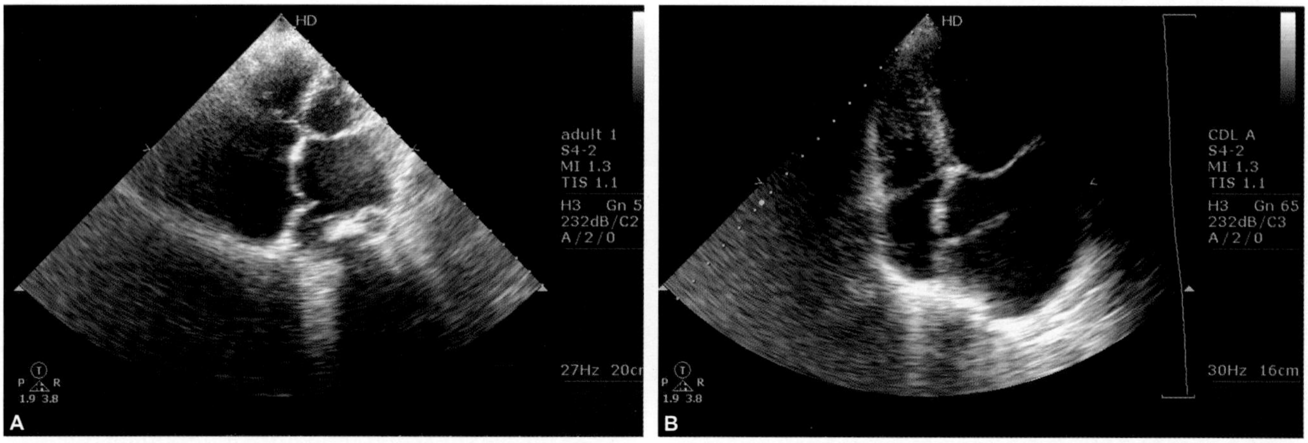

Figs. 11A and B: Transseptal puncture guided by echocardiography. (A) Transthoracic echocardiography. Tenting of interatrial septum by the Brockenbrough needle in the fossa ovalis. (B) Following successful TSP. (TSP: transseptal puncture).

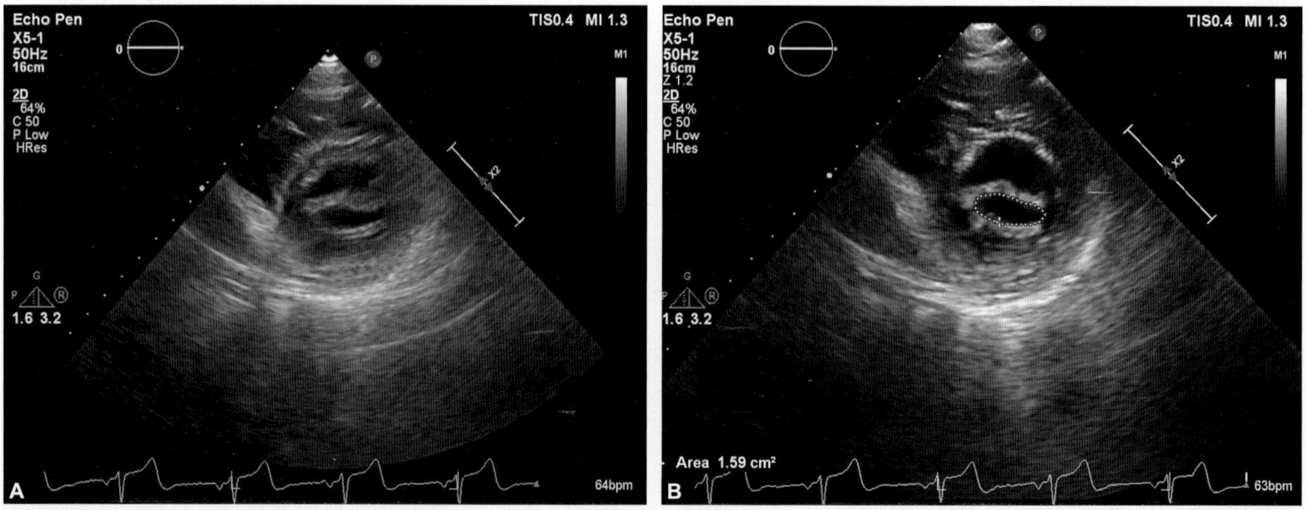

Figs. 12A and B: Parasternal short axis after BMV—the lateral commissure is completely split, and the medial commissure is partially split (A). The MVA by planimetry is 1.6 cm^2 (B). (BMV: balloon mitral valvotomy; MVA: mitral valve area).

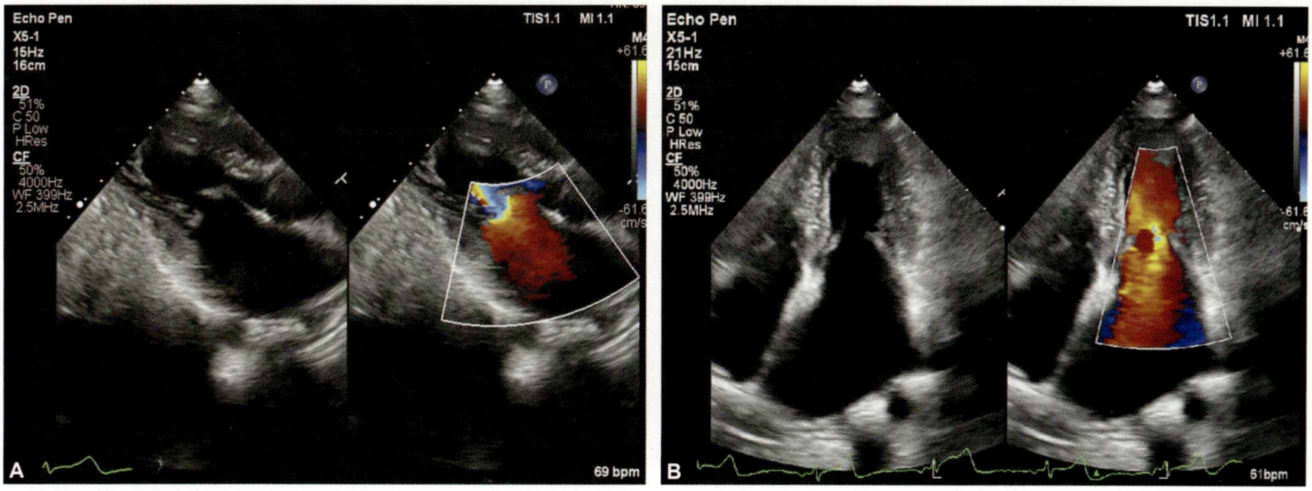

Figs. 13A and B: Color compare after successful BMV showing laminar flow across the mitral valve and straightening of the anterior mitral leaflet (no longer showing doming). (A) Parasternal long-axis view, and (B) apical four-chamber view. (BMV: balloon mitral valvotomy).

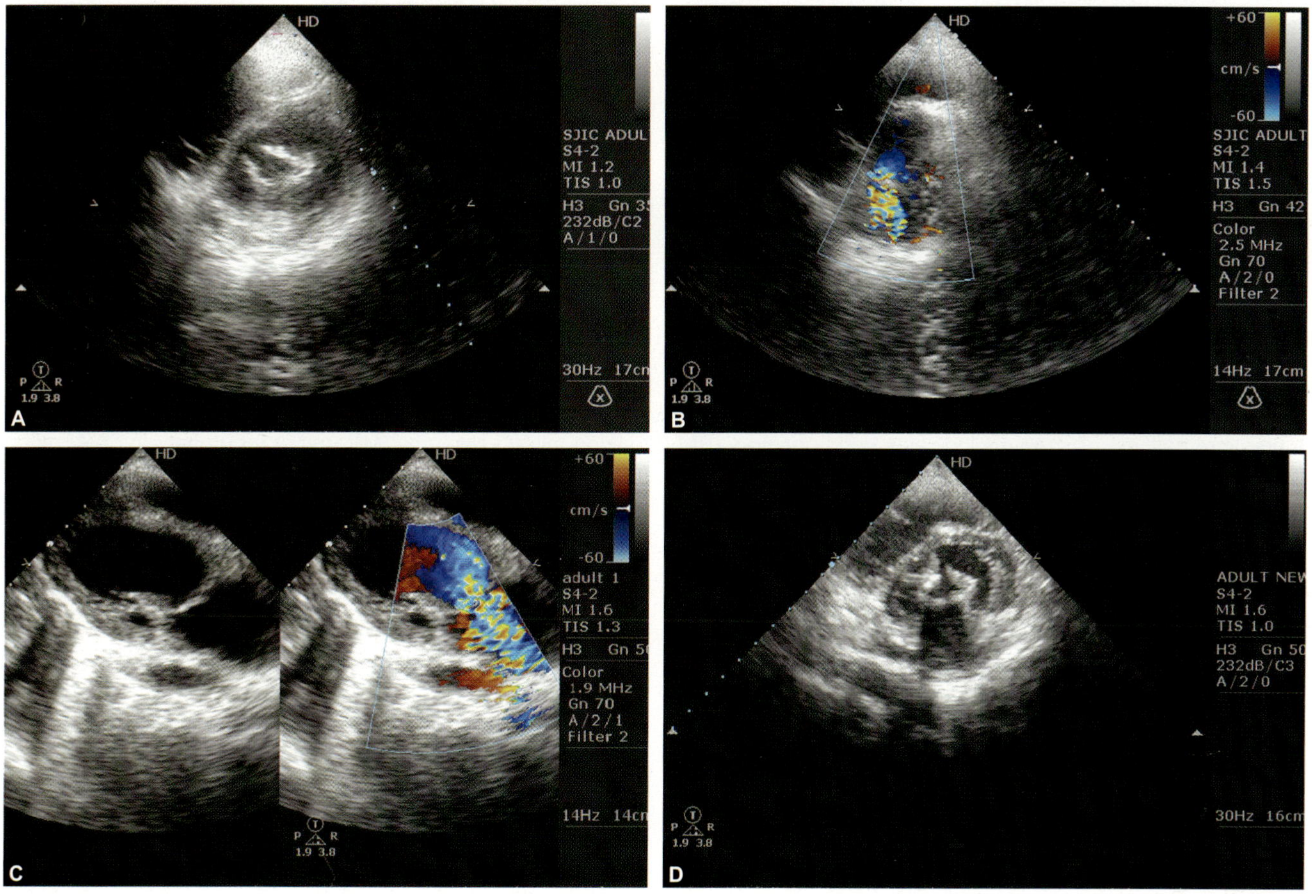

Figs. 14A to D: Mitral regurgitation following BMV. (A and B) Medial commissure split, commissural MR from the medial commissure. (C) AML tear leading to severe leaflet MR. (D) AML tear. (AML: anterior mitral leaflet; BMV: balloon mitral valvotomy; MR: mitral regurgitation).

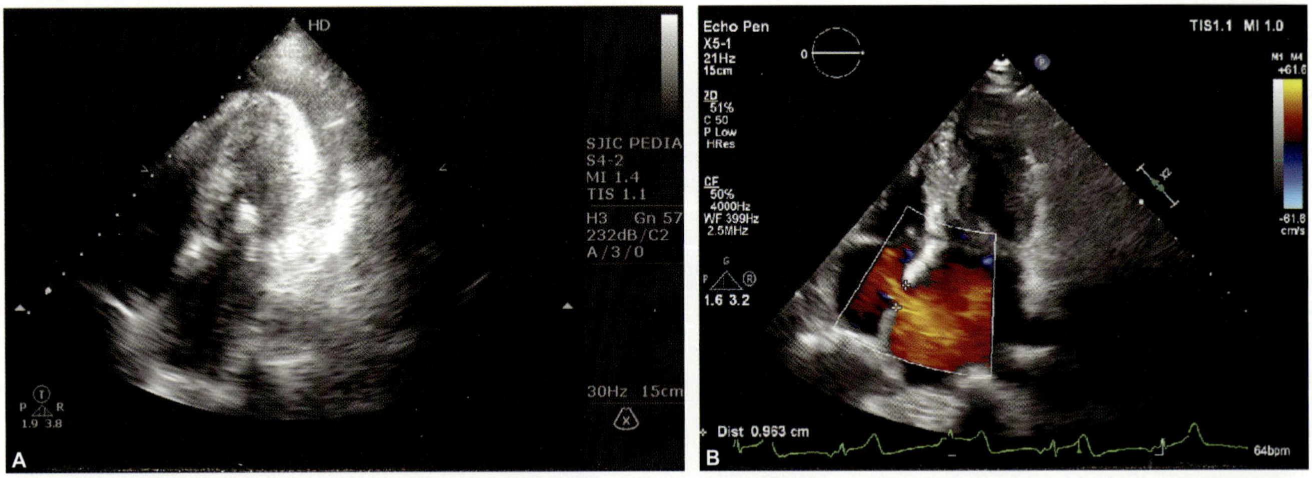

Figs. 15A and B: (A) Pericardial effusion and tamponade following TSP. (B) 9 mm atrial septal defect following BMV. (BMV: balloon mitral valvotomy; TSP: transseptal puncture).

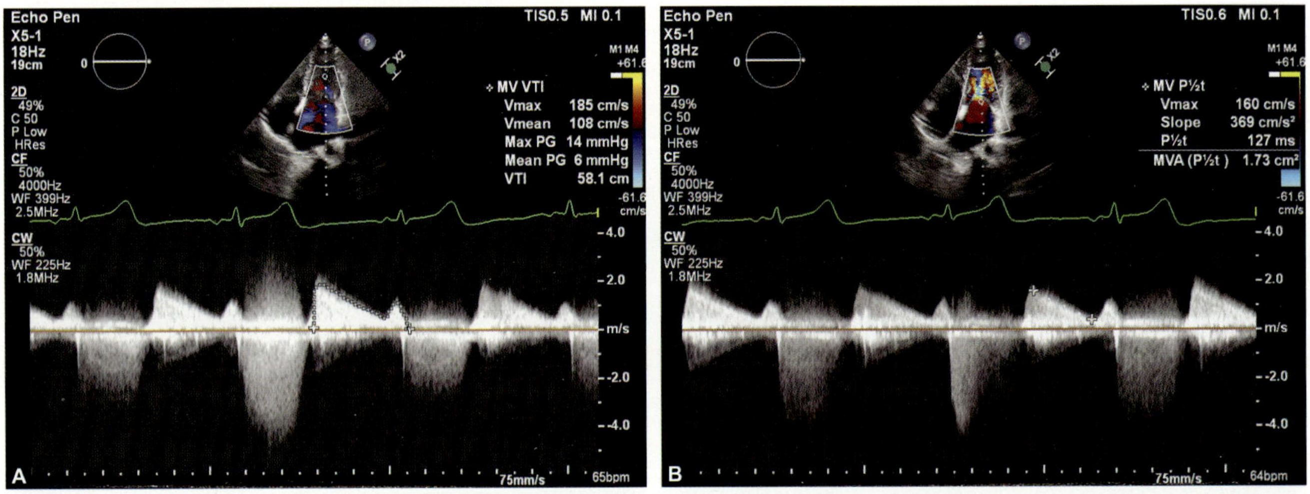

Figs. 16A and B: Continuous wave Doppler after BMV. (A) There is reduction in transmitral gradient (from 14 mm Hg to 6 mmHg). Mild MR is noted. (B) Pressure halftime method for estimating MVA after BMV. This method is not reliable after BMV. However, a pressure halftime of <130 ms indicates good opening. (BMV: balloon mitral valvotomy; MR: mitral regurgitation; MVA: mitral valve area).

and fibrosis in MV. Commissural MR is best appreciated in a parasternal short-axis view. Given the supine position of the patient, it may be difficult to exactly quantify the degree of MR or its origin. Multiple and unorthodox views may need to be used. Any rise in the LA pressure above the baseline or the appearance/increase in "v" wave should be considered to indicate the development of significant MR, and all attempts should be made to identify this. Unexpected hemodynamic collapse should lead to an echocardiogram to rule out cardiac tamponade (Fig. 15A).

ECHOCARDIOGRAPHY AFTER BALLOON MITRAL VALVOTOMY

Following BMV, in the immediate postprocedure period, the best method to assess MVA by echocardiography is planimetry. Up to 72 hours after BMV, due to large and unpredictable changes in atrial and ventricular compliance, the PHT method for MVA estimation is unreliable. Usually PHT underestimates the MVA during this period. However, a PHT of less than 130 ms (Figs. 16A and B) has been shown to correlate with a good valve opening.

Subsequently, 2D echocardiography is used to follow-up patients for the development of restenosis, progression or regression of MR, atrial septal defect (Fig. 15B), biventricular function, and PAP. Follow-up echocardiography is recommended among asymptomatic individuals at the intervals of 3–5 years in those with MVA > 1.5 cm^2, every 1–2 years with MVA ≤ 1.5 cm^2, and yearly in those with MVA < 1 cm^2.[1] Once restenosis develops, it is important to identify the predominant mechanism of restenosis as this will determine the treatment approach. While fusion

TABLE 6: Role of echocardiography in BMV.

Preprocedure	Etiology and severity of MS
	Level of obstruction (valvular/subvalvular)
	Mitral valve area and transmitral gradient
	Degree of mitral regurgitation
	LA/LAA thrombus
	LV/RV function
	Preprocedural pulmonary artery systolic pressure
	Preprocedure pericardial effusion/fat
	Associated valvular lesions
	Commissural morphology
	Subvalvular apparatus
During BMV	Interatrial septal bulge/aneurysm
	Site of TSP
	Assessment of MVA/transmitral gradients
	Assessment of mitral regurgitation
	Assessment of commissural splitting
	Pericardial effusion/tamponade
Postprocedure	Mitral restenosis
	Mechanism of mitral restenosis
	Evaluation of residual ASD/MR
	Regression of TR and PAH
	LV/RV function
	Associated valvular diseases

(ASD: atrial septal defect; BMV: balloon mitral valvotomy; LA: left atrium; LAA: left atrial appendage; LV: left ventricular; MR: mitral regurgitation; MS: mitral stenosis; MVA: mitral valve area; PAH: pulmonary artery hypertension; RV: right ventricular; TR: tricuspid regurgitation; TSP: transseptal puncture)

of commissures can be treated with a redo PTMC, severe subvalvular disease forming the effective stenotic orifice or severe valvular rigidity with split commissures should be offered MV surgery.

Another important aspect that needs to be followed up is regression of concomitant TR and PAH. Most often TR is functional, resulting from RV dilatation secondary to pulmonary hypertension. Once the MS is relieved and pulmonary hypertension disappears, the TR also improves. At times, this may not happen and, in such patients, TV repair may be needed. If the patient needs to undergo MV surgery, it is preferable to perform TV annuloplasty even if the TR is mild when the tricuspid annulus is dilated (>40 mm or >21 mm/m^2 BSA) or if there is prior recent history of right heart failure.[1] Table 6 summarizes the role of echocardiography in BMV.

REFERENCES

1. Nishimura RA, Otto CM, Bonow RO, et al. 2014 AHA/ACC guideline for the management of patients with valvular heart disease: a report of the American College of Cardiology/American Heart Association Task Force on Practice Guidelines. J Am Coll Cardiol. 2014;63:e57-185.
2. Edler I. The use of ultrasonic reflectoscope for the continuous recording of the movements of heart walls. Kungl Fysiogr sallsk i Lund forhandl. 1954;24:1-9.
3. Bonow RO, Carabello BA, Kanu C, et al. ACC/AHA 2006 guidelines for the management of patients with valvular heart disease. Circulation. 2006;114:e84-231.
4. Holmin C, Messika-Zeitoun D, Mezalek AT, et al. Mitral leaflet separation index: a new method for the evaluation of the severity of mitral stenosis? Usefulness before and after percutaneous mitral commissurotomy. J Am Soc Echocardiogr. 2007;20:1119-24.
5. Hatle L, Brubakk A, Tromsdal A, et al. Noninvasive assessment of pressure drop in mitral stenosis by Doppler ultrasound. Br Heart J. 1978;40:131.
6. Wilkins GT, Weyman AE, Abascal VM, et al. Percutaneous balloon dilatation of the mitral valve: an analysis of echocardiographic variables related to outcome and the mechanism of dilatation. Br Heart J. 1988;60:299-308.
7. Nunes MC, Tan TC, Elmariah S, et al. The echo score revisited: impact of incorporating commissural morphology and leaflet displacement to the prediction of outcome for patients undergoing percutaneous mitral valvuloplasty. Circulation. 2014;129;886-95.
8. Lung B, Cormier B, Ducimetiere P, et al. Immediate results of percutaneous mitral commissurotomy. A predictive model on a series of 1514 patients. Circulation. 1996;94:2124-30.
9. Cannan CR, Nishimura RA, Reeder GS, et al. Echocardiographic assessment of commissural calcium: a simple predictor of outcome after percutaneous mitral balloon valvotomy. J Am Coll Cardiol. 1997;29:175-80.
10. Padial LR, Freitas N, Sagie A, et al. Echocardiography can predict which patients will develop severe mitral regurgitation after percutaneous mitral valvotomy. J Am Coll Cardiol. 1996;27:1225-31.
11. Bhalgat P, Karlekar S, Modani S, et al. Subvalvular apparatus and adverse outcome of balloon valvotomy in rheumatic mitral stenosis. Indian Heart J. 2015;67:428-33.
12. Anwar AM, Attia WM, Nosir YF, et al. Validation of a new score for the assessment of mitral stenosis using real-time three-dimensional echocardiography. J Am Soc Echocardiogr. 2010;23:13-22.
13. Manjunath CN, Srinivasa KH, Ravindranath KS, et al. Balloon mitral valvotomy in patients with mitral stenosis and left atrial thrombus. Catheter Cardiovasc Interv. 2009;74(4):653-61.
14. Zamorano J, Cordeiro P, Sugeng L, et al. Real-time three-dimensional echocardiography for rheumatic mitral valve stenosis evaluation: an accurate and novel approach. J Am Coll Cardiol. 2004;43:2091-6.
15. Nunes MC, Nascimento BR, Lodi-Junqueira L, et al. Update on percutaneous mitral commissurotomy. Heart. 2016;102:500-7.

SECTION 9

Atrial Fibrillation

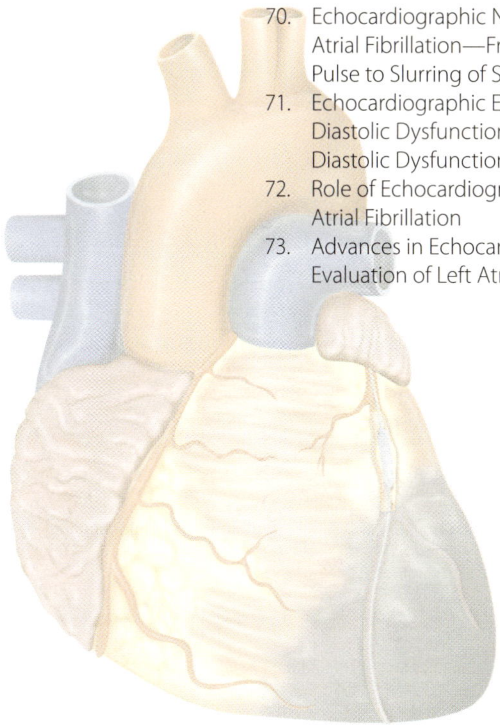

70

CHAPTER

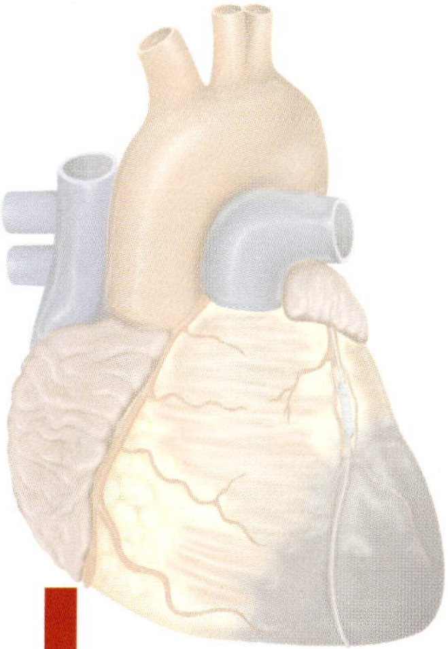

Echocardiographic Navigation in Atrial Fibrillation—From Irregular Pulse to Slurring of Speech

Shraddha Ranjan, Manish Bansal, Ravi R Kasliwal, HK Chopra

INTRODUCTION

Atrial fibrillation (AF) is the most common cardiac arrhythmia which any physician comes across in his clinical practice. Though this arrhythmia may not be usually life-threatening in emergency room, patients are at increased risk of death, heart failure, hospitalization, and thromboembolic events. The worldwide prevalence and incidence of AF is progressively increasing with significant effects on associated morbidity and mortality, findings that have massive implications for public health policy and healthcare costs. Echocardiography has a unique and important role in the assessment of cardiac structure and function and how it affects or gets affected by AF. In these patients, it has also been shown to be useful in risk stratification and guiding the management and has now been well established in guidelines. Transesophageal echocardiography (TEE) has been an irreplaceable tool particularly to guide direct cardioversion or detect cardiac sources of embolism for few years now, and recently indispensable for interventionists dealing with left atrial (LA) appendage (LAA) closure devices. Moreover, the role of intracardiac echocardiography (ICE) has led to real-time guidance of percutaneous interventions done for the management of AF, including radiofrequency ablation and LAA closure. In this chapter, we will discuss how echocardiography, especially transthoracic [transthoracic echocardiographic (TTE)] and TEE, helps in different aspects of management in a patient of AF. A systematic review done in 2010 of the current worldwide epidemiological data on AF confirmed the emergence of this condition as a global epidemic with significant and progressive effects on estimated disability and mortality. The Framingham Heart Study had already suggested that AF leads to approximate doubling of both overall and cardiovascular mortality leading to major implications on healthcare costs.[1] The annual new cases of AF globally in 2010 were estimated at close to 5 million which were much more than those in the 1990s.[2] The increase in AF burden increases with age from 2% incidence in population less than 40 years of age to approximately five times more in that with population more than 80 years.[3,4] This rapid increase can be explained by aging trends along with increased prevalence of hypertension, atherosclerosis, obesity, and other cardiovascular risk factors, which increase arterial stiffness, cause diastolic dysfunction and atrial volume overload, resulting in AF. These alterations can be observed as part of the aging process but are also likely to be involved independently of aging.[5] The arrhythmia is characterized by erratic electrical activity due to change in atrial structure and mechanical function that can further lead to electrical and structural remodeling of the atria, which in turn reinforces the chronicity of AF. Once gross, they can visibly be detected by echocardiography but with recent advances of strain even subclinical and subtle changes can be detected which enables proactive management of this disabling disease. Nearly all patients presenting with their first episode of AF will benefit from TTE evaluation of LA size and function, left ventricular (LV) cavity size, and systolic/diastolic function, along with the diagnosis of valvular, myocardial, pericardial, and congenital heart disease which may predispose to AF. A more selected subgroup may benefit from the additional

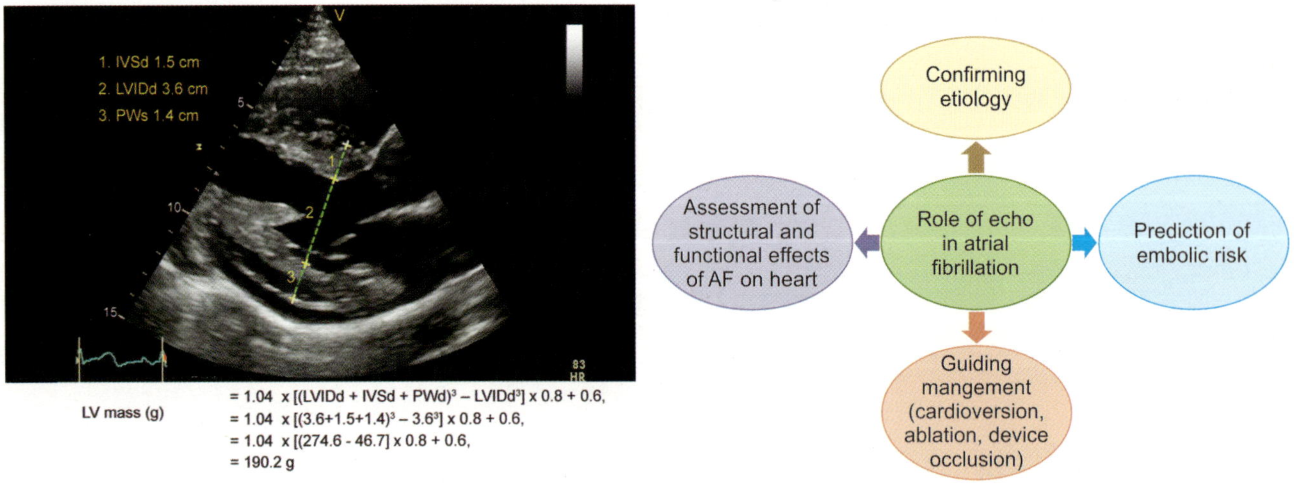

Fig. 1: Schematic depicting role of echocardiography in the evaluation and management of atrial fibrillation.

information obtained from TEE evaluation for LA thrombi to allow for early cardioversion if no thrombi are identified. For better understanding the role of echocardiographic imaging among patients with AF can be divided according to the objective of imaging (Fig. 1).

ETIOLOGY OF ATRIAL FIBRILLATION

Causes of AF can be separated into cardiac and noncardiac causes by routine blood tests and echocardiography. Noncardiac causes are usually electrolyte imbalance, thyrotoxicosis, sepsis, pharmacological or recreational drug use, and alcohol intake. These are usually reversible also, and AF reverts as primary pathology is treated. The cardiac causes of AF include few reversible causes, such as postcardiac surgery or myocarditis, but mostly are irreversible chronic pathologies resulting in structural and functional changes in the heart. These along with their salient echocardiographic features are enumerated in Table 1. Whatever be the etiology leading to AF, the fundamental abnormality is usually structural and functional changes in the left atrium. Hence, the need arises to understand the particulars of echocardiographic evaluation of LA which will be discussed subsequently in this chapter.

ATRIAL FIBRILLATION–RELATED CHANGES IN STRUCTURE AND FUNCTION OF HEART

Left Ventricular Systolic Function

Atrial fibrillation is associated with impaired ventricular function, with a spectrum of severity ranging from congestive heart failure to subtle subclinical changes in LV performance. Causation is much more challenging to establish, mostly when the index presentation is with both AF and LV dysfunction. It's possible that AF may promote ventricular dysfunction by increasing the ventricular rate also known as tachycardia-induced cardiomyopathy, or by other mechanisms, such as endothelial dysfunction and impaired myocardial perfusion. Instead, a preexisting cardiomyopathy may lead to AF because of atrial dysfunction and altered myocardial intracellular calcium handling. This can only be confirmed retrospectively when LV dysfunction in a patient improves after the conversion of AF to sinus rhythm. Echocardiography helps in the assessment of this systolic LV dysfunction. The evaluation is done on the lines of any case of LV dysfunction in sinus rhythm but reproducibility may not be absolute, especially at different heart rates and cycle lengths.

Left Ventricular Diastolic Function

It's known that the presence and severity of diastolic dysfunction are associated with an increased risk for AF in patients with sinus rhythm. In addition, the risk for heart failure is markedly increased once AF develops, and if a patient of HFpEF (heart failure with preserved ejection fraction) initially in sinus rhythm develops AF, his symptoms significantly worsen. So, it wouldn't be wrong to say that these two pathologies are intertwined in a way that is still not well understood. This relationship has garnered lots of attention, and echocardiography has been the sole contributor to this new understanding. The evaluation of diastolic function in patients with AF is complicated as usual methods involving LA mechanical function don't apply here, and the variable cycle lengths make it even more

TABLE 1: Key echocardiography findings in relation to the etiology of AF.[6-15]

Etiology	*Echocardiographic findings*
Hypertensive heart disease	LV hypertrophy + diastolic LV dysfunction, dilated LA
Coronary artery disease	Regional wall motion abnormality, systolic/diastolic LV dysfunction + LA dysfunction
Valvular heart disease (RHD and others)	Mitral stenosis/Regurgitation
Restrictive cardiomyopathy	LV hypertrophy + diastolic LV dysfunction + biatrial enlargement
Hypertrophic cardiomyopathy	Asymmetric septal hypertrophy, left ventricular outflow tract obstruction and dilated LA
Heart failure	Systolic/Diastolic LV dysfunction + changes in LA structure and function
Congenital heart diseases	Atrial septal defect, Ebstein's anomaly and corrected/uncorrected complex congenital heart disease
Obesity	Diastolic LV dysfunction + changes in LA structure and function
Diabetes	Increased LV mass and probable diastolic LV dysfunction
Chronic kidney disease	Diastolic LV dysfunction + changes in LA structure and function
Metabolic syndrome	Diastolic LV dysfunction + changes in LA structure and function
Chronic lung diseases	Right atrial strain, RV dysfunction, pulmonary artery hypertension
Obstructive sleep apnea	LV hypertrophy, pulmonary artery hypertension, dilated LA

(AF: atrial fibrillation; LA: left atrial; LV: left ventricular; RHD: rheumatic heart disease; RV: right ventricular)

difficult. Several new methods have been introduced to be useful in measuring diastolic dysfunction of patients with AF. All echocardiographic parameters have to be measured and averaged from 5 to 10 cardiac cycles, and care should be taken that cycles with approximately same R-R interval are chosen.

Transmitral flow deceleration time (DT) provides relatively accurate assessment of LV diastolic function in the setting of AF. Matsukida et al. demonstrated that a cutoff value of mitral DT ≤ 100 ms predicted a mean of pulmonary capillary wedge pressure (PCWP) ≥18 mm Hg with more than 80% sensitivity and specificity.[16] Peak E velocity can be combined with tissue Doppler (TD) early diastolic mitral annular motion velocity (e') to obtain a ratio (E/e') (Fig. 2). TD imaging (TDI) assessment of e' velocity is relatively independent of LA pressure. E/e' (septal) >15 and E/e' (lateral) >10 have been shown to be highly specific for elevated LV filling pressure and has been validated for LV diastolic filling pressure. The isovolumic relaxation time (IVRT) is the time from the aortic valve closure to the onset of mitral inflow and has been shown to be a strong negative correlation with mean PCWP in AF. Increased IVRT is a marker of impaired LV relaxation, and a shortened IVRT reflects the increased LV chamber stiffness.

In AF, there could be regional differences in diastolic filling depending on the LV response to the fibrillating atria. Therefore, regional strain rate imaging is expected to be a promising technique for assessing diastolic dysfunction in AF. However, more studies will be needed before its application to the clinical practice in patients with AF.

Left Atrial Size

It is a known fact that with the development of LV diastolic dysfunction, or a mitral valve pathology, there is progressive increase in mean LA pressure. This is because LA takes all the burden of hemodynamic tensions taking place during LV diastole as it is in direct communication with the LV. This increase in mean LA pressure eventually leads to an increase in the LA size.[17,18] LA size is assessed by either measuring its anteroposterior diameter, area, or volume at the end of the ventricular systole when the chamber size is maximum. LA diameter and area are simple to measure; the technique is less demanding and provides quick estimate of LA size. However, they may not be accurate in disease states as the LA often enlarges nonuniformly.[19,20] Therefore, measurement of volume is considered to be the most accurate and hence preferred for the estimation of LA size in American Society of Echocardiography recommendations.[21]

The normal value of indexed LA volume is ≤34 mL/m^2. LA volume can be calculated either by the biplane area-length method based on ellipsoid model or by the Simpson's method. Although the latest guidelines recommend Simpson's method because of the ease of measurement,

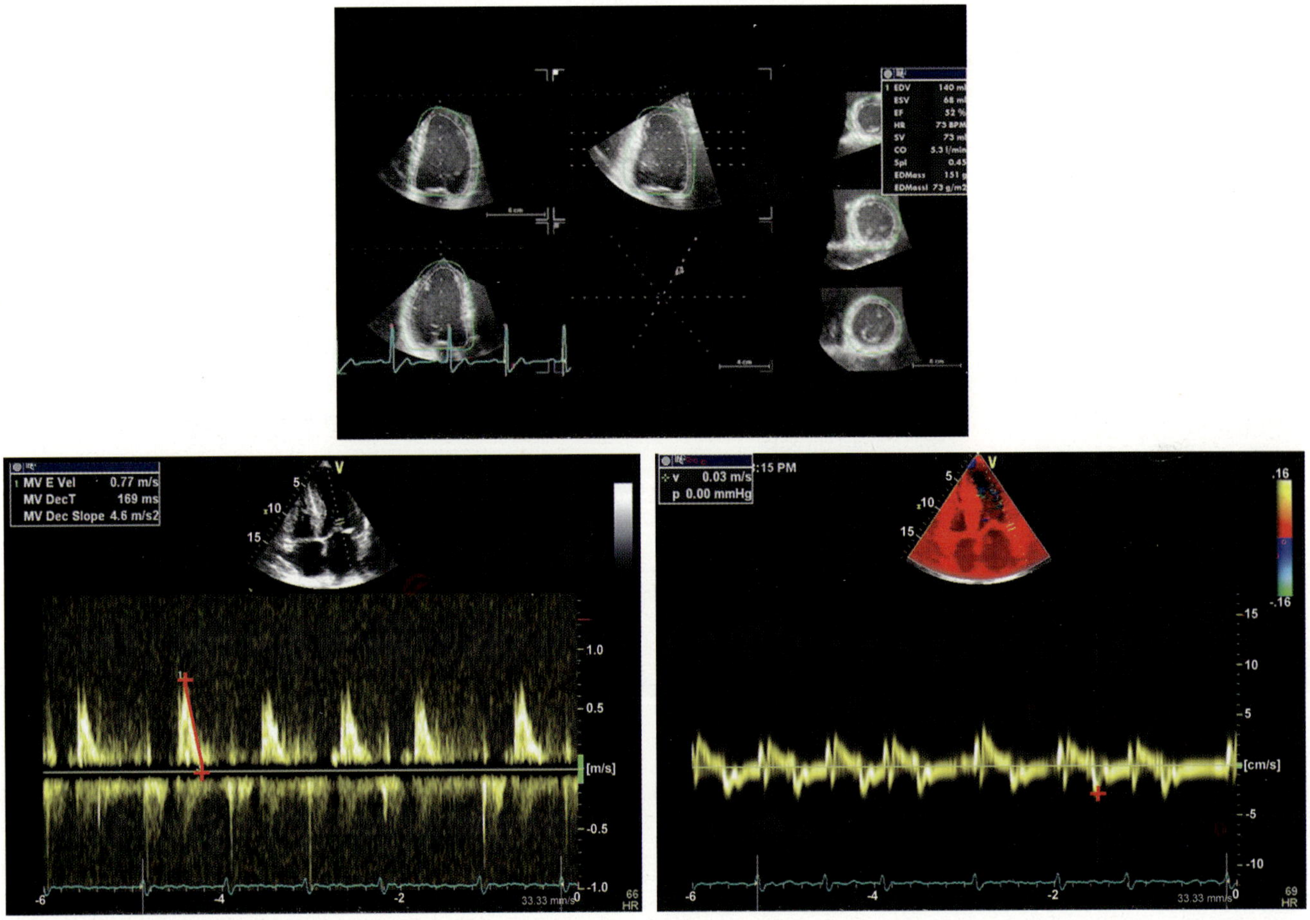

Fig. 2: Assessment of left ventricular diastolic function in the presence of atrial fibrillation. Left—early diastolic mitral inflow velocity and its deceleration time; right—early diastolic mitral annular tissue velocity.

most of the data about LA volume has been derived using the biplane area-length method (Fig. 3). Using the latter method, LA volume can be calculated as

> Left atrial volume = $8/3\pi$ {A_1 (planimetric LA area in the four-chamber view × A_2 (planimetric LA area in the two-chamber view)}/L (length of the LA from midpoint of mitral annular plane to the superior aspect of the left atrium)

While doing measurements, foreshortening should be avoided and pulmonary veins and the LAA should be excluded from the planimetry. Irrespective of the method, the estimated LA volume should always be indexed to the body surface area. There is now sufficient evidence to suggest that the LA size is an independent predictor of the recurrence of AF, risk of stroke, heart failure-related hospitalization, and risk of overall mortality.[22-34]

Left Atrial Function Assessment

The recent advent of speckle-tracking echocardiography (STE) with its application for LA strain measurement has made it practical to measure LA function in clinical practice. LA function, in addition to LA size, is also an important determinant of adverse outcomes in various disease states that directly or indirectly affect the left atrium. Moreover, in some situations, LA function may even have superior prognostic value than LA size alone.[35] Strain is basically a measure of myocardial deformation and is defined as the percent change in the length of a myocardial segment during a given phase of cardiac cycle. When the myocardial segment contracts, it undergoes shortening, and strain is depicted as a negative value, whereas lengthening would result in positive strain (Fig. 4). When done for LV as myocardial deformation is multidirectional, strain is described along three principle directions—longitudinal, radial, and circumferential. However, in the case of LA, most of the shortening and lengthening occurs in longitudinal directional only; and therefore, only longitudinal strain is measured. Strain can be measured by two methods—Doppler-based or STE-based.[36] Doppler-based strain is technically more time consuming and less accurate. In

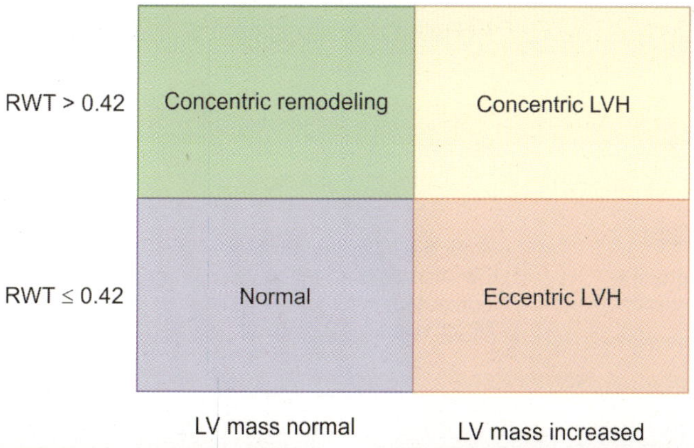

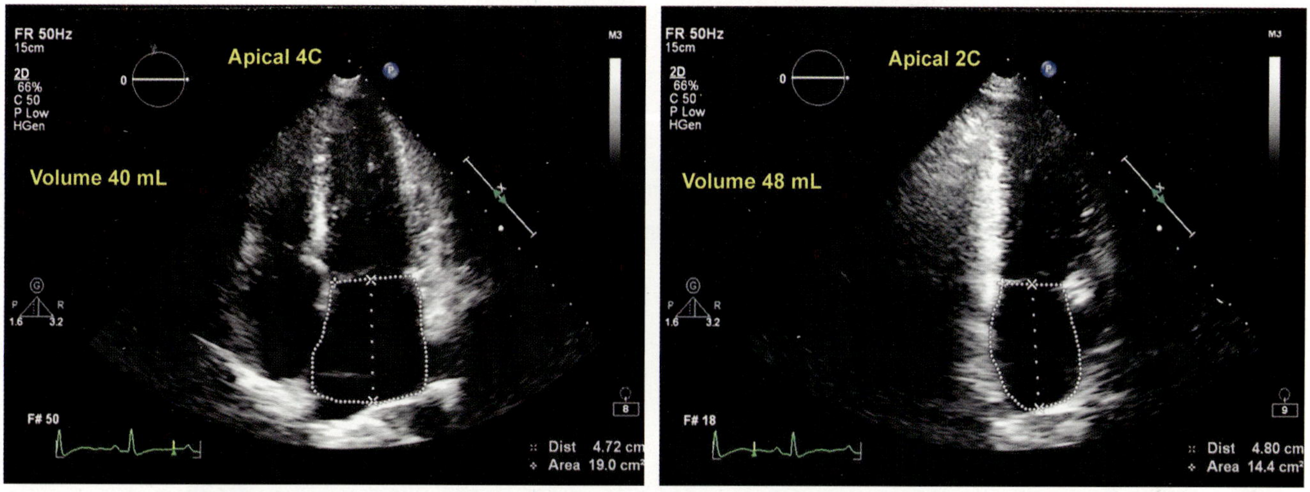

Fig. 3: Measurement of left atrial volume by the biplane area–length method. Left atrial area and length are measured in both the apical four- and two-chamber views and used in the equation (please see the text for details).

comparison, STE is simpler to use, and the measurement is relatively angle independent. This makes it apt for strain measurement in any cardiac chamber and in any direction, hence preferred for the measurement of LA strain. When evaluating LA strain, first step is to acquire grayscale good-quality moving images in apical four-chamber and two-chamber views along its maximal dimensions preferably during breath-holding with a stable electrocardiographic (ECG) recording. These images are analyzed using the same speckle-tracking software which are used for LV strain analysis. The operator has to trace LA endocardial border manually in the end-systolic frame, excluding pulmonary vein ostia and LA appendage. The software then automatically generates epicardial border tracing and creates a region of interest which can be manually adjusted according to the contour of the LA wall by the operator. The software then divides LA circumference into six segments and tracks myocardial motion for each segment frame by frame and generates strain curves for each myocardial segment. It is repeated for both the four-chamber and the two-chamber views; thus, 12 of segmental strain curves are reported. LA strain curve is measured taking QRS onset, that is the beginning of ventricular systole and the time when the left atrium is smallest in size as a reference point. During the progression of ventricular systole, the left atrium increases in size resulting in positive strain that reaches its peak just before the mitral valve opening. Once mitral valve opens, the left atrium rapidly decreases in size, resulting in reduction in strain. This early rapid emptying phase is followed by a phase of diastasis in which the strain curve plateaus. With the onset of atrial contraction, marked by P-wave on the ECG, the left atrium shortens again, resulting in the second phase of strain reduction. The strain curve eventually reaches the baseline by the onset of QRS (Fig. 5).[37] LA strain curves can be described as follows:

- Peak atrial longitudinal strain (PALS)—measured at the end of the ventricular systole representing the reservoir function of the LA

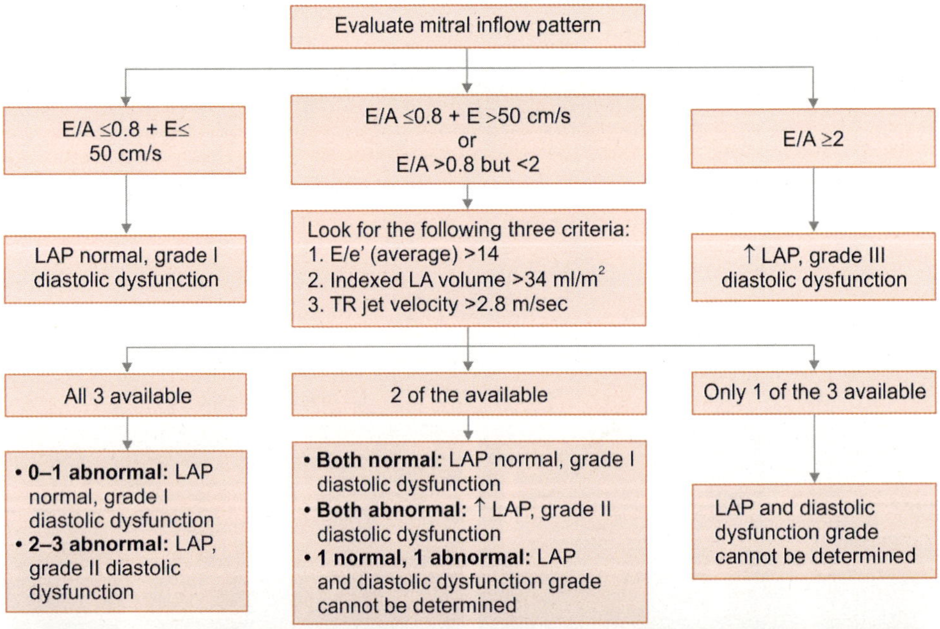

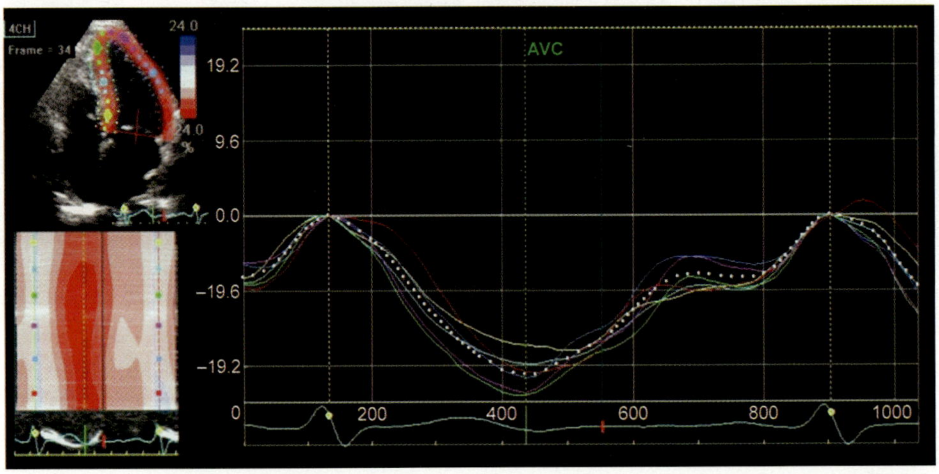

Fig. 4: Measurement of left ventricular longitudinal strain by speckle-tracking echocardiography. The colored curves depict segmental strain, whereas the white-dotted curve depicts the average of all the segments. Since the left ventricle shortens longitudinally during systole, left ventricular longitudinal strain is in negative and is depicted below the baseline.

- Reduction in strain from above peak to the plateau phase indicating the conduit function
- Peak atrial contraction strain (PACS)—final phase of LA strain reduction during atrial contraction representing the booster function

Peak atrial longitudinal strain and PACS averaged for all 12 segments (or all analyzed segments) are used as global LA strain. In addition, LA contraction strain index can also be calculated (global PACS × 100/global PALS) and represents the contribution of the LA contraction to the total LV filling. In a meta-analysis of 40 studies with approximately 2,542 healthy subjects computed a normal reference range for reservoir strain of 39%, for conduit strain of 23%, and for contractile strain of 17%.[38]

Left atrial strain is transiently reduced in patients with short-duration AF but gradually recovers with time.[39,40] If AF becomes chronic, there is structural and functional remodeling of left atrium characterized by increased fibrosis of LA myocardium. LA strain is persistently reduced in these patients and is a poor prognostic indicator. In a study, patients with persistent AF were found to have greater degree of fibrosis than those with paroxysmal AF.[41] Apart from AF, LA remodeling also occurs whenever the left atrium is chronically exposed to elevated LV filling

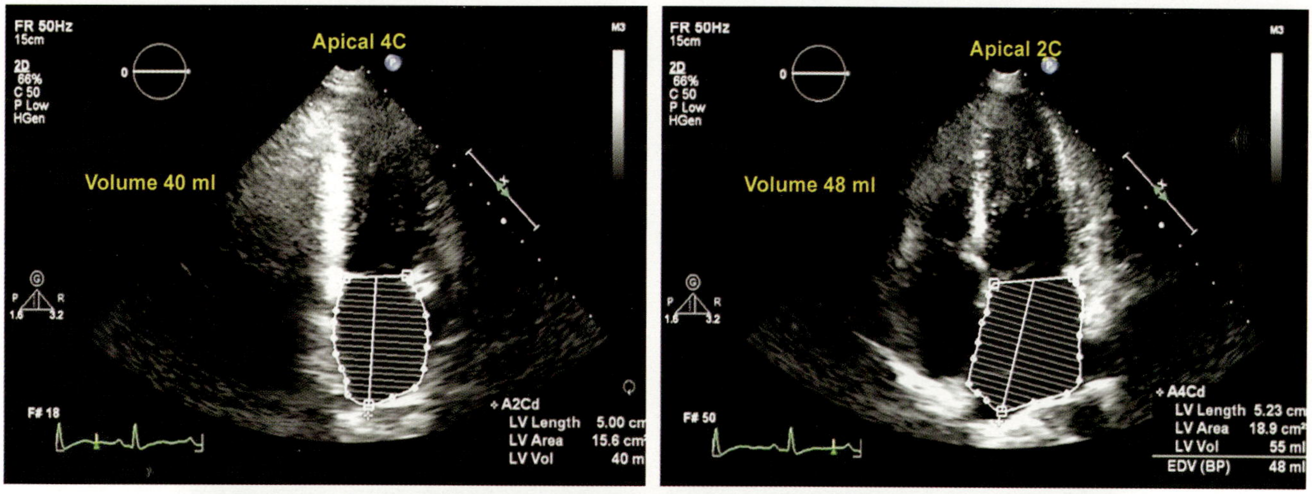

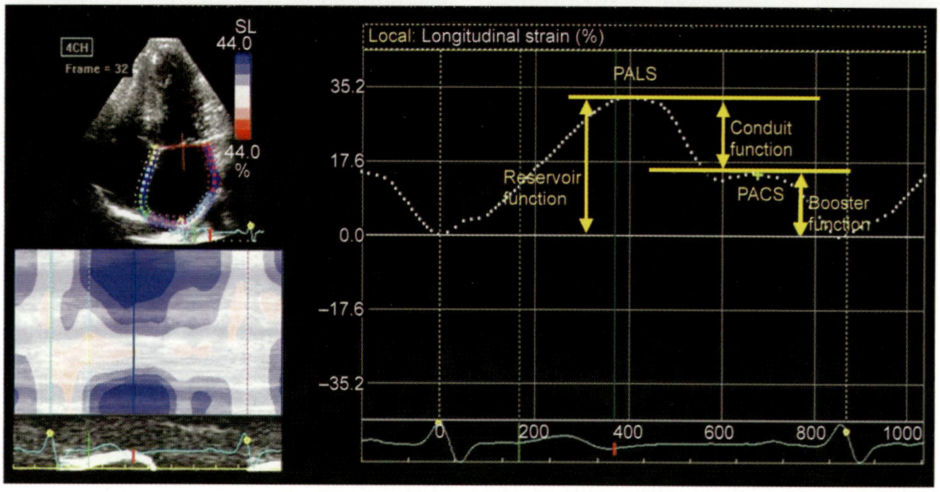

Fig. 5: Left atrial strain waveform using QRS as the reference point. There is an initial positive wave during ventricular systole which is followed by reduction in strain during early rapid filling phase and subsequently during active atrial contraction. (PACS: peak atrial contraction strain; PALS: peak atrial longitudinal strain).

pressures, and LA strain has been shown to be impaired, before other echocardiographic manifestations of LA structural remodeling appear in patients with hypertension, diabetes, and heart failure with preserved LV ejection fraction.[42]

Pulmonary Venous Flow Assessment

Echocardiography helps to define characteristic flow patterns of pulmonary veins in AF. The disappearance of atrial reverse flow, a decrease in systolic flow with a greater diastolic than systolic flow, a prolonged onset of systolic flow, and the appearance of an early systolic reverse flow are characteristic findings in AF. The disappearance of atrial reverse flow can be explained by the loss of active LA contraction. A decrease in systolic PVF has also been found to correspond closely to LAA dysfunction and spontaneous echocardiographic contrast (SEC) formation. The change of PVF in AF seems to reflect alteration in LA function, mainly atrial compliance, and reservoir function.[43]

Prediction of Risk of Thromboembolism

Stroke is the most morbid but possibly preventable complication of AF. Echocardiography, both transthoracic and transesophageal, plays a crucial role in the identification of patients at increased risk for thromboembolic complications of AF before cardioversion and also in patients with chronic AF. Studies from the stroke prevention in AF investigators confirmed the usefulness of TEE for predicting thromboembolism. LAA dysfunction has been shown to be a strong predictor of thrombus formation and the risk of embolic events, even if no clot is found at the time of initial examination.[44-47] The thromboembolic risk is greater with AF than with flutter for the same degree of LAA dysfunction.[48,49] LAA dysfunction is severely marked in patients with rheumatic mitral stenosis in AF, who typically have very low or even absent LAA velocities.[50] LAA dysfunction can be a predictor of stroke risk in sinus rhythm also as shown in a mitral stenosis study.[51] Other than LAA, LA strain can also be a useful parameter along with the validated risk scores when prevention of stroke is the matter on hand. In two studies with approximately 200 patients of paroxysmal or persistent AF with or without acute embolism, global LA strain was found to be lower not only in patients with acute embolism, it had an incremental value over the CHA_2DS_2–VASc score.[52,53] Cardioembolic strokes account for ≥15% of all ischemic strokes[54] among which LAA is the source of embolus in majority of the cases. Approximately 90% of intracardiac thrombi in nonrheumatic AF and 60% in patients with rheumatic mitral valve disease form within the LAA.[55] In patients with recent embolic event and AF, LAA thrombus is found in roughly 14% patients with short-duration AF (started <3 days before) and in roughly 27% patients with longer duration of AF.[56] TEE becomes empirical in ruling out thrombus or SEC in patients suspected to be having cardioembolic stroke (Fig. 6). The presence of SEC alone may be enough to label it a cardioembolic stroke in this context (Table 2).[57,58]

Once we look at the causes and predictors of thromboembolism, it is clear that LAA evaluation has become a necessity to predict and hence prevent this complication in AF patients. So, once thought to be a token part of LA, LAA has gained a lot of respect and attention in this aspect. This has been possible with the advancements of echocardiographic techniques, and now it has been proven that the LAA is an actively contracting structure which plays an important role in cardiac hemodynamics. More importantly, any dysfunction of LAA is the substrate for thrombus formation which can lead to potentially devastating embolic complications.[44-46,59,60] Therefore, a comprehensive assessment of LAA structure and function along with the confirmation of presence or absence of thrombus should be done to guide management in an AF patient. With the development of LA ablation techniques and the widespread presence of LAA occlusion devices, LAA imaging techniques have evolved as per requirement. Echocardiography, particularly TEE, is at present the modality of choice for the evaluation of the LAA. We will discuss here how it allows complete differentiation of the LAA anatomy along with detailed assessment of its function in most of the patients.

Left Atrial Appendage Structure and Function

Complete structural and functional assessment of LAA requires appreciating the complexity of internal LAA anatomy and relationship to surrounding structures, evaluating the ostium size and shape, morphology, detection of SEC or thrombus, and characterization of flow velocity. The LAA is a small, pyramidal muscular extension of LA which is usually multilobed and lies in the left atrioventricular sulcus in close proximity to the circumflex coronary artery. On X-ray, it constitutes part of the normal left cardiac border between the left ventricle and pulmonary outflow tract. It has been described to be mainly of four shapes—chicken wing, windsock, multilobed, or broccoli shaped—and size can also vary among individuals and pathologies. Internally LAA is trabeculated with the trabeculations, known as pectinate muscles which run parallel to each other, giving it a comb-like structure. In an autopsy study of 500 normal human hearts the LAA was bilobed in 54% and multilobed (≥2 lobes) in 80% of hearts.[61] Usefulness of TTE in LAA assessment should not be undermined as it can be really helpful in those centers where TEE is not available. LAA can be seen by two-dimensional (2D) TTE, especially in AF patients, as LAA and LA are usually enlarged, and so every effort should be made to do so. It is best seen in following standard views: parasternal short-axis at the level of aortic and pulmonic valves with slight clockwise rotation or downward tilt of the transducer; apical five-chamber view with upward tilting of the transducer; and the apical two-chamber view with a slight lateral tilt or clockwise rotation of the transducer. The ability of TTE to detect LAA thrombi is limited, with a reported sensitivity of 33% to 60%. Though seen on TTE also, TEE with the close proximity of the transducer to the LAA remains the modality of choice and is compulsory for LAA assessment. On TEE the LAA is best visualized in the midesophageal two-chamber view (80–1,000°) and the midesophageal aortic valve short-axis view (30–60°) and are therefore the recommended views for this purpose.[62] However, to exclude thrombus, it is essential to image the LAA from multiple imaging planes, midesophageal aortic valve short-axis view (30–60°) and then anteflexing the transducer and rotating the multiplane angle from 0° to 180° (Fig. 7).

Transesophageal echocardiography permits detection of thrombus in both the left atrium and the LAA with good precision. The sensitivity and specificity of TEE for LA thrombi in patients who were operated and LAA was checked on grossly was 93–100% and 99–100%, respectively, which is quite impressive.[63] Occasional visualization of pectinate muscles or artifacts make it very difficult to confirm clot where the administration of ultrasound contrast can be of great help.[64-66] The advent of live three-dimensional TEE should render imaging of the complex LAA anatomy much easier now.[67] TEE is also helpful in the detection of LAA SEC. SEC is a smoke-like swirling pattern seen on 2D imaging and is thought to reflect rouleaux formation, resulting from stasis of the blood.

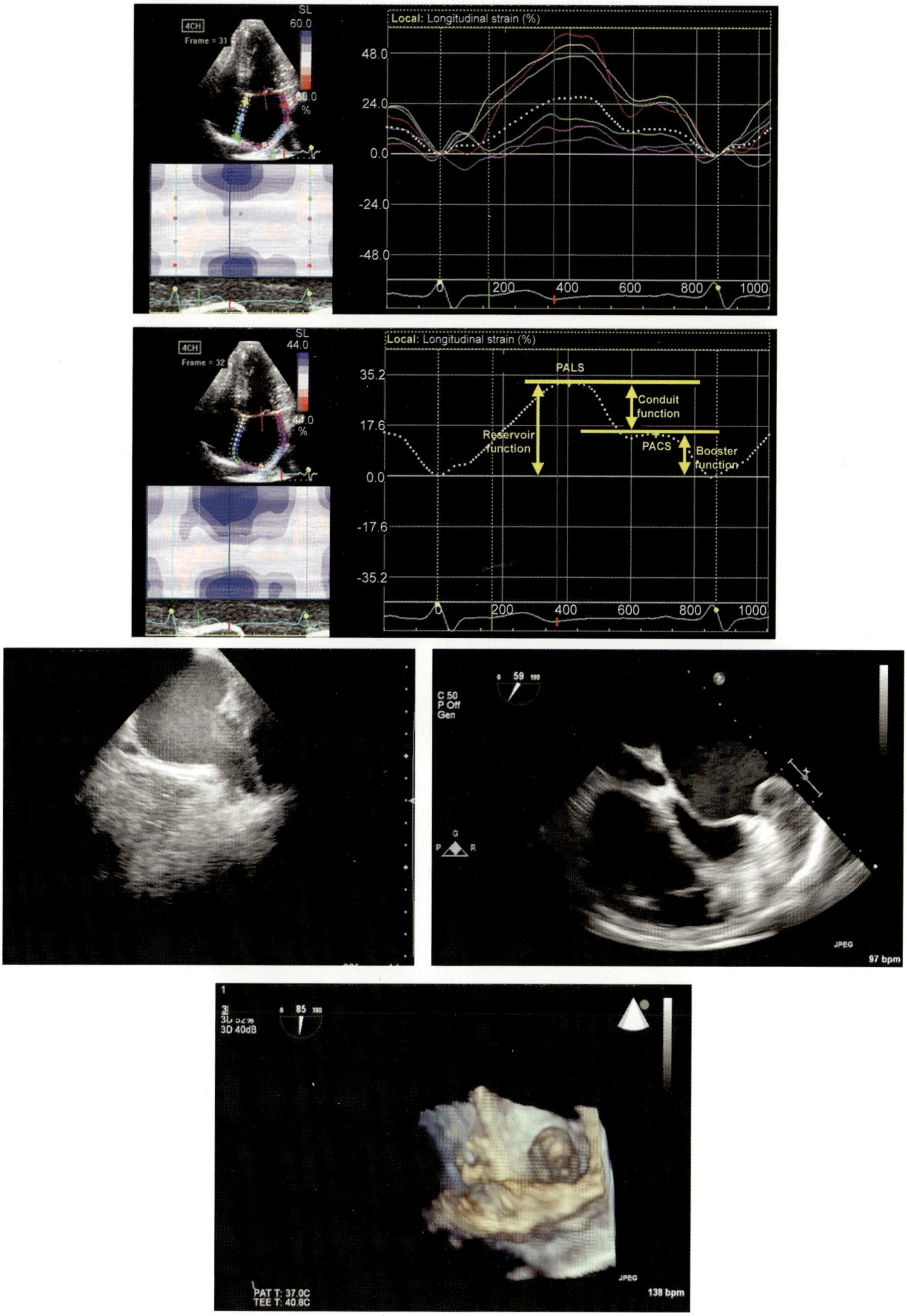

Fig. 6: Spontaneous echo contrast in the left atrium and left atrial appendage; left atrial appendage seen in two-dimensional and three-dimensional echocardiographic imaging.

SEC has been shown to be the predecessor of thrombus formation and, therefore, a predictor of thromboembolic risk in many studies.[57,58,68] With increasing knowledge about AF pathophysiology and risk of stroke, it became evident that an estimate of LAA function can provide incremental information about the risk of clot formation, embolic events, success of cardioversion, etc. Physiologic changes of the LAA emptying velocity flow signals are also seen with age or heart rate but are more pronounced once LAA dysfunction occurs. LAA dysfunction occurs as a consequence of histopathological changes in AF, including fibrosis, loss of atrial muscle mass, remodeling and changes in electrical properties which result in decreased flow within the LAA. This causes the development of a prethrombotic state which can culminate from SEC to thrombus and ultimately to a full-blown embolic event. Therefore, evaluation of the LAA function by Doppler measurement of LAA flow velocities is at present the preferred method of assessment of LAA function.[69] The LAA flow velocities by pulsed-wave Doppler can be obtained from any of the standard imaging planes on TEE by keeping the pulsed-wave sample volume in the proximal one-third segment (toward LA) of the LAA.[69,70] In patients with sinus rhythm, a typical quadriphasic flow pattern can be seen (Fig. 8) consisting of

- Early diastolic emptying velocity—low-velocity outflow seen immediately after mitral inflow E wave.
- Late diastolic emptying velocity or LAA contraction flow which results from active LAA contraction during atrial systole and is thus a marker of LAA contractile function. It is a significant predictor of thromboembolic risk.[71]
- LAA filling inflow velocity negative waves.

TABLE 2: Echocardiographic predictors of thromboembolism in AF.

- TEE evidence of left atrial appendage thrombus > dense SEC
- Reduced (<20 cm/s) left atrial appendage peak ejection velocity
- Left atrial dilatation
- Left ventricular systolic dysfunction
- Valvular pathology
- Complex aortic atheroma

(AF: atrial fibrillation; SEC: spontaneous echocardiographic contrast; TEE: transesophageal echocardiography)

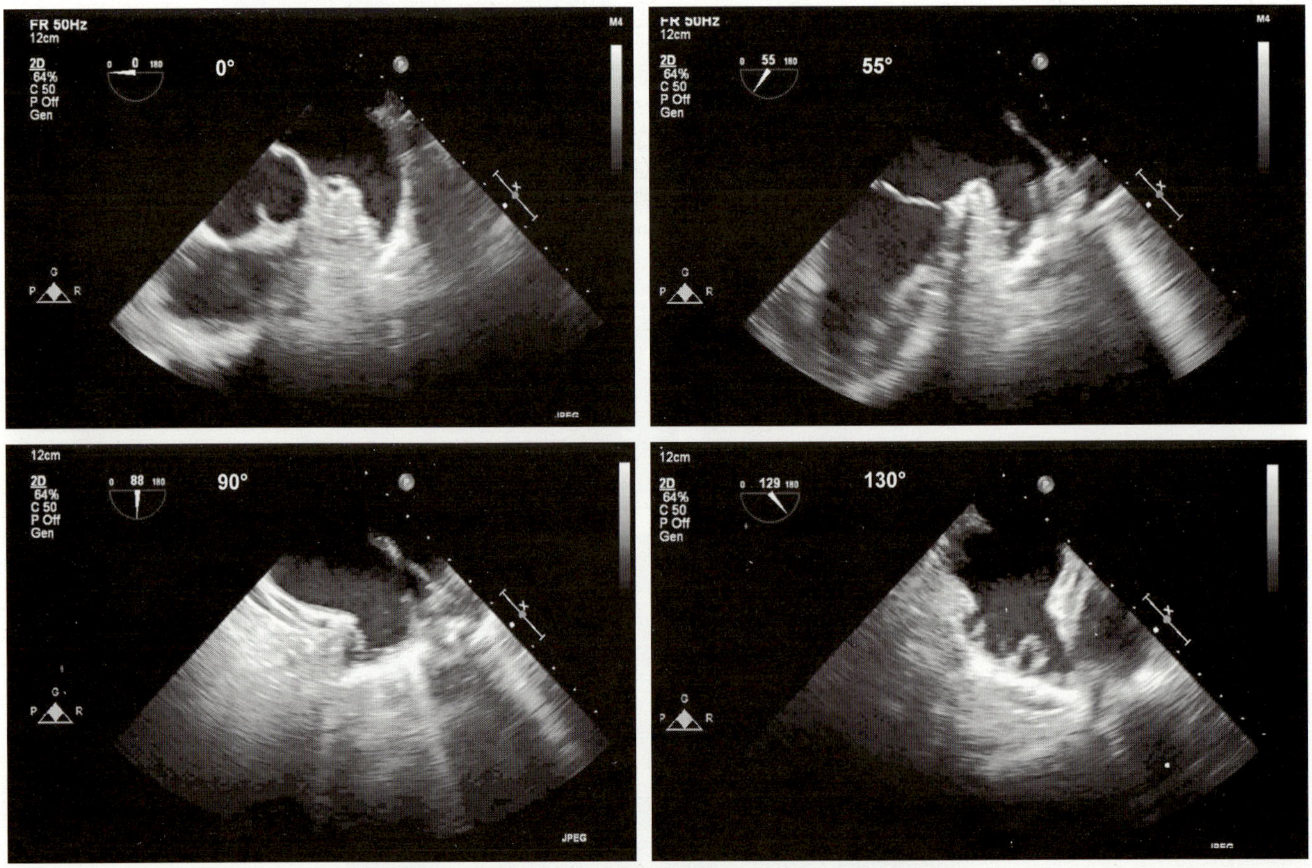

Fig. 7: During transesophageal echocardiography, left atrial appendage is visualized in different projections to ensure complete visualization of all the different lobes of the appendage.

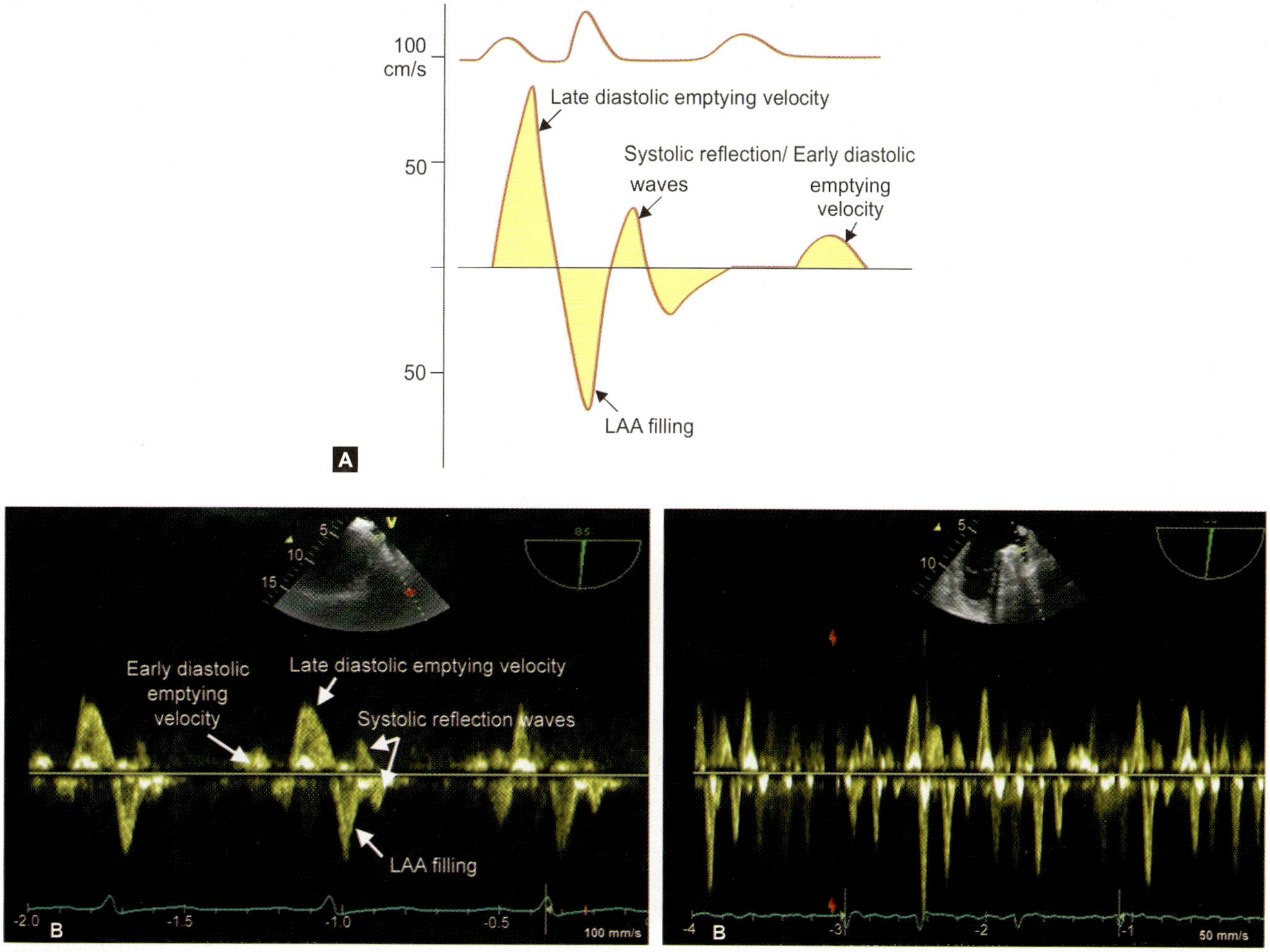

Figs. 8A to C: LAA flow pattern. (A) Schematic diagram showing different flow waves during sinus rhythm; (B) Pulsed-wave Doppler tracing of LAA flow in sinus rhythm; (C) Pulsed-wave Doppler tracing of LAA flow in atrial fibrillation. (LAA: left atrial appendage).
Source: Modified from Bansal M, Kasliwal RR. Echocardiography for left atrial appendage structure and function. Indian Heart J. 2012;64:469-75.

- Multiple low-velocity systolic reflection waves due to passive flow during the remainder of systole.

Left atrial appendage flow velocity, though informative, is an indirect measure of LAA function. It is practical and correlates well with the presence of LAA SEC or thrombus and history of thromboembolic events, but a strong limitation to this modality is that it depends on movement of heart, thus not a true measure of contractility. Other imaging techniques that improve the evaluation of LAA include TD and strain imaging because measurement of tissue velocity provides direct estimate of the LAA contractility. TDI offers the advantage of evaluating LAA myocardial regional function with additional information about risk stratification for thrombi. TDI of LAA is taken from LAA long-axis view with the sample size of 2.5 mm placed at the lateral wall (TDI-L), and septal wall (TDI-S). LAA TDI signals are composed of three waves: (1) early atrial systole, (2) high amplitude late systolic wave, and (3) a late diastolic wave occurring during LAA filling. In AF patients, TDI waves are irregular with disappearance of the early atrial systolic wave.

As discussed above, exclusion of LA/LAA thrombi is obligatory when planning intervention procedures, such as balloon mitral valvotomy, radiofrequency ablation of atrial arrhythmias, and also prior to cardioversion for AF of >48 hours duration in patients who have not been on adequate anticoagulation.

GUIDING THE MANAGEMENT

In an AF patient, the role of echocardiography in management can be understood if divided in these three headings:

1. Transesophageal echocardiography-guided direct current (DC) cardioversion/stratification for anticoagulation
2. Transesophageal echocardiography guidance of percutaneous or surgical LAA closure
3. Intracardiac echocardiography-guided radiofrequency ablation procedures

CARDIOVERSION IN ATRIAL FIBRILLATION

A mainstay of treatment in patients of AF is rhythm control, i.e. restoration to sinus rhythm. DC cardioversion for AF offers the opportunity to restore sinus rhythm, optimize cardiac performance, and potentially reduce the risk of thromboembolic events and bleeding complications caused by prolonged anticoagulation. Cardioversion of AF to sinus rhythm can be performed with high rates of immediate success but unfortunately it may be complicated by embolic events in up to 7% of patients if not preceded by several weeks of anticoagulation. Conventional care of patients with AF of prolonged (more than 48 hours) or unknown duration requires at least 4 weeks of anticoagulation. Though this approach is time tested and significantly lowers the risk of stroke, there are many disadvantages as well. Treatment course is prolonged by 2 months which also increases the bleeding risk and, moreover, being in AF rhythm potentially decreases the functional capacity and, in some cases, can be detrimental for patient care. This has promoted the recent suggestion of alternative escalated approaches, such as TEE-guided early cardioversion (Fig. 9). The advantages of TEE-guided early cardioversion are that in patients without LAA thrombus period of anticoagulation and bleeding risks can be minimized. It is more cost effective also, owing to less laboratory monitoring and reduced complications, and last but not the least, earlier cardioversion has been shown to be linked with successful return and better maintenance of sinus rhythm.[72,73] Even though the long-term value of DC cardioversion has been brought into question by the recent findings of the Atrial Fibrillation Follow-up Investigation of Rhythm Management study,[74] it is clear that symptomatic patients and a proportion of those who are asymptomatic also will continue to receive benefit from this treatment. Now, from some time, TEE has been used before cardioversion when available, and escalated treatment is desirable. It is to be noted that TEE-guided approach to DC cardioversion does not avoid the need for therapeutic anticoagulation. Thromboembolic events have been documented following cardioversion from AF among patients with no thrombus on TEE possibly caused by tiny thrombi not seen at TEE or as a result of thrombus formation caused by LAA stunning following cardioversion.

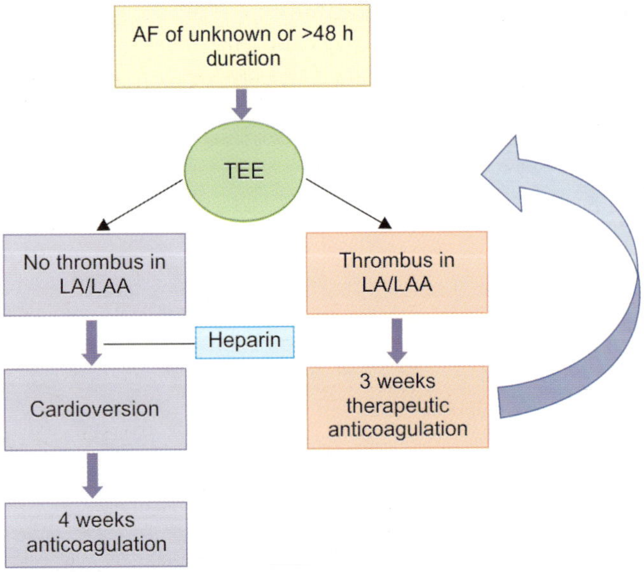

Fig. 9: Approach for transesophageal echocardiography–guided cardioversion of atrial fibrillation. (AF: Atrial fibrillation; LA: left atrium; LAA: left atrial appendage; TEE: transesophageal echocardiography).

Cardioversion can be performed with intravenous heparin or nonvitamin K oral anticoagulant (NOAC) if no thrombi are seen, and this is followed by a month of warfarin or NOAC therapy to prevent new thrombus formation after cardioversion. On the other hand, cardioversion should be delayed, if thrombi are seen in any cardiac chamber, anticoagulation is initiated, and if cardioversion is desired, a repeat TEE should be performed to confirm thrombus resolution prior to cardioversion. In patients presenting with a shorter duration of AF (<48 hours) the risk of thromboembolism following cardioversion is low. While anticoagulation before cardioversion is recommended in these patients, TEE is not usually mandated unless patients are at high-risk for thromboembolism.

Percutaneous Closure of the Left Atrial Appendage

Percutaneous occlusion of the LAA by an expandable occluder device is a new approach in the treatment of embolic complications of AF. As 90% of thrombi occur in the LA appendage, occlusion of the LAA could potentially reduce the rate of thromboembolic complications in high-risk patients or those where anticoagulation is relatively contraindicated or not desired for a long-term. Echocardiography is indispensable in the planning and guiding percutaneous device closure of the LAA (Figs. 10 and 11). Accurate echocardiographic measurement of the LAA anatomy, especially of the ostium, is critically important for successful LAA ostial closure using the Watchman device. Multiplanar TEE assessment is currently the main modality used to screen suitable candidates for device closure of the LAA as it cannot be fully examined by TTE. The presence of thrombus is an absolute contraindication, whereas the presence of dense SEC or valvular pathology is also to be watched for. Baseline LA dimensions in the anteroposterior and craniocaudal planes (0° and 120°, respectively) are noted, and an assessment of the ostial dimensions of the LAA is performed to provisionally determine the size of the device required. Typically, a device with a diameter larger than the LAA ostium is chosen to ensure sufficient anchoring for stable positioning. Device sizing is crucial to ensure device stability, optimum sealing of the LAA ostium, and minimize the risk of leakage, which could provide a new source of future thromboembolism, and it cannot be done without TEE. Echocardiography is invaluable when guiding the transseptal puncture, in verifying position of the delivery sheath and aiding delivery and deployment of the device at the LAA ostium. Color-flow Doppler is used to detect any leaks into the LA, which may suggest an undersized implant, and complete seal of the LAA orifice should be confirmed before release. Any interference with surrounding structures resulting in the disruption of mitral inflow and pulmonary vein flow is confirmed by TEE before irretrievable device deployment. The echocardiography grading system is

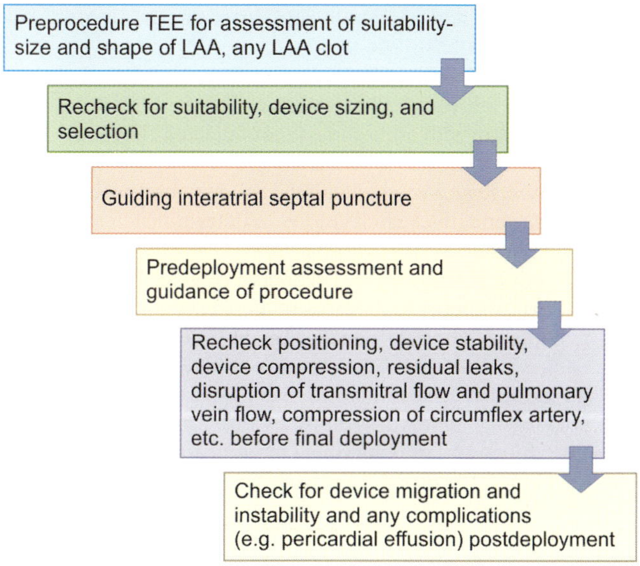

Fig. 10: Role of transesophageal echocardiography in planning and guiding percutaneous left atrial appendage occlusion. (LAA: left atrial appendage; TEE: transesophageal echocardiography).

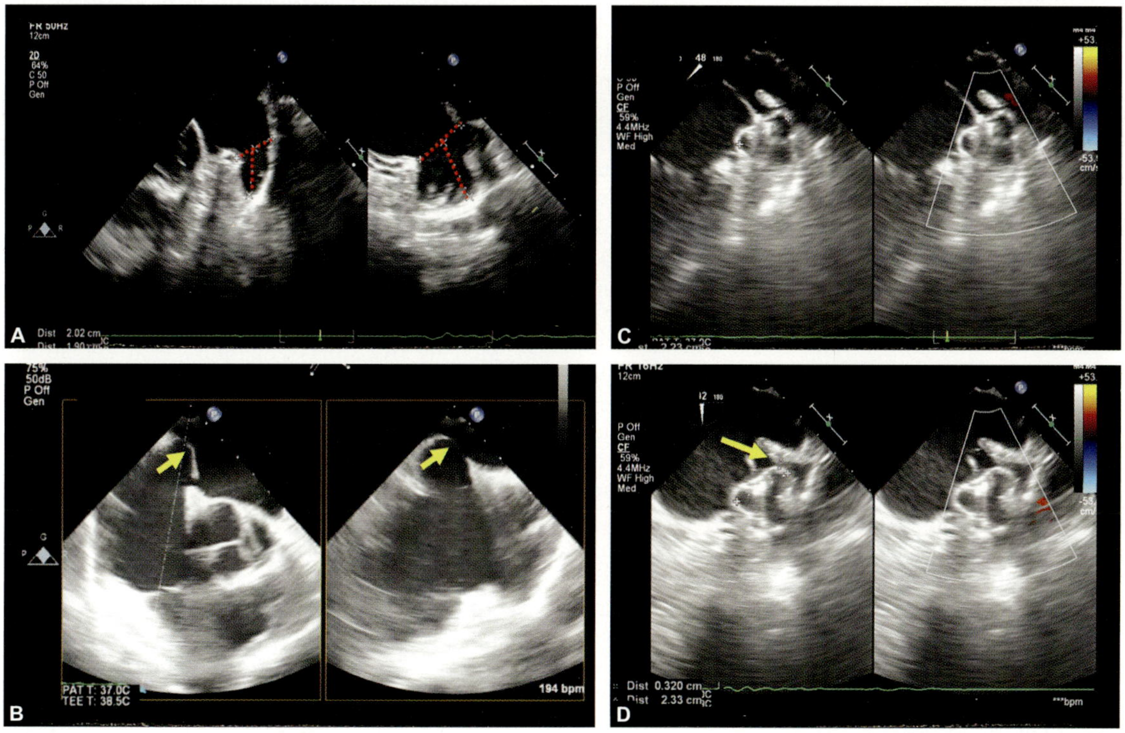

Figs. 11A to D: An illustrative example demonstrating utility of transesophageal echocardiography in guiding percutaneous left atrial appendage occlusion. (A) Measurement of the left atrial appendage for device selection. (B) Guiding transseptal puncture, which is a crucial step in this procedure. The puncture needle is seen indenting the interatrial septum in its posterior and inferior part. (C and D) Assessment of device positioning, compression, residual leak if any (arrow), pulmonary venous flow, etc. immediately before device release.

then used to assess the success of occlusion immediately postprocedure and at follow-up, with successful occlusion being defined as Grade 3 or higher.[75]

REFERENCES

1. Vaziri SM, Larson MG, Benjamin EJ, et al. Echocardiographic predictors of nonrheumatic atrial fibrillation. The Framingham Heart Study. Circulation. 1994;89:724-30.
2. Chugh SS, Havmoeller R, Narayanan K, et al. Worldwide epidemiology of atrial fibrillation: a Global Burden of Disease 2010 Study. Circulation. 2014;129:837-47.
3. Mathur R, Pollara E, Hull S, et al. Ethnicity and stroke risk in patients with atrial fibrillation. Heart. 2013;99:1087-92.
4. Kirchhof P, Benussi S, Kotecha D, et al. 2016 ESC guidelines for the management of atrial fibrillation developed in collaboration with EACTS. Eur Heart J. 2016;37: 2893-962.
5. Kannel WB, Wolf PA, Benjamin EJ, et al. Prevalence, incidence, prognosis, and predisposing conditions for atrial fibrillation: population-based estimates. Am J Cardiol. 1998;82:2N-9N.
6. Krahn AD, Manfreda J, Tate RB, et al. The natural history of atrial fibrillation: incidence, risk factors, and prognosis in the Manitoba Follow-Up Study. Am J Med. 1995;98:476-84.
7. Probst P, Goldschlager N, Selzer A. Left atrial size and atrial fibrillation in mitral stenosis. Factors influencing their relationship. Circulation. 1973;48:1282-7.
8. Santhanakrishnan R, Wang N, Larson MG, et al. Atrial fibrillation begets heart failure and vice versa: temporal associations and differences in preserved versus reduced ejection fraction. Circulation. 2016;133:484-92.
9. Cecchi F, Olivotto I, Montereggi A, et al. Hypertrophic cardiomyopathy in Tuscany: clinical course and outcome in an unselected regional population. J Am Coll Cardiol. 1995;26:1529-36.
10. Tikoff G, Schmidt AM, Hecht HH. Atrial fibrillation in atrial septal defect. Arch Intern Med. 1968;121:402-5.
11. Devereux RB, Roman MJ, Paranicas M, et al. Impact of diabetes on cardiac structure and function: the strong heart study. Circulation. 2000;101:2271-6.
12. Grundy SM, Cleeman JI, Daniels SR, et al. Diagnosis and management of the metabolic syndrome: an American Heart Association/National Heart, Lung, and Blood Institute Scientific Statement. Circulation. 2005;112:2735-52.
13. Watanabe H, Watanabe T, Sasaki S, et al. Close bidirectional relationship between chronic kidney disease and atrial fibrillation: the Niigata preventive medicine study. Am Heart J. 2009;158:629-36.
14. Nalliah CJ, Sanders P, Kalman JM. Obstructive sleep apnea treatment and atrial fibrillation: a need for definitive evidence. J Cardiovasc Electrophysiol. 2016;27:1001-10.
15. Nalliah CJ, Sanders P, Kottkamp H, et al. The role of obesity in atrial fibrillation. Eur Heart J. 2016;37:1565-72.
16. Matsukida K, Kisanuki A, Toyonaga K, et al. Comparison of transthoracic Doppler echocardiography and natriuretic peptides in predicting mean pulmonary capillary wedge pressure in patients with chronic atrial fibrillation. J Am Soc Echocardiogr. 2001;14:1080-7.
17. Tsang TS, Barnes ME, Gersh BJ, et al. Left atrial volume as a morphophysiologic expression of left ventricular diastolic dysfunction and relation to cardiovascular risk burden. Am J Cardiol. 2002;90:1284-9.
18. Simek CL, Feldman MD, Haber HL, et al. Relationship between left ventricular wall thickness and left atrial size: comparison with other measures of diastolic function. J Am Soc Echocardiogr. 1995;8:37-47.
19. Lester SJ, Ryan EW, Schiller NB, et al. Best method in clinical practice and in research studies to determine left atrial size. Am J Cardiol. 1999;84:829-32.
20. Loperfido F, Pennestri F, Digaetano A, et al. Assessment of left atrial dimensions by cross sectional echocardiography in patients with mitral valve disease. Br Heart J. 1983;50:570-8.
21. Lang RM, Bierig M, Devereux RB, et al. Recommendations for chamber quantification: a report from the American Society of Echocardiography's Guidelines and Standards Committee and the Chamber Quantification Writing Group, developed in conjunction with the European Association of Echocardiography, a branch of the European Society of Cardiology. J Am Soc Echocardiogr. 2005;18:1440-63.
22. Abhayaratna WP, Seward JB, Appleton CP, et al. Left atrial size: physiologic determinants and clinical applications. J Am Coll Cardiol. 2006;47:2357-63.
23. Benjamin EJ, D'Agostino RB, Belanger AJ, et al. Left atrial size and the risk of stroke and death. The Framingham Heart Study. Circulation. 1995;92:835-41.
24. Bouzas-Mosquera A, Broullon FJ, Alvarez-Garcia N, et al. Left atrial size and risk for all-cause mortality and ischemic stroke. CMAJ. 2011;183:E657-64.
25. Di Tullio MR, Sacco RL, Sciacca RR, et al. Left atrial size and the risk of ischemic stroke in an ethnically mixed population. Stroke. 1999;30:2019-24.
26. Dini FL, Cortigiani L, Baldini U, et al. Prognostic value of left atrial enlargement in patients with idiopathic dilated cardiomyopathy and ischemic cardiomyopathy. Am J Cardiol. 2002;89:518-23.
27. Modena MG, Muia N, Sgura FA, et al. Left atrial size is the major predictor of cardiac death and overall clinical outcome in patients with dilated cardiomyopathy: a long-term follow-up study. Clin Cardiol. 1997;20:553-60.
28. Moller JE, Hillis GS, Oh JK, et al. Left atrial volume: a powerful predictor of survival after acute myocardial infarction. Circulation. 2003;107:2207-12.
29. Nagarajarao HS, Penman AD, Taylor HA, et al. The predictive value of left atrial size for incident ischemic stroke and all-cause mortality in African Americans: the Atherosclerosis Risk in Communities (ARIC) Study. Stroke. 2008;39:2701-6.
30. Ristow B, Ali S, Whooley MA, et al. Usefulness of left atrial volume index to predict heart failure hospitalization and mortality in ambulatory patients with coronary heart disease and comparison to left ventricular ejection fraction (from the Heart and Soul Study). Am J Cardiol. 2008;102:70-6.
31. Sabharwal N, Cemin R, Rajan K, et al. Usefulness of left atrial volume as a predictor of mortality in patients with ischemic cardiomyopathy. Am J Cardiol. 2004;94:760-3.

32. Takemoto Y, Barnes ME, Seward JB, et al. Usefulness of left atrial volume in predicting first congestive heart failure in patients > or = 65 years of age with well-preserved left ventricular systolic function. Am J Cardiol. 2005;96:832-6.
33. Tsang TS, Barnes ME, Bailey KR, et al. Left atrial volume: important risk marker of incident atrial fibrillation in 1655 older men and women. Mayo Clin Proc. 2001;76:467-75.
34. Tsang TS, Barnes ME, Gersh BJ, et al. Risks for atrial fibrillation and congestive heart failure in patients >/=65 years of age with abnormal left ventricular diastolic relaxation. Am J Cardiol. 2004;93:54-8.
35. Yasuda R, Murata M, Roberts R, et al. Left atrial strain is a powerful predictor of atrial fibrillation recurrence after catheter ablation: study of a heterogeneous population with sinus rhythm or atrial fibrillation. Eur Heart J Cardiovasc Imaging. 2015;16:1008-14.
36. Mor-Avi V, Lang RM, Badano LP, et al. Current and evolving echocardiographic techniques for the quantitative evaluation of cardiac mechanics: ASE/EAE consensus statement on methodology and indications endorsed by the Japanese Society of Echocardiography. J Am Soc Echocardiogr. 2011;24:277-313.
37. Cameli M, Lisi M, Righini FM, Mondillo S. Novel echocardiographic techniques to assess left atrial size, anatomy and function. Cardiovasc Ultrasound. 2012;10:4.
38. Pathan F, D'Elia N, Nolan MT, et al. Normal ranges of left atrial strain by speckle-tracking echocardiography: a systematic review and meta-analysis. J Am Soc Echocardiogr. 2017;30:59-70.e8.
39. Donal E, Ollivier R, Veillard D, et al. Left atrial function assessed by trans-thoracic echocardiography in patients treated by ablation for a lone paroxysmal atrial fibrillation. Eur J Echocardiogr. 2010;11:845-52.
40. Kaya EB, Tokgozoglu L, Aytemir K, et al. Atrial myocardial deformation properties are temporarily reduced after cardioversion for atrial fibrillation and correlate well with left atrial appendage function. Eur J Echocardiogr. 2008;9:472-7.
41. Kuppahally SS, Akoum N, Burgon NS, et al. Left atrial strain and strain rate in patients with paroxysmal and persistent atrial fibrillation: relationship to left atrial structural remodeling detected by delayed-enhancement MRI. Circ Cardiovasc Imaging. 2010;3:231-9.
42. Mondillo S, Cameli M, Caputo ML, et al. Early detection of left atrial strain abnormalities by speckle-tracking in hypertensive and diabetic patients with normal left atrial size. J Am Soc Echocardiogr. 2011;24:898-908.
43. Bollmann A, Binias KH, Grothues F, et al. Left atrial appendage function and pulmonary venous flow in patients with nonrheumatic atrial fibrillation and their relation to spontaneous echo contrast. Echocardiography. 2002;19: 37-43.
44. Zabalgoitia M, Halperin JL, Pearce LA. Transesophageal echocardiographic correlates of thromboembolism in high-risk patients with nonvalvular atrial fibrillation. The Stroke Prevention in Atrial Fibrillation Investigators Committee on Echocardiography. Ann Intern Med. 1998;128:639-47.
45. Mugge A, Kuhn H, Nikutta P, et al. Assessment of left atrial appendage function by biplane transesophageal echocardiography in patients with nonrheumatic atrial fibrillation: identification of a subgroup of patients at increased embolic risk. J Am Coll Cardiol. 1994;23:599-607.
46. Li YH, Lai LP, Shyu KG, et al. Clinical implications of left atrial appendage flow patterns in nonrheumatic atrial fibrillation. Chest. 1994;105:748-52.
47. Li YH, Hwang JJ, Lin JL, et al. Importance of left atrial appendage function as a risk factor for systemic thromboembolism in patients with rheumatic mitral valve disease. Am J Cardiol. 1996;78:844-7.
48. Santiago D, Warshofsky M, Li Mandri G, et al. Left atrial appendage function and thrombus formation in atrial fibrillation-flutter: a transesophageal echocardiographic study. J Am Coll Cardiol. 1994;24:159-64.
49. Grimm RA, Stewart WJ, Arheart K, et al. Left atrial appendage "stunning" after electrical cardioversion of atrial flutter: an attenuated response compared with atrial fibrillation as the mechanism for lower susceptibility to thromboembolic events. J Am Coll Cardiol. 1997;29:582-9.
50. Hwang JJ, Li YH, Lin JM, et al. Left atrial appendage function determined by transesophageal echocardiography in patients with rheumatic mitral valve disease. Cardiology. 1994;85:121-8.
51. Reddy VG, Rajasekhar D, Vanajakshamma V. Effect of percutaneous mitral balloon valvuloplasty on left atrial appendage function: transesophageal echo study. Indian Heart J. 2012;64:462-8.
52. Obokata M, Negishi K, Kurosawa K, et al. Left atrial strain provides incremental value for embolism risk stratification over CHA(2)DS(2)-VASc score and indicates prognostic impact in patients with atrial fibrillation. J Am Soc Echocardiogr. 2014;27:709-716.e4.
53. Hsu PC, Lee WH, Chu CY, et al. Prognostic role of left atrial strain and its combination index with transmitral E-wave velocity in patients with atrial fibrillation. Sci Rep. 2016;6:17318.
54. [No authors listed]. Cardiogenic brain embolism. Cerebral Embolism Task Force. Arch Neurol. 1986;43:71-84.
55. Odell JA, Blackshear JL, Davies E, et al. Thoracoscopic obliteration of the left atrial appendage: potential for stroke reduction? Ann Thorac Surg. 1996;61:565-9.
56. Manning WJ, Silverman DI, Gordon SP, et al. Cardioversion from atrial fibrillation without prolonged anticoagulation with use of transesophageal echocardiography to exclude the presence of atrial thrombi. N Engl J Med. 1993;328:750-5.
57. Kasliwal RR, Mittal S, Kanojia A, et al. A study of spontaneous echo contrast in patients with rheumatic mitral stenosis and normal sinus rhythm: an Indian perspective. Br Heart J. 1995;74:296-9.
58. Black IW, Hopkins AP, Lee LC, et al. Left atrial spontaneous echo contrast: a clinical and echocardiographic analysis. J Am Coll Cardiol. 1991;18:398-404.
59. Saygi S, Turk UO, Alioglu E, et al. Left atrial appendage function in mitral stenosis: is it determined by cardiac rhythm? J Heart Valve Dis. 2011;20:417-24.
60. Tenekecioglu E, Karabulut A, Yilmaz M. Comparison of tissue Doppler dynamics with Doppler flow in evaluating left atrial appendage function by transesophageal

echocardiography in prehypertensive and hypertensive patients. Echocardiography. 2010;27:677-86.
61. Veinot JP, Harrity PJ, Gentile F, et al. Anatomy of the normal left atrial appendage: a quantitative study of age-related changes in 500 autopsy hearts: implications for echocardiographic examination. Circulation. 1997;96:3112-5.
62. Shanewise JS, Cheung AT, Aronson S, et al. ASE/SCA guidelines for performing a comprehensive intraoperative multiplane transesophageal echocardiography examination: recommendations of the American Society of Echocardiography Council for Intraoperative Echocardiography and the Society of Cardiovascular Anesthesiologists Task Force for Certification in Perioperative Transesophageal Echocardiography. J Am Soc Echocardiogr. 1999;12:884-900.
63. Manning WJ, Weintraub RM, Waksmonski CA, et al. Accuracy of transesophageal echocardiography for identifying left atrial thrombi. A prospective, intraoperative study. Ann Intern Med. 1995;123:817-22.
64. Ruiz-Arango A, Landolfo C. A novel approach to the diagnosis of left atrial appendage thrombus using contrast echocardiography and power Doppler imaging. Eur J Echocardiogr. 2008;9:329-33.
65. von der Recke G, Schmidt H, Illien S, et al. Use of transesophageal contrast echocardiography for excluding left atrial appendage thrombi in patients with atrial fibrillation before cardioversion. J Am Soc Echocardiogr. 2002;15:1256-61.
66. von der Recke G, Schmidt H, Illien S, et al. Transesophageal contrast echocardiography distinguishes a left atrial appendage thrombus from spontaneous echo contrast. Echocardiography. 2002;19:343-4.
67. Shah SJ, Bardo DM, Sugeng L, et al. Real-time three-dimensional transesophageal echocardiography of the left atrial appendage: initial experience in the clinical setting. J Am Soc Echocardiogr. 2008;21:1362-8.
68. Jaber WA, Prior DL, Thamilarasan M, et al. Efficacy of anticoagulation in resolving left atrial and left atrial appendage thrombi: a transesophageal echocardiographic study. Am Heart J. 2000;140:150-6.
69. Agmon Y, Khandheria BK, Gentile F, et al. Echocardiographic assessment of the left atrial appendage. J Am Coll Cardiol. 1999;34:1867-77.
70. Donal E, Yamada H, Leclercq C, et al. The left atrial appendage, a small, blind-ended structure: a review of its echocardiographic evaluation and its clinical role. Chest. 2005;128:1853-62.
71. Agmon Y, Khandheria BK, Meissner I, et al. Left atrial appendage flow velocities in subjects with normal left ventricular function. Am J Cardiol. 2000;86:769-73.
72. Weinberg DM, Mancini J. Anticoagulation for cardioversion of atrial fibrillation. Am J Cardiol. 1989;63:745-6.
73. Arnold AZ, Mick MJ, Mazurek RP, et al. Role of prophylactic anticoagulation for direct current cardioversion in patients with atrial fibrillation or atrial flutter. J Am Coll Cardiol. 1992;19:851-5.
74. Wyse DG, Waldo AL, DiMarco JP, et al. A comparison of rate control and rhythm control in patients with atrial fibrillation. N Engl J Med. 2002;347:1825-33.
75. Chue CD, de Giovanni J, Steeds RP. The role of echocardiography in percutaneous left atrial appendage occlusion. Eur J Echocardiogr. 2011;12:i3-10.

71

CHAPTER

Echocardiographic Evaluation of LV Diastolic Dysfunction and Drugs that Modify Diastolic Dysfunction

Hanumanth K Reddy, Ravi Komatireddy, Thirupathi K Reddy, Raghuveer Kura

INTRODUCTION

With aging population and increasing risk factor burden, diastolic heart failure is becoming more prevalent, occurring in 50% of total heart failure patients. These patients have mortality and morbidity similar to those of systolic heart failure patients.[1] Furthermore, no appropriate treatment is available for these patients. Prevention of diastolic congestive heart failure (CHF) is feasible with early diagnosis and aggressive risk factor modification. Therefore, there is a need for accurate noninvasive diagnosis of left ventricular diastolic dysfunction (LVDD) with echocardiography (Echo). Other modes of tests such as CTA, MRI and invasive cardiac catheterization are available. However, echocardiographic parameters based on Doppler measurements are often used for clinical diagnosis of LV diastolic dysfunction. These Doppler based parameters do not necessarily reflect the intrinsic LV diastolic properties of the left ventricle. Therefore, it is recommended that the diagnosis of LV diastolic dysfunction and diastolic heart failure (HF) should be based on an aggregate of clinical and echocardiographic variables including HF in the presence of normal left ventricular ejection fraction (LVEF) and the relevant echo-Doppler variables. In any given patient, a single echocardiographic parameter may not be reliable. Based on the clinical situation one or more measurements should be used in concert with the relevant clinical information in order make a diagnosis of LV diastolic dysfunction.

PATHOPHYSIOLOGY OF LV DIASTOLIC DYSFUNCTION

Left ventricular diastolic dysfunction is due to increased LV stiffness producing higher diastolic pressure at the normal ranges of LV diastolic volume as shown on the pressure/volume curve in Figure 1. Delayed myocardial relaxation in the elderly causes a decrease in mitral E/A ratio and in E' velocity (Fig. 2).

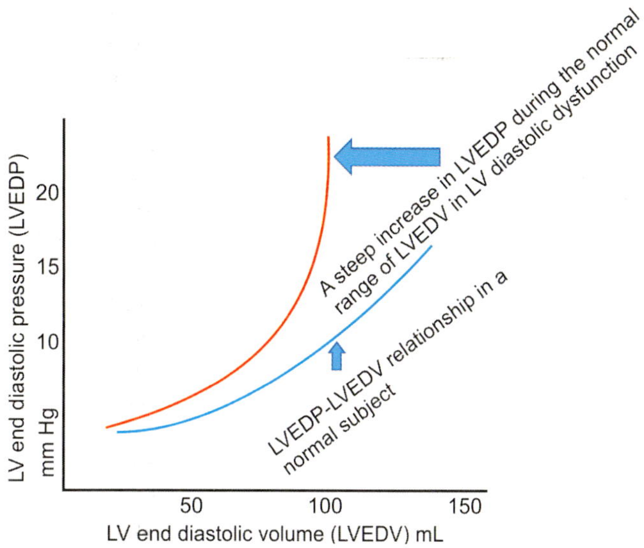

Fig. 1: Abnormal pressure-volume relationship in left ventricular diastolic dysfunction (LVDD).

ECHOCARDIOGRAPHIC PARAMETERS OF LV DIASTOLIC DYSFUNCTION (TABLE 1)

E/A Ratio

The most commonly used Doppler measurement of LVDD is E/A ratio, E reflecting the pressure gradient between the left atrium (LA) and the left ventricle and A representing peak of late diastolic mitral flow velocity during atrial contraction. In a normal person with normal LV diastolic function and normal pressures, early mitral inflow is rapid and predominant followed by late diastolic mitral flow with atrial contraction. In patients with impaired LV relaxation, early diastolic mitral inflow velocity (E) is slower occurring over a longer period of time. The late diastolic atrial contraction velocity (A) increases leading to reversal of E/A (Fig. 2).[2] However, LA to LV gradient varies with the degree of LV relaxation and LA pressure. Therefore E/A ratio, although easily obtainable and readily useful in clinical practice, is fraught with the following confounding variables. Preload, tachycardia and moderate diastolic dysfunction influence E/A ratio. For this reason, the American Society of Echocardiography, and the European Association of Echocardiography recommend the usage of an algorithm that includes E/A ratio.[3] In patients with increased LV diastolic pressure, E velocity increase and A velocity decreases giving the appearance of so-called pseudonormalization (Figs. 3 and 4). As LV diastolic dysfunction worsens, LA pressure and LA-LV pressure gradient increase significantly, causing a marked increase in E and E/A ratio of greater than 1.7.

As expected in patients with LVDD, measures of LV diastolic relaxation such as isovolumic relaxation time (IVRT) and mitral E velocity deceleration time (DT) are prolonged (Fig. 5).

TABLE 1: Echocardiographic parameters of LV diastolic dysfunction.

Category	*Abnormal changes*	*Grade of LV diastolic dysfunction*
Mitral valve velocities		
	Initial reversal of E/A ratio	Grade I LVDD
	Pseudonormalization of E/A	Grade II LVDD
	• Associated reduction in e′ • More prominent reversal of pulmonary venous velocity • Inversion of pseudonormalization with Valsalva	
	Reversal of pulmonary venous velocity	Grade III LVDD
	E/A >2 in grade III LVDD	
	IVRT >70 ms	
	DT >240 ms or <140 ms	
Tissue Doppler imaging		
	Annular septal E′ velocity	<7 cm/s
	Annular lateral velocity	<10 cm/s
	E/e′ ratio >14 indicates elevated left ventricular end-diastolic pressure	
Pressure and volume overload changes		
	Left atrial volume index	$>34/m^2$
	Biatrial dilatation	
	RV pressure overload and pulmonary hypertension	

(E/A: early diastolic velocity/atrial contraction velocity; LVDD: left ventricular diastolic dysfunction; IVRT: isovolumetric relaxation time; DT: mitral E wave deceleration time)

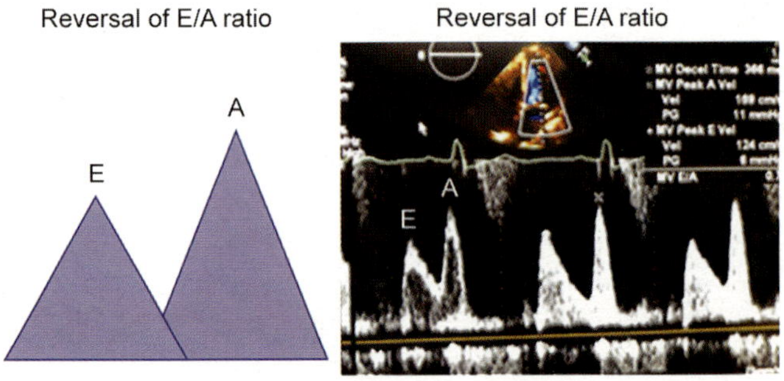

Fig. 2: Mitral inflow velocity pattern in grade I left ventricular diastolic dysfunction (LVDD).

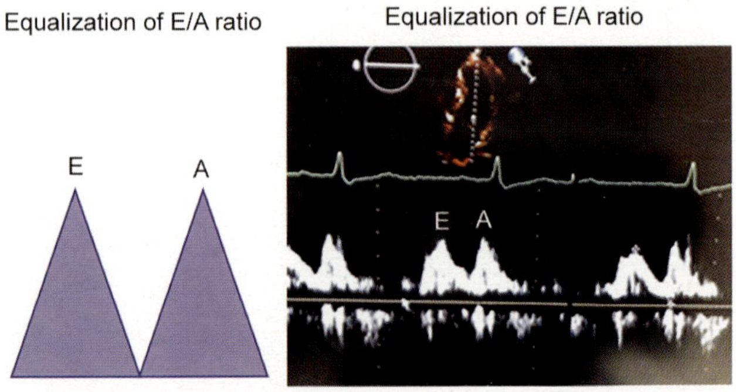

Fig. 3: Mitral inflow velocity pattern in grade II left ventricular diastolic dysfunction (LVDD).

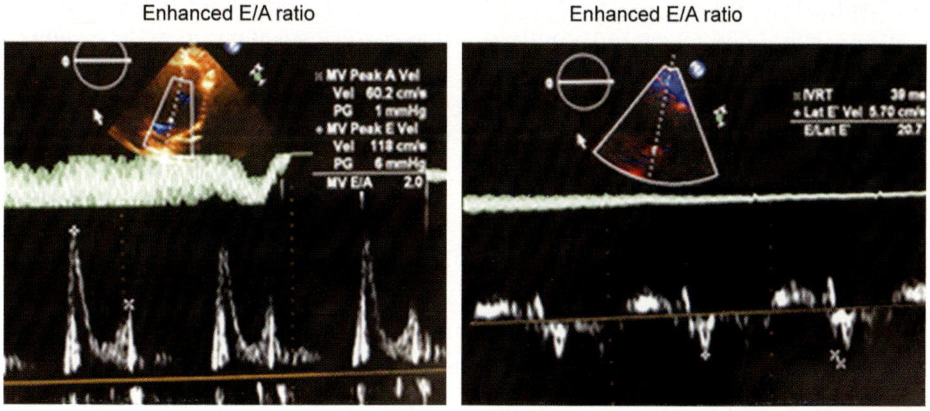

Fig. 4: Mitral inflow velocity pattern in grade III left ventricular diastolic dysfunction (LVDD).

Isovolumic Relaxation Time

It is the period of cardiac cycle from the closure of the aortic valve to the opening of the mitral valve. With impaired myocardial relaxation, IVRT is usually prolonged. Normal IVRT is 70 + 12 ms and 10 ms longer in people over the age of 40 years. In patients with LVDD, IVRT is longer than 110 ms. However, in patients with advanced LVDD, with restrictive filling it is significantly shortened to 60 ms or under.

Deceleration Time

It is the duration of time between maximal mitral E velocity and its zero. Normal DT ranges from 140 ms to 240 ms. Deceleration time is age dependent and increases with age.

In grade I LVDD, E wave DT time is more than 200 ms. However E/e' ratio is normal. In grade II LVDD, deceleration time becomes normal (160–200 ms). However, E/e' ratio is abnormally increased. In grade III LVDD, DT further decreases below 160 ms and E/e' ratio remains elevated (Fig. 4). In grade IV LVDD, a pattern of DT and E/e' is similar to that of grade III LVDD with higher severity.

STRUCTURAL SUBSTRATES OF LEFT VENTRICULAR DIASTOLIC DYSFUNCTION

LV Hypertrophy

Left ventricular hypertrophy (LVH) with increased LV mass is most commonly associated with LV diastolic dysfunction. With advanced age and hypertension, LVH is quite common in the elderly and so is LVDD. Although, LVDD may occur in patients without LVH, it is far more common in patients with LVH and therefore provides an initial clue for further echocardiographic evaluation of LVDD. Using American Society of Echocardiography guidelines, LV mass can be estimated in most patients with 2-D echocardiography.[4]

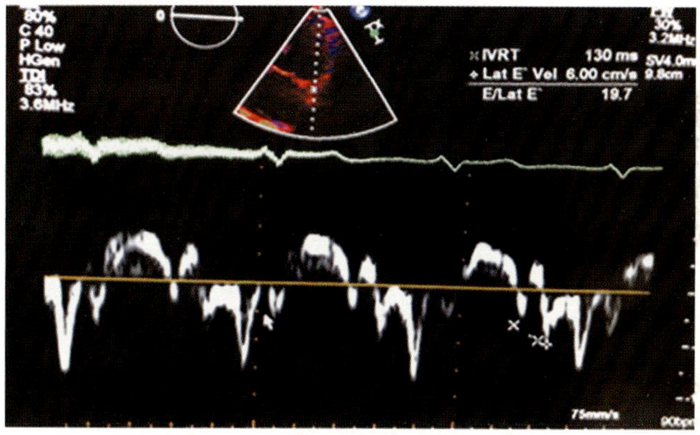

Fig. 5: Tissue Doppler imaging showing decreased E' and increased E/E'.

LA Volume

Left atrium remodeling in chronic LV diastolic dysfunction is associated with pressure overload in patients with LV diastolic dysfunction. In fact, a good correlation between LA remodeling and echocardiographic indices of diastolic function has been reported.[5] LA dilatation may occur in many other conditions, however, the most common cause is LVDD in the elderly population. However, LA assessment in LVDD should be placed in the clinical context.

In patients with suspected LVDD, measurement of LA volume index should be an integral part of routine echocardiography. LA dilatation has a significant prognostic value. LA volume index more than or equal to 34 mL/m^2 was reported to predict atrial fibrillation, ischemic stroke, CHF and death.[6]

LA Function

Through its triphasic role as a reservoir, a conduit, and a pumping chamber, left atrium plays a significant role in the facilitation and completion of LV diastole. With progressive impairment of left atrial conduit and booster functions in patients with LVDD, diastolic heart failure gets worse due to impaired LV filling with decreased cardiac output, or complete LV filling at the cost of increased LV end diastolic pressure and right sided pressures. In patients with severe LVDD, LA contractility decreases and therefore decreased LV filling and increased pulmonary and right sided congestion.

To further elucidate LA function, LA stroke volume, LA ejection force, LA strain and strain rate can be estimated with echo, Doppler and strain measurements. However, clinical utility of these complex set of measurements is yet to be determined in various conditions associated with diastolic heart failure. Therefore, detailed discussion of these parameters is beyond the scope of this chapter.[7-10]

Biatrial Dilatation

It is fairly common to find marked dilatation of both the atrial chambers in patients with advanced LVDD (Fig. 6). With pressure-volume overload of the ventricular chambers, the thin walled and flexible atria undergo marked dilatation and often larger than the ventricles themselves in patients with advanced LVDD.

Tissue Doppler Imaging and Estimation of LV Filling Pressures

During longitudinal contraction of left ventricle mitral annulus moves towards the fixed LV apex and conversely, during LV relaxation mitral annulus moves away from LV apex. For the most part, mitral annular velocities are considered to represent an average summation of myocardial segmental velocities. Early diastolic velocity (Ea) correlates with transmitral E wave and its magnitude decreases with worsening of LV diastolic dysfunction.

Pulsed wave TDI is obtained by placing 2–5 mm sample volume at the lateral or septal border of the mitral annulus in apical 4-chamber view and lateral annular Ea is more commonly used than the color tissue Doppler.

With progressive worsening of LV diastolic dysfunction, left atrial pressure increases and so is E velocity. On the other hand, Ea velocity decreases and E/Ea ratio was shown to correlate with mean left atrial pressure (*see* Fig. 5).[11]

Pulmonary Hypertension

Patients with chronic progressive LVDD, develop elevation of left ventricular end-diastolic pressure, left atrial pressure and compensatory right ventricular and pulmonary artery pressures (Fig. 7). Patients with diastolic heart failure have increased pulmonary artery (PA) pressures. In the absence of other confounding variables, Doppler derived pulmonary hypertension in LVDD patients reflects elevated left ventricular end-diastolic pressure. Bouchard et al. reported a significant correlation between PA systolic pressure and pulmonary artery wedge pressure.[12]

In routine clinical practice, using modified Bernoulli equation, PA pressures are derived from reliably obtained peak velocity of the tricuspid regurgitation (*see* Fig. 5).

Patients with pulmonary hypertension due to advanced LV diastolic dysfunction have increased E/e' ratios more than 8 in contrast to the patients with noncardiac pulmonary hypertension. Mitral lateral annular E velocity increases with elevated LA pressure, and lateral e' velocity decreases with myocardial disease.[13]

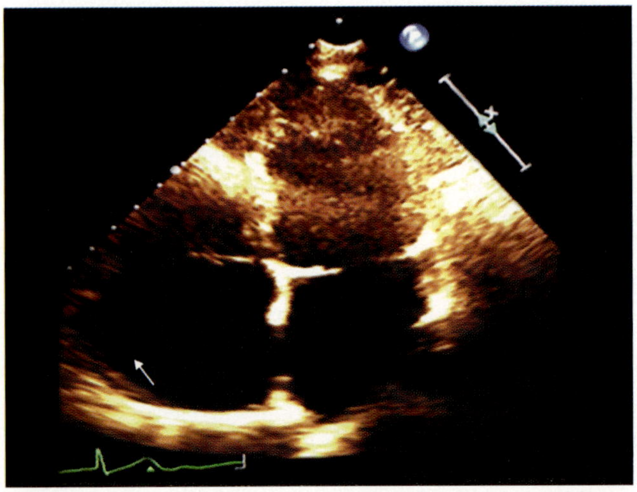

Fig. 6: Biatrial dilatation in severe left ventricular diastolic dysfunction (LVDD).

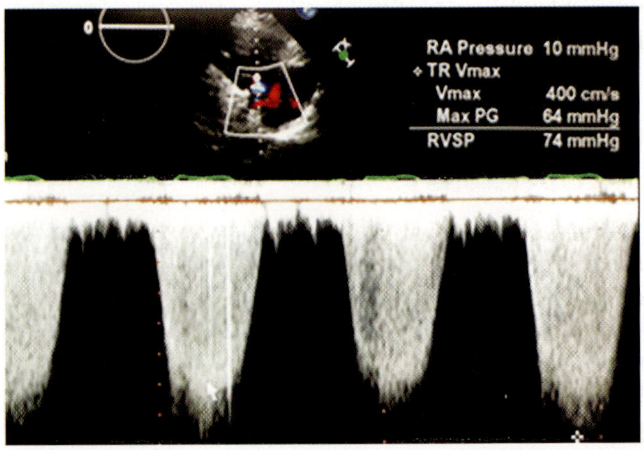

Fig. 7: Echocardiographic evidence of pulmonary hypertension in severe left ventricular diastolic dysfunction (LVDD).

Pulmonary Venous Flow

Doppler recordings of pulmonary venous flow patterns are quite useful in hemodynamic profiling of LVDD patients. Best waveforms are obtained by placing a 2–3 mm sample volume more than 0.5 cm into the right pulmonary vein.

Doppler velocity recordings of pulmonary flow waves reflect atrial and ventricular relaxation and the forward flow patterns of pulmonary vein blood flow to LA and then onto the left ventricle in health and disease. These flow waves are categorized as antegrade S1, S2 and D waves and retrograde atrial reversal wave (Ar). S1 velocity is dependent on LA relaxation, contraction and pressure. S2 is related to RV contraction, forward pulsatile flow from the PA tree. D velocity mimics E velocity and therefore is dependent on left ventricular compliance and relaxation, LA reservoir function and AV pressure gradient during early diastole.[14,15]

Pulmonary venous A wave reversal flow (Ar) velocity and duration are related to LA contractility, and LV late diastolic pressures. Peak pulmonary venous reversal flow (Ar) parallels peak atrial contraction. Ar velocity and duration increase in patients with LVDD with elevated LVEDP. As expected Ar wave disappears in patients with atrial fibrillation. Increased LA pressure and decreased LA compliance cause decreased S velocity and increased D velocity, leading to S/D ratio less than 1, and shortening of the DT of D velocity less than 150 ms.

MANAGEMENT OF LV DIASTOLIC DYSFUNCTION (TABLE 2)

Currently, no good treatment is available for LV diastolic dysfunction. Steps to delay and possibly prevent LVDD are available. Management of exacerbating conditions and symptomatic therapies should be pursued. No good randomized placebo controlled studies targeting LVDD are available at the present time. Enlisted in the following paragraphs are measures, drugs and devices aimed at improving LVDD.

Physiological Approach to LV Diastolic Dysfunction

Left ventricular diastolic dysfunction sets in early in life in certain individuals due to genetic predisposition and environmental factors foster it to make it an irreversible condition associated with diastolic heart failure. The structural and pathophysiological changes of diastolic heart failure take several years. Therefore, an early detection and prevention of structural changes in these patients is critical.

Healthy body maintains a normal range of homeostasis with maintenance of optimal body weight, adequate nutrition, oxygenation, fluid balance, heart rate, blood pressure and sane and peaceful mentation.

TABLE 2: Management of patients with LV diastolic dysfunction.

Lifestyle change	
	Obesity control
	Exercise conditioning
	Management of sleep apnea
	Salt restriction
Blood pressure control	
	Diuretics
	ARBs
	ACE inhibitors
	Calcium channel blockers
	Beta blockers
Atrial fibrillation	
	Rate control
	Ablation with pacing if needed
	Rhythm control
Pharmacology	
	Givinostat: Cardiac relaxer, currently in experimental stage

Lifestyle Modification

Healthy diet with avoidance of obesity and excessive salt, regular exercise conditioning, limiting excessive alcohol intake, smoking cessation, stress control are critical to preventing LVDD.

Management of Comorbid Conditions

Optimal management of weight, hypertension, diabetes mellitus, hyperlipidemia and coronary artery disease play a major role in delaying LVDD.

Drug Therapy

No single drug or group of drugs have so far been proven to have a major beneficial effect on LVDD. However, several drugs are available to control precipitating factors of LVDD.

Medications with Influence on Ventricular Remodeling and Fluid Homeostasis

- Angiotensin-converting enzyme (ACE) inhibitors[16]
- Angiotensin receptor blockers[17]
- Aldosterone antagonists
- Beta blockers.

Drugs, Diet and Devices Controlling Excessive Volume Overload

- Restriction of excessive salt and fluid intake
- Diuretics and dialysis
- ACE inhibitors
- Angiotensin receptor blockers
- Aldosterone antagonists.

Drugs to Relax and Regress LVH

- ACE inhibitors and ARBs
- Calcium channel blockers
- Beta blockers.

Drugs to Maintain and Control Rate and Rhythm

- Calcium channel blockers
- Beta blockers
- Digoxin
- Amiodarone.

Catheter-based and Surgical Approaches

- Atrial fibrillation ablation
- Maze Procedure
- AV nodal ablation.

Nitric Oxide Donors

Nitric oxide donors such as sildenafil and statins were shown to relax myocardial myocytes and help patients with LVDD.[18]

Novel Experimental Treatment

Givinostat: Jeong et al. demonstrated that givinostat, an inhibitor of histone deacetylase (HDAC) catalytic activity, prevented LV diastolic dysfunction due to hypertension in Dahl salt-sensitive (DSS) rats and suppressed aging-induced diastolic dysfunction in normotensive mice. This agent has a good potential to be a good therapeutic agent for patients with LVDD.[19]

Mechanical Circulatory Support Devices

In patients with severe LVDD and diastolic heart failure, miniaturized mechanical circulatory support devices to pump blood from left atrium to subclavian artery are in investigational stage.

REFERENCES

1. Redfield MM, Jacobsen SJ, Burnett JC Jr, et al. Burden of systolic and diastolic ventricular dysfunction in the community: appreciating the scope of the heart failure epidemic. JAMA. 2003;289:194-202.
2. Appleton CP, Hatle LK, Popp RL. Relation of transmitral flow velocity patterns to left ventricular diastolic function: new insights from a combined hemodynamic and Doppler echocardiographic study. J Am Coll Cardiol. 1988;12:426-40.
3. Nagueh SF, Smiseth OA, Appleton CP, et al. Recommendations for the Evaluation of Left Ventricular Diastolic Function by Echocardiography: An Update from the American Society of Echocardiography and the European Association of Cardiovascular Imaging. J Am Soc Echocardiogr. 2016;29: 277-314.
4. Lang RM, Bierig M, Devereux RB, et al. American Society of Echocardiography's Nomenclature and Standards Committee; Task Force on Chamber Quantification; American College of Cardiology Echocardiography Committee; American Heart Association; European Association of Echocardiography, European Society of Cardiology recommendations for chamber Quantification. Eur J Echocardiogr. 2006;7:79-108.
5. Prioli A, Marino P, Lanzoni L, et al. Increasing degrees of left ventricular filling impairment modulate left atrial function in humans. Am J Cardiol. 1998;82:756-61.
6. Abhayaratna WP, Seward JB, Appleton CP, et al. Left atrial size: physiologic determinants and clinical applications. J Am Coll Cardiol. 2006;47; 2357-6.
7. Manning WJ, Silverman DI, Katz SE, et al. Atrial ejection force: a noninvasive assessment of atrial systolic function. J Am Coll Cardiol. 1993;22; 221-5.
8. Stefanadis C, Dernellis J, Lambrou S, et al. Left atrial energy in normal subjects, in patients with symptomatic mitral stenosis, and in patients with advanced heart failure. Am J Cardiol. 1998;82:1220-23.
9. Inaba Y, Yuda S, Kobayashi N, et al. Strain rate imaging for noninvasive functional quantification of the left atrium: comparative studies in controls and patients with atrial fibrillation. J Am Soc Echocardiogr. 2005;18:729-36.
10. Di Salvo G, Caso P, Lo Piccolo R, et al. Atrial myocardial deformation properties predict maintenance of sinus rhythm after external cardioversion of recent-onset lone atrial fibrillation. Circulation. 2005;112:387-95.
11. Nagueh SF, Middleton KJ, Kopelen HA, et al. Doppler tissue imaging: a noninvasive technique for evaluation of left ventricular relaxation and estimation of filling pressures. J Am Coll Cardiol. 1997;30:1527-33.
12. Bouchard JL, Aurigemma GP, Hill JC, et al. Usefulness of the pulmonary arterial systolic pressure to predict pulmonary arterial wedge pressure in patients with normal left ventricular systolic function. Am J Cardiol. 2008;101:1673-6.
13. Ruan Q, Nagueh SF. Clinical application of tissue Doppler imaging in patients with idiopathic pulmonary hypertension. Chest. 2007;131:395-40.
14. Appleton CP. Hemodynamic determinants of Doppler pulmonary venous flow velocity components: new insights from studies in lightly sedated normal dogs. J Am Coll Cardiol. 1997;30:1562-74.

15. Smiseth OA, Thompson CR, Lohavanichbutr K, et al. The pulmonary venous systolic flow pulse—its origin and relationship to left atrial pressure. J Am Coll Cardiol. 1999;34:802-9.
16. Brilla CG, Funck RC, Rupp H. Lisinopril-mediated regression of myocardial fibrosis in patients with hypertensive heart disease. Circulation. 2000;102:1388-93.
17. Yusuf S, Pfeffer MA, Swedberg K, et al. Effects of candesartan in patients with chronic heart failure and preserved left-ventricular ejection fraction: the CHARM Preserved Trial. Lancet. 2003;362:777-81.
18. Fukuta H, Sane DC, Brucks S, et al. Statin therapy may be associated with lower mortality in patients with diastolic heart failure: a preliminary report. Circulation. 2005;112:357-63.
19. Jeong MY, Lin YH, Wennersten SA, et al. Histone deacetylase activity governs diastolic dysfunction through a nongenomic mechanism. Sci Trans Med. 2018;10:427.

72

CHAPTER

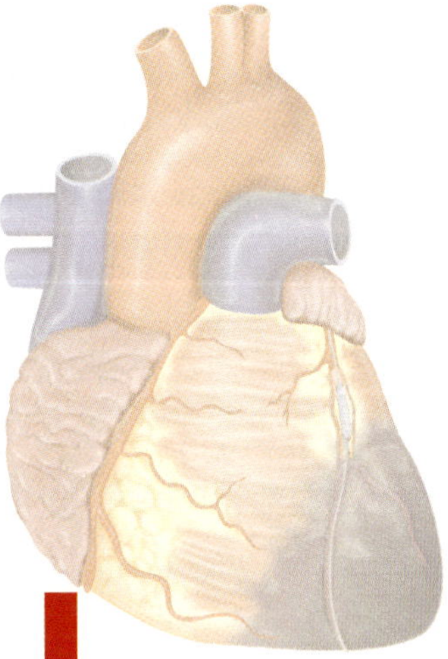

Role of Echocardiography in Atrial Fibrillation

Soumitra Kumar

INTRODUCTION

The most frequently encountered arrhythmia in clinical practice is atrial fibrillation (AF) affecting about 0.4% of the general population.[1] Aging is associated with increasing prevalence of AF, so that 3.8% of people aged 60 years and above and 9% of people 80 years and above are affected.[2,3] Significant clinical problems that are associated with AF are systemic thromboembolism and hemodynamic deterioration. The net effect is near doubling of both overall and cardiovascular mortality.[4] Among the various imaging modalities, echocardiography has a key role in the evaluation of cardiac structure and function and risk stratification in AF. This article reviews the role of echocardiography in complete evaluation and management of patients with AF.

TRANSTHORACIC ECHOCARDIOGRAPHY

Anatomical Assessment of Left Atrium

The shape of the left atrium (LA) is not spherical and its enlargement is often asymmetrical. Hence, measurement of LA anteroposterior diameter in parasternal long-axis or short-axis window employing M-mode echocardiography usually underestimates the true LA size. The two-dimension (2D) derived LA volume assessment using biplane area-length method or the Simpson's method provides more accurate measures of LA size.[5] The method is illustrated schematically in Figure 1. More recently, measurement of LA volume by three-dimensional (3D) echocardiography is being done and it has shown good correlation with biplane 2D measurements.[6] Increased LA volume and dimension is predictive of AF recurrence,[7] including recurrence after radiofrequency catheter ablation (RFCA).[8] AF begets further LA enlargement and on the contrary cardioversion and restoration of sinus rhythm may reverse this cycle.[9,10]

Functional Assessment of Left Atrium

With onset of AF, there is a reduction in both LA compliance and volume. This alters cardiac hemodynamics and increases the risk of thromboembolism. Late diastolic

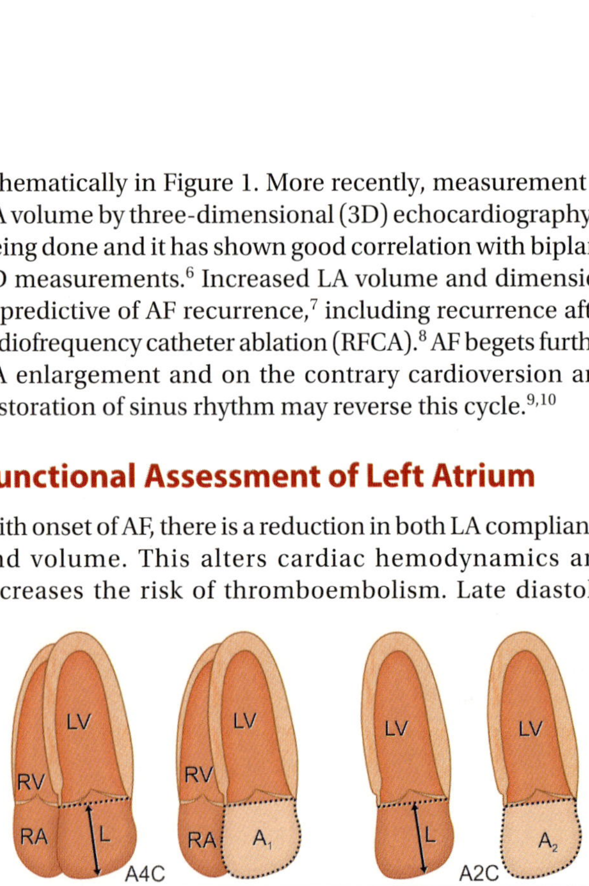

$$\text{Left atrial volume} = 8/3\text{TT}\left[\frac{(A_1)(A_2)}{(L)}\right]$$

L - the shorter of either the **A4** or **A2** lengths
A_1 and A_2 - left atrial areas on **A4C** and **A2C**

Fig. 1: Left atrial volume. (LV: left verticle; RA: right atrium; RV: right ventricle) filling wave (A) wave commonly depicts LA mechanical function, but it is conspicuous by its absence in AF. The ratio of time-velocity integral of the mitral A wave to that of total diastolic transmitral flow may be used as a measure of LA function.[11] Tissue Doppler imaging (TDI) provides a load-independent measure of both LV systolic and diastolic function. Atrial contraction (A[1] or Aa) velocity by TDI at the mitral annulus in late diastole can be utilized as a rapid and accurate marker of atrial function. The value of LA strain has been recently underscored for assessment of LA remodeling, thromboembolic risk and prognostication in patients with AF.[12] Assessment of LA function by speckle tracking echocardiography is still confined to the arena of research and observational studies and further work is required to establish its unique value in AF assessment.

Assessment of Left Ventricular Diastolic Function in Atrial Fibrillation

Atrial fibrillation and diastolic dysfunction are related to each other in a vicious cycle, i.e. diastolic dysfunction is associated with an increased risk for AF and risk of heart failure is markedly accentuated once AF develops. Standard parameters of diastolic function assessment such as early transmitral flow deceleration time (DT), E/E[1] velocity by Dokiaki TDJ, color M-mode mitral inflow propagation velocity (Vp) and isovolumic relaxation time are applicable to AF as well.[13] Like all other echocardiographic parameters which are analyzed in the context of AF, these parameters should be measured and averaged from 5 to 10 cardiac cycles. Low systolic pulmonary venous blood flow (PVF) during AF (precardioversion) as well as that obtained postcardioversion, i.e. during sinus rhythm is predictive of AF recurrences.[14,15] Pulmonary venous diastolic DT has very useful correlation with diastolic LV filling pressure in AF;[16] a value of DT less than and equal to 150 ms is associated with pulmonary capillary wedge pressure more than 18 mm Hg with 100% sensitivity and 96% specificity in patients with AF and is a better parameter than transmitral DT.[16] Another utility of monitoring PVF is detection of pulmonary venous (PV) stenosis that may occur in 1–3% cases after RFCA for AF. However, both transthoracic echocardiography (TTE) and transesophageal echocardiography (TEE) are constrained by the inability to image all four PVs adequately and hence are not fully reliable in describing the extent and location of PV stenosis.

IDENTIFICATION AND RISK STRATIFICATION OF LA/LAA THROMBUS BY TEE

Atrial fibrillation accounts for almost half of all cardiogenic thromboembolism and hence one of the prime goals of AF management is prevention of thromboembolism. While TTE has a low sensitively for detection of thrombi in LA (Fig. 2) and especially in left atrial appendage (LAA), TEE in contrast has a sensitivity and specificity of approximately 95–100% in detecting LA or LAA thrombi[17] (Fig. 3).

Even in absence of a demonstrable thrombus, dense "spontaneous echo contrast (SEC)" is associated with an annual thromboembolic event rate of 12% as compared to 3% in patients without it.[18] Apart from visualization of thrombus in the LAA, TEE can also assess its mechanical function by way of measuring the LAA emptying and filling velocities (Fig. 4). While normal peak emptying velocity is more than 50 cm/s,[19] a low velocity (<20 cm/s) in AF correlate strongly with presence of SEC and thrombus formation. In patients with AE, TEE risk factors that are harbingers of clinical thromboembolism are: (1) LAA thrombus, (2) severe SEC, (3) low (<20 cm/s) flow velocities

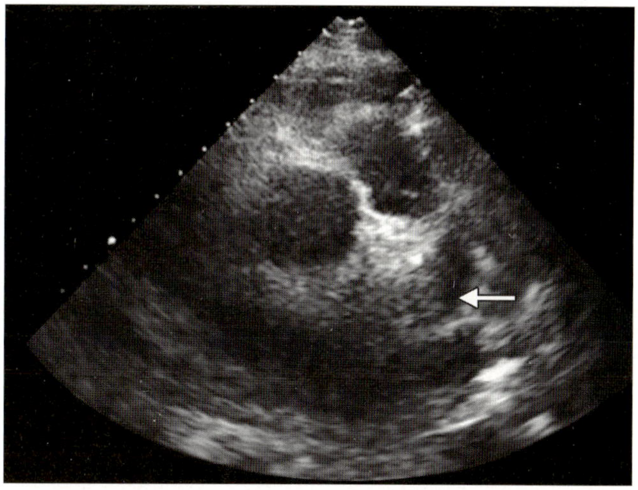

Fig. 2: Transthoracic echocardiography short-axis: Thrombus in LAA. (LAA: left atrial appendage)

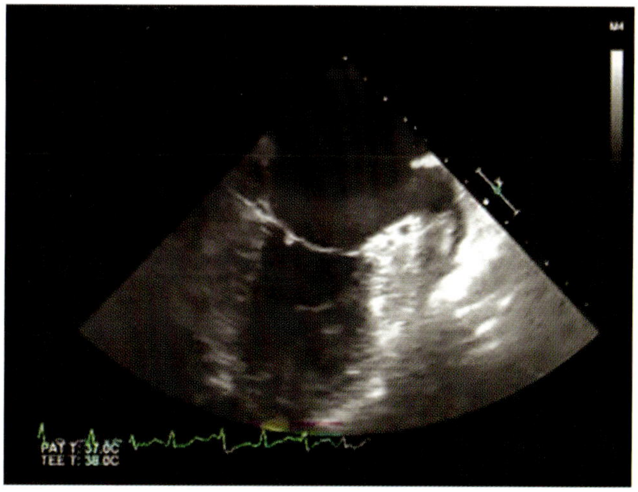

Fig. 3: Transthoracic echocardiography: Thrombus in LAA. (LAA: left atrial appendage)

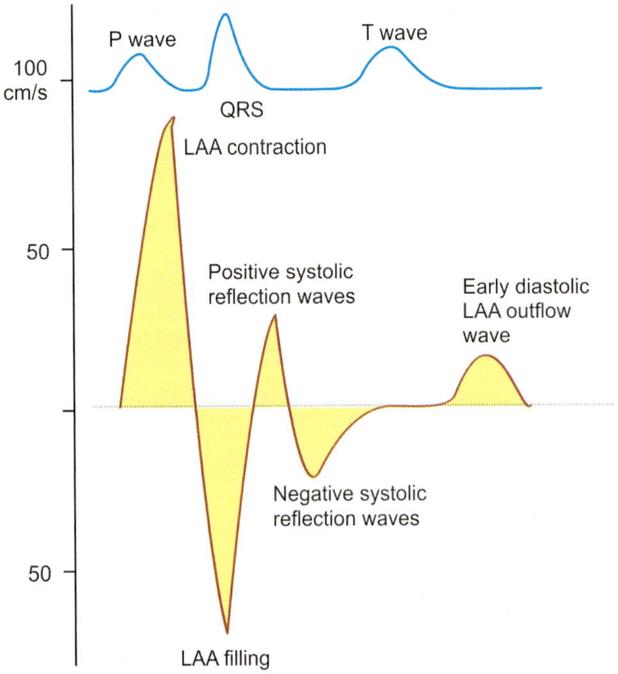

Fig. 4: Schematic representation of pulmonary venous blood flow. (LAA: left atrial appendage)

Flowchart 1: Transthoracic echocardiography-guided early cardioversion of AF algorithm.

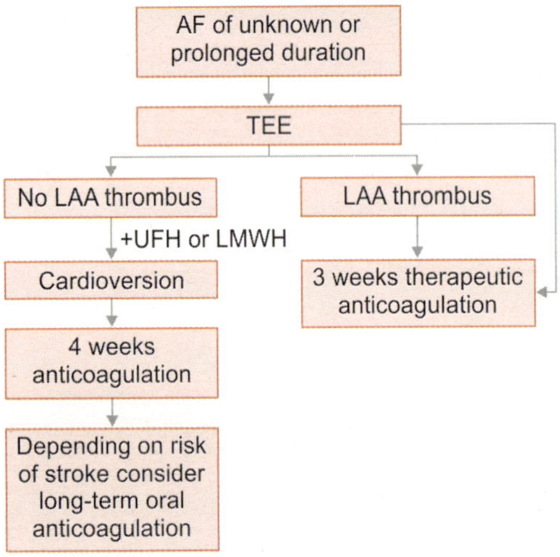

(AF: atrial fibrillation; TEE: transesophageal echocardiography; LAA: left atrial appendage; UFH: unfractionated heparin; LMWH: low molecular weight heparin).

at LAA ostium, and (4) complex aortic atheroma. Long-term anticoagulation is still indicated in a patient 3–6 months after AF ablation if TEE demonstrates these risk factors. Apart from assessment of LAA emptying velocity, measurement of LAA area and ejection fraction by TDI and 3D-TEE are emerging as potential modalities.[20]

Current practice for TEE guided early cardioversion includes exclusion of an existing thrombus by TEE, therapeutic anticoagulation at the time of TEE as well as postcardioversion anticoagulation prophylaxis to avoid new thrombus formation because of LA or LAA stunning (Flowchart 1).

ROLE OF INTRACARDIAC ECHOCARDIOGRAPHY IN AF

Intracardiac echocardiography (ICE) plays a valuable role during electrophysiologic procedures including RFCA in AF. ICE facilitates ready detection of anatomic variations of LA like pulmonary venous and interatrial septal anatomy. It also facilitates a suitable transseptal puncture in the posterior region of the fossa ovalis. It enables prevention of life-threatening complications like perforation of LA lateral wall or aortic root.[21] ICE also allows early identification of RFCA-related complications like thrombus formation, PV stenosis, damage to intracardiac structures and pericardial effusion.[22]

CONCLUSION

Transthoracic echocardiography, TEE and ICE together constitute the complete package that echocardiography offers in AF management by way of anatomical and functional information, prognostication, prevention of thromboembolic complications and electrophysiologic therapy facilitation. Further advancements in imaging acquisition and analysis will increase the popularity of echocardiography in evaluation and management of patients with AF.

REFERENCES

1. Peters NS, Shilling RJ, Kangaratnam P, et al. Atrial fibrillation: strategies to control, combat and care. Lancet. 2002;359:593-603.
2. Go AS, Hylek EM, Phillips KA, et al. Prevalence of diagnosed atrial fibrillation in adults: national implications for rhythm management and stroke prevention: the Anticoagulation and Risk Factors in Atrial Fibrillation (ATRIA) Study. JAMA. 2001;295:2370-5.
3. Lloyd-Jones DM, Wang TJ, Leip EP, et al. Lifetime risk for development of atrial fibrillation: the Framingham Heart Study. Circulation. 2004;110:1042-6.
4. Vaziri SM, Larson MG, Benjamin EJ, et al. Echocardiographic predictors of nonrheumatic atrial fibrillation: the Framingham Heart Study. Circulation. 1994;89:724-30.
5. Long RM, Bierig M, Devereux RB, et al. Recommendations for chamber quantification: a report from the American Society of Echocardiography's Guidelines and Standards Committee and the Chamber Quantification Writing Group, developed in conjunction with the European Association of Echocardiography, a branch of the European Society of Cardiology. J Am Soc Echocardiogr. 2005;18:1440-63.

6. Jenkins C, Bricknell K, Marwick TH. Use of real-time three-dimensional echocardiography to measure left atrial volume: comparison with other echocardiographic techniques. J Am Soc Echocardiogr. 2005;18:991-7.
7. Tani T, Tanabe K, Ono M, et al. Left atrial volume and the risk of paroxysmal atrial fibrillation in patients with hypertrophic cardiomyopathy. J Am Soc Echocardiogr. 2004;17:644-8.
8. Shin SH, Park MY, Oh WJ, et al. Left atrial volume as a predictor of atrial fibrillation recurrence after catheter ablation. J Am Soc Echocardiogr. 2008;21:697-702.
9. Van Gelder IC, Crijns HJ, Van Gilst WH, et al. Decrease of right and left atrial sizes after direct-current electrical cardioversion in chronic atrial fibrillation. Am J Cardiol. 1991;67:93-5.
10. Reant P, Lafitte S, Jais P, et al. Reverse remodeling of the left cardiac chambers after catheter ablation after 1 year in a series of patients with isolated atrial fibrillation. Circulation. 2005;112:2896-903.
11. Manning WJ, Silverman DI, Katz SE, et al. Impaired left atrial mechanical function after conversion: relation to the duration of atrial fibrillation. J Am Coll Cardiol. 1994;23:1535-40.
12. Donel E, Lip GY, Golderisi M, et al. EACVI/EHRA Expert Consensus Document on the role of multimodality imaging for the evaluation of patients with atrial fibrillation. Eur Heart J Cardiovasc Imaging. 2016;17:355-83.
13. Nagueh SF, Kopelen HA, Quinones MA. Assessment of left ventricular filling pressures by Doppler in the presence of atrial fibrillation. Circulation. 1996;83:724-7.
14. Okcin B, Yigit Z, Kucukogl MS, et al. Predictors for maintenance of sinus rhythm after cardioversion in patients with nonvalvular atrial fibrillation. Echocardiography. 2002;19:351-7.
15. Paraskevaidis IA, Theodorakis GN, Katritsis DG, et al. Pulmonary vein flow analysis by transesophageal echocardiography in patients with chronic atrial fibrillation; 1 year follow-up after cardioversion. Eur Heart J. 1999;20:375-85.
16. Chirillo F, Brunazzi MC, Barbiero M, et al. Estimating mean pulmonary wedge pressure in patients with chronic atrial fibrillation from transthoracic Doppler indexes of mitral and pulmonary venous flow velocity. J Am Coll Cardiol. 1997;30:19-26.
17. Klein AL, Murray RD, Grimm RA. Role of transesophageal echocardiography guided cardioversion of patients with atrial fibrillation. J Am Coll Cardiol. 2001;37:691-704.
18. Leung DY, Black IW, Cranney GB, et al. Prognostic implications of left atrial spontaneous echo contrast in nonvalvular atrial fibrillation. J. Am Coll Cardiol. 1994;24:755-62.
19. Jue J, Winslow T, Fazio G, et al. Pulsed Doppler characterization of left atrial appendage flow. J Am Soc Echocardiogr. 1993;6:237-44.
20. Agmon Y, Khandheria BK, Gentile F, et al. Echocardiographic assessment of the left atrial appendage. J Am Coll Cardiol. 1999;34:1867-77.
21. Ran JF, Marchlinski FF. Utility of intracardiac echocardiography in left heart ablation for tachyarrhythmias. Echocardiography. 2007;24:533-40.
22. Saliba W, Thomas J. Intracardiac echocardiography during catheter ablation of atrial fibrillation. Europace. 2008;10(Suppl 3):42-7.

73

CHAPTER

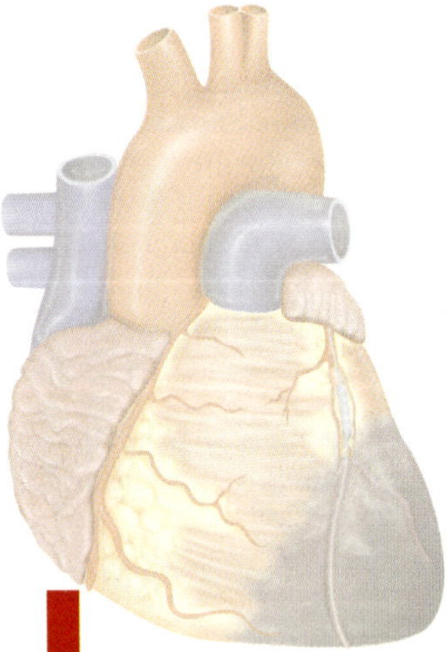

Advances in Echocardiographic Evaluation of Left Atrial Appendage

Krishnam Raju P, Chandramukhi Sunehra

INTRODUCTION

The left atrial appendage (LAA) is a finger-like projection extending from the main body of the left atrium (LA). It is not just an embryonic remnant or a vestigial appendage, but it is an important endocrine organ. LAA has an important role in the fluid balance and the regulation of heart rate. LAA endothelial cells produce the atrial natriuretic peptide and possibly the brain natriuretic peptide. LAA dysfunction is associated with increased brain natriuretic peptide levels. LAA is the most frequent source of cerebral thromboembolism in patients with cardioembolic stroke. Meticulous imaging of LAA is important for identification or exclusion of LAA thrombus in patients with atrial fibrillation (AF) before cardioversion. In current clinical era of novel transcatheter therapies, such as pulmonary vein isolation, LAA device occlusion, balloon mitral valvuloplasty, and MitraClip valve repair noninvasive echocardiographic evaluation of LAA is mandatory to guide the therapy and also to assess the results of intervention. Knowledge of LAA anatomy and function is crucial to choose the optimal imaging modality. The imaging modalities utilized in the evaluation of LAA include echocardiography, multidetector computerized tomography (MDCT), and cardiac magnetic resonance imaging (CMR). The echocardiographic techniques have gradually evolved from basic two-dimensional (2D) echocardiography (2DE) to complex three-dimensional (3D) echocardiography (3DE), tissue Doppler imaging (TDI), strain rate imaging (SRI), and intracardiac echocardiography (ICE).

ANATOMY OF LEFT ATRIAL APPENDAGE

Left atrial appendage is a conical structure situated between the lateral and anterior walls of LA and extends anterosuperiorly between the pulmonary trunk and the left main coronary artery or the left circumflex artery.[1] It is located in the left atrioventricular groove adjacent to the left circumflex coronary artery and lateral to the mitral valve annulus and medial to the left phrenic nerve. The left upper pulmonary vein is located posterior to the LAA (Fig. 1).[2]

Anatomically, LAA consists of three regions, (1) ostium, (2) neck, and (3) lobar region or the body. The ostium of the LAA is separated from the ostium of the left upper lobe pulmonary vein by the endocardial ridge or protrusion.

The ostium of LAA is usually oval, but it may be round, triangular, or tear-drop shaped. The ostium leads to neck which opens into the body, which is lobular. LAA may have single or multiple lobes. The more the number of lobes the higher the risk of thrombus formation independent of clinical risk.[3] The endocardium of LAA is lined by pectinate muscles, which may run parallelly resembling a comb or ramify like a feather-type palm-leaf pattern.[4]

ECHOCARDIOGRAPHIC IMAGING OF LEFT ATRIAL APPENDAGE

Left atrial appendage can be visualized on transthoracic echocardiography (TTE) in the modified parasternal short-axis view at the level of aortic valve and also in the

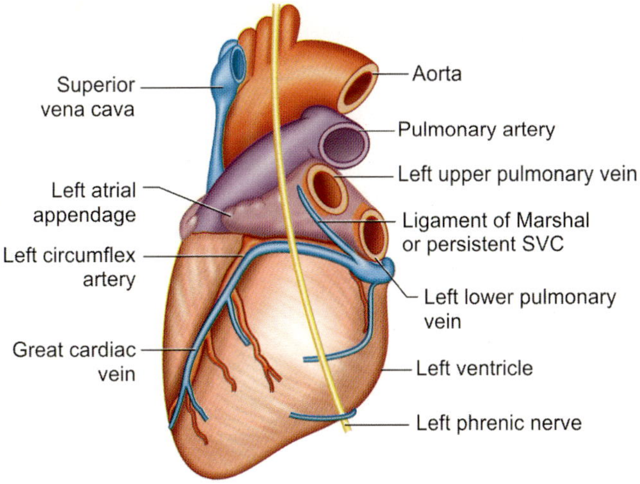

Fig. 1: Spatial relationship of left atrial appendage with surrounding structures. The LAA is in close proximity with the left upper and lower pulmonary veins and ligament of Marshal, which lie close to its posterior aspect. The superior aspect of LAA is adjacent to the pulmonary trunk. The inferior aspect of LAA overlies the LV, the left circumflex coronary artery and the great cardiac vein. The left phrenic nerve runs over the posterolateral aspect of LAA. (LAA: left atrial appendage, LV: left ventricle).

apical two-chamber view and sometimes in the apical four-chamber view. LAA is usually visible on TTE when it is enlarged as in patients with rheumatic mitral valve disease or patients with AF. However, TTE imaging of LAA is usually inadequate in majority of the patients, and transesophageal echocardiography (TEE) is mandatory for meticulous assessment of LAA anatomy and function. Currently, TEE is the preferred imaging modality for the assessment of LAA anatomy and function.

KEY POINT 1

The left atrial appendage has complex structure and anatomically divided into ostium, neck, and lobar region. The lobar region has a variable morphology. LAA lies in close relation with various vascular structures and phrenic nerve.

Transesophageal Echocardiography in Assessment of Left Atrial Appendage

Transesophageal echocardiography evaluation of LAA should involve an integrated approach including 2D imaging for assessment of size, morphology, contractility, and presence of spontaneous echo contrast (SEC), thrombus, and pulsed wave Doppler imaging to measure LAA flow velocity for the quantitative assessment of LAA function. Recent advances with 3DE and SRI are also incorporated in TEE evaluation of LAA, which have an incremental value in guiding the interventions and assessment of LAA function.

Two-dimensional Echocardiography

The most common indication for TEE evaluation of LAA is to identify or exclude a thrombus in patients with AF or patients with stroke. Imaging of the LAA is best accomplished by profiling the LAA at midesophageal level in both the short-axis and long-axis views and scanning through multiple planes from 0° to 110°. 2D TEE provides high-resolution images, but it has limitations like inadequate imaging planes for assessment of complex 3D morphology of LAA and its relation with adjacent structures. 3D TEE complements 2D TEE imaging by overcoming these limitations and allows better visualization of LAA and delineation of adjacent structures. Thus, 3D TEE provides a comprehensive evaluation of the LAA enabling the assessment of its complex morphology and relation with the surrounding structures. Comprehensive evaluation of LAA should also include the assessment of mitral valve, LA and left ventricle (LV) in order to identify the underlying cause of abnormalities of LAA structure and function. LAA varies in size, morphology, number of lobes, and pectinate muscle pattern. In patients with AF, LA and LAA are the most prominent sites for thrombus formation. Structural remodeling of the LA and LAA occurs in patients with AF, systemic hypertension, and patients with left ventricular dysfunction and heart failure, and this results in LA and LAA dilatation and dysfunction. This results in reduced contractility of LAA with subsequent stasis of blood and clot formation. The characteristic anatomic feature of LAA with dense trabeculations also predispose to thrombus formation.[1] TEE is the gold standard for the detection of LA and LAA thrombus. Manning et al.[5] studied the accuracy of TEE for detection of LAA thrombus through comparison with direct visualization of LAA during valve surgery. They concluded that TEE has a very high sensitivity and specificity of 92% and 98%, respectively, for detection of LAA thrombi and high negative and positive predictive values of 100% and 86%, respectively. Thus, TEE facilitates early and safe cardioversion by identifying or excluding the thrombus and determining whether anticoagulation is required before cardioversion. LAA should be scanned systematically in multiple planes including images at (1) 0° at high midesophageal level with slight anteflexion of the probe (Fig. 2A), (2) 45° to 60° profiling the short axis at midesophageal level (Fig. 2B), and (3) 90° to 110° profiling the long axis at midesophageal level (Fig. 2C). The LAA images profiled beyond 100° at higher angles are helpful in profiling the LAA with enhanced visualization of trabeculations. The three characteristics of LAA, which

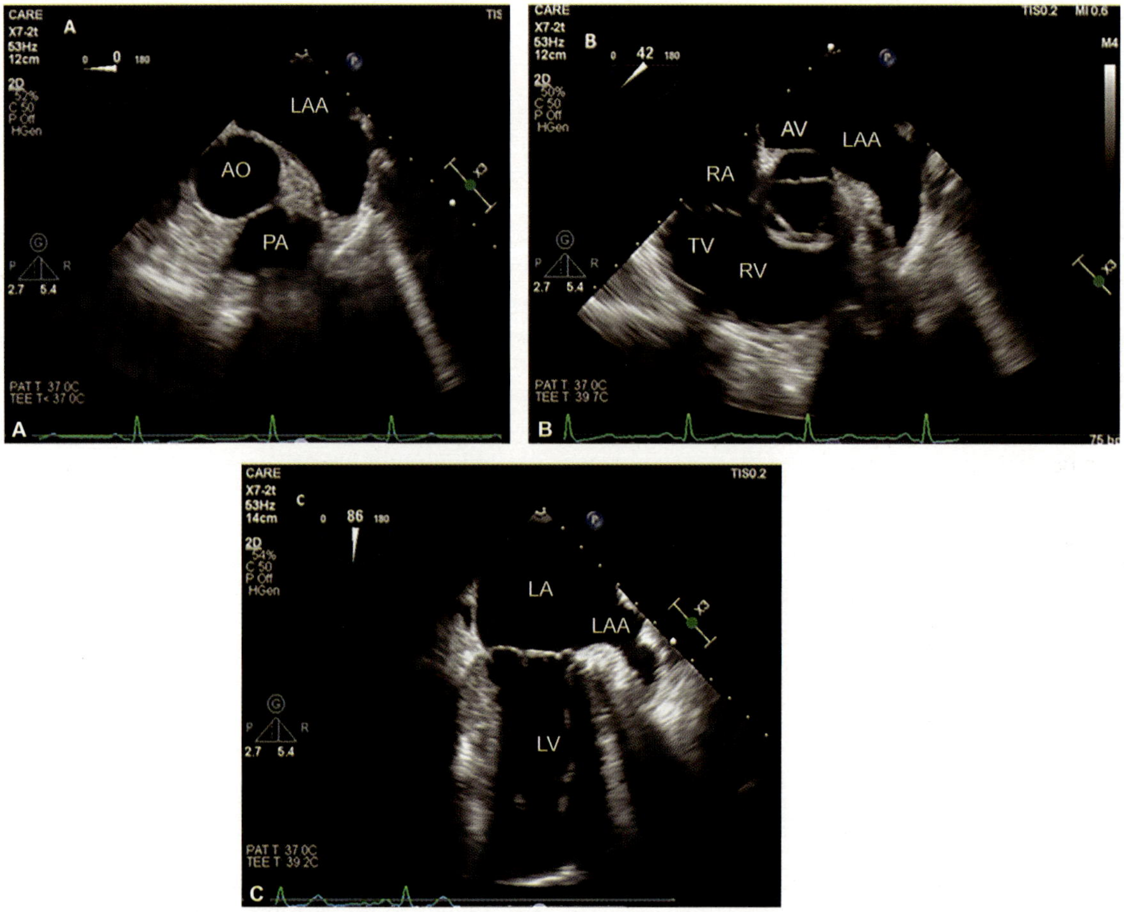

Figs. 2A to C: Two dimensional transesophageal echocardiography of left atrial appendage at various angles. (A) 2D TEE at high midesophageal level at 0° demonstrating LAA , aorta and PA; (B) 2D TEE at 42° profiling short axis view and demonstrating LAA, Aortic valve, RA,TV and RV; (C) 2D TEE at 86° profiling long axis view and demonstrating LAA, LA and LV (2D TEE: two dimensional transesophageal echocardiography, LAA: left atrial appendage, AO: aorta, PA: pulmonary artery, RA: right atrium, TV: tricuspid valve, RV: right ventricle, LA: left atrium, LV: left ventricle)

influence the risk for thrombus formation are LAA size, blood flow pattern in LAA, and the velocity of LAA flow.[6] In AF, the remodeling process results in dilatation and reduced contractility of LAA and LAA functions as a static pouch predisposing to stasis and thrombus formation. The LAA size correlates with the risk of thrombosis. LAA area >6 cm^2 predicts high risk for thrombosis.[7] LAA volume index >34 mL is associated with high risk of thromboembolic stroke.[8] LAA is a complex 3D structure; hence, 2DE-derived LAA area and volume may be inaccurate, and here comes the role of 3D TEE. Reduced LAA contractility and LAA dilatation is associated with high risk of LAA thrombosis in patients with AF as well as patients with sinus rhythm. In sinus rhythm, the elevated filling pressure is supposed to be the predisposing factor.

Spontaneous echo contrast is the precursor of thrombus and is associated with high risk of thromboembolism. SEC is defined as an amorphous, light-gray hazy, smoke-like swirling pattern visualized on 2D imaging. It results from rouleaux formation due to stasis of blood. SEC is strongly associated with thrombus formation. Four grades of SEC have been described which correlate with the LAA dilatation and reduced LAA contractility as assessed by LAA ejection velocity by Doppler imaging.[9]

- 0—Absence of echogenicity
- 1—Mild: Minimal movement of echogenic particles only transiently visible during the cardiac cycle with optimal gain settings
- 2—Mild-to-moderate: Transient movement of echogenic particles visualized without gain amplification, but more dense than mild SEC and with a clear picture
- 3—Moderate: Dense echogenic swirling pattern throughout the cardiac cycle

- 4—Severe: Dense echodensity and very slow swirling flow in the LAA, usually with similar echodensity in the main LA cavity.

Sludge is defined as echodensity within the LA or LAA which is visualized throughout the cardiac cycle and has viscid gelatinous appearance with an impression of impending precipitation but without a discrete organized mass. It has layered appearance and is more dense than severe SEC. It represents intermediate stage between SEC and thrombus.[10] Sludge is independently associated with high risk of cardioembolic events.

Thrombus is identified as a well-circumscribed echodensity with echotexture distinct from the atrial endocardium or pectinate muscles. Thorough imaging of LAA should be done to identify the thrombus, its location, size, and mobility. Additional echo features, such as echogenicity, should also be described. Thrombus with central echolucency is described as endolytic or ghost thrombus and usually indicates fresh forming thrombus or lysing thrombus, whereas thrombus with patchy hyperechogenicity indicates calcification and the layering of the thrombus point toward organized thrombus. The mobile elements projecting from the thrombus predict high risk of embolism. Thrombus with a maximum dimension of >1.5 cm[11] and pedunculated thrombus were also associated with high risk of thromboembolism. Many a times, mobile echodensities resembling thrombus will be noted in the LAA on 2D imaging. In such situations, 3D imaging with combined biplane imaging provides images of LAA in two orthogonal planes with better resolution of the structures. This helps in differentiating the echodensities visualized in LAA as thrombus or pectinate muscles or artifacts. Also in few cases, the 2D images may be suboptimal. In these cases, the use of ultrasound contrast agents can be utilized for contrast echocardiography which enhances the visualization of LAA. Contrast echocardiography opacifies the LAA, and many of the artifacts will be eliminated, pectinate muscles will be clearly visualized, and thrombus will be delineated as a filling defect. The color scale adjustment to low Nyquist limits facilitates the visualization of color flow in LAA and helps in exclusion or detection of LAA thrombus. Lack of color flow at the site of echodensity in the distal tip of LAA or in the side lobe indicates the presence of thrombus.

KEY POINT 2

Transesophageal echocardiography with 2D and 3D imaging is the basic imaging modality for the structural assessment of LAA and identification of LAA SEC or thrombus. LAA dilatation—increased area and volume—is associated with the risk of thrombus formation. LAA should be evaluated thoroughly in multiple planes, so as to evaluate each lobe, and pectinate muscles should not be mistaken for thrombus.

Left Atrial Appendage Function Assessment

Assessment of LAA function gives incremental information and predicts the risk of LAA thrombus formation, cardioembolic events, and success rate of cardioversion. Thus, LAA function assessment has now become an integral part of standard TEE assessment of LAA. Doppler-derived LAA flow velocity measurement is the preferred method for the assessment of LAA function. It is technically simple to perform, highly reproducible, and most validated method for LAA function assessment.[4] LAA function can also be assessed by LAA ejection fraction(LAA-EF), which is calculated with the help of the following equation[12]:

$$\text{LAA}-\text{EF}(\%)=\left\{\frac{\text{Maximum LAA area}-\text{Minimum LAA area}}{\text{Maximum LAA area}}\right\}\times 100$$

Maximum LAA area is measured during LAA diastole at the onset of the P wave on electrocardiogram (ECG), and the minimum LAA area is measured at the end of LAA systole, at or just after the QRS complex on ECG. LAA area is assessed by planimetry by tracing the LAA endocardial border starting from the top of the limbus of the left upper pulmonary vein along the endocardial border of the whole appendage. Shimizu et al.[13] studied the LAA function by LAA-EF by TEE in patients with acute ischemic stroke. They reported that the LAA-EF was significantly lower (8.0- 29.8%) in patients with AF, low in patient with paroxysmal AF (17–51%), and in patients with sinus rhythm LAA-EF was 43.4–76.2%. Gölbaşi et al.[14] compared LAA function in patients with rheumatic mitral stenosis in sinus rhythm and normal healthy subjects. They reported that patients with mitral stenosis had significantly low LAA-EF (36–66%) as compared to control group (63–77%).

Doppler Evaluation of Left Atrial Appendage

The LAA flow velocity and pattern can be evaluated by analysis of the pulsed-wave Doppler of the flow in the LAA cavity. The sample volume should be placed within the proximal third of LAA cavity. The pulsed wave Doppler signal should be appropriately aligned parallel to the color flow in LAA. In patients with sinus rhythm, LAA flow velocity shows regular pattern with emptying and filling velocities. During sinus rhythm, LAA contraction occurs during ventricular diastole, follows the starting point of the P wave on ECG and is represented by the diastolic emptying wave (Fig. 3),[15] which is positive with velocity varying from 50 cm/s to 64 cm/s. LAA relaxation occurs during ventricular systole, coincides with the QRS complex on ECG, and is represented by the systolic filling wave. It is a negative

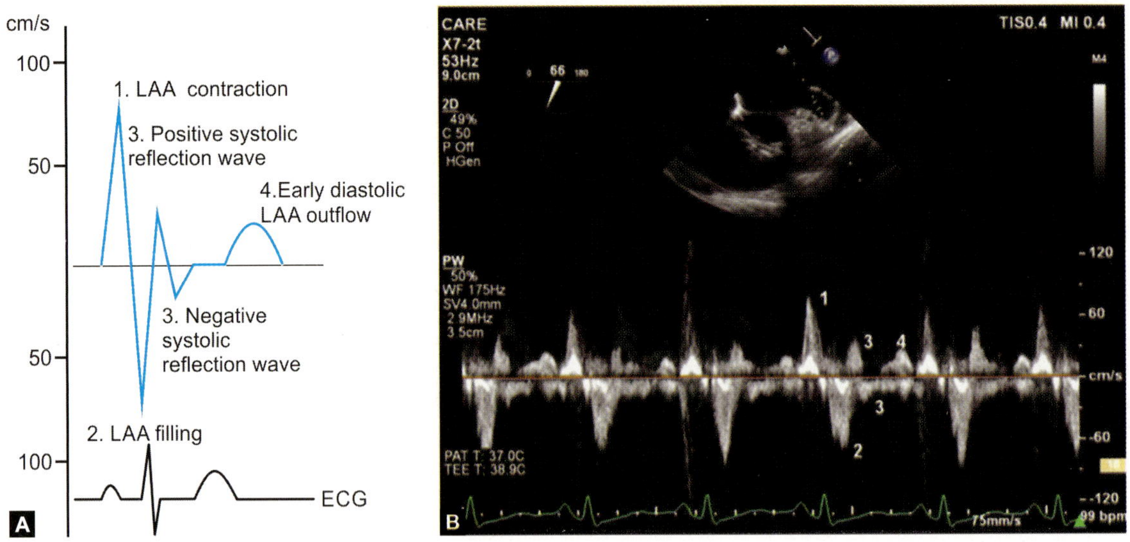

Figs. 3A and B: Left atrial appendage flow pattern assessment with pulsed wave Doppler in sinus rhythm. (A) shows schematic representation of LAA flow pattern in sinus rhythm. 1: Positive wave representing LAA contraction. 2: Negative wave due to LAA filling. 3: Systolic reflection waves which occur as

wave with velocity varying between 46 and 58 cm/s.[16-18] This is followed by a variable number of systolic reflection velocities of low amplitude which occur as alternating positive and negative waves, and represent passive flow in LAA during the remainder of systole. This is followed by the low-velocity early diastolic LAA flow velocity, and it occurs due to passive emptying of LAA simultaneous with the LA emptying during the early diastolic filling of LV. The early diastolic flow velocities are significantly low ranging from 20 cm/s to 38 cm/s[19] during active contraction of LAA but are important during LAA dysfunction. In sinus rhythm, the flow velocities may be reduced in the presence of increased left ventricular end-diastolic pressure and elevated LA pressure. In AF, the LAA flow pattern exhibits saw tooth appearance with alternate positive and negative waves of varying amplitude or the LAA flow may be chaotic with no identifiable waves. LAA peak outflow velocity correlates with the presence and severity of SEC. Decrease in the velocities is associated with increasing grades of SEC or thrombus.[17]

Handke et al.[20] assessed the LAA flow velocity and the presence of SEC or thrombus during TEE in 500 patients with stroke. Significant variations were noted in LAA velocity in patients with sinus rhythm (71 ± 16 cm/s), paroxysmal AF with sinus rhythm during TEE (46 ± 13 cm/s), paroxysmal AF with AF during TEE (32 ± 12 cm/s), and chronic AF (27 ± 9 cm/s). The LAA velocity <55 cm/s was associated with increased risk of SEC or thrombus independent of the rhythm. LAA velocity ≥55 cm/s had very low risk of SEC or thrombus with a 99% predictive value and 100% predictive value for thrombus. Antonielli et al.[21] assessed clinical and echo parameters for prediction of long-term maintenance sinus rhythm in patients with nonvalvular AF who underwent successful cardioversion. The investigators reported that the mean LAA peak emptying velocity >40 cm/s predicts the maintenance of sinus rhythm for 1 year after successful cardioversion with 66% negative and 73% positive predictive values. Kanda et al.[22] evaluated various clinical and echocardiographic parameters in 53 patients AF who underwent catheter ablation. They reported that LAA velocity <28 cm/s during preprocedure TEE predicted high risk of recurrence of AF during 1-year follow-up with 62% sensitivity and 69% specificity.

KEY POINT 3

Left atrial appendage flow velocity is technically easy and highly reproducible measure of LAA function, and it predicts the risk of thromboembolism and also the success and durability of cardioversion or RFA in patients with AF.

Tissue Doppler Imaging and Strain Rate Imaging

Recently, TDI and SRI have been utilized in the assessment of LAA function. These are the evolving techniques for the assessment of LAA function and require validation. The remodeling of LAA occurs in conditions such as hypertrophic cardiomyopathy or conditions with left ventricular dysfunction with raised LA pressure, e.g. dilated cardiomyopathy, ischemic cardiomyopathy or in patients with restrictive cardiomyopathy, or hypertrophic cardiomyopathy (HCM) with diastolic dysfunction and

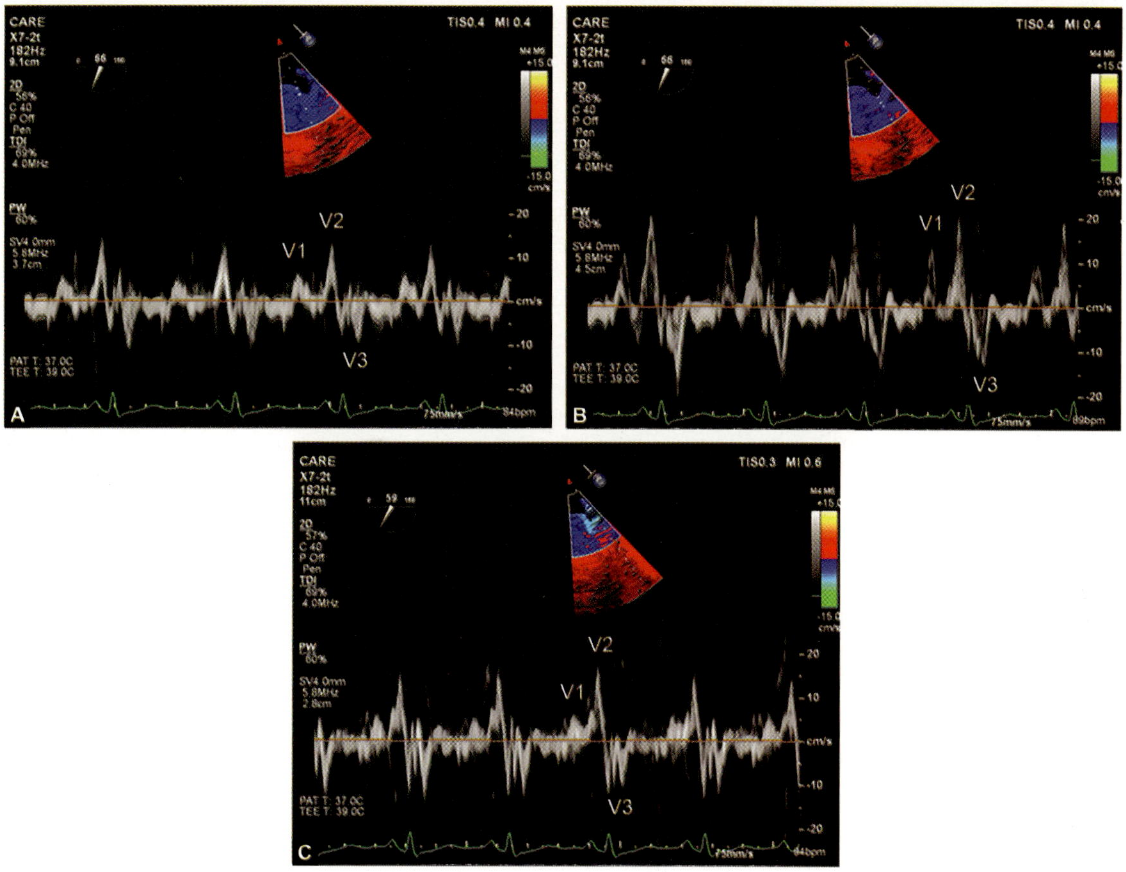

Figs. 4A to C: Assessment of tissue velocities of the left atrial appendage wall. (A) TDI of LAA at the basal medial wall; (B) Apex of LAA; and (C) Basal lateral wall. V1 : early diastolic positive wave preceding the P wave on ECG, V2 : positive emptying velocity corresponding to the LAA emptying velocity on pulsed wave Doppler V3 : negative filling velocity corresponding to the LAA filling velocity on pulsed wave Doppler. (TDI: tissue Doppler imaging; LAA: left atrial appendage).

raised LA pressure or in patients with AF. The structural remodeling and depressed LAA contractile function is associated with reduced tissue velocities of LAA wall as assessed by TDI. LAA wall tissue velocity includes a triphasic flow pattern with early diastolic positive wave V1 preceding the P wave on ECG, the positive emptying velocity V2 corresponding to the LAA emptying velocity on pulsed wave Doppler and negative filling velocity V3 corresponding to the LAA filling velocity on pulsed wave Doppler.[23] The LAA wall tissue velocities gradually increased from base of LAA to apex. The lateral LAA wall had slightly higher tissue velocities than the medial wall (Fig. 4).

Tuluce et al.[23] evaluated the LAA function in patients with HCM in sinus rhythm in a case-control study. TDI analysis was done assessing the tissue velocities of LAA walls at five points—the basal and mid points of the medial and lateral walls of LAA and the tip of LAA. In control group, V1 was 4–9 cm/s, V2 was 12–26 cm/s, and V3 was 8–17 cm/s. HCM patients had significantly reduced LAA wall tissue velocities as compared to the control group with V1: 2–6 cm/s, V2: 8–20 cm/s, and V3: 4–12 cm/s. The depressed LAA function in patients with HCM as indicated by reduced LAA tissue velocities points toward the intrinsic atrial myopathy and the predisposition to SEC and thrombus formation. Thus, TEE evaluation of LAA function with the help of LAA flow velocities and LAA tissue velocities provides incremental information regarding the tendency of SEC or thrombus formation and subsequent risk of thromboembolism.

Strain Rate Imaging of Left Atrial Appendage

Two-dimensional speckle-tracking-derived LAA strain is a novel technique for the assessment of LAA function. It evaluates the regional lengthening and shortening of LAA expressed as positive and negative values, respectively. Strain is the measure of regional deformation and strain rate is the measure of deformation with respect to time.

LAA strain is significantly low in patients with LAA SEC and thrombus. Sevimli et al. studied LAA flow velocity and strain and strain rate of LAA during TEE in 57 patients with sinus rhythm using TEE, and SRI was done in the upper esophageal transverse view at 30°–40° and the mid segment of LAA lateral wall strain was assessed. Significantly low values of strain (2.42 ± 0.98) and strain rate (0.97 ± 0.54) values were noted in patients with LAA SEC as compared to strain (13.12 ± 5.8) and strain rate (3.36 ± 1.1) in patients without LAA SEC. In patients with normal LAA function as defined by LAA emptying velocity of >50 cm/s, the strain and strain rates were 13.12 ± 5.8% and 3.36 ± 1.1, respectively.[24] Extensive validation studies are required to assess whether the diagnostic sensitivities and specificities of SRI in the assessment of LAA function are superior and acceptable.

KEY POINT 4

Tissue Doppler imaging and strain-rate imaging of LAA are novel robust methods for the assessment of LAA function. But further extensive validation studies are required to prove the superiority of these technics.

Three-dimensional Echocardiography

Two-dimensional TEE provides LAA images with high resolution; still it has certain limitations due to inadequate imaging planes to assess the complex 3D anatomy of LAA. 3D TEE overcomes this limitation and provides comprehensive evaluation of the LAA. In addition, it provides better delineation of surrounding structures.

Three-dimensional TEE enables thorough evaluation of complex LAA geometry. 3D imaging with combined biplane imaging with lateral tilt (Figs. 5A and B) provides imaging in two orthogonal planes and facilitates differentiation of a thrombus from pectinate muscle. 3D imaging is superior to 2D imaging for assessing the mobility of the thrombus and the changes in echotexture of thrombus, e.g. calcification, lysis, or degeneration.[25] It aids in the evaluation of associated intracardiac masses regarding the location, attachment, surface features, and spatial relationship to neighboring structures.

Three-dimensional imaging involves acquisition of full-volume pyramidal dataset covering the entire LAA at end expiration at midesophageal level at 0° or 45°. Real-time 3D TEE pyramidal data set should be acquired at 0° or 45° or 100° or 120° taking care to include the entire LAA. These pyramidal datasets can be cropped and entire LAA can be assessed (Fig. 6). Acquisition of full volume and real-time 3D dataset enables reconstruction of different planes of LAA in short axis and long axis at various phases of cardiac cycle. It also enables visualization and alignment of the LAA in the three different dimensions. Offline analysis of various LAA measurements includes LAA orifice diameter and LAA area tracings with automatic slicing at various levels, LAA depth from the center of LAA orifice to tip of LAA, and LAA volume tracings can be accurately assessed from the 3D dataset.[26]

KEY POINT 5

Three-dimensional TEE with multiplanar reconstruction of LAA images provides accurate measure of LAA dimensions and comprehensive assessment of LAA morphology and its relation with adjacent structures. 3D TEE is complementary to 2D TEE. 3D TEE is superior to 2D TEE in the identification or exclusion of LAA thrombus.

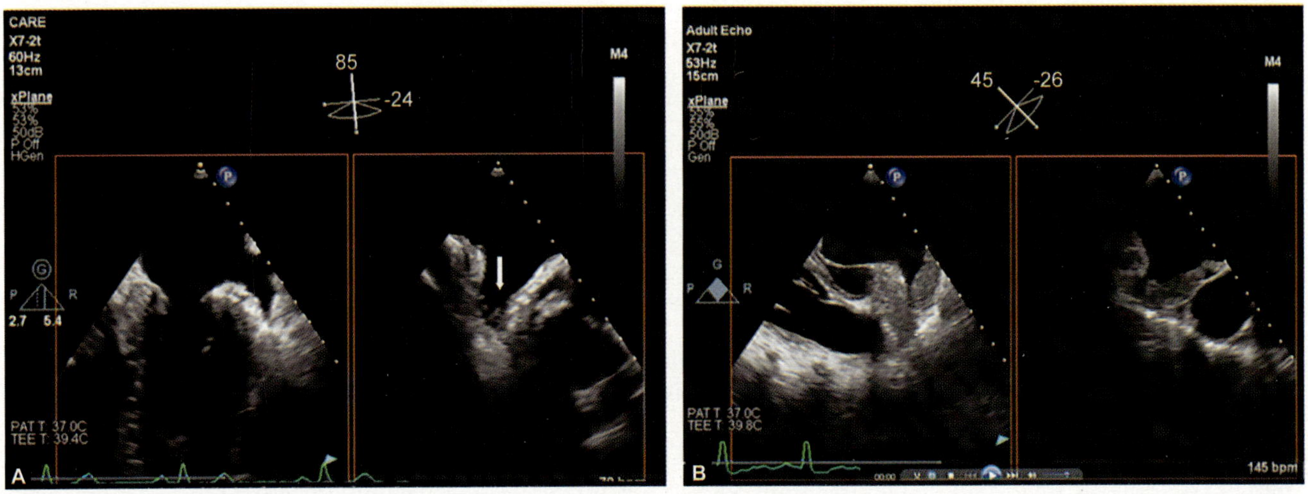

Figs. 5A and B: Three dimensional echocardiographic biplane imaging of left atrial appendage. 3D TEE with biplane imaging with lateral tilt demonstrates (A) prominent pectinate muscles (arrow) in LAA and (B). layered thrombus filling the LAA (3D TEE: three dimensional transesophageal echocardiography, LAA: left atrial appendage).

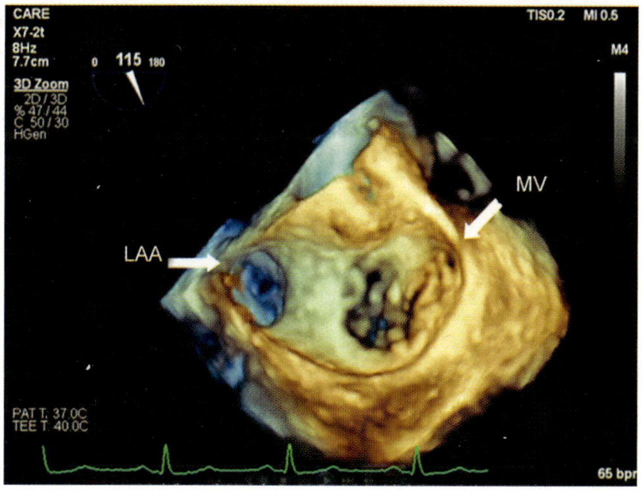

Fig. 6: Three dimensional echocardiographic imaging demonstrating enface view of left atrial appendage and mitral valve. Real time 3D TEE imaging demonstrating the enface view of mitral valve (MV) and left atrial appendage (LAA). (3D TEE: three dimensional transesophageal echocardiography).

Left Atrial Appendage Echocardiographic Imaging for Device Closure

In the current era of interventional therapies, radiofrequency ablation is the preferred modality of treatment in AF refractory to pharmacotherapy. TEE plays an important role in excluding LAA thrombus and assessing the LAA function and predicting the success and durability of radiofrequency ablation. Device closure of LAA is rapidly gaining popularity. Various imaging modalities utilized in the evaluation of LAA before device closure are 2D and 3D TEE, MDCT, and CMR. Of these, 2D and 3D TEE are the basic fundamental imaging modalities, which are widely and readily available and cost effective. Comprehensive evaluation of LAA with detailed assessment of morphology and accurate measurement of LAA dimensions is mandatory before LAA device closure. 2D TEE underestimates the LAA orifice diameter and area, while 3D measurements correlate closely with MDCT-derived measurements of LAA. Both 2D and 3D imaging should be done for comprehensive evaluation of LAA to assess the feasibility for device closure and selection of appropriate device. Evaluation of LA volume, left ventricular function (predisposing factor for thromboembolism), and exclusion of contraindications for device closure, such as mitral valve disease—valvular AF or mechanical valve disease requiring anticoagulation.[3] There is wide variation in the LAA size, shape, and number of lobes. LAA morphology has been classified according to the shape and number of lobes. LAA morphology can be better evaluated with the help of MDCT and CMR. Di Biase et al.[27] investigated LAA by MDCT and CMR and described four types of LAA morphologies (Fig. 7):

1. *Chicken wing:* Central lobe with an obvious severe bend in the proximal or midportion and which folds back at some point, secondary lobes may be present
2. *Cactus:* Central lobe with multiple secondary lobes superior and inferiorly
3. *Windsock:* Central dominant lobe with variations in secondary lobe location and number, tertiary lobes may be present
4. *Cauliflower:* Short central lobe with complex internal structure multiple lobes leading to a wider distal tip, lack of dominant lobe, and irregular orifice

Chicken wing morphology is most commonly observed morphology and occurring in (48%) cases, followed by "cactus" (30%), "windsock" (19%), and "cauliflower" (3%) cases.[27] Cauliflower morphology is most frequently associated with embolism. These varied LAA morphologies can be understood with the help of 3D imaging.

Rarely an accessory LAA may be present. Duerinckx et al.[28] reported two types of accessory LAA on MDCT: type 1: long, slender, diverticulum-like structures, and type 2: abnormalities of LA contour with a larger base.

Accessory LAA is important as it may be a source of thromboembolism and should be kept in mind while evaluating patients with AF. Also accessory LAA should be looked for during preprocedural evaluation for radiofrequency ablation of LA or device closure of LAA. During LAA closure, accessory LAA may be left unsealed and may contribute to incomplete sealing of LAA by the device. LAA is conical and its dimensions progressively reduce from the orifice to the distal tip. Assessment of three anatomical regions is very important—(1) *Ostium:* opening of LA into LAA; (2) *Neck:* tubular junction connecting the ostium and lobar region; and (3) *Lobar region:* most distal and variable part of LAA. LAA ostium is usually oval but may be eccentric. Ostial diameter measures 10–40 mm.

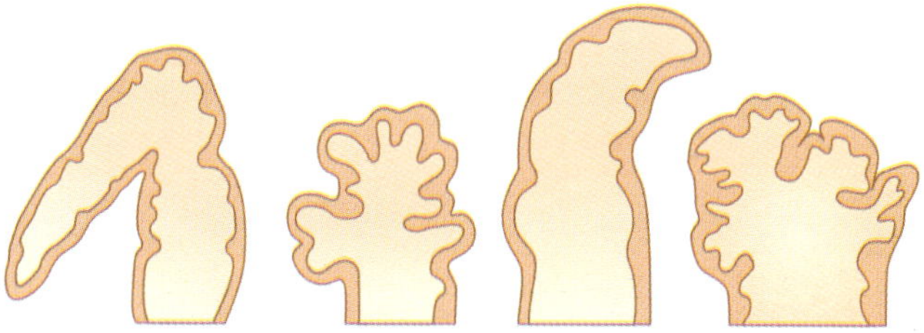

Fig. 7: Various morphologies of LAA as visualized on MDCT[27]. (LAA: left atrial appendage; MDCT: multidetector computerized tomography).

The borders of ostium may be very thin. Very eccentric ostium may pose problems during device closure due to the predisposition to peridevice leak, while thin-walled ostium is prone for perforation. Mitral valve and left upper lobe pulmonary vein are in close relation with the ostium, and care has to be taken not to interfere with them during deployment of device. The LAA neck is tubular, but there may be severe angulation between the neck and ostium, which leads to technical difficulties during device closure. A secondary lobe may arise near the ostium and may remain unsealed. The left circumflex artery and the diagonal are adjacent to the neck and are at risk during device closure. The lobar region is at the tip of LAA and curves around the base of the pulmonary trunk, left anterior descending artery, or the first diagonal and the great cardiac vein. The left phrenic nerve overlays the LAA. Care should be taken not to harm the neighboring coronary arteries or the great cardiac vein or the left phrenic nerve. The dominant lobe should be of sufficient length to accommodate the device.[29]

Appropriate selection of the LAA device requires precise measurement of LAA ostial diameter, area, landing zone diameter and the depth of the dominant anchoring lobe, and defining the orientation of anchoring lobe and origin and number of secondary lobes. For accurate sizing of device, LAA ostial diameter is measured in multiple imaging planes at midesophageal level and at all angles—0°, 45°, 60°, 90°, 110°, and 135°, and the maximum diameter is determined. The measurement of LAA ostial diameter and area of the ostium should be done at the ventricular end-systole when the ostium has the largest diameter. The maximal LAA ostial diameter is measured in the plane at the level of the left circumflex coronary artery up to a point at 1–2 cm from the tip of the left upper pulmonary vein rim. The measurement of maximal LAA depth is done from the ostium line to the apex of the LAA in the expected axis of LAA occluder device.[30] 2D TEE imaging has limitations due to foreshortening of images and limited imaging planes, and the LAA ostial diameter measurement may be inaccurate. These limitations of 2D TEE can be overcome by 3D TEE, utilizing the multiplane 3D reconstruction of images or using the enface 3D zoom images.[31] The maximum LAA ostial diameter and maximum depth of the dominant anchoring lobe determine the device size. Usually the device is sized a few millimeters larger than the LAA orifice diameter.[32] The angle between the LAA ostium and the neck, and the orientation of dominant anchoring lobe should be assessed as these are important in determining the transseptal puncture site and the choice of curve of the delivery sheath during deployment of the device. The additional LAA lobes should also to be assessed with regards to number and origin.

Periprocedural Echocardiographic Imaging during Left Atrial Appendage Device Closure

Percutaneous LAA occlusion is performed using LAA occluders, such as Watchman LAA occluder device and other models. The procedure is done under fluoroscopy and TEE guidance. 2D and 3D TEE complements fluoroscopy and guides the interatrial septal puncture, enhancing the safety, delivery of the device, and accurate positioning of the device in the LAA. The left circumflex artery, mitral valve annulus, and the limbus of left upper pulmonary vein serve as anatomical landmarks to guide the accurate positioning of the device. Following the deployment of device, the appropriate size, position, seal, and stability are ensured by fluoroscopy and 2D and 3D TEE imaging in multiplane planes and then only the device is released. Color Doppler interrogation, especially using low Nyquist limit, can confirm the adequate sealing of LAA by excluding peridevice leak (Fig. 8). Adequate sealing of LAA is established when the occlude device excludes all the lobes from communication with LA and if the peridevice leak is <5 mm in diameter.[32]

Post-procedure Imaging for Detection of Complications

Echocardiography promptly detects acute and delayed complications of LAA exclusion. Pericardial effusion with tamponade is the most life-threatening complication, which can be promptly detected by TTE or TEE. Other complications, such as residual flow in LA, alteration in left upper lobe pulmonary vein, mitral annulus or left circumflex coronary artery, or thrombus formation over the device can also be diagnosed by echocardiography.

KEY POINT 6

Transesophageal echocardiography is the preferred imaging modality for LAA device closure. TEE is crucial in the assessment of suitability for device closure and the selection of device. TEE is gold standard for the detection of LAA thrombus, which is a contraindication for device closure. It supplements other imaging modalities during the procedure and enhances the safety and success of LAA device closure. Postprocedure, it evaluates the success of procedure and detects the procedural complications and assists in the treatment of complications.

Checklist for Echocardiographic Evaluation of Left Atrial Appendage

- Left atrial appendage size, shape, and morphology
- Presence of SEC and its grading

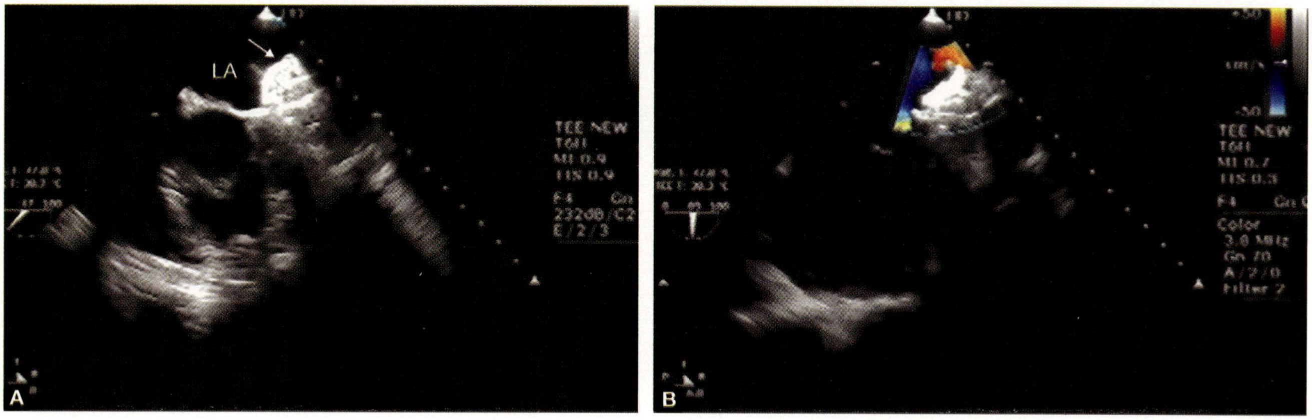

Figs. 8A and B: Two dimensional transesophageal echocardiographic imaging during the device closure of left atrial appendage. (A) Two dimensional transesophageal imaging after the release of left atrial appendage occluder device – Amplatzer cardiac plug (indicated by arrow)- after ensuring PASS (position, anchor, size, seal) criteria were fulfilled; (B) Color Doppler interrogation to assess the adequate sealing of left atrial appendage. No evidence of residual leak ensures complete seal of the left atrial appendage by the occluder device.

- Presence of thrombus and its characteristics, such as size and mobility
- Left atrial appendage flow velocities
- Tissue Doppler imaging for assessing the LAA wall tissue velocities, wherever required and feasible
- Strain rate imaging to assess LAA strain, wherever required and feasible
- Assessment of associated diseases, such as mitral valvular disease, HCM, dilated cardiomyopathy with LV dysfunction, restrictive cardiomyopathy which may result in LAA dilatation, and LAA dysfunction
- Interatrial septum anatomy, thickness, aneurysm, septal pouch, split atrial septum, patent foramen ovale
- Pulmonary venous anatomy: number and anomalous connections
- Three-dimensional TEE for assessment of LAA ostial diameter, LAA depth, and the assessment of LAA morphology, lobes, and thrombus
- Three-dimensional TEE/MDCT/magnetic resonance imaging for assessment of relationship of LAA with pulmonary veins, left circumflex artery, and great cardiac vein and aortic root (Table 1).

TABLE 1: Normal reference values for the various echocardiographic variables of left atrial appendage function in healthy individuals.

Echocardiographic variable of Left atrial appendage function	*Reference range in healthy individuals*
1. LAA ejection fraction	63–77%[14]
2. LAA flow velocity	
a. Emptying velocity (positive)	50–64 cm/s[16-18]
b. Filling velocity (negative)	46–58 cm/s[16-18]
c. Early diastolic flow velocity (positive)	20–38 cm/s[19]
3. LAA tissue velocity	
a. Early diastolic positive velocity (V1)	4–9 cm/s[23]
b. LAA emptying positive velocity (V2)	12–26 cm/s[23]
c. LAA filling negative velocity (V3)	8–17 cm/s[23]
4. LAA strain	7.32–18.92%[24]

(LAA: left atrial appendage)

Intracardiac Echocardiography

Intracardiac echocardiography is mainly utilized in the catheterization laboratories to guide the percutaneous interventions, especially electrophysiology procedures, such as radiofrequency ablation of arrhythmias and also in the percutaneous valve procedures or device closure of septal defects or LAA. The "home view" with the ICE catheter placed in right atrium depicts the right heart anatomy and enables the visualization of fossa ovalis region to guide the transseptal puncture. LAA anatomy and dimensions can be assessed to guide the selection of device and deployment of device and assess the LAA seal and stability of device. But the right atrial views are inadequate to visualize the detailed anatomy of the LAA and the positioning of delivery sheaths, catheters or devices, and color Doppler assessment for identification of peridevice leak. A near-field imaging is required which can be done with the ICE catheter placed in left pulmonary artery.[33] Also ICE can be used as an alternative method for preprocedure evaluation of LAA when TEE could not be done. But ICE is an invasive procedure, and hence, it is mainly utilized in the catheterization laboratory to guide the percutaneous intervention.

Multidetector Computerized Tomography and Cardiac Magnetic Resonance Imaging of Left Atrial Appendage

The MDCT and CMR provide detailed information of the varied morphology of LAA, *accessory LA appendages* and the relation of LAA with adjacent structures, such as mitral valve annulus, left superior pulmonary vein, left circumflex artery, the great cardiac vein, and the aortic root. This information is important during the selection of the device and also it dictates the outcome of LAA device closure. MDCT 3D multiplanar reconstruction allows the precise measurement of LAA dimensions which are more accurate than the 2D TEE-derived LAA dimensions. In few cases, it may be difficult to differentiate LAA thrombus from prominent pectinate muscles. MDCT or *contrast CMR* will be helpful in these cases to confirm or exclude the thrombus. But MDCT and CMR have limitations of cost burden and availability and MDCT imposes radiation exposure.

Advanced Technology: Fusion Imaging with Integration of Echocardiography and Fluoroscopy Imaging

Recently, advanced techniques have developed a novel imaging modality through automated real-time integration of 2D and 3D TEE and fluoroscopy imaging. Philips Healthcare has recently introduced the EchoNavigator system (EN), an innovative tool, which enables real-time overlay of echocardiographic and fluoroscopic images. The movement of the C-arm is synchronized with the TEE probe and the different echocardiographic projections are sliced according to the position of the X-ray source. The soft tissue landmarks are marked on TEE images and these appear automatically on the fluoroscopy screen and a single imaging screen can be observed during intervention. Thus, EN integrates real-time information from 2D/3D TEE and fluoroscopy in the same anatomical alignment and facilitates improved visualization of guidewires, catheters, and devices in relation to adjacent structures.[34] Fusion imaging with integration of TEE and fluoroscopy imaging reduces the radiation exposure to both patient and intervention team.

CONCLUSION

Left atial appendage has complex structure, and it is the common site for thrombus formation in patients with AF. Comprehensive echocardiographic evaluation of LAA for structure and function should include integration of various techniques like 2DE, 3DE, color Doppler interrogation, pulsed wave Doppler, TDI and SRI. TEE is the basic fundamental imaging modality for structural and functional evaluation of LAA. 2D and 3D TEE provides morphological information while pulsed wave Doppler, TDI and SRI imaging are valuable in the functional assessment of LAA. TEE with ultrasound contrast enhancement is helpful when conventional 2D TEE images are suboptimal for identification or exclusion of LAA thrombus. 2D and 3D TEE enhance the efficacy and safety of LAA device closure. ICE can be used as an alternative imaging modality in evaluation of LAA. But ICE is invasive imaging modality, and hence, it is reserved for guiding the percutaneous device closure of LAA. Fusion imaging with real-time integration of echocardiography and fluoroscopy imaging is a recent development used in the catheterization laboratory to guide the percutaneous interventions such as device closure of LAA, and it reduces the radiation exposure.

REFERENCES

1. Beigel R, Wunderlich NC, Ho SY, et al. The left atrial appendage: anatomy, function, and noninvasive evaluation. JACC Cardiovasc Imaging. 2014;7(12):1251-65.
2. Naksuk N, Padmanabhan D, Yogeswaran V, et al. Left atrial appendage: embryology, anatomy, physiology, arrhythmia and therapeutic intervention. JACC Clin Electrophysiol. 2016;2(4):403-12.
3. Wunderlich NC, Beigel R, Swaans MJ, et al. Percutaneous interventions for left atrial appendage exclusion: options, assessment, and imaging using 2D and 3D echocardiography. JACC Cardiovasc Imaging. 2015;8(4):472-88.
4. Bansal M, Kasliwal RR. Echocardiography for left atrial appendage structure and function. Indian Heart J. 2012;64(5):469-75.
5. Manning WJ, Weintraub RM, Waksmonski CA, et al. Accuracy of transesophageal echocardiography for identifying left atrial thrombi. A prospective, intraoperative study. Ann Intern Med. 1995;123:817-22.
6. Al-Saady NM, Obel OA, Camm AJ. Left atrial appendage: structure, function, and role in thromboembolism. Heart. 1999;82:547-55.
7. [No authors listed]. Predictors of thromboembolism in atrial fibrillation: II. Echocardiographic features of patients at risk. The Stroke Prevention in Atrial Fibrillation Investigators. Ann Intern Med. 1992;116(1):6-12.
8. Burrell LD, Horne BD, Anderson JL, et al. Usefulness of left atrial appendage volume as a predictor of embolic stroke in patients with atrial fibrillation. Am J Cardiol. 2013;112:1148-52.
9. Donal E, Yamada H, Leclercq C, et al. The left atrial appendage, a small, blind-ended structure: a review of its echocardiographic evaluation and its clinical role. Chest. 2005;128(3):1853-62.
10. Lowe BS, Kusunose K, Motoki H, et al. Prognostic significance of left atrial appendage "sludge" in patients with atrial

fibrillation: a new transesophageal echocardiographic thromboembolic risk factor. J Am Soc Echocardiogr. 2014;27(11):1176-83.

11. Leung DY, Davidson PM, Cranney GB, et al. Thromboembolic risks of left atrial thrombus detected by transesophageal echocardiogram. Am J Cardiol. 1997;79(5):626-9.
12. Pollick C, Taylor D. Assessment of left atrial appendage function by transesophageal echocardiography. Implications for the development of thrombus. Circulation. 1991;84(1): 223-31.
13. Shimizu T, Takada T, Shimode A, et al. Association between paroxysmal atrial fibrillation and the left atrial appendage ejection fraction during sinus rhythm in the acute stage of stroke: a transesophageal echocardiographic study. J Stroke Cerebrovasc Dis. 2013;22(8):1370-6.
14. Gölbaşi Z, Çiçek D, Canbay A, et al. Left atrial appendage function in patients with mitral stenosis in sinus rhythm. Eur J Echocardiogr. 2002;3(1):39-43.
15. Delgado V, Di Biase L, Leung M, et al. Structure and function of the left atrium and left atrial appendage: AF and stroke implications. J Am Coll Cardiol. 2017;70(25):3157-72.
16. Abdelmoneim SS, Mulvagh SL. Techniques to improve left atrial appendage imaging. J Atr Fibrillation. 2014;7(1):1059.
17. Mügge A, Kühn H, Nikutta P, et al. Assessment of left atrial appendage function by biplane transesophageal echocardiography in patients with nonrheumatic atrial fibrillation: identification of a subgroup of patients at increased embolic risk. J Am Coll Cardiol. 1994;23(3): 599-607.
18. Mikael Kortz RA, Delemarre BJ, van Dantzig JM, et al. Left atrial appendage blood flow determined by transesophageal echocardiography in healthy subjects. Am J Cardiol. 1993;71(11):976-81.
19. Agmon Y, Khandheria BK, Gentile F, et al. Echocardiographic assessment of the left atrial appendage. J Am Coll Cardiol. 1999;34(7):1867-77.
20. Handke M, Harloff A, Hetzel A, et al. Left atrial appendage flow velocity as a quantitative surrogate parameter for thromboembolic risk:' determinants and relationship to spontaneous echocontrast and thrombus formation—a transesophageal echocardiographic study in 500 patients with cerebral ischemia. J Am Soc Echocardiogr. 2005;18(12): 1366-72.
21. Antonielli E, Pizzuti A, Pálinkás A, et al. Clinical value of left atrial appendage flow for prediction of long-term sinus rhythm maintenance in patients with nonvalvular atrial fibrillation. J Am Coll Cardiol. 2002;39(9):1443-9.
22. Kanda T, Masuda M, Sunaga A, et al. Low left atrial appendage flow velocity predicts recurrence of atrial fibrillation after catheter ablation of persistent atrial fibrillation. J Cardiol. 2015;66(5):377-81.
23. Tuluce SY, Kayikcioglu M, Tuluce K, et al. Assessment of left atrial appendage function during sinus rhythm in patients with hypertrophic cardiomyopathy: transesophageal echocardiography and tissue Doppler study. J Am Soc Echocardiogr. 2010;23(11):1207-16.
24. Sevimli S, Gundogdu F, Arslan S, et al. Strain and strain rate imaging in evaluating left atrial appendage function by transesophageal echocardiography. Echocardiography. 2007;24(8):823-9.
25. Anwar AM, Nosir YFM, Ajam A, et al. Central role of real-time three-dimensional echocardiography in the assessment of intracardiac thrombi. Int J Cardiovasc Imaging. 2010;26: 519-26.
26. Agoston I, Xie T, Tiller FL, et al. Assessment of left atrial appendage by live three-dimensional echocardiography: early experience and comparison with transesophageal echocardiography. Echocardiography. 2006;23(2):127-32.
27. Di Biase L, Santangeli P, Anselmino M, et al. Does the left atrial appendage morphology correlate with the risk of stroke in patients with atrial fibrillation? Results from a multicenter study. J Am Coll Cardiol. 2012;60:531-8.
28. Duerinckx AJ, Vanovermeire O. Accessory appendages of the left atrium as seen during 64-slice coronary CT angiography. Int J Cardiovasc Imaging. 2007;24(2):215-21.
29. Su P, McCarthy KP, Ho SY. Occluding the left atrial appendage: anatomical considerations. Heart. 2008;94:1166-70.
30. Regazzoli D, Ancona F, Trevisi N, et al. Left atrial appendage: physiology, pathology, and role as a therapeutic target. BioMed Res Int. 2015;2015:205013.
31. Laura DM, Chinitz LA, Aizer A, et al. The role of multimodality imaging in percutaneous left atrial appendage suture ligation with the LARIAT device. J Am Soc Echocardiogr. 2014;27(7):699-708.
32. Lockwood SM, Alison JF, Obeyesekere MN, et al. Imaging the left atrial appendage prior to, during, and after occlusion. JACC Cardiovasc Imaging. 2011;4(3):303-6.
33. Bartel T, Müller S, Biviano A, et al. Why is intracardiac echocardiography helpful? Benefits, costs, and how to learn. Eur Heart J. 2014;35(2):69-76.
34. Jungen C, Zeus T, Balzer J, et al. Left atrial appendage closure guided by integrated echocardiography and fluoroscopy imaging reduces radiation exposure. PLoS One. 2015;10(10):e0140386.

74

CHAPTER

Advances in Echocardiographic Evaluation of Left Atrial Strain in Atrial Fibrillation

Nitin J Burkule

INTRODUCTION

Atrial fibrillation (AF) is a common arrhythmia encountered in the elderly population. The risk factors for AF are hypertension (HT), diabetes mellitus, ischemic heart disease, congestive heart failure (CHF), obstructive sleep apnea, and obesity. In younger population, AF risk factors include mitral valve disease or thyrotoxicosis. AF leads to significant morbidity and mortality due to cardioembolic cerebrovascular stroke (CVA) and CHF. The AF may be considered a marker of advanced fibrotic atrial cardiomyopathy (FAC). The underlying FAC leads to atrial mechanical dysfunction, atrial structural and electrical remodeling, atrial blood stasis, thrombogenic environment, and heart failure[1]. There is an increased risk of embolic CVA regardless of whether or not the arrhythmia is sustained. The temporal association of paroxysmal AF (PAF) with CVA is also inconsistent. The extent of left atrial (LA) and right atrial (RA) fibrosis is associated with adverse LA remodeling and reduction in LA function.

STRAIN AND STRAIN RATE IMAGING

The LA function (reservoir, conduit, and contractile functions) and LA volumes (LAV) can be assessed by echocardiography in AF. Progressive deterioration of LA function is the early marker of progressive LA fibrosis compared to LAV or LA remodeling.[2] The LA function is calculated by LA volumetric assessment at three timepoints in a cardiac cycle, viz. LA maximum (at end-systole, just before mitral valve opening) and LA minimum (at end-diastole, when the mitral valve closes) and LA pre-A (immediately before atrial systole, before the electrocardiographic P wave). LA total (reservoir), passive (conduit), and active emptying (contractile) fractions are calculated from these volume datasets.[3] These measurements are time consuming to perform in day-to-day practice in high-volume echocardiography laboratories. The LA myocardial deformation parameters by speckle-tracking echocardiography (STE), viz. strain (*S*) and the strain rate (SR), can be used as surrogate markers for the LA function. Six *S* parameters can be derived to evaluate the contractile (S_a, SR_a), conduit (S_{con}, SR_{con}), and reservoir (S_R, SR_R) function of the LA[4] (Figs. 1A and B and 2A and B). The *S* and SR are calculated either by Doppler tissue imaging or by grayscale two-dimensional (2D) *S* imaging using 2D STE imaging or velocity vector imaging (VVI). There is a good correlation of *S* and SR values with the LA fractional emptying on volumetric analysis, tissue Doppler–derived mitral annular velocity, and mitral and pulmonary venous Doppler velocities.[5] The LA *S* and SR measurements are comparable when measured with either VVI or 2D STE techniques.[6] The LA three-dimensional (3D) STE–measured area *S* values, at end-systole and before atrial systole, are reproducible and comparable with LA emptying and LA active ejection fractions.[7] The normal values of LA *S* are as follows[4]: S_a 15.3 ± 2.9, S_R 35.7 ± 5.8, and S_{con} 20.4 ± 5.0. The normal values of LA SR are as follows: SR_a −1.95 ± 0.33, SR_R 1.43 ± 0.24, and SR_{con} −1.65 ± 0.37. The reservoir, conduit, and contractile LA *S* decreases with aging, while SR during the contractile phase increases with aging.[4] All the *S* and SR indices are lower in patients with recurrent AF than in those

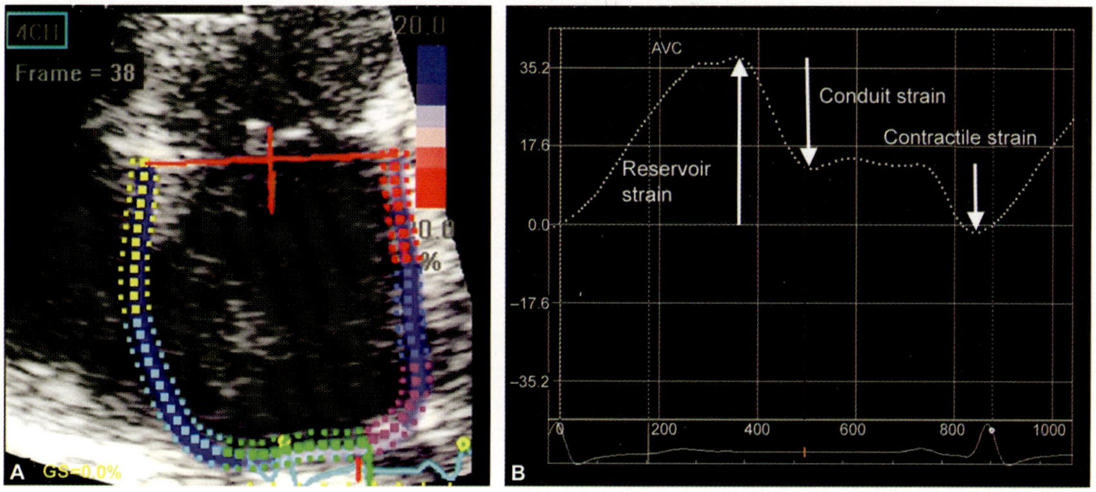

Figs. 1A and B: Normal 2D speckle-tracking *strain* imaging of LA. (A) LA four-chamber parametric view for region of interest. (B) The measurements of LA strains, viz. reservoir S_R, conduit S_{con}, contractile S_a function. (2D: two-dimensional; LA: left atrial)

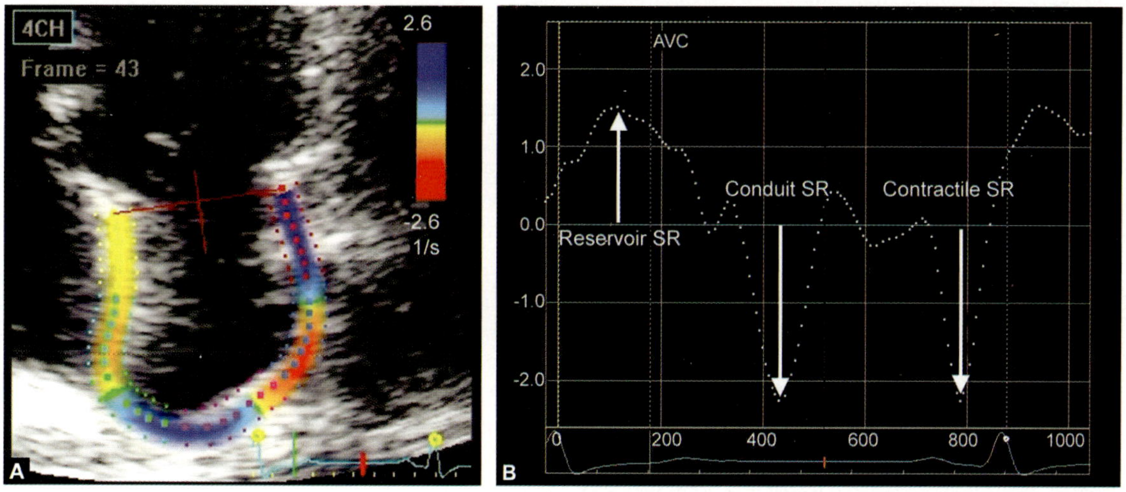

Figs. 2A and B: Normal 2D speckle-tracking *strain rate* imaging of LA. (A) LA four-chamber parametric view for region of interest. (B) The measurements of LA strain rates, viz. reservoir SR_R, conduit SR_{con}, contractile SR_a function. (2D: two-dimensional; LA: left atrial).

with the first episode of AF suggesting advanced FAC in the former. The *S* and SR values may be helpful in appropriate selection of patients for anticoagulation, cardioversion, or radiofrequency (RF) catheter ablation.[2]

STRAIN AND STRAIN RATE IMAGING IN ATRIAL FIBRILLATION

Patients with AF have lower LA *S* and SR values than the age, sex-matched healthy controls. In a study[8] of 27 AF patients of mean age of 62 ± 12 years the mean LA SR_R was 1.7 ± 0.8 compared to 2.9 ± 0.9 in controls. In another study[9] of 36 patients with AF the LA S_R was 17.7 ± 9.5% compared to 35.5 ± 14.0% in controls. Peak SR_R and SR_{con} were also reduced in patients with AF compared with controls (1.46 ± 0.73 vs 0.74 ± 0.32 for SR_R, and 1.77 ± 0.9 vs 1.01 ± 0.5 for SR_{con}). Similarly, in a study[10] of 57 low-risk AF patients, both peak S_a (3.2 ± 1.2% vs 6.9 ± 4.2%) and peak S_R (14 ± 11% vs 25 ± 12%) were significantly reduced in patients compared with healthy controls. The reduction in LA *S* and SR is related to AF burden, LA remodeling, and fibrosis. LA contractile function is lost during persistent AF. The LA reservoir and conduit functions are progressively reduced as the PAF progresses to persistent AF (Figs. 3 and 4). Patients with persistent AF have longer "total atrial conduction time" than patients with PAF. The LA S_R and increasing AF burden are independently correlated with "total atrial

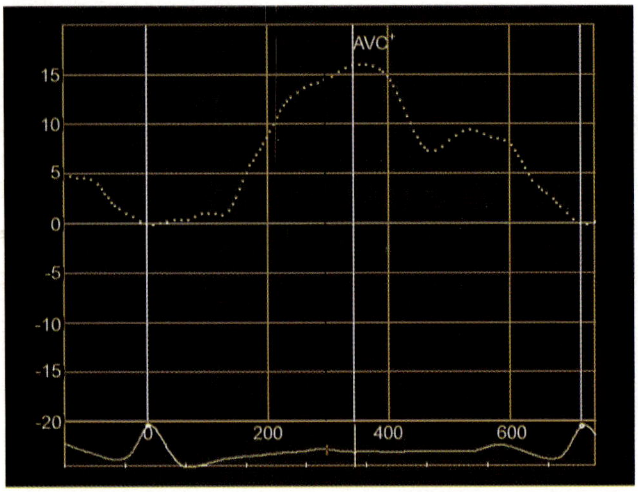

Fig. 3: 2D speckle-tracking *strain* imaging of LA in patient with hypertension and paroxysmal AF shows reduced values of LA strains, viz. reservoir S_R, conduit S_{con}, contractile S_a function. (2D: two-dimensional; AF: atrial fibrillation; LA: left atrial)

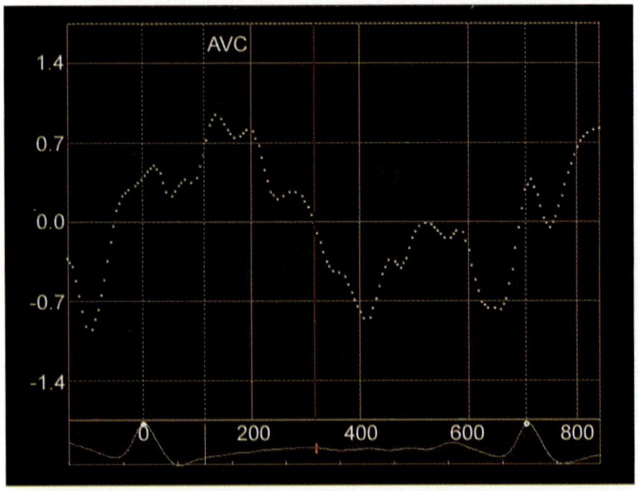

Fig. 4: 2D speckle-tracking *strain rate* imaging of LA in patient with hypertension and paroxysmal AF shows reduced values of LA strain rates, viz. reservoir SR_R, conduit SR_{con}, contractile SR_a function. (2D: two-dimensional; AF: atrial fibrillation; LA: left atrial)

conduction time." This underlines the role of progressively worsening FAC and LA structural remodeling in the natural history of progression of AF from paroxysmal to persistent AF.[11] The correlation of AF burden, LA *S* indices, and the LA fibrosis on gadolinium 3D magnetic resonance imaging (MRI) were evaluated in 65 patients (aged 61.2 ± 14.2 years) with paroxysmal (44%) or persistent (56%) AF.[12] Patients with persistent AF as compared with PAF had more fibrosis (22 ± 17% vs 14 ± 9%), lower midseptal (27 ± 14% vs 38 ± 16%), and midlateral (35 ± 16% vs 45 ± 14% *P* 0.03) S_R. The LA midlateral S_R and SR_R inversely predicted the extent of fibrosis independent of other echocardiographic parameters and the electrocardiography rhythm. In a study[13] of patients undergoing coronary artery bypass graft surgery the histopathological extent of fibrosis in the RA appendage was correlated with LA S. The extent of fibrosis in RA appendage specimen was studied by Masson's trichrome staining and was correlated with *S* values obtained preoperatively during sinus rhythm. The LA S_R during sinus rhythm was significantly reduced in patients with history of paroxysmal or persistent AF compared to the non-AF group. The reduced LA S_R values in the AF group showed good correlation to higher degree of fibrosis in RA appendage on histopathology. The patients with no AF showed normal LA S_R and absence of fibrosis in RA appendage.

PREDICTIVE POWER OF STRAIN AND STRAIN RATE IMAGING FOR INCIDENCE OF NEW ATRIAL FIBRILLATION

The patients are at a heightened risk of cardioembolic stroke with the onset of undetected paroxysmal or permanent AF. A large number of patients present with CVA as their first manifestation of paroxysmal or persistent AF without getting the benefit of anticoagulation. The guidelines for anticoagulation in AF require documentation of paroxysmal or persistent AF rhythm. The LA *S* and SR values, which reflect the extent LA fibrosis, may help to predict the future AF events. In a 3D-STE study[14] of 47 patients with AF (31 with PAF and 16 with permanent AF) the LA S_R, circumferential SR (CS_R), and area SR (AS_R) were reduced in patients with PAF compared with controls, and further reductions of these parameters were observed in patients with permanent AF. The standard deviations (SDs) of S_R, CS_R, AS_R, which are the markers of LA dissynchrony, were larger in patients with PAF and in those with permanent AF compared with controls. The 2D STE S_R, 3D STE S_R, AS_R, and CS_R were independent predictors of PAF irrespective of LA size. The 3D STE may help us to identify patients with normal LA sizes but increased risk for PAF. In rheumatic mitral stenosis (MS) the increased LA pressure causes structural and electrophysiologic remodeling which leads to early reduction in *S* and SR values and finally permanent AF in advanced stages. In a prospective study[15] of 101 asymptomatic patients with pure rheumatic MS, there was no significant differences in LA dimensions, volumes, ejection fraction, and LA compliance index between patients who developed or did not develop AF on follow-up. Over 55 months of follow-up the survival free of AF was 90% in patients with $S_R > 17.4\%$ compared to 40% in patients with mean $S_R < 17.4\%$.

The reduced global longitudinal *S* (GLS) of the left ventricular (LV) is a strong predictor of cardiovascular (CV) events and also predict new-onset AF. In Northern Manhattan Study,[16] 675 subjects in sinus rhythm with mean age 71 ± 9 years were followed for 63.6 ± 18.7 months. Lower GLS and increased LAV index (LAVi) were significantly associated with incident AF (4.7% of the cohort). Abnormal GLS (>–14.7%) was associated with 3.2-fold high risk of new-onset AF. Subjects with the presence of both "abnormal GLS and abnormal LAVi" had 28.6% incidence of AF compared to 2% in the absence of both. AF incidence was intermediate in those with either abnormal GLS or abnormal LAVi. Patients receiving dual-chamber (DDD) pacemakers are also at a risk of developing AF. In a study[17] of 146 patients on DDD implantation the risk of AF was associated with LA size, LA contractile function, and systolic blood pressure. The LA S_a < 8.6% had sensitivity of 52% and specificity of 83% to predict AF. Similarly the LAV < 62 mL had sensitivity of 69% and specificity of 61% for predicting AF.

PREDICTIVE POWER OF STRAIN AND STRAIN RATE IMAGING FOR PROGRESSION OF PAROXYSMAL TO PERMANENT ATRIAL FIBRILLATION

The PAF frequently, but not always, progresses to persistent or permanent AF. In a study[18] of 313 patients with PAF, progression to persistent or permanent AF occurred in 52 patients (16.6%) during a median follow-up period of 26 months. LA S_R was a powerful predictor of progression to permanent AF. LA S_R < 30.9% was associated with fourfold increase in AF progression. Compared to that the LA diameter >39 mm and maximal LAVi > 34.2 mL/m^2 were associated with a twofold increase in AF progression from paroxysmal to permanent.

PREDICTIVE POWER OF STRAIN AND STRAIN RATE IMAGING FOR THROMBOEMBOLIC RISK IN ATRIAL FIBRILLATION

The thromboembolic risk stratification in patients with AF is based on clinical features included in $CHADS_2$ or CHA_2DS_2–VASc score. This score is pivotal in decision of initiation of anticoagulation therapy. The cardioembolic stroke risk persists in patients with AF even after cardioversion to sinus rhythm. In patients with PAF the index stroke more often occurs during sinus rhythm and does not always chronologically follow PAF incidence. AF is considered a marker of stroke risk regardless of whether or not the arrhythmia is sustained.[1] Therefore *S* imaging being a sensitive marker of FAC has a potential to further risk stratify the AF patients with CHA_2DS_2–VASc score <2. The impaired LA *S* and SR values show good correlation with transesophageal findings of LA appendage thrombus and LA spontaneous echocardiographic contrast.[19] The lower mean LA S_R is associated with LA appendage flow velocities <20 cm/s.[20] The LA S_R and SR_R are inversely related to $CHADS_2$ score and are independent predictors of stroke after adjustment for age and LAV.[21] In a study[9] of 36 AF patients and 41 controls, LA S_R reduced with increasing $CHADS_2$ score. LA S_R was the only echocardiographic predictor of a high risk of stroke in patients with $CHADS_2$ score ≥ 2. A study[22] of *S* and SR evaluation in 66 permanent AF patients showed that patients with stroke/transient ischemic attack (TIA) had lower LA S_R (10.44% ± 4.2% vs 15.69% ± 5.1%), lower SR_R (1.09 ± 0.27 vs 1.37 ± 0.32), and lower SR_{con} (–1.28 ± 0.38 vs –1.62 ± 0.43) compared to the patients without stroke. The S_R and SR_R were independently associated with CVA, irrespective of age, LAVi, and LV ejection fraction. In AF patients with low $CHADS_2$ score (<2), there was no significant differences in rates of stroke between patients with S_R > 13.5% and <13.5% (stroke rate 12.5% vs 27.3%, respectively). However, in patients with high $CHADS_2$ score (≥ 2), there was significant difference in rates of stroke between patients with S_R > 13.5% and <13.5% (stroke rate 12.5% vs 61.9%, respectively). The advanced atrial remodeling and impaired atrial contractility indicated by low S_R may lead to greater LA stasis and greater risk for thromboembolism (Figs. 5 and 6). In AF patients with CHA_2DS_2–VASc score 0 or 1 the decision of anticoagulation can be tailored by the LA *S* data. A retrospective, registry-based, case-control study[10] evaluated *S* and SR imaging in 57 patients with PAF, low-risk $CHADS_2$ score (1 before their index CVA or TIA) and stroke/TIA and 57 controls with PAF, low $CHADS_2$ score but no stroke. The reduced LA S_a and S_R were strong predictors of stroke risk. Both LA S_a (3.2 ± 1.2% vs 6.9 ± 4.2%) and LA S_R (14 ± 11% vs 25 ± 12%) were significantly reduced in patients with the history of stroke compared with no history of stroke. A cutoff value for S_a ≤ –5.0% had sensitivity 93%, specificity 60%, positive-predictive value 71%, and negative-predictive value 92% to predict CVA/TIA in low-risk subgroup. LA *S* may help in deciding for or against oral anticoagulation in patients with $CHADS_2$ scores ≤1.

PREDICTIVE POWER OF STRAIN AND STRAIN RATE IMAGING FOR MAINTENANCE OF SINUS RHYTHM AFTER CARDIOVERSION OR RADIOFREQUENCY ABLATION

The electrical cardioversion or catheter RF ablation is often attempted to convert AF to sinus rhythm. The magnitude of

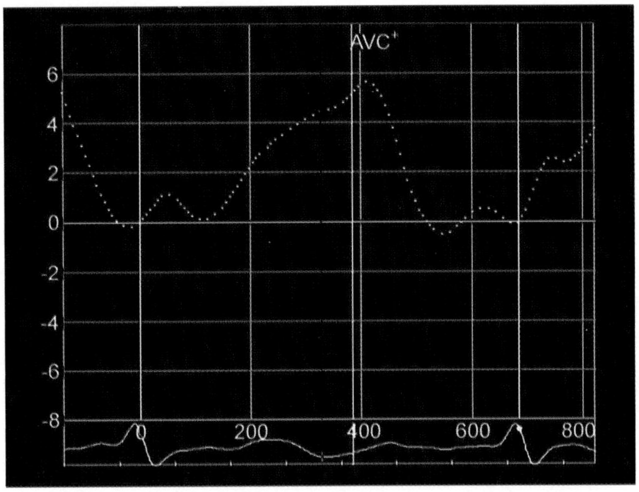

Fig. 5: 2D speckle-tracking *strain* imaging of LA in patient with AF and cardioembolic stroke shows severely reduced values of LA strains, viz. reservoir S_R, conduit S_{con} function. (2D: two-dimensional; AF: atrial fibrillation; LA: left atrial)

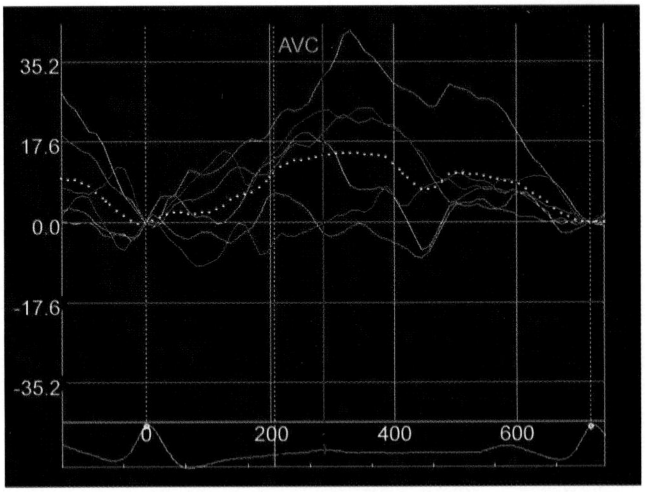

Fig. 7: 2D speckle-tracking strain imaging of LA shows dispersion of strain curves in patient with hypertension and paroxysmal AF. (2D: two-dimensional; AF: atrial fibrillation; LA: left atrial)

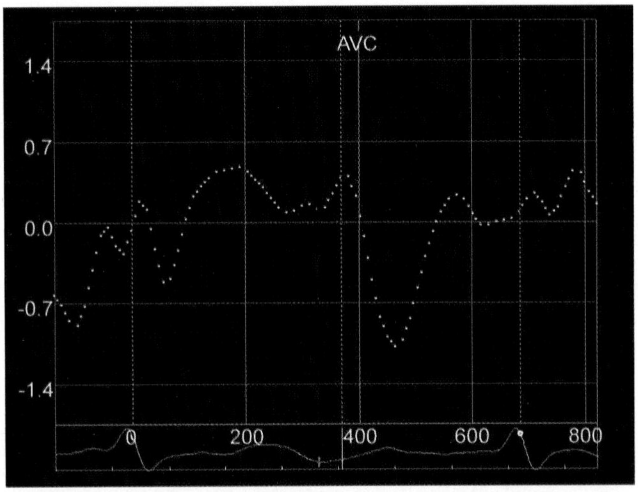

Fig. 6: 2D speckle-tracking *strain rate* imaging of LA in patient with AF and cardioembolic stroke shows severely reduced values of LA strain rates corresponding to reservoir SR_R, conduit SR_{con} function. (2D: two-dimensional; AF: atrial fibrillation; LA: left atrial)

LA remodeling and fibrosis decides the acute success of the procedure and the long-term maintenance of sinus rhythm. A 3D MRI study showed that patients with mild (<10%) LA fibrosis had greater postablation increase in LA S_R and SR_R and less recurrences of AF at 12 months compared with the patients with moderate-to-severe (>10%) LA fibrosis.[12] The postcardioversion LA stunning results in lower LA S_R, SR_R, S_{con}, SR_{con} values than the baseline, 1-day postprocedure, which improves over the next 10 days.[20] In a study[23] of global *S* assessed by 3D *S* the LA dissynchrony [SD of time to peak (TP) of area tracking, TP-SD of 16 segments of LA] and LA S_R significantly improved 3 months after pulmonary vein isolation by RF ablation (10.0 ± 5.2% to 6.8 ± 3.0%, for TP-SD; and 48.2 ± 20.2% to 58.1 ± 21.2%, for LA S_R, respectively). A lower LA SR_{con} and an enlarged LA are independent predictors of reduced success of cardioversion and a shorter duration of the maintenance of sinus rhythm. In a study[24] of 42 AF patients and 27 controls baseline, LA SR_{con} > 2.18 s had sensitivity of 83% and specificity of 64.3% to predict the maintenance of sinus rhythm at 4 weeks after cardioversion. The baseline LA S_R and SR_R are independent predictors of maintenance of sinus rhythm for as long as 9 months after cardioversion. Baseline LA S_R > 22% had sensitivity of 77% and specificity of 86% and baseline SR_R > 1.8 had sensitivity of 92% and specificity of 79% to predict the maintenance of sinus rhythm at 9 months.[25] The atrial dissynchrony is measured as the SD of the time to peak S_R in six segments of the LA (Fig. 7). In a prospective study[26] of 130 patients undergoing cardioversion for AF, atrial dissynchrony was an independent predictor of recurrence of AF. The RA mechanical function may contribute to maintenance sinus rhythm. In a study[27] of 30 patients with AF, RA and RV *S* was evaluated precardioversion, and the patients were followed up for 1-year postcardioversion. Patients who remained in sinus rhythm had significantly greater RV longitudinal S, RA reservoir, and RA booster *S* compared with patients who reverted to AF at the end of 1 year. RA booster *S* was the strongest predictor for the maintenance of sinus rhythm. The *S* and SR imaging is more useful to predict long-term outcome in patients undergoing RF catheter ablation for AF. In a study[2] of 148 AF patients undergoing RF ablation, followed for 13 months, 93 patients (63%) were classified as responders, and 55 patients (37%) were classified as nonresponders. At baseline, LA S_R was significantly higher in the responders as compared with the nonresponders (19 8% vs 14 6%). The responders had a significant increase in LA S_R, SR_R, S_a, SR_a at 13 months compared to no change in the nonresponders. The LA S_R at baseline was an independent predictor of LA reverse remodeling (LAV reduction >15%) after catheter ablation. Similar findings of improvements in LA S_R and SR_R were noticed in patients with AF who underwent minimally invasive surgical RF ablation.[28] In a study[29] of 118 AF patients, baseline (preablation) $S_R > 20\%$ had sensitivity of 57% and specificity of 56% to predict maintenance of sinus rhythm after AF catheter ablation up to 3 months. However, 24-hours postablation LA $S_R > 20.5\%$ had sensitivity of 99% and specificity of 78%, to predict the maintenance of sinus rhythm at 3 months. LA S_R, SR_R, and SR_a values 24 hours after RF catheter ablation were all predictors of the maintenance of sinus rhythm. This suggests that post-RF ablation and immediate recovery of *S* values strongly predict long-term maintenance of sinus rhythm.

PREDICTIVE POWER OF STRAIN AND STRAIN RATE IMAGING FOR HEART FAILURE AND CARDIOVASCULAR MORTALITY IN ATRIAL FIBRILLATION

The progressive LA remodeling and fibrosis in AF increase the risk of thromboembolism and heart failure. In patients with AF the LA S_R with LAV have incremental value over and above $CHADS_2$ score to predict mortality and future hospitalization for cardiac causes.[9,22] In a study[30] of 190 patients with persistent AF, increased mitral inflow velocity (E) to LA reservoir S (S_R) ratio was strongly associated with CV events. The E/LA S_R had an incremental value in predicting CV events over and above CHA_2DS_2-VASc score, LAVi, and LV systolic and diastolic function. The LV GLS is a powerful predictor of clinical adverse events in AF. Measuring LV GLS in AF entails averaging of more than 13 beats and is cumbersome to utilize in day-to-day clinical practice. An index beat is defined as the cardiac cycle which has nearly equal preceding two cardiac cycles (RR1 and RR2). The RR1 and RR2 intervals of the index beat must be >500 ms, and the difference between them must be <60 ms. Measuring LV GLS in the index beat gives near identical values as measured by more laborious conventional method.[31] The LV GLS measured by index beat has inverse relationship with the $CHADS_2$ scores or CHA_2DS_2-VASc scores.[31] The ratio of early mitral inflow velocity (E) to global LV early diastolic SR (E_{SR}) has good correlation with LV filling pressure. In a study[32] of 190 patients with persistent AF, LV E_{SR} was calculated by using the index beat method. During a follow-up period of 20 months, 22 deaths and 28 hospitalizations for heart failure were observed. The increased E/E_{SR} ratio was associated with increased cardiac events. The cutoff value of $E/E_{SR} > 64$ had the best sensitivity and specificity in predicting adverse cardiac events. There was incremental value for addition of E/E_{SR} ratio to the model, including age, chronic heart failure, diabetes, HT, LAVi, LV ejection fraction, and E/e' to predict adverse cardiac events.

REFERENCES

1. Hirsh BJ, Copeland-Halperin RS, Halperin JL, et al. Fibrotic atrial cardiomyopathy, atrial fibrillation, and thromboembolism mechanistic links and clinical inferences. J Am Coll Cardiol. 2015;65:2239-51.
2. Tops LF, Delgado V, Bertini M, et al. Left atrial strain predicts reverse remodeling after catheter ablation for atrial fibrillation. J Am Coll Cardiol. 2011;57:324-31.
3. Hoit BD. Left atrial size and function: role in prognosis. J Am Coll Cardiol. 2014;63:493-505.
4. Vieira MJ, Teixeira R, Goncalves L, et al. Left atrial mechanics: echocardiographic assessment and clinical implications. J Am Soc Echocardiogr. 2014;27:46378.
5. Saraiva RM, Demirkol S, Buakhamsri A, et al. Left atrial strain measured by two-dimensional speckle tracking represents a new tool to evaluate left atrial function. J Am Soc Echocardiogr. 2010;23:172-80.
6. Motoki H, Dahiya A, Bhargava M. Assessment of left atrial mechanics in patients with atrial fibrillation: comparison between two-dimensional speckle-based strain and velocity vector imaging. J Am Soc Echocardiogr. 2012;25:428-35.
7. Ebato M, Maezawa H, Tanabe A, et al. Left atrial area strain measured by three dimensional speckle tracking echocardiography represents global and regional left atrial function at once. J Am Coll Cardiol. 2012;59:E1269.
8. Inaba Y, Yuda S, Kobayashi N. Strain rate imaging for noninvasive functional quantification of the left atrium: comparative studies in controls and patients with atrial fibrillation. J Am Soc Echocardiogr. 2005;18:729-36.
9. Saha SK, Anderson PL, Caracciolo G, et al. Global left atrial strain correlates with CHADS2 risk score in patients with atrial fibrillation. J Am Soc Echocardiogr. 2011;24:506-12.
10. Azemi T, Rabdiya VM, Ayirala SR, et al. Left atrial strain is reduced in patients with atrial fibrillation, stroke or TIA, and low risk CHADS2 scores. J Am Soc Echocardiogr. 2012;25:1327-32.
11. Leung M, Abou R, Van Rosendael P, et al. Echocardiographic markers of left atrial fibrosis associated with the severity of atrial fibrillation. JACC. 2016;67(13)
12. Kuppahally SS, Akoum N, Burgon NS, et al. Left atrial strain and strain rate in patients with paroxysmal and persistent atrial fibrillation: relationship to left atrial structural remodeling detected by delayed-enhancement MRI. Circ Cardiovasc Imaging. 2010;3:231-9.
13. Mirza M, Jiamsripong P, Belohlavek M. Atrial mechanical abnormalities on speckle tracking echocardiography

correlate with degree of fibrosis in patients with atrial fibrillation. JACC. 2012;59(13).
14. Mochizuki A, Yuda S, Oi Y, et al. Assessment of left atrial deformation and synchrony by three-dimensional speckle-tracking echocardiography: comparative studies in healthy subjects and patients with atrial fibrillation. J Am Soc Echocardiogr. 2013;26:165-74.
15. Ancona R, Comenale Pinto S, Caso P, et al. Two-dimensional atrial systolic strain imaging predicts atrial fibrillation at 4-year follow-up in asymptomatic rheumatic mitral stenosis. J Am Soc Echocardiogr. 2013;26:270-7.
16. Russo C, Jin Z, Sera F, et al. Left ventricular systolic dysfunction by longitudinal strain is an independent predictor of incident atrial fibrillation: a community-based cohort study. Circ Cardiovasc Imaging. 2015;8:e003520.
17. Kosmala W, Saito M, Kaye G, et al. Incremental value of left atrial structural and functional characteristics for prediction of atrial fibrillation in patients receiving cardiac pacing. Circ Cardiovasc Imaging. 2015;8:e002942.
18. Yoon YE, Oh IY, Kim SA, et al. Echocardiographic predictors of progression to persistent or permanent atrial fibrillation in patients with paroxysmal atrial fibrillation (E6P Study). J Am Soc Echocardiogr. 2015;28:709-17.
19. Providencia R, Trigo J, Paiva L, et al. The role of echocardiography in thromboembolic risk assessment of patients with nonvalvular atrial fibrillation. J Am Soc Echocardiogr. 2013;26:801-12.
20. Kaya EB, Tokgozoglu L, Aytemir K, et al. Atrial myocardial deformation properties are temporarily reduced after cardioversion for atrial fibrillation and correlate well with left atrial appendage function. Eur J Echocardiogr. 2008;9:472-7.
21. Mochizuki A, Yuda S, Ohi Y, et al. Assessment of left atrial dysfunction and dyssynchrony by 3 dimensional speckle tracking in patients with atrial fibrillation. J Am Coll Cardiol. 2012;59:E1266.
22. Shih JY, Tsai WC, Huang YY, et al. Association of decreased left atrial strain and strain rate with stroke in chronic atrial fibrillation. J Am Soc Echocardiogr. 2011;24:513-9.
23. Kobayashi Y, Yamamoto K, Kobayashi Y, et al. Impact of pulmonary vein isolation to paroxismal atrial fibrillation for atrial asynchrony and global strain assessed by 3d strain echocardiography. JACC. 2013;61(10).
24. Wang T, Wang M, Fung JW, et al. Atrial strain rate echocardiography can predict success or failure of cardioversion for atrial fibrillation: a combined transthoracic tissue Doppler and transoesophageal imaging study. Int J Cardiol. 2007;114:202-9.
25. Di Salvo G, Caso P, Lo Piccolo R, et al. Atrial myocardial deformation properties predict maintenance of sinus rhythm after external cardioversion of recent-onset lone atrial fibrillation. Circulation. 2005;112:387-95.
26. Rondano E, Dell'Era G, De Luca G, et al. Left atrial asynchrony is a major predictor of 1-year recurrence of atrial fibrillation after electrical cardioversion. J Cardiovasc Med. 2010;11: 499-506.
27. Saha SK, Govindan M, Kiotsekoglou A, et al. Right atrial booster strain during an index beat is the strongest predictor of maintenance of sinus rhythm one year post cardioversion in subjects with paroxysmal atrial fibrillation. JACC. 2013;61(10).
28. La Meir M, Gelsomino S, Luca F, et al. Improvement of left atrial function and left atrial reverse remodeling after minimally invasive radiofrequency ablation evaluated by two-dimensional speckle tracking echocardiography. J Thorac Cardiovasc Surg. 2011;146:72-7.
29. Schneider C, Malisius R, Krause K, et al. Strain rate imaging for functional quantification of the left atrium: atrial deformation predicts the maintenance of sinus rhythm after catheter ablation of atrial fibrillation. Eur Heart J. 2008;29:1397-409.
30. Su HM, Lin FH, Hsu PC. The ratio of transmitral E-wave velocity to left atrial strain and left atrial strain itself can respectively predict cardiovascular and subsequent stroke outcomes in patients with atrial fibrillation. JACC. 2015;65(10S).
31. Lee CS, Lin TS, Hsu PC. Measuring left ventricular peak longitudinal systolic strain from a single beat in atrial fibrillation: validation of the index beat method. J Am Soc Echocardiogr. 2012;25:945-52.
32. Hsu PC, Lee WH, Chu CY. The ratio of early mitral inflow velocity to global diastolic strain rate as a useful predictor of cardiac outcomes in patients with atrial fibrillation. J Am Soc Echocardiogr. 2014;27:717-25.

75

CHAPTER

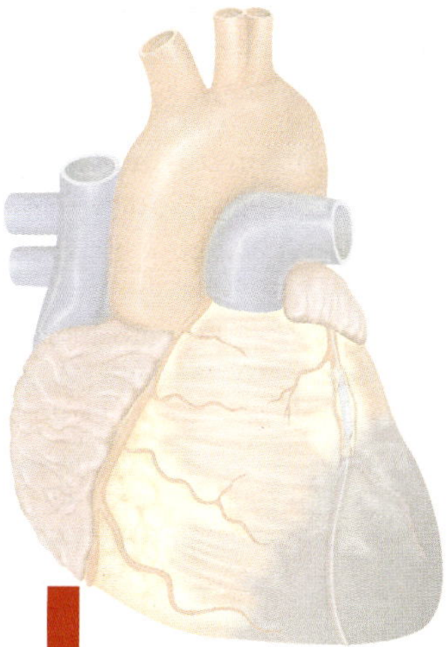

Non-Vitamin-K Oral Anticoagulant Effect and Outcome Evaluation in Echocardiography

Tapan Sinha, Mrinal Kanti Das

INTRODUCTION

Incidence of thrombotic stroke increase many times over in patients with atrial fibrillation (AF) especially in those or states with sluggish flow velocity in left atrium (LA). They have considerable morbidity and mortality with huge socioeconomic implications. Over the last 10 years, through a large body of evidences, it has been conclusively shown that non-vitamin-K oral anticoagulants (NOACs) are superior in efficacy and safer to vitamin K anticoagulants (VKAs). However, it is imperative that indications for NOACs need to be established first by electrocardiographic evidence of AF and then by transthoracic echocardiogram (TTE) or transesophageal echocardiogram (TEE), of which TEE is more sensitive and specific, and thereafter, follow-up of the efficacy may be done with echocardiography. There are very sparse reports in the literature regarding all these aspects. Hence the aim of the present article is to explore the NOACs effects, outcome evaluation by echocardiography, and to find out any statistical relevance in terms of predictability, sensitivity, and specificity (Table 1).

NON-VITAMIN-K ORAL ANTICOAGULANT EFFECT

Anecdotal Data

Atrial fibrillation is most commonly occurring tachyarrhythmia affecting 5% of people >65 years and nearly 10% of those over 80 years. AF is associated with cerebral and peripheral thromboembolism. There is four–five times increase of incidences of cerebral thromboembolism or stroke in all age-group with AF.[1] Risk of ischemic stroke is three–seven times higher in patients with mitral stenosis (MS) in AF in comparison to those in sinus rhythm.[2] In 1998, a subgroup analysis of five randomized studies (AFASAC, SPAF, BAATF, ACFCA, and SPINAF), it was agreed that incidences of ischemic stroke in nonvalvular AF (NVAF) are not less than 5%.[3] These are landmark studies which conclusively identified the following: (1) that NVAF, such as valvular diseases with AF and prosthetic valves, is associated with high incidences of thrombotic stroke; (2) that incidences are even higher in high-risk groups, e.g. chronic or paroxysmal AF with hypertension, diabetes, structural cardiomyopathy, previous history of stroke, and age >65 years; (3) that it recommended or oral

TABLE 1: TEE observation and correlates of thromboembolic risk.

TEE observation	*Low risk (%)*	*Moderate risk (%)*	*High risk (%)*
LAA area >8.4 cm^2	26	21	25
Dense SEC	4	10	20
LAA thrombus	3	8	15
LAA flow velocity ≤20 cm/s	19	28	37
Complex aortic plaque	15	16	35
Any aortic plaque	48	54	63
Moderate-to-severe MR	11	14	19

(MR: mitral regurgitation; SEC: spontaneous echocardiographic contrast; TEE: transesophageal echocardiogram)

anticoagulation for patients with NVAF; and (4) "Obesity paradox"—obesity is an independent risk factor for stoke in AF but has lower mortality.

Oral VKAs, acenocoumarol, and subsequently Warfarin are in the market since 1940s. In 1983, doses were standardized for use in deep venous thrombosis. In 1998, metanalysis[3] showed decreased risk of ischemic stroke, primary and secondary, in patients with NVAF, with a relative risk reduction in the range of 33–75%, mean 62% [95% confidence interval (CI) 48% to 72%]. Since 1950s, difficulties with monitoring for narrow therapeutic window, fatal gastrointestinal, cerebral bleedings, and other complications were identified with acenocoumarol and Warfarin.[4] It has been also documented in Randomized Evaluation of Long-term Anticoagulant Therapy (RE-LY) Study that treatment with VKA with target international normalized ratio (INR) 2–3 was superior to aspirin 75 mg daily in decreasing incidences of fatal and disabling stroke in population >65 years of age with AF. A subgroup analysis of the same study showed INR control within therapeutic range with Warfarin is lower in Asian patients in comparison to non-Asians (54.5% vs 66.2%). In addition to this, treatment time above and below therapeutic range was unfavorable to Asians in comparison to non-Asians, 10.1% versus 14.0% and 35.4% versus 19.8%, respectively.[5] However, with VKA, there was increased incidence of bleeding, allergic reaction, skin necrosis, nephropathy, teratogenicity, cholesterol embolism, vascular complications, drug-diet and drug-drug interactions.[4,6] In contrast to VKAs, regarding these drawbacks, NOACs came out to be boons producing favorable results in *NVAF*.

Mechanism and classification of NOACs: This discussion is relevant in view of the varying sites of actions of the NOACs and understanding and ramification of the whole process of anticoagulation. Figure 1 highlights the same as given below:

- Direct thrombin (factor IIa) inhibitor—Dabigatran
- Direct factor Xa inhibitor—Apixaban, Rivaroxaban, Edoxaban

Non-vitamin-K oral anticoagulants have been studied in mega trials and in clinical practice.[7-9] Years 2009 to 2013 had been particularly productive in this regard.

Indications for Echocardiography on Patients Under Non-Vitamin-K Oral Anticoagulants[10,11]

Patients with NVAF with prior history of thrombotic stroke of transient ischemic attack (TIA) being the strongest independent predictor for repeat attacks. In addition to this, deterioration of chronic heart failure, hypertension, diabetes, liver disease, peripheral vascular disease, renal transplant and dialysis, and aging are identified as compounding factors emphasizing role of echocardiography in those clinical setups.

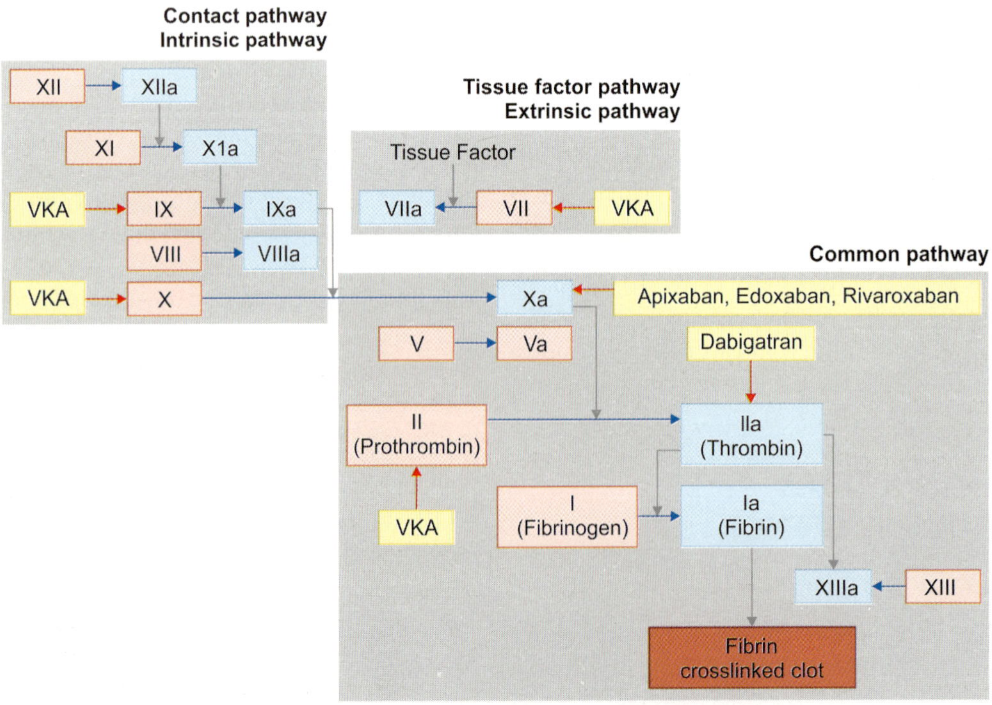

Fig. 1: Three important pathways for blood coagulation.

Summary of major trials on non-vitamin-K oral anticoagulants and 2018 European Heart Rhythm Association practical guideline[12]*:*

Randomized Evaluation of Long-term Anticoagulant Therapy (Dabigatran vs Warfarin), ROCKET-AF (Rivaroxaban vs Warfarin), Apixaban for Reduction in Stroke and Other Thromboembolic Events in Atrial Fibrillation(ARISTOTLE) (Apixaban vs Warfarin), ENGAGE AF—TIMI—48 (Edoxaban vs Warfarin), PETRO PHASE II trial, and J-ROCKET AF study highlighted the following:

- Eligibility of NVAF as the criteria. The data were reliable only in AF with mild-to-moderate aortic stenosis (AS)/ aortic regurgitation (AR) and degenerative mitral regurgitation (MR). However, recommendations extrapolated NVAF in general. Moderate-to-severe MS of rheumatic origin and mechanical valve prosthesis cases are excluded.
- All NOACs have lesser or comparable incidence of intracerebral bleeding in comparison to Warfarin. Apixaban 2.5 mg bis die (BD) and Dabigatran 110 mg BD had lesser major gastrointestinal bleeding than Warfarin, whereas incidences were similar with Rivaroxaban and Edoxaban.
- Only Apixaban has all case mortality benefit over Warfarin.
- Dabigatran showed that marginal rise of myocardial infarction (MI) in RE-LY trial is possibly due the study design. A massive study conducted by Food and Drug Administration[13] on safety issues of Dabigatran on 134,000 Medicare patients, 65 years or older, with 110 mg BD dose, found that among new users with AF for 6 months or more, Dabigatran was associated with a lower risk of clot-related strokes, bleeding in the brain, and death, than Warfarin. The study also found an increased risk of major gastrointestinal bleeding with the use of Dabigatran as compared to Warfarin. The MI risk was similar for the two drugs.
- However, none of the studies gave any indication of methodology (echocardiography) for the identification of state of cardiac valves, cardiac function status, and prior existence of cardiac thrombus or wall motion abnormality. Most importantly, 2018 European Heart Rhythm Association Practical Guideline on the use of NOACs in patients with AF does not include the identification of low-flow state in LA as selection or assessment criteria for patient selection for the use of NOACs.

In addition to these, ischemic strokes may result from number of other conditions e.g. presence atherosclerotic plaques in carotid, cerebral arteries, etc. Those subgroups may have been presented along with AF but were ignored in selection criteria and subsequent data analysis.

Based on above observations, we recommend that pretreatment and follow-up echocardiographic assessment by TEE should be recommended for all patients with AF receiving NOACs.

Implication of Nonvalvular Atrial Fibrillation

Definition of valvular and NVAF has been a matter of debate. American College of Cardiology/American Heart Association Guidelines on AF in 2014 define NVAF as AF in the absence of rheumatic MS, mechanical or bioprosthetic heart valve, or mitral valve repair, whereas NVAF is associated with other valve diseases, e.g. AS, AR, MR. *We observe that the purpose of this definition is not for etiological diagnosis of AF but for classification of high-risk cases of thromboembolism associated with low-flow states in LA.*[14]

The distinction between "valvular" AF and "NVAF," however, remains uncertain, with variable definitions adopted in the NOAC trials. This has led to therapeutic confusion, illustrated by a web-based survey among over 500 Italian physicians mainly involved in the prescription of anticoagulants to AF patients. Here, only 57.1% of the cardiologists and 67.9% of the internists agreed that the existing definitions of NVAF (e.g. from Guidelines) were sufficiently clear.[15]

ECHOCARDIOGRAPHY-BASED TRIAGING IN MECHANICAL VALVE PROSTHESIS

The RE-ALIGN[16] was a multicentric trial conducted for 12 weeks on 405 patients. Dosing algorithm for Dabigatran was based on a pharmacokinetic model developed in the RE-LY trial, which studied the characteristics of Dabigatran in a different population. It is of interest to note that most thromboembolic events occurred among patients of the Dabigatran arm when it was the initial anticoagulant, with fewer events occurring in patients who started Dabigatran after 3 months of Warfarin therapy in patients with mechanical valve prosthesis. This might be due to inadequate plasma levels of the Dabigatran during the first few weeks after surgery, which might have allowed for early formation of blood clots that were not clinically manifested until later. However, increasing the dose can lead to increased bleeding episodes, which was already higher in this group. The composite of stroke, TIA, systemic embolism, myocardial infarction, or death occurred in 4 patients (5%) in the Warfarin group and 15 patients (9%) in the Dabigatran group. Most thromboembolic events among patients in the Dabigatran group occurred in mechanical valve replacement in the aortic or mitral position or both within the past 7 days. The pathogenesis of thrombosis is likely to be different for blood coming into contact with the artificial surface of a prosthetic valve vis-a-vis what occurring in common types of AF with or without valvular disease. In patients with a mechanical prosthetic valve, even in the absence of AF, the results of the only intervention trial so far performed with a NOAC demonstrate that Warfarin is more effective and also safer than the relatively high doses of Dabigatran (RE-ALIGN study).[16]

Rivaroxaban in Mechanical Valves Study (Andre Duraes et al.) is an ongoing trial without any early bird information till the date of writing this article.

MODERATE-TO-SEVERE MITRAL STENOSIS

American College of Cardiology/American Heart Association Guidelines on AF in 2014 define NVAF on flow status in LA (<15 cm/s) designed for the identification of a subgroup for treatment. NVAF consists of those cases of AF in the presence of valvular heart disease and nonvalvular heart diseases which has higher flow rate in LA (>15 cm/s) than observed in moderate-to-severe MS with AF and as evidenced by echocardiography.[17]

The risk of thromboembolism is particularly high in AF accompanying moderate-to-severe MS as in mechanical prosthetic valve. Since MS, especially in Indian subcontinent, with or without other associated valvular disease, is most of the time rheumatic, the terms "AF with MS" and "rheumatic AF" are often used interchangeably. It is not clear, however, whether the pathogenesis of thrombosis in AF accompanying MS with lower velocity of flow in LA is qualitatively different from those of most common forms of NVAF. Warfarin has been used for decades at higher doses for satisfactory reduction of thrombotic stroke in *valvular AF*. NOACs, in higher doses when used in patients with *valvular AF* for comparable efficacy, are associated with similar or higher incidences of fatal bleedings than Warfarin.[18,19] It is therefore imperative to pick up these cardiac conditions early by echocardiography to avoid catastrophic management.

OUTCOME EVALUATION OF NOACS IN ECHOCARDIOGRAPHY: THE MOOT IDEAS ARE TO FIND OUT

- Evidence of thrombus dissolution or regression with NOACs and prognosticate
- Negating requirement of echocardiography in outcome evaluation in NOACs therapy

Methodology and Outcome

- Transesophageal echocardiogram has strong predictive power of thromboembolism in AF.[20] Sensitivity and specificity of TEE for LA thrombi are 93–100% and 99–100%, respectively.
- Main advantage of TEE is in superior visualization of posterior structures e.g. left atrial appendage.
- Four types of LA appendage (LAA) morphology have been by TEE [(preferably by magnetic resonance imaging (MRI)][21]: (1) chicken wing (48%), (2) cactus morphology (30%), (3) windsock (19%), and (4) cauliflower (3%). Incidences of thrombus in relation to morphological classes are not well studied.
- Left atrium size assessment, LA area measurements, and LA volume estimation by TEE have contributed enormously in outcome evaluation of NOAC. Three-dimensional (3D)-TTE imaging may be more informative but limited by less availability of instrumentation and expertise and is also time consuming. Reduced global longitudinal LA strain is associated with NVF and greater chance of $CHADS_2$ score >2.[22]
- Classification of low-flow-velocity state in heart, especially in LA, can be better assessed. Low flow velocity (<20 cm/s) in LAA is associated with higher incidences of thrombus. It is even higher if flow is <15 cm/s (Fig. 2).[23]
- In NVAF patient for 3 days or more, LAA thrombus is detected in about 13% patients by TEE.[24] The incidences are higher in association with moderate-to-severe MS (33%),[25] LV systolic dysfunction, enlarged LA and LAA, spontaneous echocardiographic contrast (SEC), recent thromboembolic event, (43%) and in association with $CHADS_2$ score >2.
- Spontaneous echocardiographic contrast is an indicator for sluggish flow state and associates with increased incidences of LAA thrombus.[26,27] Patients with LA SEC, compared with those without LA SEC, were characterized by more frequent advanced New York Heart Association class, AF, smaller mitral valve area, and larger LA size. By multivariate regression analysis, AF and LA end-systolic area were factors related to both LA thrombus and LA SEC, whereas mitral area was related only to LA SEC.[28]
- Classification of SEC: Four grades of SEC (Figs. 3A to D).[29] The article by Ji et al.[30] is important for quantification of SEC by TEE (Figs. 4A and B). The result shows that quantification of LASEC by video intensity value is the most favorable predictor of stroke in patients with NVAF.
- Right atrial thrombus is clearly seen by TEE. It is much less common than LA thrombus in AF occurring in 3–6% of cases. It is associated with right ventricular failure.

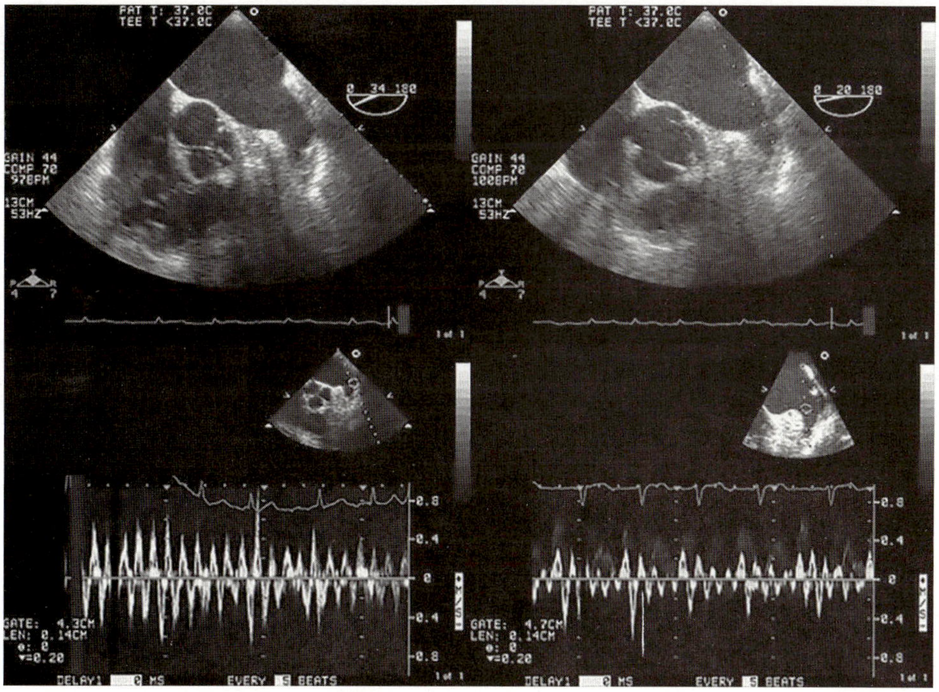

Fig. 2: TEE image of the left atrial appendage (upper, left). The upper right picture illustrates the position at the base of the appendage of the pulsed Doppler. The lower panel illustrates spectral Doppler flow from the left atrial appendage in a patient with high flow velocities (left) and low flow velocities (right), respectively. (TEE: transthoracic echocardiogram)

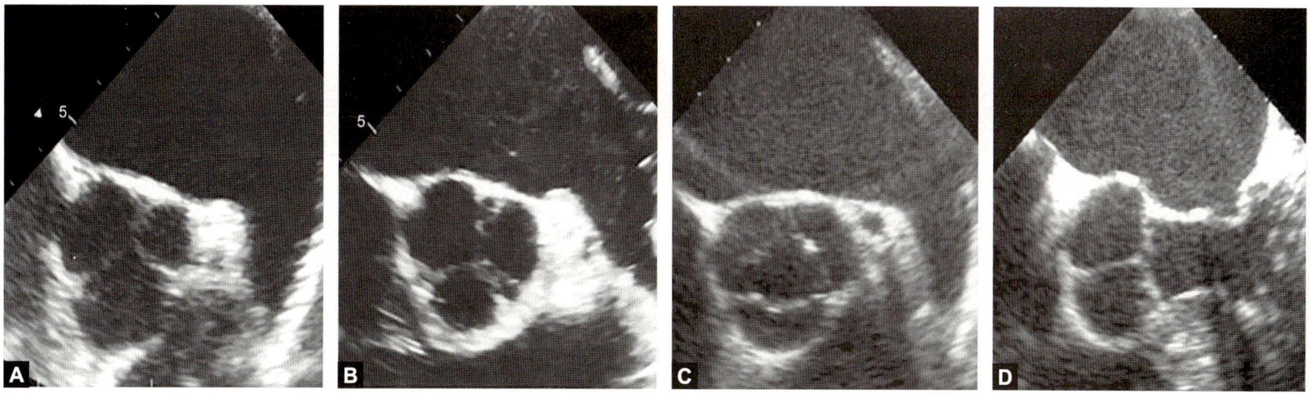

Figs. 3A to D: The intensity of left atrial SEC was classified into four grades, from 0 to 3. (A) Grade 0 was no SEC, (B) grade 1 mild, (C) grade 2 moderate, and (D) grade 3 severe. (SEC: spontaneous echo contrast)

Protocol of cardioversion with NOAC is same as in LA thrombus albeit less validated (*see* Table 1).[31]

Evidence of Thrombus Dissolution or Regression with Non-Vitamin-K Oral Anticoagulants

The major trials clinching the issue of anticoagulation for NOACs over Warfarin include a wide range of age-group, from 62 years (25th percentile) to 79 years (75th percentile). Unifying issue in all trials is the origin of thrombus from heart, resulting in thrombotic stroke. Trials (RE-LY, ARISTOTLE, and ROCKET-AF) include a heterogenous population of NVAF patients, predominantly with MR (72–89%).[19] But none of the trials give much importance in methodology of diagnosis (echocardiographic) of MR or NVAF. Thus none had any scope of identification of the presence or absence of thrombus or spontaneous echocardiographic shadow (SEC) in heart prior to administration of NOACs and in follow-up. In a very important study published in 2016, Reers,[32] including a small number of patients with AF or atrial flutter (total 306) for 6 weeks, showed that under TEE structural

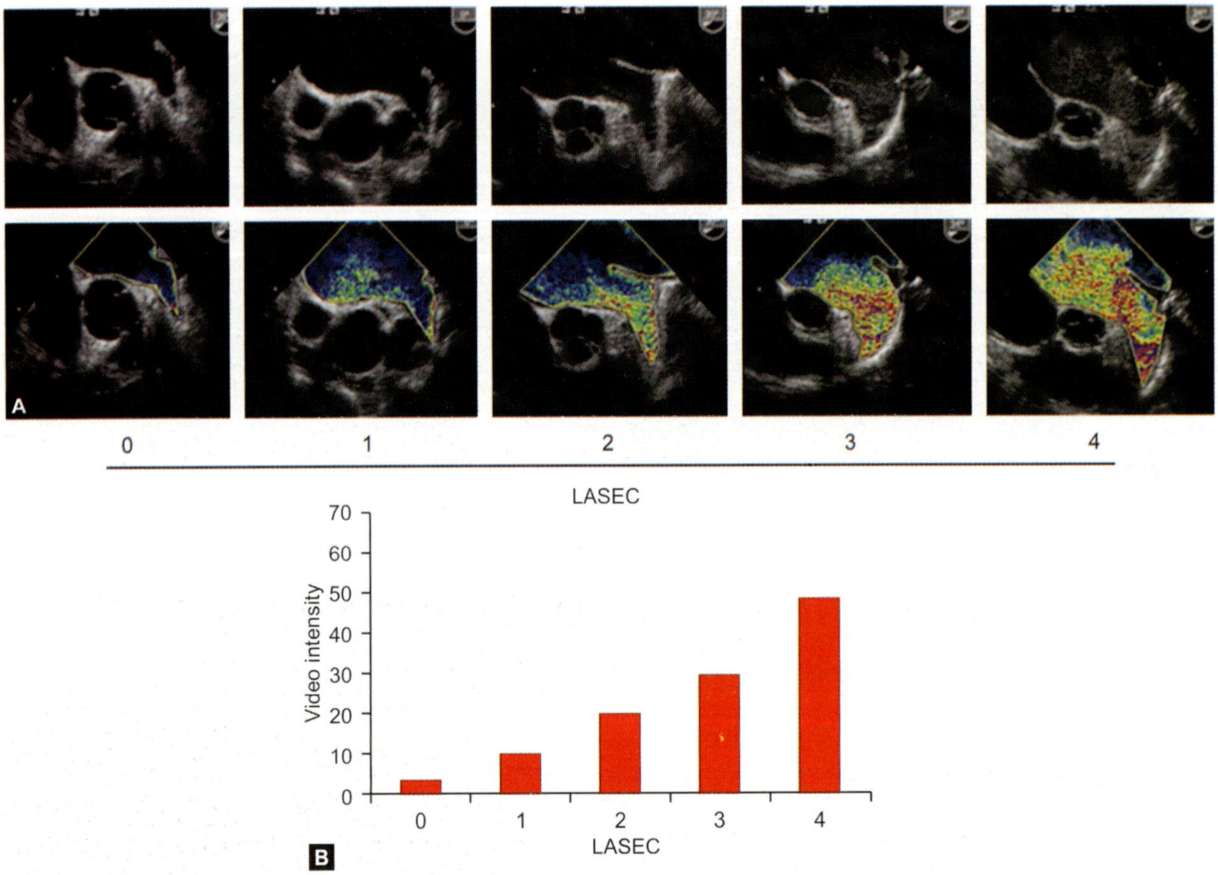

Figs. 4A and B: Two-dimensional ultrasonogram and the corresponding color-coded map of different grades of LASEC (A). Quantification of VI value in patients with each of five grades of LASEC; (B). *P <0.05. (LASEC: left atrium spontaneous echocardiographic contrast; VI; video intensity)

abnormality of LA was observed only in 3% to 9% patients receiving VKA, Dabigatran, and Rivaroxaban. When LAA flow velocity was >20 cm/s, incidences of thrombus were lower (VKA: 4%, Dabigatran: 0%, Rivaroxaban: 2% groups) in comparison to when LAA flow velocity was <20 cm/s (VKA: 4%, Dabigatran: 1%, Rivaroxaban: 2%), followed by dense SEC (VKA: 2%, Dabigatran: 1%, Rivaroxaban: 2%). However, results of uni- and multivariate analyses revealed a numerically lower but not significantly different frequency of any LA thrombus under Dabigatran [odds ratios (OR) 0.4, 95% CI 0.08–1.88, $P = 0.25$] and Rivaroxaban (OR 0.65, 95% CI 0.22–1.98, $P = 0.45$) compared to VKA. This is the first study addressing the incidence of LA/LAA thrombus formation in a predominantly low- to mid-risk patients cohort (CHA_2DS_2–VAS_c score ≥2) being treated with Dabigatran or Rivaroxaban compared with VKAs at a time in therapeutic range of >65%. The study also shows that with respect to the incidence of echocardiographic (TEE) risk factors for thromboembolic events, both Dabigatran and Rivaroxaban are not inferior to VKA. Dabigatran has been most extensively studied NOAC (Fig. 6).[31,33,34]

Resolution of Left Atrial-Appendage Thrombus—Effects of Dabigatran in Patients with Atrial Fibrillation trial is to assessed whether Dabigatran resulted in a faster complete LAA thrombus resolution as compared to vitamin K antagonist within 6 weeks of treatment and change in LAA thrombus volume under treatment as observed by TEE. This was the first prospective, multicenter, randomized controlled clinical trial investigating safety and efficacy of a NOAC for the resolution of LAA thrombi in patients with NVAF.[33]

However, efficacy of NOACs has not been sufficiently evaluated by 3D-TTE or 3D-TEE.

Negating Requirement of Echocardiography in Outcome Evaluation in Non-Vitamin-K Oral Anticoagulants Therapy

By normal logic, it should appear that prior evaluation and subsequent follow-up with TEE should influence treatment outcome in all the cases of NVAFs on NOACs. But there

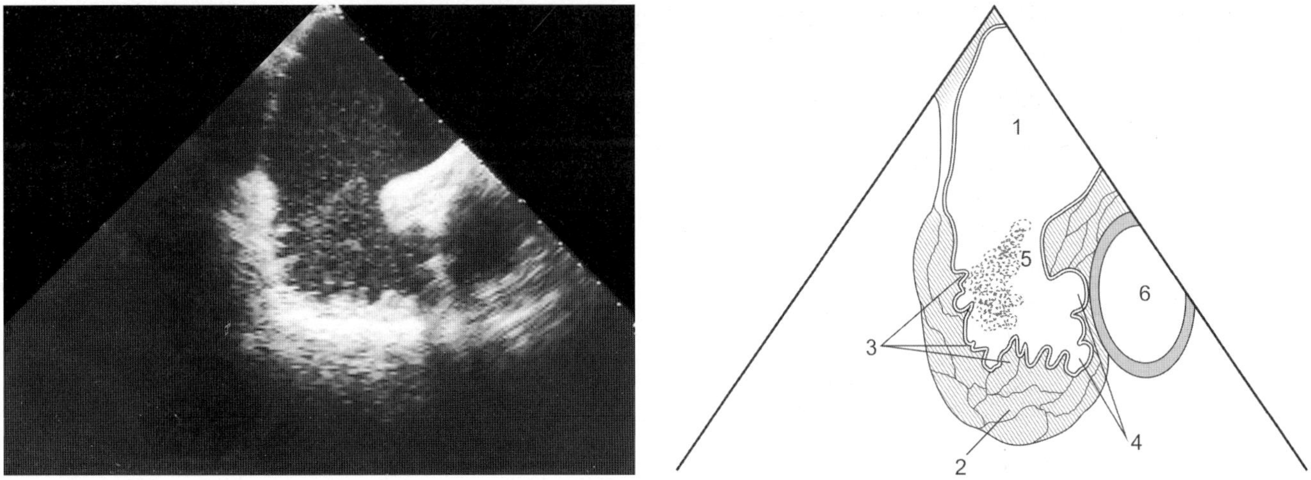

Fig. 5: SEC in LAA in midesophageal view: (1) LA, (2) LAA, (3) Pectinate muscle, (4) Lobules of LAA, (5) SEC, and (6) Pulmonary trunk. (LA: left atrium; LAA: left atrial appendage; SEC: spontaneous echocardiographic contrast)

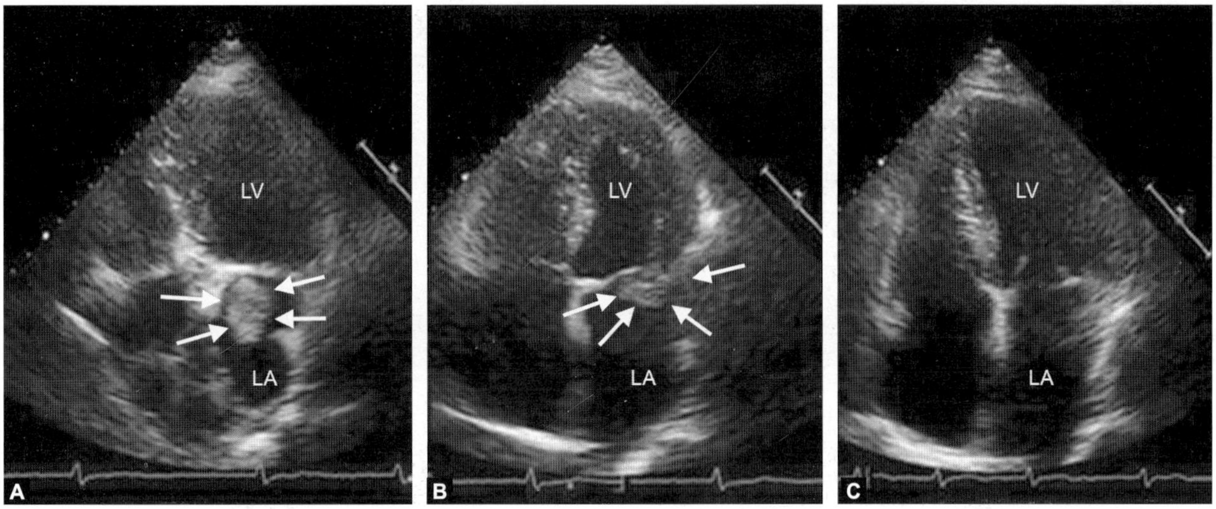

Fig. 6: TTE demonstrated a mobile high echoic mass of 2.6 × 3.0 cm in the left atrium (LA) (A), white arrows; LA; LV]. We administered heparin and warfarin, and TTE after 1 month showed that the LA mass had shrunk to 1.7 × 1.0 cm, confirming that it was thrombus [(B), white arrows]. Warfarin was changed to dabigatran 300 mg/day because she had a delusional disorder. She has remained on dabigatran for 4 months without any serious bleeding complications, and TTE confirmed that the thrombus had disappeared (C). (LA: left atrium; LV: left ventricle; TTE: transthoracic echocardiography)

are number of studies indicating that it is not necessary to examine those patients routinely by TEE.

- Di Biase L et al. published a secondary analysis of data from a multicenter registry of 970 AF patients undergoing radiofrequency catheter ablation on uninterrupted Apixaban and Rivaroxaban with the detection of SEC in 42% of cases on admission. They observed that the procedure was safe without preoperative TEE. The average CHA_2DS_2-VASc score was 3.01 ± 1.3 and $CHADS_2$ score was ≥2 in 609 (62.8%) patients. This has been observed despite silent cerebral ischemia was detected in 2.3% of patients who underwent postprocedure MRI. This study illustrates that performing AF ablation while on uninterrupted Apixaban and Rivaroxaban without TEE is feasible and safe. Finding has important clinical and economical relevance.[35]
- Patients from the ARISTOTLE trial (Apixaban vs Warfarin) with SEC, LA/LAA thrombus, or complex aortic plaque (CAP) diagnosed by either TTE or TEE were compared with patients with none of these findings on TEE. A total of 1251 patients were included: 217 had SEC, 127 had LA/LAA thrombus, 241 had CAP, and 746 had none. The rates of stroke/systemic embolism were not significantly different among patients with and without these echocardiographic findings.[36]

- Rowe et al. in 2017 evaluated whether a structured, nurse-led assessment of compliance to NOAC treatment prior to elective external direct current cardioversion (EDCCV) ensures safety without the need for routine TEE. A standardized, verbal questionnaire was administered to detect NOAC (Apixaban, Dabigatran, and Rivaroxaban) noncompliance in patients undergoing EDCCV. With appropriate compliance assessment, a nurse-led EDCCV without routine TEE did not significantly compromise safety in this study group.[37]

CONCLUSION

Anticoagulation by NOACs for thrombotic stroke prevention is limited by our understanding of pathophysiological mechanism for the formation of thrombus in NVAF and valvular AF (moderate-to-severe MS and prosthetic valves). Though mechanism for formation of thrombus is different in these two groups, in their classification, primary emphasis is given to the low-flow state in LA. For stroke prevention, in comparison to Warfarin, all NOACs, with exception of Rivaroxaban, are found to be statistically more efficacious. Dabigatran, the most extensively studied molecule, Apixaban, and Edoxaban, all are associated with lesser incidences of fatal hemorrhages while reducing incidences of thrombotic stroke in comparison to Warfarin. Apixaban is associated with most significant reduction of all-cause mortality. Efficacy of NOACs in reduction of thrombus load and eventual dissolve of thrombus is proven by TEE. However, there are some studies negating routine use of TEE in anticoagulation therapy in NVAF without compromising with safety of the patient. Further studies are needed before NOACs could be recommended for use in both NVAF and valvular AF though there is every potential of more extensive use of NOACs in coming years. In some situations, cost of NOACs is limiting factor. Taking above issues on board, we observe that Echo-Doppler evaluation of flow states in LA and also structural evaluation should have been the inclusion criteria of patients in NOACs trials. Interestingly enough, none of the trials validating use of NOACs mention such screening in inclusion criteria. Treatment outcome evaluation of NOACs by echocardiography is an interesting proposition for evidence-based medical practice.

REFERENCES

1. Lip GY, Boos CJ. Antithrombotic treatment in atrial fibrillation. Heart. 2006;92;155-61.
2. Kulo A, Mulabegovic N, Kusturica J, et al. Outpatient management of oral anticoagulation therapy in patients with non-valvular atrial fibrillation. Bosn J Basic Med Sci. 2009;9:313-9.
3. Transesophageal echocardiography correlates of clinical risk of thromboembolism in high-risk patients with non-valvular atrial fibrillation. Stroke Prevention in Atrial Fibrillation Investigators Committee on Echocardiography. Ann Intern Med. 1998;128-639.
4. Dentali F, Ageon W, Crowther M. Treatment of coumarin-associated coagulopathy: a systematic review and proposed treatment algorithms. J Thromb Haemost. 2006;4:1853.
5. Connolly SJ, Ezekowitz MD, Yusuf S, et al. Dabigatran versus warfarin in patients with atrial fibrillation. N Engl J Med. 2009;361:1139-51.
6. Garcia D, Crowther MA, Ageno W. Practical management of coagulopathy associated with Warfarin. BMJ. 2010;340:c1813.
7. Granger CB, Alexander JH, McMurray JJ, et al. Apixaban vs warfarin in patients with AF. N Eng J Med. 2011;365:981-92.
8. Patel MR, Mahaffey KW, Garg J, et al. Rivaroxaban vs warfarin in NVAF. N Eng J Med. 2011;365:883-91.
9. Giugliano RP, Ruff CT, Braunwald E, et al. Endoxan vs warfarin in patients with AF. N Eng J Med. 2013;369:2093-104.
10. Keogh C, Wallace E, Dillon C, et al. Validation of the CHADS2 clinical prediction rule to predict ischemic stroke: a systematic review and meta-analysis. Throm Haemost. 2011;106:528-38.
11. Pisters R, Lane DA, Nieuwlaat R, et al. A novel user friendly score (HAS-BLED) to assess 1-year risk of major bleeding in patients with atrial fibrillation: the European Heart Survey. Chest. 2010;138:1093-100.
12. Steffel J, Verhamme P, Potpara TS, et al. The 2018 European Heart Rhythm Association Practical Guide on the use of non-vitamin K Antagonist Oral anticoagulants in patients with atrial fibrillation. EHJ. 2018;39(16):1330-93.
13. FDA Drug Safety Communication. Update on the risk for serious bleeding events with the anticoagulant Pradaxa (dabigatran). 5.13.2014.
14. AgnerBF, Kuhl JT, Linde JJ, et al. Assessment of the LA volume and function in patients with permanent AF: Comparison of Cardiac MRI, 320 slice multidetector CT and transthoracic echocardiography. Eur Heart J Cardiovascular Imaging. 2014;15(5):532-40.
15. Molteni M, Polo Friz H, Primitz L, et al. The definition of valvular and non-valvular atrial fibrillation: results of a physicians' survey. Europace. 2014;16(12):1720-5.
16. Shazly A, Afifi A. RE-ALIGN: first trial of novel oral anticoagulant in patients with mechanical heart valves—the search continues. Glob Cardiol Sci Pract. 2014;2014(1):88-9.
17. Shively BK, Gelgand EA, Crawford MH, et al. Regional LA stasis during atrial fibrillation and flutter: determinants and relation to stroke. J Am Coll Cardiol. 1996;27:1722.
18. Eikelboom JW, Connolly SJ, Brueckmann M, et al. Dabigatran versus warfarin in patients with mechanical heart valves. N Engl J Med. 2013;369:1206-14.
19. Pan KL, Singer DE, Ovbiagele B, et al. Effects of non–vitamin K antagonist oral anticoagulants versus warfarin in patients with atrial fibrillation and valvular heart disease: a systematic review and meta-analysis. J Am Heart Assoc. 2017;6:e005835.

20. Zabalgoitia M, Halperin JL, Pearce LA et al. TEE correlates of clinical risk of thromboembolism in NVAF. SPAF III investigators. Am Heart J. 1999;137:494.
21. Masoudi FA, Calkin H, Kavinsky CJ, et al. 2015 ACC/HRS/SCAI appendage occlusion overview. JACC.2015;66:1498-513.
22. Tardif JC, Schwartz SL, Vannan MA, et al. Clinical usefulness of multiplane TEE in comparison to biplane imaging. Am Heart J. 1994;128:156.
23. Klein AL, Grimm RA, Murray M, et al. Use of TEE to guide cardioversion in patients with AF. N Engl J Med. 2001;344:1411.
24. Srimannarayana J, Varma RS, Satheesh S, et al. Prevalence of left atrial thrombus in rheumatic mitral stenosis with atrial fibrillation and its response to anticoagulation: a transesophageal echocardiographic study. Indian Heart J.2003;55:358-61.
25. Ayirala S, Kumar S, O'Sullivan DM, et al. Echocardiographic predictors of LAA thrombus formation. J Am Soc Echocardiogr. 2011;24:499.
26. Fatkin D, Kelly RP, Feneley MP. Relations between LAA blood flow velocity, SEC and thromboembolic risk in vivo. J Am Coll Cardiol. 1994;23;961.
27. Black IW, Hopkins AP, Lee LC, et al. Left atrial spontaneous echo contrast: a clinical and echocardiographic analysis. J Am Coll Cardiol. 1991;18:398-404.
28. Vigna C, de Rito V, Criconia GM, et al. Left atrial thrombus and spontaneous echo-contrast in nonanticoagulated mitral stenosis: a transesophageal echocardiographic study. Chest. 1993;103;2:348-52.
29. Watanabe T, Shinoda Y, Ikeoka K, et al. Dabigatran exhibits low intensity of left atrial spontaneous echo contrast in patients with nonvalvular atrial fibrillation as compared with warfarin. Heart Vessels. 2017;32(3):326-32.
30. Zhao Y, Ji L, Liu J, et al. 2016. Intensity of left atrial spontaneous echo contrast as a correlate for stroke risk stratification in patients with nonvalvular atrial fibrillation. Sci Rep. 2016;6:27650.
31. Manning WJ, Silerman DI, Keighley CS, et al. TEE facilitated early cardioversion from AF using short term anticoagulation: final result of a prospective 4.5 years study. J Am Cardiol. 1995;25:1354.
32. Reers S, Agdirlioglu T, Kellner M, et al. Incidence of left atrial abnormalities under treatment with dabigatran, rivaroxaban, and vitamin K antagonists. Eur J Med Res. 2016;21:41.
33. Ferner M, Wachtlin D. Rationale and design of the RE-LATED AF—AFNET 7 trial: REsolution of left atrial-appendage thrombus—effects of dabigatran in patients with atrial fibrillation. Clin Res Cardiol. 2016;105(1):29-36.
34. Parikh MG, Aziz Z. Usefulness of transesophageal echocardiography to confirm clinical utility of CHA2DS2-VASc and CHADS2 scores in atrial flutter. AJC. 2012;109(4):550-5.
35. Di Biase L, Briceno DF, Trivedi C, et al. Is transesophageal echocardiogram mandatory in patients undergoing ablation of atrial fibrillation with uninterrupted novel oral anticoagulants? Heart Rhythm. 2016;13(6):1197-202.
36. Vinereanu D, Lopes RD, Mulder H, et al. Echocardiographic risk factors for stroke and outcomes in patients with atrial fibrillation anticoagulated with apixaban or warfarin. Stroke. 2017;48(12):3266-73.
37. Rowe MK, Lollback N, Slater L, et al. Elective cardioversion in the era of novel oral anticoagulants—does a nurse administered verbal questionnaire for compliance negate the need for routine transoesophageal echocardiography? Heart Lung Circ. 2018;27(8):989-994.

76

CHAPTER

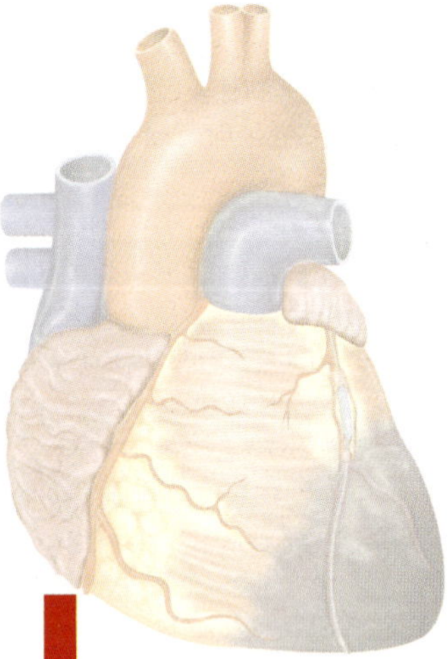

Electrophysiology Mapping in Atrial Fibrillation

Shafiq Ahmed Zargar, Aparna Jaswal

INTRODUCTION

Atrial fibrillation (AF) is the most common chronic tachycardia. Population studies have shown that prevalence of AF is increasing over the past 30 years, with projections for the growth to continue. AF causes loss of effective atrial contraction and rapid ventricular rate, which result in depressed cardiac function and formation of intracardiac thrombi. This makes AF the most common cardiac cause of stroke. AF requires a trigger that initiates the arrhythmia and substrate that favors perpetuation. Substrate for AF is created by both the changes in myocyte electrophysiology and tissue structure, such as atrial dilatation, fibrosis, fatty infiltration, and inflammation, leading to local conduction disturbances, and conduction block that are known to facilitate reentry and AF sustenance. Both this structural and electrical remodeling is much more prevalent in more persistent forms of AF. Cardiac mapping is necessary to locate triggers and substrate so that an ablation strategy can be optimized. In 1998, Haissaguerre et al.[1] for the first time showed in their seminal paper, the role of pulmonary vein (PV) ectopics in initiating paroxysmal AF. They studied 45 patients of paroxysmal AF and found a single point of origin of atrial ectopic beats in 29 patients, two points of origin in 9 patients, and three or four points of origin in 7 patients. In 94% of patients, ectopic foci were located in PVs, and among these, approximately 50% were located in left superior PV. During a mean follow-up, a period of 8 ± 6 months (median, 7), triggering foci ablation, eliminated AF completely in 62% of patients without the use of antiarrhythmic therapy. Following the role of PV ectopics, in generating AF, various technique of PV isolation (PVI) have been studied and widely used to treat AF. Although complete PVI is quite effective and recommended treatment in symptomatic paroxysmal AF, it is not effective as a sole ablation strategy in persistent AF. In paroxysmal AF, 60–80%[2,3] patients have been reported to maintain sinus rhythm (SR) following PVI, while in persistent AF, only 50%[4] patients maintain SR. Moreover, despite good single procedural success rate of PVI in paroxysmal AF, about 30% of patients develop recurrence and undergo a repeat ablation procedure.[3] As a result, cardiac mapping to locate the substrate involved in AF perpetuation and also understand the electrophysiological mechanisms involved in the maintenance of AF are of critical importance in improving outcome of ablative procedures. Two main hypotheses involved in maintaining have been extensively debated. First, the multiwavelet hypothesis proposes that spatially meandering electrical waves are responsible for causing AF.[5,6] Second, the localized source hypothesis, according to which high-frequency sources, namely rotors or focal impulses, cause AF when rapid impulses cannot be uniformly propagated and break into fibrillatory conduction.[7,8] Various mapping technics have been developed based on the understanding of AF sustenance and will be discussed under the following headings: Classical five-element acupuncture mapping, dominant frequency (DF) mapping, and focal impulse and rotor modulation (FIRM) mapping.

CLASSICAL FIVE-ELEMENT ACUPUNCTURE MAPPING

Fractionated electrograms represent dissociated electrical activity, which occurs because of asynchronous activation of muscle bundles through a fibrotic myocardium. A fractionated electrogram shows more than one deflection per activation cycle length (CL). Structural remodeling in patients with structural heart disease or in chronic AF may increase transverse fiber separation and may decrease the number of side-to-side connections throughout the free walls. This causes more frequent and more widespread distribution of fractionated electrograms. Complex fragmented atrial electrograms (CFAEs) are defined as (1) atrial electrograms with low-voltage (0.06–0.25 mV) signals with two or more deflections and/or perturbations of the baseline with continuous deflection of a prolonged activation complex and (2) a very short CL (≤120 ms), with or without multiple potentials.[9] Several studies have indicated that these CFAE sites may represent areas which may play a role in AF maintenance.[10,11] Nademanee et al.[12] first showed ablating sites that display CFAEs result in eliminating AF. They found that CFAEs were frequently localized at the septum, PVs, left atrial roof, posteroseptal mitral annulus, and coronary sinus ostium. With CFAEs ablation alone, 68% of patients were converted to SR, and in 26% of patients, conversion required a combination of ablation and ibutilide. At 1-year follow-up, approximately 90% of patients were free of AF. The same author in another study reported long-term success of CFAE ablation in high-risk AF. They found at 2.3-year mean follow-up, 89% of patients with paroxysmal AF and 85% of patients with persistent AF were in SR, while in permanent AF, SR was restored in 71% of the cases.[13] Subsequent studies showed CFAE ablation as a single strategy is associated with low success, especially in persistent AF, while when used as an adjuvant to PVI had better outcome.[14,15] A meta-analysis conducted by Hayward et al.[16] reported that in patients with nonparoxysmal AF, adding CFAE ablation to PVI results in greater improvement in freedom from AF. Adjunct CFAE ablation resulted in a significant increase in freedom from atrial tachycardia (62% for PVI + CFAE versus 47% for PVI alone). But in paroxysmal AF, this combined approach was observed to provide no additional benefit. Despite these initial encouraging results, especially in nonparoxysmal AF, recent studies have failed to replicate the benefit of additional CFAE ablation. Not all CFAE sites represent critical sites crucial to AF perpetuation, but some may represent sites of passive wavefront collision, which have no role to play in the maintenance of AF.[17] Substrate and Trigger Ablation for Reduction of Atrial Fibrillation Part II trial,[18] which is one of the largest randomized multicenter studies of persistent AF, evaluated PVI alone, PVI plus CFAE ablation, PVI plus linear ablation across the roof of the left atrium (LA) and in the mitral valve isthmus in 589 patients. This study found no reduction in the rate of recurrent AF with addition of either linear ablation or ablation of CFAE to PVI. Moreover, approximately only half of the patients were free of recurrent AF after 18 months of follow-up. Catheter Ablation of Persistent Atrial Fibrillation trial[19] is another randomized trial that again showed additional biatrial ablation of CFAEs, and linear ablation lines do not provide any benefit in persistent AF over PVI alone. CFAE ablation in most of the trials is guided by recording fractionated electrograms by a single intracardiac electrode. Multiple studies have suggested that multipolar electrode mapping as compared to single-electrode catheter mapping helps identifying critical CFAEs by differentiating CFAE regions into passive or driver regions.

DOMINANT FREQUENCY MAPPING

Recently, there is cumulative evidence that localized high-frequency sources, namely rotors producing rapid impulses that result in fibrillatory conduction to the rest of the atria, are believed to be responsible for the maintenance of AF.[20,21] This theory fueled research into accurate mapping and representation of atrial rate throughout the atria during AF because sites of high atrial rate might represent structures critical to AF maintenance and amenable to ablation. These sites of high atrial rate can be identified by measuring and averaging the CL of atrial activation at different sites across the atria in the time domain. But the recordings during ongoing AF are fragmented and irregular, and their time-domain analysis is often difficult and subjective, and thus resulting in inaccurate activation pattern characterization. As a result, another approach that uses spectral analysis of atrial electrograms and representation of local activation rate in the frequency domain is being used. DF mapping discussed later is aimed at identifying localized sites of maximal DF (DF_{max}) during AF. Frequency-domain analysis is based on a series of mathematical formulas that comprise the Fourier transform. According to this, a continuous signal can be decomposed into a sum of weighted sinusoids with different frequency, amplitude, and phase. Recorded electrogram signals are broken down by Fourier transformation into a number of constituent sinusoidal functions. Next, the magnitude of these sine waves is plotted against the frequency in a "power spectrum". The DF is the highest peak in this power spectrum.[22] Data from many animal and human studies showed that during the arrhythmia, the activation frequencies in certain areas of the LA were faster than those in any other areas.[23] Mansour et al.[23] showed using DF maps of the left and right atrium

(RA) that the LA is activated at a higher frequency, with a left-to-right decrement in DFs. The reason for this frequency gradient is the failure of both atria to be activated in 1:1 fashion at that short CL; as a result, LA activation above breakdown frequency leads to wave breakdown because of intermittent block and resulting in fibrillatory conduction. Lazar et al.[24] analyzed DF distribution in patients with paroxysmal and persistent AF by recording electrograms from all the four PV ostia, coronary sinus, and posterior RA. They found that in paroxysmal AF, DFs are highest at the PV/LA junction, intermediate in the coronary sinus, and slowest in the posterior RA. In contrast, patients with long-lasting (1 month) persistent AF did not show a consistent DF gradient between these sites. Another similar, but more detailed, study conducted by Sanders et al.[25] found that high DF sites in paroxysmal AF patients were often localized to the PVs, while in permanent AF, DF sites were more often localized to the atria, including RA. Ablation at these sites resulted in the prolongation of the AFCL and termination of paroxysmal AF. Same author in another study found, PVI in paroxysmal AF led to a significant decrease in the average atrial DF, while in persistent AF, there was no such decrease.[26] Atienza et al. performed real-time DF mapping and ablation of DF sites in AF with left-to-right frequency gradients. They reported that DF_{max} sites ablation followed by circumferential PVI results in long-term SR maintenance in 75% of paroxysmal and 50% of persistent AF patients in the absence of antiarrhythmic therapy. Some studies have shown that a left-to-right gradient may also be present in persistent AF.[27-29] Lazar et al.[30] showed that PVI alone was more successful in patients of persistent AF who had a baseline left-to-right DF gradient as compared with patients without a DF gradient.

Radiofrequency Ablation of Drivers of Atrial Fibrillation (RADAR-AF) trial[31] is the only randomized trial that compared DF ablation versus circumferential PVI. The trial was aimed to compare the efficacy and safety of the circumferential PVI with DF ablation alone in paroxysmal AF or combined with circumferential PVI in persistent AF. DF ablation alone in paroxysmal AF did not achieve noninferiority at 6 months after a single procedure, but after redo procedures, it was noninferior to circumferential PVI at 12 months, while in persistent AF, circumferential PVI + DF ablation offered no additional value. Gadenz et al.[32] performed a systematic review on clinical role of DF mapping in AF ablation. They reviewed 10 studies, which included one randomized controlled trial, and nine nonrandomized studies and concluded that current literature supports DF as a useful marker of ablation outcome, and more research is needed to further evaluate the role of DF ablation.

FOCAL IMPULSE AND ROTOR MODULATION MAPPING

Focal impulse and rotor modulation mapping system is a novel computational mapping system that was developed to identify local AF sources either reentrant or focal impulses and then tested whether ablation of these sources can acutely modulate AF (by terminating or consistently slowing AF) and improve the long-term success. The FIRM mapping system uses 64-pole basket catheter for mapping of both atria. This method involves using pacing to initiate AF, if it is not present at baseline, followed by the advancement of single or two catheters into the RA and LA for data acquisition. Patient-specific non-PV AF sources are identified using software that analyzes electrograms through phase mapping, and rate-dependent atrial repolarization and conduction dynamics. Propagation movies (FIRM maps) of electrogram amplitude at each electrode are then created and projected onto a grid. The grid represents RA opened along its meridian, with the lateral half of tricuspid valve opened laterally and the septal half opened medially. The LA is opened horizontally along the mitral annulus, with its superior and inferior halves folded upward and downward.[33,34] Rotors (spiral waves) are identified during AF as sequential clockwise or counterclockwise activation contours (isochrones) around a fixed center of rotation. Focal impulses are identified as sites with centrifugal activation to surrounding atrium. The ablation procedure typically involves FIRM-identified non-PV sites ablation, followed by PVI. Initial study results achieved with FIRM mapping were positive. The pivotal Comparison of Faslodex in Recurrent or Metastatic Breast Cancer (CONFIRM) trial[34] was a 92-patient multicenter study in which FIRM-guided ablation, followed by conventional ablation, was compared with conventional ablation alone. Conventional ablation in FIRM-blinded group comprised wide area circumferential PVI, with the verification of PVI using a circular mapping catheter. In this study, localized sources, namely rotors or focal impulses, were detected in 97% of patients with sustained AF, with an average of approximately two sources per patient. The majority of AF sources (76%) were localized to LA, which sites outside the PVs, posterior, inferior, roof, and anterior regions, while the rest 24% of sources were found the RA, including the inferolateral, posterior, and septal regions. The number of sources was higher for persistent than for paroxysmal AF (2.2 ± 1.0 versus 1.7 ± 0.9; median 2.0 versus 1.0). FIRM-guided ablation resulted in acute AF termination or consistent slowing in 86% of patients, while the same result was achieved in only 20% of FIRM-blinded cases. FIRM ablation, in addition to conventional ablation, resulted in an almost doubling of the long-term success rate. Single-procedure freedom from

AF was 82.4% versus 44.9% after median 273 days. As per Indiana University, FIRM Registry,[35] which is the largest series so far, has reported freedom from AF after a single-FIRM procedure for the entire series was 95% (paroxysmal AF), 83% (persistent AF), and 82% (long-standing persistent AF) at 1 year, and freedom from all atrial arrhythmias was 77% (paroxysmal AF), 75% (persistent AF), and 57% (long-standing persistent AF).

Unfortunately, these positive results are not replicated in other studies. In a multicenter study, conducted by Buch et al.,[36] following FIRM-guided ablation at 18 ± 7 months of follow-up, only a mere 37% of patients were free of documented recurrent AF. Similar poor results were also reported by other studies, where success rate has varied from 21% to 45%.[37,38] The exact reason for these differences is not clear. In accurate rotor site identification because of poor electrogram resolution as a result of poor basket electrode-myocardial contact, or an underlying technical software deficiency may be possible reasons for these varied results.

CONCLUSION

Significant advancements have been made in our understanding of mechanisms responsible for AF initiation and maintenance, which has led to the development of various technics for AF ablation. Complete PVI remains the best ablation therapy in paroxysmal AF, and other ablation technics have not been shown to be superior over PVI in paroxysmal AF. More persistent AF still remains a challenge because of non-PV sources of AF. Various mapping technics at present being used have improved our understanding of persistent AF. DF and FIRM mappings have led to our understanding that localized high-frequency sources (drivers) in atria, namely focal impulses and rotors, are responsible for AF sustenance. Unfortunately, available data on ablation of these localized sources has shown mixed results. RADAR-AF trial[31] showed DF ablation did not improve results in persistent AF. Despite the initial encouraging results on FIRM ablation in CONFIRM trial,[34] many other trials have not shown FIRM ablation to be that effective. Future studies are required to evaluate the usefulness of the mapping and ablation technics in more persistent forms of AF.

REFERENCES

1. Haissaguerre M, Jais P, Shah DC, et al. Spontaneous initiation of atrial fibrillation by ectopic beats originating in the pulmonary veins. N Engl J Med.1998;339:659-66.
2. Dewire J, Calkins H. Catheter ablation of atrial fibrillation to maintain sinus rhythm. J Atr Fibrillation. 2013;5:739.
3. Fichtner S, Sparn K, Reents T, et al. Recurrence of paroxysmal atrial fibrillation after pulmonary vein isolation: is repeat pulmonary vein isolation enough? A prospective, randomized trial. Europace. 2015;17:1371-5.
4. Kirchhof P, Benussi S, Kotecha D, et al. 2016 ESC guidelines for the management of atrial fibrillation developed in collaboration with EACTS. Eur Heart J. 2016;37:2893-962.
5. Konings K, Kirchhof C, Smeets J, et al. High density mapping of electrically induced atrial fibrillation in humans. Circulation. 1994;89:1665-80.
6. Allessie MA, de Groot NM, Houben RP, et al. The electropathological substrate of longstanding persistent atrial fibrillation in patients with structural heart disease: longitudinal dissociation. Circ Arrhythm Electrophysiol. 2010;3:606-15.
7. Skanes AC, Mandapati R, Berenfeld O, et al. Spatiotemporal periodicity during atrial fibrillation in the isolated sheep heart. Circulation. 1998;98:1236-48.
8. Vaquero M, Calvo D, Jalife J. Cardiac fibrillation: from ion channels to rotors in the human heart. Heart Rhythm. 2008;5:872-9.
9. Nademanee K, Schwab M, Porath J, et al. How to perform electrogram-guided atrial fibrillation ablation. Heart Rhythm. 2006;3:981-4.
10. Konings KT, Smeets JL, Penn OC, et al. Configuration of unipolar atrial electrograms during electrically induced atrial fibrillation in humans. Circulation. 1997;95:1231-41.
11. Morillo CA, Klein GJ, Jones DL, et al. Chronic rapid atrial pacing. Structural, functional, and electrophysiological characteristics of a new model of sustained atrial fibrillation. Circulation. 1995;91:1588-95.
12. Nademanee K, McKenzie J, Kosar E, et al. A new approach for catheter ablation of atrial fibrillation: mapping of the electrophysiologic substrate. J Am Coll Cardiol. 2004;43:2044-53.
13. Nademanee K, Schwab MC, Kosar EM, et al. Clinical outcomes of catheter substrate ablation for high-risk patients with atrial fibrillation. J Am Coll Cardiol. 2008;51:843-9.
14. Verma A, Mantovan R, Macle L, et al. Substrate and trigger ablation for reduction of atrial fibrillation (STAR AF): a randomized, multicentre, international trial. Eur Heart J. 2010;31:1344-56.
15. Oral H, Chugh A, Good E, et al. Radiofrequency catheter ablation of chronic atrial fibrillation guided by complex electrograms. Circulation. 2007;115:2606-12.
16. Hayward RM, Upadhyay GA, Mela T, et al. Pulmonary vein isolation with complex fractionated atrial electrogram ablation for paroxysmal and nonparoxysmal atrial fibrillation: a meta-analysis. Heart Rhythm. 2011;8:994-1000.
17. Narayan SM, Wright M, Derval N, et al. Classifying fractionated electrograms in human atrial fibrillation using monophasic action potentials and activation mapping: evidence for localized drivers, rate acceleration, and nonlocal signal etiologies. Heart Rhythm. 2011;8:244-53.
18. Atul Verma A, Jiang CY, Betts TR, et al. Approaches to catheter ablation for persistent atrial fibrillation. N Engl J Med. 2015;372:1812-22.

19. Vogler J, Willems S, Sultan A, et al. Pulmonary vein isolation versus defragmentation: the CHASE-AF clinical trial. J Am Coll Cardiol. 2015;66:2743-52.
20. Mandapati R, Skanes AC, Chen J, et al. Stable microreentrant sources as a mechanism of atrial fibrillation in the isolated sheep heart. Circulation. 2000;101:194-9.
21. Berenfeld O, Zaitsev AV, Mironov SF, et al. Frequency-dependent breakdown of wave propagation into fibrillatory conduction across the pectinate muscle network in the isolated sheep right atrium. Circ Res. 2002;90:1173-80.
22. Ng J, Goldberger JJ. Understanding and interpreting dominant frequency analysis of AF electrograms. J Cardiovasc Electrophysiol. 2007;18:680-5.
23. Mansour M, Mandapati R, Berenfeld O, et al. Left-to-right gradient of atrial frequencies during acute atrial fibrillation in the isolated sheep heart. Circulation. 2001;103:2631-6.
24. Lazar S, Dixit S, Marchlinski FE, et al. Presence of left-to-right atrial frequency gradient in paroxysmal but not persistent atrial fibrillation in humans. Circulation. 2004;110:3181-6.
25. Sanders P, Berenfeld O, Hocini M, et al. Spectral analysis identifies sites of high-frequency activity maintaining atrial fibrillation in humans. Circulation. 2005;112:789-97.
26. Sanders P, Nalliah CJ, Dubois R, et al. Frequency mapping of the pulmonary veins in paroxysmal versus permanent atrial fibrillation. J Cardiovasc Electrophysiol. 2006;17:965-72.
27. Dibs SR, Ng J, Arora R, et al. Spatiotemporal characterization of atrial activation in persistent human atrial fibrillation: multisite electrogram analysis and surface electrocardiographic correlations—a pilot study. Heart Rhythm. 2008;5:686-93.
28. Sahadevan J, Ryu K, Peltz L, et al. Epicardial mapping of chronic atrial fibrillation in patients: preliminary observations. Circulation. 2004;110:3293-9.
29. Wu TJ, Doshi RN, Huang HL, et al. Simultaneous biatrial computerized mapping during permanent atrial fibrillation in patients with organic heart disease. J Cardiovasc Electrophysiol. 2002;13:571-7.
30. Lazar S, Dixit S, Callans DJ, et al. Effect of pulmonary vein isolation on the left-to-right atrial dominant frequency gradient in human atrial fibrillation. Heart Rhythm. 2006;3:889-95.
31. Atienza F, Almendral J, Ormaetxe JM, et al. Comparison of radiofrequency catheter ablation of drivers and circumferential pulmonary vein isolation in atrial fibrillation: a noninferiority randomized multicenter RADAR-AF trial. J Am Coll Cardiol. 2014;64:2455-67.
32. Gadenz L, Javad Hashemi J, Shariat H, et al. Clinical role of dominant frequency measurements in atrial fibrillation ablation—a systematic review. J Atr Fibrillation. 2017;9:1548.
33. Narayan SM, Krummen DE, Rappel WJ. Clinical mapping approach to diagnose electrical rotors and focal impulse sources for human atrial fibrillation. J Cardiovasc Electrophysiol. 2012;23:447-54.
34. Narayan SM, Krummen DE, Shivkumar K, et al. Treatment of atrial fibrillation by the ablation of localized sources: CONFIRM (Conventional Ablation for Atrial Fibrillation With or Without Focal Impulse and Rotor Modulation) trial. J Am Coll Cardiol. 2012;60:628-36.
35. Miller JM, Kalra V, Das MK, et al. Clinical benefit of ablating localized sources for human atrial fibrillation: the Indiana University FIRM Registry. J Am Coll Cardiol. 2017;69:1247-56.
36. Buch E, Share M, Tung R, et al. Long-term clinical outcomes of focal impulse and rotor modulation for treatment of atrial fibrillation: a multicenter experience. Heart Rhythm. 2016;13:636-41.
37. Steinberg JS, Shah Y, Bhatt A, et al. Focal impulse and rotor modulation: acute procedural observations and extended clinical follow-up. Heart Rhythm. 2017;14:192-7.
38. Balouch M, Gucuk Ipek E, Chrispin J, et al. Impact of rotor temperospatial stability on acute and one-year atrial fibrillation ablation outcomes. Clin Cardiol. 2017;40:383-9.

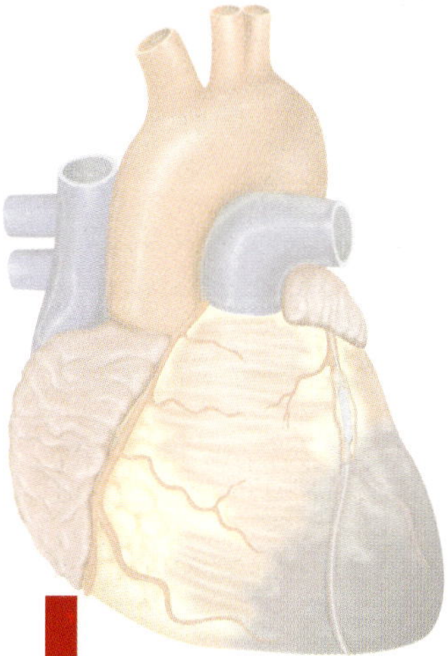

77

CHAPTER

Echocardiographic Navigation for Radiofrequency Ablation

Ajit Thachil

INTRODUCTION

In addition to assessing the anatomy prior to radiofrequency ablation in order to plan the procedure strategy,[1] echocardiographic guidance has a definite role to play during radiofrequency ablation. Owing to the presence of electrocardiography leads and defibrillation and mapping patches [for three-dimensional (3D) mapping-guided radiofrequency ablation] on the chest, as well as the requirement of movement of the C-arm for fluoroscopy, the role of transthoracic echocardiography is limited. The modes of echocardiography that are most commonly used for assistance during radiofrequency ablation are intracardiac echocardiography and transesophageal echocardiography. Both will be discussed separately.

ROLE OF INTRACARDIAC ECHOCARDIOGRAPHY DURING RADIOFREQUENCY ABLATION

The commonly used intracardiac echocardiography catheters are 8-Fg or 10-Fg, 160° bidirectionally steerable catheters mounted at the tip with a side viewing, 64-element, 5.5–10-MHz linear phased array probe capable of generating two-dimensional (2D) ultrasound as well as conventional and color Doppler images (Fig. 1).[2] The most commonly used catheters are the SoundStar (Biosense Webster, Diamond Bar, CA, USA), the Siemens Acunav, and the Abbott-St. Jude Viewflex catheters. A previously used forward-viewing intracardiac echocardiography catheter using a 9–12-MHz rotating probe at the tip, with continuous automated tip rotation and capable of forming a reconstructed 3D image (ClearView Ultra System, Boston Scientific, USA), is no longer used due to its poor depth of beam penetration. Two approaches to 3D intracardiac echocardiography are being explored. One of them involves the development of a real-time 3D volumetric intracardiac echocardiography probe.[3] The other approach involves creation of real-time reconstructed 3D anatomy from 2D intracardiac echocardiographic images obtained from a probe that automatically rotates 360° at a fixed speed.[4] A real-time 3D intracardiac echocardiography catheter (AcuNav® V catheter; Siemens, Inc., Mountain View, CA, USA) is commercially available, but only limited use has been reported. Intracardiac echocardiography catheters are introduced transfemorally through 9-Fg or 11-Fg sheaths and can be connected to selected cardiac echocardiography machines (the St. Jude Viewflex catheter to the Philips CX 50™ and the Abbott-St. Jude Zoneare™ machines, the Siemens Acunav catheter to the Siemens Acuson™ machine, and the SoundStar catheter to the CARTO 3 electroanatomical mapping system) using dedicated connecting modules. The SoundStar™ catheter is an intracardiac echocardiography catheter that can be integrated into a 3D electroanatomic mapping system (the Carto 3™ mapping system, Biosense Webster, Diamond Bar, CA, USA) used for electrophysiology procedures. This allows the integration of multiple images [preprocedure computed tomography (CT), intraprocedural 3D electroanatomical map, and intraprocedural intracardiac echocardiography] to enhance the accuracy of the

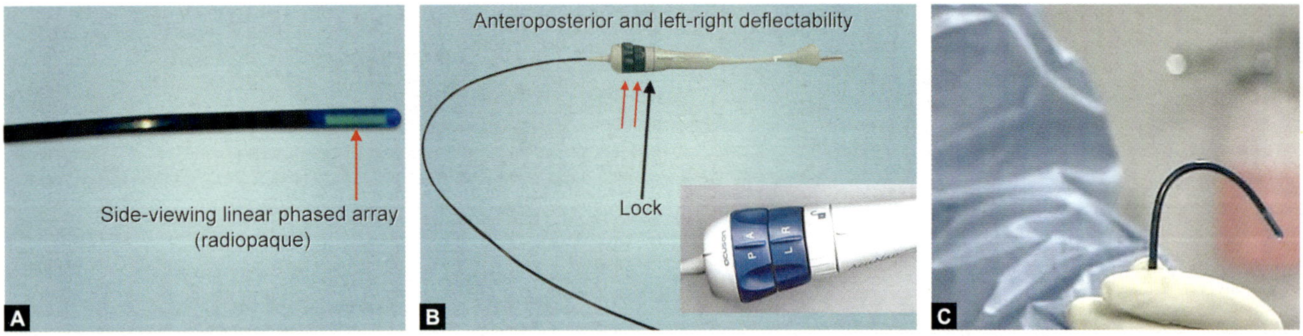

Figs. 1A to C: (A) Shows the tip of a commonly used intracardiac echocardiography catheter (Siemens Accunav) showing the side viewing transducer; (B) Shows the controls; and (C) Shows the range of deflection of this catheter.

procedure. This system allows the creation of real-time 3D intracardiac echocardiographic images by plotting multiple 2D intracardiac echocardiographic images onto previously acquired cardiac CT images or 3D electroanatomical maps.

The most common use of intracardiac echocardiography is guidance during radiofrequency ablation; other uses include guidance during lead extraction, permanent pacemaker implantation in pregnant patients, percutaneous closure of atrial septal defects and other intracardiac defects, percutaneous transaortic valve replacement, and percutaneous mitral valve clipping.[2] During electrophysiology studies and radiofrequency ablation, intracardiac echocardiography is most commonly used for transseptal puncture and visualization of pulmonary veins and the left atrial appendage. Intracardiac echocardiography can also be used to visualize virtually any structure in the heart with great clarity without the intervening air interface associated with transthoracic echocardiography. The following sections will illustrate these in detail.

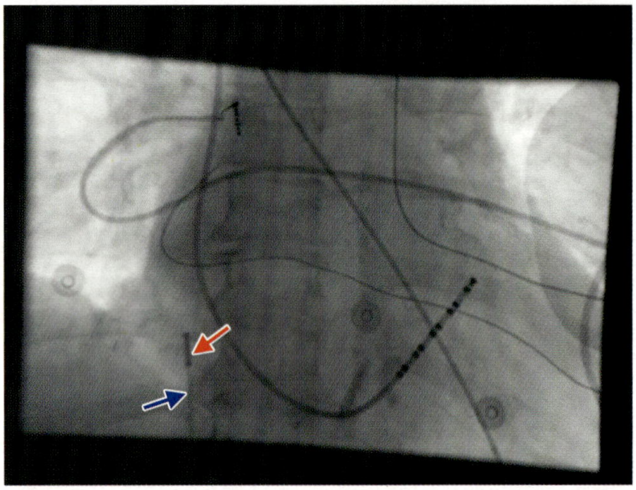

Fig. 2: Fluoroscopic orientation of the intracardiac echocardiography catheter (shown in anteroposterior projection) to obtain the "home view". A slight tilt/rotation (as shown in the figure) may sometimes be required to obtain an adequate home view. Blue arrow = catheter shaft; red arrow = ultrasound transducer.

Intracardiac Echocardiography-guided Septal Puncture

For intracardiac echocardiography-guided septal puncture, the intracardiac echocardiography catheter is usually introduced into the right atrium from where the interatrial septum and the left atrial structures can be visualized. The catheter can be left in place throughout the electrophysiology procedure. The intracardiac echocardiography catheter is initially positioned in the mid-right atrium with the controls in neutral position to view the tricuspid valve and the right ventricle. This view is called the "home view" (Fig. 2).

Gradual clockwise rotation from the home view allows sequential visualization of anterior to posterior structures starting with the aortic root and the pulmonary artery, followed by the mitral valve and the left atrial appendage along with the anterior aspect of the fossa ovalis, and finally the pulmonary venous ostia along with the posterior aspect of the fossa ovalis. Slight posterior and/or leftward deflection of the transducer tip may be required for adequate visualization of the fossa ovalis. Septal puncture must be accomplished in a plane posterior to the plane of the aortic root, at an area where there is adequate space from the interatrial septum to the posterior wall of the left atrium. The site of puncture should also be a relatively thin area of the interatrial septum. With the needle tip just inside the dilator the appropriate site in the septum is engaged by the septal puncture assembly under intracardiac echocardiography guidance. Tenting of the septum at this area is visualized on snugly engaging the septum. Subsequently the septum is punctured with the needle, at which point sudden loss of resistance is felt on the needle, and the tented part of the septum abruptly collapses back onto the needle (Fig. 3).

There are certain advantages to intracardiac echocardiography-guided transseptal access as compared to fluoroscopy-guided transseptal access. Intracardiac

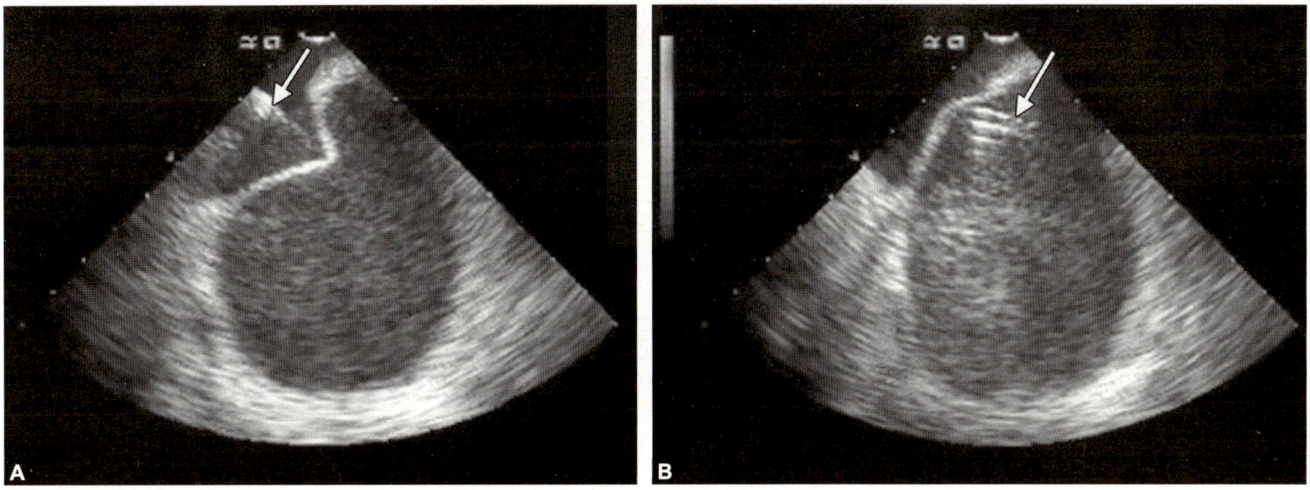

Figs. 3A and B: Intracardiac echocardiography guided trans-septal access. (A) Tenting of the interatrial septum by the septal puncture needle just before puncture; (B) The interatrial septum falling back on to the needle at the point of puncture.

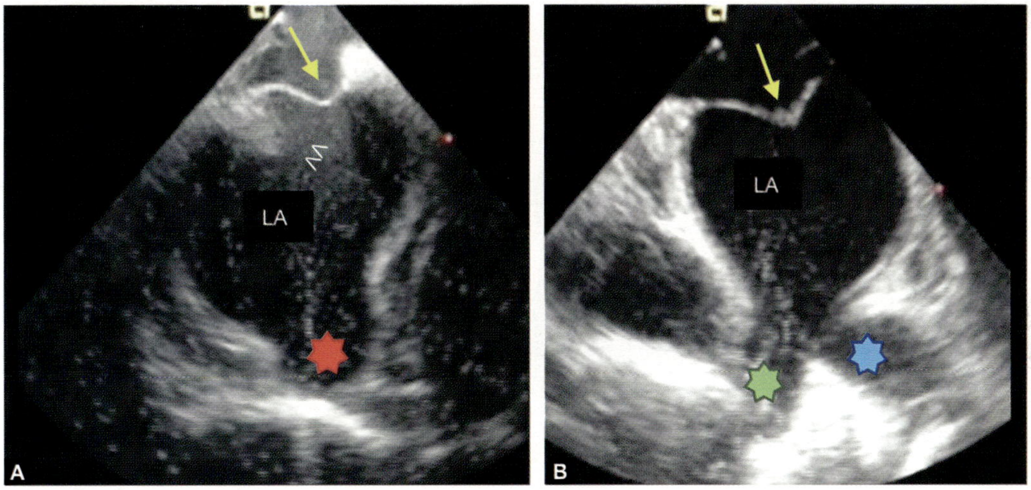

Figs. 4A and B: Intracardiac echocardiography to tailor the site of septal puncture. (A) Tenting of the interatrial septum (yellow arrow) in the plane of the left atrial appendage (red star). This is a very anterior plane; access to structures in the posterior left atrium can be difficult if puncture is performed in this plane; (B) Tenting of the interatrial septum (yellow arrow) in the plane of the left superior pulmonary vein (blue star) and the left inferior pulmonary vein (green star). This is a more posterior plane, and is the best plane to access the pulmonary veins. (LA = left atrium).

echocardiography-guided puncture allows more precise tailoring of the site of puncture within the fossa ovalis (Fig. 4), though an experienced operator may be able to do the same without the aid of intracardiac echocardiography.

In some situations, upon attempted septal puncture, the needle slides up the fossa ovalis rather than puncture the septum at the site of initial engagement. Too much sliding up can result in puncture beyond the fossa ovalis and should be avoided. Sliding movement on attempted septal puncture is often due to a slightly tangential engagement of the septum by the needle. This can be readily visualized on intracardiac echocardiography (Fig. 5).

The interatrial septum is thick in certain patients. Puncturing a thick septum may require considerably more force than the usual. Visualization of the position of the septal puncture needle provides the operator with a greater degree of confidence while using more force against a thick interatrial septum (Fig. 6).

The interatrial septum is aneurysmal in certain patients. During attempted puncture an aneurysmal septum may stretch a long distance into the left atrium. Continuous intracardiac echocardiographic guidance ensures that a safe distance is maintained from the free wall of the left atrium while puncturing a stretching, aneurysmal interatrial septum (Fig. 7).

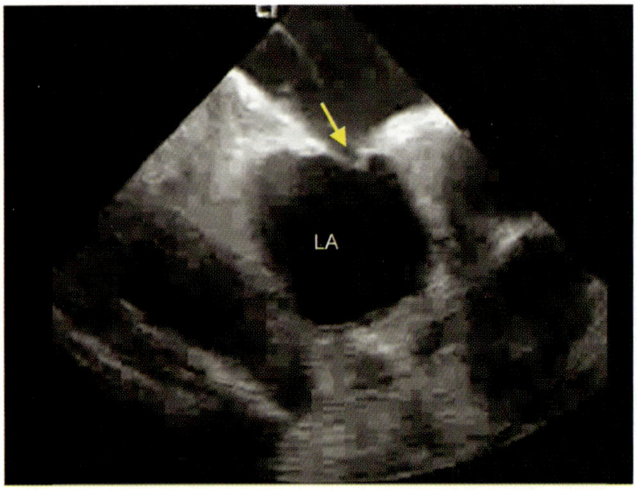

Fig. 5: Tangential engagement of the interatrial septum by the septal puncture needle (yellow arrow) causing the needle to slide up the fossa ovalis. Contrast the angle of tenting in this figure with that in Figures 3 and 4, which show a more perpendicular engagement of the interatrial.

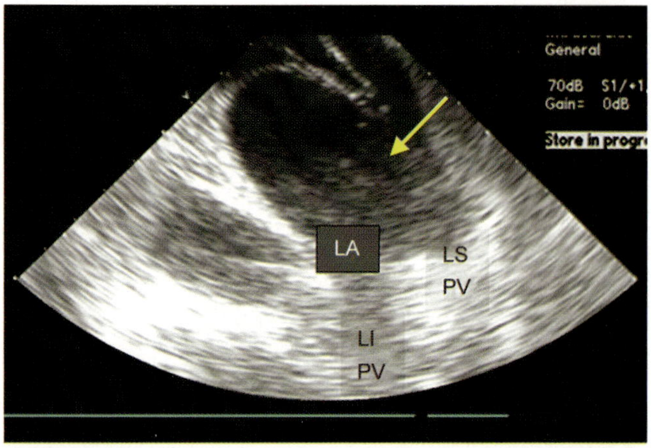

Fig. 7: Intracardiac echocardiography guidance to aid puncture of an aneurysmal interatrial septum. The aneurysmal interatrial septum (yellow arrow) is being stretched a long distance into the left atrium prior to puncture. Intracardiac echocardiography guidance ensures that there is still a safe distance from the left atrial free wall and the site of puncture. Also note that the needle tip is oriented towards the pulmonary veins rather than the left atrial free wall. (LA = left atrium, LSPV = left superior pulmonary vein, LIPV = left inferior pulmonary vein).

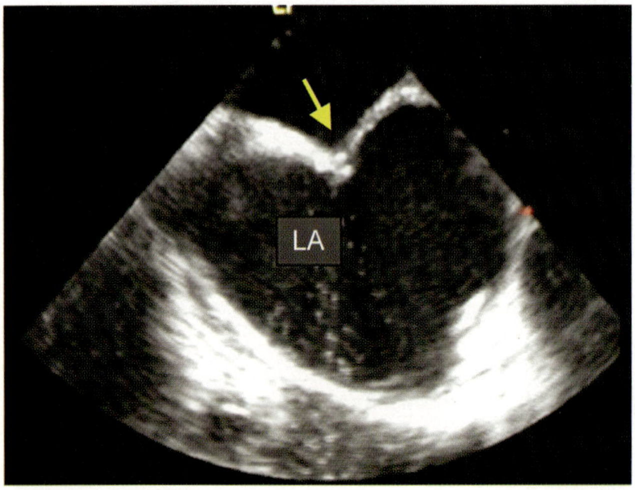

Fig. 6: Intracardiac echocardiography to visualize the septal puncture needle tenting (yellow arrow) a thick interatrial septum (compare the thickness of the interatrial septum to the examples in Figures 3 to 5).

In addition to the above situations, intracardiac echocardiographic guidance can be useful to guide septal puncture when the anatomy of the interatrial septum is altered such that the conventional fluoroscopic landmarks are less reliable. Thus, in the electrophysiology laboratory, it is useful to have intracardiac echocardiography as a standby option to guide difficult transseptal accesses.

Intracardiac Echocardiography for the Visualization of Pulmonary Veins and Esophagus

During radiofrequency ablation for atrial fibrillation, a spiral-shaped catheter is introduced sequentially into each of the pulmonary veins to record electrical activity from the vein (Fig. 8). This helps to guide radiofrequency ablation.

It is important to position the spiral catheter accurately in the pulmonary vein to be isolated. Intracardiac echocardiography helps to do this without the aid of fluoroscopy. As mentioned previously, gradual clockwise rotation of the intracardiac echocardiography catheter from the home view allows sequential visualization of anterior to posterior structures starting with the aortic root and the pulmonary artery, followed by the mitral valve and the left atrial appendage along with the anterior aspect of the fossa ovalis, and finally the pulmonary venous ostia along with the posterior aspect of the fossa ovalis. Among the pulmonary veins, the first ostium to be visualized is that of the left superior pulmonary vein, followed by (on continuing the clockwise rotation ± slight posterior tilt as required) the left inferior pulmonary vein, then the right superior pulmonary vein, and finally the posteriormost ostium, that of the right inferior pulmonary vein. While rotating posteriorly (clockwise) from the left inferior pulmonary vein ostium, before the right-sided venous ostia are visualized, the posterior wall of the left atrium and the esophagus will be

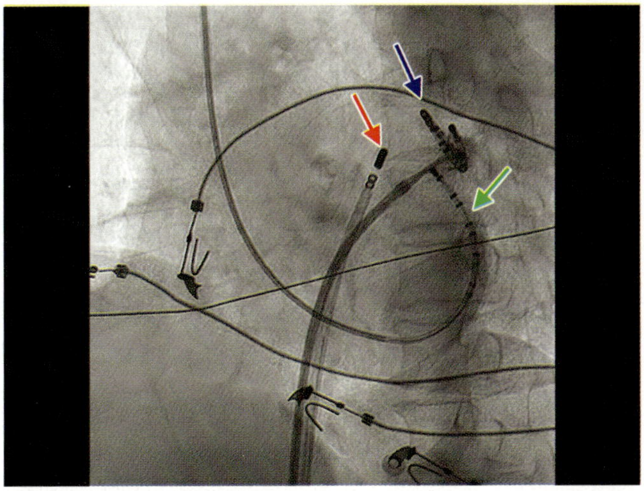

Fig. 8: Left anterior oblique fluoroscopic projection showing catheter positioning for pulmonary vein isolation during radiofrequency ablation for atrial fibrillation. Red arrow = ablation catheter in left atrium, blue arrow = spiral catheter in the pulmonary vein to be electrically isolated (the left superior pulmonary vein in this case), green arrow = decapolar catheter in the coronary sinus.

visualized (Figs. 9A to H). It is important to reduce ablation power when ablating adjacent to the esophagus. Figure 10 shows an example of intracardiac echocardiography-guided accurate placement of the spiral catheter in the desired pulmonary vein.

The structures closest to the right atrium, viz. the right pulmonary veins, may sometimes be difficult to visualize by progressive clockwise rotation from the initial location. Tilting the transducer downward provides a better view of the right superior pulmonary vein (Fig. 11).

Intracardiac Echocardiography for the Visualization of Structures outside the Left Atrium

Intracardiac echocardiography can be used for high-resolution visualization of virtually any intracardiac structure. It also helps to ensure adequate contact of the ablation catheter with the tissue being ablated. This is particularly important when the structure to be ablated is an intracavitary structure, such as a false tendon or a papillary muscle, or on an intracavitary projection, such as the eustachian ridge, or the ridge between the left atrial appendage and the left superior pulmonary vein. It can also help to guide catheter navigation in highly trabeculated areas. On the safety front, intracardiac echocardiography helps to monitor continuously for complications, such as pericardial effusion during the procedure. Similarly, visualization of an intracardiac thrombus on intracardiac echocardiography performed just prior to ablation may prompt the operator to call off the ablation procedure. Small-blinded studies have found intracardiac echocardiography to be superior to transesophageal echocardiography in detecting thrombi in the right and left atrial appendages.[5] The following illustrations provide examples for these (Figs. 12 to 17).

ROLE OF TRANSESOPHAGEAL ECHOCARDIOGRAPHY DURING RADIOFREQUENCY ABLATION

The requirement for general anesthesia limits the role of continuous transesophageal echocardiography guidance for radiofrequency ablation. Transesophageal echocardiography is still useful in the following situations:

- Single time requirement for echocardiographic guidance for only a short duration;
- Longer time echocardiographic guidance for patients who undergo radiofrequency ablation under general anesthesia;
- Requirement for echocardiographic guidance in small children in whom it may be desirable to avoid the 9-Fg or 11-Fg femoral venous sheath required for introduction of the intracardiac echocardiography catheter;
- Requirement for echocardiographic guidance in situations where intracardiac echocardiography is not available.

Figure 18 provides an example of transesophageal echo to guide a difficult transseptal access in a 4-year-old girl with tachycardiomyopathy due to an incessant atrial tachycardia ablated in the left atrial appendage.

CONCLUSION

Transthoracic and transesophageal echocardiography have definite but limited roles to play in electrophysiology and radiofrequency ablation. Intracardiac echocardiography is an important addendum to any electrophysiology laboratory, and it can sometimes be the crucial element deciding the success or failure of an ablation performed in the presence of a complex anatomy. Its applications are limited only by imagination and logistics.

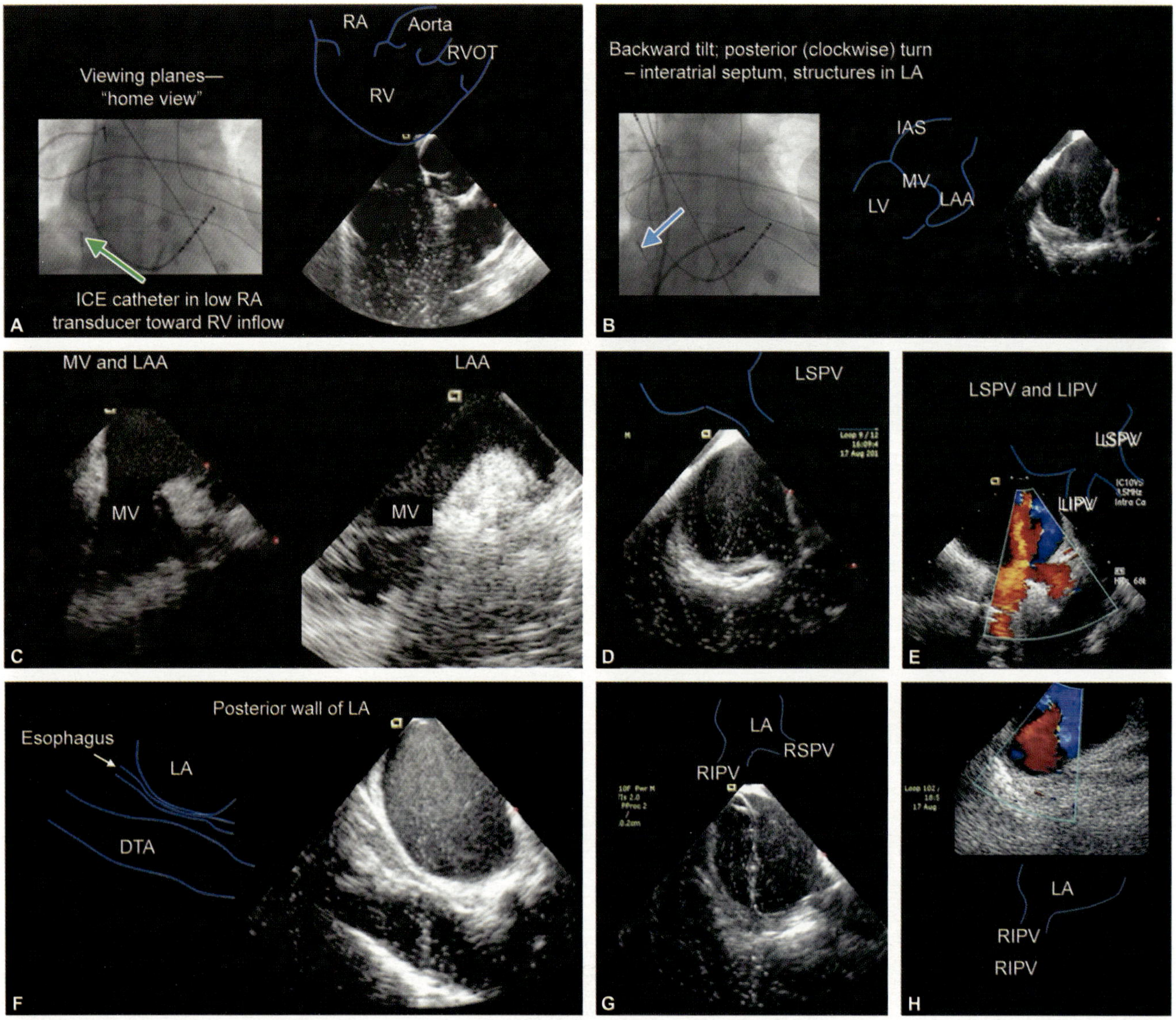

Figs. 9A to H: (A) The "home view" before comencing visualizaton of the interatrial septum and left atrial structures; (B) The catheter is locked in a position of slight backward tilt and a clockwise rotation of the shaft is made. This makes the catheter view slightly posteriorly. From this location, the anterior part of the interatrial septum is visualized, along with the anteriormost structure in the left atrium, viz., the left atrial appendage; (C) Further clockwise turn of the catheter shaft visualizes progressively more posterior structures. The structure to appear after the left atrial appendage is the mitral valve; (D and E) On further clockwise rotation from the mitral valve plane, the ostia of the left sided pulmonary veins appear, the superior followed soon after by the inferior; (F) Further clockwise rotation from the left pulmonary vein ostial plane visualizes the posterior wall of the left atrium, the esophagus and the descending thoracic aorta; (G and H) Further clockwise rotation, usually along with a slight rightward and additional posterior tilt, first visualizes the ostium of the right superior pulmonary vein followed by the right inferior pulmonary vein. (RSPV = Right superior pulmonary vein, RIPV = right inferior pulmonary vein. RA= right atrium, RV = right ventrcile, RVOT = right ventricular outflow tract, IAS = interatrial septum, MV = mitral valve, LAA = left atrial appendage, LV = left ventricle, LAA = left atrial appendage, MV = mitral valve, LSPV = left superior pulmonary vein, LIPV = left inferior pulmonary vein, LA = left atrium, DTA = descending thoracic aorta)

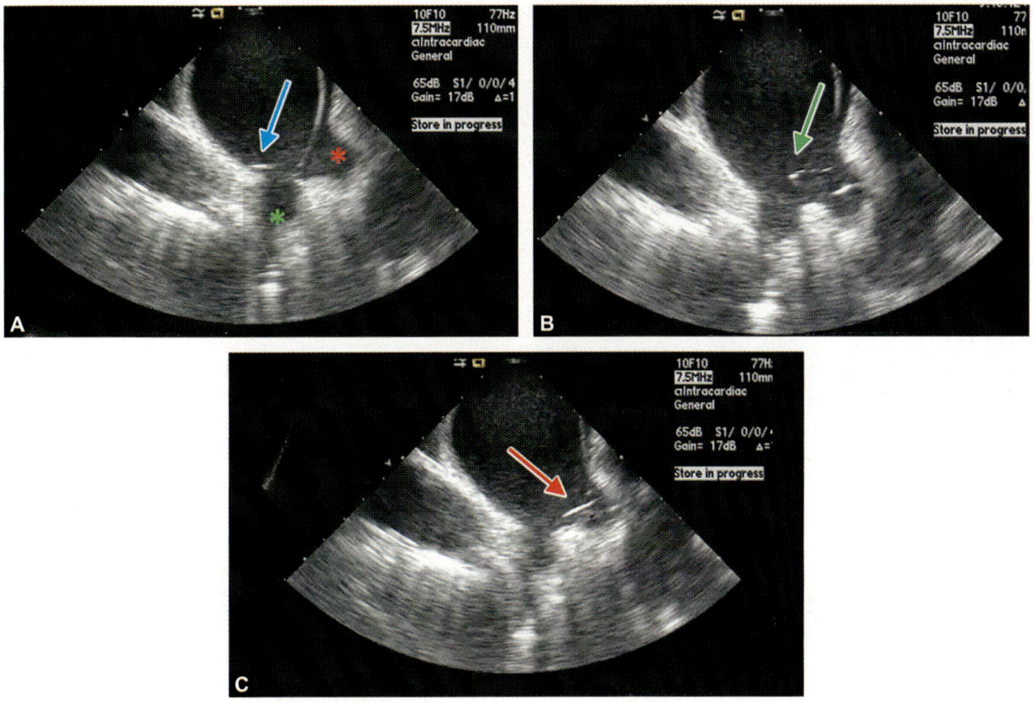

Figs. 10A to C: Intracardiac echocardiography to guide placement of the spiral catheter (blue arrows) within the desired pulmonary vein. (A) Catheter lying just outside the ostium of the left inferior pulmonary vein (green star); (B) It is being moved towards the left superior pulmonary vein (red star in A); (C) It has been placed just within the left superior pulmonary vein. The catheter location in panel C corresponds to the fluoroscopic location in Figure 8.

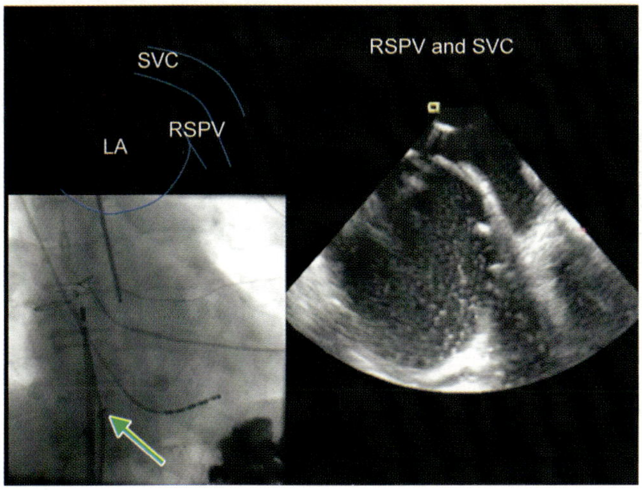

Fig. 11: Tilting the transducer down (green arrow) to take it away from the intended structure to be viewed provides better visualization. In this example, the SVC is visualized through the right superior pulmonary vein. (RSPV: right superior pulmonary vein; SVC: superior vena cava; LA = left atrium).

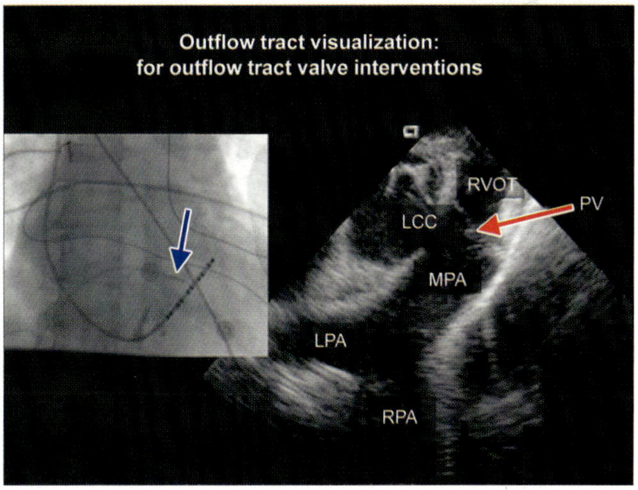

Fig. 12: View of the aortic cusps, distal RVOT and pulmonary arteries from the right ventricular inflow to guide radiofrequency ablation. Blue arrow shows transducer position. The transducer may be placed in a lower location for visualization of more of the outflow tract, and in a higher location (see next figure) for visualization of more of the coronary cusps. (RVOT: right ventricular outflow tract, NCC: noncoronary cusp, PV: pulmonary valve, MPA: main pulmonary artery, RPA: right pulmonary artery, LPA: left pulmonary artery).

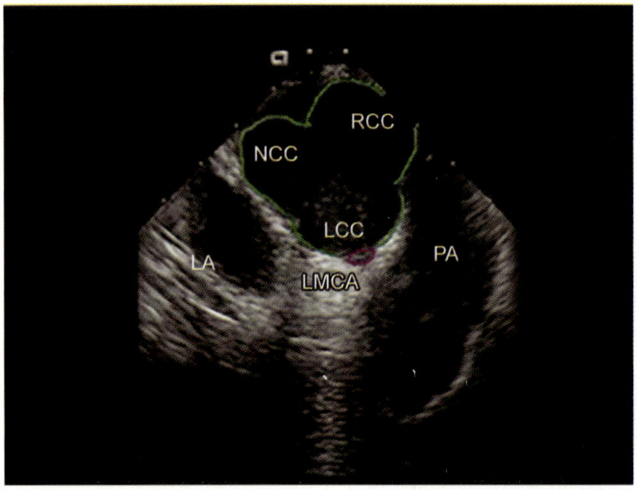

Fig. 13: View of the aortic cusps from the right ventricular outflow tract to guide radiofrequency ablation in the coronary cusps. (NCC: non coronary cusp; LCC: left coronary cusp; RCC: right coronary cusp; PA = Pulmonary artery; LA = left atrium).

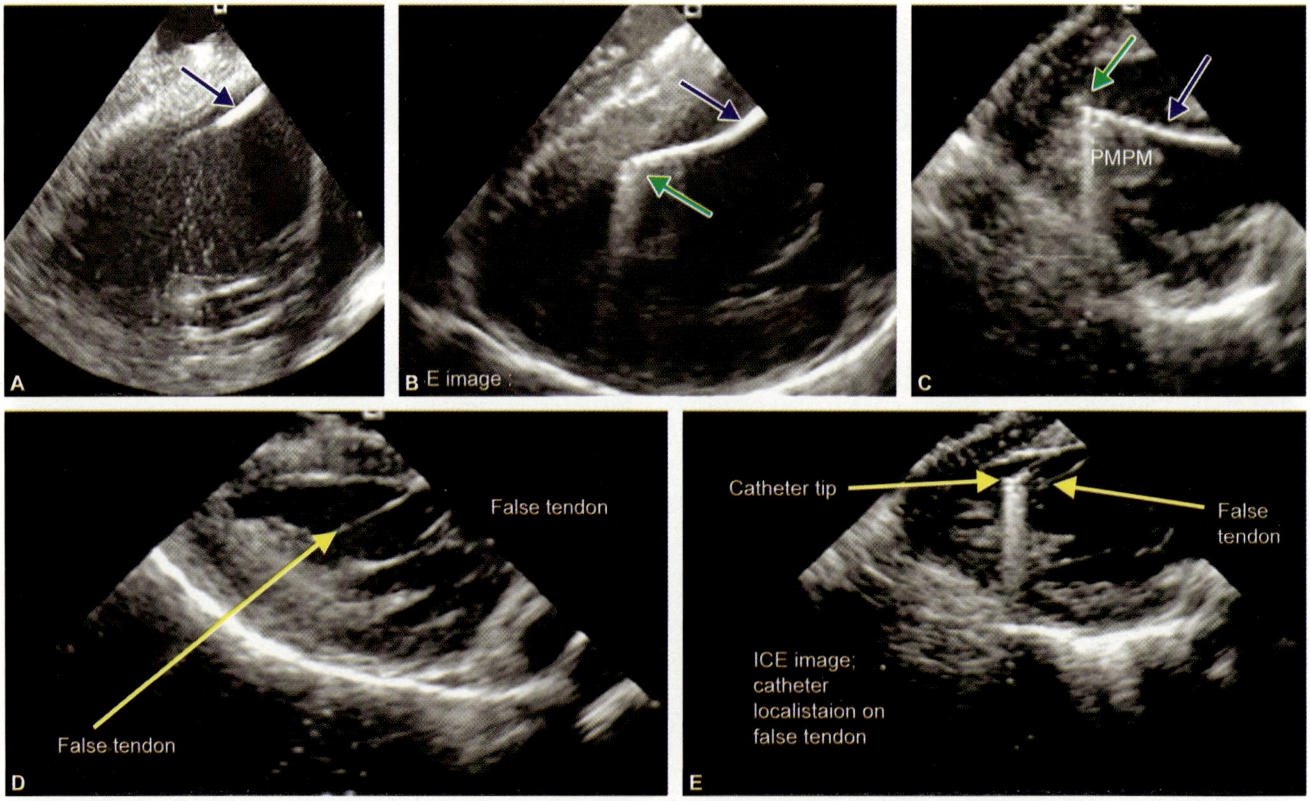

Figs. 14A to E: Long axis view of the left ventricle, from a transducer placed distally in the right ventricle. (A) Inadequate contact of the ablation catheter (blue arrow) with the septum; (B) The ablation catheter in good contact with the septum. The location of the tip of an irrigated ablation catheter can be accurately made out by noting the point from which the irrigation spray emanates (green arrow); (C) Intracardiac echocardiography shows contact of the ablation catheter (blue arrow) with the posteromedial papillary muscle (PMPM) for ablation of ventricular tachycardia from the papillary muscle. Green arrow denotes the tip of the ablation catheter; (D) A prominent false tendon in the left ventricle; (E) Contact of the ablation catheter tip with the false tendon to ablate a fascicular VT circuit where the critical elements of the circuit were localized to the false tendon; ablation on the false tendon terminated the VT. The catheter locations depicted in panels A to E are very close to each other, and would be very difficult to distinguish without the aid of intracardiac echocardiography.

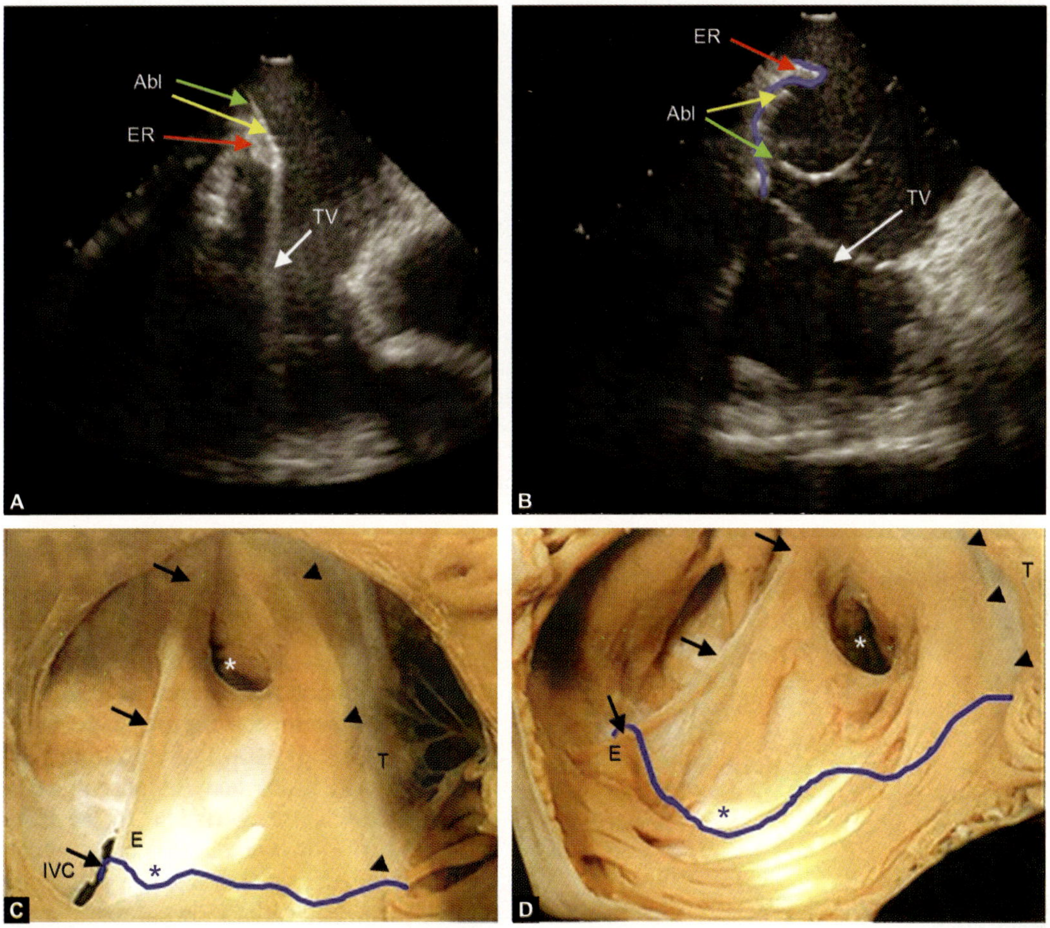

Figs. 15A to D: Use of intracardiac echocardiography to ensure tissue contact during ablation of cavotricuspid-isthmus dependent atrial flutter in presence of a prominent eustachian ridge and a large subeustachian pouch in the right atrium. (A and B) Intracardiac echocardiography images. (A) Shows contact being ensured against the large eustachian ridge; (B) Shows the ablation catheter being curled into the subeustachian pouch to ensure contact. (yellow arrow = tip of ablation catheter, from where ablation energy is delivered; green arrow = shaft of ablation catheter; blue line = intended ablation line to transect the cavo-tricuspid isthmus;[6] (C and D) Show a trans-illuminated dissection in a heart with a prominent eustachian ridge similar to that depicted in panels A and B. Explanations for panels C. (ER = Eustachian ridge; Abl = Ablation catheter; TV = tricuspid valve)

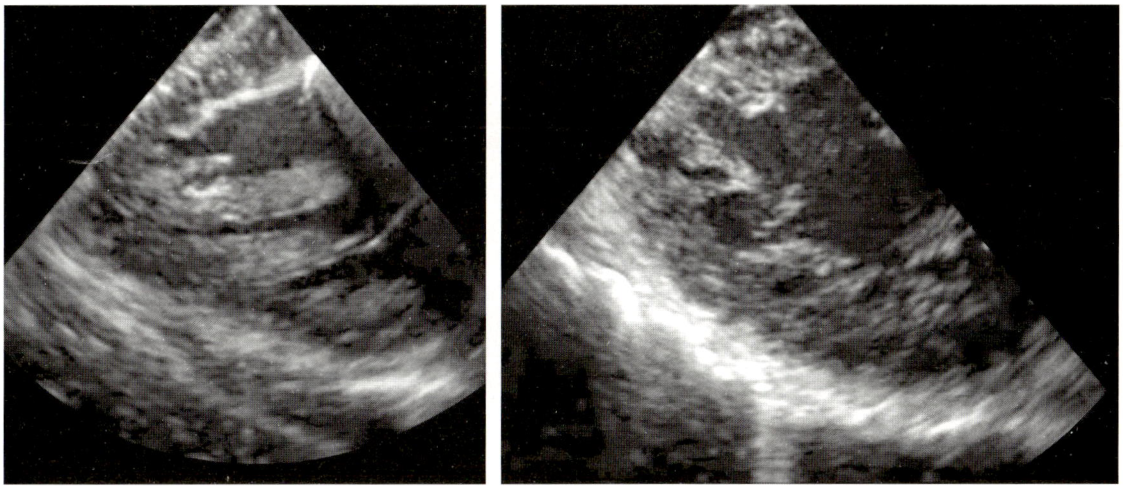

Fig. 16: Intracardiac echocardiography shows an unusually heavily trabeculated left ventricle. Intracardiac echocardiography guidance would be valuable in navigating the catheters within such a left ventricle.

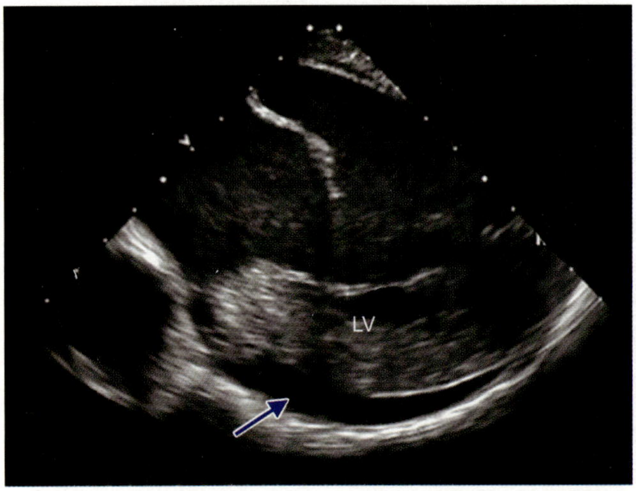

Fig. 17: Continuous intracardiac echocardiography monitoring shows a small, fresh pericardial effusion (blue arrow) that has appeared posterior to the left ventricle (LV) during ablation. At this point, there were no hemodynamic changes. Prompt detection of this effusion helped to adopt remedial measures in a timely manner to avoid any catastrophe.

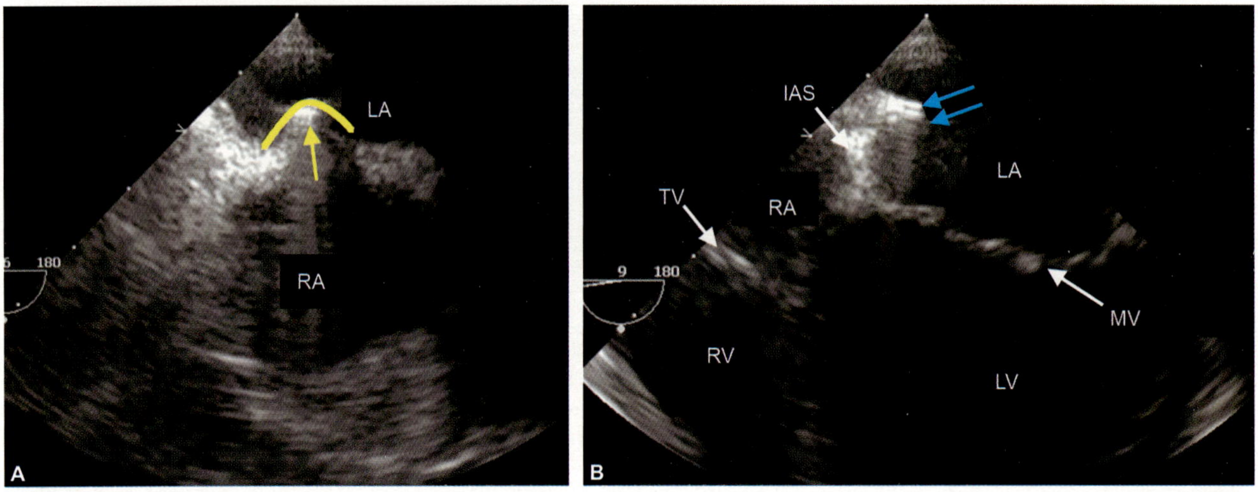

Figs. 18A and B: Images of transesophageal echo to guide transseptal access in pediatric electrophysiology. (A) Tenting of the interatrial septum (yellow arrow and yellow arc) by the transseptal needle just before puncture. (B) A Mullin's sheath (twin blue arrows) across the interatrial septum. (The transducer orientations are approximately at 90 degrees to each other in the two panels) (RA = right atrium, LA = left atrium, RV = right ventricle, LV = left ventricle, TV = tricuspid valve, MV = mitral valve, IAS = intertarial septum.

REFERENCES

1. Chen J-Y, Lin K-H, Liou Y-M, et al. Usefulness of pre-procedure cavotricuspid isthmus imaging by modified transthoracic echocardiography for predicting outcome of isthmus-dependent atrial flutter ablation. J Am Soc Echocardiogr. 2011;24:1148-55.
2. Enriquez A, Saenz LC, Rosso R, et al. Use of intracardiac echocardiography in interventional cardiology: working with the anatomy rather than fighting it. Circulation. 2018;137:2278-94.
3. Dausch DE, Castellucci JB, Gilchrist KH, et al. Live volumetric imaging (LVI) intracardiac ultrasound catheter. Cardiovasc Revasc Med. 2013;14(3):157-9.
4. Stapf D, Franke A, Schreckenberg M, et al. Beat to beat 3-dimensional intracardiac echocardiography: theoretical approach and practical experiences. Int J Cardiovasc Imaging. 2013;29(4):753-64.
5. Anter E, Silverstein J, Tschabrunn CM, et al. Comparison of intracardiac echocardiography and transesophageal echocardiography for imaging of the right and left atrial appendages. Heart Rhythm. 2014;11:1890-7.
6. Karanam S. Intracardiac echo imaging guided ablation of cavotricuspid isthmus-dependent atrial flutter. J Innov Card Rhythm Manag. 2014;5:1661-7.
7. Waki K, Saito T, Becker AE. Right atrial flutter isthmus revisited: normal anatomy favors nonuniform anisotropic conduction. J Cardiovasc Electrophysiol. 2000;11:90-4.

SECTION 10

Ventricular Tachycardia Storm

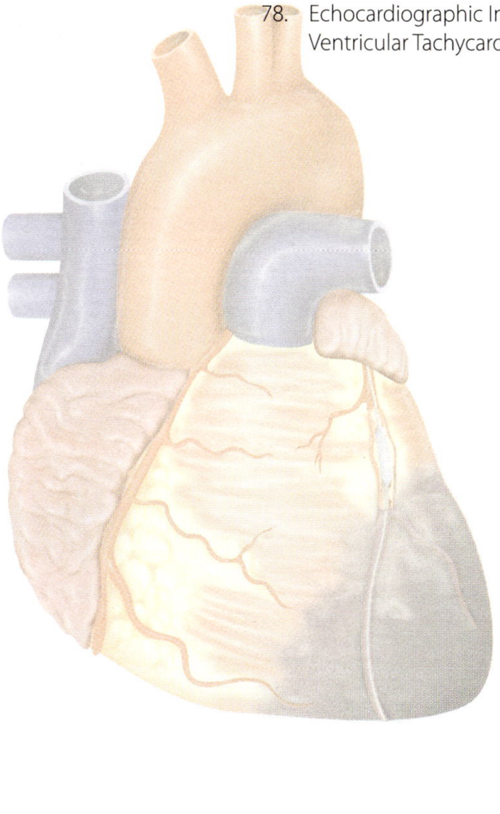

78

CHAPTER

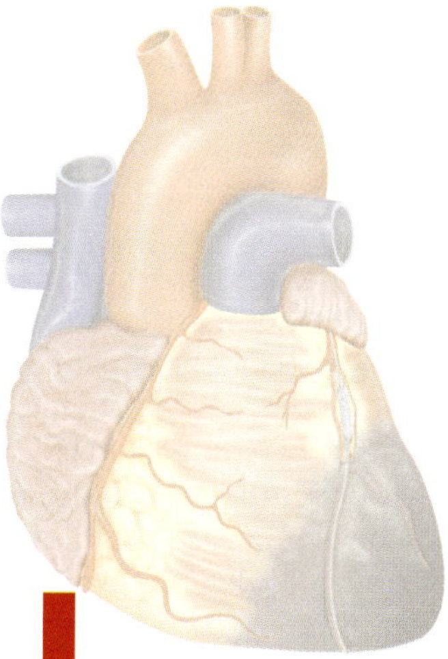

Echocardiographic Imaging in Ventricular Tachycardia Storm

Ashish Nabar, Goutam Vaggar, Varun Deokate

INTRODUCTION

Ventricular tachycardia (VT) storm is arbitrarily defined as three or more episodes of VT or ventricular fibrillation (VF) within 24 hours, and usually coexists with advanced heart failure (HF) in patients with structural heart disease (SHD). In the Nippon Storm Study, involving patients with SHD who had received an implantable cardioverter defibrillator (ICD) for sudden cardiac death (SCD) prevention, VT storm (cluster of ICD shocks) occurred in 6.6% patients over a median follow-up of 28 months.[1] In this study, the incidence of VT storm was not different, whether the underlying SHD was ischemic (ICM) or nonischemic (dilated) cardiomyopathy (DCM). Further, irrespective of the nature of SHD, the subsequent mortality tends to be higher in survivors of VT storm than those without VT storm. If the initial treatment with sotalol is ineffective in suppressing VT, then switching to amiodarone or catheter ablation (CAB) is a reasonable option.[2] However, in patients with VT storm who have an amiodarone-refractory VT, it would seem appropriate to opt for CAB rather than further escalating antiarrhythmic drug (AAD) therapy.[3] In one large VT-CAB study, patients enduring VT storm were frequently older men who had a lower left ventricular ejection fraction (LVEF), more advanced HF and higher prevalence of cardiovascular comorbidities.[4] Not surprisingly then, VT recurrence, in-hospital mortality and 1-year mortality were higher in these patients. Yet, CAB may not be declined, even to the elderly, because ablation is found to be safe and feasible, and successful CAB is associated with an improved survival.[5] In CAB studies concerning patients with VT storm; lack of amiodarone usage before ablation, long procedure times and incomplete procedural success determined the risk of early VT recurrences and the consequent high-risk of all-cause death.[6] Repeat CAB procedures could be required, particularly in patients with DCM, due to more number of inducible, unmappable and/or epicardial VTs; and particularly when VT remains inducible after the index procedure.[7] An alternate approach that can reduce the burden of appropriate ICD shocks is cardiac sympathetic denervation (CSD). Recently, an International collaborative group reported a moderate success with CSD; 1-year freedom from sustained VT/ICD shock and ICD shock, transplant, and death as 58% and 50%, respectively.[8] Bilateral CSD seems to score over left-sided-only procedure. An interesting conclusion was brought forth by the OBSERVO-ICD registry wherein patients receiving cardiac resynchronization therapy (CRT-D) had 45% relative risk reduction in VT storm occurrence when compared to patients with ICD alone, the lower risk accruing to "responders".[9] Further observations from this registry suggest that even the sporadic VT/VF therapies delivered by the device were lesser in clinical and ECHO responders. It can be easily derived from all the above-mentioned facts that a detailed echocardiographic (ECHO) evaluation, initially and repeatedly, would guide management of our sick VT storm patients. ECHO would be useful for diagnostic (evaluate for SHD), therapeutic (periprocedural assessment), and prognostication (early and late results of therapeutic interventions) purposes. We aim to elaborate these aspects in the present article.

ROLE OF ECHO IN DIAGNOSIS

Ventricular tachycardia storm may have differing triggers, including ischemia, dyselectrolytemia, sympathetic stimulation and medication toxicities; as well as varying myocardial substrates (Table 1),[10] like ICM, DCM congenital heart disease or rare genetic conditions such as long QT syndrome (LQTS) and Brugada syndrome. In general, monomorphic VT (MMVT), whether spontaneous or inducible single or pleomorphic, would suggest a scar VT, imperative therewith an underlying SHD; whereas a polymorphic VT (PMVT) or VF is more often seen in the setting of acute coronary syndrome or primary electrical disorders like LQTS or Brugada syndrome. Nonreentrant VTs, suspected when antitachycardia pacing is ineffective or reinitiations are observed repeatedly after ICD shocks, may present with electrical storm, usually in patients without SHD or in a few patients with DCM. While a detailed scrutiny of the VT ECG and the ECG recorded in sinus rhythm could point to the etiopathogenesis, ECHO is required as a first-line imaging technique to uncover SHD. It is important to realize that patients with primary electrical disorders would have normal ECHO study, those with infiltrative cardiomyopathies may show restrictive features without significant systolic dysfunction, and those with myocarditis or tachycardiomyopathy could have a transiently impaired left ventricular (LV) systolic function. Amiodarone-refractory VT storm is often noted in patients with acute myocardial infarction (AMI). Low LVEF (<30–35%) has remained the most easily quantifiable parameter to identify high-risk candidates for prophylactic ICD implantation. However, patients with low LVEF and an ICD implanted for secondary SCD prevention are more prone to VT storm. In patients with ICM, the extent of ECHO wall motion abnormalities, as measured by the global wall motion score index, has been used as a prognostic index for the composite endpoint of appropriate ICD therapy and all-cause mortality.[11] A greater number of scarred segments, preferentially involving anterior, septal and apical endocardial LV scar has been observed in ICM patients developing VT storm.[12] Relative wall thickness (RWT) reflects LV geometry and reduced RWT is associated with an increased risk of VTs and VT-related deaths in patients with either ICM or DCM. Infact, one study suggests that VT storm in these patients with negatively remodeled LV is a sign of worsening HF.[13] Some researchers have claimed that CRT-D therapy in responders showed increased RWT and thereby reduced the risk of VT/VF and death. Advanced ECHO techniques based on deformation imaging assess the tissue heterogeneity of myocardial function, focusing on the mechanical and electrical properties. Ersboll et al. showed that, in a population of 988 patients after acute myocardial infarction, LV global longitudinal strain (GLS) was independently associated with occurrence of the composite endpoint of SCD, VT/VF, or appropriate ICD shocks.[14] Mechanical dispersion reflects the heterogeneity of myocardial contraction as a product of electrical alterations and tissue abnormalities. It is defined as the standard deviation of time to peak negative strain from the 16 LV segments and could be a novel risk stratifying parameter of VT/VF events, independent of LVEF. In a prospective, multicenter study, Haugaa et al. evaluated 569 patients more than 40 days after acute myocardial infarction and showed that a combination of mechanical dispersion and global strain may improve the selection of patients for ICD therapy, particularly in those with LVEF more than35% who did not fulfill current ICD indications (Fig. 1). These two parameters, quantifying deformation, should also be studied in patients with VT storm.[15] Despite its lesser efficacy, a successful prophylactic CAB, prior to ICD implantation in patients with DCM and clinical MMVT, can prevent VT storm.[16] However, unlike in ICM patients, ECHO has a limited role in DCM patients in defining the scar burden, which are the source of MMVT and a certain predictor of 1-year mortality following CAB.[17] In DCM patients, VT from inferolateral scar often requires epicardial CAB, while an anteroseptal scar is associated with intramural substrate and consequently higher postprocedure VT recurrences.[18] In patients with sarcoidosis and VT storm, scar predilection has been noted quite extensively in LV basal septum, anterior wall and perivalvular regions. Furthermore, the confluent right ventricular (RV) scarring is more epicardial than endocardial.[19] Resultingly, in sarcoidosis patients, CAB may control VT storm, but multiple residual VTs after index CAB leads to higher recurrence rates. Based on this

TABLE 1: Causes of ventricular tachycardia storms.

- Structural heart diseases
  - Ischemic heart diseases
  - Nonischemic cardiomyopathy
  - Dilated cardiomyopathy
  - Hypertrophic cardiomyopathy
  - Arrhythmogenic right ventricular dysplasia/cardiomyopathy
  - Cardiac sarcoidosis
  - Myocarditis
  - Valvular heart diseases
  - Corrected congenital heart diseases
- Structurally normal heart (Abnormal electrical substrate)
  - Idiopathic
  - Brugada syndrome
  - Early repolarization syndrome
  - Long QT syndrome
  - Short QT syndrome
  - Catecholaminergic polymorphic ventricular tachycardia

experience, it is better to image myocardial scarring in DCM patients by contrast-enhanced MRI, FDG-PET or electro-anatomical voltage mapping. In patients with hypertrophic cardiomyopathy (HCM) developing VT storm, mechanical overload due to severe mid-septal hypertrophy and apical ballooning/wall motion abnormalities has been found.[20] Patients who have worsened to a dilated phase of HCM, have recurrent scar VT emanating from the basal septal and anterolateral LV, thereby leading to a stormy course.[21] VT storm occurs in approximately 30% of patients with arrhythmogenic RV cardiomyopathy (ARVC) and could well be the initial presentation.[22] Unless an ECHO is carefully done in all patients with LBBB-VT, ARVC could be missed. In the long-term, 20% ARVC patients with ICD experience a VT storm. CAB, in these patients is effective in short-term, but amiodarone works better to restrict long-term VT recurrences.[23] VT storm is considerably infrequent in adults with congenital heart disease. ECHO being normal, ECG diagnosis is critical to avoid misguided therapy in patients with primary electrical disease developing PMVT storm. For example, sympathetic blockade is effective in controlling electrical storm in patients with LQTS and catecholaminergic PMVT, whereas sympathetic stimulation using isoproterenol will contain storm in patients with Brugada syndrome, early repolarization syndrome and SQTS.

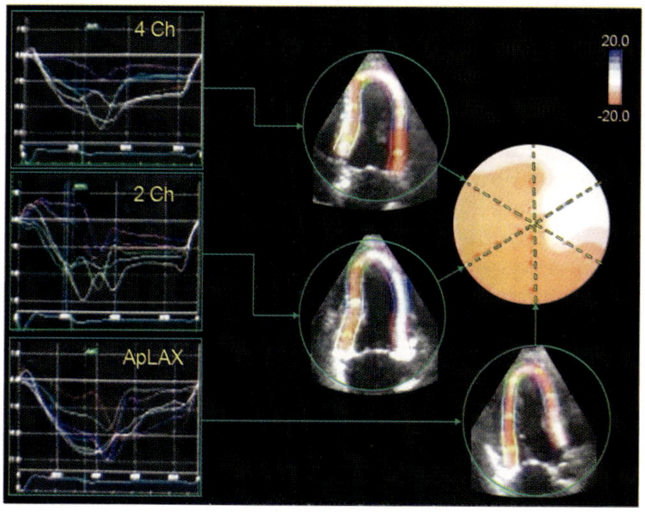

Fig. 1: Transthoracic echocardiography showing four chamber, two chamber, PLAX to show Mechanical dispersion of strain curves indicative of contraction heterogeneity in patient with ventricular tachycardia storm patient.

ROLE OF ECHO IN THERAPY

With its due limitations, ECHO identification of scar is based on recognizing the extent of wall motion abnormalities, which can be improved by using myocardial contrast echocardiography. CAB technique relying on substrate modification involves identification and ablation of, as many, local abnormal ventricular activities within the scar. This approach results in a substantial reduction of VT storm and ICD shocks and up to 49% of patients are free from arrhythmia at 5 years after a single CAB procedure.[24] In ICM patients with ICD having recurrent VT despite AAD, endocardial CAB is a superior option than escalation of AAD, probably because of better scar delineation.[25] However, in patients with DCM, because of difficulty in outlining the scar extent, epicardial CAB may be required, if endocardial CAB fails or even primarily CAB in DCM is less gratifying. LV cavitary thrombus is more common in ICM (after anterior wall AMI) then in DCM. Transthoracic ECHO with contrast (Fig. 2) would be sufficient to detect LV thrombus, and transesophageal ECHO would not be

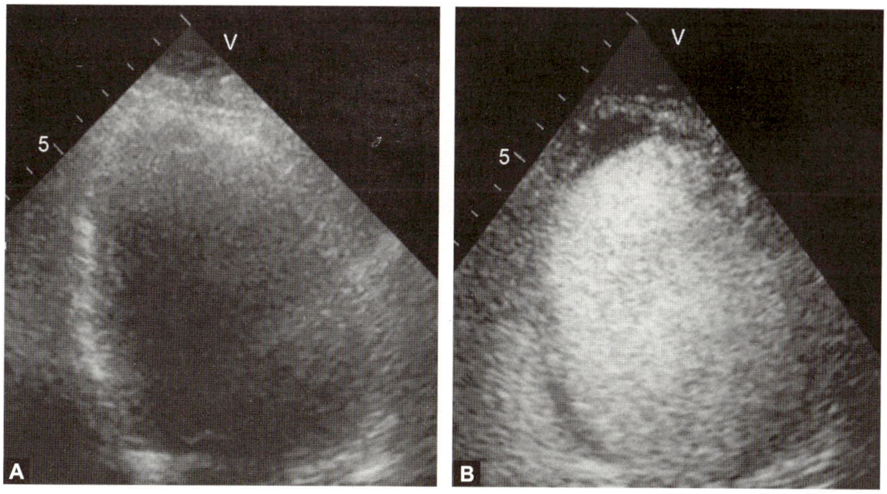

Figs. 2A and B: Echocardiography shows a left ventricular (LV) apical thrombus on an apical four-chamber view (A) and contrast echocardiography confirms a filling defect of the LV thrombus (B).

considered mandatory, as in case of left atrial thrombi. Soft, mobile protruding LV thrombi, early after AMI would suggest higher embolic risk precluding CAB. However, a small study by Rao et al.[26] suggests that a laminated thrombus detected in the setting of VT storm should not deter CAB, by whichever approach, endo- or epicardial, that is considered effective. In fact, successful CAB may prevent recurrent ICD shocks and attendant embolic risk. Transesophageal or intracardiac echocardiography would be helpful during epicardial ablation to monitor pericardial fluid that may accumulate while using an irrigated tip catheter, as well as to recognize complications like intrapericardial hemorrhage.

ROLE OF ECHO IN PROGNOSTICATION

Quelling the VT storm by successful CAB, using multiple or epicardial procedures, is definitely more promising in ICM patients providing freedom from VT recurrences in the immediate period.[27] In comparison, DCM patients remain prone to early VT recurrence despite CAB. Among different clinical variables that determine early post-CAB mortality, in patients with VT storm and SHD, the risk looms large in patients with low LVEF. [28] In our own study,[29] higher LV end diastolic volume and end systolic diameter in effect the extent of negative LV remodeling predicted lower survival following CAB. In patients with ARVC, VT storm can often be easily resolved with intravenous amiodarone.[30] Lamin A/C DCM patients with VT storm have moderate LV systolic dysfunction and fare poorly after CAB.[31]

CONCLUSION

In patients presenting with MMVT storm, a careful ECG analysis should be followed by ECHO evaluation directed at understanding the nature (ICM versus DCM) of underlying SHD. ECHO is likely to be normal in patients with primary electrical disease presenting with recurrent PMVT. Defining myocardial scar is based on recognizing the extent of wall motion abnormalities in patients with ICM. In contrast, echocardiographic recognition of scar presence and its extent has limitations in DCM patients, and would be better with other imaging modalities like contrast-enhanced MRI, FDG-PET or electroanatomical voltage mapping. Resultingly, procedural and short-term CAB results based on scar (substrate) modification are better in patients with ICM than DCM. Among different clinical variables, low LVEF dictates late mortality after VT storm even after a CAB or CSD procedure.

REFERENCES

1. Noda T, Kurita T, Nitta T, et al. Significant impact of electrical storm on mortality in patients with structural heart disease and an implantable cardiac defibrillator. Int J Cardiol. 2018;255:85-91.
2. Abdel Wahab A, Sapp J. Ventricular tachycardia with ICD shocks: when to medicate and when to ablate. Curr Cardiol Rep. 2017;19:105.
3. Parkash R, Nault I, Rivard L, et al. Effect of baseline antiarrhythmic drug on outcomes with ablation in ischemic ventricular tachycardia: a VANISH Substudy (Ventricular Tachycardia Ablation Versus Escalated Antiarrhythmic Drug Therapy in Ischemic Heart Disease). Circ Arrhythm Electrophysiol. 2018;11(1):e005663.
4. Vergara P, Tung R, Vaseghi M, et al. Successful ventricular tachycardia ablation in patients with electrical storm reduces recurrences and improves survival. Heart Rhythm. 2018;15:48-55.
5. Vakil K, Garcia S, Tung R, et al. Ventricular tachycardia ablation in the elderly: an International Ventricular Tachycardia Center Collaborative Group Analysis. Circ Arrhythm Electrophysiol. 2017;10(12). pii:e005332.
6. Jin Q, Jacobsen PK, Pehrson S, et al. Prediction and prognosis of ventricular tachycardia recurrence after catheter ablation with remote magnetic navigation for electrical storm in patients with ischemic cardiomyopathy. Clin Cardiol. 2017;40:1083-9.
7. Tzou WS, Tung R, Frankel DS, et al. Outcomes after repeat ablation of ventricular tachycardia in structural heart disease: an analysis from the International VT Ablation Center Collaborative Group. Heart Rhythm. 2017;14:991-7.
8. Vaseghi M, Barwad P, Lokhandwala Y, et al. Cardiac sympathetic denervation for refractory ventricular arrhythmias. J Am Coll Cardiol. 2017;69:3070-80.
9. Guerra F, Palmisano P, Dell' Era G et al. Cardiac resynchronization therapy and electrical storm: results of the Observational registry on long-term outcome of ICD patients (OBSERVO-ICD). Europace.2018;20:979-85.
10. Maruyama M. Management of electrical storm: the mechanism matters. J Arrhythmia. 2014;30:242-9.
11. Mahenthiran J, Das MK, Bhakta D, et al. Prognostic importance of wall motion abnormalities in patients with ischemic cardiomyopathy and an implantable cardioverter-defibrillator. Am J Cardiol. 2006;98:1301-6.
12. Kumar S, Fujii A, Kapur S, et al. Beyond the storm: comparison of clinical factors, arrhythmogenic substrate, and catheter ablation outcomes in structural heart disease patients with versus those without a history of ventricular tachycardia storm. J Cardiovasc Electrophysiol. 2017;28:56-67.
13. Biton Y, Goldenberg I, Kutyifa V, et al. Relative wall thickness and the risk for ventricular tachyarrhythmias in patients with left ventricular dysfunction. J Am Coll Cardiol. 2016;67:303-12.

14. Ersbøll M, Valeur N, Mogensen UM, et al. Prediction of all-cause mortality and heart failure admissions from global left ventricular longitudinal strain in patients with acute myocardial infarction and preserved left ventricular ejection fraction. J Am Coll Cardiol. 2013;61:2365-73.
15. Haugaa KH, Grenne BL, Eek CH, et al. Strain echocardiography improves risk prediction of ventricular arrhythmias after myocardial infarction. JACC Cardiovasc Imaging. 2013;6(8):841-50.
16. Suzuki A, Yoshida A, Takei A, et al. Prophylactic catheter ablation of ventricular tachycardia before cardioverter-defibrillator implantation in patients with non-ischemic cardiomyopathy: clinical outcomes after a single endocardial ablation. J Arrhythmia. 2015;31:122-9.
17. Kojodjojo P, Tokuda M, Bohnen M, et al. Electrocardiographic left ventricular scar burden predicts clinical outcomes following infarct-related ventricular tachycardia ablation. Heart Rhythm. 2013;10:1119-24.
18. Piers SR, Tao Q, van Taxis CF, et al. Contrast-enhanced MRI-derived scar patterns and associated ventricular tachycardias in nonischemic cardiomyopathy: implications for the ablation strategy. Circ Arrhythm Electrophysiol. 2013;6(5):875-83.
19. Kumar S, Barbhaiya C, Nagashima K, et al. Ventricular tachycardia in cardiac sarcoidosis: characterization of ventricular substrate and outcomes of catheter ablation. Circ Arrhythm Electrophysiol. 2015;8(1):87-93.
20. Hwang ES, Pak HN. Mid-septal hypertrophy and apical ballooning; potential mechanism of ventricular tachycardia storm in patients with hypertrophic cardiomyopathy. Yonsei Med J. 2012;53:221-3.
21. Ueda A, Fukamizu S, Soejima K, et al. Clinical and electrophysiological characteristics in patients with sustained monomorphic reentrant ventricular tachycardia associated with dilated-phase hypertrophic cardiomyopathy. Europace. 2012;14(5):734-40.
22. Gulgun M, Fidanci MK, Genç AF, et al. Electrical storm might be the initial presentation of arrhythmogenic right ventricular cardiomyopathy. Anatol J Cardiol. 2016;16(3):218-9.
23. Carbucicchio C, Santamaria M, Trevisi N, et al. Catheter ablation for the treatment of electrical storm in patients with implantable cardioverter-defibrillators: short-and long-term outcomes in a prospective single-center study. Circulation. 2008;117:462-9.
24. Wolf M, Sacher F, Cochet H, et al. Long-term outcome of substrate modification in ablation of post–myocardial infarction ventricular tachycardia. Circ Arrhythm Electrophysiol. 2018;11(2):e005635.
25. Sapp JL, Wells GA, Parkash R, et al. Ventricular tachycardia ablation versus escalation of antiarrhythmic drugs. N Engl J Med. 2016;375:111-21.
26. Rao HB, Yu R, Chitnis N, et al. Ventricular tachycardia ablation in the presence of left ventricular thrombus: safety and efficacy. J Cardiovasc Electrophysiol. 2016;27:453-9.
27. Russo AD, Casella M, Pelargonio G, et al. Feasibility and safety of catheter ablation of electrical storm in ischemic dilated cardiomyopathy. J Cardiovasc Med. 2016;17:425-32.
28. Santangeli P, Frankel DS, Tung R, et al. Early mortality after catheter ablation of ventricular tachycardia in patients with structural heart disease. J Am Coll Cardiol. 2017;69:2105-15.
29. Nabar A, Rodriguez LM, Batra RK, et al. Echocardiographic predictors of survival in patients undergoing radiofrequency ablation of postinfarct clinical ventricular tachycardia. J Cardiovasc Electrophysiol. 2002;13:118-21.
30. Yin K, Ding L, Hua W, et al. Electrical storm in ICD recipients with arrhythmogenic right ventricular cardiomyopathy. Pacing and Clinical Electrophysiology. 2017;40:683-92.
31. Kumar S, Androulakis AF, Sellal JM et al. Multicenter experience with catheter ablation for ventricular tachycardia in lamin A/C cardiomyopathy. Circ Arrhythm Electrophysiol. 2016;9(8). pii:e004357.

79

CHAPTER

Cryoballoon Ablation for Atrial Fibrillation

Jayakeerthi Yoganarasimha

"Any sufficiently advanced technology is indistinguishable from magic."

—Sir Arthur C Clarke

INTRODUCTION

We have realized the importance of pulmonary veins in the origin of atrial fibrillation (AF). Pulmonary vein isolation (PVI) by radiofrequency ablation (RFA) is established as a cornerstone therapy both in paroxysmal and persistent AF. Cryoballoon ablation (CRAB) was introduced for PVI more than a decade ago. With sufficient expertise and clinical evidence, CRAB is fast becoming the first modality for PVI.

PROCEDURE

Under general anesthesia/deep sedation, a 6-Fr quadripolar catheter is inserted in the right jugular vein and advanced to the coronary sinus. A single trans-septal puncture is then performed under fluoroscopic guidance, using the right femoral venous approach. After gaining left atrial access, bolus heparin followed by supplements is given to maintain an ACT ~300 seconds throughout the procedure. A 0.32-Fr guide wire is advanced in the left superior pulmonary vein and a steerable 15-Fr over-the-wire sheath (FlexCath, Cryocath) is positioned in the left atrium. A circular mapping catheter is then advanced in each pulmonary vein (PV) ostium to obtain baseline electrical information. After withdrawing the mapping catheter, a 28 or 23mm double-walled cryoballoon (Arctic Front, Cryocath) is advanced over the wire up to the left atrium, inflated, and positioned in the pulmonary vein ostium of each vein. Optimal vessel occlusion is considered to have been achieved when selective contrast injection shows total contrast retention with no backflow to the atrium. For each vein, CRAB consists of a minimum of two applications lasting at least 4 min each or one 3 min uninterrupted freeze. In order to avoid phrenic nerve injury (PNI), a complication observed during right sided PV ablation with the cryoballoon, a quadripolar catheter is inserted in the superior vena cava, and diaphragmatic stimulation is achieved by pacing the ipsilateral phrenic nerve. Ablation is stopped at the first evidence of PNI, to avoid long-term palsy.

EQUIPMENT

Cryoballoon ablation involves a console with the settings control, N_2O cylinder and monitoring mechanisms (Fig. 1A). The fluoroscopic appearance during ideal positioning of the balloon (Fig. 1B). The first-generation cryoballoon (CB1) is available in 2 sizes: 23 mm and 28 mm diameter. In August 2012, a redesigned second-generation balloon catheter (CB2) was introduced in the same sizes. Important differences include more number of refrigerant ports on the injection coil, a more distal injection coil in the balloon, and increased N_2O flow rates in the larger balloon.

EVIDENCE

The relevance of PVs as the trigger for AF is well established.[1] This is amenable to RFA which is the cornerstone modality for PVI in both paroxysmal AF (PAF) and persistent AF (PstAF). Cryoballoon technique for PVI was introduced a decade ago with the initial report of efficacy[2] paving way

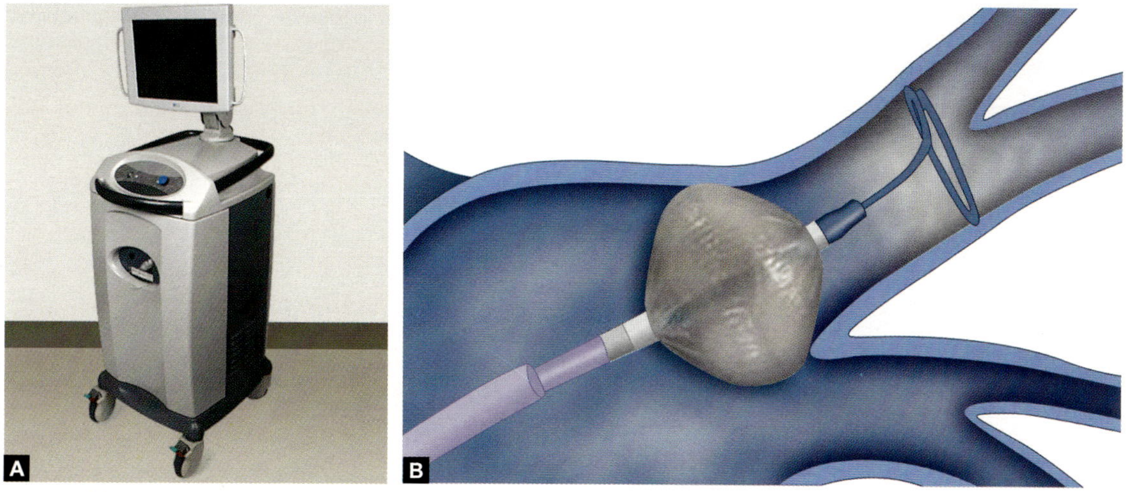

Figs. 1A and B: (A) Cryoconsole which houses the N_2O and controls. (B) Cryoballoon at the PV ostium with Grade 4 occlusion, along with Achieve^{TM} multipolar catheter for assessment of real-time PVI.
Source: www.medtronic.com

for further evaluation. CRAB was proven to be effective and safe with acceptable short-term outcomes.[3] Various groups reported the outcomes of CRAB in the long term including up to 3 years.[4,5] CRAB using CB1 has been evaluated in both PAF and PstAF with favorable outcomes, yet there was scope for better success rates (Table 1). With an aim to perform faster and more lasting PV isolation, the CB2 was introduced with some fundamental changes. These modifications create a broader, more uniform freezing zone almost across the entire distal half of the balloon surface. Technically CB2 has advantages and significantly reduced the procedural time, fluoroscopy times and improved procedural success as shown by Sergio Conti et al.[6] Liu et al.[7] and others. There is a steep learning curve for optimal usage of cryoballoon and fluoroscopy times were shorter in experienced centers. In PAF, CRAB with CB2 was similar in efficacy to next generation contact force sensing ablation catheters (Smart Touch, Biosense-Webster, Inc.) as demonstrated by Cardoso R et al.[8] For 2 years, freedom from atrial arrhythmias after a single procedure was around 72% with either modality, but CRAB procedure time was shorter by 60 minutes. Meta-analysis of CRAB compared to RF ablation showed similar rates of AF free interval. Analysis by Liu et al. showed CRAB significantly decreased the procedural time compared to RFA and the difference was more marked with CB2. AF recrudescence was significantly lower with CRAB using CB2 than RF ablation. Also, acute PVI, procedure time, fluoroscopy time, and energy delivery time were significantly shorter with CRAB compared to RFA or MESH catheter. Major complications favor the use of CB2 over RF ablation. Many investigators studied the safety and efficacy of the second-generation balloon. Meta-analysis by Buiatti A et al.[9] comparable freedom from any atrial arrhythmia (~70% at 16 months) with either CRAB or RF ablation. However, the procedure time was lower with CRAB. Similar results were reported in the largest meta-analysis of CRAB versus RFA in PAF by Garg J et al.[10] They found no difference in terms of efficacy, procedural times, and overall complications. There was also no difference between CB1 and CB2 in terms of efficacy. The multicenter randomized FIRE and ICE study[11] provided the most robust data comparing the two modalities of ablation in drug refractory PAF. It showed noninferiority of CRAB versus RFA, with no difference between the groups either in primary efficacy end point or primary safety end point. Evidence on the efficacy of AF ablation using either CB1 and CB2 alone, or versus RFA in the medium and longer terms are enlisted in the Table 1.[12-19] Traditionally, 2–3 freezes of 2 minutes each for each PV was practiced. But data on the appropriate number and duration of freeze was lacking. To bridge this gap, Aryana A et al.[20] conducted the Cryo-Dosing study in which the duration and number of freezes were based on the rapidity of disappearance of the PV potentials. This was compared to the standard conventional approach for CRAB using two 2-minute freezes or single 3-minute freeze. They demonstrated Cryo-AF_{Dosing} arm resulted in shorter and fewer cryoapplications, reduced overall procedure, ablation, fluoroscopy and LA dwell times. Twelve-month atrial arrhythmia free rates were similar but significantly lower atypical atrial flutter/tachycardias were noted in Cryo-AF_{Dosing} arm.

CRAB as Index Modality of PVI in AF

Our group conducted one of the early long term follow up studies using CRAB as the index procedure instead of RFA for PVI in cases of drug refractory PAF. This study involved CB1 and conventional 2 freeze regimen. In 3 years, 57.5% sinus rhythm off antiarrhythmic drugs[5] was maintained Ciconte et al.[21] studied the efficacy of CRAB as the index

TABLE 1: Studies performed with the two generations of balloon and their efficacy over follow-up compared to radiofrequency ablation.

			AT/AF free over medium to long-term follow-up		
1st generation balloon (CB1)			*1 year*	*2 years*	*3 years*
CRAB	Van Belle et al.[4]	PAF	59% off AADs after 1, 2 procedures 41% on AAD with reduced AF burden		
	Luik A et al.[12]	PAF	73.6% CB vs. 70.7% with RFA. 19% had redo ablations		
	Sergio C et al.[6]	PAF		68.3%	
	Cardoso R et al.[8]	PAF/PstAF Meta-analysis	57.9% CB1 vs. 58.1% Regular RF catheter		
	Rao J Y et al.[5]	PAF		60%	57.5% off AAD
	Namdar M et al.[22]	Lone AF–First Line therapy	89%		
2nd generation balloon (CB2)			*1 year*	*2 years*	*3 years*
CRAB	Tscholl V et al.[13]	PAF/PstAF>75 years age	70%		
	Akkaya E et al.[14]	PsyAF. PVI + roof line where indicated			70.3%
	Takarada K et al.[15]	PAF			71.5%
	Sergio C et al.[6]	PAF		86.7%	
	Heeger CH et al.[16]	PAF/PstAF			60.2% after single CRAB vs. 78.6% after mean of 1.37 procedures
	Tondo C et al.[17]	PstAF/ Long standing PstAF	63.9%	51.5% at 18 months	
	Yalin K et al.[18]	PstAF	67%		
CRAB vs. RFA	Kuck HK et al. FIRE and ICE study[11]	PAF/ PstAF		65% CRAB vs. 64% with RFA	
	Cardoso et al.[8]	PAF/PstAF Meta-analysis	78.1% CB2 vs. 78.2% Contact force RF catheter		
	Buiatti et al.[9]	PAF Meta-analysis		71% CRAB vs. 72% RFA at 16 months. No difference between CB1 and CB2	
	Ciconte G et al.[19]	PstAF	60% CB2 vs. 56% with RFA		

(CRAB: cryoballoon ablation; RFA: radiofrequency ablation; PAF: paroxysmal atrial fibrillation)

method for PVI in persistent AF using CB2. In that study, 41% were in AF at the time of procedure and 26% converted to sinus during CRAB. 60% remained arrhythmia free at 12 months. Frontiers were extended when CRAB was evaluated as first line therapy in patients with symptomatic lone PAF who opted for the procedure overlong term drugs. A large proportion of patients (89%) in this relatively small study by Namdar et al.[22] remained in sinus rhythm off drugs at 1-year follow-up.

COMPLICATIONS

Meta-analysis has shown that the major complication rates between CRAB and RFA are similar but the types of complications vary. Whereas, the most common major complication observed during CRAB is PNI during right sided PVI (2.7–11%), it is pericardial perforation and tamponade that is more common with RF ablation. Most often PNI is transient and recovery can sometimes take up to 6 months. Progression to permanent PNI is noted in ~0.3–1% of cases. Other complications remain similar between CRAB and RFA in the range of 1–4%.

GUIDELINES

Although, guidelines clearly recommend AF ablation in drug refractory PAF as class I indication and Class IIa indication in persistent AF, there is no specific recommendation on which modality of catheter ablation is preferred over the other for the first procedure. This is based on the evidence presented which shows similar safety and efficacy of CRAB or RF ablation in rhythm control of PVI. However, for redo procedures and touch up during the first procedure in cases of nonisolated PVs, RF ablation is preferred. Further improvement in technology and longer term data showing sustainable results, should pave way for larger utilization of CRAB in atrial fibrillation.

REFERENCES

1. Haissaguerre M, Jais P, Shah DC, et al. Spontaneous initiation of atrial fibrillation by ectopic beats originating in the pulmonary veins. N Engl J Med. 1998;339(10):659-66.
2. Van Belle Y, Janse P, Rivero-Ayerza MJ, et al. Pulmonary vein isolation using an occluding cryoballoon for circumferential ablation: feasibility, complications, and short-term outcome. Eur Heart J. 2007;28(18):2231-7.
3. Klein G, Oswald H, Gardiwal A, et al. Efficacy of pulmonary vein isolation by cryoballoon ablation in patients with paroxysmal atrial fibrillation. Heart Rhythm. 2008;5(6):802-6.
4. Van Belle Y, Janse P, Theuns D, et al. One year follow-up after cryoballoon isolation of the pulmonary veins in patients with paroxysmal atrial fibrillation. Europace. 2008;10(11):1271-6.
5. Rao JY, Chierchia GB, de Asmundis C, et al. Cryoballoon ablation as index procedure for paroxysmal atrial fibrillation: long-term results from a single center early experience. J Cardiovasc Med (Hagerstown). 2014;15(3):194-8.
6. Conti S, Moltrasio M, Fassini G, et al. Comparison between first- and second-generation cryoballoon for paroxysmal atrial fibrillation ablation. Cardiol Res Pract. 2016;2016:5106127.
7. Liu XH, Chen CF, Gao XF, et al. Safety and efficacy of different catheter ablations for atrial fibrillation: a systematic review and meta-analysis. Pacing Clin Electrophysiol. 2016;39(8):883-99.
8. Cardoso R, Mendirichaga R, Fernandes G, et al. Cryoballoon versus radiofrequency catheter ablation in atrial fibrillation: A Meta-Analysis. J Cardiovasc Electrophysiol. 2016;27(10):1151-9.
9. Buiatti A, von Olshausen G, Barthel P, et al. Cryoballoon versus radiofrequency ablation for paroxysmal atrial fibrillation: an updated meta-analysis of randomized and observational studies. Europace. 2017;19(3):378-84.
10. Garg J, Chaudhary R, Palaniswamy C et al. Cryoballoon versus radiofrequency ablation for atrial fibrillation: a meta-analysis of 16 clinical trials. J Atr Fibrillation. 2016;9(3):29.
11. Kuck KH, Brugada J, Fürnkranz A, et al. Cryoballoon or Radiofrequency Ablation for Paroxysmal Atrial Fibrillation. N Engl J Med. 2016; 374:2235-45.
12. Luik A, Radzewitz A, Kieser M, et al. Cryoballoon versus open irrigated radiofrequency ablation in patients with paroxysmal atrial fibrillation: the prospective, randomized, controlled, noninferiority freeze AF study. Circulation. 2015;132(14):1311-9.
13. Tscholl V, Lin T, Lsharaf AK, et al. Cryoballoon ablation in the elderly: one year outcome and safety of the second-generation 28 mm cryoballoon in patients over 75 years old. Europace. 2018;20(5):772-7.
14. Akkaya E, Berkowitsch A, ZaltsbergS, et al. Second-generation cryoballoon ablation for treatment of persistent atrial fibrillation: three-year outcome and predictors of recurrence after a single procedure. J Cardiovasc Electrophysiol. 2018;29(1):38-45.
15. Takarada K, Overeinder I, de Asmundis C, et al. Long-term outcome after second-generation cryoballoon ablation for paroxysmal atrial fibrillation—a 3-years follow-up. J Interv Card Electrophysiol. 2017;49(1):93-100.
16. Heeger CH, Wissner E, Knöll M, et al. Three-year clinical outcome after 2nd-generation cryoballoon-based pulmonary vein isolation for the treatment of paroxysmal and persistent atrial fibrillation. Circ J. 2017;81(7):974-980.
17. Tondo C, Iacopino S, Pieragnoli P, et al. Pulmonary vein isolation cryoablation for patients with persistent and longstanding persistent atrial fibrillation: Clinical outcomes from the real-world multicenter observational project. Heart Rhythm. 2018;15(3):363-8.
18. Yalin K, Abdin A, Lyan E, et al. Safety and efficacy of persistent atrial fibrillation ablation using the second-generation cryoballoon. Clin Res Cardiol. 2018;107(7):570-7.
19. Ciconte G, Baltogiannis G, de Asmundis C, et al. Circumferential pulmonary vein isolation as index procedure for persistent atrial fibrillation: a comparison between radiofrequency catheter ablation and second-generation cryoballoon ablation. Europace. 2015;17(4):559-65.
20. Aryana A, Kenigsberg DN, Kowalski M, et al. Verification of a novel atrial fibrillation cryoablation dosing algorithm guided by time-to-pulmonary vein isolation: Results from the Cryo-DOSING Study (Cryoballoon-ablation DOSING Based on the Assessment of Time-to-Effect and Pulmonary Vein Isolation Guidance). Heart Rhythm. 2017;14(9):1319-25.
21. Ciconte G, Ottaviano L, de Asmundis C, et al. Pulmonary vein isolation as index procedure for persistent atrial fibrillation: One-year clinical outcome after ablation using the second-generation cryoballoon. Heart Rhythm. 2015;12(1):60-6.
22. Namdar M, Chierchia GB, Westra S, et al. Isolating the pulmonary veins as first-line therapy in patients with lone paroxysmal atrial fibrillation using the Cryoballoon. Europace. 2012;14(2):197-203.

SECTION 11

Dilated Cardiomyopathy

80

CHAPTER

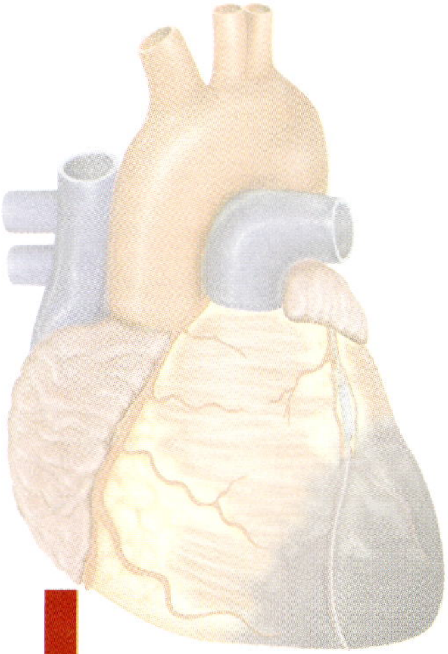

Advances in Echocardiographic Navigation in Dilated Cardiomyopathy

Vivek Tandon

INTRODUCTION

The cardiomyopathies are a diverse group of diseases, difficult to define in one line. This is why there are a number of definitions of these diseases. The two most widely accepted definitions are from respected cardiological societies from the US and Europe.

The American Heart Association (AHA) defines cardiomyopathies as "a heterogeneous group of diseases of the myocardium associated with mechanical and/or electrical dysfunction that usually (but not invariably) exhibits inappropriate ventricular hypertrophy or dilatation and are due to a variety of causes that frequently are genetic. Cardiomyopathies either are confined to the heart or are part of generalized systemic disorders, often leading to cardiovascular death or progressive heart failure related disability".[1]

The European Society of Cardiology (ESC) defines cardiomyopathies as "a myocardial disorder in which the heart muscle is structurally and functionally abnormal, in the absence of coronary artery disease, hypertension, valvular disease and congenital heart disease sufficient to cause the observed myocardial abnormality."[2]

Dilated cardiomyopathy (DCM) is a progressive disease of heart muscle. It is characterized by chamber enlargement and contractile dysfunction of the left ventricle (LV) in the absence of chronic pressure and/or volume overload.[3] This excludes the occurrence of a dilated and failing LV due to hypertension, valvular heart disease, congenital heart disease or ischemic heart disease. The right ventricle (RV) may be similarly affected, but this is not essential for the diagnosis.

Dilated cardiomyopathy is the commonest type of cardiomyopathy, and a leading cause of heart failure. The prevalence is estimated at about 1:2,500. It is the third most common cause of heart failure, and the most common cause of heart transplantation.[1] It may first become manifest in a wide range of age groups, even in children. It usually presents with symptoms of heart failure, causing severe restriction of the patient's lifestyle.

The phenotype of a dilated, failing heart may be the end result of a variety of pathological conditions, such as infections, toxins or autoimmune diseases. However, it is now recognized that between 20% and 35% of idiopathic cases may be due to an inherited gene background.[4] The various primary and secondary causes of the DCM phenotype are shown in Flowchart 1.

DIAGNOSIS

Most patients present with DCM in the fourth or fifth decades of life, though the disease may present in childhood. The presenting symptoms include features of low cardiac output or frank heart failure, with increasing degrees of breathlessness and swelling. Signs of heart failure will be detected on examination, including edema, an elevated jugular venous pressure, an enlarged heart on palpation, with an S3 gallop and murmurs of mitral regurgitation (MR) and/or tricuspid regurgitation (TR) on auscultation.

The ECG in patients of DCM may vary from normal to an ECG with mild nonspecific ST segment and T wave changes to an ECG with pronounced conduction abnormalities and various arrhythmias. The chest X-ray will reveal cardiomegaly, and usually features of increased pulmonary

Flowchart 1: Causes of dilated cardiomyopathy.

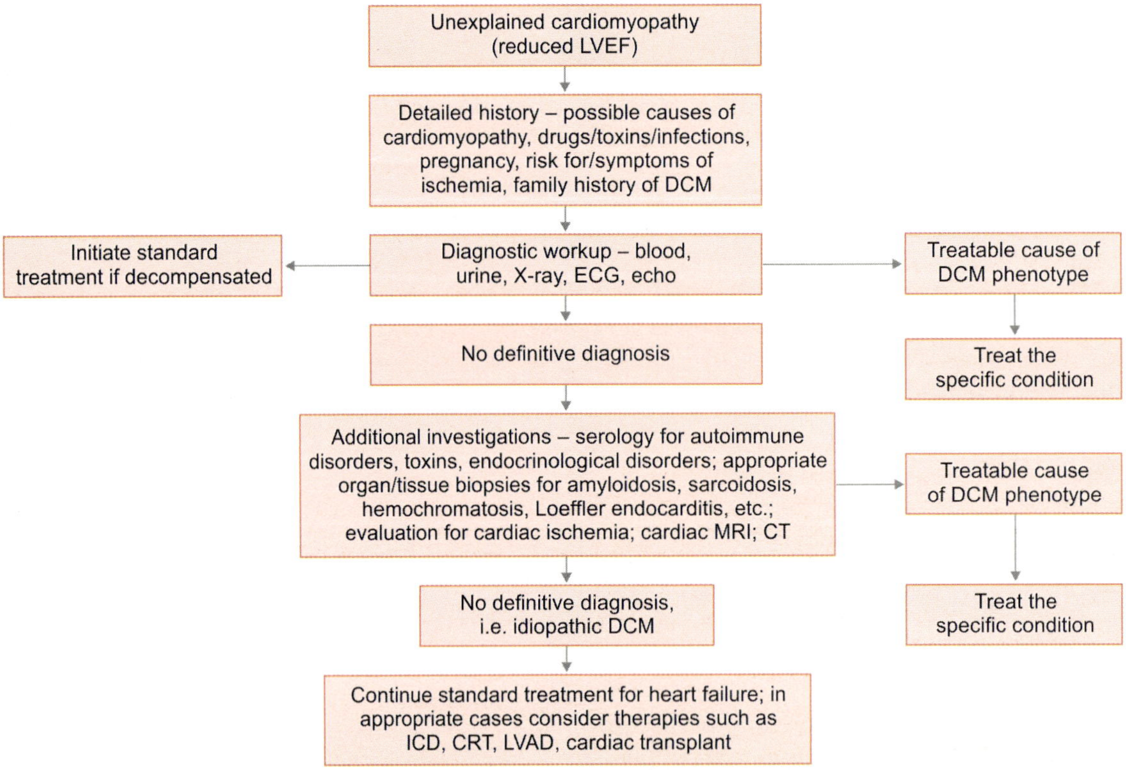

(LVEF: left ventricular ejection fraction; DCM: dilated cardiomyopathy; ECG: electrocardiography; MRI: magnetic resonance imaging; CT: computed tomography; ICD: implantable cardioverter defibrillators; CRT: cardiac resynchronization therapy; LVAD: left ventricular assist device)

venous pressure. Pleural and pericardial effusions may also be present in patients with severe and long-standing heart failure.

The cornerstone for the diagnosis of DCM is the echocardiographic examination. The ACC/AHA guidelines for the management of heart failure include echocardiography as a class IC recommendation in this context.[5] This one test will not only provide diagnostic and prognostic information, it will also help guide therapy, especially if serial examinations are conducted over the course of the treatment of the patient. Other imaging modalities are available and are very useful in many cases. However, echocardiography being a relatively inexpensive test with no side effects or exposure to ionizing radiation, can be repeated as frequently as required. It can also be used as a tool for screening family members of the patient, if a familial/genetic form of DCM is suspected.

Echocardiographic Examination in DCM

All the modes of echocardiography including motion (M) mode echocardiography, two dimensional (2D) imaging, pulsed wave (PW) Doppler, continuous wave (CW) Doppler, color Doppler, tissue Doppler imaging (TDI),[6] three dimensional (3D) imaging, and speckle tracking echocardiography (STE) are useful in the evaluation of a suspected or known case of DCM. In addition, in certain cases, the use of ultrasound enhancing agents (previously referred to as ultrasound contrast agents) may help resolve various diagnostic dilemmas.

The echocardiographic examination in a case of suspected or known DCM should focus on the following issues:
- Chamber dimensions and volumes
- Myocardial thickness
- Global LV and RV systolic function
- Doppler evaluation of degree of diastolic dysfunction, assessment of LV filling pressure and RA pressure, assessment of pulmonary artery pressure, LV dp/dt, and degree of mitral regurgitation (MR)
- Calculation of stroke volume and cardiac output
- Myocardial dyssynchrony
- Presence of intracardiac thrombus.

In addition, the echocardiographic examination may also reveal ancillary evidence of heart failure, such as pleural and pericardial effusions.

M mode Echocardiography

- With its high temporal resolution, M mode echocardiography provides accurate measurements of chamber dimensions, provided the M mode cursor can be aligned in the correct plane recommended for obtaining these measurements.[7]

- Mitral valve motion can be studied in detail using M mode and may reveal an increased E point septal separation (EPSS) (Fig. 1). This is indicative of the LV dilatation accompanied by reduced motion of the mitral valve due to reduction in the cardiac output. Because of these factors, the distance between the maximum excursion of the anterior mitral leaflet during early diastole (E point) and the interventricular septum is increased as compared to the normally functioning heart. The overall excursion of the mitral leaflets is also reduced, leading to a reduced separation of the two leaflets. The anterior motion of the root of the aorta with systole is also reduced in DCM and can be demonstrated by M mode (Fig. 2).

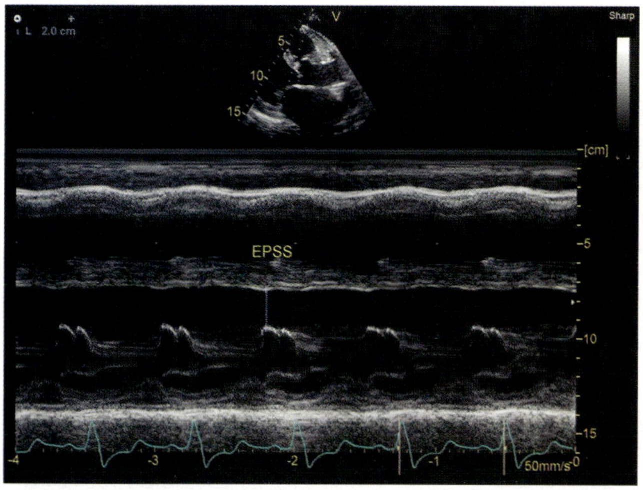

Fig. 1: M mode through the LV and mitral valve, showing reduced excursion of the mitral valve, and increased E point septal separation (EPSS).

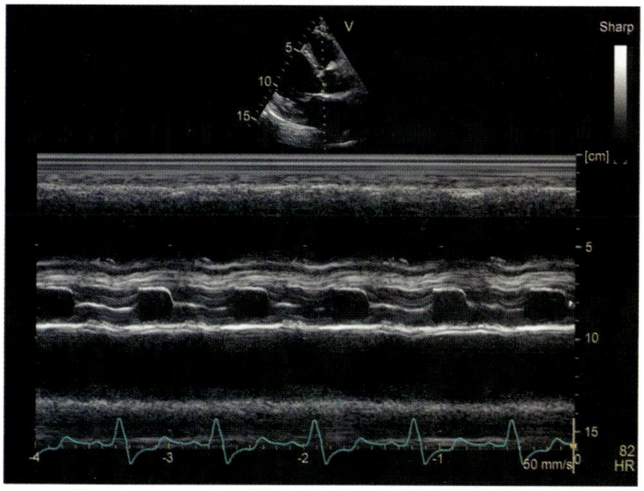

Fig. 2: M mode through the root of aorta and LA showing reduced motion of the aortic root with systole.

- A B-bump sometimes appears in the terminal part of the closing motion of the mitral valve, indicative of elevated LV filling pressure.
- Premature closure of the mitral valve may be seen in patients who have severe elevation of LV filling pressure.
- Premature closure of the aortic valve (AV) may be identified on M mode, suggesting severely reduced LV output.
- With the help of color M mode, diastolic mitral regurgitation (MR) may be visualized, in the presence of severe elevation of LV diastolic pressure (Fig. 3).
- Though LV volumes and LV mass can be calculated using linear dimensions measured by M mode, these calculations rely on various assumptions regarding the geometry of the ventricle. They are thus liable to have a wide margin of errors and should be avoided in favor of measurements and calculations made from 2D or 3D examinations.
- The tricuspid annular plane systolic excursion (TAPSE) can be measured for evaluating RV systolic function (Fig. 4). This single measurement has good correlation with RV systolic function evaluated by other means.

2D Echocardiography

- In patients where an adequate echocardiographic window is not available for accurate measurements of chamber dimensions using M mode, 2D echocardiography can be used for these measurements (Fig. 5).[7]
- 2D echocardiography allows accurate assessment of LV size, volume, and contractility, visually as well as by direct measurement (Fig. 6). For calculation of LV volumes and ejection fraction, a biplane method of discs

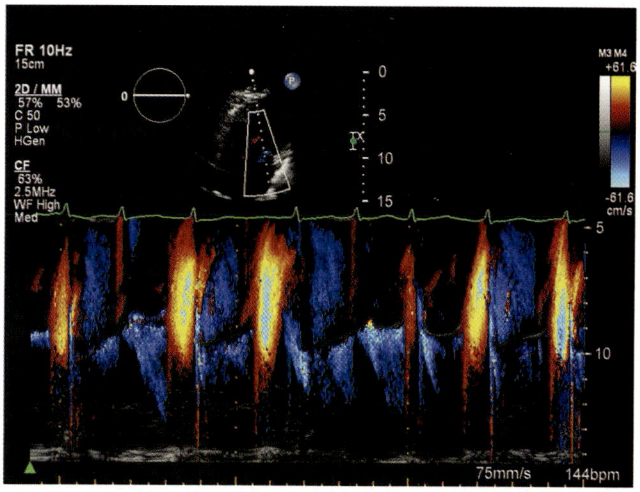

Fig. 3: A patient with DCM in atrial fibrillation showing diastolic MR using color M mode. Note that the blue flow of MR starts before the QRS complex in some cardiac cycles, demonstrating elevated LV diastolic pressure.

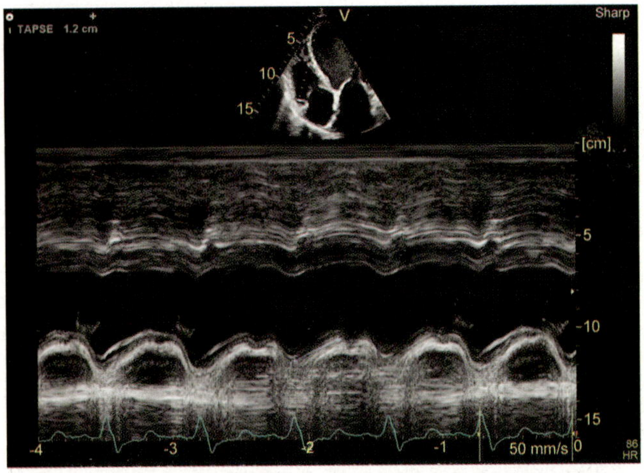

Fig. 4: Using M mode to measure tricuspid annular plane systolic excursion (TAPSE). This simple and reproducible measurement is a reasonably accurate measure of RV systolic function.

(modified Simpson's method) is best. LV mass can also be calculated from 2D echocardiography. The chamber volumes and mass will be increased in cases of DCM, and the systolic function will be reduced.

- All the cardiac structures, especially the valves, can be assessed by 2D echocardiography (Fig. 7). Valvular heart diseases or other cardiac abnormalities, which could be contributing to the DCM phenotype (congenital heart diseases, ischemic heart disease, and hypertensive heart disease), can be excluded. Additional abnormalities such as myocardial noncompaction, which can contribute to systolic dysfunction, can also be visualized (Fig. 8).
- Additional findings such as intracardiac thrombi, which can complicate a case of DCM, can be visualized (Figs. 9 and 10).

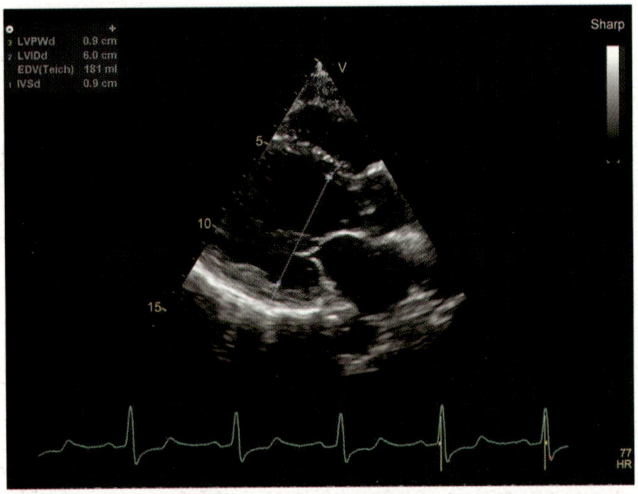

Fig. 5: 2D measurement of LV dimensions (diastolic) showing increased chamber size.

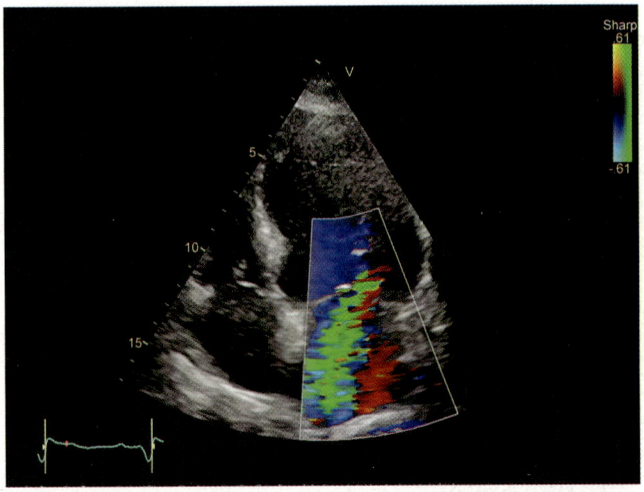

Fig. 7: Color flow imaging shows a jet of severe MR in the case of DCM.

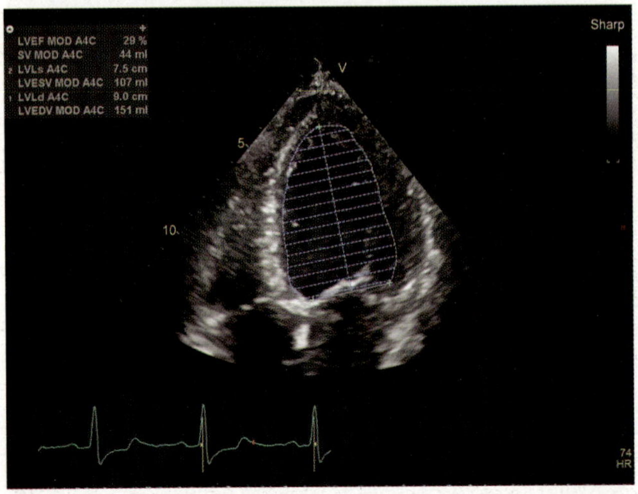

Fig. 6: Measurement of LV ejection fraction by Simpson's method in 2D echocardiography. The LVEF is markedly reduced in this case of DCM.

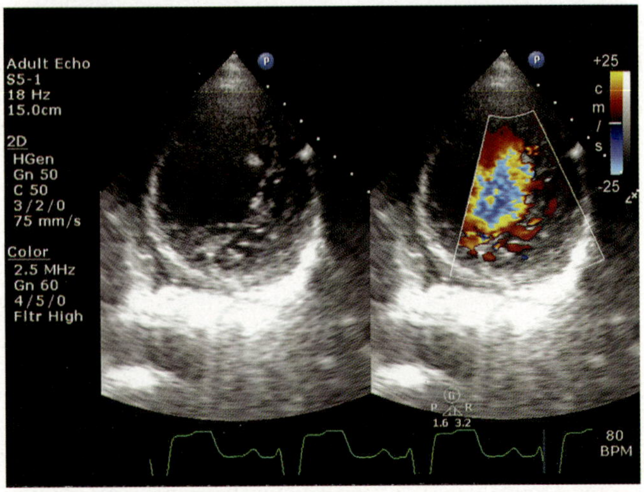

Fig. 8: Short axis view through the LV apex recorded as a dual image with 2D and color Doppler, showing multiple communicating sinusoids in noncompacted myocardium with color flow visible inside the sinusoids.

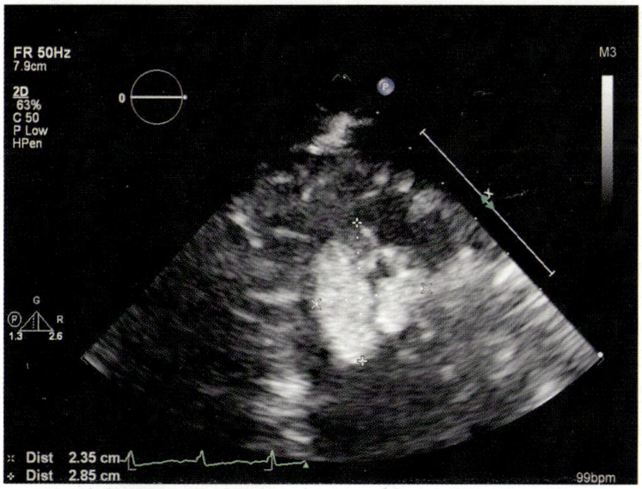

Fig. 9: A zoomed view of the LV apex showing an organized thrombus in a case of DCM (the same patient as in Fig. 8).

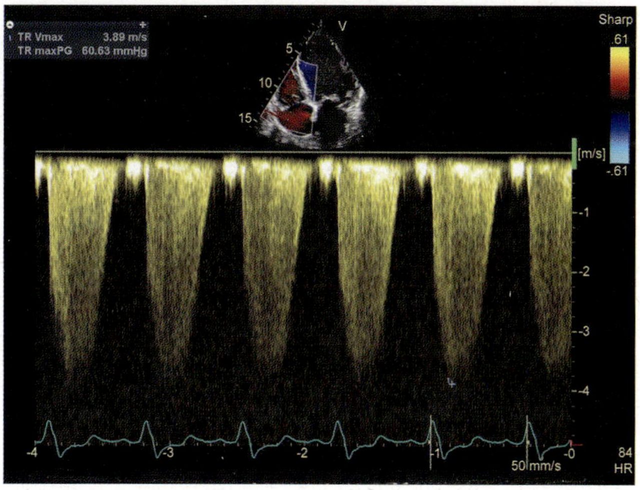

Fig. 11: CW Doppler recording of the velocity/gradient of the TR jet in the case of DCM. This gradient can be used to calculate the PA systolic pressure (which is elevated in this case).

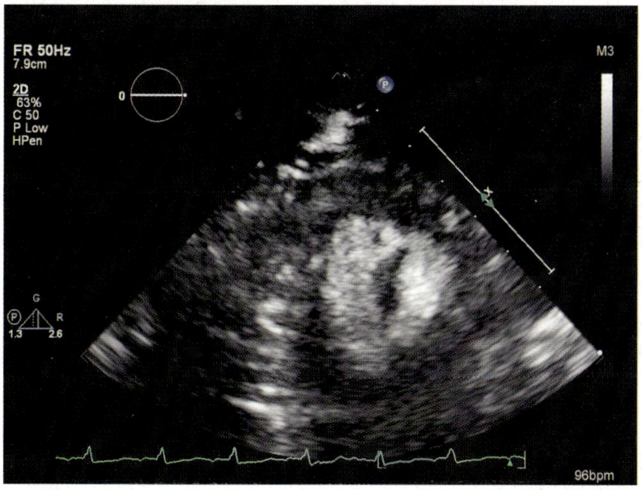

Fig. 10: A zoomed view of the RV apex showing an organized thrombus (the same patient as in Fig. 7).

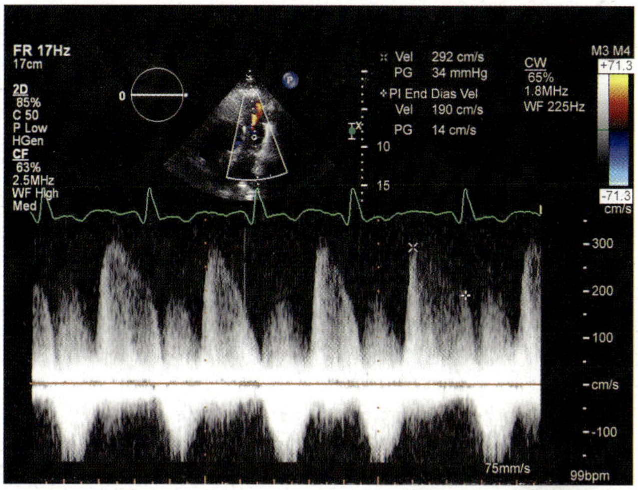

Fig. 12: CW Doppler recording of the PR jet in the case of DCM to calculate the mean PA pressure and the PA diastolic pressure.

Doppler Echocardiography

- Color Doppler echocardiography can be used to detect the presence of mitral regurgitation (MR) and tricuspid regurgitation (TR) and assess their severity.
- A combination of PW Doppler and CW Doppler will allow measurement of the velocities of flow and pressure gradients across the valves. Stroke volume and cardiac output can be calculated using these values in combination with 2D measurements and the heart rate at the time of the examination.
- Doppler measurement of TR and PR velocities/gradients allows the calculation of pulmonary arterial systolic, diastolic, and mean pressures (Figs. 11 and 12).
- PW Doppler and tissue Doppler imaging (TDI) should be used to assess the degree of diastolic dysfunction (Figs. 13 to 15).[8]

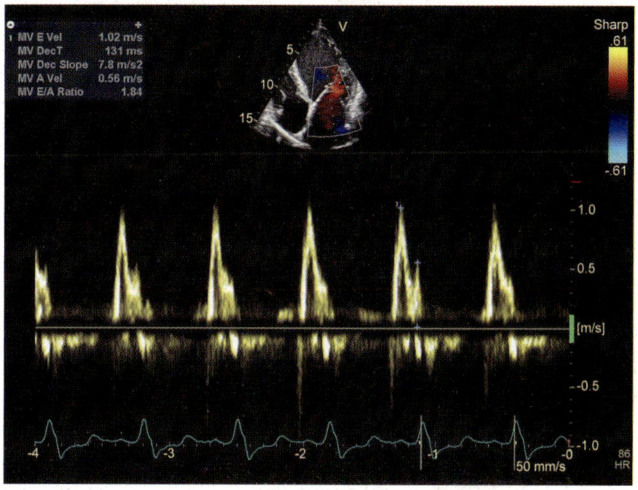

Fig. 13: PW Doppler recording of the flow across the MV showing a restrictive pattern of flow.

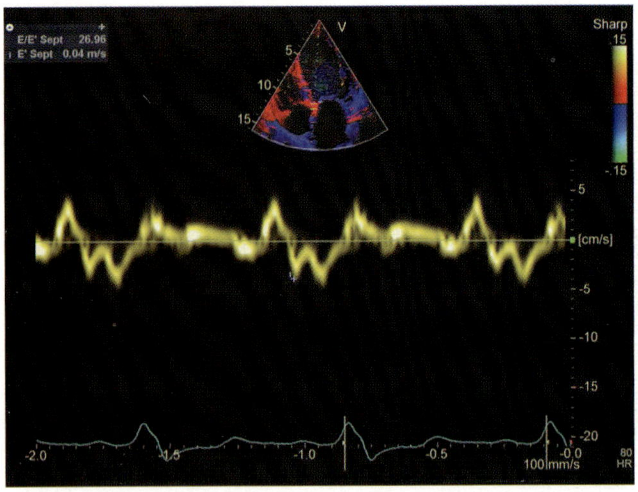

Fig. 14: Tissue Doppler imaging (TDI) of the medial mitral annular velocities in the same patient as in Figure 13, showing reduced diastolic velocities.

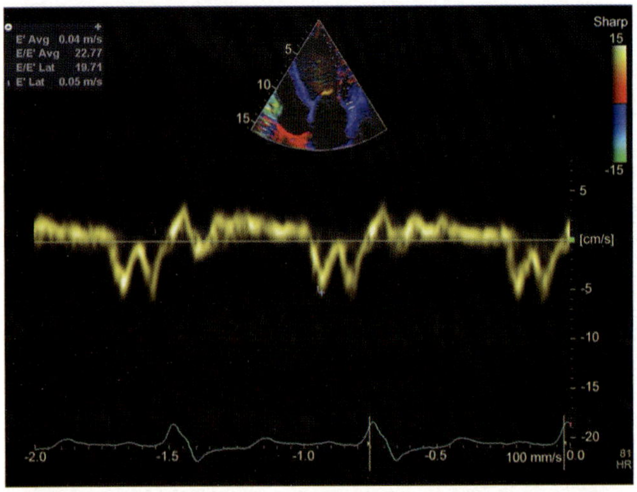

Fig. 15: TDI of the lateral mitral annular velocities in the same patient as in Figure 13 and Figure 14 showing reduced diastolic velocities. The E/E' ratio calculated from the average of the medial E' and lateral E' velocities is elevated indicating elevated left sided diastolic pressure.

- TDI measurement of the S' (systolic) velocity of the tricuspid valve annulus provides a simple and reproducible measure of RV systolic function (Fig. 16).
- Sometimes the Doppler recording of the flow across a valve provides additional insight into the hemodynamics of the patient, such as the presence of mechanical alternans in patients with severe systolic dysfunction (Fig. 17).

3D Echocardiography

- 3D echocardiography facilitates a better understanding of the anatomy of the heart, especially the valves. The

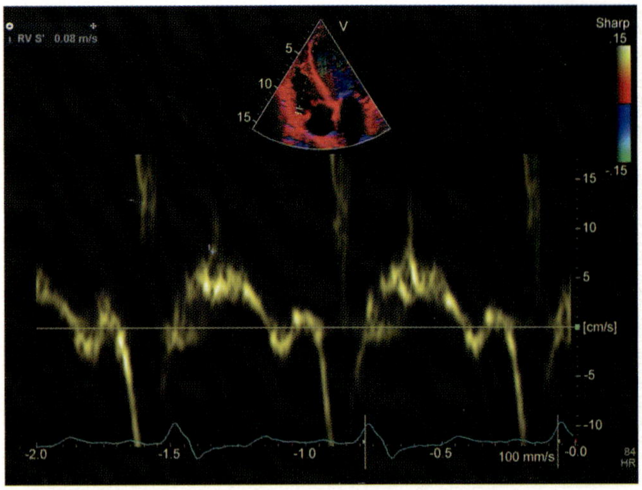

Fig. 16: TDI of the tricuspid annular velocities showing reduced S' (systolic) velocity in a case of DCM with reduced RV systolic function.

mechanisms of MR and TR can be better evaluated using 3D echocardiography, especially using en face views of these valves which are often not obtainable with conventional 2D echocardiography.
- 3D echocardiography allows more comprehensive evaluation of intracardiac thrombi (or any other masses), and myocardial noncompaction.
- 3D echocardiography provides the most accurate evaluation of LV ejection fraction, as compared to all other echocardiographic methods (Fig. 18). This technique also allows the calculation of RV ejection fraction, which is not possible by other echocardiographic methods.

Speckle Tracking Echocardiography

- The use of speckle tracking echocardiography (STE) allows the study of myocardial mechanics, providing greater insight into abnormalities of myocardial contraction and relaxation.
- In general, the global longitudinal strain will be reduced in all myocardial segments of the LV, though in some cases, there may be marked regional variations in the segmental strain values (Fig. 19).
- Disrupted myocardial mechanics may be evident in the form of post systolic strain developing in some myocardial segments. There may also be marked variations in the time to peak systolic strain in various segments, reflecting pronounced myocardial dyssynchrony.

Ultrasound Enhancing (Contrast) Agents

- Agitated saline contrast can be used to study the right sided chambers, to better visualize their dimensions in

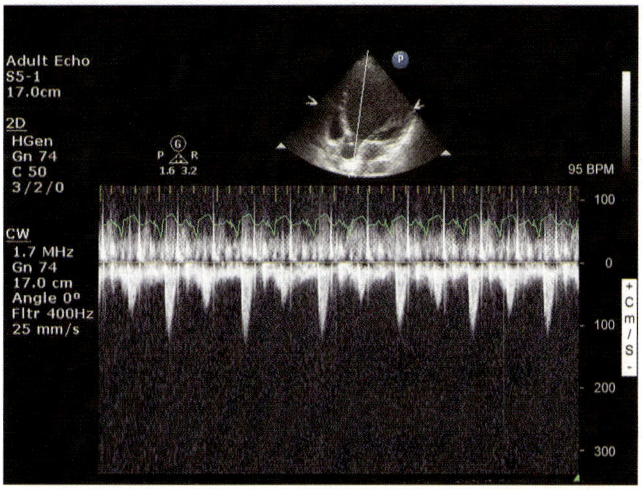

Fig. 17: CW Doppler across the aortic valve showing alternating higher and lower velocities due to mechanical alternans in the case of DCM with severe LV systolic dysfunction.

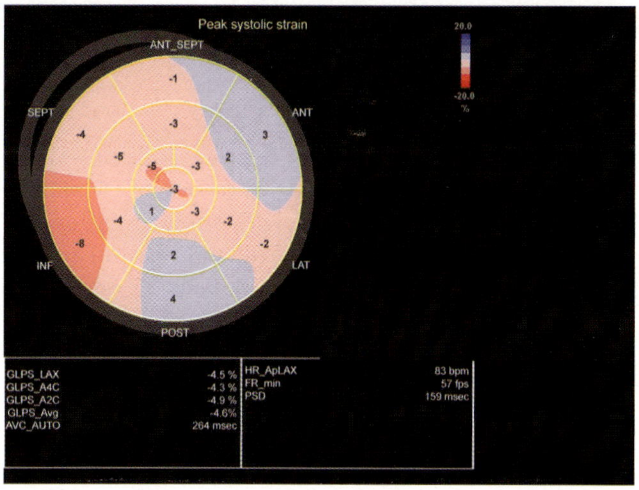

Fig. 19: Using speckle tracking echocardiography to calculate global longitudinal strain (GLS), in this patient with DCM, the GLS is 4.6%, which is severely reduced.

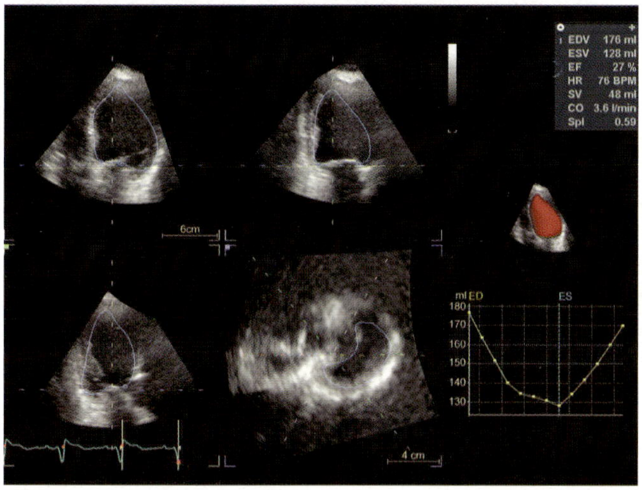

Fig. 18: 3D calculation of LV ejection fraction in the case of DCM. This is the most accurate echocardiographic technique for the calculation of LVEF.

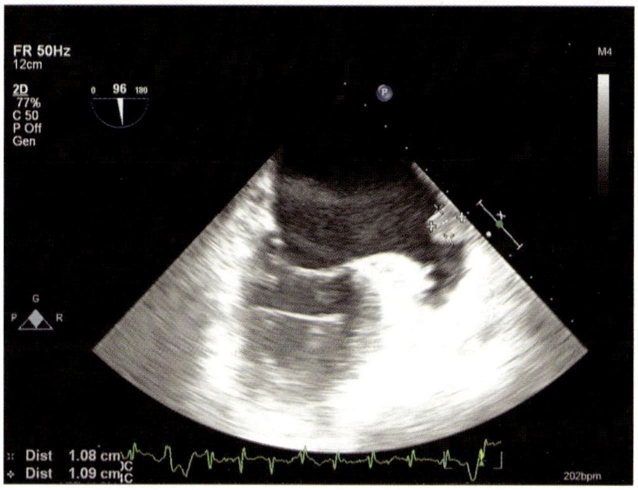

Fig. 20: LA appendage thrombus detected by TEE.

patients with limited acoustic windows. Any thrombi or other masses in the right sided chambers may be better visualized using an injection of agitated saline. The velocity and gradient of a TR jet can also be more accurately measured using this technique if a clear signal of TR cannot be obtained without the use of contrast. Unsuspected patent foramen ovale (PFO) or shunts at the atrial, ventricular or pulmonary vascular level may also be unmasked. [9]

- Ultrasound enhancing agents who can pass through the pulmonary circulation to the left side of the heart after an intravenous injection are useful for allowing endocardial surface definition in patients with suboptimal acoustic windows (LV opacification, LVO). More accurate calculation of LV volumes and ejection fraction thus become possible. Intracardiac masses such as thrombi, and LV noncompaction can also be more easily identified.[10]

Transesophageal Echocardiography

- Transesophageal echocardiography (TEE) is particularly useful for assessment of valvular abnormalities, especially the MV and TV. The mechanism of valvular regurgitation can be confirmed, especially with 3D TEE.
- The presence of thrombi or vegetations can be confirmed (Fig. 20).
- In patients with prosthetic valves, TEE allows superb visualization of the valves and their functioning.

Echocardiography in a Few Specific Variants of DCM

Familial DCM

It is now recognized that 20–35% of all cases of DCM may have a familial background.[4] The expression of DCM may vary among family members, with some manifesting the disease, while others may have a normal heart. Echocardiography provides a readily available screening tool for families where the disease is suspected.

Left Ventricular Noncompaction

Ventricular myocardial noncompaction occurs most commonly in the left ventricle, though, it may involve both ventricles or rarely may involve only the right ventricle. Criteria for the diagnosis of left ventricular noncompaction have been described.[11] These criteria help in the echocardiographic diagnosis of LV noncompaction. The condition may have a genetic cause,[12] however, the mere presence of noncompaction may not be associated with the DCM phenotype. 3D echocardiography provides additional help in the diagnosis of LV noncompaction,[13] as does the use of ultrasound enhancing agents.[10]

Chemotherapy-induced Cardiomyopathy

The anthracyclines are well known as cardiotoxic agents. It is incumbent upon treating physicians to monitor cardiac functions for any deterioration during chemotherapy with such agents. While a multimodality imaging approach is recommended in this situation[14] echocardiography is the most easily available imaging modality which can also be used for serial follow-up of such patients. With the advent of speckle tracking echocardiography for evaluation of myocardial strain using 2D echocardiography, it has become possible to detect subclinical myocardial toxicity before there are obvious changes in LV systolic function or chamber dimensions.[15]

IMPLICATIONS FOR FURTHER INVESTIGATIONS AND MANAGEMENT

- Cardiac magnetic resonance (CMR) imaging can help confirm the diagnosis of DCM. It can also be used to detect the presence of myocardial inflammation, as in viral myocarditis, and track the regression of the inflammation with treatment.[16] It is also helpful in the diagnosis of conditions such as amyloidosis, sarcoidosis, storage disorders, hemochromatosis, etc., which can present with the DCM phenotype.
- Exercise testing can document the exercise capacity of patients of DCM, and serial testing can be used to assess improvement or deterioration. It is also helpful in deciding the timing of heart transplantation.
- Cardiac catheterization is useful in selected cases to confirm pulmonary artery pressures and assess reversibility of elevated PA pressure in candidates being considered for cardiac transplantation. Coronary angiography will be useful in excluding coronary artery disease as a cause of the dilated cardiomyopathy.
- Endomyocardial biopsy is useful in patients where there is a suspicion of sarcoidosis, storage disorders, malignant disorders or hemochromatosis. It is also useful in patients after cardiac transplantation for early detection of graft rejection.
- Standard treatment for heart failure should be instituted including diuretics, angiotensin converting enzyme inhibitors (ACEI) or angiotensin receptor blockers (ARB), beta blockers, and digoxin in selected cases. Antiarrhythmics and anticoagulants should be used where indicated.
- In selected patients, the use of cardiac resynchronization therapy (CRT) devices, with or without defibrillator function, can provide substantial benefits.[17] Echocardiography can provide evidence of cardiac dyssynchrony, using M mode, 2D, tissue Doppler and STE parameters. Implantable cardioverter defibrillators (ICD) are now a recommended therapy in patients with DCM and poor LV systolic function, especially those with nonsustained VT or survivors of cardiac arrest.
- Left ventricular assist devices (LVAD) can help reduce the burden on the failing left ventricle. These devices can be used as a bridge to recovery in patients with a reversible cause of DCM, or as a bridge to transplantation in patients awaiting cardiac transplantation. Echocardiography is an essential part of the LVAD implantation process. Candidate selection is dependent on echocardiography. TEE is used in the preimplantation period, in the perioperative period, and during initial LVAD activation and speed optimization. Echocardiography is also routinely used after LVAD implantation for surveillance of LVAD function, and to monitor cardiac function during speed changes.[18]
- In end stage cardiac failure, cardiac transplantation provides the only hope. However, availability of organs for transplantation and facilities where these surgeries can be carried out are a limiting factor.

PROGNOSIS

Many options are now available for the treatment of DCM. Newer drugs allow better control of heart failure and improve the quality of life. The advent of devices such as CRT-D, ICD, and LVAD can improve the quality of life and decrease mortality. Cardiac transplantation, though, not easily available, can give a new lease of life to patients who are fortunate enough to be able to have the surgery.

REFERENCES

1. Maron BJ, Towbin JA, Thiene G, et al. Contemporary definitions and classification of the cardiomyopathies. An American Heart Association Scientific Statement From the Council on Clinical Cardiology, Heart Failure and Transplantation Committee; Quality of Care and Outcomes Research and Functional Genomics and Translational Biology Interdisciplinary Working Groups; and Council on Epidemiology and Prevention. Circulation. 2006;113:1807-16.
2. Elliott P, Andersson B, Arbustini E, et al. Classification of the cardiomyopathies: a position statement from the European Society of Cardiology working group on myocardial and pericardial diseases. Eur Heart J. 2008;29(2):270-6.
3. Mathew T, Williams L, Navaratnam G, et al. Diagnosis and assessment of dilated cardiomyopathy: a guideline protocol from the British Society of Echocardiography. Echo Res Pract. 2017;4(2):G1-G13.
4. Hershberger RE, Morales A, Siegfried JD. Clinical and genetic issues in dilated cardiomyopathy: a review for genetics professionals. Genet Med. 2010;12(11):655-67.
5. Yancy CW, Jessup M, Bozkurt B, et al. 2013 ACCF/AHA guideline for the management of heart failure. J Am Coll Cardiol. 2013;62(16):e147-239.
6. Mathew T, Williams L, Navaratnam G, et al. Diagnosis and assessment of dilated cardiomyopathy: a guideline protocol from the British Society of Echocardiography. Echo Res Pract. 2017;4(2):G1-G13.
7. Lang RM, Badano LP, Mor-Avi V, et al. Recommendations for cardiac chamber quantification by echocardiography in adults: an update from the American Society of Echocardiography and the European Association of Cardiovascular Imaging. J Am Soc Echocardiogr. 2015;28(1):1-39.
8. Nagueh SF, Smiseth OA, Appleton CP, et al. Recommendations for the evaluation of left ventricular diastolic function by echocardiography: an update from the American Society of Echocardiography and the European Association of Cardiovascular Imaging. J Am Soc Echocardiogr. 2016; 29:277-314.
9. Porter TR, Abdelmoneim S, Belcik JT , et al. Guidelines for the cardiac sonographer in the performance of contrast echocardiography: a focused update from the American Society of Echocardiography. J Am Soc Echocardiogr. 2014; 27:797-810.
10. Porter TR, Mulvagh SL, Abdelmoneim SS, et al. Clinical applications of ultrasonic enhancing agents in echocardiography: 2018 American Society of Echocardiography Guidelines Update. J Am Soc Echocardiogr. 2018; 31(3):241-74.
11. Jenni R, Oechslin E, Schneider J, et al. . Echocardiographic and pathoanatomical characteristics of isolated left ventricular non-compaction: a step towards classification as a distinct cardiomyopathy. Heart 2001; 86:666-71.
12. Arbustini E, Favalli V, Narula N, et al. Left ventricular noncompaction A distinct genetic cardiomyopathy? J Am Coll Cardiol. 2016;68(9):949-66.
13. Bodiwala K, Miller AP, Nanda NC, et al. Live three - dimensional transthoracic echocardiographic assessment of ventricular non compaction. Echocardiography. 2005: 22(7):611-20.
14. Plana JC, Galderisi M, Barac A, et al. Expert consensus for multimodality imaging evaluation of adult patients during and after cancer therapy: a report from the American Society of Echocardiography and the European Association of Cardiovascular Imaging. J Am Soc Echocardiogr. 2014; 27(9):911-39.
15. Thavendiranathan P, Poulin F, Lim KD, et al. Use of myocardial strain imaging by echocardiography for the early detection of cardiotoxicity in patients during and after cancer chemotherapy: a systematic review. J Am Coll Cardiol. 2014;63:2751-68.
16. Olimulder M A, van ES J, Galjee M A. The importance of cardiac MRI as a diagnostic tool in viral myocarditis induced cardiomyopathy. Neth Heart J. 2009;17:481-6.
17. Bristow MR, Saxon LA, Boehmer J, et al. Cardiac-resynchronisation therapy with or without an implantable defibrillator in advanced chronic heart failure. N Engl J Med. 2004;350:2140-50.
18. Stainback RF, Estep JD, Agler DA, et al. Echocardiography in the management of patients with left ventricular assist devices: recommendations from the American Society of Echocardiography. J Am Soc Echocardiogr. 2015;28: 853-909.

CHAPTER 81

ICD/CRT Evaluation in DCMP by Echocardiography

Nitin Burkule

The present evidence-based guidelines for selection of patients for cardiac resynchronization therapy (CRT), from various cardiology, electrophysiology and heart failure societies are concurrent on following criteria:[1]

- QRS ≥ 130 msec with left bundle branch block (LBBB) morphology
- QRS ≥ 150 msec with non-LBBB morphology
- NYHA class II-III or ambulatory class IV on optimal guideline directed medical therapy
- Left ventricular ejection fraction (LVEF) ≤ 35.

The echocardiographic criteria of CRT response are LV reverse remodeling (RR) measured as more than 15% reduction in LV end-systolic volume (LVESV) and improvement in LVEF more than 10% point. The clinical criteria of CRT response are improved by more than 10% in Minnesota living with heart failure questionnaire score, peak oxygen consumption (VO_2 max), or 6 minutes walking distance.

The current selection criteria do not need echocardiographic dyssynchrony assessment and rely entirely on QRS duration. The electrocardiographic (ECG) criteria based on QRS duration are not robust. The CRT responder rate can vary from 50–70% for different QRS intervals (Fig. 1).[2] Across 15 large, randomized control trials of CRT, the average responder rate was 66.9% by clinical criteria and 56.9% by echocardiographic criteria.

The earlier echocardiographic dyssynchrony imaging criteria used following time delay indices for assessing intraventricular, interventricular and atrioventricular dyssynchrony:

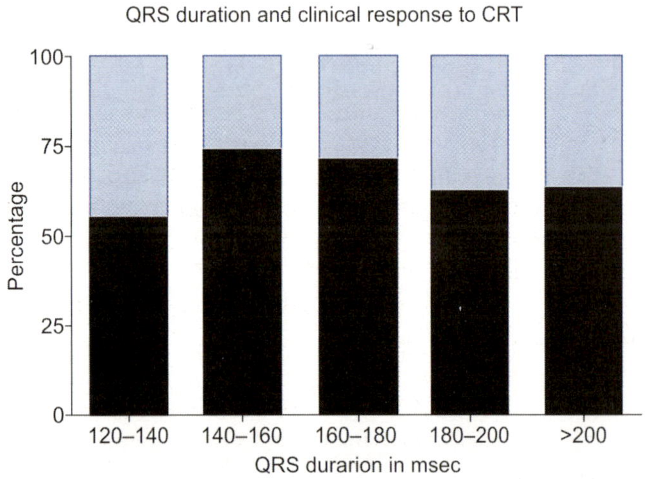

Fig. 1: The CRT responder rate depending upon QRS duration. The black shaded column represent percentage of patients with clinical response to CRT. Adapted from Bax et al.[2]

- M-Mode (Septal-posterior wall delay)
- Tissue Doppler imaging (TDI) peak velocity or strain delays in septum-posterolateral wall or standard deviation (SD) for 12 segments.
- Two-dimensional (2D) peak strain delays in septum-posterolateral wall: Longitudinal strain (LS), Radial strain (RS), Circumferential strain (CS)
- 3D-minimal volume time delays in 12 segments.
- Pulse wave (PW) Doppler intervals: Aortic and pulmonary preejection periods (PEP)/isovolumic contraction time (IVCT)/isovolumic relaxation time (IVRT)

The most comprehensive single center, single reader study, performed by Miyazaki et al.,[3] prospectively evaluated 131 patients, pre-and post-CRT implantation for the prognostic value of all these parameters for the CRT response. The overall CRT responder rate in their study was 55%. The various parameters performed poorly with the true positive rates varying from 60-80% and false negative rates varying from 20% and 50%, thereby showing no clinical utility (Fig. 2). The multicenter PROSPECT trial,[4] prospectively evaluated 498 patients by 12 echocardiographic time delay dyssynchrony parameters. The echo parameters failed to predict CRT clinical response (sensitivity 6–74%, specificity 35–91% for various parameters) or echocardiographic response of reverse remodeling (sensitivity 9–77%, specificity 31–93% for various parameters).

The classical LV apical rocking motion in LBBB, perceived visually in four chamber views on echocardiography has been shown to be a simple predictor of CRT response. The apical rocking integrates information on mechanical dyssynchrony and scar burden and is predictive of clinical response and long-term survival following CRT. The Apical rocking is quantified as percentage of cardiac cycle when TDI displacement curves of septal and lateral walls show discordance. Apical rocking more than 31% or diastolic filling time less than or equal to 39% showed sensitivity of 95%, specificity of 80%, positive predictive value (PPV) of 83% and negative predictive value (NPV) of 94% for predicting CRT response.[5] In another study,[6] the apical rocking more than 1.5 mm at baseline, predicted CRT response with sensitivity of 92%, specificity of 84%, PPV of 92%, and NPV of 84%. Interestingly, the quantitative increase in apical rocking by dobutamine stress echocardiography was also a strong predictor of CRT response and long-term survival.[6]

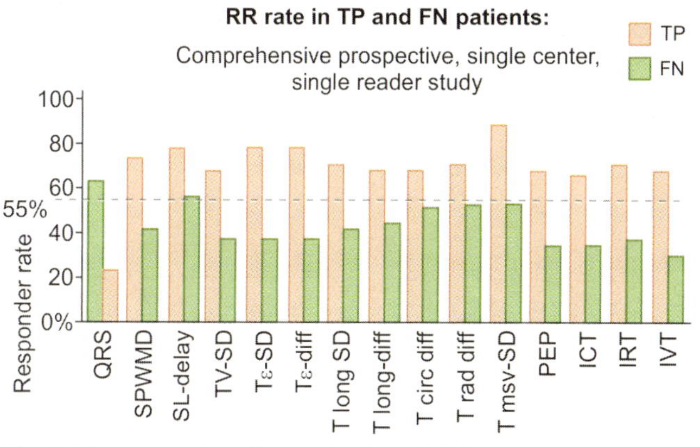

Fig. 2: The comprehensive evaluation of all the echocardiographic time delay parameters for prediction of CRT response. The X-axis shows the various parameters evaluated and Y-axis shows the percentage. The red bars denote False Negative rates and the light green bars denote True Positive rates for each parameter.

The radial strain delay parameters appear to be more robust than TDI derived time delay indices. In Speckle Tracking and Resynchronization (STAR) study[7] of 132 patients with NYHA class III and IV, LV EF less than or equal to 35% and QRS more than or equal to 120 milliseconds, undergoing CRT implantation, the radial, circumferential and transverse and longitudinal strains were analyzed. The Radial, and transverse strain delay more than or equal to 130 milliseconds in septal-posterolateral walls was predictive of CRT response and clinical outcome. The patients with radial and transverse strain delay more than 130 milliseconds predicted EF rise more than 15% with sensitivity of 86% and specificity of 67%. On Post-CRT follow up clinical adverse events (death, need of heart transplant or LV assist device) were 12 % if pre-CRT Radial and Transverse strain delays were more than 130 milliseconds compared to 53% if strain delays were less than 130 msec. The radial strain delay more than 130 msec is also a useful parameter for predicting CRT response across various wide QRS morphologies. In a study[8] of 254 patients, the radial strain delay was present in 85% of 128 patients with LBBB, 59% of 81 patients with intraventricular conduction delay (IVCD), 40% of 45 patients with RBBB. As expected, post-CRT clinical outcome was progressively worse in the three groups of patients with LBBB, IVCD and RBBB. However, the post-CRT reduction in clinical adverse events (death, heart transplant or LV assist device implantation) and positive echocardiographic response (increase in LV EF and reduction in LV ESV) was equivalent in patients with LBBB and patients with non-LBBB QRS widening but with radial strain delay more than 130 msec.

Despite the inconsistent results of various echocardiographic mechanical dyssynchrony measurements to predict CRT response, there is strong evidence to suggest that CRT works through correcting mechanical dyssynchrony itself (Figs. 3A and B). In the posthoc analysis[9] of MADIT-CRT trial, for every quartile reduction of post-CRT mechanical dyssynchrony there was progressively increasing gain in the LV global longitudinal strain. For every 20 msec reduction in post-CRT dyssynchrony, there was 7% reduction in congestive heart failure (CHF) and death. In the STARTER trial[10] the event free survival (freedom from CHF hospitalization or death) over 2 years was approximately 90% for patients who showed post-CRT more than 50% reduction in mechanical dyssynchrony (assessed by radial strain delays) compared to approximately 60% event free survival for patients who showed post-CRT less than 50% reduction in mechanical dyssynchrony. The Echo-CRT trial[11] showed no benefit of CRT in patients with QRS duration less than 130 msec and

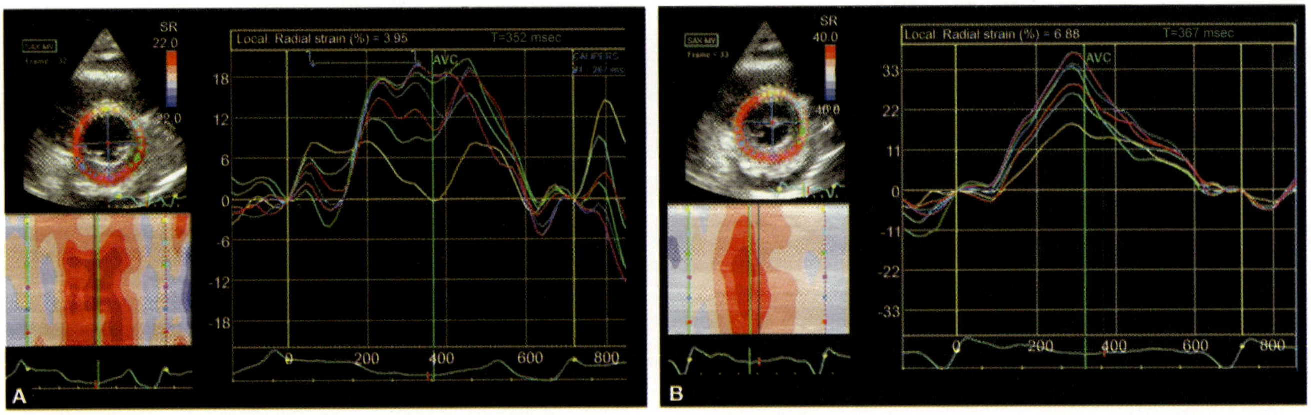

Figs. 3A and B: The 2D strain curves of 6 LV basal segments in a patient with dilated cardiomyopathy, LBBB and CRT implantation with (A) CRT turned off, (B) CRT turned on. There is immediate complete restoration of synchrony of all the strain curves when CRT is turned on suggesting that CRT works through restoration of mechanical synchrony.

echo derived mechanical dyssynchrony. However, post-CRT TDI derived longitudinal velocity delay more than or equal to 80 msec or 2D strain imaging derived radial strain delay more than or equal to 130 msec in opposite walls was strongly associated with death and HF hospitalizations.

The 2D Strain derived dyssynchrony delays are longer than electrical delays. There are following components of electro-mechanical delay as measured by strain over time curves:[12]

- Electrical conduction delay "primary electrical dyssynchrony"
- Excitation–contraction coupling
- Regional delay in time to peak shortening "primary mechanical dyssynchrony"

Only electrical delays are corrected favorably by CRT implantation. There are several conjectural reasons for the inconsistency of mechanical dyssynchrony measured by echocardiography in predicting CRT response:[13]

1. The time-delay indices measured by Doppler, TDI, 2D strain are suboptimal due to technical factors. The time-delay indices also do not account for the recruitable work of the early or late contracting segments.
2. It is highly likely that in many cases, the CRT delivery is suboptimal due to technical reasons thereby defeating the purpose of stimulating the delayed contracting segments.
3. The CRT may not be beneficial in patients with very advanced LV remodeling. A multiparametric Echo-score[14,15] has been proposed to predict the advanced LV remodeling unsuitable for CRT. The echo parameters, their threshold values, and assigned score are shown in Table 1. A score more than 17 predicts post CRT reverse remodeling with sensitivity of 84% and specificity of 79%.

TABLE 1: Multiparametric ECHO score to predict CRT response.

Parameter	Cut off	Score
LV end-diastolic diameter	<3.1 cm/m^2	6
LV global longitudinal	< 7%	6
Strainleft atrial area	< 26 cm^2	1
RV end-diastolic area	< 10 cm^2/m^2	2
RV fractional area change	> 35%	20
RA area	< 20 cm^2	2

4. CRT corrects only the electrical delays in activation of various LV segments. However, after electromechanical coupling, the LV segments have variable time to peak strain depending upon the variable extent of myopathic process in these segments (Figs. 4A and B).
5. As underlying disease progresses the electromechanical coupling to peak strain delays in different LV segments change over time causing loss of CRT response (Figs. 5A to C).

The focus for echo evaluation has shifted to two different aspects of dyssynchrony as follows:

1. The measurement of wasted or nonejection work which takes into account not only the time delays of these LV segments but also the contractility status and viability of these segments.
2. Identification of the latest activating LV segment and its contractile status and viability to guide the LV lead placement to target the latest activating.

There is growing realization of the uneven distribution of work due to dyssynchrony.[12] The septum due to early activation faces the lowest wall stress and performs significant nonejection work before the opening of the aortic valve. The posterolateral wall due to delayed activation faces higher wall stress and performs significant nonejection work

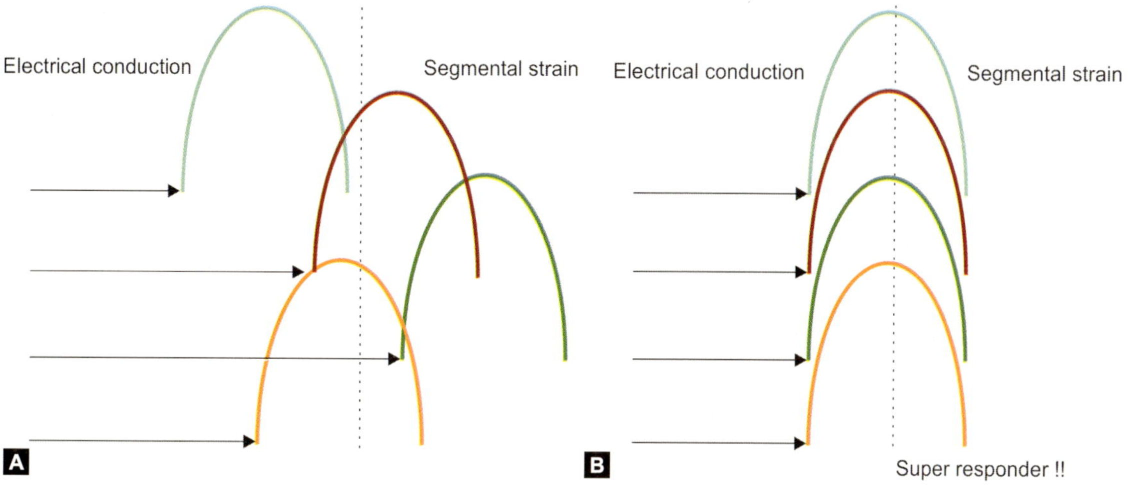

Figs. 4A and B: The concept of primary electrical and primary mechanical delay. CRT corrects electrical delays and if time to peak strain after electromechanical coupling is similar in various segments complete mechanical synchronization can be achieved. (A) Pre-CRT (B) Post-CRT

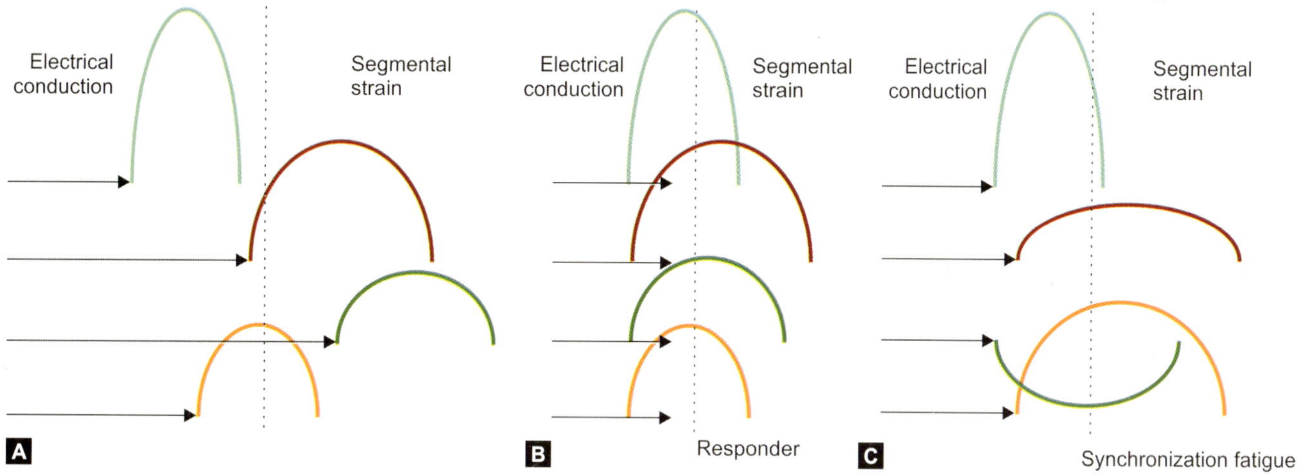

Figs. 5A to C: The concept of variable primary electrical and primary mechanical delays (time to peak strain after electromechanical coupling) in various LV segments in advanced cardiomyopathy. (A) Pre-CRT. (B) Immediate Post-CRT near total resynchronization. (C) Post-CRT late follow-up complete loss of synchrony due to variable extent of myopathic process in various segments.

or postsystolic shortening after the closure of the aortic valve (Fig. 6). If the nonejection work gets synchronized, the overall LV performance can improve.

The surrogate measure for the delay and contractility of all the LV segments is called Strain-delay index (SDI) either measured for longitudinal strain (Fig. 7) or radial strain (Fig. 8). The difference in the peak strain and end-systolic strain (at aortic valve closure) for each of the 6 basal and 6 mid LV segments are calculated and then summated to get the Strain delay index. The segment generating good strain but an early or a delayed strain peak has higher recruitable work to contribute to global LV function after resynchronization. Lim et al.[16] showed SDI for longitudinal strain more than 25% identified 82% responders and 92% nonresponders for CRT. Kydd et al.[17] showed SDI for radial strain more than 40% had Sensitivity 89%, Specificity 84%, PPV 84%. NPV 85% in predicting CRT responders. The wasted work can also be calculated more objectively by subtracting the strain time integral[18] at end systole (aortic valve closure) from the strain time integral at peak strain for every LV segment (Fig. 9).

Systolic rebound stretch in the septal wall (SRS) in LBBB is the sum of the positive strains (stretch) which develop during systole in the septum before aortic valve closure (Fig. 10). It measures the amount of premature termination of systolic shortening and the post-shortening systolic stretching in the early activated segments. It is highly specific for asynchronous activation of septum and gives better differentiation between ischemic and nonischemic

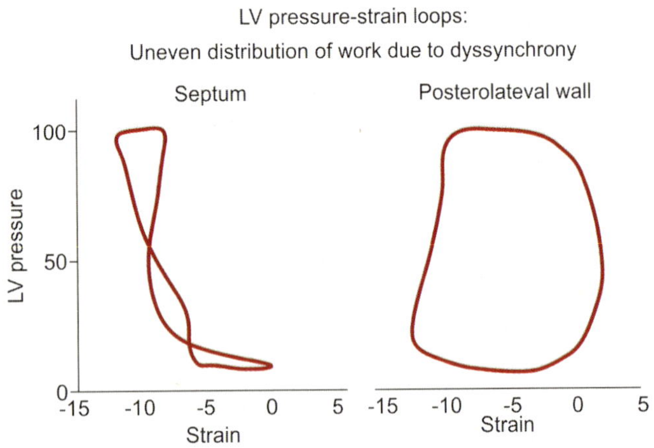

Fig. 6: LV pressure-strain loop during cardiac cycle in septum and posterolateral wall showing nonuniform distribution of work and wall stress in patient with LBBB.

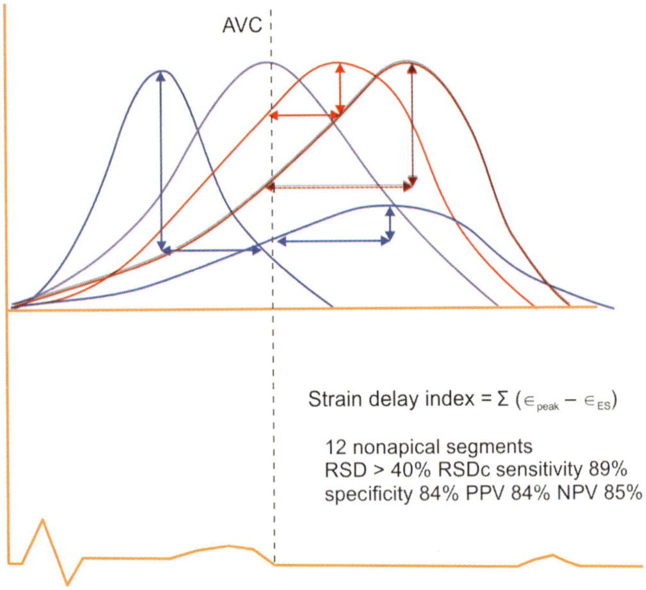

Fig. 8: Schematic drawing of LV radial strain-time curves. The Strain Delay Index is better predictor of recruitable work after re-synchronization.

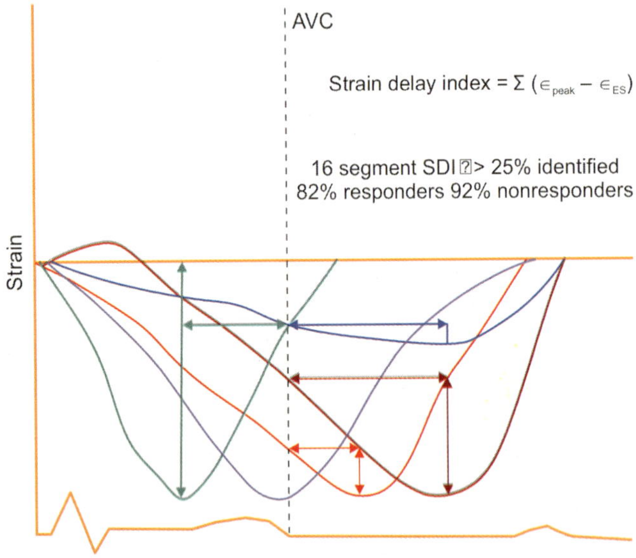

Fig. 7: Schematic drawing of LV longitudinal strain-time curves. The Strain Delay Index is better predictor of recruitable work after re-synchronization.

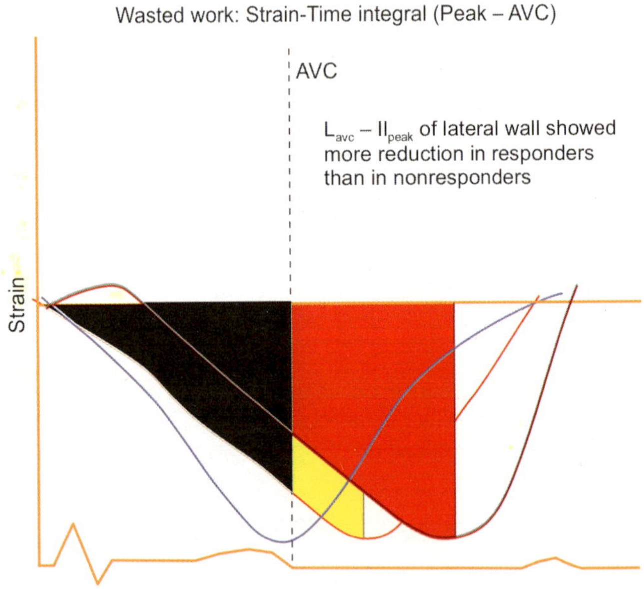

Fig. 9: Schematic drawing of LV longitudinal strain-time integrals. The shaded area red and yellow shows wasted post systolic work which is recruitable after resynchronizations.

cause of LV dysfunction. SRS more than 4.7% was strongly associated with LV reverse remodeling compared to time delay indices.[19]

In conventional CRT implantation, the LV lead is positioned under fluoroscopic guidance in the available coronary sinus tributary draining from the remote posterolateral wall. The concept of identifying latest activating segment with good contractile reserve by 2D strain echocardiography before CRT implantation can help in attempting to target the LV lead precisely to this segment. The LV basal and midsegment radial strain maps can identify the latest activating segment (Fig. 11).

The LV short Axis images are analyzed by 2D strain at mid and basal segments. The radial strain curves are inspected for the latest activating segment with radial strain >10%. The left anterior oblique (LAO) view on fluoroscopy

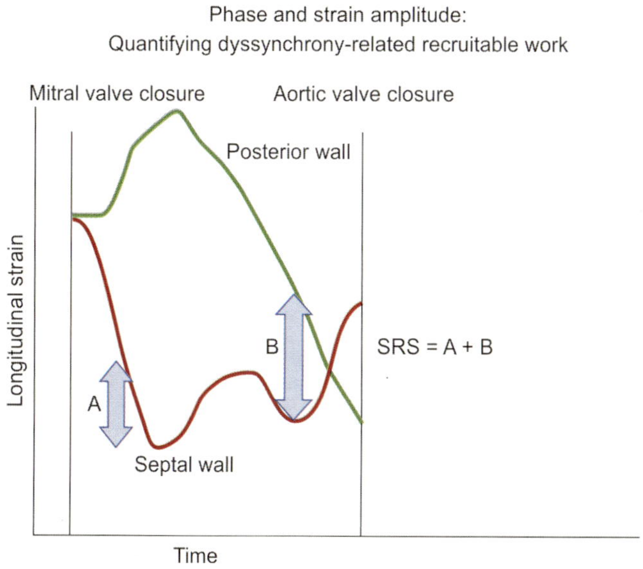

Fig. 10: Schematic diagram showing systolic rebound stretch on septal wall strain-time curve in patient with LBBB. The sum of positive strains in midsystole (A) and late systole (B) gives SRS value.

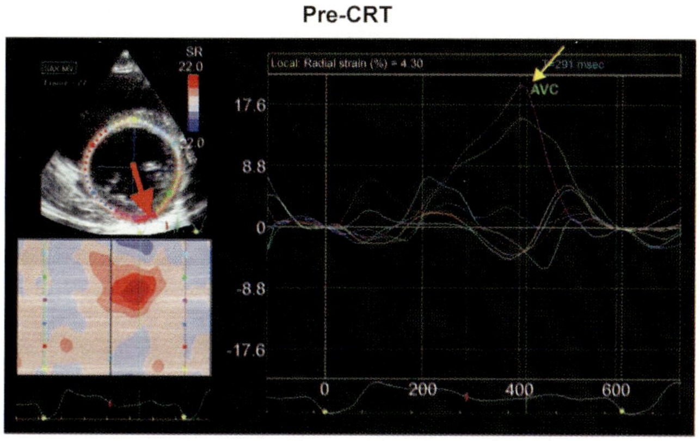

Fig. 11: The radial strain curves from 6 LV basal segments. The yellow arrow shows the strain curve and the red arrow shows the location of the latest activating segment with good contractility.

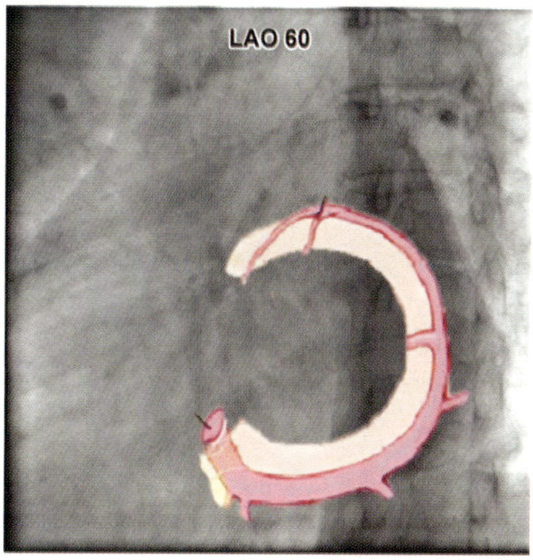

Fig. 12: The left anterior oblique (LAO) view on fluoroscopy profiles the coronary sinus in the atrioventricular groove.

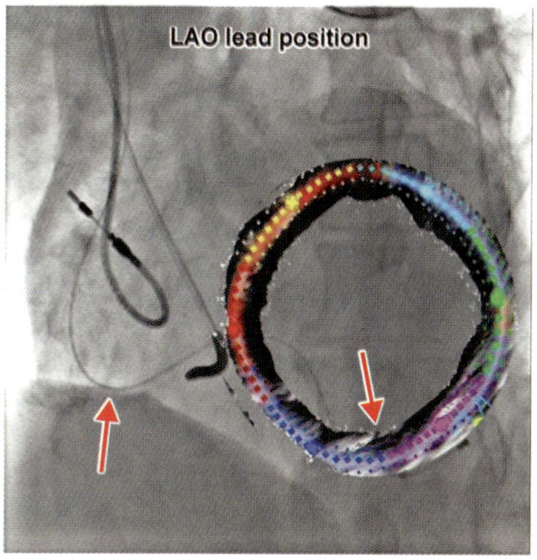

Fig. 13: The superimposition of the LV short axis parametric strain image on fluoroscopic LAO view. The red arrows show the positioning of the LV lead.

corresponds to the LV short Axis view and also profiles the coronary sinus in the atrioventricular groove (Fig. 12). The approximate location of the target tributary, draining from the desired segment, for lodging the LV lead can be identified. (Fig. 13). The right anterior oblique view (RAO) on fluoroscopy corresponds to the long axis view of the LV and profiles the tributaries of the coronary sinus (Fig. 14). The desired basal or midsegment location can be ascertained in this view (Fig. 15).

The radial strain less than10% has been shown to correlate with no Technetium sestamibi uptake on nuclear SPECT (sensitivity 77% and specificity 89%).[20] The latest activating segment should have at least more than 10% radial strain to avoid scar and have meaningful recruitment of myocardial work. Pacing in the scar has been shown to be associated with higher mortality.[20] In one post-CRT study,[21] if LV Pacing was achieved concordant to latest activating segment with contractile reserve the CRT responder rate was as high as 90%. However, LV pacing in nonconcordant segment with no contractile reserve, the CRT nonresponder rate was as high as 90%.

In the STARTER trial[22] (187 patients) and TARGET trial[23] (220 patients) Echo-guidance achieved higher rates of concordant or adjacent LV lead placements in latest

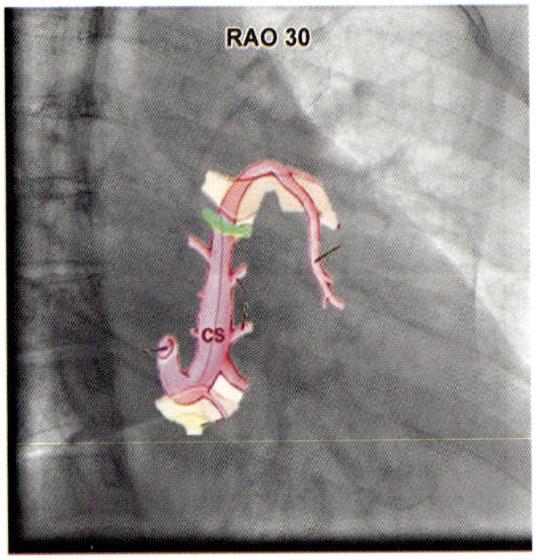

Fig. 14: The right anterior oblique view (RAO) on fluoroscopy profiles the tributaries of the coronary sinus.

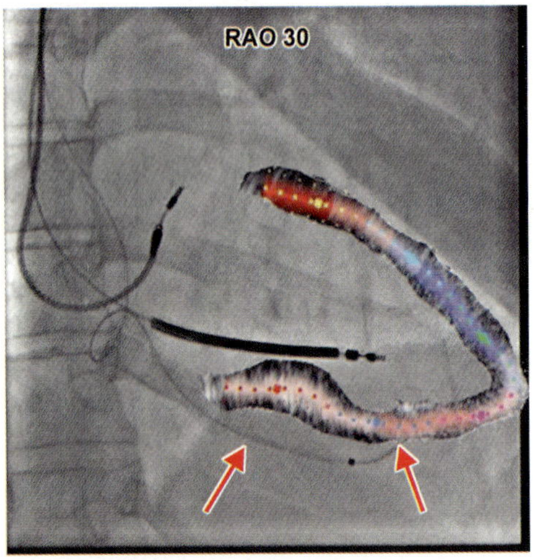

Fig. 15: The superimposition of the LV long axis parametric strain image on fluoroscopic RAO view. The red arrows show the positioning of the LV lead.

activating viable segments (Table 2). It is interesting to note the distribution of latest activating segment on 2D radial strain analysis of LV basal and midsegments in both the trials. Approximately 22% and 28% latest activating segments in TARGET and STARTER trials respectively were not mid and basal lateral or posterolateral locations often targeted blindly by fluoroscopic guidance (Table 3). The echo guided LV lead strategy achieved resynchronization (> 50% reduction in radial strain delays) in 70% patients as opposed to only 48% by fluoroscopic guidance.[22] This translated into event free survival (freedom from CHF and death) 77% for Echo guided group versus 57% in fluoroscopy guided group over next 2 years (26% reduction in event). The overall 2 years event-free survival for the entire study population was 73% in all concordant or adjacent lead

TABLE 2: LV lead position achieved either by echo guidance or by fluoroscopy with respect to the latest activating segment on radial strain imaging.

STARTER trial			*TARGET trial*		
LV lead	Echo	Fluoroscopy	LV lead	Echo	Fluoroscopy
Concordant	30%	12%	Concordant	61%	45%
Concordant or adjacent	85%	66%	Concordant or adjacent	86%	73%
Remote	15%	33%	Remote	10%	24 %

TABLE 3: The frequency of latest activating LV segments on 2D radial strain imaging in pre-CRT assessment.

Starter Trial Latest Activating Segment		*Target Trial Latest Activating Segment Echo Fluoroscopy*		
Basal Anterolateral	(4%)	Basal Anterolateral	(3%)	(3%)
Basal Lateral	(12%)	Basal Lateral	(13%)	(11%)
Basal Posterolateral	(20%)	Basal Posterolateral	(14%)	(15%)
Basal Posterior	(11%)	Basal Posterior	(4%)	(5%)
Mid-Anterolateral	(3%)	Mid-Anterolateral	(6%)	(4%)
Mid-Lateral	(15%)	Mid-Lateral	(19%)	(20%)
Mid-Posterolateral	(25%)	Mid-Posterolateral	(24%)	(26%)
Mid-Posterior	(10%)	Mid-Posterior	(9%)	(9%)

placements versus 46% in all remote lead placements irrespective of the echo or fluoroscopy strategy (37% reduction in event rates).[22]

The exact concordant LV leads may not be achieved in 30% of patients due to various factors:[24]

- Lack of suitable coronary veins (68%)
- LV lead instability (13%)
- Phrenic nerve stimulation (10%)
- Insufficient LV pacing capture (10%)
- Excluded LV target segments due to low-amplitude ST-RS signals anterior (7%), lateral (1%) posterior (7%).

Post-CRT implantation, Echo Doppler assessment can help fine tune the CRT pacing parameters like atrioventricular (AV) interval or interventricular (V-V) interval. This may help to get maximal LV stroke volume as measured by Doppler LV outflow (LVOT) velocity time integral (VTI) multiplied by LVOT cross-sectional area. The optimal AV delay in CRT patients exhibits great variability from patient to patient. AV optimization will not convert a nonresponder to a responder, but it may convert an under-responder to an improved status.[25] The optimal AV delay should provide the following:

- The best left atrial (LA) contribution to LV filling as seen by nontruncated and separate A wave on mitral flow spectral Doppler
- The maximum stroke volume as calculated by LVOT VTI
- Shortening of the isovolumic contraction phase as measured by PW spectral Doppler with sample volume placed at the interface of LV inflow and outflow.
- The longest diastolic filling time on mitral flow spectral Doppler
- No diastolic mitral regurgitation (MR).
- Maximal dP/dt on systolic MR.

Optimized AV synchrony is achieved by adjusting the AV delay by the external programmer and simultaneously performing Echo-Doppler study. Iterative method is the most commonly employed method for optimizing CRT pacing delays. This method involves programming a long AV delay and then shortening it by 20 millisecond increments, with simultaneously monitoring PW Doppler mitral flow until truncation of the A wave is noted. Optimal AV delay is then identified by lengthening the AV delay in 10 ms increments until A wave truncation is no longer present. Similar principle is used to optimize the V-V delay to shorten the bi-ventricular activation time. Generally, there is significant latency in activation of LV myocardium compared to RV. The RV lead is activated 20–40 millisecond later than the LV lead. The delay is adjusted progressively to get maximal stroke volume by LVOT VTI.

The RV dysfunction has powerful adverse effect on clinical outcome post-CRT.[26] The low tricuspid annular plane systolic excursion (TAPSE) values are associated with lower survival rates after CRT implantation. In the MADIT-CRT trial, the CRT-induced reduction of LV mechanical dyssynchrony was associated with reduction of ventricular tachycardia (VT) or ventricular fibrillation (VF) in patients with LBBB as compared to ICD patients.[27]

The present literature evidence suggests that the CRT response depends on many clinical, cardiac pathophysiological and procedural factors and not on single imaging parameter. The major factors determining the responder rates are as follows:[28,29]

- Morphology of QRS complex
- Substantial recruitable pre or postejection work due to mechanical dyssynchrony
- Global scar burden
- Lead position *vis-a-vis* Scar location and delayed activation
- Irreversibly advanced LV and RV remodeling
- AV and VV interval device optimization

A multimodality imaging approach may be useful to reduce the high number of nonresponder rate in CRT.[30] The Echocardiography can help in defining mechanical dyssynchrony in patients with wide QRS ECG and in ruling out advanced LV and RV remodeling. The latest activating LV segment can be identified on radial strain imaging. The cardiac magnetic resonance can quantify the total scar burden and can delineate the extent of transmural scarring in the segment of interest. The CT angiography of the coronary sinus can predefine the availability, take-off and tortuosity of the tributary located in the segment of interest and its proximity to phrenic nerve.[31] Such multimodality approach for pre-CRT evaluation should be prospectively tested for clinical efficacy and cost effectiveness.

We are still in search for echocardiography parameter with high specificity or high negative predictive value, on the basis of which CRT can be avoided in patients who qualify by conventional selection criteria.[13,15,32,33] The TDI or strain echo parameters have significant variability, poor reproducibility, and low positive predictive value. However, for health care cost savings and to avoid the unnecessary exposure to periprocedural complications, it is imperative to identify nonresponders prospectively. The current guidelines of CRT implantation are unlikely to be a sustainable strategy in the present global scenario of ever increasing health care expenditure.

CONCLUSION

In the patients with postmyocardial infarction (MI) LV dysfunction or nonischemic dilated cardiomyopathy (DCM) current indications of implantable cardioverter defibrillator ICD depend upon presence of LVEF less than 35%, nonsustained VT (NSVT) on 24 hour Holter, resuscitated cardiac arrest or unexplained syncope. The contraction heterogeneity in LV segments, seen on longitudinal strain analysis, is equivalent to inhomogeneous electrical conduction and repolarization in the myocardium (Fig. 16). The mechanical dispersion index can be derived from the time to peak strain analysis for all the LV myocardial segments. In a study[34] of 569 patients, 40 days after first MI, the mechanical dispersion index more than 75 msec was associated with significantly higher incidence of ventricular tachycardia or fibrillation. The global longitudinal strain numerically lower than 16% and mechanical dispersion index more than 75 msec increased the positive predictive value for occurrence of arrhythmia to 21% compared to 11% when only LVEF less than 35% parameter is considered. Similarly, in patients with nonischemic, DCM global longitudinal strain is numerically lower than 7% and mechanical dispersion index more than 72 msec was associated with significantly lower cumulative arrhythmia free survival and showed better area under the curve than the LVEF in predicting ventricular arrhythmia.[35]

LV mechanical dispersion

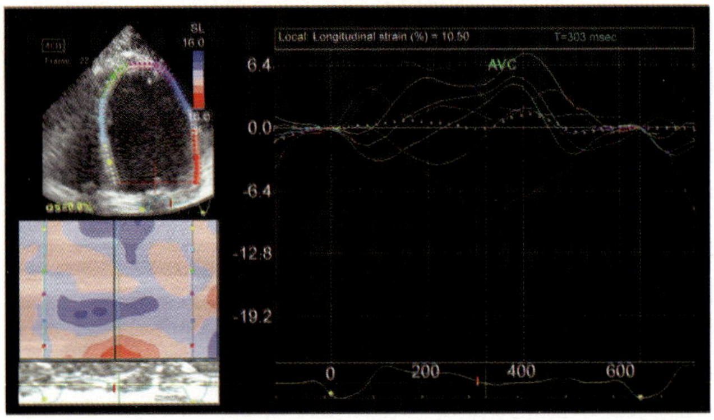

Fig. 16: The LV longitudinal strain-time curves in four chamber view. There is severe dispersion in time to peak strain (Mechanical dispersion) in the six LV segments.

REFERENCES

1. Normand C, Linde C, Singh J, et al. Indications for Cardiac Resynchronization Therapy A Comparison of the Major International Guidelines. J Am Coll Cardiol HF. 2018; 6:308-16.
2. Bax JJ, Gorcsan J. Echocardiography and Noninvasive Imaging in Cardiac Resynchronization Therapy Results of the PROSPECT (Predictors of Response to Cardiac Resynchronization Therapy) Study in Perspective. J Am Coll Cardiol. 2009;53:1933-43.
3. Miyazaki C, Redfield MM, Powell BD, et al. Dyssynchrony Indices To Predict Response to Cardiac Resynchronization Therapy A Comprehensive Prospective Single-Center Study. Circ Heart Fail. 2010;3:565-73.
4. Chung ES, Leon AR, Tavazzi L, et al. Results of the Predictors of Response to CRT (PROSPECT) Trial. Circ. 2008; 117: 2608-16.
5. Tournoux F, Singh JP, Chan RC, et al. Absence of left ventricular apical rocking and atrial-ventricular dyssynchrony predicts non-response to cardiac resynchronization therapy. Eur Heart J Cardiovasc Imaging . 2012;13(1):86-94.
6. Stankovic I, Aarones M, Smith HJ, et al. Dynamic relationship of left-ventricular dyssynchrony and contractile reserve in patients undergoing cardiac resynchronization therapy. Eur Heart J. 2014;35(1):48-55.
7. Tanaka H, Nesser HJ, Buck T, et al. Dyssynchrony by speckle-tracking echocardiography and response to cardiac resynchronization therapy: results of the Speckle Tracking and Resynchronization (STAR) study. Eur Heart J. 2010;31(14):1690-700.
8. Hara H, Oyenuga OA, Tanaka H, et al. The relationship of QRS morphology and mechanical dyssynchrony to long-term outcome following cardiac resynchronization therapy. Eur Heart J. 2012;33(21):2680-91.
9. Pouleur AC, Knappe D, Shah AM,, et al. Relationship between improvement in left ventricular dyssynchrony and contractile function and clinical outcome with cardiac resynchronization therapy: the MADIT-CRT trial. Eur Heart J. 2011;32(14):1720-9.
10. Saba S, Marek J, Schwartzman D, et al. Echocardiography-Guided Left Ventricular Lead Placement for Cardiac Resynchronization Therapy Results of the Speckle Tracking Assisted Resynchronization Therapy for Electrode Region Trial. Circ Heart Fail. 2013;6:427-34.
11. Gorcsan J, Sogaard P, Bax JJ et al. Association of persistent or worsened echocardiographic dyssynchrony with unfavourable clinical outcomes in heart failure patients with narrow QRS width: a subgroup analysis of the EchoCRT trial. Eur Heart J. 2016;37(1):49-59.
12. Smiseth OA, Russell K, Skulstad H. The role of echocardiography in quantification of left ventricular dyssynchrony: state of the art and future directions. Eur Heart J Cardiovasc Imaging. 2012;13(1):61-8.
13. Cleland JG, Tageldien A, Buga L, et al. Should We Be Trying to Define Responders to Cardiac Resynchronization Therapy? JACC Cardiovasc Imaging. 2010;3(5):541-9.
14. Park JH, Negishi K, Grimm RA, et al. Echocardiographic Predictors of Reverse Remodeling After Cardiac Resynchronization Therapy and Subsequent Events. Circ Cardiovasc Imaging. 2013;6(6):864-72.
15. Marwick TH. Selection for Cardiac Resynchronization Therapy All in a Flash? JACC Cardiovasc Imaging. 2014;7(10):980-2.
16. Lim P, Buakhamsri A, Popovic ZB, et al. Longitudinal Strain Delay Index by Speckle Tracking Imaging A New Marker of Response to Cardiac Resynchronization Therapy. Circulation. 2008;118(11):1130-7.
17. Kydd AC, Khan FZ, O'Halloran D, et al. Radial Strain Delay Based on Segmental Timing and Strain Amplitude Predicts Left Ventricular Reverse Remodeling and Survival After Cardiac Resynchronization Therapy. Circ Cardiovasc Imaging. 2013;6(2):177-84.
18. Bernard A, Donal E, Leclercq C, et al. Impact of Cardiac Resynchronization Therapy on Left Ventricular Mechanics: Understanding the Response through a New Quantitative Approach Based on Longitudinal Strain Integrals. J Am Soc Echocardiogr. 2015;28(6):700-8.
19. Chan YH, Wu LS, Kuo CT, et al. Incremental Value of Inefficient Deformation Indices for Predicting Response to Cardiac Resynchronization Therapy. J Am Soc Echocardiogr. 2013;26(3):307-15.
20. Sade LE, Saba S, Marek JJ, et al. The Association of Left Ventricular Lead Position Related to Regional Scar by Speckle-Tracking Echocardiography with Clinical Outcomes in Patients Receiving Cardiac Resynchronization Therapy. J Am Soc Echocardiogr. 2014;27(6):648-56.
21. Khan FZ, Virdee MS, Read PA, et al. Effect of Low-Amplitude Two-Dimensional Radial Strain at Left Ventricular Pacing Sites on Response to Cardiac Resynchronization Therapy. J Am Soc Echocardiogr. 2010;23(11):1168-76.
22. Saba S, Marek J, Schwartzman D, et al. Echocardiography-Guided Left Ventricular Lead Placement for Cardiac Resynchronization Therapy Results of the Speckle Tracking Assisted Resynchronization Therapy for Electrode Region Trial. Circ Heart Fail. 2013;6(3):427-34.

23. Khan FZ, Virdee MS, Palmer CR, et al. Targeted Left Ventricular Lead Placement to Guide Cardiac Resynchronization Therapy The TARGET Study: A Randomized, Controlled Trial. J Am Coll Cardiol. 2012;59(17):1509-18.
24. Kristiansen HM, Vollan G, Hovstad T, et al. The impact of left ventricular lead position on left ventricular reverse remodelling and improvement in mechanical dyssynchrony in cardiac resynchronization therapy. Eur Heart J Cardiovasc Imaging. 2012;13(12):991-1000.
25. Barold SS, Ilercil A, Herweg B. Echocardiographic optimization of the atrioventricular and interventricular intervals during cardiac resynchronization. Europace. 2008;10(Suppl 3):iii88-95.
26. Damy T, Ghio S, Rigby AS, et al. Interplay Between Right Ventricular Function and Cardiac Resynchronization Therapy An Analysis of the CARE-HF Trial (Cardiac Resynchronization–Heart Failure). J Am Coll Cardiol. 2013;61(21):2153-60.
27. Kutyifa V, Pouleur AC, Knappe D, et al. Dyssynchrony and the Risk of Ventricular Arrhythmias. JACC Cardiovasc Imaging. 2013;6(4):432-44.
28. Prinzen FW, Vernooy K, Auricchio A. Cardiac Resynchronization Therapy State-of-the-Art of Current Applications, Guidelines, Ongoing Trials, and Areas of Controversy. Circulation. 2013;128(22):2407-18.
29. Marwick TH. Use of Speckle-Strain in a Multiparametric Approach to Dyssynchrony Imaging. JACC Cardiovasc Imaging. 2011;4(4):375-7.
30. Sanderson JE. Echocardiography for Cardiac Resynchronization Therapy Selection Fatally Flawed or Misjudged? J Am Coll Cardiol. 2009;53(21):1960-4.
31. Van de Veire NR, Schuijf JD, De Sutter J, et al. Non-Invasive Visualization of the Cardiac Venous System in Coronary Artery Disease Patients Using 64-Slice Computed Tomography. J Am Coll Cardiol. 2006;48(9):1832-8.
32. Anderson LJ, Miyazaki C, Sutherland GR et al. Patient Selection and Echocardiographic Assessment of Dyssynchrony in Cardiac Resynchronization Therapy. Circulation. 2008;117(15):2009-23.
33. Hawkins NM, Petrie MC, Burgess MI, et al. Selecting Patients for Cardiac Resynchronization Therapy The Fallacy of Echocardiographic Dyssynchrony J Am Coll Cardiol. 2009;53:1944-59
34. Haugaa KH, Grenne BL, Eek CH, et al. Strain Echocardiography Improves Risk Prediction of Ventricular Arrhythmias After Myocardial Infarction. JACC Cardiovasc Imaging. 2013;6(8):841-50.
35. Haugaa KH, Goebel B, Dahlslett T, et al. Risk Assessment of Ventricular Arrhythmias in Patients with Nonischemic Dilated Cardiomyopathy by Strain Echocardiography. J Am Soc Echocardiogr. 2012;25(6):667-73.

82

CHAPTER

Echo-guided Dyssynchrony Evaluation in Dilated Cardiomyopathy

Rahul Mehrotra, Raj Kumar

INTRODUCTION

Heart failure (HF) is currently a major public health problem, with an estimated prevalence of 5.8 million in the United States and 23 million worldwide.[1] HF is a condition associated with significant mortality, morbidity, and healthcare expenditure, particularly among those aged more than or equal to 65 years of age.[1] Recurrent hospitalization is another major issue in patients surviving with HF. Despite the progress made in managing HF, hospitalizations for HF remain frequent and rates of readmissions continue to rise. Along with coronary artery disease related HF, dilated cardiomyopathy (DCM) is one of the most common causes of HF. DCM is defined as left ventricular (LV) dilation and systolic dysfunction in the absence of coronary artery disease or abnormal loading conditions proportionate to the degree of LV impairment.[2] DCM predominantly affects younger adults and is the most frequent indication for cardiac transplantation. Echocardiography is a key diagnostic tool in diagnosing and following up patients with DCM. The first step for the treatment of DCM is the identification and appropriate treatment of the underlying disease or condition. Apart from that, the drug treatment for DCM consists of guideline-directed medical therapy centered on addressing fluid overload, improving hemodynamics (inhibition of renin-angiotensin-aldosterone axis and sympathetic nervous system), and reducing heart rate. Often the patients of HF continue to deteriorate in spite of optimal medical therapy and carry a substantial risk of sudden cardiac death. Device therapy in the form of implantable cardioverter defibrillator (ICD), cardiac resynchronization therapy (CRT), alone or in combination is then required. End-stage heart failure patients also require surgical treatment in the form of ventricular assist devices (VAD) and heart transplantation.[2] CRT is a therapy known to improve functional capacity, quality of life and even survival, when given to carefully selected patients of HF. It has been shown to be effective for patients of heart failure with reduced ejection fraction (HFrEF) whom have presence of ventricular dyssynchrony. Despite various efforts to improve the effectiveness of CRT delivery, a significant number of patients (approximately 30%) are nonresponders[3] and fail to benefit from this expensive and technically demanding therapy. As such, it becomes imperative to identify the subset of patients who are most likely to benefit from this treatment beforehand. In the following paragraphs, we discuss the current role of echocardiography in evaluating the patients of DCM for CRT.

ECHOCARDIOGRAPHY IN CARDIAC RESYNCHRONIZATION THERAPY

As discussed earlier, CRT is an interventional technique used for patients of HFrEF, refractory to optimal, guideline-directed medical therapy. The criteria for selection of patients for CRT are based on symptomatology, functional class, ECG, and left ventricular ejection fraction (LVEF) derived by echocardiography, on the basis of evidence developed for the patients who are most likely to respond. As per the most recent guidelines, CRT is recommended for symptomatic patients with HFrEF in sinus rhythm with a QRS duration more than or equal to 150 milliseconds (ms) and left bundle branch block (LBBB) morphology on ECG and with LVEF less than or equal to 35%, despite optimal medical treatment to improve symptoms and reduce morbidity and mortality (class I, level A). At the same time, CRT is contraindicated (class III, level A), in those patients with a QRS duration less than 130 ms.[4] Echocardiography remains an important and indispensable tool in providing valuable information in patients with HF. Echocardiography not only helps in identifying the structural heart disease responsible for HF, it is fundamental to categorizing the patients into those with reduced, preserved and mid-range EF and provides valuable information related to prognosis, disease progression, and response to therapy. In candidates of DCM slated for CRT too, echocardiography plays a pivotal role in patient selection, predicting outcome, and optimization of device settings after implantation.[5] Though echocardiography is a versatile, safe, cost-effective, and accurate tool for evaluation of cardiac structure and function, the fundamentals in acquiring good quality imaging for collecting the required information cannot be overemphasized. For this subset of patients, it should be ensured that good quality ECG with a stable baseline and clear delineation of the onset of QRS complex is displayed on the echocardiography machine. This is very useful in accurate measurement of time periods. Besides, an ectopic free sequence of at least 3–5 beats, with breath held in expiration should be acquired and used for measurements. The echocardiographer should use all available modalities [M-mode, two-dimensional (2D), Doppler, three-dimensional (3D)] required for the particular information. When using 3D imaging, optimum gain settings with clear delineation of the endocardial border, especially at the apex should be ensured. It should be remembered that no single parameter alone is predictive and there is no standard recommended approach for all patients. Hence, all the possible parameters depending on the laboratory, machines and expertise should be evaluated in each patient.[6] Echocardiography is broadly utilized on two occasions in these patients—before, and after CRT is done. The following sections describe the role of echocardiography under these broad headings.

Echocardiography before Cardiac Resynchronization Therapy Implantation

Before CRT implantation, in symptomatic patients, echocardiography is initially used to confirm and assess the severity of LV systolic dysfunction and to detect other associated abnormalities like mitral regurgitation, right ventricular systolic function, intracardiac pressures, diastolic dysfunction, etc. A comprehensive study should be performed at this stage as this will also serve as the baseline for comparison after CRT is done. Evaluation of LV systolic function is the most important parameter as discussed earlier. A variety of echocardiography techniques are currently available to assess LV systolic function. If the expertise is available, 3D echocardiography is the recommended way of calculating LV end-diastolic and end-systolic volumes and ejection fraction accurately. It has been shown to be a rapid, reliable, and reproducible measure of these parameters, comparable to cardiac MRI. Besides, it also provides certain parameters related to cardiac dyssynchrony, which are discussed here. In the absence of 3D echocardiography, biplane Simpson's method by 2D echocardiography is the recommended method for this purpose. Right ventricular systolic function should also be assessed routinely during dyssynchrony analysis and the findings should be reported. Color flow imaging is used to detect the presence and estimate the severity of regurgitant lesions. Pulsed wave Doppler is particularly useful in these patients to assess LV diastolic function, calculate diastolic filling time, and detect the presence of diastolic mitral regurgitation. Although, the presence of mechanical dyssynchrony by echocardiography is not a prerequisite for use of CRT as discussed earlier, its use may further help in decision making for the careful selection of patients who are likely to respond. The three types of dyssynchrony described are: (1) atrioventricular (AV) dyssynchrony, (2) interventricular (VV) dyssynchrony, and (3) intraventricular dyssynchrony.

Atrioventricular Dyssynchrony

Atrioventricular dyssynchrony is a measure of the adequacy of diastolic filling of the LV. It is measured by dividing diastolic filling time (time from onset of "E" wave to end of "A" wave measured by pulse wave Doppler placed at the tips of mitral valve in diastole) by R-R interval (from the ECG displayed on the screen), also known as diastolic filling fraction (DFF). DFF value less than 0.40 is considered to represent significant AV dyssynchrony.

Interventricular Dyssynchrony

Interventricular dyssynchrony represents the time discordance between right ventricle and left ventricle contractions determined by the difference between the right and left ventricular pre-ejection periods. The pre-ejection period is determined by measuring the time interval from the onset of Q wave on the ECG tracing to onset of ventricular outflow tract tracing obtained by placing the pulse Doppler cursor in left and right ventricular outflow tracts.[5] The difference between RV and LV pre-ejection periods is normally less than 40 ms.[7] Also, if LV pre-ejection period is greater than 140 ms, it is considered prolonged.[8]

Intraventricular Dyssynchrony

Intraventricular dyssynchrony is the most important parameter used for assessment of dyssynchrony and can be measured by different echocardiography methods. LV septal and posterior wall motion recorded by color M-mode echocardiography is one of the most useful methods for determining LV intraventricular dyssynchrony (Fig. 1). An anteroseptal and posterior wall contraction delay longer than 130 ms is considered to represent presence of significant dyssynchrony.[7]

Tissue Doppler imaging (TDI), which measures the velocity of the myocardial muscle in a relatively load-independent manner, has been used extensively for assessment of intraventricular dyssynchrony. Several indices have been proposed based on comparison of time to peak systolic contraction of different myocardial segments. In a normal myocardium, the basal and midsegments contract simultaneously and thus, have similar time to peak systolic contraction. On the other hand, in an LV with significant dyssynchrony, considerable heterogeneity is observed in the time to reach peak contraction in systole. TDI offers the advantage of excellent temporal resolution and the contraction pattern of different segments are represented in the form of color-coded waveforms wherein the difference in timings between segments can be easily measured (Fig. 2). One very reliable and commonly used parameter is septal to lateral delay in the four basal and midsegments in apical four-chamber view. The normal delay should be *less than 65 ms*. Another index, known as the *Yu index,* calculates the standard deviation of time to peak systolic velocity in basal and midsegments of all the three apical views (four-, two-, and three-chamber views). A standard deviation value of *more than or equal to 33 ms* of these 12 segments is considered indicative of presence of dyssynchrony.[9] A maximal delay of *more than or equal to 100 ms* in the time to peak systolic velocity of these 12 segments is also a useful parameter. Tissue synchronization imaging (TSI) is a related modality, which is also useful in this regard and makes available septal posterior wall delay also. Similar indices of mechanical dyssynchrony are also made possible by 2D speckle-tracking based strain imaging. Radial strain is most useful in this regard and a time to peak systolic radial strain in the six segments of mid-LV cavity is used for this purpose. Septal to posterior delay of *more than or equal to 130 ms* is a useful parameter of dyssynchrony (Fig. 3). Strain imaging has also been shown to be useful in selecting the site for LV lead positioning. It has been shown that if LV lead is positioned at the most delayed site of by strain imaging, the benefit of pacing is maximal.[10] Strain imaging also has the capability to determine the degree of mechanical dyssynchrony and possibly, predicts likelihood of benefit with CRT.[11]

Three-dimensional echocardiography (3DE) has also been used for evaluation of left ventricular mechanical dyssynchrony. It is an accurate and reproducible method of estimation of LV dyssynchrony along with providing global LV volumes, EF and LV mass in very less time. The most validated parameter for LV dyssynchrony is the systolic dyssynchrony index (SDI), which is based on the calculation of the time required for each myocardial segment to reach its minimum volume. It indicates the degree of global LV dyssynchrony and correlates with LVEF (Fig. 4). Other parameters like maximum segmental dyssynchrony (MSD) and opposite segment dyssynchrony (OSD) have also recently been reported but have not been well validated.[12]

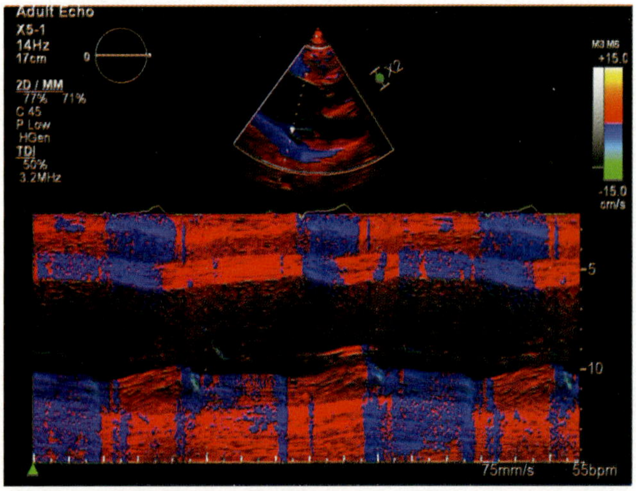

Fig. 1: M-mode with color tissue Doppler to detect septal-posterior wall mechanical delay. Sharp color transition makes detection of myocardial velocity easier.

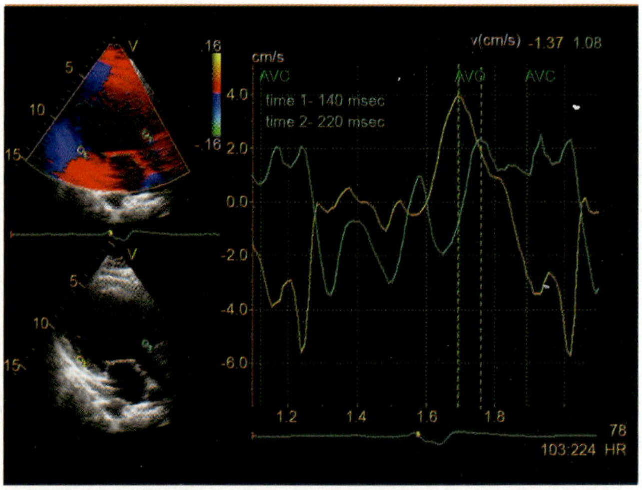

Fig. 2: Color tissue Doppler imaging in apical long-axis view. There is significant delay (80 ms) in time-to-peak-systolic velocity between basal posterior wall (yellow curve) and basal anterior septum (blue curve).

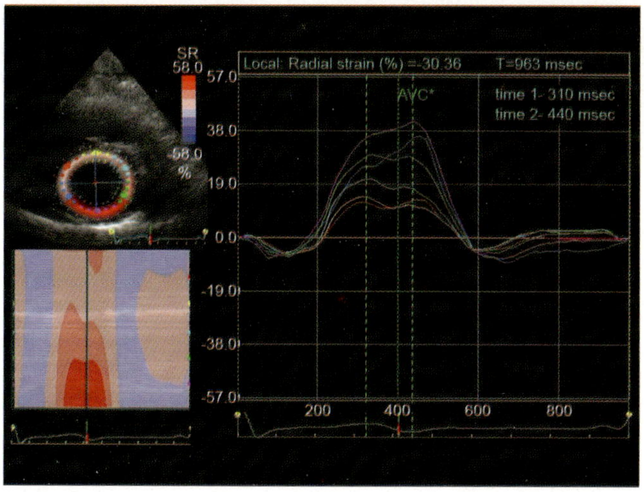

Fig. 3: Radial strain measurement at mid-papillary level using two-dimensional speckle tracking. Significant intraventricular dyssynchrony is indicated by septal-posterior delay. The pink curve (mid-posterior segment) is significantly delayed as compared to yellow curve (mid-anterior septum).

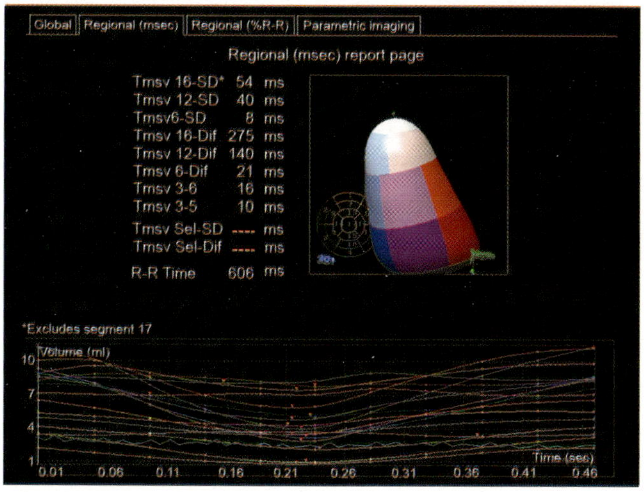

Fig. 4: Three-dimensional echocardiography showing segmental time to minimum volumes (shell view) and regional curves (below) for each segment.

For determining SDI, a full volume data set of the LV is acquired from the apical window and analyzed with the help of dedicated software. The LV cast made by the software for calculating LV volumes and EF is divided into 16 segments as proposed by the American Society of Echocardiography and the time to minimum systolic volume (Tmsv) is plotted for the entire cardiac cycle for each segment, as percentage of cardiac cycle. In a normal LV, all the segments will have almost same Tmsv but in an LV with significant dyssynchrony, there will be considerable variability in Tmsv. The degree of this variability in Tmsv (dispersion) is calculated by the standard deviation of Tmsv of all the segments and is a measure of the degree of dyssynchrony. Greater the degree of LV dysfunction, greater the SDI, independent of the QRS duration. A value greater than 8.3% is considered to represent significant dyssynchrony.[13] SDI also has been shown to be a good predictor of response to CRT and it improves in responders with reverse remodeling. Table 1 summarizes various echocardiography indices of dyssynchrony.

Echocardiography after Cardiac Resynchronization Therapy Implantation

Echocardiography continues to guide optimal utilization of CRT even after the device implantation has been successfully done. Sometimes, even during the procedure, echo (transesophageal or transthoracic), is called for to help in difficult coronary sinus cannulation and for guiding lead placement in the most delayed LV segment. Echocardiography is also used soon after the procedure to look for the presence of any pericardial effusion, particularly, after a prolonged procedure. Changes in degree of MR, in LV volumes and EF are also evaluated routinely but the most common utilization of echocardiography is for optimization of the AV delay and VV delays. The echocardiography-guided approach for AV and VV optimization can improve the acute hemodynamic response of CRT and also result in long-term clinical improvement.

Atrioventricular Delay

Improvement of AV synchrony is an important part of CRT. The AV interval is optimized to ensure adequate time that is available for LV filling to occur and the presystolic time is truncated to eliminate the chances of diastolic MR. This also results in improved cardiac output (CO).[11] Generally, this is done before discharge but also may be required at follow-up 3 months or even later, to improve cardiac performance.

Pulse wave Doppler echocardiography is generally used for this purpose with AV optimization being performed before VV optimization. Two approaches are used for AV optimization: (1) diastolic filling—based on ensuring optimal ventricular filling in diastole and (2) reiterative method of getting maximal cardiac output.[14] For diastolic filling approach, two methods are available: (1) Ritter's and (2) Ishikawa methods. Ritter's method is generally used in most laboratories and it relies on the availability of an A wave on pulse wave Doppler of transmittal flow in the apical four-chamber view. Other parameters required are the programmed long and short AV intervals and their corresponding QA intervals (onset of Q wave to end of A wave). All these parameters are put in an equation to derive the optimal AV delay.[15]

TABLE 1: Different modes of echocardiography with the various indices used for dyssynchrony assessment.

Echo modality	*Index*	*Cutoff value for dyssynchrony*	*Types of dyssynchrony*
M-mode	Septal-posterior wall mechanical delay (SPWMD)	≥130 millisecond (ms)	Intraventricular
Pulse wave Doppler	DFP/R-R interval	<40%	Atrioventricular
Doppler echo	Interventricular mechanical delay	>40 ms	Interventricular
Tissue Doppler imaging	Septal to lateral delay	≥65 ms	Intraventricular
Tissue Doppler imaging	Yu index (Ts-SD)	≥33 ms	Intraventricular
Tissue Doppler imaging	Maximal delay in six basal and six midsegments	≥100 ms	Intraventricular
2D speckle tracking (radial strain)	Septal-to-posterior delay	≥130 ms	Intraventricular
3D echocardiography	Systolic dyssynchrony index (SDI)	>8.3%	Intraventricular

When a clear A wave is not available, optimal AV interval is decided based on the reiterative method which calculates the CO using the velocity-time integral and cross-sectional area at the LV outflow tract. The AV interval is step-by-step increased and CO calculated for each increment. An AV interval providing maximal CO is chosen. This method is considered a better determinant of the optimal AV delay for CRT, because it represents direct systolic performance of the LV rather than the diastolic filling alone.

Interventricular Delay

Optimization of VV interval is also important to improve cardiac output and to reduce the severity of MR. The reiterative method as discussed earlier is used for this purpose. Different VV interval settings are tried (20–40 ms apart) with either LV first or right ventricle first or simultaneous pacing of both chambers and CO calculated to find the VV interval, which results in maximum CO.[16] It is a time-consuming method but should be done *after* adjusting the AV delay. As discussed earlier, echocardiography is routinely performed after CRT device implantation, any time before discharge to optimize the AV, and VV intervals for maximal cardiac output. Apart from this, the AV and VV intervals can further be optimized during follow-up visits at 3–6 months or any time later.

Echocardiography-derived LV volumes and EF is to be carefully calculated at each visit and they also form the basic determinants of differentiating responders from nonresponders to CRT.

Limitations

In spite of the enormous strides made in developing CRT and defining the criteria for patient selection, the responder rate has remained largely unchanged over the years. Echocardiography has contributed majorly in this, but none of echocardiography criteria is currently recommended for selection of candidates for CRT. Many new methods for AV and VV optimization have been proposed and acute improvements in systolic and diastolic function of LV are obtained by these methods but none has shown to help improve the nonresponder rate. There are no guidelines-based recommendations for these parameters also. Besides, differences in echocardiography software and the expertise of echocardiographers with these parameters also result in substantial difference in the evaluation of these patients before and after CRT device implantation.

CONCLUSION

Cardiac resynchronization therapy is an established therapy for improving symptoms, quality of life, and survival in patients of DCM in HF with reduced EF. However, approximately one-third of patients do not respond to this therapy in spite of careful selection. Echocardiography, with all its attendant modalities, plays a crucial role in all stages of this therapy. Echocardiography offers the advantages of versatility, portability, widespread availability at low cost, and being virtually free of any side effects. Echocardiography is the key modality for calculating LV volumes, EF and thus, selecting eligible patients for CRT. It can even contribute further in defining the candidates most likely to respond based on demonstrating significant mechanical delay in the LV, defining the scar burden and location, guide in targeting most appropriate LV segment for lead placement and has an indispensable role postprocedure for device optimization, and defining the response during follow-up. However, in spite of this, the responder rates have remained unchanged and newer approaches need to be worked out and new parameters need to be evaluated to further explore the role of echocardiography in this area.

REFERENCES

1. Roger VL. Epidemiology of heart failure. Circ Res. 2013;113(6):646-59.

2. Japp AG, Gulati A, Cook SA, et al. The diagnosis and evaluation of dilated cardiomyopathy. Circ Res. 2017;121(7):731-48.
3. Brugada J, Brachmann J, Delnoy PP, et al. Automatic optimization of cardiac resynchronization therapy using SonR—rationale and design of the clinical trial of the SonRtip lead and automatic av-vv optimization algorithm in the Paradym RF SonR CRT-D(RESPOND CRT) Trial. Ochsner J. 2014;14(4):596-607.
4. Ponikowski P, Voors AA, Anker SD, et al. 2016 ESC Guidelines for the diagnosis and treatment of acute and chronic heart failure: the task force for the diagnosis and treatment of acute and chronic heart failure of the European Society of Cardiology (ESC). Developed with the special contribution of the Heart Failure Association (HFA) of the ESC. Eur J Heart Fail. 2016;18(8):891-975.
5. Mazur W, Chung ES. The role of echocardiography in cardiac resynchronization therapy. Curr Heart Fail Rep. 2009;6(1): 37-43.
6. Mehrotra R, Bansal M, Chopra HK, et al. Echocardiography for Assessment of Electromechanical Dyssynchrony. Indian Heart J. 2009;61(2):218-22.
7. Chen CH, Ko WC, Chin CH, et al. The role of echocardiography in cardiac resynchronization therapy. J Med Ultrasound. 2008;16(1):1-6.
8. Cazeau S, Bordachar P, Jauvert G, et al. Echocardiographic modeling of cardiac dyssynchrony before and during multisite stimulation: a prospective study. Pacing Clin Electrophysiol. 2003;26(1 Pt 2):137-43.
9. Yu CM, Zhang Q, Fun JWH, et al. A novel tool to assess systolic asynchrony and identify responders of cardiac resynchronization therapy by tissue synchronization imaging. J Am Coll Cardiol. 2005;45:677-84.
10. Ansalone G, Giannantoni P, Ricci R, et al. Doppler myocardial imaging to evaluate the effectiveness of pacing sites in patients receiving biventricular pacing. J Am Coll Cardiol. 2002;39(3):489-99.
11. Mehrotra R, Kumar R, Maheshwari M. Echo-guided CRT in cardiodiabetes. Cardiodiabetes Update. 2017;1:227-32.
12. Bhambhani A, John N, Kumar B, et al., Three-dimensional echocardiographic evaluation of mechanical dyssynchrony in systolic heart failure with narrow QRS complex. Indian Heart J. 2018;70(3):387-93.
13. Kapetanakis S, Kearney MT, Siva A, et al. Real-time three-dimensional echocardiography: a novel technique to quantify global left ventricular mechanical dyssynchrony. Circulation. 2005;112(7):992-1000.
14. Faddis MN, Waggoner AD, Garhwal S, et al. AV delay optimization by aortic VTI is superior diabetes to the pulsed Doppler mitral inflow method for cardiac resynchronization therapy. Pacing Clin Electrophysiol. 2003;26(4):1042-5.
15. Ritter P, Padeletti L, Gillio-Meina L, et al. Determination of the optimal Atrioventricular delay in DDD pacing. Comparison between echo and peak endocardial acceleration measurements. Europace. 1999;1(2):126-30.
16. Agler DA, Adams DB, Waggoner AD. Cardiac resynchronization therapy and the emerging role of echocardiography (part 2): the comprehensive examination. J Am Soc Echocardiogr. 2007;20(1):76-90.

83

CHAPTER

Myocardial Perfusion Single-photon Emission Computed Tomography in Assessment of Left Ventricular Dyssynchrony

Chetan D Patel, Anirban Mukherjee

INTRODUCTION

Mechanical dyssynchrony refers to the abnormal prolongation of the timing of contraction or relaxation between the atria and ventricle (atrioventricular dyssynchrony), between the ventricles (interventricular dyssynchrony), or between myocardial segments within the left ventricle (LV) termed as intraventricular or LV dyssynchrony (LVD).[1] LV dyssynchrony is frequently observed in patients with heart failure (HF).[2] Due to its wide availability, echocardiography is most commonly used to measure mechanical dyssynchrony. However, it has limited reproducibility and high operator dependency. The result of PROSPECT trial had revealed the limitations of echocardiography for routine clinical practice in the assessment of LVD.[3] In post-PROSPECT era, studies using newer echocardiography techniques have shown more promising results in assessment of LVD and predicting response to cardiac resynchronization therapy (CRT).[4,5] Apart from echocardiography, in recent years, nuclear medicine techniques have also gained considerable attention in assessment of cardiac mechanical dyssynchrony. In the last decade, several researchers have established the utility of gated myocardial perfusion SPECT (GMPS) in assessment of cardiac synchrony and have suggested its potential clinical applications.[6-8] Gated myocardial perfusion SPECT has been a mainstay investigation in management of patients with coronary artery disease (CAD) for the last 3–4 decades. In 2005, Chen et al. developed a diagnostic tool for the assessment of LVD using phase analysis of GMPS.[9] GMPS has widespread availability and has advantage of superior reproducibility, permits retrospective analysis of acquired data and can simultaneously assess LV perfusion, function, and LVD. In GMPS, Fourier analysis converts regional myocardial counts, which relates to regional wall thickening into a continuous function to calculate a phase angle for each region. Phase angles of all regions of LV are obtained; to generate a phase distribution from which parameters to quantify LVD can be obtained.[9]

DIAGNOSTIC CRITERION

Cardiac quantitative softwares for assessment of cardiac dyssynchrony on GMPS are commercially available providing objective parameters for assessment of LVD and the normal values of synchrony have been established.[10-12] The two parameters commonly used to assess LVD on GMPS are phase standard deviation (PSD) and phase histogram bandwidth (PHB). At our center, we established the normal values of synchrony [(male: stress PSD 14.3 ± 4.7, rest PSD 8.9 ± 2.9, stress PHB 40.1 ± 11.9, and rest PHB 30.6 ± 7.6), (female: stress PSD 11 ± 4, rest PSD 7.7 ± 2.7, stress PHB 34.7 ± 12.6, and rest PHB 25.3 ± 8.6)] and established cutoff values of LVD [(male: stress PSD 23.7, rest PSD 14.7, stress PHB 63.9, and rest PHB 45.8), (female: stress PSD 19, rest PSD 13.1, stress PHB 59.9, and rest PHB 42.5)] in our population (Figs. 1 and 2).[11]

PROGNOSTIC IMPLICATIONS

The prognostic implication of assessment of cardiac dyssynchrony on GMPS has been evaluated by several

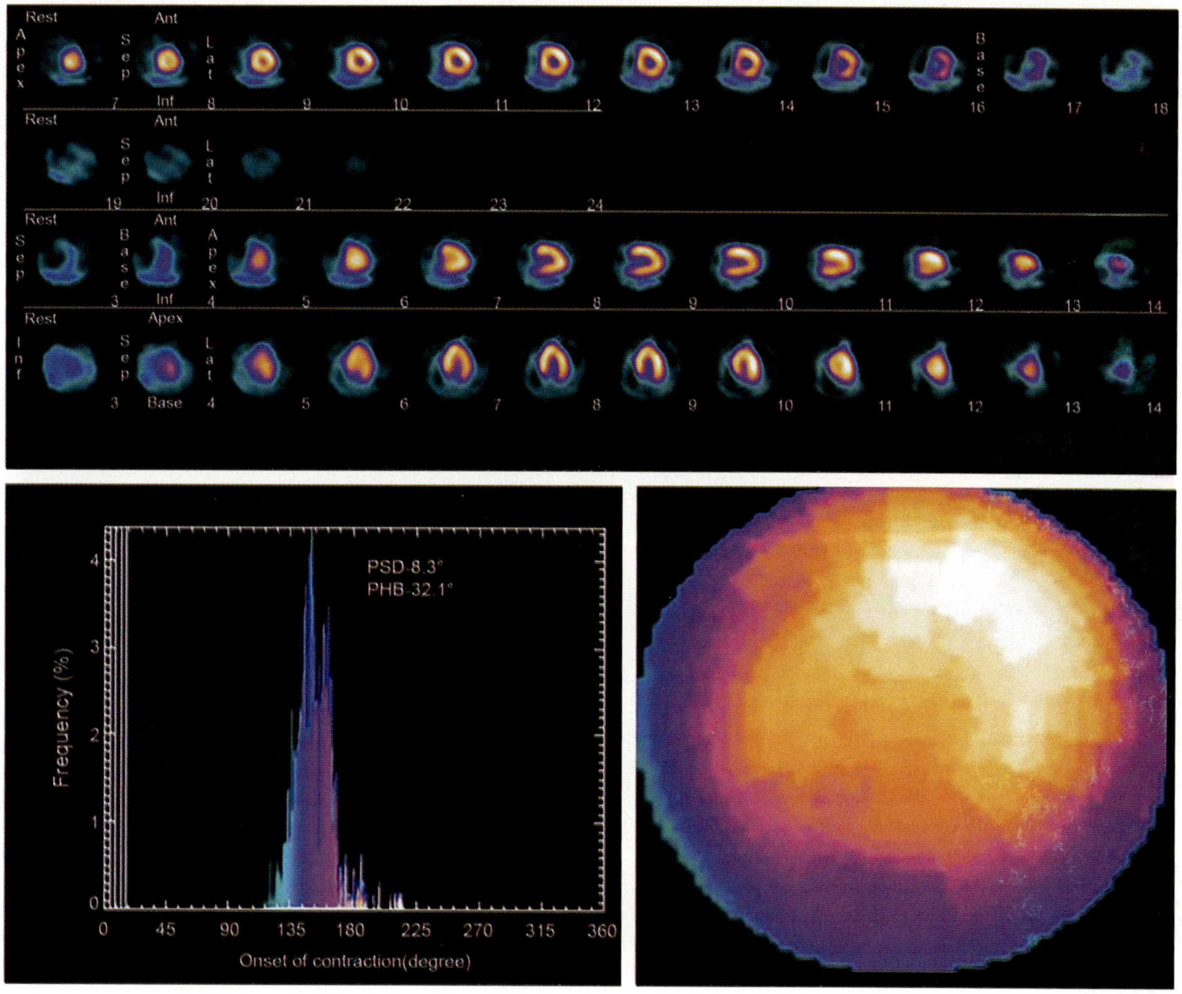

Fig. 1: Gated myocardial perfusion SPECT: represents a normal study with normal perfusion in the left ventricle. The phase analysis shows synchrony with values of phase standard deviation (PSD) and phase histogram bandwidth (PHB) within normal range.

authors in patients with CAD,[7] heart failure,[13] patients submitted to CRT,[14] nonischemic cardiomyopathy (NICM),[15] implantable cardiac defibrillator,[16] and end-stage renal disease.[17] Pazhenkottil et al. in a series of 202 patients of CAD who underwent stress-rest GMPS noted that presence of LVD was significantly associated with major adverse cardiac events (MACE).[7] Zafrir et al. followed 787 CAD patients with LV dysfunction for mean duration of 18.3 ± 6.2 months and observed that LVD can predict cardiac death in conjunction with the New York Heart Association (NYHA) class.[18] In another study, LVD was found as an independent predictor of death in patients with known CAD.[19] Hess et al. in their study of 1,244 patients observed that in CAD patients, mechanical LVD measured by GMPS has a stronger relationship with major cardiac events than electrical dyssynchrony measured by QRS duration.[20] Also, the prognostic value of LVD in predicting MACE was demonstrated in patients with acute myocardial infarction and multivessel disease (MVD).[21] Similar association of LVD with poor prognosis has been observed in patients of NICM, in patients with implantable cardiac defibrillator, and end-stage renal disease.[15-17]

THERAPEUTIC IMPLICATIONS

Prediction of Response to Cardiac Resynchronization Therapy

The results of CRT have shown moderate success, in spite of selection of patients according to the conventional criteria,[22] with about 20–40% of patients not showing favorable response to CRT.[23,24] Since it is associated with high cost and procedural complications, it is important to find out an objective parameter which can accurately

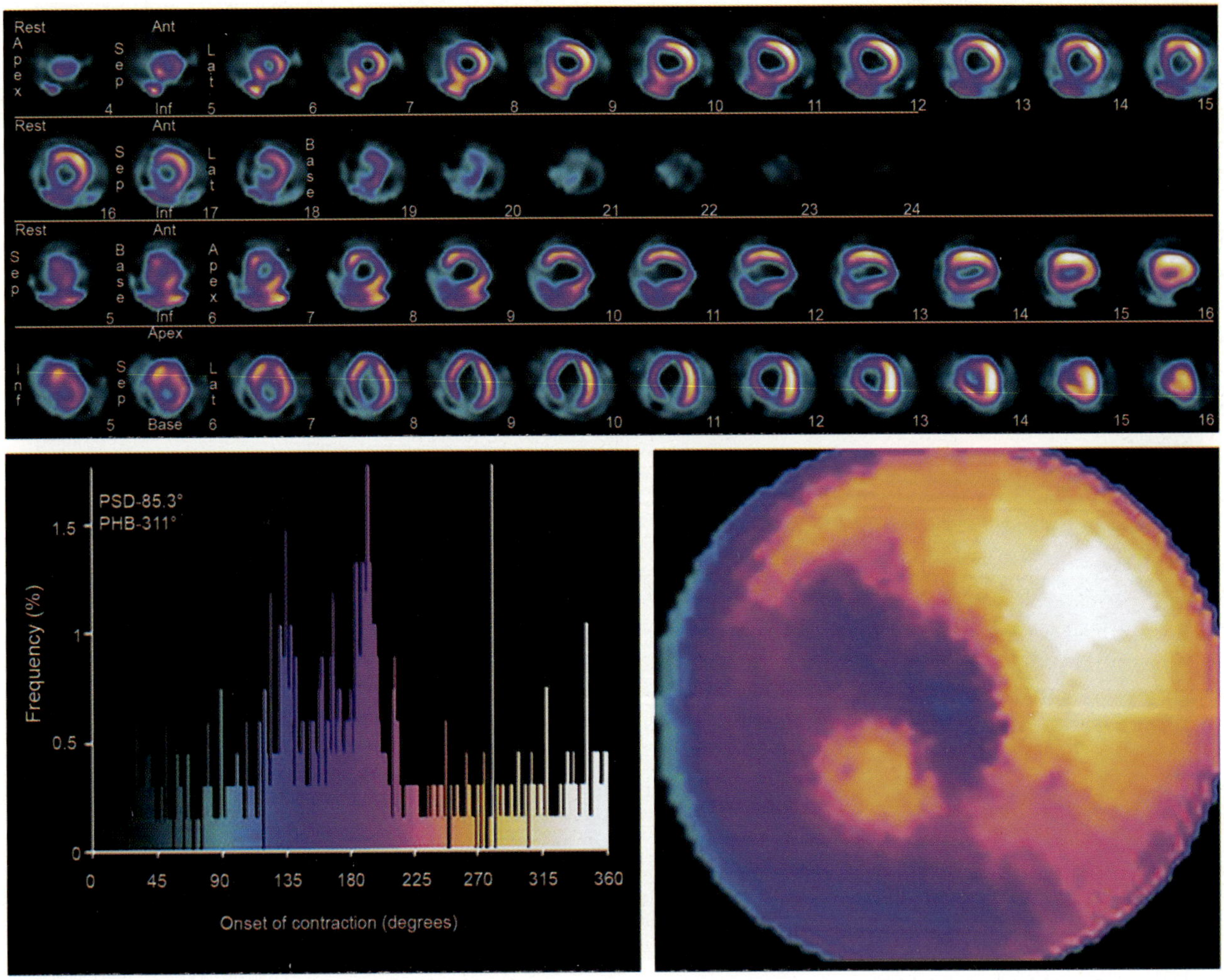

Fig. 2: Gated myocardial perfusion SPECT: shows perfusion defects in the distal anteroseptal wall, apical region, and proximal inferoseptal wall of the left ventricle. The phase analysis shows presence of LVD with values of PSD and PHB above the normal range. (PHB: phase histogram bandwidth; PSD: phase standard deviation; LVD: left ventricular dyssynchrony)

predict the response to therapy prior to device implantation. Mechanical cardiac dyssynchrony has been recognized as an additional and essential criterion for response to CRT.[25,26] Henneman et al.[8] demonstrated the clinical utility of mechanical LVD assessed on GMPS in prediction of response to CRT. They proposed cutoff value of 43 for PSD and 135 for PHB to predict response to CRT. Mukherjee et al.[27] in their study of 32 NICM patients noted that responders had significantly higher dyssynchrony indices compared to nonresponders. A cutoff value of 128 for PHB and 43 for PSD (86% sensitivity and 80% specificity) can predict response to CRT with maximum accuracy. Recently, there has been a lot of interest in using imaging modalities especially GMPS to guide LV lead placement in CRT. The rationale is to identify the site of latest mechanical activation, which is viable where the lead can be placed to improve the success rate of CRT.[28,29]

DISCUSSION

Since its inception, phase analysis of GMPS has shown tremendous promise in assessment of dyssynchrony. Most of the studies have evaluated the role of GMPS in CRT and majority has reported good sensitivity and specificity in predicting response to CRT.[8,27,30-35] An important issue related to CRT response is the position of the LV pacing lead. Ypenburg et al. showed that pacing at the site of latest mechanical activation resulted in superior response to CRT after 6 months and better prognosis during long-term follow-up, as compared to pacing outside the site of latest mechanical activation.[36] Another study showed that CRT resulted in clinical and echocardiographic nonresponse when there was myocardial scar in the lateral or inferolateral wall, which is the most commonly, used position of the LV pacing lead.[37] These studies suggest that the optimal

LV pacing lead position should be outside myocardial scar and the site of latest mechanical activation. Also, GMPS studies have shown that response to CRT is more favorable in NICM compared to ischemic cardiomyopathy (ICM) patients with scarred myocardium and that patients with lower scar burden have better outcome post-CRT.[38] Boogers et al. evaluated the relationship between the site of latest mechanical activation on GMPS, LV lead position, and response to CRT in 90 patients with advanced HF. The site of latest mechanical activation was correlated to LV lead position on fluoroscopy. The LV lead was considered concordant if positioned at the site of latest mechanical activation and discordant if placed outside. CRT response was significantly better in patients with concordant than in patients with discordant LV lead position (79% versus 26%, $p < 0.01$) and showed significant improvement in LV function after 6 months.[39] Recently, Tao et al. evaluated the role of left ventricular contraction pattern in predicting response to CRT. Apart from analyzing PSD and PHB, the mean phase angle of each segment was displayed on a 13-segmentation polar map to generate different contraction patterns termed U-shape and non-U-shape patterns. On 6 months follow-up, 90% of those with U-shape contraction pattern responded to CRT compared to 50% with non-U-shape pattern. The patients with U-shape who did not respond, included those with either phase SD less than 43, significant scar burden, or nonconcordant LV lead. Multivariate analysis revealed U-shape contraction pattern as an independent predictor of CRT response.[35] Another major role of assessment of dyssynchrony using GMPS is in the settings of CAD. Apart from prognostication and risk stratification, it is also helpful in determining extent of CAD.[7,18-21] Several studies have demonstrated the relation of LVD with myocardial ischemic and/or scar burden, relation of poststress LVD with stress-induced ischemia, and CAD extent.[40-42] Chen et al. observed association between stress-induced ischemia and early poststress LVD. The authors suggested that stress-induced myocardial ischemia caused dyssynchronous contraction in the ischemic region, leading to deterioration in LV synchrony and this pattern may aid the diagnosis of CAD.[40] Huang et al.[41] observed that patients with MVD had significantly more global and territorial dyssynchrony at early poststress than at rest on Thallium-201 study. Another study, using Tc-99m tetrofosmin, observed higher prevalence of MVD disease in patients with LVD at rest than those without dyssynchrony.[42] At present, assessment of LV diastolic dyssynchrony is most commonly performed using echocardiography. Studies have shown the feasibility of phase analysis of GMPS in evaluation of LV diastolic dyssynchrony with results comparable to echocardiography.[43,44]

Flowchart 1: Proposed algorithm to optimize patient selection for CRT based on GMPS.

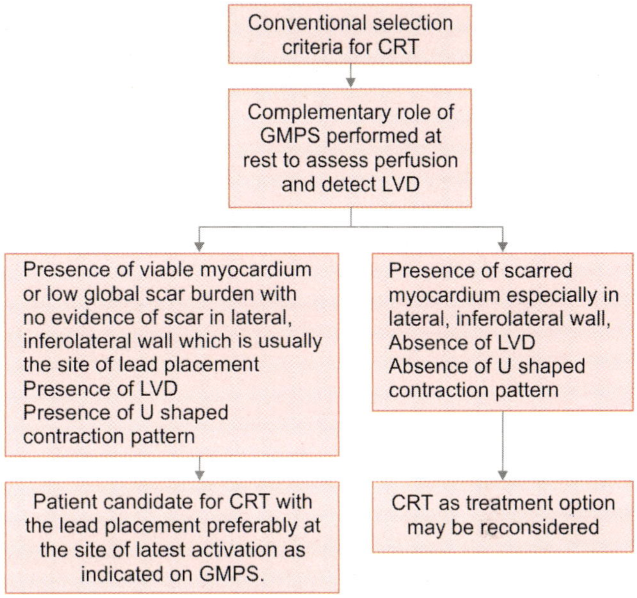

(CRT: cardiac resynchronization therapy; GMPS: gated myocardial perfusion SPECT; LVD: left ventricular dyssynchrony)

LIMITATIONS

Despite its widespread availability and utility, GMPS has few disadvantages. It has limited temporal resolution with associated noise and artifact from areas with significantly reduced perfusion due to scar. Most of the studies performed to assess its role in prediction of response to CRT are single center study with limited number of patients. A large multicenter trial can prove the value of GMPS in selection of patients and predicting outcome in patients submitted for CRT (Flowchart 1). Also, unlike echocardiography, there is limited data available as GMPS is not performed routinely prior to CRT.

CONCLUSION

Accurate and reproducible assessment of cardiac mechanical dyssynchrony can be performed with GMPS. It has gained considerable attention in prediction of response to CRT. Studies in literature have also shown the utility of gated SPECT in assessment of cardiac dyssynchrony in CAD and other varied clinical settings.

REFERENCES

1. Gorcsan J, Abraham T, Agler DA, et al. Echocardiography for cardiac resynchronization therapy: recommendations for performance and reporting—a report from the American Society of echocardiography dyssynchrony writing group endorsed by the heart rhythm society. J Am Soc Echocardiogr. 2008;21(3):191-213.

2. Yu CM, Lin H, Zhang Q, et al. High prevalence of left ventricular systolic and diastolic asynchrony in patients with congestive heart failure and normal QRS duration. Heart. 2003;89(1):54-60.
3. Chung ES, Leon AR, Tavazzi L, et al. Results of the Predictors of Response to CRT (PROSPECT) trial. Circulation. 2008;117(20):2608-16.
4. Zhang Q, Yu CM. Is mechanical dyssynchrony still a major determinant for responses after cardiac resynchronization therapy? J Cardiol. 2011;57(3):239-48.
5. Galli E, Leclercq C, Donal E. Mechanical dyssynchrony in heart failure: still a valid concept for optimizing treatment? Arch Cardiovasc Dis. 2017;110(1):60-8.
6. Chen J, Garcia EV, Bax JJ, et al. SPECT myocardial perfusion imaging for the assessment of left ventricular mechanical dyssynchrony. J Nucl Cardiol. 2011;18(4):685-94.
7. Pazhenkottil AP, Buechel RR, Husmann L, et al. Long-term prognostic value of left ventricular dyssynchrony assessment by phase analysis from myocardial perfusion imaging. Heart. 2011;97(1):33-7.
8. Henneman MM, Chen J, Dibbets P, et al. Can LV dyssynchrony as assessed with phase analysis on gated myocardial perfusion SPECT predict response to CRT? J Nucl Med. 2007;48(7):1104-11.
9. Chen J, Garcia EV, Folks RD, et al. Onset of left ventricular mechanical contraction as determined by phase analysis of ECG gated myocardial perfusion SPECT imaging: Development of a SPECT myocardial perfusion imaging diagnostic tool for assessment of cardiac mechanical dyssynchrony. J Nucl Cardiol. 2005;12(6):687-95.
10. Romero-Farina G, Aguadé-Bruix S, Candell-Riera J, et al. Cut-off values of myocardial perfusion gated-SPECT phase analysis parameters of normal subjects, and conduction and mechanical cardiac diseases. J Nucl Cardiol. 2015;22(6):1247-58.
11. Mukherjee A, Singh H, Patel C, et al. Normal values of cardiac mechanical synchrony parameters using gated myocardial perfusion single-photon emission computed tomography: impact of population and study protocol. Indian J Nucl Med. 2016;31(4):255-9.
12. AlJaroudi W, Jaber WA, Grimm RA, et al. Alternative methods for the assessment of mechanical dyssynchrony using phase analysis of gated single photon emission computed tomography myocardial perfusion imaging. Int J Cardiovasc Imaging. 2012;28(6):1385-94.
13. Malhotra S, Pasupula DK, Sharma RK, et al. Relationship between left ventricular dyssynchrony and scar burden in the genesis of ventricular tachyarrhythmia. J Nucl Cardiol. 2018;25(2):555-69.
14. Tsai SC, Chang YC, Chiang KF, et al. Dyssynchrony is helpful in predicting ventricular arrhythmia in ischemic cardiomyopathy after cardiac resynchronization therapy: a preliminary study. Medicine (Baltimore). 2016;95(7):e2840..
15. Goldberg AS, Alraies MC, Cerqueira MD, et al. Prognostic value of left ventricular mechanical dyssynchrony by phase analysis in patients with non-ischemic cardiomyopathy with ejection fraction 35-50% and QRS<150 ms. J Nucl Cardiol. 2014;21(1):57-66.
16. Aljaroudi WA, Hage FG, Hermann D, et al. Relation of left-ventricular dyssynchrony by phase analysis of gated SPECT images and cardiovascular events in patients with implantable cardiac defibrillators. J Nucl Cardiol. 2010;17(3):398-404.
17. Aggarwal H, Aljaroudi WA, Mehta S, et al. The prognostic value of left ventricular mechanical dyssynchrony using gated myocardial perfusion imaging in patients with end-stage renal disease. J Nucl Cardiol. 2014;21(4):739-46.
18. Zafrir N, Nevzorov R, Bental T, et al. Prognostic value of left ventricular dyssynchrony by myocardial perfusion-gated SPECT in patients with normal and abnormal left ventricular functions. J Nucl Cardiol. 2014;21(3):532-40.
19. Uebleis C, Hellweger S, Laubender RP, et al. Left ventricular dyssynchrony assessed by gated SPECT phase analysis is an independent predictor of death in patients with advanced coronary artery disease and reduced left ventricular function not undergoing cardiac resynchronization therapy. Eur J Nucl Med Mol Imaging. 2012;39(10):1561-9.
20. Hess PL, Shaw LK, Fudim M, et al. The prognostic value of mechanical left ventricular dyssynchrony defined by phase analysis from gated single-photon emission computed tomography myocardial perfusion imaging among patients with coronary heart disease. J Nucl Cardiol. 2017;24(2):482-90.
21. Cho SG, Jabin Z, Park KS, et al. Clinical values of left ventricular mechanical dyssynchrony assessment by gated myocardial perfusion SPECT in patients with acute myocardial infarction and multivessel disease. Eur J Nucl Med Mol Imaging. 2017;44(2):259-66.
22. Yancy CW, Jessup M, Bozkurt B, et al. 2013 ACCF/AHA guideline for the management of heart failure: a report of the American College of Cardiology Foundation/ American Heart Association Task Force on Practice Guidelines. J Am Coll Cardiol. 2013;62(16):e147-239.
23. Abraham WT, Fisher WG, Smith AL, et al. Cardiac resynchronization in chronic heart failure. N Engl J Med. 2002;346(2):1845-53.
24. Fox DJ, Fitzpatrick AP, Davidson NC. Optimization of cardiac resynchronization therapy: addressing the problem of 'nonresponders'. Heart. 2005;91(8):1000-2.
25. Bax JJ, Bleeker GB, Marwick TH, et al. Left ventricular dyssynchrony predicts response and prognosis after cardiac resynchronization therapy. J Am Coll Cardiol. 2004;44(9):1834-40.
26. Leclercq C, Faris O, Tunin R, et al. Systolic improvement and mechanical resynchronization does not require electrical synchrony in the dilated failing heart with left bundle-branch block. Circulation. 2002;106(14):1760-3.
27. Mukherjee A, Patel CD, Naik N, et al. Quantitative assessment of cardiac mechanical dyssynchrony and prediction of response to cardiac resynchronization therapy in patients with nonischaemic dilated cardiomyopathy using gated myocardial perfusion SPECT. Nucl Med Commun. 2015;36(5):494-501.
28. Lin X, Xu H, Zhao X, et al. Repeatability of left ventricular dyssynchrony and function parameters in serial gated myocardial perfusion SPECT studies. J Nucl Cardiol. 2010;17(5):811-6.

29. Sommer A, Kronborg MB, Poulsen SH, et al. Empiric versus imaging guided left ventricular lead placement in cardiac resynchronization therapy (ImagingCRT): study protocol for a randomized controlled trial. Trials. 2013;14(2):113.
30. Nakamura K, Takami M, Shimabukuro M, et al. Effective prediction of response to cardiac resynchronization therapy using a novel program of gated myocardial perfusion single photon emission computed tomography. Europace. 2011;13(12):1731-7.
31. Kiso K, Imoto A, Nishimura Y, et al. Novel algorithm for quantitative assessment of left ventricular dyssynchrony with ECG-gated myocardial perfusion SPECT: useful technique for management of cardiac resynchronization therapy. Ann Nucl Med. 2011;25(10):768-76.
32. Azizian N, Rastgou F, Ghaedian T, et al. LV Dyssynchrony assessed with phase analysis on gated myocardial perfusion spect can predict response to CRT in patients with end-stage heart failure. Res Cardiovasc Med. 2014;3(4):e20720.
33. Qin S, Shi H, Su Y, et al. Can the prognosis of cardiac resynchronization therapy be predicted by gated SPECT? Clin Nucl Med. 2015;40(10):786-92.
34. Gendre R, Lairez O, Mondoly P, et al. Research of predictive factors for cardiac resynchronization therapy: a prospective study comparing data from phase-analysis of gated myocardial perfusion single-photon computed tomography and echocardiography : trying to anticipate response to CRT. Ann Nucl Med. 2017;31(3):218-26.
35. Tao N, Qiu Y, Tang H, et al. Assessment of left ventricular contraction patterns using gated SPECT MPI to predict cardiac resynchronization therapy response. J Nucl Cardiol. 2017. [Epub ahead of print].
36. Ypenburg C, van Bommel RJ, Delgado V, et al. Optimal left ventricular lead position predicts reverse remodeling and survival after cardiac resynchronization therapy. J Am Coll Cardiol. 2008;52(4):1402-9.
37. Bleeker GB, Kaandorp TA, Lamb HJ, et al. Effect of posterolateral scar tissue on clinical and echocardiographic improvement after cardiac resynchronization therapy. Circulation. 2006;113(7):969-76.
38. Adelstein EC, Tanaka H, Soman P, et al. Impact of scar burden by single-photon emission computed tomography myocardial perfusion imaging on patient outcomes following cardiac resynchronization therapy. Eur Heart J. 2011;32(1):93-103.
39. Boogers MJ, Chen J, van Bommel RJ, et al. Optimal left ventricular leads position assessed with phase analysis on gated myocardial perfusion SPECT. Eur J Nucl Med Mol Imaging. 2011;38(2):230-8.
40. Chen CC, She TY, Chang MC, et al. Stress-induced myocardial ischemia is associated with early post-stress left ventricular mechanical dyssynchrony as assessed by phase analysis of 201 T1 gated SPECT myocardial perfusion imaging. Eur J Nucl Med Mol Imaging. 2012;39(12):1904-9.
41. Huang W, Huang C, Lee C, et al. Relation of early post-stress left ventricular dyssynchrony and the extent of angiographic coronary artery disease. J Nucl Cardiol. 2014;21(6):1048-56.
42. Gimelli A, Liga R, Giorgetti A, et al. Determinants of left ventricular mechanical dyssynchrony in patients submitted to myocardial perfusion imaging: a cardiac CZT study. J Nucl Cardiol. 2016;23(4):728-36.
43. Hsu TH, Huang WS, Chen CC, et al. Left ventricular systolic and diastolic dyssynchrony assessed by phase analysis of gated SPECT myocardial perfusion imaging: a comparison with speckle tracking echocardiography. Ann Nucl Med. 2013;27(8):764-71.
44. Boogers MJ, Chen J, Veltman CE, et al. Left ventricular diastolic dyssynchrony assessed with phase analysis of gated myocardial perfusion SPECT: a comparison with tissue Doppler imaging. Eur J Nucl Med Mol Imaging. 2011;38(11):2031-9.

84

CHAPTER

Left and Right Ventricular and Atrial Strain Evaluation by Two-dimensional Speckle Tracking Echocardiography

Sudhir Wahi, Adrian Chong, Tony Stanton, Liza Thomas

LEFT VENTRICULAR STRAIN

Ischemic Cardiomyopathy

The measurement of ejection fraction (EF) has been central to the practice of cardiology for many decades. Its calculation continues to act as a gatekeeper for patients to access potentially lifesaving medications and devices, such as implantable defibrillators. Cardiac contraction is, however, a complex process involving motion in numerous geometric planes. EF is a volume-based measurement where numerous geometrical assumptions are made which can contribute to large errors being made, especially in patients with difficult or foreshortened left ventricular (LV) windows. Advances in computing power are now allowing the accurate quantification of myocardial mechanics by speckle tracking echocardiography (STE). STE can measure myocardial motion in longitudinal, circumferential, radial (expansion) planes and quantifying twist (torsion). To date, the most robust clinical data exists for longitudinal and circumferential strain. The myocardium shortens in these planes during systole and thus both are expressed as negative numbers. In clinical practice however, the negative prefix is often omitted.

Global Left Ventricular Function

Global longitudinal strain (GLS) is calculated by measuring the longitudinal contraction of the LV from the three standard apical windows. It has been shown to be a superior predictor of both morbidity and mortality in both unselected populations (Fig. 1)[1] and in those with ischemic cardiomyopathy.[2] A particular benefit of GLS over EF is in its prognostic superiority in heart failure (HF) patients with either a mid-range (40–49%) or preserved (≥50%) EF.[1] GLS can also reliably delineate subclinical LV dysfunction theoretically allowing earlier diagnosis and initiation of appropriate therapy. Concerns about the intervendor differences in GLS measures have largely been allayed with GLS now being considered a reliable and less variable measure than EF.[3] Standard reference ranges for GLS were

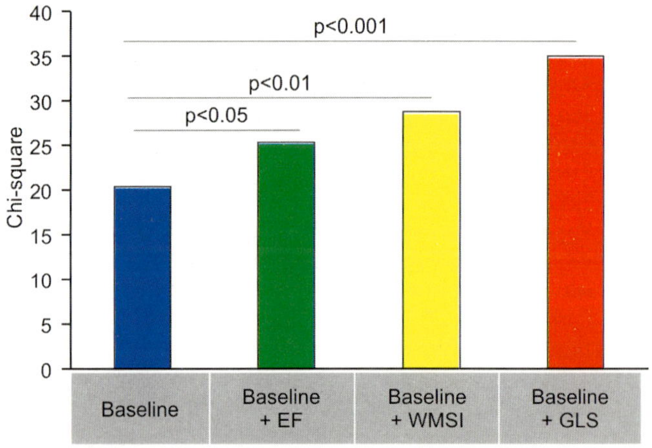

From Stanton et al[1]. Reproduced with permission.
(EF = ejection fraction; WMSI = wall motion scoring index; GLS=global longitudinal strain)

Fig. 1: The addition of three different measures of LV function (EF, WMSI and GLS) in a series of Cox Models added to patient baseline characteristics for the prediction of outcome in an unselected patient population. GLS is superior to WMSI and EF.

published in 2013.[4] A recent large analysis of patients with acute HF and subsequent poor outcome (4,172 consecutive patients; mean EF - 40%, 5-year mortality - 40.4%) showed that GLS was independently predictive of mortality but EF was not. For each reduction in GLS of 1%, there was a 5% worsening of 5-year mortality.[5] In addition, global circumferential strain has also been shown to be prognostic in populations with acute ischemic HF (mean EF - 34 ± 13%)[6] and chronic ischemic cardiomyopathy (mean EF - 41 ± 7%).[7]

Regional Left Ventricular Function

In myocardial ischemia, GLS is frequently affected early in the disease process as the subendocardial fibers is longitudinally orientated. In clinical practice, the assessment of regional wall motion abnormalities (RWMA) is typically based on the subjective assessment of the reading clinician. Longitudinal strain can be used reliably to diagnose RWMA even in the presence of normal EF with no RWMA apparent to the naked eye.[8] As regional longitudinal strain is reduced, it follows that this contributes to a reduction in the global value also, with GLS of less than 21% having a negative-predictive value of 92% for significant coronary artery disease.[9] In patients with stable coronary artery disease, global peak systolic longitudinal strain has been shown to be an independent predictor of significant coronary stenosis (≥70%) and to be incremental when combined with a standard exercise stress ECG. This raises the possibility of adding global STE, rather than regional STE which is more variable, into the standard workup of the stable chest pain patient.[10]

Acute Myocardial Ischemia

End-systolic, rather than peak, strain should be used as a measure of acute myocardial ischemia due to the affected myocardial segments showing systolic lengthening and postsystolic shortening. Two-dimensional STE (2D STE) can be utilized to identify acute coronary vessel occlusion in non-ST elevation myocardial infarction (NSTEMI). A GLS value of less than 13.8% has been shown to have an area under the receiver operating curve (ROC) of 0.95 to identify a significant myocardial infarction (MI) defined as more than and equal to 12% of total myocardium involved (Fig. 2).[11] It is conceivable that STE may be of benefit in identifying those with NSTEMI who would benefit from urgent revascularization despite a relative lack of ECG abnormalities on presentation. GLS is also a significant predictor of LV remodeling and significant adverse events postprimary percutaneous coronary intervention in patients with STEMI. In a prospective study of 97 patients with 6 month and then 3 year follow-up, GLS was identified to be a significant independent predictor of both LV remodeling and significant adverse events, superior to peak troponin or EF. Optimal cutoffs of less than 12.5% and less than 9.3% were identified respectively for LV remodeling and future significant adverse events.[12]

Chronic Myocardial Ischemia, Scar and Viability

After an acute infarct myocardial segments can become stunned (with recovery taking place over the next few weeks or months), hibernate (a state of chronic downregulation of myocardial contraction due to ongoing chronic ischemia) or form scar (irreversible necrosis with permanent akinesia). The identification of each of these states is critical in the consideration of further treatment and amelioration of ongoing cardiovascular risk. Sudden cardiac death remains a devastating and unpredictable cause in ischemic cardiomyopathy. Although implantable cardioverter defibrillators have a class 1 indication in symptomatic patients with an EF less than 35% on optimal medical

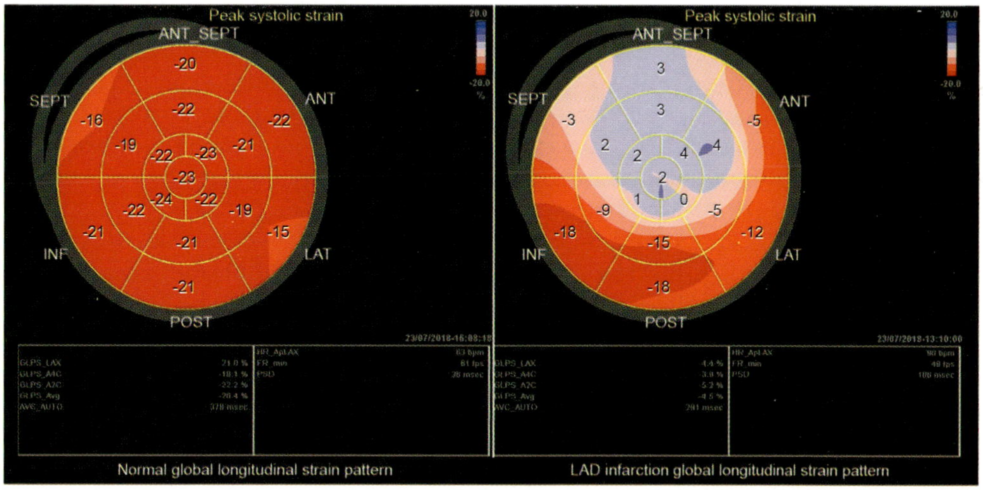

Fig. 2: GLS bull's eye plots from 2 different patients (recorded in the same echocardiography laboratory on the same day) showing a normal GLS pattern (left) and a patient who has suffered an extensive LAD infarction (right).

therapy for three months,[13] the fact remains that most patients who die suddenly post-MI have a left ventricular ejection fraction (LVEF) more than 35%.[14] Given the limitations of LVEF as a risk-stratifying parameter, Haugaa and colleagues investigated the use of STE in a prospective, multicenter study of 569 patients (268 STEMI, 301 NSTEMI) over a month after an acute MI.[15] They showed that GLS was a superior predictor of significant ventricular arrhythmias compared to EF, especially in those with LVEF more than 35%. STE was also used to estimate the contractile heterogeneity of the LV, termed mechanical dispersion, which is the standard deviation of the time to peak negative strain from the 16 LV segments. Mechanical dispersion (>75 ms) was an independent predictor of arrhythmic events and, when combined with GLS (<16%), had best positive-predictive value for arrhythmic events (21% PPV vs. 11% for LVEF alone). Late gadolinium-enhanced cardiac magnetic resonance (LGE-CMR) is the gold standard for the identification of myocardial viability and scar. The advent of layer specific strain raised the possibility of utilizing STE to differentiate subendocardial, and so possibly viable, scar from transmural scar. To date however, STE has only been shown to reliably identify transmural scar. A study by Tarascio and colleagues found that a peak end-systolic cutoff of worse than 9.6% discriminated normal myocardium from scar. A circumferential strain of worse than 12.1% had similar sensitivity and specificity.[16] One further use of STE in ischemic cardiomyopathy has been to assist in the identification of the optimal placement of the LV pacing lead tip. Pacing of a segment with the greatest mechanical delay that is not identified as scar has been shown to both improve cardiac resynchronization therapy (CRT) response and reduce HF morbidity and mortality.[17,18]

Nonischemic Cardiomyopathy

Distinguishing physiological from pathological LV hypertrophy (LVH) remains a diagnostic challenge with significant clinical implications. The "athlete's" heart has been used to describe myocardial hypertrophy and cardiac enlargement in response to exercise.[19-21] However, the differential diagnosis also includes pathological hypertrophic cardiomyopathies (HCM) defined by the presence of increased LV wall thickness (end-diastolic LV segmental thickness ≥15 mm) in the absence of abnormal loading conditions or coexistent systemic hypertension or aortic stenosis,[22-24] metabolic disorders (e.g. Anderson-Fabry disease) or infiltrative diseases (e.g. cardiac amyloidosis). Despite an apparently preserved LVEF, the hypertrophied LV may have a reduced stroke volume due to the small chamber size. Myocardial strain imaging has been shown to be able to detect subclinical LV dysfunction in the setting of the misleading "normal" LVEF, and providing incremental prognostic value.[25] Features favoring HCM over the athlete's heart include the presence of sarcomeric mutations, family history of HCM, smaller LV cavity (<45 mm), unusual or noncontiguous patterns of LVH, lack of LVH regression postcessation of exercise, and diastolic dysfunction.[26,27] Compared to sedentary controls, competitive athletes showed no difference in the GLS and peak systolic strain, which were markedly reduced in HCM (GLS <-10% has a sensitivity of 80% and specificity of 95%).[28] A reduced GLS (<10%) combined with tissue Doppler imaging of the mitral annulus (S' and E' velocities less than 9 cm per sec; global function index = [(E/E')/S) >1.77], increased the sensitivity and specificity to 100% and 95%, respectively. These findings were confirmed in another larger study, revealing a significantly lower GLS (11.2 ± 4.2%) in HCM compared to athletes (17.8 ± 2.2%) and hypertensive patients (17.8 ± 3.1%).[29] Endocardial longitudinal and radial strain remain significantly reduced in HCM patients even with septal thickness in the grey zone of 12–16 mm.[30] It has also been demonstrated that all components of 2D STE strain were significantly reduced in familial HCM patients when compared to controls, despite normal LVEF (mean 69.3 ± 6.4%).[31] Myocardial fibrosis predisposes HCM patients to a higher risk of ventricular arrhythmias independent of septal thickness. GLS by 2D STE appears to correlate with the burden of fibrosis and in turn, ventricular arrhythmias, potentially influencing decisions regarding prophylactic defibrillator implantation.[32,33] In an observational cohort study of 472 HCM patients (mean follow-up 4.3 years), GLS was also an independent predictor of heart failure, with increased risk at a GLS threshold of less than and equal to 15.6%.[34] Anderson-Fabry or Fabry disease, is an X-linked lysosomal storage disorder caused by a deficiency in the alpha-galactosidase A enzyme, resulting in the multisystem intracellular accumulation of glycosphingolipids. Cardiac involvement typically mainfests as concentric LVH with "preserved" LVEF despite the development of myocardial replacement fibrosis. In Fabry cardiomyopathy, GLS was lower in affected males (males: 15.4 ± 3.6% vs. females: 17.7 ± 3.2%; $p < 0.001$) and in those with MRI-proven myocardial fibrosis (fibrosis: 14.8 ± 3.5% vs. no fibrosis: 18.9 ± 2.1%; $p < 0.001$).[35] GLS correlated with the degree of LGE and regional strain was lowest in the basal posterolateral segments (in keeping with the distribution of mid-myocardial replacement fibrosis of Fabry disease) (Fig. 3). Cardiac amyloidosis (CA) is characterized by extracellular deposition of insoluble β-pleated fibrillar proteins in the myocardium resulting in progressive increase in biventricular wall thickness rather than true hypertrophy per se.[36] The subendocardium is diffusely affected by the amyloid deposition in primary

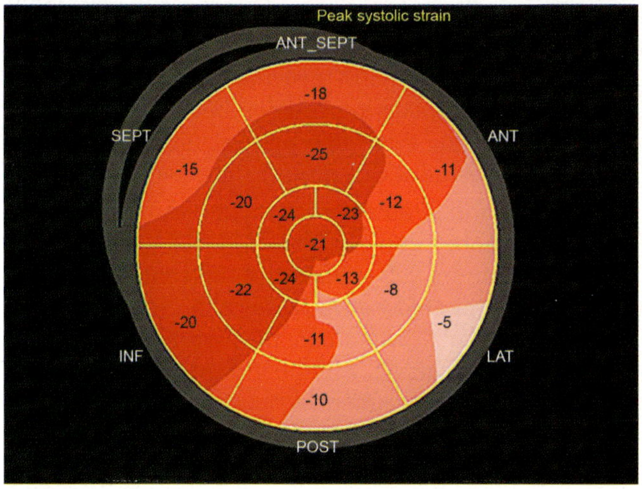

Fig. 3: Reduced regional longitudinal in the basal inferolateral segments (with normal LVEF - 56%) that would be in keeping with the typical distribution of mid-myocardial replacement fibrosis in Fabry disease.

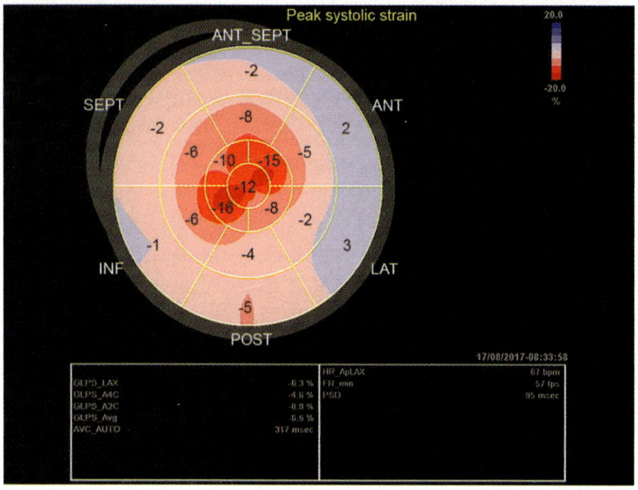

Fig. 4: Example of an apical sparing pattern 2D STE bull's eye plot from a 65-year-old male patient with biopsy-proven CA from primary (AL) amyloidosis (Relative apical sparing index: 1.59).

amyloid light-chain (AL) amyloidosis resulting in early impairment of longitudinal myocardial performance. GLS values are significantly lower in comparison to familial HCM and hypertension-related LVH.[37] 2D STE-GLS of less than 11.78% was independently associated with poorer survival in patients with AL-CA.[38] It is now well-recognized the relative "apical sparing" pattern of LV regional longitudinal strain (LS) is a reproducible and accurate technique for differentiating CA from other phenotypic "hypertrophic" cardiomyopathies (Fig. 4).[39] A relative apical sparing index [average apical LS (average basal LS + average mid LS)] of more than and equal to 1.0 was able to discriminate CA from HCM and LVH due to aortic stenosis (AS) with a sensitivity of 93% and specificity of 82%. Higher values were associated with worse outcomes.[40] An additional observation that may also discriminate CA from HCM is the proposed LVEF/GLS ratio where a value of more than and equal to 4.1 was more suggestive of CA [ROC-area under the curve (AUC) = 0.91 (CI: 0.88-0.97); $p < 0.005$].[41]

Chemotherapy offers a potential increase in life expectancy for patients with malignancies. However, this may be accompanied by an increased risk of early or delayed cardiovascular toxicities. A decline in LVEF is a late marker of cardiotoxicity, as sufficient myocyte damage has already developed and irreversible LV systolic dysfunction has occurred. Despite this major limitation, LVEF remains the key parameter in the consensus definition of cancer therapeutics-related cardiac dysfunction (CTRCD), where the diagnosis is based upon a reduction in LVEF of more than 10% to below 53%, and the change confirmed by repeat imaging within 2–3 weeks.[42] A systemic review of 1,504 patients confirmed that changes in GLS preceded alterations in LVEF consistent with the onset of subclinical LV systolic dysfunction, and a 10–15% decrease in 2D STE-GLS during treatment was predictive of future cardiotoxicity.[43] The prototypical agents causing type 1 CTRCD (cell apoptosis) are anthracyclines that are associated with the development of dose-dependent cardiotoxicity. Preanthracycline GLS less than 17.5% was associated with a sixfold increase in cardiac events (symptomatic HF or cardiac death), independent of a normal baseline LVEF, potentially offering a window of opportunity to tailor treatments and minimize the risk of cardiotoxicity.[44] GLS of less than 19% postcompletion of anthracycline treatment also predicted future development of heart failure.[45] Trastuzumab is commonly used as adjuvant treatment for breast cancer and may result in type 2 CTRCD that is often reversible. A relative reduction of GLS by 11% (95% CI: 8–15%) was predictive of decrease in LVEF (sensitivity: 65%, specificity: 94%) due to Trastuzumab therapy.[46] From the clinical perspective, a more than 15% relative decrease in GLS from baseline is regarded as significant and may imply the development of cardiotoxicity.[42,47]

Valvular Heart Disease

Echocardiography is often relied upon as the primary imaging modality for defining both the mechanism and the severity of valvular heart disease. Optimal timing for intervention remains a difficult decision as symptoms can be nonspecific and over-reliance on LVEF may fail to detect subclinical dysfunction where progressive myocardial remodelling and fibrosis has already begun. As strain imaging is now able to detect early LV systolic dysfunction despite a "preserved" LVEF, the impetus for earlier referral for surgical or transcatheter treatments warrants further consideration.

Mitral regurgitation: Chronic severe mitral regurgitation (MR) provides an alternative path of low impedance to offload the LV, thereby inciting a state of "increasing" LVEF with increased preload and reduced afterload, and in doing so masking the signs of LV systolic dysfunction.[48,49] The ability to detect insidious LV contractile dysfunction may trigger earlier and more optimal timing of surgery, avoiding irreversible LV dysfunction and ultimately offering a survival advantage.[50-52] Risk stratification for latent LV systolic dysfunction has previously been undertaken using exercise stress echocardiography where the lack of contractile reserve (defined as a failure to increase the LVEF by >4% with exercise) predicted the development of postoperative deterioration of LVEF and congestive cardiac failure.[53,54] However, this approach would still be limited by LVEF quantification in a volume-overloaded ventricle. Baseline LV-GLS measured by 2D STE in patients with moderate-severe valvular MR and LVEF more than 60% undergoing mitral valve repair was found to be an independent predictor of postoperative long-term LV systolic dysfunction (LVEF < 50%).[55] GLS less than 19.9% was the best cutoff value with a sensitivity and specificity of 90% and 79%, respectively. Exercise-induced increase in GLS of less than 1.9% was also suggestive of resting preclinical LV dysfunction and was predictive of postoperative decline of LVEF to less than 50%.[56] These findings were reconfirmed in another larger cohort of 135 patients, where the lack of improvement of GLS more than 2% postexercise independently predicted future cardiac events and/or mitral valve surgery.[57]

Aortic stenosis: In asymptomatic severe AS, LV systolic dysfunction (LVEF < 50%) or an abnormal hemodynamic exercise response (LVEF ≥ 50%) carries a class 1C recommendation for surgical aortic valve replacement (AVR).[58] However, LVEF is insensitive and can remain "normal" until late in the disease process where transition from compensatory concentric hypertrophy to permanent myocardial damage and decompensation occurs. 2D STE-GLS has been shown to decrease as the severity of AS progresses with no change in LVEF (mild AS: 17.1 ± 3.0%; moderate AS: 16.4 ± 3.0%; severe AS: 14.5 ± 3.9%; *ANOVA* $p = 0.003$).[59] There also appears to be a sequential progression of impairment in multidirectional strain on 2D STE in parallel with increasing severity of AS, starting with the subendocardium (LS) in mild AS, mid-wall (CS) in moderate AS, and ultimately transmural (remodeling strains) involvement in severe AS.[60] This highlights the concept that subclinical myocardial dysfunction develops early in the disease process, predating onset of symptoms or change LVEF, and can be better assessed using myocardial deformation imaging. A mean absolute GLS; less than 15% assessed with VVI in asymptomatic severe AS patients with LVEF more than 50% provided independent and incremental prognostic information beyond clinical risk scores in predicting event-free survival, further validating the prognostic value of GLS despite the preserved LVEF.[61]

The echocardiographic assessment of AS has become increasingly more complex especially when discrepancies between measured valve gradients and calculated valve areas are encountered.[62] A reclassification scheme for AS with integration of flow-gradient parameters [normal flow (NF) vs. low flow: stroke volume index (SVi) ≥35 mL/m^2 vs. <35 mL/m^2; high-gradient vs. low-gradient (LG) mean gradient: ≥40 mm Hg vs. <40 mm Hg] has been proposed for more comprehensive characterization of patients with asymptomatic severe AS and LVEF more than 55% and improved prognostication.[63] Paradoxical low flow low gradient aortic stenosis (PLFLGAS) patients have significantly lower basal LS in comparison to those with NF/LG-AS (11.6 ± 3.4% vs. 14.8 ± 3%, $p < 0.001$) in addition to higher Z_{Va} or global afterload (5.5 ± 1.1 vs. 4 ± 0.8 mm Hg/mL/m^2, $p < 0.001$) and systemic vascular resistance.[64] Both baseline SVi ≤ 35 mL/m^2 and GLS <15% were independent predictors of increased mortality in an observational study of 134 PLFLGAS patients undergoing AVR, suggesting that this subset of patients were at a more advanced stage of the disease.[65] Assessment of myocardial mechanics may therefore identify patients who would most benefit from preemptive aortic valve intervention.

Aortic regurgitation: Chronic severe aortic regurgitation (AR) imposes both a pressure and volume load on the LV with compensatory concentric and eccentric hypertrophy to "normalize" filling pressures and maintain an adequate forward stroke volume. As afterload excess continues to increase, LVEF begins to fall but the remodeling remains reversible following AVR. When preload compensation is depleted, progressive LV cavity dilatation develops and impaired myocardial contractility is responsible for further deterioration in LV systolic function. The progression to this later stage may occur before development of symptoms in more than 25% of patients, may not be fully reversible postsurgery, and therefore mitigate the prognostic benefits of AVR. Reduced GLS as a marker of subclinical myocardial dysfunction has been demonstrated in patients with isolated chronic severe AR with a normal LVEF.[66] Symptomatic patients with moderate-severe AR (LVEF >50%) had significantly more impaired baseline multidirectional strain in comparison to asymptomatic cases.[67] 2D STE-GLS more than and equal to 17.4% (sensitivity: 77%, specificity: 57%, AUC = 0.70, $p = 0.008$) was predictive of progression to AVR in the asymptomatic group while GLS more than and equal to 19.3% had a 100% negative-predictive value for patients remaining free of symptoms and need for surgery. Resting GLS values have also been independently associated in another study with the need for earlier surgery.[68,69] In addition to disease progression (onset of symptoms, LV dilatation by >15%, or deterioration in LVEF by >10%), a preoperative reduction in myocardial strain portends a poorer outcome post-AVR [persistent symptoms (New York Heart Association Class ≥2) or LV dilatation (LV diastolic volume indexed for body surface area ≥87 mL/m^2), and LVEF <50%].[70]

RIGHT VENTRICULAR STRAIN

Right ventricle (RV) contractility and function are well-recognized as an important prognostic factor in cardiovascular diseases. Due to its shape, the assessment of RV contractility had been difficult until the advent of MRI. RV EF by MRI is considered the default "gold standard". As echocardiography remains a cost-effective and widely practiced imaging modality, and many echocardiographic parameters correlate well with MRI measures, it is recognized as an important diagnostic tool for the assessment of RV function. Majority of the RV subendocardial fibers are oriented longitudinally and the long-axis contraction (or piston movement) is a major contributor to RVEF. The current measures of RV function include tricuspid annular plane systolic excursion (TAPSE), peak systolic velocity [right ventricular systolic (RVS)], RV fractional area change (RVFAC) and RV dP/dt. TAPSE uses the M-mode motion of the tricuspid annulus while the RVS' is derived from the RV myocardial velocities using tissue Doppler imaging.[71,72] These correlate moderately with the RVEF on MRI. RVFAC remains a 2D measure for a three-dimensional (3D) structure, however, there is prognostic data supporting its use. The rate of rise in RV pressure (RV dP/dt) can be measured noninvasively on echocardiography and a value less than 400 mm Hg/sec correlates with a reduced RVEF on MRI[73] and a poorer prognosis.[74] 2D STE is emerging as a standard measurement of RV function. Strain and strain rate are representative of the myocardial contractility. Similar to the left ventricle, the RV peak longitudinal strain is derived from the apical views. In some studies, RV longitudinal strain is measured from the three segments of the RV free wall, while others have included the interventricular septum in the measurement. While not completely defined, consensus seems to be settling in excluding the septum as part of the LV myocardium and using just the three segments of the RV free wall in the strain measurement. The chamber quantification guidelines from the American Society of Echocardiography and European Association of Cardiovascular Imaging, describe an absolute cutoff of more than 20% as normal RV longitudinal strain.[72] In another study, prospectively screening patients with pulmonary hypertension defined the normal range between 24% and 29%.[75,76] Studies which include the septum along with the RV free wall in the strain measurement had a slightly lower strain value when compared to those with the RV free wall strain alone. RV strain can be reduced in many cardiopulmonary conditions and correlates with functional and prognostic measurements in HF and pulmonary hypertension.[77,78]

Two-dimensional Speckle Tracking Strain and Atrial Function

Evaluation of left atrial (LA) strain is an emerging area with clinical utility particularly in specific patient subsets. LA function is complex, comprising of a reservoir phase in systole, conduit phase in early diastole and contractile phase in late diastole.[79] Evaluation of LA strain permits measurements of phasic LA function throughout the cardiac cycle. While tissue Doppler derived LA strain was initially used, it was time consuming with difficulties sampling from the LA roof and basal segments.[79] 2D speckle tracking strain being semiautomated and angle independent, made evaluation of LA strain more feasible, and reproducible. However, LA strain measurements are currently performed using a strain measurement package developed for LV strain evaluation. Importantly, after tracking the LA endocardium in systole, the region of interest should be minimized for the thin-walled LA. Strain measurements are obtained from unzoomed apical four- and two-chamber views, maximizing the LA volume, that are used (Figs. 5A and B).

Normal Left Atrial Strain

The pattern of the LA strain curve corresponds to the ECG gating that has been utilized. Typically, R-R gating is used and this permits measurement of LA strain even in patients in atrial fibrillation.[79] In this instance, the positive wave is LA reservoir function which then plateaus and represents LA contractile function, with the difference in the two measurements being LA conduit strain (Fig. 6). More recently P-P gating has been used, and this is thought to perhaps be a more accurate measure of LA contractile function. With P-P gating, the first wave is negative and represents LA contractile function while the peak-positive wave is a measure of LA conduit function, and their sum representing LA reservoir function (Fig. 6). Normal LA strain values have been reported. In a multicenter study involving 329 healthy subjects, Morris et al. reported normal LA reservoir strain to be 45.5 ± 11.4% and LA strain rate during late diastole to be – 2.11 ± 0.61 s-1. The lowest expected values (using mean – 2SD) was 23.1% for LA reservoir strain and –0.91 s-1 for A sr in late diastole.[80] More recently

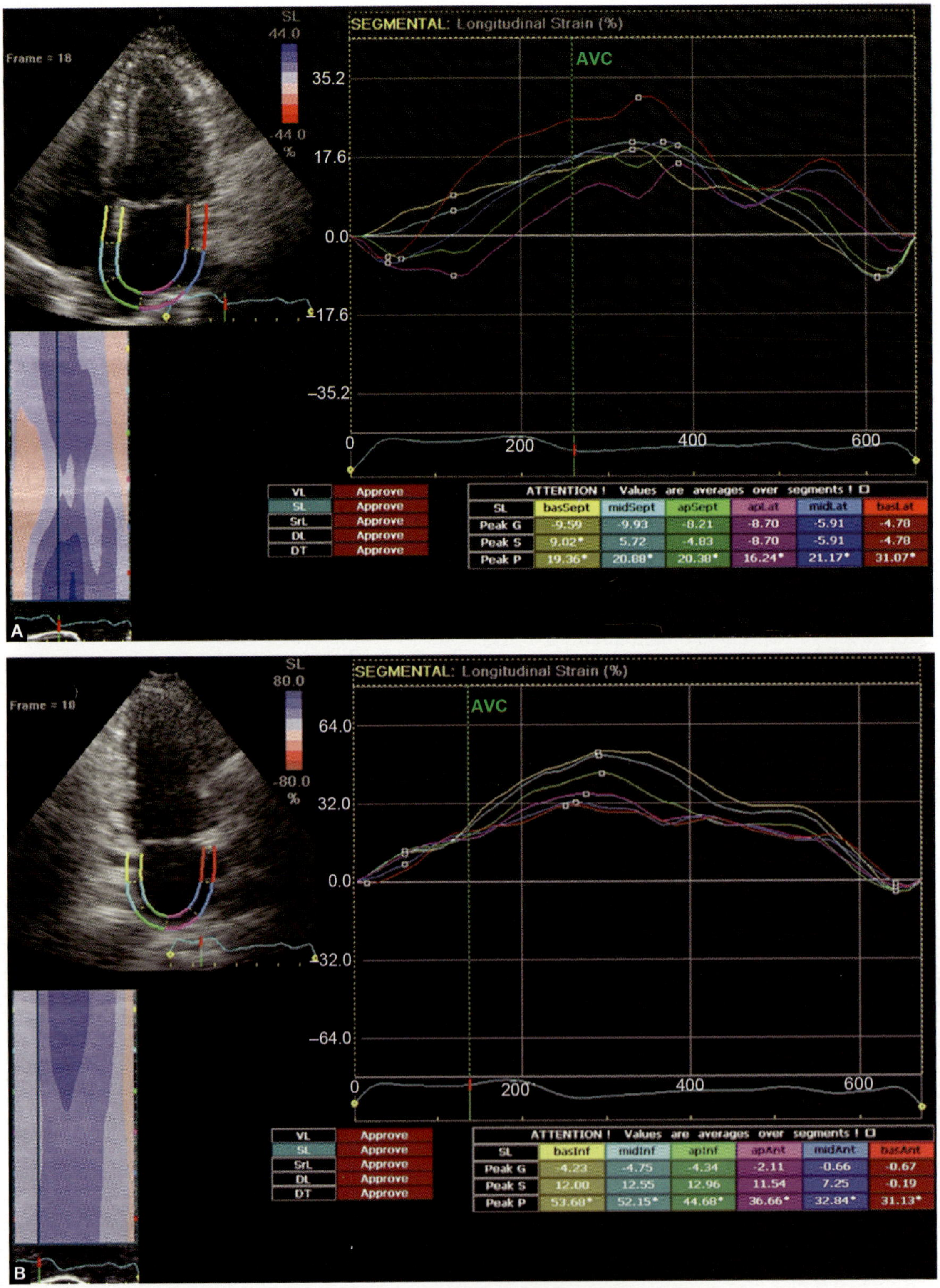

Figs. 5A and B: Phasic left atrial strain measured using global longitudinal strain, from apical four-chamber and two-chamber views.

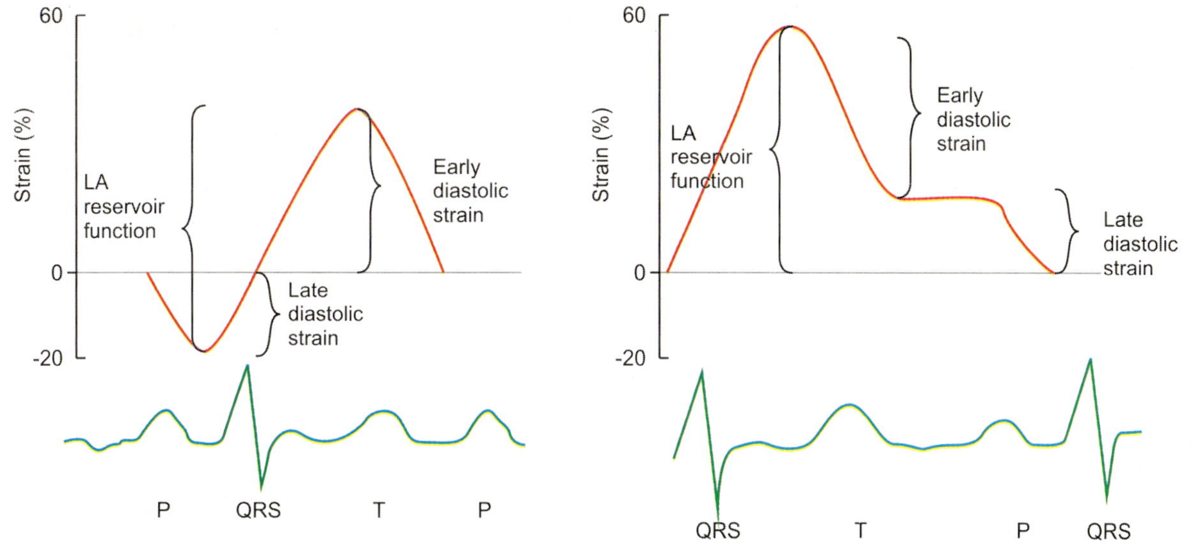

Fig. 6: Left atrial strain patterns based on electrographic gating from P – P wave or R – R wave (Modified from Hoit et al.)

a metanalysis of 40 studies (37 with R-R gating and 3 with P-P gating), reported a mean LA reservoir strain of 39.4% (38–41%), conduit LA strain of 23% (21-25%) and contractile LA strain of 17.4% (16–19%).[81] Both heart rate and body surface area contribute to heterogeneity of LA strain.[81] There have been reports of age related reduction in LA strain using both tissue Doppler[82] and 2D strain,[80,83] with a decline in LA strain values with increasing age. Changes in LA strain have been demonstrated before volumetric changes in the left atrium are apparent.[82] There are also reports that suggest that gender may alter LA strain. Gender differences were observed with strain being higher in younger women (<55 years) in a group of healthy individuals.[84]

LA strain and Diastolic Function

Left atrial strain is increasingly being demonstrated to be a useful parameter for grading diastolic dysfunction. Morris et al. demonstrated that LA strain correlated inversely to LV filling pressure (E/e') and with grade of diastolic dysfunction.[85] The Berlin Female Risk Evaluation trial demonstrated that LA reservoir strain decreased with worsening grades of diastolic function, while LA contractile strain was increased in those with grade 1 diastolic dysfunction as compared to those with normal diastolic function, as a compensatory mechanism.[86] LA systolic strain also correlated with invasively determined LV end-diastolic pressure as well as levels of N-terminal pro-B-type natriuretic peptide.[87] In a group of 517 patients, LA strain was altered even before LA enlargement was manifested in patients with diastolic dysfunction.[85] Additionally, a lower LA strain was associated with increased hospitalization with heart failure. In 308 HF with preserved ejection fraction (HFpEF) patients, LA strain was reduced, correlated with adverse events, and was independently associated with the composite endpoint of hospitalization from cardiovascular events and death.[88]

Left Atrial Strain with Cardiovascular Risk Factors: Hypertension, Diabetes and Chronic Kidney Disease

Left atrial strain alterations have been reported in hypertension even prior to LA enlargement.[89] Improved LA strain was demonstrated with blood pressure lowering therapy with renin angiotensin receptor blockers and beta blockers in mild to moderate hypertension.[90] Altered LA strain has also been observed in patients with diabetes mellitus, independent of hypertension, LV hypertrophy and altered diastolic dysfunction suggesting an independent effect of diabetes on LA function.[91,92] Chronic kidney disease (CKD) is increasingly being realised as a significant risk factor for adverse cardiovascular events. LA strain added incremental value to the C statistic, when stage 3 CKD patients were compared to risk factor matched controls. In CKD patients, LA strain was altered before LA enlargement occurred.[93]

Ischemic Heart Disease and Heart Failure

Two-dimensional LA strain was an independent predictor of all cause mortality, HF hospitalization and reinfarction following MI.[94] However, the independent prognostic value of LA strain was not demonstrated in a larger cohort.[95] LA strain improved in patients with cardiac rehabilitation following a MI.[96] LA strain was an independent predictor for the development of atrial fibrillation (AF) following coronary artery bypass grafting.[97] LA strain has particular value in the evaluation and treatment of HF patients, as it is a surrogate of LV filling pressure (e/e'). LA systolic strain had the highest diagnostic accuracy in predicting elevated LV filling pressure, and was the best determinant of pulmonary capillary wedge pressure.[98] Kurt et al. demonstrated correlations with invasively estimated LV filling pressure, B-type natriuretic peptide levels and demonstrated that LA strain derived LA stiffness index could differentiate patients with diastolic dysfunction from diastolic HF.[87,99] In HFpEF patients, LA strain was a marker of reduced exercise capacity.[100] In heart failure with reduced ejection fraction patients, LA strain also correlated with metabolic equivalents at exercise.[101] A differential reduction in LA strain was observed in idiopathic versus ischemic cardiomyopathies, demonstrating a coexisting atrial myopathy in the former group.[101] LA strain was a predictor of improvement where CRT has been successful in treating HF patients.[102]

Valvular Heart Disease

Left atrial strain has demonstrated utility in both mitral and aortic valve disease. In MR-LA strain decreased with increasing MR severity[103] and could identify patients requiring mitral valve surgery and those with increased mortality.[104] LA strain was also an independent predictor of post op AF following mitral valve surgery.[105] Similar utility was seen in patients with mitral stenosis, with LA strain being a predictor of adverse events as well as postoperative AF.[106] In patients with aortic stenosis, LA strain was an independent predictor of post op AF.[107] Additionally, a low LA strain was associated with increased adverse events including HF hospitalization and mortality.[108]

Atrial Fibrillation

Atrial fibrillation is of particular relevance in terms of evaluation of LA strain. Tissue Doppler strain was a predictor of patients who maintained sinus rhythm postcardioversion.[109] A reduced LA strain was the strongest predictor for the progression of paroxysmal AF to persistent AF.[110] LA strain was predictive of paroxysmal AF in a cohort of patients with cryptogenic stroke.[111] Catheter ablation is used as therapy for AF, and LA strain is an independent predictor for maintenance of sinus rhythm post ablation,[112,113] with both global and regional LA strain (i.e. lateral LA strain) being predictors. Thus, LA strain may be utilized as a tool for selection of patients for ablation.

Stroke

Left atrial strain evaluation in ischemic stroke is an emerging area as an atrial myopathy (independent of associated AF) is thought to contribute, in a proportion of patients with ischemic strokes. LA strain was an independent predictor of stroke in patients with paroxysmal and persistent AF,[114] providing incremental value over the CHA2DS2 VaSc score. Similarly, reduced LA strain was predictive of stroke in patients with paroxysmal AF and low CHADS score[115] as well as in patients with permanent AF.[116] Hsu et al. demonstrated the incremental value of LA strain over the CHA2DS2 VaSc score and LV function for subsequent strokes.[117] Others have demonstrated reduced LA strain in stroke patients who subsequently develop AF.[118,119] However, future prospective studies are required to evaluate the role of LA strain and its utility in stroke patients.

CONCLUSION

Myocardial strain imaging using 2D STE is rapidly emerging as true index of myocardial function. It is a relatively load independent measure of myocardial performance. GLS is recognized as a sensitive marker of early or subclinical myocardial dysfunction, and is effect much before a deterioration in global LVEF occurs. GLS is finding clinical application in numerous myocardial diseases, including ischemic and nonischemic cardiomyopathies, infilterative cardiomyopathies, chemotherapy induced cardiomyopathy, valvular heart disease, and in multisystem disease like diabetes, renal failure, hypertension and pulmonary hypertension. It now has applications in the assessment of both systolic and diastolic function. The normative data for GLS has been established and the earlier intervendor variation in the assessment of GLS has largely been resolved with good test-retest reproducibility. The clinical applications are likely to steadily increase further in the coming years.

REFERENCES

1. Stanton T, Leano R, Marwick TH. Prediction of all-cause mortality from global longitudinal speckle strain: comparison with ejection fraction and wall motion scoring. Circ Cardiovasc Imaging. 2009;2(5):356-64.
2. Hung CL, Verma A, Uno H, et al. Longitudinal and circumferential strain rate, left ventricular remodeling, and prognosis after myocardial infarction. J Am Coll Cardiol. 2010;56(22):1812-22.
3. Farsalinos KE, Daraban AM, Ünlü S, et al. Head-to-head comparison of global longitudinal strain measurements among nine different vendors: The EACVI/ASE inter-vendor comparison study. J Am Soc Echocardiogr. 2015;28(10): 1171-81.
4. Yingchoncharoen T, Agarwal S, Popovic ZB ,et al. Normal ranges of left ventricular strain: a meta-analysis. J Am Soc Echocardiogr. 2013;26(2):185-91.
5. Park JJ, Park J-B, Park JH, et al. Global longitudinal strain to predict mortality in patients with acute heart failure. J Am Coll Cardiol. 2018;71(18):1947-57.

6. Cho GY, Marwick TH, Kim HS, et al. Global 2-dimensional strain as a new prognosticator in patients with heart failure. J Am Coll Cardiol. 2009;54(7):618-24.
7. Hamada S, Schroeder J, Hoffmann R, et al. Prediction of outcomes in patients with chronic ischemic cardiomyopathy by layer-specific strain echocardiography: A proof of concept. J Am Soc Echocardiogr. 2016;29(5):412-20.
8. Choi JO, Cho SW, Song YB, et al. Longitudinal 2D strain at rest predicts the presence of left main and three vessel coronary artery disease in patients without regional wall motion abnormality. Eur J Echocardiogr. 2009;10(5):695-701.
9. Dahlslett T, Karlsen S, Grenne B, et al. Early assessment of strain echocardiography can accurately exclude significant coronary artery stenosis in suspected non-ST-segment elevation acute coronary syndrome. J Am Soc Echocardiogr. 2014;27(5):512-9.
10. Biering-Sørensen T, Hoffmann S, Mogelvang R, et al. Myocardial strain analysis by 2-dimensional speckle tracking echocardiography improves diagnostics of coronary artery stenosis in stable angina pectoris. Circ Cardiovasc Imaging. 2014;7(1):58-65.
11. Eek C, Grenne B, Brunvand H, et al. Strain echocardiography and wall motion score index predicts final infarct size in patients with non-ST-segment-elevation myocardial infarction. Circ Cardiovasc Imaging. 2010;3(2):187-94.
12. Lacalzada J, la Rosa de A, Izquierdo MM, et al. Left ventricular global longitudinal systolic strain predicts adverse remodeling and subsequent cardiac events in patients with acute myocardial infarction treated with primary percutaneous coronary intervention. Int J Cardiovasc Imaging. 2015;31(3):575-84.
13. Priori SG, Blomström-Lundqvist C, Mazzanti A, et al. 2015 ESC Guidelines for the management of patients with ventricular arrhythmias and the prevention of sudden cardiac death: The Task Force for the Management of Patients with Ventricular Arrhythmias and the Prevention of Sudden Cardiac Death of the European Society of Cardiology (ESC). Endorsed by: Association for European Paediatric and Congenital Cardiology (AEPC). Eur Heart J. 2015;36:2793-867.
14. Buxton AE, Lee KL, Hafley GE, et al. Limitations of ejection fraction for prediction of sudden death risk in patients with coronary artery disease: lessons from the MUSTT study. J Am Coll Cardiol. 2007;50(12):1150-7.
15. Haugaa KH, Grenne BL, Eek CH, et al. Strain echocardiography improves risk prediction of ventricular arrhythmias after myocardial infarction. JACC Cardiovasc Imaging. 2013;6(8):841-50.
16. Tarascio M, Leo LA, Klersy C, et al. Speckle-tracking layer-specific analysis of myocardial deformation and evaluation of scar transmurality in chronic ischemic heart disease. J Am Soc Echocardiogr. 2017;30(7):667-75.
17. Saba S, Marek J, Schwartzman D, et al. Echocardiography-guided left ventricular lead placement for cardiac resynchronization therapy: Results of the speckle tracking assisted resynchronization therapy for electrode region trial. Circ Heart Fail. 2013;6(3):427-34.
18. Kydd AC, Khan FZ, Watson WD, et al. Prognostic benefit of optimum left ventricular lead position in cardiac resynchronization therapy: follow-up of the TARGET Study Cohort (Targeted Left Ventricular Lead Placement to guide Cardiac Resynchronization Therapy). JACC Heart Fail. 2014;2(3):205-12.
19. Naylor LH, George K, O'Driscoll G, et al. The athlete's heart: a contemporary appraisal of the 'Morganroth hypothesis'. Sports Med. 2008;38(1):69-90.
20. Baggish AL, Wood MJ. Athlete's heart and cardiovascular care of the athlete: Scientific and clinical update. Circulation. 2011;123(23):2723-35.
21. Paterick TE, Gordon T, Spiegel D. Echocardiography: profiling of the athlete's heart. J Am Soc Echocardiogr. 2014;27(9):940-8.
22. Maron BJ, Towbin JA, Thiene G, et al. Contemporary definitions and classification of the cardiomyopathies: an American Heart Association Scientific Statement from the Council on Clinical Cardiology, Heart Failure and Transplantation Committee; Quality of Care and Outcomes Research and Functional Genomics and Translational Biology Interdisciplinary Working Groups; and Council on Epidemiology and Prevention. Circulation. 2006;113(14):1807-16.
23. Elliott PM, Anastasakis A, Borger MA, et al. 2014 ESC Guidelines on diagnosis and management of hypertrophic cardiomyopathy: The task force for the diagnosis and management of hypertrophic cardiomyopathy of the European Society of Cardiology (ESC). Eur Heart J. 2014;35(39):2733-79.
24. Marian AJ, Braunwald E. Hypertrophic cardiomyopathy: Genetics, pathogenesis, clinical manifestations, diagnosis, and therapy. Circ Res. 2017;121(7):749-70.
25. Habib G, Bucciarelli-Ducci C, Caforio ALP, et al. Multimodality imaging in restrictive cardiomyopathies: An EACVI expert consensus document in collaboration with the "Working Group on myocardial and pericardial diseases" of the European Society of Cardiology Endorsed by The Indian Academy of Echocardiography. Eur Heart J Cardiovasc Imaging. 2017;18(10):1090-121.
26. Afonso LC, Bernal J, Bax JJ, et al. Echocardiography in hypertrophic cardiomyopathy: the role of conventional and emerging technologies. JACC Cardiovasc Imaging. 2008;1(6):787-800.
27. Gersh BJ, Maron BJ, Bonow RO. 2011 ACCF/AHA guideline for the diagnosis and treatment of hypertrophic cardiomyopathy: a report of the American College of Cardiology Foundation/American Heart Association Task Force on Practice Guidelines. J Am Coll Cardiol. 2011;58(25):2703-38.
28. Butz T, van Buuren F, Mellwig KP, et al. Two-dimensional strain analysis of the global and regional myocardial function for the differentiation of pathologic and physiologic left ventricular hypertrophy: a study in athletes and in patients with hypertrophic cardiomyopathy. Int J Cardiovasc Imaging. 2011;27(1):91-100.
29. Afonso L, Kondur A, Simegn M, et al. Two-dimensional strain profiles in patients with physiological and pathological

hypertrophy and preserved left ventricular systolic function: a comparative analyses. BMJ Open. 2012;2(4):e001390.
30. Kansal MM, Lester SJ, Surapaneni P, et al. Usefulness of two-dimensional and speckle tracking echocardiography in "Gray Zone" left ventricular hypertrophy to differentiate professional football player's heart from hypertrophic cardiomyopathy. Am J Cardiol. 2011;108(9):1322-6.
31. Serri K, Reant P, Lafitte M, et al. Global and regional myocardial function quantification by two-dimensional strain: application in hypertrophic cardiomyopathy. J Am Coll Cardiol. 2006;47(6):1175-81.
32. Popovic ZB, Kwon DH, Mishra M, et al. Association between regional ventricular function and myocardial fibrosis in hypertrophic cardiomyopathy assessed by speckle tracking echocardiography and delayed hyperenhancement magnetic resonance imaging. J Am Soc Echocardiogr. 2008;21(12):1299-305.
33. Haland TF, Almaas VM, Hasselberg NE, et al. Strain echocardiography is related to fibrosis and ventricular arrhythmias in hypertrophic cardiomyopathy. Eur Heart J Cardiovasc Imaging. 2016;17(6):613-21.
34. Reant P, Mirabel M, Lloyd G, et al. Global longitudinal strain is associated with heart failure outcomes in hypertrophic cardiomyopathy. Heart. 2016;102(10):741-7.
35. Krämer J, Niemann M, Liu D, et al. Two-dimensional speckle tracking as a non-invasive tool for identification of myocardial fibrosis in Fabry disease. Eur Heart J. 2013;34(21):1587-96.
36. Fadel B, Baldini L, Pergola V. Myocardial deformation imaging and rare cardiomyopathies with hypertrophic phenotype: a review focused on Fabry disease, Friedreich ataxia and amyloidosis. Cardiogenetics. 2013;3:e4.
37. Sun JP, Stewart WJ, Yang XS, et al. Differentiation of hypertrophic cardiomyopathy and cardiac amyloidosis from other causes of ventricular wall thickening by two-dimensional strain imaging echocardiography. Am J Cardiol. 2009;103(3):411-5.
38. Buss SJ, Emami M, Mereles D, et al. Longitudinal left ventricular function for prediction of survival in systemic light-chain amyloidosis: incremental value compared with clinical and biochemical markers. J Am Coll Cardiol. 2012;60(12):1067-76.
39. Phelan D, Collier P, Thavendiranathan P, et al. Relative apical sparing of longitudinal strain using two-dimensional speckle-tracking echocardiography is both sensitive and specific for the diagnosis of cardiac amyloidosis. Heart. 2012;98(19):1442-8.
40. Senapati A, Sperry BW, Grodin JL, et al. Prognostic implication of relative regional strain ratio in cardiac amyloidosis. Heart. 2016;102(10):748-54.
41. Pagourelias ED, Duchenne J, Mirea O, et al. The Relation of Ejection Fraction and Global Longitudinal Strain in Amyloidosis: Implications for Differential Diagnosis. JACC Cardiovasc Imaging. 2016;9(11):1358-9.
42. Plana JC, Galderisi M, Barac A, et al. Expert consensus for multimodality imaging evaluation of adult patients during and after cancer therapy: a report from the American Society of Echocardiography and the European Association of Cardiovascular Imaging. J Am Soc Echocardiogr. 2014;27(9):911-39.
43. Thavendiranathan P, Poulin F, Lim KD, et al. Use of myocardial strain imaging by echocardiography for the early detection of cardiotoxicity in patients during and after cancer chemotherapy: a systematic review. J Am Coll Cardiol. 2014;63(25 Pt A):2751-68.
44. Ali MT, Yucel E, Bouras S, et al. Myocardial strain is associated with adverse clinical cardiac events in patients treated with anthracyclines. J Am Soc Echocardiogr. 2016;29(6):522-3.
45. Sawaya H, Sebag IA, Plana JC, et al. Assessment of echocardiography and biomarkers for the extended prediction of cardiotoxicity in patients treated with anthracyclines, taxanes, and trastuzumab. Circ Cardiovasc Imaging. 2012;5(5):596-603.
46. Negishi K, Negishi T, Hare JL. Independent and incremental value of deformation indices for prediction of trastuzumab-induced cardiotoxicity. J Am Soc Echocardiogr. 2013;26(5):493-8.
47. Zamorano JL, Lancellotti P, Rodriguez Muñoz D, et al. 2016 ESC Position Paper on cancer treatments and cardiovascular toxicity developed under the auspices of the ESC Committee for Practice Guidelines: The Task Force for cancer treatments and cardiovascular toxicity of the European Society of Cardiology (ESC). Eur Heart J. 2016;37(36):2768-801.
48. Starling MR, Kirsh MM, Montgomery DG, et al. Impaired left ventricular contractile function in patients with long-term mitral regurgitation and normal ejection fraction. J Am Coll Cardiol. 1993;22(1):239-50.
49. Lee R, Marwick TH. Assessment of subclinical left ventricular dysfunction in asymptomatic mitral regurgitation. Eur J Echocardiogr. 2007;8(3):175-84.
50. Enriquez-Sarano M, Tajik AJ, Schaff HV, et al. Echocardiographic prediction of left ventricular function after correction of mitral regurgitation: Results and clinical implications. J Am Coll Cardiol. 1994;24(6):1536-43.
51. Enriquez-Sarano M, Tajik AJ, Schaff HV, et al. Echocardiographic prediction of survival after surgical correction of organic mitral regurgitation. Circulation. 1994;90(2):830-7.
52. Starling MR. Effects of valve surgery on left ventricular contractile function in patients with long-term mitral regurgitation. Circulation. 1995;92(4):811-8.
53. Leung DY, Griffin BP, Stewart WJ, et al. Left ventricular function after valve repair for chronic mitral regurgitation: Predictive value of preoperative assessment of contractile reserve by exercise echocardiography. J Am Coll Cardiol. 1996;28(5):1198-205.
54. Lee R, Haluska B, Leung DY, et al. Functional and prognostic implications of left ventricular contractile reserve in patients with asymptomatic severe mitral regurgitation. Heart. 2005;91(11):1407-12.
55. Witkowski TG, Thomas JD, Debonnaire PJMR, et al. Global longitudinal strain predicts left ventricular dysfunction after mitral valve repair. Eur Heart J Cardiovasc Imaging. 2013;14(1):69-76.

56. Lancellotti P, Cosyns B, Zacharakis D, et al. Importance of left ventricular longitudinal function and functional reserve in patients with degenerative mitral regurgitation: Assessment by two-dimensional speckle tracking. J Am Soc Echocardiogr. 2008;21(12):1331-6.
57. Magne J, Mahjoub H, Dulgheru R, et al. Left ventricular contractile reserve in asymptomatic primary mitral regurgitation. Eur Heart J. 2014;35(24):1608-16.
58. Baumgartner H, Falk V, Bax JJ, et al. 2017 ESC/EACTS Guidelines for the management of valvular heart disease. Eur Heart J. 2017;38(36):2739-91.
59. Miyazaki S, Daimon M, Miyazaki T, et al. Global longitudinal strain in relation to the severity of aortic stenosis: A two-dimensional speckle-tracking study. Echocardiography. 2011;28(7):703-8.
60. Ng ACT, Delgado V, Bertini M, et al. Alterations in multidirectional myocardial functions in patients with aortic stenosis and preserved ejection fraction: a two-dimensional speckle tracking analysis. Eur Heart J. 2011;32(12):1542-50.
61. Yingchoncharoen T, Gibby C, Rodriguez LL, et al. Association of myocardial deformation with outcome in asymptomatic aortic stenosis with normal ejection fraction. Circ Cardiovasc Imaging. 2012;5(6):719-25.
62. Minners J, Allgeier M, Gohlke-Baerwolf C, et al. Inconsistencies of echocardiographic criteria for the grading of aortic valve stenosis. Eur Heart J. 2008;29(8):1043-8.
63. Lancellotti P, Magne J, Donal E, et al. Clinical outcome in asymptomatic severe aortic stenosis: insights from the new proposed aortic stenosis grading classification. J Am Coll Cardiol. 2012;59(3):235-43.
64. Adda J, Mielot C, Giorgi R, et al. Low-flow, low-gradient severe aortic stenosis despite normal ejection fraction is associated with severe left ventricular dysfunction as assessed by speckle-tracking echocardiography: a multicenter study. Circ Cardiovasc Imaging. 2012;5(1):27-35.
65. Kamperidis V, van Rosendael PJ, Ng ACT, et al. Impact of flow and left ventricular strain on outcome of patients with preserved left ventricular ejection fraction and low gradient severe aortic stenosis undergoing aortic valve replacement. Am J Cardiol. 2014;114(12):1875-81.
66. Smedsrud MK, Pettersen E, Gjesdal O, et al. Detection of left ventricular dysfunction by global longitudinal systolic strain in patients with chronic aortic regurgitation. J Am Soc Echocardiogr. 2011;24(11):1253-9.
67. Ewe SH, Haeck MLA, Ng ACT, et al. Detection of subtle left ventricular systolic dysfunction in patients with significant aortic regurgitation and preserved left ventricular ejection fraction: speckle tracking echocardiographic analysis. Eur Heart J Cardiovasc Imaging. 2015;16(9):992-9.
68. Kusunose K, Agarwal S, Marwick TH, et al. Decision making in asymptomatic aortic regurgitation in the era of guidelines: incremental values of resting and exercise cardiac dysfunction. Circ Cardiovasc Imaging. 2014;7(2):352-62.
69. Kusunose K, Goodman A, Parikh R, et al. Incremental prognostic value of left ventricular global longitudinal strain in patients with aortic stenosis and preserved ejection fraction. Circ Cardiovasc Imaging. 2014;7(6):938-45.
70. Olsen NT, Sogaard P, Larsson HBW, et al. Speckle-tracking echocardiography for predicting outcome in chronic aortic regurgitation during conservative management and after surgery. JACC Cardiovasc Imaging. 2011;4(3):223-30.
71. Ghio S, Pica S, Klersy C, et al. Prognostic value of TAPSE after therapy optimisation in patients with pulmonary arterial hypertension is independent of the haemodynamic effects of therapy. Open Heart. 2016;3(1):e000408.
72. Lang RM, Badano LP, Mor-Avi V, et al. Recommendations for cardiac chamber quantification by echocardiography in adults: an update from the American Society of Echocardiography and the European Association of Cardiovascular Imaging. J Am Soc Echocardiogr. 2015;28(1):1-39.
73. Singbal Y, Vollbon W, Huynh LT, et al. Exploring Noninvasive Tricuspid dP/dt as a Marker of Right Ventricular Function. Echocardiography. 2015;32(9):1347-51.
74. Ameloot K, Palmers PJ, Vande Bruaene A, et al. Clinical value of echocardiographic Doppler-derived right ventricular dp/dt in patients with pulmonary arterial hypertension. Eur Heart J Cardiovasc Imaging. 2014;15(12):1411-9.
75. Fine NM, Chen L, Bastiansen PM, et al. Reference values for right ventricular strain in patients without cardiopulmonary disease: A prospective evaluation and meta-analysis. Echocardiography. 2015;32(5):787-96.
76. Fine NM, Chen L, Bastiansen PM, et al. Outcome prediction by quantitative right ventricular function assessment in 575 subjects evaluated for pulmonary hypertension. Circ Cardiovasc Imaging. 2013;6(5):711-21.
77. Donal E, Coquerel N, Bodi S, et al. Importance of ventricular longitudinal function in chronic heart failure. Eur J Echocardiogr. 2011;12(8):619-27.
78. Wright L, Negishi K, Dwyer N, et al. Afterload dependence of right ventricular myocardial strain. J Am Soc Echocardiogr. 2017;30(7):676-684.
79. Hoit BD. Left atrial size and function: role in prognosis. J Am Coll Cardiol. 2014;63(6):493-505.
80. Morris DA, Takeuchi M, Krisper M, et al. Normal values and clinical relevance of left atrial myocardial function analysed by speckle-tracking echocardiography: multicentre study. Eur Heart J Cardiovasc Imaging. 2015;16(4):364-72.
81. Pathan F, D'Elia N, Nolan MT, et al. Normal ranges of left atrial strain by speckle-tracking echocardiography: A systematic review and meta-analysis. J Am Soc Echocardiogr. 2017;30(1):59-70.
82. Boyd AC, Richards DAB, Marwick T, et al. Atrial strain rate is a sensitive measure of alterations in atrial phasic function in healthy ageing. Heart. 2011;97(18):1513-9.
83. Meel R, Khandheria BK, Peters F, et al. Effects of age on left atrial volume and strain parameters using echocardiography in a normal black population. Echo Res Pract. 2016;3(4):115-23.
84. Miglioranza MH, Badano LP, Mihăilă S, et al. Physiologic determinants of left atrial longitudinal strain: A two-dimensional speckle-tracking and three-dimensional echocardiographic study in healthy volunteers. J Am Soc Echocardiogr. 2016;29(11):1023-3.
85. Morris DA, Belyavskiy E, Aravind-Kumar R, et al. Potential usefulness and clinical relevance of adding left atrial

strain to left atrial volume index in the detection of left ventricular diastolic dysfunction. JACC Cardiovasc Imaging. 2018;11(10):1405-15.
86. Brecht A, Oertelt-Prigione S, Seeland U, et al. Left atrial function in preclinical diastolic dysfunction: Two-dimensional speckle-tracking echocardiography-derived results from the BEFRI Trial. J Am Soc Echocardiogr. 2016;29(8):750-8.
87. Kurt M, Tanboga IH, Aksakal E, et al. Relation of left ventricular end-diastolic pressure and N-terminal pro-brain natriuretic peptide level with left atrial deformation parameters. Eur Heart J Cardiovasc Imaging. 2012;13(6):524-30.
88. Freed BH, Daruwalla V, Cheng JY, et al. Prognostic utility and clinical significance of cardiac mechanics in heart failure with preserved ejection fraction: Importance of left atrial strain. Circ Cardiovasc Imaging. 2016;9(3):e003754.
89. Mondillo S, Cameli M, Caputo ML, et al. Early detection of left atrial strain abnormalities by speckle-tracking in hypertensive and diabetic patients with normal left atrial size. J Am Soc Echocardiogr. 2011;24(8):898-908.
90. Degirmenci H, Duman H, Demirelli S, et al. Assessment of effect of irbesartan and nebivolol on the left atrium volume and deformation in the patients with mild-moderate hypertension. Eur Rev Med Pharmacol Sci. 2014;18(6):781-9.
91. Kadappu KK, Boyd A, Eshoo S, et al. Changes in left atrial volume in diabetes mellitus: More than diastolic dysfunction? Eur Heart J Cardiovasc Imaging. 2012;13(12):1016-23.
92. Muranaka A, Yuda S, Tsuchihashi K, et al. Quantitative assessment of left ventricular and left atrial functions by strain rate imaging in diabetic patients with and without hypertension. Echocardiography. 2009;26(3):262-71.
93. Kadappu KK, Abhayaratna K, Boyd A, et al. Independent echocardiographic markers of cardiovascular involvement in chronic kidney disease: The value of left atrial function and volume. J Am Soc Echocardiogr. 2016;29(4):359-67.
94. Antoni ML, Brinke ten EA, Atary JZ, et al. Left atrial strain is related to adverse events in patients after acute myocardial infarction treated with primary percutaneous coronary intervention. Heart. 2011;97(16):1332-7.
95. Ersbøll M, Andersen MJ, Valeur N, et al. The prognostic value of left atrial peak reservoir strain in acute myocardial infarction is dependent on left ventricular longitudinal function and left atrial size. Circ Cardiovasc Imaging. 2013;6(1):26-33.
96. Deniz Acar R, Bulut M, Ergün S, et al. Effect of cardiac rehabilitation on left atrial functions in patients with acute myocardial infarction. Ann Phys Rehabil Med. 2014;57(2):105-13.
97. Verdejo HE, Becerra E, Zalaquet R, et al. Atrial function assessed by speckle tracking echocardiography is a good predictor of postoperative atrial fibrillation in elderly patients. Echocardiography. 2016;33(2):242-8.
98. Cameli M, Lisi M, Mondillo S, et al. Left atrial longitudinal strain by speckle tracking echocardiography correlates well with left ventricular filling pressures in patients with heart failure. Cardiovasc Ultrasound. 2010;8:14.
99. Kurt M, Wang J, Torre-Amione G, et al. Left atrial function in diastolic heart failure. Circ Cardiovasc Imaging. 2009;2(1):10-5.
100. Kusunose K, Motoki H, Popovic ZB, et al. Independent association of left atrial function with exercise capacity in patients with preserved ejection fraction. Heart. 2012;98(17):1311-7.
101. D'Andrea A, Caso P, Romano S, et al. Association between left atrial myocardial function and exercise capacity in patients with either idiopathic or ischemic dilated cardiomyopathy: a two-dimensional speckle strain study. Int J Cardiol. 2009;132(3):354-63.
102. D'Andrea A, Caso P, Romano S, et al. Different effects of cardiac resynchronization therapy on left atrial function in patients with either idiopathic or ischaemic dilated cardiomyopathy: a two-dimensional speckle strain study. Eur Heart J. 2007;28(22):2738-48.
103. Cameli M, Lisi M, Giacomin E, et al. Chronic mitral regurgitation: Left atrial deformation analysis by two-dimensional speckle tracking echocardiography. Echocardiography. 2011;28(3):327-34.
104. Debonnaire P, Leong DP, Witkowski TG, et al. Left atrial function by two-dimensional speckle-tracking echocardiography in patients with severe organic mitral regurgitation: association with guidelines-based surgical indication and postoperative (long-term) survival. J Am Soc Echocardiogr. 2013;26(9):1053-62.
105. Borg AN, Pearce KA, Williams SG, et al. Left atrial function and deformation in chronic primary mitral regurgitation. Eur J Echocardiogr. 2009;10(7):833-40.
106. Ancona R, Comenale Pinto S, Caso P, et al. Two-dimensional atrial systolic strain imaging predicts atrial fibrillation at 4-year follow-up in asymptomatic rheumatic mitral stenosis. J Am Soc Echocardiogr. 2013;26(3):270-7.
107. Imanishi J, Tanaka H, Sawa T, et al. Left atrial booster-pump function as a predictive parameter for new-onset postoperative atrial fibrillation in patients with severe aortic stenosis. Int J Cardiovasc Imaging. 2014;30(2):295-304.
108. Galli E, Fournet M, Chabanne C, et al. Prognostic value of left atrial reservoir function in patients with severe aortic stenosis: a 2D speckle-tracking echocardiographic study. Eur Heart J Cardiovasc Imaging. 2016;17(5):533-41.
109. Di Salvo G, Caso P, Piccolo Lo R, et al. Atrial myocardial deformation properties predict maintenance of sinus rhythm after external cardioversion of recent-onset lone atrial fibrillation: a color Doppler myocardial imaging and transthoracic and transesophageal echocardiographic study. Circulation. 2005;112(3):387-95.
110. Yoon YE, Oh IY, Kim SA, et al. Echocardiographic predictors of progression to persistent or permanent atrial fibrillation in patients with paroxysmal atrial fibrillation (E6P Study). J Am Soc Echocardiogr. 2015;28(6):709-17.
111. Pagola J, González-Alujas T, Flores A, et al. Left atria strain is a surrogate marker for detection of atrial fibrillation in cryptogenic strokes. Stroke. 2014;45(8):e164-6.
112. Mirza M, Caracciolo G, Khan U, et al. Left atrial reservoir function predicts atrial fibrillation recurrence after catheter

ablation: a two-dimensional speckle strain study. J Interv Card Electrophysiol. 2011;31(3):197-206.
113. Yasuda R, Murata M, Roberts, et al. Left atrial strain is a powerful predictor of atrial fibrillation recurrence after catheter ablation: Study of a heterogeneous population with sinus rhythm or atrial fibrillation. Eur Heart J Cardiovasc Imaging. 2015;16(9):1008-14.
114. Obokata M, Negishi K, Kurosawa K, et al. Left atrial strain provides incremental value for embolism risk stratification over CHA_2DS_2-VASc score and indicates prognostic impact in patients with atrial fibrillation. J Am Soc Echocardiogr. 2014;27(7):709-16.
115. Azemi T, Rabdiya VM, Ayirala SR, et al. Left atrial strain is reduced in patients with atrial fibrillation, stroke or TIA, and low risk CHADS(2) scores. J Am Soc Echocardiogr. 2012;25(12):1327-32.
116. Shih JY, Tsai WC, Huang YY, et al. Association of decreased left atrial strain and strain rate with stroke in chronic atrial fibrillation. J Am Soc Echocardiogr. 2011;24(5):513-9.
117. Hsu PC, Lee WH, Chu CY, Lee, et al. Prognostic role of left atrial strain and its combination index with transmitral E-wave velocity in patients with atrial fibrillation. Sci Rep. 2016;6:17318.
118. Olsen FJ, Jørgensen PG, Mogelvang R, et al. Predicting paroxysmal atrial fibrillation in cerebrovascular ischemia using tissue doppler imaging and speckle tracking echocardiography. J Stroke Cerebrovasc Dis. 2016;25(2):350-9.
119. Kim D, Shim CY, Cho IJ, et al. Incremental value of left atrial global longitudinal strain for prediction of post stroke atrial fibrillation in patients with acute ischemic stroke. J Cardiovasc Ultrasound. 2016;24(1):20-7.

85

CHAPTER

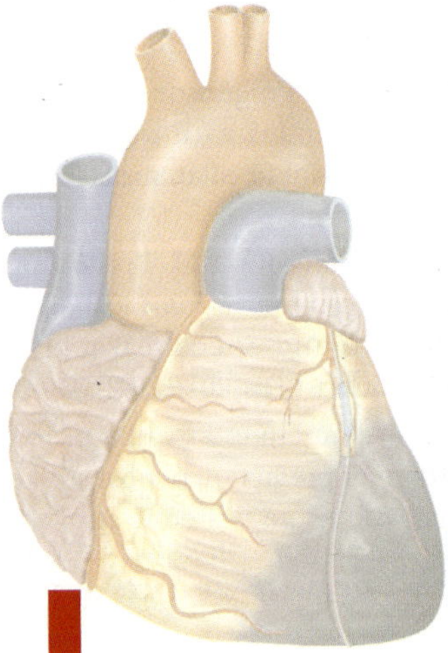

Echo-guided PPI Evaluation in Dilated Cardiomyopathy by Echocardiography

Soumitra Kumar

INTRODUCTION

Dual chamber (Bicameral) and biventricular pacing devices need optimization of pacing parameters to suit the individual patient's electrophysiological variables. Such optimization is particularly important in cardiac resynchronization therapy (CRT) to influence morbidity and mortality in patients with severe heart failure and increased QRS duration. However, optimization of AV delay in particular may also be important in bicameral devices especially in patients with left-ventricular systolic dysfunction as in dilated cardiomyopathy (DCMP). This chapter will deal with programming of bicameral devices only.

THE RATIONALE BEHIND OPTIMIZATION OF ATRIOVENTRICULAR DELAY

The left atrium (LA) and left ventricular (LV) are not electrically connected in series, yet cardiac output is affected by their synchronization. During paced cardiac rhythm, the impulse neither arises from the sinus node nor travels through fibres of Bachmann's bundle to LA. Consequently, interatrial conduction time (IACT) and left atrial systolic (LAS) are delayed.[1] This actual delay in left atrial systole during DDD pacing is longer than a shorter empirically set AV delay. The net result may be systolic AV asynchrony[2] whereby left atrium and left ventricle contract simultaneously or in unphysiological sequence. The whole period of atrial systolic electromechanical action (AEA) can be measured in case of sequential pacing by echo-Doppler coupled with electrocardiogram (ECG) (Fig. 1).

In bicameral (DDD) pacing, the rule to programming of an optimal AV delay is to correlate the end of LA emptying with the onset of LV contraction (Fig. 2). The optimal AV delay is directly proportional to the atrial electromechanical action (AEA); longer the AEA, longer is the AV interval.[3]

METHODS TO PROGRAM ATRIOVENTRICULAR DELAY

The various proposed methods can be divided into three groups: (1) predefined, (2) iterative, and (3) automatic. Of these methods, only those applicable to programming

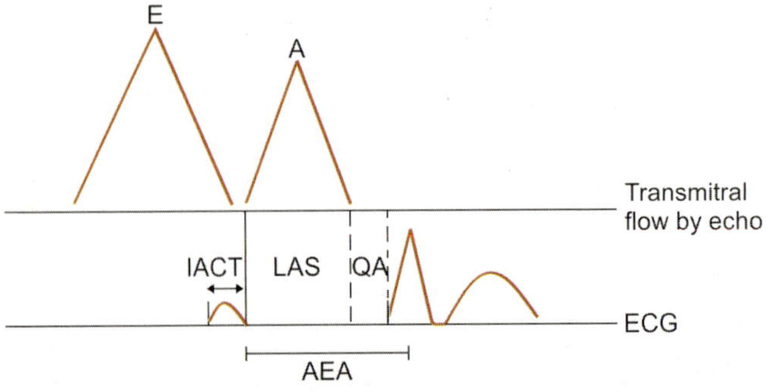

Fig. 1: Atrial electromechanical action. (IACT: interatrial conduction time; IAS: left atrial systole; AEA: atrial electromechanical action; QA: interval between Q wave and end of A-wave)

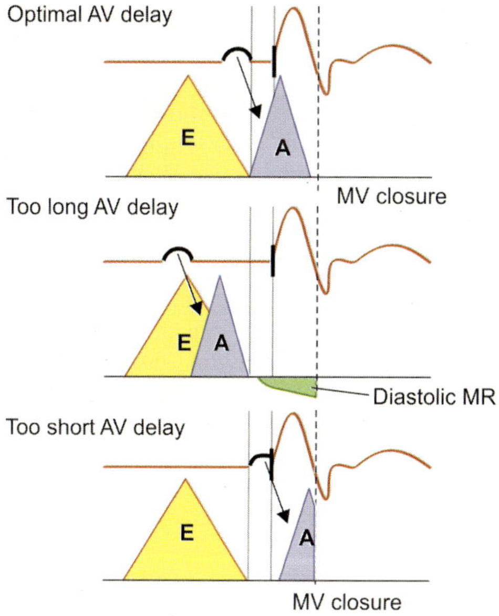

Fig. 2: Effect of atrioventricular delay on transmitral flow.

of AV delay in DDD pacing and those which utilize echocardiography will be discussed here.

Ismer's Formula

Ismer proposed a method for programming AV delay in DDD pacing by using simultaneous filtered bipolar esophageal electrogram and echo-Doppler transmitral flow.[4] The formula is as following:

Optimal AV delay = IACT + LAS – LVEC = AEA – LVEC (LVEC = latency time between the first ventricular potential or the pacing of ventricular artifact and left-ventricular contraction) (Fig. 3).

Left ventricular ejection fraction (LVEF) that resulted with the calculated optimal AV delay in VDD mode was significantly higher than the shorter value (optimal AV delay—50 ms) (28 ± 12 vs 20 ± 7 p = 0.03). No difference was found with the longer optimal AV delay, 23 ± 7%, p = 0.11.

Ritter's Formula

Ritter originally proposed use of an echo Doppler method to obtain an optimal AV delay in DDD pacing in subjects with normal LV function and complete AV block.[5] Two extreme AV intervals are programmed as per Ritter's method: (1) a short one (30 ms) with truncated A-wave and (2) a long one (200 ms) without A-wave attenuation.

The optimal AV delay is given by: AV long – (QA short – QA long).

A modified Ritter's formula (AV long – QA long) – QA short is equivalent to Ismer's formula (AEA – LVEC).

Melzer et al.[6] evaluated the application of Ritter's method to patients with reduced LV function and compared

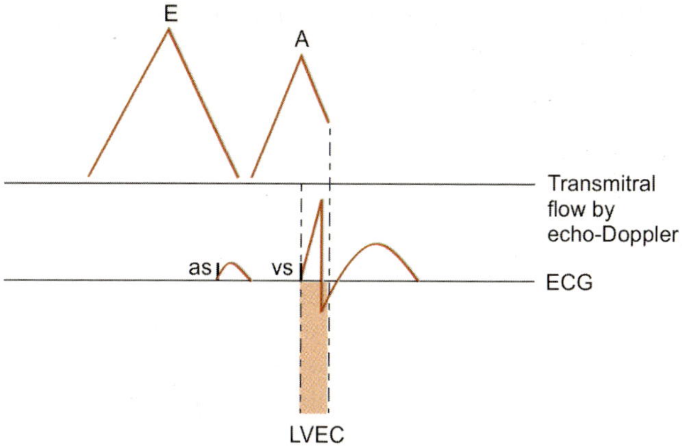

Fig. 3: Calculation of LVEC. (LVEC: latency time between the first ventricular potential or the pacing of ventricular artifact and left-ventricular contraction)

the method with an empirical setting (AV range: 100–250 ms) utilizing radionuclide ventriculography as a marker of LV systolic performance.

The advantages of Ritter's method are: (1) short time required, (2) noninvasive, (3) cost-effective, and (4) MV inflow profile detection. Ritter's method was found to be well correlated with best systolic performance, especially in patients with reduced LVEF.

Ishikawa's Formula

Ishikawa[7] proposed a formula for programming bicameral devices based on echo-Doppler mitral regurgitation detection, especially diastolic mitral regurgitation.

Diastolic Filling Time Method

Diastolic filling time (DFT) is measured from onset of the E-wave of transmitral flow until the end of a nontruncated A-wave. The method comprises of starting with a long AV delay and then reducing it by 20 ms steps until A-wave truncates. The interval is then increased in 10 ms steps and shortest AV delay without A-wave truncation is considered.[8]

The method was compared with Ritter's method and empirical setting (AV 100–120 ms) in a retrospective analysis of 215 patients who underwent optimization within 30 days of CRT implantation.[9] 9% of 215 patients had improvement in diastolic function following optimization and LVEF was found to increase by more than or equal to 5% in 46 patients (21%). 51% of subjects had improvement of the New York Heart Association (NYHA) functional class by at least one level. The method is recommended by the American Society of Echocardiography as a simplified screening technique.[8]

Other Doppler parameters which are used for echo Doppler-guided AV delay optimization include aortic VTI,[10]

VTI of mitral inflow,[11] Doppler-derived dp/dt,[12] tissue Doppler imaging,[13] LV and RV preejection delays, and myocardial performance index.[14]

ATRIOVENTRICULAR OPTIMIZATION AND RIGHT VENTRICULAR FUNCTION

A study by Koneru et al.[15] reported that a significant improvement in RV ejection fraction was noted in the AV delay optimized group. As in the case of LV, optimal AV interval should allow completion of end-diastolic filling of the RV prior to ventricular contraction. An approximately timed atrial systole improves RV filling and hence the stroke volume or cardiac output of RV by virtue of the Frank-Starling law.

A PRACTICAL APPROACH TO ECHOCARDIOGRAPHIC OPTIMIZATION OF ATRIOVENTRICULAR DELAY

- Paced AV delay to be increased successfully from 80 ms to 200 ms at 20 ms stepwise intervals; for sensed AV delay, step-up should at 30 ms.
- At each value, pulsed Doppler transmitral flow is to be recorded and compared with each other.
- Optimum AV delay show:
  - Good E-A separation
  - No (or trivial) mitral regurgitation
  - No A-wave truncation.

Limitations of this method in DCMP patients with LV diastolic dysfunction (in addition to systolic dysfunction) is that mitral A-wave may be severely attenuated or abbreviated by early mitral valve closure. Nevertheless, all DCMP patients with DDD pacemakers should be subjected to echo-guided AV delay optimization as this is likely to have beneficial effects on systolic function and symptomatology.

REFERENCES

1. Bernheim A, Ammann P, Stichrling C, et al. Right atrial pacing impairs cardiac function during resynchronization therapy : acute effects of DDD pacing compared to VDD pacing. J Am Coll Cardiol. 2005;45(9):1482-7.
2. Antonini L, Pasceri V, Aeillo A, et al. Asincronie atrioventricolari e-pacing. G. Ital Cardiol. 2010;11(2):28-34.
3. Antonini L, Greeco S, Santini M, et al. Optimization of DDD pacing programming by rest and stress echocardiography. Progress in Clinical Pacing. New York: Future Medica Services; 1994. pp. 925-6.
4. Ismer B, Von Knorre GH, Voss W, et al. Definition of the optimal atrioventricular delay by simultaneous measurement of electrocardiographic and Doppler echocardiographic parameters. Prog Biomed Res. 2002;202(1):116-20.
5. Ritter P, Dib JC, Lelievre T, et al. Quick determination of the optimal AV delay at rest in patients paced in DDD mode for complete AV block. Eur JCPE. 1994;4(3):163.
6. Melzer C, Borges AC, Richter WS, et al. Echocardiographic AV interval optimization in patients with reduced left ventricular function. Cardiovasc Ultrasound. 2004;2(4):30.
7. Ishikawa T, Sumita S, Kimura K, et al. Prediction of optimal atrioventricular delay in patients with implanted DDD pacemakers. Pacing Clin Electrophysiol. 1999;22(9):1365-71.
8. Gorscan J, Abraham T, Agler DA, et al. Echocardiography for cardiac synchronization therapy; recommendation for performance and reporting—a report from the American Society of Echocardiography Dyssynchrony. Writing Group endorsed by the Heart Rhythm Society. J Am Soc Echocardiogr. 2008;21(3):191-213.
9. Kedia N, Kenneth Ng, Apperson-Hausen C, et al. Usefullness of atrioventricular delay optimization using Doppler assessment of mitral inflow in patients undergoing cardiac reshychronization therapy. Am J Cardiol. 2006;98(6):780-5.
10. Kerlan JE, Sawhney NS, Waggoner AD, et al. Prospective comparison of echocardiographic atrioventricular delay optimization methods for cardiac resynchronization therapy. Heart Rhythm. 2006;3(2):148-54.
11. Jansen AH, Bracke FA, van Dantzig JM, et al. Correlation of echodoppler optimization of atrioventricular delay in cardiac resynchronization therapy with invasive hemodynamics in patients with heart failure secondary to ischemic or idiopathic dilated cardiomyopathy. Am J Cardiol. 2006;97(4):552-7.
12. Morales MA, Startari U, Panchetti L, et al. Atrioventricular Delay Optimization by Doppler-derived left-ventricular dp/dt improves 6-month outcome of resynchronized patients. Pacing Clin Electrophysiol. 2006;29(6):564-8.
13. Bordachar P, Stephane L, Sylvain R, et al. Bientricular pacing and left ventricular pacing in heart failure. J Cardiovascl Electrophysiol. 2004;15(12):1342-47.
14. Stockburger M, Fateh-Moghadam S, Nitardy A, et al. Optimization of cardiac resynchronization guided by Doppler echocardiography: hemodynamic improvement and intraindividual variability with different pacing configuration and atrioventricular delays. Europace. 2006;8(10):881-6.
15. Koneru S, Zoran P, Patrick T, et al. Echo-guided arioventricular delay optimization in patients undergoing cardic resynchronization therapy: single center experience in 2196 patients. J Am Coll Cardiol. 2015;65(10):A912.

SECTION 12

Hypertrophic Obstructive Cardiomyopathy

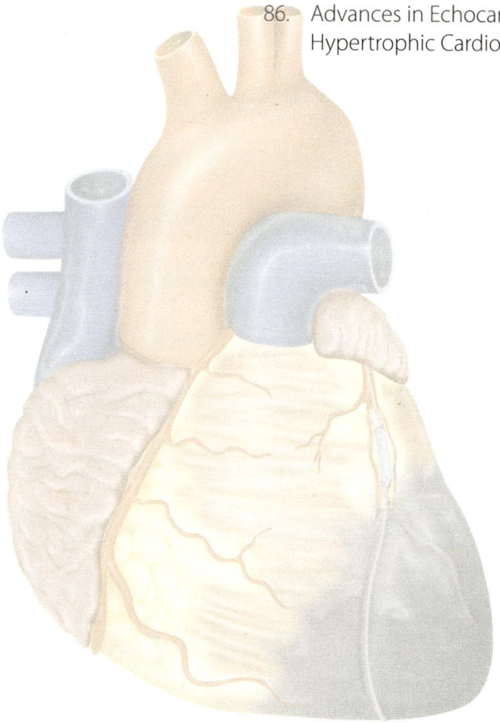

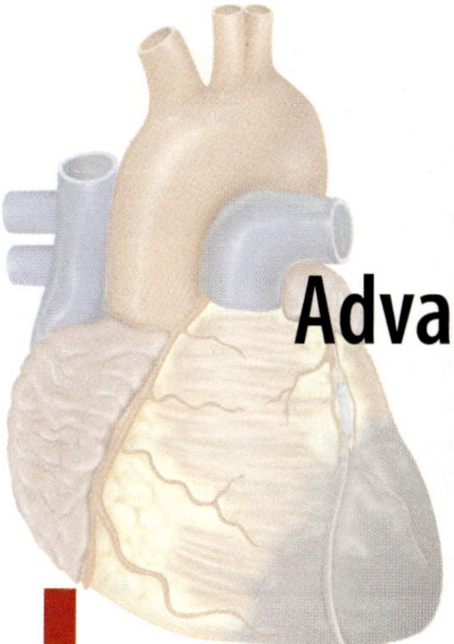

CHAPTER 86

Advances in Echocardiographic Navigation in Hypertrophic Cardiomyopathy

Rahul Mehrotra, Showkat Hussain Bhat, Raj Kumar, Bharat Bansal

INTRODUCTION

Hypertrophic cardiomyopathy (HCM) is a genetic disorder that is characterized by unexplained left ventricular hypertrophy and a nondilated left ventricle with preserved or increased ejection fraction. Any part of the left ventricle can be involved or there can be generalized hypertrophy but commonly hypertrophy is asymmetrical with basal interventricular septum being the most commonly involved segment. In the past, HCM was considered a rare disorder associated with a poor prognosis but recent population screening studies suggest that it is actually common with an estimated prevalence of 1/500 individuals.[1] The genes most commonly involved are the—*MYH7* and *MYBPC3*, coding for β-myosin heavy chain and myosin-binding protein C, respectively (accounting for almost 50% of HCM families). The inheritance of HCM is typically autosomal dominant; therefore, children of a single HCM parent have 50% chance of inheriting the disease-causing mutation. The histological features of HCM include myocyte hypertrophy, disarray, and interstitial fibrosis. The diagnosis of HCM may be initially suspected because of a heart murmur, positive family history, new symptoms or abnormal ECG pattern showing LV hypertrophy, and abnormal Q waves. This is usually followed by transthoracic echocardiography for establishing the diagnosis. Cardiac magnetic resonance imaging (MRI) and genetic testing are also sometimes utilized for prognostication and confirmation of diagnosis. However, echocardiography remains the single most useful modality for comprehensive evaluation of a patient of HCM. In the following pages we describe the role of echocardiography with recent advances in HCM.

ECHOCARDIOGRAPHY IN HYPERTROPHIC CARDIOMYOPATHY

A systematically performed transthoracic echocardiogram is the most useful tool for evaluation of a patient with HCM. All routine modes contribute to the gamut of information obtained in a patient of HCM. A comprehensive echocardiogram provides information not only related to the diagnosis but also helps in prognostication and evaluating response to therapy. Echocardiography is also the key supporting modality utilized for guiding the interventions—percutaneous transluminal septal myocardial ablation (PTSMA) and septal myomectomy. A description of each modality with its utility is given in the following sections.

M-mode Echocardiography

The first echocardiographic diagnostic criteria in HCM were historically established using M-mode imaging, which included asymmetrical septal hypertrophy, systolic anterior motion of the mitral valve (SAM), small LV cavity, septal immobility, and premature closure of aortic valve.[2] LV thickness, evaluated at septum and free wall level at end-diastole, is considered diagnostic when there is unexplained thickness more than or equal to 15 mm, and is considered asymmetrical in presence of a septal to posterior wall thickness ratio of 1.3:1 in normotensive patients.

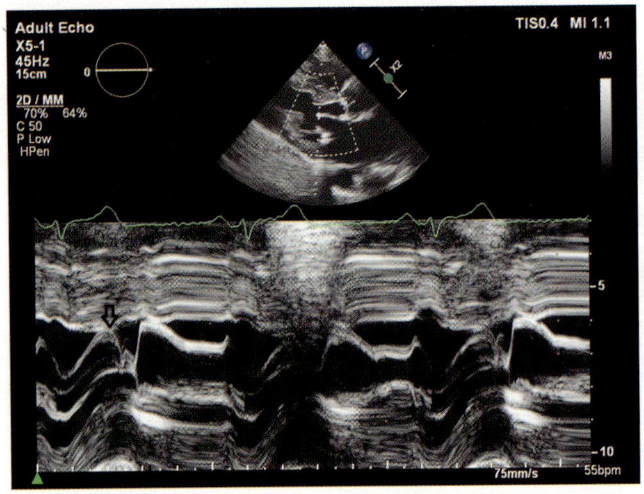

Fig. 1: M-mode echocardiogram of a patient with hypertrophic cardiomyopathy (HCM) showing systolic anterior motion of mitral valve (arrow).

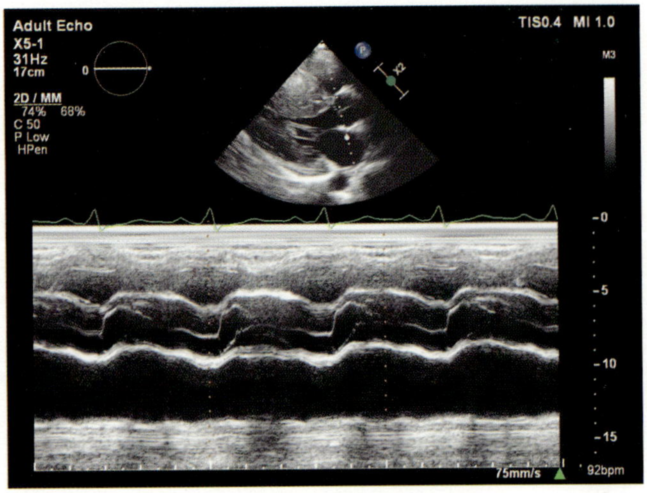

Fig. 2: M-mode echocardiogram of the same patient through the aortic valve showing coarse fluttering and midsystolic closure.

In hypertensive patients, septal/posterior wall thickness ratio more than 1.5 is diagnostic. SAM is characterized by an abrupt anterior movement of the mitral valve reaching its peak before maximum movement of the posterior wall (Fig. 1); this characteristic helps to differentiate true SAM from "pseudo-SAM"—produced by an exaggerated anterior motion of the mitral valve which reaches its peak after the full contraction of the posterior wall. The severity of SAM can be inferred from the duration of leaflet/chordal contact with the septum, being mild if contact occurs for less than 10% of systole, and severe if it is for more than 30% of systole. There is a positive correlation between the severity of SAM and the severity of obstruction evaluated invasively.[3] These findings, once considered pathognomonic of HCM, can also be seen in other forms of secondary and primary hypertrophy, like hypertension, Fabry's disease, Friedreich ataxia, and some other situations like postcardiac surgery, posterior wall infarction, etc.

M-mode of aortic valve reveals coarse fluttering of the aortic leaflets and midsystolic closure—a feature of obstructive HCM (Fig. 2).

Left atrial (LA) diameter is usually increased in patients with HCM because of diastolic dysfunction and raised left ventricular end-diastolic pressure (LVEDP). LA diameter gives information about the risk of atrial fibrillation, heart failure, and cardiac mortality (which is particularly high in patients with an LA diameter > 48 mm). Finally, LA fractional shortening evaluated as [(maximal diameter-minimum diameter)/maximal diameter × 100], an estimate of end-diastolic pressure in HCM, is directly related to exercise tolerance, and its reduction to less than 16% represents an independent risk for development of atrial fibrillation.[4]

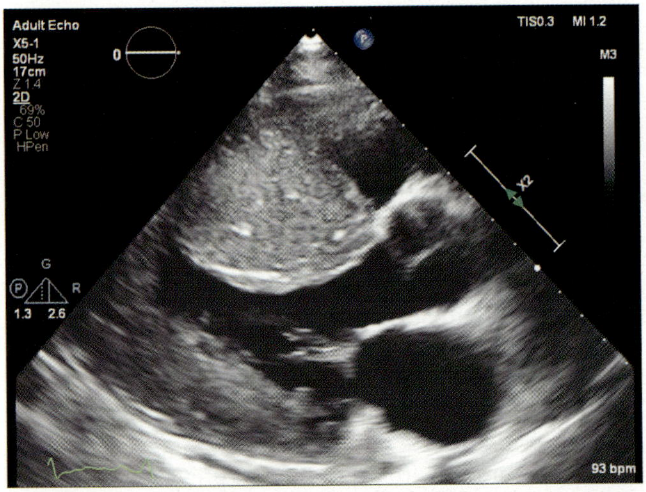

Fig. 3: Two-dimensional (2D) echocardiogram (parasternal long-axis view) of a patient with asymmetrical septal hypertrophy along with typical ground-glass appearance of myocardium.

Two-dimensional Echocardiography

The myocardium typically gives a ground-glass appearance in patients with HCM. This should alert the echocardiographer to the presence of HCM (Fig. 3).

The two-dimensional (2D) echocardiographic criteria used to diagnose HCM are the same as in M-mode.

The distribution of hypertrophy should also be carefully delineated in different views. Although, HCM is commonly characterized by asymmetric septal hypertrophy (ASH), almost any myocardial segment may be involved. Apart from the presence and distribution, the degree of hypertrophy is also important to document. Excessive myocardial hypertrophy (defined as ≥ 30 mm), though seen in around 10% of patients, is also associated with adverse prognosis[5] while in some cases, where the hypertrophy is localized to the apex, the prognosis remains excellent.

Left atrial volume measured by two-dimensional echocardiography has some clinical and prognostic implications. The American Society of Echocardiography recommends indexing LA volume (derived from biplane area length or method of disks) to body surface area (normal indexed LA volume = 22 ± 6 mL/m^2). It has been shown that LA remodeling, measured by LA volume, correlates directly with exercise capacity in these patients.[6] Moreover, patients with normal LA volume which show dilatation during follow-up, i.e. more than 3 mL/year, have a worse outcome compared to patients with normal and stable LA volume during follow-up.

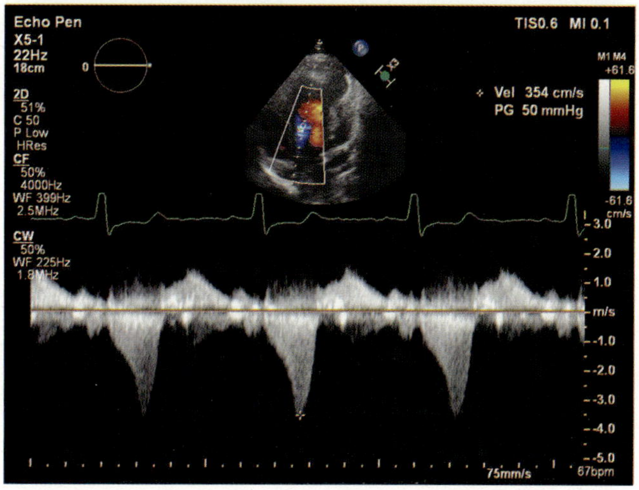

Fig. 4: Continuous wave Doppler beam passing left ventricular outflow tract (LVOT) producing a characteristic dagger-shaped trace with a peak gradient of 50 mm Hg.

Doppler Echocardiography

Each Doppler technique provides useful information in the analysis of patients with HCM.

Color Doppler Echocardiography

Evaluation of the presence and degree of mitral regurgitation (MR) is performed by color Doppler echocardiography. Posteriorly directed jet of MR occurs in almost all patients with obstructive HCM as a consequence of SAM, which induces abnormal mitral leaflet coaptation and may be an important cause of dyspnea. The direction of the mitral regurgitation jet is useful in identifying patients with associated mitral valve disease, since presence of an anteriorly directed jet in HCM usually indicates other pathologies. Color Doppler is also useful in localizing the site of maximal obstruction in the LV cavity as discussed here.

Continuous Wave Doppler Echocardiography

Approximately 25% of patients with HCM have a significant resting pressure gradient (≥30 mm Hg), between the body and LV outflow tract. This is almost always accompanied by SAM. Continuous wave (CW) Doppler interrogation, guided by turbulence in color Doppler, across the LVOT, results in a characteristic signal with a late peaking dagger-shaped appearance in obstructive HCM (Fig. 4). A midsystolic decrease in LV ejection velocity is sometimes observed in patients with severe obstruction, giving rise to the characteristic "Lobster-claw" tracing abnormality, caused by an interruption of LV longitudinal segmental shortening. In some patients without outflow obstruction at rest, gradients can be provoked by physiological and pharmacological interventions that diminish LV end-diastolic volume or augment LV contractility. The term labile obstruction has been used to describe the spontaneous appearance and disappearance of obstruction and latent obstruction to describe gradients that only appear with provocation. A number of methods can provoke obstruction in the echocardiography laboratory, including Valsalva maneuver, amyl nitrite, and dobutamine. However, these methods are not standardized and can underestimate the degree of obstruction (Valsalva maneuver) or have low specificity (dobutamine). Exercise is a physiologic means of provoking latent LVOT gradients. Over 50% of HCM patients without significant outflow tract obstruction at rest demonstrate outflow gradients over 30 mm Hg with exercise. Right ventricular outflow tract obstruction may also coexist with LVOT gradient in a minority of patients with massive septal hypertrophy and occasionally, it may even be isolated.

Pulse Doppler Echocardiography

Pulsed Doppler at mitral and pulmonary vein level is used to assess the presence and the degree of diastolic dysfunction. Almost all patients with HCM have some degree of LV diastolic dysfunction. Isovolumic relaxation is prolonged, the rate of rapid filling is diminished, and atrial contribution to filling is increased.

Systolic function: Systolic function is typically normal or supranormal in both obstructive and nonobstructive HCM when assessed using conventional echocardiographic indices such ejection fraction, or fractional shortening. Ejection fraction is typically preserved (or increased) despite an impairment of long-axis function, as demonstrated by the tissue Doppler-derived mitral annular velocities. Systolic dysfunction occurs in a small subset (10–15%) of patients as a natural course, often termed end-stage or "burnt-out HCM". This transformation occurs as a result of wall thinning, cavity dilation, and fibrosis and is associated with increased mortality (up to 11% annual risk) and risk of sudden cardiac death (SCD).[7]

Novel echocardiographic technologies

Tissue Doppler imaging: This Doppler-based technique allows real-time quantification of axial or longitudinal myocardial function. Mitral annular displacements toward the apex in systole and away from the apex during diastole, measured by tissue Doppler imaging (TDI) represents surrogate marker of longitudinal ventricular contraction and relaxation, respectively. Systolic and diastolic myocardial velocities are recorded by placing a pulsed TDI sample volume within the ventricular myocardium immediately adjacent to either the medial or lateral mitral annulus.

Systolic myocardial velocity (Sa), has been shown to be attenuated in HCM, even in nonhypertrophied ventricular segments.[8] Mutation positive subjects without echocardiographic evidence of LVH have been accurately identified by an Sa TDI velocity less than 13 cm/s in the lateral mitral annulus with a sensitivity of 100% and specificity of 93%. A mean of four systolic annular velocities (medial, lateral, anterior, and inferior) less than 9 cm/s has been proposed for differentiating between pathological LVH from physiological LVH (diagnostic accuracy of 92%).[9] In a recent report of patients with established HCM, low lateral mitral annular velocity less than 4 cm/s was found to have prognostic value and independently predicted death or hospitalization for worsening heart failure.[10]

Utility of pulsed wave TDI in the assessment of regional longitudinal myocardial function is restricted to the apical views only, as being a Doppler based technique, it is limited by its inherent inability to appraise regions nonparallel to the ultrasound beam (angle dependence). Although TDI provides an assessment of regional myocardial function, it is influenced by cardiac translational motion and tethering.

Two-dimensional strain imaging: Two-dimensional strain allows spatial and temporal tracking of longitudinal, circumferential, and radial myocardial deformation. Studies in patients with HCM have demonstrated a reduction in longitudinal strain (LS), an increase in circumferential strain, and normal systolic twist or torsion,[11] but a reduction in untwisting in diastole (Fig. 5). Significant reductions in LS in the septal segments (particularly the midseptal segment), correlate with the septal/posterior wall ratio.[12] Longitudinal deformation abnormalities are often focal or subsegmental and may be underestimated if careful spatial mapping is not used. Of note, the ability of 2D strain to assess myocardial shortening in the apical segments (particularly relevant in apical HCM variants) represents yet another advantage of this modality. Serri et al.[12] applied 2D strain echocardiography to a subset of patients with

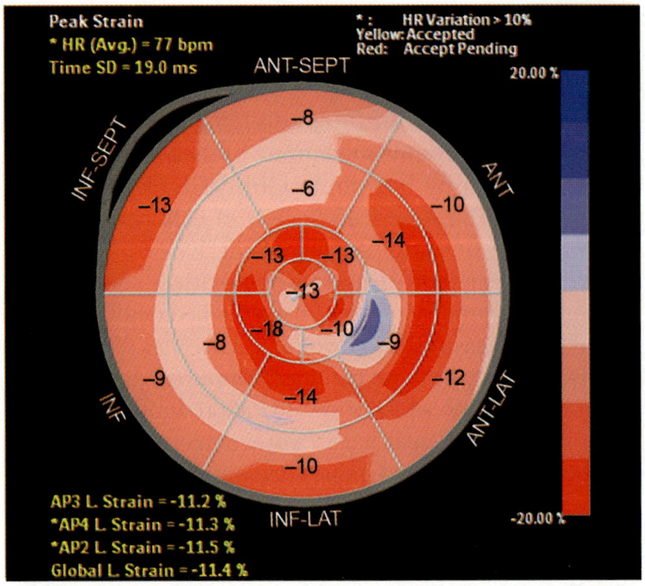

Fig. 5: Bull's eye map showing significant reduced average global longitudinal strain (–11.4%) in a patient with normal ejection fraction.

familial nonobstructed HCM. Interestingly, average global longitudinal strain was reduced in affected individuals compared with healthy controls (–15.1 ± 6.2% vs. –20.3 ± 5.6%), despite apparently normal systolic function.

Three-dimensional Echocardiography

Three-dimensional echocardiography (3D-E) can help in aiding diagnosis, assessing systolic function, and understanding the mechanics of SAM and LVOTO in HCM. It also improves recognition of location and extent of LV cavity obliteration. 3D-E can also provide volumetric data for accurate assessment of systolic function and has been shown to correlate well with magnetic resonance imaging for the assessment of LV volumes, ejection fraction, and LV mass. 3D-E also provides more information about the distribution of hypertrophy within the LV myocardium than 2D echocardiography. A novel 3D-E-derived mass dispersion index (MDI) has been used in differentiation of HCM from other forms of LVH. The MDI equates to the average of the standard deviations of the segmental mass volumes. The authors demonstrated that the MDI was significantly greater in patients with HCM than those with hypertension or athlete's heart, owing to the asymmetric nature of the hypertrophy.

Contrast Echocardiography

Contrast echocardiography currently is used to enhance endocardial definition, Doppler signals, and to evaluate myocardial perfusion during PTSMA. PTSMA is a catheter interventional technique, which entails injection of absolute alcohol into a septal perforator branch of the left anterior descending coronary artery to produce a myocardial infarction within the hypertrophied proximal ventricular septum. The introduction of the echo contrast has resulted in reduced side effects by helping select the appropriate septal perforator branch for injection. A potential role for contrast enhancement in the diagnosis of apical HCM has been demonstrated,[13] although systematic studies have not been yet performed.

Assessment of Intraventricular Dyssynchrony

Intraventricular and interventricular delay is commonly encountered in patients with HCM, despite the absence of conduction abnormalities on surface electrocardiogram and appears to correlate with the degree of septal LVH and the presence of LV outflow obstruction.[14] The authors of a study of 123 patients with HCM assessed systolic intraventricular dyssynchrony by using tissue Doppler and identified a strong association between the degree of intraventricular dyssynchrony and extent of LVH. In this study, an intraventricular delay of more than 45 ms, predicted an increased risk for ventricular tachyarrhythmias and sudden cardiac death at 5-year follow-up.[15]

Stress Echocardiography

Exercise stress echo is safe and commonly used to assess inducible LVOTO, especially in patients with equivocal symptoms, and for risk stratification. Guidelines recommend exercise echocardiography in symptomatic patients if bedside maneuvers fail to induce LVOTO more than or equal to 50 mm Hg. Of note, pharmacological provocation with dobutamine is not recommended, as it is not physiological, can be poorly tolerated, and can induce LVOTO even in normal subjects.[16] In patients with equivocal symptoms, if exercise stress echo does not produce LVOTO gradients, assessment for postexercise standing gradients should be considered as upright position after exercise causes a greater decrease in preload.

A limited exercise capacity, an abnormal blood pressure response (hypotensive or blunted response), significant ST-depression, inducible wall motion abnormalities, exercise LVOTO more than 50 mm Hg, and blunted systolic function reserve are all parameters of worse prognosis.[17-20] Blunted increase in global longitudinal strain (limited contractile reserve) favors diagnosis of HCM rather than athlete's heart. Intriguingly, some patients can display a paradoxical decrease in LVOTO during exercise, which is associated with a more favorable outcome and suggests alternative reasons for dyspnea.[21]

CONCLUSION

Echocardiography with all its attendant modalities is the most useful tool for patients with HCM. It is useful for screening the family members, differentiating from other entities with hypertrophy (athlete's heart), determination of type (obstructive/labile/latent/nonobstructive), distribution of hypertrophy (apical or septal), assessing response to drug therapy, guiding interventions, and risk stratification. A thorough knowledge of all the tools available along with their utility in patients in HCM is, thus, imperative for appropriate evaluation of these patients.

REFERENCES

1. Maron BJ, Gardin JM, Gidding SS, et al. Prevalence of hypertrophic cardiomyopathy in a general population of young adults. Echocardiographic analysis of 4111 subjects in the CARDIA STUDY. Coronary Artery Risk Development in (Young) Adults. Circulation. 1995;92(4):785-9.
2. Maron BJ, Towbin JA, Thiene G, et al. Contemporary definitions and classification of the cardiomyopathies: an American Heart Association Scientific Statement from the Council on Clinical Cardiology, Heart Failure and Transplantation Committee; Quality of Care and Outcomes Research and Functional Genomics and Translational Biology Interdisciplinary Working Groups; and Council on Epidemiology and Prevention. Circulation. 2006;113(14):1807-16.
3. Elliot P, Andersson B, Arbustini E, et al. Classification of the cardiomyopathies: a position statement from the European Society of Cardiology Working Group on Myocardial and Pericardial Diseases. Eur Heart J. 2008;29(2):270-6.
4. Losi MA, Betochhi S, Aversa M, et al. Determinants of atrial fibrillation development in patients with hypertrophic cardiomyopathy. Am J Cardiol. 2004;94(7):895-900.
5. Spirito P, Bellone P, Harris KM, et al. Magnitude of left ventricular hypertrophy and risk of sudden death in hypertrophic cardiomyopathy. N Engl J Med. 2000;342(24):1778-85.
6. Sachdev V, Shizukuda Y, Brenneman CL, et al. Left atrial volumetric remodelling is predictive of functional capacity in nonobstructive hypertrophic cardiomyopathy. Am Heart J. 2005;149(4):730-6.
7. Harris KM, Spirito P, Maron MS, et al. Prevalence, clinical profile and significance of left ventricular remodelling in the end stage phase of hypertrophic cardiomyopathy. Circulation. 2006;114(3):216-25.
8. Cardim N, Oliveira AG, Longo S, et al. Doppler tissue imaging; regional myocardial function in hypertrophic cardiomyopathy and in athlete's heart. J Am Soc Echocardiogr. 2003;16(3):223-32.
9. Vinereanu D, Florescu N, Sculthorpe N, et al. Differentiation between pathological and physiological left ventricular hypertrophy by tissue Doppler assessment of long-axis function in patients with hypertrophic cardiomyopathy

or systemic hypertension and in athletes. Am J Cardiol. 2001;88(1):53-8.
10. Bayrak F, Kahveci G, Mutlu B, et al. Tissue Doppler imaging to predict clinical course of patients with hypertrophic cardiomyopathy. Eur J Echocardiogr. 2008;9(2):278-83.
11. Carasso S, Yang H, Woo A, et al. Systolic myocardial mechanics in hypertrophic cardiomyopathy: novel concepts and implications for clinical status. J Am Soc Echocardiogr. 2008;21(6):675-83.
12. Serri K, Reant P, Lafitte M, et al. Global and regional myocardial function quantification by two dimensional strain: application in hypertrophic cardiomyopathy. J Am Coll Cardiol. 2006;47(6):1175-81.
13. Soman P, Swinburn J, Callister M, et al. Apical hypertrophic cardiomyopathy: bedside diagnosis by intravenous contrast echocardiography. J Am Soc Echocardiogr. 2001;14(4):311-3.
14. D'Andrea A , Caso P, Severino S, et al. Association between intraventricular myocardial systolic dyssynchrony and ventricular arrhythmias in patients with hypertrophic cardiomyopathy. Echocardiography. 2005;22(7):571-8.
15. D'Andrea A, Caso P, S Cuomo, et al. Prognostic value of intra-left ventricular electromechanical asynchrony in patients with mild hypertrophic cardiomyopathy compared with power athletes.. Br J Sports Med. 2006;40(3):244-50.
16. Pellika PA, Oh JK, Bailey KR, et al. Dynamic intraventricular obstruction during dobutamine stress echocardiography: a new observation. Circulation. 1992;86(5):1429-32.
17. Cardim N, Galderisi M, Edvardsen T, et al. Role of multimodality cardiac imaging in the management of patients with hypertrophic cardiomyopathy: an expert consensus of the European Association of Cardiovascular Imaging Endorsed by the Saudi Heart Association. Eur Heart J Cardiovasc Imaging. 2015;16(3):280.
18. Gersh BJ, Maron BJ, Bonow RO, et al. 2011 ACCF/AHA guideline for the diagnosis and treatment of hypertrophic cardiomyopathy: executive summary: a report of the American College of Cardiology Foundation/American Heart Association Task Force on Practice Guidelines. Circulation. 2011;124(24):2761-96.
19. Maron BJ, Maron MS, Wigle ED, et al. The 50year history, controversy and clinical implications of left ventricular outflow tract obstruction in hypertrophic cardiomyopathy from idiopathic subaortic stenosis to hypertrophic cardiomyopathy: from idiopathic hypertrophic subaortic stenosis to hypertrophic cardiomyopathy. J Am Coll Cardiol. 2009;54(3):191-200.
20. Peteiro J, Fernandez X, Bouzas MA, et al. Exercise echocardiography and magnetic resonance imaging to predict outcome in patients with hypertrophic cardiomyopathy. Eur Heart J Cardiovasc Imaging. 2015;16(4):423-32.
21. Lafitte S, Reant P, Touche C, et al. Paradoxical response to exercise in asymptomatic hypertrophic cardiomyopathy: a new description of outflow tract obstruction dynamics. J Am Coll Cardiol. 2013;62(9):842-50.

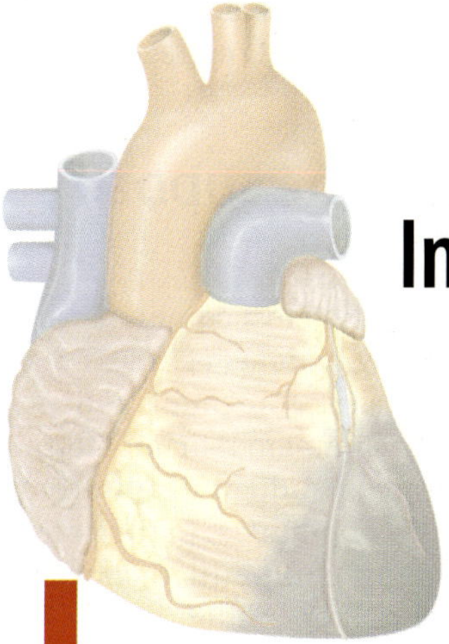

87

CHAPTER

Implantable Cardioverter Defibrillator for Sudden Death Prevention in Hypertrophic Cardiomyopathy

Surendra Chutani, Arti Shah, Arun Chutani, Bharat Kantharia

INTRODUCTION

Hypertrophic cardiomyopathy (HCM) is the most common genetic cardiomyopathy with prevalence in the general population of 1:500, although possibly even more common. Mutations in genes encoding proteins of the cardiac sarcomere are responsible for HCM and result in a diverse pattern of phenotypic expression and clinical course. HCM occurs equally in both sexes as well as in many races. HCM is the most common cause of sudden death in young people and can also lead to heart failure symptoms and stroke at any age.[1-3]

ROLE OF ECHOCARDIOGRAPHY

A clinical diagnosis of HCM is confirmed when unexplained increased LV wall thickness is imaged, range 13–60 mm, with average 22 mm, in the presence of a nondilated LV chamber. The most common location for LV hypertrophy is the basal anterior septum in continuity with the anterior free wall, with the posterior septum (at the mid-LV level) the third most common location. Although, LV hypertrophy often involves a substantial portion of the LV wall, an important minority of HCM patients (10%) have increased wall thickness confined to only one or two LV segments. Although, typically asymmetric in distribution, any pattern of LV wall thickening can be seen in HCM, including apical and concentric LV hypertrophy in a small minority (1%). Systolic anterior motion (SAM) of the mitral valve is not a requisite for a diagnosis of HCM, although the presence of SAM-septal contact producing outflow obstruction at rest or with provocation is present in the majority of patients. A number of other morphologic abnormalities are also not diagnostic of HCM, but can be part of the phenotypic expression of the disease, including: (1) hypertrophied and apically displaced papillary muscles, (2) anomalous insertion of the papillary muscle directly in the anterior leaflet of the mitral valve (in the absence of chordae tendineae), and (3) elongated mitral valve leaflets.[4-6]

HISTOPATHOLOGY RELEVANT TO SUDDEN CARDIAC DEATH

Hypertrophic cardiomyopathy is characterized by myocardial disarray, an abnormal histology including myocyte hypertrophy with cells arranged in a disorganized and chaotic pattern with increased amounts of interstitial fibrosis. In addition, the intramural coronary arterioles are structurally abnormal, with decreased luminal cross-sectional area and impaired vasodilatory capacity resulting in blunted myocardial blood flow during stress, i.e. "small vessel ischemia". Over a time, repetitive bouts of small vessel ischemia lead to myocyte cell death and ultimately repair in the form of replacement fibrosis. Although, these are common histopathologic findings in patients with HCM, right ventricular myocardial biopsy is not recommended for diagnostic purposes in patients suspected of HCM, due to a high rate of sampling error.[7-9]

INTRACARDIAC DEFIBRILLATOR FOR PREVENTION OF SUDDEN CARDIAC DEATH

For patients considered at high risk, the intracardiac defibrillator (ICD) is the only proven therapy to prevent sudden death. In this regard, there is no compelling evidence that medical therapy with beta-blockers and other antiarrhythmic drugs, such as amiodarone, can provide an appropriate level of protection against lethal ventricular tachycardia (VT). In a recent multicenter study with more than 500 primarily adult HCM patients, the ICD delivered an appropriate shock for VT and ventricular fibrillation (VT/VF) in 20% of patients over a follow-up period of less than 4 years. Appropriate device interventions occurred at a rate of 11% per year for secondary prevention and 4% per year for primary prevention.[1-5]

ECHOCARDIOGRAPHIC SCREENING

In the absence of genetic testing, current guidelines recommend that all relatives of patients with HCM undergo echocardiographic screening, starting at the onset of puberty and continuing every 1–1.5 years through the end of adolescence, ages 12–18 years. Screening in preadolescence is optional, unless family history is malignant, participation in particularly intense competitive sports is anticipated, or early onset disease is suspected. Although uncommon, some sarcomere mutations can result in delayed phenotypic expression; therefore, echocardiographic screening should continue every 5–7 years through midlife in family members who remain phenotypically negative by early adulthood. HCM family members who carry a disease-causing mutation, but remain phenotype negative at the end of puberty, should have echocardiographic screening continued for several years during adulthood.

HYPERTROPHIC CARDIOMYOPATHY VERSUS ATHLETE HEART

The most common cause of sudden death in young competitive athletes in North America is HCM, with close to one-third of all athletic field deaths attributed to this disease. The diagnosis of HCM in athletes may be challenging, particularly when the extent of LV hypertrophy is mild, falling into the so-called "gray-zone", i.e. 13–15 mm of LV wall thickness, between physiologic LV hypertrophy and mild phenotypic expression of HCM. This differential diagnosis is relevant because of the therapeutic, ethical, and social implications that a diagnosis of HCM conveys in young individuals participating in organized sports activity. Sex also plays a role, as maximal LV wall thickness measurements almost never exceed 11 mm in women. Therefore, measurements within the gray zone of 13–15 mm in female athletes almost always suggest HCM. Finally, SAM with ventricular septal contact and an outflow tract gradient at rest is strongly supportive of HCM.

RISK STRATIFICATION FOR SUDDEN CARDIAC DEATH

Hypertrophic cardiomyopathy is the most common cause of sudden cardiac death in young patients ages less than 35 years, with the highest prevalence in young patients, and the risk decreasing (but not eliminated) in midlife and beyond. Although, the majority of sudden death events in HCM occur under sedentary conditions, participation in intense physical activity and competitive sports is associated with an increased risk of sudden death. The mechanism of sudden death in HCM is VT emanating from an abnormal myocardial substrate consisting of myocyte disarray and interstitial and replacement fibrosis.[1-5]

RISK MARKERS FOR SUDDEN CARDIAC DEATH

A number of noninvasive clinical risk markers are currently available to help identify HCM patients at increased risk of sudden death, and who therefore may be a candidate for ICD therapy for primary prevention. The five primary risk factors include:

1. Family history of premature HCM-related death, particularly if sudden death, and in close or multiple relatives
2. Unexplained syncope judged non-neurocardiogenic, particularly if recent, in young patients
3. Nonsustained VT on serial ambulatory ECGs, particularly when bursts are multiple, repetitive, or prolonged
4. Hypotensive or attenuated blood pressure response to exercise, and
5. Extreme LV hypertrophy (wall thickness ≥ 30 mm).

Patients with a history of prior cardiac arrest or spontaneous, sustained VT are candidates for ICD therapy for secondary prevention. Patient age remains an important determinant influencing sudden death risk in this disease, with the noninvasive risk markers most applicable to young and middle-aged HCM patients, while the achievement of advanced age (>60 years) is associated with low risk, even in the presence of one or more of the conventional risk factors. For this reason, aggressive prophylactic ICD therapy in HCM patients with advanced ages is not warranted. Of note, given the unpredictability of the HCM disease process and the inevitable changes which occur due to the underlying abnormal myocardial substrate, risk stratification should occur for most patients on a regular (usually annual) basis, with surveillance to monitor potential clinical changes and/or risk profile with imaging and ambulatory monitoring.[1-6] Due to the heterogeneous and complex nature of HCM, it is not possible to give equal weighting to each of the five primary prevention risk factors. As a result, adding risk factors to generate a score that could be used to identify patients at future risk of sudden death is not feasible. Although, HCM patients with multiple risk factors, two or more are at greatest risk for sudden death, the presence of one risk factor alone may be sufficient to consider an individual patient as being in a high-risk category, particularly a patient with massive LV hypertrophy, family history of sudden death, or a recent, unexplained syncope.

SUDDEN DEATH RISK CALCULATOR

Most recently, the European Society of Cardiology has advanced a novel strategy incorporating a range of clinical and demographic information to generate an individualized risk score, using highly mathematical and statistical modeling techniques to identify patients most likely to benefit from ICD therapy. However, it remains unclear whether the new risk score will actually recognize individual young patients at risk for sudden death who are not currently identified with the current consensus guideline (2011 ACC/AHA guideline), or will reliably eliminate from consideration patients who will not benefit from an ICD. For these reasons, risk stratification in HCM still appears to require analysis of the conventional noninvasive risk factors, with a measure of individualized physician judgment in the framework of shared decision-making with fully informed HCM patients.[8-10]

CONCLUSION

Hypertrophic cardiomyopathy remains the most common cause of sudden death in young patients including athletes. Patients with one or more of the five primary sudden death risk factors may be considered at increased risk and considered for ICD therapy for primary prevention. For patients considered at high risk, i.e. with one or more primary risk factors described earlier, the ICD is the only proven therapy to prevent sudden death. In this regard, there is no compelling evidence that medical therapy with beta-blockers and other antiarrhythmic drugs, such as amiodarone, can provide an appropriate level of protection against lethal VT. Evidence for the efficacy of the defibrillator also has been demonstrated in children and adolescents with HCM, in which similar intervention rates for potentially life-threatening VT were observed. With the current generation of devices and contemporary programming strategies, device-related complications, including inappropriate shocks, is low in patients with HCM (5% per year). Therefore, the decision to undergo ICD therapy for primary prevention has to be balanced with the possibility of incurring device-related issues over what can often be long implant times. The vast majority of HCM patients can be treated with single-chamber ICDs. Dual-chamber devices are largely reserved for those with a history of supraventricular tachyarrhythmias, and/or patients in whom a trial of forced atrioventricular pacing is indicated to treat symptoms related to LV outflow obstruction. Although there is a number of potential advantages to applying the subcutaneous defibrillators in patients with HCM, including avoiding long-term lead and vascular complications, caution is warranted in considering implantation in patients with this disease, because long-term efficacy data are not yet available.

REFERENCES

1. Gersh BJ, Maron BJ, Bonow RO, et al. 2011 ACCF/AHA guideline for the diagnosis and treatment of hypertrophic cardiomyopathy: a report of the American College of Cardiology Foundation/American Heart Association Task Force on Practice Guidelines Developed in Collaboration With the American Association for Thoracic Surgery, American Society of Echocardiography, American Society of Nuclear Cardiology, Heart Failure Society of America, Heart Rhythm Society, Society for Cardiovascular Angiography and Interventions, and Society of Thoracic Surgeons. J Am Coll Cardiol. 2011;58(25):e212-60.
2. Maron BJ, Ommen SR, Semsarian C, et al. Hypertrophic cardiomyopathy: present and future, with translation into contemporary medicine. J Am Coll Cardiol. 2014;64(1):83-99.
3. Semsarian C, Ingles J, Maron MS, Maron BJ. New perspectives on the prevalence of hypertrophic cardiomyopathy. J Am Coll Cardiol. 2015;65(12):1249-54.
4. Alcalai R, Seidman JG, Seidman CE. Genetic basis of hypertrophic cardiomyopathy: from bench to the clinics. J Cardiovasc Electrophysiol. 2008;19(1):104-10.
5. Shirani J, Pick R, Roberts WC, et al. Morphology and significance of the left ventricular collagen network in young patients with hypertrophic cardiomyopathy and sudden cardiac death. J Am Coll Cardiol. 2000;35(1):36-44.
6. O'Mahony C, Jichi F, Pavlou M, et al. A novel clinical risk prediction model for sudden cardiac death in hypertrophic cardiomyopathy (HCM Risk-SCD). Eur Heart J. 2014;35(30):2010-20.
7. Maron BJ, Spirito P, Shen WK, et al. Implantable cardioverter-defibrillators and prevention of sudden cardiac death in hypertrophic cardiomyopathy. JAMA. 2007;298(4):405-12.
8. Bos JM, Towbin JA, Ackerman MJ. Diagnostic, prognostic, and therapeutic implications of genetic testing for hypertrophic cardiomyopathy. J Am Coll Cardiol. 2009;54(3):201-11.
9. Maron BJ, Spirito P, Ackerman MJ, et al. Prevention of sudden cardiac death with implantable cardioverter-defibrillator in children and adolescents with hypertrophic cardiomyopathy. J Am Coll Cardiol. 2013;61(14):1527-35.
10. Elliott PM, Poloniecki J, Dickie S, et al. Sudden death in hypertrophic cardiomyopathy: identification of high risk patients. J Am Coll Cardiol. 2000;36(7):2212-8.

SECTION 13

Restrictive Cardiomyopathy

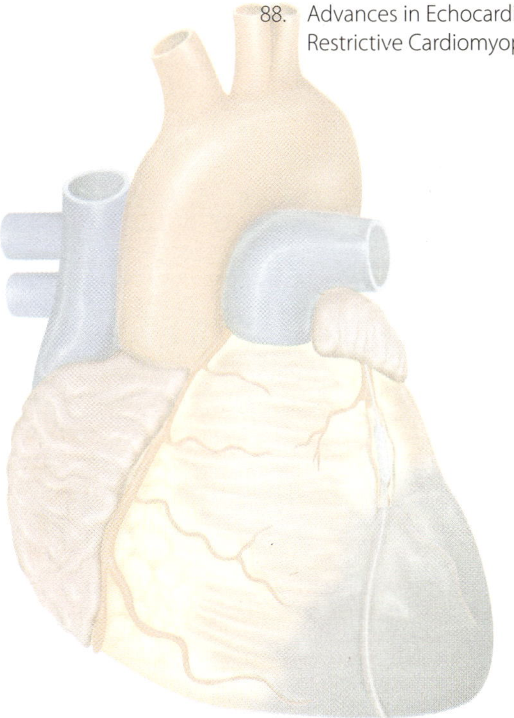

88

CHAPTER

Advances in Echocardiographic Navigation in Restrictive Cardiomyopathies

S Sivasankaran, G Vijayaraghavan

INTRODUCTION

Restrictive cardiomyopathy is a functional diagnosis in subjects presenting with heart failure when filling abnormalities are demonstrated with near normal ventricular wall thickness and pumping function.[1-3] Majority of restrictive cardiomyopathies are secondary to systemic disorders like amyloidosis, sarcoidosis, eosinophilic heart disease, or after irradiation therapy and rarely due to primary myocardial diseases. Primary myocardial diseases need myocardial biopsy and molecular studies for a definite diagnosis.[4] Many subjects the diagnosis is made after the onset of complications like atrial or ventricular arrhythmias or after a stroke, and in a minority, on targeted screening or incidental echocardiography.[5,6] The heart is unique in its ability to modulate the cardiac output to match the systemic demands within physiological range, facilitated by the sequential filling, and ejection, termed as the diastolic and systolic functions of the pumping chambers, the ventricles.[7,8] The filling function of the heart is facilitated by gravity, respiration, venous and skeletal muscular tone, in addition to the lusitropic or relaxing function of the myocardium. Restraining effect of the fibrous pericardium limits acute dilatation of the cardiac chambers by an additional 20% in the acute setting. Normal diastole or filling of the ventricle occupies two-thirds of the cardiac cycle because of the small venous pressure head, aided by large atrioventricular orifices which offer little restraint. Primary myocardial disorders which interfere with compliance of the heart either because of endocardial involvement, myocardial or interstitial involvement form the restrictive cardiomyopathies.[3] Reduced compliance of the heart results in disproportionate elevation of ventricular filling pressures to unit increase in volume. This forms the hemodynamic hallmark of restrictive cardiomyopathies represented by the square root sign in the ventricular diastolic pressure tracings. This is compensated by atrial dilatation and venous congestion and abnormal filling patterns across the atrioventricular valves and venoatrial junctions. Echocardiographic evaluation defines these hemodynamic features by documenting the near normal ventricular systolic functions with minimal or no hypertrophy, disproportionate atrial dilatation (Figs. 1 to 3), and abnormal filling patterns.[9] Thus, echo evaluation is the simple bedside evaluation which is fundamental in the diagnosis and prognostication of subjects with restrictive cardiomyopathies.[10] This chapter deals with these restrictive cardiomyopathies and the disorders of ventricular filling arising from the pericardial disorders that are dealt within the subsequent chapters.

PHASES OF DIASTOLE AND PATTERNS OF DIASTOLIC DYSFUNCTION[11-13]

Ventricles being muscular are unable to distend at low filling pressure and hence, the nature designed the thin-walled roomy atria to receive the blood at lower venous pressures. The atria facilitate the ventricular filling by an atrial booster function which can contribute up to one-third of the ventricular filling when needed. Atrial systole precedes ventricular systole to ensure appropriate

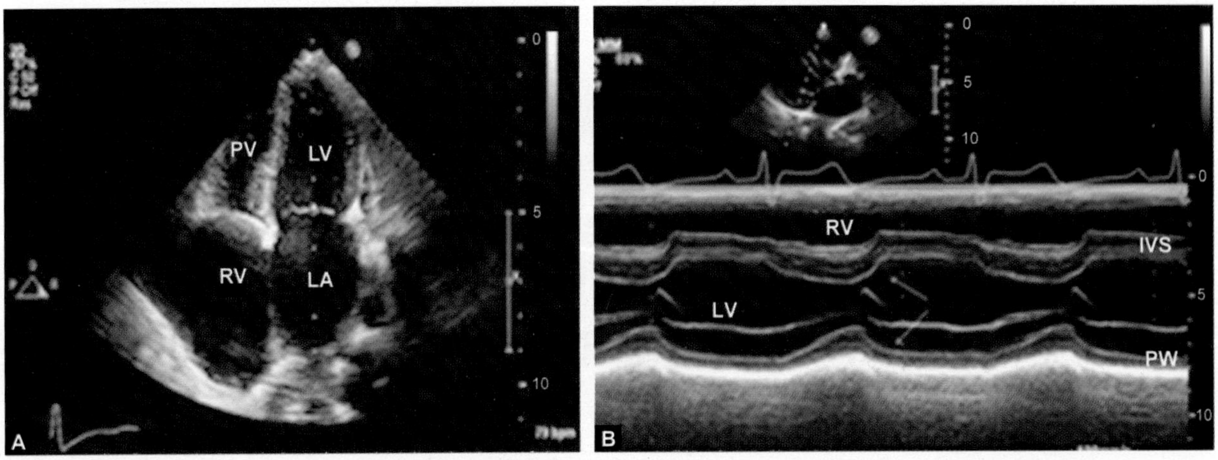

Figs. 1A and B: Two-dimensional (left A) and M-mode (right B) echocardiogram, the diagnostic hallmark of restrictive cardiomyopathy. Note the normal ventricular dimension, wall thickness and function, dilated atrial chambers, and near normal looking atrioventricular valves (RA—right atrium, RV—right ventricle, LA—left atrium, LV—left ventricle, IVS—interventricular septum). Abrupt posterior wall and septal motion (white arrows in B) corresponds to rapid early diastolic filling of the left ventricle followed by a straight course reflecting the dip and plateau demonstrated at cardiac catheterization is diagnostic of restrictive physiology.

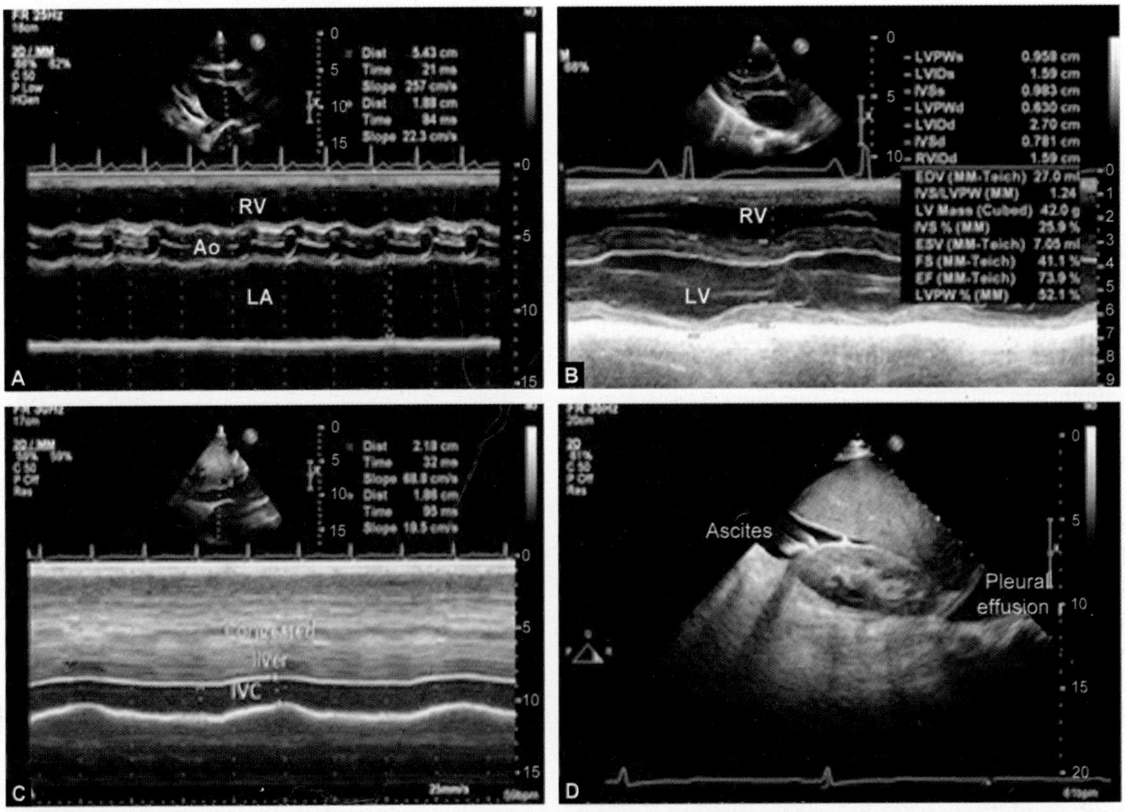

Figs. 2A to D: Typical indirect echocardiographic features of restrictive cardiomyopathy. (A) Shows the M mode across the aorta (AO) and left atrium (LA) showing normal aortic valve and dilated left atrium; (B) Shows the M mode of the nondilated nonhypertrophied left ventricle (LV) with normal mitral valve movement and good systolic function; (C) Shows the congested liver with dilated inferior vena cava (IVC); and (D) Shows the other consequences like ascites and pleural effusion on tilting the transducer to abdomen.

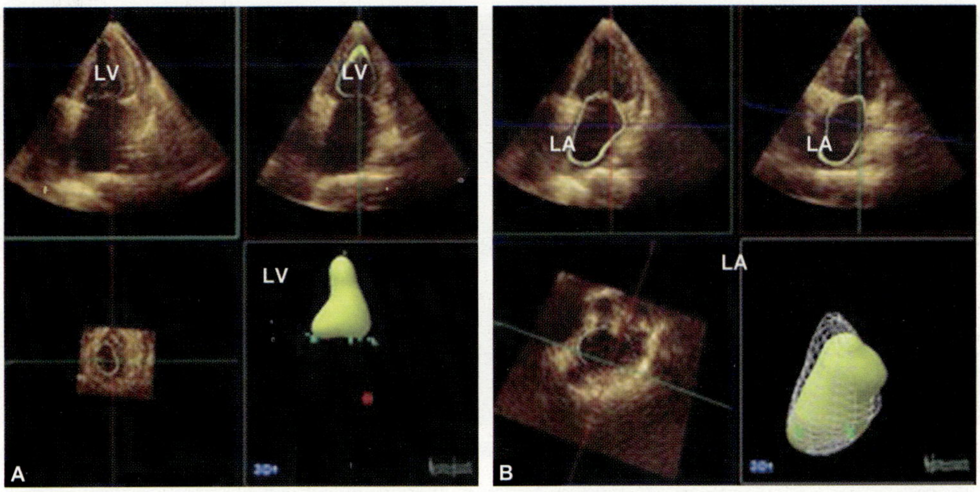

Figs. 3A and B: Three-dimensional volume rendered images in restrictive cardiomyopathy Left ventricular (LV) volume measurements in panel A shows good left ventricular function and the left atrial (LA) volume measures on the right panel B shows the disproportionate atrial dilatation with left atrial systolic volume index more than 34 mL/m^2.

ventricular filling and large atrioventricular orifices facilitate it, irrespective of the low pressures in the venous system, when the ventricle actively relaxes by the lusitropic function of myocardium. Aquatic to terrestrial migration demanded more muscular left ventricle to pump against the gravity, doubling the average pressure needed to fill on the left side when compared to the right ventricle. Conversely, the right ventricle pumping the cardiac output to the low pressure pulmonary circuit, essentially halves the systemic venous pressures. Simultaneous closure of the semilunar valve marks the onset of ventricular diastole. The initial phase of diastole is the isovolumic relaxation period, when the myocardium actively relaxes from the high end-systolic pressures to a value, lower than the left atrial pressure, facilitating the opening of the atrioventricular valves. This allows the free flow of blood from atrium to ventricle, initiating the rapid, reduced and atrial systolic filling phases. The onset of ventricular systole abolishes the flow gradient across the atrioventricular valves, which makes the valve float back and close to mark the onset of isovolumic contraction phase. Normally, majority of the ventricular filling occur in the early rapid filling phase, initiated by the lusitropic or suction function of the ventricle, represented by the "E" waves across the atrioventricular valves. This is followed by the delayed filling "A" or atrial systolic wave.[14] The period of reduced filling between the two phases is called the diastasis, which essentially is a reserve period to facilitate increase in heart rate. Hence, diastolic dysfunction of the ventricles is reflected in the filling patterns by abnormalities of early diastolic filling and evidence of atrial compensation characterized by the disproportionate dilatation of the atria, and atrial arrhythmias, with evidence for systemic or pulmonary venous congestion. Similar to flow across the atrioventricular valves, the flow of blood across the venoatrial junction also indirectly reflects the filling abnormalities of the heart. Venoatrial junction orifices are small and are not guarded by the valves. Hence, venoatrial filling occurs throughout the cardiac cycle but for a transient flow reversal with atrial systole. Maximal atrial filling occurs during ventricular systole when the volume of the heart inside the pericardial space is minimal allowing maximal space for the atrium to expand. The atrial filling is further facilitated by the pulling down of the atrioventricular rings at early ventricular ejection. Four phases of evolution of diastolic function are described based on the early and late filing patterns of the ventricles, correlating with the compensatory increase in filling pressures.[15]

Doppler and Color Doppler in Deciphering Restrictive Filling

The important Doppler features of restrictive filling are:[12,16-19]

- Large early filling wave with E/A ratio more than 2 (Figs. 4A and C) in the absence of atrioventricular valve regurgitation
- Mitral early filling (E) divided by the mitral annular e' ratio is more than 15 suggesting high ventricular filling pressures (Figs. 4A to D)[18,19]
- Mitral inflow velocity will show less than 25% variation during phases of respiration (Fig. 4B)
- Short isovolumic relaxation time less than 60 milliseconds, essentially because the elevated atrial pressures initiate forward flow early in diastole

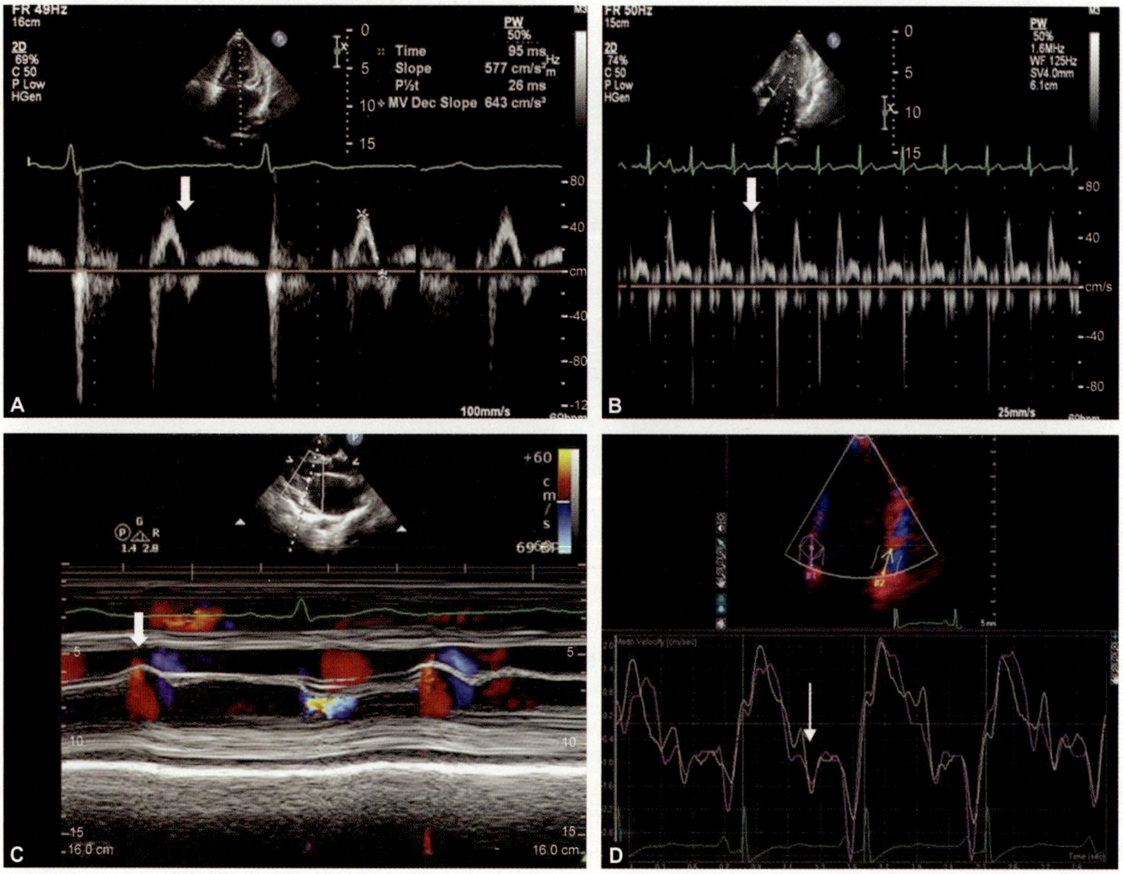

Figs. 4A to D: Mitral valve Doppler features of restrictive physiology. Panel A shows prominent filling E waves (broad arrow) and declaration time is less than 130 milliseconds. Panel B shows a slow speed recording to document minimal variation in mitral inflow during respiration. Panel C: Color M mode across the mitral valve, shows monophasic mitral flow only in early diastole though the valve is open during most of the diastole reflecting pressure equalization between the atria and the ventricle. Panel D shows the tissue Doppler characteristics of the septal (violet) and lateral (yellow) mitral annulus. Contrary to blood flow, the tissue movement during early diastole (e') (slender arrow) is minimal with high E/e' ratio is more than 15 reflecting high filling pressures which rapidly drives the initial blood flow into the ventricle. In contrast, tissue annular e' velocity is high in constrictive pericarditis.

- Short deceleration time less than 150 milliseconds (Fig. 4A), where the noncompliant ventricle causes rapid elevation of ventricular filling pressures causing more rapid deceleration of antegrade filling
- Pulmonary and hepatic venous flow showing large atrial flow reversal and systolic to diastolic wave ratio less than 0.5 (Fig. 5)
- Color Doppler echocardiography helps to quantitate the atrioventricular valve regurgitation and color M-mode echocardiography demonstrates the restrictive inflow filling pattern as reduction of flow propagation velocity of less than 35 cm/s[16] as illustrated in Figure 6.

Patterns of Diastolic Dysfunction

Restrictive physiology across the mitral valve demonstrated by Doppler is classified into four stages.[16] Stage 1 is early restriction due to relaxation or lusitropic abnormalities where the atrial compensation takes over the compensatory function. Atrial filling pressures are near normal thought ventricular end-diastolic pressures are elevated.[20] Early filling velocity gets (E) reduced and its duration is prolonged. Atrial filling (A) velocity is increased so that E/A ratios are one or less (Fig. 7). Mitral propagation velocity is normal and mitral annular velocity shows diminished e' velocities. Many of these patients present with large "a" waves in the jugular venous pulse when right heart is involved or on hemodynamic studies and loud fourth heart sound on cardiac ausculatation.[20]

Type II diastolic dysfunction is characterized by increasing atrial filling pressures so that the E wave velocity is increased and the mitral Doppler appears almost normal, called pseudonormalization. This phase can be differentiated from normal by Valsalva maneuver release

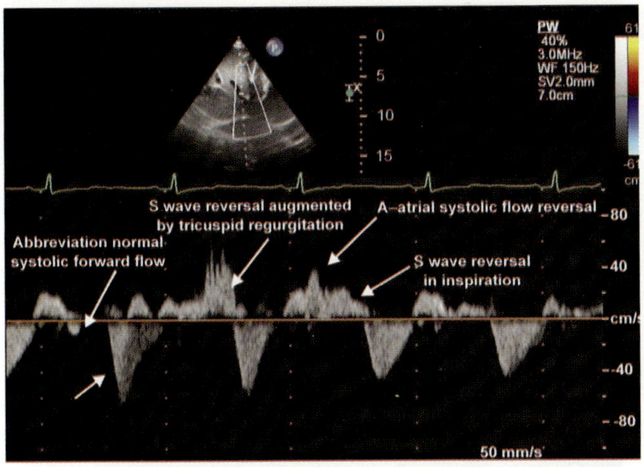

Fig. 5: Hepatic venous flow pattern in restrictive cardiomyopathy. In restrictive physiology, the normal large systolic (s) flow into atria compared to diastolic flow (D) is lost. Diastolic flow (D) is almost double the systolic flow reflecting the sharp Vy collapse in the Jugular venous pulse. S waves are diminutive show flow reversal in inspiration and superadded tricuspid regurgitation will make them more prominent.

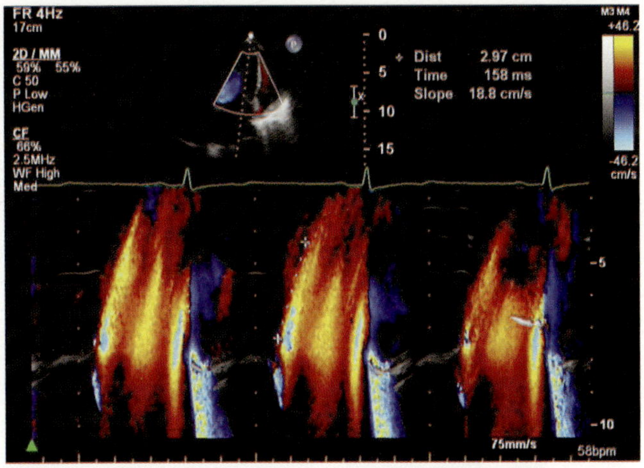

Fig. 6: Color Doppler M-mode across the mitral orifice to measure the mitral propagation velocity. Velocity is measured along the aliasing border 4 cm into the left ventricle, with optimal gain setting around 40–50 cm. Propagation velocity less than 35 cm/s is diagnostic of restrictive left ventricular filling. The red forward flow shows three phases corresponding to E, L, and A wave atrial filling consistent with the diagnosis of advanced diastolic dysfunction. In contrast, mitral propagation velocity is typically more than 50 cm in constrictive pericarditis.

phase when the filling pressures are reduced, and the type 1 pattern is restored. In addition, the e' generated by the tissue Doppler at the mitral annulus will be small so that the E/e' ratio will be more than 15, suggesting elevated filling pressures. Similarly, A wave reversal in the pulmonary veins will be more than 30 milliseconds wider than the A wave duration across the mitral valve. These typical features are illustrated in Figure 8. The clinical counterparts are large Vy descend in the jugular venous pressure when right heart is involved and a loud third heart sound on cardiac auscultation.

Stage III restriction is typical with mitral E deceleration time less than 150 milliseconds, mitral E propagation velocity less than 35 cm/s and with E/A ratio more than two. Advanced restrictive physiology across the mitral valve has documented a triphasic filling wave called the L wave during mid-diastole as illustrated in Figure 9.[21] In case of treatable restrictive cardiomyopathies, the early stage III changes return back to normal and the terminal irreversible changes in others are sometimes referred to as stage IV restrictive changes. Here, the atrial impression causes no forward flow but only venous flow reversal and presystolic forward flow across the pulmonary valve if pulmonary diastolic pressures are really low. These preterminal echocardiographic features are complicated by atrial fibrillation, wherein a wave parameters are no longer measurable, atrioventricular valve regurgitation and progressive ventricular systolic dysfunction, and varying grades of pericardial effusion.

In summary, type I diastolic dysfunction essentially denotes the relaxation abnormalities of the myocardium whereas type 2 signifies the elevation of left atrial pressures and type 3 cardiac restraint to ventricular filling, and type 4 advanced irreversible reduction in stroke volume because of diastolic dysfunction. The echo parameters like medial e' velocity less than 7 cm/s, lateral e' velocity less than 10 cm/s, and left atrial systolic volume index more than 34 mL/m^2 are definite hallmarks of diastolic dysfunction.[13]

Other Echocardiographic Measures of Diastolic Dysfunction

Diastolic dysfunction of the myocardium can be evaluated by the isometric relaxation indices like the duration and negative dp/dt when there is a regurgitant jet. The elevation of ventricular diastolic pressures above the atrial pressure during the presystolic phase, especially when the PR interval is prolonged allowing the relaxation of atria ahead of onset of ventricular systole, generates the presystolic low pressure atrioventricular valve regurgitation, the hallmark of atrioventricular **dyssynchrony**. Since the diastolic blood pressure, the pulmonary arteries are lower, elevation of right ventricular diastolic pressures in pulmonary stenosis

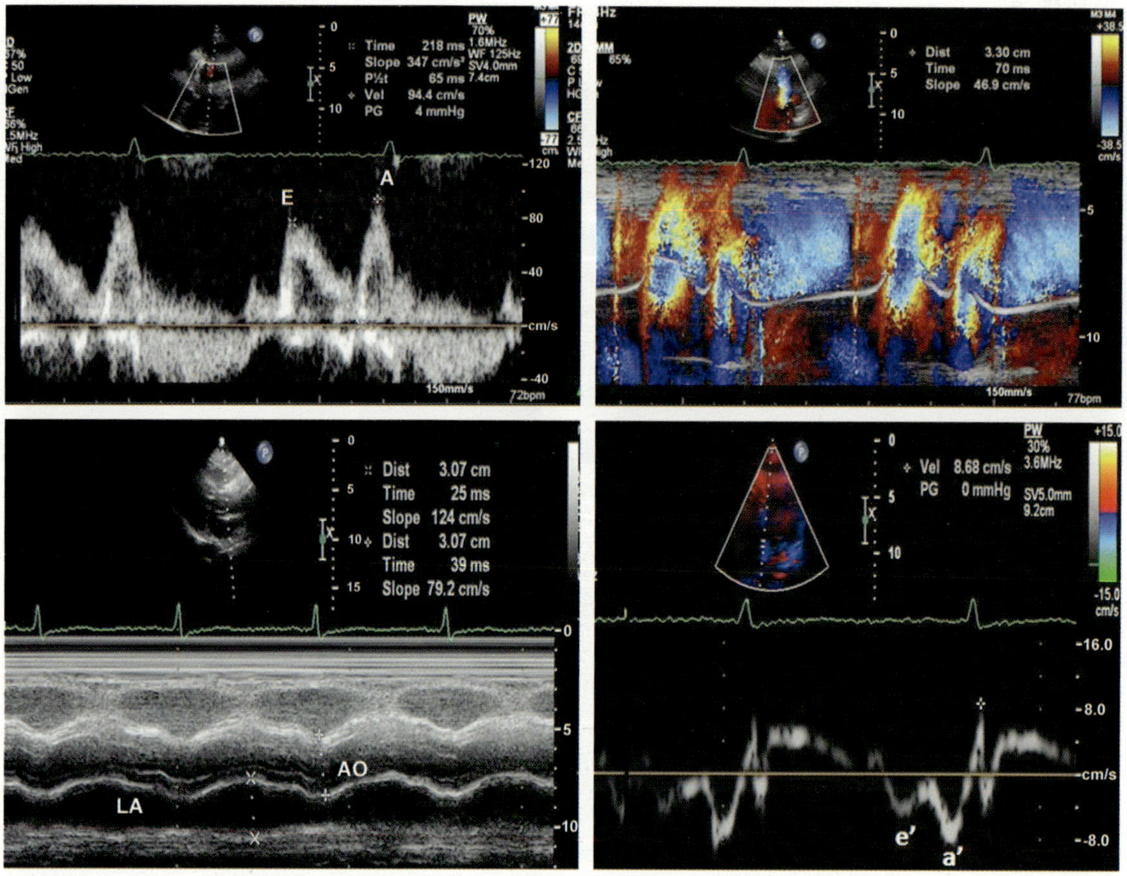

Fig. 7: Type I early diastolic dysfunction. Panel A shows reversal of early (E) to late (A) mitral inflow velocities with normal mitral propagation velocity by color Doppler M mode (Panel B). Left atrial dimensions are normal on M mode at the level of aorta (Panel C) and mitral annular tissue Doppler velocities show reduced early (e') and increased atrial (a') velocities.

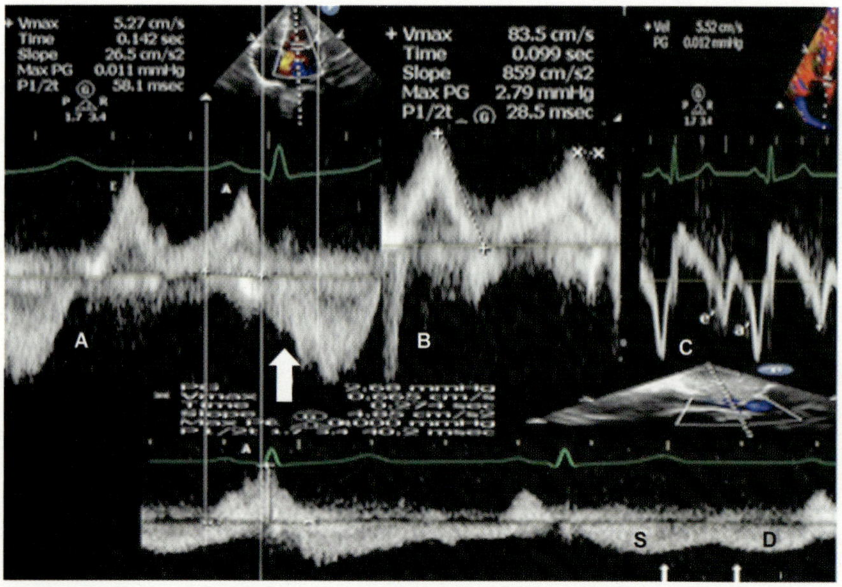

Fig. 8: Pseudonormal mitral inflow pattern in early restrictive cardiomyopathy. Early inflow mitral velocities in a panel A (E) is larger than the late (A) velocities, but mitral valve deceleration time is less than 150 milliseconds (panel B), and mitral annular inflow early (e') velocities are smaller than the late (a) velocities on tissue Doppler evaluation (panel C). Pulmonary venous flow in Panel D from the subcostal window shows diastolic D waves becoming as large as the systolic S waves, and atrial reversal duration exceed the mitral inflow A wave duration by more than 30 milliseconds. Bold white arrow shows the diastolic mitral regurgitation correlating with elevated ventricular end-diastolic pressures which exceed the left atrial pressures as the atria starts relaxing.

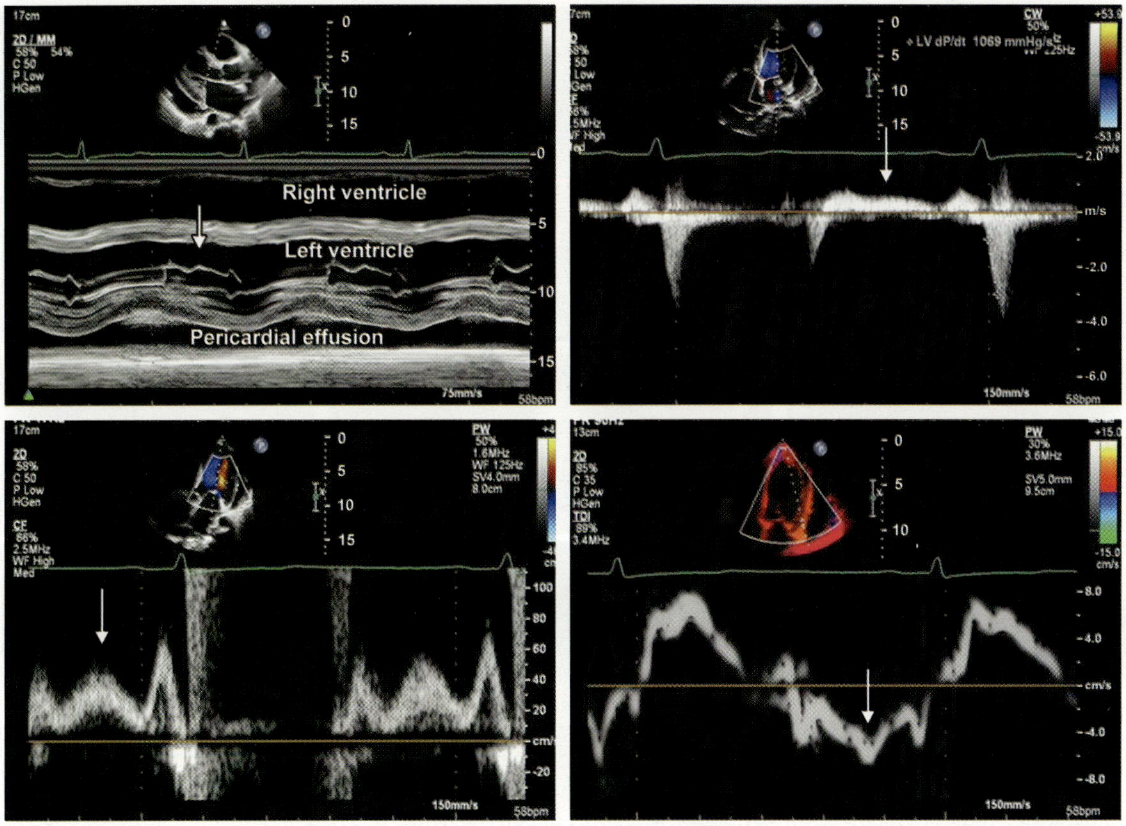

Fig. 9: Triphasic inflow pattern in advanced restrictive cardiomyopathy. In between the early filling E and late filling, A waves, an additional mid-diastolic filling occurs represented by broad arrows, best seen when the heart rates are slow. They are known as L waves. Panel A shows the mitral valve M-mode impression of L wave, panels B and C, the continuous and pulse wave Doppler velocities of the L wave across the mitral valve, and panel D the tissue Doppler impression. Note the dp/dt in continuous Doppler and the S waves on tissue Doppler reflects good ventricular systolic function.

and right-sided cardiomyopathies can lead to presystolic forward flow into pulmonary arteries. Total loss of right ventricular systolic function in certain cardiomyopathies can generate spontaneous Fontan paradox, where systemic venous pressures exceed the pulmonary venous mean pressures, identified by the forward flow into pulmonary arteries during the preatrial systolic or diastatic phase.[22,23] But in many patients' development of significant atrioventricular valve regurgitation, atrial fibrillation, pericardial effusion, progressive fibrosis, and ventricular systolic dysfunction in late stages, will make the Doppler features less useful. Doppler flow across the pulmonary valve (Fig. 10), shows the presystolic forward flow across the pulmonary valve during atrial systole, when the right ventricular diastolic pressures exceed the pulmonary diastolic pressures. Other features are sudden early diastolic termination of pulmonary regurgitation which could be a marker of the abrupt elevation of right ventricular end-diastolic pressure reflecting the square root sign during cardiac catheterization.

Ventricles of the adult human heart on an average have a volume of 120 mL which ejects 80 mLin the ensuing systole at a heart rate of 60 beats/min. The ejection fraction is 66% in this situation. 20% increase in ventricular volume is permitted by the pericardial stretching and improvement in contractile function achieves an 80% ejection. Thus, the maximal increase in cardiac output to five times the basal state is possible by a tripling in heart rate when the diastolic duration declines to 200 milliseconds beyond which further increase in cardiac output is compromised by the impaired filling. The disappearance of diastasis in diastole sets the limit for compensation in diastolic function. Thus, fusion of early filling and atrial booster waves are the evidences for maximal heart rate compensation for diastolic function. Prolongation of PR interval and prolongation of systole by bundle branch block, or prolonged ejection as in heart failure and outflow tract obstructions further reduces the range of this heart rate compensation (Fig. 11).[24] Presence of diastatic ventricular filling wave, the L wave, and diastolic flow reversal from ventricle to atria, i.e. mid-diastolic

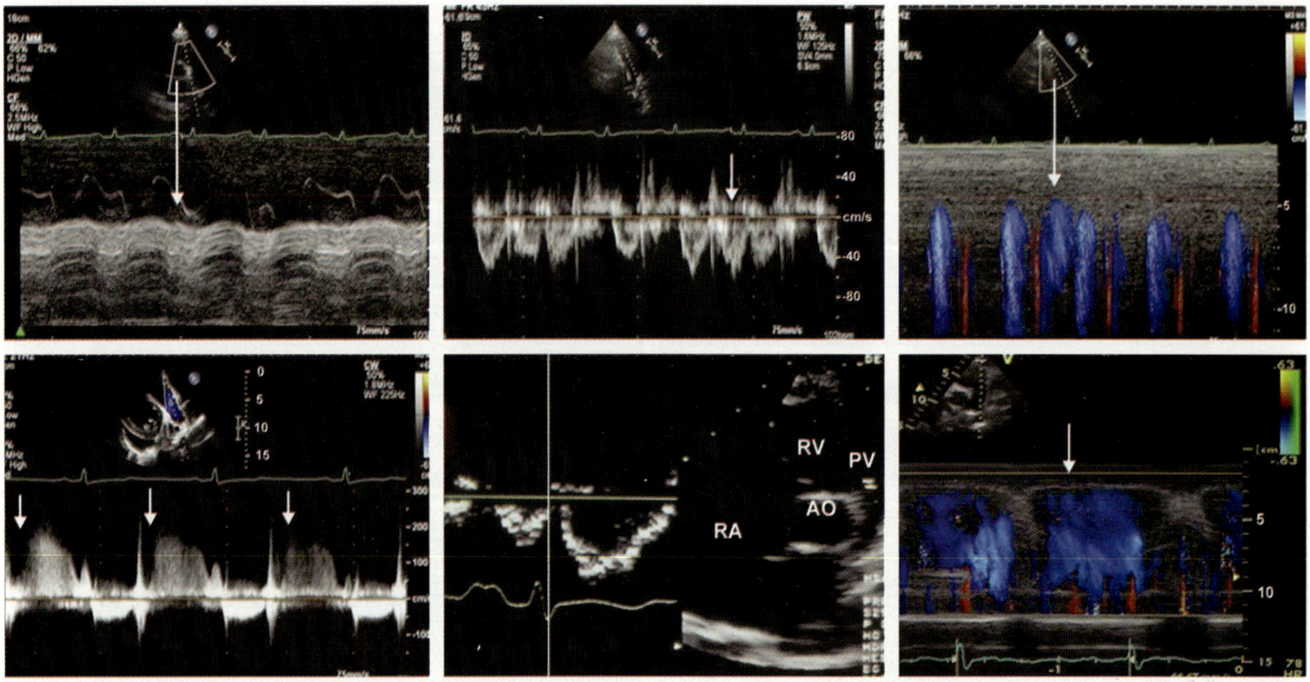

Fig. 10: M-mode and Doppler flow across the pulmonary valve in restrictive cardiomyopathy: Panel A shows the presystolic opening of the pulmonary valve indicated by the long white arrows demonstrated by M-mode. Pulse Doppler in panel B and color Doppler M-mode across the pulmonary valve in panel C shows the presystolic forward flow. Panel D shows continuous wave Doppler signal of pulmonary regurgitation showing early diastolic loss of gradient, reflecting the sudden increase in the right ventricular diastolic pressures (short arrows). Panel E illustrates expanded single beat Doppler forward flow into pulmonary artery to illustrate the atrial systolic forward flow into pulmonary artery preceding the QRS complex (vertical line). Panel F shows the pandiastolic forward flow into pulmonary artery, illustrating elevation of systemic venous pressures above the pulmonary artery diastolic pressures, the Fontan paradox which is peculiar for isolated right ventricular cardiomyopathy.

atrioventricular valve regurgitation (Fig. 12), are other hallmarks of diastolic dysfunction in relation to diastasis.[25,26]

PROGNOSTIC IMPLICATIONS

Unlike dilated and hypertrophic cardiomyopathies, where the definition is morphological, the definitions of restrictive cardiomyopathy are based on the hemodynamic abnormality.[27] Some have even questioned the need for identifying this entity but all the recent reviews on classification have retained this diagnosis.[4,28] Left ventricular involvement produces pulmonary venous congestion and dyspnea, while the right-sided disease presents with signs of systemic venous congestion like jugular venous distension, tender hepatomegaly, and pedal edema. Over a period of time, atrial fibrillation with thromboembolic episodes leads to a rapid downhill course. Prognoses of individuals diagnosed with primary restrictive cardiomyopathies are worse than the more common variety of diastolic heart failure, unless they receive a cardiac transplant.[29,30] A myocardial relaxation abnormality coupled with interstitial fibrosis with or without calcification forms the fundamental abnormality of restrictive cardiomyopathies. As a result, there is progressive restriction of the ventricular filling. The pressure volume loop of restrictive physiology is, therefore, shifted upward and to the left.[31-33] The myocardium, which can no longer benefit from the Frank-Starling mechanism, heavily depends on the atrial booster function and on rate and rhythm to improve the cardiac output.[32] The ventricle fills rapidly in the early filling phase, which is halted abruptly in mid to late diastole, so that the ventricular stroke volume is almost fixed. Cardiac output can be increased by a small increase in heart rate but a further increase hampers the diastolic duration and ventricular filling. Chronically decreased cardiac output leads to cardiac anasarca and cachexia. Symptoms of any associated systemic disorder may also be present.[34,35] Elevation of atrial natriuretic polypeptides in circulation can be a marker of the existence and a measure of the severity of the condition.[36] Demonstration of restrictive filling of the ventricles in a patient with heart failure portends a poor prognosis but demonstration of restrictive physiology early in the natural history of systemic disorders leading to restrictive heart disease can favorably modify the outcome.[37,38]

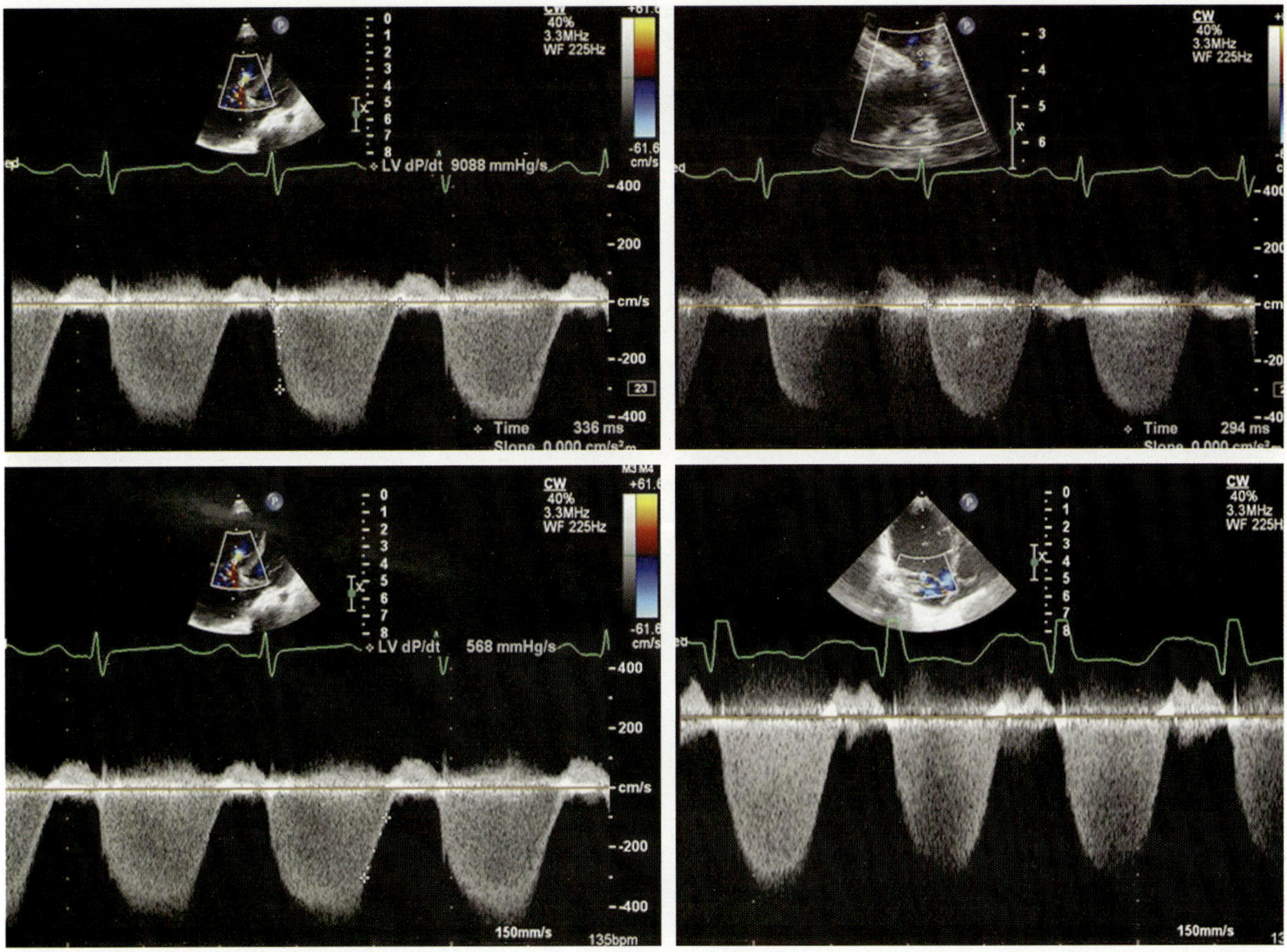

Fig. 11: Heart rate limitation of diastolic duration evidence (disappearing diastasis): note the EA fusion. Panels A to C, EA fusion occurs at a heart rate of 135 beats/min in a patient with severe valvar pulmonary stenosis. Systolic ventricular function is good as evidences by good positive dp/dt of the tricuspid regurgitation get in panel A. Other evidences of diastolic dysfunction because of the hypertrophied right ventricle are the steep deceleration pulmonary regurgitation jet with a pressure half time of 50 milliseconds in panel B and 20 times lower –dp/dt of the regurgitation get in the isometric relaxation period of 25 milliseconds duration, panel C. Tricuspid valve closure to opening time is 336 milliseconds in panel A whereas pulmonary ejection time is 294 milliseconds in panel B and myocardial performance of right ventricle is 336 – 296/296 = 0.14. Panel D shows EA fusion on the left heart at similar heart rates, but with prolongation of QRS complex and PR interval, with slurred positive and negative dp/dt of mitral regurgitation secondary to left ventricular dysfunction.

THERAPEUTIC IMPLICATIONS

The major advantage of echocardiogram is not only in deciphering the hemodynamic abnormality but also in defining probable etiology which has major therapeutic implications. Endocardial restriction is typical of hyper eosinophilic syndromes and tropical endomyocardial fibrosis. The morphology of the ventricles is diagnostic because of the hyperechogenic endocardium, which in late phases shows calcification. In the early thrombogenic phase, layered thrombi can be demonstrated (Fig. 13), which, when recognized helps in avoiding catastrophic thromboembolic complications and necessitates adequate anticoagulation. Late phases of endomyocardial fibrosis (EMF) with atrioventricular valve regurgitation can be managed surgically be endocardial resection and atrioventricular valve replacement. Though several patients had mitral and tricuspid valve replacement during 1980–1991 for EMF in certain centers, this is now rarely offered because of the poor long-term outcome for mechanical prosthetic valves especially placed in the tricuspid position.[39] Bidirectional Glenn's shunt is offered only to patients with isolated RVEMF (Figs. 14 and 15), with no pulmonary hypertension, mitral incompetence, or left

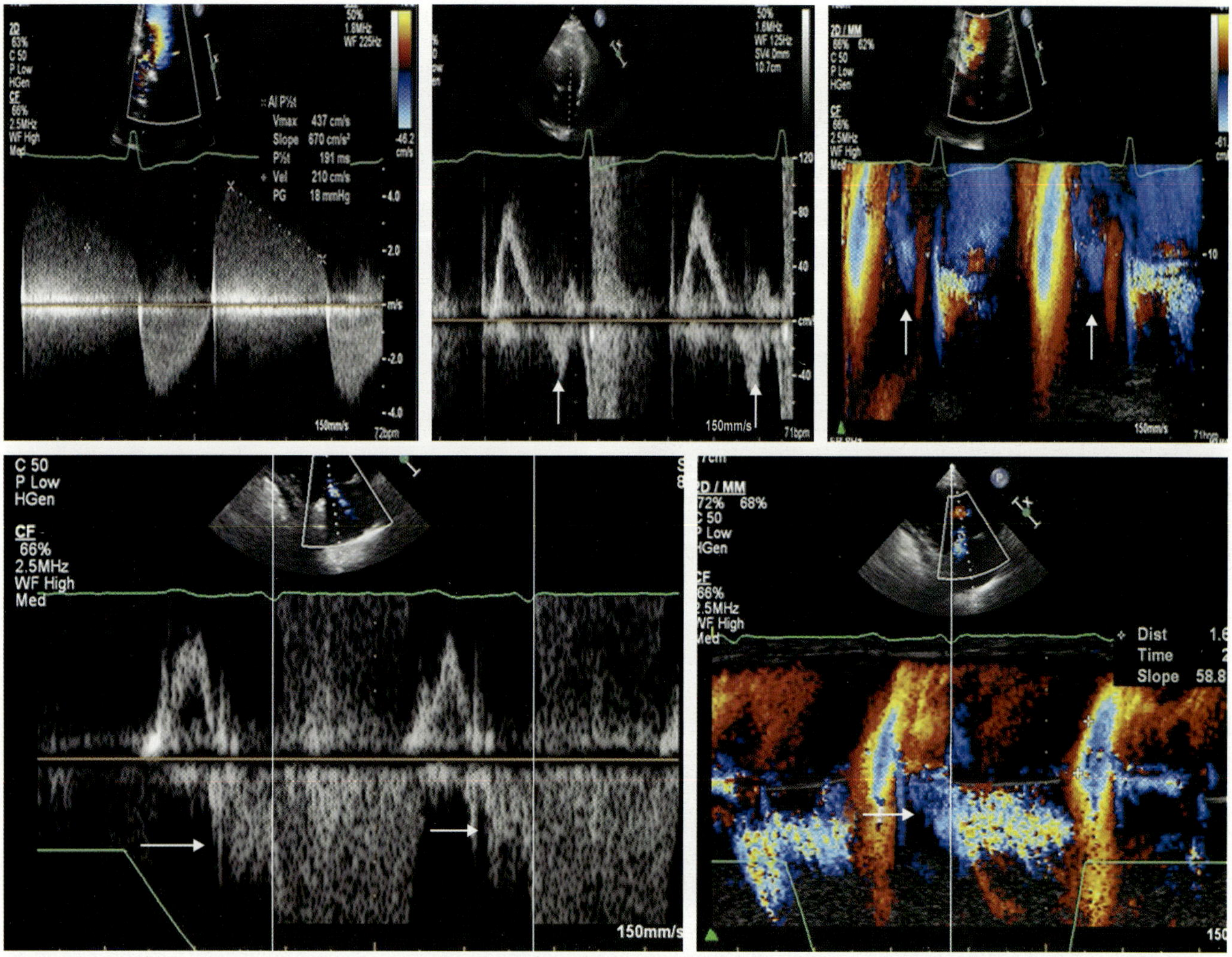

Fig. 12: Diastolic atrioventricular valve regurgitation as a cause of increasing atrial pressures. Panel A: shows severe aortic regurgitation with a pressure half time of 210 milliseconds, which elevates the left ventricular diastolic pressures above the atrial pressures in mid-diastole causing reversal of e' wave in mid-diastole causing mitral regurgitation in diastasis, shown by pulse Doppler and color M-mode Doppler in panel B and C indicated by vertical blue arrows. Presystolic low pressure tricuspid regurgitation is illustrated in panel D and E by pulse Doppler and color Doppler M-mode in a person with prolonged PR interval and restrictive heart disease by horizontal white arrows. Vertical white line shows the peak of QRS complex.

ventricular diastolic dysfunction. The delineation of isolated right ventricular involvement needs detailed evaluation like contrast echo, 3D studies, and transesophageal echo study, if precordial echo window is poor. Hemodynamic study and angiographic evaluation are a must as a part of presurgical workup, though many of the patients attend surgical centers in the burned-out phase.[40] Surgical treatment has always been contemplated only for NYHA class III and IV patients. A careful 2D echo Doppler examination can identify surgical candidates with EMF with a fair amount of certainty. Figures 16A to D illustrates the echocardiographic features of left ventricular endomyocardial fibrosis (LVEMF).

Amyloidosis,[41] sarcoidosis,[42,43] cardiomyopathy after cancer treatment,[44] and storage diseases[45] like hemochromatosis[1,46] are other disorders where both systolic and diastolic dysfunction coexists, which are more common in adults and old age. Many a times, multimodality imaging and cardiac muscle biopsy are needed to come to a correct diagnosis. Early detection and prompt treatment favorably alters the natural history.[47] Recent advances in understanding the specific patterns of systolic dysfunction by strain imaging has contributed a lot for noninvasive characterization of amyloid heart disease avoiding the risk involved in undertaking a cardiac biopsy.[48] Figure 17 illustrates the classical echo features of systemic amyloidosis in the late stage.

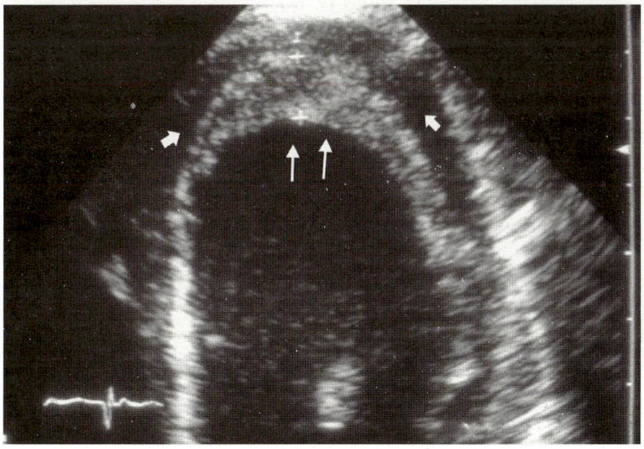

Fig. 13: Loeffler's endocarditis. Note the layering of the left ventricular apex by thrombus (thin arrows). Thick arrows show the normal myocardium.

LIMITATIONS

Subjects with poor echo window or having overlap of pericardial and valvular heart diseases, necessitates additional evaluation. Restrictive cardiomyopathy in late stages does have arrhythmias, valve regurgitations, impaired systolic function, and varying grades of pericardial effusion, which make the echo studies nondiagnostic. When precordial echo window is poor, transesophageal echocardiography though useful, may need general anesthesia for a complete study.

CONCLUSION

Echocardiography, because of the easy availability, repeatability, low cost, and noninvasive nature is at present the best bedside modality for early recognition, diagnosis, prognostication, and follow-up of patients with restrictive cardiomyopathy. Good temporal resolution provides excellent edge over other modalities. Mastering of the

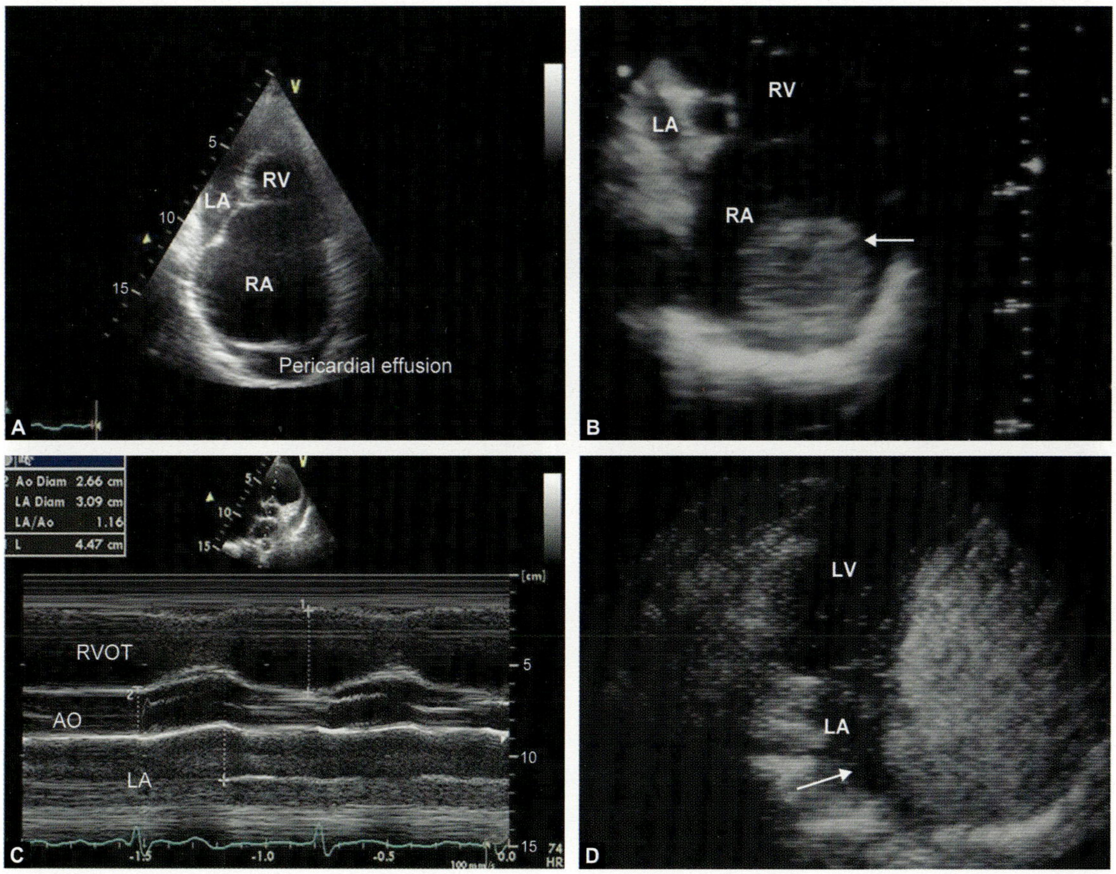

Figs. 14A to D: Echocardiographic features of right ventricular endomyocardial fibrosis. (A) Note the aneurysmal right atrium (RA), distorted right ventricle (RV), and the small pericardial effusion; (B) Thin white arrow shows a large right atrial thrombus; (C) Dilated hyperdynamic right ventricular outflow tract (RVOT); and (D) Contrast filled large right atrium with stretched open foramen ovale with small right to left shunt (note the right-sided chambers are on the right-hand side in this display).

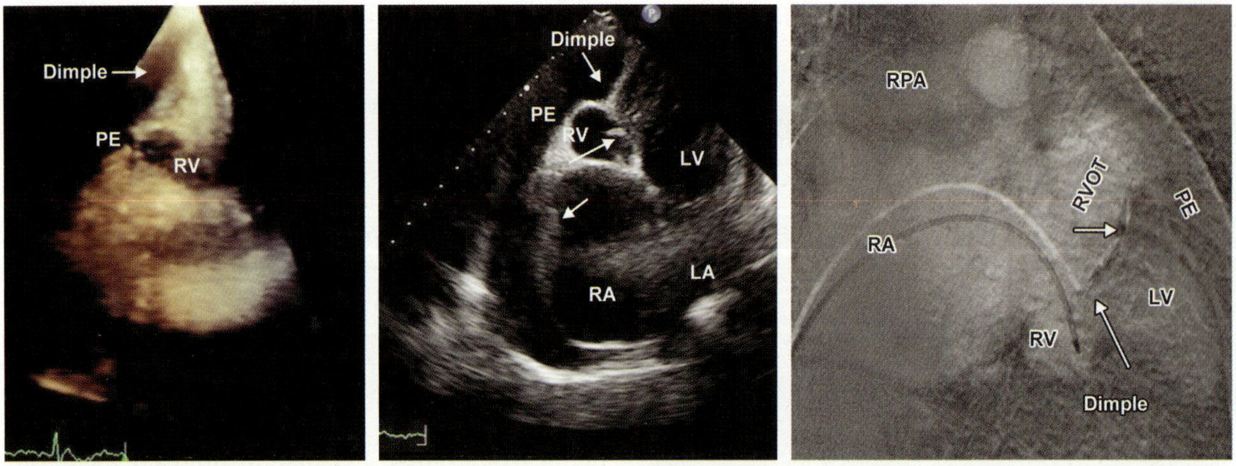

Fig. 15: Ventricular dimple in right ventricular endomyocardial fibrosis. The reduction of long axis of the right ventricle because of fibrotic obliteration from apex leads to dimple-like retraction of the free wall which can be delineated by three-dimensional (A) and two-dimensional (B) echocardiography in presence of moderate pericardial effusion. Panel C shows the digital subtraction of the right ventricular angiogram in levo phase to delineate the relation of the dimple compared to the cardiac apex. Horizontal dense arrows in panels B and C show the right ventricular calcium and the small arrow in the right atrium in panel B shows the layered thrombus in the free fall. (RA: right atrium; RV: right ventricle; LA: left atrium; LV: left ventricle; RPA: right pulmonary artery; RVOT: right ventricular outflow tract; PE: pericardial effusion)

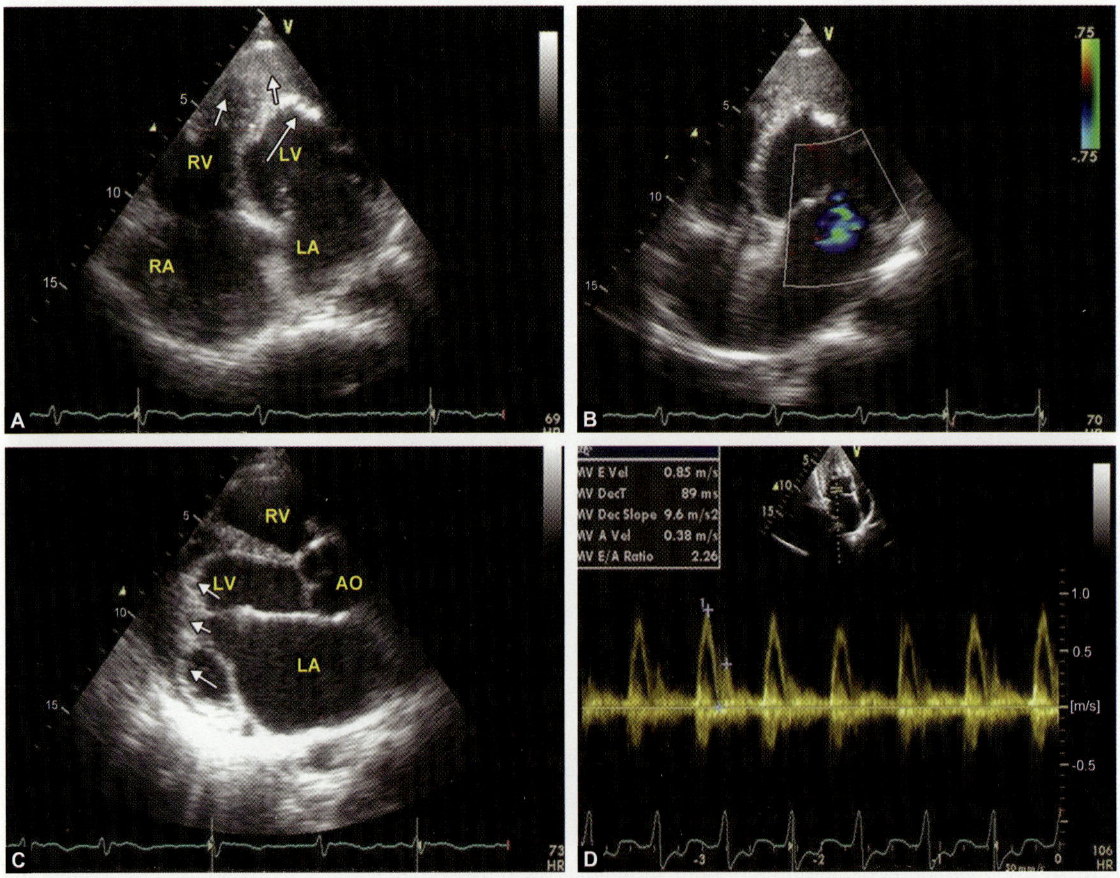

Figs. 16A to D: Echo Doppler features of left ventricular endomyocardial fibrosis. (A) Apical four-chamber view showing apical fibrosis (short arrows) and endocardial calcification (long arrows); (B and C) Mitral valve leaflets are only minimally involved with mild regurgitation; and (D) Restrictive filling pattern with e/a ratio more than 2 and mitral deceleration time of 89 milliseconds. (RA: right atrium; LA: left atrium; RV: right ventricle; LV: left ventricle)

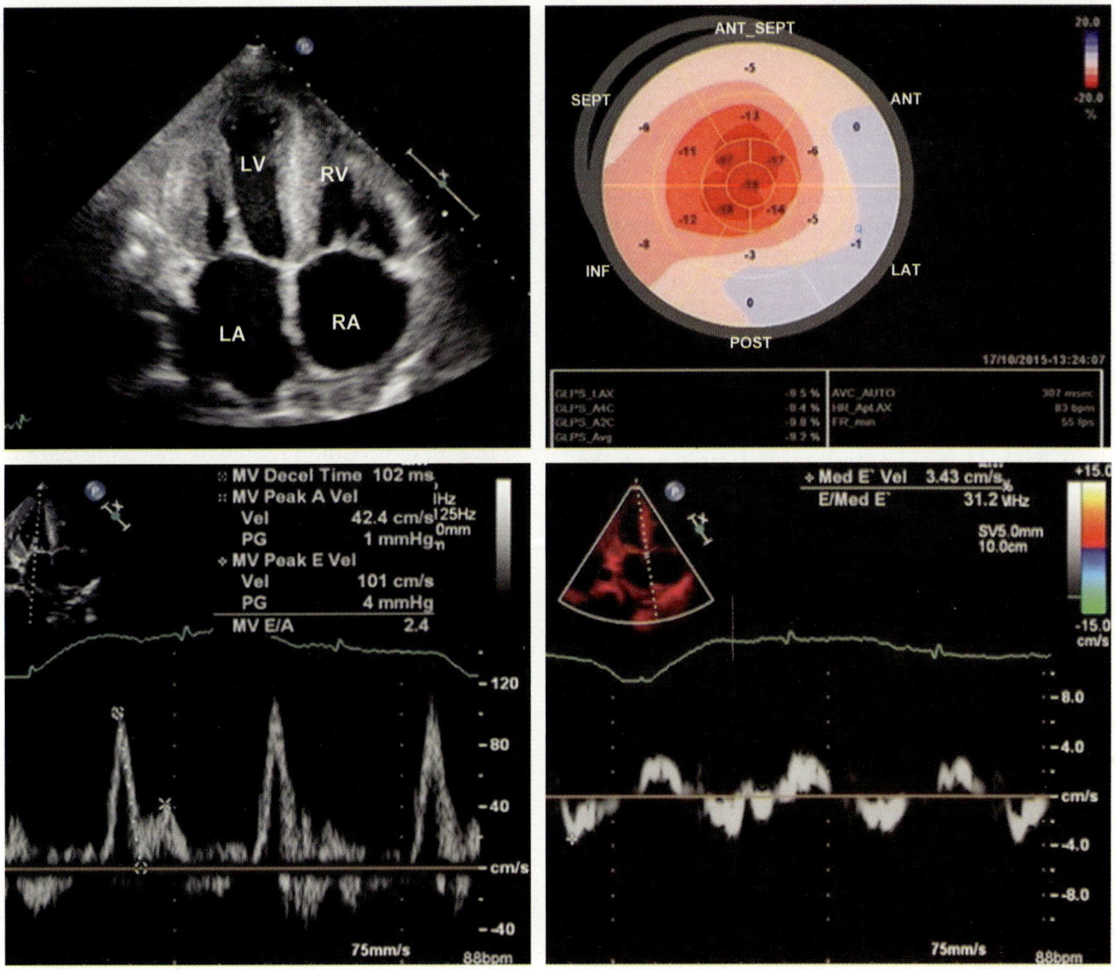

Fig. 17: Typical echocardiographic features of cardiac amyloidosis. Panel A shows the four-chamber view, thickened nondilated ventricles with granular sparkling appearance, dilated atria, giving the owl eye appearance, with interatrial septal thickening. Panel B shows the Bulls eye map of the longitudinal strain of the left ventricle by speckle tracking, the apical strain parameters are preserved, whereas basal segments where the infiltration is more affected, making a cherry red pattern. Panel C shows the typical mitral inflow pattern of restriction with dominant E waves with E deceleration time of 102 milliseconds. Panel D shows the tissue Doppler evaluation of mitral annulus with poor e' velocities and typical E/e' ratio of 31 reflecting high filling pressures.

various modalities of measurement and parameters is a must for the appropriate use of this technology.

REFERENCES

1. Nihoyannopoulos P, Dawson D. Restrictive cardiomyopathies. Eur J Echocardiogr. 2009;10(8):iii23-33.
2. Sisakian H. Cardiomyopathies: Evolution of pathogenesis concepts and potential for new therapies. World J Cardiol. 2014;6(6):478-94.
3. Mogensen J, Arbustini E. Restrictive cardiomyopathy. Curr Opin Cardiol. 2009;24(3):214-20.
4. Arbustini E, Narula N, Dec GW, et al. The MOGE(S) Classification for a Phenotype-Genotype Nomenclature of Cardiomyopathy: Endorsed by the World Heart Federation. J Am Coll Cardiol. 2013;62(22):2046-72.
5. Wood MJ, Picard MH. Utility of echocardiography in the evaluation of individuals with cardiomyopathy. Heart. 2004;90(6):707-12.
6. Kuznetsova T, Herbots L, Jin Y, et al. Systolic and diastolic left ventricular dysfunction: from risk factors to overt heart failure. Expert Rev Cardiovasc Ther. 2010;8(2):251-8.
7. Daneshvar D, Wei J, Tolstrup K, et al. Diastolic dysfunction: improved understanding using emerging imaging techniques. Am Heart J. 2010;160(3):394-404.
8. Murakami T, Kawai C. Advances in the understanding of systolic and diastolic functions of the heart. Int J Cardiol. 1991;32(2):149-73.
9. Appleton CP, Firstenberg MS, Garcia MJ, et al. The echo-Doppler evaluation of left ventricular diastolic function. A current perspective. Cardiol Clin. 2000;18(3):513-46.
10. Nagueh SF, Smiseth OA, Appleton CP, et al. Recommendations for the Evaluation of Left Ventricular Diastolic Function by

Echocardiography: An Update from the American Society of Echocardiography and the European Association of Cardiovascular Imaging. J Am Soc Echocardiogr. 2016;29(4):277-314.
11. Luers C, Maisch B. Echocardiography: future developments. What is diastole and how to assess it? Impaired left ventricular systolic function. Minerva Cardioangiol. 2011;59(4):331-47.
12. Ogunyankin KO. Assessment of left ventricular diastolic function: the power, possibilities, and pitfalls of echocardiographic imaging techniques. Can J Cardiol. 2011;27(3):311-8.
13. Morrissey C. Echo for diastology. Ann Card Anaesth. 2016;19(Suppl 1):S12-8.
14. Nishimura RA, Tajik AJ. Evaluation of diastolic filling of left ventricle in health and disease: Doppler echocardiography is the clinician's Rosetta Stone. J Am Coll Cardiol. 1997;30(1):8-18.
15. Lester SJ, Tajik AJ, Nishimura RA, et al. Unlocking the mysteries of diastolic function: deciphering the Rosetta Stone 10 years later. J Am Coll Cardiol. 2008;51(7):679-89.
16. Gillebert TC, De Pauw M, Timmermans F. Echo-Doppler assessment of diastole: flow, function and hemodynamics. Heart. 2013;99(1):55-64.
17. Vasan RS, Levy D. Defining diastolic heart failure: a call for standardized diagnostic criteria. Circulation. 2000;101(17):2118-21.
18. Little WC, Oh JK. Echocardiographic evaluation of diastolic function can be used to guide clinical care. Circulation. 2009; 120(9):802-9.
19. Tschöpe C, Paulus WJ. Is echocardiographic evaluation of diastolic function useful in determining clinical care? Doppler echocardiography yields dubious estimates of left ventricular diastolic pressures. Circulation. 2009;120(9):810-20.
20. Gopalakrishnan A, Nair KK, Ganapathi S. Hemodynamic challenge in nonrestrictive atrial septal defect. Heart Asia. 2018;10(2):e011014.
21. Ha JW, Ahn JA, Moon JY, et al. Triphasic mitral inflow velocity with middiastolic flow: The presence of middiastolic mitral annular velocity indicates advanced diastolic dysfunction. Eur J Echocardiogr. 2006;7(1):16-21.
22. Narayan GS, Sivasubramonian S. Spontaneous Fontan Physiology in Burnt-Out Endomyocardial Fibrosis. Circulation. 2012;125(4):e296-7.
23. Saran M, Sivasubramonian S, Abhilash SP, et al. Acquired Fontan paradox in isolated right ventricular cardiomyopathy. Ann Pediatr Cardiol. 2016;9(3):251-3.
24. Kampaktsis PN, Kokkinidis DG, Wong SC, et al. The role and clinical implications of diastolic dysfunction in aortic stenosis. Heart. 2017;103(19):1481-7.
25. Sivasubramonian S, Gopalakrishnan A, Sasidharan B, et al. Role of Diastology in Transcatheter Aortic Valve Implantation. J Invasive Cardiol. 2018;30(3):E23-4.
26. Kumar V, Jose J, Jose VJ. L wave in echo Doppler. Indian Heart J. 2014;66(3):392-3.
27. Maisch B, Noutsias M, Ruppert V, et al. Cardiomyopathies: Classification, Diagnosis, and Treatment. Heart Fail Clin. 2012;8(1):53-78.
28. Ginghină C, Mihalache R, Popescu BA, et al. Restrictive cardiomyopathy—an outdated concept. Rom J Intern Med. 2010;48(4):293-8.
29. Bograd AJ, Mital S, Schwarzenberger JC, et al. Twenty-year experience with heart transplantation for infants and children with restrictive cardiomyopathy: 1986-2006. Am J Transplant. 2008;8(1):201-7.
30. Franklin KM, Aurigemma GP. Prognosis in diastolic heart failure. Prog Cardiovasc Dis. 2005;47(5):333-9.
31. Asher CR, Klein AL. Diastolic heart failure: restrictive cardiomyopathy, constrictive pericarditis, and cardiac tamponade: clinical and echocardiographic evaluation. Cardiol Rev. 2002;10(4):218-29.
32. Packer M. Abnormalities of diastolic function as a potential cause of exercise intolerance in chronic heart failure. Circulation. 1990;81(2 Suppl):III78-86.
33. Maurer MS, King DL, El-Khoury Rumbarger L, et al. Left heart failure with a normal ejection fraction: identification of different pathophysiologic mechanisms. J Card Fail. 2005;11(3):177-87.
34. Stöllberger C, Finsterer J. Extracardiac medical and neuromuscular implications in restrictive cardiomyopathy. Clin Cardiol. 2007;30(8):375-80.
35. Restrictive cardiomyopathy or constrictive pericarditis. Lancet. 1987;2(8555):372-4.
36. Parekh N, Maisel AS. Utility of B-natriuretic peptide in the evaluation of left ventricular diastolic function and diastolic heart failure. Curr Opin Cardiol. 2009;24(2):155-60.
37. Bejar D, Colombo PC, Latif F, et al. Infiltrative Cardiomyopathies. Clin Med Insights Cardiol. 2015;9(Suppl 2):29-38.
38. Sperry BW, Tang WHW. Amyloid heart disease: genetics translated into disease-modifying therapy. Heart. 2017; 103(11):812-7.
39. TharakanJ, Bohora S. (2010). Current perspective on endomyocardial fibrosis. [online] Available from www.ias.ac.in/currsci/aug102009/405.pdf. [October, 2018].
40. Vijayaraghavan G, Sivasankaran S. Tropical endomyocardial fibrosis in India: A vanishing disease. Indian J Med Res. 2012;136(5):729-38.
41. Falk RH, Quarta CC, Dorbala S. How to Image Cardiac Amyloidosis: A Focused Practical Review. Circ Cardiovasc Imaging. 2014;7(3):552-62.
42. Guleria R Sharma R, Mohan A, et al. Cardiac Sarcoidosis, an uncommon presentation of sarcoidosis in India. Indian J Chest Dis Allied Sci. 2006;48(2):133-7.
43. Sharma SK, Soneja M, Sharma A, et al. Rare manifestations of sarcoidosis in modern era of new diagnositic tools. Indian J Med Res. 2012;135(5):621-9.
44. Barbero U, Destefanis P. An Indian-look right into restrictive cardiomyopathies. Indian Heart J. 2015;67(6):512-3.
45. Selthofer-Relatic K. Time of Anderson-Fabry Disease Detection and Cardiovascular Presentation. Case Rep Cardiol. 2018;2018:6131083.
46. Kremastinos DT, Farmakis D, Aessopos A, et al. Beta-thalassemia cardiomyopathy: history, present considerations, and future perspectives. Circ Heart Fail. 2010;3(3):451-8.
47. Siddiqi OK, Ruberg FL. Cardiac amyloidosis: An update on pathophysiology, diagnosis, and treatment. Trends Cardiovasc Med. 2018;28(1):10-21.
48. Piper C, Butz T, Farr M, et al. How to diagnose cardiac amyloidosis early: impact of ECG, tissue Doppler echocardiography, and myocardial biopsy. Amyloid. 2010;17(1):1-9.

89

CHAPTER

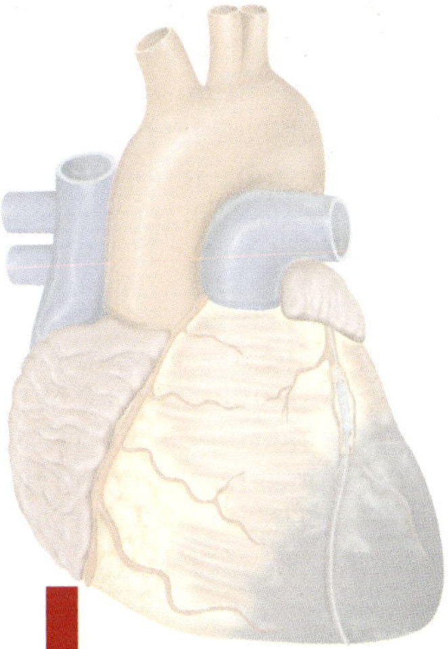

Restrictive Cardiomyopathies

Krishnam Raju P, Chandramukhi Modi

INTRODUCTION

Cardiomyopathy was defined by Goodwin in 1951 as a subacute or chronic disorder of heart muscle of unknown etiology and often associated with involvement of endocardium and sometimes pericardial involvement and not atherosclerotic in origin. Cardiomyopathies were then classified according to the disorder of structure and function into hypertrophic, congestive, restrictive, and obliterative. European Society of Cardiology statement is as follows: Definition of Cardiomyopathy, "A myocardial disorder in which the heart muscle is structurally and functionally abnormal in the absence of coronary artery disease, hypertension, valvular disease and congenital heart disease sufficient to explain the observed myocardial abnormality." Restrictive cardiomyopathy (RCM) is a rarely encountered form of cardiomyopathy. It is characterized by increased stiffness of the ventricles with elevated diastolic filling pressures and impaired ventricular filling, with normal or decreased diastolic volume of either or both ventricles. Systolic function usually remains normal, at least early in the disease. Although therapy is generally unsatisfactory for RCM, the importance of an accurate diagnosis lies in distinguishing RCM from constrictive pericarditis, which can also present with "restrictive physiology" but which is often cured surgically by pericardiectomy.[1]

EPIDEMIOLOGY

Restrictive cardiomyopathy is the least common of the cardiomyopathic disorders. Cardiac amyloidosis is the most thoroughly studied RCM. Endomyocardial fibrosis (EMF) is endemic in parts of Africa, India, South and Central America, and Asia, and it occurs sporadically throughout the world.[2] The disease occurs in its classical endemic form in the selected coastal belt in Kerala, India, affecting young people of lower socioeconomic families. Over the past four decades, there has been a tremendous change in socioeconomic and health status in Kerala and a corresponding decline in new cases of EMF in the younger age-group. At present, the number of new cases diagnosed has declined significantly to 10 new cases a year in the past decade. Furthermore, the mean age at presentation has also changed by a decade from 25 years to 33 years, suggesting late recognition of asymptomatic cases and possible decline in the incidence of new cases. In the current era, patients with EMF have relatively stable symptomatic course on follow-up with mortality of around 10% on 3-year follow-up.[3]

GENETICS

In 1992, Feld and Caspi reported a family with mixed features of RCM and hypertrophic cardiomyopathy (HCM). The histopathology of a deceased individual at necropsy with RCM showed typical features of HCM with myocyte disarray.[4] Mogensen and Arbustin[5] performed mutation analysis in nine unrelated RCM patients with unexplained restrictive filling patterns, gross atrial dilatation, normal systolic function, and normal wall thickness. The study concluded that mutations in cardiac troponin I were responsible for the development of RCM in a significant proportion of patients. Additional mutations in sarcomeric genes including troponin T: *TNNT2, TNNI3*; beta-myosin heavy chain: *MYH7*; and alpha-cardiac actin have been shown to be associated in patients with idiopathic RCM. De novo mutations appear to be prevalent findings, especially in children and young adults, suggesting that they are associated with a more severe disease expression. Autosomal dominant RCM with atrioventricular (AV) block and skeletal myopathy has been reported in five generations of an Italian family. Symptoms developed in the third to fourth decade of life, with the eventual appearance of AV block and skeletal-muscle weakness.[6] Other familial disorders associated with RCM include amyloidosis, hemochromatosis, Anderson-Fabry's disease. In patients with cardiac amyloidosis, ChfuuLubitz et al.[7] reported mutations in the genes for transthyretin and apolipoprotein A1. Hemochromatosis is an autosomal recessive disorder leading to iron deposition in multiple organs resulting in widespread damage, few patients have cardiac involvement. Hoedemaekers et al.[8] reported that the major cardiomyopathies are genetically heterogeneous diseases for which the causative genes are partially overlapping. The phenotypic variability of sarcomeric mutations is illustrated by *MYH7* mutations, known to be involved in HCM, dilated cardiomyopathy (DCM), RCM, and noncompaction cardiomyopathy (NCCM). The genetic heterogeneity of NCCM and the identification of *MYH7* defects in familial NCCM suggest that NCCM may be part of a cardiomyopathy spectrum including HCM, RCM, and DCM. However, it is not clear whether these are different diseases or rather different manifestations (phenotypes) of the same pathological mechanism. It is important to realize that transitional forms of the conditions frequently appear even within the same family affected by the same mutation. Therefore, the diagnosis of any condition likely to be a cardiomyopathy should lead to family screening for a potential hereditary disorder. Identification and risk stratification of affected relatives is important to avoid adverse disease complications and diminishes the rate of sudden death. Genetic testing is now available on a clinical basis for several of the genes responsible for cardiomyopathies. However, it has its limitations and challenges. Testing sensitivity is low, and there may be more than one genetic variant in an affected patient or within a single family.

The "restrictive phenotype" in isolation is an uncommon presentation of the clinical spectrum of HCM and is associated with severe symptoms and poor prognosis. This phenotype may be associated with beta-myosin heavy chain and cardiac troponin I mutations. Kubo et al.[9] studied the prevalence, clinical significance, and genetic basis of HCM with "restrictive phenotype" characterized by restrictive filling and minimal or no left ventricular (LV) hypertrophy (LVH). HCM is associated with diastolic abnormalities in the majority of patients, and diastolic dysfunction has long been recognized as a determinant of symptoms and exercise limitation. The diastolic abnormalities are usually mild and consist of impaired relaxation and slow LV filling, but some patients exhibit more severe diastolic abnormalities with rapid early filling and restrictive physiology. Kubo et al.[9] reported a family with disease caused by a mutation in cardiac troponin I; in which, 12 individuals had typical HCM and 3 others exhibited a "restrictive phenotype" characterized by restrictive filling and minimal or no LVH which (if seen in isolation) resembled idiopathic RCM. They noticed that in addition to mutations in *TNNI3*, *MYH7* mutations are also associated with HCM characterized by "restrictive phenotype." The main cause of death in "restrictive phenotype" patients was related to heart failure: 42% developed signs of right heart failure, including edema, abdominal discomfort, and ascites. "Restrictive phenotype" patients were also more prone to atrial fibrillation/flutter and stroke, presumably as a consequence of elevated filling pressure and left atrial enlargement. Thus, HCM patients who exhibit RCM phenotype have grade III or more advanced diastolic heart failure and high rates of atrial fibrillation/flutter and stroke. This phenotype seems to be related to mutations in beta-myosin heavy chain and cardiac troponin I. Prognosis is poor, and the patients may ultimately require cardiac transplantation.

CLINICAL PRESENTATION

Restrictive cardiomyopathy can present at any age but its incidence is increased in the elderly. It is more common in elderly females than males. The clinical course can be variable. The clinical diagnosis is difficult to establish early in the clinical course due to the lack of symptoms. Therefore, in many cases, this diagnosis is made only after the patient presents with symptoms and signs of right ventricular (RV) or LV failure. Symptoms are due to increase in the left atrial and pulmonary venous pressure and an inability to increase the cardiac output with exercise. Patients may present with signs and symptoms of both pulmonary and systemic congestion, such as dyspnea, paroxysmal nocturnal dyspnea, orthopnea, peripheral edema, palpitations, syncope, fatigue, weakness, and exercise intolerance. Some patients may give past history of chemotherapy or systemic disease involving myocardium. In advanced cases, there may be raised jugular venous pressure (JVP) with prominent Y descent, Kusmaul's sign: an inspiratory increase in venous pressure, third heart sound (S3) gallop, soft systolic murmurs of functional mitral regurgitation (MR) or tricuspid regurgitation (TR), hepatosplenomegaly, ascites, and anasarca.

EVALUATION

Once suspected, meticulous evaluation with investigations, such as electrocardiogram (ECG), chest radiograph, echocardiogram and cardiac magnetic resonance (CMR) imaging, and finally cardiac catheterization, help confirm the diagnosis of RCM.

- *Electrocardiogram:* It may show nonspecific abnormalities and include either large P waves indicating enlarged atria or atrial fibrillation, ST-T wave abnormalities, premature atrial and ventricular beats, AV block, and intraventricular (IV) conduction delay. A case report suggested that significant ST depression with T inversion mimicking subendocardial ischemia is a potential predictor of sudden cardiac death[10]
- *Chest radiograph:* It is usually characterized by significant atrial enlargement with pulmonary venous congestion and pleural effusions. Endomyocardial calcium may be found which is characteristic of EMF
- *Echocardiogram:* Echocardiogram is the most commonly performed and most useful imaging modality in the evaluation and management of patients suspected to have RCM. Echocardiography with its multimodality imaging techniques, including two-dimensional (2D) echocardiography, M mode, Doppler evaluation, and color Doppler imaging, gives a comprehensive description of cardiac involvement with detailed structural and hemodynamic assessment. An integrated approach with the combination of all these echocardiography modalities is important to identify specific features of RCM. Novel echocardiography techniques, such as tissue velocity imaging and speckle tracking, which analyzes strain and strain rate, provide information regarding ventricular myocardial properties and can detect the disease in its early course. These techniques also help in differentiating RCM from constrictive pericarditis (Table 1)

  The characteristic echocardiography features of RCM include:
  - *Two-dimensional echocardiography features:*
    - Biatrial enlargement
    - Normal or small ventricular cavity size with generally preserved or mildly reduced systolic ventricular function
    - In RCM, wall thickness is typically normal, though it may be increased with certain infiltrative processes (e.g. amyloidosis) or storage disease (e.g. Fabry disease)
    - Raised right atrial (RA) pressures as evidenced by dilated inferior vena cava (IVC)
    - Valve thickening, interatrial septal thickening, or pericardial effusion may be present and are suggestive of cardiac amyloidosis.
  - *Doppler echocardiography:*
    Abnormal diastolic function, frequently with a restrictive filling pattern as evidenced by
    - Increased early diastolic filling velocity (E)
    - Decreased atrial filling velocity (A)
    - $E/A \geq 1.5$
    - Decreased E-wave deceleration time (Edt) < 150 ms
    - Decreased isovolumic relaxation time (IVRT)
    - Significant decrease in the ratio of systolic (S) and diastolic (D) wave velocities in pulmonary venous flow, i.e. S/D ratio
    - Augmented atrial reversal velocity in the pulmonary venous flow and pulmonary arterial hypertension, which can be assessed by TR jet velocity providing RV systolic pressure (RVSP) or pulmonary regurgitation velocity providing pulmonary arterial mean pressure and pulmonary arterial diastolic pressure.
  - *Tissue velocity imaging:*
    - Markedly reduced mitral annular tissue velocities: Early diastolic medial mitral annular tissue velocity e′ and late diastolic medial mitral annular tissue velocity a′ and systolic medial mitral annular tissue velocity s′ are all significantly reduced
    - Evaluation of segmental myocardial tissue velocities of LV and RV shows significantly reduced segmental myocardial tissue velocities. Tissue velocity imaging identifies the subclinical ventricular dysfunction even before the reduction in ejection fraction occurs. It also helps in distinguishing RCM from constrictive pericarditis, with a mitral annular diastolic velocity $e' \leq 8$ cm/s, a good discriminator for restrictive physiology while constrictive pericarditis is characterized by normal or elevated mitral annular tissue velocities.
  - *Two-dimensional speckle-tracking echocardiography: strain and strain rate imaging:*
    - Markedly reduced global strain rate of left and right ventricle
    - Specific longitudinal strain rate pattern, such as reduced longitudinal strain rate with relative apical sparing as seen in amyloidosis.

KEY POINT 1

RCM should be considered in patients presenting with heart failure in the presence of a nondilated, nonhypertrophied LV with preserved contractility but abnormal diastolic function and dilated atria. Echocardiography is the preferred imaging modality for assessing the morphological and functional characteristics of RCM.

TABLE 1: Features differentiating restrictive cardiomyopathy from constrictive pericarditis.

	Restrictive cardiomyopathy	*Constrictive pericarditis*
History	• Systemic disease involving myocardium, amyloid, chemotherapy, radiotherapy	• Previous pericarditis, cardiac surgery, chest trauma, systemic disease involving pericardium, radiotherapy, connective tissue disorder
Physical examination	• Kussmaul's sign may be present • Apical impulse may be prominent • S3 may be present, rarely S4 may be present • Regurgitant murmurs common	• Kussmaul's sign usually present • Apical impulse usually not palpable • Pericardial knock may be present • Regurgitant murmurs are extremely uncommon
ECG	• P waves—LAO/RAO/BAO • AV/IV conduction delay common • Atrial fibrillation—early • Low-voltage complexes: Amyloid • Pseudo-MI pattern	• P waves—Intra-atrial conduction delay • AV/IV conduction delay rare • Atrial fibrillation—late • Low-voltage complexes, T wave inversion, conduction abnormalities if present indicate myocardial involvement
Chest X-ray	• Absence of pericardial calcification but presence of endomyocardial calcium (EMF) • Massive atrial enlargement	• Pericardial calcification (20%), moderate atrial enlargement
Echocardiogram	• Marked biatrial enlargement • Increased ventricular wall thickness, altered myocardial echotexture • Increased thickness of interatrial septum (in cardiac amyloid) • Significantly reduced myocardial tissue velocities and mitral annular tissue velocities (e′ < 8 cm/s) • Reduced strain rate • Inspiratory increase in diastolic flow reversal in hepatic veins • LV/RV apical obliteration (EMF) • Torsion and twist: Marked endocardial dysfunction with relatively normal epicardial function leads to abnormal longitudinal mechanics and relatively normal circumferential and twist mechanics	• Moderate biatrial enlargement • Normal ventricular wall thickness with normal myocardial echotexture • Respirophasic interventricular septal motion, prominent early diastolic filling with abrupt displacement of interventricular septum interventricular septal bounce, diastolic septal notch • Normal myocardial tissue velocities • Mitral annular tissue velocities are exaggerated (e′ > 12 cm/s) with annulus paradox, normal strain rate • >25% expiratory increase in mitral inflow tissue velocities • Normal strain rate • Expiratory increase in diastolic flow reversal in hepatic veins • *Torsion and twist:* Marked epicardial dysfunction leads to impairment of circumferential shortening and twist mechanics, whereas the subendocardial longitudinal mechanics are relatively spared
CMR/MDCT	• LGE CMR: Myocardial fibrosis, scarring, or necrosis • MDCT: Pericardium is usually normal	• LGE CMR: Myocardium is normal • MDCT: Pericardium may be thickened or calcified
Hemodynamics	• RVEDP < one-third of RVSP • No interventricular dependence • LVEDP is typically greater than RVEDP by 5 mm Hg • Separation of LVEDP from RVEDP with volume challenge if equalization present	• RVEDP > one-third of RVSP • Interventricular dependence+ • LVEDP is typically equal to RVEDP or LVEDP and RVEDP vary by less than 5 mm Hg • RVSP < 50 mm Hg • Dip and plateau pattern on cardiac catheterization
Endomyocardial biopsy	• Fibrosis, hypertrophy, infiltration (yield is low)	• Normal

(AV: atrioventricular; BAO: biatrial atrial overload; CMR: cardiac magnetic resonance imaging; ECG: electrocardiogram; EMF: endomyocardial fibrosis; IV: intraventricular; LAO: left atrial overload; LGE: late gadolinium enhancement; LV: left ventricular; LVEDP: LV end-diastolic pressure; MDCT: multidetector computed tomography; MI: myocardial infarction; RAO: right atrial overload; RV: right ventricular; RVEDP: RV end-diastolic pressure; RVSP: RV systolic pressure; S3: third heart sound; S4: fourth heart sound)

Echocardiography is a multimodality imaging technique that when used appropriately and expertly in its full capacity allows for the comprehensive description of cardiac involvement in RCM. Other imaging modalities, particularly CMR, may be complementary to echocardiography in that it is the only method that can depict the presence of myocardial fibrosis.

- *Plasma brain natriuretic peptide:* In patients with suspected RCM, brain natriuretic peptide (BNP) levels help distinguish RCM from constrictive pericarditis and noncardiac causes of dyspnea. BNP levels are significantly elevated in RCM and may be higher than 400 pg/mL.[11] But BNP levels may be elevated in patients with renal failure and has limited value in the diagnosis of RCM in these patients
- *Multidetector computed tomography:* It is especially helpful in excluding constrictive pericarditis, which is a very deceptive mimic of RCM. The evidence of pericardial thickening and calcification on computed tomography (CT) favor constrictive pericarditis, though not conclusive
- *Cardiac magnetic resonance imaging:* It has a specific ability of tissue characterization, which provides incremental information to that obtained from echocardiography, and helps in the identification or exclusion of various causes of RCM.[12] Cardiac magnetic resonance imaging (CMR) yields characteristic findings in amyloidosis and facilitates the early detection of cardiac involvement. Late gadolinium enhancement (LGE) enables identification of myocardial fibrosis, scar, necrosis, or infiltration. Characteristic patterns of LGE help the diagnosis of certain characteristic disease processes. In sarcoidosis, there is often patchy enhancement, such as at the base of the septum and base of the inferolateral wall, frequently not consistent with any coronary artery distribution. Myocardial iron overload can be assessed by cardiac T2 measurements. In addition, similar to echocardiography, CMR-based tissue tracking can be used to differentiate RCM from constrictive pericarditis
- *Cardiac catheterization:* It is indicated in patients in whom the evaluation by noninvasive imaging modalities, such as echocardiography or CMR, is inconclusive for the diagnosis of RCM. The characteristic features on cardiac catheterization diagnostic of RCM include:
  - Elevated RA pressure with prominent x and y descent
  - Classic square root sign
  - Right ventricular systolic pressure more than or equal to 50 mm Hg
  - Right ventricular end-diastolic pressure (RVEDP) less than one-third of RVSP
  - Left ventricular end-diastolic pressure (LVEDP) is typically greater than RVEDP by 5 mm Hg or more
  - Separation of LVEDP from RVEDP with volume challenge if equalization present
  - Absence of discordance in RVSP and LVSP during respiration (absence of ventricular interdependence), this being a very important differentiator.

DIFFERENTIAL DIAGNOSIS

Restrictive cardiomyopathy and constrictive pericarditis have close resemblance as both have the common hemodynamic abnormality of diastolic dysfunction. However, a meticulous evaluation will help differentiating RCM from constrictive pericarditis.

Endomyocardial biopsy (EMB): It is suggested in selected patients with RCM if the preliminary evaluation is inconclusive.[13] EMB can help identify or exclude specific conditions, such as amyloidosis, sarcoidosis, and hemochromatosis. However, it is now rarely done as part of evaluation of RCM as the diagnostic yield is suboptimal.

KEY POINT 2

Constrictive pericarditis with significant myocardial involvement with fibrosis may have mixed features suggestive of myocardial abnormality.

CLASSIFICATION

Unlike the other cardiomyopathies that are classified according to morphological criteria, i.e. HCM, DCM, or RV cardiomyopathy, RCM is a functional classification, which is based on the hemodynamic consequences of diastolic dysfunction. This automatically represents a challenge as many anatomical variants may have a common denominator—the restrictive physiology (Flowchart 1).

Restrictive myocardial disease may result from various local and systemic disorders and can be classified according to the causative factors as enlisted in Table 2. Conditions,

Flowchart 1: Classification of RCM.[14]

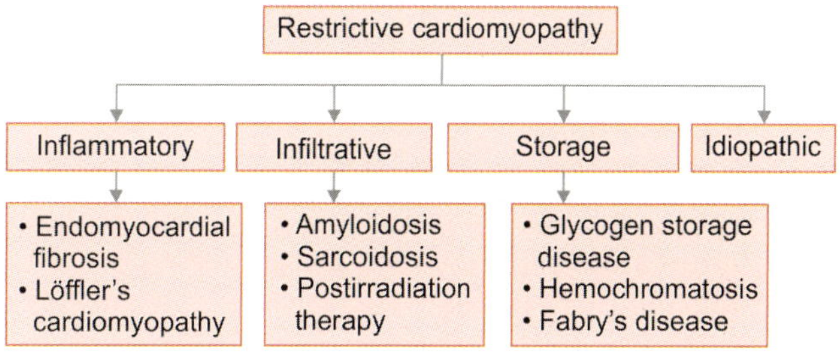

(RCM: restrictive cardiomyopathy)

TABLE 2: Classification of types of restrictive cardiomyopathy according to cause.[2]

I. *Myocardial:*
   1. *Noninfiltrative:* Idiopathic cardiomyopathy,* familial cardiomyopathy, hypertrophic cardiomyopathy, scleroderma, pseudoxanthoma elasticum, diabetic cardiomyopathy
   2. *Infiltrative:* Amyloidosis,* sarcoidosis,* Gaucher's disease, Hurler's disease, fatty infiltration, storage diseases, hemochromatosis Fabry's disease, glycogen storage disease

II. *Endomyocardial:* Endomyocardial fibrosis,* hypereosinophilic syndrome

III. *Carcinoid heart disease*

IV. *Metastatic cancers*

V. *Radiation**

VI. *Toxic effects of anthracycline* (chemocardiotoxicity)*

VII. *Drugs causing fibrous endocarditis:* Serotonin, methysergide, ergotamine, mercurial agents, busulfan

VIII. *Miscellaneous: Reversible RCM in hypercoagulable states*—some patients typically present with vague symptoms of exertional dyspnea or transient giddiness or syncope. On evaluation, these patients are found to have various features suggestive of primary hypercoagulation disorder, such as hypereosinophilia or antiphospholipid antibody syndrome. Echocardiogram typically demonstrates thrombus at the LV or RV apex or both apices, no wall motion abnormality, and restrictive filling pattern. When treated with appropriate anticoagulation, the thrombus disappears and also the filling pattern improves from restrictive filling pattern to grade II or grade I diastolic dysfunction

(LV: left ventricular; RCM: restrictive cardiomyopathy; RV: right ventricular)

*This condition is more likely than the others to be encountered in clinical practice.

TABLE 3: Distribution of various types of restrictive cardiomyopathy in 73 patients with restrictive cardiomyopathy out of total 71,587 patients in our echocardiography laboratory the 3-year period from January 2013 to December 2015.

Type of RCM	*Number of patients with echocardiographic features of RCM*	*Number of patients with echocardiographic diagnosis of RCM confirmed by CMR*
Amyloidosis	30	24 (Remaining 4 had nonspecific features with CKD and 2: no CMR)
Idiopathic	23	19 (Remaining 1 had amyloid, 2 had inflammatory RCM, 1: no CMR)
Löffler's	2	2
EMF	2	2

(CMR: cardiac magnetic resonance imaging; EMF: endomyocardial fibrosis; RCM: restrictive cardiomyopathy)

such as amyloidosis, are more common. In idiopathic RCM, the hemodynamic abnormalities occur in the absence of specific histopathological changes.[14]

Incidence of RCM in the patients referred to our echocardiography laboratories during the period of 3 years from January 2013 to December 2015.

In our institution, we performed 71,587 transthoracic echocardiograms in our inpatient and outpatient echocardiography laboratories during the 3-year period from January 2013 to December 2015. A total of 73 (0.10 %) cases were reported to have features of RCM. Out of these 73 cases, 30 were reported to have features of cardiac amyloid. CMR was done in 28 cases, and 24 cases were confirmed by CMR, while 4 cases were found to have nonspecific features with chronic kidney disease with myocardial edema. Out of the remaining 43 cases with echocardiographic features of RCM, 23 had features suggestive of RCM but not specific to any form of RCM and reported as idiopathic RCM. CMR confirmed the diagnosis of idiopathic RCM in 19 of these 23 cases, while one case was reported as cardiac amyloid, two cases were reported as inflammatory cardiomyopathy, and remaining one case did not undergo CMR. Out of the remaining 20 patients with RCM on echocardiography, two patients had features of Löffler's endocarditis (confirmed by CMR), two cases had EMF—one had LVEMF and other had biventricular EMF: both confirmed by CMR, seven were reported to have nonspecific features, and the remaining nine patients did not undergo CMR. Table 3 shows the various types of RCM encountered in our patient population.

Idiopathic Restrictive Cardiomyopathy

Idiopathic or primary RCM is an uncommon disorder that is manifested by characteristic morphologic and hemodynamic changes of RCM in the absence of any identifiable cause.[12] Morphologic changes include nondilated ventricles with typically normal wall thicknesses but rigid walls, resulting in stiff ventricles with severe diastolic dysfunction and restrictive filling with elevated filling pressures and dilated atria. Generally, the LV systolic function is preserved or mildly decreased. Idiopathic or primary RCM is a rare and poorly characterized entity. It is a diagnosis of exclusion because restrictive physiology is also seen in a number of other disorders, including several systemic conditions. Restrictive hemodynamics can occur with many advanced primary or secondary cardiac diseases, such as ischemic, valvular, or infiltrative conditions, such as amyloidosis. Primary RCM may affect both children and adults. Both familial and sporadic cases have been described. Familial cases are usually characterized by autosomal dominant inheritance with incomplete penetrance.[15] Genetic mutations encoding the sarcomeric proteins troponin I, troponin T, alpha-cardiac actin, and beta-myosin heavy chain, which are similar to those associated with HCM, are implicated.[16,17] Fitzpatrick et al.[6] studied five generations of an Italian family with autosomal dominant RCM and found that symptoms usually developed in the third or fourth decade but the disease did occur in childhood. Bundle branch blocks, leading to complete AV block, were the early manifestations, while skeletal myopathy developed late in the course of disease. Cooke et al.[18] reported the association of primary, familial, non-HCM with echocardiographic and hemodynamic features of restrictive pathophysiology in three family members with classic Noonan's phenotype. These associations suggest that there is a genetic predisposition to idiopathic RCM, and in some cases, the genetic locus is associated with skeletal myopathy. Some cases are sporadic and possibly the result of spontaneous mutation (Fig. 1).

The condition is usually detected in advanced stages, and the patient typically presents with congestive heart failure with symptoms and signs of systemic and pulmonary venous congestion. Echocardiographic evaluation reveals severe left atrial and moderate RA dilation with normal ventricular dimensions and function. The disease can involve both the LV and RV. Ventricular wall thickness is usually normal, but in some cases, it is possible to detect mild hypertrophy. However, various degrees of systolic dysfunction with diffuse hypokinesia can be found in more advanced disease. Functional mild-to-moderate MR and TR are frequent. Elevated RA pressure will be evident by dilated IVC (Fig. 2).

Treatment

There is no specific therapy for idiopathic RCM. Patient is treated with supportive therapy aimed at reducing

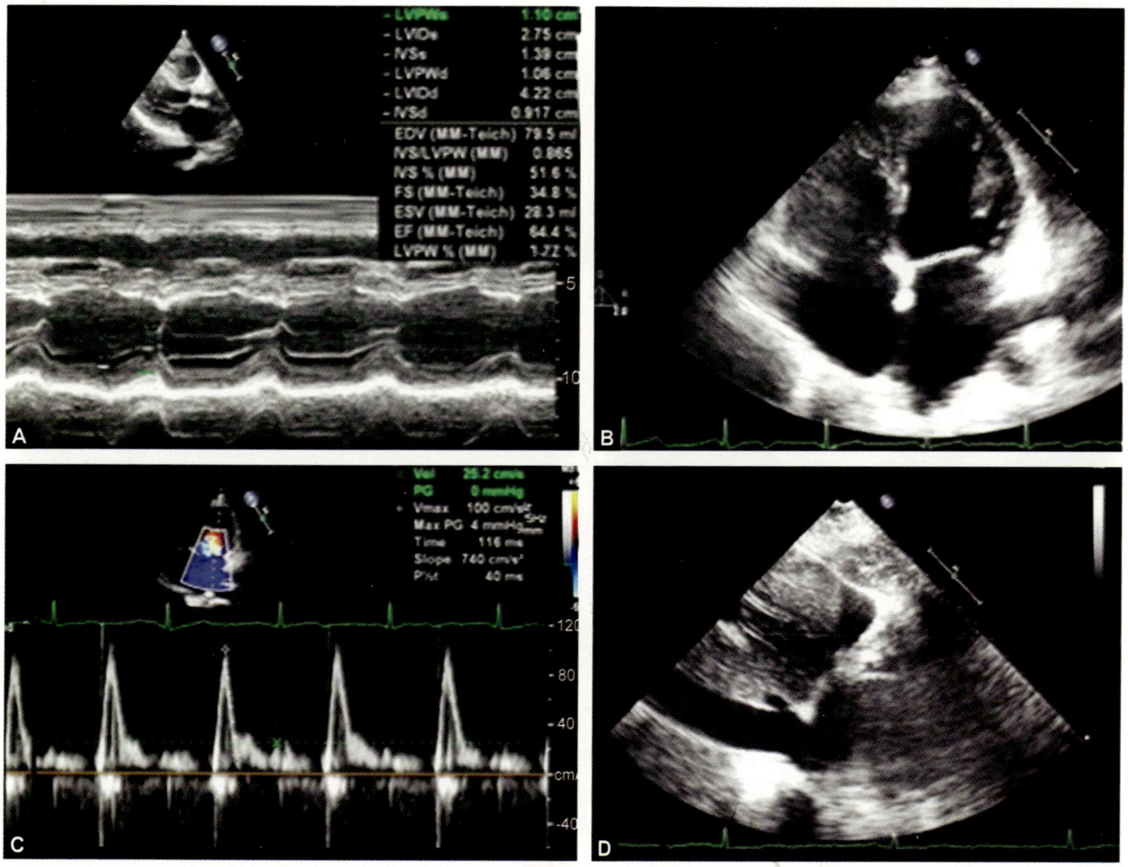

Figs. 1A to D: Echocardiographic features in a patient with idiopathic RCM. (A) M-mode assessment of LV ejection fraction shows normal LV systolic function; (B) Apical four-chamber view shows dilated atria with normal size ventricles; (C) Pulsed wave Doppler across mitral inflow shows restrictive filling pattern; (D) IVC is dilated. These features should raise the suspicion of RCM—idiopathic. (IVC: inferior vena cava; LV: left ventricular; RCM: restrictive cardiomyopathy)

pulmonary and systemic congestion, lowering the venous pressure, controlling heart rate, maintenance of atrial contractions, correction of AV conduction disturbances, correction of anemia, nutritional deficiency, calcium overload, and electrolyte imbalance. Oral anticoagulants are instituted particularly in patients with RCM and atrial fibrillation. Heart transplantation is an effective therapy for patients with end-stage primary RCM, but severe pulmonary hypertension usually present at this stage is a contraindication for heart transplant (Fig. 3).

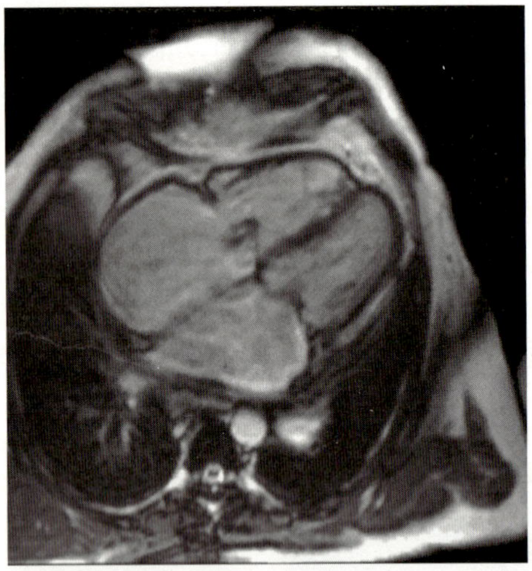

Fig. 2: Cardiac MRI with LGE in a patient with idiopathic RCM. Apical four-chamber view shows marked enlargement of both the atria with normal size ventricles. There is enhancement of the left atrial wall suggestive of fibrosis. CMR provides incremental information to that obtained from echo and helps in the confirmation of diagnosis of RCM and identification or exclusion of various causes of RCM. (CMR: cardiac magnetic resonance; LGE: late gadolinium enhancement; MRI: magnetic resonance imaging; RCM: restrictive cardiomyopathy)

Amyloidosis

Amyloidosis is a systemic disorder characterized by extracellular deposition of insoluble fibrillar protein in the interstitial space in the liver, kidney, heart, bowel, nerves, skin, and tongue. Cardiac amyloidosis is the commonest cause of RCM. However, it results in both diastolic and systolic LV dysfunction. Cardiac involvement is the primary determinant of prognosis in systemic amyloidoses. It is characterized by infiltration of myocardium by amyloid protein resulting in cardiomyopathy and conduction disturbances. Cardiac involvement is primarily encountered in immunoglobulin amyloid light-chain (AL) and transthyretin-associated (hereditary/familial and senile) amyloidoses. Five major clinical types of cardiac amyloidosis are recognized, as shown in Table 4, each associated with a different precursor protein.[19]

Primary or systemic AL amyloidosis is the most common form of amyloidosis involving the heart in 90% of the cases,[20] and heart failure is the common presentation, and it is associated with monoclonal gammopathy of undetermined significance or plasma cell dyscrasias, such as multiple myeloma. Cardiac involvement is associated with a poor prognosis, with a median survival from diagnosis of 1 year.[21] Hence, early detection of cardiac amyloidosis is critical. The initial presentation of systemic amyloidosis is vague with nonspecific systemic symptoms, such as dizziness, ankle swelling, bruising, "frothy" urine, diarrhea, numbness, shortness of breath, weight loss, poor appetite,

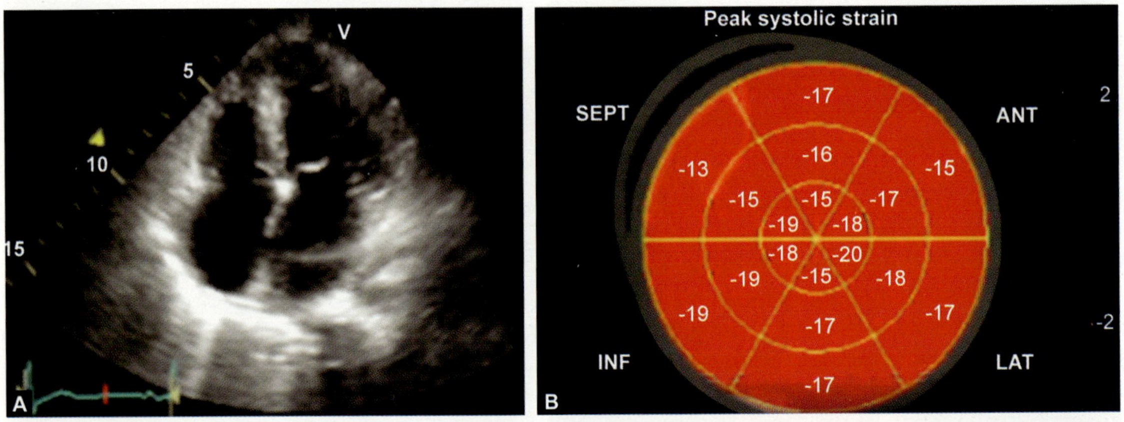

Figs. 3A and B: Strain rate imaging to assess the subclinical LV systolic dysfunction in idiopathic RCM. (A) Apical four-chamber view shows dilated atria with normal size ventricles. This patient had normal LV ejection fraction with restrictive filling pattern, mild pulmonary arterial hypertension with mildly reduced myocardial tissue velocities; (B) Strain rate imaging with Bull's eye plot showing mildly reduced global longitudinal strain. Echocardiographic diagnosis of idiopathic RCM was proposed which was confirmed by CMR. (LV: left ventricular; RCM: restrictive cardiomyopathy)

TABLE 4: Classification of cardiac amyloid.[19]

Amyloidosis type	Precursor	Comment
Light chain or light chain/heavy chain	Immunoglobulin light chain	Systemic plasma cell dyscrasia
Mutant transthyretin-related	TTR point mutation	Inherited autosomal-dominant mutation, expressed after the fifth decade
Wild-type TTR	None	Formerly known as senile cardiac amyloidosis
Amyloid A	Serum amyloid A	Sustained inflammatory process, cardiac involvement rare
Isolated atrial amyloid	Atrial natriuretic factor	Diagnosis before death rare, features atrial fibrillation

nausea, diarrhea, dizziness, and collapse. The nonspecific presenting features hamper the initial suspicion of amyloidosis. Macroglossia, which is pathognomonic of AL amyloid (excluding acromegaly and myxedema), occurs in around 10% of cases.[22] Vascular manifestations, such as periorbital purpura ("racoon" or "panda" eyes) and other major bleeding complications, occur as a result of vascular fragility and are seen in around one third of patients with AL amyloid, while recurrent petechial lesions of the eyelids and periorbital area caused by rubbing the area, or coughing and sneezing are more commonly seen. The initial workup in suspected cases should include serum and urine analysis for the presence of a monoclonal immunoglobulin, in addition to standard blood tests, such as complete blood picture, urea and electrolytes, liver function tests, clotting screen, and glucose and thyroid function tests. The standard serum protein electrophoresis may fail to detect a monoclonal band in a significant number of cases, hence immunofixation which is more sensitive and should be performed whenever amyloidosis is suspected.[23] The next stage in the evaluation is determining the involvement of heart by amyloid deposition and then defining the exact type of amyloid so that specific treatment can be initiated and prognosis can be determined. The treatment options are dictated by the type of amyloid, extent of organ involvement, and the individual mutation, and it should be formulated within a specialist unit with the appropriate expertise.

Diagnosis

Cardiac amyloidosis must be suspected when systemic features are present and patient has symptoms of congestive heart failure, such as dyspnea, paroxysmal nocturnal dyspnea, ankle swelling, abdominal distension, or other symptoms, such as syncope or angina. There may be family history of heart failure, conduction disease, pacemaker implantation, or neuropathy. On clinical examination the classic stigmata (panda eyes, macroglossia, and skin features) should be sought, but are often absent. Cardiovascular examination reveals raised JVP, edema, ascites, hepatomegaly, low blood pressure, postural hypotension, atrial fibrillation, or cardiac cachexia. Despite the stiff ventricle, a fourth heart sound is rarely present, due to atrial dysfunction. A formal diagnosis of amyloid requires a biopsy specimen, which stains with Congo red dye to produce an apple-green birefringence when viewed under polarized light. A screening biopsy should be taken from an easily accessible, safe, and likely site of involvement. In clinical practice, this is frequently done by an abdominal fat aspiration (capillaries in the subcutaneous fat are often involved) but can also be done from kidney, heart, peripheral nerve, salivary gland, stomach, liver, or bone marrow.

The diagnosis of cardiac amyloidosis is established directly by EMB or indirectly by echocardiographic evidence of amyloidosis and histologic confirmation of amyloid on noncardiac tissue. Several other investigations, including a 12-lead ECG and cardiac biomarkers, further corroborate cardiac involvement, but are not specific when interpreted in isolation.[23]

Electrocardiography: The characteristic ECG patterns diagnostic of cardiac amyloidosis are:

- *Low-voltage complexes:* The low-voltage complexes in precordial and limb leads are primarily due to the destruction and replacement of myocytes by the electrically inert amyloid. This ECG pattern is exhibited by approximately 70% of AL-associated cardiac amyloidosis, and only one third of patients with hereditary amyloidosis and senile systemic amyloidosis show low voltage
- *Pseudoinfarction pattern:* It is evidenced by QS waves in two consecutive leads and commonly seen in AL amyloid. It usually involves the precordial ECG leads (V1-V3), but can also occur in the inferior leads (II, III, and arteriovenous fistula)[24]
- *Large P waves* due to biatrial enlargement
- *Conduction abnormalities:* IV conduction delays or blocks, such as incomplete right bundle branch block or left anterior fascicular block, may be present
- *Arrhythmia and long QTc:* Usually the rhythm is sinus rhythm but atrial fibrillation usually occurs in the advanced stages and may be responsible for rapid clinical deterioration
- *Fragmented QRS complexes*

- *Reduced heart rate variability* on a 24-hour Holter predicts high short-term mortality
- *Late after potentials* on signal averaged ECG.

Echocardiography: The characteristic echocardiographic features suggestive of amyloid infiltration of the heart consist of:

- *Dilated atria,* which are immobile and often described to have owl's eye appearance.
- *Normal sized ventricles or small ventricles.*
- *Increased thickness of the ventricular wall, mitral and tricuspid leaflets, and interatrial septum.* The thickening of the ventricular walls is due to amyloid infiltration and not due to myocyte hypertrophy. A distinctive characteristic inverse relationship between ECG voltage and LV mass with a low voltage on the ECG and increased septal and posterior LV wall thickness on the echocardiogram are highly specific for cardiac amyloidosis. Low voltage on ECG and interventricular septal (Sep) thickness of more than 19.8 mm on echocardiography together have a sensitivity of 72% and specificity of 91% for cardiac amyloidosis.[25]
- *"Granular" or "sparkling" (ground-glass) appearance of the myocardium.*
- *Left ventricular function* may be normal in early stages but it is usually reduced in advanced stages.
- *Small pericardial effusion* is often present.
- *Mild valvular regurgitation* is quite common, but severe regurgitation is rare.
- *Diastolic dysfunction* is the hallmark and is present in all patients. *Restrictive filling pattern* is evident on the transmitral pulsed wave Doppler interrogation. The transmitral velocities exhibit high early diastolic (E-wave) and low late diastolic (A-wave) filling wave and short deceleration time suggestive of elevated filling pressures. In clinical practice, it is important to remember that in some patients with RCM, treatment with diuretics may normalize the filling pattern. In this situation, restrictive filling pattern can be unmasked after a fluid challenge.
- *Tissue velocity imaging* has shown reduced diastolic and systolic velocities in both early and late cardiac amyloid, so even early diastolic dysfunction could be identified (when wall thickening is minimal). The segmental evaluation of various segments of LV and RV in apical views can be done with color tissue Doppler imaging. It reveals significantly reduced segmental myocardial tissue velocities of LV and RV, and it provides information on subclinical ventricular dysfunction before any changes in ejection fraction occur. It also helps in distinguishing amyloid and other RCMA from constrictive pericarditis, with a mitral annular diastolic velocity E less than or equal to 8 cm/s, a good discriminator for restrictive physiology (Fig. 4).[26]
- High E/e′ ratio suggestive of elevated LV filling pressure.
- *Two-dimensional speckle-tracking echocardiography: strain and strain rate imaging.*

Strain rate imaging reveals markedly reduced global strain—both longitudinal and radial strains of LV—in the disease state.[27] The clinical use of such finding in the diagnosis of cardiac amyloidosis is difficult due to overlap of diseases that are also associated with reduced global strain.

Phelan et al.[28] reported characteristic regional patterns in longitudinal strain (LS) using 2D speckle-tracking echocardiography with regional variations in LS from base to apex with relative apical sparing. A relative *apical sparing* pattern of LS is an easily recognizable, accurate, and reproducible method of differentiating cardiac amyloidosis from other causes of LVH. This characteristic regional pattern of LS can be easily identified on strain polar maps or "Bull's eye" plots. It typically displays marked decrease in LS in the basal- and midwall segments with relative apical sparring of LS. This characteristic pattern of apical sparing is typically called *cherry on the top* by some authors. This is in contradistinction to HCM, where there is preferential decrease in longitudinal strain at the site of greatest hypertrophy. This pattern was integrated into a relative apical LS formula as relative apical LS = average apical LS/(average of basal + mid LS).

A score of >1 was associated with an impressive 93% sensitivity and 82% specificity for the diagnosis of cardiac amyloidosis. However, patients with known coronary artery disease were excluded from this study (Fig. 5).

Today strain imaging has become a standard of care in patients with RCM or other features suggestive of cardiac amyloidosis in many echocardiography laboratories. Furthermore, new data have shown promising role of RV strain in the diagnosis of AL cardiac amyloidosis. But it is worth noting that strain rate imaging cannot differentiate between different types of cardiac amyloidosis.[29]

However, the characteristic echocardiographic features of amyloid infiltration of the heart are present in the advanced stages of the disease, but early cardiac infiltration may produce a mixed and confusing picture. This makes the diagnosis of cardiac amyloid challenging in early stages. There are many echocardiographic features commonly seen in amyloid, though none are highly specific individually, and a combination of several is helpful in achieving a diagnosis. LV wall thickness more than or equal to 15 mm, restrictive filling on Doppler echocardiography with an early mitral inflow Edt less than 150 ms, and reduced LV ejection fraction have been associated with poor prognosis.[30,31]

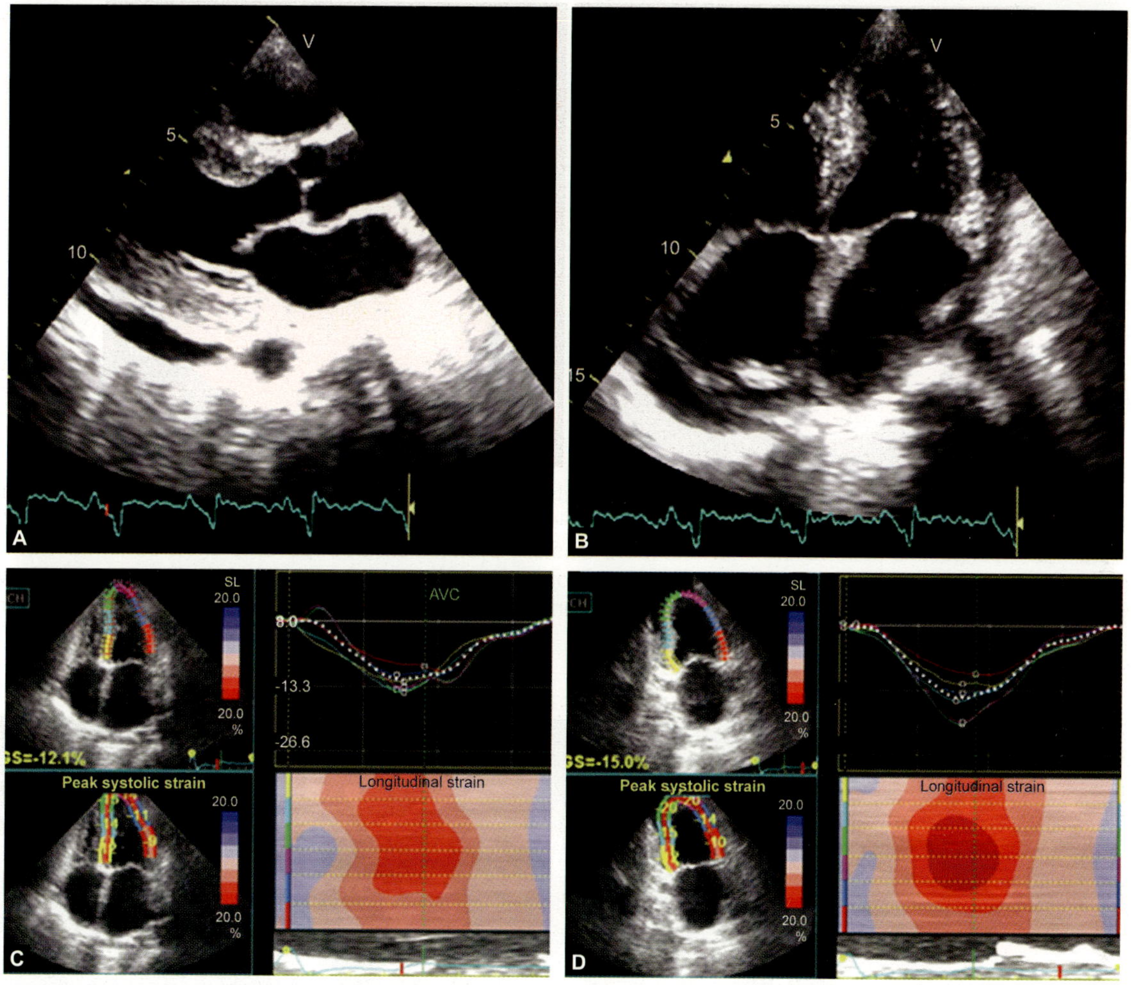

Figs. 4A to D: Echocardiographic features of cardiac amyloidosis. (A) Parasternal long-axis view shows thickened interventricular septum and posterior wall with sparkling appearance of myocardium, dilated LA, and small posterior pericardial effusion; (B) Apical four-chamber view shows normal size LV and RV, dilated atria, thickened and sparkling interventricular septum. This patient had atrial fibrillation on ECG and E/e′ ratio was 20 and had significantly reduced segmental myocardial tissue velocities of LV and RV on tissue velocity imaging; (C) Strain rate imaging in apical four-chamber view shows reduced longitudinal peak systolic strain; (D) Strain rate imaging in apical two-chamber view also shows reduced longitudinal peak systolic strain of basal and midsegments. Typically note that the mid and basal segments have low strain rate as compared to the apical segments in the apical four-chamber and two-chamber views and also apical segments in two-chamber view show normal strain of 20%. This is the characteristic relative *apical sparing* pattern of longitudinal strain which is diagnostic of cardiac amyloidosis. (ECG: electrocardiogram; LA: left atrium; LV: left ventricular; RV: right ventricular)

Reduced global LS has been shown to be a strong predictor of reduced survival.

KEY POINT 3

Echocardiography is the noninvasive diagnostic test of choice in cardiac amyloidosis. The characteristic features include increased ventricular wall thickness, "granular sparkling" appearance of the myocardium, valvular thickening with regurgitation, interatrial septal thickening, normal or decreased LV cavity size, dilated atria, and small-to-moderate pericardial effusion. Tissue velocity imaging, myocardial strain, and strain rate imaging are more sensitive.

KEY POINT 4

An ECG finding of low voltage in a patient with preserved LV ejection fraction and increased LV wall thickness by echocardiography should raise the clinical suspicion for cardiac.

KEY POINT 5

Strain echocardiography aids in early identification of the regional impairment in systolic function. A relative *apical sparing* pattern of LS is an easily recognizable, accurate, and reproducible method of differentiating cardiac amyloidosis from other causes of LV hypertrophy.

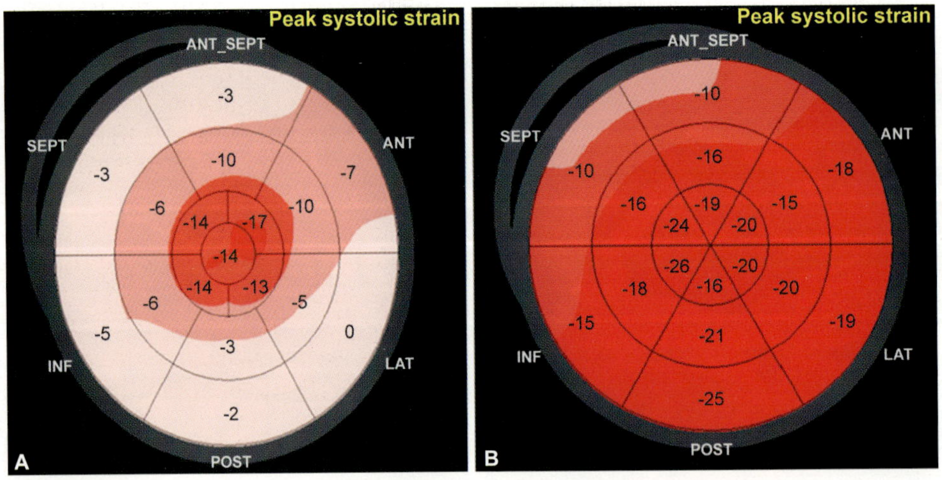

Figs. 5A and B: Bull's eye plot depicting LS pattern in patients with cardiac amyloidosis and hypertrophic cardiomyopathy. Global LS pattern on Bull's eye plot: Global LS with Bull's eye plot in two patients with increased LV wall thickness, LV ejection fraction of 55% and congestive heart failure with restrictive diastolic dysfunction. Both patients show abnormal LS. However, (A) shows apical sparing pattern typically called *cherry on the top* which is very characteristic of cardiac amyloidosis, while the (B) shows decreased strain in the basal inferior septum and anterior septum that is suggestive of hypertrophic cardiomyopathy.[29] (LS: longitudinal strain; LV: left ventricular)

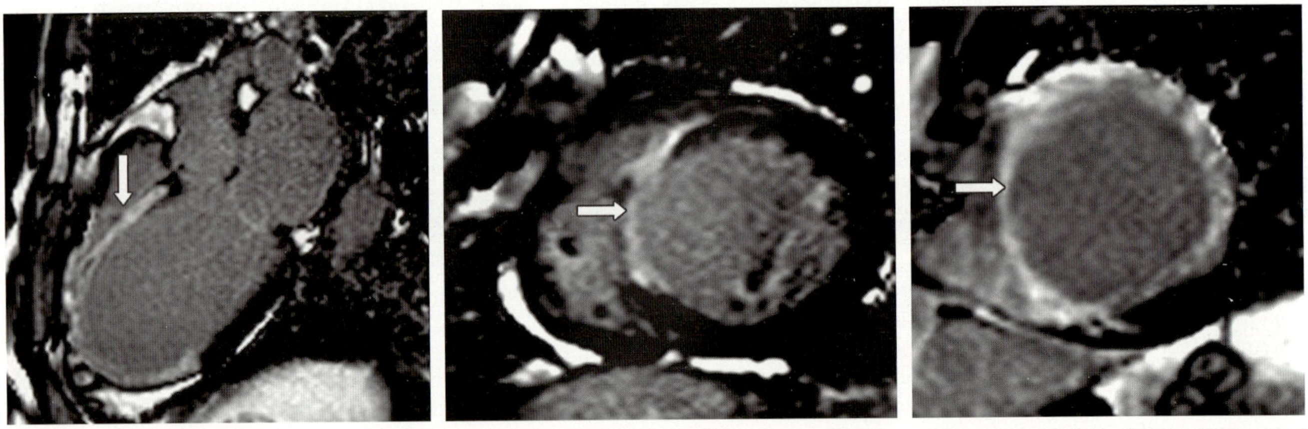

Fig. 6: CMR features of cardiac amyloidosis. CMR with late gadolinium enhancement images depicting diffuse transmural enhancement of LV (as indicated by arrows), a diagnostic feature of cardiac amyloidosis. (CMR: cardiac magnetic resonance; LV: left ventricle)

Cardiac magnetic resonance imaging: Cardiac magnetic resonance imaging provides incremental information in the identification or exclusion of various causes of RCM. Delayed post-gadolinium enhancement images reveal the characteristic diffuse subendocardial enhancement with diffuse LV subendocardial or transmural LGE, which may also involve the right ventricle and atrial walls and aid in the diagnostic confirmation of cardiac amyloidosis. This characteristic pattern of global transmural or diffuse subendocardial LGE can detect the disease early when significant increase in LV wall thickness is not present, and it correlates with disease severity (Fig. 6).[32]

Late gadolinium enhancement enables identification of myocardial fibrosis, scar, necrosis, or infiltration. In this disease, LGE CMR typically shows diffuse transmural enhancement of LV. The degree of enhancement depends on the ventricular mass and global ventricular systolic function. RV enhancement is seen in transthyretin-related amyloidosis (ATTR) and less commonly in AL amyloidosis. Austin et al.[33,34] showed that LGE CMR had a sensitivity of 88%, specificity 95%, positive predictive value of 93%, and negative predictive value of 90% in patients with biopsy proven amyloidosis. Recent data have shown promising role for equilibrium contrast CMR for the quantification of extracellular volume fraction as a more robust method that correlates with amyloid burden, and hence quantify it objectively. T1 and T2 kinetics seem to provide more robust prognostic data. Left atrial LGE is a useful evidence of cardiac amyloidosis and predicts atrial fibrillation.

KEY POINT 6

In cardiac amyloidosis, there is interstitial expansion from the amyloid deposit that avidly picks up and retains gadolinium, resulting in signal enhancement of the tissue and fast blood-pool washout. In addition, patients have abnormal myocardial and blood-pool gadolinium kinetics. Together, these findings have 97% accuracy for diagnosing cardiac amyloidosis.[34]

However, there are few limitations to LGE CMR:

- Patchy myocardial involvement is also seen in some cases and can be easily missed
- Underestimation of the degree of disease burden as compared to technetium-99m (^{99m}Tc) diphosphonate nuclear imaging due to diffuse nature of LGE on conventional CMR. This can happen because normal reference myocardium—used to provide context for setting pulse sequence parameters and for visual interpretation—may be absent[29]
- Does not differentiate AL amyloidosis from ATTR. However, one characteristic feature is that ATTR subtype almost always has LGE of the right ventricle, while almost one third of patients with AL do not.[35]

KEY POINT 7

CMR aids in the diagnostic confirmation of cardiac amyloidosis. Delayed postgadolinium enhancement images reveal the characteristic diffuse subendocardial enhancement and atrial and valvular uptake as well. This characteristic pattern of global transmural or diffuse subendocardial LGE can detect the disease early.

Radionuclide imaging: Serum amyloid P component has been used to assess amyloidosis for the last few decades. All amyloid deposits contain serum amyloid P component and, therefore, radioiodination allows visualization of the distribution of deposits. Unfortunately, this technique cannot be used for imaging of the myocardium because of the distribution properties of the radionuclide and the kinetics of cardiac function.[36] ^{99m}Tc-phosphate derivatives—^{99m}Tc—3,3-diphosphono-1,2-propanodicarboxylic acid and ^{99m}Tc-pyrophosphate—selectively bind ATTR,[37] but not AL subtype. Positive scans on scintigraphic imaging of cardiac amyloid can, therefore, be used to identify wild-type and mutant ATTR. By contrast, cardiac localization of amyloid deposits occurs in only a small proportion of patients with AL amyloidosis, and usually to a lesser degree than in patients with ATTR. Consequently, negative scans are predictive of AL amyloidosis.[38] This technique is cheap and widely available and can be used as best noninvasive tool to distinguish transthyretin-related cardiac amyloidosis from other forms (Fig. 7).[39]

Cardiac catheterization and endomyocardial biopsy: Although EMB with staining techniques is the gold standard for diagnosis, it is suggested in selected patients with RCM if other workup is inconclusive. It has limitations because of the issues of uneven distribution. Definitive diagnosis is established by the mere demonstration of apple-green birefringence with Congo red under polarized light microscopy. It can help identify or exclude specific conditions, such as amyloidosis, sarcoidosis, and hemochromatosis. Cardiac catheterization with hemodynamic pressure recording reveals the characteristic pattern with elevated LVEDP and "dip and plateau" or "square root" pattern of diastolic pressure tracings, similar to those in constrictive pericarditis. A screening biopsy from

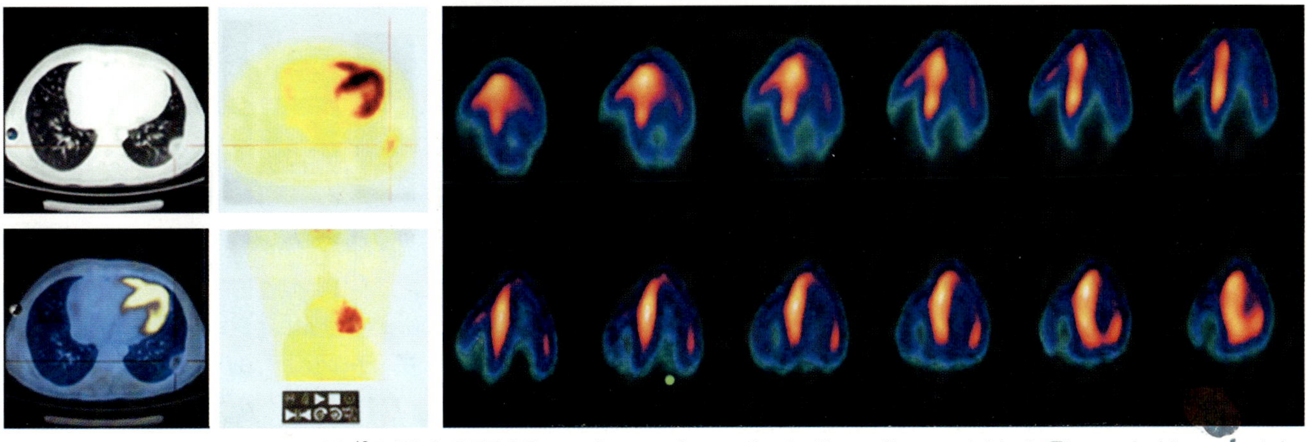

Fig. 7: *Radionuclide imaging with ^{18}F-FDG:* PET-CT scan images in a patient with cardiac amyloidosis. It revealed tracer uptake in thickened LV and RV myocardium. Patchy low-grade uptake is seen in thickened wall of dilated RA. (FDG: fluorodeoxyglucose; LV: left ventricular; RA: right atrial; RV: right ventricular)

an easily accessible, safe, and likely site of involvement, such as abdominal fat aspiration (capillaries in the subcutaneous fat are often involved) or bone marrow aspiration, is routinely used in clinical practice for diagnosis (Fig. 8).

Treatment

Early unequivocal diagnosis and prompt therapy are warranted to arrest or reverse AL-related cardiac dysfunction. In the late stages, poor cardiac reserve severely limits the management options. In general, the goal of therapy is twofold: (1) light-chain suppression for AL amyloidosis and (2) supportive care. The concept of eliminating clonogenic light chain-producing plasma cells in AL amyloidosis has gained acceptance over the years. It improves patients' performance status, and quality of life. Corticosteroids, alkylators, immunomodulating agents, and proteasome inhibitors are active agents. The median time taken to respond to an alkylator-based regimen, melphalan-prednisone, is approximately 1 year, and only one third respond. The cardiotoxicity of doxorubicin and neuropathy of vincristine limit their use. Dexamethasone-related fluid retention can potentially exacerbate heart failure.[40]

The primary goal of treatment in cardiac amyloidosis remains relief of symptoms. Diuretic therapy relieves congestion, but needs to be monitored closely due to the risk of hypotension and renal failure. Digoxin and calcium channel blockers are contraindicated due to the high risk of heart block.[41,42] Beta-blockers and angiotensin-converting enzyme inhibitors are poorly tolerated. Chemotherapy and stem cell transplantation for AL amyloid may prolong survival and increase quality of life if started early. Stem cell transplantation has shown some promise for the treatment of primary amyloidosis. However, compared with other hematologic malignancies, the early postprocedural mortality is significantly higher in patients with amyloidosis.[43,44] Bortezomib-based regimens have shown near complete remission of plasma cell dyscrasias and are now considered to be the preferred treatment option.[45] Clinical trials of several drugs that seek to reduce amyloid protein production in transthyretin monomer

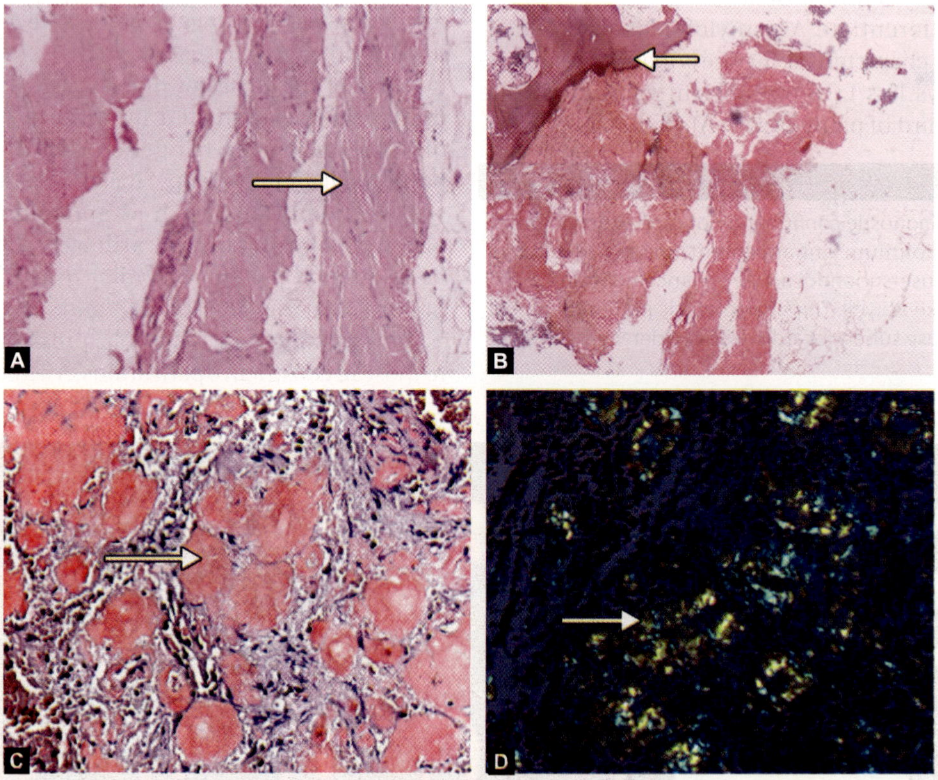

Figs. 8A to D: Tissue diagnosis in amyloidosis—histopathology in cardiac amyloidosis. (A) Fat pad biopsy (H and E stain) shows adipose tissue with vessels showing thickening of wall by pink waxy material—amyloid deposit; (B) Bone marrow biopsy with Congo red stain shows deposits of congophilic material—amyloid in the vessel walls; (C) Endomyocardial biopsy shows typical amorphous extracellular Congo red-stained positive deposits; (D) Congo red-stained endomyocardial biopsy examined under polarized light shows characteristic apple-green birefringence confirming the amyloid nature of deposits. (H&E: hematoxylin and eosin)

(m-TTR) are currently in progress.[46] Recent data support the benefit of implantable cardioverter-defibrillators for primary prevention of sudden cardiac death.[47] Cardiac transplantation may be effective in patients with m-TTR amyloid if there is limited hepatic and nerve involvement. Liver and combined liver-cardiac transplantation may improve survival in these patients when there is significant liver involvement.

Endomyocardial Fibrosis

Endomyocardial fibrosis is endemic in tropical and subtropical Africa, Asia, and South America, but occasional cases are reported outside the tropics.[48] It is typically characterized by endocardial involvement with the deposition of fibrous tissue in the endomyocardium, endocardial calcification of LV or RV, or both, leading to restrictive physiology and endemicity in certain geographical pockets and propensity to affect the poor. A few decades ago, it used to be the most common form of RCM observed in India. The disease used to occur in its classical endemic form in the selected coastal belt in Kerala, affecting young people of lower socioeconomic families. Several environmental/toxic factors, such as magnesium deficiency, cerium toxicity, the cyanogenic glycosides, high vitamin D, serotonin toxicity, and, more recently, the potential effect of certain herbal preparations, have been advocated in the pathogenesis. Malnutrition may also contribute to the pathogenesis of EMF by increasing susceptibility to parasitic infections. The disease has gradually disappeared from Kerala with improving socioeconomic and health status, and this finding adds credence to the nutritional and inflammatory components postulated in its genesis. Sivasankaran[3] reported decline in the incidence of EMF in Kerala to 10 new cases a year in the past decade from 20 cases seen in the previous decade. Moreover, a relatively stable symptomatic course on follow-up with mortality of around 10% at 3 years was reported. EMF can be defined as an obliterative cardiomyopathy characterized by fibrotic thickening and obliteration of either of the ventricles or both with selective involvement of the ventricular apices and inflow region sparing the outflow tract.[49] Various stages of EMF have been described which are as follows:

- Stage of endocardial inflammation
- Stage of necrosis
- Stage of thrombosis
- Stage of fibrosis.

The fibrotic process does not affect the valve leaflets, the atria, or the great vessels, and extracardiac involvement is not known. Clinical recognition of EMF depends on the degree of ventricular involvement. The biventricular nature of the disease is seen in more than 50% patients with the remainder having isolated RV or LV involvement. Most patients are diagnosed in the burnt-out stage of the disease. When either LV or RV is affected in isolation, long-term follow-up usually does not show further extension of the disease process to the other.[50] The papillary muscles may be fibrosed and affect the function of the AV valves by plastering the valve to the wall, resulting in AV valve regurgitation. Dilated atria may cause atrial fibrillation with consequent thromboembolic complications, which may be the initial presentation. The exact etiopathogenesis of EMF is not clearly understood. The peculiar geographical distribution suggests malnutrition and infections as the cause.

Clinical Presentation

It may vary from asymptomatic incidental detection to cardiac cachexia, resulting from end-stage disease with refractory heart failure. EMF usually starts with a febrile illness associated with pancarditis and eosinophilia, dyspnea, itching, and periorbital swelling. The fibrosis and apical obliteration results in reduced ventricular compliance and diastolic dysfunction. The restrictive physiology leads to aneurismal dilatation of the atria and pulmonary venous congestion together with pulmonary hypertension when the left ventricle is affected and systemic venous congestion when the right ventricle is involved. The triad of elevated JVP, ascites, and hepatomegaly formed the hallmark of RV EMF, which can present with cyanosis and clubbing because of stretch opening of foramen ovale.[51] Ascites is usually disproportionate to the pedal edema and may be inflammatory. Mild cardiomegaly, loud LV S3, short systolic murmur, and severe pulmonary hypertension formed the hallmark for the diagnosis of LV EMF.[52]

Evaluation of Patients with Endomyocardial Fibrosis

Electrocardiogram: Electrocardiogram shows low voltages, some features of ventricular hypertrophy with IV conduction defects and nonspecific ST-T changes. RV EMF with severe RA dilatation is reflected in the ECG as qR pattern in V1.[53] Atrial fibrillation may be seen late in the course of disease.

Chest X-ray: Varying degree of cardiomegaly and at times typical endocardial calcification can be evident on chest X-ray.

Echocardiography: Echocardiographic features of EMF include:

- Ventricular apex is typically blunted or obliterated with endocardial thickening and calcification or thrombus may be present at the apex. A distinct highly echogenic line is seen covering the endocardial surface of the left and right ventricles. This echo-dense area lining the endocardium corresponds to the areas of fibrosis

extending from the apex to the bases of the ventricles and the papillary muscles
- Marked biatrial enlargement
- Pericardial effusion is often present
- Ventricular systolic function (including the apex) is usually spared, but in the late stages, there may be severe systolic dysfunction
- Restriction of mobility of mitral and tricuspid valve due to plastering of leaflets with inadequate coaptation and resultant regurgitation, which is often moderate or severe
- Restriction to ventricular filling is manifested by an early diastolic halt on the M-mode echocardiogram
- A typical RV apical obliteration with apical dimpling
- Diastolic dysfunction as evidenced by restrictive filling pattern with E/A ratio > 1.5 and reduced Edt < 150 ms. E/e′ ratio > 15 suggestive of significantly elevated LV filling pressures with estimated LVEDP > 25 mm Hg
- Tissue velocity imaging reveals significantly reduced segmental tissue velocities of LV and RV
- Thrombi may be found in left atrium or right atrium or both or the left atrial appendage or the RA appendage.

Treatment and Prognosis

Typically, the disease has an insidious onset, with the development of increasing severe right- or left-sided heart failure. Most patients are treated symptomatically with supportive care with diuretics, and rate control measures with or without anticoagulant agents. Massive ascites is relieved by intermittent tapping. In addition to medical management of heart failure, early open heart surgery (endocardectomy and valve repair/replacement) appears to improve outcomes to some extent; however, surgery is technically challenging. About one third of the most symptomatic patients benefit from surgery, which carries 30% mortality.[54] Patients with end-stage cardiac failure can be offered cardiac transplantation.[3] The overall prognosis of patients with EMF is poor and depends on the degree and location of involvement in the heart (Fig. 9).

Cardiac magnetic resonance imaging: Cardiac magnetic resonance imaging often provides additional diagnostic information due to its ability to detect subendocardial fibrosis and its greater sensitivity for ventricular thrombus detection. It gives additional functional information and tissue characterization. Apical obliteration seen by echocardiography may be due to thrombosis, fibrosis, tumor, calcification, or myohypertrophy. Patterns of fibrosis, myohypertrophy, and thrombosis can be differentiated by tissue characterization and delayed enhancement on contrast studies using gadolinium. CMR, therefore, could offer an excellent opportunity to identify the disease in the early stages (Fig. 10).[3]

KEY POINT 8

Endomyocardial fibrosis has peculiar characteristics with specific endocardial involvement with typical endocardial fibrosis and calcification of one or both the ventricles, localization to certain geographical pockets, and propensity to affect the poor. It has gradually disappeared from Kerala with improving socioeconomic and health status. Treatment includes management of heart failure and oral anticoagulants in patients with atrial fibrillation. Surgery with endocardectomy and valve repair/replacement which improves outcomes to some extent and can be done in some patients; however, surgery is technically challenging.

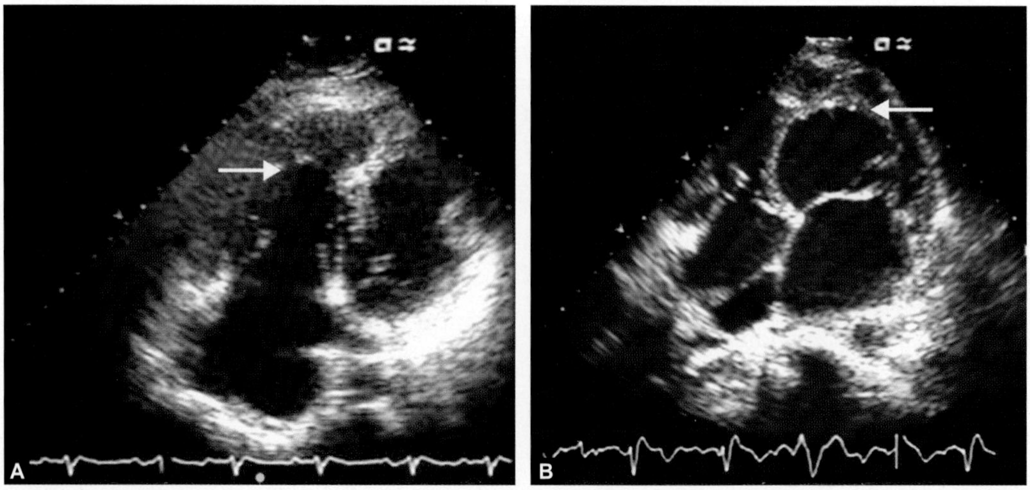

Figs. 9A and B: Echocardiographic features in EMF. (A) Apical four-chamber view in a patient with RV EMF. RA is dilated, and RV apex shows echogenicity with blunting suggestive of apical obliteration and endocardial calcium as shown by arrow; (B) Apical four-chamber view in a patient with LV EMF. RA and LA are dilated, and LV apex shows echogenicity with blunting suggestive of apical obliteration and endocardial calcium as shown by arrow. (EMF: endomyocardial fibrosis; LA: left atrium; LV: left ventricular; RA: right atrial; RV: right ventricular)

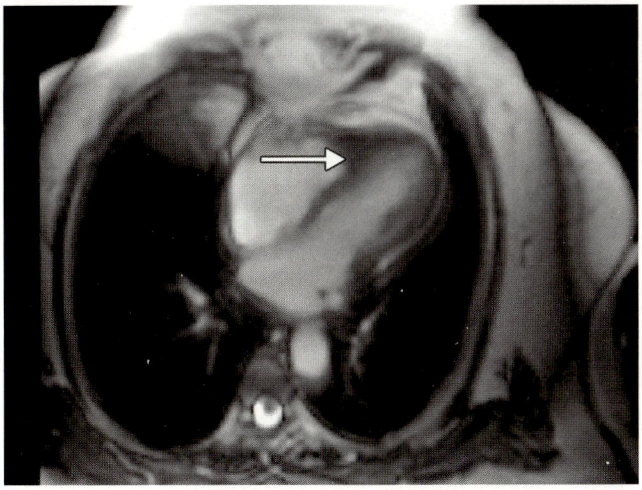

Fig. 10: Cardiac MRI cine image in patient with RV EMF shows dilated RA and RV apical obliteration with a large thrombus (arrow) attached to the fibrotic endocardium. (EMF: endomyocardial fibrosis; MRI: magnetic resonance imaging; RA: right atrial; RV: right ventricular)

Löffler's Endocarditis (Eosinophilic Cardiomyopathy)

Loffler's endocarditis is a relatively rare condition that was first described in 1936 by Wilhelm Löffler. He referred to it as "fibroplastic parietal endocarditis with blood eosinophilia."[55] It is a manifestation of hypereosinophilia, and morphologic abnormalities of eosinophils have been noted in patients with Löffler's endocarditis. It is thought that the intracytoplasmic granular content of activated eosinophils is responsible for the toxic damage to the heart.[56] Hypereosinophilic syndrome (HES) is a rare disorder that is characterized by persistent and marked eosinophilia combined with organ system dysfunction. HES can be fatal without treatment, especially in patients who present with a myelodysplastic variant of the disorder. Chusid et al.[57] established empirical diagnostic criteria for idiopathic HES that are used still today.

- Blood eosinophilia exceeding 1,500/mm^3 for more than 6 consecutive months with signs and symptoms of hypereosinophilic disease
- Absence of an underlying cause of hypereosinophilia despite extensive diagnostic evaluation
- Organ damage or dysfunction as a result of local release of toxic contents of eosinophils.

Mild eosinophilia is defined by a level of 500–1,500 eosinophils/mm^3. A count of 1,500–5,000 eosinophils/mm^3 is considered moderate, and more than 5,000 eosinophils/mm^3 is a significant eosinophilia.[58] The most characteristic cardiac abnormality in HES is EMF. About 50–60% of patients with HES show cardiovascular manifestations.[59] The cardiac involvement in HES follows three stages:[60]

1. *Acute necrotic stage:* Eosinophilic infiltration of the myocardium associated with myocardial necrosis due to the release of toxic cationic proteins from degranulating eosinophils
2. *Intermediate phase:* Mural thrombi and thrombus formation along the damaged endocardium (thrombotic stage). This is followed by the organization of the thrombus into a thick layer of granulation tissue, which replaces the normal endocardium
3. *Fibrotic stage:* The granulation tissue is changed into hyaline fibrosis.

As mural fibrosis develops, the LV compliance decreases, resulting in an RCM. Fibrosis affecting the papillary muscle and chordae tendinae may produce papillary dysfunction and MR. As a consequence, in such patients, symptoms and signs of heart failure can be present. The structural changes of the myocardium can provoke arrhythmias. Embolic events originating from the intracardiac thrombus are seen in up to 25%.[61]

Clinical Manifestations

The patients with Löffler's endocarditis present with the symptoms of heart failure, intracardiac thrombus, myocardial ischemia or arrhythmias, and rarely pericarditis. The presenting symptoms may be dyspnea, paroxysmal nocturnal dyspnea, cough, chest pain, palpitations or thromboembolic phenomenon, such as syncope.

Diagnostic Evaluation

Electrocardiogram: Most frequent ECG finding is T-wave inversions, and these represent subendocardial injury due to endocardial fibrosis. Premature ventricular beats or LVH pattern may be present.

Echocardiography: The characteristic echocardiographic features of Löffler's endocarditis include (Fig. 11):

- Endomyocardial thickening with apical obliteration due to thrombus formation, especially in the absence of any regional wall motion abnormality. Rarely focal involvement of other segments of LV can be seen
- Posterior mitral leaflet involvement with tethering of the leaflet and MR
- Doppler echocardiography can show diastolic dysfunction, often a restrictive LV filling pattern
- Pericardial effusion may be present
- Preserved LV systolic function (including the apex)
- Right ventricular thrombus may be present, and tricuspid valve may be involved with restricted mobility and resultant TR.

Cardiac magnetic resonance imaging: Cardiac magnetic resonance is highly sensitive and specific for detecting apical thrombi. Delayed enhancement gadolinium

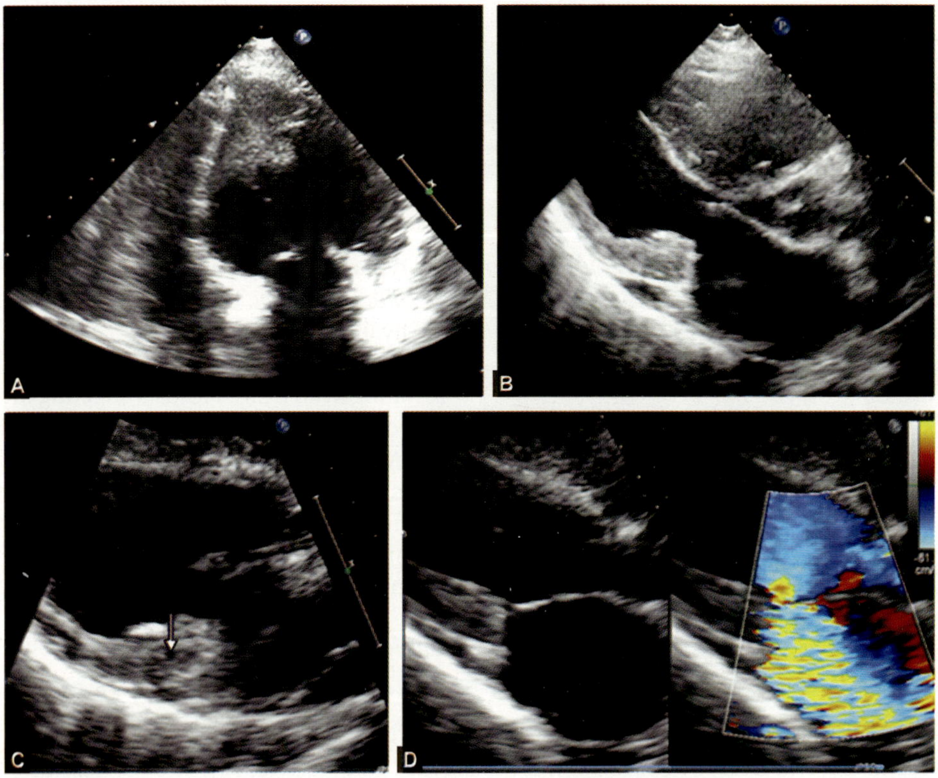

Figs. 11A to D: Echocardiographic features in patients with Löffler's endocarditis. (A) Apical four-chamber view shows LV apical obliteration with echogenic mass with central echolucency and a projection from the mass in LV cavity. LV apex had normal contractility; (B) Parasternal long-axis view shows focal thickening and hyperechogenicity of basal posterior wall in a patient with congestive heart failure and hypereosinophilia. This focal area of increased echo density denotes thrombus and/or fibrosis; (C) Zoomed view of part (B) showing the echogenic layering (arrow) over the basal posterior wall indicating fibrosis and thrombus formation; (D) Color Doppler interrogation showing severe mitral regurgitation. (LV: left ventricular)

imaging is capable of detecting myocardial fibrosis and inflammation. Overlying thrombus is identifiable as a low signal mass on the delayed enhancement images, which does not deform on tagged images. A characteristic three-layered image can be seen: a hypointense inner rim of thrombus adjacent to a hyperenhancement of the endocardium compared with the rest of the myocardium. Despite the convincing diagnostic information available from the noninvasive imaging modalities, EMB remains the diagnostic gold standard.[62]

The differential diagnosis of Löffler's endocarditis includes (Fig. 12):

- Apical HCM (typical ECG pattern of apical HCM with LVH pattern with giant T-wave inversions may help differentiation). CMR imaging is very useful in differentiating the Löffler's endocarditis from apical HCM. The use of transpulmonary contrast is also a good option for differentiating the two conditions
- Apical infarct with thrombus (ECG pattern of anterior wall myocardial infarction and wall motion abnormality on echocardiography may help differentiation)
- Noncompaction of the myocardium (color Doppler interrogation at the apex with decrease in the Nyquist limits will demonstrate the color flow in the crevices in noncompaction or use of contrast echocardiography will help).[63]

Treatment

Early treatment can limit irreversible damage; hence, echocardiography should be systematically performed in the cases of eosinophilia, especially if it is prolonged. In the absence of etiology, first-line treatment should include antihelminthic therapy, corticosteroid therapy, and anticoagulant therapy. The goal of this therapeutics is to rapidly lower the eosinophil count and prevent thromboembolic events. Conventional therapy with treatment of heart failure with diuretics and rate-controlling measures—beta-adrenergic blockers, angiotensin-converting enzyme inhibitors, angiotensin II receptor blockers—should be initiated in patients presenting with heart failure. Thromboembolism is seen in about 25% cases with Löffler's endocardial disease. Recurrence may

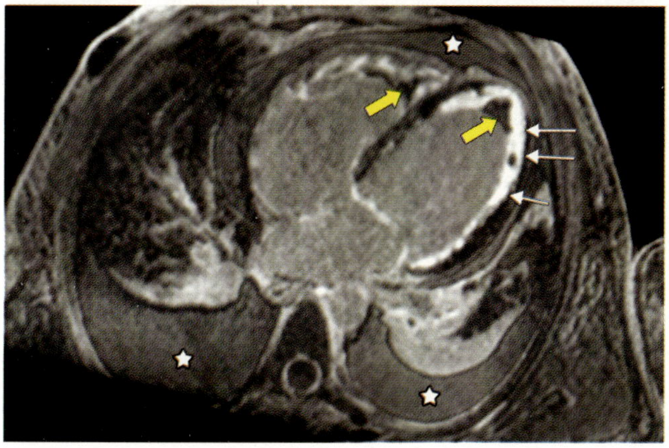

Fig. 12: CMR features in Löffler's endocardial disease. CMR high-resolution delayed-enhancement four-chamber view showing "three-layered" appearance of the ventricular walls: the middle layer (thin white arrows) shows hyperenhancement secondary to fibrosis; the innermost layer consists of nonenhancing endocardial thrombus (thick yellow arrows) and mainly affects apices; pericardial and bilateral pleural effusions are also well depicted (stars)(CMR: cardiac magnetic resonance).[63]

occur despite therapeutic international normalized ratio (INR). INR should be maintained around 3.0 and bridged with heparin for those with thrombus. Prophylactic anticoagulation is not recommended for patients without thrombus.[64]

As second-line treatment, specific treatment of eosinophilia must be conducted depending on the cause. Steroids remain the mainstay of treatment for the most patients with Löffler's endocarditis. Cytotoxic drugs, such as hydroxyurea, have shown good results. Immunomodulatory drugs, interferon alpha, intravenous immunoglobulin, cytoxan, cyclosporine, and methotrexate, are used in refractory cases. Treatment with tyrosine kinase inhibitors—imatinib—is indicated for patients with proven myeloproliferative HES.[65] Novel monoclonal antibody therapies, especially anti-interleukin-5 antibodies targeting eosinophils, show promise for the treatment of Löffler's disease. Bone marrow transplantation may be required in imatinib-resistant cases. Finally, surgery may be necessary at the fibrotic stage of the disease with decortication for apical obliteration and/or chordal entrapment with valve replacement (bioprosthesis) in patients with significant regurgitant lesions.[66] Cardiac transplantation may be considered for the most severe cases.

KEY POINT 9

Endomyocardial fibrosis and Löffler's endocarditis are thought to be different manifestations of restrictive obliterative cardiomyopathy, both associated with eosinophilia. Löffler's endocardial disease is characterized by hypereosinophilia and endocardial fibrosis and thrombus formation. The management of this disease includes normalization of the peripheral eosinophil count, and treating the underlying disorder causing hypereosinophilia, initiating anticoagulant therapy in patients with or at risk for thrombotic complications, and considering heart transplantation for patients with progressive cardiac disease despite conventional management.

Sarcoidosis

It is a systemic inflammatory disorder characterized by noncaseating granulomas in lungs, spleen, lymph nodes, skin, liver, parotid glands, and heart. It can affect patients of all ages but most commonly develops before the age of 50 years. The precise etiology is unknown. Sarcoidosis often is clinically suspected when abnormalities are detected on a chest X-ray during routine screening. Patient may present with nonspecific symptoms, such as fatigue, night sweats, and weight loss. The organ system that is most affected varies with the given patient. Cardiac granulomas are found in approximately 25% of autopsy patients but cardiac sarcoidosis is clinically apparent in only about 5% of all patients. Cardiac involvement is patchy with the most common locations of granulomas found in the LV free wall and basal ventricular septum, often involving the conducting system. Cardiac sarcoidosis is increasingly recognized and is associated with poor prognosis. Clinically, it is manifested as a cardiomyopathy, usually RCM, with the loss of muscle function or tachyarrhythmias, including heart block, syncope, and sudden death. Clinical presentation may range from asymptomatic conduction abnormalities to fatal ventricular arrhythmias, depending upon the location and extent of granulomatous inflammation. Complete heart block is the most common finding in patients with clinically evident cardiac sarcoidosis and is reported in 23–30% of patients.[67] First-degree heart block and bundle branch block also often occur, due to the involvement of the basal septum by scar tissue or granulomas or the involvement of the nodal artery causing ischemia in the conduction system. Sarcoid granulomas in the ventricular myocardium can become foci for abnormal automaticity, increasing the likelihood of reentrant tachyarrhythmias. Ventricular tachycardia (VT) is the most frequent arrhythmia noted in cardiac sarcoidosis with a reported incidence of 23%.[68] Other clinical manifestations include chest pain, electrocardiographic changes that may mimic transmural myocardial infarction, and pericardial abnormalities, such as pericardial effusion or constrictive pericarditis.

Diagnosis

Electrocardiogram: An ECG should be performed in every patient with sarcoidosis (systemic or cardiac) to detect subtle or overt conduction or repolarization abnormalities.

Many patients may have splintered QRS complexes, AV or IV conduction abnormalities. In patients with suspected or known cardiac sarcoidosis, 24-hour ECG monitoring should be performed to document and define subclinical rhythm disturbances that may be missed on ECGs and to aid risk estimation of sudden death.

Echocardiography: Characteristic echocardiographic findings are:

- Systolic function may be normal initially but it is usually severely impaired late in the course of the disease when it usually comes to clinical attention due to symptoms of heart failure
- Global hypokinesia of LV or regional wall motion abnormalities not consistent with vascular territory
- Focal thinning, hyperechogenicity or scarring of myocardium, usually basal septum is affected while apex is spared
- Pulmonary involvement is frequently noted with resultant pulmonary hypertension or right heart failure
- Left ventricular aneurysms
- Valvular regurgitation
- Septum or LV free wall may appear hyperechogenic
- Diastolic dysfunction of LV, usually grade III.

Cardiac magnetic resonance: Cardiac magnetic resonance imaging reveals dilated LV with diffuse hypokinesis with LV wall thinning and LV dysfunction. The very important CMR finding is patchy pattern of delayed enhancement. CMR imaging enables fast, accurate, high-resolution, and noninvasive diagnosis of subclinical or clinical cardiac sarcoidosis and is currently the technique of choice in the evaluation of sarcoidosis. Sensitivity has been shown to be much higher than with radionucleotide methods. CMR uses T2-weighted imaging and early gadolinium images to detect acute inflammation (edema). T1-weighted (cine) imaging illustrates wall motion abnormalities, hypertrophy due to possible infiltrative disease, wall thinning, or heart failure. LGE assesses fibrosis or scar and may represent chronic rather than active disease 9.[69] Typical patterns of enhancement on CMR are nonvascular in territory, midmyocardial, and subepicardial, although many patients have patterns in a coronary distribution with subendocardial involvement similar to myocardial infarction.

Positron emission tomography: ^{18}F-Fluorodeoxyglucose (FDG) positron emission tomography (PET) appears to detect active cardiac sarcoidosis with high sensitivity. FDG PET is more sensitive than gallium-67 scintigraphy, thallium-201, or ^{99m}Tc single-photon emission computed tomography (SPECT).[70] It can also be combined with myocardial perfusion imaging to detect fibrogranulomatous replacement. However, PET is nonspecific for sarcoidosis and uptake of ^{18}F-FDG is seen in other inflammatory myocardial diseases also. The actual specificity of FDG PET perfusion imaging is uncertain. Reported specificity has ranged from 38% to 90%; in which, the lower range may be due to detection of early subclinical disease (Fig. 13).

Treatment

Corticosteroids are the cornerstone in the treatment of cardiac sarcoidosis. Alternative agents, such as chloroquine, hydroxychloroquine, cyclosporine, and methotrexate, may be given to patients who do not respond to glucocorticoids or who cannot tolerate their side effects. Antiarrhythmic treatment and beta-blockers are also often needed in the management. Supportive therapy with diuretics and rate-

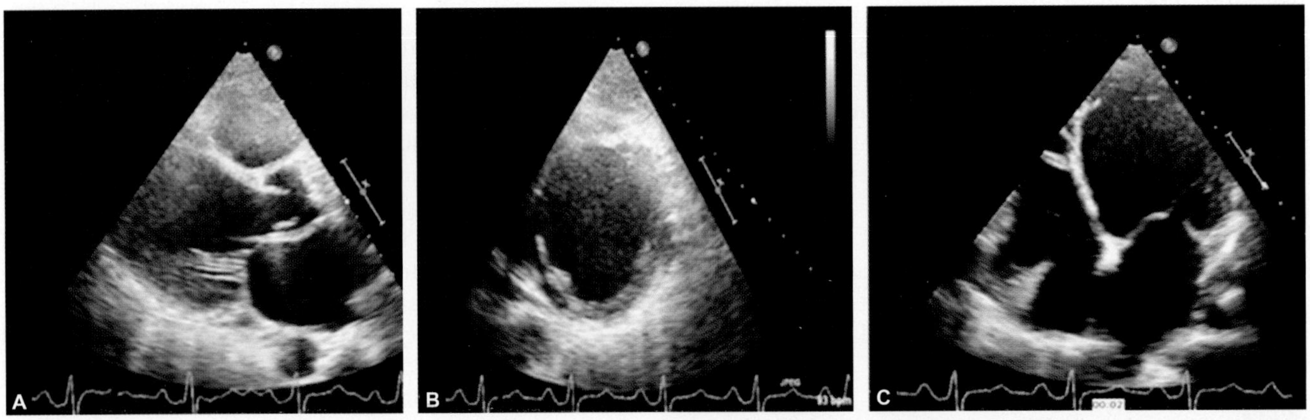

Figs. 13A to C: Characteristic echocardiographic features in cardiac sarcoidosis. (A) Parasternal long-axis view shows dilated LA and LV with hyperechoic and thinned-out basal anterior septum; (B) Parasternal short-axis view of LV at the level of papillary muscles shows dilated LV with thinning of inferior and anterior septum; (C) Apical four-chamber view shows dilated all four cardiac chambers with focal thinning and hyperechogenicity of basal and mid inferior septum. This focal thinning and hyperechogenicity is not consistent with any vascular territory and is diagnostic of cardiac sarcoidosis. (LA: left atrium; LV: left ventricular)

controlling drugs is initiated in patients with heart failure. Catheter radiofrequency ablation may be effective in eliminating or reducing VT in some patients with cardiac sarcoidosis not controlled by antiarrhythmic drug therapy. A permanent pacemaker is indicated when there is evidence of complete AV block or other high-grade conduction system disease is present. Intracardiac defibrillator (ICD) device therapy is recommended in patients with inducible VT at electrophysiologic study performed for symptoms (palpitations, syncope, presyncope) and/or nonsustained ventricular arrhythmias.[71] ICD therapy can be considered in patients with an established diagnosis of sarcoidosis who have extensive cardiac magnetic resonance LGE of the left ventricle or PET abnormalities, particularly in those requiring a permanent pacemaker.[72] Cardiac transplantation is considered in patients with refractory heart failure.

KEY POINT 10

Cardiac sarcoidosis is usually detected late in the stages of heart failure in daily clinical practice. The echocardiographic features typical of cardiac sarcoidosis are focal thinning and scarring of myocardium which is not consistent with vascular territory, and the diagnosis can be confirmed by CMR or nuclear imaging—PET scan.

Hemochromatosis

Hemochromatosis is a storage disorder that results from increased iron deposition in the sarcoplasmic reticulum of cells in various organs, such as liver, pancreas, heart, and gonads. It is a rare disorder characterized by cirrhosis, diabetes, changes in skin pigmentation, endocrine failure, heart failure, and arthropathy. Primary, or hereditary, hemochromatosis is a relatively common autosomal recessive disorder and results in increased intestinal absorption of iron.[73] Secondary hemochromatosis results from receiving multiple blood transfusions in conditions where there is ineffective erythropoiesis, such as thalassemia major, sideroblastic anemia, and myelodysplastic syndrome. Repeated transfusion leads to rapid iron loading and iron deposition in various organs known as "transfusional siderosis". Cardiomyopathy is more prominent in patients with transfusional iron overload than in those with hemochromatosis, probably because of rapid iron loading. Approximately 15% of patients with hemochromatosis present with cardiac symptoms.[74]

Early in the course of the disease, iron overload may cause diastolic dysfunction, including restrictive physiology.[75] The right ventricle may also be involved with normal size but increased thickness. Most patients with clinical heart failure, however, exhibit a DCM phenotype. When patients become symptomatic with breathlessness and edema, the left atrium may be enlarged. The key diagnosis here is the elevated pulmonary pressures, due to high filling pressures. It is therefore crucial to measure the tricuspid regurgitant velocity during echocardiographic evaluation in these patients. Rhythm disorders, such as supraventricular arrhythmias—as atrial fibrillation, may occur.[76]

Cardiac magnetic resonance has high accuracy in the diagnosis of myocardial iron overload. Myocardial iron deposition results in lower T2 times, with decreased myocardial signals on T2-weighted images. CMR is superior to serum ferritin levels for determination of the extent of cardiac involvement. Cardiac biopsy shows abnormal deposits of granular, yellow-gray material within the sarcoplasm of the myocytes under light microscopy, and Prussian blue stains positive for iron, which is diagnostic of iron overload.[77] Phlebotomy is the first-line treatment for primary hemochromatosis. In patients who are anemic, iron chelation therapy with either deferoxamine, deferasirox, or deferiprone is the treatment of choice. Cardiac transplantation is an option in patients who have advanced HF refractory to medical therapy.

Radiation-induced Cardiomyopathy

Cardiac toxicity is one of the most concerning side effects of anticancer therapy. The gain in life expectancy obtained with anticancer therapy can be compromised by increased morbidity and mortality associated with its cardiac complications. Radiosensitivity of the heart is regarded as one of the most critical dose-limiting organs in radiotherapy.[78] A high-dose radiation exposure on the thorax is mainly used in the context of adjuvant radiotherapy after conservative or radical breast surgery, adjuvant or exclusive radiotherapy of lung and esophageal cancer, and as a complement to systemic treatment in lymphoma. Radiation-induced heart disease is generated by total cumulative dosage of radiotherapy potentiated by the adjunctive chemotherapy. Radiation affects all tissues, including the coronary vessels, heart valves, and pericardium, and may result in pericarditis, myocardial fibrosis, muscular dysfunction, valvular abnormalities, and conduction disturbances. Pericarditis, with pericardial thickening, may lead to constriction. Extensive fibrous thickening, adhesions, chronic constriction, and chronic pericardial effusion can occur. It is observed in up to 20% of patients within 2 years following irradiation. Constrictive pericarditis can be observed in 4–20% of patients and appears to be dose-dependent and related to the presence of pericardial effusion in the delayed acute phase.[79]

In more advanced instances, radiotherapy may induce myocardial fibrosis, which will lead to RCM. Postradiation cardiomyopathy is a noninfiltrative disorder that occurs as a result of endothelial cell damage and subsequent microvascular dysfunction due to fibrosis.[80] Pericardial constriction and RCM may both coexist and may pose diagnostic challenges. However, both can be differentiated by systematic evaluation using various imaging modalities, such as echocardiography, multidetector computed tomography (MDCT), and CMR, as delineated in Table 1 earlier. Echocardiography is the most useful, noninvasive, and first-line investigation to identify and monitor LV systolic and diastolic dysfunctions.

It is worth noting that primary cardiac lymphoma may sometimes present as RCM when there is invasion in the LV or RV myocardium. It may impair the ventricular compliance and cause diastolic dysfunction and may result in restrictive filling pattern and mimic RCM. Moreover, rarely the lymphoma may encase the heart and may cause diastolic dysfunction and can be mistaken for constrictive pericarditis. In such cases, further evaluation with MDCT, CMR, or PET–CT will be useful. Moreover, when lymph nodes are enlarged, lymph node biopsy may lead to the diagnosis (Flowchart 2).

Dobutamine stress echocardiography can be used to check contractile reserve in order to identify and follow subclinical LV dysfunction over time. CMR is the method of choice in patients with poor acoustic windows, while cardiac CT and RNV represent potential alternatives. However, LV ejection fraction alone does not provide all the relevant clinical information. In patients with the preserved LV ejection fraction, reduced longitudinal function as evaluated by 2D speckle-tracking global strain,[81] patchy distribution of myocardial fibrosis on CMR,[82] and abnormal myocardial perfusion on SPECT,[83] all represent markers of an intrinsic myocardial disease progression. Early detection of these abnormalities may allow the initiation of tailored treatment. A pretreatment cardiovascular screening for risk factors and a careful clinical examination should be performed in all patients who are planned for radiotherapy. A baseline comprehensive echocardiographic evaluation is warranted in all the patients before initiating the radiotherapy to identify any cardiac abnormalities. During follow-up, a yearly history and physical examination with close attention to symptoms and signs of heart disease that might otherwise be overlooked in this generally young population is essential. The development of either new cardiopulmonary symptoms or new suggestive physical examination findings, such as a new murmur, should prompt transthoracic echocardiography examination.

Flowchart 2: Pathophysiological manifestations of radiation-induced cardiac tissue injury.[79]

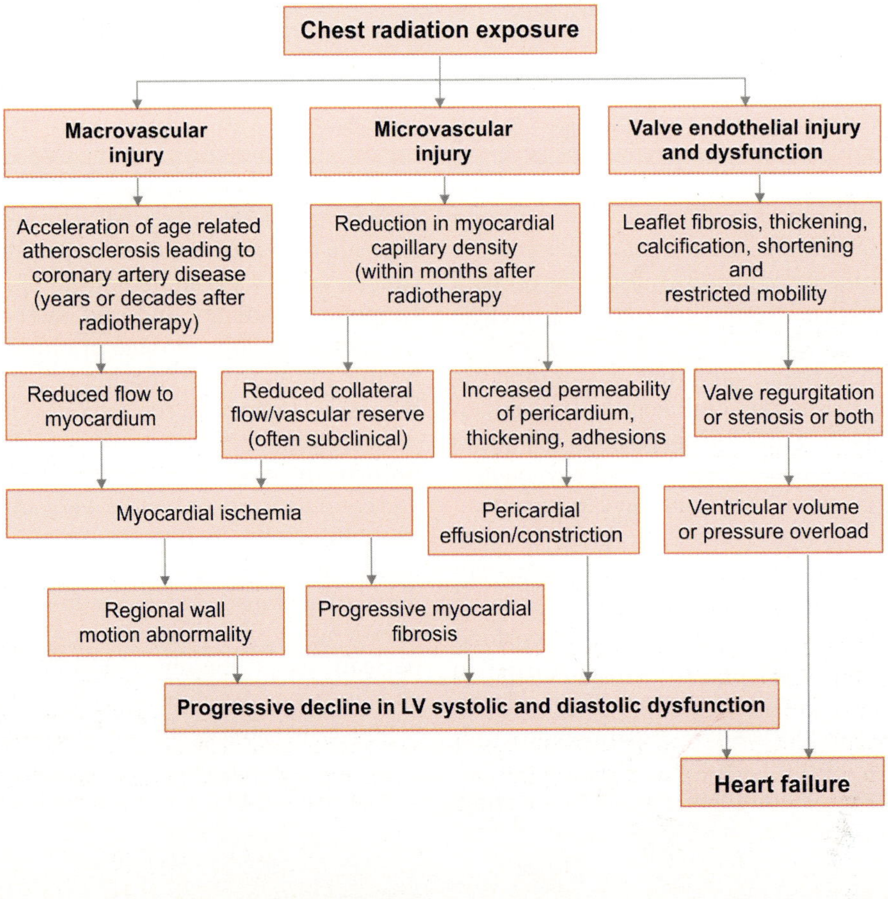

Drug-induced Restrictive Cardiomyopathy

Drug-induced RCM is a result of many systemically administered chemotherapeutic and biologic agents that may cause cardiovascular complications. The combination of increased use of chemotherapy, overall increased survival and development of newer agents have led to the emergence of chemotherapy-induced cardiotoxicity as a major health issue. Cardiotoxicity can manifest as an acute, reversible impairment of myocardial systolic function during or immediately after the initial infusion, although acute cardiotoxicity occurs very rarely. The cessation of therapy usually improves myocardial function, though this depends on the cumulative dose experienced by patients. The acute or subacute cardiotoxicity may cause abnormalities in ventricular repolarization and the QT-interval (supraventricular and ventricular arrhythmias), acute coronary syndromes, and pericarditis or myocarditis, such as syndromes, which can occur at the initiation of chemotherapy or up to 2 weeks after its termination.[84] Early cardiotoxicity can occur within 12 months of treatment, and late cardiotoxicity can occur beyond 12 months. Early toxicity has been noted to occur in up to 2.1% of children treated with anthracyclines, with a peak incidence at 3–4 months. The concomitant use of trastuzumab has been shown to potentiate the cardiotoxic effects of anthracyclines. The cardiotoxicity occurs as a result of the primary myocyte insult mediated via free radical (via both mitochondrial and iron-dependent pathways) in response to oxidative stress. The free radical production can self-propagate and persist even after treatment. There is resultant apoptosis of the myocytes and thinning of the left ventricle. Elevated afterload and decreased contractility follow, leading to the deterioration of LV function that characterizes cardiomyopathy. Chronic cardiotoxicity is characterized by asymptomatic systolic or diastolic LV dysfunction leading to severe congestive cardiomyopathy. In addition to causing DCM, anthracyclines can also cause EMF and diastolic dysfunction with restrictive filling pattern. The risk of restrictive cardiac failure is greatly increased when there is a history of irradiation. Therefore, substantial abnormalities of diastolic function occur after treatment with anthracyclines, even administered many years previously, and the abnormalities appear not to be correlated with the dose.[85] The regular monitoring of heart function during chemotherapy is of major importance so that cardiac dysfunction can be detected. Biomarkers, such as N-terminal-pro-BNP and troponin I, may help in detecting myocyte damage very early after chemotherapy. Three-dimensional echocardiography has been validated as the accurate echocardiographic modality for the calculation of LV ejection fraction. Two-dimension-based strain and strain rate imaging identifies abnormalities in myocardial mechanics early during cardiotoxicity, allowing the prediction of later overt systolic dysfunction. These parameters may be useful in the detection of patients treated with chemotherapy who could benefit from alternate therapies, thereby decreasing the incidence of cardiotoxicity and its associated morbidity and mortality. Exercise and pharmacologic stress testing has been studied as a way to unmask subclinical abnormalities of LV function induced by chemotherapeutic agents.[86]

Acute Cardiac Allograft Rejection

Acute cardiac allograft rejection is characterized by pathological alterations, including microvascular antigen deposition, myocyte edema, interstitial hemorrhage, inflammatory cellular infiltration, and varying degrees of myocardial necrosis. These alterations will impair myocyte function, especially diastolic function,[87] and may mimic RCM in the early stage. Diastolic function is impaired as a result of ventricular wall stiffness through inflammatory cellular infiltration and myocardial edema, thus causing a reduction of LV compliance. Echocardiography indices of diastolic dysfunction, including Edt, IVRT, early diastolic mitral inflow velocity (E wave), late diastolic mitral inflow velocity (A wave), E/A, e′, E/e′, are the most commonly used parameters for screening for acute cardiac allograft rejection. RV myocardial biopsy and histological evaluation of obtained samples constitute the gold standard for the detection of acute rejection in patients who have undergone heart transplantation but it is associated with major complications. Roshanali et al. studied novel echocardiography parameters derived from tissue velocity imaging and strain rate imaging for the detection of cardiac allograft rejection. In the study, the peak systolic strain of the three segments—RV base, Sep base, and lateral LV (Lat) base—strain (RV-S, Lat-S, and Sep-S) was measured from the apical four-chamber view. In addition, time to systole (TS) was measured at the same three segments, yielding the three variables of RV-TS, Sep-TS, and Lat-TS. They reported that an increase in the LV mass index and the posterior wall thickness correlated with rejection and a decrease in the Lat-S and the Sep-TS correlated with rejection.[88]

CONCLUSION

Restrictive cardiomyopathy is the least common of the cardiomyopathic disorders. It may result from various local and systemic disorders, many of them rarely seen in clinical practice. Other conditions, such as amyloidosis, are more common and may present with symptoms and signs of congestive heart failure. EMF used to be endemic in the coastal belt of Kerala and other tropical countries.

But it has gradually disappeared over the last two decades, and at present, primary RCM has become more common. RCM is diagnosed based on detailed history, thorough clinical examination and tests, such as blood tests, ECG, chest X-ray, echocardiography and magnetic resonance imaging, and PET, in some cases. With its wide availability, echocardiography is probably the most important investigation to identify the LV diastolic and systolic dysfunction and should be performed early. Finally, on rare occasions, the differential diagnosis from constrictive pericarditis is mandatory as it can also present with "restrictive physiology" but which is often cured surgically by pericardiectomy.

LIST OF ABBREVIATIONS

2D: Two dimensional
a′: Medial mitral annular late diastolic tissue velocity
AL: Amyloid light-chain
ATTR: Transthyretin-related
AV: Atrioventricular
BAO: Biatrial overload
BNP: Brain natriuretic peptide
CKD: Chronic kidney disease
CMR: Cardiac magnetic resonance
DCM: Dilated cardiomyopathy
e′: Medial mitral annular early diastolic tissue velocity
ECG: Electrocardiogram
Edt: E-wave deceleration time
EMB: Endomyocardial biopsy
EMF: Endomyocardial fibrosis
FDG: ^{18}F-Fluorodeoxyglucose
HCM: Hypertrophic cardiomyopathy
HES: Hypereosinophilia syndrome
ICD: Intracardiac defibrillator
IV: Intraventricular
IVC: Inferior vena cava
IVRT: Isovolumic relaxation time
LAO: Left atrial overload
LGE: Late gadolinium enhancement
LS: Longitudinal strain
LV: Left ventricle
LVEDP: Left ventricular end-diastolic pressure
LVH: Left ventricular hypertrophy
MDCT: Multidetector computed tomography
MI: Myocardial infarction
MR: Mitral regurgitation
NCCM: Noncompaction cardiomyopathy
Nt: N terminal
PET: Positron emission tomography
RA: Right atrial
RAO: Right atrial overload
RCM: Restrictive cardiomyopathy
RIHD: Radiation-induced heart disease
RV: Right ventricular
RVEDP: Right ventricular end-diastolic pressure
RVSP: Right ventricular systolic pressure
s′: Medial mitral annular systolic tissue velocity
S3: Third heart sound
S4: Fourth heart sound
SPECT: Single-photon emission computed tomography
TR: Tricuspid regurgitation
VT: Ventricular tachycardia

ACKNOWLEDGMENTS

Authors are thankful to Management of Care Hospitals, Banjara Hills, Hyderabad; Department of Telemedicine—Mr SG Prasad; Noninvasive Cardiac Imaging Laboratory—Prof Mandapal, Dr Johann, Mr Shiva for providing MDCT and CMR images; Department of Pathology—Dr Vijaya Tourani; Department of Biochemistry—Dr Shanti Naidu; and Echocardiography Laboratory—Dr Raghu for the important support.

REFERENCES

1. Schoenfeld MH, Supple EW, Dec GW Jr., et al. Restrictive cardiomyopathy versus constrictive pericarditis: role of endomyocardial biopsy in avoiding unnecessary thoracotomy. Circulation. 1987;75:1012-7.
2. Kushwaha SS, Fallon JT, Fuster V. Restrictive cardiomyopathy. N Engl J Med. 1997;336:267-76.
3. Sivasankaran S. Restrictive cardiomyopathy in India: the story of a vanishing mystery. Heart. 2009;95:9-14.
4. Feld S, Caspi A. Familial cardiomyopathy with variable hypertrophic and restrictive features and common HLA haplotype. Isr J Med Sci. 1992;28:277-80.
5. Mogensen J, Arbustini E. Restrictive cardiomyopathy. Curr Opin Cardiol. 2009:214-20.
6. Fitzpatrick AP, Shapiro LM, Rickards AF, et al. Familial restrictive cardiomyopathy with atrioventricular block and skeletal myopathy. Br Heart J. 1990;63:114-8.
7. ChfuuLubitz SA, Goldbarg SH, Mehta D. Sudden cardiac death in infiltrative cardiomyopathies: sarcoidosis, scleroderma, amyloidosis, hemachromatosis. Prog Cardiovasc Dis. 2008;51:58-73.
8. Hoedemaekers YM, Caliskan K, Majoor-Krakauer D, et al. Cardiac beta-myosin heavy chain defects in two families with non-compaction cardiomyopathy: linking non-compaction to hypertrophic, restrictive, and dilated cardiomyopathies. Eur Heart J. 2007;28(22):2732-7.
9. Kubo T, Gimeno JR, Bahl A, et al. Prevalence, clinical significance, and genetic basis of hypertrophic cardiomyopathy with restrictive phenotype. J Am Coll Cardiol. 2007;49:2419-26.

10. Selvaganesh M, Arul AS, Balasubramanian S, et al. An unusual ECG pattern in restrictive cardiomyopathy. Indian Heart J. 2015;67:362.
11. Reddy PR, Dieter RS, Das P, et al. Utility of BNP in differentiating constrictive pericarditis from restrictive cardiomyopathy in patients with renal insufficiency. J Card Fail. 2007;13:668.
12. Karamitsos TD, Francis JM, Myerson S, et al. The role of cardiovascular magnetic resonance imaging in heart failure. J Am Coll Cardiol. 2009;54:1407.
13. UpToDate. (2016). Idiopathic restrictive cardiomyopathy. [online]. Available from: https://www.uptodate.com/contents/idiopathic-restrictive-cardiomyopathy. [Accessed October, 2018]
14. Topol EJ (Ed). Textbook of Cardiovascular Medicine. Philadelphia, PA: Lippincott Williams and Wilkins; 2007. p. 430.
15. Katritsis D, Wilmshurst PT, Wendon JA, et al. Primary restrictive cardiomyopathy: clinical and pathologic characteristics. J Am Coll Cardiol. 1991;18:1230-5.
16. Ware SM, Quinn ME, Ballard ET, et al. Pediatric restrictive cardiomyopathy associated with a mutation in beta-myosin heavy chain. Clin Genet. 2008;73:165-70.
17. Kaski JP, Syrris P, Burch M, et al. Idiopathic restrictive cardiomyopathy in children is caused by mutations in cardiac sarcomere protein genes. Heart. 2008;94:1478-84.
18. Cooke RA, Chambers JB, Curry PV. Noonan's cardiomyopathy: a non-hypertrophic variant. Br Heart J. 1994;71:561-5.
19. Gertz MA, Dispenzieri A, Sher T. Pathophysiology and treatment of cardiac amyloidosis. Nat Rev Cardiol. 2015;12:91-102.
20. Nihoyannopoulos P, Dawson D. Restrictive cardiomyopathies. Eur J Echocardiogr. 2009;10:iii23-33.
21. Dubrey SW, Cha K, Anderson J, et al. The clinical features of immunoglobulin light-chain (AL) amyloidosis with heart involvement. QJM. 1998;91:141-57.
22. Connors LH, Lim A, Prokaeva T, et al. Guidelines on the diagnosis and management of AL amyloidosis. Br J Haematol. 2004;125:681-700.
23. Gertz MA, Comenzo R, Falk RH, et al. Definition of organ involvement and treatment response in immunoglobulin light chain amyloidosis (AL): a consensus opinion from the 10th International symposium on Amyloid and Amyloidosis, Tours, France: 18e22 April 2004. Am J Hematol. 2005;79:319-28.
24. Dubrey SW, Hawkins PN, Falk RH. Amyloid diseases of the heart: assessment, diagnosis, and referral. Heart. 2011;97:75-84.
25. Rahman JE, Helou EF, Gelzer-Bell R, et al. Noninvasive diagnosis of biopsy-proven cardiac amyloidosis. J Am Coll Cardiol. 2004;43:410-5.
26. Ha JW, Ommen SR, Tajik AJ, et al. Differentiation of constrictive pericarditis from restrictive cardiomyopathy using mitral annular velocity by tissue Doppler echocardiography. Am J Cardiol. 2004;94:316-9.
27. Bellavia D, Pellikka PA, Abraham TP, et al. Evidence of impaired left ventricular systolic function by Doppler myocardial imaging in patients with systemic amyloidosis and no evidence of cardiac involvement by standard two-dimensional and Doppler echocardiography. Am J Cardiol. 2008;101:1039-45.
28. Phelan D, Collier P, Thavendiranathan P, et al. Relative "apical sparing" of longitudinal strain using 2-dimensional speckle-tracking echocardiography is both sensitive and specific for the diagnosis of cardiac amyloidosis. Heart. 2012;98:1442-8.
29. AlJaroudi WA, Desai MY, Tang WHW, et al. Role of imaging in the diagnosis and management of patients with cardiac amyloidosis: state of the art review and focus on emerging nuclear techniques. J Nucl Cardiol. 2014;21:271-83.
30. Cueto-Garcia L, Reeder GS, Kyle RA, et al. Echocardiographic findings in systemic amyloidosis: spectrum of cardiac involvement and relation to survival. J Am Coll Cardiol. 1985;6:737-43.
31. Klein AL, Hatle LK, Taliercio CP, et al. Prognostic significance of Doppler measures of diastolic function in cardiac amyloidosis. A Doppler echocardiography study. Circulation. 1991;83:808-16.
32. Syed IS, Glockner JF, Feng D, et al. Role of cardiac magnetic resonance imaging in the detection of cardiac amyloidosis. JACC Cardiovasc Imaging. 2010;3:155-64.
33. Austin BA, Tang WH, Rodriguez ER, et al. Delayed hyper-enhancement magnetic resonance imaging provides incremental diagnostic and prognostic utility in suspected cardiac amyloidosis. JACC Cardiovasc Imaging. 2009;2:1369-77.
34. Maceira AM, Joshi J, Prasad SK, et al. Cardiovascular magnetic resonance in cardiac amyloidosis. Circulation. 2005;111:186-93.
35. Banypersad SM, Sado DM, Flett AS, et al. Quantification of myocardial extracellular volume fraction in systemic al amyloidosis: an equilibrium contrast cardiovascular magnetic resonance study. Circ Cardiovasc Imaging. 2013;6:34-9.
36. Hazenberg BP, van Rijswijk MH, Lub-de Hooge MN, et al. Diagnostic performance and prognostic value of extravascular retention of 123I-labeled serum amyloid P component in systemic amyloidosis. J Nucl Med. 2007;48:865-72.
37. Sachchithanantham S, Wechalekar AD. Imaging in systemic amyloidosis. Br Med Bull. 2013;107:41-56.
38. Bokhari S, Castano A, Pozniakoff T, et al. 99mTc-pyrophosphate scintigraphy for differentiating light-chain cardiac amyloidosis from the transthyretin-related familial and senile cardiac amyloidoses. Circ Cardiovasc Imaging. 2013;6:195-201.
39. Gertz MA, Brown ML, Hauser MF, et al. Utility of technetium Tc99m pyrophosphate bone scanning in cardiac amyloidosis. Arch Intern Med. 1987;147:1039-44.
40. Kapoor P, Thenappan T, Singh E, et al. Cardiac amyloidosis: a practical approach to diagnosis and management. Am J Med. 2011;124:1006-15.
41. Gertz MA, Falk RH, Skinner M, et al. Worsening of congestive heart failure in amyloid heart disease treated by calcium channel-blocking agents. Am J Cardiol. 1985;55:1645.
42. Griffiths BE, Hughes P, Dowdle R, et al. Cardiac amyloidosis with asymmetrical septal hypertrophy and deterioration after nifedipine. Thorax. 1982;37:711-2.

43. Moreau P, Leblond V, Bourquelot P, et al. Prognostic factors for survival and response after high-dose therapy and autologous stem cell transplantation in systemic AL amyloidosis: a report on 21 patients. Br J Haematol. 1998;101:766-9.
44. Comenzo RL, Vosburgh E, Simms RW, et al. Dose-intensive melphalan with blood stem cell support for the treatment of AL amyloidosis: one-year follow-up in five patients. Blood. 1996;88:2801-6.
45. Mikhael JR, Schuster SR, Jimenez-Zepeda VH, et al. Cyclophosphamide-bortezomib-dexamethasone (CyBorD) produces rapid and complete hematologic response in patients with AL amyloidosis. Blood. 2012;119:4391-4.
46. Ackermann EJ, Guo S, Booten S, et al. Clinical development of an antisense therapy for the treatment of transthyretin-associated polyneuropathy. Amyloid. 2012;19(Suppl. 1): 43-4.
47. Varr BC, Zarafshar S, Coakley T, et al. Implantable cardioverter-defibrillator placement in patients with cardiac amyloidosis. Heart Rhythm. 2014;11:158-62.
48. Hassan WM, Fawzy ME, Al Helaly S, et al. Pitfalls in diagnosis and clinical, echocardiographic, and hemodynamic findings in endomyocardial fibrosis: a 25-year experience. Chest. 2005;128:3985-92.
49. Vijayaraghavan G, Balakrishnan M, Sadanandan S, et al. Patterns of calcification in tropical endomyocardial fibrosis. Heart Vessels. 1990;5:S4-7.
50. Anbarasu M, Manohar SR, Titus T, et al. One-and-a-half ventricular repair for right ventricular endomyocardial fibrosis. Asian Cardiovasc Thorac Ann. 2004;12:363-5.
51. Cox PR. Endomyocardial fibrosis and restrictive cardiomyopathy: pathologic and clinical features. J Vet Cardiol. 2004;6:25-31.
52. Padmakumar R, Rao N, Tharakan J. A clinical overview of endomyocardial fibrosis. In: Radhakrishnan K (Ed). Silver Lines. Thiruvananthapuram, India: Sree Chitra Tirunal Institute for Medical Sciences and Technology; 2004. pp. 133-40.
53. Vijayaraghavan G, Sivasankaran S. Tropical endomyocardial fibrosis in India: a vanishing disease. Indian J Med Res. 2012;136(5):729-38.
54. Freers J, Mayanja-Kizza H, Rutakingirwa M, et al. Enodomyocardial fibrosis: why is there striking ascites with little or no pedal edema? Lancet. 1996;347:197.
55. Löffler W. Endocarditis parietalis fibroplastica mit bluteosinophilie. Ein eigenartiges Krankheitsbild. Schweiz MedWochenschr. 1936;66:817-20.
56. Tai PC, Ackerman SJ, Spry CJ, et al. Deposits of eosinophil granule proteins in cardiac tissues of patients with eosinophilic endomyocardial disease. Lancet. 1987;1:643-7.
57. Chusid MJ, Dale DC, West BC, et al. The hypereosinophilic syndrome: analysis of fourteen cases with review of the literature. Medicine (Baltimore). 1975;54(1):1-27.
58. Chusid MJ. Eosinophilia in childhood. Immunol Allergy Clin North Am. 1999;19:327-46.
59. Sheikh J, Weller PF. Clinical overview of hypereosinophilic syndromes. Immunol Allergy Clin North Am. 2007;27:333-55.
60. Brockington IF, Olsen EG. Löffler's endocarditis and Davies' endomyocardial fibrosis. Am Heart J. 1973;85:308-22.
61. Parillo JE, Borer JS, Henry WL, et al. The cardiovascular manifestations of the hypereosinophilic syndrome. Prospective study of 26 patients, with review of the literature. Am J Med. 1979;67:572-82.
62. ten Oever J, Theunissen LJHJ, Tick LW, et al. Cardiac involvement in hypereosinophilic syndrome. J Med, Netherlands. 2011;69(5):240-44.
63. Séguélaa PE, Iriart X, Acar P, et al. Eosinophilic cardiac disease: molecular, clinical and imaging aspects. Arch Cardiovasc Dis. 2015;108:258-68.
64. Ogbogu P, Rosing DR, Horne MK, III. Cardiovascular manifestations of hypereosinophilic syndromes. Immunol Allergy Clin North Am. 2007;27(3):457-75.
65. Klion AD, Bochner BS, Gleich GJ, et al. Approaches to the treatment of hypereosinophilic syndromes: a workshop summary report. J Allergy Clin Immunol. 2006;117(6): 1292-302.
66. Boustany CW Jr., Murphy GW, Hicks GL Jr. Mitral valve replacement in idiopathic hypereosinophilic syndrome. Ann Thorac Surg. 1991;51(6):1007-9.
67. Roberts WC, McAllister HA Jr., Ferrans VJ. Sarcoidosis of the heart. A clinicopathologic study of 35 necropsy patients (group 1) and review of 78 previously described necropsy patients (group 11). Am J Med. 1977;63:86-108.
68. Sekiguchi M, Numao Y, Imai M, et al. Clinical and histopathological profile of sarcoidosis of the heart and acute idiopathic myocarditis. Concepts through a study employing endomyocardial biopsy. I. Sarcoidosis. Jpn Circ J. 1980;44:249-63.
69. Sharma S. Cardiac imaging in myocardial sarcoidosis and other cardiomyopathies. Curr Opin Pulm Med. 2009;15:507.
70. Ishimaru S, Tsujino I, Sakaue S, et al. Combination of 18F-fluoro-2-deoxyglucose positron emission tomography and magnetic resonance imaging in assessing cardiac sarcoidosis. Sarcoidosis Vasc Diffuse Lung Dis. 2005; 22:234.
71. Aizer A, Stern EH, Gomes JA, et al. Usefulness of programmed ventricular stimulation in predicting future arrhythmic events in patients with cardiac sarcoidosis. Am J Cardiol. 2005;96:276.
72. Betensky BP, Tschabrunn CM, Zado ES, et al. Long-term follow-up of patients with cardiac sarcoidosis and implantable cardioverter-defibrillators. Heart Rhythm. 2012;9:884.
73. McCarthy GM, Crowe J, McCarthy CJ, et al. Hereditary hemochromatosis: a common, often unrecognized, genetic disease. Cleve Clin J Med. 2002;69:224-6, 229-30, 232-3.
74. Cecchetti G, Binda A, Piperno A, et al. Cardiac alterations in 36 consecutive patients with idiopathic haemochromatosis: polygraphic and echocardiographic evaluation. Eur Heart J. 1991;12:224-30.
75. Palka P, Macdonald G, Lange A, et al. The role of Doppler left ventricular filling indexes and Doppler tissue echocardiography in the assessment of cardiac involvement in hereditary hemochromatosis. J Am Soc Echocardiogr. 2002;15:884-90.

76. Case records of the Massachusetts General Hospital. Weekly clinicopathological exercises. Case 31-1994. A 25-year-old man with the recent onset of diabetes mellitus and congestive heart failure. N Engl J Med. 1994;331:460-6.
77. Olson LJ, Edwards WD, Holmes DR Jr, et al. Endomyocardial biopsy in hemochromatosis: clinicopathologic correlates in six cases. J Am Coll Cardiol. 1989;13:116-20.
78. Carver JR, Shapiro CL, Ng A, et al., ASCO Cancer Survivorship Expert Panel. American Society of Clinical Oncology clinical evidence review on the ongoing care of adult cancer survivors: cardiac and pulmonary late effects. J Clin Oncol. 2007;25:3991-4008.
79. Lancellotti P, Nkomo VT, Badano LP, et al. Expert consensus for multi-modality imaging evaluation of cardiovascular complications of radiotherapy in adults: a report from the European Association of Cardiovascular Imaging and the American Society of Echocardiography. Eur Heart J Cardiovasc Imaging. 2013;14:721-40.
80. Chello M, Mastroroberto P, Romano R, et al. Changes in the proportion of types I and III collagen in the left ventricular wall of patients with post-irradiative pericarditis. Cardiovasc Surg. 1996;4:222-6.
81. Tsai HR, Gjesdal O, Wethal T, et al. Left ventricular function assessed by two-dimensional speckle tracking echocardiography in long-term survivors of Hodgkin's lymphoma treated by mediastinal radiotherapy with or without anthracycline therapy. Am J Cardiol. 2011;107:472-7.
82. Martin J, Narula J, Marwick T. Assessment of nonischemic myocardial fibrosis. J Am Coll Cardiol. 2010;56:89-97.
83. Marks L, Yu X, Prosnitz R, et al. The incidence and functional consequences of RT-associated cardiac perfusion defects. Int J Radiat Oncol Biol Phys. 2005;63:214-23.
84. Sawaya H, Plana JC, Scherrer-Crosbie M. Newest echocardiographic techniques for the detection of cardiotoxicity and heart failure during chemotherapy. Heart Failure Clin. 2011;7:313-21.
85. Khawaja MZ, Cafferkey C, Rajani R, et al. Cardiac complications and manifestations of chemotherapy for cancer. Heart. 2014;100:1133-40.
86. Cottin Y, L'Huillier I, Casasnovas O, et al. Dobutamine stress echocardiography identifies anthracycline cardiotoxicity. Eur J Echocardiogr. 2000;1:180.
87. Miller CA, Fildes JE, Ray SG, et al. Non-invasive approaches for the diagnosis of acute cardiac allograft rejection. Heart. 2013;99(7):445-53.
88. Roshanali F, Mandegar MH, Bagheri J, et al. Echo rejection score: new echocardiographic approach to diagnosis of heart transplant rejection. Eur J Cardiothorac Surg. 2010;38: 176-180.

SECTION 14

Pericardial Effusion

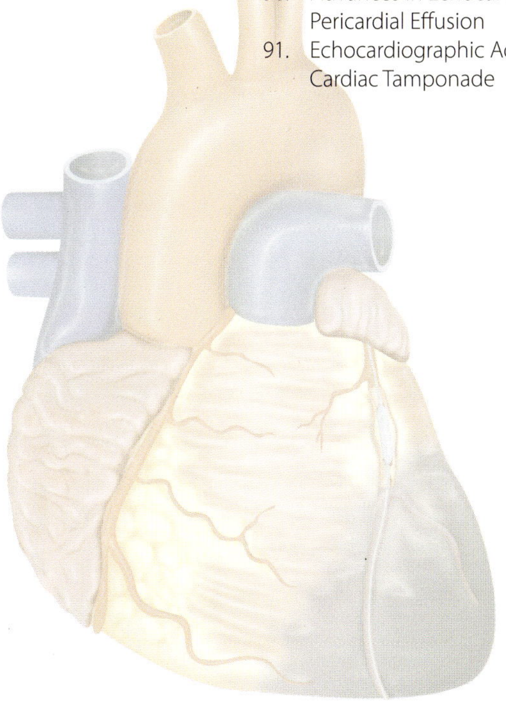

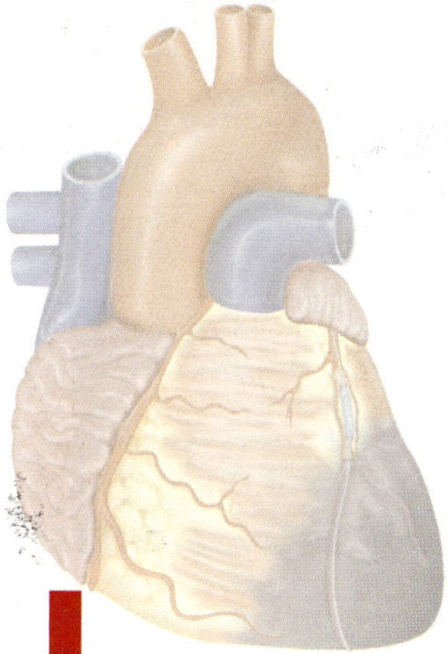

90

CHAPTER

Advances in Echocardiographic Navigation in Pericardial Effusion

Sakhalesh Patil, S Sivasankaran, G Vijayaraghavan

INTRODUCTION

Pericardial disorders include diverse group of pathologies ranging from congenital absences of pericardium to pericarditis, asymptomatic pericardial effusion, and life-threatening conditions such as constrictive pericarditis and pericardial tamponade.[1] Normal intrapericardial pressure ranges from +3 mm Hg (end expiration) to –6 mm Hg (end inspiration) and is influenced by factors which increase intrathoracic pressure.[2] Pericardial diseases are not uncommon in daily practice, but familiarity with diagnosis and managing these diseases appears to be less with treating physicians. Even though, pericardium is not essential for life, but prevents the overdistension of cardiac chambers and prevents lung infections spreading to the heart.[3-5] Any inflammatory process involving pericardium, causes pericardial effusion (exudate) due to increased production of pericardial fluid. Another mechanism of production of pericardial fluid may be due to decreased reabsorption because of increased systemic venous pressure generally as a result of congestive cardiac failure or pulmonary hypertension (transudate).[6-9] If pericardial fluid is free to move within the pericardial sac following the gravity forces, it usually starts accumulating posteriorly to the left ventricle when the patient is lying on his/her left side for echocardiographic evaluation (mild effusion detected initially as posterior), then circumferentially in the case of moderate-to-large pericardial effusions. A mild pericardial effusion may also be detected around the right atrium because this is the cardiac chamber with the lowest pressure during the cardiac cycle and thus pericardial fluid accumulation is most evident around this chamber. Transthoracic echocardiography (TTE) is considered as the first-line imaging modality in the assessment of pericardial effusion, as it is simple and quick to perform.[6] However, 2D echocardiography has limitation of not imaging the entire pericardium. This chapter includes focused echocardiographic approach to pericardial effusion and its management. We have incorporated the American Society of Echocardiography (ASE), 2013 and the European Society of Cardiology (ESC) guidelines, 2015 for the diagnosis and management of pericardial diseases.[6,10]

DIAGNOSTIC CRITERIA

Presence of more than 40–50 mL of fluid in the pericardial cavity is abnormal and is diagnostic of pericardial effusion. It may occur following infections, blunt trauma of chest, myocardial infarction, hypothyroidism, and invasive cardiac interventions such as coronary angioplasty and electrophysiologic studies. Rough quantitative estimation of pericardial fluid may be made by measuring the width of the pericardial fluid in end diastole of M-mode echocardiogram. When the effusion collects slowly over weeks to months, the pericardial cavity stretches to a flask-shaped structure and the intrapericardial pressure is only moderately increased. When the effusion is large, the heart could be seen as a swinging structure within the pericardial cavity (Figs. 1A to C).[11] Echocardiography is the initial procedure of choice to detect the presence of a pericardial effusion, as it can be performed with minimal delay and has an accuracy of nearly 100%. It is also the best diagnostic tool for assessing the physiologic and hemodynamic effects of a pericardial effusion.[12]

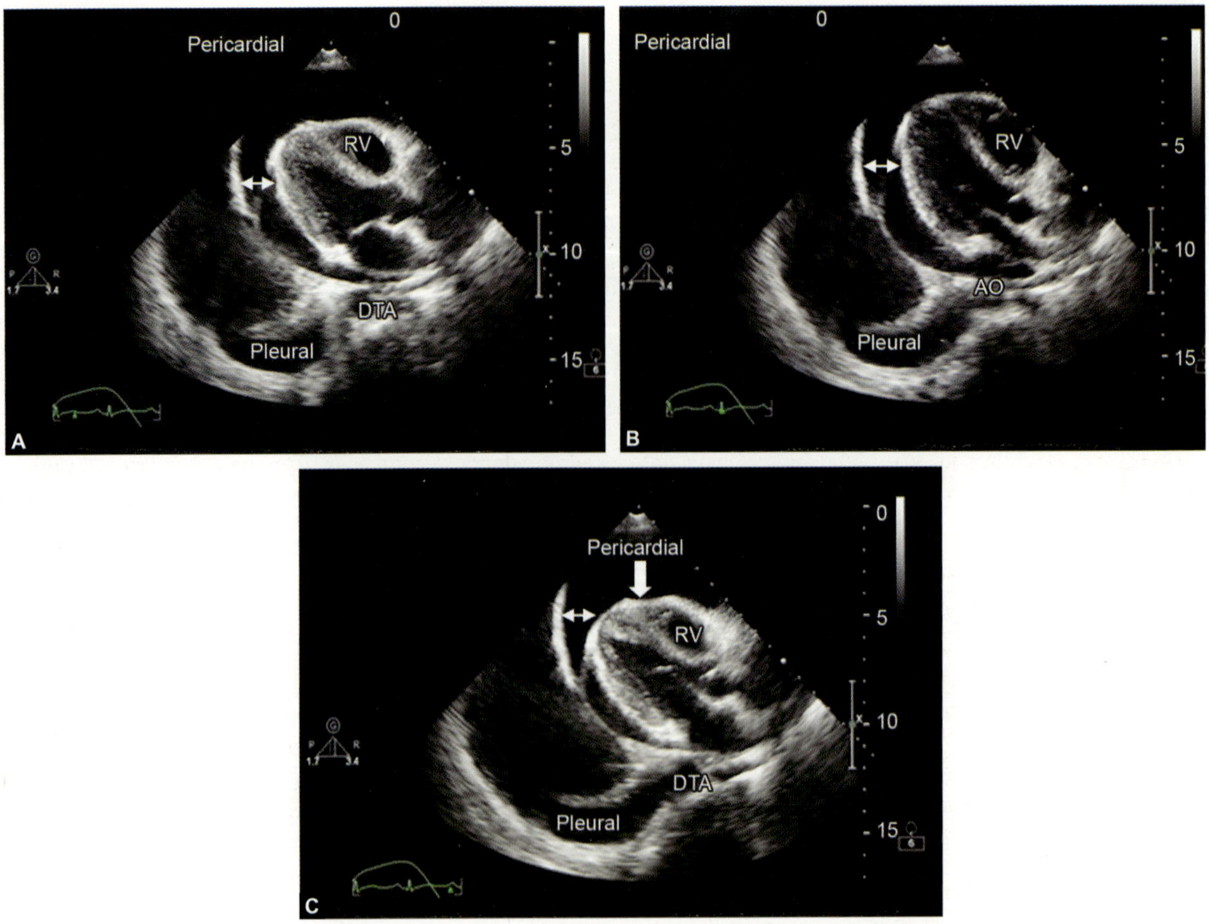

Figs. 1A to C: Two-dimensional echocardiogram showing swinging/flip flop heart in a patient with large pericardial and pleural effusion. Note the pericardial effusion is anterior to descending thoracic aorta (DTA) compared to pleural effusion which is posterior. Small vertical arrows in the lower left-hand corner show the phases of respiration and cardiac cycle. (A) The end-systolic frame in inspiration; (B) Shows the end-diastolic frame in inspiration; and (C) Shows the preatrial systolic frame in expiration. Bidirectional arrows show the variation in posterior pericardial space consistent with swinging movement of the heart in relation to respiration and cardiac cycle. Vertical stout arrow in (C) illustrates the diastolic right ventricular (RV) collapse.

ESTIMATION OF PERICARDIAL EFFUSION

M-mode echocardiography shows the persistence of an echo-free space between the visceral and parietal pericardium throughout the cardiac cycle. Separation of the two layers that is seen only in systole represents a normal phenomenon or clinically insignificant (trivial pericardial effusion), whereas separation that is present throughout the cardiac cycle (in systole and diastole) is associated with effusions of more than 50 mL (small pericardial effusion) (Figs. 2A and B). Most importantly, all measurements of pericardial effusion should be made at the end of diastole.[9]

- *Mild:* Less than 1 cm (approximately 300 mL)
- *Moderate:* 1–2 cm (approximately 500 mL)
- *Large:* More than 2 cm (typically > 700 mL).

In asymptomatic individuals with chronic pericardial effusion, there are no guidelines, how often an echocardiogram should be repeated. Apical four-chamber view and subcostal view are extremely important in the assessment of pericardial effusion more so, detecting pericardial tamponade.[12,13]

DIFFERENTIATION BETWEEN PLEURAL EFFUSION AND PERICARDIAL EFFUSION

Often the left-sided pleural effusion is confused with pericardial effusion. In the left parasternal view, the descending thoracic aortic image separates the two effusions. In pericardial effusion, you will find the descending thoracic

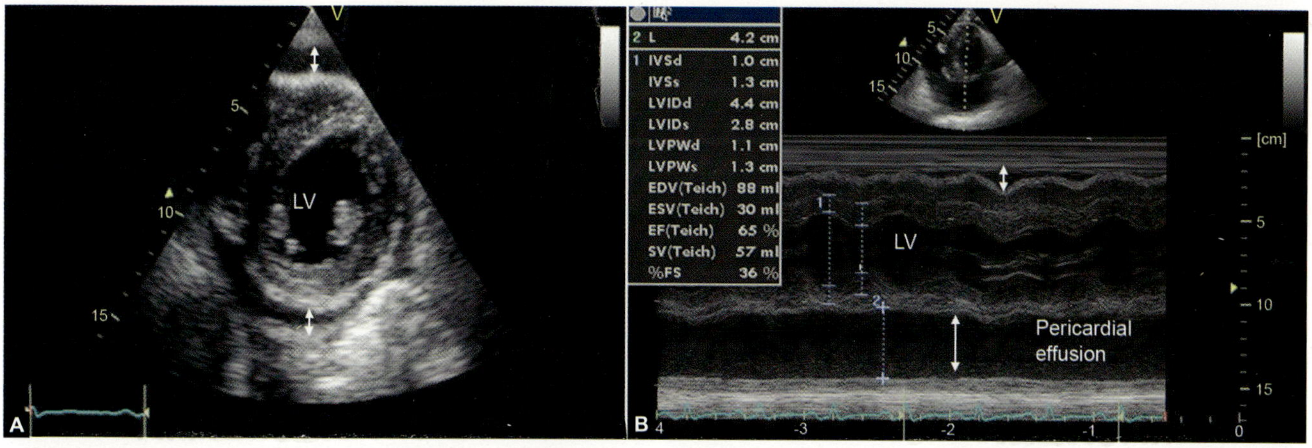

Figs. 2A and B: Moderate and large pericardial effusion, anterior and posterior separation of the parietal and visceral pericardium is shown by the vertical double headed arrows. (A) Two-dimensional echocardiogram in the parasternal short-axis view in a subject with mild-to-moderate pericardial effusion; (B) Shows the M-mode echocardiogram in a subject with large pericardial effusion where the posterior pericardial separation measures more than 4 cm. (LV: left ventricle).

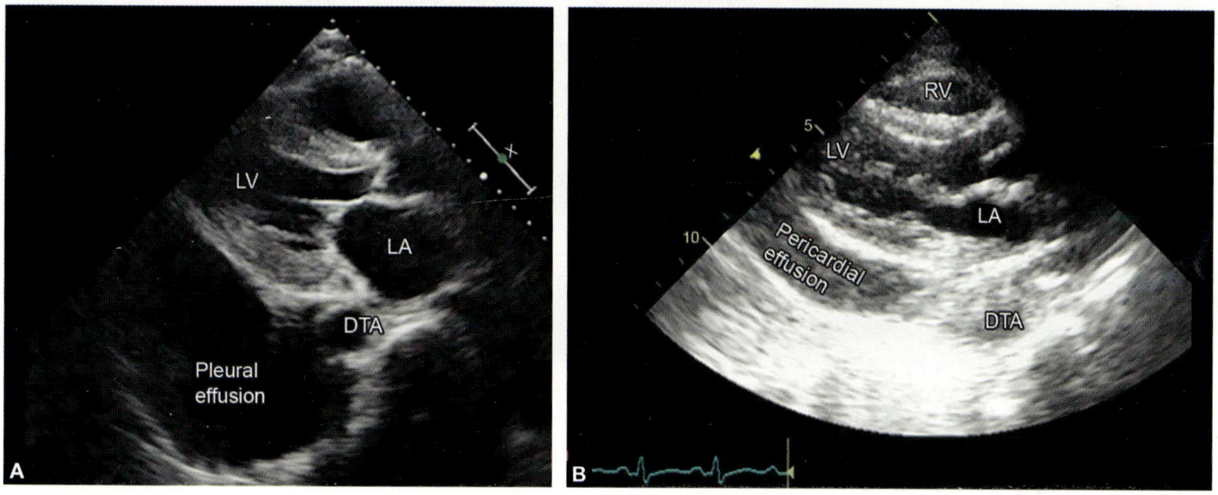

Figs. 3A and B: Differentiating left-sided pleural effusion and pericardial effusion by two-dimensional echocardiography in the parasternal long-axis view. (A) Left-sided pleural effusion with thoracic descending aorta, DTA anterior to the effuse ion. (B) Pericardial effusion with thoracic descending aorta posterior to effusion. (LV: left ventricle; RV: right ventricle; LA: left atrium)

aorta posterior to the effusion, while the aorta will be anterior to the left pleural effusion. Large pericardial effusions will continue all around the heart except behind the left where there is very little pericardial cavity (Figs. 3A and B). But large pleural effusions can increase the intrathoracic pressures and mimic cardiac tamponade.

CAUSES OF PERICARDIAL EFFUSION

Pericardial effusion may occur as a part of many viral fevers such as dengue fever, may remain asymptomatic and disappear when the febrile illness subsides.[14] However, acute benign pericarditis with effusion is the most common one which may present to the clinician as a clinical dilemma and diagnosis can be confirmed by a detailed echocardiography.[15] The pericardium may be thin and effusions may often be mild or moderate subsiding with rest and analgesics.[7] Rarely, they develop tamponade. Rheumatic pericarditis may be seen with pericardial edema and effusion. All varieties of dyscollagenosis may develop pericarditis during their natural history.[16] Often the pericardium is thickened in an uneven manner due to edema and fibrosis. Presence of associated pulmonary hypertension in some of these patients is independent of the pericardial pathology.[17] The effusion may contain amorphous material due to high fibrin content. Response to steroids or drugs such as methotrexate may be dramatic in these patients. Some of them may progress on to constriction. Pericardial effusion secondary to malignancy

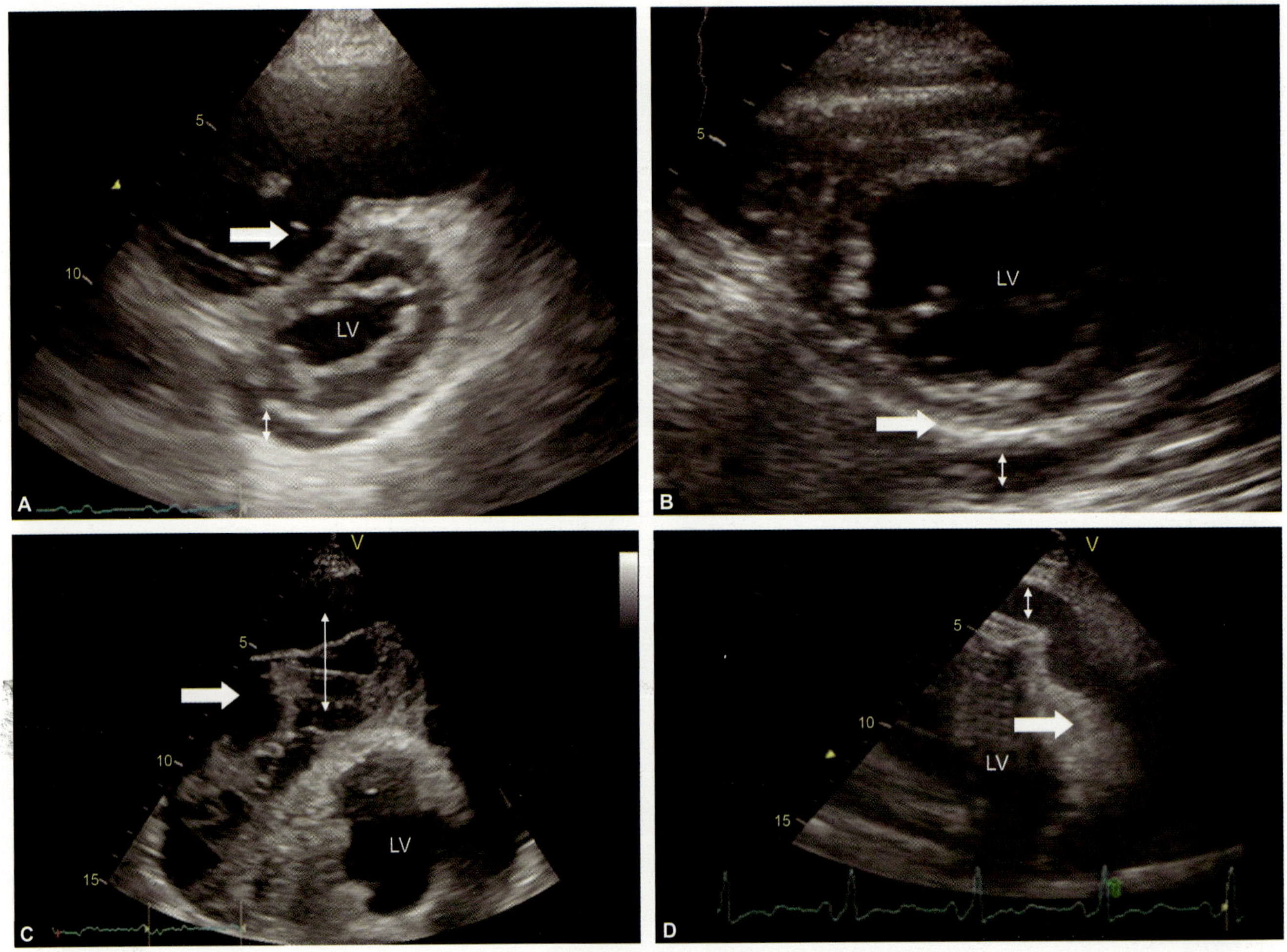

Figs. 4A to D: *Causes and patterns of pericardial effusion:* Vertical double headed arrows show the pericardial separation. (A to D) Two-dimensional echocardiogram in parasternal short-axis view: (A) Mild pericardial effusion in a subject with systemic sclerosis: Horizontal thick arrow shows the bowing of the interventricular septum due to pulmonary hypertension. (B) Moderate pericardial effusion in a subject with systemic lupus erythematosus, horizontal arrow shows the thickening and edema of visceral pericardium. (C) Shows the fibrinous strands in a large pericardial effusion. (D) Thick irregular thickening of pericardium could suggest secondary deposits in a subject with malignant pericardial effusion.

may recur and needs frequent pericardiocentesis to prevent tamponade. Lund malignancies are notorious to develop malignant pericardial effusion which may be difficult to treat. Rarely, one may be able to see secondary deposits on the epicardial surface of the heart. Primary malignancy of the pericardium-like mesothelioma is rare (Figs. 4A to D).

Chylous Pericardial Effusion

It is a milky-white pericardial effusion comprising of chyle, normal content of lymphatics of small intestine passing up the thoracic duct (Fig. 5).[18] It generally follows trauma or surgical injury to the thoracic duct but may occur without a clear etiology. The effusion could be large to produce to tamponade and may require multiple aspirations.[19] As the effusion is rich in triglycerides, it may form webs within the pericardial cavity and amorphous material may be seen floating within the pericardial cavity. The pericardial fluid characteristic will be milky white in color and will have a few white cells (Fig. 4D). The triglyceride content will be very high; however, the protein level will be less than 1.5 g. Teleologically, pericardium is equated to a large lymphatic channel and lymphangiography with three-dimensional CT could help in video-assisted correction.[20,21]

Pericardial Tamponade

Pericardial tamponade is a medical emergency, characterized by hypotension, sweating and the patient often goes into shock. The characteristic paradoxical pulse

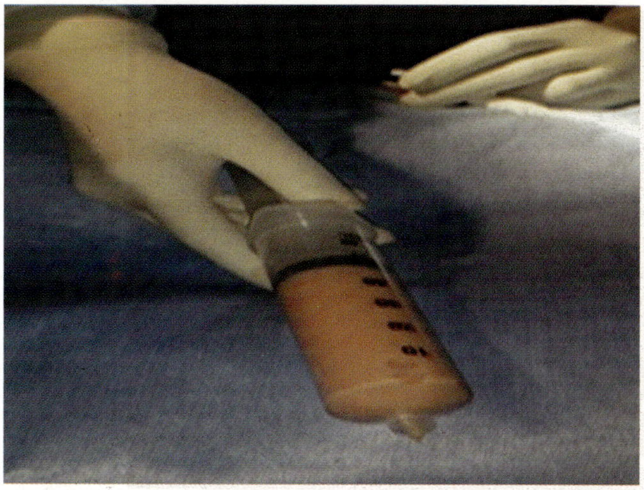

Fig. 5: Chylous pericardial effusion. Milky white aspirate from the pericardial cavity in chylous pericardial effusion.

and abnormal jugular pulse may be diagnostic. Figures 6A and B illustrate the Doppler evidence for decline in pulse pressure velocity with inspiration and inspiratory distension of inferior vena cava. Urgent echocardiography in emergency room will clarify the diagnosis and immediate treatment can be instituted.[22-24]

ECHOCARDIOGRAPHIC FINDINGS IN PERICARDIAL TAMPONADE

Since diastolic pressures of right heart are lower than the left, RA and RV are the first chambers to exhibit evidence of raised intrapericardial pressure. Inversion of RA wall during atrial systole and right ventricle outflow tract compression during diastole are the earliest sign of pericardial tamponade.[25] Right ventricle is the next chamber to get compressed.[26] Left ventricular compression could occur in localized pericardial effusion or when the right ventricle is more hypertrophied in subjects with severe pulmonary hypertension.[27,28] When there is hypovolemia or in acute situations even minimal accumulation of fluid will result in tamponade physiology when fluid resuscitation and echo-guided pericardiocentesis is life-saving (Figs. 7A and B).[29]

Right Atrial and Right Ventricle Inversion

Right atrial could be seen collapsing during ventricular systole.[30] This RA inversion lasting for more than one-third of ventricular systole has sensitivity of 94% and specificity of 100% for the diagnosis of tamponade (Fig. 8).[10] This sign can be best detected in apical four-chamber view, subcostal four-chamber view, and parasternal short-axis view at the level of great vessels.[6]

Right Atrial Inversion Time Index

It is calculated as the number of frames during which RA is inverted and divided by the number of frames per cardiac cycle. Index value of 0.33 is associated with clinical evidence of pericardial tamponade. This index has 95% sensitivity and 100% specificity.[30]

Right Ventricular Diastolic Inversion

Diastolic collapse or inversion of the RV free wall is a more specific sign of tamponade and can be appreciated both on

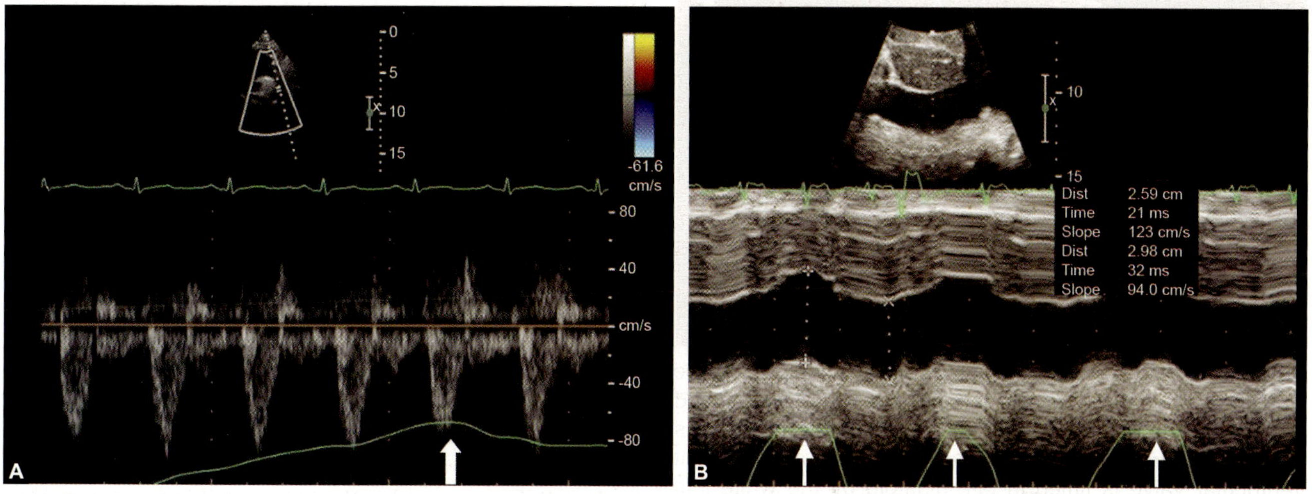

Figs. 6A and B: Echocardiographic illustration of Kussumaul's sign, the vertical broad arrows point to peak inspiration in respirometer. (A) Doppler echo of descending aortic flow from suprasternal window shows declining velocity in peak inspiration and sinus tachycardia @ 116/mt. (B) Shows M-mode echocardiography of inferior vena cava, recorded at slow speed, shows plethora and inspiratory expansion, since the increased inspiratory venous return is no longer accommodated by the heart which is under high pressure compression by the pericardial fluid.

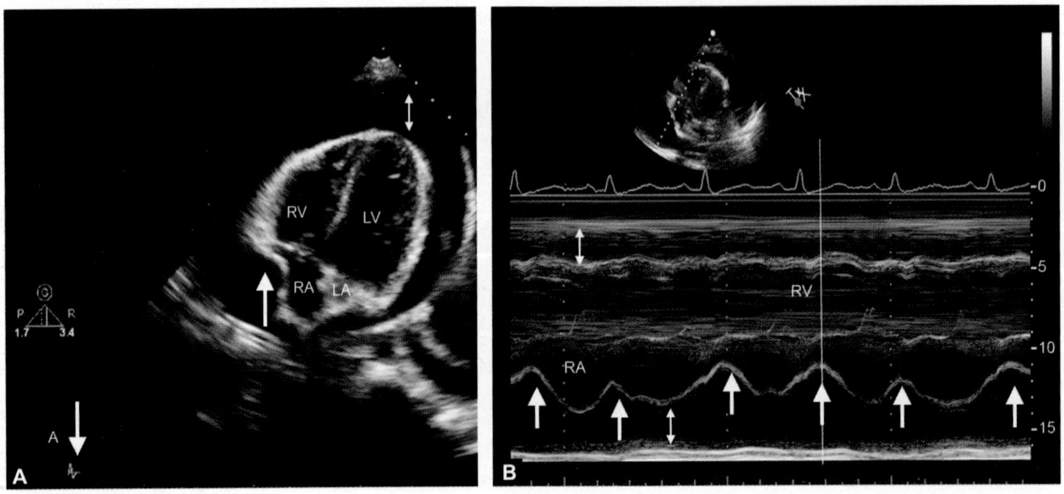

Figs. 7A and B: Systolic inversion of right atrium shown by two-dimensional, (A) and M-mode echocardiography, (B) Vertical upward arrows show the inversion of the right atrial free wall, double headed arrows show the pericardial effusion. Systole in marked by the electrocardiographic ST segment and closed atrioventricular valves in the apical four-chamber view. The RV inversion index, the number of cycles with inversion divided by the total QRS complex in the M-mode panel is 100%. Vertical downward arrow in (B) denotes diastolic right ventricular collapse. (LA: left atrium; LV: left ventricle; RA: right atrium; RV: right ventricle).

2D and M-mode imaging (Fig. 8). Right ventricular outflow tract (RVOT) with its thin wall is the most compressible area of RV and is the first one to collapse. This is best appreciated in the parasternal long-axis view (PLAX view) and short-axis views (PSAX), with a sensitivity of 82–94% and specificity of 88–100%.[23,26,30]

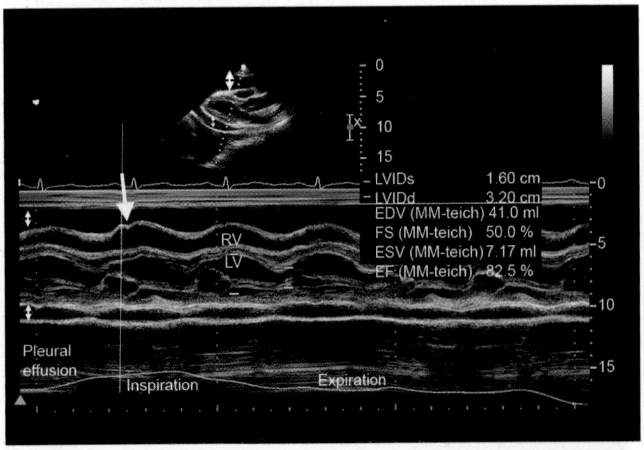

Fig. 8: Diastolic inversion of the right ventricular outflow, specific sign of cardiac tamponade is illustrated by arrow. A high-speed M-mode recording at the mitral valve level with simultaneous electrocardiogram and respirometer. Dip in the anterior right ventricular valve is timed in late diastole by the white line correlating with the electrocardiogram and open mitral valve. Note the sinus tachycardia of 117/mt, good ejection fraction, 2 cm anterior and 1 cm posterior pericardial effusion, (double headed arrows) 4 cm posterior pleural effusion, smaller cardiac chamber dimensions in expiration.

Swinging Heart

Detection of swinging heart is a marker of massive pericardial effusion in which all the cardiac chambers are free to float within the pericardial space in a phasic manner. This sign may not always indicate the presence of pericardial tamponade.[11]

Inferior Vena Cava Plethora

Dilatation of inferior vena cava with reduced inspiratory collapse is another useful sign of cardiac tamponade.[31] A dilated inferior vena cava with less than 50% inspiratory reduction in diameter near IVC-RA junction, is a nonspecific sign of tamponade.[32]

Doppler Findings

Normally mitral inflow varies by 15% or less with respiration and tricuspid inflow by 25% or less. Variation in peak velocity in aortic and pulmonary flow profiles is normally less than 10%. In presence of tamponade, exaggerated ventricular interdependence develops as illustrated in Figures 9A and B. Respiratory variation in filling is exaggerated and inspiration produces a significant decrease in left-sided filling. Accordingly, mitral and aortic the flow is reduced by more than 40%. Tricuspid inflow velocities are easily demonstrable in presence of pericardial tamponade. There is a striking exaggeration inflow velocities and the "E" waves may be more prominent when compared to "E" wave in expiration. An inspiratory increase in velocity of 40% from expiratory velocity is diagnostic of tamponade.[33]

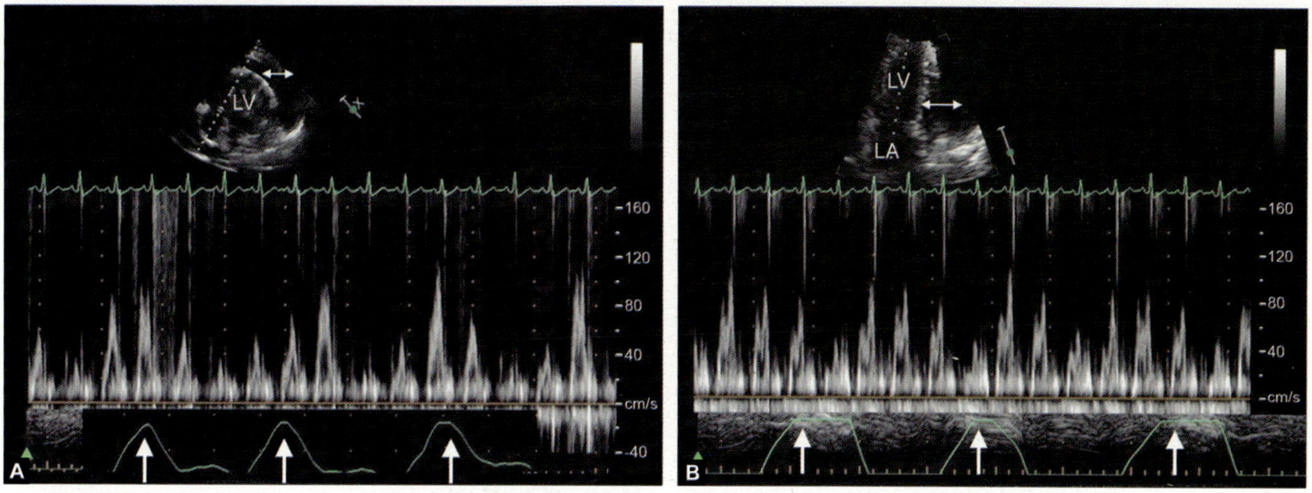

Figs. 9A and B: Exaggerated variation in ventricular inflow velocities in inspiration across the left atrioventricular valve, (A) and in expiration across the right atrioventricular valve, (B) in a subject admitted in cardiac tamponade. Vertical upward arrows show the inspiratory phase of respiration trace, and double-headed horizontal arrow shows the pericardial effusion. (LV: left ventricle; LA: left atrium)

Low Pressure Tamponade (Cheshire Cat Tamponade)

In certain clinical settings such as hypovolemia may lead to end-diastolic collapse of RA, RV, and rarely LA and even LV. These patients will not have any other clinical sign of pericardial tamponade, but echocardiographic signs may show the presence of pericardial tamponade.[34] Correction of dehydration will make all the signs of pericardial tamponade disappear.[35] This type of echocardiographic picture of tamponade mainly seen in the emergency room is like the Cheshire Cat, a fictional cat popularized in the novel "Alice Adventures in Wonderland" is known for its mischievous grin, the whiskers and the bright eyes (Cheshire cat tamponade term contributed by G Vijayaraghavan).

Loculated Effusion

Diagnosing loculated effusion is important because of hemodynamic compromise that can occur with even small, strategically located fluid collection especially in the postoperative or post traumatic intensive care units.[36] Echocardiography is crucial in both the situations where both clinical and imaging presentations are atypical. It is always difficult to explore loculated effusions and in such situations modified apical, subcostal, and posterior views are useful in confirming the diagnosis. Postoperative cardiac tamponade may be suspected in the presence of loculated effusions along the right atrium and /or along its junction with superior vena cava, with left atrial, or biatrial compression. When in doubt, or if the precordial echo windows are not accessible, proceed with Transesophageal or intracardiac echocardiography.[37,38] Pericardial effusions are usually more common with valve replacement surgery than coronary artery bypass grafting. After valve replacement surgery, diffuse fluid accumulations were more common than loculated effusions. After coronary artery bypass grafting, loculated effusions are more common. In conditions where pericardial tamponade is strongly suspected and transthoracic echocardiography does not provide complete imaging of the pericardial sac transesophageal echocardiography (TEE) should be considered.[39,40]

RECOMMENDATIONS: ESC 2015 GUIDELINES[6]

- TTE is recommended in all patients with suspected pericardial effusion—class I, LOE-C
- Admission is recommended for high-risk patients with pericardial effusion—class I, LOE-C.
- In patient with clinical suspicion of cardiac tamponade, echocardiography is recommended as the first imaging technique to evaluate the size, location and degree of hemodynamic impact of the pericardial effusion—class I, LOE-C.
- A judicious clinical evaluation including echocardiographic finding is recommended to treat cardiac tamponade—Class I, LOE-C.
- Pericardiocentesis or cardiac surgery is indicated for cardiac tamponade or for symptomatic moderate-to-large pericardial effusion not responsive to medical therapy, and for suspicion of unknown bacterial or neoplastic etiology—Class I, LOE-C.

LIMITATIONS

Bedside echocardiography is the most sensitive and specific tool to identify and understand the pathophysiology of a pericardial collection. Limitation set by the poor echo or inaccessible echo window in the intensive care unit or theater, is now overcome by transesophageal echo Doppler techniques.

PROGNOSIS AND MANAGEMENT OF PERICARDIAL EFFUSION

Prognosis depends on the size and the rate of fluid accumulation. Moderate-to-large effusions are more common in conditions such as neoplastic, bacterial, or related to a systemic inflammatory disease.[9] For idiopathic moderate effusions, an appropriate timing for echocardiographic follow-up may be an echocardiogram every 6 months. For a severe effusion, an echocardiographic follow-up may be necessary every 3–6 months. Asymptomatic small pericardial effusion may be left alone with follow-up imaging. Managing chylous pericardial effusion is challenging.[21] Recurrence of pericardial effusion in spite of repeated pericardiocentesis, with episodes of tamponade will it make imperative that definitive surgical procedure is warranted? Pericardial aspirations or pericardial window may result in progressive cachexia and wasting. Thoracic duct ligation or creating adhesions by injecting irritant drugs are the only definitive treatment in many patients.[41,42]

Early diagnosis and treatment of all patients with suspected tamponade represents an important clinical goal. Once diagnosis is confirmed, decompression by safe, simple, and rapid method is required.[10] The treatment of choice is drainage of pericardial fluid, preferably by needle paracentesis, or by inserting a pigtail catheter into the pericardial cavity. Echocardiography or fluoroscopy or CT should guide the operator. Transient left ventricular dysfunction is also reported after pericardiocentesis.[43] Mortality rates from blind pericardiocentesis had complications ranging from 6% to 70% and mortality of up to 6%. Drainage may be performed in catheterization laboratory when the diagnosis is uncertain. Pericardial effusions with echocardiographic evidence of tamponade are usually treated with echo-guided pericardiocentesis because the balance of risks and benefits generally in favor of drainage. Echo-guided pericardiocentesis is simple, safe, and very effective in removing the fluid.[6]

COMPLICATIONS OF PERICARDIOCENTESIS

- Inadvertent puncture of a coronary artery, right ventricle, or liver
- Hemopericardium, hemoperitoneum
- Liver hematoma
- Air embolism
- Right ventricle pseudoaneurysm.

CONCLUSION

Echocardiographic imaging is a simple bedside procedure and has contributed substantially to our understanding of pericardial pathology. It is useful in the diagnosis, assessment, and treatment of pericardial effusion. One should concentrate not only on the size of pericardial effusion but also on pericardial pathology and the hemodynamics, which could be delineated in most subjects.

REFERENCES

1. Hoit BD. Pathophysiology of the Pericardium. Prog Cardiovasc Dis. 2017;59(4):341-8.
2. Gowani SA, Danielian A, Villaneuva J, et al. Large pleural effusions causing cardiac tamponade: a case report and review of the literature. Conn Med. 2014;78(3):149-52.
3. Spodick DH. The normal and diseased pericardium: current concepts of pericardial physiology, diagnosis and treatment. J Am Coll Cardiol. 1983;1(1):240-51.
4. Shabetai R. Function of the normal pericardium. Clin Cardiol. 1999;22(1 Suppl 1):I4-5.
5. Jaworska-Wilczynska M, Trzaskoma P, Szczepankiewicz AA, et al. Pericardium: structure and function in health and disease. Folia Histochem Cytobiol. 2016;54(3):121-5.
6. Adler Y, Charron P, Imazio M, et al. 2015 ESC Guidelines for the Diagnosis and Management of Pericardial Diseases. Rev Esp Cardiol (Engl Ed). 2015;68(12):1126.
7. Xu B, Harb SC, Cremer PC. New Insights into Pericarditis: Mechanisms of Injury and Therapeutic Targets. Curr Cardiol Rep. 2017;19(7):60.
8. Shabetai R. Pericardial effusion: hemodynamic spectrum. Heart. 2004;90(3):255-6.
9. Imazio M, Gaido L, Battaglia A, et al. Contemporary management of pericardial effusion: practical aspects for clinical practice. Postgrad Med. 2017;129(2):178-86.
10. Klein AL, Abbara S, Agler DA, et al. American Society of Echocardiography clinical recommendations for multimodality cardiovascular imaging of patients with pericardial disease: Endorsed by the Society for Cardiovascular Magnetic Resonance and Society of Cardiovascular Computed Tomography. J Am Soc Echocardiogr. 2013;26(9):965-1012.e15.
11. Ambardekar AV, Krantz MJ. Medical images. Flip-flop heart. Mayo Clin Proc. 2010;85(1):103.
12. D'Cruz IA, Constantine A. Problems and pitfalls in the echocardiographic assessment of pericardial effusion. Echocardiography. 1993;10(2):151-66.
13. Gunasegaran K, Yao J, De Castro S, et al. Large Pericardial Effusions. Curr Treat Options Cardiovasc Med. 2000;2(4):357-64.
14. Imazio M, Gaita F. Diagnosis and treatment of pericarditis. Heart. 2015;101(14):1159-68.

15. Imazio M, Gaita F. Acute and Recurrent Pericarditis. Cardiol Clin. 2017;35(4):505-13.
16. Lee KS, Kronbichler A, Eisenhut M, et al. Cardiovascular involvement in systemic rheumatic diseases: An integrated view for the treating physicians. Autoimmun Rev. 2018;17(3):201-14.
17. Vandecasteele EH, De Pauw M, Brusselle G, et al. The heart and pulmonary arterial hypertension in systemic sclerosis. Acta Clin Belg. 2016;71(1):1-18.
18. Lippmann M, Gupta K. Chylous pericardial effusion resulting in cardiac tamponade. Indian Heart J. 2016;68 (Suppl 2):S161-2.
19. Alsmady MM, Aladaileh MA, Al-Zaben K, et al. Chylopericardium presenting as cardiac tamponade secondary to mediastinal lymphangioma. Ann R Coll Surg Engl. 2016;98(8):e154-6.
20. Cerra MC, Amelio D, Tavolaro P, et al. Pericardium of the frog, Rana esculenta, is morphologically designed as a lymphatic space. J Morphol. 2003;257(1):72-7.
21. Rosa GM, Campisi C, Bioccardo F, et al. Chylopericardium: a case report demonstrating utility of lymphography combined with 3D computed tomography for corrective surgical treatment using VATS. Lymphology. 2014;47(1):40-3.
22. Kronzon I, Cohen ML, Winer HE. Contribution of echocardiography to the understanding of the pathophysiology of cardiac tamponade. J Am Coll Cardiol. 1983;1(4):1180-2.
23. Argulian E, Messerli F. Misconceptions and facts about pericardial effusion and tamponade. Am J Med. 2013;126(10):858-61.
24. Pérez-Casares A, Cesar S, Brunet-Garcia L, et al. Echocardiographic evaluation of pericardial effusion and cardiac tamponade. Front Pediatr. 2017;5:79.
25. Gillam LD, Guyer DE, Gibson TC, et al. Hydrodynamic compression of the right atrium: a new echocardiographic sign of cardiac tamponade. Circulation. 1983;68(2):294-301.
26. Fast J, Wielenga RP, Jansen E, et al. Abnormal wall movements of the right ventricle and both atria in patients with pericardial effusion as indicators of cardiac tamponade. Eur Heart J. 1986;7(5):431-6.
27. Gollapudi RR, Yeager M, Johnson AD. Left ventricular cardiac tamponade in the setting of cor pulmonale and circumferential pericardial effusion. Case Report and Review of the Literature. Cardiol Rev. 2005;13(4):214-7.
28. Chuttani K, Pandian NG, Mohanty PK, et al. Left ventricular diastolic collapse. An echocardiographic sign of regional cardiac tamponade. Circulation. 1991;83(6):1999-2006.
29. Tsang TS, Freeman WK, Barnes ME, et al. Rescue echocardiographically guided pericardiocentesis for cardiac perforation complicating catheter-based procedures. The Mayo Clinic experience. J Am Coll Cardiol. 1998;32(5):1345-50.
30. Kearns MJ, Walley KR. Tamponade: Hemodynamic and Echocardiographic Diagnosis. Chest. 2018;153(5):1266-75.
31. Fowler NO. Inferior vena cava plethora as an echocardiography sign of cardiac tamponade. J Am Coll Cardiol. 19881;12(6):1478-9.
32. Stone MB, Huang JV. Inferior Vena Cava Assessment: Correlation with CVP and Plethora in Tamponade. Glob Heart. 2013;8(4):323-7.
33. Shaver JA, Reddy PS, Curtiss EI, et al. Noninvasive/invasive correlates of exaggerated ventricular interdependence in cardiac tamponade. J Cardiol. 2001;37 (Suppl 1):71-6.
34. Restrepo JA, Martinis G, Diego G, et al. Low-pressure cardiac tamponade: A case report. J Cardiol Cases. 2016;14(1):8-10.
35. Sagristà-Sauleda J, Angel J, Sambola A, et al. Low-Pressure Cardiac Tamponade: Clinical and Hemodynamic Profile. Circulation. 2006;114(9):945-52.
36. Syros G, Maysky M. High-Pressure Loculated Pericardial Effusion in Postpericardiotomy Syndrome. Circulation. 2012;125(21):2677-8.
37. Berge KH, Lanier WL, Reeder GS. Occult cardiac tamponade detected by transesophageal echocardiography. Mayo Clin Proc. 1992;67(7):667-70.
38. Weintraub AR, Schwartz SL, Smith J, et al. Intracardiac two-dimensional echocardiography in patients with pericardial effusion and cardiac tamponade. J Am Soc Echocardiogr. 1991;4(6):571-6.
39. Kronzon I, Tunick PA, Freedberg RS. Transesophageal echocardiography in pericardial disease and tamponade. Echocardiography. 1994;11(5):493-505.
40. Saito Y, Donohue A, Attai S, et al. The syndrome of cardiac tamponade with "small" pericardial effusion. Echocardiography. 2008;25(3):321-7.
41. Nath DS, Savla J, Khemani RG, et al. Thoracic Duct Ligation for Persistent Chylothorax After Pediatric Cardiothoracic Surgery. Ann Thorac Surg. 2009;88(1):246-52.
42. Maruyama R, Yokoyama H, Seto T, et al. Catheter drainage followed by the instillation of bleomycin to manage malignant pericardial effusion in nonsmall cell lung cancer: a multi-institutional phase II trial. J Thorac Oncol. 2007;2(1):65-8.
43. Belluschi I, Cioni M, Moriggia S, et al. Takotsubo Cardiomyopathy Following Pericardiocentesis After Aortic Valve Repair and Ascending Aorta Replacement. Ann Thorac Surg. 2016;102(4):e291-3.

91

CHAPTER

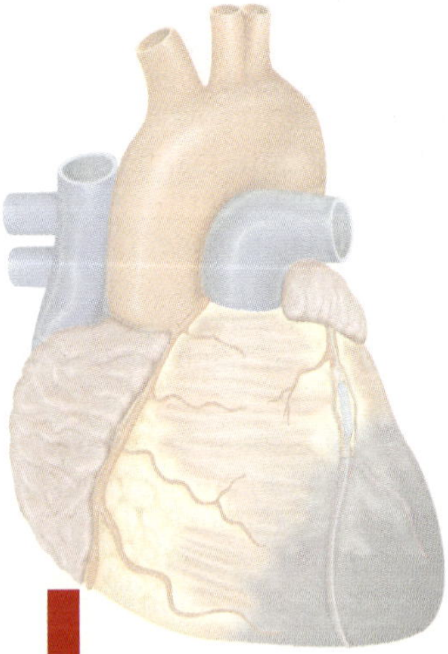

Echocardiographic Advances in Evaluation of Cardiac Tamponade

S Shanmugasundaram, U Ilayaraja, K Rajeswari

INTRODUCTION

Pericardium assumes importance only when it is diseased. Though it is claimed to possess certain physiological functions, absence of pericardium (congenital or postsurgical) is compatible with normal performance of the heart. Apart from providing a lubricating insulation for the heart and acting as a barrier against invasion of organisms, pericardium limits excessive distension of heart in case of acute overload states and modulates ventricular interaction. It has an inelastic, relatively thicker external layer called parietal pericardium which is rich in collagen with few elastic fibers and an inner serosal layer which is a thin layer of fibrous tissue lined by mesothelium. Serosal layer has a visceral component adherent over the underlying myocardium and a parietal component adherent with the fibrous layer.[1] There is a potential space between the parietal and the visceral layer which normally has minimal fluid, often not exceeding 20–50 mL. Excessive fluid accumulation in the pericardial cavity may be in the form of a transudate due to defective clearance by lymphatics as a result of elevated systemic venous pressure typical of heart failure or an exudate due to infective, inflammatory or malignant diseases. Progressive accumulation of fluid can increase the intrapericardial pressure (IPP) which eventually leads to restriction of ventricular filling. Cardiac tamponade is a form of compressive disorder of the heart, wherein accumulation of fluid, blood, pus or gas or a combination any of these would result in extrinsic compression on the cardiac chambers leading to progressive limitation of filling of heart. The other form of compressive disorder of the heart is constrictive pericarditis, wherein thick adherent inelastic layers of the pericardium cause impediment to cardiac filling. In between tamponade and constriction, there may be some intermediate compressive syndromes like effusive constrictive pericarditis and subacute elastic compression of the heart, which share the hemodynamic features of both tamponade and constriction, either simultaneously or sequentially. Cardiac tamponade is a medical emergency and failure to provide timely relief by pericardial aspiration may lead to cardiovascular collapse and death. An astute physician can make a bedside diagnosis but only when the altered hemodynamics is quite advanced. Because of its inexpensiveness, widespread availability, easy accessibility and portability, Echocardiography plays a cardinal role in early and rapid diagnosis and appropriate management of pericardial diseases including tamponade. Historically, the initial attempts of echocardiography to diagnose cardiac diseases were performed for mitral valve diseases and pericardial disease. It is not an exaggeration to say that echocardiography has improved our understanding of hemodynamics of pericardial diseases over the last many years. What was an abstract postulation in the past and what was based on experimental animal studies in the previous years, became an easily understood scientific fact with the bedside usage of two-dimensional (2D) and Doppler echocardiography in the present era.

PHYSIOLOGY OF TAMPONADE

Despite many advances in our understanding of physiology of pericardium in health and disease, based on numerous clinical and experimental studies, it still remains elusive and complex. The complexities start with the most basic question of what is normal intrapericardial pressure. There is a difference between the pericardial pressure recorded by a needle or catheter attached to fluid filled system (called as fluid pressure) and that is recorded by a flat balloon (contact pressure). The fluid pressure reflects the hydrostatic pressure and it corresponds to the intrapleural pressure, i.e. -2 to -3 mm Hg in expiration and -5 to -6 mm Hg in inspiration. In contrast, the contact pressure is the pressure exerted on the surface (surface pressure) that closely follows the right atrial (RA) pressure and may be little less than that. It tends to remain positive throughout the respiratory cycle, less positive in inspiration (say + 2 mm Hg) and more positive in expiration (say + 6 mm Hg). It is argued that the pericardial cavity is just a potential space and pressure recording by flat balloon is the best way to know the true pressure. It may be true in the absence of fluid or with little fluid (say 20–30 mL). However with pathological fluid accumulation, there is no difference of IPP obtained by these two methods.[2] Though the absolute values of normal IPP differ between the two techniques, the noncontroversial fact is that there is a gradient of pressure between the ventricles and the pericardial cavity in diastole—the transmural gradient that allows the ventricle to fill optimally. When the ventricular filling (distension) reaches the pericardial limits, the transmural gradient becomes 0 and no further filling occurs. When progressive accumulation of fluid increases the intrapericardial pressure, the transmural gradient decreases and gets reversed at one point of time. Since at this stage, IPP is more than the chamber pressure, compression of ventricles occurs in diastole with reduction of ventricular filling. Since right ventricular (RV) is thin-walled and more compliant with the resultant lower filling pressures, right heart chambers get compressed initially. IPP and RV filling pressures continue to increase further and match up with the left heart filling pressures. At this stage, the typical hemodynamic abnormality manifests, namely elevation and equalization of pressures in the cardiac chambers and pericardial cavity in diastole. Decline in stroke volume is compensated by increase in peripheral arterial resistance and an increase in heart rate in an attempt to maintain cardiac output and adequate tissue perfusion. At extremes, near total compression of the heart impairs diastolic filling totally which may finally lead on to bradycardia, hypotension and cardiovascular collapse. Previously, it was believed that cardiac tamponade is an all or none phenomenon and when it occurs, it does so abruptly. Such a definition was adopted because frank clinical expression of tamponade in the form of pulsus paradoxus and elevated jugular venous pressure was required to diagnose tamponade. However, if one accepts that any form of hemodynamic alteration caused by the compressive effect of pericardial fluid indicates tamponade then it is more appropriate to consider cardiac tamponade as a continuum (Fig. 1). In stage 0, pericardial fluid accumulates without increase in IPP. In stage 1, IPP is increased but is still less than right heart filling pressures. In stage 2, IPP increases further and approaches right heart filling pressures. In stage 3, IPP is more than that of right heart filling pressures, but still lesser than left heart filling pressures. In stage 4, IPP and right heart filling pressures increase further to reach left heart filling pressures. It is very likely that in stage 1 itself, the earliest echocardiographic sign namely flow paradoxus may manifest. Further in stage 1, cardiac output starts declining, but marginally. In stage 2, RA and RV collapse may manifest and cardiac output may decline further. Even in this early stage, inspiratory reduction of arterial pressure starts occurring but not to the arbitrary level of definition, i.e. more than 10 mm Hg drop in pressure in inspiration. The reduction of cardiac output and inspiratory reduction of arterial pressure continue to worsen

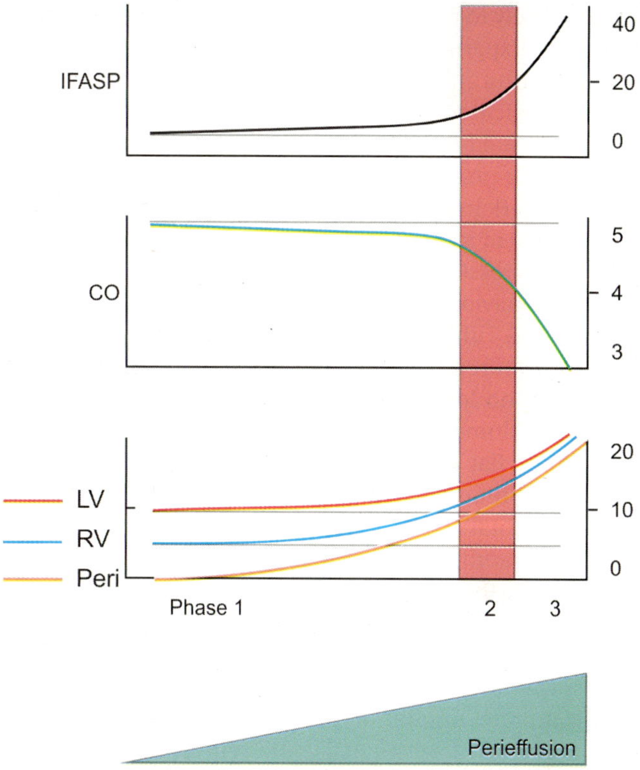

Fig. 1: Cardiac tamponade viewed as a continuum. Note pulsus paradoxus and decline in cardiac output occurring gradually from stage 1. Conventionally defined tamponade occurs in stage 3.

progressively to reach the levels of conventional definition at stage 4. Experimental animal studies and hemodynamic studies in humans during pericardial aspiration have clearly indicated that cardiac output starts decreasing before elevated right heart pressures reach the level of left heart filling pressures and well before pulsus paradoxus manifests. Echocardiography thus helps in diagnosing tamponade in its early stages itself, much before the frank clinical expression manifests.

The behavior of the pericardium is somewhat similar to that of a rubber band which when stretched yields with little force initially and when the elastic limit is reached it no longer yields despite maximum force. The pressure volume relationship of pericardium is nonlinear, it is nearly flat at lower volumes and hence increase in pericardial fluid volume occurs initially at the expense of no or minimal increase in pressure. Once the reserve is exhausted, addition of even little amount of fluid increases the pressure to much greater levels, as the pressure volume curve becomes steeper at this point (Fig. 2). Hence at this maximal reserve volume, addition of even a drop of fluid may markedly increase the pressure and similarly letting out even little amount of fluid brings down the pressure to much lower levels quickly and relieves tamponade—the last drop phenomenon. Because the pericardium is noncompliant, IPP rises steeply with rapid accumulation of as little as 150–200 mL of fluid. The usual causes for such rapid collection of fluid in pericardial cavity are iatrogenic [during invasive procedures like percutaneous transluminal coronary angioplasty (PTCA), percutaneous transvenous mitral commissurotomy (PTMC)], dissection and trauma. Because of the nature of causes and the need for early surgical intervention, they are grouped under the category of surgical tamponade. When the fluid accumulates slowly over weeks and months, as in viral or idiopathic pericarditis, tuberculosis, malignancy, etc., the pericardium has enough time to stretch itself slowly so that IPP does not increase with accumulation of much larger volumes of fluid, as much as 1–2 liters. Once the pericardial stretch capacity reaches its maximal values, IPP increases to cause tamponade. This category is called as medical tamponade. In the hemodynamic sense, the pressure volume curve is shifted to right in such slowly accumulating effusions.

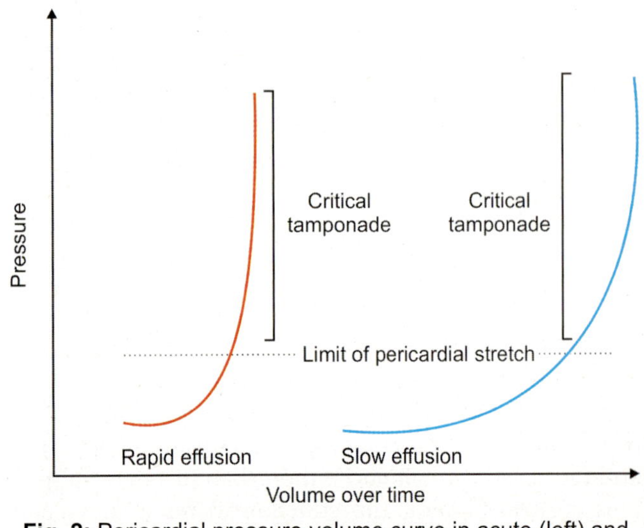

Fig. 2: Pericardial pressure volume curve in acute (left) and chronic (right) tamponade.

Pericardial recesses and sinuses provide the initial reserve volume for the pericardium. Ventricular filling in normal individuals occurs without increase in intrapericardial pressure because of this reserve volume. During inspiration, when right heart filling is increased, the physiological fluid gets redistributed to these reserve spaces, thereby allowing the pricardium to accommodate the increased intracardiac volume without restraint. Similarly, small pathological effusions that collect in the main pericardial cavity may also use this reserve volume during diastole and hence the normal transmural pressure gradient is preserved. In the next phase of adaptation, the wavy collagen in parietal pericardium straighten out to increase the pericardial volume thereby accommodating some more fluid without increase in pressure. In the final stage of accommodation, the pericardium has to undergo "creep" phenomenon, by which new connective tissue develops and increases the elasticity of pericardium.

When the IPP equals or exceeds the intra cardiac pressure, the total cardiac volume (pericardial + intracardiac) becomes fixed. In a noncompliant (maximally stretched) pericardial sac, the cardiac chambers tend to compete with pericardial fluid. Hence, the ventricular interaction becomes more pronounced when the expected respirophasic changes occur in the ventricular volumes. Augmentation of ventricular volume on one side tends to occur at the expense of reduction of volume of the contralateral ventricle. Thus, the ventricular filling becomes reciprocal and is achieved by shift of the ventricular septum.

ECHOCARDIOGRAPHIC FEATURES OF TAMPONADE

Progressively increasing intrapericardial pressure due to the accumulating fluid initially approximates with the RV filling pressures both of which may continue to increase to approximate with the left ventricular (LV) filling pressures. The transmural filling pressures in the ventrices initially decrease and finally get reversed. The reversed transmural pressures result in compression of cardiac chambers, which could be recognized by echocardiography. Moreover, transmission of respiration induced fluctuations of intrathoracic pressure to the cardiac chambers alters the filling pattern of the ventricles. These hemodynamic alterations result in characteristic changes in 2D and Doppler echocardiography which help the clinician to diagnose tamponade with reasonable accuracy. Standard views of 2D echocardiography should be used to assess pericardial effusion and its hemodynamic consequences. Parasternal long-axis, short-axis, apical 4-chamber (A4C) and subcostal imaging should be done for all patients, except in postoperative cardiac surgery patients in whom the imaging has to be restricted to subcostal and A4C views or nonconventional windows. The comprehensive assessment of pericardial effusion should be done in terms of rough quantification of fluid, identification of nature of fluid, distribution of fluid in the pericardial cavity, whether it is uniform or loculated and finally the hemodynamic consequences. When fluid accumulates in the pericardial cavity, the parietal pericardium and visceral pericardium separate out with echo free space in between. Rough quantification may be done as follows: (1) negligible—when pericardial separation is seen only in systole (may be normal fluid in the pericardium); (2) minimal—when the pericardial layers are separated throughout the cardiac cycle and maximal fluid width in diastole is less than 5 mm (roughly equivalent to a volume of 50–100 mL); (3) small if it is 5–10 mm (100–250 mL); moderate if it is 10–20 mm (250–500 mL) and (4) large when it is more than 20 mm (>500 mL) (Fig. 3). Quantification of fluid is an important step in evaluation of patients with pericardial effusion as the amount of pericardial effusion turned out to be the best predictor of prognosis when compared to other echo variables in a study[3] and nearly one-third with large effusion may develop tamponade sooner or later. The quantity may also give a clue about the possible etiology. Small effusions are likely to be viral or idiopathic; moderate effusions occur in a variety of medical conditions; large effusions are mostly due to tuberculosis, neoplasm or hypothyroidism.

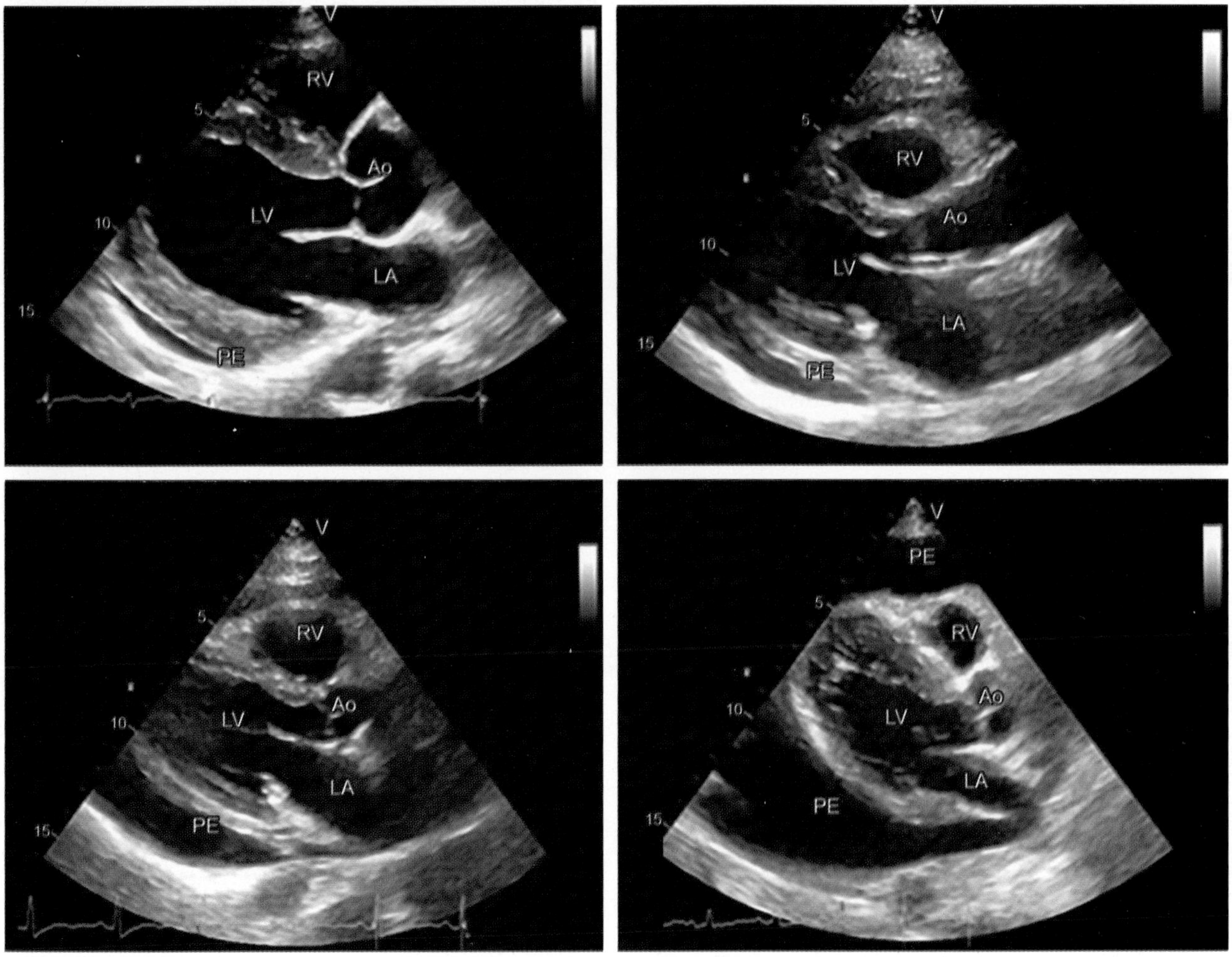

Fig. 3: Pericardial effusion of varying severity.

Though the diagnosis of pericardial effusion is straightforward, certain conditions may pose diagnostic challenge. A large left-sided pleural effusion may give an appearance suggestive of fluid behind the LV posterior wall. In pericardial effusion, quantity will be more toward LV apex and less toward left atrium (LA) and fluid behind LA is uncommon. Moreover, descending aorta in cross-section will be posterior to the fluid in pericardial effusion in parasternal long-axis view and will be anterior to the fluid in pleural effusion. In pleural effusion, the quantity is likely to be more toward LA and less toward cardiac apex and fluid behind LA is commonly seen. Absence of fluid anteriorly may also suggest pleural effusion. Certain other conditions that present with echo free spaces like aneurysm of LA appendage, submitral aneurysms and hydatid cyst should be considered if echo appearances are not typical. Large epicardial pad of fat may mimic pericardial fluid but it is likely to be located anterior to RV alone. In case of adiposus cordis, where thick pad fat is present all around, computed tomography (CT) or magnetic resonance (MR) imaging will be of help to make the differentiation. Moreover, total echolucency is not a feature of fat in the pericardium. If the echo free space is clear with no added echogenicity on the epicardium or parietal pericardium, the fluid is likely to be serous—either a transudate or an exudate with less fibrin content. If there are fimbriae like structures extending from epicardium or if there is echo dense layer over epicardium or parietal pericardium it is serofibrinous exudative effusion, which may occur with tuberculous, idiopathic or viral pericardial effusion, connective tissue disorders, uremia, etc. (Fig. 4). Abundant fibrinous strands, particularly thicker ones, frond like masses, strands crossing the pericardial cavity (Fig. 5), fibrinous coating and thick deposits and thickened pericardium are encountered more frequently with tuberculous rather than viral or idiopathic effusions.[4] Pyopericardium is notorious to have numerous such strands crossing the pericardial cavity, giving rise to a vivid sunray appearance. At times tumor deposits over the epicardium with infiltration of adjacent myocardium may be identified (Fig. 6). Blood in the pericardium (as in iatrogenic or traumatic effusions) may also give rise to turbid fluid in the pericardial cavity which may exhibit swirling echoes of autocontrast or slow snake like movement of echoes in the pericardial cavity. A localized organizing hematoma, may take the shape of a mass and could cause symptoms and signs of tamponade. If the fluid is distributed all around with most of the fluid in the dependent position (maximal amount of fluid behind posterior wall of LV and least amount anteriorly, in supine posture), there is free fluid in the cavity. If the fluid accumulation is in pockets of different sizes and shoes or when the fluid appears maximal

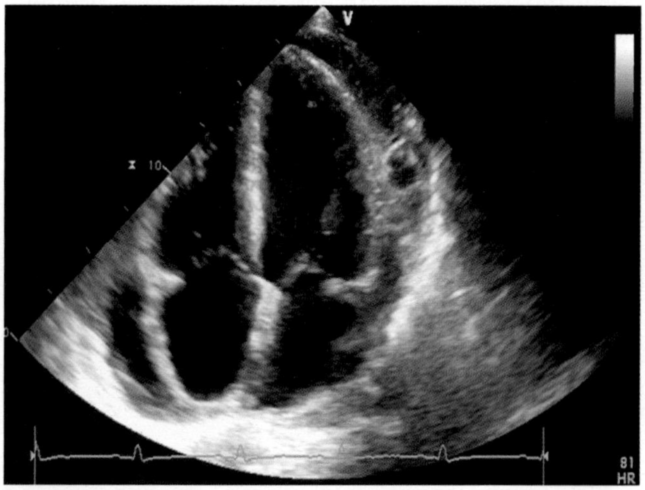

Fig. 5: Fibrinous strands extending from LV lateral wall.

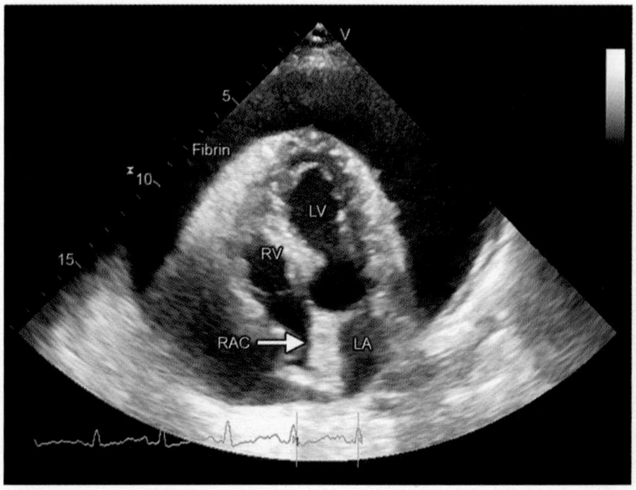

Fig. 4: Fibrin deposits over RV free wall.

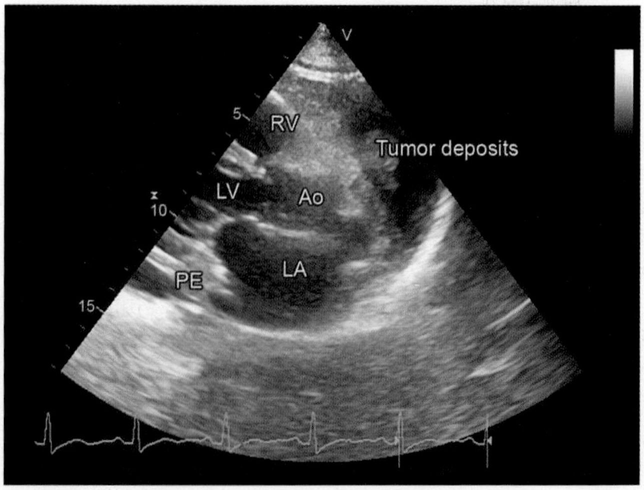

Fig. 6: Tumor deposits in malignant effusion.

anteriorly and less posteriorly, one may consider loculation. The hemodynamic consequences of tamponade result in the following echocardiographic findings that help the clinician to diagnose this condition early in the disease process. The echocardiographic features of tamponade can be made out in 2D echo in the form of: (1) RA and RV collapse; (2) reduction of the size of ventricles and reciprocal filling (RV size increases in inspiration with simultaneous decrease of LV dimension; the reverse happens in expiration) and (3) inferior vena cava (IVC) plethora. Doppler echo may reveal: (1) marked respiratory variation of mitral and tricuspid velocities; (2) predominant systolic flow in systemic and pulmonary veins with expiratory decrease or reversal of flow in diastole in systemic veins and inspiratory reduction or reversal of diastolic flow in pulmonary veins and (3) inspiratory augmentation of pulmonary flow with simultaneous decrease of aortic flow.

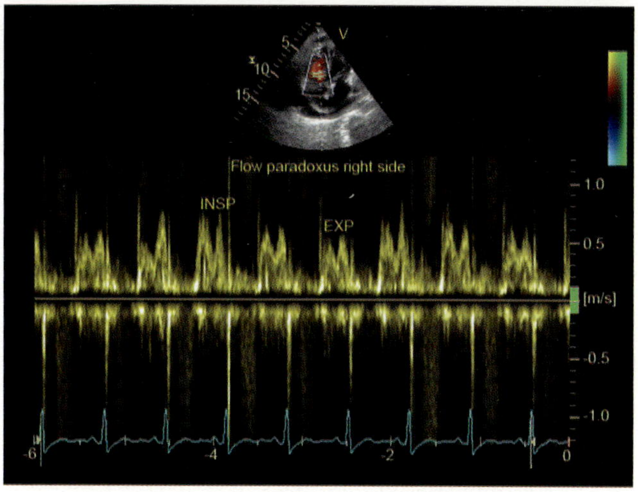

Fig. 7: Flow paradoxus across tricuspid valve.

Flow Paradoxus

Respiratory variation of transmitral and transtricuspid flow occurs in normal individuals, but to a minimal extent. The transtricuspid flow velocities [or velocity-time integral (VTI) increase slightly and transmitral velocities (or VTI)] decrease slightly in inspiration and converse occurs in expiration. The lowered intrathoracic pressure during inspiration is passively transmitted to the cardiac chambers. When the right heart pressures decrease in inspiration due to this effect, the gradient between the extrathoracic systemic veins and right heart increases and hence the flow across tricuspid valve increases. The pressures in the pulmonary veins, being intrathoracic structures, also decrease in inspiration, along with simultaneous reduction of left heart filling pressures and hence the gradient between pulmonary veins and left heart does not change. Thus, in normal individuals, increased flow into right heart occurs due to the increased gradient between extrathoracic systemic veins and right heart, while a similar phenomenon does not happen on the left side due to the anatomical location of pulmonary veins. Augmentation of right heart filling in inspiration may shift the ventricular septum subtly to the left and may decrease LV compliance which in turn may elevate left ventricular filling pressures. This results in inspiratory reduction of LA-LV gradient in diastole and hence the flow velocities recorded across mitral valve decrease.

The situation is little different in the presence of tense fluid around the heart. Though changes in intrathoracic pressure are transmitted to the pericardial fluid, the changes in IPP are of lesser magnitude because of tense fluid in pericardium. In inspiration, IPP decreases slightly and right heart filling pressures also decrease to a similar extent. Since the systemic venous pressures are already elevated due to the restraining effect of pericardial fluid, the gradient between the already elevated extrathoracic systemic venous pressures and decreased right heart pressures drives more blood across tricuspid valve than in normal individuals (Fig. 7). On the contrary, decreased intrathoracic pressure in inspiration is transmitted to the pulmonary veins as well as to the left heart, both being intrathoracic structures. Due to the tense nature of pericardial fluid, reduction of IPP occurs to a lesser degree than reduction of pulmonary venous pressures. Hence, the gradient between pulmonary veins and LA may be lesser than in normal and at times the gradient may even get reversed in inspiration. This could be responsible for reduction of left heart filling in inspiration. It is likely that both the mechanisms could contribute to mitral flow paradoxus, i.e. inspiratory reduction of mitral flow is due to leftward septal shift and lesser or reversed gradient between pulmonary vein (PA) and LA. Reverse happens in expiration, i.e. decreased RV filling in expiration may allow the septum to get shifted toward right. This rightward septal shift increases LV compliance and reduces filling pressures promoting increased flow across mitral valve. Moreover, expiration increases intrathoracic pressure which in turn increase pulmonary venous pressure. Because of the tense pericardial fluid the left heart filling pressures do not increase to that extent. Then, the gradient between pulmonary veins and left heart may increase which may contribute to the expiratory increase in mitral flow (Fig. 8). In an elegant study done by Appleton,[5] it was observed that in normal, the tricuspid E velocity increased in inspiration but not more than 25% and the mitral E velocity decreased in inspiration but not more than 10%. In tamponade, the mitral E velocity decreased by 43 ± 9% and the tricuspid E velocity increased by 85 ± 53%. The changes across tricuspid valve are more than that of changes across mitral valve.

The first beat in inspiratory phase exhibited the maximum change. The above said percentage of difference was derived by comparing the first beat of expiration and the first beat of inspiration. LV isovolumic relaxation time showed a significant increase in inspiration (85 ± 14%) in tamponade while in normal it was not more than 5%. Though similar flow paradoxus occurs in obstructive airway disease, the changes seem to occur in the second beat of inspiration or expiration unlike in tamponade wherein the first beat exhibits the maximum change.

Altered aortic and pulmonary flow: Similar mechanism, described above is responsible for an exaggerated decrease in aortic velocity (or VTI) during inspiration (Fig. 9). In the study quoted above,[5] LV ejection time decreased by 21 ± 3% and aortic flow velocity decreased by 26 ± 6% (Doppler equivalent of pulsus paradoxus) in the first beat of inspiration, while the magnitude of change was less than 5% after pericardocentesis. Pulmonary flow velocity increased by 40 ± 25% in tamponade while it was 13 ± 14% after pericardiocentesis (Fig. 10).

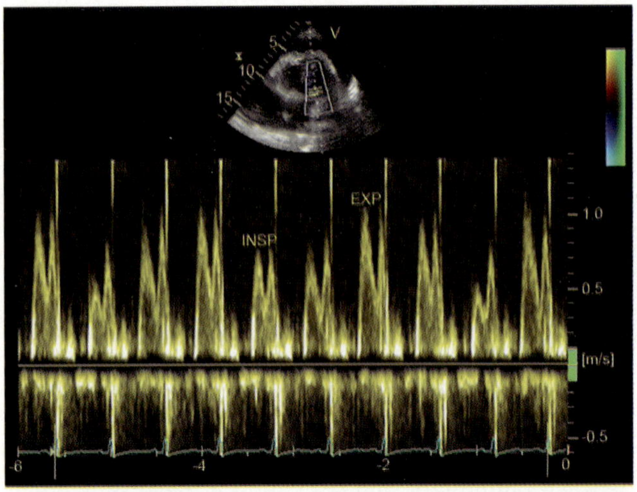

Fig. 8: Flow paradoxus across mitral valve.

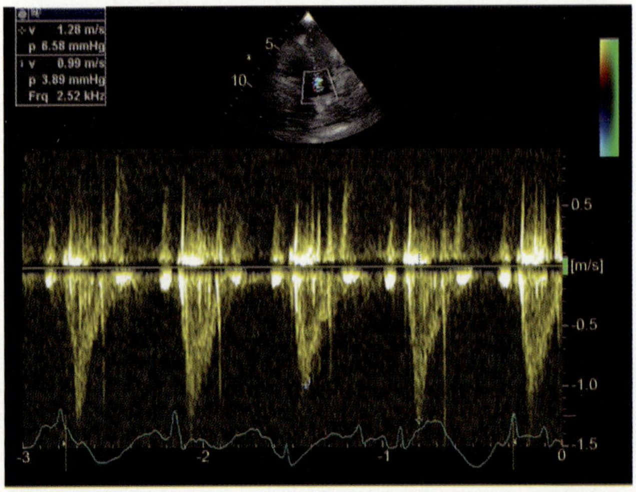

Fig. 9: Inspiratory increase in pulmonary velocity.

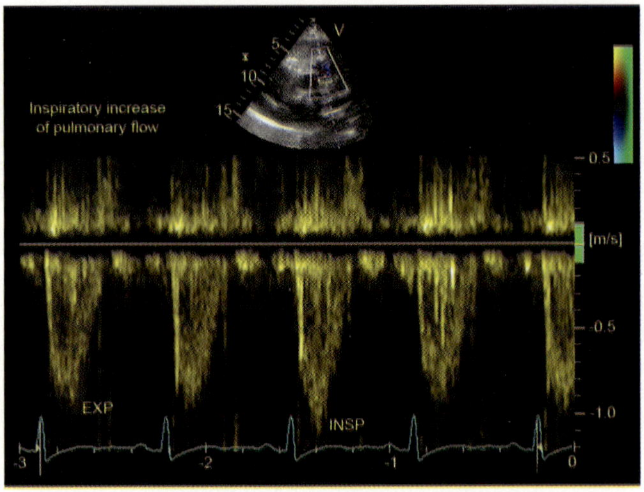

Fig. 10: Inspiratory decrease of aortic velocity (echo equivalent of pulsus paradoxus).

Altered systemic venous flow: Reciprocal changes in the systemic and PV flow with respiration seem to be the basic hemodynamic change in tamponade with all other Doppler findings being considered to be secondary to it. However in the practical sense, it is hard to obtain good quality Doppler recordings of venous flow and the respiratory behavior may be inconsistent at times. Information about systemic venous flow may be obtained from superior vena cava (suprasternal widow) or hepatic veins. In normal, systolic flow is generally more than diastolic flow (or equal) with a slight increase of systolic and diastolic velocities in inspiration. In tamponade, both systolic and diastolic velocities show overall decrease but systolic forward velocity dominates with a distinct diminution of diastolic velocity[6] (Doppler counterpart of shallow y descent in RA wave form). There may be an exaggeration of decrease in diastolic flow in expiration and at times expiratory flow reversal may be demonstrable (Fig. 11).[7] Though analysis of hepatic vein flow is quite useful in diagnosing tamponade with high positive- and negative-predictive values (82% and 88%), it is technically more challenging and in one-third of patients, it cannot be properly evaluated.[8]

Altered pulmonary venous flow: The pulmonary venous flow may show systolic dominance, particularly during inspiration. In systole, as the ventricular emptying occurs, the intracardiac volume decreases. Hence the IPP decreases which leads to reduction of LA pressure so as to promote flow from pulmonary veins to LA, an echo equivalent of prominent x descent. In diastole, right from the onset, the ventricles face the compressive effect of fluid around and hence the gradient between pulmonary veins and LA

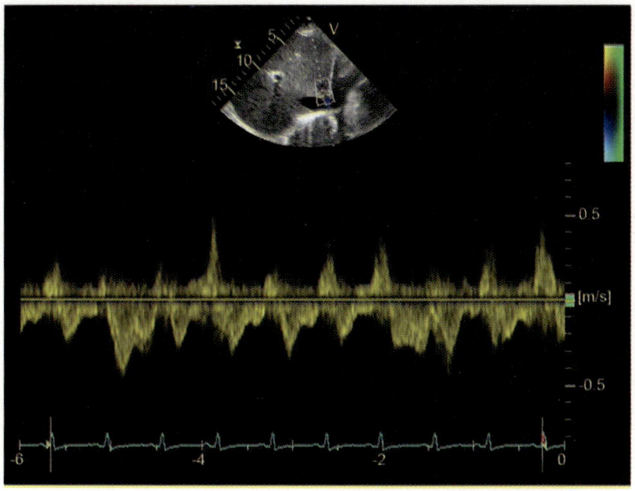

Fig. 11: Hepatic vein Doppler: Dominant systolic flow, expiratory flow reversal.

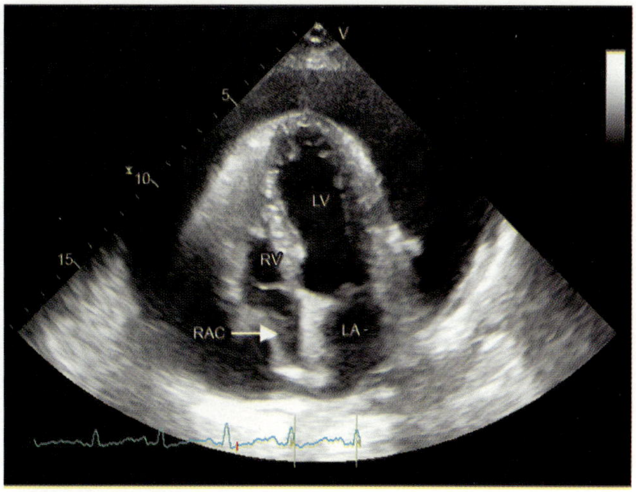

Fig. 12: RA collapse in A4C view.

decrease. This is responsible for smaller diastolic component in PV flow, an echo equivalent of shallow y descent. This tends to become more prominent in inspiration wherein the pulmonary venous pressure decreases to a greater extent than LA pressure and at times the PV-LA gradient may get reversed thereby completely obliterating the flow in diastole. In an animal experimental study, instillation of fluid into pericardium causing tamponade resulted in overall decrease of both systolic and diastolic peak velocities and integral, more so the diastolic velocity. The ratio of systolic or diastolic pulmonary venous flow velocity integral increased significantly (1.65 ± 0.24 at baseline and 2.77 ± 0.43 after tamponade). Distinct inspiratory decrease in the ratio occurred with tamponade (at baseline 1.74 ± 0.46 in expiration and 1.60 ± 0.39 in inspiration; with tamponade 4.06 ± 1.12 in expiration and 3.0 ± 0.9 in inspiration).[9]

Chamber collapse or inversion: Chamber collapse or more appropriately chamber inversion is an important echocardiographic sign that occurs in many patients with tamponade. The inversion of atrial or ventricular wall is due to the mechanical compressive effect of tense pericardial fluid and the inversion occurs at a time in cardiac cycle, when the IPP exceeds the intracardiac pressure. Hence chamber inversion is a dynamic phenomenon. Right atrium and right ventricle are thin-walled compliant structures and moreover the right heart filling pressures are lower than that of left-sided chambers. Hence, chamber inversion involves mostly RA and RV. Right atrium normally has a smooth contour with convexity facing outside, and even during atrial contraction this configuration is preserved. With progressive accumulation of pericardial fluid, there is initially flattening or brief inversion of RA wall and later frank sustained inversion with convexity facing the cavity manifests. Since RA volume and pressure are least during atrial relaxation and initial ventricular systole, RA wall inversion is prominent during this part of the cardiac cycle (Fig. 12). It is a very sensitive sign of tamponade but lacks specificity. In the early report of this finding,[10] RA collapse was found to have a sensitivity of 100%, a specificity of 82% and a predictive value of 50%. The specificity of RA collapse increases if there is sustained RA inversion—starting in late diastole and extending into variable duration of ventricular systole, with the duration of atrial inversion exceeding 35% of cardiac cycle. This value, called as right atrial inversion index is calculated by dividing the frames manifesting RA inversion by the number of frames in one cardiac cycle. A value of more than 0.34 was found to increase the specificity and predictive value to 100% in the study done by Gillam.[10] Documentation of just the presence of RA collapse without considering the duration had a specificity of 82% and a predictive value of 50%. In that study, the degree or the extent of inversion did not seem to increase the specificity of this sign for diagnosis of tamponade. RA inversion is better visualized in A4C or subcostal or parasternal short-axis view.

Right ventricular wall inversion is also a dynamic phenomenon occurring in early diastole, as the intracardiac pressure in RV is at its minimum in this phase of cardiac cycle. It starts during isovolumic relaxation phase extending into variable portion of early diastole. Being a relatively thinner part of RV, it is the outflow tract region that exhibits this sign frequently. The outflow tract buckles in early diastole with convexity facing inward which is better documented in parasternal long or short-axis views (Figs. 13A to C). An M mode study may be helpful to confirm the temporal sequence and the duration of inversion; RV free wall moves in during systole which is followed by another inward movement in early diastole (Fig. 14). At times, RV inward movement in systole may continue with early diastolic compression and appear as a single

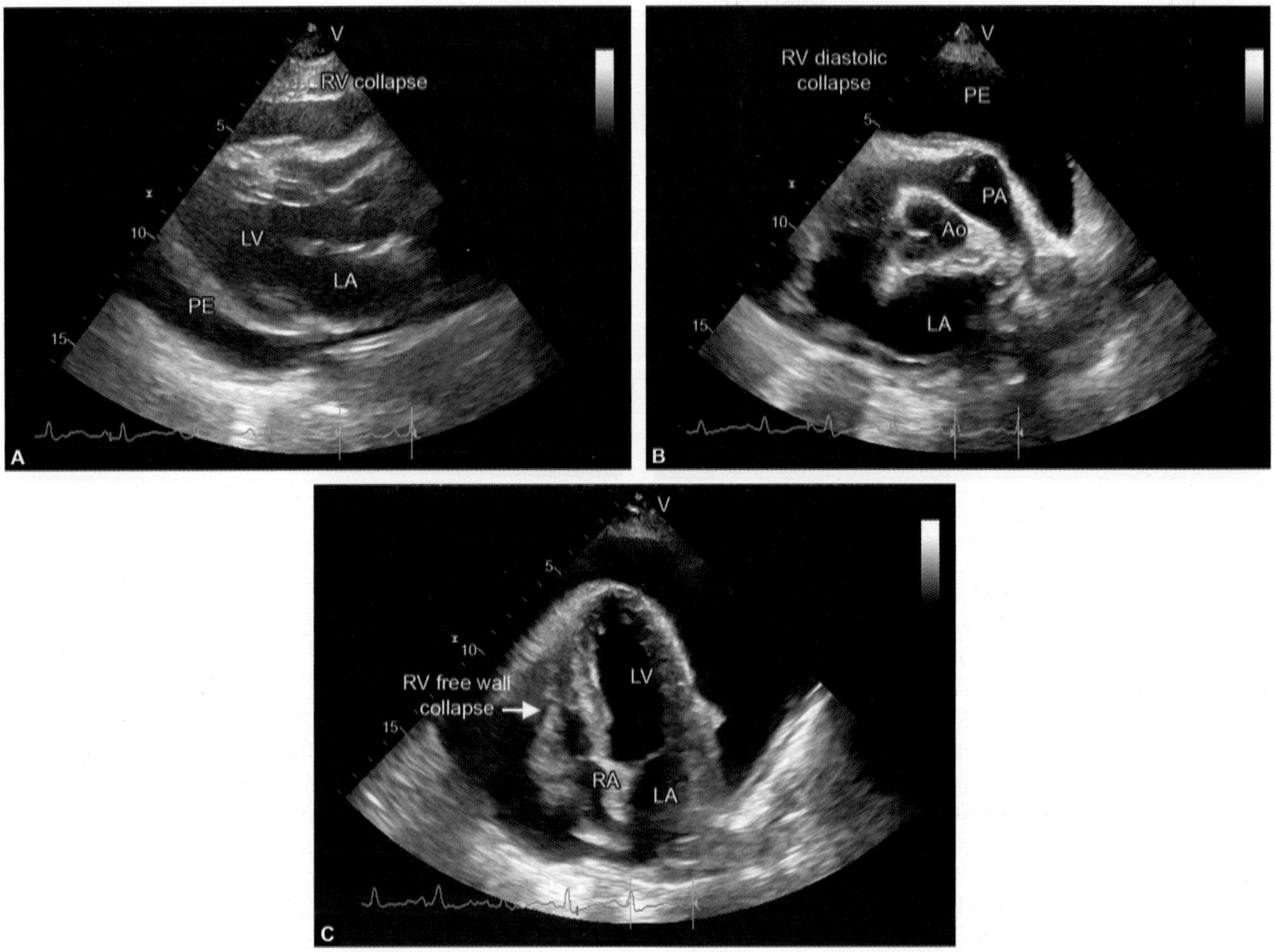

Figs. 13A to C: RV Collapse—(A) Long axis; (B) Short axis (C) A4C.

inflection. In advanced tamponade, even the RV free wall could be seen to get inverted in early diastole which can be documented in A4C or subcostal view. Generally, the RV collapse may manifest only in expiratory phase during early tamponade and subsequently present throughout the respiratory cycle. In a study of 86 patients with pericardial effusion, tamponade was present in 17 patients, 15 of which demonstrated RV inversion. Seven of 69 patients without evidence of tamponade, also exhibited this sign. This study also highlighted that when RV compression is absent, pericardial effusion is exerting little effect on cardiac function.[11] RV inversion is a less sensitive sign of tamponade but it carries higher specificity. Longer the duration of RV collapse, the more severe the tamponade.

Singh[12] has reported that the sensitivity of RV inversion for diagnosis of tamponade was 92% with a specificity of 100%, accuracy of 94% and a predictive value of 100%. In the same study, the sensitivity, specificity and predictive value

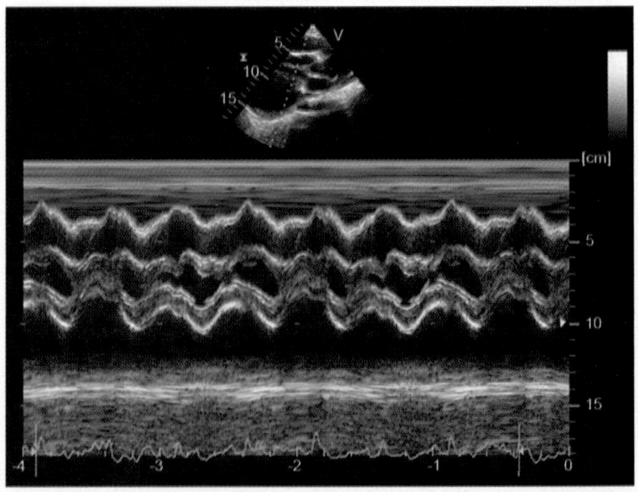

Fig. 14: M mode at mid LV— note the early diastolic RV inversion.

for RA inversion was 64%, 100% and 100%, respectively. Though this study has given lower sensitivity rate and higher specificity rate for RA inversion, RA inversion is generally more sensitive and less specific. Moreover in the combined hemodynamic and echocardiographic study of Singh, RV inversion disappeared first and then RA inversion during pericardial aspiration, thereby meaning that RA inversion may be the first to appear in early phases of tamponade. When there is RV hypertrophy with decreased compliance and elevated filling pressures, as in pulmonary hypertension (PH), RA and RV inversion fail to manifest because of thicker incompressible wall and or higher intracardiac pressures. Similarly, RV compression may not manifest in RV myocardial infarction despite normal RV wall thickness. It is the markedly elevated RV filling pressure that prevents RV collapse from manifesting in this condition. On rare occasions, RA and RV collapse may not manifest despite normal RV wall thickness and filling pressures. The later finding is attributed to adhesions preventing the RA and RV free wall to get inverted. Importantly, the absence of RA and RV inversion in a patient with moderate to large pericardial effusion and normal right heart, implies that the IPP is not elevated. LA inversion is rare, not merely because of little higher pressures in LA than in RA, but mainly because of the reflections of pericardium. Since the pericardium gets reflected around the pulmonary veins, large area of posterior wall of LA is not covered by pericardium. Anteriorly between LA and aorta, there is only a thin recess which gets filled up with large effusions. Though in a report of small series of nine patients, five had LA inversion,[13] the occurrence of this sign is generally very rare. It is considered that not more than 25% of patients with tamponade may exhibit LA compression and it is generally present when the amount of pericardial fluid is quite large. LA compression when present is better documented in long-axis view and A4C view and has a similar timing as that of RA inversion (Fig. 15).

LV compression manifesting as diastolic inward bowing of LV posterior wall is typically caused by a loculated effusion behind LV posterior wall (more of blood and hematoma). The common clinical setting in which such regional collection of fluid (blood) occurs is the early postcardiac surgery period (Figs. 16A and B). Somewhat similar to RA and RV collapse, LV compression may also be dynamic, occurring in early to mid-diastole with the usual contour of LV getting restored in late diastole and maintained in systole. At times, LV compression may present with persistent bowing of LV inferior wall so that the endocardial aspect is convex toward the LV cavity throughout the cardiac cycle. Adhesions between RA and RV anterior wall with pericardium may prevent fluid to accumulate anteriorly and hence the loculation preferentially occurs behind posterior wall. When there is loculated collection of pericardial blood, IPP increases locally and LV gets compressed as the pericardium becomes nonyielding. In a report of 18 patients with postoperative cardiac tamponade, three had circumferential effusion, 10 had localized effusion behind LV posterior wall and five had local collection laterally or inferiorly.[14] Rarely, in patients with severe PH with right ventricular hypertrophy, tamponade may manifest in the form of isolated LV collapse. This type of regional phenomenon occurs despite circumferential fluid accumulation, as the elevated IPP could compress LV but not the hypertrophied noncompliant RV. Rarely LV compression (along with RA and RV inversion) has been reported in low pressure tamponade as well.[15] In regional tamponade, classic signs of tamponade at the bedside and in echocardiography may be lacking. However, this condition may be an important reason for early postoperative decline in cardiac output or arterial pressure. If not recognized and treated with surgical exploration, fatal outcome is likely. In an experimental study,[16] it was demonstrated that when a regional fluid accumulation was induced, diastolic inversion occurred when the IPP exceeded LV diastolic pressure by approximately 3 mm Hg. This sign occurred before the onset of hypotension and occurrence of pulsus paradoxus, meaning that recognition of LV inversion in regional tamponade could help the clinician to relieve the compression well before hemodynamic deterioration.

Reduction of ventricular volumes: Because of tense fluid around the heart exerting a restraining effect on the heart chambers, LV and RV volumes are reduced in the presence of tamponade. Because the cavity size is decreased, LV retaining the same mass, may look hypertrophied (pseudohypertrophy).[17]

Reciprocal filling of ventricles: Since the ventricles compete for their respective place inside the pericardium when there

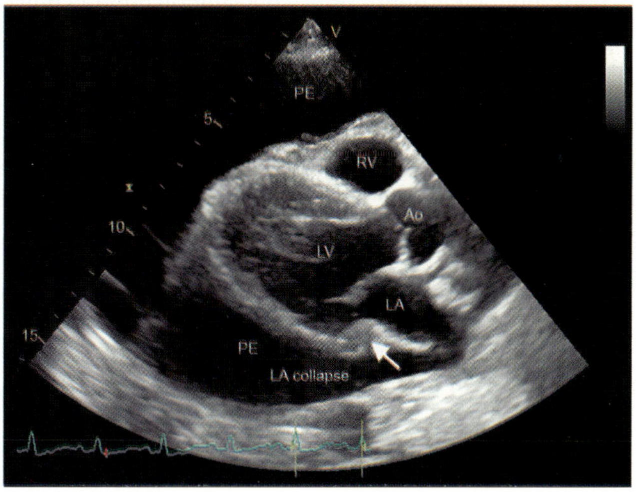

Fig. 15: LA collapse—long axis view.

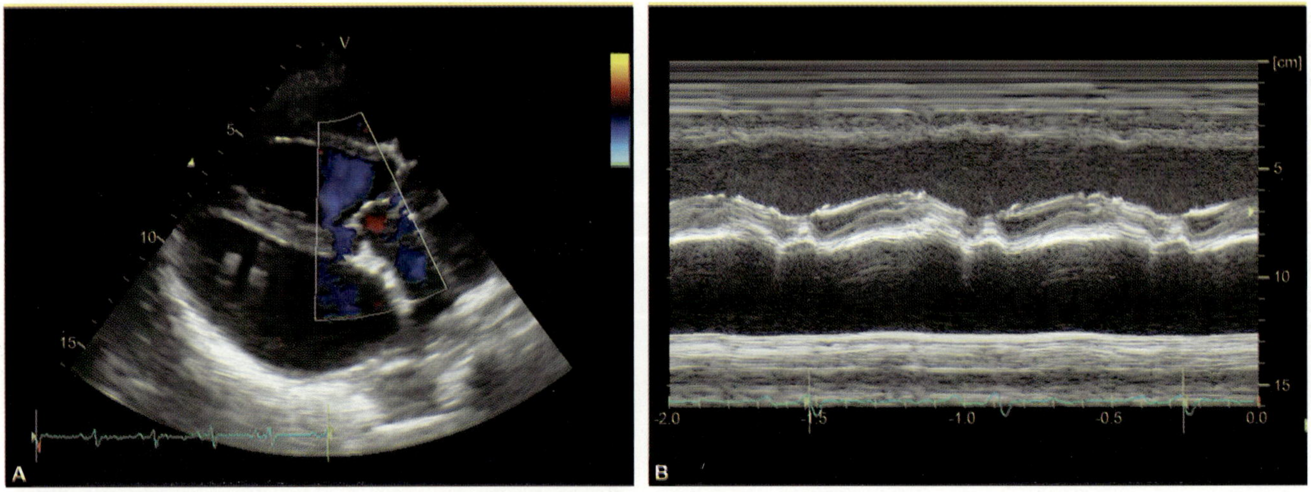

Figs. 16A and B: (A) Regional tamponade; fluid behind posterior wall of LV with inversion. (B) M mode of LV posterior wall depicting prolonged LV diastolic collapse.

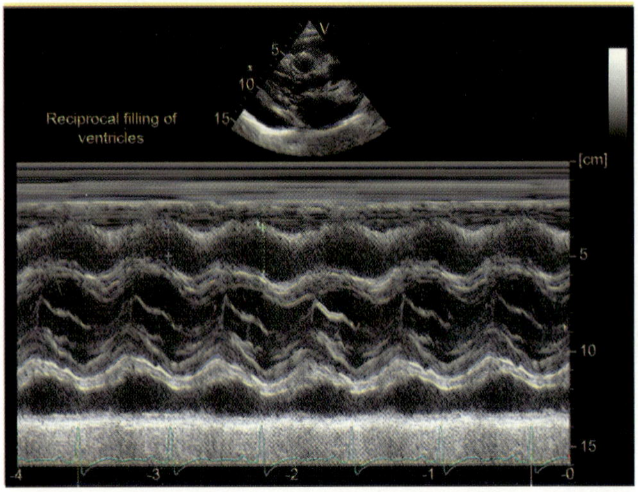

Fig. 17: Reciprocal filling of ventricles.

is tense fluid all around, ventricular interaction becomes more pronounced. Augmented filling of the RV during inspiration at the expense of reduction of LV filling is demonstrated in the simple M mode study obtained at the level of mitral valve tip (Fig. 17). In one of the earlier studies done by Settle,[18] there was an average inspiratory increase of RV internal dimension (measured at end-diastole) was 10 mm and to a similar degree, LV internal dimension decreased. In normal individuals, the mutual alteration of size of the ventricles in respiratory phases does not generally exceed 5 mm. In tamponade, diastolic excursion (DE) amplitude and E-F slope of anterior mitral leaflet show decline in inspiration indicating LV underfilling. Reciprocal filling of ventricles is a feature of constriction as well and the classical septal bounce (jerky leftward shift of septum in inspiration) which occurs in constriction may not be seen in tamponade. The possible reasons are that the magnitude of septal shift is more in constriction and rapid early diastolic filling of ventricles coming to an abrupt halt afterward (equivalent of square root sign) occurs in constriction but not in tamponade. In tamponade, the RV size increases in inspiration and decreases in expiration but with smooth transitions. It may be more appropriately called as septal bulge or deviation rather than bounce based on the less abruptness of the septal shift. Such septal shift may occur in other conditions that cause pulsus paradoxus namely, obstructive airway disease, pulmonary embolism, acidotic breathing, etc. Septal shift may be absent inspite of tamponade physiology if there is LV hypertrophy or LV dysfunction.

Echocardiographic equivalents of pulsus Paradoxus: Pulsus paradoxus is a bedside clinical sign of tamponade which is merely an exaggeration of the normal phenomenon of inspiratory reduction of systolic arterial pressure. In Doppler echocardiography, it manifests in the form of significant inspiratory reduction of left ventricular outflow tract (LVOT) peak velocity or more appropriately the VTI. In contrast, the pulmonary flow may show marked increase in inspiration. An inspiratory drop in aortic velocity of more than 10% and an inspiratory increase in pulmonary velocity is abnormal and indicative of tamponade in the presence of moderate to large effusion. Apparently, the mechanisms implicated in atrioventricular (AV) valve flow paradoxus are responsible for the inspiratory reduction of aortic or LVOT velocities. In an animal experimental study,[19] it was found that RV diastolic collapse was much more sensitive than invasively measured pulsus paradoxus. It is due the fact that tamponade is a continuum and chamber collapse occurred chronologically well ahead of appearance of puslus paradoxus. Once IPP approaches RV filling pressures, RA and RV collapse start manifesting along with reduction of cardiac output. But, pulsus paradoxus as defined conventionally (>10 mm Hg drop in systolic arterial pressure in inspiration), occurs subsequently when there is elevation and equalization of pressures in the pericardial cavity and cardiac chambers.

Echocardiographic equivalents of pulsus paradoxus may be absent in atrial septal defect, aortic regurgitation and conditions in which LV diastolic impairment exists. Similar to the clinically observed pulsus paradoxus, echocardiographic signs of reciprocal filling and output of ventricles with respiratory phases may be present in other conditions like subacute constriction, acute severe asthma, RV infarction, acute AV valve regurgitations, acute pulmonary embolism and marked obesity.

Swinging heart: In the presence of a massive fluid accumulation, the heart with the smaller size and augmented contractility of both ventricles swings anteroposteriorly (Fig. 18). When this phenomenon occurs, other echocardiographic signs of tamponade are generally present. At times, the extent of anteroposterior swinging may alternate which is responsible for alternans in ECG. When there is swinging heart, certain other features coexist—namely hypercontractile ventricles, paradoxically moving LV inferior wall, pseudoprolapse of mitral valve and midsystolic notching of aortic valve in M-mode.

Inferior vena cava plethora: Dilated IVC with reduced or absent collapsibility in inspiration indicate elevated systemic venous pressure as a result in increased IPP causing tamponade.[20] IVC dimension often exceeds 20 mm with less than 50% inspiratory collapse (Fig. 19). IVC plethora is present in more than 90% of patients with tamponade. It is however not specific for tamponade and occurs in any condition characterized by the presence of RA hypertension. In case of difficulty in imaging IVC, dilated hepatic veins may serve as a surrogate.

Chronology of echocardiographic signs: Though different echocardiographic signs of tamponade have been described in literature, only few studies looked at the chronological sequence of signs manifesting during progressive fluid accumulation. Both animal studies and studies in patients with tamponade undergoing pericardiocentesis, have indicated that tamponade is a continuum. Gonzalez[21] had looked at the different hemodynamic variables and echocardiographic findings in 11 sedated dogs and concluded that with progressive increase in pericardial fluid volume, parameters like heart rate, filling pressures of both ventricles and the magnitude of inspiratory fall in systolic arterial pressure showed a progressive (linear) increase, while blood pressure, cardiac output and mitral velocities showed a decrease. The exaggerated respiratory variation of mitral E velocity and isovolumic relaxation time (IVRT) occurred almost with an increase in IPP and persisted at all stages of increasing pericardial effusion. Occurrence of this finding preceded right heart collapse in echo and well before equalization of pressures in cardiac chambers. The magnitude of respiratory variation of was not predictive of pericardial pressure or the severity of tamponade. Thus, flow paradoxus is an initial finding occurring in early (mild) tamponade. Since mitral and tricuspid flow paradoxus are essentially due to the changes in systemic and pulmonary venous flow pattern, they all occur together in stage 1. In stage 2A, RA collapse occurs, in stage 2B, RV diastolic collapse occurs . In stage 3–4, distinct inspiratory reduction of LV stroke volume occurs (equivalent of clinical pulsus paradoxus). Cardiac output starts decreasing gradually from stage 1 and when RV diastolic collapse occurs, there is already a reduction of cardiac output by 15–20%, though arterial pressure is normal.

Which echo finding is the most reliable? If one considers that tamponade is diagnosed clinically (pulsus paradoxus), then

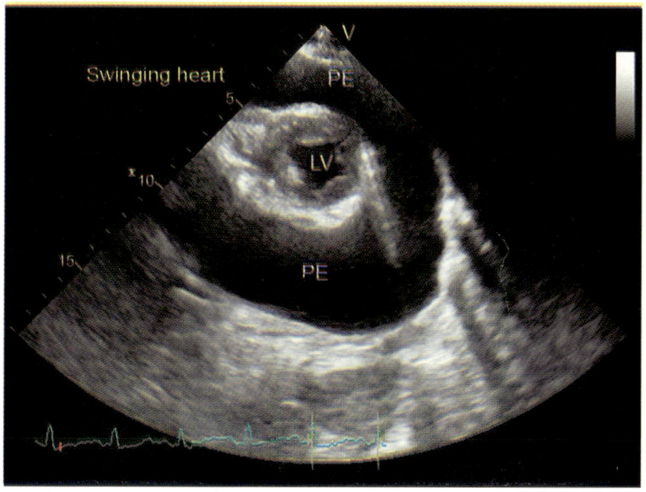

Fig .18: Swinging heart.

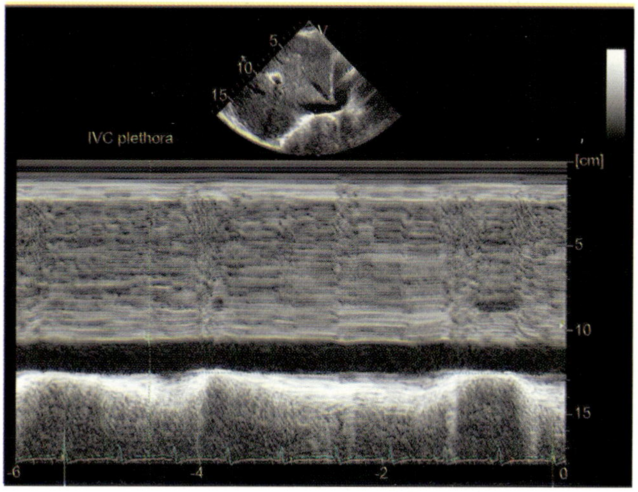

Fig. 19: IVC plethora.

the sensitivity and specificity would be 90% and 65% for the presence of any chamber collapse, 68% and 66% for RA collapse, 60% and 90% for RV collapse, 45% and 92% for both chamber collapse and 75% and 91% for abnormal venous flow.[22] This tells us that no single finding is diagnostic and constellation of multiple signs improves the diagnostic accuracy. If one accepts that cardiac tamponade is a continuum with pulsus paradoxus appearing toward the end and if any hemodynamic derangement is considered as indicative of tamponade (for example: reduction of cardiac output occurring early in the spectrum) the sensitivity and specificity of these signs would be totally different. Ideally, the signs like flow paradoxus and RA collapse may suggest early tamponade, RV collapse an intermediate stage and marked inspiratory reduction of aortic velocities (Doppler equivalent of pulsus paradoxus) as an advanced stage.

Regional Tamponade: Somewhat similar to loculated pleural effusion, localized collection of fluid or hematoma in the pericardial cavity may induce some of the echocardiographic signs. Though this variety may occur in any situation that leads to pericardial adhesions leading to loculation, it is typically encountered in postcardiac surgery patients. Quite often the bloody effusion or hematoma tends to occur behind the LV inferior wall in this setting. Rarely, the localized collection may occur posteriorly, near the AV groove, near the right atrium or anterior to RV free wall. Depending on the location and the extent of compression of adjacent segments, hemodynamic compromise and clinical expression are variably present.

Low Pressure Tamponade: It is a form of cardiac tamponade in which comparatively low pericardial pressure results in cardiac compression in the setting of lower filling pressures in the heart. Lower filling pressures are generally caused by dehydration or hypovolemia, but may occur without these clinical conditions. Clinical conditions like traumatic hemorrhage, poor oral intake or vomiting (patients with malignancies), hemodialysis or ultrafiltration (excessive fluid removal) or overdiuresis are responsible for this hemodynamic subtype of tamponade. Such patients lack the typical clinical presentation; jugular venous pressure is normal and pulsus paradoxus absent in majority. Sagrista-Salueda[23] has suggested a hemodynamic definition, namely intrapericardial pressure being less than 7 mm Hg before pericardiocentesis and right atrial pressure less than 4 mm Hg postpericardiocentesis, when the IPP got lowered to nearly 0. In the clinical sense, there is lowered filling pressure of the heart and hence tamponade tends to occur even with modest elevations of IPP. In his series of 279 cases of tamponade, nearly 10% of patients had low pressure tamponade. When patients with adequate hemodynamic data were available, 20% satisfied the hemodynamic criteria laid down by him. Interestingly, echocardiographically determined quantity of pericardial effusion, presence of right atrial collapse (RAC) and right ventricular collapse (RVC) and flow paradoxus did not differ between the garden variety of tamponade and low pressure tamponade. Though IPP is only modestly elevated cardiac compression results because of low filling pressures in the heart—IPP is relatively higher than intra cardiac pressures. Thus this entity should be considered in patients who exhibit echocardiographic features but without typical clinical signs.

Isolated RA Collapse with minimal effusion: It is common to encounter brief RA collapse, in some patients presenting with small pericardial fluid. Generally the fluid is < 2 mm behind LV posterior wall and A4C view may show little more fluid near RA. If the temporal sequence of RA inversion is analyzed, it is often confined to late diastole. The author had observed this finding not infrequently in those with recent myocardial infarction associated with minimal pericardial effusion. The mechanism is somewhat similar to the finding of an experimental study wherein acute constriction of descending thoracic aorta in animals had produced RV collapse in the presence of even small amount of fluid instilled into the pericardium.[24] Acute rise in LV filling pressures may get transmitted to the pericardial cavity which in turn compresses the thin walled compliant RV. Similarly, increased LV filling pressure due to acute ischemic LV dysfunction may mediate RA collapse by transmitting the elevated LV diastolic pressure into the pericardial cavity. RA being thinner than RV that too with lower pressures, readily collapses but the briefness of RA collapse and smallness of pericardial effusion should alert the investigator that it is not tamponade in true sense.

Gas/Air in the pericardium: Gas may accumulate inside the pericardium whenever gas producing organisms enter after penetrating injuries or when esophageal malignancy erodes into pericardial cavity or rarely when air gets sucked into pericardium during attempts of pericardiocentesis. If the gas is under tension, tamponade may happen. Since air is a poor conductor of ultrasound, one may not be able to visualize cardiac structures from conventional thoracic windows—all will appear white on the screen. At the most plethoric IVC may be visualized from subxiphoid window. Making the patient to lie one one side and viewing from opposite site, may allow cardiac structures to be visualized. Fluoroscopy is however confirmatory and is needed for confirmation.

Pleural effusion causing tamponade: Clinical observation of patients with large bilateral pleural effusion and mild pericardial effusion manifesting RV collapse had motivated investigators to perform an animal experimental study to identify the mechanism of such observation.[25] Hemodynamics and echo findings were analyzed in conscious chronically instrumented dogs, during instillation of saline into pericardial space and into both pleural spaces fluid after draining most of the pericardial fluid but leaving a minimal amount. In both situations RA collapse was noticed when IPP rose to similar values (8–9 mm Hg). But there were some differences namely the RV collapse was more prominent in expiration with large pericardial effusion and overall hemodynamic derangement was much worse. With bilateral pleural effusion and minimal pericardial effusion the RV collapse was more prominent in inspiration and overall hemodynamic perturbation was mild. Large pleural effusion with elevated intra pleural pressure probably exerts its effect on pericardium provided it is compliant and contains some fluid. Hence RV collapse in the presence of large bilateral effusion but with small pericardial effusion is a false positive sign and does not require separate treatment of pericardial effusion in the form of drainage.

The need for TEE: TTE is often enough to make the diagnosis of tamponade. One would need TEE if the precordial windows are poor or inaccessible (post cardiac surgery). Transmitral and trans tricuspid velocities and most importantly pulmonary venous flow velocities are better recorded through TEE. Regional tamponade, particularly those which occur in unusual sites, may also require TEE for confirmation.

Echo to guide Pericardiocentesis: Safe removal of pericardial fluid may be done at bedside with echo guidance. First of all, the access site for aspiration may be determined from the distribution and location of maximal amount of fluid by echo. The needle tip may be visualized as it enters the pericardial cavity and injecting air (ideally CO_2) will allow the physician to ascertain the needle position in the pericardial cavity. Whether done at bedside or in the cathlab with fluoroscopic guidance, echocardiography may allow the operator to achieve dry tap. The later is more likely to allow adhesions to form between the visceral and parietal layer thereby minimizing the chances for fluid re-accumulation. Echo may also help to decide when to remove the indwelling catheter, based on the daily drain volume (<25 mL/d) and absence or minimal fluid detectable by echo. Theoretically echo should help in locating loculated fluid and for draining it percutaneously if present in accessible location. Echocardiography may also help in identifying the some of the unusual cardiac events that may happen after removal of pericardial fluid. It is not uncommon to see acute LV dysfunction following rapid removal of large volume of fluid. Rarely reversible acute RV dysfunction may also occur after RV dysfunction, as seen in one of the patients of author (Fig. 20).

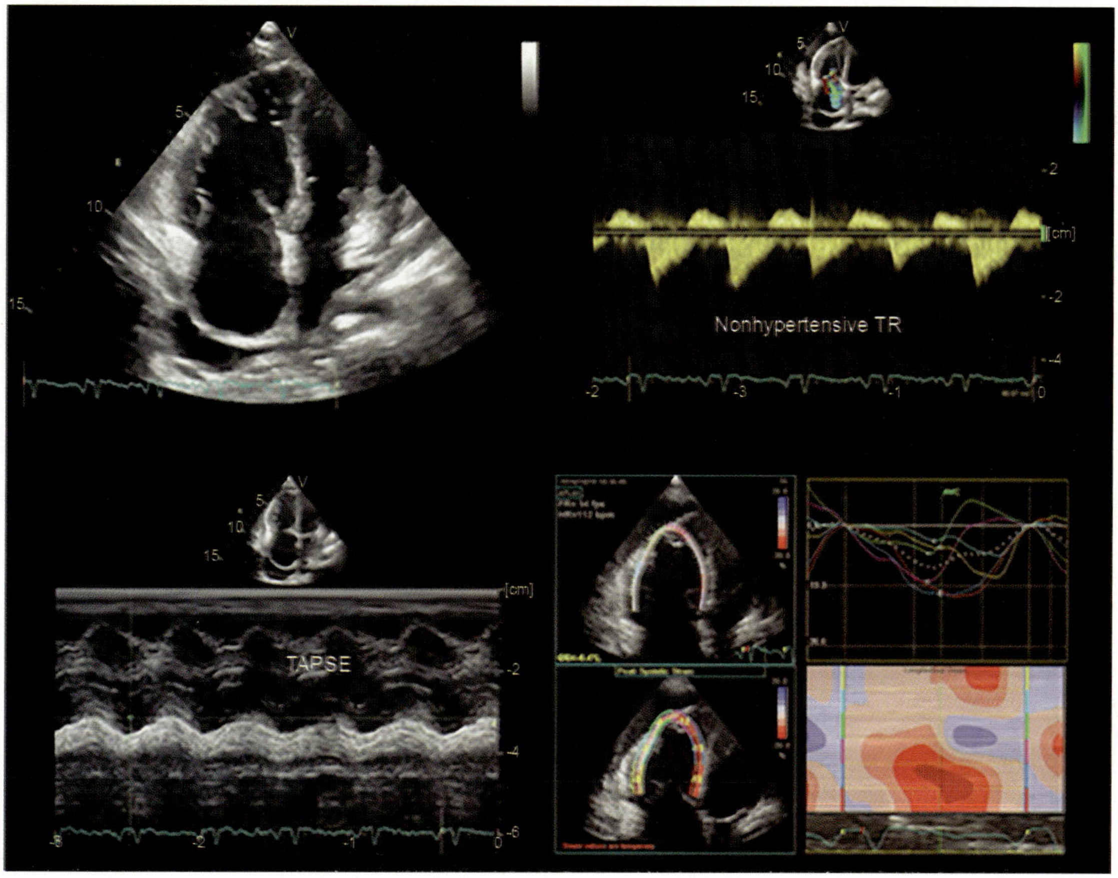

Fig. 20: Post aspiration reversible RV dysfunction and TR.

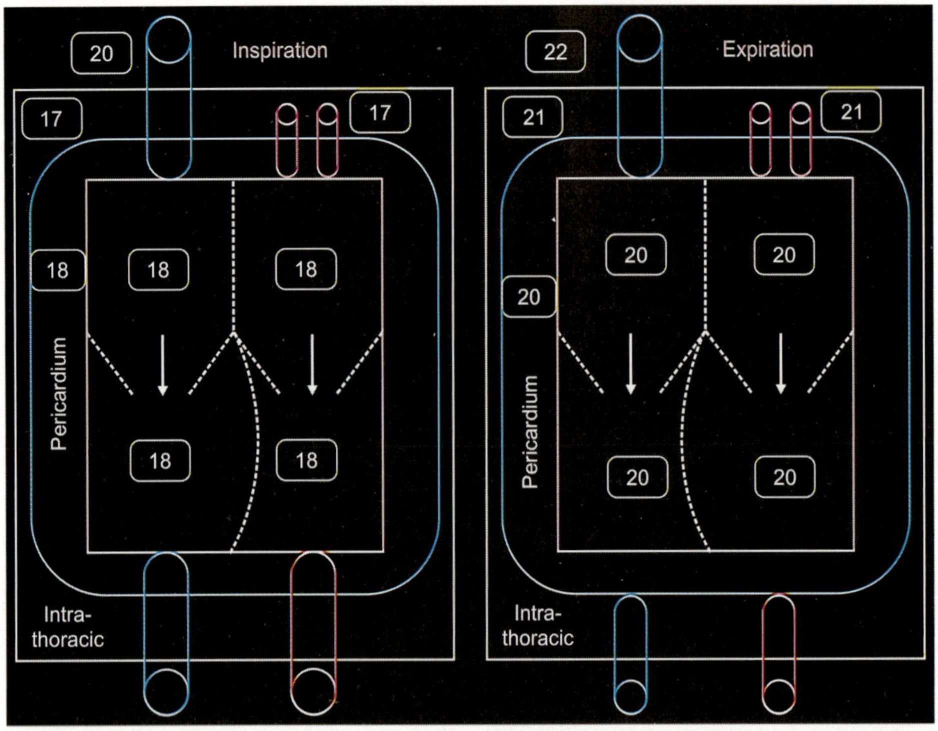

Fig. 21: Conceptualizing hemodynamics of tamponade.

CONCLUSION

Echocardiography has a versatile role in management of pericardial effusion, right from making the diagnosis to quantification, inferring the nature of fluid, measuring its hemodynamic consequences upto its use in therapeutic intervention. A thorough understanding of the hemodynamics of tamponade is essential to understand the Echocardiographic features (Figs. 21 and 22) Diagnosis should not be based on a single echocardiographic sign but the entire imaging findings should be taken together into account, as each sign has limited sensitivity and specificity, though high. For example, flow paradoxus in the absence of chamber collapse should alert the clinician to look for other potential causes for respiratory variation, considering pericardial effusion as an innocent bystander. Assessment should be comprehensive and include quantification of fluid, identification of nature of fluid and presence of loculation before the echocardiographic signs of tamponade are sought. For identifying chamber collapse, multiple windows should be used, observation is done in both phases of respiration and duration of inversion is measured on frame count. One should look for Flow paradoxus across all valves, it should be done during quite breathing and the first beat in each respiratory phase should be carefully analyzed for making out this valid sign. Echocardiography should preferably be done during fluid aspiration to ensure dry tap and immediately after aspiration to look for the rare occurrence of effusive constrictive pericarditis and follow up study is needed to identify re accumulation.

"Exploit Echo for Excellence"

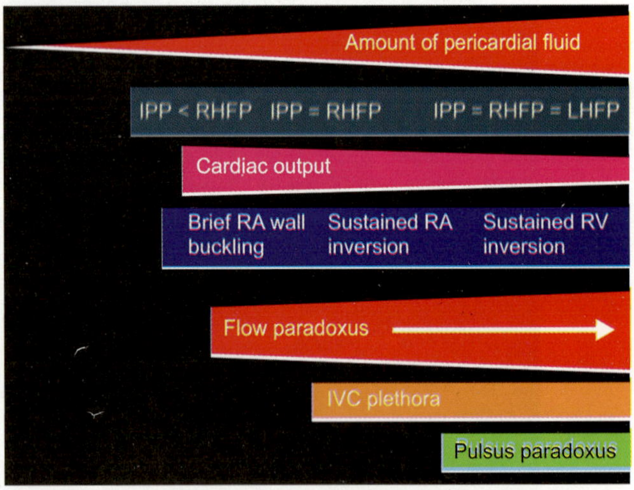

Fig. 22: Chronology of Echo features and hemodynamics in tamponade.

REFERENCES

1. Hoit JP. The normal pericardium. Am J Cardiol. 1970;26:455-65.

2. Smiseth OA, Frais MA, Kingma I. et al. Assessment of pericardlal constraint: the relation between right ventricular filling pressure and pericardial pressure measured after pericardiocentesis. J Am Coll Cardiol. 1986;7:307-14.
3. Eisenberg MJ, Oken K, Guerrero S et al. Prognostic value of echocardiography in hospitalized patients with pericardial effusion. Am J Cardiol. 1992;70:934-39.
4. George S, Salama AL, Uthaman A, et al. Echocardiography in differentiating tuberculous from chronic idiopathic pericardial effusion. Heart. 2004;90:1338-9.
5. Appleton CP, Hatle LK, Popp RL. Cardiac tamponade and pericardial effusion: Respiratory variation in transvalvular flow velocities studied by Doppler Echocardiography. J Am Coll Cardiol. 1988;11:1020-30.
6. Zhang S, Kerins DM, Byrd III BF. Doppler echocardiography in cardiac tamponade and constrictive pericarditis. Echocardiography. 1994;11:507-21.
7. Burstow DJ, Oj JK, Bailey KR et al. Cardiac Tamponade: Characteristic Doppler observations. Mayo Clin Proc. 1989;64:312-24.
8. Merce J, Sagrista-Sauleda J, Permanyer-Mirlda G, et al. Correlation between clinical and Doppler echocardiographic findings in patients with moderate and large pericardial effusion: implications for the diagnosis of cardiac tamponade. Am Heart J. 1999;138:759-64.
9. Hoit BD, Ramrakhyani K. Pulmonary venous flow in cardiac tamponade: Influence of left ventricular dysfunction and the relation to pulsus paradoxus. J Am Soc Echocardiogr. 1991;4:559-70.
10. Gillam LD, Guyer DE, Gibson TC, et al. Hydrodynamic compression of right atrium: a new echocardiographic sign of tamponade. Circulation. 1983;68(2):294-301.
11. Armstrong WF, Schilt BF, Helper DJ et al. Diastolic collapse of the Right Ventricle with Cardiac Tamponade: An Echocardiographic study. Circulation. 1982;65:1491-96.
12. Singh S, Wann S, Schuchard GH et al. Right ventricular and right atrial collapse in patients with cardiac tamponade–a combined radiographic and hemodynamic study. Circulation 1984;70:966-71.
13. Kronzon I, Cohen ML, Winer HE et al. Diastolic atrial compression: A sensitive echocardiographic sign of cardiac tamponade. J Am Coll Cardiol. 1983;2:770-5.
14. Chuttani K, Pandian NG, Mohanty PK et al. Left ventricular diastolic collapse. An echocardiographic sign of regional tamponade. Circulation. 1991;83:1999-2006.
15. Dwivedi S, Saran R, Narain VS. Left ventricular diastolic collapse in low pressure cardiac tamponade. Clin Cardiol. 1998;21:224-26.
16. Schwartz SL, Pandian NG, Cao QL, et al. Left ventricular diastolic collapse in regional left heart tamponade. An experimental echocardiographic and hemodynamic study. J Am Coll Cardiol. 1993;22:907-13.
17. Di Segni E, Feinberg MS, Sheinowitz M et al. Left ventricular pseudo hypertrophy in cardiac tamponade: an echocardiographic study in canine model. J Am Coll Cardiol 1993;21:1286-94.
18. Settle HP, Adolph RJ, Fowler NO, et al. Echocardiographic study of Cardiac Tamponade. Circulaton. 1977;56:951-59.
19. Loppenstein HS, Schuchard GH, Wann LS, et al. The relative merits of pulsus paradoxus and right ventricular diastolic collapse in the early detection of cardiac tamponade: an experimental study. Circulation. 1985;71:829-33.
20. Himelman RB, Kircher B, Rockey DC, et al. Inferior vena cava plethora with blunted respiratory response: a sensitive echocardiographic sign of cardiac tamponade. J Am Coll Cardiol. 1988;12:1470-7.
21. Gonzalez MS, Basnight MA, Appleton CP, et al. Experimental Pericardial Effusion: Relation of Abnormal Respiratory variation in mitral flow velocity to Hemodynamics and Diastolic Right heart collapse. J Am Coll Cardiol. 1991;17:239-48.
22. Merce J, Sagrista-Sauleda J, Permanyer-Mirlda G, et al. Correlation between clinical and Doppler echocardiographic findings in patients with moderate and large pericardial effusion: implications for the diagnosis of cardiac tamponade. Am Heart J. 1999;138:759-64.
23. Sagrista-Salueda J, Angel J, Sambola A, et al. Low Pressure Cardiac Tamponade: Clinical and Hemodynamic profile. Circulation. 2006;114:945-952.
24. Cogswell T, Bernath GA, Keelan MH, et al. The shift in the relationship between intra pericardial fluid pressure and volume induced by acute left ventricular pressure overload during cardiac tamponade. Circulation. 1986;74:173-80.
25. Vaska K, Wann LS, Sagar K, et al. Pleural effusion as a cause of right ventricular collapse. Circulation. 1992;86:609-17.

92

CHAPTER

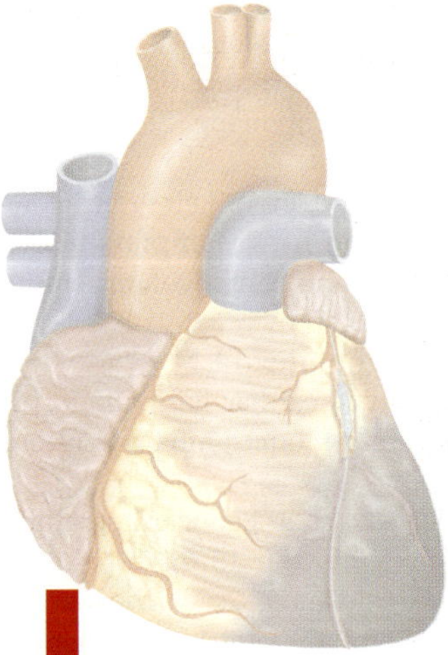

Multimodality Imaging of Pericardium

Vidyut Jain, Avani Jain, Ravi Masand

INTRODUCTION

Heart remains the most vital organ of the body and it is protected by pericardium all-around. In addition to protection of heart, pericardium dynamics also control intracardiac pressures. Pericardium has two layers, i.e. visceral and parietal which wrap the heart and the origin of great vessels. The pericardium may be affected by various disease processes and can lead to significant morbidity and mortality. To diagnose pericardial diseases remains a challenge but substantial advancement in various imaging methods has proved to be great help. Echocardiography, developed in 1970, was the earliest imaging technique utilized for examination of patients suspected of having or known to have pericardial disease. Echocardiography is capable of diagnosing structural changes of pericardium and functional impairment of ventricle due to pericardial fibrosis. In last 2 decades with emergence of, cardiac computed tomography (CT) and magnetic resonance (MR) additional information on pericardial diseases could be obtained and thus, a positive impact on clinical management of such patients has been seen. All these diagnostic modalities are easy to perform, noninvasive, and are known to have high sensitivity. In present era, the multimodality imaging is considered to be ideal approach for diagnosing pericardial diseases. This review elucidates the role of different imaging techniques for the assessment of pericardium in health and pathological state.[1] Pericardial diseases are the important cause of cardiac morbidity and mortality by adversely affecting cardiac hemodynamic in addition to their own pathological outcome. Pericardium may be involved commonly by many acquired disease and rarely congenital defects are seen. Spectrum of acquired disease ranges from infective, neoplastic, autoimmune, traumatic, postmyocardial infarction, etc. Pericardium may be involved in radiation injury, occasionally after cardiac surgery and cardiac interventions. Echocardiography as noninvasive tool and has helped a lot in understanding pericardial disease but more comprehensive information is obtained with multidetector computed tomography (MDCT) and MRI, hence. In true sense, multimodality imaging is better option for the diagnosis of pericardial diseases.

ANATOMY AND PHYSIOLOGY OF PERICARDIUM

The first sign of formation of heart *in utero* is found at the end of 6 weeks. The heart-forming cells appear as irregular clusters in the cephalic part of the embryo between the endoderm of the yolk sac and the splanchnic mesoderm which later form the basis of pericardium. Pleuropericardial membrane is supplied blood from cardinal vessels during embryogenesis. Richard Lower (1631–1691) was first to note intermittent pulse in constrictive pericarditis, later on William Harvey, and Norman Chevars described several cases of constrictive pericarditis.[2] The pericardium is composed of fibroserous tissue that surrounds the heart and the roots of the great blood vessels arising from heart. A void space found among the two linings of serous pericardium is called pericardial cavity. The parietal layer of pericardium is thicker than the visceral pericardium.[3] The normal combined pericardial thickness is 2 mm or less the inner serosa (also referred as the visceral pericardium or the epicardium) and the outer fibrosa (also referred as the parietal pericardium).[4] The serosa forms a complete sac filled with small quantity (40–50 mL) in adult of plasmatic ultrafiltrate and is separated from the heart by loose epicardial connective tissue and a single layer of mesothelial cells. Like visceral abdominal fat, the thickness of the epicardial fat is increased in obesity. There is accumulating evidence that epicardial fat can directly influence coronary atherogenesis, because there is no fibrous layer to impede diffusion to the underlying coronary arteries of the free fatty acids and adipokines that modulate atherothrombosis.[5,6] The fat distribution is usually uneven more on right ventricular surface than on left ventricle (LV) surface.[7] Pericardial membranes have simple microscopic architecture, crucial but has complex role in ensuring the normal performance of the heart. It has mechanical, membranous, and ligamentous component over heart and controls normal ventricular compliance to minimize ventricular dilatation and protect the heart by means of the production of lubricating fluid and surfactants. It also prevents displacement of the heart in the mediastinum.[8] As pericardium is partially elastic, it allows both the ventricle to work with minimal mutual interaction, a phenomenon defined as "ventricular coupling" or "ventricular interdependence." The over distension of one ventricle compresses the other one and would lead to poor diastolic relaxation of other ventricle.[9] Presence and severity of ventricular coupling, and the effect of respiration, be altered due to disease states like constrictive pericarditis.[10]

COMPUTED TOMOGRAPHY SCAN

Multidetector CT scan has revolutionized the CT imaging of pericardium using a high-resolution volumetric acquisition with a section thickness of greater than 3 mm emit usually offer adequate anatomical imaging of the pericardium.[3] Artifacts caused by body movement is a limitation however, can be reduced by using electrocardiography (ECG)-synchronized acquisitions, it improves imaging of the pericardial sinuses and recesses and thus, reduces the risk of misinterpretation can be avoided which sometimes mimic as enlarged lymph nodes or focal aortic disease.[11] To avoid artifacts distorting images, ECG-synchronized real-time functional images are obtained.[12] Adequate dynamic evaluation of ventricular septal motion to evaluate constrictive physiology is theoretically possible only with ECG-synchronized CT, real-time functional imaging.[4] In present era with multidetector scanners and gated electrocardiographically-synchronized data acquisition enables accurate assessment of the coronary arteries and the remainder of the heart and pericardium, including functional cardiac analysis thus, increases the utility of CT chest evaluation.[13]

MAGNETIC RESONANCE IMAGING

Magnetic resonance imaging is a noninvasive technique which very accurately complements imaging pericardium. In addition to pericardial imaging one can evaluate morphologic assessment of adjacent structure of the mediastinum, and heart. MR also gives insights into hemodynamic abnormalities of both ventricles. The change in tissue characterization helps to understand pericardial diseases better. It also helps in evaluation of pericardial mobility and fusion of pericardial layers. Acquisition of fast MR sequences allow helps in analysis of cardiac motion and inflow patterns in real-time during free breathing, which allows identification of constrictive physiology pattern better.[14,15] Newer technique of delayed (or late) gadolinium-enhanced MR imaging is useful for the detection of active pericardial inflammation and assess the effects of medical treatment.[16,17]

IMAGING OF NORMAL PERICARDIUM

The normal pericardium appears as thin layers of membrane on CT and MR images which encircles the myocardial contours. Epicardial fat can also be seen. Thickness of epicardial fat is variable and is more in female and possibly more with coronary artery disease. Pericardial membranes are better seen near right ventricle, however, it is difficult to get good images of pericardium along lateral margins and posterior border of LV due to close proximity of pulmonary parenchyma.[18] There is a marginal difference in normal pericardial thickness measured by CT and MRI. The normal thickness of pericardium by CT is in the range of 0.7–2 mm, however, by MRI it is 1.2–1.7 mm.[19,20] This difference may be due difference in variability of resolution in the two methods of imaging where in fluid content may be taken as thickness on MR.[21] Pericardial recesses can be seen in nearly 20–43% of cases by CT examination.[22]

CONGENITAL PERICARDIAL DEFECT

Relative rare occurrence and may be isolated or associated with other congenital heart defects. Larger defect may remain asymptomatic in majority, however, smaller defects

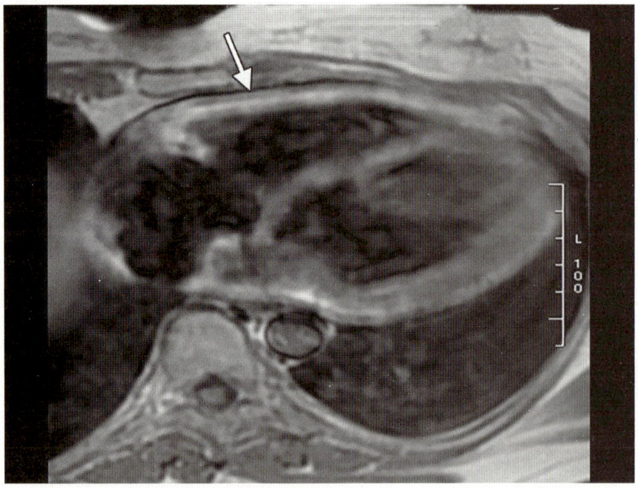

Fig. 1: Cardiac magnetic resonance imaging: Congenital absence of pericardium, pericardium is missing posteriorly (arrow).

of congenital absence of pericardium may present as acute emergency as cardiac structures may get herniated or strangulate through these defects. Occasionally, patient may come for angina due to compression of coronary arteries. These defects are usually due to premature closure of cardinal vessels supplying blood to pleuropericardial folds. These defects are more on left side of heart. A strong clinical suspicion and radiological chest X-ray finding of "snoopy sign" with heart deviated to the left with the left-heart border straightening and elongation should be evaluated initially by echocardiography. Echocardiographic finding of excessive motion of left ventricular posterior wall on M-mode echocardiography and marked changes in position of heart. Cardioptosis should raise further suspicion and needs to be confirmed by MR examination (Fig. 1).[23]

Pericardial Cyst and Diverticulum

Relatively rare and may be a surprise finding on CT and MR imaging. They may represent about 13–17% of all cystic findings in mediastinum.[24] Usually pericardial cyst appears as unilocular mass which is of caloric origin embryologically without any septa and occasionally may be pedunculated. These cysts may remain asymptomatic and rarely may cause symptoms and sign clinically by compressing nearby intrathoracic structures.[25] More commonly in the right cardiophrenic angle (70% of cases), and less in the left cardiophrenic angle (20% of cases).[26] Pericardial diverticulum may be considered to be focal out pouching of the pericardial sac, which has direct communication with the pericardial cavity, usually identified by changes in its morphology with change in position of body.[25]

ACQUIRED PERICARDIAL DISEASES

Pericardial Effusion

It is a commonly encountered problem of pericardium. It may be of heterogeneous etiology in which pericardial sac contains abnormal fluid collection. This abnormal fluid collection may be due to chronic diseases or may be result of acute etiology. Collection of fluid in pericardium may be due to diseases of pericardium itself, adjacent structure or other systemic illness such as acute infection, inflammatory diseases, heart failure, renal and liver insufficiency, neoplastic disease, trauma, myocardial infarction, and hypothyroidism, etc.[4]

Transthoracic echocardiography imaging is often very informative in diagnosing and assessing the severity of pericardial effusion. Content of pericardium like fibrinous stranding and presence of clot can also be identified. Routine monitoring along with information on associated cardiac problem can also be detected. Echocardiography has almost 98% accuracy in diagnosing pericardial effusion.[27] However CT imaging further helps to confirm the diagnosis, and in addition information on nature fluid content is obtained with more specificity (Figs. 2 and 3). More importantly diseases of adjacent structure, i.e. mediastinum, lung parenchyma, and aorta can be assessed. It also informs about the chronicity of disease, associated neoplastic masses, etc. It can also give information on hemodynamic compromise.

Computed tomography and MR information on pericardial thickness, and exact extension of pericardial collection and localization of loculated collection is more sensitive and specific than echocardiography.[28] Nature of pericardial fluid whether it is exudate or transudate can

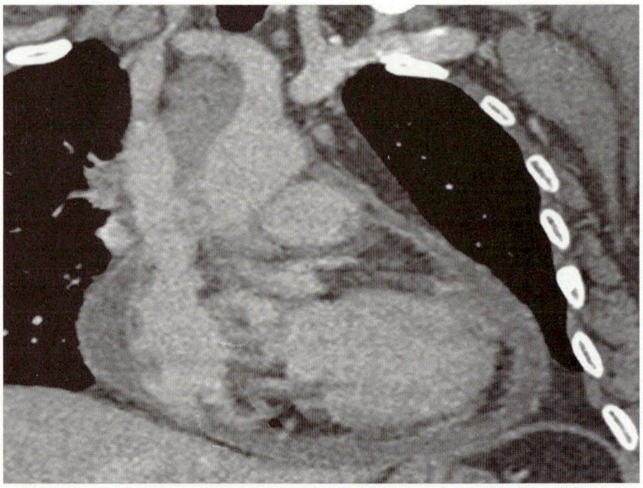

Fig. 2: Computed tomography scan showing pericardial effusion with thickening of pericardium.

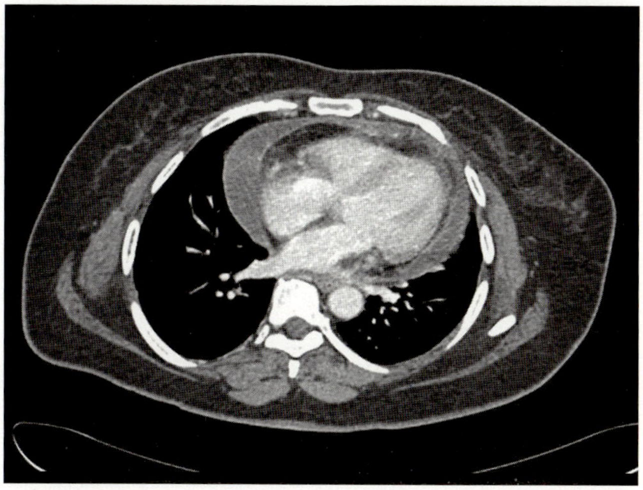

Fig. 3: Computed tomography scan showing pericardial effusion.

be roughly guessed by measuring attenuation values on CT images and signal intensity on MR images. Higher CT attenuation value usually seen in fluid due to pyogenic process, posttrauma, and in malignancy.[11] In general, these imaging modalities are used to supplement the information obtained by routine echocardiography which can be done bedside in emergency and is affordable without any limitation. Echocardiographic signs of dilated inferior vena cava along with absence of inspiratory collapse and low stroke output by Doppler favors significant pericardial effusion. Right ventricular collapse also guides to presence of temponade, however in presence of right ventricular hypertrophy or severe pulmonary hypertension, this sign may not be detactable.[29,30] MR detected low-attenuation pericardial effusions can be seen due to chylopericardium.[14] Intrapericardial content can be imaged better by dynamic cine MR imaging.[31] Pericardial layer thickness and inflammatory nature can also be assessed better with MRI and CT imaging.

Acute Pericarditis

Acute pericarditis which often present as acute chest pain, pyrexia and few clinical signs is not easy to diagnose clinically, because most of these markers are nonspecific. However, a strong clinical suspicion and supportive clinical signs of tachycardia, pericardial rub, may raise its possibility. Initial imaging method is always echocardiography and presence of abnormal fluid in pericardium will be helpful but often echocardiography may be unremarkable.[32-34] CT scan is not usually a primary imaging modality in acute pericarditis as it may be normal; however, increased thickness along with presence of fluid may be supportive to clinical diagnosis.[34] In acute pericarditis, MR imaging may prove sensitive diagnostic modality. Increased thickness and presence of fluid is easily picked up and enhanced gadolinium imaging can suggest inflammatory state. The degree of inflammation can be seen as increased signal on T2-weighted short tau inversion recovery sequence on CMR.[35] Utilizing pericardial late gadolinium enhancement imaging the sensitivity is as high as 96–100% for detection of pericardium inflammation suggestive of increased permeability and neovascularization. Persistence of MR signs of inflammation suggest that treatment needs to up titrated and to be continued further as there is no response.[36]

Constrictive Pericarditis

Constrictive pericarditis often poses diagnostic and management challenges. Constrictive pericarditis reflects a condition disease leading to fibrosis of pericardial layer thereby it becomes less elastic and compliance of the pericardium is reduced. This loss of elasticity and invasion by fibrosis of epicardium leads to poor relaxation of ventricle and impaired ventricular filling, which clinically manifest as severe diastolic dysfunction, and right heart failure.[8,33]

As this disease entity runs as a slow progressive disorder with minimal clinical signs in initial clinical course and often diagnosed late stage with clinical deterioration. In countries like India, most common cause for pericardial effusion is tuberculosis. However other causes are like postviral, postcardiac surgery, and postradiation and may be of idiopathic etiology.[19,37] Once clinically this disease is suspected, next step to supplement the diagnostic workup is echocardiography, which gives lot of information. Increased pericardial thickness with calcification can be seen often. M-mode echocardiographic signs of abnormal septal motion, diastolic septal bounce, and other important clues may be significant respiratory variation in transmitral inflow, increased inspiratory mitral E wave velocity by 25%, and decreased tricuspid E wave velocity by 40% often helps in establishing diagnosis.[38,39] Study on tissue Doppler imaging show normal or enhanced mitral early diastolic velocity (e') from medial annulus and sometimes higher than lateral annulus.[40] After obtaining information with echocardiography, additional information on extent of pericardial thickness, calcification can be obtained with MDCT (Fig. 4) and MR imaging. Increased thickness of pericardium up to 20 mm has been often noted on MDCT, but absence of thickness cannot rule out constrictive pericarditis, and is reported normal in 18% cases of surgical operated.[19]

It is also reported that toward an end-stage irreversible chronic fibrosing pericarditis, there is thinning of the chronically inflamed pericardium.[41] Observations made by Feng et al. pericardial thickness was significantly less

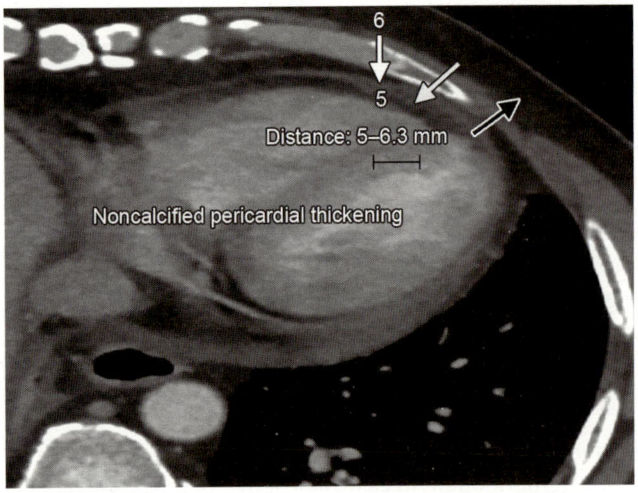

Fig. 4: Noncalcified pericardial thickening (arrows).

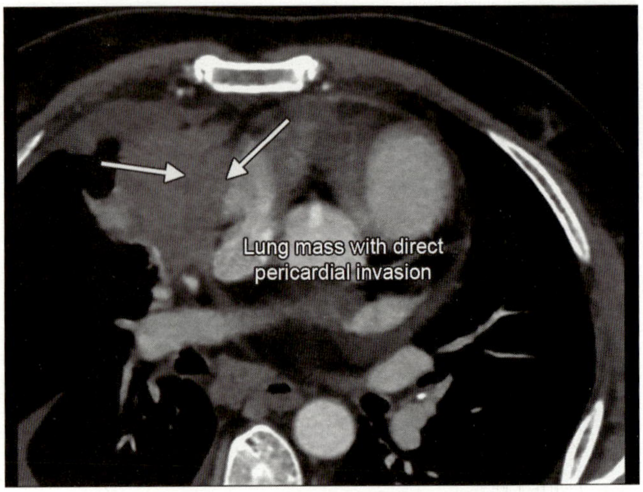

Fig. 5: CT scan showing lung mass invading pericardium (arrows).

in patients with persistent constrictive pericarditis than in those with reversible constrictive pericarditis (2 mm ± 1 vs 4 mm) in a study of 21 patients with end-stage constrictive pericarditis than in those with evidence of persistent chronic inflammation (3.1 mm ± 1.7). This may be postulated that not all patients of constrictive pericarditis will require surgery.[42] Hemodynamic signs of constrictive pericarditis are often picked on MR also. Reduction in pericardial stretch in constrictive pericarditis leads to increased ventricular coupling, which is characterized by septal flattening or inversion ("septal bounce") at early diastolic ventricular filling on MR examination.

Pericardial Masses

Pericardial masses may be primary or secondary tumors that can have mass effect on heart. Multimodality imaging has tremendously improved our experience in their detection, localization, and extension using CT and MR imaging (Fig. 5). Primary tumors of pericardium are rare, secondary tumors may be seen in 10% of cases.[42-44] Common primary tumors are mesothelioma, lymphoma, and liposarcoma. Benign tumors include fibroma, teratoma, hemangioma, and lipoma are extremely rare. Malignant mesothelioma is the most common primary lesion and is usually characterized by the presence of hemorrhagic effusion with pericardial nodular lesions or plaques.[45]

Pericardial masses are usually associated with a variable amount of effusion that is disproportionally greater than the size of the solid lesion, and often may be hemorrhagic, and are therefore, characterized by inhomogeneous high signal intensity on both T1-weighted and T2-weighted MR images and high attenuation on unenhanced CT images.[44]

Pericardial involvement may occur by direct invasion from tumor of adjacent structures such as lung, mediastinum, or heart or by hematologic spread, e.g. malignant melanoma, lymphoma, breast cancer, and rarely by direct venous extension of hepatocellular carcinomas and renal cell carcinoma. Malignant invasion can result in focal interruption of pericardial layers invading the pericardium from outside by lung cancer or inside angiosarcoma arising from the right atrium which rapidly invades the pericardium. Mass-like appearance has been misinterpreted may due to hematoma.[45] The CT and MR characteristics of hematoma depend upon the duration of hematoma imaging characteristics of foreign body granulomas, postsurgical or post-traumatic can be occasionally seen on CT and MR study as tumor mass. A final entity to be mentioned is pericardial fat necrosis. This benign entity of unknown cause typically manifests with sudden onset of chest pain, mimicking other diseases such as myocardial ischemia, in which only CT scan give clue by lesion of fat attenuation surrounded by the increased attenuation of the anterior mediastinal paracardiac fat adjacent to the pericardium can help in diagnosis.[46]

CONCLUSION

Pericardium is a very thin but very important structure. Various types of pathological processes may involve it, may be local diseases, diseases of adjacent structure, or remote systemic diseases. Any abnormal collection in pericardium or reduced compliance of pericardium can lead to serious adverse effect on cardiac hemodynamic in addition to basic disease. Imaging of pericardium is challenging but multimodality imaging has helped our understanding of various pericardial diseases better. In future, further advances in imaging will enhance our understanding.

REFERENCES

1. Bogarrt J, Francone M. Pericardial disease: value of CT and MR imaging. Radiology. 2013;267(2):340-56.
2. Spodick DH. Medical history of the pericardium. The hairy hearts of hoary heroes. Am J Cardiol. 1970;26(5):447-54.
3. Bull RK, Edwards PD, Dixon AK. CT dimensions of the normal pericardium. Br J Radiol. 1998;71(849):923-5.
4. Groell R, Schaffler GJ, Rienmueller R. Pericardial sinuses and recesses: findings at electrocardiographically triggered electron-beam CT. Radiology. 1999;212(1):69-73.
5. Rabkin SW. Epicardial fat: properties, function and relationship to obesity. Obes Rev. 2007;8(3):253-61.
6. Iacobellis G, Corradi D, Sharma AM. Epicardial adipose tissue: anatomic, biomolecular and clinical relationships with the heart. Nat Clin Pract Cardiovasc Med. 2005;2(10):536-43.
7. Sacks HS, Fain JN. Human epicardial adipose tissue: a review. Am Heart J. 2007;153(6):907-17.
8. Spodick DH. The Pericardium: A Comprehensive Textbook. New York: Marcel Dekker; 1997.
9. Ivens EL, Munt BI, Moss RR. Pericardial disease: what the general cardiologist needs to know. Heart. 2007;93(8):993-1000.
10. Nishimura RA. Constrictive pericarditis in the modern era: a diagnostic dilemma. Heart. 2001;86(6):619-23.
11. O'Leary SM, Williams PL, Williams MP, et al. Imaging the pericardium: appearances on ECG-gated 64-detector row cardiac computed tomography. Br J Radiol. 2010;83(987):194-205.
12. Groell R, Schaffler GJ, Rienmueller R. Pericardial sinuses and recesses: findings at electrocardiographically triggered electron-beam CT. Radiology. 1999;212(1):69-73.
13. Achenbach S, Raggi P. Imaging of coronary atherosclerosis by computed tomography. Eur Heart J. 2010;31(12):1442-8.
14. Wang ZJ, Reddy GP, Gotway MB, et al. CT and MR imaging of pericardial disease. Radiographics. 2003;23 Spec No:S167-80.
15. Giorgi B, Mollet NR, Dymarkowski S, et al. Clinically suspected constrictive pericarditis: MR imaging assessment of ventricular septal motion and configuration in patients and healthy subjects. Radiology. 2003;228(2):417-24.
16. Taylor AM, Dymarkowski S, Verbeken EK, et al. Detection of pericardial inflammation with late-enhancement cardiac magnetic resonance imaging: initial results. Eur Radiol. 2006;16(3):569-74.
17. Zurick AO, Bolen MA, Kwon DH, et al. Pericardial delayed hyperenhancement with CMR imaging in patients with constrictive pericarditis undergoing surgical pericardiactomy: a case series with histopathological correlation. JACC Cardiovasc Imaging. 2011;4(11):1180-91.
18. Bogaert J, Dymarkowski S, Taylor AM, et al. Clinical Cardiac MRI, 2nd edition. Germany: Springer; 2012.
19. Talreja DR, Edwards WD, Danielson GK, et al. Constrictive pericarditis in 26 patients with histologically normal pericardial thickness. Circulation. 2003;108(15):1852-7.
20. Im JG, Rosen A, Webb WR, et al. MR imaging of the transverse sinus of the pericardium. Am J Roentgenol. 1988;150(1):79-84.
21. McMurdo KK, Webb WR, von Schulthess GK, et al. Magnetic resonance imaging of the superior pericardial recesses. AJR Am J Roentgenol. 1985;145(5):985-8.
22. Kodama F, Fultz PJ, Wandtke JC. Comparing thin-section and thick-section CT of pericardial sinuses and recesses. Am J Roentgenol. 2003;181(4):1101-8.
23. Abbas AE, Appleton CP, Liu PT, et al. Congenital absence of the pericardium: case presentation and review of literature. Int J Cardiol. 2005;98(1):21-5.
24. Akiba T, Marushima H, Masubuchi M, et al. Small symptomatic pericardial diverticula treated by video-assisted thoracic surgical resection. Ann Thorac Cardiovasc Surg. 2009;15(2):123-5.
25. Feigin DS, Fenoglio JJ, McAllister HA, et al. Pericardial cysts. A radiologic-pathologic correlation and review. Radiology. 1977;125(1):15-20.
26. Jeung MY, Gasser B, Gangi A, et al. Imaging of cystic masses of the mediastinum. Radiographics. 2002;22 Spec No:S79-93.
27. Klein AL, Abbara S, Agler DA, et al. American Society of Echocardiography clinical recommendation for multimodality cardiovascular imaging. J Am Soc Echocardiogr. 2013;26(9):965-1012.
28. Frank H, Globits S. Magnetic resonance imaging evaluation of myocardial and pericardial disease. J Magn Reson Imaging. 1999;10(5):617-62.
29. Hoit BD, Gabel M, Fowler NO. Cardiac tamponade in left ventricular dysfunction. Circulation. 1990;82(4):1370-6.
30. Hoit BD, Gabel M, Fowler NO. Influence of acute right ventricular dysfunction on cardiac tamponade. JACC. 1991;18(7):1787-93.
31. Bogaert J, Francone M. Cardiovascular magnetic resonance in pericardial diseases. J Cardiovasc Magn Reson. 2009;11:14.
32. Khandaker MH, Espinosa RE, Nishimura RA, et al. Pericardial diseases: diagnosis and management. Myo Clin Proc. 2010;85(6);572-93.
33. Troughton RW, Asher CR, Klein AL. Pericarditis. Lancet. 2004;363(9410):717-27.
34. Hall WB, Truitt SG, Scheunemann LP, et al. Prevalence of clinically relevant incidental findings on chest computed tomographic angiograms ordered to diagnose pulmonary embolism. Arch Intern Med. 2009;169(21):1961-5.
35. Young PM, Glockner JF, Williamson EE, et al. MR imaging finding in 76 consecutive surgically proven cases of pericardial disease with CT scan and pathological correlation. Int J Cardiovasc Imaging. 2012;28(5);1099-109.
36. Taylor AM, Dymarkowski S, Verbeken EK, et al. Detection of pericardial inflammation with late-enhancement cardiac magnetic resonance imaging: initial results. Eur Radiol. 2006;16(3):569-74.
37. Lieng LH, Oh JK, Schaff HV, et al. Constrictive pericarditis in modern era. Circulation. 2003;108(5):1852-7.
38. Hatle LK, Appelton CP, Popp RL. Differentiation of constrictive pericarditis and restrictive cardiomyopathy by Doppler echocardiography. Circulation. 1989;79(2):357-70.
39. Oh JK, Hatle JB, Seward JB, et al. Diagnostic role of Doppler echocardiography in constrictive pericarditis. J Am Coll Cardiol. 1994;23(1):154-62.

40. Choi JH, Choi JO, Ryu DR, et al. Mitral and tricuspid valve annular velocity in constrictive pericarditis and restrictive cardiomyopathy: correlation with pericardial thickness on computed tomography. JACC Cardiovasc Imaging. 2011;4(6):567-75.
41. Cremer PC, Kumar A, Kontzias A, et al. Complicated pericarditis: Understanding risk factors and pathophysiology to inform imaging and treatment. J Am Coll Cardiol. 2016;69(21):2311-28.
42. Syed IS, Feng D, Harris SR, et al. MR imaging of cardiac masses. Magn Reson Imaging Clin North Am. 2008;16(2):137-64.
43. Fussen S, De Boeck BW, Zellweger MJ, et al. Cardiovascular magnetic resonance imaging for diagnosis and clinical management of suspected cardiac masses and tumours. Eur Heart J. 2011;32(12):1551-60.
44. Maksimović R, Dill T, Seferović PM, et al. Magnetic resonance imaging in pericardial diseases. Indications and diagnostic value. Herz. 2006;31(7):708-14.
45. Grebenc ML, Rosado de Christenson ML, Burke AP, et al. Primary cardiac and pericardial neoplasms: radiologic-pathologic correlation. Radiographics. 2000;20(4):1073-103.
46. Hernandez D, Galimany J, Pernas JC, et al. Case 170: Pericardial fat necrosis. Radiology. 2011;259(3):919-22.

SECTION 15

Constrictive Pericarditis

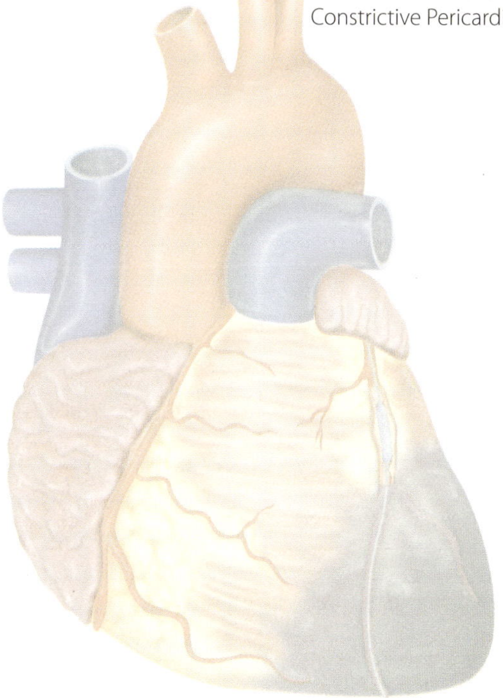

93

CHAPTER

Advances in Echocardiographic Evaluation of Constrictive Pericarditis

G Vijayaraghavan, S Sivasankaran, Sakhalesh Patil

INTRODUCTION

Constrictive pericarditis (CP) is the end result of many pericardial diseases, which has thickened, scarred, inelastic and often calcified, noncompliant pericardium limiting diastolic filling of cardiac chambers.[1] The etiology of CP are diverse, including tuberculosis, postirradiation, postcardiac surgery, dyscollagenosis, viral pericarditis, uremic pericarditis and sometimes idiopathic.[2] Tuberculosis is the most common cause before the advent of effective drug therapy and still remains important in the developing countries.[3]

PATHOPHYSIOLOGY

The pathophysiology of CP relates to the elevated and equalized cardiac pressures, because the total cardiac volume is determined by the scarred, fibrotic, and inelastic pericardium and should be considered in every patient presenting with congestive cardiac failure, because of the treatable option.[1] The unique pathophysiologic feature is the dissociation of intrathoracic and intracardiac pressures and enhanced ventricular interaction.[4] Like tamponade, this causes the heart chambers to operate in a "fixed" and noncompliant space and systemic and pulmonary venous pressures rises in an attempt to maintain cardiac filling. Contrast to cardiac tamponade, early part of diastolic filling in CP is more rapid than the normal because the restraining effects of the pericardium is minimal until mid-diastole, after which little ventricular filling is possible even during atrial contraction. As CP becomes more severe and total cardiac volume is reduced further, cardiac output becomes lower and systemic venous pressures become high with ascites and cachexia.

Radiological features of constrictive pericardial diseases are fairly classical in the late stage, as shown in Figures 1A to E, when the surgical outcome is unpredictable.[5] Echocardiography on the other hand is a simple bedside tool, to delineate the early stages as well as the hemodyamics of this often clinically missed disorders.[6] Pericardial thickening and calcification leads to abnormal ventricular filling produce characteristic changes in M-mode echocardiography.[7] Increased pericardial thickness will be noted as parallel motion of the visceral and parietal pericardium, which is separated by a relatively echo-free space as in Figures 2A to C. It is surprising that in 18% of patients constriction may happen with a normally looking pericardium.[8]increased pericardial thickness has been considered an essential diagnostic feature of constrictive pericarditis. Although constriction with a normal-thickness pericardium has been demonstrated clinically by noninvasive imaging, the details of clinicopathological correlates have not been described. A total of 143 patients with proven constriction underwent pericardiectomy at Mayo Clinic between 1993 and 1999. Their baseline characteristics, operative data, and pathological specimens were reviewed retrospectively. The pericardium was of normal thickness (≤2 mm Echocardiographic signs of the hemodynamic abnormalities of CP include abrupt posterior motion followed by diastolic flattening of the left ventricular (LV) posterior wall endocardium, abrupt

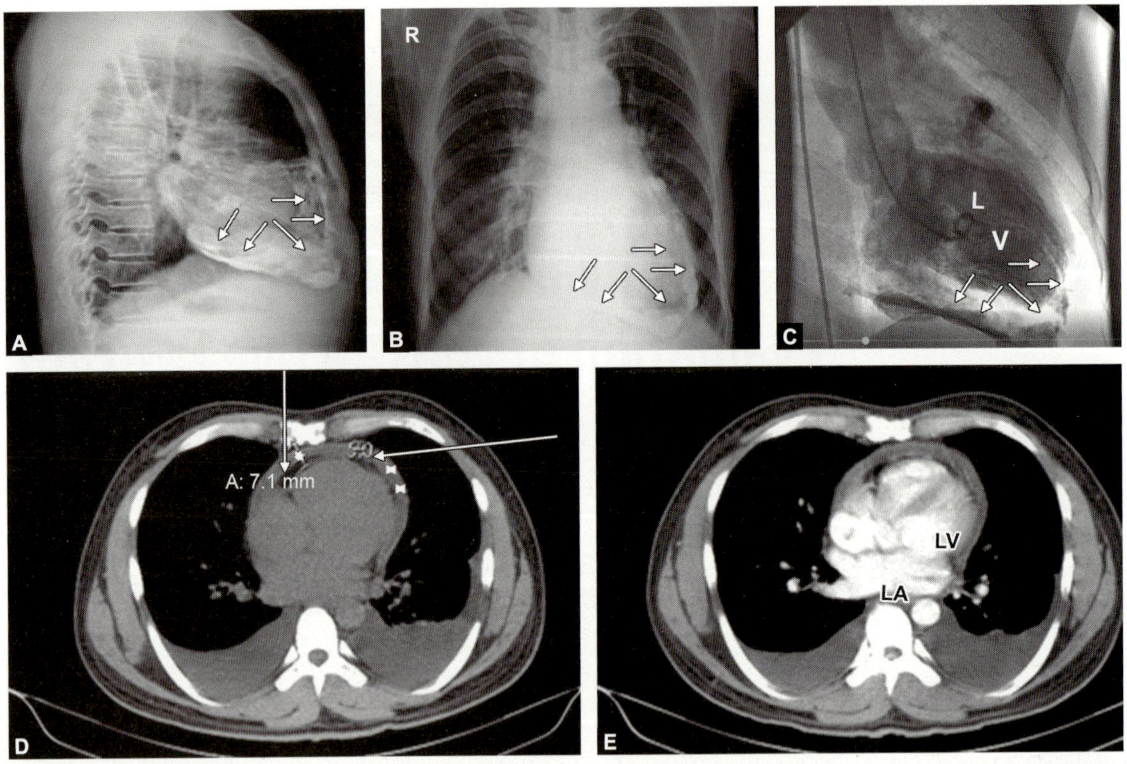

Figs. 1A to E: Radiologic feature of late stage pericardial disease. (A and B) X-ray of chest lateral and posteroanterior (PA) views showing eggshell-type calcified pericardium, small radiating arrows, in constrictive pericarditis; (C) Left ventricular (LV) angiogram showing marked thickening of the pericardium with calcification. Note the distance from the LV endocardium to the calcific epicardium; (D and E) Plain and contrast computed tomography (CT) images of the heart in a patient showing effusive constrictive pericarditis. Effusion is seen as the white ring around the heart, then thin long arrows showing the visceral and parietal pericardium on either side. Bilateral pleural effusions are seen suggesting elevated systemic venous pressures. Contrast CT in (E) also shows normal LV size, dilated left atrium (LA) with congested pulmonary veins.

posterior motion of the ventricular septum in early diastole with inspiration (septal shudder and bounce).[9] The diseased pericardium insulates the heart from the intrathoracic pressure changes of respiration. As a result, the right heart chambers have to accommodate the inspiratory increase in venous flow by pushing the septum and reducing the LV filling.[4] Recording the M-mode at slow speed of 25 mm/s with respirometer trace to identify the respiratory variation in the ventricular volumes is needed to define these.[9]

Two-dimensional (2D) echocardiography reveals dilation or diminished collapse of the inferior vena cava (IVC) and hepatic veins [plethora, a sign of elevated right atrial (RA) pressure], moderate biatrial enlargement (Figs. 3A to D).[10] Inspiratory expansion of the IVC, Kussmaul's sign, and prominent VY collapse in diastole in the absence of significant tricuspid regurgitation are useful Doppler signs which get augmented in inspiration.[11] Expiratory augmentation of the venous flow reversal is another useful sign to differentiate CP from restrictive cardiomyopathy.[12] Most patients with CP will have elevated venous pressures except in early disease, or when the venous filling pressures are low, like in occult CP, where a fluid challenge will reveal the physiology.[13]

Since the ventricles can no longer fill after the initial rapid filling the atrial systole pushes the blood forward into the low pressure pulmonary artery which can be demonstrated by M-mode, pulse Doppler, and color M-mode echocardiogram as in Figures 4A to D.

ATRIOVENTRICULAR INFLOW VELOCITIES

They are typically characterized by the very rapid early inflow filling reflecting the high filling pressures which facilitates rapid filling of the ventricles with the onset of ventricular diastole.[14] No further ventricular filling is possible even with atrial systole as a result the E/A ratio is more than one with short deceleration times of less than 150 ms and propagation velocities are fast more than 40 cm/s.[15] The annular velocities are also large more than 8 cm/s because of the rapid myocardial relaxation.[16] Doppler

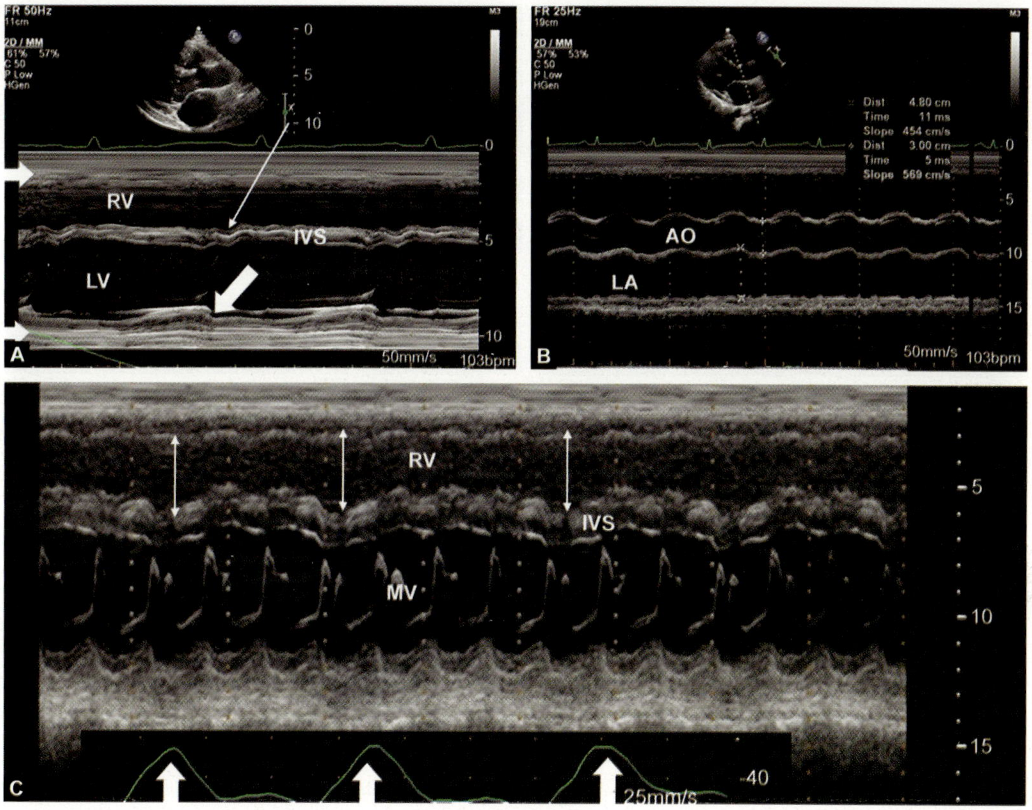

Figs. 2A to C: M-mode echocardiographic signs of constrictive pericarditis. (A) Horizontal thick arrows indicate thickened pericardium with no pericardial separation. Ventricular dimensions and function are normal, abrupt posterior motion of the posterior wall with flattening in diastole is indicated by oblique thick arrow. Thin oblique arrow shows the septal shudder; (B) The dilated left atria, indicating high filling pressures; (C) The classical inspiratory dilatation of the right ventricle, shown by double-headed arrows, recorded at slow speed of 25 mm/s. Vertical thick arrows indicate inspiration. (AO: aorta; IVS: interventricular septum; LA: left atrium; LV: left ventricle; MV mitral valve; RV: right ventricle)

echocardiography is essential for establishing the diagnosis and usually shows a restrictive LV and right ventricular (RV) diastolic filling pattern, characterized by a high early (E) velocity, a shortened deceleration time, and a reduced atrial (A) wave.[17] Mitral inflow velocity usually, but not always, falls by as much as 25–40%, and tricuspid velocity greatly increases (>40–60%) in the first beat after inspiration.[18] The respiratory variation and the mitral annular motion and the increased propagation velocity are the distinguishing features from restrictive cardiomyopathy.[19] At times, the respiratory variations can be provoked.[20] Presence of associated congenital heart disease or valve pathology may interfere with proper understanding of the hemodynamic changes (Figs. 5A to D).[21]

Combination of more than 25% variation in mitral inflow E-wave velocity and expiratory reversal of hepatic venous flow identifies patients with CP.[4] Restrictive cardiomyopathy is more often associated with severe atrial enlargement, a sharp halt in ventricular diastolic filling, and abnormal ventricular septal motion that results from interventricular dependence.[12] Figures 6A and B depicts the respiratory inflow velocity change between the right and left atrioventricular valves.

INTERVENTRICULAR SEPTAL MOVEMENTS IN CONSTRICTIVE PERICARDITIS

There is early rapid filling and equalization of both RV and LV diastolic pressures, findings which are seen in both constrictive and restrictive diseases. However, there is abrupt rise in RV pressure curve above the LV pressure curve during early diastole in CP.[22] This causes the early diastolic posterior movement of the ventricular septum called "septal bounce". M-mode shows interventricular septum (IVS) shifting briskly from the RV into the LV. As RV pressure plateaued, filling of the LV led to increased LV pressure, shifting the septum back (Fig. 7).[23] These findings were not seen in patients with restrictive cardiomyopathy. Septal bounce is a sign of exaggeration of respiratory ventricular

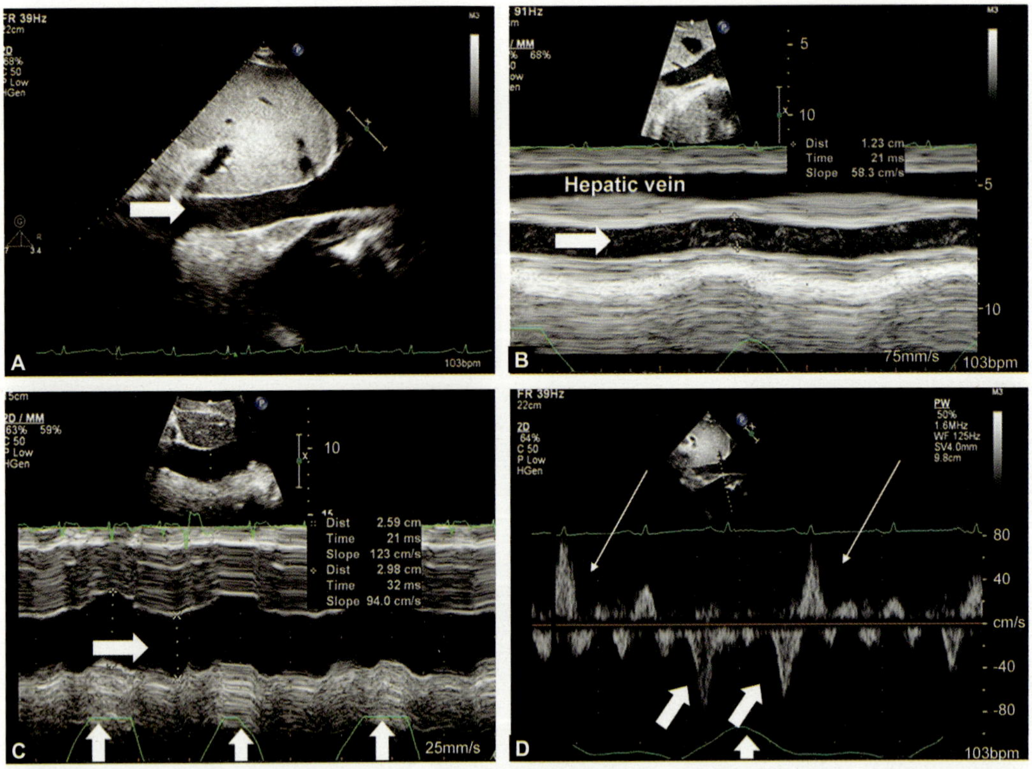

Figs. 3A to D: Inferior vena cava (IVC) signs of cardiac constriction. Horizontal thick arrows indicate dilated congested IVC in two-dimensional long-axis view in (A) and in M-mode in (B) and (C); (B) Spontaneous intravascular contrast, as echo shadows inside the IVC, reflecting sluggish flow, the traffic jam sign; (C) Inspiratory expansion, Kussmaul's sign; and (D) Finer details of Doppler interrogation, prominent VY collapse in the absence of significant tricuspid regurgitation, in inspiration, and prominent end-diastolic a wave reversal in expiration. Vertical thick arrow shows the inspiratory phase of respiration.

interdependence on echocardiography, cardiac computed tomography (CT), and cardiac magnetic resonance imaging (MRI).[9] There is reduced or paradoxical IVS movement during early diastole (i.e. initial septal movement toward and then away from the LV) secondary to marked restricted ventricular filling, seen mainly in constriction. In mild cases of constriction, a single wobble of the IVS was seen during normal inspiration. In more moderate cases a double motion of the septum (termed "double wobble") was seen where the septum bowed initially into the LV cavity in diastole then relaxed to the middle only to deviate again into the LV cavity late in diastole after atrial contraction (atrial systolic notch). In severe cases, the septum bowed into the LV cavity for the full duration of diastole (pan-diastolic motion). Inspiration also helped to characterize the severity of constriction especially in mild-to-moderate cases. The RV pressure may be higher than the LV pressure from the middle of the P wave owing to earlier activation and contraction of the RA producing the atrial systolic notch. Color M-mode Doppler is extremely sensitive to delineate this septal motion as shown in Figure 8. Essentially, the IVS being intracardiac is not involved in the fibrotic restraint of the pericardium like the free myocardial walls and so, truly oscillates with the transient intracardiac pressures shifts in diastole along with respiratory changes.

Abnormal septal motion (ASM) can be also seen in patients who underwent pericardiotomy during open heart surgery.[24] Valve surgery is more likely to cause ASM than coronary artery bypass surgery. Interestingly, it appeared about 70% of patients immediately after the open-heart surgery. It was associated with lower LV ejection fraction and late mitral filling velocity. It was not associated with myocardial ischemia and disappears with time (25% at 3–6 months and 15% after 1 year). ASM can be associated with the pericardial incision and resultant acute pericardial inflammation. As pericardial inflammation resolved gradually, the incidence of ASM decreased. Persistent ASM after 1 year might be associated with the pericardial adhesion. In addition to CP, pericardial tamponade, pulmonary hypertension, left bundle branch block, RV apical pacing are diseases which may show ASM.

ANNULUS PARADOXUS AND REVERSUS

It has been well established that the E/e' of more than 15, using mitral diastolic E wave and the mitral annular tissue

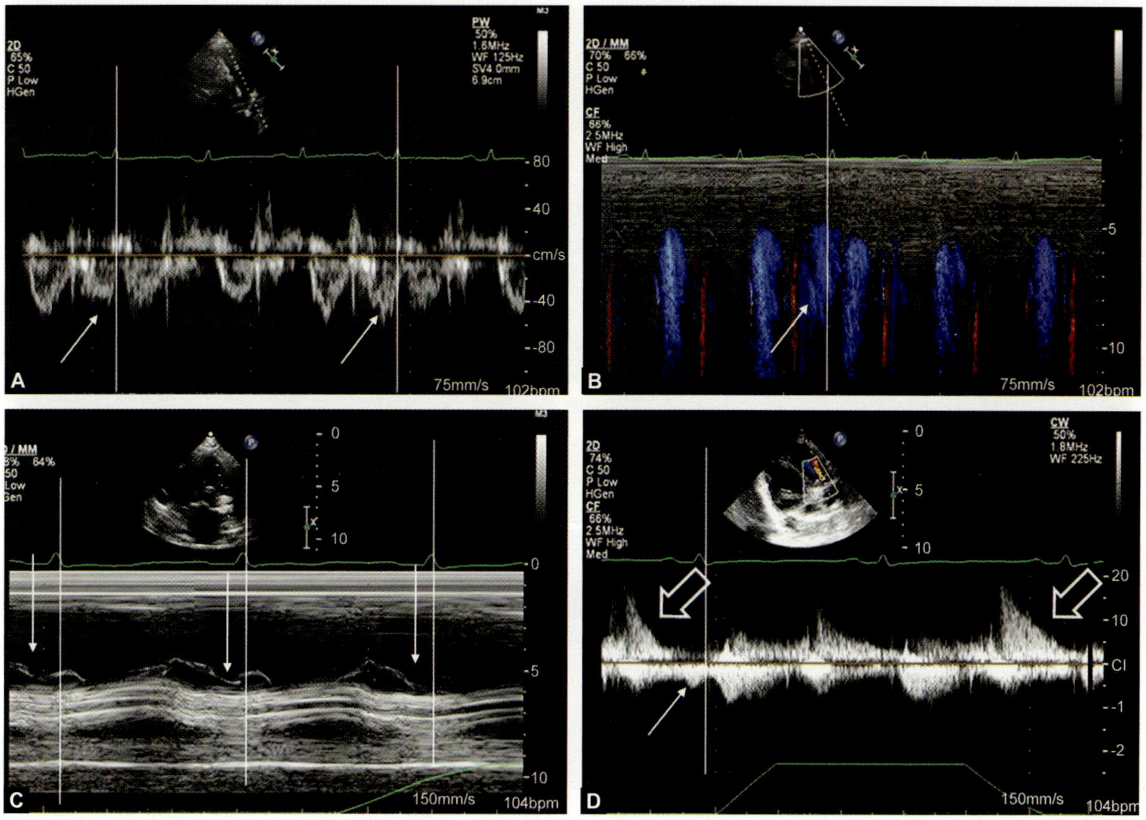

Figs. 4A to D: Atrial systolic forward flow into pulmonary artery shown by thin oblique arrows and the subsequent QRS complex is delineated by the vertical white line. (A) Pulse Doppler echo across the pulmonary valve; (B) Color M-mode Doppler across the pulmonary valve; (C) M-mode echocardiogram of the pulmonary valve showing the atrial systolic opening of the valve; and (D) Continuous wave Doppler echo across the pulmonary valve shows sharp deceleration time of the regurgitant jet coinciding with the atrial systolic elevation of right ventricular pressures.

Doppler E' wave, reflect elevated LV diastolic pressure of more than 20 mm Hg.[25] In patients with CP, mitral annular E' is well-preserved, despite increased filling pressures (Fig. 9), due to greater contribution by the longitudinal movement of the LV for diastolic filling and normal LV relaxation.[19] Hence E/e' remains low or normal and do not reflect the elevated LV diastolic or filling pressure.[26] This is called the annulus paradoxus.

Similarly, the amplitude of movement of lateral mitral annulus is more than the medial mitral annulus in normal individuals. The lateral annulus being adherent to the thickened pericardium in patients CP, may move less than the medial mitral annulus an abnormality unique for pericardial constriction (Figs. 10A and B). Reuss et al. noted the absolute difference of the averaged lateral and medial E' velocities for CP was –0.55 ± –2.57 cm/s and 2.27 ± –2.79 cm/s in controls. This relationship represents a reversal of the typical lateral and medial E' velocities observed in controls, hence termed "annulus reversus".[27]

EFFUSIVE CONSTRICTIVE PERICARDITIS

It is the most uncommon form of pericardial constraint syndromes. It occurs when pericardial fluid accumulates between a thickened, edematous or fibrotic parietal and visceral pericardium.[28] Infection, chest radiation, neoplasia, and connective tissue disorders are common causes.[29] Hallmark of this condition is similar to CP with hemodynamic occurrence of an elevated RA pressure, RV pressure, and LV end-diastolic pressure.[30] Echocardiographic features depend on the stage of disease. Most often M-mode, 2D, and Doppler features are consistent with a sizable pericardial effusion and cardiac tamponade, whereas later stage may have features suggestive of CP. Visceral pericardial thickening and irregularities may be appreciated at times (Fig. 11).[31]

Echocardiographic features of effusive CP, as illustrated, shows pericardial effusion, which could be echogenic, and may show organized strands. These bands could traverse

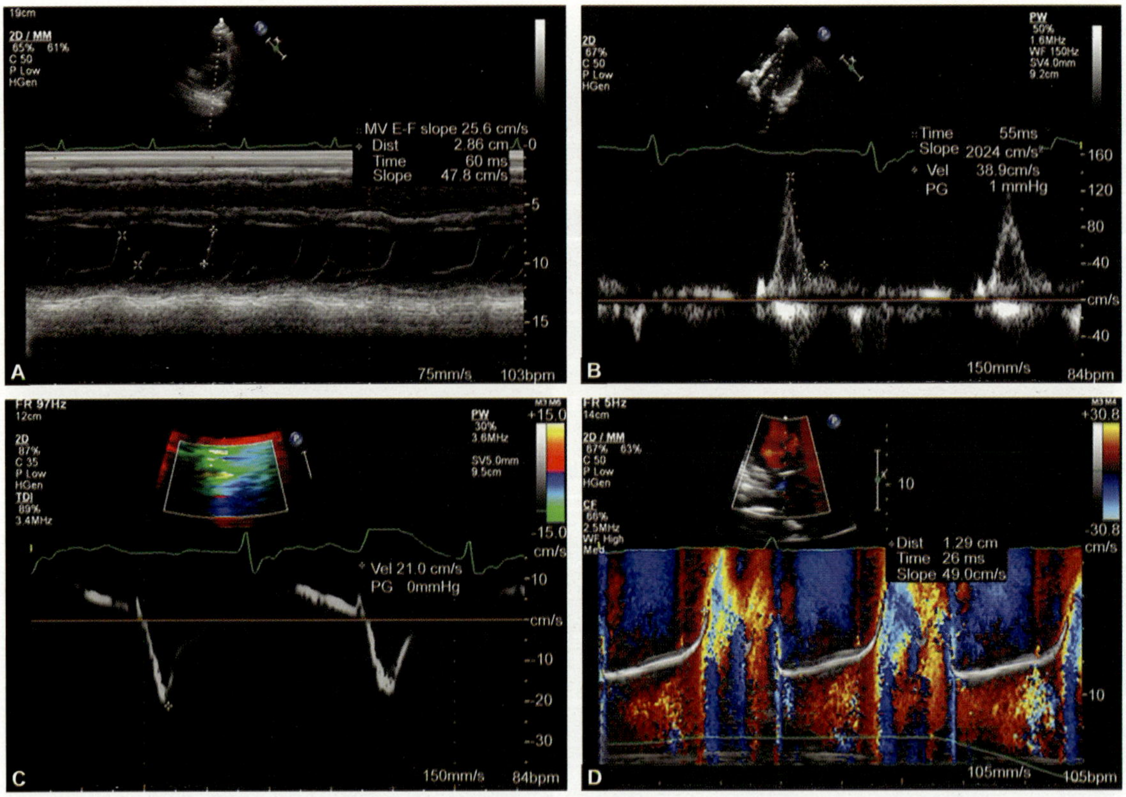

Figs. 5A to D: Echocardiographic features across the mitral inflow in constrictive pericarditis. (A) M-mode echo shows the rapid DE excursion and fast EF slope, with very little a wave excursion; (B) The pulse Doppler with a large E wave with a very short deceleration time and a diminutive atrial filling; (C) The tissue Doppler across the medial mitral annulus which shows an exaggerated e' wave of 21 cm/s; and (D) Illustrates the mitral propagation velocity which is 49 cm/s in the illustration.

the pericardial space from visceral to parietal surface.[32] Because of the effusion, thickening irregularities on the surface of the visceral pericardium can be better imaged. Loculation of the effusion is usual, and some features of tamponade illustrated at admission. Failure of reduction of diastolic intracardiac pressure after pericardial tapping unmasks the underlying constrictive physiology. Presence of effusion in addition helps to measure the visceral and parietal pericardial thickening.

CONSTRICTIVE PERICARDITIS AND RESTRICTIVE CARDIOMYOPATHY

Constrictive pericarditis and restrictive cardiomyopathy are challenging entities for echocardiographers to differentiate; however, advances in tissue Doppler imaging technology have led to more sophisticated methods to distinguish these cardiac conditions.[12] Both these conditions result in diastolic heart failure. Myocardial diastolic heart failure due to a stiff noncompliant ventricular myocardium causes restrictive cardiomyopathy while thickened noncompliant pericardium causes impaired diastolic filling of cardiac chambers results in CP.[33] Restrictive filling pattern due to stiff ventricle with normal or reduced RV and LV volumes.[34] When echocardiographic findings are similar tissue Doppler demonstration of low "S" waves and blunted E prime waves with no annulus paradoxus may identify restrictive cardiomyopathy.[35] CP with normal myocardium will always show normal "S" waves (Figs. 12A to C) and annulus reverses. Finer details of tissue motion and mitral annular studies and respiratory variation helps to differentiate both the entities.[16] But in some subset of patients especially after irradiation both constrictive pericardial and restrictive myocardial pathology could coexist which manifests as persistent heart failure post successful pericardiectomy.[34]

THREE-DIMENSIONAL AND SPECKLE TRACKING ECHO

Three-dimensional and speckle tracking echocardiography with advances computer software are useful in precisely estimating chamber volumes and function and understanding the torsional movements of the ventricles which have prognostic implications (Figs. 13 and 14).[36-38] Because

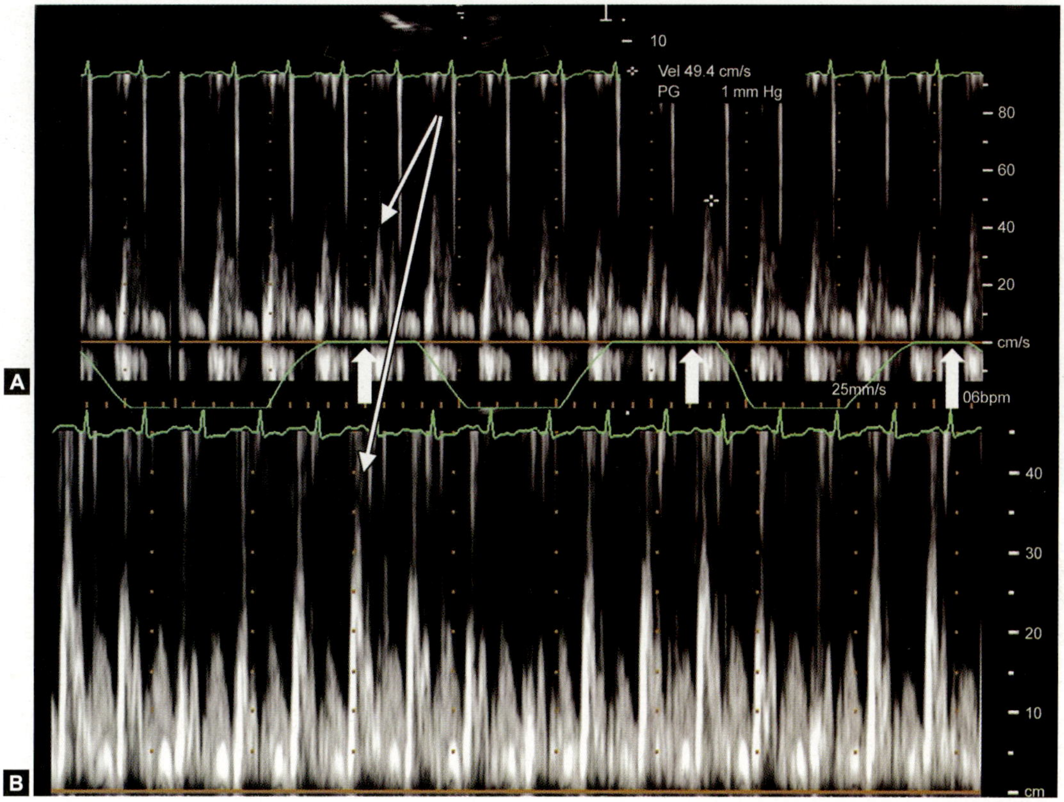

Figs. 6A and B: Exaggeration of inflow velocities with respiration on pulse Doppler interrogation. (A) The flow pattern across mitral valve, short-thin arrow, which declines more than 25% on inspiration, thick-white arrows; and (B) The flow pattern across the tricuspid valve which shows more than 33% increase in E wave velocities, thin-long arrow, during inspiration.

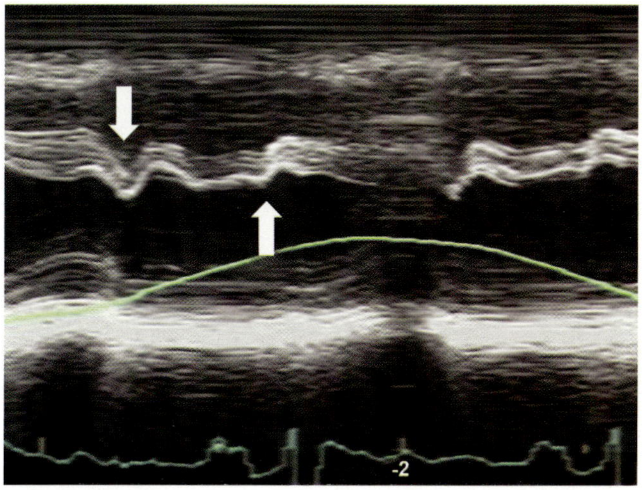

Fig. 7: Interventricular septum (IVS) movements in constrictive pericarditis. There is an abrupt posterior movement of the IVS (downward arrow) due to sudden rise of right ventricular pressure in early systole called the septal bounce. Later after the P of the electrocardiogram a short lived posterior movement of IVS is seen (upward arrow) due to earlier right atrial contraction.

of its limited availability in dedicated echo laboratories at research centers, the observations have not translated into routine clinical practices.[39,40]

LIMITATIONS

Those subjects who have difficult transthoracic echo window often restricts the information that can be generated to confidently identify the pericardial function problem. In the intensive care setting transesophageal echo is useful for bedside evaluation of pericardial problems.[41]

DIAGNOSTIC ALGORITHM

Good ventricular function with dilated atria and congested veins are the diagnostic hallmarks of diastolic heart failure. Restrictive filling of the ventricle is further confirmed by the prominent mitral E waves with short deceleration time less than 150 ms. The next stage is to differentiate between the restrictive cardiomyopathy and CP. The most useful pointers for the diagnosis of CP are the septal bounce, prominent E prime waves more than 8 cm at the mitral

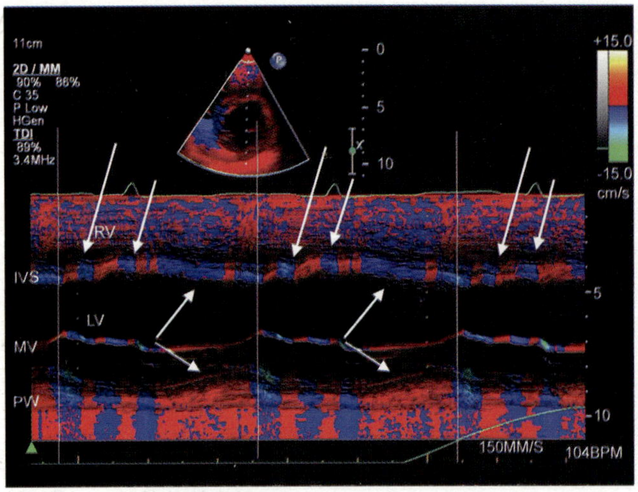

Fig. 8: Color M-mode echocardiogram of septal bounce in constrictive pericarditis. Motion away from the transducer is depicted blue and toward is depicted red. White lines show the end of ventricular systole. Diverging arrows inside the left ventricle (LV) show that the septum, interventricular septum (IVS), and the posterior wall, PW move toward each other in systole, reducing the ventricular volume, where in the septal movement is blue and the posterior wall red. In early diastole, the initial red movement of the septum depicting LV expansion is punctuated by the septal bounce, blue notch representing rapid right ventricular filling, (long white oblique arrow), followed by another blue notch corresponding with the atrial filling of the right ventricle, short oblique arrow.

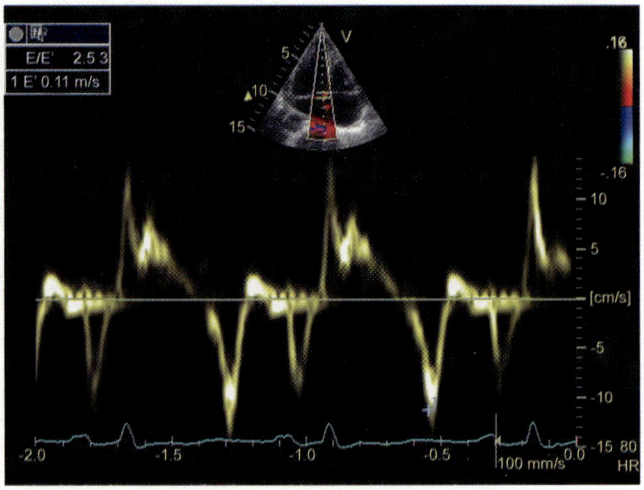

Fig. 9: Pulse tissue Doppler tracing from a patient with constrictive pericarditis. Movement of the medial annulus of the mitral valve showing prominent mitral E'. With normal E wave of mitral valve the E/e' is less than 7 in presence elevated pulmonary wedge or left atrial (LA) pressure. Measured pulmonary capillary wedge pressure was 28 mm Hg and E/e' is only 2.53.

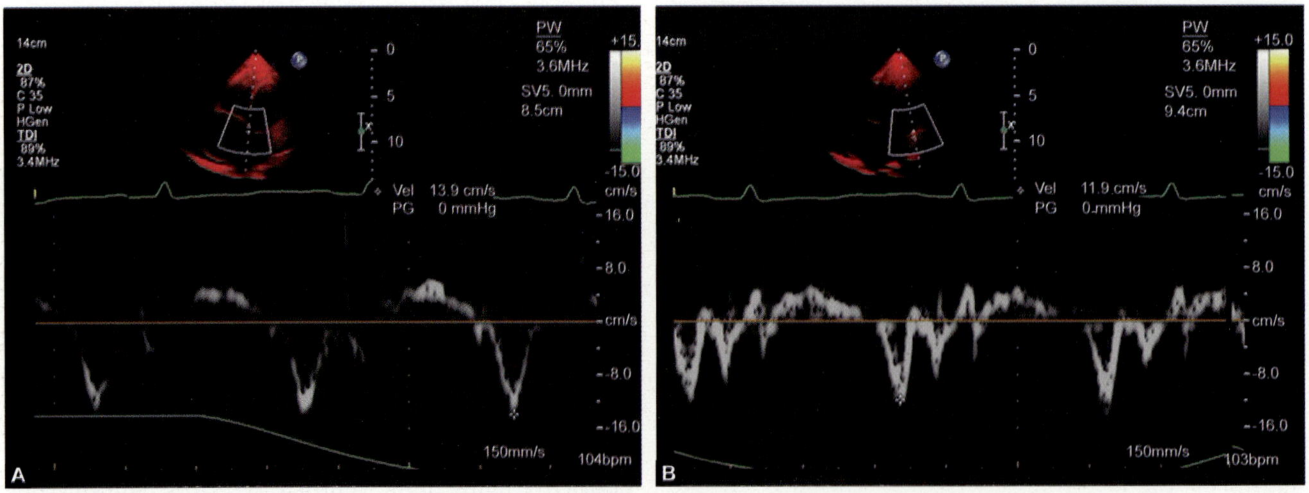

Figs. 10A and B: Annulus reverses demonstrated by pulse tissue Doppler evaluation in a subject with constrictive pericarditis. (A) The medial mitral annulus with E' prime of 13.9; and (B) Lateral mitral annular velocity is 11.9 cm/s.

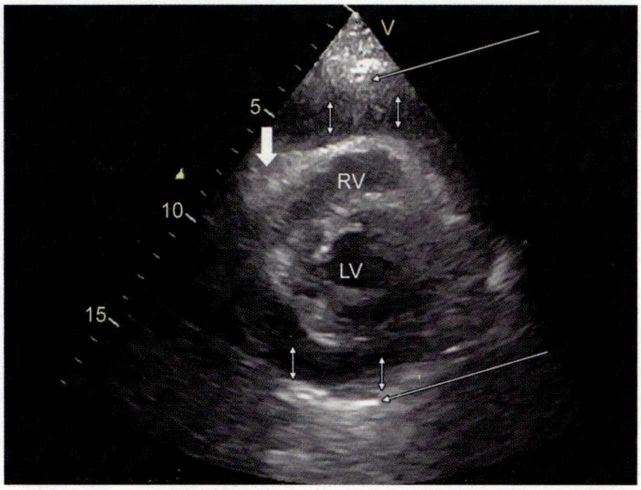

Fig. 11: Effusive constrictive pericarditis showing thickening of visceral shown by thick vertical arrows and parietal pericardium, shown by long oblique arrows with pericardial effusion illustrated by vertical double-headed arrows. (LV: left ventricle; RV: right ventricle)

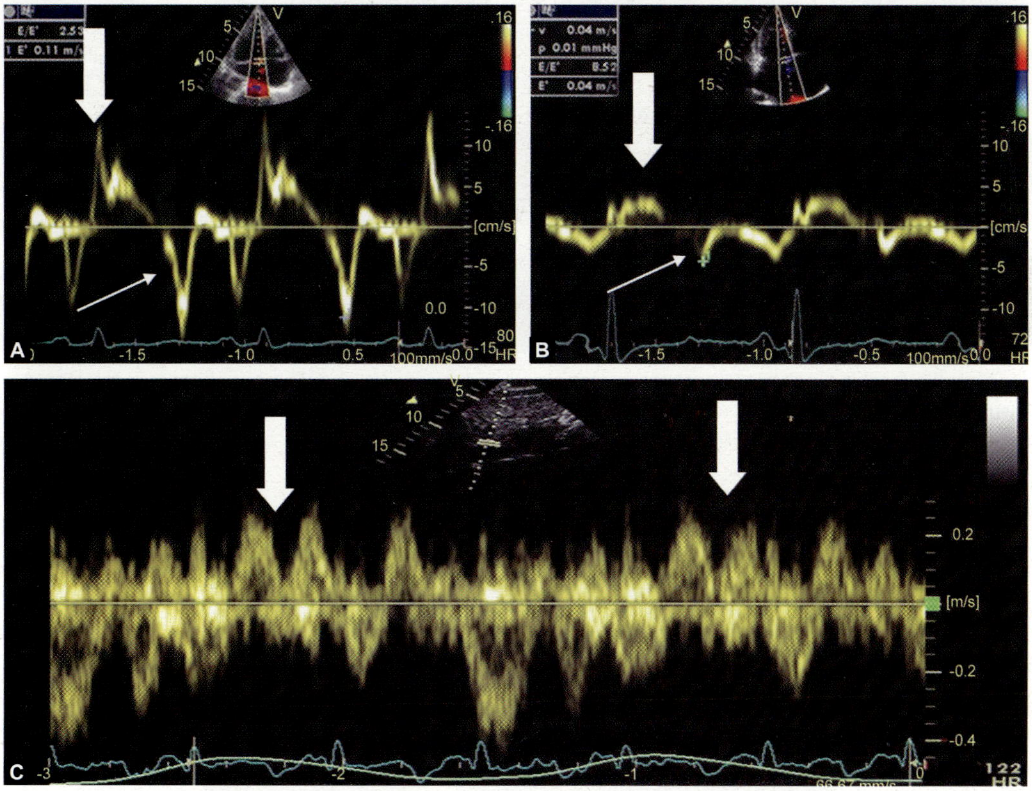

Figs. 12A to C: Selected Doppler studies to differentiate constrictive pericarditis from restrictive cardiomyopathy. Tissue Doppler tracings from the medial mitral annulus. (A) Normal S wave velocity (arrow) and good E' prime velocity consistent with constrictive pericarditis; (B) Contrasts the same in restrictive cardiomyopathy. S waves (arrow) are of low velocity due to myocardial involvement. Note the poor E' prime velocity also; and (C) The exaggerated flow reversal in early expiration in the subject with restrictive cardiomyopathy.

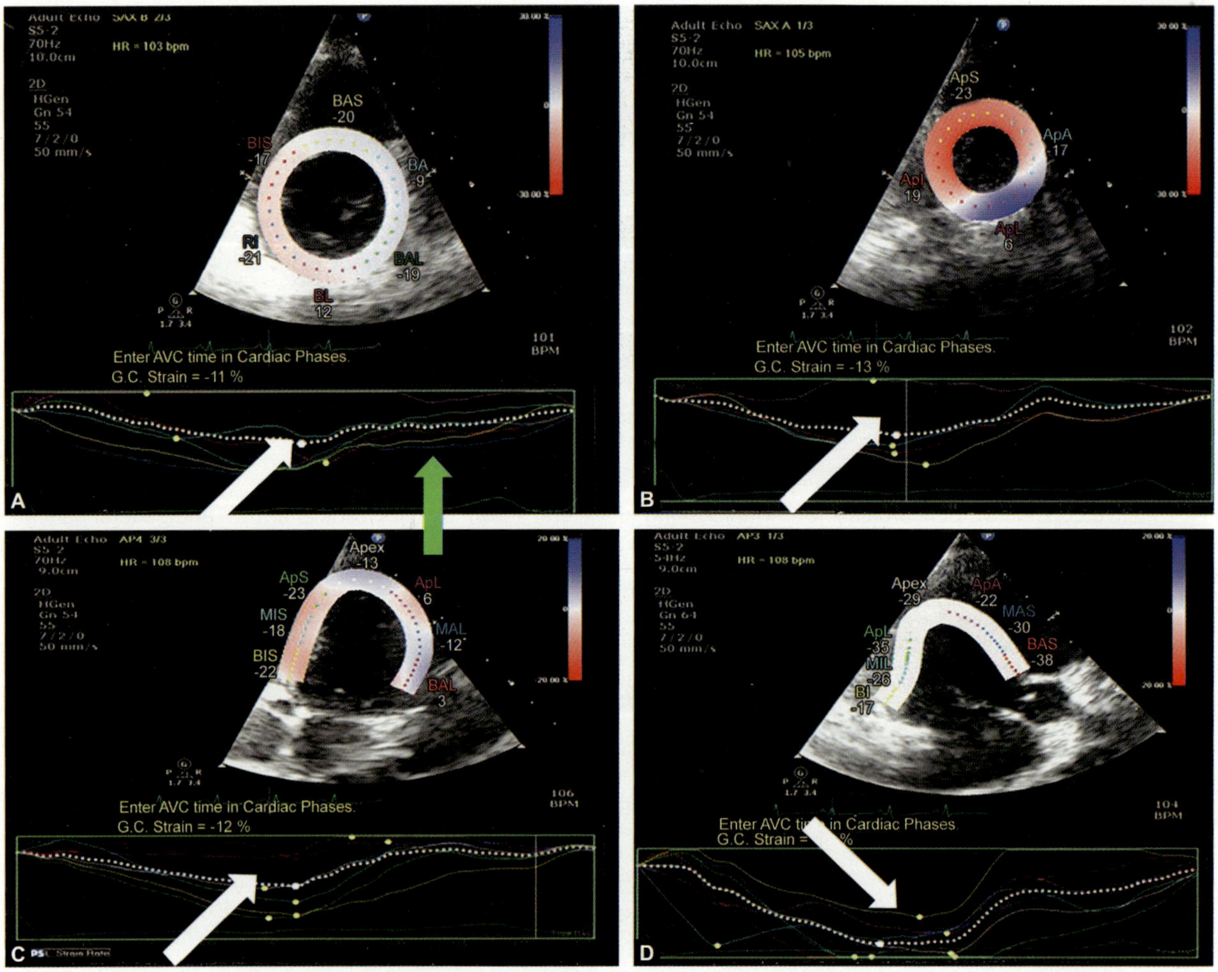

Figs. 13A to D: Speckle tracking echocardiography in constrictive pericarditis showing synchronous movements of the septal and adjacent structures which are not involved in the fibrous constriction compared to reduced or dyskinetic movement of the adherent lateral wall. (A) Cross-section at the base; (B) Cross-section at the apex; (C) Long-axis four-chamber view; and (D) Apical three-chamber view.

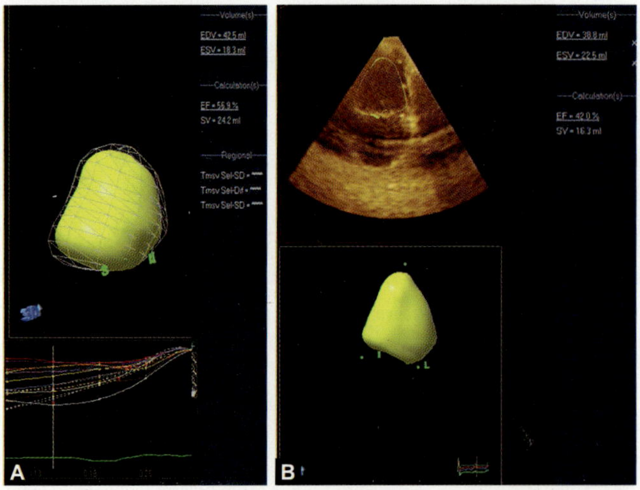

Figs. 14A and B: Volume estimation using Q-Lab of three-dimensional echocardiographic surface rendered images. (A and B) A large left atrial volume compared to left ventricle in (B). Systolic function of both the chambers is good. 2 mL higher stroke volume of the left atrium signifies the mild regurgitant volume of atrioventricular valve regurgitation.

annulus and mitral propagation velocity more than 40 cm/s in the absence of any major atrioventricular regurgitation.[6]

CONCLUSION

Bedside Doppler echocardiography is the simple cheap, evaluation to delineate the constrictive pericardial physiology which can be repeated serially, to understand its clinical course.[42] Hence many patients with transient pericardial constriction are now identified and medically managed avoiding years of mistaken diagnosis.[43] Mastering the finer echocardiographic details of the diagnostic algorithm is therefore the crux in identifying CP.[4]

REFERENCES

1. Syed FF, Schaff HV, Oh JK. Constrictive pericarditis—a curable diastolic heart failure. Nat Rev Cardiol. 2014;11(9):530-44.
2. Fowler NO. Constrictive pericarditis: its history and current status. Clin Cardiol. 1995;18(6):341-50.
3. Sultan FAT, Tariq MU. Clinical features, management and outcome of patients with constrictive pericarditis—experience from a third world country. J Saudi Heart Assoc. 2018;30(1):9-13.
4. Welch TD, Oh JK. Constrictive pericarditis: old disease, new approaches. Curr Cardiol Rep. 2015;17(4):20.
5. Nachum E, Sternik L, Kassif Y, et al. Surgical pericardiectomy for constrictive pericarditis: a single tertiary center experience. Thorac Cardiovasc Surg. 2018. [Epub ahead of print].
6. Welch TD, Ling LH, Espinosa RE, et al. Echocardiographic diagnosis of constrictive pericarditis: Mayo Clinic criteria. Circ Cardiovasc Imaging. 2014;7(3):526-34.
7. Engel PJ, Fowler NO, Tei C, et al. M-mode echocardiography in constrictive pericarditis. J Am Coll Cardiol. 1985;6(2):471-4.
8. Talreja DR, Edwards WD, Danielson GK, et al. Constrictive pericarditis in 26 patients with histologically normal pericardial thickness. Circulation. 2003;108(15):1852-7.
9. Walker CM, Chung JH, Reddy GP. "Septal bounce". J Thorac Imaging. 2012;27(1):W1.
10. Himelman RB, Kircher B, Rockey DC, et al. Inferior vena cava plethora with blunted respiratory response: a sensitive echocardiographic sign of cardiac tamponade. J Am Coll Cardiol. 1988;12(6):1470-7.
11. Spodick DH. Cardiac tamponade and Kussmaul's sign. Circulation. 1981;64(5):1078-8.
12. Zwas DR, Gotsman I, Admon D, et al. Advances in the differentiation of constrictive pericarditis and restrictive cardiomyopathy. Herz. 2012;37(6):664-73.
13. Goten C, Murai H, Takashima S-I, et al. Occult constrictive pericardial disease emerging 40 years after chest radiation therapy: a case report. BMC Cardiovasc Disord. 2018;18(1):107.
14. Sohn DW. Constrictive pericarditis as a never ending story: what's new? Korean Circ J. 2012;42(3):143-50.
15. Napolitano G, Pressacco J, Paquet E. Imaging features of constrictive pericarditis: beyond pericardial thickening. Can Assoc Radiol J. 2009;60(1):40-6.
16. Liu S, Ren W, Zhang J, et al. Incremental value of the tissue motion of annular displacement derived from speckle-tracking echocardiography for differentiating chronic constrictive pericarditis from restrictive cardiomyopathy. J Ultrasound Med. 2018;37(11):2637-45.
17. Oh JK, Hatle LK, Seward JB, et al. Diagnostic role of Doppler echocardiography in constrictive pericarditis. J Am Coll Cardiol. 1994;23(1):154-62.
18. Sohn DW, Kim YJ, Kim HS, et al. Unique features of early diastolic mitral annulus velocity in constrictive pericarditis. J Am Soc Echocardiogr. 2004;17(3):222-6.
19. Ha JW, Oh JK, Ommen SR, et al. Diagnostic value of mitral annular velocity for constrictive pericarditis in the absence of respiratory variation in mitral inflow velocity. J Am Soc Echocardiogr. 2002;15(12):1468-71.
20. Oh JK, Tajik AJ, Appleton CP, et al. Preload reduction to unmask the characteristic Doppler features of constrictive pericarditis. A new observation. Circulation. 1997;95(4):796-9.
21. Gupta SK, Ramakrishnan S, Kothari SS, et al. Hemodynamics of large ventricular septal defect and coexisting chronic constrictive pericarditis masquerading as Eisenmenger's syndrome. Catheter Cardiovasc Interv. 2014;83(2):263-9.
22. Tei C, Child JS, Tanaka H, et al. Atrial systolic notch on the interventricular septal echogram: an echocardiographic sign of constrictive pericarditis. J Am Coll Cardiol. 1983;1(3):907-12.
23. Coylewright M, Welch TD, Nishimura RA. Mechanism of septal bounce in constrictive pericarditis: a simultaneous cardiac catheterisation and echocardiographic study. Heart. 2013;99(18):1376.
24. Park JH. Incidence and fate of the abnormal septal motion after open heart surgeries. J Cardiovasc Ultrasound. 2014;22(1):6-7.
25. Matsushita K, Minamishima T, Goda A, et al. Comparison of the reliability of E/E' to estimate pulmonary capillary wedge pressure in heart failure patients with preserved ejection fraction versus those with reduced ejection fraction. Int J Cardiovasc Imaging. 2015;31(8):1497-502.
26. Welch TD, Oh JK. Constrictive pericarditis: the mitral annulus remains paradoxical. Am J Cardiol. 2015;115(5):704.
27. Reuss CS, Wilansky SM, Lester SJ, et al. Using mitral "annulus reversus" to diagnose constrictive pericarditis. Eur J Echocardiogr. 2009;10(3):372-5.
28. Sagristà-Sauleda J, Angel J, Sánchez A, et al. Effusive-constrictive pericarditis. N Engl J Med. 2004;350(5):469-75.
29. Hancock EW. A clearer view of effusive-constrictive pericarditis. N Engl J Med. 2004;350(5):435-7.
30. Syed FF, Ntsekhe M, Mayosi BM, et al. Effusive-constrictive pericarditis. Heart Fail Rev. 2013;18(3):277-87.
31. Klein AL, Cremer PC. Ephemeral effusive constrictive pathophysiology. JACC Cardiovasc Imaging. 2018;11(4): 542-5.
32. Mohanan Nair KK, Ganapathi S, Sivadasanpillai H, et al. A case of rheumatic fibrinous pericarditis. Circ Cardiovasc Imaging. 2016;9(12):e005399.

33. Ardhanari S, Yarlagadda B, Parikh V, et al. Systematic review of non-invasive cardiovascular imaging in the diagnosis of constrictive pericarditis. Indian Heart J. 2017;69(1):57-67.
34. Geske JB, Anavekar NS, Nishimura RA, et al. Differentiation of constriction and restriction: complex cardiovascular hemodynamics. J Am Coll Cardiol. 2016;68(21):2329-47.
35. Chhabra L, Azeem AA, Spodick DH, et al. Revisiting annulus paradoxus in constrictive pericarditis. Int J Cardiol. 2015;195(1):288-9.
36. Choudhry MW, Homsi M, Mastouri R, et al. Prevalence and prognostic value of right ventricular systolic dysfunction in patients with constrictive pericarditis who underwent pericardiectomy. Am J Cardiol. 2015;116(3):469-73.
37. Liu S, Ma C, Ren W, et al. Left atrial systolic and diastolic dysfunction in patients with chronic constrictive pericarditis: a study using speckle tracking and conventional echocardiography. PLoS ONE. 2013;8(6):e68718.
38. Sudhakar S, Nanda NC. Role of live/real time three-dimensional transthoracic echocardiography in pericardial disease. Echocardiography. 2012;29(1):98-102.
39. Choudhury A, Magoon R, Malik V, et al. Studying diastology with speckle tracking echocardiography: the essentials. Ann Card Anaesth. 2017;20(Suppl):S57-60.
40. Sengupta PP, Krishnamoorthy VK, Abhayaratna WP, et al. Disparate patterns of left ventricular mechanics differentiate constrictive pericarditis from restrictive cardiomyopathy. JACC Cardiovasc Imaging. 2008;1(1):29-38.
41. Scohy TV, Maat APWM, McGhie J, et al. Three-dimensional transesophageal echocardiography: diagnosing the extent of pericarditis constrictiva and intraoperative surgical support. J Card Surg. 2009;24(3):305-8.
42. Kytö V, Sipilä J, Rautava P. Chronic constrictive pericarditis in general adult population. Int J Cardiol. 2014;176(3):1158-60.
43. Gentry J, Klein AL, Jellis CL. Transient constrictive pericarditis: current diagnostic and therapeutic strategies. Curr Cardiol Rep. 2016;18(5):41.

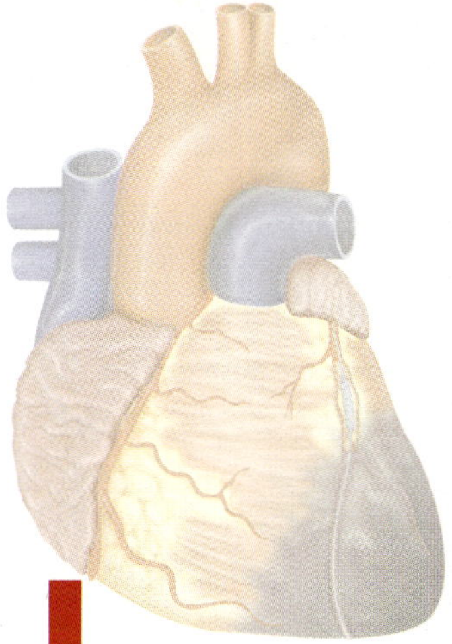

94

CHAPTER

Computed Tomography and Magnetic Resonance Imaging in Pericardial Diseases

Tarun Mittal

INTRODUCTION

The role of multimodality imaging for pericardial diseases has been emerging in recent years and has been recommended both by the American Society of Echocardiography as well as the European Society of Cardiovascular Imaging.[1,2] Although echocardiography is the first line of imaging technique in patients suspected with pericardial diseases and plays an important role in assessment of pericardial effusion and diagnosis of constrictive pericarditis as well as tamponade, both computed tomography (CT) and magnetic resonance imaging (MRI) are complementary in diagnosis and management of pericardial diseases. The role of CT and MRI in pericardial diseases emerged in 1970s,[3,4] but has been enhanced with advances in electrocardiography (ECG)-gating and increased spatial resolution with cardiac CT,[5] and faster sequences and tissue characterization with MRI.[6,7] Both CT and MRI have the advantage of providing a wider perspective of the heart, surrounding mediastinum, and chest irrespective of patient's body size and chronic obstructive pulmonary disease.

TECHNICAL ASPECTS AND PROTOCOL

Computed Tomography

Computed tomography can be performed with or without intravenous contrast, and with or without ECG-gating. For best demonstration of pericardium, CT is best performed with ECG-gating. Initially, the scan is performed without contrast for assessment of calcification followed by contrast in a delayed phase. To reduce the radiation dose, prospective ECG-gating protocols are employed with body mass index (BMI) adjusted milliampere second (mAs) and peak kilovoltage (kVp). However, functional assessment of the ventricles can also be obtained by using retrospective ECG-gating along with ECG-modulation to reduce the radiation dose. Although, optimal demonstration of the pericardium is obtained with ECG-gating, simple nongating CT can also suffice in some cases. Modern multislice CT scanners (64-slice or more) can acquire the whole scan in 10–20 seconds breath-hold with high spatial resolution (0.3–0.5 mm). The images are acquired in axial plane but as the data is volumetric, it is easily displayed on postprocessing software in sagittal and coronal planes as well as different cardiac long and short-axis planes for easier interpretation. Although 64-slice or more CT scanners are recommended for CT coronary angiography, a scan for the pericardium can also be performed with lower slice scanners at a cost of increased breath holding time. As CT scanning uses ionizing radiation to produce images, patient receives a radiation dose ranging from 1 mSv to 15 mSv depending upon the scanner and protocol used.

Magnetic Resonance Imaging

Magnetic resonance imaging scan does not involve ionizing radiation and provides anatomy of the heart and pericardium, functional assessment, as well as tissue characterization.[1,7] MRI of the heart is typically performed with ECG-gating in axial and different cardiac-axis planes.

TABLE 1: Comparison of CT and MRI for pericardial diseases.

Technical parameters and findings	*CT*	*MRI (sequences)*
Imaging time	<10 minutes for whole scan	30–60 minutes
Ionizing radiation	Radiation dose 1–15 mSv	None
Spatial resolution	0.3–1 mm	5–8 mm
Demonstration of pericardial thickness	Easy, with higher spatial resolution	Easy, but less spatial resolution (T1- and T2-weighted)
Demonstration of calcification	Very sensitive	Difficult (same)
Demonstration of inflammation	With contrast in delayed phase	Easier (T2-weighted, pre- and postcontrast T1-weighted)
Demonstration of effusion	Easy, particularly with contrast	Easy (T1- and T2-weighted)
Characterization of effusion	Based on density	Based on signal intensity (T1- and T2-weighted)
Assessment of ventricular function	Only possible with retrospective ECG-gating	Standard (cine sequences)
Assessment of ventricular coupling and septal bounce	Only possible with retrospective ECG-gating	Easy (cine sequences with free-breathing)
Demonstration of associated myocarditis	Difficult	Easily performed (STIR and late gadolinium enhancement)
Demonstration of lung parenchyma	Gold standard technique	To some extent (T1-weighted)

(CT: computed tomography; ECG: electrocardiography; MRI: magnetic resonance imaging; STIR: short tau inversion recovery)

Different sequences are employed to demonstrate anatomy (black blood, fast spin echo T1- and T2-weighted images) and function of the heart [cine balanced steady-state free precession (SSFP) sequence]. Latter is typically performed with breath-holding in expiratory phase, but free-breathing sequences can be performed to evaluate septal bounce. Fat suppressed T2-weighted short tau inversion recovery (STIR) images help in detecting edema while delayed enhancement (DE) after contrast (gadolinium chelates) administration may demonstrate inflammation or fibrosis.[8] Although MRI allows imaging of the heart and pericardium in different planes, the images can only be viewed as acquired and no further reconstructions can be performed once images are obtained.

A 1.5-T MRI scanner with ECG-gating facility and surface coils are considered to be best for imaging the heart.

Although, CT and MRI are different technically in terms of how images are produced and visualized, both techniques have their advantages and limitations for different pathologies and can be complementary in the diagnosis of pericardial diseases (Table 1).

ANATOMY OF PERICARDIUM ON CT AND MRI

The outer parietal and the inner visceral layers of pericardium are normally apposed to each other appearing as a single layer on CT and MRI separated by a layer of fat from the underlying myocardium (Fig. 1).[1,7] Between the two layers is a potential pericardial space which becomes evident with accumulation of fluid and separation of the two layers (Figs. 3D and 4). The combined pericardium is up to 2 mm thick and is readily visible as a thin curvilinear structure with intermediate density on CT images or low signal intensity of T1- or T2-weighted MRI images, sandwiched between the two layers of fat. There is no enhancement of a normal pericardium after contrast on either CT or MRI. A small amount of fluid (up to 50 mL) can normally be seen in the dependent inferior pericardial space which acts as a lubricant between the two layers. The layer of fat between the pericardium and the underlying myocardium is called epicardial fat, while the layer of fat outside the pericardium is also called pericardial fat (Fig. 1).[1] The fat appears much darker than the pericardium on CT while it appears brighter than the pericardium on MRI sequences (when not suppressed), thus making the pericardium easily visible on both scans. The pericardium is best visible along the anterior surface of the right ventricle and atrium due to larger amount of fat, and less so along the posterior and lateral surfaces where lack of visualization should not be mistaken as absent pericardium (Fig. 1A). The pericardium surrounds the heart expect where it reflects due to insertion of veins and arteries forming sinuses (Figs. 1B and C). There is an oblique sinus on the posterior aspect of the left atrium due to insertion of the pulmonary veins, and a transverse sinus formed between ascending aorta and main

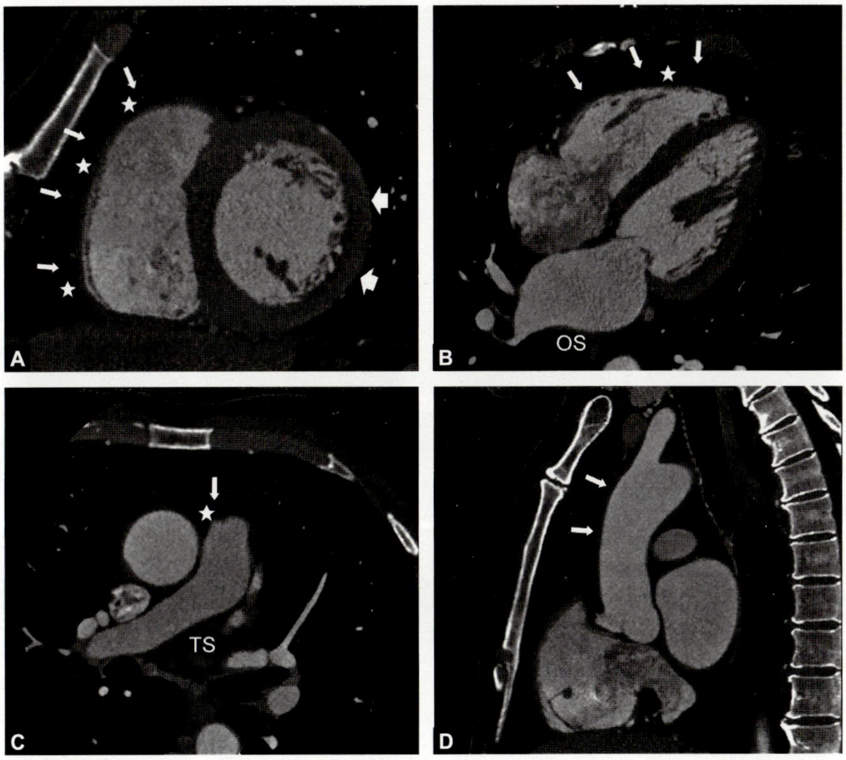

Figs. 1A to D: Cardiac CT scan with contrast in arterial phase demonstrates normal pericardium as thin curvilinear structure (white arrows, comprising of both parietal and visceral layers) in short-axis (A) and four-chamber views (B). Pericardium surrounds the heart except at the oblique sinus (OS, B) and transverse sinus (TS, C), and extend superiorly to cover the anterior aspects of the ascending aorta (C and D) as well as main pulmonary artery (C). Epicardial layer of fat (white asterisk) lies between the pericardium and myocardium, while pericardial fat lies outside. *Note*: Lack of visualization of the pericardium on the posterior surface of the left ventricle due to relative lack of fat (wide arrow, A).

pulmonary artery anteriorly and superior vena cava (SVC) and superior pulmonary veins posteriorly. The pericardium extends along the ascending aorta, sometimes to the aortic arch ending proximal to the origin of the brachiocephalic trunk. In some patients, the pericardium forms pouches along the proximal parts of ascending aorta, pulmonary arteries, and superior venae cava, and pulmonary veins called recesses, which are a normal finding but mistaken for lymphadenopathy and other pathologies.[9]

DIAGNOSIS OF PERICARDIAL DISEASES ON CT AND MRI

Pericardial diseases may be considered as acquired or congenital. Of the acquired conditions, pericarditis, pericardial effusion, cardiac tamponade, and constrictive pericarditis comprise the "pericardial syndrome".[10] The etiology of pericardial diseases is varied and can be broadly classified as infectious and noninfectious, with viruses being most common cause in developed countries and tuberculosis being common in developing ones.

Pericarditis

The diagnosis of pericarditis is generally clinical, but certain findings on CT and MRI which can support the clinical diagnosis. Diffuse thickening of the pericardium on either CT or MRI to more than or equal to 4 mm with or without pericardial effusion in a patient with clinical suspicion of acute or chronic pericarditis can be highly supportive (Fig. 2).[1,5] Enhancement of pericardium may not be present in all cases but when present has been shown to be characteristic of inflammation, increased granulation tissue, and neovascularization.[8,11] On MRI, morphology of the pericardium can be easily demonstrated on black-blood T1- and T2-weighted images. To demonstrate inflammation, both STIR (Fig. 2E) and DE sequences (Fig. 2F) have been shown to be helpful.[6,8,11] The latter sequences are also useful to demonstrate associated myocarditis if present, when the pericarditis is termed as myopericarditis and is associated with raised troponin and ST-elevation, mimicking acute myocardial infarction. Myocardial involvement in

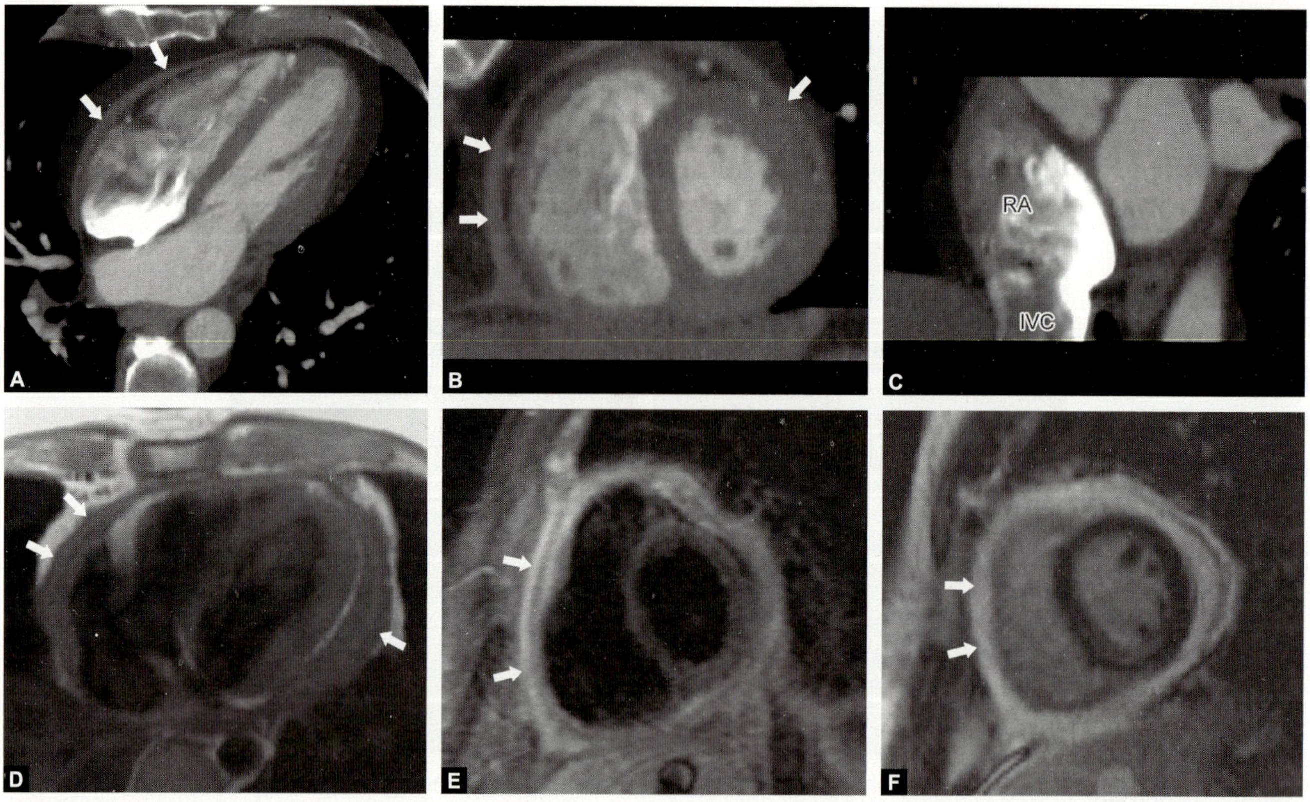

Figs. 2A to F: Cardiac computed tomography angiogram (upper row) of a 34-year-old man presenting with chest pain and shortness of breath showing diffuse thickening of the pericardium on four-chamber (arrows, A) and short-axis views (B). Note the tubular shape of the heart (A) along with dilatation of the right atrium (RA) and inferior vena cava (IVC, C) suggesting constrictive pericarditis. Cardiac magnetic resonance imaging scan (lower row) of a 22-year-old man with pyrexia and breathlessness demonstrate irregular thickening of the pericardium to varying degree on four-chamber view (arrows, D), edema on the short-axis (arrows, E), and generalized enhancement on the delayed postcontrast images (arrows, F).

pericarditis can be seen in almost one-third of cases and carries a relatively benign prognosis.[12] CT or MRI are indicated in pericarditis where there is ongoing clinical concern and echocardiographic findings are inconclusive,[1] failure of response to anti-inflammatory therapy, to search for a specific cause (i.e. tuberculosis or malignancy), or in patients with associated trauma.

Pericardial Calcification

Calcification in the pericardium is characteristic of tuberculous infection, a common cause of pericarditis in developing countries. However, calcification can also be idiopathic, occur following viral pericarditis, chronic purulent pericarditis, hemopericardium, previous cardiac surgery or radiotherapy, or collagen diseases.[5,13] Calcification in the pericardium is best seen with CT (Fig. 3), which is the most sensitive noninvasive technique to demonstrate calcification. Calcification can be focal involving any part of the pericardium or be more diffuse almost encasing the heart. Presence of calcification by itself does not necessarily means constriction,[14] a diagnosis that requires other clinical and imaging features to be present.

Constrictive Pericarditis

Constrictive pericarditis is characterized by impaired diastolic filling of the ventricles due to pericardial disease[10] with diagnosis made on clinical features and echocardiography. Both CT and MRI can demonstrate the thickened pericardium, pericardial effusion, pleural effusion, dilatation of atria, and that of inferior vena cava (IVC; greater than descending aorta at the level of esophageal hiatus), which are more common in patients with constriction compared to those without constriction (Figs 2A to C).[6,13,15] CT readily demonstrates calcification which can be focal or extensive (Fig. 3) and is present in about 50% of patients with constriction.[1] CT may assist in the preoperative planning of pericardiectomy by detailing the location and severity of pericardial thickening and calcification.[1] It can also detect the presence of fibrosis in the

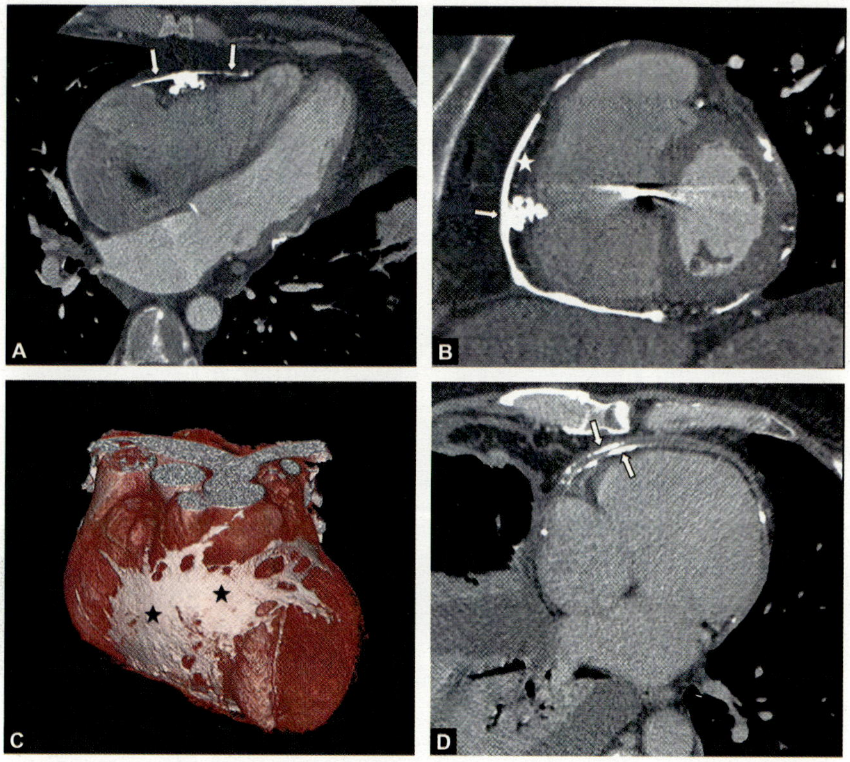

Figs. 3A to D: Extensive pericardial calcification (A to C) in a 49-year-old man with progressive shortness of breath and history of previous myopericarditis. Calcification is most pronounced anteriorly (arrows) and cross the anterior atrioventricular (A and B) and anterior interventricular grooves (C) with florid focal calcification extending into the myocardium. Elsewhere calcified pericardium is separate from underlying myocardium anteriorly by epicardial fat (white asterisk, B). Also seen is tubular-shaped heart with enlargement of right ventricle and atrium with bowing of septum toward left ventricle (A and B). Another patient with calcification separately in the two layers of pericardium (arrows, D).

adjacent lung parenchyma due to radiotherapy which may have a bearing on surgical approach. Another characteristic appearance of constrictive pericarditis is that of tube-like configuration of one or more ventricles on both CT and MRI in patients with advanced pericardial constriction (Figs 2A and 3A).[13] Septal bounce is best shown on cine MRI, particularly with free breathing. Presence of delayed contrast enhancement on MRI has been shown in constrictive pericarditis to represent inflammatory component,[6,11] but constriction can occur without enhancement due to chronic fibrosing pericarditis. Inflammatory edema is similarly less frequent in constrictive pericarditis. Although increased pericardial thickening of more than or equal to 4 mm is one of the characteristic features of constriction, normal thickness of pericardium has been reported in up to 18% of patients[16] in pericardial constriction generally caused by previous thoracotomy and irradiation.

Pericardial Effusion

Both loculated and generalized pericardial effusions are easily demonstrable on CT and MRI due to larger field of view (Fig. 4). However, smaller effusions of less than 5 mm which are associated with thickening of pericardial layers may be difficult of identify on CT without delayed phase contrast.[1] MRI may more readily demonstrate small effusions from surrounding pericardium without contrast. The size of the effusion is quantified in the same way as on echocardiography with less than 10 mm depth being classified as small, between 10 mm and 20 mm being moderate, and larger than 20 mm being classified as large.[10] Pericardial effusions are characterized by their density on CT, with lower density (<20 HU) representing serous or transudate collection from any cause and moderate density (20–60 HU) representing purulent, malignant, myxedematous cause (Fig. 4B).[1] Acute hemorrhage from trauma or other causes could have a much higher density (>60 HU). Transudate fluid on MRI would have signal intensity similar to clear fluid, being low on T1-weighted images and bright on T2-weighted images. Increasing degree of exudative content would increase the signal on T1-weighted images as well as on T2-weighted images. Appearance of hemorrhage would depend upon its duration.

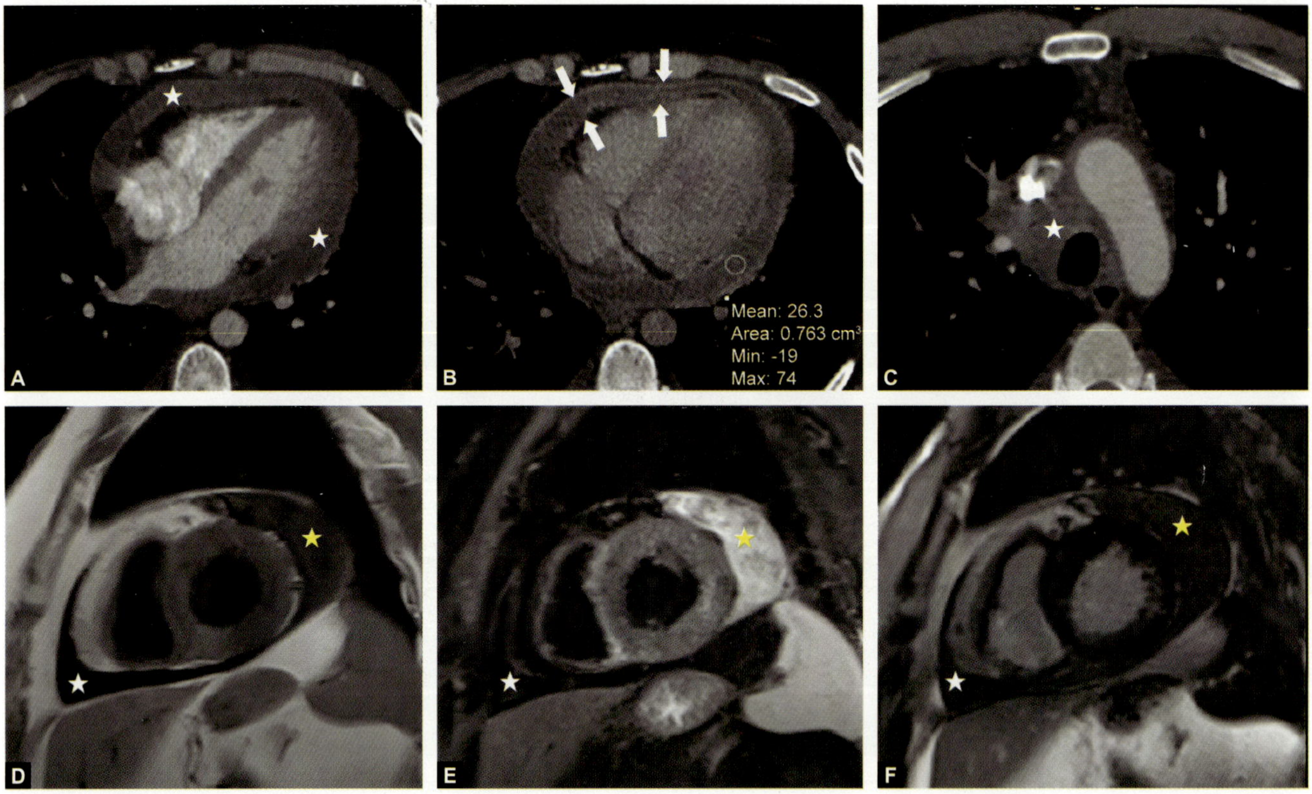

Figs. 4A to F: Arterial (A) and delayed phase (B) CT scan images of a 32-year-old man of Asian origin presented with breathless and low-grade pyrexia, demonstrating generalized pericardial effusion (white asterisk) with mean density of 26 HU representing exudate and enhancement of pericardial layers (arrows, B), and mediastinal lymphadenopathy (asterisk, C). A 65-year-old women with pericardial effusion on MRI scan (C to E) with different compositions anteriorly (white asterisk) and posteriorly (yellow asterisk). The anterior effusion is low signal intensity in both T1-weighted (D) and short tau inversion recovery (STIR, E) images while posterior one has intermediate signal in T1 and is bright on STIR images, with none of them showing enhancement on delayed postcontrast image (F).

Pericardial Tamponade

Cardiac tamponade is a life-threatening condition caused by rapid or slow accumulation of fluid, pus, blood, gas, or neoplastic tissue within the pericardial sac that compresses the cardiac chambers and inhibits normal ventricular filling.[1] Echocardiography is the initial imaging technique in cases of suspected tamponade for both diagnosis and therapeutic drainage. While both CT and MRI can readily demonstrate pericardial effusion, role of MRI is limited in acute cases as patient would have to be in the scanner for longer duration. CT can be helpful in subacute tamponade which is due to loculated or complex effusion and help in determining feasibility of percutaneous versus surgical drainage.[1] Signs of tamponade on CT include a "flattened heart" due to compression of the anterior surface of right ventricle by fluid, air, or connective tissue,[17] compression of the coronary sinus, and bowing of interventricular septum correlating to the septal bulge or "bounce".[18] Besides, there would be dilatation of the right atrium and enlargement of IVC and SVC compared to the adjacent aorta.

Pericardial Neoplasms

Tumors of the pericardium can be primary (benign or malignant) or metastatic.[1] Benign primary pericardial tumors include teratoma, lipoma, fibroma, hemangioma, and lymphangioma. These can grow to sizeable lesions before causing symptoms. The most common malignant primary tumor of the pericardium is mesothelioma followed by angiosarcoma. Secondary tumors are 20–40 times more common than the primary and include metastasis from lymphoma, melanoma, lung, and breast carcinomas.[19] Both CT and MRI provide valuable information about the morphology, location, extent, and characterization of pericardial tumors. CT in addition is more robust in identifying pulmonary and other body abnormalities including primary tumors elsewhere and is much faster to perform compared to MRI. Positron emission tomography (PET) with 18F-fluorodeoxyglucose (18F-FDG) now complements CT in identifying active tracer uptake in the abnormal pericardium or cardiac mass and elsewhere in the body that may represent primary or secondary

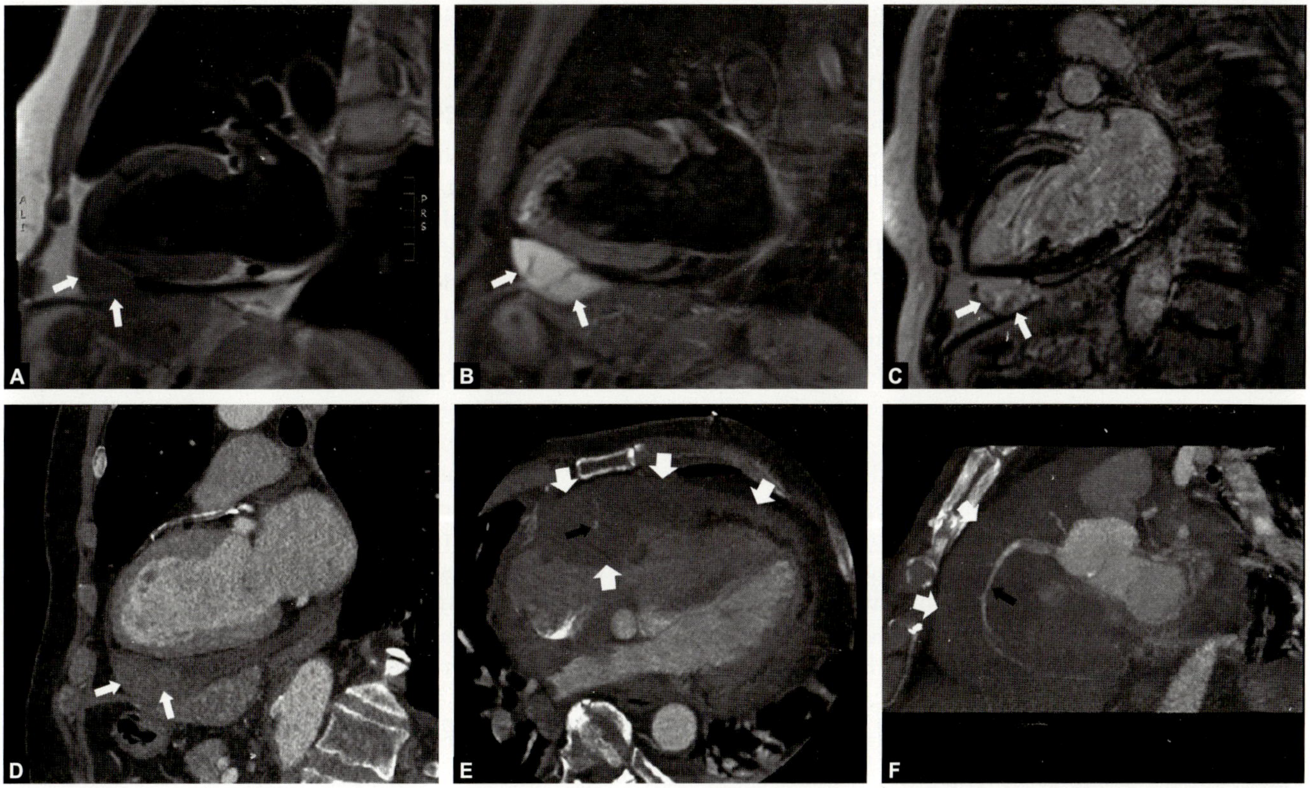

Figs. 5A to F: MRI scan (A to C) of a patient with well-defined mass in the apical inferior aspect of the pericardium (arrows) which has intermediate signal on T1-weighted images (A), bright on STIR (B), and shows enhancement on delayed gadolinium images (C). Computed tomography scan on the same patient (D) shows mild enhancement of the mass in arterial phase (arrows). Another patient with an irregular mass infiltrating both myocardium and the pericardium (arrows) on CT scan (E and F) with encasement of the right coronary artery (black arrows). Histology revealed the mass to be an aggressive B-cell lymphoma.

neoplastic tissue.[20] Benign tumors appear as well-defined localized soft tissue masses (Figs 5A to D) while malignant ones as infiltrating or invasive masses (Figs 5A to D) or simply as thickened pericardium with regions of nodularity related to tumor deposition. Malignant tumors can also demonstrate disruption of the pericardial sac, invasion into the epicardial fat plane, myocardium, or even the cardiac chambers, along with complex or hemorrhagic pericardial effusion. The density or signal intensity of the tumor could be characteristic of their predominant tissue component and may show varying degree of enhancement with contrast on both CT and MRI. Cine MRI can be used to identify involvement of underlying myocardium by a pericardial tumor and help in surgical resection. Lipomas demonstrate low-attenuation (in the region of 100 HU) due to fat on CT scans while would be bright on T1- and T2-weighted MRI images with signal reducing on fat-suppressed images. Teratomas with their varying tissue components would demonstrate low attenuating fat and high-attenuating calcium on CT, while high signal of fat and very low of calcium on T1-weighted MRI imaging. Fibromas on the other hand would have soft tissue density on CT and low signal intensity on MRI, with more intense contrast enhancement on delayed phase. A malignant pericardial mesothelioma may present as thickened pericardium with nodules and calcification, and pericardial effusion. These features may cause encasement of the heart and pericardial constriction. Lymphomas on the other hand present as irregular soft tissue masses with infiltration of pericardium to varying degree and may also involve the underlying myocardium (Figs. 5E and F). They have similar density and signal characteristics to that of myocardium and demonstrate varying degree of enhancement. Lymphomas may also encase the epicardial coronary arteries rather than obstructing them, a feature that is typical of lymphatic infiltration in other parts of the body. Although most malignant tumors on MRI would have signal-intensity similar to that of myocardium, metastasis from melanoma have high signal due to melanin.

Congenital Pericardial Conditions

Pericardial Cysts

The majority of pericardial cysts are congenital malformations, while some, such as hydatid cysts, are infectious in nature. Congenital pericardial cysts are fluid-filled, unilocular sacs lined by mesothelial cells, and do not communicate with the pericardial space. They are generally detected between the 3rd decades and 4th decades as incidental findings on chest X-rays, echocardiography, or CT, mostly in the right cardiophrenic angle but may be found elsewhere around the heart. The appearance on both CT and MRI is that of well-defined, smooth bordered, encapsulated lesions abutting the pericardium with density or signal-intensity similar to that of water with no enhancement on contrast (Figs. 6A to C). Occasionally, they may have high proteinaceous content causing higher density on CT and high signal-intensity on MRI images.

Pericardial Diverticula

Pericardial diverticula are very rare and can be congenital or acquired malformations. They form as outpouching or herniation through a defect in the parietal pericardium and occur most often at the costophrenic angles. Unlike pericardial cysts, diverticula communicate with the pericardial sac and can, thus, change in size. Their appearance of diverticula on CT and MRI is similar to that of cysts except that a communication with pericardial scan can be identified.

Congenital Absence of Pericardium

Congenital absence of pericardium is one of the rarest cardiac congenital abnormalities. Five types have been identified: complete absence of the entire pericardium, complete absence of left or right side, and partial absence of the left or right side of pericardium, with complete absence of left pericardium being the most common.[1,21] Defect size may vary from small foraminal types to extensive. Identification of congenital absence of the pericardium is mostly incidental during surgery or on imaging. Those with complete absence are usually asymptomatic, while those with partial absence may present with nonspecific symptoms of chest pain, dyspnea, or palpitations, and have risk of compression, herniation, or strangulation of cardiac chambers. The pericardium on both CT and MRI is easily demonstrated in regions with presence of fat but may be difficult along the posterior aspect or in patients with minimal pericardial fat. However, there are indirect

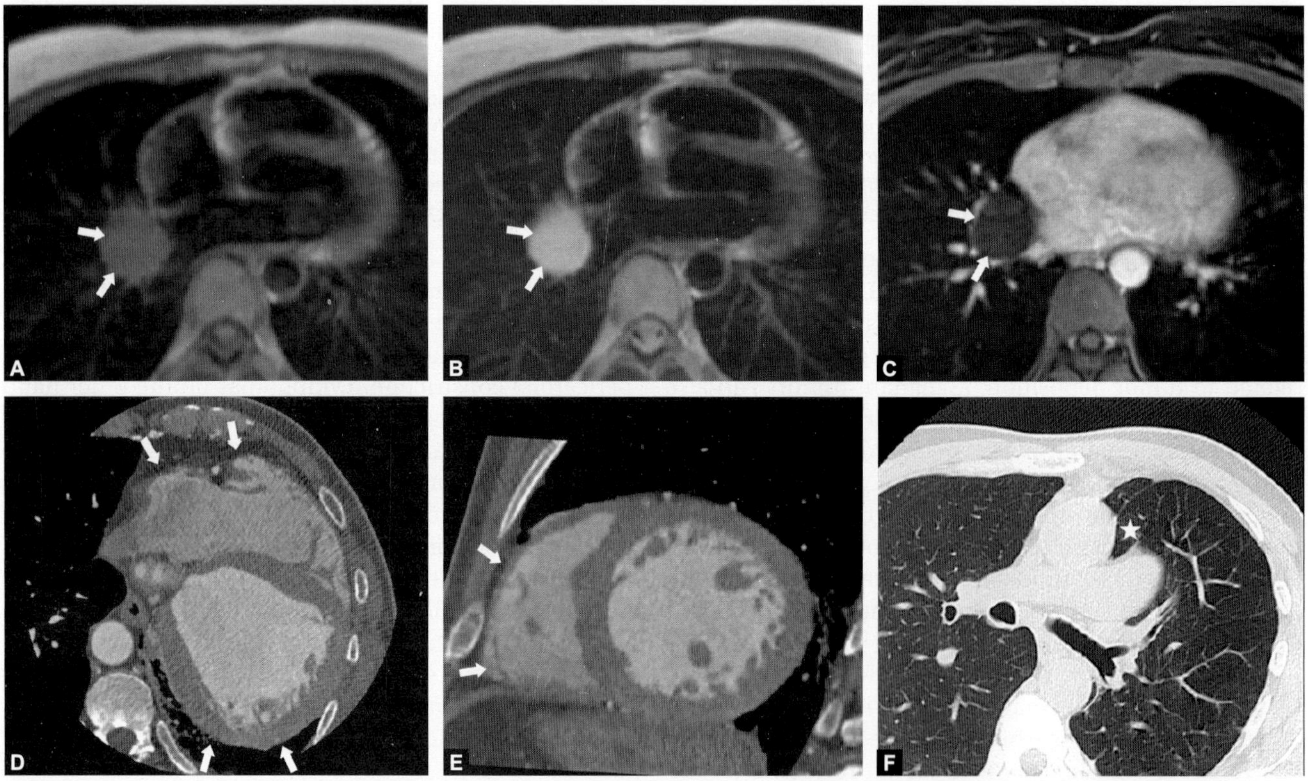

Figs. 6A to F: Cardiac magnetic resonance imaging (MRI) images of a 28-year-old woman showing a well-defined round lesion in the right paracardiac region showing intermediate signal-intensity on T1-weighted images (arrows, A), bright on T2-weighted images (arrows, B) with no enhancement on postcontrast T1-weighted images (arrows, C). Cardiac CT scan images of a 35-year-old man presenting with shortness of breath demonstrating displacement of heart toward the left hemithorax on axial images (D) with no visible pericardium on both axial and short-axis images (arrows, A and B), and invagination of lung between the ascending aorta and main pulmonary artery (asterisk, F), all features of complete absence of pericardium.

signs that can be helpful in making the diagnosis. The displacement of the heart to the left side (levorotation) in the absence of other pulmonary or thoracic abnormality can be due to complete absence of left pericardium (Figs. 6D to F). A specific sign of complete left-sided absence is interposition of lung tissue between the ascending aorta and main pulmonary artery, a space typically covered with pericardium (Figs. 1C and 6F), or between the diaphragm and the base of the heart.

CONCLUSION

Both CT and MRI are complementary to echocardiography in the diagnosis and management of pericardial diseases. Due to their wider field of view and ability of characterize abnormalities, multimodality international guidelines recommend their use for localization, identifying specific cause such as inflammation and neoplasia, extracardiac abnormalities, and congenital conditions.

REFERENCES

1. Klein AL, Abbara S, Agler DA, et al. American Society of Echocardiography clinical recommendations for multimodality cardiovascular imaging of patients with pericardial disease: endorsed by the Society for Cardiovascular Magnetic Resonance and Society of Cardiovascular Computed Tomography. J Am Soc Echocardiogr. 2013;26(9):965-1012.e15.
2. Cosyns B, Plein S, Nihoyanopoulos P, et al. European Association of Cardiovascular Imaging (EACVI) position paper: Multimodality imaging in pericardial disease. Eur Heart J Cardiovasc Imaging. 2015;16(1):12-31.
3. Isner JM, Carter BL, Bankoff MS, et al. Computed tomography in the diagnosis of pericardial heart disease. Ann Intern Med. 1982;97(4):473-9.
4. Sechtem U, Tscholakoff D, Higgins CB. MRI of the abnormal pericardium. AJR Am J Roentgenol. 1986;147(2):245-52.
5. Rajiah P, Kanne JP. Computed tomography of the pericardium and pericardial disease. J Cardiovasc Comput Tomogr. 2010;4(1):3-18.
6. Young PM, Glockner JF, Williamson EE, et al. MR imaging findings in 76 consecutive surgically proven cases of pericardial disease with CT and pathologic correlation. Int J Cardiovasc Imaging. 2012;28(5):1099-109.
7. Bogaert J, Francone M. Pericardial disease: value of CT and MR imaging. Radiology. 2013;267(2):340-56.
8. Taylor AM, Dymarkowski S, Verbeken EK, et al. Detection of pericardial inflammation with late-enhancement cardiac magnetic resonance imaging: initial results. Eur Radiol. 2006;16(3):569-74.
9. Truong MT, Erasmus JJ, Gladish GW, et al. Anatomy of pericardial recesses on multidetector CT: implications for oncologic imaging. AJR Am J Roentgenol. 2003;181(4):1109-13.
10. Adler Y, Charron P, Imazio M, et al. 2015 ESC Guidelines for the diagnosis and management of pericardial diseases: The Task Force for the Diagnosis and Management of Pericardial Diseases of the European Society of Cardiology (ESC) Endorsed by: The European Association for Cardio-Thoracic Surgery (EACTS). Eur Heart J. 2015;36(42):2921-64.
11. Zurick AO, Bolen MA, Kwon DH, et al. Pericardial delayed hyperenhancement with CMR imaging in patients with constrictive pericarditis undergoing surgical pericardiectomy: a case series with histopathological correlation. JACC Cardiovasc Imaging. 2011;4(11):1180-91.
12. Imazio M, Brucato A, Barbieri A, et al. Good prognosis for pericarditis with and without myocardial involvement: results from a multicenter, prospective cohort study. Circulation 2013;128(1):42-9.
13. Reinmuller R, Gurgan M, Erdmann E, et al. CT and MR evaluation of pericardial constriction: a new diagnostic and therapeutic concept. J Thorac Imaging. 1993;8(2):108-21.
14. Nguyen T, Phillips C, Movahed A. Incidental findings of pericardial calcification. World journal of clinical cases 2014;2(9):455-8.
15. Hanneman K, Thavendiranathan P, Nguyen ET, et al. Cardiovascular CT in the diagnosis of pericardial constriction: predictive value of inferior vena cava cross-sectional area. J Cardiovasc Comput Tomogr. 2014;8(2):149-57.
16. Talreja DR, Edwards WD, Danielson GK, et al. Constrictive pericarditis in 26 patients with histologically normal pericardial thickness. Circulation. 2003;108(15):1852-7.
17. Hernandez-Luyando L, Calvo J, Gonzalez de las Heras E, et al. Tension pericardial collections: sign of 'flattened heart' in CT. Eur J Radiol. 1996;23(3):250-2.
18. Restrepo CS, Lemos DF, Lemos JA, et al. Imaging findings in cardiac tamponade with emphasis on CT. Radiographics. 2007;27(6):1595-610.
19. Luk A, Ahn E, Vaideeswar P, et al. Pericardial tumors. Seminars in diagnostic pathology. 2008;25:47-53.
20. Rahbar K, Seifarth H, Schafers M, et al. Differentiation of malignant and benign cardiac tumors using 18F-FDG PET/CT. J Nucl Med. 2012;53(6):856-63.
21. Lopez D, Asher CR. Congenital absence of the pericardium. Prog Cardiovasc Dis. 2017;59(4):398-406.

SECTION 16

Infective Endocarditis

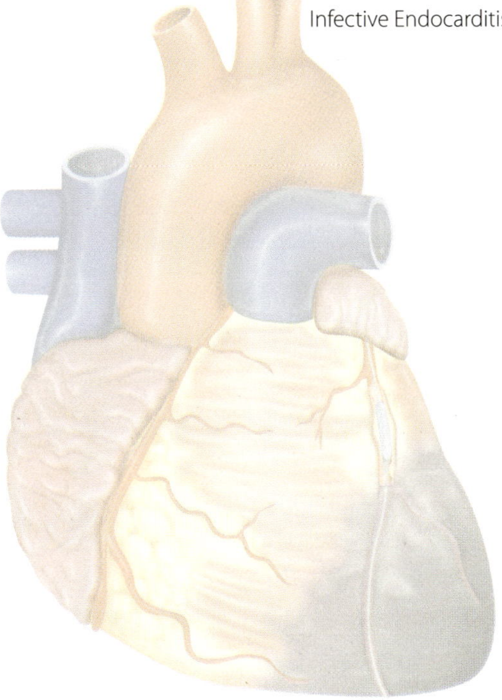

95

CHAPTER

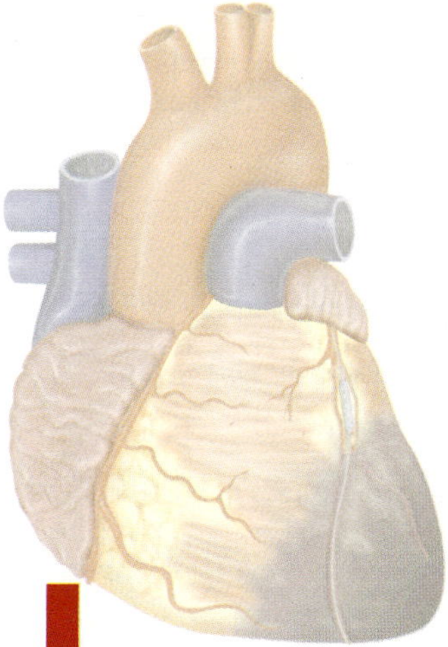

Advances in Echocardiographic Navigation of Infective Endocarditis

Krishnam Raju P, Chandramukhi Sunehra

INTRODUCTION

Infective endocarditis (IE) primarily involves the endocardium of heart valves or congenital defects but can affect any cardiac structure. It can affect the prosthetic valves or implanted cardiac devices. Rarely, it affects the walls of the great arteries or the cardiac chambers. The epidemiology of IE has significantly changed IE, since the first description of IE by Sir William Osler in 1885. Valvular heart disease—degenerative and rheumatic valve disease—is still the common predisposing factor for IE. At present, hemodialysis, immunosuppressive therapy, or prolonged intravenous drug therapy, such as chemotherapy and intravenous drug abuse are the major predisposing factors for IE. *Staphylococcus aureus* is the common causative organism in these patients. Thus the microbiological trends are shifting from the streptococcus group to the more virulent *S. aureus* group of organisms. These evolving trends in the epidemiology and microbiology of IE have significant influence on the evaluation, management, and outcome of IE. The diagnosis of IE requires multidisciplinary approach and is based on the modified Duke criteria. These criteria include clinical findings, microbiology and histopathology data, and supportive evidence from the imaging modalities, such as echocardiography, multidetector computed tomography (MDCT), or 2-deoxy-2-[fluorine-18] fluoro-D-glucose-positron emission tomography-computed tomography (^{18}F-FDG PET/CT). Echocardiography is the basic fundamental imaging modality for the diagnosis and management of IE. The diagnosis of IE requires a very high index of clinical suspicion. IE should be suspected in any one of the following clinical situations:[1]

- Sepsis of unknown origin (especially when associated with IE-related causative organism)
- Fever in patient with predisposing cardiac or noncardiac risk factors for IE, or history of recent dental or surgical procedure
- Detection of new regurgitant murmur
- Embolic events without evident etiology
- Development of new conduction abnormalities in a patient with fever
- Identification of focal neurological deficit or nonspecific neurological symptoms or development of signs of pulmonary embolism or pulmonary infarction in a patient with fever (right-sided endocarditis)

The diagnosis of IE is based on the modified Duke criteria as illustrated in Table 1.[2]

Elderly individuals and immune-compromised hosts frequently have atypical presentation. Fever is typically absent in these cases, and very high index of clinical suspicion and low threshold for transthoracic echocardiography (TTE) or transesophageal echocardiography (TEE) are required to clinch the diagnosis.

Whenever there is clinical suspicion of IE, echocardiographic evaluation is mandatory for the confirmation of the diagnosis and prompt initiation of treatment. Initial TTE should be performed to have a baseline data, and TEE is must in all cases with positive TTE, especially in patients with intracardiac device or

TABLE 1: Modified Duke criteria for the diagnosis of infective endocarditis.[2]

1. *Pathological criteria:*
   Pathological material sought from autopsy or cardiac surgery (vegetations, valve tissue, embolic fragments, or contents obtained from intracardiac abscess) showing features of active endocarditis on histology or microorganisms demonstrated by culture
2. *Major criteria:*
   i. *Blood cultures positive for microorganisms typical for IE (any one of the following)*
      a. *Two separate sets of blood cultures positive for microorganisms typical for IE:*
         I. *Staphylococcus aureus;*
         II. Viridans streptococci, *Streptococcus gallolyticus*, including nutritional variant strains (*Granulicatella* spp. and *Abiotrophia defectiva*);
         III. HACEK group: *Haemophilus* spp., *Aggregatibacter*, *Cardiobacterium hominis*, *Eikenella* spp., and *Kingella kingae*; and
         IV. Community-acquired enterococci, in the absence of a primary focus; *OR*
      b. *Persistently positive blood culture:*
         I. At least two sets of blood cultures positive for organisms that are typical causes of IE, the two samples of blood culture being drawn >12 h apart
         II. Three or more separate blood cultures (with the first and the last samples drawn at least 1 h apart) positive for less specific organisms that are more commonly skin contaminants
      c. *Single positive blood culture for Coxiella burnetii or phase I IgG antibody titer >1:800*
      Clinical manifestations resolve within ≤4 days of antibiotic treatment OR
      Alternate diagnosis is established beyond doubt OR
   ii. *Evidence of endocardial involvement:*
      I. *Echocardiogram positive for IE:* Vegetation *OR* New valvular regurgitation *OR*
      II. Periannular or intracardiac abscess *OR* New partial dehiscence of prosthetic valve
   iii. *In patients with prosthetic valve endocarditis, detection of abnormal activity or ^{18}F-FDG uptake around the site of prosthetic valve implantation on evaluation by ^{18}F-FDG PET/CT (the prosthesis being implanted for >3 months) or radiolabeled leukocytes SPECT/CT.*[3]
   iv. *Detection of definite paravalvular lesions by cardiac MDCT.*[3]
3. *Minor criteria:*
   i. Presence of predisposing cardiac risk factors, such as valvular disease with significant regurgitation or stenosis or prosthetic heart valve or congenital heart disease or noncardiac risk factor, such as intravenous drug use
   ii. *Fever:* Defined as body temperature ≥38.0°C (100.4°F)
   iii. *Vascular phenomena:* Janeway lesions or major arterial emboli, conjunctival hemorrhages, septic pulmonary infarcts, mycotic aneurysm, or intracranial hemorrhage
   iv. *Immunologic phenomena:* Osler nodes, glomerulonephritis, Roth spots, or rheumatoid factor
   v. *Microbiologic evidence:* Positive blood cultures not satisfying major criteria *OR* serologic evidence of active infection with organism consistent with IE

(^{18}F-FDG: ^{18}F-Fluorodesoxyglucose; CT: computed tomography; IE: infective endocarditis; IgG: immunoglobulin G; MDCT: multidetector computed tomography; PET: positron emission tomography; SPECT: single-photon emission computed tomography)

prosthetic valves. However, in the cases, with low clinical probability of IE, a good-quality TTE will be sufficient to rule out the diagnosis of IE. TTE has 70% and 50% sensitivity for the detection of vegetation in native and prosthetic valves, respectively, while TEE has a better sensitivity of 96% and 92% for the diagnosis of vegetation in native and prosthetic valves, respectively.[4] The specificity for the detection of vegetation is 90% for both TTE and TEE. However, echocardiography may be false positive in approximately 15% of cases. False-positive results are common in myxomatous valves with redundant tissue or degenerative and calcified valves or prosthetic valves and intracardiac devices. TEE with better resolution will be helpful in these cases. Moreover, TEE is useful in patients with difficult TTE window, e.g. in obese patients or patients with emphysematous chest or chest wall deformity.

Various categories in IE can be established depending on the criteria illustrated in Table 2.[5]

ECHOCARDIOGRAPHY IN INFECTIVE ENDOCARDITIS

Echocardiography plays an important role across all stages of the disease, and the various roles of echocardiography are as follows:

- Identifying predisposing cardiac condition
- Establish diagnosis
- Risk stratification
- Detect complications
- Treatment plan—planning perioperative intervention
- Determine prognosis (risk of complications)
- Assessment of response to therapy and serial evaluation
- Follow-up after the completion of definitive therapy.

Echocardiographic evaluation of IE should involve a systematic approach, including both TTE and TEE as per the demand of the clinical situation (Flowchart 1[5] and Table 3[6]).

TABLE 2: Various categories in establishing the diagnosis of IE.[5]

1. *Definite IE is established if any of the following is present:*
   i. *Pathologic criteria:*
      a. Pathologic lesions: Vegetation or intracardiac abscess showing active endocarditis on histology *OR*
      b. A vegetation or intracardiac abscess showing microorganism by culture or histology
   ii. *Clinical criteria:*
      a. 2 major clinical criteria *OR*
      b. 1 major and 3 minor clinical criteria *OR*
      c. 5 minor clinical criteria
2. *Possible IE:*
   i. Presence of 1 major and 1 minor clinical criterion *OR*
   ii. The presence of 3 minor clinical criteria
3. *Rejected IE*
   i. Alternate diagnosis is established beyond doubt *OR*
   ii. Clinical manifestations resolve within ≤4 days of antibiotic treatment *OR*
   iii. Pathologic evidence of infective endocarditis is not found at surgery or autopsy after antibiotic therapy of ≤4 days duration
4. Lack of clinical criteria favoring possible or definite IE

(IE: infective endocarditis)

Echocardiographic Features of Infective Endocarditis

The characteristic anatomic features diagnostic of IE on echocardiography are as follows:

- Vegetations
- Lesions, as a result of destruction of leaflet, such as perforation, aneurysm or prolapse of leaflets or rupture of chordae, or less frequently rupture of papillary muscle
- Abscess formation
- New dehiscence of prosthetic valve
- Less common echocardiographic features of IE include pseudoaneurysm or fistula

Echocardiographic evaluation of IE has evolved from the basic motion-mode (M-mode) and two-dimensional (2D) imaging to three-dimensional (3D) imaging, including 3D TTE and 3D TEE.

Motion-mode Echocardiography in Infective Endocarditis

Motion-mode echocardiography was first utilized in 1973 for the diagnosis of IE by Dillon et al.[7] M-mode findings included irregular thickening of valve leaflets with unrestricted mobility. The abnormal echoes responsible for

Flowchart 1: Approach to the echocardiographic evaluation in a patient with clinical suspicion of IE.[5] (IE: infective endocarditis)

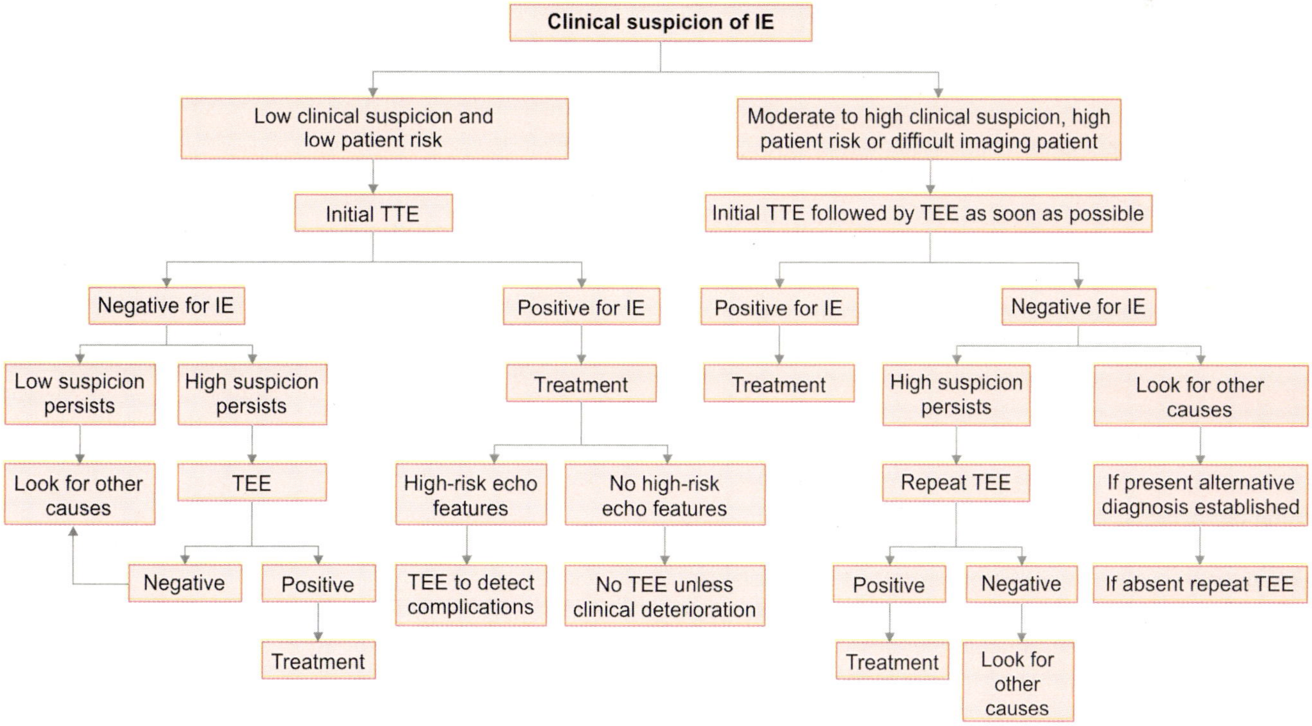

TABLE 3: Algorithm for echocardiographic evaluation in patients with clinical suspicion of IE.[6]

1. TTE should be done in all patients with *Staphylococcus aureus* bacteremia to confirm or rule out the diagnosis of IE. In addition to TTE, TEE should also be done in patients with prosthetic valves or intracardiac devices
2. Despite negative baseline TTE, TEE should be done in patients with high clinical suspicion of endocarditis
3. Repeat evaluation should be done within 7 days to 10 days when baseline TEE is negative but there is high clinical suspicion of IE. TEE should be repeated earlier for patients with *Staphylococcus aureus* bacteremia
4. Perform TEE in all patients with positive baseline TTE. TEE is helpful for further evaluation as TEE has better specificity for the diagnosis of both IE and its complications
5. Evaluation should be done in multiple views including subcostal views and imaging in off-axis planes in patients with prosthetic valves and intracardiac devices. TEE is preferred over TTE in this subset of patients
6. Repeat echocardiographic evaluation by TTE/TEE if complications of IE are suspected and also to monitor the response to antibiotic therapy.

(IE: infective endocarditis; TEE: transesophageal echocardiography; TTE: transthoracic echocardiography)

leaflet thickening had a shaggy appearance. High-frequency oscillatory motion of the vegetation could be appreciated on M-mode echo (Fig. 1A).

Two-dimensional Echocardiography in Infective Endocarditis

Gilbert et al.[8] in 1977 assessed the utility of 2D echocardiography (2DE) in the documentation and characterization of vegetation. On 2D imaging, vegetations appeared as rapidly oscillating masses attached to the valve tissue (Fig. 1B). Morphologically, vegetations varied from a small, pedunculated mobile mass to a relatively large immobile mass. 2DE provides spatial information and enables the reliable assessment of the location and the size of vegetation. 2DE became the preferred method for the evaluation of the morphological changes in the vegetation and assess the efficacy of the antibiotic therapy.

Vegetation

Vegetation is defined as a discrete, irregular shaped, oscillating, or nonoscillating mass attached to valve or other endocardial structures or intracardiac device implant material.[9] It is the hallmark lesion of IE. Vegetation is visualized consistently throughout the cardiac cycle and in multiple views and multiple planes. Vegetation has low reflectance and a shaggy appearance with inhomogeneous echogenicity. The echotexture may be heterogeneous with the areas of hyperechogenicity or echolucency. It may be sessile or pedunculated. The characteristic oscillatory motion of vegetation is independent of the valve motion. The vegetation is characteristically attached on the low-pressure side of the valve structure—the ventricular side of the aortic and pulmonary valves, while on the atrial side of the mitral (Figs. 2A and B) and tricuspid valves. It may be attached anywhere on the valvular or subvalvular apparatus. Rarely, it may be located on the mural endocardium of the cardiac chambers or the great arteries—ascending aorta or pulmonary trunk. Vegetation is frequently found in the path of turbulent blood flow from valvular regurgitation (jet lesion) or a shunt lesion. It may be located on adjacent structures by direct contact of the high-velocity jet with the leaflets or chordate tendinae or the vascular endocardium ("satellite lesion" or "kissing lesion"). The vegetation should be assessed with regard to location, attachment, size, echotexture, mobility, and relation with adjacent structures. Vegetations usually result in regurgitation (Fig. 2C). Few vegetations may have mobile elements which have very high-risk for embolism. Moreover, large and mobile vegetations are prone for embolism and rarely cause obstruction to the valve.

Vegetation size >10 mm carries higher risk of systemic embolism.[10] Large vegetations are usually seen with fungal endocarditis. The maximum size of the vegetation—linear dimensions and area by planimetry—should be assessed carefully at the time of initial evaluation, so that it facilitates risk stratification and also helps in assessing the response to antibiotic therapy. Some vegetations decrease in size and show increase in echogenicity with calcified foci suggestive of healing process during the course of antibiotic treatment. Very small vegetations <2 mm may not be visualized on TTE. In such cases, repeat evaluation by TTE or TEE can be performed after 7–10 days in patients with high clinical suspicion of IE.

Technical tricks facilitating the accurate diagnosis of vegetations on TTE and TEE:

- The valves should be thoroughly examined in all the views and in all planes by slowly tilting the transducer and panning through cardiac valves during TTE. During TEE the valve should be profiled in all the angles with slow angulation. This facilitates imaging all aspects of these 3D structures in minor details.
- Appropriately zoomed images should be utilized to search a vegetation and assess the minor details of vegetation.
- The zone of focus should be placed at the level of valves to optimize the resolution of the image.

Mimics of Vegetations

- Ruptured or redundant chordate or redundant tissue over the myxomatous valves
- Focal thickening or calcium deposits on the leaflet

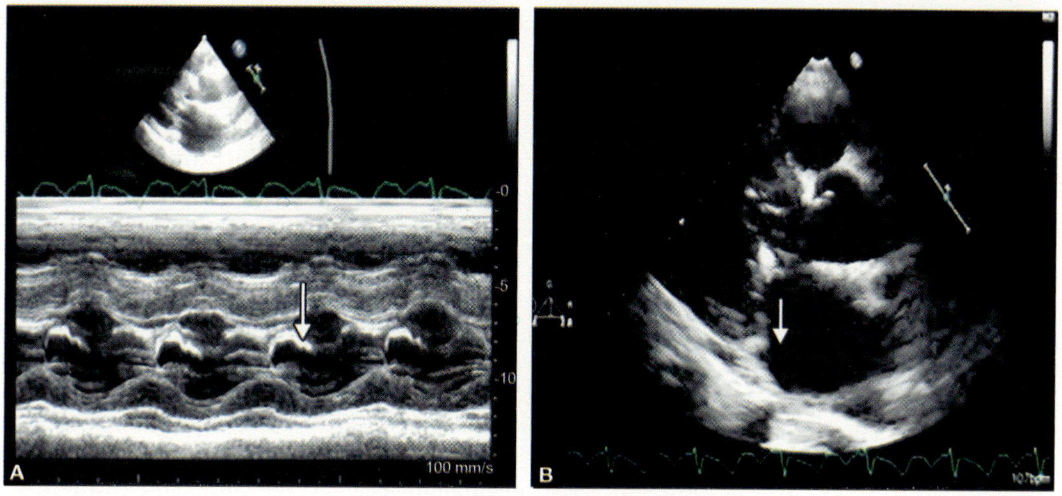

Figs. 1A and B: Motion-mode and two-dimensional echocardiographic views of vegetation. Parasternal long-axis view depicts (A) motion mode across the mitral valve showing the mobile vegetation with shaggy appearance (arrow) attached to the anterior mitral leaflet; (B) Two-dimensional imaging showing the echodense mobile nodular element (arrow) suggestive of vegetation.

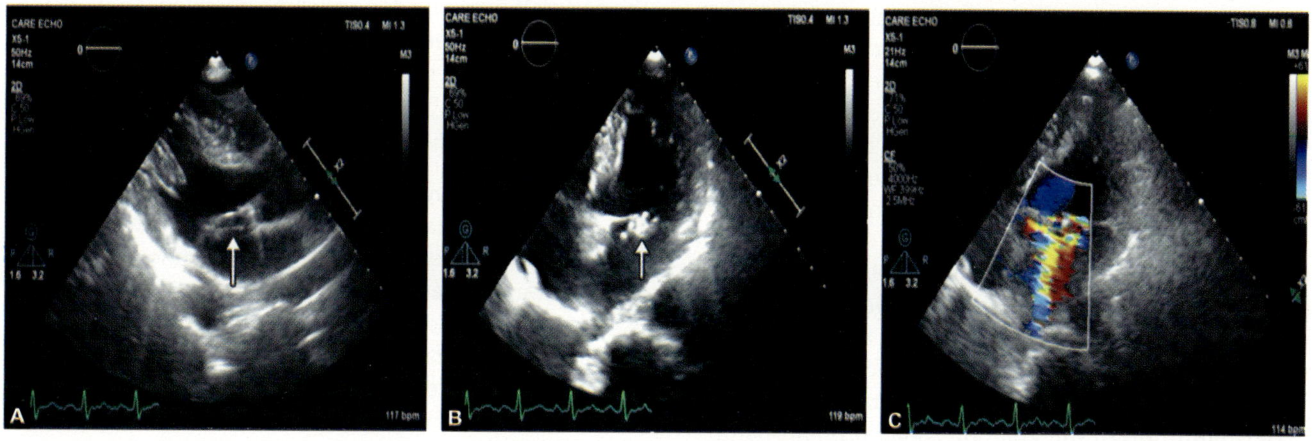

Figs. 2A to C: Transthoracic echocardiogram depicting vegetation over the mitral valve. Transthoracic echocardiogram shows (A) parasternal long-axis view demonstrating mobile element attached to the anterior mitral leaflet on the atrial side (arrow) diagnostic of vegetation; (B) Apical four-chamber view showing the same vegetation (arrow) attached to the anterior mitral leaflet and having multiple mobile fragments; and (C) Color Doppler interrogation showing severe mitral regurgitation.

- Lambl's excrescences
- Small thrombus or tumor (especially papillary fibroelastoma)
- Retained mitral valve chordae postmitral valve surgery
- Sutures or strands on prosthetic valves.

Few echocardiographic characteristics will help differentiation of a vegetation from a thrombus. The thrombi usually have a central echolucency and may be mobile or static. The clinical features of IE will be absent and the blood cultures will be nonproductive in the cases with thrombi, while a vegetation has a low reflectance and a shaggy appearance and frequently has oscillatory motion.

Nonbacterial Thrombotic Endocarditis

In few instances the vegetation may not be infective, and it is then referred to as nonbacterial thrombotic endocarditis or Libman-Sacks endocarditis. These noninfective vegetations are characteristically seen in patients with autoimmune disorders—systemic lupus erythematosus or antiphospholipid syndrome. Most commonly, the mitral valve is involved; other valves may also be affected. These are usually small, immobile with heterogeneous appearance and irregular borders and are associated with valve leaflet thickening and regurgitation, and very rarely stenosis.

Three-dimensional Echocardiography in Infective Endocarditis

The major benefit of 3D echocardiographic (3DE) imaging is the visualization of the entire valve, the annulus and periannular structures in a single beat. This enables the visualization of eccentrically located vegetations which may be missed on 2D imaging. Moreover, when vegetations are very large or multiple in number, 3DE enables better localization and morphological characterization of lesions compared to 2D imaging. Moreover, 3DE *x*-plane imaging with lateral tilt is very useful in improved visualization of the attachment of the vegetation and its relationship with surrounding structures. 3D TEE can delineate vegetations located at atypical sites. 3D TEE is superior to 2D TEE in diagnosing the complications of IE, especially chordal rupture, leaflet perforation, localization and evaluation of perivalvular extension in the form of abscess or prosthetic valve dehiscence. This complementary data provides incremental information and aids in decision-making with regard to both timing and planning of surgery. 3D imaging involves acquisition of full-volume pyramidal and real-time 3D pyramidal dataset profiling the entire valve at end expiration. This enables reconstruction of different planes of the valve and enables visualization in three different dimensions. These dataset should be acquired in different views and multiple angles. These pyramidal datasets can be cropped, and minor details of the entire valve and the attached vegetation and any associated perivalvular lesions can be assessed. Reconstruction and cropping provides enface view of the valves which is identical with the surgical view. 3D imaging facilitates superior visualization and identification of perivalvular complications with better definition of the anatomy; spatial relationship to neighboring structures; and accurate definition of the location, size, and extent of the lesion in paravalvular region. In prosthetic valves the vegetations may be obscured by reverberation and acoustic shadowing on 2D imaging. But 3D imaging overcomes this limitation and is superior in localization of vegetations in prosthetic valves. Thus 3D TEE with its superior resolution has the advantage of identifying smaller lesions which occur in the early course of IE.

KEY POINT 1

Three-dimensional TEE with multiplanar reconstruction of valve images provides comprehensive assessment of valve morphology and the attached vegetation and its relation with adjacent structures. 3D TEE is complementary to 2D TEE. 3D TEE is superior to 2D TEE in the identification of complications of infective endocarditis.

Complications of Infective Endocarditis

Leaflet Perforation

Leaflet perforation is defined as a defect in the body of leaflet due to the interruption of endocardial tissue continuity and evidence of color flow across it on color Doppler interrogation.[9] The defect is surrounded by the endocardium in its entirety, and this differentiates it from a cleft. Leaflet perforation frequently involves the anterior mitral leaflet. It is usually associated with significant regurgitation—acute mitral regurgitation. The perforation is visualized as a dropout and discontinuity of the leaflet tissue on 2D imaging. 3D TEE clearly demonstrates the punched-out defect of the leaflet perforation on the enface view. The regurgitant jet is eccentric originating away from the point of coaptation of the leaflets. Using color comparison imaging helps in identifying the origin of the regurgitant jet from the perforation site away from the leaflet coaptation point. (Figs. 3A to E). Valve sparing surgery through the patch repair of the perforation can be done after the infection is adequately treated with antibiotic therapy, and valve replacement may be avoided.

Perivalvular Involvement and Abscess

Extension of the infection beyond the valve annulus to the surrounding tissues results in perivalvular abscess. Periannular abscess is the second major echocardiographic criterion for the diagnosis of IE. In native valves, it occurs as the valve infection gives way through the weakest part of the annulus near the membranous septum and the atrioventricular node. Thus conduction abnormalities with atrioventricular blocks are a common complication associated with periannular abscess. Perivalvular abscess occurs more frequently in prosthetic valve endocarditis (PVE) with an incidence rate of 56–100%,[11,12] and aortic valve is most often involved. The incidence of root abscess in native valve endocarditis is 10–40%. *S. aureus (especially coagulase negative)* is the most common organism associated with periannular abscess. Clinical diagnosis of root abscess requires exceptional clinical skills and a very high index of suspicion. Periannular abscess is a likely complication when a patient with IE appropriately treated with antibiotics develops congestive heart failure, prolonged PR interval or complete heart block on electrocardiography, new regurgitant murmur, recurrent embolic events. Moreover, persistent fever or bacteremia should raise the suspicion. Prompt evaluation by TTE and TEE is mandatory as it is a life-threatening complication.

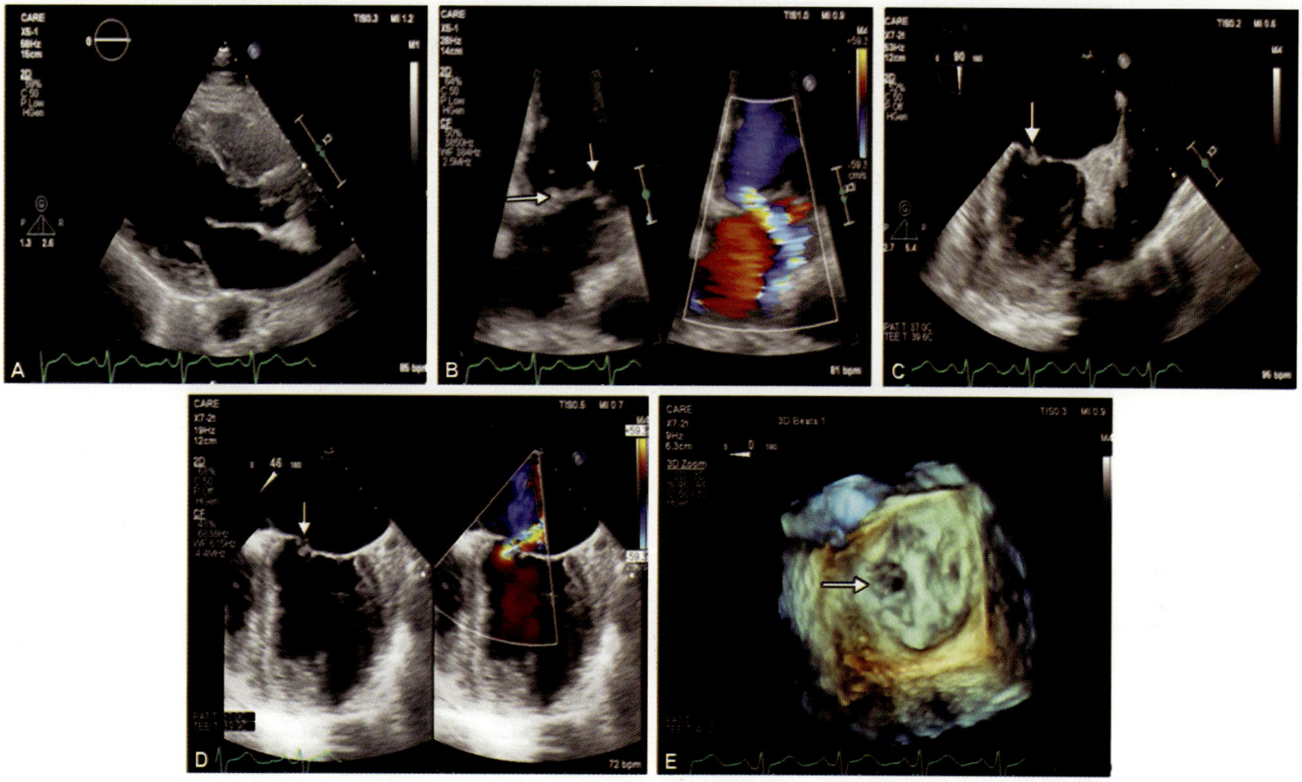

Figs. 3A to E: Transthoracic and transesophageal echocardiogram with 3D imaging demonstrating infective endocarditis of mitral valve with perforation of leaflet. Transthoracic and transesophageal echocardiograms with 3D echocardiographic views demonstrating infective endocarditis in a patient with history of fever for 1 month and signs of heart failure. (A) Parasternal long-axis view profiling the mitral valve with thin leaflets without any mobile elements; (B) Apical four-chamber view with color comparison shows the mitral regurgitation which is eccentric and originating at a point away from the point of leaflet coaptation (arrows); (C) Transesophageal echocardiography profiling the two-chamber view and demonstrating a small linear mobile element (arrow)—vegetation attached to the anterior mitral leaflet; (D) Transesophageal echocardiography at 46° with color comparison shows vegetation attached to anterior mitral leaflet with a dropout visualized in the anterior mitral leaflet and the mitral regurgitation originating from the same site suggestive of perforation; (E) 3D transesophageal echocardiographic image showing enface view of the mitral valve with the punched-out lesion (arrow) in anterior mitral leaflet—A1 scallop indicating perforation of anterior mitral leaflet. (3D: three-dimensional)

Echocardiographic Features of Periannular Abscess

Thickening of aortic root identified as a circular or more irregularly delineated area of echolucency or increased echodensity is the initial echocardiographic feature of periannular abscess on TTE. Once periannular lesion is identified, meticulous evaluation should be performed through manipulation of the transducer across multiple planes and angles to assess the location, size, and spatial relation to adjacent structures. The abscess cavity will be devoid of blood flow in its interior on color Doppler interrogation.[9] The abscess cavity dimensions—largest diameter and largest area by planimetry—should be determined and documented. Ellis et al.[13] reported following echocardiographic features suggestive of the presence of perivalvular abscesses on TTE:

- Thickening of the aortic root wall ≥10 mm measured 1.0 cm from the aortic valve plane.
- Rocking motion of the prosthetic valve sewing ring.
- Formation of aneurysm of sinus of Valsalva.
- Perivalvular density in the interventricular septum of ≥14 mm measured 1.0 cm from the aortic valve plane. The individual echocardiographic characteristic has a low sensitivity but combined together have a very high sensitivity of 86%, specificity of 88%, and positive predictive value of 86% for the diagnosis of periannular abscess in an adequately performed TTE.

In the initial stages of perivalvular abscess when there is just thickening of the aortic root wall and it may be difficult to be identified on TTE. But later, during the course of the disease with progressive infection, a well-defined abscess cavity will be visualized as echo-free space in the region of aortic root, and the diagnosis of perivalvular abscess is confirmed (Figs. 4A to D). Both TTE and TEE are mandatory in the evaluation of a patient with IE with the

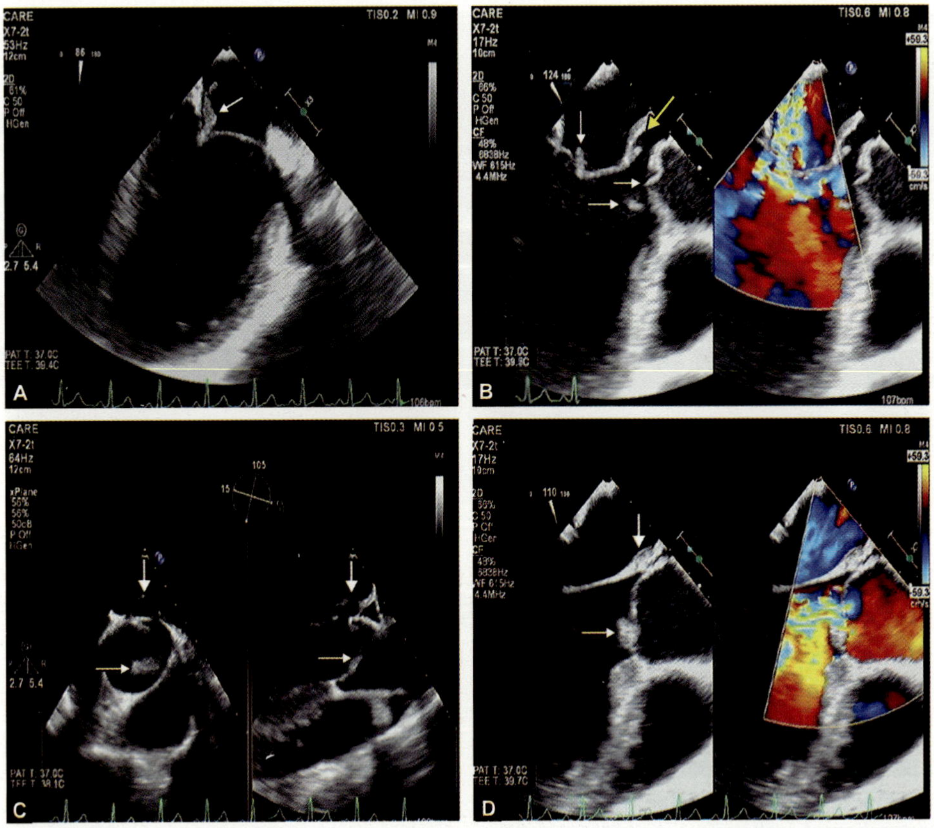

Figs. 4A to D: Transesophageal echocardiographic pictures depicting infective endocarditis of mitral and aortic valves with aortic periannular abscess and severe mitral regurgitation and severe aortic regurgitation. (A) Two-dimensional transesophageal echocardiogram shows the two-chamber view profiling the large, shaggy mobile element—vegetation (arrow) attached to the anterior mitral leaflet; (B) Long-axis view at 124° with color comparison shows the vegetations (white arrows) attached to the anterior mitral leaflet and aortic valve and a large echolucent space (yellow arrow) in the region of noncoronary sinus of Valsalva suggestive of abscess cavity. Color Doppler shows severe mitral regurgitation; (C) Two-dimensional imaging with x-plane (lateral tilt) imaging shows the vegetation attached to the aortic valve with the echolucent pouch at the mitral annulus suggestive of anterior mitral leaflet aneurysm (vertical arrow); (D) Imaging with color comparison shows the vegetation and the thickened aortic wall suggestive of root abscess on two-dimensional imaging and color Doppler shows severe aortic regurgitation.

suspicion of periannular abscess as both the modalities of echocardiography are complementary to each other. The baseline TTE serves as baseline data reference for quick comparison of change in vegetation size, severity of valvular regurgitation, or change in the abscess cavity during the follow-up studies of the individual during therapy and after the completion of therapy. However, TEE is superior (76–100% sensitivity) to TTE (50% sensitivity) in the detection of periannular abscess. TEE also has a very high specificity of 95% and high positive and negative predictive values of 87% and 89%,[14] respectively, for the diagnosis of periannular abscess. Traditional 2D TEE may be inadequate to provide complete anatomical information and the spatial relationship of the periannular lesions with adjacent structures.

Three-dimensional echocardiography has advantage of better visualization of structures in multiple planes with improved identification and characterization of the morphology, and it provides incremental information with clear demarcation of periannular abscess.

In mechanical prosthetic aortic valves, prosthetic aspect of the valve ring lies in the far field in the acoustic shadow of the mechanical prosthesis and poses challenges during imaging. TEE overcomes this limitation of TTE due to the proximity of the transducer to the heart and a higher signal to noise ratio and has superior resolution for better identification of lesions. In instances, when TEE is also negative in the diagnosis of root abscess, repeat evaluation by TEE should be done a week or 10 days later in search of echolucent abscess cavity—a hallmark of periannular abscess. Small abscess cavities located anteriorly may be difficult in visualization by TEE, and TTE is preferred over TEE in such situations. The periannular abscess located at the posterior mitral annulus lies in the far field of echocardiography, and very often, it is missed by TTE. These lesions are likely to be picked up by TEE. When the periannular lesions are associated with a large calcification, the calcium may interfere with abscess detection. In such situations, ^{18}F-FDG PET–CT and single-photon emission computed tomography fused with conventional computed tomography (SPECT/CT) will be helpful in arriving at the diagnosis.

The abscess cavity may rupture into adjacent structures and result in the formation of fistulae or pseudoaneurysms. Color Doppler interrogation in combination with pulsed-wave Doppler and continuous wave Doppler assessment will establish the distinctive flow pattern of fistulae and pseudoaneurysm.

KEY POINT 2

The clinical suspicion of periannular extension in IE should initiate prompt evaluation by both TTE or TEE. TTE may yield better images of an anterior root abscess, while TEE is better for posterior root abscess. 3D TEE provides complementary information regarding the extent of abscess and its relationship with neighboring structures. A normal TEE does not rule out periannular abscess, and alternate modes of diagnosis should be utilized in the evaluation.

Leaflet Aneurysm

The progressive infection in IE results in the formation of an abscess over the leaflet with local weakening of underlying tissue and results in a sac-like bulging and eventually aneurysm formation.[15] It is a rare complication of IE and frequently affects the mitral valve, though other valves may be affected. The perforation of leaflet aneurysm results in acute severe regurgitation with resultant heart failure and hemodynamic deterioration. On echocardiography, leaflet aneurysm appears as localized saccular bulging of the leaflet with systolic expansion and diastolic collapse.

Pseudoaneurysm

Pseudoaneurysm due to complicated IE is defined as a perivalvular cavity communicating with the cardiovascular lumen. On color Doppler interrogation, color flow is detected into this perivalvular cavity, and it appears as a pulsatile echo-free perivalvular pouch.[4]

Fistulae

Fistula develops as a result of rupture of the abscess cavity leading to an abnormal communication between two neighboring cardiac cavities through perforation or nonanatomic channel.[4,16] Color Doppler interrogation demonstrates color flow between the two cavities indicating a communication between two neighboring cavities.

Intervalvular Fibrosa Pseudoaneurysm

It is a deadly complication of IE and requires urgent surgery. It frequently occurs as a complication of aortic valve endocarditis. Rarely the periannular infection extends to the mitral aortic intervalvular fibrosa and may result in the formation of pseudoaneurysm. On TEE the pseudoaneurysm appears as a pulsatile saccular pouch in the region between posterior aortic annulus and the anterior wall of left atrium.[17] If surgery is delayed the pseudoaneurysm may rupture into the pericardial space resulting in acute cardiac tamponade, or it may rupture into left atrium causing acute severe mitral regurgitation, or it may lead to the formation of fistulous tract from left ventricular outflow to left atrium. The enlarging pseudoaneurysm may lead to coronary artery compression and acute myocardial infarction.

Dehiscence of a Prosthetic Valve

Prosthetic valve dehiscence is defined as a rocking motion of prosthetic valve greater than 15° in any one plane on echocardiography. It is one of the major diagnostic criteria for IE. It indicates late stage of the infection or aggressive infection. Extensive endocarditis results in suture destruction and valve dehiscence. It invariably results in significant paravalvular leak and hemodynamic compromise and is an indication for emergency surgical intervention. In severe cases, it results in gross separation of prosthetic annulus from the native tissue and results in tilting or rocking motion of the valve annulus.

Congestive Heart Failure

Heart failure is the most frequent indication for urgent surgery in IE. It usually occurs due to acute severe aortic or mitral insufficiency as a result of valve destruction—mitral chordal rupture, leaflet rupture, or perforation or the vegetation interfering with the coaptation of leaflets. Rare complications of IE, such as sudden intracardiac shunt lesions or fistulae, prosthetic valve dehiscence, and more rarely valve obstruction due to a large vegetation present with heart failure. Associated myocarditis and myocardial infarction due to the embolic obstruction of the coronary artery are other rare causes of heart failure in IE. Congestive heart failure carries a very high mortality and morbidity and is an independent strong predictor of inhospital and 1-year mortality. However, early detection and prompt surgery significantly improves the outcome and survival.

Embolic Events

Embolic events result from the embolization of the vegetations or fragments of vegetation via the vascular bed. Vegetations located on the mitral valve, particularly the anterior mitral leaflet, are more prone for embolization. Large vegetations, freely mobile vegetations, multivalvular vegetations, and vegetations due to specific organisms, such as *Staphylococci*, *Streptococcus bovis*, and *Candida* spp. carry high-risk for embolization. Embolic events occur in 20–50% of cases with IE and predispose to morbidity and mortality. Initiation of antibiotic therapy reduces the risk of new embolic event reduces to 6–21%.[5] Large vegetations more than 10 mm in length carry very high-risk of embolism, and surgery is recommended in these patients following more than one embolic episodes.[1]

Mycotic Aneurysm

Mycotic aneurysm is a rare but important complication of IE. It occurs as a result of septic arterial embolization of vegetation. The intracranial arteries are most commonly involved, followed by the visceral arteries. The upper and lower limb arteries are very rarely involved. Computed tomography and magnetic resonance angiography can reliably diagnose mycotic aneurysm. The mycotic aneurysms have a tendency to rupture, and ruptured aneurysms carry poor prognosis.

Integrated approach involving 2D imaging, color Doppler interrogation, pulsed- and continuous-wave Doppler assessment, and 3D imaging utilizing, both TTE and TEE play a crucial role in the prompt detection of complications of IE and the subsequent hemodynamic consequences (Table 4).

Very rarely IE may involve multiple valves (Figs. 5A to C) and usually occurs in multivalve disease, such as rheumatic valvular disease with the involvement of multiple valves.

TABLE 4: Role of echocardiography in identification of complications of endocarditis.[18]

1. *Uncontrolled infection with persistent pyrexia and bacteremia:*
   i. Check for periannular complications, abscess, fistula, perforation, increase in vegetation size
   ii. Detection and assessment of the severity of regurgitation or obstruction of aortic or mitral valve
2. *Identification of cause of heart failure which may be in the form of pulmonary edema, or cardiogenic shock:*
   i. Check for acute aortic or mitral regurgitation, or obstruction
   ii. Search for fistula into intracardiac chamber or pericardium
   iii. Assess signs of hemodynamic intolerance: Pulmonary arterial hypertension, left or right ventricular systolic dysfunction, premature mitral valve closure
3. *Detection of prosthetic valve dysfunction:*
   i. Severe regurgitation which may be valvular due to vegetation interfering with leaflet coaptation or paravalvular leak due to periannular complications
   ii. Periannular abscess
   iii. Valve dehiscence indicating by the rocking motion of the valve ring
   iv. Prosthetic valve obstruction due to large vegetation
4. *Assessment of risk of embolism: Echocardiographic features predicting high-risk for peripheral embolism:*
   i. Large vegetation or increasing vegetation size carries high-risk for embolic events
   ii. Very large vegetation >15 mm is highly susceptible for embolism
   iii. Persistent large vegetation >10 mm after previous embolism despite initiation of antibiotic therapy
   iv. Large vegetation >10 mm associated with other risk factors, e.g. heart failure, abscess, persistent infection
5. *Detection of rare complications, such as pericardial effusion or myocarditis.*

Indications for Surgery in Infective Endocarditis

The three different categories of indications for surgery in IE are hemodynamic, infectious, and embolic indications (Table 5). Valvular dysfunction with acute severe regurgitation, either valvular or paravalvular, usually results in ventricular dysfunction and heart failure and requires early surgery. Occasionally large vegetation can cause valve obstruction and heart failure requiring surgery. Heart failure is the most common indication for surgery in IE. Large size of the vegetation >10 mm, and particularly when located on mitral valve, poses high-risk for embolism. Moreover, increasing size of vegetation despite appropriate antibiotic therapy carries high-risk of systemic embolization and should be treated by surgery. Uncontrolled infection with valve destruction or extension of infection to periannular region results in complications, such as periannular abscess, fistula, or pseudoaneurysm formation. These complications are associated with high mortality and morbidity and should be treated with urgent surgery. We need to be aware that not infrequently there may be asymptomatic systemic embolization to clinically silent areas, such as spleen, liver, and some regions of brain.

Preoperative Echocardiography

Preoperative TTE and TEE provide comprehensive assessment of the valve morphology, appropriate annulus size, mechanism of valve dysfunction, and any associated periannular lesions. Thus it facilitates the surgical planning and determines whether IE can be treated with valve repair or valve replacement. Leaflet perforation or chordal rupture with severe mitral regurgitation can be treated successfully with valve repair techniques involving pericardial patch

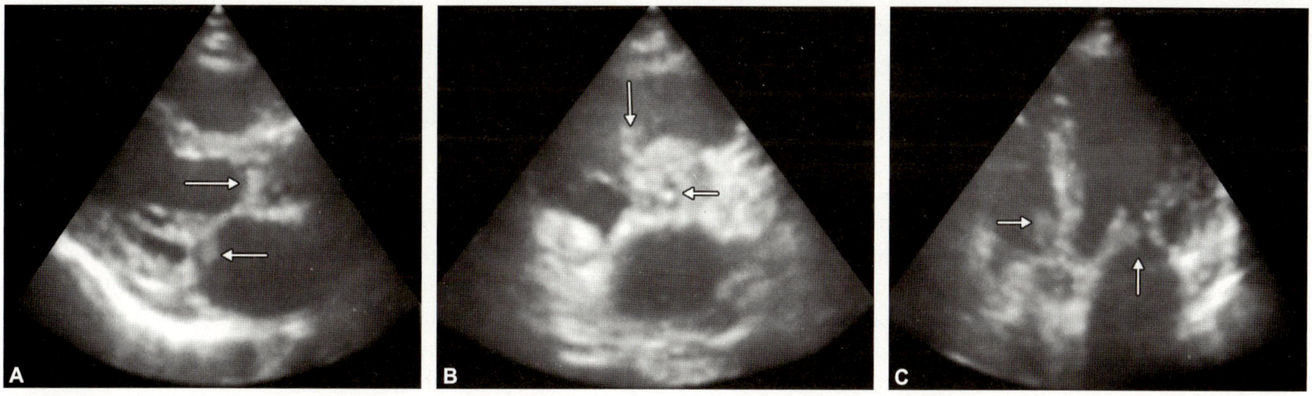

Figs. 5A to C: Transthoracic echocardiographic images in multivalvular infective endocarditis. Infective endocarditis involving multiple valves. (A) Transthoracic echocardiographic image showing parasternal long-axis view profiling shaggy masses—vegetations (arrows) attached over the anterior mitral leaflet and noncoronary cusp of the aortic valve; (B) Parasternal short-axis view showing vegetation attached to the aortic valve and the septal leaflet of tricuspid valve; (C) Apical four-chamber view showing the vegetation attached to the anterior mitral leaflet and the septal leaflet of the tricuspid valve.

TABLE 5: Role of echocardiography in assessing the potential need for surgical intervention.[20]

- *Valvular dysfunction with heart failure:*
  - Acute severe regurgitation of aortic or mitral valve with the signs of ventricular dysfunction and heart failure
  - Valve leaflet perforation or chordal rupture with severe regurgitation
  - Vegetation causing valve obstruction and pulmonary edema
  - Vegetation or periannular abscess resulting in rupture of sinus of Valsalva into right heart
  - Prosthetic valve instability
  - Fistula or pseudoaneurysm formation
- *Persistent infection with perivalvular extension:*
  - Large abscess or extension of abscess despite appropriate antimicrobial therapy
  - Valvular abscess dehiscence, rupture, or fistula
- *Vegetation with features of increased susceptibility for embolic events:*
  - Persistence of vegetation even after systemic embolization
  - Large and mobile anterior mitral leaflet vegetation, particularly ≥10 mm
  - ≥1 embolic events during initial 2 weeks of antimicrobial treatment
  - Increasing size of vegetation even after appropriate antimicrobial treatment.

repair of perforation or replacement of ruptured chordae with neochordae. If valve replacement is contemplated, it enables appropriate selection of prosthetic valves and aortic homografts.

Intraoperative Echocardiography

Intraoperative TEE provides the cardiothoracic surgeon with a final anatomical picture of valvular and perivalvular damage and identification of complications and guides the decision regarding the best surgical approach. It is especially useful to assess the adequacy of valve repair and the result of complex perivalvular repair.[21] At the completion of corrective procedure, it is crucial to assess the result by acquiring postcardiopulmonary bypass images. During postpump imaging the afterload frequently requires augmentation to reach representative ambulatory levels for accurate estimation of regurgitant jet severity and significance.

These images will decide the success of the repair or replacement of valve and the closure of fistulous tracts and repair of pseudoaneurysm. Thus intraoperative TEE improves the success rate of surgical intervention. Perivalvular leaks, if present, should be assessed for severity and the responsible mechanism and dictate any corrective measures, if required. Hemodynamically insignificant perivalvular leak related to technical factors should be identified and documented. It can also serve as reference data for future follow-up of and prevent the confusion whether the leaks are the result of recurrent infection during follow-up.

Echocardiography at the Completion of Therapy

Serial echocardiographic evaluation is essential during the antibiotic therapy to assess the changes in the characteristics of the endocarditis lesions, valve morphology, ventricular function, and valvular insufficiency and to assess the response to therapy. All patients who had IE carry high-risk for recurrent infection indefinitely. Thus, close follow-up with thorough clinical examination and serial echocardiographic assessment is mandatory at intervals of 1, 3, 6, and 12 months after the end of antibiotic treatment or following surgery in order to rule out the recurrence of IE.

Echocardiography in Specific Clinical Situations of Infective Endocarditis

Prosthetic Valve Endocarditis

Prosthetic valve endocarditis constitutes 10–30% of all cases of endocarditis and occurs in 1–6% of patients with valve prostheses. Both mechanical prosthetic and bioprosthetic valves are equally affected. PVE is typically more severe than native valve endocarditis due to frequent periannular complications and associated with very high inhospital mortality rate of 20–40%.[22] The *early-onset* PVE occurs within 60 days of valve replacement surgery, *intermediate-onset* PVE occurs from 60 days to 365 days, and *late-onset* PVE occurs 365 days after the valve surgery. In mechanical prostheses the infection usually arises from the junction between the sewing ring and the annulus or from the thrombi located near the sewing ring. Therefore perivalvular abscess, dehiscence, perivalvular leak (Figs. 6A to C), pseudoaneurysms, and fistula occur more frequently. Conversely the infection is usually localized to leaflet cusps in bioprosthetic valves, and there is a relatively low risk for perivalvular complications. PVE usually results in prosthetic regurgitation or perivalvular leak causing heart failure. Rarely large vegetations may cause obstruction of the prosthetic valve.

Echocardiographic imaging is more challenging in PVE, especially with mechanical valves, due to reverberation and acoustic shadowing. Imaging of perivalvular complications may be obscured by acoustic shadowing from the valve prosthesis during TTE. TEE has a higher sensitivity of 92% as compared with 50% for TTE in the diagnosis of PVE.[23] Therefore TEE is preferred in PVE for the detection of vegetations and periannular complications. Both the structural lesions and their hemodynamic consequences can be completely evaluated by echocardiography through integrated approach using 2D, 3D, color Doppler and spectral Doppler echocardiographic techniques.

Although TEE plays an important role in the diagnosis of PVE, echocardiography is inconclusive in the initial stages. Thus alternative imaging modalities, such as PET-CT, can identify the site of infection due to the uptake of positron-labeled glucose by the inflammatory leukocytes. Moreover, MDCT may yield diagnostic evidence of infection where TEE has been nondiagnostic. However, MDCT and PETCT should be used judiciously because these imaging modalities are expensive and associated with radiation exposure and contrast-related complications.

The 2015 European Society of Cardiology guidelines for the management of IE[3] have proposed the inclusion of these imaging modalities in the diagnostic criteria of IE. The three new points included are as follows:

1. Detection of definite paravalvular lesion by cardiac MDCT as a major criterion
2. Detection of abnormal activity around the site of implantation of prosthetic valve by ^{18}F-FDG PET-CT (only after 3 months of prosthesis implantation) or radiolabeled leukocyte SPECT-CT as a major criterion
3. Detection of recent embolic episodes or infectious aneurysms by imaging only as a minor criterion

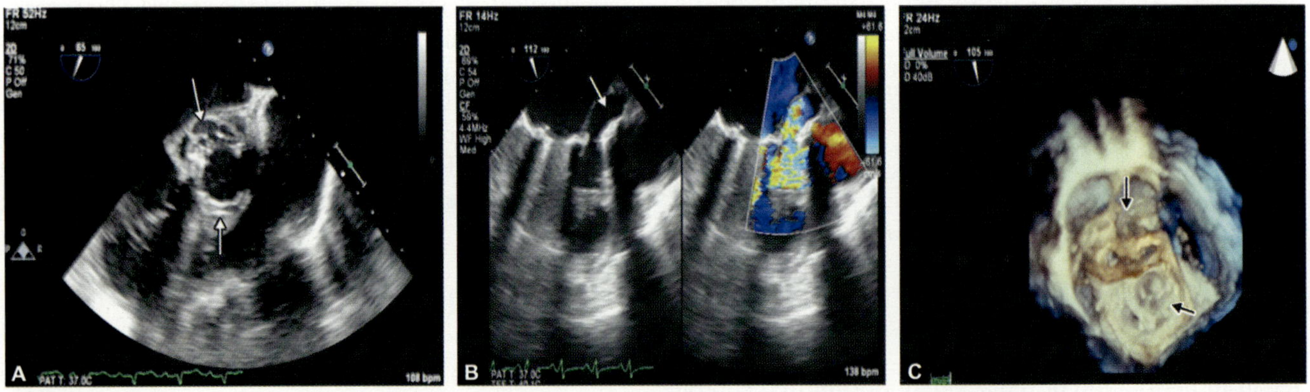

Figs. 6A to C: Transesophageal echocardiography evaluation of prosthetic valve endocarditis complicated with periannular abscess and valve dehiscence. Transesophageal echocardiography in a patient with double-valve replacement with early infective endocarditis involving the prosthetic valve in aortic position with periannular abscess and valve dehiscence. (A) Two-dimensional imaging at 65° shows the short-axis of the aortic valve. The arrow indicates a large echolucent space in the region of noncoronary sinus of Valsalva with multiple septations representing periannular abscess, and the thickening of the aortic wall in the region of right coronary cusp is also a sign of periannular abscess; (B) Long-axis view at 112° with color comparison demonstrated severe paravalvular leak. Two-dimensional images showed echolucent abscess cavity (arrow) in the noncoronary sinus region and the mechanical prosthetic valve in the mitral position; (C) Three-dimensional imaging shows large periannular abscess cavity (vertical arrow) encircling the valve ring and causing extensive destruction, the cavity has multiple septations. The mechanical prosthesis is visualized in the mitral position.

Right-Sided Endocarditis

Infective endocarditis involving the right side of the heart primarily affects patients with intravenous drug abuse, implanted cardiac devices, central venous catheters, or congenital heart disease (CHD). Right-sided IE (RIE) is encountered rarely in general population and seen in <5% of IE cases.[24] Tricuspid valve is most commonly affected. As right is a relatively low-flow and low-pressure zone, vegetations grow faster and are relatively larger. Vegetations are typically located over the atrial side of the tricuspid valve, cardiac device leads, and less frequently over the right ventricular side of pulmonary valve. The usual clinical presentation of RIE includes persistent fever and bacteremia. RIE is often complicated with multiple septic pulmonary emboli, which may manifest with chest pain, cough, or hemoptysis. Pulmonary septic emboli may be complicated by pulmonary infarction, abscess, pneumothorax, and purulent pleural effusion.[25] Right heart structures are located anteriorly and in proximity to the TTE transducer; hence, TTE can adequately profile the tricuspid valve for the visualization of vegetations. Modified off-axis parasternal long-axis profiling the right ventricular inflow view, short-axis, apical four-chamber, and subcostal views may be necessary to get a clear visualization of the right ventricular inflow and outflow tracts, the Eustachian valve and the posterior leaflet of the tricuspid valve. Sometimes, it becomes difficult to differentiate normal structural variants, such as Chiari network or prominent Eustachian valve, from vegetations. Very rarely vegetations are also found on the Eustachian valve. Moreover, vegetations on pacing lead or intracardiac defibrillator lead, indwelling catheters, and right-sided prostheses are particularly difficult to diagnose with TTE because of the reverberation and shadowing artifacts. In these cases, TEE yields images with superior resolution, and tricuspid and pulmonary valves and the intracardiac devices may be better visualized in the transgastric views at 90°–100° profiling right atrium, tricuspid valve, right ventricle, and the right ventricular outflow tract. 3D TEE may provide better visualization of vegetations located over the intracardiac pacing leads or defibrillator leads. Figures 7A to F illustrate the TTE images in a patient with the history of persistent fever for 2 months, New York Heart Association functional class III dyspnea, and paroxysmal nocturnal dyspnea. On examination, he was febrile with tachycardia and continuous murmur in the left second and third parasternal region. Echocardiographic evaluation revealed ruptured sinus of Valsalva and ventricular septal defect with IE involving the tricuspid valve, aneurysm of Valsalva, and the interventricular septum.

Cardiac Device–Related Infective Endocarditis

The diagnosis and treatment of cardiac device infection is challenging and is associated with the increase in morbidity and mortality. In some instances the imaging of the cardiac devices—pacemaker leads, intracardiac defibrillator lead, and septal occluder—is difficult on TTE due to the acoustic shadowing. TEE is mandatory in such situations. Usually pacemaker or the defibrillator lead vegetation is located over the lead, frequently in the right atrial portion than the right ventricular portion of the lead, and rarely over the tricuspid valve.

Figures 8A and B demonstrate TEE images of lead endocarditis in a patient with permanent pacemaker implant. In challenging cases, ^{18}F-FDG PET/CT can detect the abnormal FDG uptake along the course of the lead and facilitate the diagnosis of lead endocarditis. It can also evaluate the extracardiac portion of leads, also has the potential ability to differentiate a vegetation from a thrombus, and can diagnose septic emboli. Thus it has incremental value over echocardiography in early recognition of lead endocarditis. SPECT may also be helpful in the early detection of cardiac device IE. Urgent removal of the infected device in adjunction to the antibiotic therapy is mandatory to treat cardiac device–related IE. After the removal of the infected device, echogenic, sleeve-like sheets may be visualized in the right atrium on TEE, and these are called "ghost" sheets. These "ghost" sheets indicate a worse outcome.

Infective Endocarditis in Congenital Heart Disease

Congenital heart disease (CHD) is a major predisposing risk factor for IE in younger individuals. Cyanotic CHD lesions, such as tetralogy of Fallot, transposition of the great arteries, endocardial cushion defects, and left-sided lesions, such as coarctation of aorta, patent ductus arteriosus, aortic valve disease, ventricular septal defect, and mitral valve disease are associated with an increased risk of IE. Some relatively low-flow lesions, such as ostium secundum atrial septal defect, carry a low-risk of IE. Surgical repair of congenital defects eliminates the risk of IE if no residual lesion is left over. But most of the operated patients with complex CHD are left with some form of residua or sequalae, many of which become targets for IE. The implanted device, the septal occlude may be a nidus for vegetation. Figures 9A and B show TEE images depicting IE involving the atrial septal defect occluder device. The clinical course of the disease and complications of IE in CHD are similar to

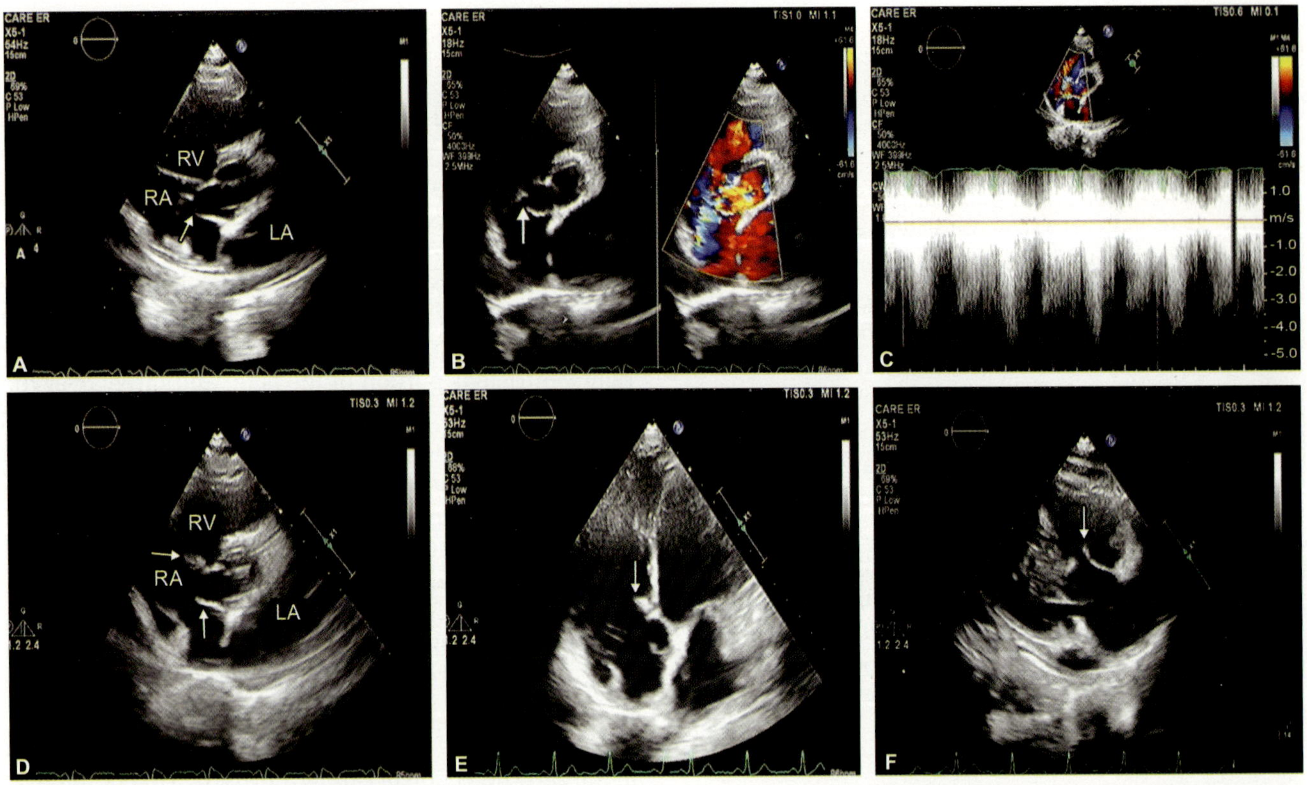

Figs. 7A to F: Transthoracic echocardiography in a patient with ruptured sinus of Valsalva and ventricular septal defect with infective endocarditis involving the tricuspid valve, aneurysm of the Valsalva, and the interventricular septum. (A) Parasternal short-axis view shows the classical windsock deformity (arrow) of aneurysm of noncoronary sinus of Valsalva with rupture into the right atrium, and the mobile element attached to the windsock deformity is also visualized; (B) Imaging with color comparison demonstrates the mosaic flow indicating left-to-right shunt across the ruptured aneurysm of noncoronary sinus of Valsalva into right atrium; (C) Continuous-wave Doppler interrogation demonstrates the continuous flow from noncoronary sinus of Valsalva to right atrium indicating the left-to-right shunt across the ruptured aneurysm of sinus of Valsalva to right atrium; (D) Parasternal short-axis view shows the vegetation (arrow) attached to the septal leaflet of the tricuspid valve; (E) Apical four-chamber view shows the vegetation attached to the interventricular septum; (F) Parasternal right ventricular inflow view shows the vegetation (arrow) attached to the anterior leaflet of tricuspid valve. (LA: left atrium; RA: right atrium; RV: right ventricle)

IE in general. Echocardiography is the mainstay in the diagnosis and management of IE in CHD. Figures 10A to D show TTE images of a patient with double-chambered right ventricle who presented with the history of fever for 4 months and treated as pulmonary kochs. TTE revealed vegetations attached to the tricuspid and pulmonary valves and the main pulmonary artery. TTE may be adequate in the identification of vegetation and sequalae of IE in pediatric population, but TEE will be complementary in patients with complex anatomy and in the presence of prosthetic valves or implanted material, particularly in the adult patients.

Infective Endocarditis in Hypertrophic Cardiomyopathy

Infective endocarditis occurs rarely in hypertrophic cardiomyopathy (HCM), but it is associated with substantial morbidity and mortality. Vegetations are frequently located on the mitral valve, characteristically on the ventricular aspect of the anterior mitral leaflet. Aortic valve—the ventricular aspect of the cusps and the adjacent surface of proximal ventricular septum are the other sites where vegetations may develop. This can be explained by the damage of mitral or aortic valve endocardium or both (Figs. 11A to F) as a consequence of turbulence of blood flow during ejection and the systolic anterior motion of anterior mitral leaflet. The main risk factors for the development of IE were the presence of outflow tract obstruction and left atrial dilation >50 mm.[26] Patients with both left ventricular outflow obstruction and dilated left atrium have the highest risk of endocarditis. The proposed explanation for dilated left atrium and increased risk of IE is that a dilated left atrial cavity may reflect more severe hemodynamic impairment, with a higher outflow gradient, more important mitral valve regurgitation, and thus, resulting in a greater damage to the valve endocardium. IE in HCM can be diagnosed by TTE,

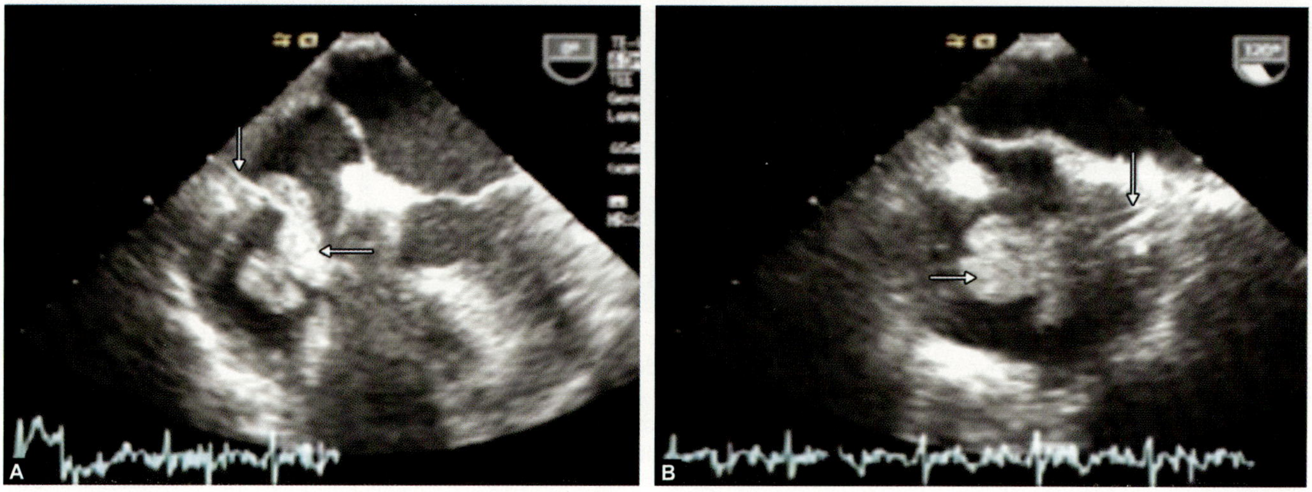

Figs. 8A and B: Transesophageal echocardiographic images of lead endocarditis in a patient with permanent pacemaker implant. Transesophageal echocardiographic images demonstrating infective endocarditis involving the pacemaker lead. (A) Transesophageal echocardiographic image at 0° profiling the four-chamber view and demonstrating the pacemaker lead (vertical arrow) in right atrium and the large homogeneous mass—vegetation (horizontal arrow) engulfing the pacemaker lead; (B) Bicaval view profiling the pacemaker lead (vertical arrow) and the large vegetation (horizontal arrow) attached to the pacemaker lead in right atrium.

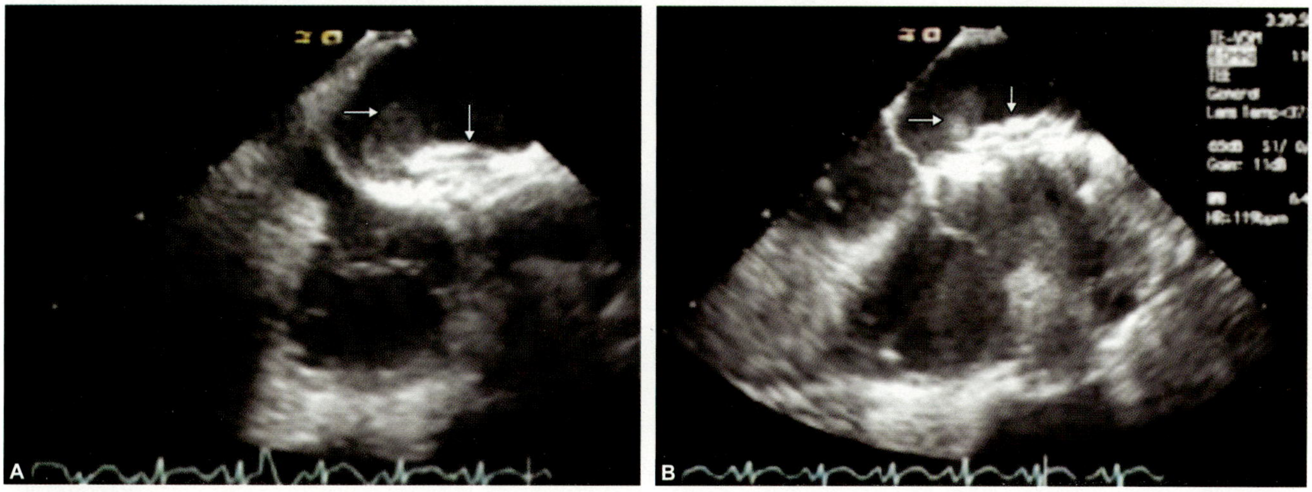

Figs. 9A and B: Transesophageal echocardiographic images depicting infective endocarditis involving the atrial septal defect occluder device. (A) Transesophageal echocardiographic image profiling the bicaval view demonstrating the atrial septal defect occluder device in position (vertical arrow). Freely mobile shaggy globular element suggestive of vegetation (horizontal arrow) is attached to the left atrial disk of the occluder device; (B) Modified four-chamber view at 145° profiling the atrial septal defect occluder device. The left atrial disk (vertical arrow) is clearly visualized and the vegetation (horizontal arrow) attached to the left atrial disk is also seen.

and if TTE is inconclusive, TEE will be required. TEE will also be mandatory if patient develops complications of IE.

KEY POINT 3

According to American college of Cardiology (ACC)/American Heart Association (AHA) guidelines, TEE has an important role in patients with prosthetic valves or intracardiac implants or inconclusive TTE and also in the assessment of complications of IE.[19]

Checklist for Echocardiographic Assessment in a Patient with Infective Endocarditis

- Number, size, location, shape, and mobility of vegetation
- Echotexture whether soft and shaggy suggestive of acute endocarditis or with focal hyperechogenicity indicating calcification and fibrosis suggestive of subacute or chronic infection

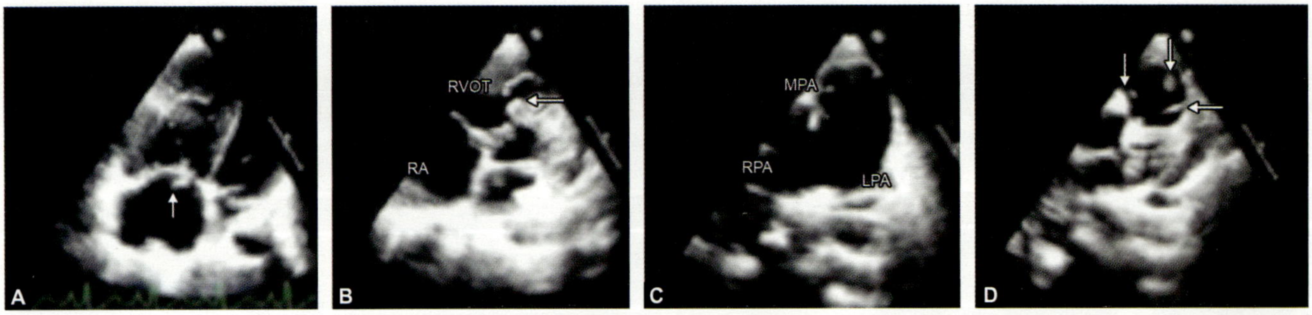

Figs. 10A to D: Transthoracic echocardiographic images of a patient with double-chambered right ventricle with infective endocarditis. Right-sided infective endocarditis in a patient with double-chamber right ventricle with vegetations attached to the tricuspid and pulmonary valves and the MPA. (A) Transthoracic echocardiographic images showing apical four-chamber view demonstrating vegetation (arrow) attached to the septal leaflet of tricuspid valve; (B) Parasternal short-axis view showing the accessory muscle bundle (arrow) in the RVOT; (C) Parasternal short-axis view profiling the MPA, RPA, and LPA. Small elements are seen suggestive of vegetations in MPA; (D) Modified short-axis view clearly delineating the pulmonary valve (horizontal arrow) and the vegetations (vertical arrows) attached to the pulmonary artery. (LPA: left pulmonary artery; MPA: main pulmonary artery; RPA: right pulmonary artery; RVOT: right ventricular outflow tract)

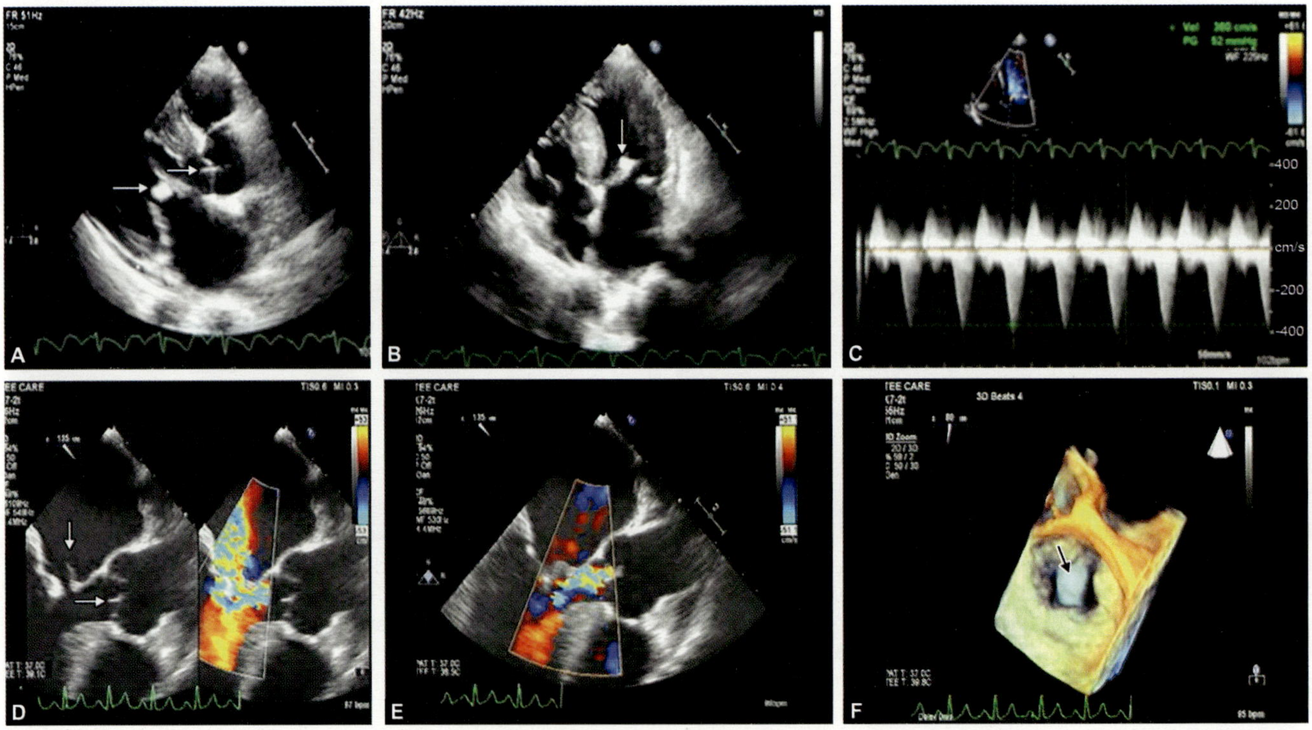

Figs. 11A to F: Transthoracic echocardiographic images in hypertrophic cardiomyopathy with infective endocarditis. Transthoracic (A to C) and transesophageal (D to F) echocardiographic images in hypertrophic obstructive cardiomyopathy with infective endocarditis. (A) Parasternal long-axis view shows asymmetric septal hypertrophy and linear vegetation (arrow) attached to the aortic valve and echodense vegetation (arrow) attached to the anterior mitral leaflet; (B) Apical four-chamber view shows the echodense vegetation attached to the tip of anterior mitral leaflet; (C) Continuous-wave Doppler interrogation shows severe left ventricular outflow tract obstruction with a peak pressure gradient of 62 mm Hg; (D) Transesophageal echocardiography with two-dimensional imaging with color comparison shows vegetations attached to the right coronary cusp of aortic valve and the anterior mitral leaflet (arrow) and severe mitral regurgitation; (E) Color Doppler interrogation in the long-axis view at 135° shows moderate aortic regurgitation; (F) Three-dimensional imaging on transesophageal echocardiography shows the large vegetation (arrow) attached to anterior mitral leaflet.

- Relationship with surrounding structures
- Check for resultant regurgitation or obstruction of the affected valve
- Assess the severity of the valvular regurgitation or obstruction
- Assess the chamber dimensions: Left ventricular and left atrial dimensions in the case of mitral or aortic endocarditis and right ventricular and right atrial dimensions in right-sided endocarditis
- Check for vegetations by profiling the valves in all possible views, including the subcostal view, especially for right-sided endocarditis; sometimes off-axis views may be required, especially in right-sided endocarditis involving the intracardiac devices
- Assess for hemodynamic consequences of the regurgitation or obstruction by assessing pulmonary arterial pressures or left ventricular filling pressure or right atrial pressure
- Check all the valves for the presence of vegetation as IE may rarely involve multiple valves
- *Assess for the complications of endocarditis:*
    - Leaflet perforation and regurgitation
    - Leaflet aneurysm with or without regurgitation
    - Satellite lesions on the neighboring structures
- *Periannular complications, such as:*
    - Aortic root abscess or
    - Pseudoaneurysm or fistula formation, mitral-aortic intervalvular fibrosa pseudoaneurysm
    - Rupture of the pseudoaneurysm into the pericardial space, resulting in acute cardiac tamponade or rupture into left atrium causing acute severe mitral regurgitation or formation of fistulous tract from left ventricular outflow to left atrium
    - The enlarging pseudoaneurysm may lead to coronary artery compression and acute myocardial infarction
    - Subvalvular left ventricular aneurysms—subaortic or submitral aneurysm
- Check for rare complications of endocarditis, such as myocarditis—regional or global left ventricular function assessment—or pericarditis
- In the case of PVE, carefully assess the vegetation, prosthetic valve stability, check for regurgitation or obstruction, paravalvular leak, periannular complications, such as periannular abscess, valve dehiscence, and other complications, such as pseudoaneurysm or fistula.

Limitations of Echocardiography in Infective Endocarditis

Echocardiography is fundamental in the evaluation of patients with IE, and it is widely accepted as the preferred imaging modality for the diagnosis, risk stratification, management, and follow-up of patients with IE. But the clinician should be aware that negative echocardiography findings do not rule out the diagnosis of IE. Echocardiography may be negative in about 15% of cases of IE. Echocardiography may be inconclusive in some clinical situations, such as prosthetic valves, intracardiac devices, the presence of pre-existing severe lesions (degenerative lesions, mitral valve prolapse), very small vegetations <2 mm, and periannular abscesses. Echocardiography may be inadequate in assessing periannular complications as it has limitations in the identification of morphological substrate or the extent of perivalvular pathology. Alternative imaging modalities will be of help in these situations.

ALTERNATIVE IMAGING MODALITIES

Cardiac Multidetector Computed Tomography, Magnetic Resonance Imaging, and Nuclear Imaging

Cardiac MDCT and magnetic resonance imaging (MRI) are becoming popular as complementary imaging modalities in the diagnosis of PVE. Electrocardiogram-gated image acquisition during MDCT enables the 3D reconstruction of images in any plane during any part of cardiac cycle. Contrast-enhanced MDCT detects prosthetic valve thrombi, pannus, vegetations, paravalvular leak, mycotic aneurysm, and periannular abscesses. The diagnosis of endocarditis is challenging in the very early stage due to subtle diagnostic features and also in patients with prosthetic valves and intracardiac devices. In these situations, nuclear imaging with PET–CT or cardiac MRI may provide the solution. In some cases the echocardiogram remains inconclusive or negative even after a repeat evaluation. Combination of MDCT and FDG PET provides high-resolution anatomical and metabolic imaging of prosthetic valves and the adjacent structures. Figures 12A to D exhibit the TTE and ^{18}F-FDG PET–CT images of early-onset PVE in a patient who underwent aortic valve replacement and developed persistent fever within 2 weeks of surgery. Echocardiography revealed a large vegetation attached to the valve ring and severe aortic regurgitation, while ^{18}F-FDG PET–CT revealed FDG uptake in the valve sewing ring and the vegetation. Echocardiography exhibits morphological changes and hemodynamic abnormalities, but the underlying pathophysiological processes at the molecular level are not addressed. This limitation of echocardiography is overcome with the advent of new molecular imaging methods, such as ^{18}F-FDG PET-CT and SPECT/CT. Of these methods, ^{18}F-FDG PET–CT carries the best promise for a future role in endocarditis. MRI and spiral CT are methods

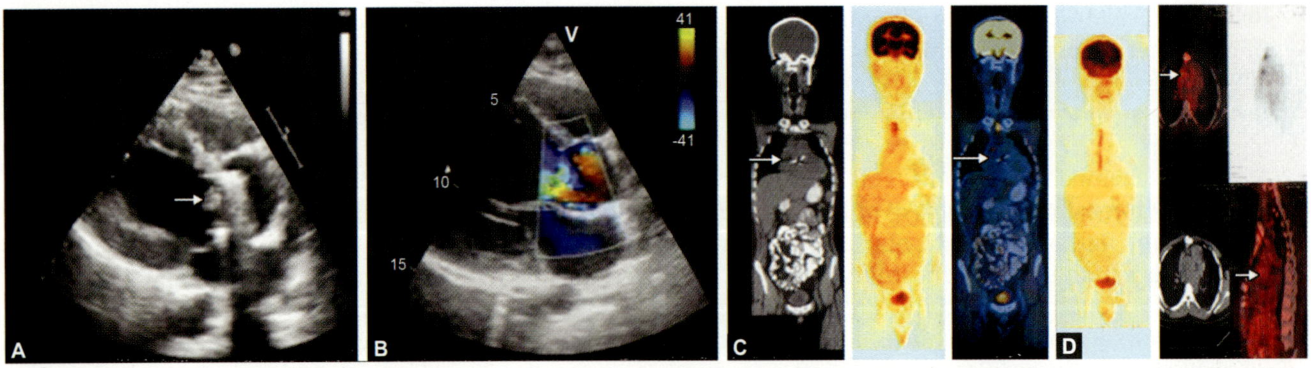

Figs. 12A to D: Transthoracic echocardiographic and ^{18}F-FDG PET-CT images in a patient with early-onset IE after aortic valve replacement. (A) Parasternal long-axis view shows the large shaggy vegetation attached to the valve sewing ring; (B) Color Doppler interrogation demonstrated severe valvular aortic regurgitation; (C) Coronal slices of whole body ^{18}F-FDG PET, CT, and fused PET/CT with abnormal FDG uptake at the aortic valve (arrow); (D) Axial slices of fused ^{18}F-FDG PET/CT, ^{18}F-FDG PET, and low-dose CT with abnormal FDG uptake at the aortic valve (arrow). (^{18}F-FDG: ^{18}F-Fluorodesoxyglucose; CT: computed tomography; IE: infective endocarditis; PET: positron emission tomography)

primarily used in the search for extra cardiac infectious foci. Inclusion of PET/CT, wherever justified, in the evaluation of IE substantially improves the sensitivity of modified Duke criteria, especially in prosthetic valves and cardiac device-related IE.

CONCLUSION

Echocardiography is the preferred imaging modality in the management of IE and plays a key role across all stages—diagnosis, risk stratification, identification of complications, treatment and prognosis of IE. The limitations of echocardiography are prominent in certain clinical situations, such as initial stages of IE, patients with prosthetic valves, or intracardiac devices or complicated IE. Multiplane TEE provides images with excellent temporal and spatial resolution and improves the accuracy of diagnosis of IE and its complications. Advanced echocardiography technique of 3D echocardiography facilitates the noninvasive and radiation-free assessment of the extent of infection and the involvement of adjacent structures and thus enables efficient treatment plan with surgical intervention. Alternative imaging modalities, such as ^{18}F-FDG PET-CT, cardiac MDCT, and cardiac MRI, are emerging as important supplementary modalities whenever echocardiography is inconclusive. These advanced imaging techniques offer new perspectives and improve the diagnostic accuracy and identification of perivalvular and extracardiac complications of IE.

ACKNOWLEDGMENT

Authors are thankful to Management of Care Hospitals, Banjara Hills, Hyderabad.

REFERENCES

1. Habib G, Hoen B, Tornos P, et al. Guidelines on the prevention, diagnosis, and treatment of infective endocarditis (new version 2009). Eur Heart J. 2009;30: 2369-413.
2. Li JS, Sexton DJ, Mick N, et al. Proposed modifications to the Duke criteria for the diagnosis of infective endocarditis. Clin Infect Dis. 2000;30:633-8.
3. Habib G, Badano L, Tribouilloy C, et al. Recommendations for the practice of echocardiography in infective endocarditis. Eur J Echocardiogr. 2010;11:202-19.
4. Baddour LM, Wilson WR, Bayer AS, et al. Infective endocarditis in adults: diagnosis, antimicrobial therapy, and management of complications. A scientific statement for healthcare professionals from the American Heart Association. Circulation. 2015;132:1435-86.
5. Bergler-Klein J. Role of echocardiography in the evaluation of patients with *Staphylococcus aureus* bacteraemia: time to look at the heart. Eur J Echocardiogr. 2011;12:411-3.
6. Dillon JC, Feigenbaum H, Konecke LL, et al. Echocardiographic manifestations of valvular vegetations. Am Heart J. 1973;86(5):698-704.
7. Gilbert BW, Haney RS, Crawford F, et al. Two-dimensional echocardiographic assessment of vegetative endocarditis. Circulation. 1977;55(2):346-53.
8. Thuny F, Gaubert JY, Jacquier A, et al. Imaging investigations in infective endocarditis: current approach and perspectives. Arch Cardiovasc Dis. 2013;106:52-62.
9. Di Salvo G, Habib G, Pergola V, et al. Echocardiography predicts embolic events in infective endocarditis. J Am Coll Cardiol. 2001;37:106976.
10. Blumberg EA, Karalis DA, Chandrasekaran K, et al. Endocarditis-associated paravalvular abscesses: do clinical parameters predict the presence of abscess? Chest. 1995;107:898-903.
11. Becher H, Hanrath P, Bleifeld W, et al. Correlation of echocardiographic and surgical findings in acute bacterial endocarditis. Eur Heart J. 1984;5(suppl C):67-70.

12. Ellis SG, Goldstein J, Popp RL. Detection of endocarditis-associated perivalvular abscesses by two-dimensional echocardiography. J Am Coll Cardiol. 1985;5:647-53.
13. Daniel WG, Mugge A, Martin RP, et al. Improvement in the diagnosis of abscesses associated with endocarditis by transesophageal echocardiography. N Engl J Med. 1991;324:795-800.
14. Tomsic A, Li WWL, van Paridon M, et al. Infective endocarditis of the aortic valve with anterior mitral valve leaflet aneurysm. Tex Heart Inst J. 2016;43(4):345-9.
15. Millar BC, Habib G, Moore JE. New diagnostic approaches in infective endocarditis. Heart. 2016;102:796-807.
16. Fazlinezhad A, Fatehi H, Tabaee S, et al. Pseudoaneurysm of mitro-aortic intervalvular fibrosa during the course of mitral valve endocarditis with aorto-left ventricle outflow tract fistula. J Saudi Heart Assoc. 2012;24:201-4.
17. Vilacosta I, Graupner C, San Román JA, et al. Risk of embolization after institution of antibiotic therapy for infective endocarditis. J Am Coll Cardiol. 2002;39(9):1489-95.
18. Nishimura RA, Otto CM, Bonow RO, et al. 2014 AHA/ACC guidelines for the management of patients with valvular heart disease. J Am Coll Cardiol. 2014;63(22):e57-185.
19. Baddour LM, Wilson WR, Bayer AS, et al. Infective endocarditis: diagnosis, antimicrobial therapy, and management of complications: a statement for healthcare professionals from the Committee on Rheumatic Fever, Endocarditis, and Kawasaki Disease, Council on Cardiovascular Disease in the Young, and the Councils on Clinical Cardiology, Stroke, and Cardiovascular Surgery and Anesthesia, American Heart Association: Endorsed by the Infectious Diseases Society of America. Circulation. 2005;111:e394-433.
20. Shapira Y, Weisenberg DE, Vaturi M, et al. The impact of intraoperative transesophageal echocardiography in infective endocarditis. Isr Med Assoc J. 2007;9:299-302.
21. Vongpatanasin W, Hillis LD, Lange RA. Prosthetic heart valves. N Engl J Med. 1996;335.
22. Habib G, Thuny F, Avierinos JF. Prosthetic valve endocarditis: current approach and therapeutic options. Prog Cardiovasc Dis. 2008;50:274-81.
23. Habib G, Lancellotti P, Antunes MJ, et al. 2015 ESC guidelines for the management of infective endocarditis: The Task Force for the Management of Infective Endocarditis of the European Society of Cardiology (ESC). Endorsed by: European Association for Cardio-Thoracic Surgery (EACTS), the European Association of Nuclear Medicine (EANM). Eur Heart J. 2015;36(44):3075-128.
24. Scudeller L, Badano LP, Crapis M, et al. Population based surveillance of infectious endocarditis in an Italian region. Arch Intern Med. 2009;169:1720-3.
25. Miro JM, del Rio A, Mestres CA. Infective endocarditis and cardiac surgery in intravenous drug abusers and HIV-1 infected patients. Cardiol Clin. 2003;21:167-84,v–vi.
26. Spirito P, Rapezzi C, Bellone P, et al. Infective endocarditis in hypertrophic cardiomyopathy prevalence, incidence, and indications for antibiotic prophylaxis. Circulation. 1999;99:2132-7.

SECTION 17

Pulmonary Embolism and Deep Vein Thrombosis

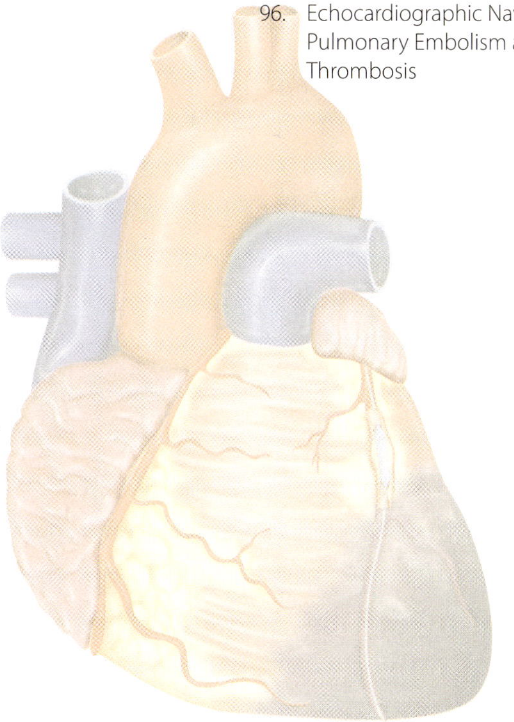

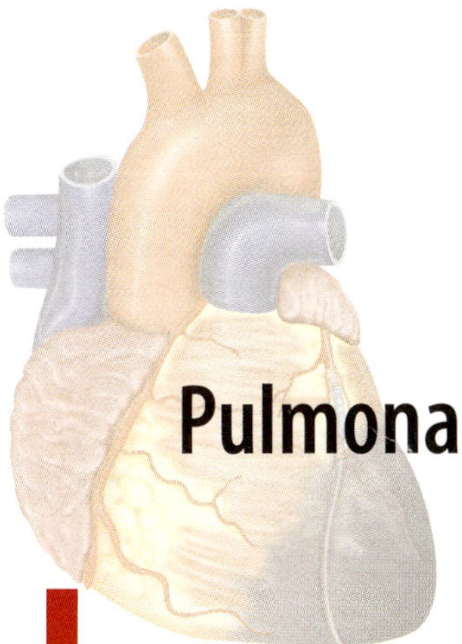

CHAPTER 96

Echocardiographic Navigation in Pulmonary Embolism and Deep Vein Thrombosis

Satish K Parashar, HK Chopra, PK Mangla

INTRODUCTION

Venous thromboembolism is a common condition encountered in clinical practice. It is a combination of deep vein thrombosis (DVT), a common association, and acute pulmonary embolism (APE). Within this combination APE accounts for almost one-third of cases. APE is a major contributor of global disease burden. Annual incidence is about 75–269 cases per 100,000 patients. Risk doubles with each decade after 40 years age. Risk is usually highest in first two postoperative weeks. Mortality for PE is about 2% in normotensive patients without evidence of right ventricular dysfunction (RVD), but rises up to 30% in patients with shock and up to 65% in patients with cardiac arrest at presentation. If left untreated, approximately one-third of patients who survive an initial PE die of a subsequent embolic episode.[1-4] The International Cooperative Pulmonary Embolism Registry (ICOPER) demonstrated 90-day mortality rates of 58.3% in patients with massive PE versus 15.1% in submassive PE. Furthermore, a small fraction (up to 4%) of surviving patients will later on develop chronic thromboembolic pulmonary hypertension (CTEPH), untreated CTEPH carries a poor prognosis, especially if associated with RVD. Its development is multifactorial like incompletely resolved thrombi, shear stress, remodeling of the pulmonary vascular bed, and microvascular inflammation.

PATHOPHYSIOLOGY

The main manifestations of major PE are acute right ventricular (RV) failure and hypoxia. The basic pathophysiology is an acutely increased pulmonary vascular resistance (PVR) which is mainly contributed by: (a) anatomical obstruction to the pulmonary vasculature; (b) pulmonary artery (PA) vasoconstriction induced by release of neurohormonal substances (serotonin from platelets, thrombin from plasma, and histamine from tissues; and (c) RV hypoxemia.

The sequence of APE is shown in Flowchart 1 and a simplified version in Flowchart 2. In brief, this acute increase

Flowchart 1: Pathophysiology of effect of acute pulmonary embolism.

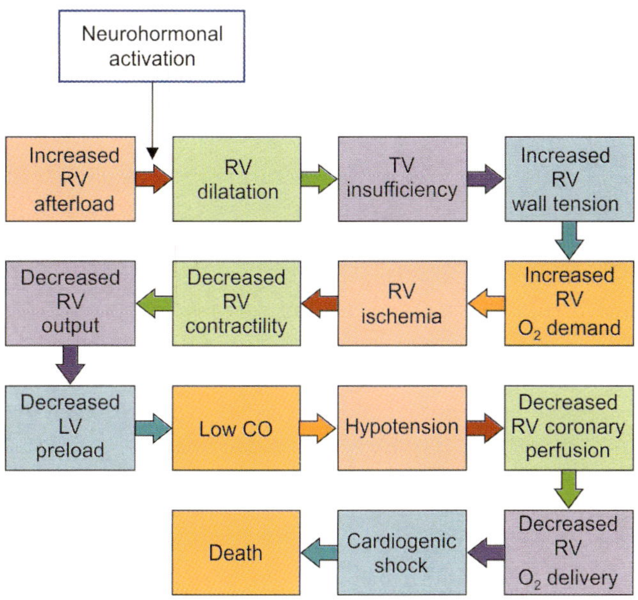

(CO: cardiac output; LV: left ventricle; RV: right ventricle)

Flowchart 2: A simplified version showing pathophysiology of right ventricular dysfunction.

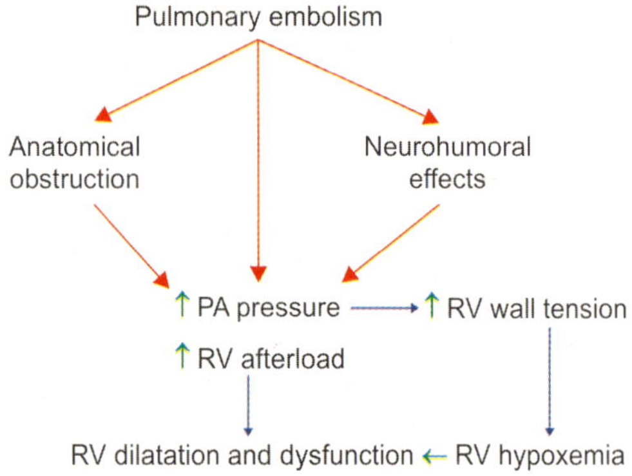

(RV: right ventricle; PA: pulmonary artery)

in PVR, which RV is not able to handle, leads to increased RV overload which in turn is manifests as RV dilatation, hypokinesis, and failure. The dilatation of RV leads to increased RV wall tension leading to increased RV oxygen consumption, further aggravated by tachycardia, resulting in RV ischemia. This in turn leads to decreased RV contractility and output. The coexisting reduced cardiac output and hypoxemia aggravates RV ischemia resulting in RV dysfunction. This dilatation of RV affects the left ventricle (LV) function due to displacement of interventricular septum (IVS) into LV cavity thereby worsening the distensibility of LV and decreases diastolic filling leading to reduced LV preload further reducing cardiac output. This in turn leads to systemic arterial hypotension, cardiogenic shock, cardiac arrest, and ultimately death.[3-5] Most of the echocardiographic findings are based on this pathophysiology and hence remains an important imaging modality in clinical categorization and management of a case of APE.

PREDISPOSING FACTORS

Some of the important risk factors for PE, as shown in Table 1, are divided into strong, moderate, or weak factors based on odds ratio for causing PE. Few of the weak factors deserve emphasis like: air travel which is increasing worldwide and involves prolonged sitting especially in long haul flights, bed rest more than 3 days, pregnancy, presence of varicose veins, etc. These risk factors must to be taken into account during history taking.[5-7] Some of the inherited major thrombotic disorders like protein C and S deficiency, antithrombin 111 deficiency, prothrombin gene mutation 20, 210 (3.7%), factor V Leiden-activated protein C resistance, and dysfibrinogenemia are getting less importance now.

TABLE 1: Various risk factors for pulmonary embolism.

Strong factors (OR > 10)	*Moderate factors (OR 2–9)*	*Weak factors (OR < 2)*
Bone fracture (hip, leg)	Arthorscopic knee surgery	Bed rest > 3 days
Hip or knee replacement	Central venous lines	Immobility due to sitting (e.g. prolonged ear or plane travel)
Major general surgery	Heart or respiratory failure	Increasing age
Major trauma	Hormone replacement and oral contraceptive therapy	Laparoscopic surgery (e.g. cholecystectomy)
Spinal cord injury	Malignancy chemotherapy	Obesity
	Immobility after stroke	Pregnancy (antepartum)
	Pregnancy (peripartum) lactation	Chronic venous insufficiency, varicose veins
	Previous VTE	
	Thrombophilia	

(OR: odds ratio for different predisposing factors; VTE: venous thromboembolism)

SEVERITY OF ACUTE PULMONARY EMBOLISM BASED ON CLINICAL PRESENTATION

The assessment of severity, based on hemodynamic status and RV involvement plays a significant role in prognosis and deciding management. These can be subdivided into the following categories.

Massive Pulmonary Embolism

This is characterized by systolic BP less than 90 mm Hg or requiring inotropic support to maintain BP more than 90 mm Hg together with features of RV involvement and dysfunction or cardiac arrest. It has an in-hospital mortality of about 25–50%.

Submassive Pulmonary Embolism

The patient is hemodynamically stable (BP >90 mm Hg) with evidence of RV dysfunction, tachycardia, tachypnea, elevated biomarkers, etc. The in-hospital mortality varies between 3% and 15%.

Nonmassive Pulmonary Embolism

There is neither systemic hypotension nor RV dysfunction and usually constitute about 95% of cases, with a mortality of less than 3%.[6-8]

DIAGNOSIS

Acute PE poses a fair amount of diagnostic problem as it masquerades many other illnesses, and it can be silent and occur concomitantly with other diseases. Some useful approaches in diagnosis are as follows:

- Having high index of suspicion
- Clinical pretest probability as assessed by modified Wells criteria
- Awareness of predisposing factors which can be present even 4–8 weeks prior to an episode of APE and not in recent past
- Careful evaluation of presenting signs and symptoms
- Other diagnostic techniques.

OTHER DIAGNOSTIC TESTS

These include: (a) plasma D-dimer assay; (b) computed tomography (CT) pulmonary angiography which has good diagnostic sensitivity, specificity, and negative predictive value; (c) ventilation-perfusion (VQ) scan which could be inconclusive in elderly patients; (d) venous Doppler of lower limbs which is mandatory in all cases of APE; and (e) echocardiography.

It may be worthwhile to mention the significance of plasma D-dimer assay which is usually the first test performed in emergency units. D-dimer is a fibrin degradation product (FDP), a small protein fragment present in the blood after a blood clot is degraded. D-dimers are not normally present in human blood plasma, except when the coagulation system has been activated, as in the presence of thrombosis or disseminated intravascular coagulation. D-dimer assays are characterized by having good sensitivity and negative predictive value, but poor specificity because elevated D-dimer may be present in various causes like liver disease, high rheumatoid factor, inflammation, malignancy, trauma, pregnancy, recent surgery as well as advanced age. The causes of false negative D-dimer results are small emboli, pretreatment with anticoagulant therapy and symptoms lasting for more than 10 days. Depending on the clinical probability of APE, it has high sensitivity (96–100%) and negative predictive value (100%), but low specificity (37.5%) and also low positive predictive value.[9] As such it alone cannot confirm or exclude APE. Despite this an absence of elevation usually favors exclusion of APE.

ROLE OF ECHOCARDIOGRAPHY IN ACUTE PULMONARY EMBOLISM

Echo is an important investigative modality due to following reasons:

- It is simple and widely available.
- Bedside modality in critically ill patients which can also assess any other cause of hemodynamic instability and identify a subset of patients who can be benefited by an aggressive therapy in the form of thrombolytics.
- Allows evaluation of RV size and function as involvement of RV, as per pathophysiology of APE, is an important component in APE in about 40–70% of cases.
- Provides immediate result.
- Risk stratification.
- Serial follow-up.

Diagnostic Accuracy of Transthoracic Echo[10-12]

Based on several studies, the sensitivity of TTE has varied between 41% and 51% and specificity between 87% and 91%. Because of the negative predictive value of 40–50%, a negative result does not exclude PE.[10-12] The diminished overall sensitivity of TTE for the diagnosis of PE limits the utility of echocardiography as a screening tool for all patients with this suspected disorder. Still it continues to be an important modality due to reasons mentioned earlier. However, in those with massive PE, echocardiographic evidence of PE may be seen in up to 80% of patients. The specificity is about 80–90%. Transesophageal echo may increase sensitivity. Despite this a combination of echo + electrocardiography (ECG) + D-dimer has a high diagnostic specificity.

Echocardiography has indirect and direct evidences in diagnosis of APE. The indirect evidences have relatively more value in presence of a nidus for APE or high pretest probability of PE.

Indirect Evidences

These evidences can be effectively utilized to give a clue to diagnosis. Some indirect evidences are as follows:

- Unexplained RV and right atrial (RA) enlargement (Fig. 1). This is because of increased RV afterload.
- Right ventricular dysfunction, if present in some cases as assessed by various parameters like RV fractional area shortening (<35%), tricuspid annular plane systolic excursion (<17 mm), tricuspid annular systolic velocity (<10 cm/sec), RV myocardial performance index [>0.40 or >0.55 by Tei index (TDI)] and abnormal RV longitudinal strain (<–20%).
- Dilated inferior vena cava (IVC) with inspiratory collapse.

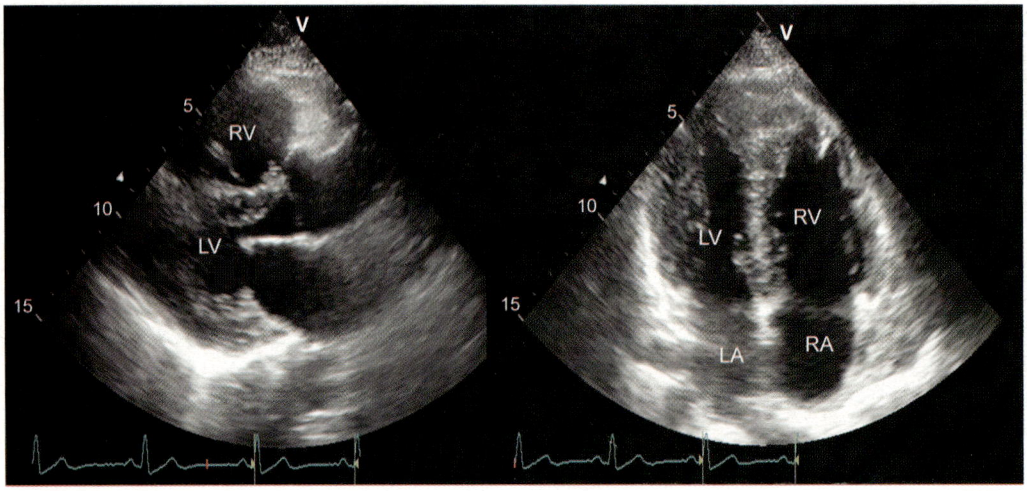

Fig. 1: Unexplained enlargement of right ventricle (RV) and right atrium (RA) and patient also had raised pulmonary artery pressure, hence was provisionally diagnosed as acute pulmonary embolism which was subsequently confirmed by CT pulmonary angiography. (LA: left atrium; LV: left ventricle)

- Pulmonary hypertension with systolic flattening of IVS due to decreased IVS gradient (Fig. 2).
- Dilated IVC with decreased inspiratory collapse due to increased RA pressure consequent to increased RV pressure.

McConnell's Sign

It is defined as a regional contractile dysfunction of RV characterized by hypokinesia or akinesia of mid and basal free wall of RV with preserved or hypercontractility of the apical segments. It is believed to be present in acute massive PE with a large thrombus in main PA or in lobar PA.[13] Its pathophysiology has been studied by various workers based on two-dimensional (2D) speckle tracking.[14-16] It has been postulated that an often hyperdynamic LV that shares the ventricular apex with the right ventricle pulls the hypocontractile RV free wall toward the left in systole in a way that tethers the RV apex and hence it appears to be contracting vigorously. McConnell's sign can be found in any cause of an acute increase in PVR with APE being the most common etiology.

Direct Evidences

These are more diagnostic as they involve direct visualization of thrombus in the venous system including various cardiac chambers. There are basically three subclassifications of right heart thrombi: Type A thrombi are morphologically serpiginous, highly mobile, and associated with DVT and PE. It is hypothesized that these clots embolize from large veins and are captured in-transit within the right heart. Predisposing factors include prominent Eustachian valves, tricuspid regurgitation, low cardiac output, and pulmonary hypertension. Type B thrombi are believed to form in situ in association with underlying cardiac abnormalities. Type C thrombi are rare, share a similar appearance to a myxoma and are highly mobile. As such, a careful evaluation should start from deep veins of leg and gradually followed in a stepwise sequence from IVC (Fig. 3), then proceed sequentially to right atrium (Fig. 4), RV outflow tract (Fig. 5), RV (Fig. 6), PAs usually at the level of bifurcation (Fig. 7), or in one of the branches (Fig. 8). This is usually possible with TTE. In the right atrium, important differential diagnosis includes prominent Eustachian valve, Chiari network, tumors, large vegetations, etc.

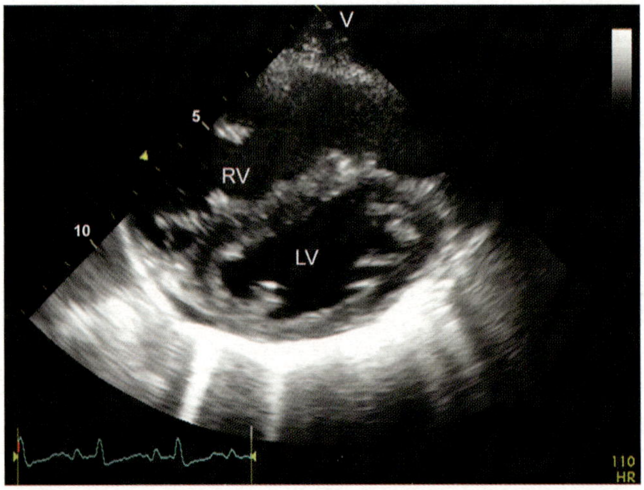

Fig. 2: There is flattening of interventricular septum due to increased pulmonary artery or RV pressure. (LV: left ventricle; RV: right ventricle)

Transesophageal Echo

This is useful in: (a) inaccessible portions of main PA; (b) significant portion of right PA until it branches to the right

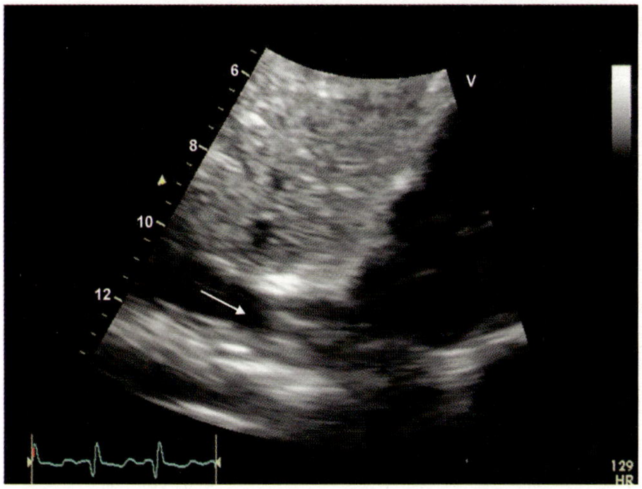

Fig. 3: A thrombus (arrow) seen in inferior vena cava (IVC).

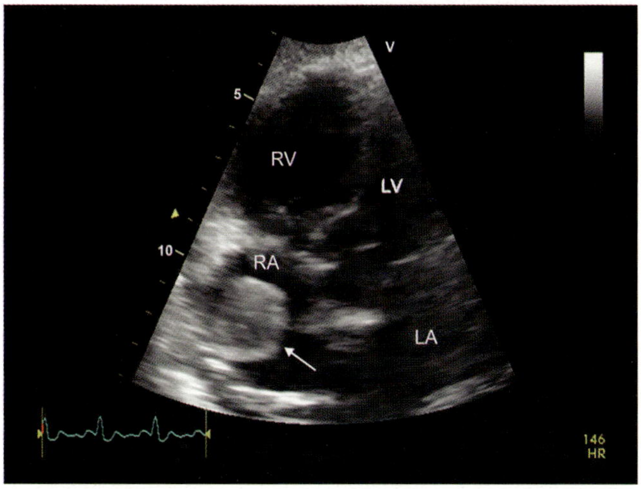

Fig. 4: A large thrombus (arrow) present in right atrium (RA) which led to acute pulmonary embolism leading to shock. (LA: left atrium; LV: left ventricle; RV: right ventricle)

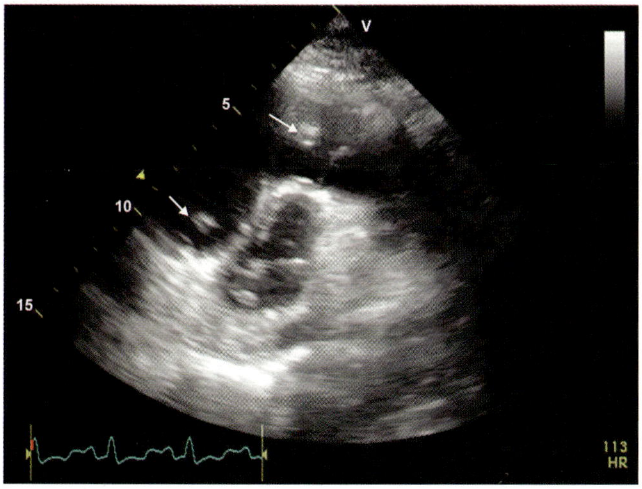

Fig. 5: Clots migrating to right ventricular outflow tract (upper arrow). Systolic flattening of interventricular septum (lower arrow) is also seen.

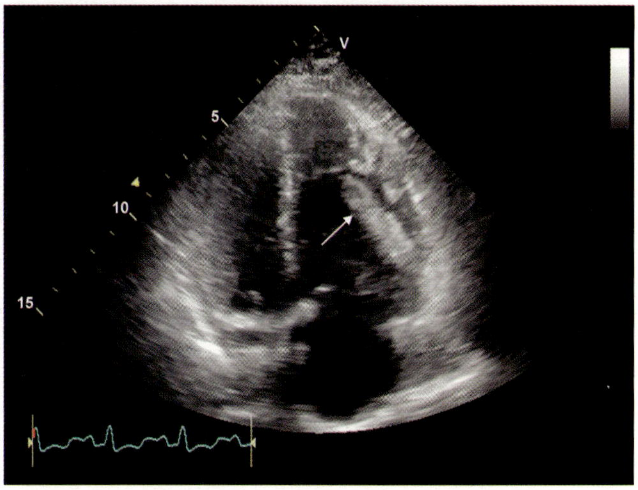

Fig. 6: A large thrombus present in right ventricle (arrow) with enlargement of right ventricle and atrium.

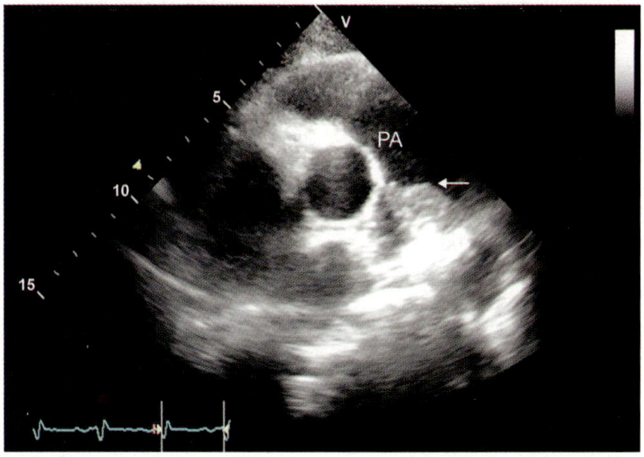

Fig. 7: A case of acute pulmonary embolism with saddle thrombus at bifurcation of pulmonary artery (PA) (arrow).

lobar PA; (c) proximal portion of left PA as interposition of the left main bronchus interferes with the ultrasound beam in the middle portion of the left PA. Therefore, thromboembolism is more difficult to detect in the left PA; and (d) in about 60–70% cases of central emboli (Fig. 9).

From a practical point of view, PE should be excluded in three unexplained situations namely: (1) RV enlargement, (2) RV dysfunction, and (3) pulmonary arterial hypertension.

Role in Prognosis

The presence of RV dilatation and systolic dysfunction has a significant impact on the outcome. Toosi et al.[17] reported their data associated with risk stratification of 159 patients with acute pulmonary thromboembolism (PTE). In their study, moderate-to-severe RV hypokinesis and RV/LV end-diastolic area ratio more than 1.0 were

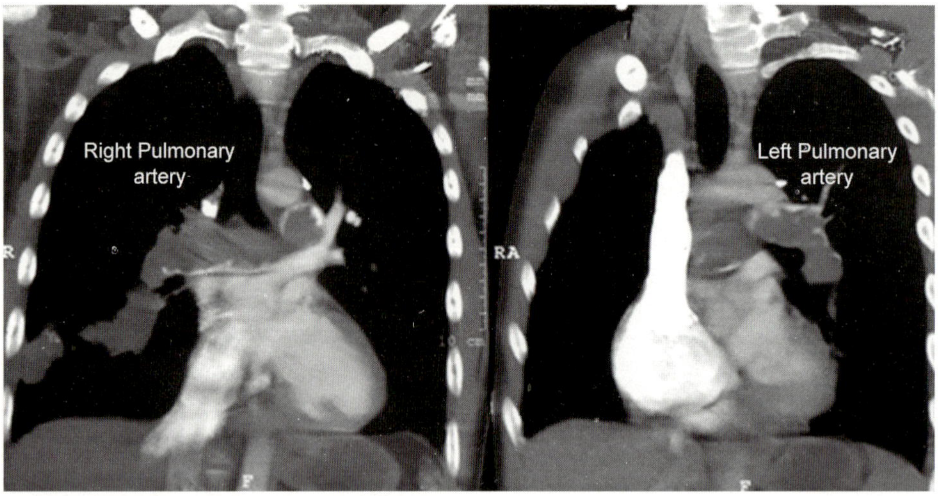

Fig. 8: Contrast-enhanced computed tomography angiography of a patient in Figure 7. The thrombus is more marked in right branch of pulmonary artery.

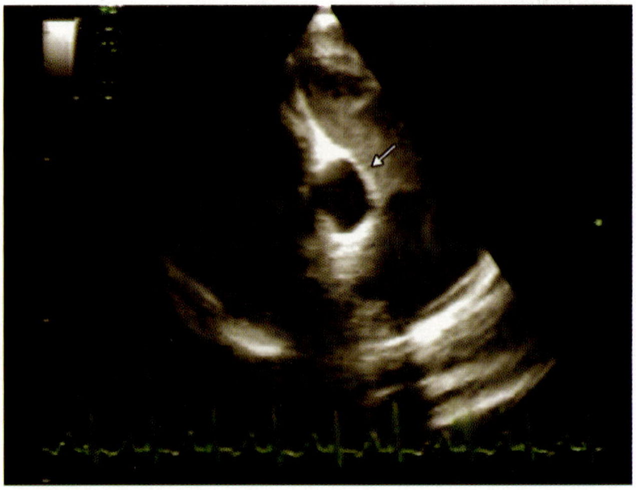

Fig. 9: Transesophageal echo (TEE) in a patient of pulmonary embolism (PE), in which spontaneous contrast echo and thrombus in right pulmonary artery (arrow) could be seen only by TEE.

Source: Courtesy by R Alagesan.

significantly associated with higher in-hospital mortality and demonstrated the best predictive values for short-term outcomes. In another prospective study of 209 consecutive patients diagnosed with an acute PTE without hemodynamic compromise, 65 patients (31%) had echo assessed RV dysfunction.[18] In these patients, the mortality rate was much higher than those patients without RV dysfunction (5% with RV dysfunction vs 1.2% without RV dysfunction). In the International Cooperative Pulmonary Embolism Registry (ICOPER)[19] which included 2,454 consecutive patients with acute PTE, 40% of the patients had RV dysfunction, and 4% had free-floating cardiac thrombi. The overall 90-day mortality was 15.3%. Multiple-regression modeling revealed that RV dysfunction was a strong and significant predictor of death.

Dahhan et al.[20] studied 69 cases of confirmed acute PE of which 14 died over a 30 days period. RV functions were studied in detail by several well-established methods including longitudinal strain of RV free wall, longitudinal strain of RV septum, and global longitudinal RV strain (RVLS). They observed that Tei index, global, and free wall RVLS were significantly different between survivors and nonsurvivors ($p \leq 0.05$). A significant proportion of nonsurvivors had global and free wall LS of more than—12.5, a value which has been demonstrated to be associated with worse outcomes in pulmonary hypertension. Tricuspid annular plane systolic excursion (TAPSE), right ventricular fractional area change (RVFAC), subjective RV dilation, and subjective RV dysfunction were not statistically different between survivors and nonsurvivors ($p > 0.05$). Similarly Vitarelli et al.[21] showed that changes in three-dimensional (3D) RV ejection fraction (EF) and mid-free wall (MFW) RVLS were the most sensitive predictors of adverse events. By multivariate analysis, RV systolic pressure ($p = 0.007$), MFW RVLS ($p = 0.002$), and 3D RVEF ($p = 0.001$) were independently associated with adverse outcomes.

Contrary to the earlier, an interesting study was performed by Khemasuwan et al.[22] on 235 confirmed cases of APE. The primary outcomes of interest were intensive care unit (ICU; death that occurred during the ICU stay), hospital (death that occurred at any point during the hospitalization, including the ICU stay). Besides the analysis of RV strain and strain rate by 2D speckle-tracking, some other measured RV parameters included RV outflow tract diameter and time-velocity integral, RV end-diastolic diameter (EDD; basal, midcavity, and longitudinal), RV end-diastolic wall thickness, RV systolic pressure, RV to LV EDD ratio (RV/LV EDD), RA midcavity diameter, and end-systolic area. TAPSE, IVC collapsibility was assessed. 13% patients died during ICU stay and 18% died during period of hospitalization with median stay of 2.8–11.1 days, respectively. The four simple parameters that measure different aspects of the right ventricle (ratio of RV to left ventricular EDD > 1.0, RV systolic pressure, tricuspid annular plane systolic excursion, and IVC collapsibility) were independently associated with mortality in patients presenting with APE who were admitted to the ICU. There was a lack of prognostic value of McConnell's sign to predict mortality, length of stay, or clinical deterioration. RV strain analysis by speckle-tracking imaging was not correlated with hospital or long-term mortality. As such more studies are needed on the prognostic information about deformation imaging.

Combining echocardiographic data and laboratory tests can give additional prognostic implications. Binder et al.[23] reported their results about the combination of echocardiographic data with either N-terminal (NT)-pro B-type natriuretic peptide (BNP) or cardiac troponin T (cTnT) in the prediction of complicated in-hospital course or death. With a positive echocardiographic results and either NT-pro BNP more than 1,000 pg/mL or cTnT more than 0.04 ng/mL, the risk of severe complication or death was approximately 38%. In another study[24] evaluating the association of RV enlargement, elevated cardiac troponin I (cTnI) and 30-day mortality in patients with acute PTE, the mortality rate for patients with cTnI more than 0.1 ng/mL was 32%, with RV enlargement 28% and for patients with both findings it was 38%.

In summary, some of the adverse echo prognostic signs are: (a) RV dilatation and hypokinesis—RV diameter/LV diameter more than 0.9; (b) interventricular septal flattening and paradoxical leftward septal motion; (c) presence of tricuspid regurgitation and pulmonary hypertension; and (d) RV free wall hypokinesis with apical sparing (McConnell's sign).

Serial Follow-up

Being a noninvasive and bedside technology, echo can be utilized in follow-up of confirmed cases of APE. The success or failure of an individual patient's therapy can be monitored by serial assessment of RV function. Following a reduction in size of embolus, the degree of RV strain will be reduced. After anticoagulation therapy, there will be a reduction in PA pressure, the RV and RA gradually reduce in size and the function of RV improves. Figure 10 shows almost a complete regression of thrombus in RV following therapy that initially had a large RV thrombus (*see* Fig. 6). On the other hand, a patient who had no response in the saddle thrombus following thrombolytic therapy (*see* Fig. 7) and patient remained hemodynamically unstable following re-evaluation by echo, a repeat CT pulmonary angio did not show any resolution. Following pulmonary embolectomy, the emboli was found to be of metastatic etiology. As such, echo can be a guide to the response to therapy.

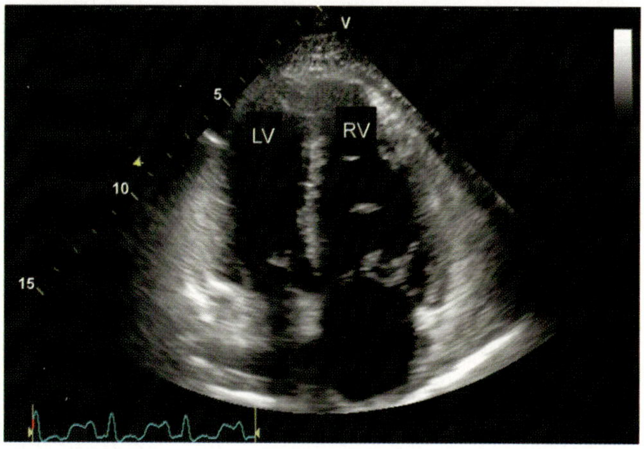

Fig. 10: A follow-up of case of acute pulmonary embolism (APE) (Fig. 6) showing almost complete resolution of RV thrombus following anticoagulation. (LV: left ventricle; RV: right ventricle)

In view of the earlier, despite variable reported sensitivity and specificity of echocardiography in PE, it still remains the first diagnostic tool in these cases. A carefully performed echo, in conjunction with clinical history, gives a useful clue in the diagnosis, as mentioned earlier, in the form of unexplained RV, RA enlargement/RV dysfunction/pulmonary hypertension. A sequential and careful examination from IVC to RA to RV to PA should always be made to see for a thrombus. Once a diagnosis is confirmed, then its prognostic role is well established.

Role in Management

This will be briefly confined to role of echo and not detailed management of APE. There are multiple strategies of treatment of APE namely:

- Anticoagulation.
- Thrombolysis.
- Percutaneous catheter-directed reperfusion techniques or clot retrieval from main PA including novel ultrasound-assisted catheter-directed thrombolysis (UA-CDT).
- Surgical embolectomy as a last resort.

Of these, the first two are more important and of practical significance. Echo plays a role in risk stratification on the basis of which the treatment strategy is based. Though it is mainly clinical, but echo parameters classifying in various categories of severity, as mentioned earlier, are crucial. Majority of the patients are beneficiary of anticoagulation, including newer oral anticoagulants. A combination of hemodynamic stability like persistent hypotension, tachypnea, echo parameters of degree of RV enlargement, RV dysfunction, and pulmonary hypertension demarcate high-risk patients. Based on these parameters of echo severity, thrombolytics, as per meta-analysis of various trials, have been found to reduce mortality in massive

APE with unstable hemodynamics. The early resolution of pulmonary obstruction leads to a prompt reduction in PA pressure and resistance, with a concomitant improvement in RV function. Accelerated regimens administered over 2 hours are preferable to prolonged infusions of first-generation thrombolytic agents over 12–24 hours. In submassive APE, rescue fibrinolysis, is employed if clinical signs of hemodynamic decompensation occur during treatment.

A highly individualized approach encompassing patient selection, type of therapy, operator and hospital level of experience should be followed to maximize the benefits of an interventional strategy as well as minimize the risk of harm. Irrespective of approach one important take home message is to avoid aggressive fluid resuscitation as it may lead to RV overstretch, leading to RV ischemia with worsening of RV failure.

In conclusion, bedside echo is very helpful for evaluation of acutely ill patients in whom diagnosis of APE is doubtful. By determining signs of RV strain and pulmonary arterial hypertension (PAH) it can be of help in these patients. It helps in excluding other causes of hemodynamic instability. It is able to assess which patient is at highest risk for adverse outcome and hence guides in pattern of management.

REFERENCES

1. White RH. The epidemiology of venous thromboembolism. Circulation. 2003;107(23 Suppl 1):I4-8.
2. American College of Emergency Physicians Clinical Policies Committee, Clinical Policies Committee Subcommittee on Suspected Pulmonary Embolism. Clinical policy: critical issues in the evaluation and management of adult patients presenting with suspected pulmonary embolism. Ann Emerg Med. 2003;41(2):257-70.
3. Goldhaber SZ, Elliott CG. Acute pulmonary embolism: part I: epidemiology, pathophysiology, and diagnosis. Circulation. 2003;108(22):2726-9.
4. Stein PD, Woodard PK, Weg JG, et al. Diagnostic pathways in acute pulmonary embolism: recommendations of the PIOPED II investigators. Am J Med. 2006;119(12):1048-55.
5. Writing Group for Christopher Study Investigators. Effectiveness of managing suspected pulmonary embolism using an algorithm combining clinical probability, D-dimer testing, and computer tomography. JAMA. 2006;295(2):172-9.
6. Le Gal G, Righini M, Roy PM, et al. Prediction of pulmonary embolism in the emergency department: the revised Geneva score. Ann Intern Med. 2006;144(3):165-71.
7. Becattini C, Agnelli G. Acute pulmonary embolism: risk stratification in the emergency department. Intern Emerg Med. 2007;2(2):119-29.
8. Torbicki A, Perrier A, Konstantinides S, et al. Guidelines on the diagnosis and management of acute pulmonary embolism of the European Society of Cardiology. Eur Heart J. 2008;29(18):2276-315.
9. Abdel Rahem I Youssi, Mohammed FM Ismail, Reda ElGhamry, et al. Diagnostic accuracy of D-dimer assay in suspected pulmonary embolism patients. Egypt J Chest Dis Tuberc. 2014;63:411-7.
10. Bova C, Greco F, Misuraka G, et al. Diagnostic utility of echocardiography in patients with suspected pulmonary embolism. Am J Emerg Med. 2003;21(3):180-3.
11. Roy PM, Colombet I, Durieux P, et al. Systemic review and meta-analysis of strategies for the diagnosis of pulmonary embolism. BMJ. 2005;331(7511): 259.
12. Konstantinides SV, Torbicki A, Agnelli G, et al. 2014 ESC guidelines on the diagnosis and management of acute pulmonary embolism. Eur Heart J. 2014;35(43):3033-69.
13. Oh SB, Bang SJ, Kim MJ. McConnells sign; a distinctive echocardiographic finding for diagnosing acute pulmonary embolism in emergency department. Crit Ultrasound J. 2015;7(Suppl 1):A20.
14. Mediratta A, Addetia K, Medvedofsky D. Echocardiographic diagnosis of acute pulmonary embolism in patients with McConnell's sign. Echocardiography. 2016;33(5):696-702.
15. López-Candales A, Edelman K, Candales MD. Right ventricular apical contractility in acute pulmonary embolism: the McConnell sign revisited. Echocardiography. 2010;27(6):614-20.
16. Platz E, Hassanein AH, Shah A, et al. Regional right ventricular strain pattern in patients with acute pulmonary embolism. Echocardiography. 2012;29(4):464-70.
17. Toosi MS, Merlino JD, Leeper KV. Prognostic value of the shock index along with transthoracic echocardiography in risk stratification of patients with acute pulmonary embolism. Am J Cardiol. 2008;101(5):700-5.
18. Grifoni S, Olivotto I, Cecchini P, et al. Short-term clinical outcome of patients with acute pulmonary embolism, normal blood pressure, and echocardiographic right ventricular dysfunction. Circulation. 2000;101(24):2817-22.
19. Goldhaber SZ, Visani L, De Rosa M. Acute pulmonary embolism: clinical outcomes in the International Cooperative Pulmonary Embolism Registry (ICOPER). Lancet. 1999;353(9162):1386-9.
20. Dahhan T, Siddiqui I, Tapson VF, et al. Clinical and echocardiographic predictors of mortality in acute pulmonary embolism. Cardiovasc Ultrasound. 2016;14(1):44.
21. Vitarelli A, Barilla F, Capotosto L, et al. Right ventricular function in acute pulmonary embolism: A combined assessment by three-dimensional and speckle-tracking echocardiography. J Am Soc Echocardiogr. 2014;27(3):329-38.
22. Khemasuwan D, Yingchoncharoen T, Klein A, et al. Right ventricular echocardiographic parameters are associated with mortality after acute pulmonary embolism. J Am Soc Echocardiogr. 2015;28(3):355-62.
23. Binder L, Pieske B, Olschewski M, et al. N-terminal pro-brain natriuretic peptide or troponin testing followed by echocardiography for risk stratification of acute pulmonary embolism. Circulation 2005;112(11):1573-9.
24. Scridon T, Scridon C, Skali H, et al. Prognostic significance of troponin elevation and right ventricular enlargement in acute pulmonary embolism. Am J Cardiol. 2005;96(2):303-5.

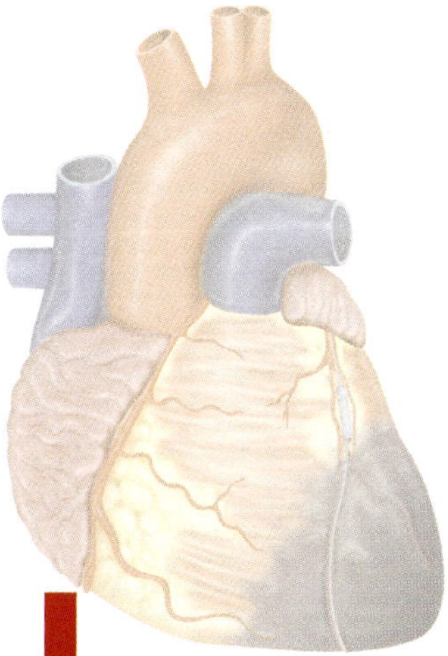

97

CHAPTER

Computed Tomography Angiographic Evaluation in Pulmonary Embolism and Deep Vein Thrombosis

Priya Jagia, Niraj Pandey

INTRODUCTION

Pulmonary embolism (PE) is the third most common acute cardiovascular emergency, after myocardial infarction and stroke.[1] It may lead to acute life-threatening right ventricular dysfunction by causing occlusion of the pulmonary arterial bed. PE and deep vein thrombosis (DVT) are two clinical presentations of venous thromboembolism, with PE being consequent to DVT in most cases. About 50% patients with proximal DVT have an associated PE although usually it is asymptomatic.[2] Conversely, in about 70% patients having PE, DVT is present in the lower limbs.[3,4] Although diagnosing PE is difficult, owing to its nonspecific clinical presentation, establishing the diagnosis accurately and reliably as early as possible and is vital to enable rapid treatment and guide patient management.[5] Pulmonary computed tomography angiography (CTA) has been firmly established as the imaging modality of choice in suspected acute PE.[6,7] Pulmonary CTA, on account of its widespread availability and recent technical advances, has surpassed nuclear scintigraphy to become the investigation of choice.[8,9] Invasive pulmonary angiography for the sole purpose of diagnosis is practically no more used in the acute setup.[10] With the widespread availability of pulmonary CTA, the threshold for ordering this test has lowered significantly resulting in a fall in the rate of positive studies. Ensuring appropriate use depends upon on stringent patient selection. For assessment of the pretest likelihood of PE, a combined approach using clinical signs and symptoms along with laboratory markers should be used.

PATHOPHYSIOLOGY

The key consequences of acute PE are primarily hemodynamic.[11] Massive PE may cause an abrupt increase in pulmonary vascular resistance which the right ventricle (RV) may not be able to overcome. It may result in sudden death or the patient may present with syncope and/or systemic hypotension, which might progress to shock and death due to acute RV failure. Systemic cardiac output is further compromised as a result of bulging of the interventricular septum causing diastolic left ventricle (LV) dysfunction.[12] Smaller and distal embolization does not cause a profound effect on hemodynamics. However, it may result in areas of alveolar pulmonary hemorrhage and infarction, resulting in hemoptysis, pleuritis, and pleural effusion.

DIAGNOSTIC CRITERIA[1]

Both acute and chronic PE are seen as filling defects having a sharp boundary with the intraluminal contrast medium.

Criteria for Diagnosing Acute Pulmonary Embolism

- Completely occluded artery with nonenhancing lumen due to a large thrombus (Fig. 1). It may also be accompanied by enlargement of the involved artery.
- Partial filling defect surrounded by intraluminal contrast (Figs. 2A and B).

- An intraluminal partial filling defect making an acute angle with the wall of the involved artery (Fig. 3).

Associated ancillary findings:
- Peripheral wedge-shaped areas of hyperattenuation or linear bands representing infarcts (Fig. 4). However, they are not specific for PE.
- *Features of right ventricular strain or failure*:
  - Dilated RV (RV diameter more than LV diameter measured on reconstructed short-axis and four chamber images) (Figs. 5A and B).
  - Bowing of the interventricular septum toward the LV.
  - Reflux of contrast into the inferior vena cava.

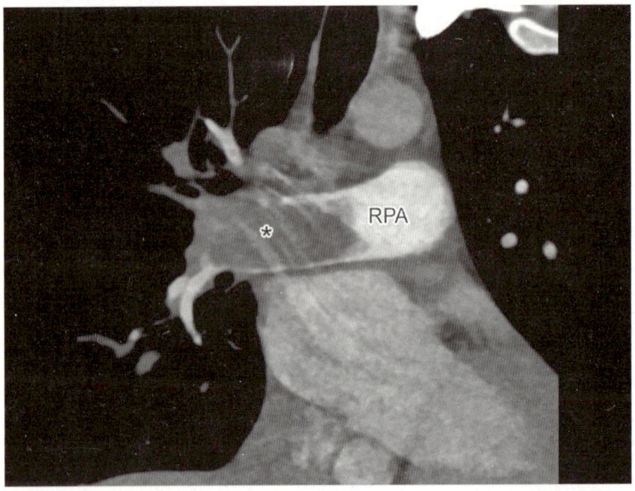

Fig. 1: Coronal oblique reconstruction of computed tomography pulmonary angiogram shows presence of a large nonenhancing filling defect (indicated by*) in the right pulmonary artery (RPA) causing complete occlusion.

Criteria for Diagnosing Chronic Pulmonary Embolism

- Completely occluded artery with nonenhancing lumen that appears to be smaller than adjacent vessels.
- Peripheral, crescent-shaped filling defect making an obtuse angle with the wall of the involved artery (Fig. 6).
- Recanalized arteries appearing as thickened, smaller vessels with intraluminal contrast opacification.
- Webs or membranes within a contrast opacified artery (Fig. 6).

Associated ancillary findings:
- Extensive bronchial or other systemic collateral vessels.
- Mosaic perfusion pattern (Fig. 7).
- Calcification within eccentric vessel thickening.
- Changes secondary to pulmonary arterial hypertension:
  - Enlarged pulmonary artery diameters.
  - Presence of pericardial effusion.

PROGNOSTICATION

Pulmonary CTA has emerged as an impressive prognostic marker to estimate the severity of hemodynamic compromise resulting from acute PE as well identifying high-risk patients for fatal or nonfatal adverse events. Thus it has evolved into an important tool helping guide clinical management.

Various methods classifying the severity and hemodynamic relevance of PE include:[13-15]
- Imaging markers of right ventricular strain or failure.
- Clot burden quantification.
- Lung perfusion measurements.

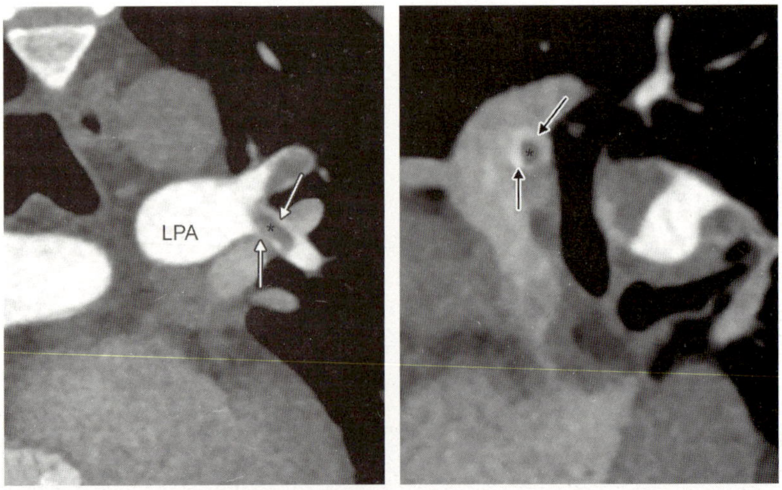

Figs. 2A and B: Computed tomography angiogram reveals partial filling defects (*) in the segmental branches (indicated by arrows) of the left upper lobe branch, with contrast material seen surrounding it, giving rise to (A) "railway track sign" (along the length of involved vessel; and (B) "polo mint" sign (in the cross-section of the vessel).

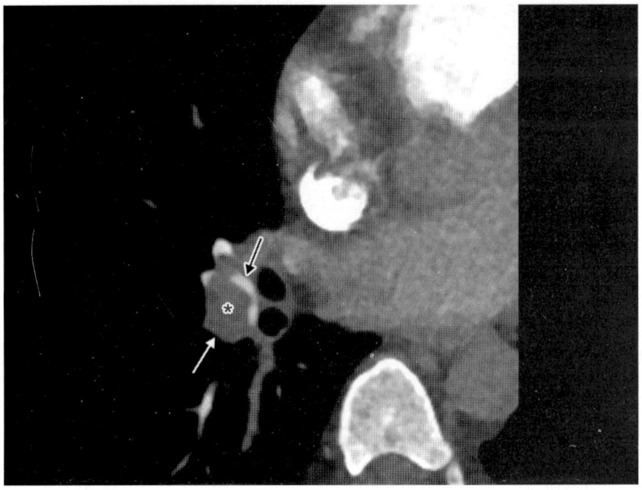

Fig. 3: Axial computed tomography (CT) angiogram image depicts enlarged right descending pulmonary artery (arrows) with an intraluminal partial filling defect (*) forming acute angles with the vessel wall.

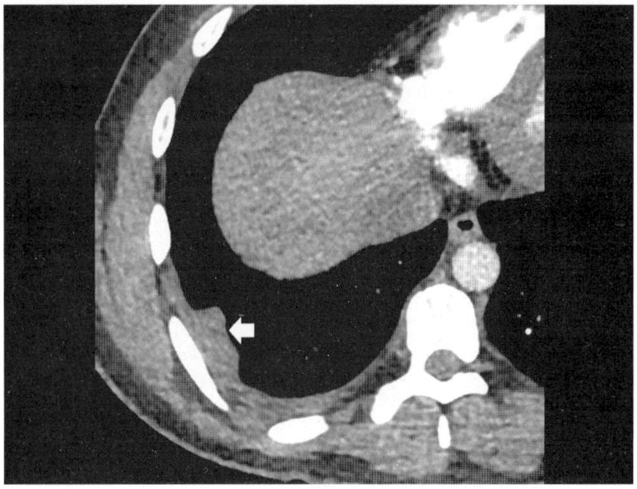

Fig. 4: In the same patient as in Figure 3, axial computed tomography (CT) scan at a lower level reveals a peripheral wedge-shaped infarct in the right lower lobe lateral basal segment.

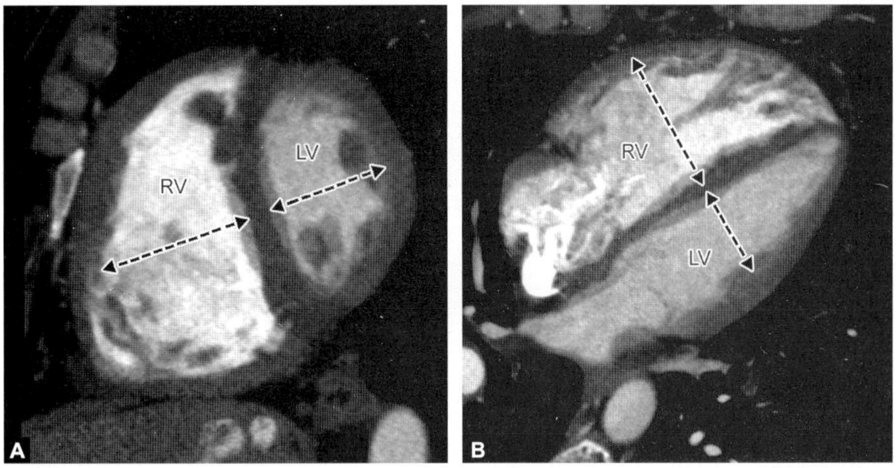

Figs. 5A and B: In a patient with acute pulmonary embolism, reconstructed short-axis (A) and four chamber (B) images shows increased diameter of the right ventricle (RV) than the left ventricle (LV) with straightening of interventricular septum.

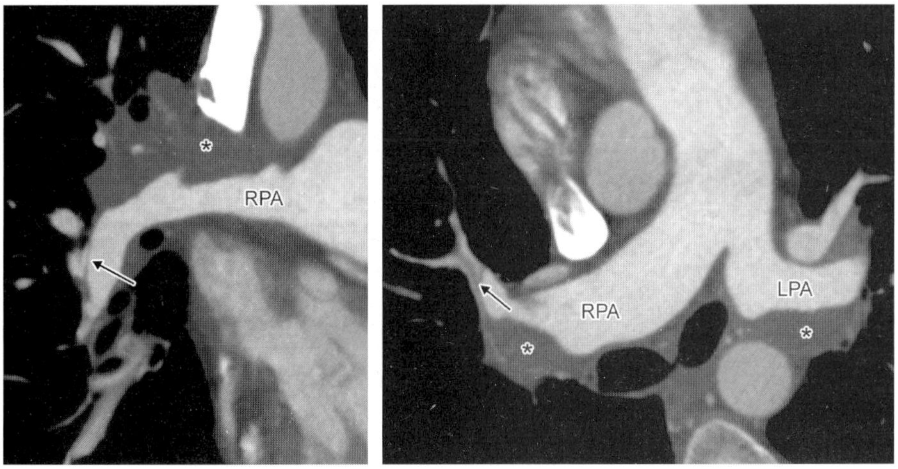

Fig. 6: Computed tomography (CT) pulmonary angiogram images reveal peripheral eccentric thrombus (*) in the right pulmonary artery (RPA) and left pulmonary artery (LPA) forming obtuse angles with the vessel wall.

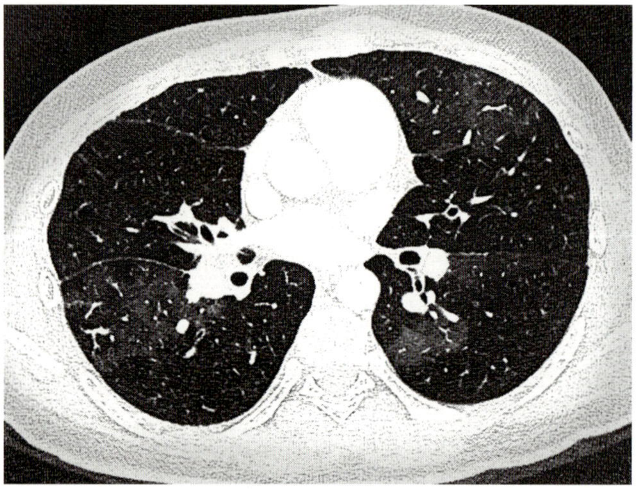

Fig. 7: In the same patient as in Figure 6, axial computed tomography (CT) image (lung window) reveals mosaic attenuation in bilateral lung parenchyma.

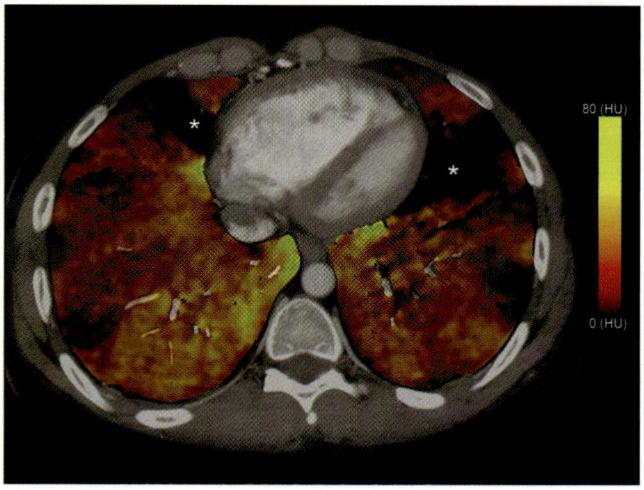

Fig. 8: Dual energy computed tomography (CT) perfusion map reveals perfusion deficits (*) in the right middle lobe and the lingular segment of the left upper lobe.

Imaging Markers of Right Ventricular Strain or Failure

Right and left ventricle (RV/LV) diameter ratio more than 1 on reconstructed short-axis images of a pulmonary CTA has the highest positive predictive value for adverse outcomes and early mortality in patients having acute PE (Fig. 5).[13,16] With advancements in technology, it is now also possible to accurately and reliably calculate the RV/LV volume ratio as well.[17] Some studies have actually demonstrated that this three-dimensional (3D) assessment of ventricular volumes is superior to measurement of ventricular diameters in diagnosing RV dysfunction.[18,19]

Other criteria based on findings on pulmonary CTA which have been proposed as markers of RV dysfunction, but not found to have significant prognostic relevance, include:[20-22]

- Bowing of the interventricular septum toward the LV.
- Pulmonary arterial diameter and aortic diameter ratio.
- Diameters of the coronary sinus, azygos vein and superior vena cava.
- Reflux of contrast into the inferior vena cava.

Clot Burden Quantification

Clot burden scores on pulmonary CTA, estimating the PE severity, have been proposed as predictor of RV dysfunction. Higher clot burden scores show a linear correlation with other pulmonary CTA markers of RV dysfunction. It has been shown that the combination of RV/LV diameter ratio more than 1 and a CT obstruction index more than 40% increases the positive predictive value for 3-month PE-related mortality to 18.8%.[23] However calculating the clot burden (i.e. CT obstruction index), e.g. using Mastora and Qanaldi scores, is cumbersome and hence has not seen much acceptance in routine clinical practice.[24,25]

Lung Perfusion Measurements

Different tissues display varying X-ray absorption characteristics at different X-ray energies. Dual energy CT (DECT) makes use of this property to identify specific materials. Thus, using DECT, an iodine overlay map can be constructed and superimposed on the routine CT images to create a perfusion map. These maps display the iodine-perfused lung tissue, allowing visual assessment of perfusion deficits distal to vessels affected by PE (Fig. 8). DECT perfusion maps may also help in the identification and assessment of nonobstructive emboli.[26]

The perfusion defect score has been shown to have good positive correlation with the RV/LV diameter ratio and a CT obstruction index.[27] With advent of automated reconstruction of perfusion maps and quantification of perfusion parameters, the interobserver variability has decreased as well as immediate reader-independent estimation has been made possible.

COMPUTED TOMOGRAPHY VENOGRAPHY: TO DO OR NOT TO DO?

Pulmonary embolism originates from DVT in a lower limb in about 90% of patients.[28] In a classic study by Hull et al. using venography, it was found that 70% of patients with proven PE had DVT.[29] Lower limb compression venous ultrasonography has largely replaced venography for diagnosing DVT, owing to its high sensitivity and specificity of over 90% and about 95% respectively for proximal DVT.[30,31]

More recently, CT venography has been proposed as an investigation to diagnose DVT in patients with suspected PE undergoing chest CTA as it can be combined into a single procedure using a single contrast injection. Adding CT venography to CTA enhances the sensitivity for diagnosing PE from 83% to 90% and has a similar specificity of about 95%, but shows no clinically significant increase in the negative predictive value.[32,33] Thus it can be inferred that CT venography only marginally increases the detection rate, albeit with the addition of a considerable amount of radiation. This is of particular concern in young patients, especially women. Therefore, compression venous ultrasonography should be used instead of CT venography, whenever indicated. CT venography may also be done for visualization of suspected iliac vein thrombus since they may not be evaluable on Doppler especially in obese patients.

RADIATION AND CONTRAST DOSE REDUCTION STRATEGIES

With increasing application of pulmonary CTA, concurrent efforts have also been made in a direction to reduce the radiation dose incurred by the patient as well the contrast load on the patient's kidneys.

Various dose reduction strategies include the use of anatomy based tube current modulation, low-tube voltage scans, use of adaptive high-pitch scanning, postprocessing of raw CT data using iterative reconstruction and limiting the scan range to the area of interest. Also, use of biphasic, triphasic or other optimized contrast injection protocols has resulted in reduced contrast dose to patients while maintaining optimum contrast opacification.[34-36]

CONCLUSION

Pulmonary CTA is well established as a rapid, accurate, and reliable investigation for diagnosing or excluding PE. For all practical purposes, pulmonary CTA has become the imaging modality of choice in patients suspected of having PE. With ongoing advancements in CT system hardware and software, the radiation dose as well as contrast load has reduced along with incremental improvement in image quality. Ability of pulmonary CTA to stratify risk as well as prognosticate individual cases has further refined its clinical value.

REFERENCES

1. Wittram C, Maher MM, Yoo AJ, et al. CT angiography of pulmonary embolism: diagnostic criteria and causes of misdiagnosis. Radiographics. 2004;24(5):1219-38.
2. Moser KM, Fedullo PF, Littejohn JK, et al. Frequent asymptomatic pulmonary embolism in patients with deep venous thrombosis. JAMA. 1994;271(3):223-5.
3. Dalen JE. Pulmonary embolism: what have we learned since Virchow? Natural history, pathophysiology, and diagnosis. Chest. 2002;122(4):1440-56.
4. Kearon C. Natural history of venous thromboembolism. Circulation. 2003;107(23 Suppl 1):I22-30.
5. Roy PM, Meyer G, Vielle B, et al. Appropriateness of diagnostic management and outcomes of suspected pulmonary embolism. Ann Intern Med. 2006;144(3):157-64.
6. Konstantinides SV, Torbicki A, Agnelli G, et al. Task force for the diagnosis and management of acute pulmonary embolism of the European Society of Cardiology (ESC). 2014 ESC Guidelines on the diagnosis and management of acute pulmonary embolism. Eur Heart J. 2014;35(43):3033-69.
7. Remy-Jardin M, Pistolesi M, Goodman LR, et al. Management of suspected acute pulmonary embolism in the era of CT angiography: a statement from the Fleischner Society. Radiology. 2007;245(2):315-29.
8. Thieme SF, Becker CR, Hacker M, et al. Dual energy CT for the assessment of lung perfusion: correlation to scintigraphy. Eur J Radiol. 2008;68(3):369-74.
9. Henzler T, Barraza JM, Nance JW, et al. CT imaging of acute pulmonary embolism. J Cardiovasc Comput Tomogr. 2011;5(1):3-11.
10. Albrecht MH, Bickford MW, Nance JW Jr, et al. State-of-the-Art Pulmonary CT Angiography for Acute Pulmonary Embolism. AJR Am J Roentgenol. 2017;208(3):495-504.
11. Wood KE. Major pulmonary embolism: review of a pathophysiologic approach to the golden hour of hemodynamically significant pulmonary embolism. Chest. 2002;121(3):877-905.
12. Jardin F, Dubourg O, Bourdarias JP. Echocardiographic pattern of acute cor pulmonale. Chest. 1997;111(1):209-17.
13. Zhang LJ, Lu GM, Meinel FG, et al. Computed tomography of acute pulmonary embolism: state-of-the-art. Eur Radiol. 2015;25(9):2547-57.
14. Meinel FG, Graef A, Bamberg F, et al. Effectiveness of automated quantification of pulmonary perfused blood volume using dual-energy CTPA for the severity assessment of acute pulmonary embolism. Invest Radiol. 2013;48(8):563-9.
15. Meinel FG, Nance JW, Schoepf UJ, et al. Predictive value of computed tomography in acute pulmonary embolism: systematic review and meta-analysis. Am J Med. 2015;128(7):747-59.
16. Schoepf UJ. Right ventricular enlargement on chest computed tomography: a predictor of early death in acute pulmonary embolism. Circulation. 2004;110(20):3276-80.
17. Kang DK, Thilo C, Schoepf UJ, et al. CT signs of right ventricular dysfunction. JACC Cardiovasc Imaging. 2011;4(8):841-9.
18. Henzler T, Krissak R, Reichter M. Volumetric analysis of pulmonary CTA for the assessment of right ventricular dysfunction in patients with acute pulmonary embolism: usefulness for predicting short-term outcome. Acad Radiol. 2010;17(3):309-15.

19. Van der Bijl N, Klok FA, Huisman MW. Measurement of right and left ventricular function by ECG-synchronized CT in patients with acute pulmonary embolism: usefulness for predicting short-term outcome. Chest. 2011;140(4):1008-15.
20. Martins SR. Pulmonary CT angiography in pulmonary embolism: beyond diagnosis. Rev Port Cardiol. 2012;31(11):697-9.
21. Araoz PA, Gotway MB, Trowbridge RL, et al. Helical CT pulmonary angiography predictors of in-hospital morbidity and mortality in patients with acute pulmonary embolism, J Thorac Imaging. 2003;18(4):207-16.
22. Ghuysen A, Ghaye B, Willems V, et al. Computed tomographic pulmonary angiography and prognostic significance in patients with acute pulmonary embolism. Thorax. 2005;60(2):956-61.
23. van der Meer RW, Pattynama PM, van Strijen MJ, et al. Right ventricular dysfunction and pulmonary obstruction index at helical CT: prediction of clinical outcome during 3-month follow-up in patients with acute pulmonary embolism. Radiology. 2005;235(3):798-803.
24. Mastora I, Remy-Jardin M, Masson P, et al. Severity of acute pulmonary embolism: evaluation of a new spiral CT angiographic score in correlation with echocardiographic data. Eur Radiol. 2003;13(1):29-35.
25. Qanadli SD, El Hajjam M, Vieillard-Baron A, et al. New CT index to quantify arterial obstruction in pulmonary embolism: comparison with angiographic index and echocardiography. AJR. 2001;176(6):1415-20.
26. Thieme SF, Johnson TR, Lee C, et al. Dual-energy CT for the assessment of contrast material distribution in the pulmonary parenchyma. AJR. 2009;193(1):144-9.
27. Chae EJ, Seo JB, Jang YM, et al. Dual-energy CT for assessment of the severity of acute pulmonary embolism: pulmonary perfusion defect score compared with CT angiographic obstruction score and right ventricular/left ventricular diameter ratio. AJR. 2010;194(3):604-10.
28. Sevitt S, Gallaher N. Venous thrombosis and pulmonary embolism. A clinico-pathological study in injured and burned patients. Br J Surg. 1961;48(2):475-89.
29. Hull RD, Hirsh J, Carter CJ, et al. Pulmonary angiography, ventilation lung scanning, and venography for clinically suspected pulmonary embolism with abnormal perfusion lung scan. Ann Intern Med. 1983;98(6):891-99.
30. Kearon C, Ginsberg JS, Hirsh J. The role of venous ultrasonography in the diagnosis of suspected deep venous thrombosis and pulmonary embolism. Ann Intern Med. 1998;129(12):1044-9.
31. Perrier A, Bounameaux H. Ultrasonography of leg veins in patients suspected of having pulmonary embolism. Ann Intern Med. 1998;128(3):243-5.
32. Goodman LR, Stein PD, Matta F, et al. CT venography and compression sonography are diagnostically equivalent: data from PIOPED II. AJR Am J Roentgenol. 2007;189(5):1071-6.
33. Stein PD, Fowler SE, Goodman LR, et al. Multidetector computed tomography for acute pulmonary embolism. N Engl J Med. 2006;354(22):2317-27.
34. Mayo J, Thakur Y. Pulmonary CT angiography as first-line imaging for PE: image quality and radiation dose considerations. AJR. 2013;200(3):522-8.
35. Sarma A, Heilbrun ME, Conner KE, et al. Radiation and chest CT scan examinations: what do we know? Chest. 2012;142(3):750-60.
36. Park CH, Lee J, Oh C, et al. The feasibility of sub-millisievert coronary CT angiography with low tube voltage, prospective ECG gating, and a knowledge-based iterative model reconstruction algorithm. Int J Cardiovasc Imaging. 2015;31(Suppl 2):197-203.

SECTION 18

Pulmonary Hypertension

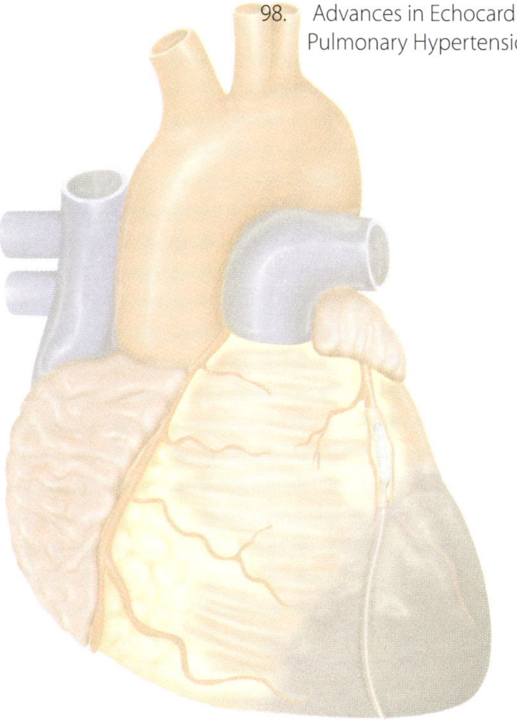

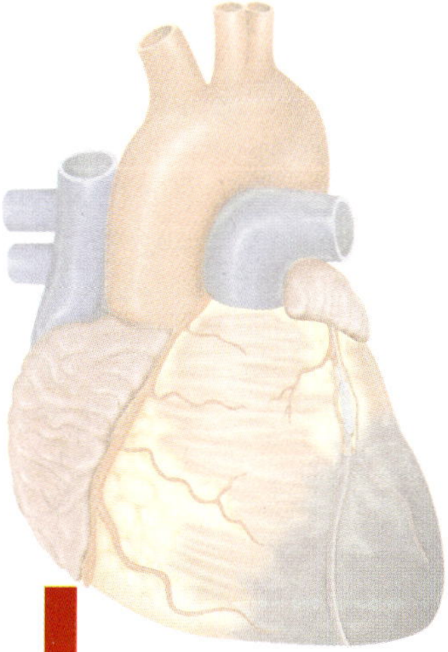

CHAPTER 98

Advances in Echocardiographic Navigation in Pulmonary Hypertension

S Shanmugasundaram, U Ilayaraja, K Rajeswari

INTRODUCTION

Pulmonary hypertension (PH) refers to a hemodynamic situation caused by many conditions, characterized by elevated pulmonary arterial pressures (PAP). Pulmonary circulation is a low pressure low resistance circuit which can accommodate nearly six-fold increase in flow with minimal rise in pressure. Numerous pathological conditions convert it into a high resistance high pressure circuit. Such conditions or diseases that cause PH are categorized into five groups. Group 1: Pulmonary arterial hypertension (PAH) which essentially includes idiopathic PH, heritable PH and PH secondary to congenital heart diseases causing left to right shunt, connective tissue disorders, portal hypertension, human immunodeficiency virus (HIV) infection, etc. The diseases that fit into this group are characterized by the typical histopathological finding of plexiform arteriopathy which involves primarily the small arteries and arterioles. Group 2: It includes left heart diseases (ischemic, myocardial, and valvular) that cause PH. The hemodynamic feature that differentiates this from other groups is the presence of elevated pulmonary artery wedge pressure (PAWP), i.e. more than 15 mm Hg. The disease starts with passive (backward) transmission of elevated left heart filling pressures which may progress to reactive (vasoconstrictive) and then obliterative phases. Because the pulmonary capillary pressures are elevated and the disease processes occur distal to pulmonary capillaries, it also called as postcapillary PH, in contrast to all other varieties that are categorized as precapillary PH. In precapillary PH, PAWP is normal, i.e. less than or equal to 15 mm Hg. Group 3: PH due to lung diseases or hypoxic conditions. Group 4: PH due to chronic thromboembolism involving predominantly the large pulmonary arteries with secondary small vessel arteriopathy. Group 5: Miscellaneous or PH due to undefined mechanisms. Whether due to inherent abnormality in the pulmonary arterial tree or secondary to congenital or acquired conditions in the heart or elsewhere, elevated PAP aggravates the symptoms, decreases the functional capacity and worsens the outlook of the patients, irrespective of management—medical, interventional or surgical. Prognosis is likely to be much worse if right ventricular dysfunction supervenes. PH is a progressive disease with a dismal prognosis, the natural history of which can be modified to a certain extent with PH specific therapies. Early diagnosis and early therapy have been found to offer favorable response and better prognosis. Echocardiography, plays a crucial role in recognition and management of the disease and is often the screening test of choice for patients with suspected PH.

DEFINITION

Pulmonary hypertension, as defined hemodynamically, is a pathophysiological state characterized by elevated mean PAP of more than or equal to 25 mm Hg, at rest when recorded in supine posture. Normally the mean PAP ranges from 9 mm Hg to 18 mm Hg, with a mean value of 14.3 ± 3.3 mm Hg. It is customary to define upper limit of normal as mean value plus 2 standard deviations and thus 20 mm Hg is kept as the upper limit. A value of 21–24 mm Hg is considered as borderline and may carry significance in the presence of certain predisposing conditions like familial occurrence, connective tissue disorders, etc. In other situations, a closer follow-up of such patients with borderline values is all that is needed. In cohort studies it has been found that there is a progressive worsening of prognosis right from a value of mean PAP of 17 mm Hg. PAH is a subset of PH being characterized by mean PAP of more than or equal to 25 mm Hg, pulmonary vascular resistance (PVR) of more than or equal to 3 Wood Units and mean pulmonary capillary wedge pressure of less than or equal to 15 mm Hg. PAH is the hemodynamic abnormality that occurs in group 1, 3, 4, and 5. Group 2 is characterized by elevated PAWP, i.e. more than 15 mm Hg. Previously exercise induced elevation of mean PAP to a value of more than or equal to 30 mm Hg was considered to be a part of definition PH. But exercise-induced elevations of PAP show wide variability among normals and may reach values of 50–55 mm Hg in elderly, athletes and obese individuals.[1] Hence it is no longer considered to be a component for defining PH. However significant exercise induced elevations of PAP in the setting of valvular diseases may be important for decision making for surgery. In familial screening and screening those with connective tissue disorders, there may be a potential advantage of identifying those who develop exercise induced PH. Though not for institution of therapy, this may be useful to select the vulnerable patients who need closer follow-up. An upper limit of 43 mm Hg may be used for exercise pulmonary artery systolic pressure (PASP), at nonextreme workloads.

JUSTIFYING THE PRIME ROLE OF ECHO

Precise diagnosis of PH, thus requires invasive estimation of PA pressures, which is considered as the gold standard. However because of the invasive nature of the investigation which carries some risk to life (though negligible), it is practically difficult to do catheterization for all in whom PH is suspected. Moreover, in the presence of significant elevation of PAP, particularly with significant tricuspid regurgitation (TR), it is often difficult to get an optimal wedge pressure resulting in fallacies. It is also expensive and unsuitable for serial testing. On the contrary, echocardiography is a simple, inexpensive test which can be done at the bedside. Moreover, access to this diagnostic modality is much easier because of the wider availability of echocardiographs and trained personnel. Catheterization is deemed necessary for diagnosing postcapillary PH with confidence and for assessing the vascular reactivity. However almost all the conditions that cause postcapillary PH, like left-sided valvular and myocardial diseases, can be diagnosed with ease by echocardiography. In certain rare diseases like pulmonary capillary hemangiomatosis (PCH) and pulmonary veno-occlusive disease (PVOD), the PAWP may be elevated and catheterization studies may give a clue regarding their presence. Though echocardiography may fail to identify these conditions, other noninvasive investigations like chest X-ray and computed tomography (CT) scan of chest can provide enough findings to suggest their presence. Thus echocardiography is not a mere screening test to identify PH, it provides reliable hemodynamic data, it helps in diagnosing secondary causes like left heart diseases and shunt lesions, it gives vivid information regarding the effect of PH on RV geometry and function and finally it helps to prognosticate. Invasive study may be reserved for research purposes or for assessing vascular reactivity.

ECHOCARDIOGRAPHIC CRITERIA FOR DIAGNOSIS OF PULMONARY HYPERTENSION

Principles Behind

In contrast to invasive studies which use mean PAP for diagnosis, in echocardiography, the diagnosis by echo is based on elevation of predicted PASP. It is because of the ease with which RV systolic pressure (RVSP) can be calculated by echo by using TR jet. By applying Hatley's modification of Bernoulli equation,[2] TR pressure gradient (TRPG) is calculated by using a simple formula: TRPG = ($4 \times TRV^2$); V is the peak velocity of TR in the Doppler spectrum recorded by continuous wave Doppler (CWD; Fig. 1). TR is demonstrable in echo in as many as 80% of normals and in more than 90% of PH patients. TRPG reflects the RV-RA gradient and RVSP is then derived by adding TRPG to RA mean pressure (RAP). RA pressure is dilated due to diastolic dysfunction of RV ± TR. Increased pressure in RA, leads to dilated plethoric inferior vena cava (IVC) and an approximation of RA pressure could be predicted based on its dimension and its variation with respiration. IVC size normally reduces by more than 50% during inspiration or sniff. The reduction of IVC size in inspiration is possibly due to fall in intrathoracic pressure allowing IVC to empty into RA. Additionally the increased intra-abdominal pressure may compress IVC and empty it. RAP is roughly assumed to be 3 mm Hg if IVC is less than 21 mm in size showing more than 50% collapsibility in inspiration or sniff and 15 mm Hg if IVC is more than 21 mm with less than 50% collapsibility. An intermediate value of 8 mm Hg is assigned if the IVC size and percentage of collapsibility do not fit into either of these criteria, i.e. IVC is less than 21 mm with inspiratory collapse being less than 50% or more than 21 mm in size but with more than 50% collapsibility.[3]

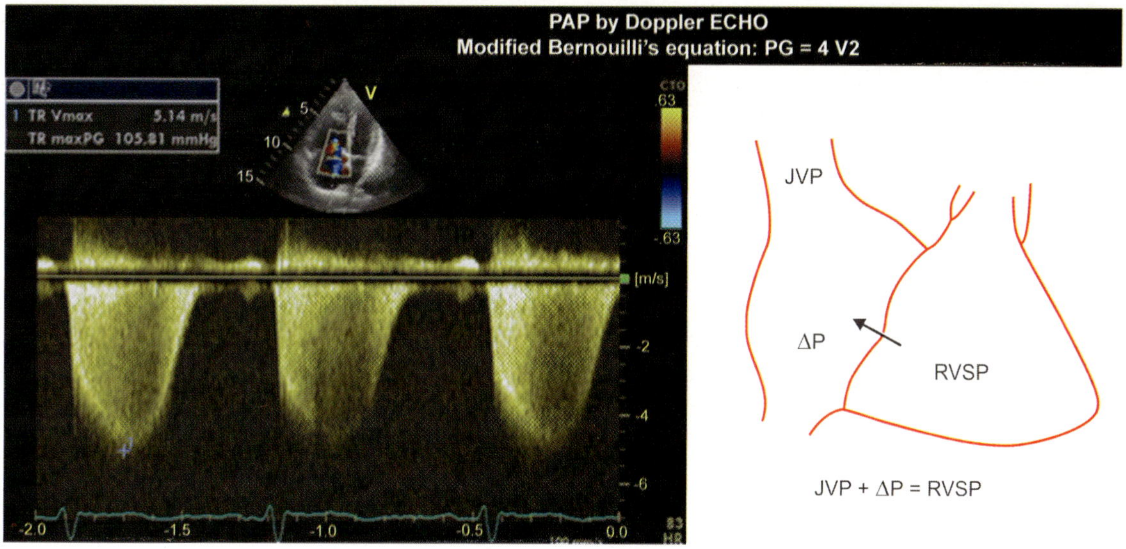

Fig. 1: Measurement of right ventricle-right atrial pressure gradient from tricuspid regurgitation velocity obtained by continuous wave Doppler (JVP: jugular venous pulse; PAP: pulmonary arterial pressures; RVSP: right ventricle systolic pressure).

If secondary indices of elevated RA pressure are present, namely restrictive filling pattern of transtricuspid flow, E/e' of RV lateral wall more than 6 and dominant diastolic flow in hepatic vein Doppler, then the intermediate category may be upgraded into the high-pressure category of 15 mm Hg. IVC is imaged in subcostal view and the dimension is measured at end expiration just proximal to entry of hepatic veins (0.5–3 cm proximal to ostium). An M-mode recording with respirometric tracing is highly desirable (Fig. 2). Once RVSP is calculated by the above method, it is expected to be equal to PASP in the absence of right ventricular outflow tract (RVOT) obstruction (Fig. 3). Ruling out valvular or subvalvular pulmonary stenosis is straight forward by echo. But peripheral pulmonary artery stenosis (PPAS) may be missed out, particularly when the stenoses are present distally, well beyond the bifurcation. A distinct, loud peripherally located delayed systolic murmur should alert the clinician regarding the presence of PPAS. Though this possibility is quite rare, every effort should be taken to rule out RVOT obstructions including PPAS, before high TRPG is attributed to PH. Personally I am aware of a patient who has been diagnosed as idiopathic PAH (IPAH) by many cardiologists right from childhood to early adulthood based on high TRPG and she was even offered lung transplantation by some. Cautioned by the presence of loud widespread murmur over precordium and elsewhere on the chest wall, a CT scan was ordered and diagnosis was established. She underwent serial balloon angioplasty which improved her symptomatic status and the hemodynamics.

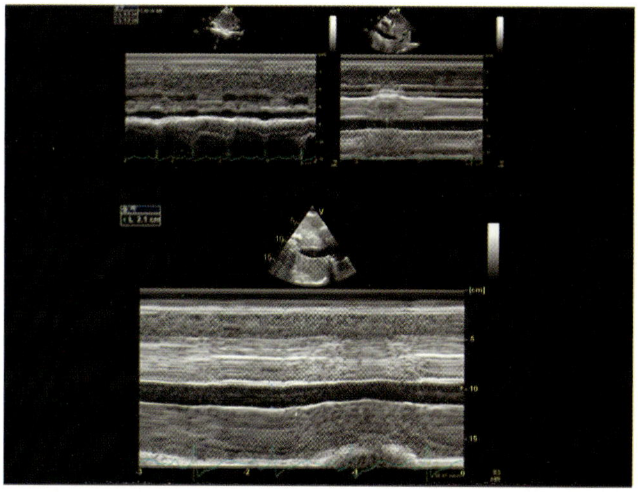

Fig. 2: Predicting right atrial pressure from inferior vena cava (IVC) size and collapsibility (top left): normal size, more than 50% collapse; (top right) intermediate behavior: normal sized IVC with less than 50% collapsibility; bottom: dilated IVC with less than 50% collapsibility.

Pulmonary arterial diastolic pressure (PADP) may be calculated from pulmonary regurgitation (PR) jet using the same principle. PADP = PG between PA and RV in end-diastole + RV end-diastolic pressure (RVEDP) = (4 × PR end-diastolic V^2) + RAP. RAP is used as a surrogate for RVEDP because it has to be equal to RV pressures in diastole. Mean PAP may be calculated from early (peak) diastolic velocity of PR: mean PAP = (4 × PR early diastolic V^2) + RAP.

Invasively recorded right heart pressures are as follows: RA 2–6 mm Hg; RV systolic 15–30 mm Hg, diastolic 2–8 mm Hg; PA systolic 15–30 mm Hg, diastolic 8–15 mm Hg, mean 9–18 mm Hg [mean pressure = systolic + (2 × diastolic)/3]; PAWP 6–2 mm Hg; PVR 67 ± 30 dynes-sec-cm^{-5} (<150 dynes-sec-cm^{-5}).

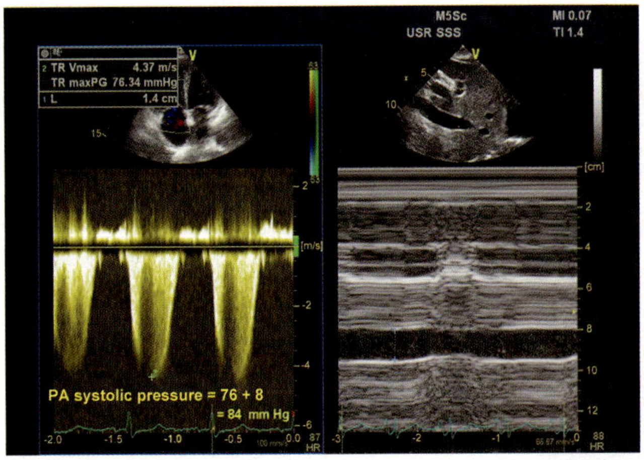

Fig. 3: Calculating right ventricle systolic pressure by adding tricuspid regurgitation pressure gradient (right ventricle-right atrial gradient) to RA pressure obtained from inferior vena cava behavior.

ACCURACY OF ECHO IN PREDICTING PULMONARY ARTERY PRESSURES

Earlier studies have indicated that a modest correlation existed between PASP obtained by invasive studies and by echo. However studies done subsequently revealed a poor correlation between the values obtained by echo and those by right heart catheterization (RHC). For example, in the study done by Fisher, Doppler echo was inaccurate (greater than ± 10 mm Hg) in 48% of cases. The magnitude of underestimation was more than overestimation (–30 ± 16 vs + 19 ± 11 mm Hg).[4] In a study done by Rich, the modest correlation between echo PASP and RHC (r 0.68) improved (r 0.71) when the invasive and echo values were simultaneously obtained. However, despite simultaneous measurements, the bias for Doppler estimates of PASP was 8 mm Hg with 95% limits of agreement ranging from –28.4 mm Hg to +44.4 mm Hg. In a systematic review of 32 studies with 2,604 patients studied by echo and RHC, the correlation was again modest (0.68 ± 0.19).[5] The correlation was much poorer with predominant right heart pathologies, particularly PH due to lung diseases as well as in normals. Somewhat better correlation occurred in PH due to left heart diseases. In the midst of such discouraging reports, a recent study, though a retrospective one, showed better correlation (r 0.80).[6] The correlation between RHC obtained mean PAP and Doppler predicted PASP of more than 38 mm Hg was even better (r 0.82). When the time interval between invasive and noninvasive studies was less than 2 days, the sensitivity and specificity significantly improved (88% and 89%). Similarly in another study by D'Alto, there was reasonably good correlation between echo and RHC derived values: PASP 59 ± 17 mm Hg by echo vs 63 ± 21 mm Hg by RHC; mean PAP 40 ± 10 mm Hg by echo vs 40 ± 12 mm Hg by RHC.[7] Thus in the real world practice, echo estimates of PAP are likely to be accurate with high degree of sensitivity and specificity and it occupies its major position as a primary noninvasive tool to evaluate PH patients. Many clinicians adopt a practical approach of using TR velocity of more than 3 m/s or derived PASP more than 40 mm Hg as indicative of PH.

To avoid over or under diagnosis, the European Society of Cardiology has recommended that other echocardiographic signs of PH should be incorporated into diagnosis instead of relying only on elevated PAP.[8] The echocardiographic features of right heart overload (presumed to be due to PH, in the absence of RVOT obstruction) include RV enlargement, D-shaped left ventricle (LV) with flat ventricular septum, RVOT Doppler exhibiting early peaking ± notching, dilated PA (>25 mm), early diastolic PR velocity more than 2.2 m/s, right atrial enlargement (RA area >18 cm^2) and plethoric IVC. The probability of PH is considered low if TR peak velocity (TRPV) is less than 2.8 m/s and signs of right heart overload are absent. The probability is likely to be intermediate if TRPV is less than 2.8 m/s but signs of right heart overload are present (such is the case in acute pulmonary embolism) or TRPV is 2.9–3.4 m/s without signs of right heart overload. The probability is high if TRPV is more than 3.4 m/s (even in the absence of signs of right heart overload) or when TRPV is 2.9–3.4 m/s with echo features of right heart overload.

POSSIBLE REASONS FOR THE "CLAIMED" INACCURACY OF DOPPLER DERIVED PULMONARY ARTERY SYSTOLIC PRESSURE

Tricuspid regurgitation pressure gradient is mostly measured from A4C view and at times from RV long-axis view with a parallel alignment of CWD cursor with the TR jet. Whenever it is difficult to align CWD cursor with the TR color jet, TRPG may be underestimated. This may happen with eccentrically directed TR jet or marked alteration of right heart geometry, particularly in those with marked RA enlargement. The simplified Bernoulli equation neglects the inertial component of the complete Bernoulli equation which may be another reason for systematic under estimation of RV-RA PG. The severity of TR assessed by color flow measurements need not correlate with the severity of PH. When significant RV remodeling does not occur and when tricuspid annulus does not dilate, TR may be mild or even trivial despite significantly elevated PAP. When the TR jet is small, TR spectral waveform is often incomplete resulting in inaccurate measurements. In such case, saline contrast may help to accentuate the TR signals so as to get a complete envelope. It should also be noted that when contrast artifacts adulterate TR spectrum, possibility of overestimation of TRPG may also happen. As the disease progresses, RV dysfunction may supervene resulting in reduction of RVSP due to its inability to generate high pressures. Moreover in advanced disease with significant TR and markedly elevated RA pressures, RV-RA pressure equalization may occur resulting in lowered TR gradient. In the presence of significant regurgitation, TRPV may show respiratory variation, being lower in inspiration and higher in expiration. In such case, TR velocity is better measured at end expiration. In the presence of atrial fibrillation (AF), at least 10 consecutive cycles should be averaged. Overestimation of RVSP may happen when higher RA pressures are assigned based on IVC behavior. Failure to measure the peak modal velocity (dense rim in TR waveform) and trying to include signals outside the modal velocity is an important reason for overestimation. Trying to extrapolate the peak of TR velocity in the presence of incomplete signals is another common reason for overestimation.

ECHO FOR PREDICTING PULMONARY ARTERY DIASTOLIC AND MEAN PRESSURES

If PR is present, CWD interrogation would offer a characteristic spectral form which is rectangular in shape with less steep deceleration of velocity from early to end-diastole. Since PR is secondary to PH, the velocities tend to be higher. In normals, PR CWD waveform is of lower velocity and rather triangular in configuration with a steep deceleration slope, at times with a notch in late diastole. The notch is caused by RA contraction halting regurgitation momentarily. By applying Bernoulli principle, the gradient between PA and RV in end-diastole can be calculated by 4 × PR end-diastolic V^2. PADP is then obtained by adding PR end-diastolic PG to RV end-diastolic pressure. Mean RA pressure, as obtained from IVC size and respiratory behavior is used as a surrogate for RVEDP PADP = (4 × PR end-diastolic V^2) + mean RAP (Fig. 4). This method may not be valid in the presence of pericardial diseases and in severe PR, wherein rapid equalization of PADP with RVEDP may result in steeper deceleration slope and lower end-diastolic velocities. Mean PAP has been found to correlate with early diastolic (peak) velocity of PR Doppler spectrum. The following formula is used to obtain mean PAP from PR Doppler waveform. PAP mean = (4 × PR early diastolic V^2) + RAP (Fig. 4).[9] Multiple derivation formulae exist for calculating PA mean pressure from other echo variables.[10]

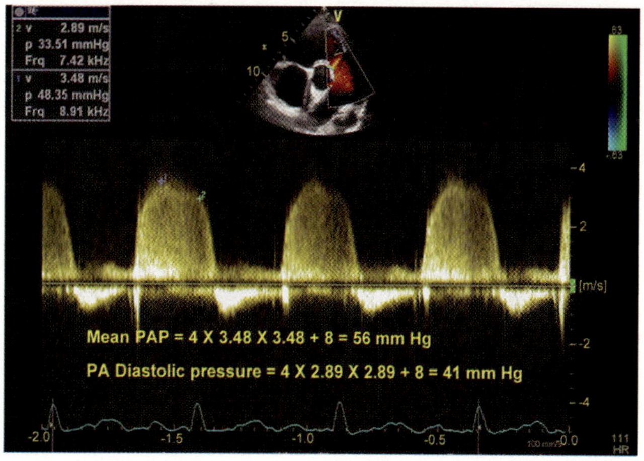

Fig. 4: Obtaining pulmonary artery (PA) diastolic pressure and mean pressure from pulmonary regurgitation (PR) Doppler signals.

From PASP: Mean PAP = 0.61 × PASP + 2 mm Hg.[11] Syyed had used a little different version of a similar formula to derive mean PAP: mPAP = 0.65 (PASP) + 0.55 mm Hg. From pulmonary acceleration time (PAccT): PAccT is the time taken for the forward flow Doppler signals to reach its peak. It is inversely proportional to PA pressure or PVR and hence the RVOT or pulmonary artery Doppler waveform tends to be asymmetrical and triangular with early peaking in PH, while in normals it is dome shaped and symmetrical. Generally PAccT is more than 130 ms in normal and a value of less than 100 ms indicates PH. This physiological fact of early peaking of RVOT flow by Doppler has been used to formulate several equations to calculate PA mean pressure, of which Mahan's equation, i.e. mean PAP = 79 – (0.45 × PAccT) is popular (Fig. 5).[12] Other formulae are: (1) 80 – ½PAccT—this formula performed better than the previous one, particularly in those with AccT of less than 120 ms;[13] (2) 90 – (0.62 × PAccT); mean PAP calculated by using PAccT is valid at heart rate (HR) between 60 and 100. From TR mean velocity: Alternatively mean PAP can be calculated from TR velocity time integral (VTI). Mean PAP = (4 × mean velocity of TR) + RAP (Fig. 6).[14]

If PR jet is not available, PADP can be indirectly obtained from CWD spectral waveform of TR. PADP corresponds to pulmonary valve (PV) opening or in other words the RV-RA PG at the time of PV opening. Hence if the time interval between R wave in electrocardiography (ECG) and the onset of forward flow into PA obtained by pulsed-wave Doppler (PWD) sample volume placed just distal to PV is known and if the HR is stable and similar, TR velocity measured at the same time interval can be used to obtain PADP (Fig. 7). PADP = 4 × TR velocity^2 at the time of PV opening. In the study done by Stephen using this principle, there was excellent correlation between this Doppler value and the value obtained by RHC.[15]

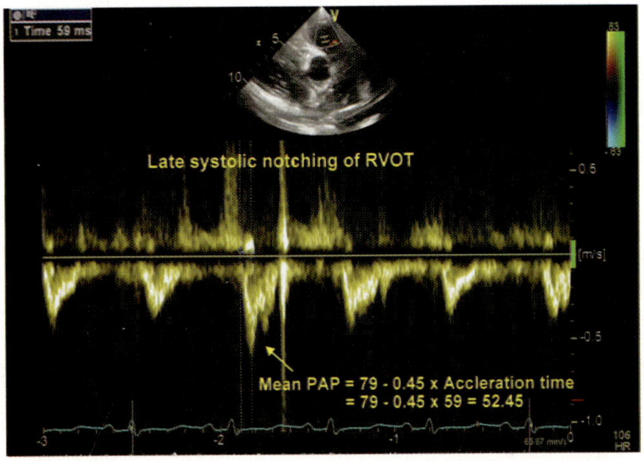

Fig. 5: Derivation of pulmonary artery (PA) mean pressure from right ventricular outflow tract (RVOT) Doppler (Mahan equation).

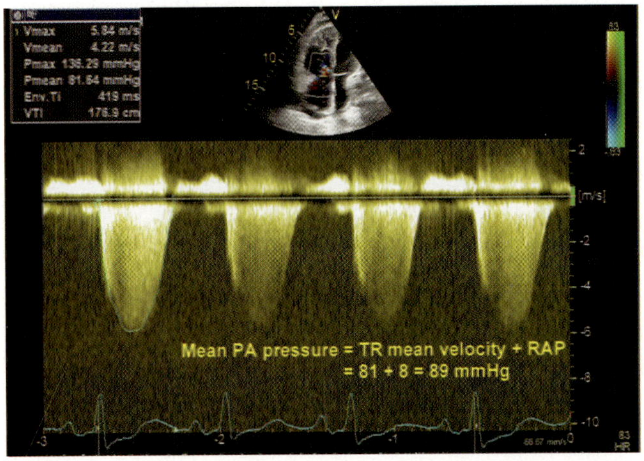

Fig. 6: Derivation of mean pulmonary arterial pressure (PAP) from mean tricuspid regurgitation (TR) velocity (RAP: right atrial pressure).

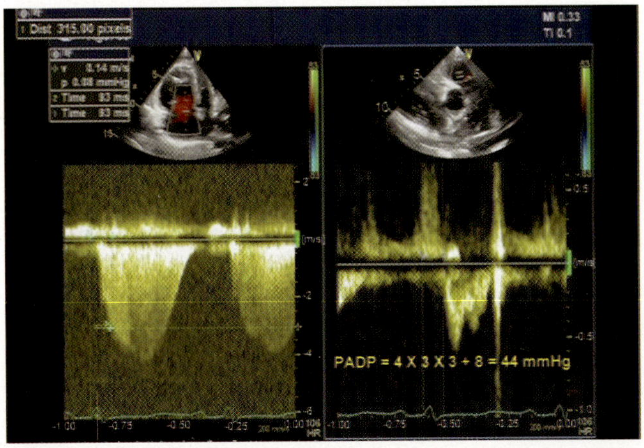

Fig. 7: Pulmonary artery diastolic pressure obtained from tricuspid regurgitation (TR) velocity, being measured at the time of pulmonary valve (PV) opening.

SEVERITY OF DISEASE AND THE ECHO CALCULATED PULMONARY ARTERIAL PRESSURE

Arbitrarily, the severity of PH may be categorized into mild (PASP 40–54 mm Hg), moderate (PASP 55–64 mm Hg) and severe (PASP ≥ 65 mm Hg). Based on mean PAP, a value of 25–35 mm Hg indicates mild PH, 35–45 mm Hg moderate PH and more than 45 mm Hg severe PH. However this hemodynamic classification of severity of disease is applicable to those with preserved RV function, but not in those with RV dysfunction. When RV dysfunction supervenes, PASP may decline in spite of progressively increasing PVR. This phenomenon is somewhat akin to what happens in patients with aortic stenosis with LV dysfunction leading to lower gradients (low-flow, low-gradient aortic stenosis with LV dysfunction). The relationship between PASP, cardiac output and PVR are diagrammatically represented in Figure 8. When RV dysfunction results in lowering of cardiac output, PASP decreases despite progressive increase in PVR. When inotropes like dobutamine were given as infusion for patients with end-stage IPAH with severe refractory RV failure, increase in PASP was witnessed because of increase in cardiac output caused by augmented RV performance.

ADDITIONAL INFORMATION OBTAINED FROM TRICUSPID REGURGITATION SPECTRAL WAVEFORM

Studies have shown that if the time to peak in TR velocity (tPTRV) exceeds 240 ms, RV dysfunction is suggested in

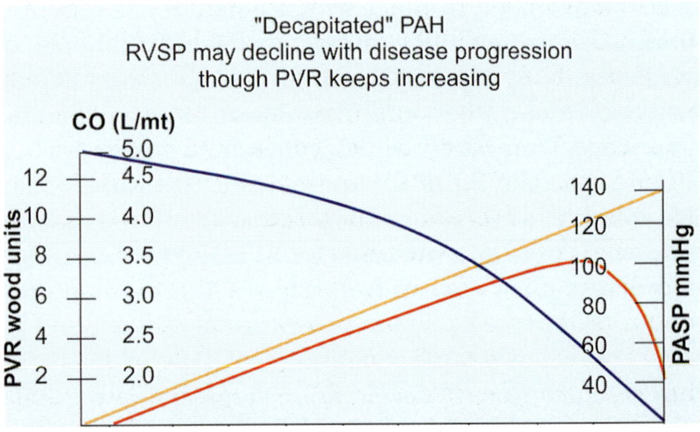

Fig. 8: As the disease progresses, PVR increases (yellow), PA pressure also increases to a certain extent and starts falling (red) with decline in CO (blue), as a result of right ventricular dysfunction (CO: cardiac output; PAH: pulmonary arterial hypertension; PASP: PA systolic pressure; PVR: pulmonary vascular resistance).

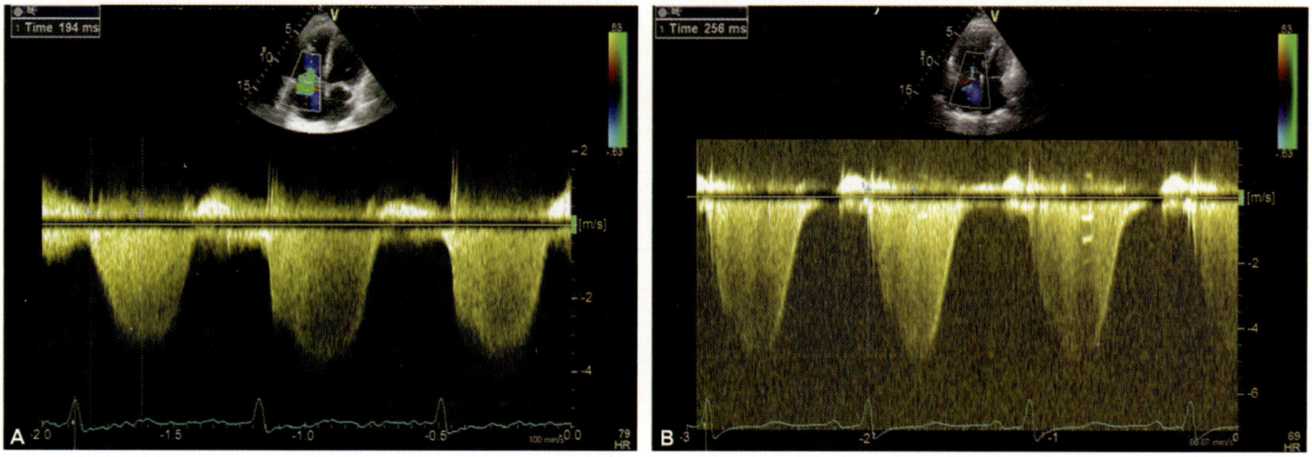

Figs. 9A and B: (A) Tricuspid regurgitation (TR) with earlier peaking implying normal right ventricle (RV) function; (B) TR with late peaking indicating that RV dysfunction is present.

the absence of PH. PH per se may increase tPTRV upto this value. When there is PH with RV dysfunction, the tPTRV approaches 300 ms. In the study of Lopez-Candales, the group with normal RV function with no PH, tPTRV was 163 ± 47 ms, in those with RV dysfunction with no PH it was 282 ± 38 ms, in PH without RV dysfunction it was 243 ± 57 ms and in those with PH and RV dysfunction, the value was 310 ± 30 ms.[16] The velocity waveform may look asymmetrical in such case with a slower descent and a steeper ascent (Figs 9A and B). Another information that can be gathered from the behavior of TR signal is its respiratory variation—if there is distinct decrease of TR velocity in inspiration it signifies severe TR.

ECHO FOR MEASUREMENT OF PULMONARY VASCULAR RESISTANCE

Since PAP is flow dependent, changes in cardiac output with unaltered constant PVR may yield differing PA pressures. In particular, PAP may decrease despite progressive increase in PVR, if flow (cardiac output) decreases thereby leading to an apparent underestimation of the severity of the disease. In such case, deriving PVR from echo variables may help to identify the true severity of the disease. TR velocity shows a positive correlation with PAP and RVOT flow (VTI) shows a negative correlation with PAP. These variables move in opposite directions with progressive increase in PVR—TRV increases and RVOT VTI decreases due to reflected waves from PA abbreviating the RVOT flow. Abbas exploited this physiological fact and formulated a noninvasive method of measuring PVR.[17] PVR (Wood Units) = [(10 × TRPV)/RVOT VTI] + 0.16 (Fig. 10). A value of more than 0.2 suggests increased PVR (>2 WU) and when the ratio is less than 0.2, PVR is likely to be normal. If PVR is normal with increased PA pressures, PH is likely to be due to due to increase in flow, as in anemic and other hyperkinetic situations. Though the ratio shows a linear relationship with PVR, absolute values are unreliable particularly at higher values. In the study done by Dahiya[18] the correlation between PVR by echo using this formula and PVR by RHC was poor beyond 5 WU. Echo was consistently under estimating the values at higher PVR. Alternatively PVR can be calculated by using the conventional formula PVR = (mean PAP – mean (PAWP) LAP)/cardiac output (Figs. 11A to C). Mean PAP is calculated by using the derivation formula 0.61 × PASP. Mean left atrial pressure (LAP) in mm Hg is obtained by using the formula (1.24 × E/e') + 1.9. Cardiac output is calculated by multiplying stroke volume (LVOT area × LVOT VTI) by HR. This formula approximates with invasively obtained PVR. Thus the assessment of PVR gives a true estimate of the severity of disease, may help to differentiate PH due to increase in flow [anemia, obesity, arteriovenous (AV) fistula] from PH caused by increased PVR and may prove to be a better index to assess therapeutic response during follow-up.

DIFFERENTIATING PRECAPILLARY FROM POSTCAPILLARY PULMONARY HYPERTENSION BY ECHO

Diagnosis of Group 2 PH is quite straight forward when elevated PAP is secondary to systolic dysfunction of LV or significant left-sided valvular diseases. However when PH occurs in the setting of heart failure with preserved ejection fraction (HFpEF), diagnosis may at times be difficult. Type II diastolic dysfunction pattern can occur in diseases causing precapillary PH (due to reduced LV filling) and may cause confusion whether diastolic dysfunction of LV could be responsible for elevation of PAP. However in diseases that cause precapillary PH, right heart dominance

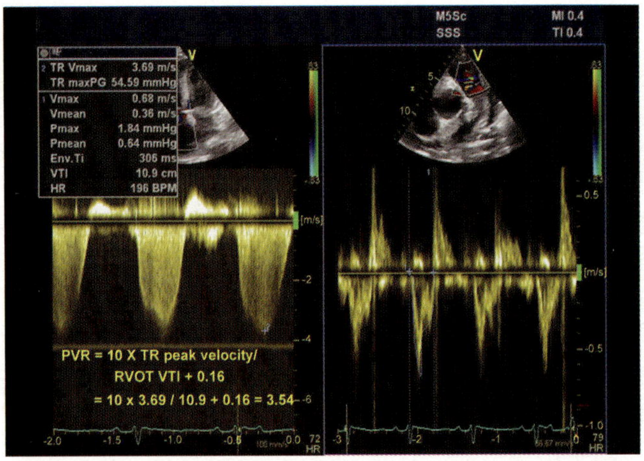

Fig. 10: Calculating pulmonary vascular resistance (PVR) from tricuspid regurgitation (TR) peak velocity and right ventricular outflow tract velocity time interval (RVOT VTI).

will be quite obvious in the form of significant right atrial and right ventricular enlargement with bowing of atrial and ventricular septa toward left, D-shaped LV with eccentricity index being more than 1.2 and RV forming the apex as identified in A4C view. Diastolic dysfunction of LV, when present is not greater than II and E/e' of LV will be less than 10. Moreover notched RVOT Doppler pattern characteristically occurs in precapillary PH particularly with advanced disease, reflecting significant increase in PVR. In contrast, the diseases that cause HFpEF leading to PH are characterized by obvious left heart dominance (enlargement of LA and LV with bowing of atrial septum toward right, presence of LVH, heart apex being formed by LV). The diastolic dysfunction is often Grade III-restrictive pattern. E/e' is abnormal, often exceeding 15 and the global longitudinal strain of LV shows a significant reduction, often less negative than 15% (Fig. 12). Notched RVOT Doppler

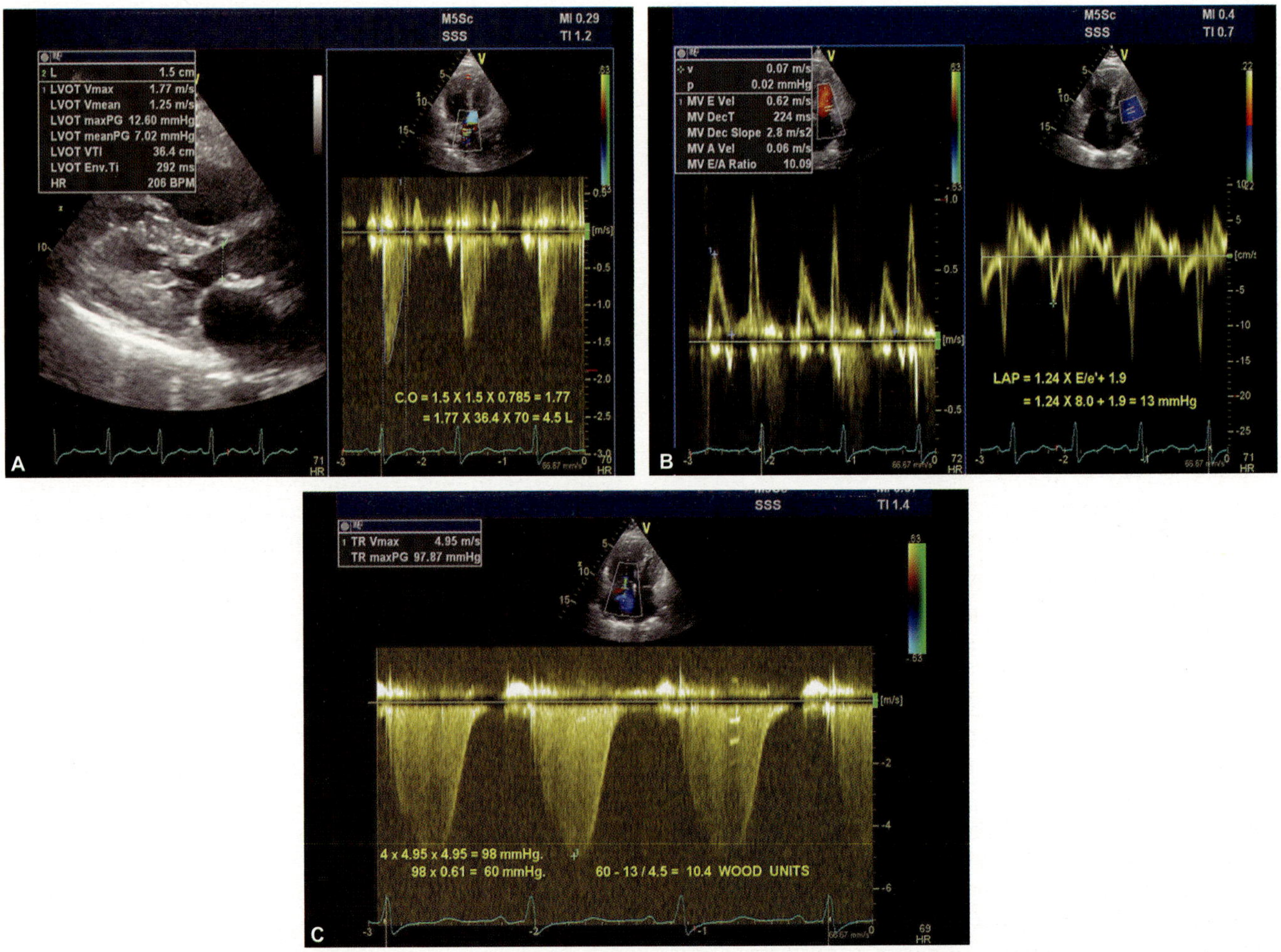

Figs. 11A to C: Steps in calculating pulmonary vascular resistance (PVR) from the formula PVR = (Mean PAP − Mean LAP)/CO; where CO: cardiac output, LAP: left atrial pressure, PAP: pulmonary arterial pressure.

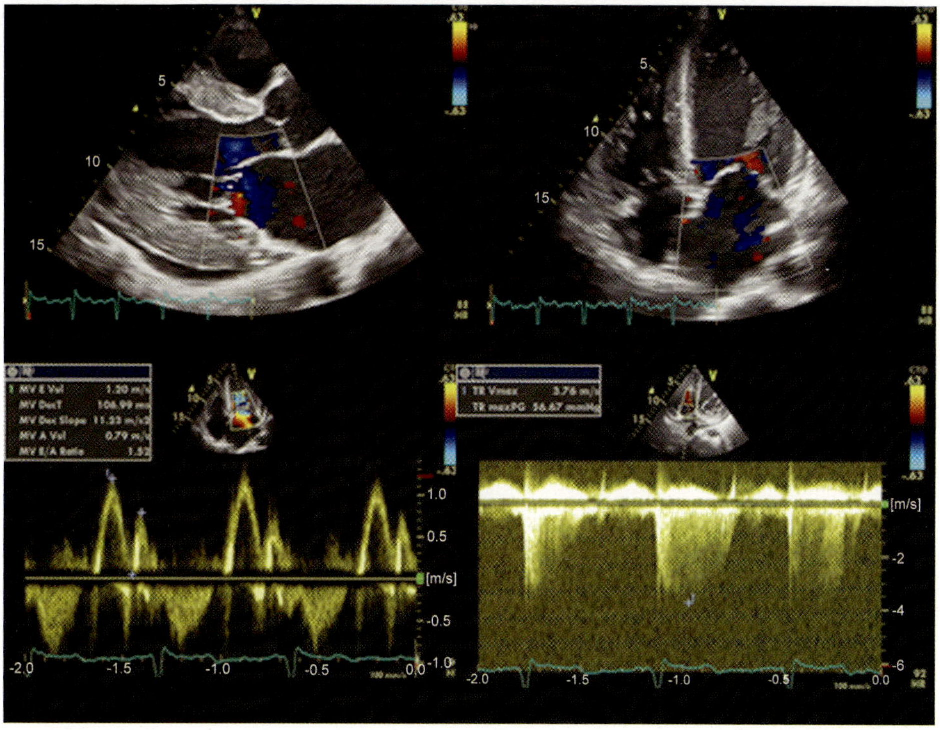

Fig. 12: Severe pulmonary hypertension in a patient with heart failure with preserved ejection fraction. Note the left heat dominance.

pattern is characteristically absent except in few patients with HFpEF with out of proportion PH.

DIAGNOSIS OF SOME SECONDARY CAUSES OF PULMONARY HYPERTENSION

Systolic dysfunction of LV causing type 2 PH, can be diagnosed with confidence by echocardiography. Usually the degree of LV dysfunction is severe, with an EF of less than 30–35%. Type III diastolic dysfunction is almost an invariable accompaniment in such case. Left-sided valve diseases particularly moderate to severe mitral stenosis or aortic stenosis and severe regurgitant lesions like mitral or aortic regurgitation can be identified and quantitated by echo. Isolated partial anomalous pulmonary venous connection is one rare cause of secondary PH, which may be missed by transthoracic echocardiogram (TTE) if an exclusive search is not made. When echo raises the possibility of presence of this condition, additional imaging like cardiovascular magnetic resonance (CMR) would be needed to confirm. children and at times even adults with this condition may be potentially curable by surgery. Diagnosis of shunt lesions, particularly ventricular septal defect (VSD) is simple by echo. Demonstration of a large defect particularly with bidirectional shunting by color Doppler study may establish the diagnosis of VSD and atrial septal defect (ASD) easily. However right to left shunt or balanced shunt across ASD may at times be difficult to diagnose by echo. Saline contrast study, particularly with transesophageal echocardiography (TEE), would be helpful in such situation. In PH with intact atrial septum, the atrial septum particularly the fossa ovalis part may distinctly bow toward left while if ASD is present it may maintain its neutral position. When severe PH occurs in patent ductus arteriosus (PDA), shunting in either direction may not be detectable by routine TTE and additional imaging like contrast CT or CMR would be required. A meticulous search may help to identify a thin nonturbulent right to left shunt from PDA traversing along the lateral wall of main pulmonary artery (MPA) in some patients. Rarely saline contrast echo may identify right to left shunt from PA to descending aorta in parasternal short-axis (PS SAX) or suprasternal window. The other uncommon diseases causing PH like aortopulmonary window, supravalvular mitral ring and cor triatriatum can also be diagnosed by TTE.

ECHO FOR ASSESSING ALTERED RIGHT VENTRICULAR GEOMETRY

Right ventricular hypertrophies (RVH) in response to chronic pressure overload. RVH is diagnosed when RV free-wall thickness measured near the base in subcostal or PS long-axis (LAX) view, is ± 5 mm. A hypertrophied RV could withstand (or generate) high pressures, as high as 100–120 mm Hg. Systolic performance of RV is preserved at least in the beginning, because increase in RV wall thickness reduces the wall stress. But with long-standing RV hypertension, decline in systolic performance may eventually occur due to afterload mismatch in the beginning and due to decline in intrinsic contractility in the later phases. Decline in systolic performance leads to increase in RV end-diastolic and end-systolic volumes with subsequent dilatation of TV annulus (TVA) causing TR. RV cavity becomes more spherical. RV starts forming the heart apex, well identified in A4C view. In SAX view, RV takes the shape of a circle because of the remodeling. The volume overload caused by TR, imposes additional burden on the dysfunctioning ventricle and a vicious cycle sets in. Moreover TR caused by dilated annulus is worsened by tethering of tricuspid leaflets caused by spherical remodeling of RV and lateral displacement of papillary muscles. Measuring TVA, tethering distance and area and the inter papillary distance would provide quantitative parameters of RV remodeling.

Right ventricular enlargement is diagnosed if RV internal minor diameter in systole exceeds 42 mm at the base or 35 mm at mid cavity or when the major dimension (apex to base) exceeds 86 mm. RV/LV ratio (measured roughly 1 cm caudal to annulus) is normally 0.6–0.8. A ratio of 0.8–1 indicates mild enlargement, 1.1–1.4 moderate enlargement and more than PR equal to 1.5 severe RV enlargement. Normally RV apex has a triangular or sickle shape with an acute angle pointing to right or just upward. With RV enlargement, the RV apex becomes more oblong and forms the heart apex with the apical angle pointing to left (Fig. 13). RA dilatation is a feature of PH, that is caused by diastolic dysfunction and TR. RA enlargement is diagnosed when RA area measured in end-systole in A4C view, exceeds 18 cm^2 (Fig. 14) or when the major (vertical) dimension is more than 53 mm or the minor dimension is more than 44 mm. RVOT is considered to be dilated if the proximal diameter exceeds 33 mm (PS LAX view) or the distal diameter (PS SAX view) exceeds 27 mm. Coronary sinus may be dilated due to RA hypertension. IVC plethora is similarly a sign of increased RAP. Pericardial effusion may be noticeable with advanced disease, as increased RA pressure may interfere with the lymphatic drainage of fluid from the cavity.

ECHO FOR EVALUATION OF STRUCTURE AND DYNAMICS OF PULMONARY ARTERIES

Proximal PAs are dilated in the presence of long-standing PH. MPA, the bifurcation and the proximal right and left PAs are better imaged by SAX imaging from high left parasternal window (Fig. 15). A slight clockwise rotation of transducer helps in bringing the bifurcation into a better view. PA dilatation may be diagnosed when the diameter of MPA measured just distal to PV is more than 25 mm or when the ratio of MPA and ascending aorta is more than 1. In CT the upper limit of MPA dimension is larger: 29 mm for men and 27 mm for women.

Normal pulmonary circulation is a low-pressure low-resistance system. Hence, reflection of incident (forward) wave may not occur or may occur in diastole. Because of elevated PVR and reduced compliance of PAs, there is an augmentation and earlier reflection of forward flow. This may be evident by documenting flow reversal in color flow mapping, a swirling red laminar flow may be detected

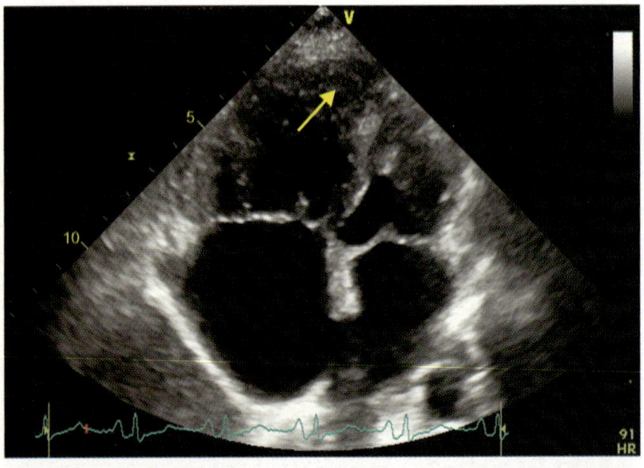

Fig. 13: Altered right ventricle (RV) geometry in pulmonary hypertension. Note the presence of RV enlargement with heart apex being formed by RV. RV apex is wide and directed toward left and RV hypertrophies.

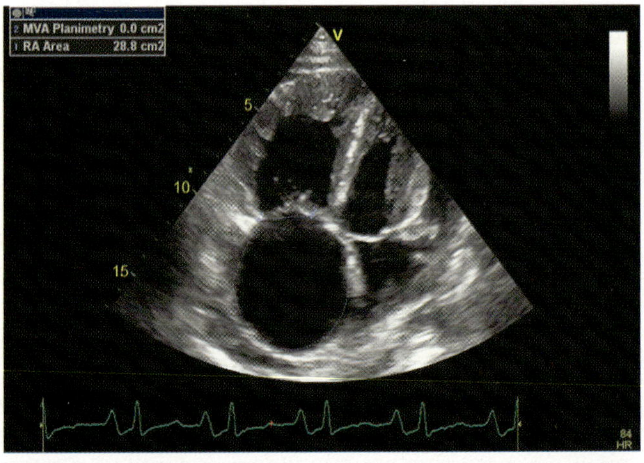

Fig. 14: Marked right atrial (RA) enlargement as quantified by RA area in systole. It is a prognosticator.

inside PA in mid-late systole. The same phenomenon is responsible for notching of Doppler flow signals in PA or RVOT (Fig. 16). The notching mostly suggests elevated PVR, earlier the notch higher will be the vascular impedance. In type 2 PH, RVOT Doppler generally does not show notching, unless there is out of proportion PH as encountered in some minority of patients in Group 2 PH. Three patterns of RVOT Doppler have been described by Arkles; a symmetrical dome shaped waveform that occurred in normals or in those with PH without increase in PVR (3.3 ± 2.4 WU), a triangular waveform with early peaking and late systolic notching which was seen in PAH patients with moderately elevated PVR (5.7 ± 3.1 WU) and a triangular waveform with early peaking and mid-systolic notch which occurred in PAH patients with markedly elevated PVR (9.2 ± 3.5 WU). More than the mere increase in PAP, the presence of elevated PVR, decreased vascular compliance and RV dysfunction seem to contribute to the notched RVOT signals.[19] In a study of chronic thromboembolic PH (CTPH), notching was found to occur early in systole while it occurred in mid-late systole in IPAH. Early reflection of forward flow due to predominant proximal pathology in CTPH may be the underlying mechanism for early occurring notch (Fig. 17). Later studies, however fail to confirm this finding. Moreover, in practice considerable overlap tends to occur between the two categories so that in an individual patient it is difficult to precisely differentiate between CTPH and IPAH based on RVOT Doppler waveform. In CTPH, pulse pressure is expected to be higher (somewhat similar to the wide pulse pressure of isolated systolic hypertension) and the ratio of pulse pressure and mean pressure called as fractional pressure is higher in CTPH. In the study done by Nakayama, fractional pressure was 0.94 ± 0.25 in IPAH and 1.65 ± 0.30 in CTPH. A cut-off value of 1.35 predicted CTPH with a sensitivity of 95% and specificity of 100%.[20] M-mode recording of PV may show distinct signs of PH—reduced or absent "a", steep "bc" segment (descending limb in early systole), flat "ef" segment and most importantly mid-systolic (cd segment) notching (Fig. 18).

The presence of an organized thrombotic fibrous material at the bifurcation or in proximal right pulmonary arteries/left pulmonary arteries (RPA/LPA) may suggest CTPH (Fig. 19). It should be noted that secondary thrombi may occur due to sluggish flow in other types of PH also. Ventilation/perfusion (V/Q) lung scan may help to differentiate between these two situations—larger perfusion defects are conspicuous by absence if thrombi are secondary to reduced flow. When PAs are imaged, a meticulous search should be done to identify a diastolic flow from descending aorta to PA (thin laminar jet along the lateral wall of PA) which will confirm the presence of PDA as the cause of PH. Unilateral absence of RPA or LPA

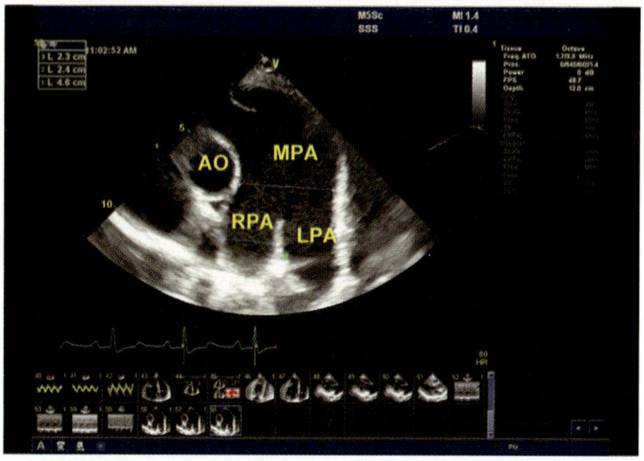

Fig. 15: Markedly dilated proximal pulmonary arteries as seen in parasternal short axis view.

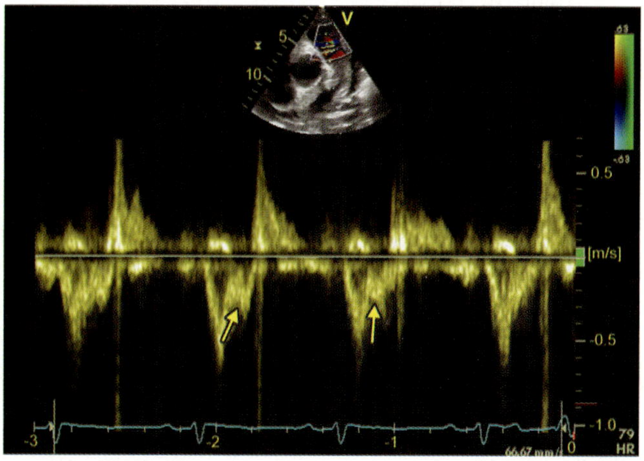

Fig. 16: Characteristic notching of right ventricular outflow tract (RVOT) Doppler signifying elevated pulmonary vascular resistance (PVR).

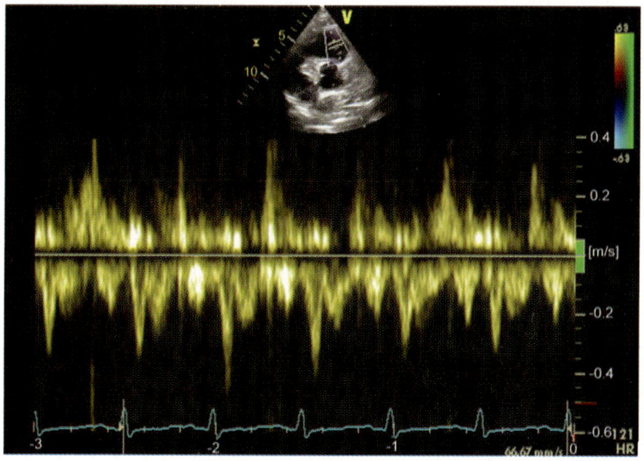

Fig. 17: Early notching of right ventricular outflow tract (RVOT) Doppler in a patient with chronic thromboembolic pulmonary hypertension.

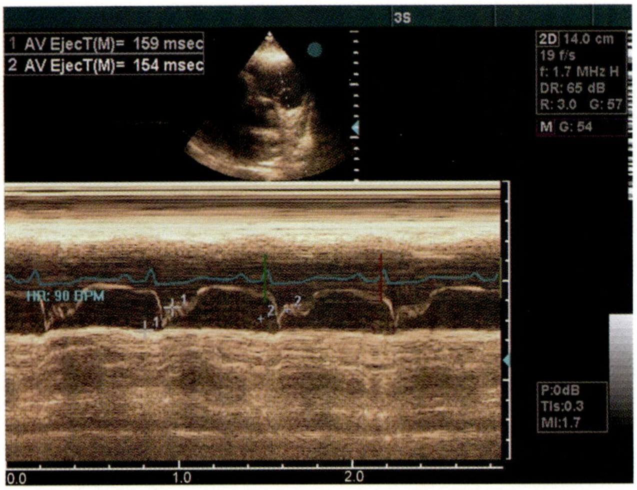

Fig. 18: Typical m-Mode signs of pulmonary hypertension. Note flat EF slope, small "a" and mid-systolic notch.

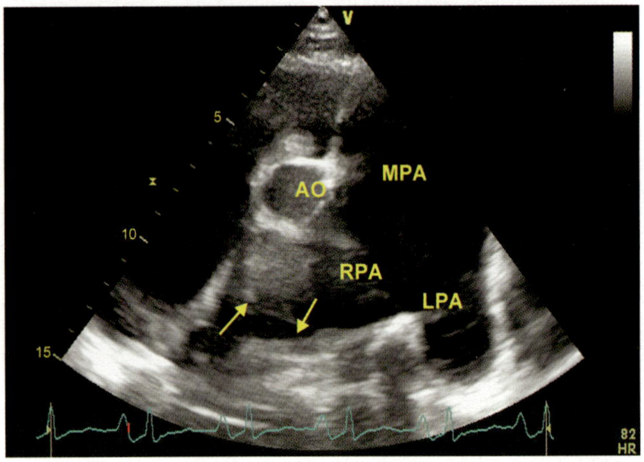

Fig. 19: Organized thrombi in right pulmonary artery in a patient with chronic thromboembolic pulmonary hypertension.

is another secondary cause of PH which can be diagnosed by careful PA imaging—this condition generally manifests in pediatric age, but rarely in adults as well. As mentioned in the previous section, aortopulmonary window, a cause of pediatric PH, may also be diagnosed by PA imaging.

ECHO FOR DETECTION OF RIGHT VENTRICULAR DYSFUNCTION

Right ventricle is a thin-walled structure with a trapezoidal external appearance and a crescentic cross sectional shape. With this anatomy, bellows type of contraction (RV free-wall moving toward the ventricular septum like a bellow) with a peristaltic pattern (from base to apex and then RVOT) makes RV well-suited for handling volume overload. But RV may poorly tolerate pressure overload and may fail quickly with a rapid rise in PA pressures as it happens in acute pulmonary

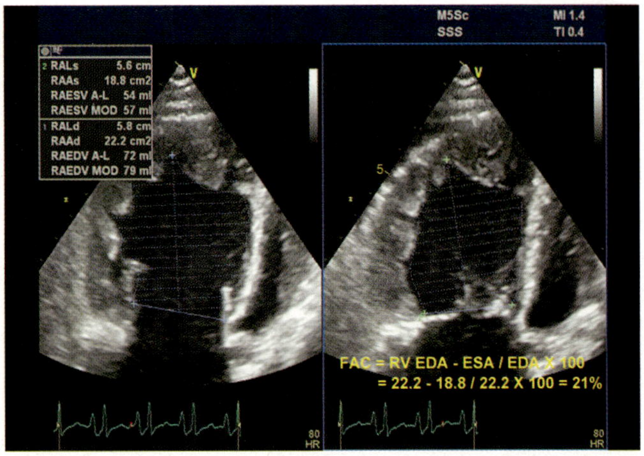

Fig. 20: Right ventricle (RV) area fractional shortening as an indicator of RV dysfunction (EDA; end-diastolic area; ESA: end-systolic area; FAC: fractional area change).

embolism. But in PH, gradually increasing PVR and PAP over a period of time allows adequate compensatory hypertrophy to occur so as to withstand the elevated pressures. But this compensatory phase does not last long and RV starts failing subsequently.

The occurrence of RV dysfunction is identified by reduction of RV fractional area change (RVFAC) from the conventional A4C or RV focused A4C view (Fig. 20). RVFAC = (RV end-diastolic area – RV end-systolic area/RV end-diastolic area) × 100. A value of less than 35% indicates RV dysfunction. When the cavity endocardium is traced, trabeculations should not be included and at the base it should be traced straight from medial to lateral annulus and not along the tricuspid leaflets. Volume calculations from two-dimensional (2-D) yield unreliable estimates because of complex shape of RV. Three-dimensional (3-D) echo, however can provide reliable estimates of end-diastolic volume (EDV), end-systolic volume (ESV), and EF. The disk summation and apical rotational methods using more than or equal to 8 equiangular planes are commonly used in 3D echo study of RV. The volumes obtained by 3-D echo correlate well with those derived from CMR. The upper limit of RV EDV is 89 mL/m^2 and RVESV is 45 mL/m^2 with indexed volumes being 10–15% lower in women than in men.[21] The lower limit of RVEF is 44% by this technique.

Right ventricle dP/dt, the rate of rise of pressure in RV during isovolumic contraction phase is validated in invasive studies as an index of RV contractility or systolic function. RV dP/dt may be noninvasively calculated from the proximal limb of TR CWD signal.[22] The time required for the TR jet to increase from 1 m/s to 2 m/s is calculated. Using Bernoulli equation this represents a 12 mm Hg rise in RV pressure. The dP/dt is then calculated by dividing 12 mm Hg by the time in seconds taken for the TR to increase from 1 m/s to 2 m/s (Fig. 21). Alternatively the time taken for the TR velocity to increase from 0.5 m/s to 2 m/s can be used with 15 mm Hg as numerator. A value of less than 400 mm Hg/s is considered as abnormal.

Tei index (TEI) or myocardial performance index (MPI) is a global estimate of both systolic and diastolic function. It is the ratio of total isovolumic time divided by ejection time: [isovolumic relaxation time (IVRT) + isovolumic contraction time (IVCT)/RV ejection time (RVET). It may be obtained by two methods, the PWD method and tissue Doppler imaging (TDI) method. In pulsed Doppler method, RVET is measured from the PWD recording of RVOT (assigned A). The tricuspid closure to opening time (assigned B) is calculated either from PWD recording of transtricuspid flow (end of A to beginning of E) or continuous-wave Doppler (CWD) recording of TR (onset to termination). TEI index = (B – A)/A. Since these two traces are obtained from different views, one should confirm that the tracings are obtained at identical HR. RV MPI may be much more easily calculated from TDI obtained from RV free-wall. IVCT and IVRT are directly calculated in the same cardiac cycle. IVCT is the time interval from end of A' to beginning of S' of next cycle. IVRT is the time interval from the end of S' to beginning of E'. ET is the time interval between the beginning and end of S' (Fig. 22). A value of more than 0.40 by PWD method and more than 0.55 by TDI method is indicative of RV dysfunction. RV MPI has prognostic significance in patients with PH.[23] It is invalid in the presence of very high RA pressures and in AF.

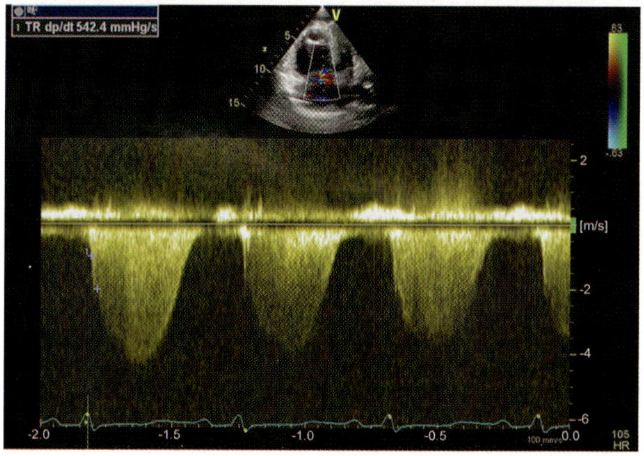

Fig. 21: Right ventricle (RV) dP/dt calculated from tricuspid regurgitation (TR) velocity.

A much more simpler method of assessing the long-axis function of RV is to measure the tricuspid annulus plane systolic excursion (TAPSE) otherwise called tricuspid annulus motion (TAM) (Fig. 23). It is obtained by M-mode recording of lateral tricuspid annulus from A4C window. TAPSE has been found to correlate with RV systolic function measured by other techniques. A value of less than 17 mm is a very specific but not very sensitive measure of RV dysfunction.[24] Angle dependency and load dependency are the disadvantages of this method.

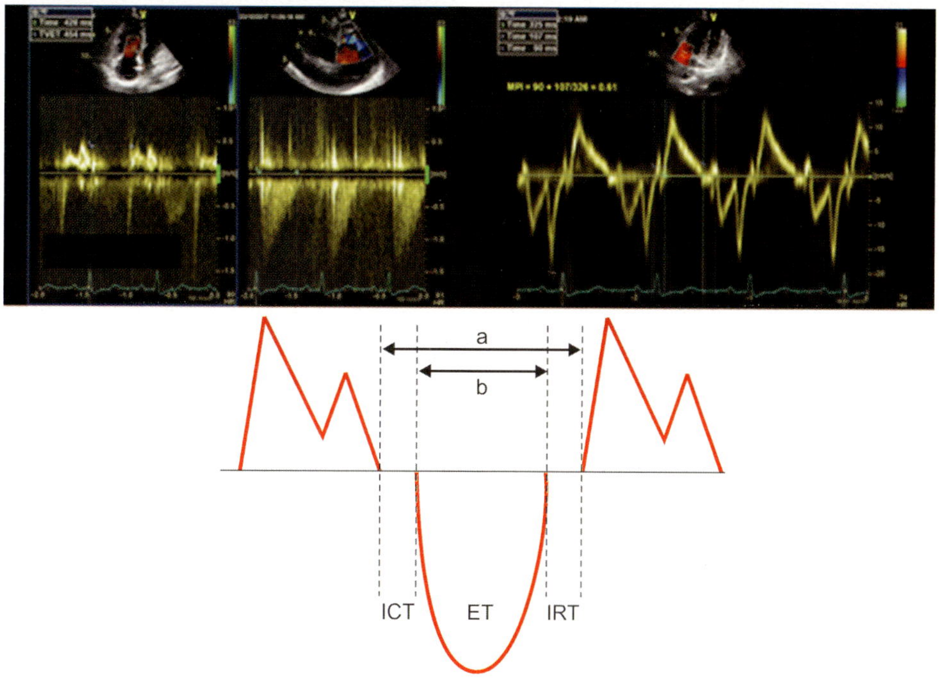

Fig. 22: Right ventricle (RV) myocardial performance index by pulsed-wave Doppler (PWD) and tissue Doppler imaging (TDI) methods.

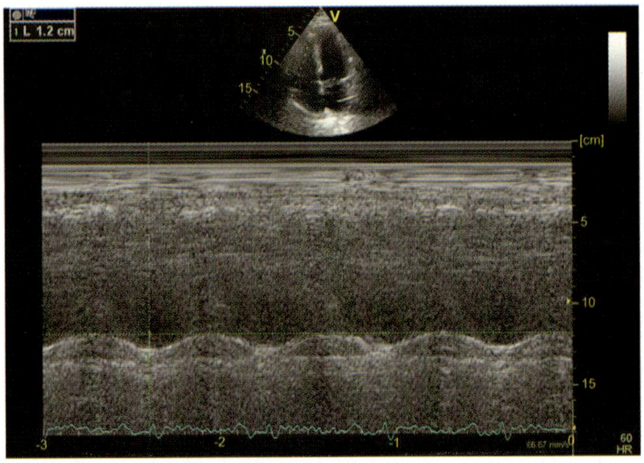

Fig. 23: Right ventricle long-axis function assessed by tricuspid annulus plane systolic excursion (TAPSE).

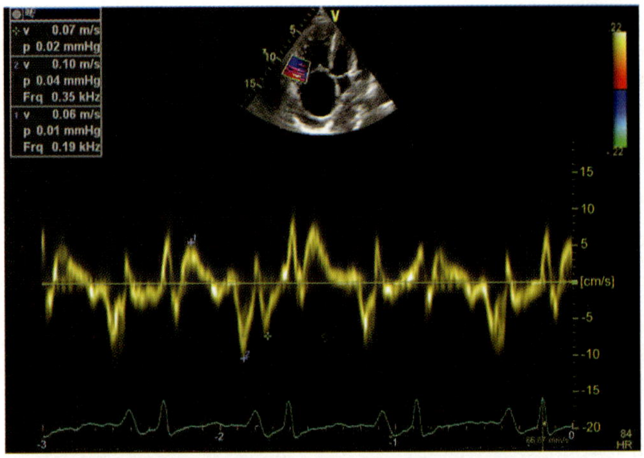

Fig. 24: Tissue Doppler imaging systolic velocity as a measure of right ventricle systolic function.

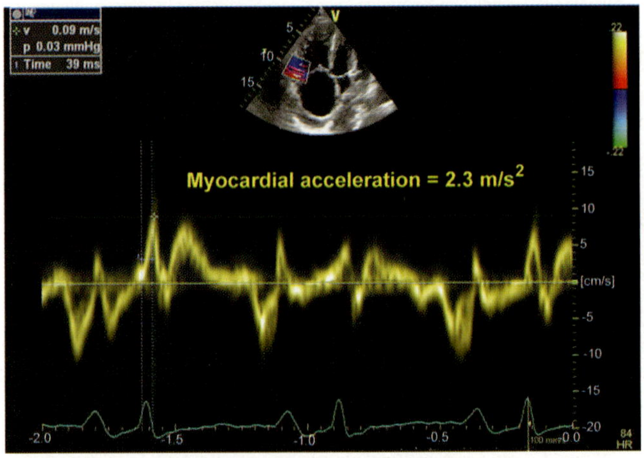

Fig. 25: Right ventricle isovolumic acceleration.

Right ventricle S' obtained by tissue Doppler interrogation (PWD) of basal RV lateral wall is a much more sensitive method of identifying RV dysfunction (Fig. 24). It is 15 cm/s on an average in general population[3] and a value of less than 10 cm/s is considered abnormal. Color coded tissue Doppler offers lower values as it provides mean velocity data unlike PWD method which gives peak velocity data. A value of less than 6 cm/s in color coded TDI indicates RV dysfunction, while the normal value ranges between 8.5 and 10. It is angle dependent and elderly may have lower values. It is influenced by tethering and translational effects. A high frame rate is desirable to obtain reliable values. Myocardial acceleration during isovolumic contraction phase is obtained in TDI of RV basal lateral wall by dividing peak isovolumic myocardial velocity by the time to peak velocity (Fig. 25). It is relatively load independent but dependent on angle of interrogation, age and HR. A value of less than 2.2 m/s^2 is considered abnormal. Strain measurement using speckle tracking echocardiography may give reliable values of RV function and appear angle independent with a better signal to noise ratio. RV focused A4C view is used for strain imaging. Frame rate must be optimized to more than 40 frames per second (fps) by narrowing the imaging sector and reducing the depth to focus on RV for optimal recording. In a study which had included Japanese and Germans, normal global RV peak systolic strain was -24.5 ± 3.8 and RV free-wall strain was –28.5 ± 4.8.[25] In a study done in 53 patients with PH, RV global peak longitudinal systolic strain (GPLSS) less negative than –19.26% predicted patients with severe PH with a mean PAP more than 45 mm Hg.[26,27] RV longitudinal global (RV free-wall + septum) strain value of less than –15% and RV longitudinal free-wall strain of less than –15.3% appear to indicate advanced RV dysfunction with reasonable sensitivity and specificity. Normally the 2-D strain value for RV exceeds (more negative than) –25%, a value of –20% to –25% may indicate mild RV dysfunction, –15% to –20% moderate RV dysfunction and less negative than –15% may indicate severe RV dysfunction (Fig. 26).[28] Diastolic function of RV may be estimated from transtricuspid flow Doppler measurements. Tricuspid E/A velocity ratio less than 0.8 suggests Grade 1 diastolic dysfunction; E/A of 0.8–2.1 with E/e' of more than 6 or diastolic flow dominance in hepatic vein Doppler indicates Grade 2 diastolic dysfunction and E/A more than 2.1 with a deceleration time of less than 120 ms indicates Grade III diastolic dysfunction. RV diastolic function abnormalities may manifest before the onset of systolic dysfunction or even before RVH or RV dilatation starts manifesting. Advanced RV diastolic dysfunction is an incremental adverse prognostic indicator. RV isovolumic relaxation time is another useful diastolic time interval that is calculated from TDI of RV free-wall, from the offset of S' to the onset of E'. A value of more than 75 ms indicates PH. However with the onset of RV dysfunction and or TR, IVRT may get shortened (pseudonormalized).

ECHO FOR ASSESSING ALTERED LEFT VENTRICULAR GEOMETRY AND FUNCTION

Left ventricle size becomes smaller and assumes a D-shape in SAX. The septum loses its curvature and becomes flat. The eccentricity index (measured at end-systole and end-diastole) is the ratio between the anteroposterior (parallel to septum) and septolateral (perpendicular to septum) dimensions of LV. It is normally 1 and in RV overload states, it exceeds 1 (Fig. 27). In RV volume overload states, the ratio is abnormal in diastole and LV becomes circular is systole. Pressure overload results in septal shift and flattening both in diastole and systole, most markedly in end-systole. In advanced PH, LV becomes crescentric and slit like. Because of reduced preload to LV, transmitral flow pattern is that of type II diastolic dysfunction.

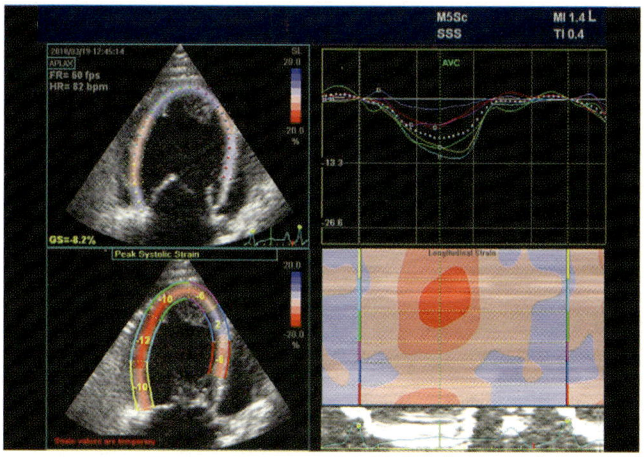

Fig. 26: Right ventricle global peak longitudinal systolic strain by speckle tracking.

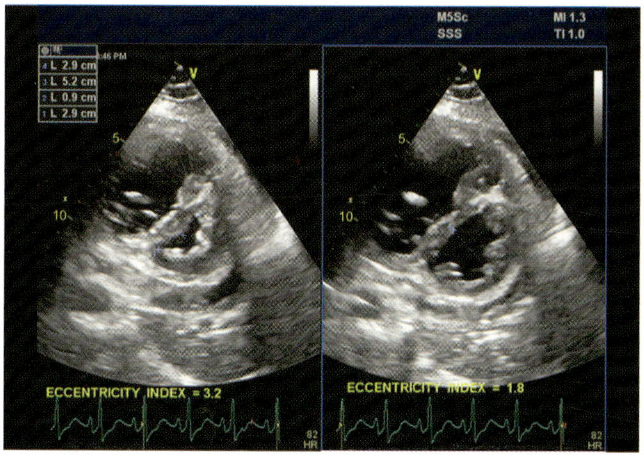

Fig. 27: Altered left ventricle geometry in pulmonary hypertension. Note D-shaped LV with flat septum and increased eccentricity index.

MEASURING CARDIAC OUTPUT

Cardiac output measured in the conventional manner, i.e. LVOT VTI × cross sectional area (CSA) of LVOT x HR, seems to correlate reasonably well with the invasively measured cardiac output (r = 0.74). A simpler alternative approach is to measure RVOT VTI and a value of less than 12 cm could predict a cardiac index less than 2.2 with a sensitivity of 86% and specificity of 71%.[29]

TRANSESOPHAGEAL ECHO

Transesophageal echo may be needed to confirm ASD, in particular superior vena caval (SVC) type, as the cause of PH, when the color Doppler TTE does not demonstrate right to left shunt across atrial septum. Combined with saline contrast study, TEE is very useful in this circumstance. For differentiation between patent foramen ovale and ASD, TEE would be required. Imaging of central PAs including the lobar branches is possible in TEE and may be useful to identify obliterative changes that occur in CTPH. However the proximal most part of LPA may be a blind spot in TEE.

CONTRAST ECHOCARDIOGRAPHY

Contrast echocardiography (CE) using agitated saline may be needed to augment incomplete TR signals so as to get a well-defined spectral waveform from which RV-RA gradient can be accurately calculated. CE may also help to document right to left shunt across ASD or PDA. Contrast swirling within PAs is a characteristic feature in PH.

ECHO FOR FOLLOW-UP OF PATIENTS WITH PULMONARY HYPERTENSION

With the introduction of disease modifying therapies, the functional capacity has been found to improve as assessed by serial assessment of 6 minutes walk distance. It is logically expected that these agents would lead to reduction of PA pressures when used for weeks to months. Invasive studies have indicated that mean PAP showed a modest decline with various disease modifying agents but reduction of PVR and improvement of cardiac output were more substantial than reduction of PAP. When PVR comes down because of pulmonary vasodilatation and reverse remodeling of pulmonary arteries, cardiac output increases which tries to negate the expected decrease in PAP. If this were the case for invasively recorded mean PAP, the situation may be worse with the systolic pressure measured by echo. This phenomenon is due to the flow dependence of pressures in the diseased pulmonary vasculature. If at all echo is used for objectively documenting the benefit of medical therapies, either PVR or the stroke volume or cardiac output measurements have to be used. Possibly, documentation of reverse remodeling of RV and improvement of RV systolic function may prove to be better indices to identify responders.

ECHO DETERMINANTS OF PROGNOSIS

The degree of RV dysfunction is the major determinant of long-term prognosis of patients with PH. TAPSE and S' by TDI are useful measures to indicate prognosis. In an echocardiographic study done on 81 patients with IPAH with a follow-up for 3–4 years, it was confirmed that simple indices like the presence of pericardial effusion (HR 4.38; Fig. 28), RA area (HR 1.24 per 5 cm^2/m increase of RA area) and the degree of septal displacement in diastole as measured by the eccentricity index are the best predictors of poor outcome. In that study, normal RA area index was 9.1 ± 1.7 cm^2/m being corrected for height.[30] It must be recalled that RVSP fails to emerge as a predictor of prognosis for the simple reason that it may decrease with decline of RV function. In that circumstance the degree of septal shift (eccentricity index) particularly in diastole, will definitely give an indication of the severity of disease. Since RVEDP will progressively increase with progression of disease and RV dysfunction, the degree of septal convexity toward LV may indicate advanced disease with poor outcome. In the study done by Brierre on 79 patients with PAH followed up for 12 months, mean PAP more than 49 mm Hg, PADP more than 29 mm Hg, abnormal end-diastolic septal curve, IVC diameter of more than 20 mm with less than 50% respiratory variation emerged as prognostic markers.[31]

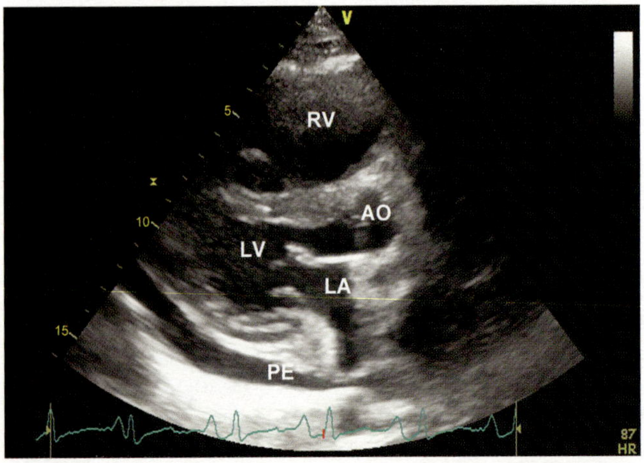

Fig. 28: Pericardial effusion in pulmonary hypertension indicated bad prognosis.

CONCLUSION

Echocardiography thus has a versatile role in evaluating patients suspected to have PH, in each and every stage: confirming the presence of elevated PAP, assessing the severity of perturbed pulmonary hemodynamics, its impact on RV geometry and function, prognostication and serial follow-up to identify responders to the disease modifying therapies. Though identification of elevated PAP is the basic requirement, echo features of right heart overload and RV dysfunction due to PH are far more important to correlate with the patient's functional capacity and future outlook. The important lesson is "look beyond pressures" for a comprehensive evaluation.

Steps to follow: In patients with suspected to have PH (usually for evaluation of dyspnea or syncope) a comprehensive echocardiography is strongly indicated.

1. Look for signs of right heart overload: RA and RV enlargement and RVH. In most of the cases of chronic PH, right heart overload signs will be prominently present. In PH of recent onset and in PH secondary to left heart disease, such signs may not be present. Remember that the presence of RA-RV enlargement and RVH are supportive findings which are useful if PA pressures are in the borderline zone. Absence of these features may not negate the diagnosis of PH, however. In case right heart overload is present with global or regional (McConnell's sign) dysfunction, but with no or mild rise in PAP, consider pulmonary embolism. Whenever RA and RV enlargement is significant, but PA pressure is normal, consider SVC ASD, PAPVC, ARVC.
2. Calculate PASP from a well-delineated TR jet, interrogate multiple windows, namely A4C, parasternal SAX and RV LAX views. Be prepared to do off axis imaging to delineate the jet better and align it with CWD cursor. If CWD signals are incomplete, do not try to calculate TRPG by extrapolating the waveform. If TR is absent, obtain mean PAP from RVOT Doppler.
3. Rule out RVOT obstruction including PPAS before attributing high TRPG (RV-RA gradient) to PH.
4. Look for PR and if present use it for measuring PADP and mean PAP.
5. Triangular RVOT Doppler waveform with short acceleration time is an important sign of PH and also seen in pulmonary embolism.
6. Look for notched RVOT Doppler as it is very suggestive of increased PVR and analyze the position of notch to estimate the disease severity.
7. Rule out secondary causes, perform a meticulous search for VSD in unusual location like mid-muscular or inflow defect, ASD particularly SVC type (TEE with contrast may be needed), left heart valve diseases and

systolic dysfunction of LV. If there is LA enlargement, LVH, AF, etc. Consider HFpEF causing PH. Appropriate laboratory testing should be done to rule out liver disease, HIV, connective tissue disorders, hypo or hyperthyroidism and certain hematological disorders.

8. Document the presence and degree of RV remodeling, particularly D-shaped septum with increased LV eccentricity index. Measure the tricuspid annulus, tethering distance and area.
9. Do not forget to analyze pulmonary arteries and PV.
10. Assess RV function by at least two of the following—TPASE, RV MPI, RV S′ by TDI, RV AF S, RV longitudinal peak systolic strain.
11. Measure cardiac output and PVR, as they will be useful to measure the response to therapy. Never rely on just the PAP changes for monitoring.
12. Look for pericardial effusion, as it is an important negative prognostic marker.

REFERENCES

1. Bossone E, Rubenfire M, Bach DS, et al. Range of tricuspid regurgitation velocity at rest and during exercise in normal adult men: implications for the diagnosis of pulmonary hypertension. J Am Coll Cardiol. 1999;33(6):1662-6.
2. Hatle L, Angelesen BA, Tromsdal A. Noninvasive estimation of pulmonary artery systolic pressure with Doppler ultrasound. Br Heart J. 1981;45(2):157-65.
3. Rudski LG, Lai WW, Afilalo J. Guidelines for the Echocardiographic Assessment of Right Heart in Adults: A report from the American Society of Echocardiography. J AM Soc Echocardiogr. 2010;23(7):685-713.
4. Fisher MR, Forfia PR, Chamera E. Accuracy of Doppler echocardiography in the hemodynamic assessment of pulmonary hypertension. Am J Respir Crit Care Med. 2009;179(7):615-21.
5. Finkelhor RS, Lewis SA, Pillai D. Limitations and strengths of Doppler/echo pulmonary artery systolic pressure-right heart catheterization correlations: a systematic literature review. Echocardiography. 2015;32(1):10-8.
6. Lafitte S, Pillois X, Reant P. Estimation of pulmonary pressures and diagnosis of pulmonary hypertension by Doppler echocardiography: A retrospective comparison of routine echocardiography and invasive hemodynamics. J Am Soc Echocardiogr. 2013;26(5):457-63.
7. D'Alto M, Romeo E, Argiento P. Accuracy and prediction of echocardiography versus right heart catheterization for the assessment of pulmonary hypertension. Intl J Cardiol. 2013;168(4):4058-62.
8. Galiie N, Humbert M, Vachiery JL, et al. 2015 ESC/ERS Guidelines for the diagnosis and treatment of pulmonary hypertension. Eur Heart J. 2016;37(1):67-119.
9. Masuyama T, Kodama K, Kitabatake A, et al. Continuous wave Doppler echocardiographic detection of pulmonary regurgitation and its application to noninvasive estimation of pulmonary artery pressure. Circulation. 1986;74(3):484-92.
10. Parasuraman S, Walker S, Loudon BL, et al. Assessment of pulmonary artery pressure by echocardiography—a comprehensive review. Int J Cardiol Heart Vasc. 2016;12:45-51
11. Chemla D, Castelain V, Humbert M. New formula for predicting mean pulmonary artery pressure using systolic pulmonary artery pressure. Chest. 2004;126(4):1313-7.
12. Mahan G, Dabestani A, Gardin J, et al. Estimation of pulmonary artery pressure by pulsed Doppler echocardiography (abstract). Circulation. 1983;68 Suppl III:III-367.
13. Dabestani A, Mahan G, Gardin JM, et al. Evaluation of pulmonary artery pressure and resistance by pulsed Doppler echocardiography. AM J Cardiol. 1987;59(6):662-8.
14. Aduen JF, Castello R, Lozano MM. An alternative echocardiographic method to estimate mean pulmonary artery pressure: diagnostic and clinical implications. J Am Soc Echocardiogr. 2009;22(7):814-9.
15. Stephen B, Dalal P, Berger M. Noninvasive estimation of pulmonary artery diastolic pressure in patients with tricuspid regurgitation by Doppler echocardiography. Chest. 1999;116(1):73-7.
16. Lopez-Candales A, Rajagopalan N, Gulyasy B, et al. A delayed time of the peak tricuspid regurgitation signal: marker of right ventricular dysfunction. Am J Med Sci. 2008;336(3):224-9.
17. Abbas AE, Fortuin D, Schiller NB. A simple method for noninvasive estimation of pulmonary vascular resistance. J Am Coll Cardiol. 2003;41(6):1021-7.
18. Dahiya A, Vollbon W, Jellis C. Echocardiographic assessment of raised pulmonary vascular resistance: application to diagnosis and follow-up of pulmonary hypertension. Heart. 2010;96(24):2005-9.
19. Arkles JS, Opotowsky AR, Ojeda J, et al. Shape of the right ventricular Doppler envelope predicts hemodynamics and right heart function in pulmonary hypertension. Am J Respir Crit Care Med. 2011;183(2):268-76.
20. Nakayama Y, Sugimachi M, Nakanishi N, et al. Noninvasive differential diagnosis between chronic pulmonary thromboembolism and primary pulmonary hypertension by means of Doppler ultrasound measurement. J Am Coll Cardiol. 1988;31(6):1367-71.
21. Tamborini G, Marsan NA, Gripari P. Reference values for right ventricular volumes and ejection fraction with real time three dimensional echocardiography: evaluation in a large series of normal subjects. J Am Soc Echocardiogr. 2010;23(2):109-15.
22. Anconina J, Danchin N, Selton-Suty C, et al. Noninvasive estimation of right ventricular dP/dt in patients with tricuspid regurgitation. Am J Cardiol. 1993;71(16):1495-7.
23. Tei C, Dujardin KS, Hodge DO, et al. Doppler echocardiographic index for assessment of global right ventricular function. J Am Soc Echocardiogr. 1996;9(6):838-47.
24. Tamborini G, Pepei M, Galli CA, et al. Feasibility and accuracy of a routine echocardiographic assessment of right ventricular function. Int J Cardiol. 2007;115(1):86-9.

25. Morris DA, Krisper M, Nakatani S, et al. Normal range and usefulness of right ventricular systolic strain to detect right ventricular systolic abnormalities in patients with heart failure: a multicentre stiudy. Eur Heart J Cardiovasc Imaging. 2017;18(2):212-23.
26. Li Y, Wang Y, Meng X, et al. Assessment of right ventricular strain by 2-D speckle tracking imaging with RV function and hemodynamics in pulmonary hypertension. Int J Cardiovasc Imaging. 2017;33(11):1737-48.
27. Li Y, Wang Y, Ye X, et al. Clinical study of right ventricular longitudinal strain for assessing right ventricular dysfunction and hemodynamics in pulmonary hypertension. Medicine. 2016;95(50):e5668.
28. Fine NM, Chen L, Bastiansen PM, et al. Outcome prediction by quantitative right ventricular function assessment in 575 subjects evaluated for pulmonary hypertension. Circ Cardiovasc Imaging. 2013;6(5):711-21.
29. Forfia PR, Fisher MR, Mathai SC, et al. Tricuspid annular displacement predicts survival in pulmonary hypertension. Am J Respir Crit Care Med. 2006;174(9):1034-41.
30. Raymond J, Hinderliter AL, Willis PW. Echocardiographic predictors of adverse outcomes in Primary Pulmonary Hypertension. J Am Coll Cardiol. 2002;39(7):1214-9.
31. Brierre G, Blot-Souletie N, Degano B, et al. New echocardiographic prognostic factors for mortality in pulmonary arterial hypertension. Eur J Echocardiogr. 2010;11(6):516-22.

SECTION 19

Aortic Disease

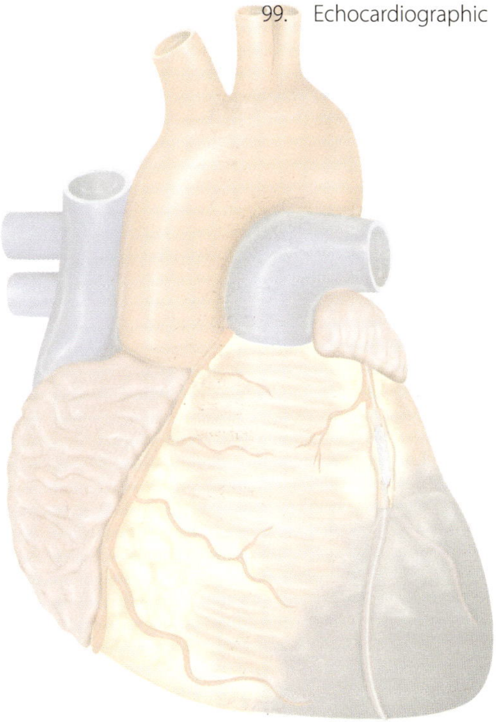

CHAPTER 99

Echocardiographic Evaluation in Aortic Disease

Anjlee M Mehta, HK Chopra, Navin C Nanda, Ahmed Y Salama, Raziye E Akdogan, Hanan Fadala

INTRODUCTION

Our knowledge regarding the pathophysiology of aortic disease continues to grow, and more data regarding risk factors, prognoses, and outcomes is now available. As such, it is imperative to review the echocardiographic evaluation of the aorta as it continues to play a key role in rapid, noninvasive diagnosis and further management. This chapter will review well-established techniques in the basic echocardiographic evaluation of the aorta and highlight echocardiographic features of aortic pathology.

TWO-DIMENSIONAL ECHOCARDIOGRAPHY

Transthoracic (Figs. 1 to 4)

As shown in Figure 1, a basic parasternal long-axis view (PLAX) can allow quick assessment of the aortic root, sinotubular junction, and proximal ascending aorta. ASE/EACVI guidelines (2015) recommend the long-axis view for measurement of the aortic root at the level of the sinuses of Valsalva from leading edge to leading edge during end-diastole.[1] However, some prefers measuring the aortic lumen. Rotation of the probe 90° from the PLAX view results in a parasternal short-axis view (PSAX) that is useful for cursory evaluation of aortic root anatomy and asymmetry. Upward and rightward angulation of the transducer from the PLAX position can bring into view a larger segment of the ascending aorta. Using a right parasternal window with the transducer kept close to the sternum and the patient positioned in the right decubitus position (to displace the right lung laterally), an even larger segment of the proximal ascending aorta (including the aortic root and sinotubular junction) can be visualized.[2-6] The descending thoracic aorta can be evaluated with posterior PLAX and PSAX views. This technique works particularly well, due to improved acoustic impedance, when a large left pleural effusion is

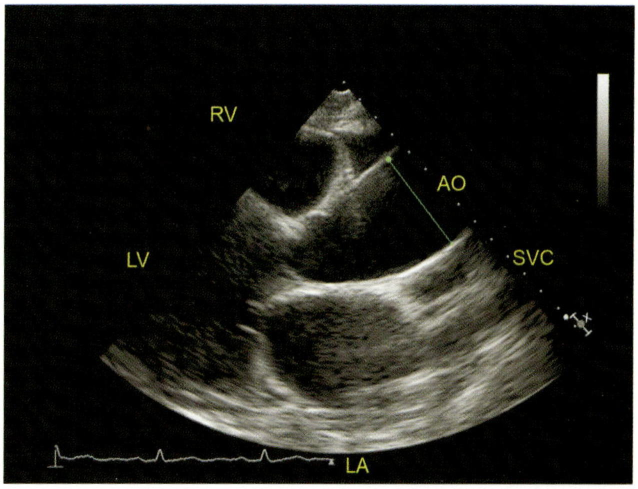

Fig. 1: Two-dimensional transthoracic echocardiography. Cranial angulations from parasternal long axis view demonstrate a dilated proximal ascending aorta (AO) measuring 44 mm. (LA: left atrium; LV: left ventricle; RV: right ventricle; SVC: superior vena cava)

Source: Reproduced with permission from Nanda NC. Interesting Cases in Echocardiography. New Delhi: Jaypee Brothers Medical Publishers; 2017.

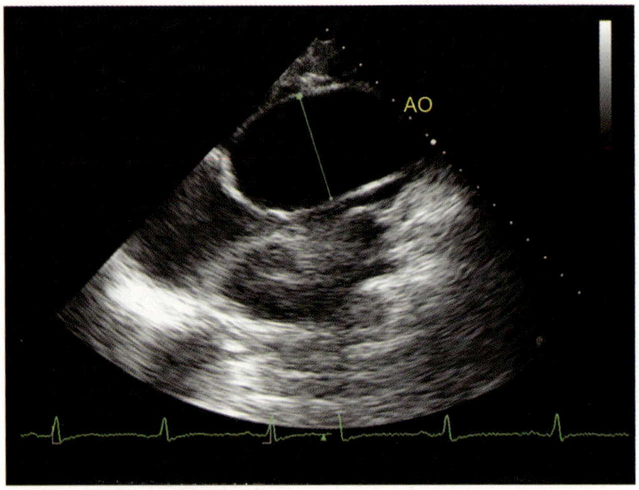

Fig. 2: Two-dimensional transthoracic echocardiography. Obtained from the same patient in Figure 1. Right parasternal approach. A large segment of the ascending aorta (AO) is imaged. The inner dimension measures 43 mm.
Source: Reproduced with permission from Nanda NC. Interesting Cases in Echocardiography. New Delhi: Jaypee Brothers Medical Publishers; 2017.

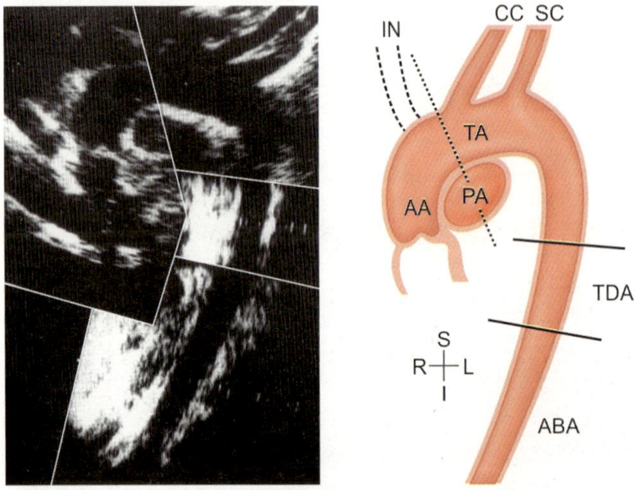

Fig. 3: Two-dimensional transthoracic echocardiography. The normal aorta reconstructed from the root level to the abdominal region by assembling two-dimensional transthoracic images of contiguous segments obtained from different transducer positions. (AA: ascending aorta; ABA: abdominal aorta; CC: common carotid artery; IN: innominate artery; PA: pulmonary artery; SC: subclavian artery; TA: transverse aorta (aortic arch); TDA: thoracic descending aorta)
Source: Reproduced with permission from Mathew T, Nanda NC. Two-dimensional and Doppler echocardiographic evaluation of aortic aneurysm and dissection. Am J Cardiol. 19841;54(3):379-85.

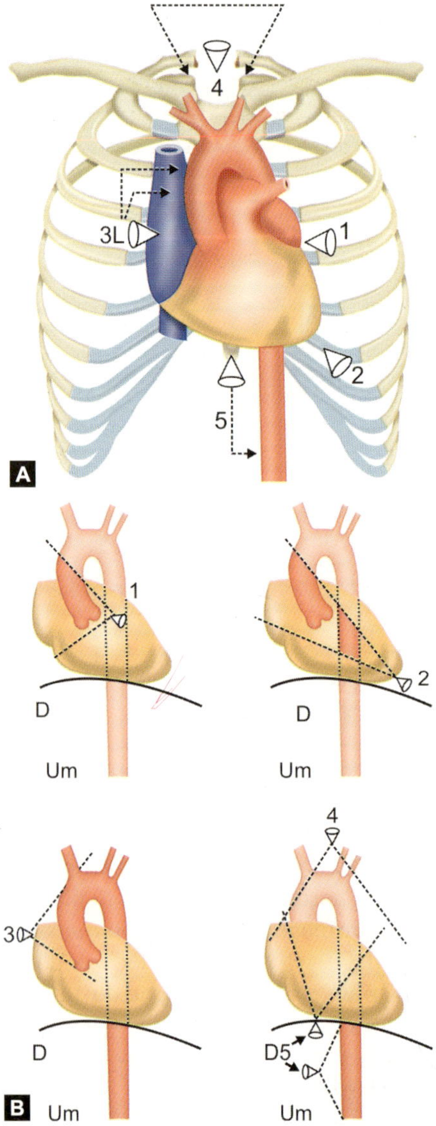

Figs. 4A and B: (A) Various transducer positions used to examine the aorta in our cases. (1 = precordial; 2 = apical: 3 = right parasternal including infraclavicular; 4 = suprasternal and supraclavicular; 5 = subcostal and abdominal). (B) Various aortic segments imaged from the transducer positions shown in A. (D = diaphragm: Um = umbilicus).
Source: Reproduced with permission from: Mathew T, Nanda NC. Two-dimensional and Doppler echocardiographic evaluation of aortic aneurysm and dissection. Am J Cardiol. 1984;54(3):379-85.

present. The transducer can be placed in a left posterior intercostal space and images can be obtained while the patient is sitting up. In the standard suprasternal notch view, the aortic arch and its major branches, the innominate, the common carotid, and the subclavian arteries along with the proximal descending aorta can be visualized. The innominate can be identified as the first branch from the aortic arch and is larger than the other branches.[2] Pulse wave Doppler can be used to differentiate the left common carotid artery from the adjacent left subclavian artery by the presence of low resistance antegrade flow signals in systole and diastole in the former and high resistance oppositely moving flow signals in systole and diastole in the latter vessel.[2] The subcostal view can also allow for visualization of the proximal abdominal aorta and its branches including the celiac and superior mesenteric arteries. Pulse wave and color flow Doppler can be used for confirmation of these pulsatile structures.

Transesophageal

The proximity of the esophagus to the aorta makes it the ideal conduit from which to image the aorta. Due to minimal interference from other anatomical structures, high quality, high-resolution images of the thoracic aorta can be obtained via the transesophageal approach. However, one exception is the distal ascending aorta and proximal aortic arch where visualization can be more challenging due to the presence of the trachea and resultant decreased penetration of ultrasound through this air-filled structure. As our laboratory has shown, with improved operator expertise and technique, this area can be successfully imaged by the transesophageal approach. As one withdraws the transesophageal probe, the aortic arch can be identified because the once circular vessel (descending thoracic aorta) becomes more tube-like (arch). A 90° rotation from this tube-like view shows a more circular (cross-sectional) view of the arch and clockwise and counter-clockwise rotation at this point allows for examination of the entire arch and identification of branch vessels in many patients.[3-8]

Transpharyngeal

By slowly withdrawing the probe from the upper esophagus to the pharynx while keeping the left carotid artery in view (with the aid of color flow Doppler), the carotid bulb, presenting as a localized dilation, and the proximal external and internal carotid arteries can be viewed.[4,9] The external carotid gives off branches through its extracranial course and this can distinguish it from the internal carotid artery which does not branch.[9] The advantage of utilizing the transpharyngeal technique to examine these vessels is the ability to place the Doppler cursor parallel to flow in the internal carotid artery thereby providing more accurate blood flow velocities that those obtained with an external surface approach from the neck. In the latter approach, the ultrasound beam is oriented at a significant angle to blood flow (usually 60°) such that even the algorithm conventionally used for angle correction does not provide the best estimation of the true velocity. Our echo laboratory initially developed the transpharyngeal technique and we have successfully used it to assess and visualize the carotid bulb, internal carotid artery stenosis, a carotid stent, and a paraganglioma.[2] Simply rotating the probe to the right allows visualization of the right carotid artery.

LIVE/REAL-TIME THREE-DIMENSIONAL ECHOCARDIOGRAPHY

Three-dimensional echocardiography (transthoracic and transesophageal) continues to provide additive value in the evaluation of the aorta as it does in many aspects of cardiac pathology. Our laboratory showed that in a study of 67 patients, 20 with aortic aneurysm without dissection, 21 with aortic aneurysm and dissection, and 26 with aortic dissection without aneurysm, live/real time three-dimensional transesophageal echocardiography (3D TEE) increased the level of confidence in the diagnosis and supplemented two-dimensional echocardiography by allowing views from multiple planes and angulations and providing en face views of the rupture site.[8] A common mimic of dissection occurs when a linear echo with minimal or no mobility is seen in the aorta. Imaging with three-dimensional echocardiography allows for differentiation of this artifact from a true dissection as a true dissection flap will be seen as a curvilinear "sheet" rather than a thin linear structure.[10-12]

Thoracic Aortic Aneurysms (Figs. 5 and 6)

An abnormal dilation of greater than 50% of the aorta is considered an aneurysm.[13] They are usually the result of a weakening in the vessel wall. Cystic medial degeneration (previously cystic medial necrosis) is one mechanism that is felt to be a possible response to shear wall stress.

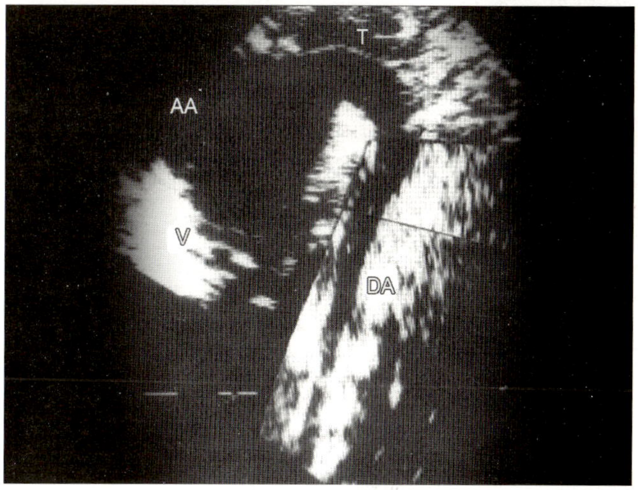

Fig. 5: Two-dimensional transthoracic echocardiography. Ascending aortic aneurysm. This composite illustration made by the reconstruction method utilized in Figure 3 to show the full extent of the aneurysm. The transverse aortic arch (T) and the descending thoracic aorta (DA) are not involved. (AA: ascending aorta; V: aortic valve)

Source: Reproduced with permission from Mathew T, Nanda NC. Two-dimensional and Doppler echocardiographic evaluation of aortic aneurysm and dissection. Am J Cardiol. 1984;54(3):379-85.

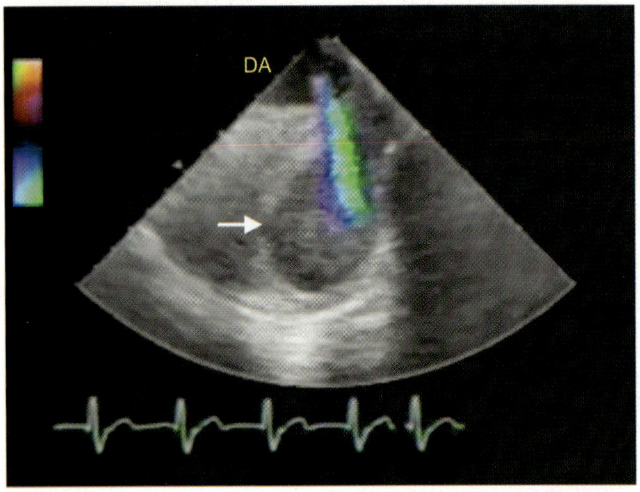

Fig. 6: Two-dimensional transesophageal echocardiography. Arrow points to a large saccular aneurysm of the descending thoracic aorta (DA).

Source: Reproduced with permission from Aaluri SR, Miller A, Nanda NC, et al. Transesophageal echocardiographic identification of a descending aortic aneurysm rupture into the left lung. Echocardiography. 2000;17(3):269-71.

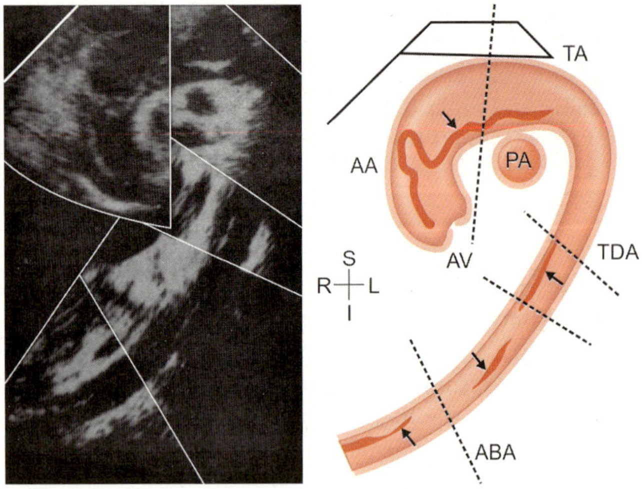

Fig. 7: Two-dimensional transthoracic echocardiography. Aortic dissection (DeBakey type I). This composite illustration was also made by the reconstruction method. The dissection flap (arrows) can be seen in the ascending aorta (AA), transverse aortic arch (TA), thoracic descending aorta (TDA) and in the abdominal segment (ABA). (A: aortic valve; PA: pulmonary artery)

Source: Reproduced with permission from: Mathew T, Nanda NC. Two-dimensional and Doppler echocardiographic evaluation of aortic aneurysm and dissection. Am J Cardiol. 1984;54(3):379-85.

Other syndromes including Marfan and Loeys-Dietz are also associated with medial degeneration. Factors such as matrix metalloproteinases 2 (MMP-2) and transforming growth factor-beta have also been implicated in aneurysm formation.[13]

Aneurysms are of two morphologies. More common are the fusiform type, described as a circumferential dilation as opposed to the saccular type, a focal bulging on one side.[1] Serial monitoring is recommended due to the risk of complications like pseudoaneurysm, penetrating atherosclerotic ulcer, dissection or most commonly, rupture. ACC/AHA guidelines recommend referral for evaluation by surgery for ascending aortic aneurysms more than 5.5 cm. Size thresholds are lower for those with certain connective tissue disorders and syndromes.[14-17]

Aortic Dissection (Figs. 7 to 12)

An aortic dissection is defined by the presence of an intimal tear that can propagate under systolic pressure with subsequent intramural hemorrhage into the medial layer. A high degree of clinical suspicion is necessary in the timely diagnosis of aortic dissection. De novo acute, severe chest pain should prompt consideration of this diagnosis. Although both TEE and computed tomography scanning are significantly more sensitive and specific, transthoracic echocardiography can still be a useful tool. It is a fast, noninvasive bedside test that can screen for dissection and associated complications. It can provide an immediate diagnosis that expedites management, particularly in the case of type A aortic dissection.[18] A PLAX view can quickly identify an ascending aorta dissection by visualization of a highly, independently mobile linear echo representing the flap. Aortic root involvement, associated aortic regurgitation, aortic valve compromise, wall motion abnormalities, coronary ostia involvement, and the presence of a pericardial effusion can also be identified with a good window. The suprasternal notch view can be used to evaluate for a flap in the aortic arch. M-mode echocardiography can also be used to confirm the presence of a true flap versus an artifact.[18] A suprasternal notch window can also be utilized to evaluate for dissection or abnormalities of the aortic arch or proximal descending thoracic aorta. Of note, focused point-of-care echocardiography is a growing area in which properly trained providers can potentially obtain images even sooner and prevent further delay in taking the patient to the operating room because studies have shown that mortality increases 1–2%/hour after the onset of symptoms in dissections that involve the ascending aorta.[12]

In describing the aortic dissection, several pieces of information should attempt to be obtained. The first is distinguishing between a Type A or a Type B dissection per the Stanford classification. A Type A dissection originates in the ascending aorta and is a surgical emergency. A Type B dissection is a tear originating in the descending aorta and can often be managed more conservatively with

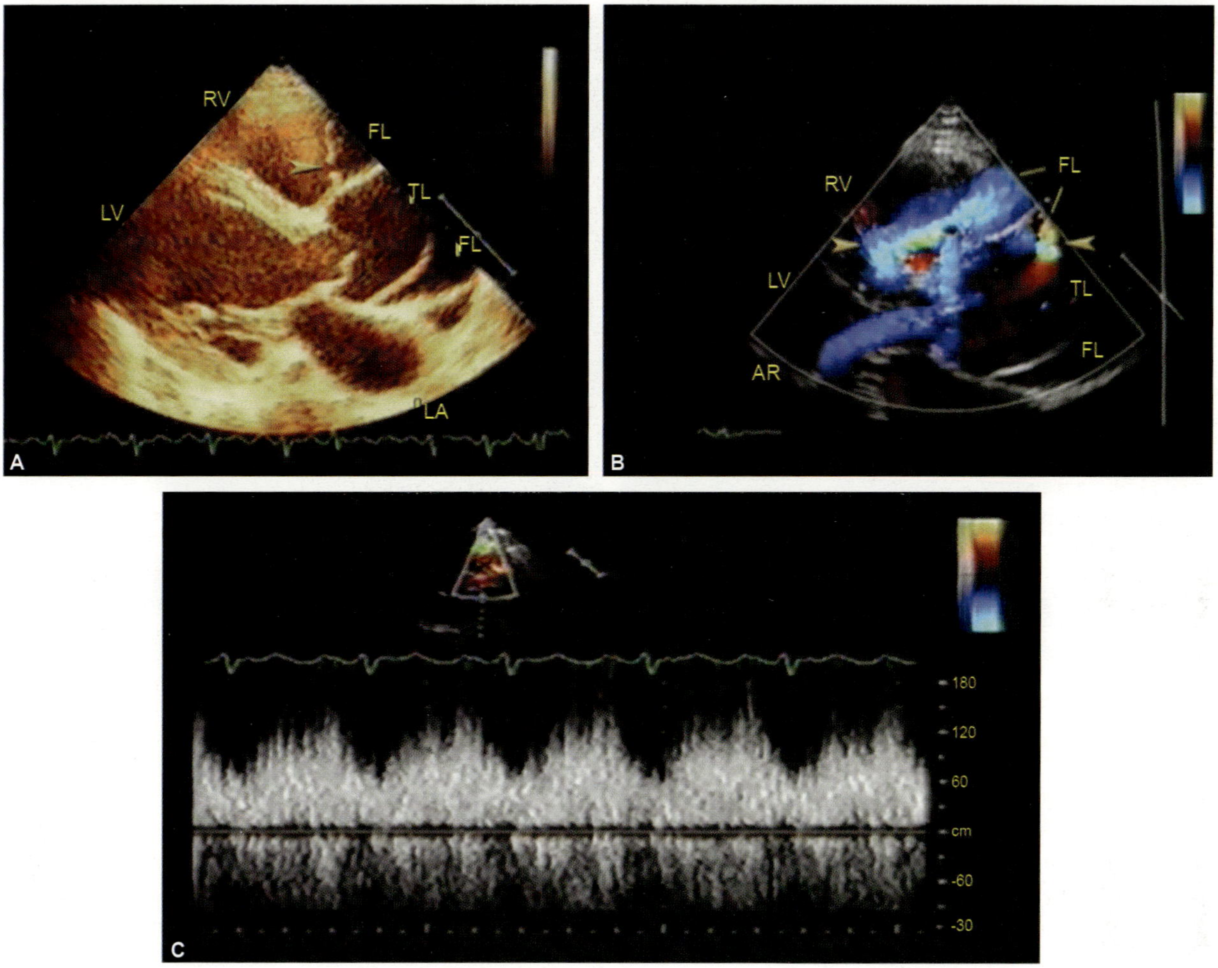

Figs. 8A to C: Two-dimensional transthoracic echocardiographic assessment of aortic dissection rupture into the right ventricular outflow tract. (A) Parasternal long axis view. The arrow head points to the site of rupture of the false lumen (FL) into the right ventricular outflow tract (RVOT). (B) Color Doppler examination. The arrow head on the right points to a communication between the true lumen (TL) and FL. The arrow head on the left shows flow signals moving from the FL to the RVOT. Moderate aortic regurgitation (AR) is also displayed. (C). Continuous wave spectral Doppler interrogation of the rupture site shows continuous flow throughout the cardiac cycle. (LV: left ventricle; LA: left atrium; RA: right atrium)

Source: Reproduced with permission from Hansalia S, Nanda NC, Bandarupalli N, et al. Live/real time three-dimensional transthoracic echocardiographic assessment of aortic dissection rupture into right ventricular outflow tract: a case report and review of the literature. Echocardiography. 2009;26(1):100-5.

medications.[12] The DeBakey classification is an alternate system in which DeBakey I describes a tear in the ascending aorta that continues into the arch and descending aorta, DeBakey II is a tear limited to the ascending aorta, and DeBakey III describes a tear in the descending aorta.[12] The intimal flap can be visualized and the true and false lumens it creates should be identified. The true lumen is often smaller and is characterized by systolic expansion and more turbulent flow on color flow Doppler. The false lumen is often larger, has lower velocity, less turbulent flow, and may contain thrombus. Tools like M-mode, color flow Doppler, and three-dimensional echocardiography can help in distinguishing a true flap from artifact.[10,11] As noted earlier, assessment for complications like tamponade from rupture into the pericardium, acute aortic insufficiency from involvement of the aortic valve, extension into the right or left coronary systems, hematomas, and thrombus should be undertaken.

Aortic Intramural Hematoma

Clinically, aortic intramural hematoma can present similarly to aortic dissection with severe, sharp chest or back pain. Echocardiographically, a characteristic of aortic intramural hematomas is a tendency to have a smoother luminal surface compared to the irregular crevices and peaks of

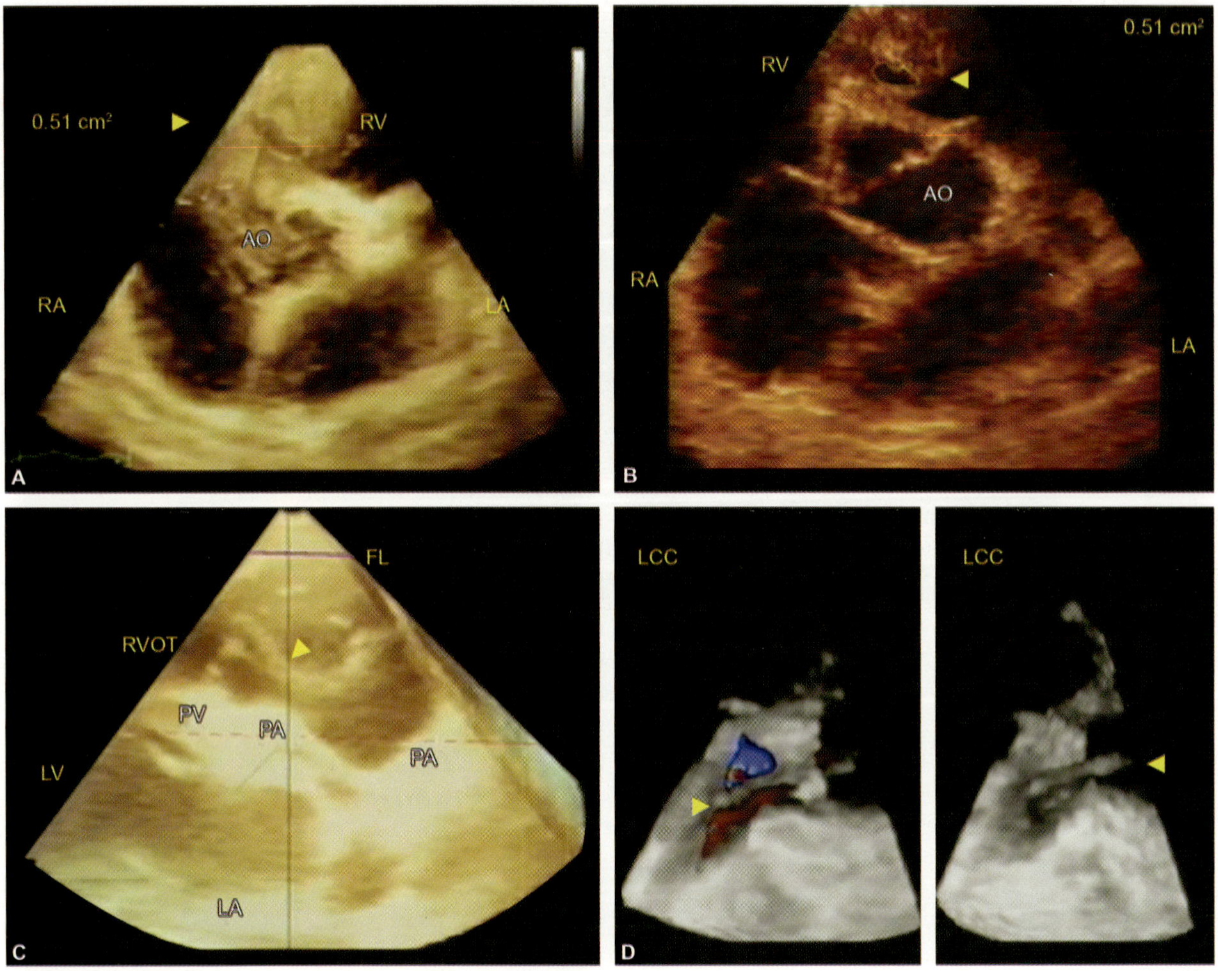

Figs. 9A to D: Live/real time three-dimensional transthoracic echocardiographic assessment of aortic dissection rupture into the right ventricle outflow tract. (A) The arrow head points to the enface view of the rupture site upon cropping of the data set. It is roughly elliptical in shape and measured 0.51 cm^2 in area (A) by planimetry. (B) Q Lab image of the same data set with the orifice (arrow head) planimetered. (C) Arrowhead points to compression of the main pulmonary artery (PA) by the false lumen. (D) Extension of the dissection (arrow head) into the left common carotid artery (LCC) is shown. (AO: aorta; PV: pulmonary valve)
Source: Reproduced with permission from Hansalia S, Nanda NC, Bandarupalli N, et al. Live/real time three-dimensional transthoracic echocardiographic assessment of aortic dissection rupture into right ventricular outflow tract: a case report and review of the literature. Echocardiography. 2009;26(1):100-5.

atherosclerotic ulcers. They appear as an echolucent, crescentic thickening of greater than 7 mm. This should be distinguished from mimics like hemiazygous vein sheath. Bleeding from rupture of the vaso vasorum perfusing the medial layer of the aortic wall is thought to be the etiology of intramural hematomas. Unlike aortic dissection, the presence of an intimal tear with communication is not the precipitating event even though compromise of the intima can be seen with hematoma progression.[19] Additionally, the hematoma is often found closer to the adventitial side and on imaging results in outward splaying of intimal calcification. The diagnosis has important clinical implications as 16% of aortic intramural hematomas develop into dissections.[19-22]

Aortic Transection (Fig. 13)

Aortic transection, a cross-sectional tear disrupting the aortic wall, is usually a consequence of acute trauma to the aorta. The area of the aorta most susceptible to this type of rupture is at the aortic isthmus which is anatomically located just after the origin of the left subclavian artery at the junction of the ligamentum arteriosum which tethers the aorta to the left pulmonary artery. With blunt thoracic trauma or sudden deceleration that can occur in motor vehicle accidents, these forces can result in shearing at this site where the mobile aortic arch meets the descending aorta. Echocardiography will show a thicker tear involving

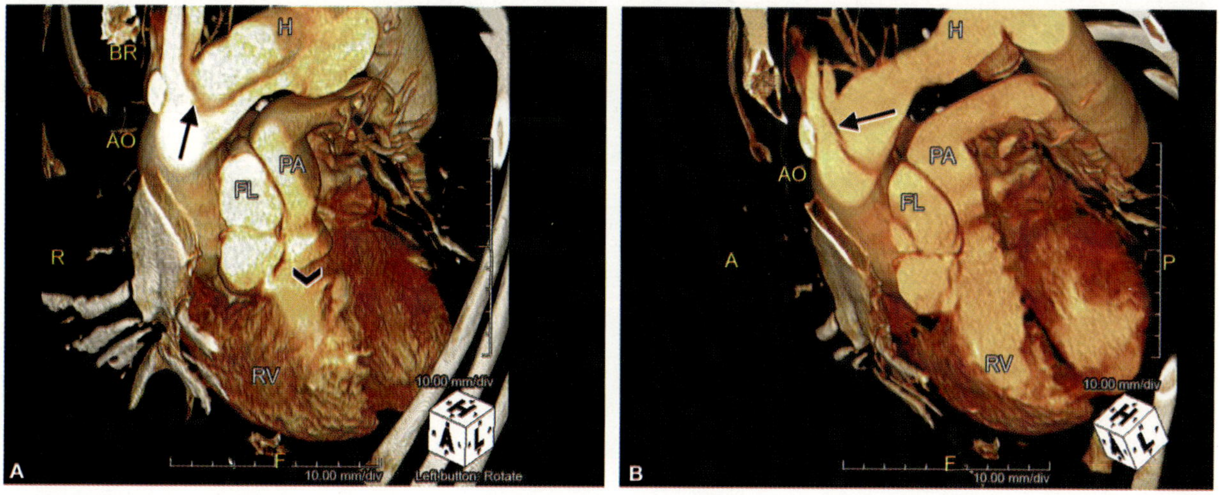

Figs. 10A and B: Computed tomography angiogram assessment of aortic dissection rupture into the right ventricular outflow tract. (A) Left anterior oblique (LAO) view demonstrating the communication (arrow head) between the FL and RVOT. (B) Cut slab volume rendered image in oblique LAO view demonstrating PA compression by the dilated FL. The arrow in figures A and B points to the dissection flap extending into the aortic arch and the brachiocephalic artery (BR). (H: head; F: foot; L: left; R: right; A: anterior; P: posterior)

Source: Reproduced with permission from Hansalia S, Nanda NC, Bandarupalli N, et al. Live/real time three-dimensional transthoracic echocardiographic assessment of aortic dissection rupture into right ventricular outflow tract: a case report and review of the literature. Echocardiography. 2009;26(1):100-5.

both the media and intima rather than just an intimal tear and the thin flap characteristic of a dissection.[23,24] The torn portion tends to be oriented perpendicular to the aortic wall unlike with a dissection where the flap is roughly parallel to the aortic wall. The torn portions may mimic a communication between true, more aptly "perfusing", and false, "non-perfusing", lumens seen with dissection, however, the flow signals in transection move in one direction during systole with minimal backward flow in diastole (due to aortic recoil) similar to normal aortic flow. Conversely, in the case of dissection, color flow signals move from the true to the false lumen in systole and back to the true lumen in diastole.

Aortic Atheromas (Fig. 14)

The presence of atheromas can also be seen on echo. Transesophageal echo provides visualization of the thoracic aorta and produces high quality images of atherosclerotic plaques. Classification based on thickness, degree of protrusion into the aortic lumen, presence of surface ulceration, and presence of mobile components can be easily assessed. Thrombus overlying complex atheroma is thought to be responsible for most embolic phenomena.[25-27] Penetrating atherosclerotic ulcer is a type of acute aortic syndrome in which a complex ulcerating atheromatous plaque penetrates the intimal layer and can progress into the media. It can be a risk factor for aortic dissection or rupture. Thoracic aortic calcification can also be evaluated using echocardiography though quantification by ultrasound has been limited. Nevertheless, the presence of thoracic aortic calcification is a marker of systemic atherosclerosis and a predictor of atherosclerotic cardiovascular disease though data do not support screening for extracardiac calcification solely for this reason.[26]

Aortic Tumors (Fig. 15)

While not as common as the other aforementioned aortic pathology, the possibility of an aortic tumor should remain on the differential. A case from our laboratory involved a patient who was initially referred from an outside hospital for suspected aortic dissection. An artifact was seen in the aorta, but no dissection was seen. A mass was seen in the descending thoracic aorta with normal velocities in the surrounding lumen making tumor higher on the differential than thrombus. The patient ultimately underwent surgical resection for a leiomyosarcoma. Methods to manage tumor infiltration from metastatic disease to the thoracic aorta with stent-grafting have also now shown safety and efficacy in facilitating metastatic tumor resection and imaging with CT for further characterization is warranted in many of these cases.[28]

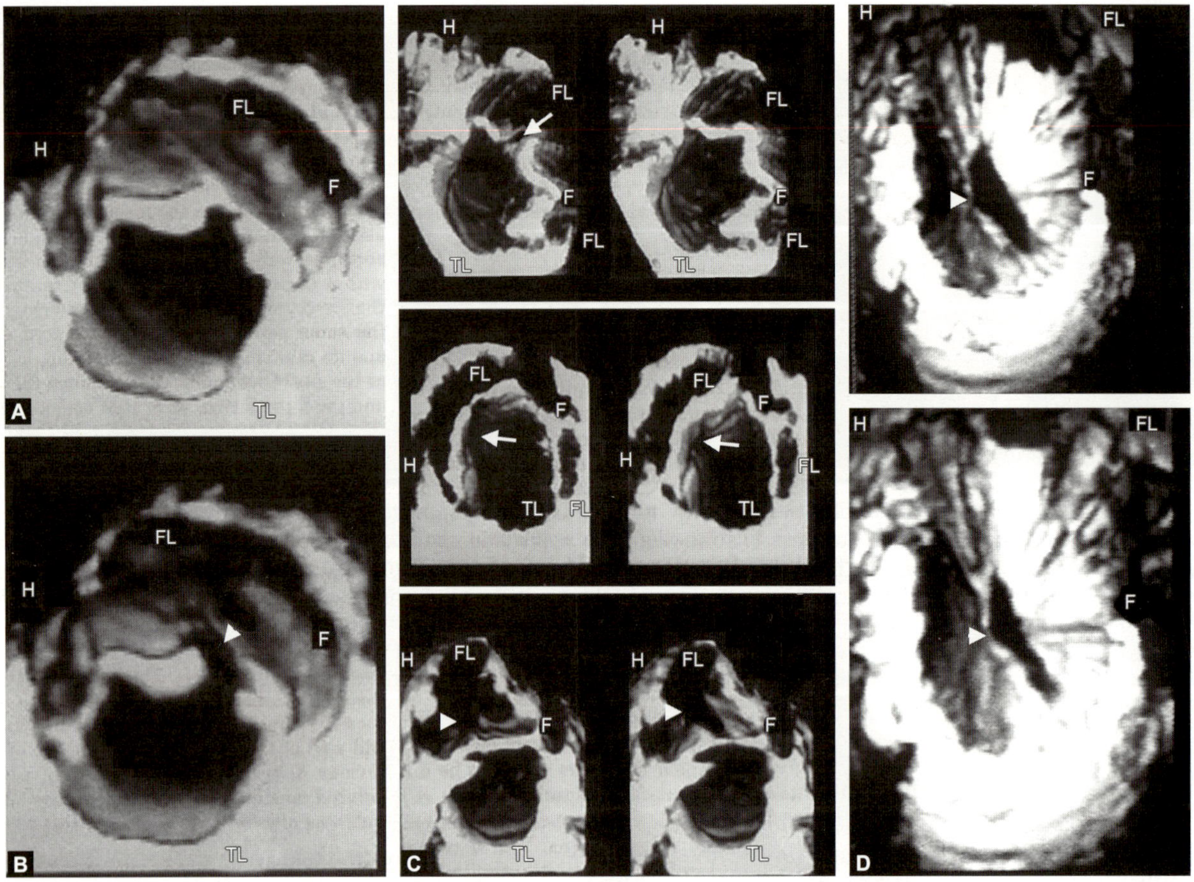

Figs. 11A to D: Transesophageal three-dimensional echocardiographic reconstruction in aortic dissection. The descending thoracic aorta was examined using multiple cut sections and various viewing angles. (A and B) Both the true (TL) and the false (FL) lumens are well visualized, and the dissection flap (F) presents as a sheet-like structure along the aortic length. (C and D) The communication (arrowheads) between the true and false lumens is viewed as en face using a transverse section. As would be expected, the communication is larger in systole than in diastole. (H: mediastinal hematoma)

Source: Reproduced with permission from: Nanda NC, Khatri GK, Samal AK, et al. Three-Dimensional Echocardiographic Assessment of Aortic Dissection. Echocardiography. 1998 ;15(8 Pt 1):745-54.

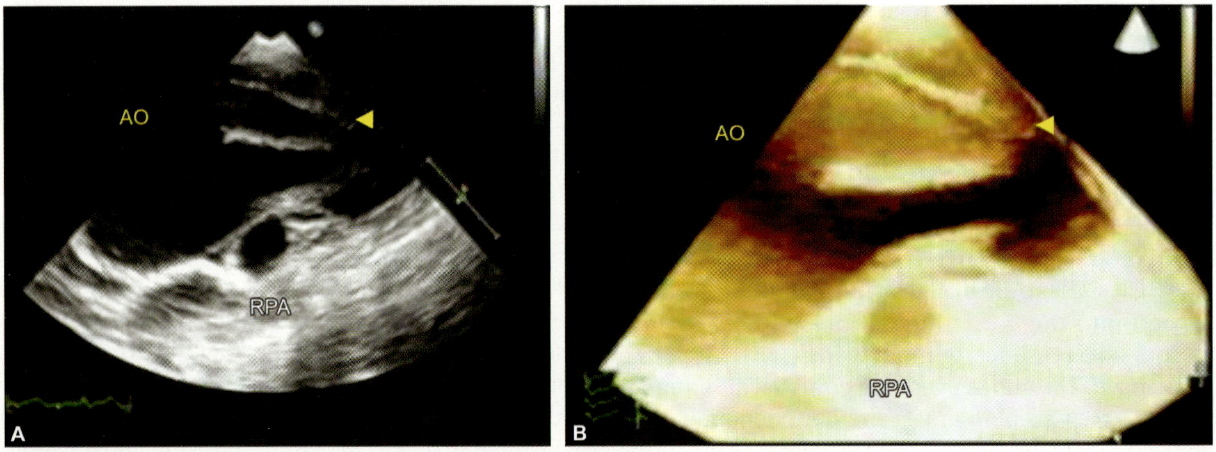

Figs. 12A and B: Comparison of two- and live/real time three-dimensional transesophageal echocardiography in the assessment of aortic dissection. (A) The dissection flap (arrowhead) appears as a linear echo in the ascending aorta (AO) using the two-dimensional technique. B. With the three-dimensional modality, the dissection flap (arrowhead) appears as a sheet of tissue. (RPA: right pulmonary artery)

Source: Reproduced with permission from Nanda NC. Comprehensive Textbook of Echocardiography. New Delhi: Jaypee Brothers Medical Publishers; 2014.

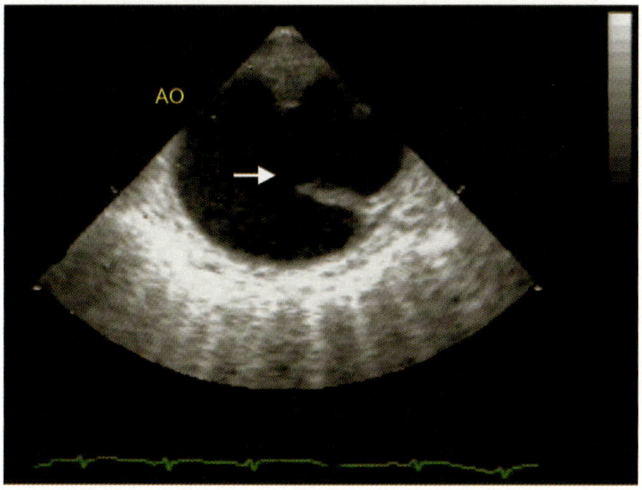

Fig. 13: Two-dimensional tranesophageal echocardiography. Aortic transection. The arrow points to a linear echo which is perpendicular to the aortic (AO) wall.

Source: Reproduced with permission from Nanda NC. Comprehensive Textbook of Echocardiography. New Delhi: Jaypee Brothers Medical Publishers; 2014.

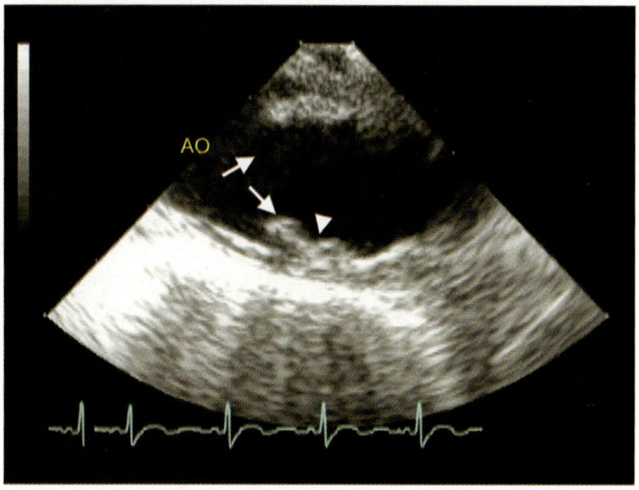

Fig. 14: Two-dimensional transesophageal echocardiography. Aortic atherosclerosis in an elderly patient. Upper arrow points to a mobile atherosclerotic plaque and the lower to a fixed one in the descending thoracic aorta (AO). Arrowhead shows prominent ulceration in the plaque.

Source: Reproduced with permission from Nanda NC. Comprehensive Textbook of Echocardiography. New Delhi: Jaypee Brothers Medical Publishers; 2014.

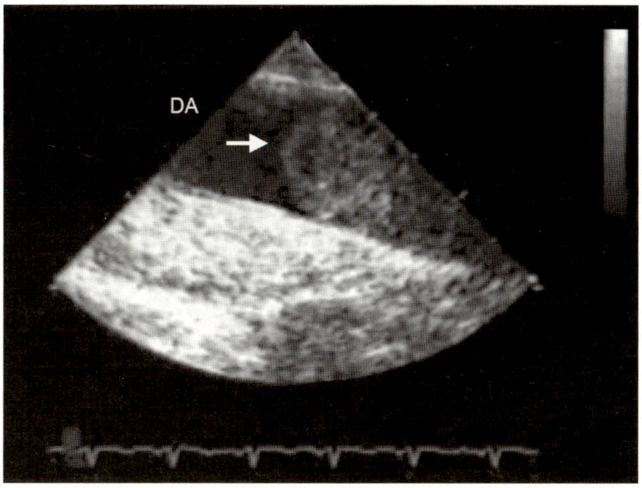

Fig. 15: Two-dimensional transesophageal echocardiography. Aortic leiomyosarcoma. The arrow points to the tumor. (DA: descending thoracic aorta)

REFERENCES

1. Goldstein SA, Evangelista A, Abbara S. Multimodality Imaging of Diseases of the Thoracic Aorta in Adults: From the American Society of Echocardiography and the European Association of Cardiovascular Imaging. J Am Soc Echocardiography. 2015;28:119-82.
2. Nanda NC. Interesting Cases in Echocardiography. New Delhi: Jaypee Brothers Medical Publishers; 2017.
3. Mathew T, Nanda NC. Two-dimensional and Doppler echocardiographic evaluation of aortic aneurysm and dissection. Am J Cardiol. 1984;54(3):379-85.
4. El-Hajj S, Nanda NC, Bhagatwala K, et al. Upper Transesophageal and Transpharyngeal Examination. In Nanda NC (Ed). Comprehensive Textbook of Echocardiography. New Delhi: Jaypee Brothers Medical Publishers; 2013. pp. 487-506.
5. Agrawal G, LaMotte LC, Nanda NC, et al. Identification of the aortic arch branches using transesophageal echocardiography. Echocardiography. 1997;14(5):461-6.
6. Nanda NC, Thakur AC, Thakur D, et al. Transesophageal echocardiographic examination of left subclavian artery branches. Echocardiography. 1999;16(3):271.

7. Aaluri SR, Miller A, Nanda NC, et al. Transesophageal echocardiographic identification of a descending aortic aneurysm rupture into the left lung. Echocardiography. 2000;17(3):269-71.
8. Joshi D, Bicer EI, Donmez C et al. Incremental value of live/real time three-dimensional transesophageal echocardiography over the two-dimensional technique in the assessment of aortic aneurysm and dissection. Echocardiography. 2012;29(5):620-30.
9. Nanda NC, Miller AP, Nekkanti R, et al Transpharyngeal echocardiographic imaging of the right and left carotid arteries. Echocardiography. 2001;18(8):711-6.
10. Htay T, Nanda NC, Agrawal G, et al. Live three-dimensional transthoracic echocardiographic assessment of aortic dissection. Echocardiography. 2003;20(6):573-7.
11. Nanda NC, Khatri GK, Samal AK, et al. Three-dimensional echocardiographic assessment of aortic dissection. Echocardiography. 1998;15(8 Pt 1):745-54.
12. Nanda NC. Comprehensive Textbook of Echocardiography. New Delhi: Jaypee Brothers Medical Publishers; 2014.
13. Goldfinger JZ, Halperin JL, Marin ML, et al. Thoracic aortic aneurysm and dissection. J Am Coll Cardiol. 2014;64(16):1725-39.
14. Bonaca MP, O'Gara PT. Diagnosis and management of acute aortic syndromes: dissection, intramural hematoma, and penetrating aortic ulcer. Curr Cardiol Rep. 2014;16(10):536.
15. Shiga T, Wajima Z, Apfel CC, et al. Diagnostic accuracy of transesophageal echocardiography, helical computed tomography, and magnetic resonance imaging for suspected thoracic aortic dissection: systematic review and meta-analysis. Arch Intern Med. 2006;166(13):1350-6.
16. Elefteriades JA. Natural history of thoracic aortic aneurysms: indications for surgery, and surgical versus nonsurgical risks. Ann Thorac Surg. 2002;74(5):S1877-80; discussion S18921878.
17. Hiratzka LF, Bakris GL, Beckman JA, et al. 2010 ACCF/AHA/AATS/ACR/ASA/SCA/SCAI/SIR/STS/SVM guidelines for the diagnosis and management of patients with thoracic aortic disease: executive summary. A report of the American College of Cardiology Foundation/American Heart Association Task Force on Practice Guidelines, American Association for Thoracic Surgery, American College of Radiology, American Stroke Association, Society of Cardiovascular Anesthesiologists, Society for Cardiovascular Angiography and Interventions, Society of Interventional Radiology, Society of Thoracic Surgeons, and Society for Vascular Medicine. Catheter Cardiovasc Interv. 2010;76(2):E43-86.
18. Hansalia S, Nanda NC, Bandarupalli N, et al. Live/Real Time Three-Dimensional Transthoracic Echocardiographic Assessment of Aortic Dissection Rupture into Right Ventricular Outflow Tract: A case report and review of the literature Echocardiography. 2009; 26(1):100-5.
19. Bhave NM, Nienaber CA, Clough RE, et al. Multimodality Imaging of Thoracic Aortic Diseases in Adults. J Am Coll Cardiol Cardiovasc Imag. 2018:11(6):902-19.
20. Evangelista A, Mukherjee D, Mehta RH, et al. Acute intramural hematoma of the aorta: a mystery in evolution. Circulation. 2005;111(8):1063-70.
21. Buckley O, Rybicki FJ, Gerson DS, et al. Imaging features of intramural hematoma of the aorta. Int J Cardiovasc Imaging. 2010;26(1):65-76.
22. Mansour M, Berkery W, Kozlowski L, et al. Mild thickening of the aortic wall: subtle intramural hematoma? Echocardiography. 2001;18(6):519-22.
23. Nzewi O, Slight RD, Zamvar V. Management of blunt thoracic aortic injury. Eur J Vasc Endovasc Surg. 2006;31(1):18-27.
24. Nanda NC, Samal AK, Bakir S, et al. Transesophageal echocardiographic diagnosis of right sided aortic arch. Echocardiography. 1998;15:409-17.
25. Thenappan T, Ali Raza J, Movahed A. Aortic atheromas: current concepts and controversies—a review of the literature. Echocardiography. 2008;25(2):198-207.
26. Desai M, Cremer P, Schoenhagen P. Thoracic aortic calcification. J Am Coll Cardiol Cardiovasc Imag. 2018:11(7):1012-26.
27. Elsayed M, Bulur S, Kalla A, et al. Incremental value of live/real time three-dimensional transesophageal echocardiography over the two-dimensional technique in the assessment of aortic atherosclerotic thrombi and ulcers. Echocardiography. 2016;33:1234-18.
28. Collaud S, Waddell TK, Yasufuku K. Thoracic aortic endografting facilitates the resection of tumors infiltrating the aorta. J Thorac Cardiovasc Surg. 2014;147(4):1178-82.

100

CHAPTER

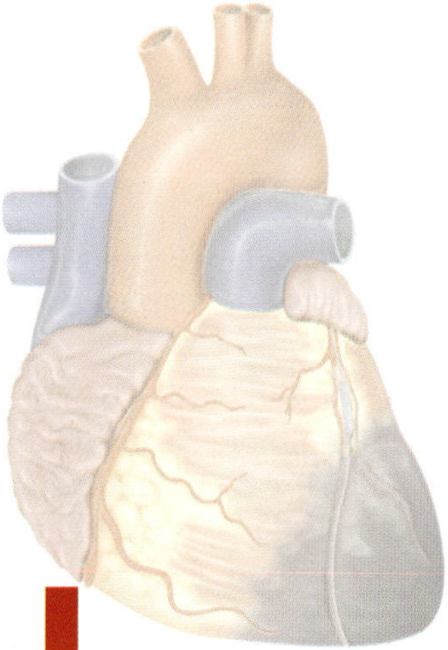

CT and MR Angiographic Evaluation of Aortic Diseases

Vineeta Ojha, Sanjeev Kumar

INTRODUCTION

Aorta is the major vessel supplying oxygenated blood from heart to different body parts. Aortic diseases are major cause of morbidity and mortality in general population. Comprehensive evaluation and early diagnosis is important for timely and appropriate treatment. Computed tomography (CT) and magnetic resonance imaging (MRI) are the most commonly used imaging examinations to evaluate variety of congenital and acquired aortic lesions. They allow for comprehensive evaluation with excellent spatial and temporal resolutions, wide fields of view, and multiplanar imaging capabilities. Multidetector CT (MDCT) is more commonly used than MRI because of faster scans and easy availability.

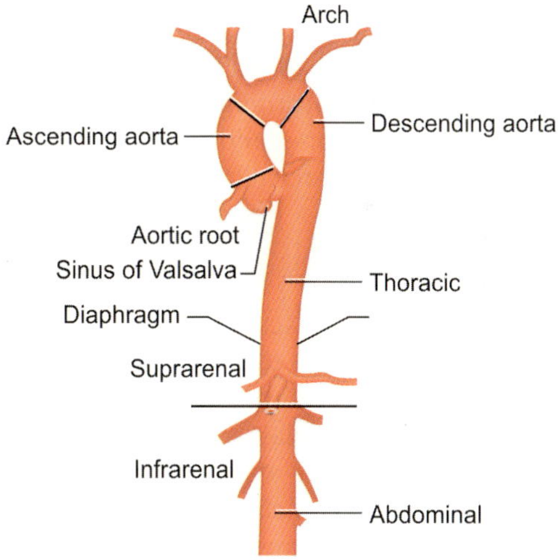

Fig. 1: Graphic showing anatomy of aorta.

NORMAL ANATOMY OF AORTA

The ascending aorta extends from the aortic valve to the origin of the brachiocephalic artery (BCA). The most proximal portion of it is referred to as aortic root which has three components: the annulus, the sinuses of Valsalva, and the sinotubular junction. The aortic arch begins at the BCA and ends at the ligamentum arteriosum. Its most distal aspect, which is slightly narrowed, is termed the "aortic isthmus". The descending thoracic aorta extends from ligamentum to diaphragmatic hiatus. The normal branching pattern [BCA, left common carotid artery (LCCA) and left subclavian artery (LSCA)] is seen in about 70% of individuals (Fig. 1). The most common variation is a combined origin of the BCA and LCCA (bovine trunk), seen in 20% of individuals. In about 5% of cases, the left vertebral artery arises directly from the aorta, between the LCCA and LSCA. Aortic arch anomalies include aberrant origin of the right subclavian artery (RSCA) as the last branch of the thoracic aorta just distal to LSCA (1%), right-sided aortic arch (1%), and aberrant origin of LSCA (1%), etc.[1] The abdominal portion of the aorta has single anterior branches-celiac trunk (D12), the superior mesenteric artery (SMA; L1), and the inferior mesenteric artery (IMA; L3), which arises just above the aortic bifurcation. The paired lateral abdominal aorta branches are the inferior phrenic artery, suprarenal and renal arteries, gonadal arteries, and several paired lumbar arteries.

AORTIC MEASUREMENTS

Aortic measurements are made in true short-axis projection acquired from double oblique views, from one blood-wall boundary to the other.[2]

Aortic Dilatation

The aortic diameter varies with body size, sex, and aging. The average mean diameter is as follows:[3,4]

- *Aortic root*: 2.6 cm (sagittal), 2.4 cm (coronal)
- *Ascending aorta*: 3.6 cm
- *Aortic arch*: 3.5 cm
- *Proximal descending aorta*: 2.6 cm
- *Distal descending aorta*: 2.4 cm
- *Abdominal aorta*: 2 cm

In adults, the aortic diameter increases by approximately 0.1 cm per decade. Table 1 gives simplified values of the maximal normal diameters of the aorta.

Computed Tomography Angiography Protocol

Aorta is well-imaged on a 64-MDCT/128-dual source CT (DSCT) with initial electrocardiography (ECG)-gated scan followed by flash scan (non-gated). The scan should cover area 3 cm above the aortic arch till the level of femoral heads. Contrast injection is with a pressure injector with saline chase with flow rate around 3–4 mL/s and volume should be calculated as follows:

Flow rate × (scan time + scan delay)

This is followed by saline chase with the same flow rate for 5–6 seconds. For acquisition, "bolus chase" technique is preferred over fixed time delay, with threshold of contrast density kept around 100 HU (at level of ascending aorta) to trigger the acquisition with delay of 4–5 seconds to achieve maximum luminal enhancement. Data thus acquired can be reconstructed in axial or three-dimensional (3D) images [maximum intensity projections (MIP), shaded surface display (SSD) or volume rendered technique (VRT)].

The major advantages of CT angiography (CTA) over a digital subtraction angiography (DSA) of the aorta are visualization of the wall and its surrounding changes, pathologies like intramural hematoma (IMH), rapid imaging, identification of branch vessels, etc. The major limitation includes lack of "flow quantification".

TABLE 1: Maximal normal aortic diameter and aneurysm size critera.[1]

Segment	*Maximal normal aortic diameter (cm)*	*Aneurysm size criteria (cm)*
Ascending	4	5
DTA	3	4
Abdominal	2	3

(DTA: descending thoracic aneurysm)

MRI and MR Angiography Protocol

Major advantages of MRI are lack of radiation (hence suited for follow-ups), flow quantification as well as identification. Several techniques are available:

- Three-dimensional contrast-enhanced MR angiography (3D CE MRA) workhorse for imaging aorta. It also allows multiplanar reformations (MPRs) like CTA. Gadolinium (0.1 mmol/kg body weight) is injected as contrast agent with a flow rate of 2–5 mL per second, followed by a saline flush of 20 mL (Fig. 2).
- *White blood imaging (static and cine):* Noncontrast 3D steady-state free-precession [SSFP; fast imaging employing steady-state acquisition (FIESTA), TrueFISP—most preferred], two-dimensional (2D) cine SSFP. It is a short repetition time (TE) and echo time (TR) sequence, which provides very high and homogenous intraluminal signal even in cases of turbulent flow.
- *Black blood imaging:* Static imaging-spin echo T2 2D images. Short tau inversion recovery (STIR) sequence is restricted for demonstration of wall edema and recommended to demonstrate aortic wall pathology such as mural hematoma and aortoarteritis.
- *Phase contrast (PC) sequences:* For flow quantification in aortic regurgitation, stenosis, congenital heart diseases, and coarctation of aorta.

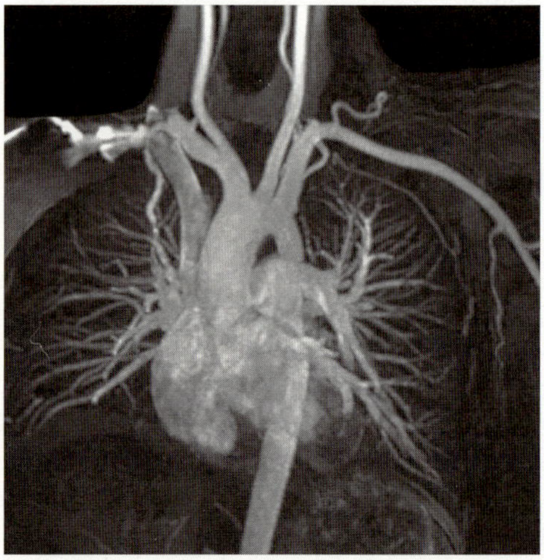

Fig. 2: Three-dimensional maximum intensity projections image at contrast-enhanced magnetic resonance angiography showing aortic arch, ascending and descending thoracic aorta and its major branches.

ACQUIRED AORTIC PATHOLOGIES

Aortic Aneurysm

Thoracic Aortic Aneurysm

Measurements: An aneurysm is defined as permanent localized dilation of the aorta, either 50% or 2 standard deviations larger than normal expected diameter at a given anatomic level.[3] Table 2 gives simplified values for diagnosis of aneurysm considering that a diameter equaling or exceeding 1.5 times the expected normal diameter is considered an aneurysm.

Epidemiology: The prevalence of aortic aneurysms increases with the age of the patient, the incidence being approximately 450/100,000 and a 3:1 male predominance. In up to one-third of cases, the abdominal aorta is also involved.[5]

Causes: Atherosclerosis is the overall most common cause of aneurysm, accounting for 70% of these cases. Cystic medial degeneration is the most common cause of ascending aortic aneurysm. It is most frequently caused by Marfan syndrome. Atherosclerosis is the most common cause of descending thoracic aneurysm (DTA). 60% of patients have systemic hypertension. Other causes of aortic aneurysm include Ehlers-Danlos syndrome, Loeys-Dietz syndrome, syphilis and other infections, arteritis, aortic dissection (AD), congenital medial degeneration, bicuspid aortic valve, or trauma.[6]

Types: In true aneurysms, all three layers of the aortic wall (intima, media, and adventitia) are involved in aneurysm formation. In false aneurysms (also referred to as pseudoaneurysms), the intima and often media is disrupted, and blood is contained by the adventitia and periadventitial tissues. Post-traumatic pseudoaneurysms are usually seen in the aortic isthmus (90%), whereas penetrating aortic ulcer (PAU) occurs in the descending aorta.[7] Syphilitic aneurysms have an incidence of 12% and they are prone to rupture.[6] In patients with bicuspid valve, an inherent aortopathy results in aortic dilatation. Aortitis in rheumatological disorders like ankylosing spondylitis, rheumatoid arthritis, etc. also involve the ascending aorta. Takayasu arteritis commonly affects the aortic arch and branches.

True aortic aneurysms are usually fusiform in shape, pseudoaneurysms are usually saccular. Mycotic aneurysms usually have a wide neck and are saccular. Because the areas affected by infective endocarditis are usually near the ascending aorta, mycotic aneurysms usually affect the ascending aorta.[7]

TABLE 2: Modified Crawford classification of thoracoabdominal aneurysms.[8]

Type	*Anatomical location involved*
Type I	DTA below the origin of the LSCA and the suprarenal abdominal aorta
Type II	Both the DTA and most of the abdominal aorta (including infrarenal)
Type III	From the level of sixth intercostal space to infrarenal abdominal aorta
Type IV	From level of 12th intercostal space to below the renal arteries (total abdominal aortic aneurysm)
Type V	From level of sixth intercostal space to above the renal arteries

(DTA: descending thoracic aneurysm; LSCA: left subclavian artery)

Abdominal Aortic Aneurysms (AAA)

Atherosclerosis is the most common cause. Diameter of more than 3 cm is considered diagnostic of an AAA. AAA most often involves the infrarenal segment of the aorta.

Thoracoabdominal Aneurysms

Thoracoabdominal aneurysms can be classified based on location using the modified Crawford classification system (Table 2).[8] Of these four types, types II and III represent the greatest therapeutic challenge.

Imaging in Aortic Aneurysms

On both MDCT and MRI, the key features for assessment of aneurysms are: (a) maximal aortic diameter; (b) shape and extent; (c) involvement of aortic branches; (d) relationship to adjacent structures, such as the bronchi and esophagus; presence of mural thrombus; (e) detection of aortic calcifications (MDCT); (f) other relevant structures, such as the coronary arteries and the intercostal arterial supply to the spinal cord at the lower thoracic-upper lumbar level. Both CT and MRI show excellent accuracy for characterizing these features.[9]

Multidetector Computed Tomography

Common techniques that should be applied to all imaging protocols to provide optimal spatial and temporal resolution are: (1) utilization of the maximum detector array; (2) bolus-timing for optimization of contrast delivery timing; (3) thin-section acquisition; and (4) administration of at least 100 mL of nonionic contrast material (preferably 350 mg I/mL) injected at rapid infusion rates (4–5 mL/s) with a target opacification of the aorta greater than 250 HU.[10] Widely available postprocessing techniques include MPR, MIP, curved planar reformation, and 3D volume rendering (Figs. 3 and 4). MPRs (curved planar reformations) are

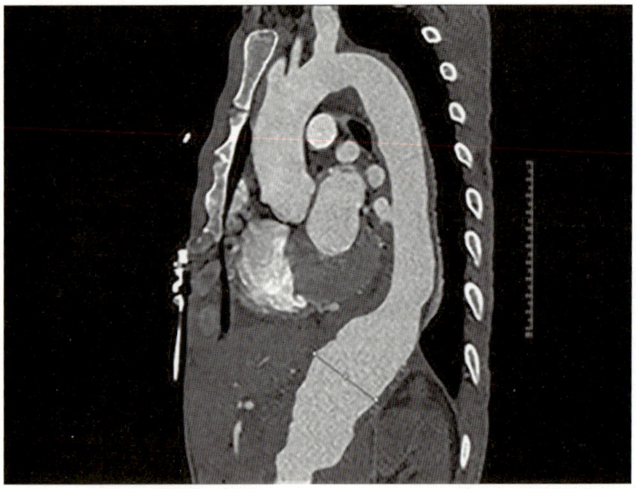

Fig. 3: Computed tomography angiography showing fusiform aneurysm of abdominal aorta.

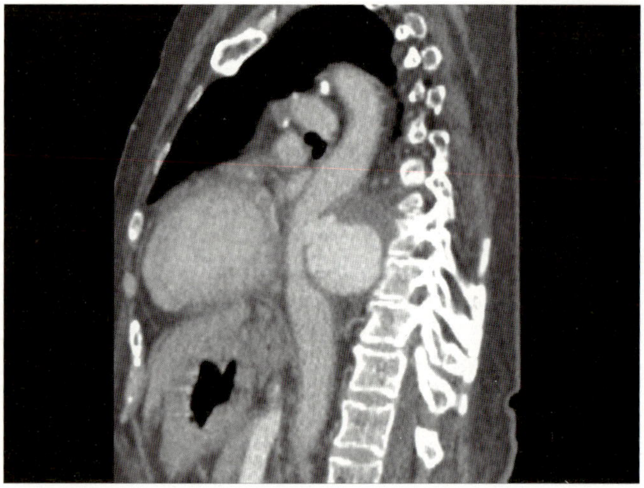

Fig. 5: Computed tomography angiography showing a saccular aneurysm of descending thoracic aneurysm.

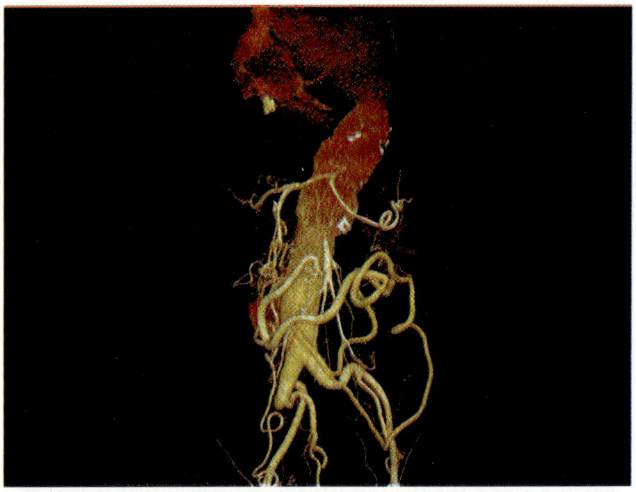

Fig. 4: Volume rendered image of computed tomography angiography showing fusiform aneurysm of abdominal aorta.

more accurate in estimating the aneurysmal diameter compared with axial images. MIP, a technique that highlights the highest-attenuation voxels, has relatively limited applications because simultaneous display and distinction of the contrast-enhanced flow lumen and mural calcifications are usually not possible. Calculation of aneurysm volume provides the most accurate measure of aneurysm size, but this method is time-consuming.[10,11]

Computed tomography clearly has advantages as it shows the presence of wall calcification as well as the low attenuation crescentic thrombus. A thrombus is usually peripheral to the patent lumen, low in density, and located internal to mural calcifications from the luminal side (Fig. 5). It can be differentiated from IMH which usually has a smooth margin, has a high attenuation and is located external to the intimal calcification (within the media).

Magnetic Resonance Imaging

Three-dimensional contrast-enhanced MRA is highly accurate at depicting the location, extent, and precise diameter of an aneurysm and its relationship to the aortic branch vessels. On spin-echo MRI images, the patent lumen has signal void and thrombus has intermediate signal intensity. However, a known pitfall of this technique is an intraluminal signal produced by slow flow that may mimic intraluminal thrombus. This problem may be avoided by combining spin-echo with gradient-recalled echo (GRE) cine MRI or contrast-enhanced MRA.[12] With MRA, particularly on MIPs, only the lumen is seen, and the aneurysm size is underestimated.[13] So, measurements should be obtained from source images on which the vessel wall is visible. Recently, real-time, bright blood, cine imaging has been introduced and is referred to as balanced SSFP, TrueFISP, and FIESTA by various vendors. Contrast enhancement is determined on the basis of the ratio of T2 to T1 rather than on the basis of inflow effects, which eliminates sensitivity to saturation effects from absent or slow flow.[14] Because of its lack of ionizing radiation, MRI is especially useful in patients with either contraindications to iodinated contrast material or in those with known aneurysms who require sequential follow-up with multiple examinations (Figs. 6 and 7).

Complications

The most frequent complications of aortic aneurysm—mass effect, dissection, and rupture—are directly related to size. The mean rate of dilatation for thoracic aortic aneurysm is 0.12 cm per year.[15] The risk of rupture increases with increasing aortic diameter as demonstrated in Table 3.

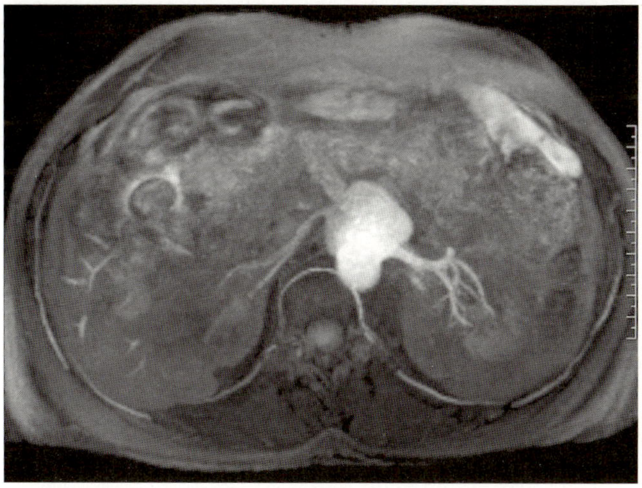

Fig. 6: Axial TrueFISP image showing abdominal aortic aneurysm.

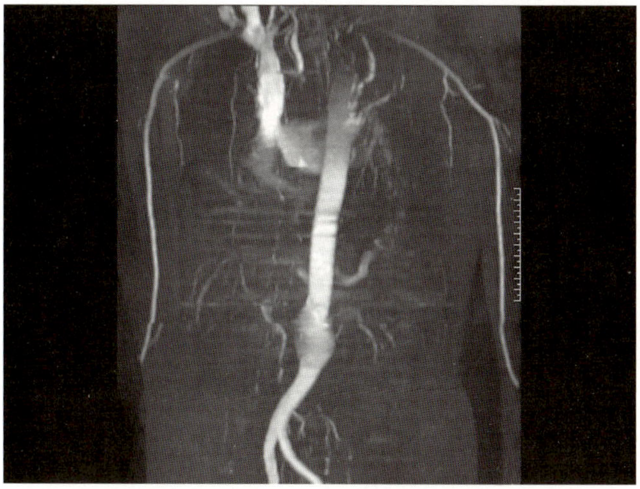

Fig. 7: Magnetic resonance angiography three-dimensional image showing abdominal aortic aneurysm.

TABLE 3: Risk of rupture of abdominal aortic aneurysms.[1]

Aneurysm size (cm)	*Yearly risk (%)*
<4	0
4–5	0.5–5
5–6	10–20
6–8	20–30
>8	30–50

Computed tomography angiography is the technique of choice for evaluation of suspected aortic rupture. Diagnostic findings include active contrast extravasation or high-attenuation collections in the pleura, pericardium, or mediastinum, retroperitoneum, etc. Enlargement of psoas shadow may be subtle and sometimes only sign of bleed. A draped aorta sign, defined as the posterior wall of the aorta closely following the contour of adjacent vertebral bodies, may be seen in a contained rupture of the posterior aortic wall. Impending rupture may be seen as a crescent of high-attenuation contrast material within the mural thrombus.[16] Another complication of AAA is aorto-duodenal fistula, which may cause catastrophic bleeding. CT shows loss of the normal fat plane between the aorta and duodenum and the presence of air in the aorta.[16]

Treatment and Outcomes

Indications for treatment of aortic aneurysms:

- Ascending or AAA more than or equal to 5.5 cm diameter, DTA aneurysm more than 6 cm.
- Symptomatic aneurysms regardless of size:
  - Contained-rupture AAA.
  - Inflammatory AAA.
- Rapidly expanding (>5 mm/6 months) AAA.
- High-risk for complication with open surgery.

In patients with Marfan syndrome, surgery is usually performed when the ascending aorta exceeds 4.5 cm. Endovascular aortic repair is increasingly used as an alternative to open surgical repair, especially among patients who are poor surgical candidates.[15]

Descending thoracic aneurysm: An attractive alternative to open surgical repair is endovascular repair where the anatomy is suited for stent graft placement. Stent-grafts function by depressurizing the aneurysm sac. CT scan is used for determining suitability for endovascular repair of descending thoracic aortic aneurysms. The prerequisites for endovascular repair are at least 15 mm distance between the origin of LSCA and the proximal end of aneurysm or between the origin of celiac artery and the distal end of aneurysm, a distance of at least 25 mm between origin of LCCA and aneurysm; maximum aortic diameter in landing zone not more than 4 cm; and absence of thrombus or atheroma in the landing zone.[6] In addition, the common femoral artery diameter of more than 7 mm is deemed suitable for device delivery. AAA-stent-graft repair of thoracoabdominal aneurysms requires either a hybrid procedure with surgical debranching of the abdominal aortic branches followed by stent-graft placement, or branched stent-grafts. Multilayered flow modulator devices and stents are currently being developed for treatment of true fusiform aneurysm and holds promise for future application. Infrarenal AAA which fulfills the criteria for treatment may be treated by placement of a stent-graft or surgery. Most patients treated with current devices receive bifurcated stent-grafts.

ACUTE AORTIC SYNDROMES

Aortic Dissection

Pathophysiology and Classification

Aortic dissection is the most common acute aortic disorder, with an incidence up to 0.2–0.8%, and also carries the highest mortality rate. It is caused by an intimal tear within an abnormal, weakened vessel wall. Classification is on the basis of Stanford or DeBakey systems (Table 4). "Stanford classification" is universally followed now. Approximately 70% of dissections are type A (those involving ascending aorta). Type A carries high mortality and morbidity and requires urgent surgical intervention.[17]

Clinical Features

Patients with acute dissection usually present with chest pain radiating to the back, syncope, and shortness of breath. Acute AD is defined as dissection detected within 2 weeks of the onset of symptoms. The major risk factor for AD is systemic hypertension, followed by cystic medial necrosis, congenital lesions (such as bicuspid aortic valve and aortic coarctation), pregnancy, smoking, trauma, and arteritis.[18]

TABLE 4: Classification of aortic dissection.

DeBakey type	*Involvement*	*Stanford type*
I	Originates in the ascending aorta and extends to a variable distance beyond the aortic arch	A
II	Confined to ascending aorta	A
III	Originates distal to the LSCA. It is subclassified into type IIIA (up to diaphragm) and type IIIB (below diaphragm)	B

Imaging in Aortic Dissection

The goal of imaging is to achieve:

- Differentiation of true and false lumen.
- Location of intimal tears.
- Precise measurements of the extent of dissection.
- Coronary artery ostia integrity.
- Identify complications: Pleural or pericardial effusion, rupture, organ malperfusion, carotid artery dissection and stroke, acute aortic insufficiency.

Computed tomography angiography: CTA begins with an noncontrast CT (NCCT) to rule out IMH, followed by gated contrast scan. Table 5 summarizes the CT imaging findings in acute aortic syndromes. Differentiation between true and false lumens of AD is important in planning of percutaneous endovascular grafts or surgical repair (Fig. 8; Table 6). It is

TABLE 5: Computed tomography imaging findings in acute aortic syndromes.

Disease	*Noncontrast CT*	*Contrast CT*
Aortic dissection	Intimal calcification is medially displaced	Intimal flap, Cobweb sign (strands) in false lumen
Intramural hematoma	High attenuation crescent in aortic wall outside intimal calcification	Aortic wall-thickening (cannot appreciate the crescent well)
Penetrating atherosclerotic ulcer	Ulcer/outpouching adjacent to plaque	Ulcer penetrating the intima into the aortic wall

(CT: computed tomography)

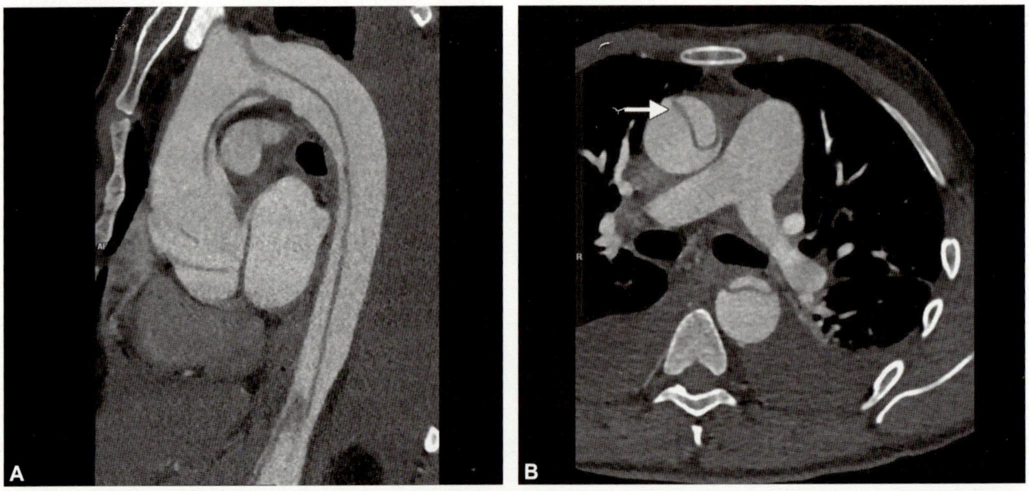

Figs. 8A and B: (A) Computed tomography angiography(CTA) oblique sagittal image showing type A aortic dissection involving both ascending and descending aorta; (B) CTA axial image showing type A aortic dissection (arrow showing dissection flap).

TABLE 6: Computed tomography features for differentiating true from false lumen.

S No	Features	True lumen	False lumen
1.	Continuity of lumen with lumen of uninvolved portion of aorta (most reliable)	+	–
2.	Direction of free edges of the dissection flap at entrance tear	–	+
3.	Aortic Cobweb	–	+
4.	Outer wall calcification	+	–
5.	Beak sign	–	+
6.	Thrombosis	–/+	+/+
7.	Peak flow	Faster	Slower
8.	Size	Smaller and compressed	Larger and toward intimal concavity

critical to identify the lumen of origin of coronary, carotid, renal, and mesenteric arteries before treatment.[17] CTA is also a useful modality to assess the remodeling of aorta after stent grafting in the follow-up period (Figs. 9 and 10).

Triple-rule out: "Triple-rule out" is a relatively new term that describes an ECG-gated 64-MDCT angiography study to evaluate patients with acute chest pain for three potential causes: AD, pulmonary embolism, and coronary artery dissection.

MRI: It has been shown to be an effective alternative technique to CT for evaluation of AD with a reported sensitivity and specificity of 98%. Black blood imaging shows the intimal flap as thin linear structure in the aortic flow void. True lumen shows preservation of the flow void whereas the false lumen is seen as area of increased signal intensity. Phase contrast images can be done to identify aortic insufficiency, intimal tear sites and to differentiate slow flow from thrombus in the false lumen. A pulsation artefact may mimic dissection (Fig. 11).

Treatment

A mnemonic-based approach to the evaluation of AD, the DISSECT (duration, intimal tear, size of aorta, segmental extend of involvement, clinical complications, and thrombosis of false lumen) classification system guides the radiologist through an assessment of characteristics that facilitate a complete description of the most salient details that currently influence the selection of a treatment (Table 7). Acute type A AD constitutes a surgical emergency since these patients are at high-risk for a life-threatening

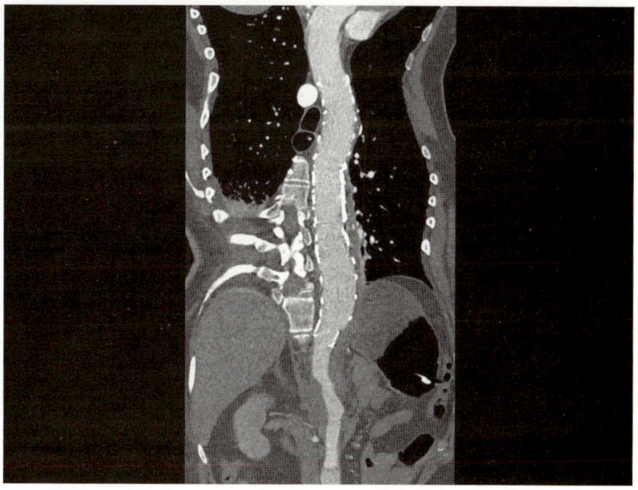

Fig. 9: Straightened multiplanar reformation of the aorta with stent-graft in situ.

complications such as aortic regurgitation, cardiac tamponade, frank rupture, and myocardial infarction. Medical management has a mortality of up to 50%. At certain centers, a hybrid approach to the repair of type A AD, referred to as the "frozen elephant trunk repair," may be attempted. This involves combination of an open approach to surgically repair the ascending aorta, while deploying a stent-graft to manage the descending aorta.

Type B dissection is generally managed initially with best medical therapy. Intervention (surgical or endovascular) for descending thoracic AD is reserved for patients who develop complications as described in Table 7. Interventional management consists of placing a stent-graft over the proximal entry tear which depressurizes the false lumen and restores normal flow in the true lumen. The endograft should be sized to the estimated diameter of the true lumen.

A summary of the prerequisites for interventional management is given in Table 8.

Successful stent-graft deployment requires proximal and distal landing zones of nondiseased aorta to be at least 15 mm. However, if the landing zones are inadequate, endovascular (use of branched stent graft, chimney, or snorkel technique) or surgical debranching techniques can be used to extend the landing zones. Using the classification proposed by Criado et al. landing zones can be classified into five types (Fig. 12). An endovascular procedure with proximal landing zones at zone 3 and 4 is a favorable situation.

Intramural Hematoma

Intramural hematoma is defined as a bleeding of the vasa vasorum in the medial layer of the aorta, with no blood flow within the media. The IMH is considered as a

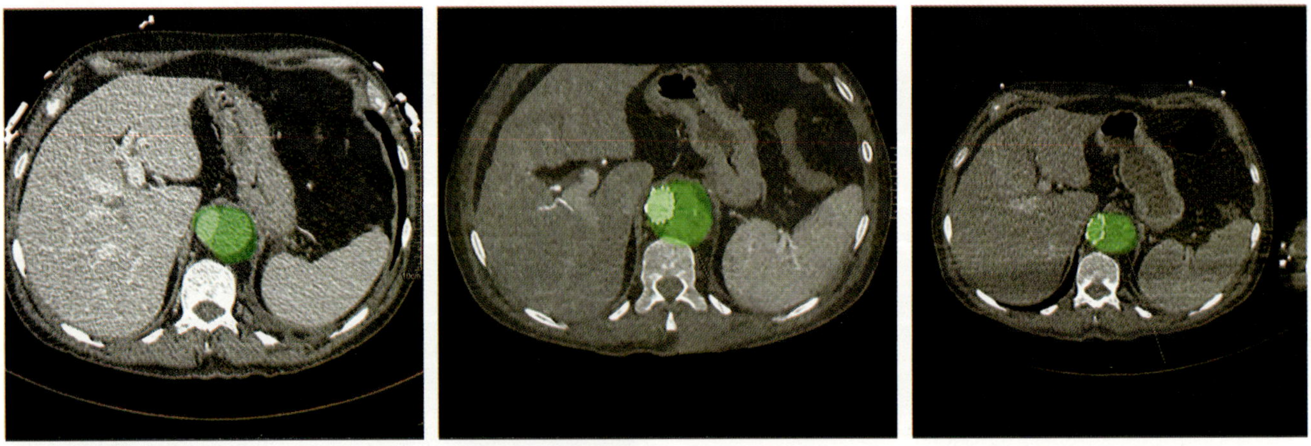

Fig. 10: Software-based calculation of the true and false lumen volumes in the follow-up scan of a stent-graft.

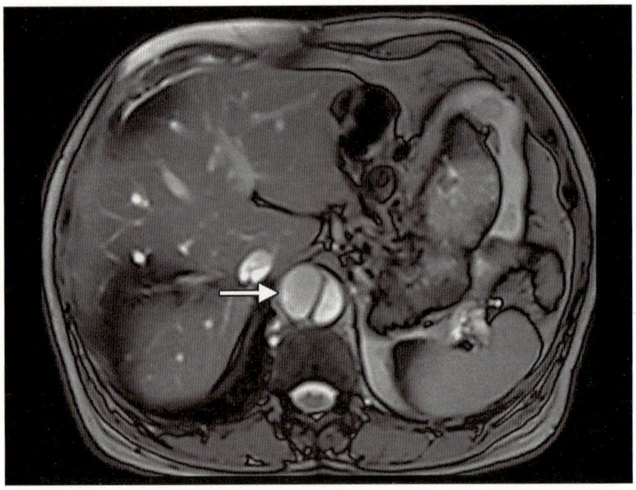

Fig. 11: Axial magnetic resonance image showing dissection flap.

TABLE 7: DISSECT classification.

D: Duration of symptoms	*Acute:* <2 weeks from onset of symptoms *Subacute:* 2 weeks to 3 months after symptom onset *Chronic:* >3 months from initial symptoms
I: Intimal tear location	Ascending aorta, aortic arch, descending aorta, abdominal aorta, unknown
S: Sizes	Maximum aortic diameter at any level
SE: Segmental extent	Proximal entry and distal re-entry tear locations
C: Complications	• Cardiac tamponade • Rupture • Branch vessel malperfusion • Static and/or dynamic branch involvement with accompanying stroke, paraplegia, coronary, mesenteric, visceral, renal, and/or extremity symptoms • Progression of aortic involvement with proximal or distal extension of dissection • Involvement of aortic valve in case of type A dissection • Others – Uncontrollable hypertension – Uncontrollable clinical symptoms – Rapid false lumen dilation – Overall transaortic enlargement of >10 mm within the first 2 weeks of initial diagnosis
T: Thrombosis of false lumen	Patent, completely or partially thrombosed

precursor of AD. This entity constitutes 10–20% of acute aortic syndromes.

Systemic hypertension is the leading risk factor for IMH. IMH most frequently involves the ascending or proximal descending aorta, up to 70% of cases. IMH is classified in the same way as AD: type A when the ascending aorta is involved and type B when involvement is limited to the descending aorta.

Imaging

Computed tomography angiography: When evaluating the aorta using MDCT, an unenhanced acquisition is crucial for diagnosis. It appears as a high-attenuation crescentic thickening in the wall of the aorta external to the intimal calcification, extending longitudinally. Infrequently, however, the differentiation of IMH from either atherosclerotic thickening of the aorta, thrombus, or thrombosed dissection may be difficult at CT. In such settings, MRI can be a valuable problem-solving tool, especially when dynamic cine gradient-echo sequences are applied. Imaging findings on CTA include: (a) Focal

TABLE 8: Prerequisites for interventional management of dissection.

Proximal landing zone	At least 1.5 cm normal aorta distal to LSCA. If unavailable debranching procedures to extend the proximal landing zone
Distal landing zone	1.5–2 cm normal aorta above celiac artery
Severe angulation of proximal or distal aorta	Longer landing zones needed which may necessitate debranching
Patency and caliber of pelvic arteries	Minimal CFA diameter required 7 mm

(CFA: common femoral artery; LSCA: left subclavian artery)

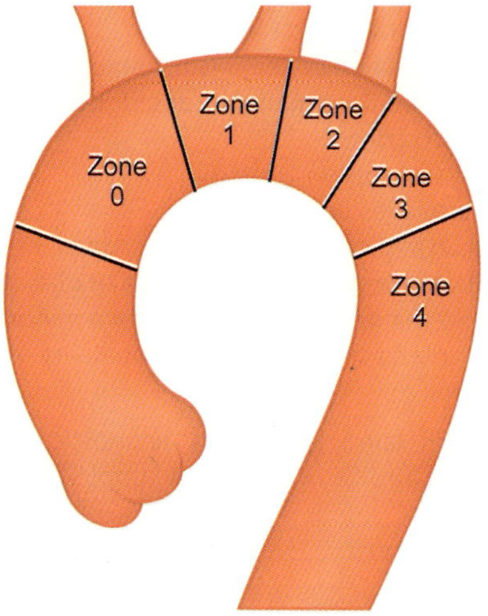

Fig. 12: Landing zones proposed by Criado.

aortic wall-thickening (crescentic more than concentric); (b) Preserved luminal shape with smooth luminal border; (c) Absence of dissection flap and false lumen; (d) Central displacement of intimal calcium. Several findings on initial CT examination have been shown to predict progression, including aneurysm formation, PAU, development of pleural effusion, and wall thickness of 10 mm or greater (Fig. 13).

Magnetic resonance imaging: MRI may also provide a determination of the age of a hematoma based on the signal characteristics of different degradation products of hemoglobin. For example, T1-weighted spin-echo images show intermediate signal intensity caused by the presence of oxyhemoglobin in the acute stage and high signal intensity caused by the presence of methemoglobin in the subacute stage.[19]

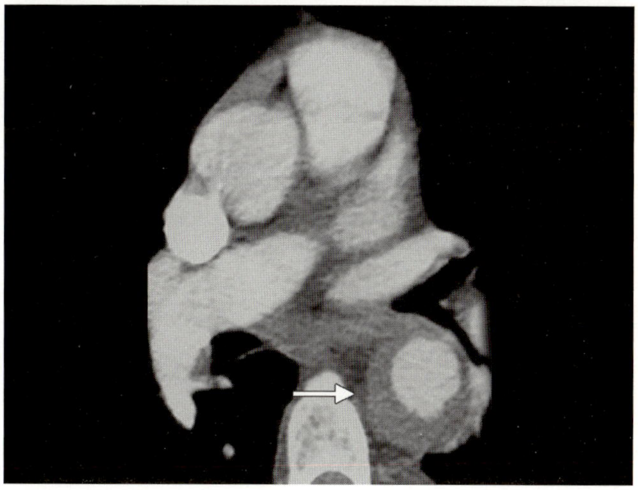

Fig. 13: Computed tomography angiography image showing acute aortic intramural hematoma (arrow).

Treatment and Clinical Outcome

Surgical management is the treatment of choice for type A IMH. As with AD, most patients with type B IMH have a good short-term outcome with aggressive control of hypertension. Close follow-up imaging during the first 30 days of presentation is recommended for all patients treated medically. Surgical or endovascular treatment is considered if there is increase in the extent of IMH, progressive dilatation of the lumen, presence of penetrating ulcer or development of dissection.

Penetrating Aortic Ulcer

Penetrating aortic ulcer occurs when ulceration of atherosclerotic plaque disrupts the intima with subsequent extension of the blood into the media. PAU can cause IMH, extend along the media, or rarely may progress into frank dissection or rupture through the adventitia. These lesions represent 2–7% of all acute aortic syndrome. Elderly hypertensive patients are most frequently affected, and the mid descending thoracic aorta is most commonly (90%) involved.

Imaging

Contrast-enhanced MDCT is the imaging modality of choice for diagnosis of PAU. A focal ulceration penetrating through the aortic intima into the media of the aortic wall is the characteristic finding. Localized high-attenuation thickening of the adjacent aorta is suggestive of associated IMH. Limitation of MRI is that it is unable to detect displacement of intimal calcification, which frequently accompanies PAU (Fig. 14).

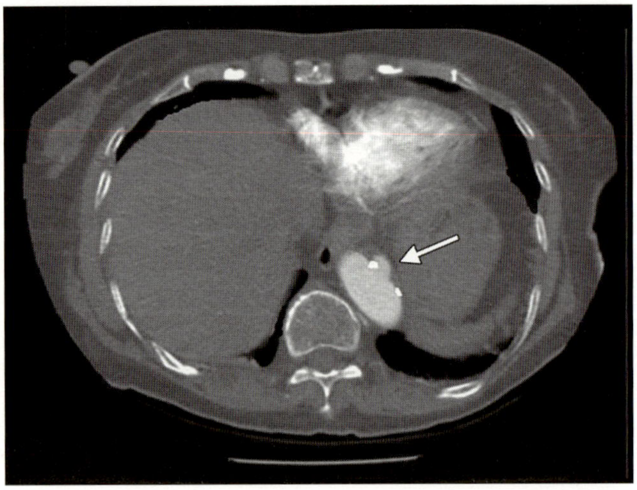

Fig. 14: Computed tomography angiography image showing penetrating aortic ulcer (arrow).

Treatment and Outcome

Surgery is advocated in patients with ascending aortic ulcerations. Although most patients with PAU in the descending aorta can be managed conservatively, progression to aneurysm formation, rupture, or dissection has been reported in up to 40% of patients. Some authors suggest that a symptomatic ulceration that is 20 mm in diameter or greater, or 10 mm in depth, should be managed aggressively.[19]

TABLE 9: Modified diagnostic criteria for Takayasu arteritis.

Three major criteria
1. Left mid subclavian artery lesion.
2. Right mid subclavian artery lesion.
3. Characteristic signs and symptoms of at least one month duration (limb claudication, pulselessness or pulse differences in limbs, an unobtainable or significant blood pressure difference (>10 mm Hg systolic blood pressure difference in limb), fever, neck, pain, transient amaurosis, blurred vision, syncope, dyspnea or palpitations).
Ten minor criteria
1. High erythrocyte sedimentation rate (ESR).
2. Carotid artery tenderness.
3. Hypertension.
4. Aortic regurgitation or annuloaortic ectasia.
5. Pulmonary artery lesion.
6. Left mid common carotid lesion.
7. Distal brachiocephalic trunk lesion.
8. Descending thoracic aorta lesion. Narrowing, dilatation or aneurysm, luminal irregularity or any combination determined by angiography: tortuosity alone is unacceptable.
9. Abdominal aorta lesion.
10. Coronary artery lesion.
Documented on angiography below the age of 30 years in the absence of risk factors like hyperlipidemia or diabetes mellitus.
Presence of two major or one major and two minor criteria or four minor criteria suggests a high probability of Takayasu arteritis.

Source: Sharma BK, Jain S, Suri S, et al. Diagnostic criteria for Takayasu arteritis. Int J Cardiol. 1996;54 Suppl:S141-7.

AORTITIS

Takayasu Arteritis

Takayasu arteritis is a large vessel panarteritis of unknown etiology that affects the aorta and its major branches including the pulmonary and coronary arteries. Young Asian women are predisposed to this disease. Modified diagnostic criteria for Takayasu arteritis by Sharma et al. have led to an early diagnosis of this condition thereby preventing high morbidity and mortality (Table 9).

Types

- *Type I*: Involves only the branches of the aortic arch.
- *Type IIa*: Involves the aorta only at its ascending portion and/or at the aortic arch. The branches of the aortic arch may be involved as well. The rest of the aorta is not affected.
- *Type IIb*: Affects the descending thoracic aorta with or without involvement of the ascending aorta or the aortic arch with its branches. The abdominal aorta is not involved.
- *Type III*: It is the concomitant involvement of the descending thoracic aorta, the abdominal aorta, and/or the renal arteries. The ascending aorta and the aortic arch and its branches are not involved.
- *Type IV*: Involves only the abdominal aorta and/or the renal arteries.
- *Type V*: It is a generalized type, with combined features of the other types.

Note: Involvement of the coronary and pulmonary arteries should be indicated as C(+) or P(+), respectively.

The commonly involved arteries are LSCA (50%), left common carotid (20%), brachiocephalic, renal arteries, celiac trunk, SMA and pulmonary arteries (50%).

Imaging Findings

The main imaging modalities are CT, MRI and /or positron emission tomography (PET) CT/MRI. Role of conventional angiography in Takayasu arteritis is now restricted for interventional procedures.

Early/acute stage: There is mural thickening that is detected on CT or MRI (fat suppressed T1-weighted postcontrast MR images) with circumferential peripheral contrast enhancement (inflamed media and adventitia).

On T2-weighted sequences wall edema is seen as high-signal intensity. PET with 2-deoxy-2-[fluorine-18]fluoro-D-glucose (^{18}F-FDG PET) with either CT or MRI is now emerging as the initial diagnosis and assessment of disease activity with high sensitivity of 60–90% and specificity of 88–100% as 18F-FDG is a surrogate marker of increased activity of inflammatory cells (Fig. 15).

Chronic stage: The disease is characterized by development of wall irregularities and stenoses. There may be long diffuse or short segmental irregular stenosis with occlusion of the major branches of the aorta near its origin. There may be presence of skip lesions, abundant collateralization, saccular or fusiform aortic aneurysm (10–15%). These findings can be depicted on conventional angiography, CTA or MRA. Cross-sectional imaging, in addition, shows arterial wall-thickening, mural calcium deposition and full thickness calcification which is very suggestive of chronic phase of disease.

Management

Active Takayasu arteritis is treated with steroids or immunosuppressants before revascularization as revascularization during the active phase can increase the risk of procedure-related complications, including restenosis and dissection. Occlusion/restenosis rates in transluminal angioplasty with or without stent implantation in active disease is reported to be as high as 71.4% after a follow-up of 1.3 years. Symptomatic Takayasu arteritis is treated with revascularization of the affected vessels. In the chronic fibrotic stage, the principle of treatment is revascularization either by surgery or balloon angioplasty.[20]

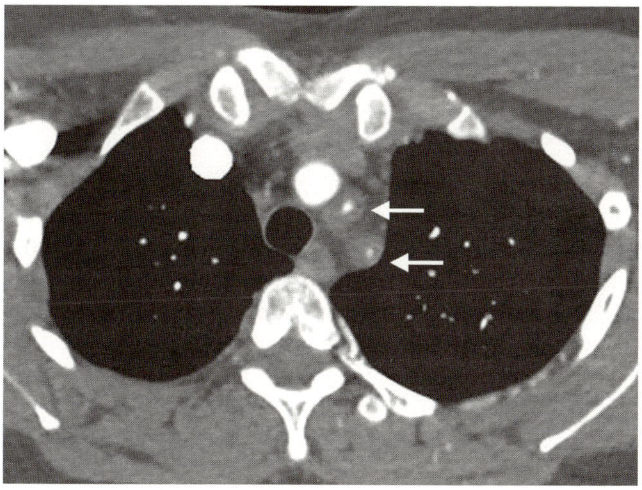

Fig. 15: Takayasu arteritis: Computed tomography angiography source image showing circumferential mural thickening of the lateral common carotid and subclavian arteries (arrows).

TUBERCULAR AORTITIS AND PSEUDOANEURYSMS

Tubercular aneurysm is a well-known complication of tuberculosis especially in Indian subcontinent where the prevalence of the disease is so high. It usually affects the young individuals in the age group of 20–50 years.

Pathology and Presentation

Aorta is involved by hematogenous route or direct extension. Direct extension appears to be the commoner route. Usually there is a focus of tuberculosis near these lesions, in the form of mediastinal nodes or pericardial/pleural involvement. Hence, tubercular pseudoaneurysms usually involve the ascending aorta (10.2%), distal arch of aorta (11.4%), DTA (28.4%), and infrarenal abdominal aorta (42%). The patients may present with fever, pain, hypovolemic shock due to rupture or enlarging paraaortic mass.

Imaging

These aneurysms are most commonly pseudoaneurysms (87%). Occasionally, true (9%) or dissecting (4%) aneurysms can also be seen. CTA findings are like other pseudoaneurysms of aorta (narrow neck, associated hematoma with or without signs of rupture-extravasation of contrast). Tell-tale signs of tuberculosis are usually present in the form of mediastinal lymphadenopathy/parenchymal lesions/pleural or pericardial lesions. 65% of tubercular pseudoaneurysms tend to rupture (Figs. 16A to C).

The management usually involves surgical repair (graft interposition, patch repair) combined with antitubercular treatment.[21]

AORTIC TRAUMA

Traumatic injuries to the aorta can be caused by either blunt or sharp (direct) trauma. Stab or bullet wounds that puncture the aortic wall are the major penetrating traumatic injuries. Blunt aortic injuries (BAIs) are most common and the aortic wall is damaged from the intima to the adventitia. High-speed accidents cause sudden deceleration which lead to torsion and a shearing stress at the isthmus where the aorta is relatively fixed, and causes traumatic injury/transection at isthumus. "Osseous pinch" effect is due to pinching of the aorta between the manubrium and medial end of clavicle anteriorly and spine posteriorly. About 90% of traumatic tears occur around the isthmus. The other sites include aortic arch with avulsion of brachiocephalic trunk (4.5%), ascending aorta (1%), and descending aorta (2.5%).

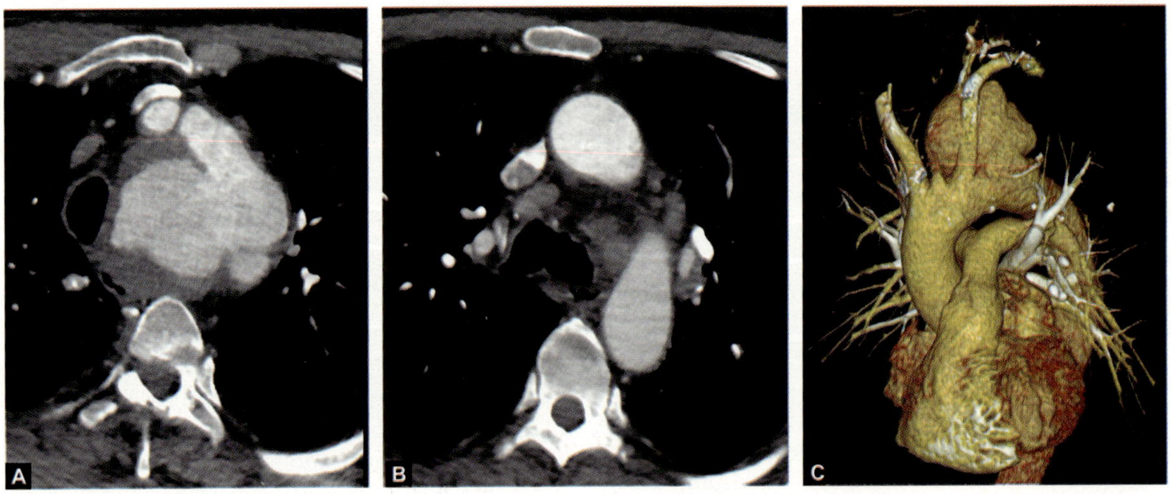

Figs. 16A to C: (A) Tubercular pseudoaneurysm of arch of aorta with adjacent hematoma; (B) Axial section in the same patient shows mediastinal lymph nodes; (C) Volume rendered technique (VRT) images show the relationship of the pseudoaneurysm with arch vessels.

Grading of aortic injuries:

- Grade 0: Normal mediastinum and normal aorta
- Grade I: Abnormal mediastinum and normal aorta
- Grade II: Minimal aortic injury
- Grade III: Confined aortic injury
- Grade IV: Aortic disruption

Imaging

Computed Tomography

Plain CT may demonstrate mediastinal hematoma. Contrast-enhanced CT (CECT) may show an abrupt change in aortic contour, intimal flap, pseudoaneurysm, pseudocoarctation, and extravasation of contrast. CTA shows 96.2% sensitivity, 99.8% specificity, and 99.7% accuracy for the diagnosis of aortic injury.

Magnetic Resonance Imaging

In an acute setting of multiple injuries, MR is not recommended.

CONGENITAL AORTIC ANOMALIES

Coarctation of Aorta

It is congenital narrowing in the region of isthumus and is more common in males. There are two types:

- *Adult or juxta-ductal type*: Most common type where there is a short-segment narrowing close to the ligamentum arteriosum.
- *Infantile or preductal type*: There is tubular hypoplasia of the aortic arch after origin of BCA. Coexistent cardiac anomalies are common.

The collateral circulation distal to the coarctation is through the subclavian arteries and its branches—internal mammary artery to intercostal arteries, scapular artery to anterior spinal artery and transverse cervical artery to lateral thoracic artery. Associated anomalies generally include bicuspid aortic valve (25–50%), cardiac shunts: patent ductus arteriosus (PDA; 33%), ventricular septal defect (VSD; 15%), Turner's syndrome (13–15%), cerebral berry aneurysms (5–7%), etc. A review of the natural history of coarctation revealed that of those patients who survived infancy, 20% were dead before the age of 20 years, 50% by 32 years, and 90% by 58 years. Most common causes of death are due to cardiac failure, aortic rupture, infective endocarditis, intracerebral hemorrhage, etc.

Role of Computed Tomography Angiography

Computed tomography angiography can depict the morphology of the coarcted segment with good spatial resolution as well as status of aortic arch vessels and collaterals. However, it is not able to measure the gradient across the lesion, nor the direction of the flow. Still it is an important adjuvant in stent-graft implantation and follow-up imaging after surgery (Figs. 17A and B).

Role of Magnetic Resonance Angiography

Phase-contrast velocity-encoded cine MR can give reliable information regarding flow velocity, flow volume, and the pressure gradient across the stenosed segment. Also, it can give information regarding the collaterals and the direction of flow in them. Though this technique is promising its use

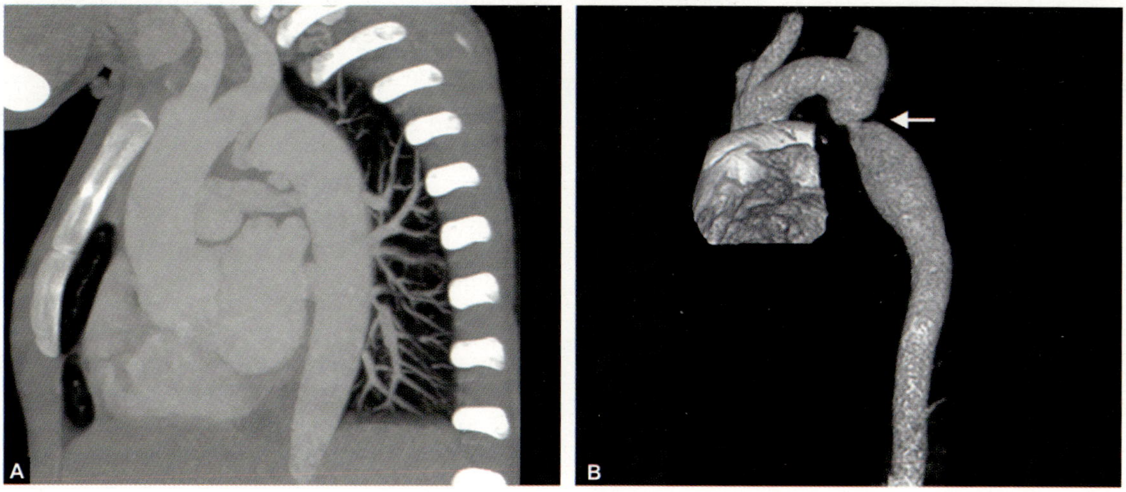

Figs. 17A and B: (A) Computed tomography angiography (CTA) maximum intensity projections image shows coarctation of aorta (postductal); (B) CTA volume rendered three-dimensional image showing coarctation of aorta (arrow).

in routine clinical practice is limited because it also suffers from certain drawbacks like underestimation of flow volume and velocity and also is poor in small vessel assessment.

Differential Diagnoses

- Pseudocoarctation is a condition that results from an elongation of the distal aortic arch which, as it is fixed at the arterial ligament, bulges backward above and below this point causing a "double-aortic" bulge. There is no hemodynamic obstruction.
- Interrupted aortic arch is a rare condition in which a localized atresia of the arch occurs distal to the LSCA (type A: 42%), distal to the LCCA (type B: 53%) or distal to the brachiocephalic trunk (type C: 5%). It is usually associated with various cardiac anomalies like PDA and VSD.

Management

Guidelines recommend that coarctation correction should be performed as early as possible (ideally as early as possible in childhood) to reduce the long-term morbidity. Percutaneous interventions and surgical correction are both acceptable options for coarctation repair.

Indications for corrective treatment include:

- Peak to peak (or maximum instantaneous) coarctation gradient more than or equal to 20 mm Hg.
- Peak to peak coarctation gradient less than 20 mm Hg in the presence of significant coarctation with imaging evidence of significant collateral flow.

CONCLUSION

Noninvasive imaging of the aorta has almost replaced invasive aortography. CECT should be used routinely both for preoperative and postoperative assessment of aortic diseases. At a reasonable cost and low-risk to patients, CT and CT-angiography can provide the diagnosis, operability, and anatomic definition including concomitant intrathoracic or intra-abdominal abnormalities. The recent advances in MR hardware can now provide all the information needed for evaluating aortic diseases, anatomic as well as functional and gadolinium enhanced 3D MRA may replace catheter angiography for both preoperative and postoperative evaluation.

REFERENCES

1. Litmanovich D, Bankier AA, Cantin L, et al. CT and MRI in diseases of the aorta. Am J Roentgenology. 2009;193(4):928-40.
2. Mao SS, Ahmadi N, Shah B, et al. Normal thoracic aorta diameter on cardiac computed tomography in healthy asymptomatic adults: impact of age and gender. Acad Radiol. 2008;15(7):827-34.
3. Aronberg DJ, Glazer HS, Madsen K, et al. Normal thoracic aortic diameters by computed tomography. J Comput Assist Tomogr. 1984;8(2):247-50.
4. Tops LF, Wood DA, Delgado V, et al. Noninvasive evaluation of the aortic root with multislice computed tomography. JACC Cardiovasc Imaging. 2008;1(3):321-30.
5. Bickerstaff LK, Pairolero PC, Hollier LH, et al. Thoracic aortic aneurysms: a population-based study. Surgery. 1982;92(6):1103-8.
6. Agarwal PP, Chughtai A, Matzinger FR, et al. Multidetector CT of thoracic aortic aneurysms. Radiographics. 2009;29(2):537-52.
7. Green CE, Klein JF. Multidetector row CT angiography of the thoracic aorta. In: Boiselle PM, White CS (Eds). New Techniques in Cardiothoracic Imaging. New York: Informa HealthCare; 2007. pp. 105-26.

8. Svensson LG, Crawford ES, Hess KR, et al. Experience with 1509 patients undergoing thoracoabdominal aortic operations. J Vasc Surg. 1993;17(2):357-68.
9. Hartnell GG. Imaging of aortic aneurysms and dissection: CT and MRI. J Thorac Imaging. 2001;16(1):35-46.
10. Tatli S, Yucel EK, Lipton MJ. CT and MR imaging of the thoracic aorta: current techniques and clinical applications. Radiol Clin North Am. 2004;42(3):565-85.
11. Yu T, Zhu X, Tang L, et al. Review of CT angiography of aorta. Radiol Clin North Am. 2007;45(3):461-83.
12. Russo V, Renzulli M, Buttazzi K, et al. Acquired diseases of the thoracic aorta: role of MRI and MRA. Eur Radiol. 2006;16(4):852-65.
13. Sakamoto I, Sueyoshi E, Uetani M. MR imaging of the aorta. Radiol Clin North Am. 2007;45(3):485-97.
14. Lohan DG, Krishnam M, Saleh R, et al. MR imaging of the thoracic aorta. Magn Reson Imaging Clin N Am. 2008;16(2):213-34.
15. Coady MA, Rizzo JA, Hammond GL, et al. What is the appropriate size criterion for resection of thoracic aortic aneurysms? J Thorac Cardiovasc Surg. 1997;113(3):476-91.
16. Frauenfelder T, Wildermuth S, Marincek B, et al. Nontraumatic emergent abdominal vascular conditions: advantages of multi-detector row CT and three-dimensional imaging. Radiographics. 2004;24(2):481-96.
17. Khan IA, Nair CK. Clinical, diagnostic, and management perspectives of aortic dissection. Chest. 2002;122(1):311-28.
18. Pretre R, Von Segesser LK. Aortic dissection. Lancet. 1997;349(9063):1461-4.
19. Eggebrecht H, Plicht B, Kahlert P, et al. Intramural hematoma and penetrating ulcers: indications to endovascular treatment. Eur J Vasc Endovasc Surg. 2009;38(6):659-65.
20. Keser G, Direskeneli H, Aksu K. Management of Takayasu arteritis: a systematic review. Rheumatology (Oxford). 2014;53(5):793-801.
21. Choudhary SK, Bhan A, Talwar S, et al. Tubercular pseudoaneurysms of aorta. Ann Thorac Surg. 2001;72(4):1239-44.

SECTION 20

Carotid Artery Disease

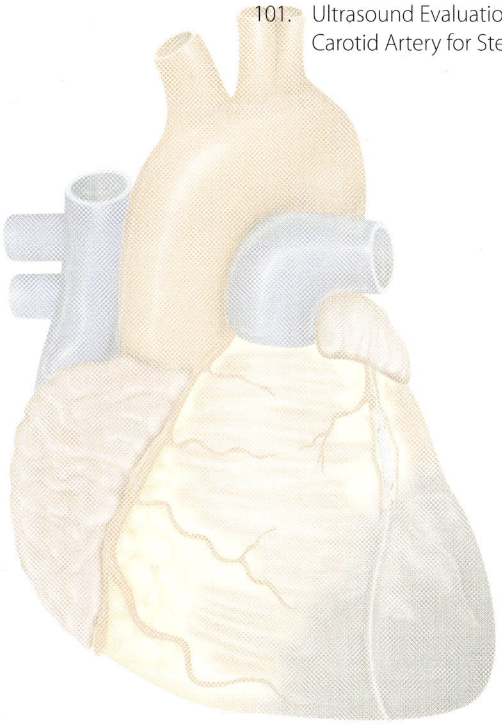

101

CHAPTER

Ultrasound Evaluation of the Carotid Artery for Stenosis

Christopher SG Murray, Tamanna Nahar, Navin C Nanda, HK Chopra

INTRODUCTION

Our aim is to first acquaint the reader with the available modalities for imaging of the carotid vasculature in the current armamentarium of diagnostic vascular imaging and measurement, before we look more specifically at the description and physical concept of carotid ultrasound (US) for the evaluation of stenotic lesions, the diagnostic criteria associated with same, advantages and disadvantages of the procedure and also at newer sonographic techniques which have demonstrated clear clinical benefit in the assessment of these vessels. Prior to this, we first make mention of a number of methods which can be used to measure stenotic severity of carotid artery, based on the interpretation of the images obtained, with three main methods predominating worldwide; namely:

1. The North American Symptomatic Carotid Endarterectomy Trial (NASCET) method, which compares stenosis to diameter of the distal normal poststenotic internal carotid artery (ICA).[1]
2. The European Carotid Surgery trial (ECST) method which compares stenosis to estimate the normal carotid bulb diameter.[2]
3. The common carotid (CC) method, which measures the diameter of the residual lumen at the portion with greatest stenosis in the vessel and then compares this to the luminal diameter in the proximal common carotid artery (CCA).[3]

It should be noted that the ECST and CC being somewhat more sensitive, estimating severe stenosis in twice as many studies as did the NASCET method, as well as generally deeming less stenoses as being mild.[4]

There are four main diagnostic modalities available to image the ICA, namely:

1. Digital subtraction angiography (DSA)
2. Computed tomography angiography (CTA)
3. Magnetic resonance angiography (MRA)
4. Duplex ultrasound (DUS).

Some of these modalities, particularly the noninvasive methods, have undergone significant development over recent years, of note, CTA and MRA in particular; however, despite these developments it should be stated that invasive DSA is still considered the gold standard. For each technique, there are distinct advantages and disadvantages.

DIGITAL SUBTRACTION ANGIOGRAPHY

Conventional DSA, despite being the most reliable modality, is not a first-line method for carotid stenotic assessment, but has its place in the process of carotid stenting, where the vessel can be visualized in several views; three or more are usually recommended, and it facilitates an accurate evaluation of both the severity as well as the morphology of the stenotic lesion, as it is able to elucidate plaque ulceration as well as thrombi when present; the former by irregular margins and the latter by intraluminal defects seen.

The main advantage of this method of carotid imaging is that it has the capability of imaging and evaluating the entire carotid arterial system, generating information about atherosclerotic disease, morphology of the plaque, collateral circulation in the vascular territory, and the presence of intracranial atherosclerotic disease associated with that vessel.

However, the main disadvantage lies in the fact that the DSA is an invasive method, which carries a complication of embolization and stroke (<1%),[5] which occurs because of the fact that the carotid has to be selectively catheterized with at least two views. Rotational angiography, which allows for multiple views and angles, will show more severe ICA stenosis as opposed to conventional DSA, and generally tends to correlate better with contrast-enhanced MRA.[6,7]

COMPUTED TOMOGRAPHY ANGIOGRAPHY

The entire course of the carotid artery from the arch of the aorta to the intracranial segments can be visualized by CTA with intravenous (IV) iodinated contrast, and the stenotic severity at all levels of the vessel is also permitted. This technique is done in multiple views, then reconstructed allowing assessment of plaque composition. Luminal area can form the basis of stenotic measurement, but NASCET or ESCT criteria are used in clinical practice, and accuracy of this CT-based method has increased with the current developments seeing the detector row number increased from 4 to 320, although a relatively recent meta-analysis showed reduction in sensitivity and specificity for milder stenoses; however a dual source CT study showed better accuracy.[7,8] The main advantages of CTA are its wide availability, with the dual utility of performing CT brain and carotid artery CTA at any time with faster, relatively operator independent acquisition. The main disadvantages are the IV use of iodine contrast and the attendant radiation involved, deeming those with impaired renal function—a common comorbidity of vascular disease—relatively contraindicated to the technique, as well as reduced accuracy in the setting of extensive calcification.

MAGNETIC RESONANCE ANGIOGRAPHY

Direct visualization of stenosis can be accomplished with this modality, which can be performed as time-of-flight (TOF-MRA), which is performed without contrast and uses features of blood flowing, or contrast-enhanced (CE-MRA), which uses IV gadolinium, with stenosis being measured using NASCET or ESCT method; this technique is not calcification-sensitive, CE-MRA being superior to TOF-MRA, the latter having a tendency to overestimation. The main advantage is a three-dimensional (3D) image of the carotid bifurcation with good sensitivity for detection of high-grade stenotic lesions.[8,9] It is also less operator dependent than DUS, and is radiation free, however, it is more expensive than DUS as well as CTA and is less available. If the patient is claustrophobic or unable to lie supine this test is precluded, as well as if a pacemaker or ferromagnetic implants are present.

CAROTID DUPLEX ULTRASOUND

Both grayscale and Doppler US can be used for assessment of extracranial segments of the carotid arteries, allowing the ability to differentiate between calcified and noncalcified portions of the plaque;[10] noncalcified and hypoechoic portions of the plaques being an independent risk factor for stroke; grayscale also permits the estimation of intima-media complex thickness, aiding in the detection of preclinical atherosclerotic disease and subsequent assessment of risk stratification.

Doppler US is based on the Doppler effect that permits measurement of flow based on the reflection of mechanical waves, with both pulse and color Doppler US both being used to evaluate vessels of interest, which are typically the cervical portions of the common carotid artery (CCA), internal carotid artery (ICA), and external carotid arteries (ECAs). The color Doppler US will visualize flow in color-coded information about both direction and velocity interposed on grayscale images, also high-grade stenotic lesions can be more easily detected with color than with pulse Doppler US although the latter allows direct measurement of the velocity of flow. The peak systolic velocity (PSV) is used for quantification of stenosis, but end-diastolic velocity, carotid index, and spectral waveform analysis are also used for assessment of stenosis. Sensitivity to stenotic lesions falls sharply by two-thirds going from severe-to-moderate stenosis, but specificity remains constant.[8]

The main advantages of carotid US are its safety, affordability, and the ability to directly visualize morphology and measure flow; the main disadvantage of this technique is that its accuracy is largely contingent on the experience and skill of the operator, with the possibility of wide interobserver variability in measurements, as well as the patient's body habitus, anatomic anomalies, and tortuous arterial courses resulting in difficult detection and flow measurement. It is important to carefully interpret the results of Doppler in patients with a carotid occlusion on the opposite side, to avoid overestimation of an ipsilateral carotid stenosis, as PSV will often be increased in the presence of a contralateral ICA occlusion; also only the cervical portion of the ICA can be studied, although added information can be gleaned from transcranial Doppler studies. It should be noted that this could be useful in cases

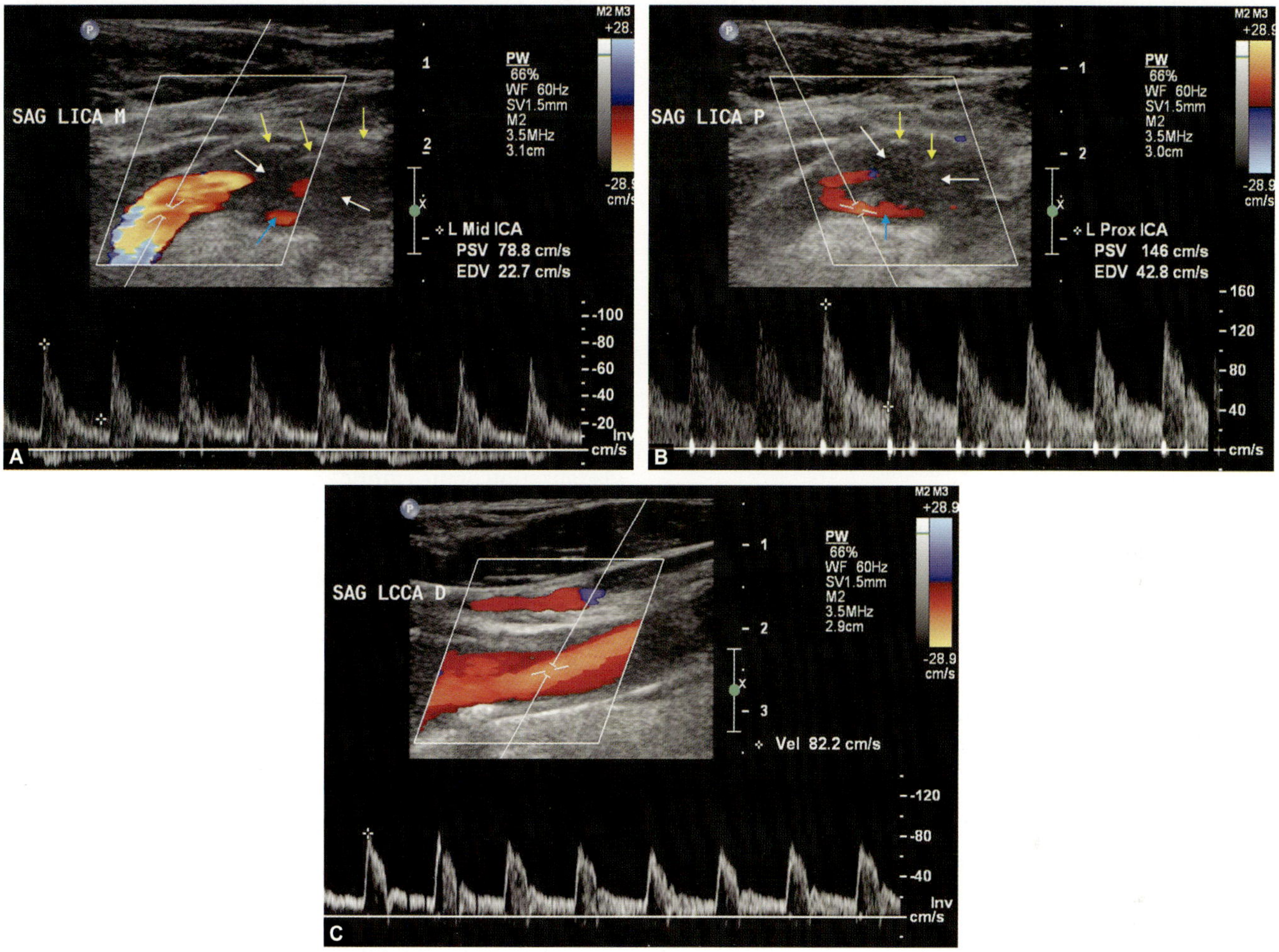

Figs. 1A to C: Duplex scans of the left carotid artery. (A) Proximal part of internal carotid artery (bulb). Color Doppler shows flow signals only in the posterior portion of the bulb (blue arrows). The remainder of the bulb is the plaque with mixed calcified areas (yellow arrows) and markedly hypoechogenic ones (white arrows). The peak systolic velocity (146 cm/s) together with spectral broadening indicates lumen stenosis of more than 50% (50–69%); (B) Middle part of the internal carotid artery (ICA) shows unobstructed flow on color Doppler, and normal velocities on spectral Doppler; and (C) Distal common carotid artery (CCA) shows a peak systolic velocity of 82.2 cm/s, and it is also diseased but there is no significant stenosis.
Source: Kalashyan H, Saqqur M, Shuaib A, et al. Comprehensive and rapid assessment of carotid plaques in acute stroke using a new single sweep method for three-dimensional carotid ultrasound. Echocardiography. 2013;30(4):414-8.

of extracranial stenosis (see criteria for stenosis in Table 1 here).[11]

It must be noted that subtotal arterial occlusion may be sometimes mistaken for total occlusion, which is of critical clinical importance. The ratio of flow velocities in the ICA and CCA may help distinguish between increased compensatory flow through collaterals and true contralateral ICA stenosis or occlusion. There are a number of pitfalls in velocity-based estimation of ICA stenosis, such as higher velocities in women, and elevated velocities where there is contralateral carotid artery occlusion.[12,13] If there is severe tortuosity of the artery, high-carotid bifurcation, obesity, and extensive vascular calcification, these will reduce the sonographic accuracy; if carotid artery stents are already *in situ*, vessel wall compliance can be diminished, accelerating flow velocity.[14] Variability in operator expertize also affects the quality of the examinations and the reliability of the results.[15-17] Despite these limitations, US performed by well-trained experienced technologists provides accurate and relatively inexpensive assessment of the cervical carotid arteries (Figs. 1A to C and Table 1).[15-19]

CAROTID ARTERIAL ANATOMY AS IT RELATES TO ULTRASOUND PROCEDURE

The right carotid A comes out of the R brachiocephalic A, with the LCCA arising from the arch of the aorta. US can

TABLE 1: Grayscale and Doppler criteria for assessment of internal carotid artery stenosis.

% stenosis	Sonographic parameters
Normal	ICA PSV <125 cm/s and none visible plaque, additionally
	ICA/CCA PSV ratio <2 and ICA EDV < 40 cm/s
<50	ICA PSV <125 cm/s and estimate plaque <50%, additionally ICA/CCA PSV ratio <2 and ICA EDV < 40 cm/s
50–69	ICA PSV 125–230 cm/s and estimate plaque 50% and more, additionally ICA/CCA PSV ratio 2–4 and ICA EDV 40–100 cm/s
>70 but less than near occlusion	ICA PSV > 230 cm/s and estimate plaque 50% and more, additionally ICA/CCA PSV ratio >4 and ICA EDV > 100 cm/s
Near occlusion	ICA PSV high, low, or undetectable, estimate plaque visible, additionally variable ICA/CCA ratio and ICA EDV
Total occlusion	Undetectable flow, visible plaque, no detectable lumen

(CCA: common carotid artery; EDV: end-diastolic velocity; ICA: internal carotid artery; PSV: peak systolic velocity)

Source: Adapted from Grant EG, Benson CB, Moneta GL, et al. Carotid artery stenosis: grayscale and Doppler ultrasound diagnosis—Society of Radiologists in Ultrasound Consensus Conference. Ultrasound Q. 2003;19(4):190-8.

show the most proximal segment of the R but not the L.[20] The examiner should have the ability to differentiate between the ICA and ECA, the former being located posterolaterally to the latter and being slightly larger as well; the ECA having branches which the ICA does not, such as the lingual artery. Also, a lower resistive pattern is seen in the Doppler spectrums, with the difference in velocity between the systolic and diastolic phases of this vessel being smaller than that of the ECA. The ECA can also be differentiated from the ICA by a useful tool known as "temporal tapping", this is an artifact specific to the ECA, generated during acquisition of the ECA Doppler spectrum, by placement of the fingertips on the temporal artery on the same side; this generates a saw tooth-like artifact on the Doppler spectrum from the ECA only.[20]

INTIMA-MEDIA THICKNESS

The intima-medial thickness (IMT), is used as a parameter of atherosclerotic burden.[21,22] It is performed perpendicular to the insonation beam in the longitudinal plane, displayed as two bright interfaces along the arterial wall, which is the blood-intima and medial-adventitial interface. The IMT is represented as the distance between these two layers and should be evaluated in areas devoid of focal lesions, best measured on the far wall of the distal CCA as it is easier to image and has less variation than the ICA due to beam angle or vessel depth, with 89% versus 38% success rate of IMT measurement respectively.[21] It should be noted that carotid artery atherosclerosis as it is measured by IMT is an independent risk factor for cerebrovascular accident (CVA) and myocardial infarction (MI).[21-23]

ASSESSMENT OF MORPHOLOGY AND VOLUME OF THE PLAQUE IN TWO-DIMENSIONAL CAROTID ULTRASOUND

As much as positioning, localization, and accurate visualization of the carotids is important, even more so an accurate estimation and assessment of the morphology and volume of the plaque is integral to a comprehensive study. Morphology of the plaque, such as its echogenicity, surface characteristics, presence or absence of ulceration, as well as presence of plaque and stenosis, is of vital importance in the prediction of future cardiovascular events.[24] A morphologic description of the plaque from grayscale imaging should include the plaque echogenicity, surface characteristics and the presence of ulceration. There are a number of ways in which the echogenicity of the plaque may be described, including echogenic, isoechoic, as well as echolucent, or heterogeneous, with isoechoic meaning that the echogenic nature of the plaque is the same as that of the intima-media complex. The plaque surface can be characterized as smooth, irregular or ulcerated, bearing in mind that plaque ulceration has been associated with an increased risk of CVA.[25,26] It should be noted that plaque ulceration is very difficult to detect by US examination without careful grayscale examination, and is also operator dependent, with sensitivities ranging from 30% to 80%.[27,28] A concerted effort should be made on the part of the examiner, to detect ulceration in the risk assessment of the patient with the carotid plaque, this being tied to the fact that ulceration does not correlate with symptomatology. A depression of the plaque surface by more than 2 mm is thought to indicate ulceration, and this ulceration may have different patterns, such as cystic, bridge-shaped, sponge-shaped, or merely a simple depression.[28-31] It has been noted that symptomatic lesions are usually associated with a higher incidence of hyperechoic plaques; the grayscale median (GSM) has been put forward by Biasi et al.[32] in an effort to quantitatively measure plaque echogenicity; this was done using longitudinal images of the plaque and vessel wall. The GSM of the blood pool was 0–5, and that of the adventitia of the wall was 185–195. These investigators found that the stroke risk during the procedure of carotid stenting was dependent on the GSM of the plaque, with values of 25 or less showing a 7.1% stroke risk, and those with values more than 25 showing only a 1.5% stroke risk, deeming echolucent plaque as having more vulnerability.[31]

THE USE OF THREE-DIMENSIONAL CAROTID ULTRASOUND

In recent times, 3D US, has been used for the measurement of plaque volume.[33-35] With a 2D grayscale image, plaque size can be measured utilizing the parameters of length and height, but it is not possible to measure the total volume of plaque by this method. 3D-US has shown good intra- and interobserver reproducibility for measuring total plaque volume.[35] This plaque volume can be used as a monitoring tool for treatment of atherosclerosis, and studies have shown it to increase without treatment as well as diminish with statin therapy.[36] It should be noted that 3D-US volume measurements are more sensitive than IMT for the evaluation of carotid plaque progression post-treatment. Also, even with a significant change in the plaque volume seen in 3D during the follow-up period, there may be no commensurate change seen in the IMT.[37] Characterization of the plaque can also be done by 3D US; the limitations of a 2D grayscale evaluation of plaque being that single or even multiple images cannot be representative of the entire plaque volume. Studies have shown that there is a higher incidence of hypoechoic plaque in symptomatic patients.[38]

CAROTID TRANSESOPHAGEAL AND TRANSPHARYNGEAL ECHOCARDIOGRAPHIC EXAMINATION

With the advent of improved echocardiographic systems as well as the multiplane probe, the methodology of transesophageal echocardiographic (TEE) examination has now been widened to involve many vascular structures such as the coronary arteries, the branches of the aortic arch, the neck veins, and the carotid arteries; this has already been shown to be of distinct clinical importance, with current utilization in the area of ascertainment of stroke etiology, as well as vascular steal syndromes. In the process, clinically useful images can be obtained.[39-48] TEE are used to evaluate a cardiac source for ischemic stroke. It has been found that toward the end of the TEE procedure, the US probe can be positioned in the upper esophagus, to evaluate the aortic arch and the proximal extent of its branches, for atherosclerotic lesions and stenosis.[39-43] Longitudinal plane examination at 90° with clockwise rotation of the probe at the level of the aortic arch will bring the origin of the innominate artery into view, which can be followed proximally, but the bifurcation cannot be imaged due to tracheobronchial tree obscuration. When the probe is rotated counterclockwise, the LCCA can be seen, as well as the L subclavian A with further rotation. This study may be further extended to the ICA and ECA for their evaluation, by further slowly withdrawing the probe into the pharynx,[42-43,47-49] keeping the color Doppler turned on during this procedure, as it is the color flow signals that are useful in the differentiation between vascular structures and soft tissue. The LCCA is generally similar in size to its subclavian counterpart, but displays low resistance Doppler signals, and it can be distinguished from the latter in that none of its branches can be visualized. With transpharyngeal echocardiography (TPE), careful, slow withdrawal of the probe from the esophagus into the pharynx while keeping the LCCA in view, may demonstrate the slight dilatation of the carotid bulb, before its bifurcation into LICA and ECA. The Doppler US beam can be aligned parallel to flow direction in the ICA, allowing for accurate velocity assessment, in contrast to the surface approach, where the Doppler beam is at an angle to the flow direction, which can cause an underestimation of velocities which in turn can lead to diagnostic errors as regards stenotic severity. It should be noted that both vessels show antegrade flow both in systole and diastole, but the waveforms from the ECA tend to be sharper as well as the diastolic antegrade flow being somewhat less prominent. In addition, the branches of the ECA are easily visualized, but the ICA has no branches in its extracranial course. With

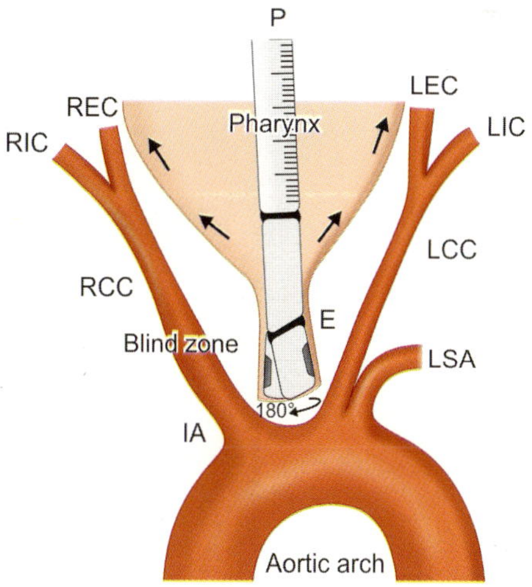

Fig. 2: Schematic demonstrating the technique of examining both the left and right-sided carotid arteries. (E: esophagus; IA: innominate artery; LCC: left common carotid artery; LEC: left external carotid; LIC: left internal carotid; LSA: left subclavian artery; P: probe; RCC: right common carotid artery; REC: right external carotid artery; RIC: right internal carotid artery)

Source: Nanda NC, Miller AP, Nekkanti R, et al. Transpharyngeal echocardiographic imaging of the right and left carotid arteries. Echocardiography. 2001;18(8):711-6.

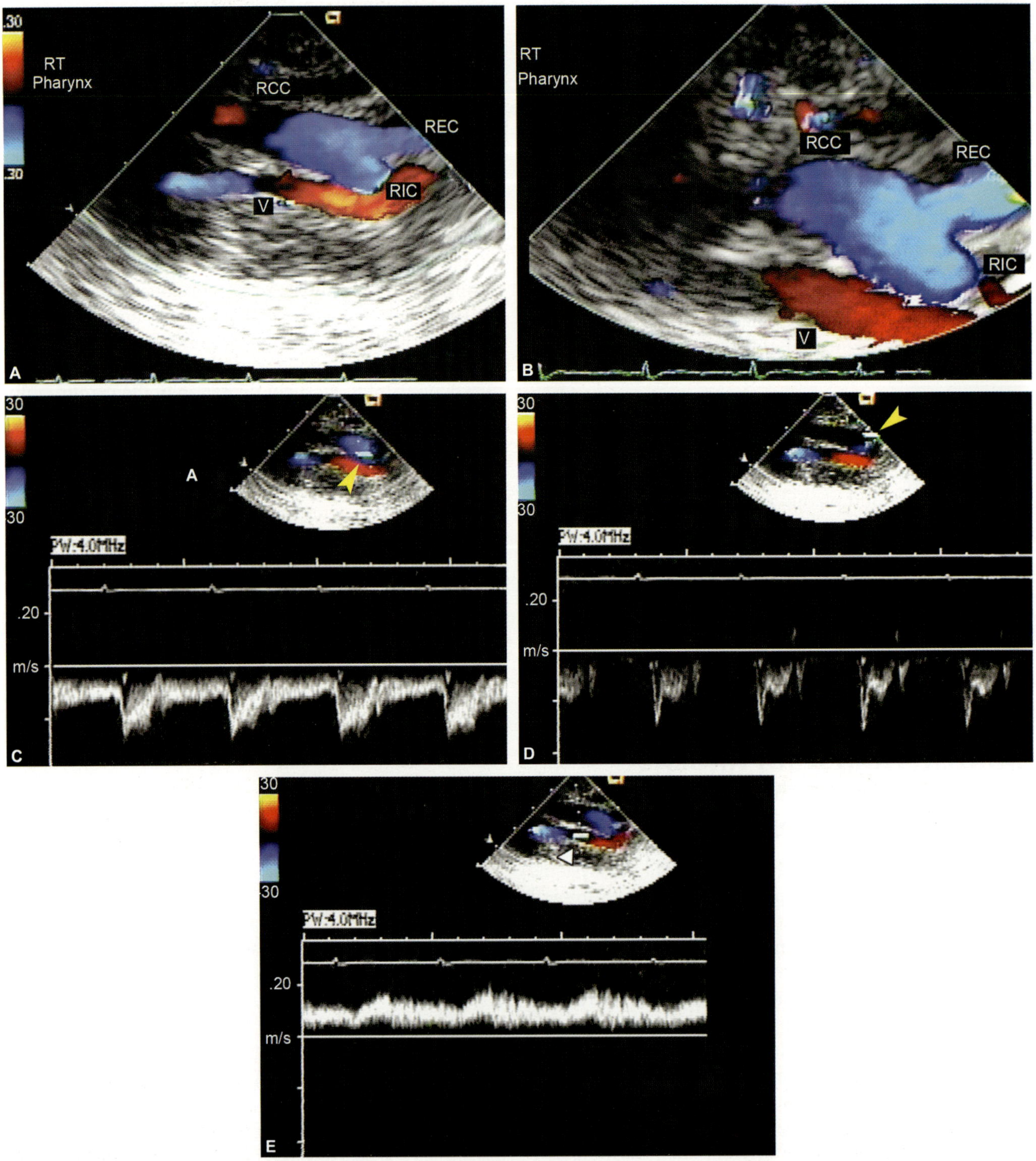

Figs. 3A to E: Transpharyngeal echocardiographic examination of right-sided carotid arteries. (A and B) The right common carotid artery (RCC) bifurcates into right internal (RIC) and right external (REC) branches; (C) Color Doppler-guided pulsed Doppler interrogation of the RIC (arrowhead) shows prominent antegrade systolic and diastolic flow signals; (D) Interrogation of the REC (arrowhead) shows much less prominent antegrade diastolic signals. Note the parallel alignment of the Doppler cursor line to flow direction in RIC in C; and (E) Pulsed Doppler interrogation of the right internal jugular vein (V; arrowhead) demonstrates flow signals typical of venous flow.

Source: Nanda NC, Miller AP, Nekkanti R, et al. Transpharyngeal echocardiographic imaging of the right and left carotid arteries. Echocardiography. 2001;18(8):711-6.

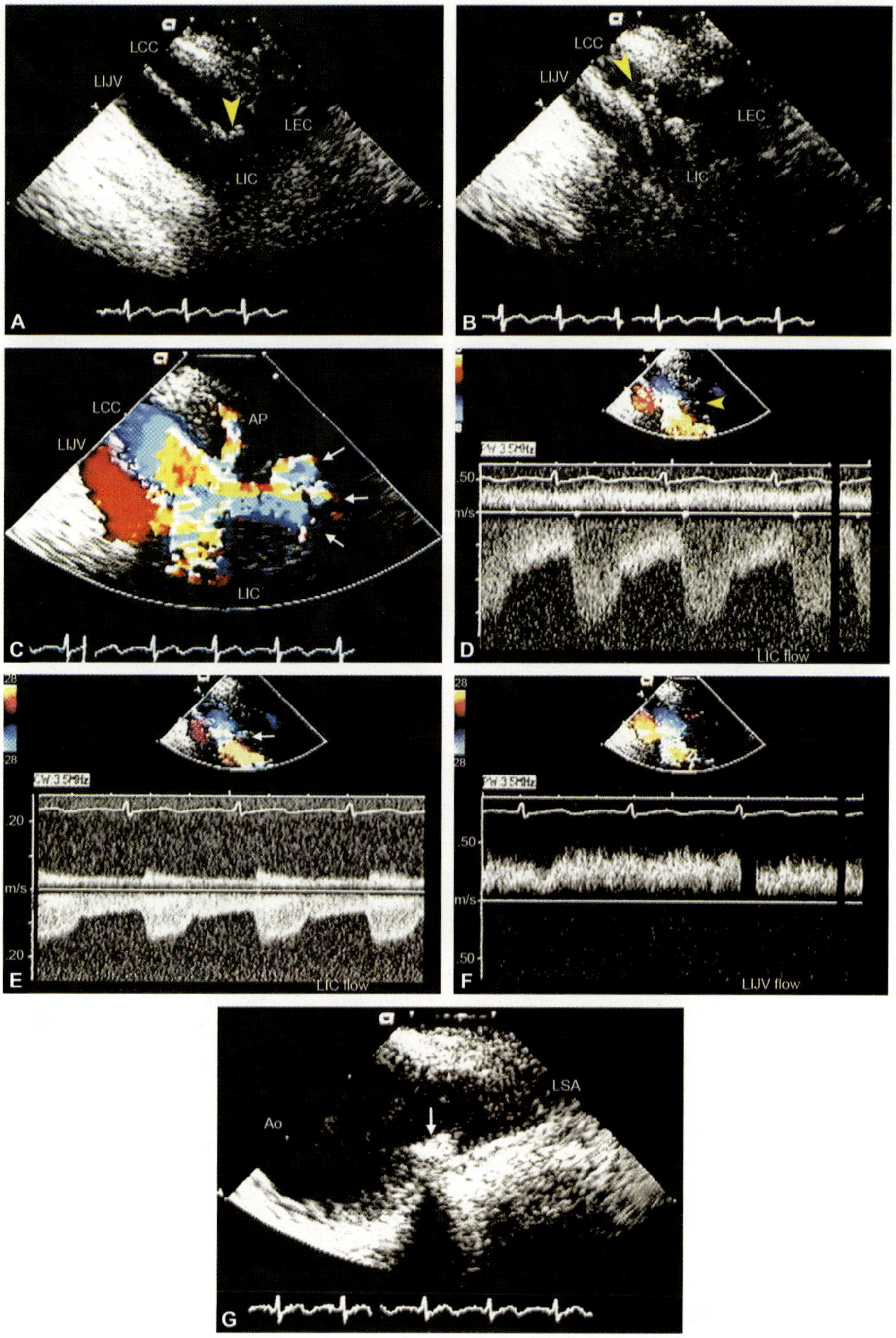

Figs. 4A to G: Transpharyngeal echocardiographic diagnosis of left carotid bulb and internal carotid artery stenosis. (A and B) The arrowheads point to a prominent calcified plaque in the bulb and proximal portion of the left internal carotid artery (LIC); (C) Color Doppler examination demonstrating the ascending pharyngeal (AP) and other branches (arrows) of the left external carotid artery. The left internal jugular vein (LIJV) is seen adjacent to the left common carotid artery (LCC); (D and E) Color Doppler-guided pulsed and continuous wave Doppler examination of the proximal left internal carotid artery shows a peak systolic velocity of 1.8 m/s and a peak diastolic velocity approaching 1 m/s, indicative of significant stenosis. Note that the Doppler beam is aligned parallel to the flow direction in the proximal LIC; and (F) Pulsed Doppler interrogation of the left internal jugular vein demonstrates continuous venous-type flow signals throughout the cardiac cycle; and (G) The arrow shows a large atherosclerotic plaque at the origin of the left subclavian artery (LSA). The probe was in the upper esophagus. (AO: aorta; LEC: left external carotid artery)

Source: Nanda NC, Gomez CR, Narayan VK, et al. Transpharyngeal echocardiographic diagnosis of carotid bulb and left internal carotid artery stenosis. Echocardiography. 1999;16(7 Pt 1):671-4.

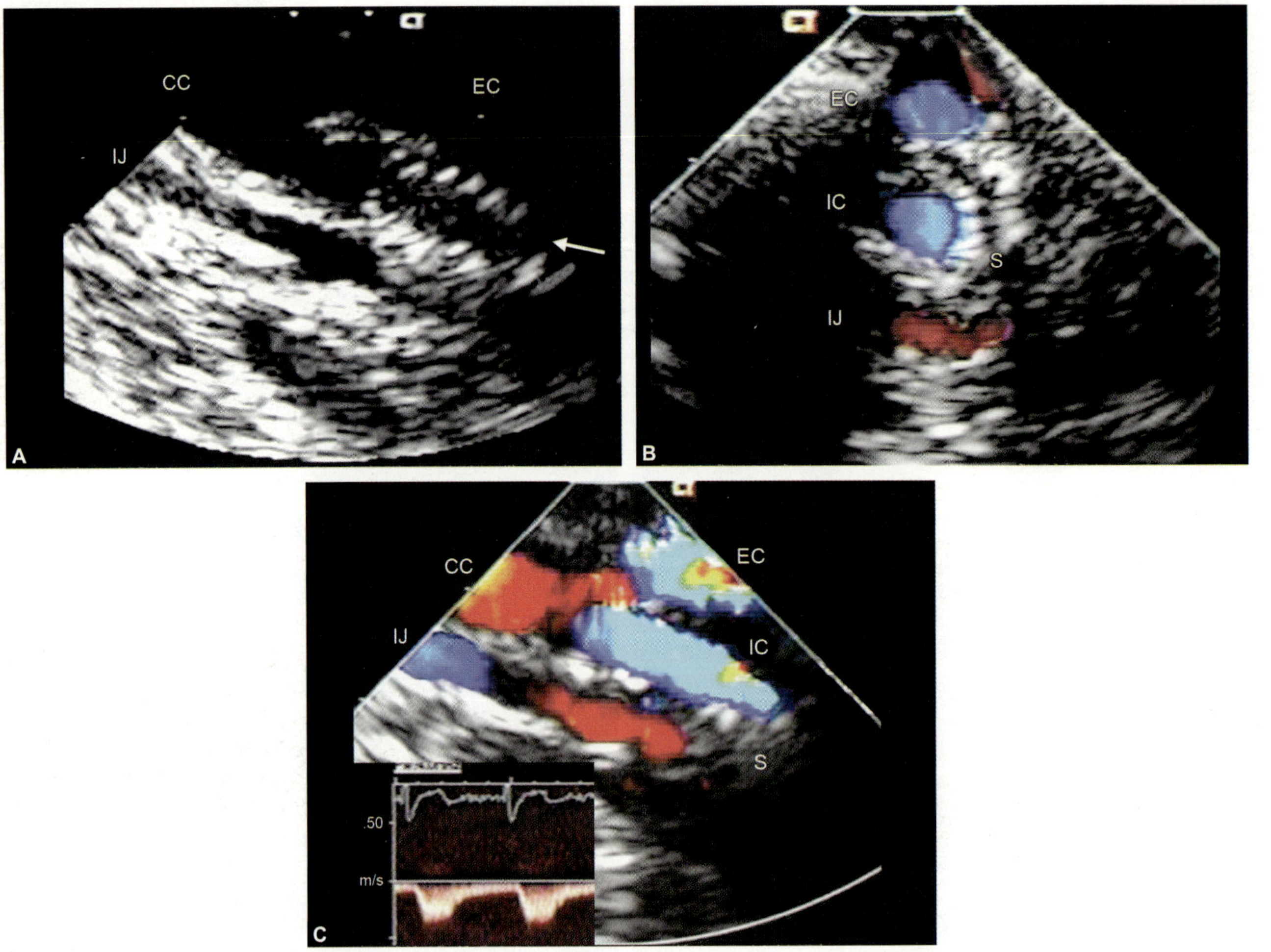

Figs. 5A to C: Transpharyngeal ultrasound evaluation of internal carotid artery stent in an octogenarian. (A) The arrow points to the stent located in the left internal carotid artery, visualized in long axis; (B) The stent (S) visualized in short axis. Note the regularly spaced coils of the stent in both A and B; and (C) Laminar flow signals with only mild aliasing are visualized within the stent (S) located in the left internal carotid artery (IC), suggesting no significant stenosis. This was confirmed by color Doppler-guided pulsed wave interrogation (inset), which also shows absence of high velocities in both systole and diastole. Peak systolic and diastolic velocities measured 0.4 m/s and 0.2 m/s, respectively. (CC: left common carotid artery; EC: left external carotid artery; IJ: left internal jugular vein)

Source: Howard JH, Dod HS, Nanda NC, et al. Transpharyngeal ultrasound evaluation of internal carotid artery stent in an octogenarian. Am J Geriatr Cardiol. 2003;12(6):375-6.

respect to the R-sided neck vessels, the probe is rotated in the upper esophagus such that the face or footprint of the transducer is turned toward the patient's right side, then gradually withdrawn and rotated slightly to identify these arteries. During probe withdrawal, there is a blind spot created by interference from the tracheobronchial tree, this extends for a few centimeters after which one or more vessels should appear with the probe still in the esophagus, and with Doppler interrogation, it can be determined whether the vessel seen is the R subclavian or the RCCA. The R vertebral A, like the RCCA will also demonstrate low-resistance Doppler signals, but this vessel is much smaller and the origin from the subclavian A may be identified. In the majority of patients, the R CCA is the only vessel visualized when the probe is facing the R side of the patient; further withdrawal into the pharynx will demonstrate its bifurcation into R internal and ECA. At this point, it is also easy to align the Doppler US beam parallel to the flow direction in the ICA. It may be impossible to see these vessels from the pharynx, as it is a considerably larger cavity than the collapsible and thin-walled esophagus, where close contact can be maintained, necessitating close contact with the pharyngeal wall. Alternatively, the probe may be placed in the tonsillar fossa, before or after the

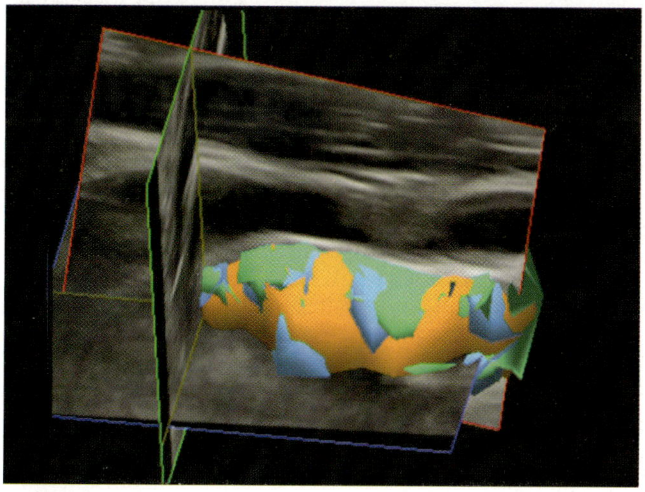

Fig. 6: Three-dimensional ultrasound reconstruction of a diseased carotid artery. Reconstructed schematic three-dimensional ultrasound representation of the plaque (green), thrombus (blue), and internal carotid artery lumen (orange). *Source:* Kalashyan H, Saqqur M, Shuaib A, et al. Comprehensive and rapid assessment of carotid plaques in acute stroke using a new single sweep method for three-dimensional carotid ultrasound. Echocardiography. 2013;30(4):414-8.

procedure. In addition to assessment of carotid A stenosis this technique is useful for detecting stent patency in the ICA, carotid body paragangliomas, distal extracranial segments of vertebral arteries, and neck vessel flow reversal in severe aortic regurgitation (AR), using color Doppler-guided pulsed-Doppler interrogation; of note TEE utility also extends to carotid surgical intra- and postoperative use (Figs. 2 to 4).[49-53]

THREE-DIMENSIONAL COLOR DOPPLER TRANSPHARYNGEAL ECHOCARDIOGRAPHIC RECONSTRUCTION OF CAROTIDS

In addition to use of 3D-(TPE), to view the above-mentioned vascular structures, which has been preceded by 2D TPE in the diagnosis of subclavian or internal carotid artery stenosis, as well as patency of ICA stents, 3D color Doppler reconstruction of 2D images of carotid arterial segments and branches has been performed using 3D color Doppler TPE, providing short and long-axis views of the vessels (Figs. 5A to C). This has been done by initially doing a TEE using a 5–7 MHz multiplane probe intraoperatively, and at the conclusion, withdrawing and rotating the probe in the pharynx from 0° to 180° with electrocardiographic and respiration gating, resulting in the acquisition and storage of 3D color Doppler TPE images, which are later reconstructed in 3D with state-of-the-art software (Fig. 6).[39-43,46,48-53]

CONCLUSION

Carotid US represents the general initial approach to patients with suspected carotid stenosis. Those with actual stenosis less than 50% are usually followed with serial examinations, to chart possible disease progression, and those with stenotic lesions greater than 50% will warrant further evaluation with the other known modalities, namely transcranial Doppler, MRA, and CTA.[54-56] This diagnostic modality, which boasts more than adequate reliability, coupled with its capability to directly view morphology and flow patterns, as well as its safe and noninvasive nature in the hands of trained personnel, and its general affordability and accessibility to the majority of any population, will continue to be widely available; it has already undergone much by way of technological advancement and is expected to further undergo more upgrades and embellishments, with continued research and review, over time.

REFERENCES

1. North American Symptomatic Carotid Endarterectomy Trial Collaborators, Barnett HJ, Taylor DW, et al. Beneficial effect of carotid endarterectomy in symptomatic patients with high-grade carotid stenosis. N Engl J Med. 1991;325(7):445-53.
2. ECST Collaborative Group. Randomised trial of endarterectomy for recently symptomatic carotid stenosis: final results of the MRC European Carotid Surgery Trial (ECST). Lancet. 1998;351(9113):1379-87.
3. Williams MA, Nicolaides AN. Predicting the normal dimensions of the internal and external carotid arteries from the diameter of the common carotid. Eur J Vasc Surg. 1987;1(2):91-6.
4. Rothwell PM, Gibson RJ, Slattery J, et al. Equivalence of measurements of carotid stenosis. A comparison of three methods on 1001 angiograms. European Carotid Surgery Trialists' Collaborative Group. Stroke. 1994;25(12):2435-9.
5. Davies KN, Humphrey PR. Complications of cerebral angiography in patients with symptomatic carotid territory ischaemia screened by carotid ultrasound. J Neurol Neurosurg Psychiatry. 1993;56(9):967-72.
6. Elgersma OE, Buijs PC, Wüst AF, et al. Maximum internal carotid arterial stenosis: assessment with rotational angiography versus conventional intraarterial digital subtraction angiography. Radiology. 1999;213(3):777-83.
7. Anzalone N, Scomazzoni F, Castellano R, et al. Carotid artery stenosis: intraindividual correlations of 3D time-of-flight MR angiography, contrast-enhanced MR angiography, conventional DSA, and rotational angiography for detection and grading. Radiology. 2005;236(1):204-13.
8. Wardlaw JM, Chappell FM, Stevenson M, et al. Accurate, practical and cost-effective assessment of carotid stenosis in the UK. Health Technol Assess. 2006;10(30):1-82.
9. Weber J, Veith P, Jung B, et al. MR angiography at 3 Tesla to assess proximal internal carotid artery stenoses: contrast-enhanced or 3D time-of-flight MR angiography? Clin Neuroradiol. 2015;25(1):41-8.

10. Polak JF, Shemanski L, O'Leary DH, et al. Hypoechoic plaque at US of the carotid artery: an independent risk factor for incident stroke in adults aged 65 years or older. Cardiovascular Health Study. Radiology. 1998;208(3):649-54.
11. Grant EG, Benson CB, Moneta GL, et al. Carotid artery stenosis: grayscale and Doppler ultrasound diagnosis: Society of Radiologists in Ultrasound Consensus Conference. Radiology. 2003;229(2):340-6.
12. Comerota AJ, Salles-Cunha SX, Daoud Y, et al. Gender differences in blood velocities across carotid stenoses. J Vasc Surg. 2004;40(5):939-44.
13. Busuttil SJ, Franklin DP, Youkey JR, et al. Carotid duplex overestimation of stenosis due to severe contralateral disease. Am J Surg. 1996;172(2):144-7.
14. Chi YW, White CJ, Woods TC, et al. Ultrasound velocity criteria for carotid in-stent restenosis. Catheter Cardiovasc Interv. 2007;69(3):349-54.
15. Howard G, Baker WH, Chambless LE, et al. An approach for the use of Doppler ultrasound as a screening tool for hemodynamically significant stenosis (despite heterogeneity of Doppler performance). A multicenter experience. Asymptomatic Carotid Atherosclerosis Study Investigators. Stroke. 1996;27(11):1951-7.
16. Kuntz KM, Polak JF, Whittemore AD, et al. Duplex ultrasound criteria for the identification of carotid stenosis should be laboratory specific. Stroke. 1997;28(3):597-602.
17. Alexandrov AV. Ultrasound and angiography in the selection of patients for carotid endarterectomy. Curr Cardiol Rep. 2003;5(2):141-7.
18. Paciaroni M, Caso V, Cardaioli G, et al. Is ultrasound examination sufficient in the evaluation of patients with internal carotid artery severe stenosis or occlusion? Cerebrovasc Dis. 2003;15(3):173- 6.
19. Filis KA, Arko FR, Johnson BL, et al. Duplex ultrasound criteria for defining the severity of carotid stenosis. Ann Vasc Surg. 2002;16(4):413-21.
20. Lee W. General principles of carotid Doppler ultrasonography. Ultrasonography. 2014;33(1):11-7.
21. Bots ML, Hoes AW, Koudstaal PJ, et al. Common carotid intima-media thickness and risk of stroke and myocardial infarction: the Rotterdam Study. Circulation. 1997;96(5):1432-7.
22. Ross R. The pathogenesis of atherosclerosis: a perspective for the 1990s. Nature. 1993;362(6423):801-9.
23. Smith SC, Greenland P, Grundy SM. AHA Conference Proceedings. Prevention conference V. Beyond secondary prevention: identifying the high-risk patient for primary prevention: executive summary. American Heart Association. Circulation. 2000;101(1):111-6.
24. Park AE, McCarthy WJ, Pearce WH, et al. Carotid plaque morphology correlates with presenting symptomatology. J Vasc Surg. 1998;27(5):872-8.
25. Gasecki AP, Eliasziw M, Barnett HJ. Risk factors for cervical atherosclerosis in patients with transient ischemic attack or minor ischemic stroke. Stroke. 1994;25(1):226.
26. Eliasziw M, Streifler JY, Fox AJ, et al. Significance of plaque ulceration in symptomatic patients with high-grade carotid stenosis. North American Symptomatic Carotid Endarterectomy Trial. Stroke. 1994;25(2):304-8.
27. O'Leary DH, Holen J, Ricotta JJ, et al. Carotid bifurcation disease: prediction of ulceration with B-mode US. Radiology. 1987;162(2):523-5.
28. O'Donnell TF Jr, Erdoes L, Mackey WC, et al. Correlation of B-mode ultrasound imaging and arteriography with pathologic findings at carotid endarterectomy. Arch Surg. 1985;120(4):443-9.
29. Comerota AJ, Katz ML, White JV, et al. The preoperative diagnosis of the ulcerated carotid atheroma. J Vasc Surg. 1990;11(4):505-10.
30. Widder B, Paulat K, Hackspacher J, et al. Morphological characterization of carotid artery stenoses by ultrasound duplex scanning. Ultrasound Med Biol. 1990;16(4):349-54.
31. Gray-Weale AC, Graham JC, Burnett JR, et al. Carotid artery atheroma: comparison of preoperative B-mode ultrasound appearance with carotid endarterectomy specimen pathology. J Cardiovasc Surg (Torino). 1988;29(6):676-81.
32. Biasi GM, Froio A, Diethrich EB, et al. Carotid plaque echolucency increases the risk of stroke in carotid stenting: the Imaging in Carotid Angioplasty and Risk of Stroke (ICAROS) study. Circulation. 2004;110(6):756-62.
33. Delcker A, Diener HC. Quantification of atherosclerotic plaques in carotid arteries by three-dimensional ultrasound. Br J Radiol. 1994;67(799):672-8.
34. Griewing B, Schminke U, Morgenstern C, et al. Three-dimensional ultrasound angiography (power mode) for the quantification of carotid artery atherosclerosis. J Neuroimaging. 1997;7(1):40-5.
35. Landry A, Spence JD, Fenster A. Measurement of carotid plaque volume by 3-dimensional ultrasound. Stroke. 2004;35(4):864-9.
36. Pollex RL, Spence JD, House AA, et al. A comparison of ultrasound measurements to assess carotid atherosclerosis development in subjects with and without type 2 diabetes. Cardiovasc Ultrasound. 2005;3:15.
37. Australasian Society for Ultrasound in Medicine (ASUM). (2015). Guidelines, Policies and Statements D14 Duplex Ultrasound: Extracranial Carotid Artery Disease. [online] Available from https://www.ultrasoundpaedia.com/uploads/53003/ufiles/Carotid/Pathology/ASUM_2015-Duplex-Ultrasound-Extracranial-Carotid-Artery-Disease.pdf. [Accessed October, 2018].
38. Heliopoulos J, Vadikolias K, Mitsias P, et al. A three-dimensional ultrasonographic quantitative analysis of non-ulcerated carotid plaque morphology in symptomatic and asymptomatic carotid stenosis. Atherosclerosis. 2008;198(1):129-35.
39. Agrawal G, LaMotte LC, Nanda NC. Identification of the aortic arch branches using transesophageal echocardiography. Echocardiography. 1997;14(5):461-6.
40. Katz ES, Koneckey E, Tunick PA, et al. Visualization and identification of the left common carotid and left subclavian arteries: a transesophageal echocardiographic approach. J Am Soc Echocardiogr. 1996;9(1):58-61

41. Nanda NC, Thakur AC, Thakur D, et al. Transesophageal echocardiographic examination of left subclavian artery branches. Echocardiography. 1999;16(3):271-7.
42. Nanda NC, Biederman RW, Thakur AC, et al. Examination of left external and internal carotid arteries during transesophageal echocardiography. Echocardiography. 1998;15(8 Pt 1):755-8.
43. Nanda NC, Gomez CR, Narayan VK, et al. Transpharyngeal echocardiographic diagnosis of carotid bulb and left internal carotid artery stenosis. Echocardiography. 1999;16(7 Pt 1):671-4.
44. Weyman AE, Feigenbaum H, Dillon JC, et al. Noninvasive visualization of the left main coronary artery by cross sectional echocardiography. Circulation. 1976;54:169-74.
45. Samdarshi TE, Nanda NC, Gatewood RP, et al. Usefulness and limitations of transesophageal echocardiography in the assessment of proximal coronary artery stenosis. J Am Coll Cardiol. 1992;19(3):572-80.
46. LaMotte LC, Nanda NC, Thakur AC, et al. Transesophageal echocardiographic identification of neck veins: Value of contrast echocardiography. Echocardiography. 1998;15(3):259-67.
47. Voros S, Nanda NC, Thakur AC, et al. Transesophageal echocardiography performed in stroke patients to exclude cardiac sources of embolism accurately detects significant coronary artery stenosis often resulting in changes of management. Circulation. 1999;l00(Suppl 1):677.
48. Mukhtar OM, Miller AP, Nanda NC, et al. Transesophageal echocardiographic identification of left subclavian artery stenosis with steal phenomenon. Echocardiography. 2000;17(2):197-200.
49. Nanda NC. Upper transesophageal and transpharyngeal examination. Comprehensive Textbook of Echocardiography, 1st edition. New Delhi: Jaypee Brothers Medical Publishers (P) Ltd; 2014.pp. 487-506.
50. Nanda NC, Miller AP, Nekkanti R, et al. Transpharyngeal echocardiographic imaging of the right and left carotid arteries. Echocardiography. 2001;18(8):711-6.
51. Miller AP, Nanda NC, Mukhtar O, et al. Transpharyngeal echocardiographic detection of a left internal carotid artery stent. Echocardiography. 2000;17(8):739-41.
52. Howard JH, Dod HS, Nanda NC, et al. Transpharyngeal ultrasound evaluation of internal carotid artery stent in an octogenarian. Am J Geriatr Cardiol. 2003;12(6):375-6.
53. Khanna D, Cheng PH, Nanda NC, et al. Transpharyngeal ultrasound detection of carotid body paraganglioma. Echocardiography. 2004; 21(3): 299-301.
54. Johnston DC, Goldstein LB. Clinical carotid endarterectomy decision making: noninvasive vascular imaging versus angiography. Neurology. 2001;56(8):1009-15.
55. Qureshi AI, Suri MF, Ali Z, et al. Role of conventional angiography in evaluation of patients with carotid artery stenosis demonstrated by Doppler ultrasound in general practice. Stroke 2001;32(10):2287-91.
56. Kalashyan H, Saqqur M, Shuaib A, et al. Comprehensive and rapid assessment of carotid plaques in acute stroke using a new single sweep method for three-dimensional carotid ultrasound. Echocardiography. 2013;30(4):414-8.

SECTION 21

Vertebral Artery Disease

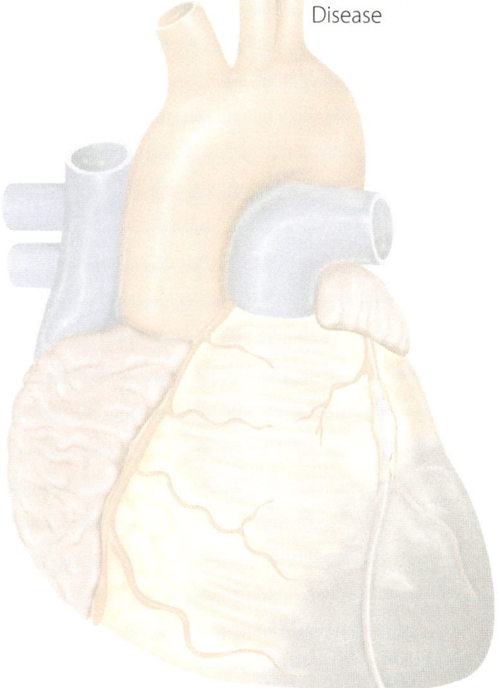

102

CHAPTER

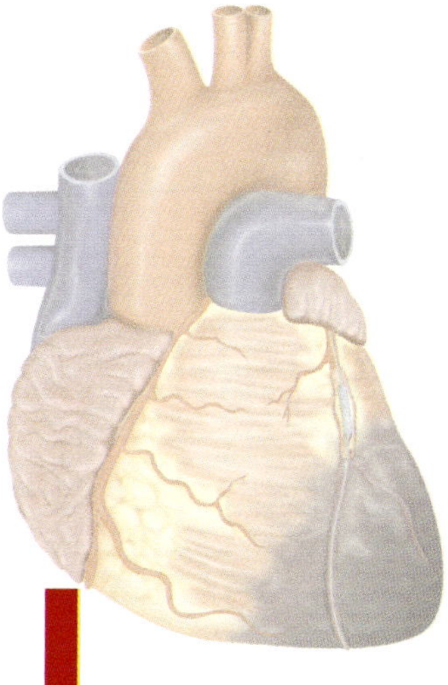

Color Doppler Evaluation of Vertebral Artery Disease

Naveen Garg, KK Kapur

VERTEBRAL ARTERIES

The brain is supplied by the four vessels, bilaterally internal carotids and vertebral artery (VA).

The VA ascends through the cervical vertebral foramina and passes through the foramen magnum. It has no major branches in the neck. After giving rise to the posterior inferior cerebellar artery, the vertebral arteries join to form the basilar artery. Excellent communications exist between the carotid and vertebral arteries systems via the circle of Willis (Figs. 1A and B).

The anatomical course of VA may be divided into four parts (Fig. 1C):

1. *V1*: The first (preforaminal) part, after its origin from subclavian artery (SA) it runs upward and backward over the transverse process of the seventh cervical vertebra (C7), to reach foramen of C6
2. *V2*: The second (foraminal) part, it runs upward through the foramina in the transverse processes of the C6 to C2 vertebra
3. *V3*: The third (extradural or atlantic) part, it emerges out from the C2 foramen moves upward to enter in the foramen of C1, and then curves medially and posteriorly to enters the vertebral canal in occiput
4. *V4*: The fourth (intradural or intracranial) part, it pierces the dura mater and at the lower border of the pons it unites with the vessel of the opposite side to form the basilar artery.[1]

Usually the first and second part is readily imaged by color Doppler. Imaging of the third part could be technically difficult while the fourth part is only imaged by transcranial Doppler.

DOPPLER ULTRASOUND IMAGING

Doppler ultrasound (US) is an established technique for evaluating extracranial portion of carotids and vertebral arteries in patients with manifested or suspected cerebrovascular diseases, not only for screening but also for preoperative assessment. The interrogation of VA is usually done by placing the US probe at rot of the neck and then moving gradually the transducer distally. The VA is located posterior to the common carotids and internal carotids. At the root of the neck with the probe oriented longitudinally, SA is visualized in cross section and VA is seen originating from the first part of SA usually at 4 o'clock position. VA is then traced distally up to the angle of jaw.[2-4] Normally, the VA is a low-resistance vessel. The Doppler waveform is monophasic with a good diastolic flow. Usual Doppler velocities are 30–60 cm/s systolic and 15–20 cm/s diastolic, and resistive index varies from 0.50 to 0.80, depending on the patients' age and dominance (one of the VA could be larger and dominant as compared to the opposite side VA; Figs. 2A and B).[5,6]

SUBCLAVIAN STEAL SYNDROME

The stenosis or occlusion proximal to the SA, results in retrograde flow in ipsilateral VA to supply the arm at expense of vertebra-basilar circulation. This is called subclavian

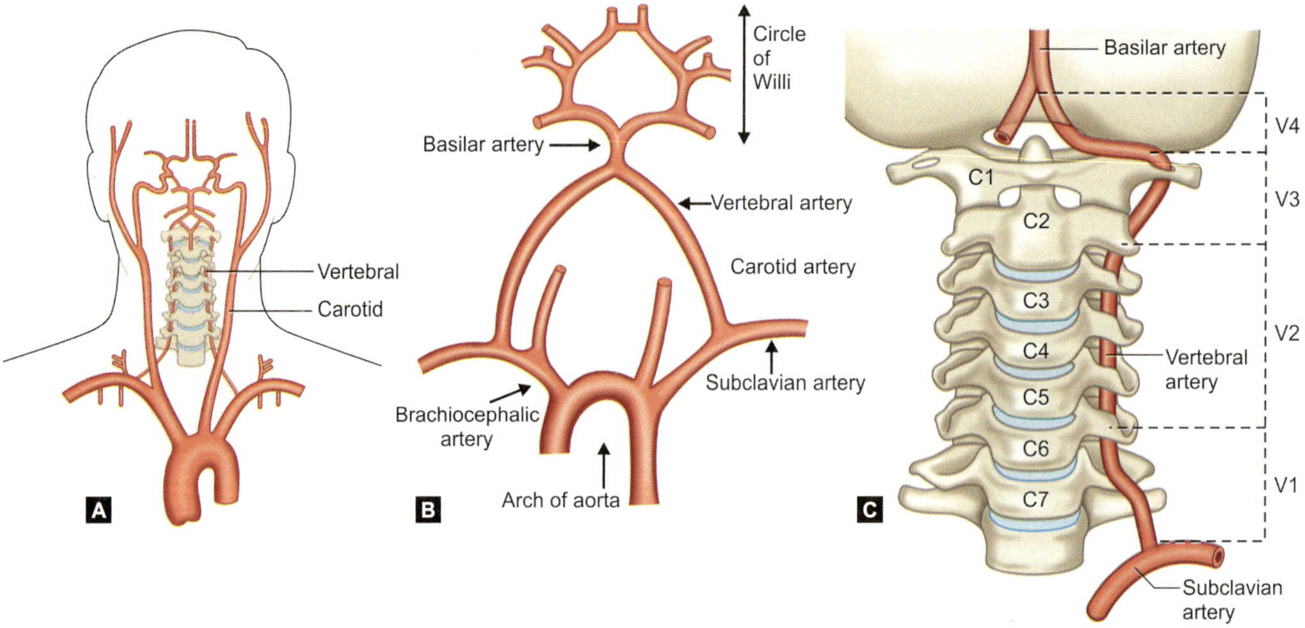

Figs. 1A to C: (A) Basic anatomy of vertebral arteries; (B) Pictorial description of vertebral arteries; (C) Anatomical parts of vertebral artery.

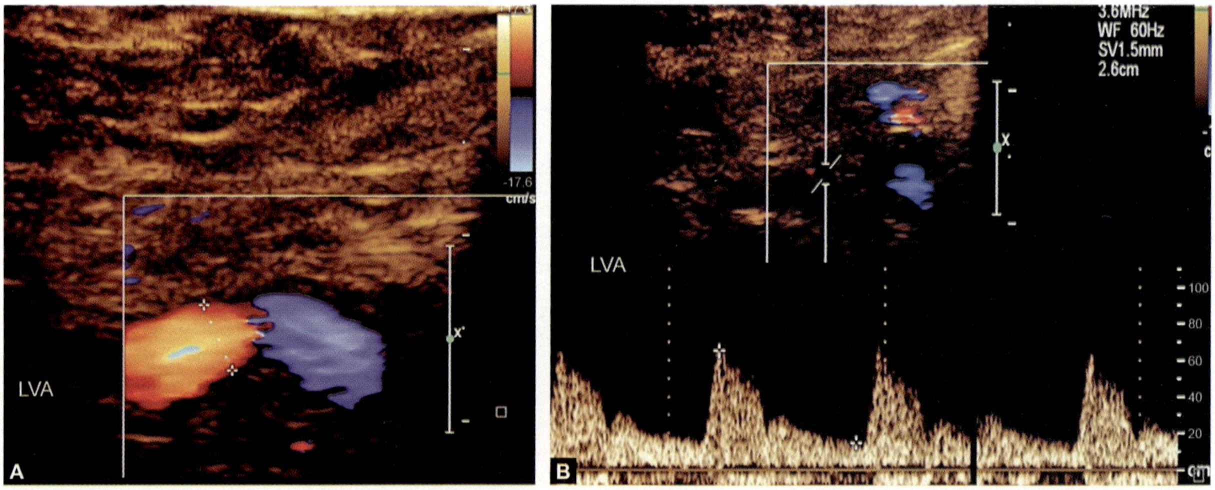

Figs. 2A and B: (A) Color Doppler of left vertebral artery; (B) Pulse Doppler of vertebral artery (LVA: left vertebral artery). Peak systolic velocity (PSV) = 65 cm/s; end-diastolic velocity (EDV) = 14.9 cm/s; resistive index (RI) = 0.77. Doppler sonogram shows waveforms resemble internal carotid artery, because vertebral artery also supplies low-resistance vascular bed of brain. Typical vertebral artery waveform shows a low-resistance pattern with antegrade diastolic flow.

steal and hence, the symptoms or signs that arise from this phenomenon is known as subclavian steal syndrome (SSS). These are depicted in Figures 3A to C.

Atherosclerosis is the most common cause of SSS, accounting for close to 100% of cases. Rarer causes include congenital atresia of the first part of the SA, interruptions due to embolic, traumatic or iatrogenic causes, inflammatory arteritis such as Takayasu arteritis. Signs and symptoms involved are of ischemic involving the central nervous system or the ipsilateral upper limb or both. The most consistent clinical findings are a diminished or an absent pulse and asymmetrical blood pressure between the upper limbs.[7-9]

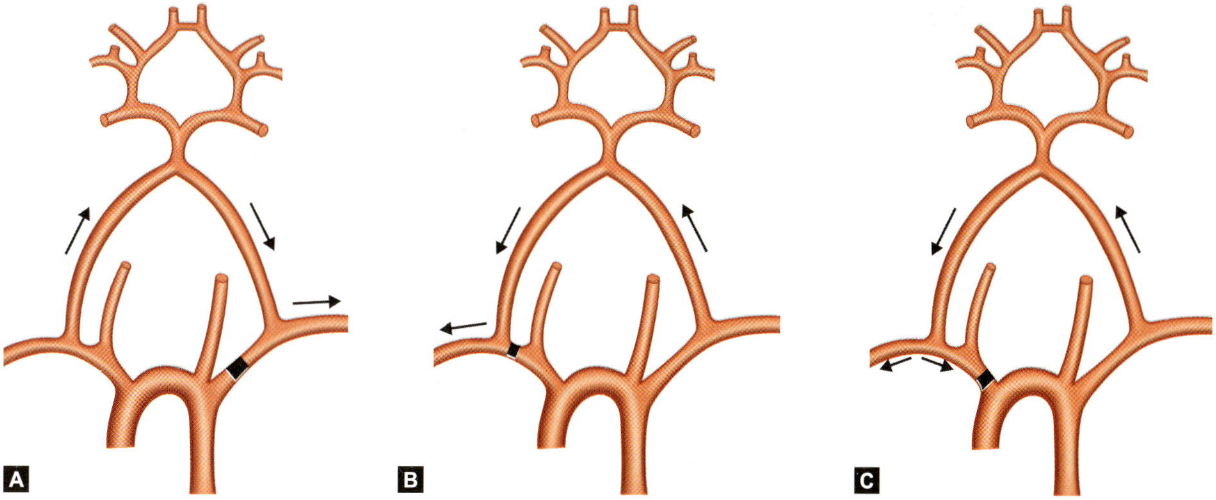

Figs. 3A to C: (A) Depicts left-sided subclavian steal syndrome. Proximal part of subclavian artery is blocked and reverse flow in left vertebral artery; (B) Similarly proximal portion of right subclavian artery is blocked after common carotid origin from brachiocephalic artery; (C) Depicts blockage at origin of brachiocephalic artery. Reverse flow can be appreciated both in right vertebral as well as in right common carotid artery.

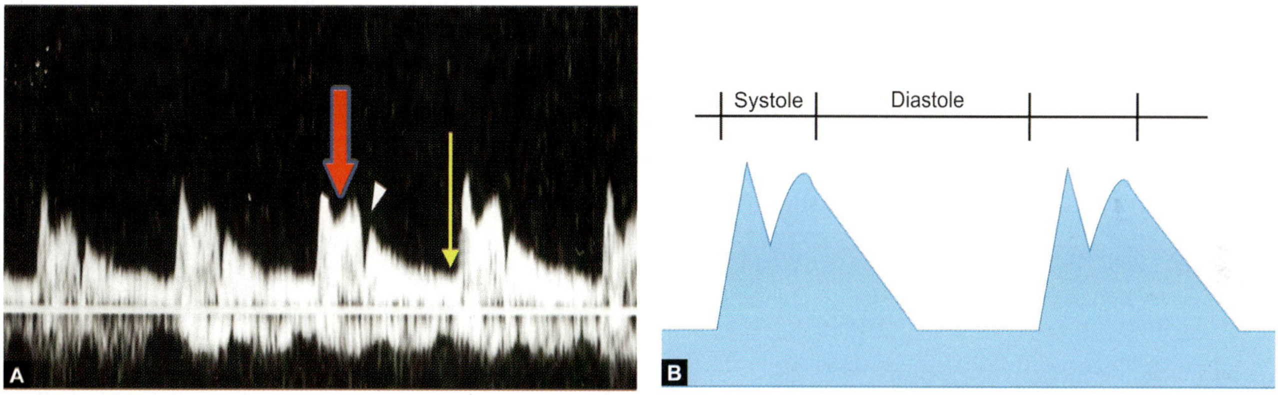

Figs. 4A and B: Double peak in systole: (A) Notch after first peak is depicted in red arrow. Incisura at the beginning of diastole is marked as white arrow head. End-diastolic velocity is marked as yellow arrow; (B) Schematic diagram showing double peak in systole.

SEVERITY OF STENOSIS AND DOPPLER WAVEFORMS IN SSS

Depending on the severity of the SA stenosis, different patterns of spectral waveforms are observed. According to the severity of stenosis prevertebral segment of SA, five spectral patterns can be seen. Systolic component of the waveform is usually notched and two distinct peaks can be discerned. The first peak is usually sharp and the second one is more blunted. The patterns of the waveform are defined by the nadir (depth) of notch between two peaks.[10-12]

- *Type 1*: The flow velocity at the nadir of the notch is more than the end-diastolic velocity (Figs. 4A and B)
- *Type 2*: The flow velocity at the nadir of the notch is equal to the end-diastolic velocity (Figs. 5A and B)
- *Type 3*: The flow velocity at the nadir of the notch is less than the end-diastolic velocity (Figs. 6A and B)
- *Type 4*: The flow velocity at the nadir of the notch is less than and seen on opposite side of the baseline to the end-diastolic velocity (Figs. 7A and B)
- *Type 5*: The flow velocity is totally reversed, below the baseline as compared to the expected direction of antegrade flow. This indicates almost total blockage (Fig. 8).

Thus, as the severity of stenosis increases, the retrograde flow in mid to end-systole increases. This can also be provoked by maneuvers causing decrease in peripheral vascular resistance in affected arm (like exercise or induced reactive hyperemia).

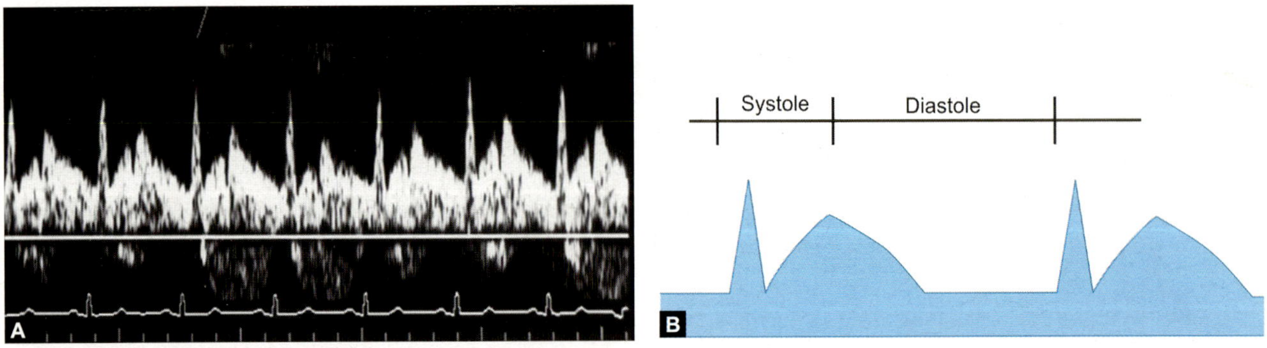

Figs. 5A and B: (A) Nadir of systrolic notch has same velocity as at of end-diastole; (B) Schematic waveform of type-2. Outline resembles body profile of rabbit and is sometimes referred to as "bunny waveform".

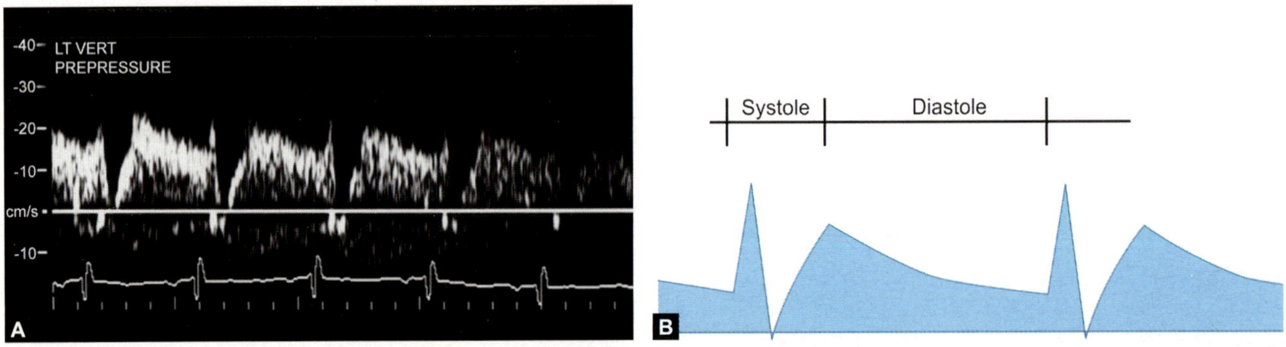

Figs. 6A and B: (A) Nadir of systolic notch touches baseline. Velocity at nadir is below of end-diastolic velocity; (B) Schematic diagram of the same.

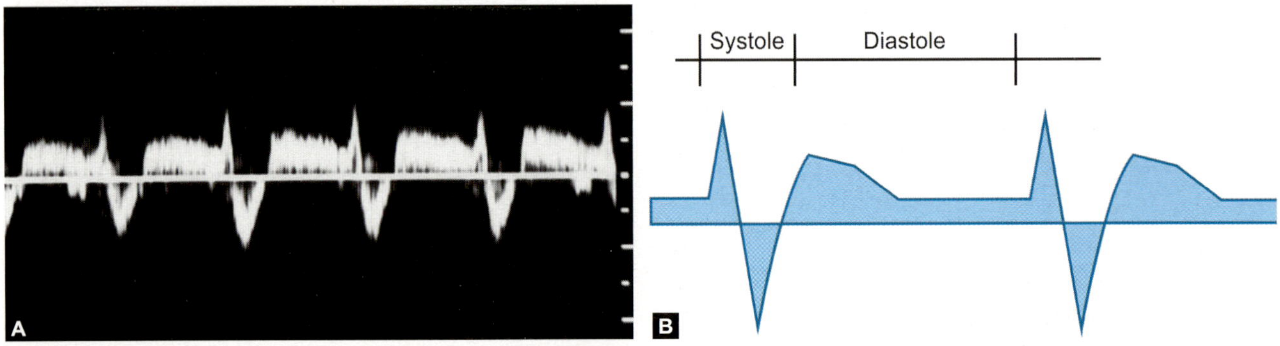

Figs. 7A and B: (A) Nadir of systolic notch is well below baseline, indicates late systolic mild retrograde flow due to significant stenosis causing drop of blood pressure in poststenotic vessel occurring due to jet effect; (B) Schematic diagram of the same.

REACTIVE HYPEREMIA INDUCTION MANEUVER

The principle behind this maneuver is to elicit a change in the direction of the spectral waveform in VA in patients with significant proximal SA stenosis. Flow in vertebral arteries is reversed only in mid to late-systolic phase as during early systole pressure is enough to cause antegrade flow. Distal to stenosis because of jet effect there is drop in pressure, and this leads to origin of mid systolic notch. Thus when the drop in pressure due to jet effect is more than the antegrade flow, reversal of flow occurs. This can be elicited by lowering the pressure (peripheral resistance) of ipsilateral arm so that more blood in withdrawn in SA and there is low blood flow (antegrade) in VA. This will lead to increased poststenotic drop in blood pressure and the reversal of blood (blood from vertebra-basilar) will occur. Induction of reactive hyperemia is either elicited by exercising the arm and then observing the effect on VA Doppler pattern. However, a more technically correct procedure is to place the

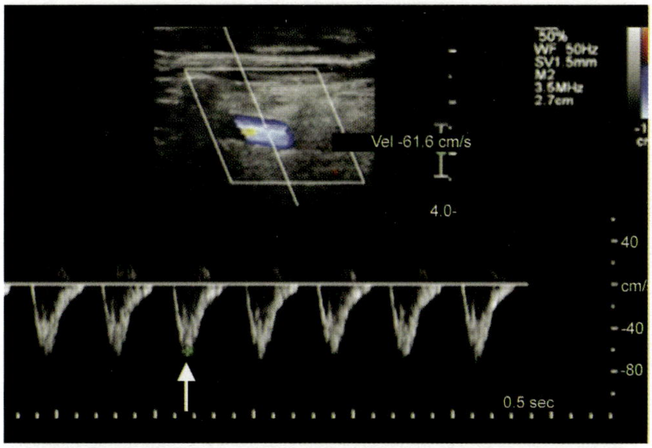

Fig. 8: Reversal flow in the vertebral artery due to total occlusion in proximal subclavian artery.

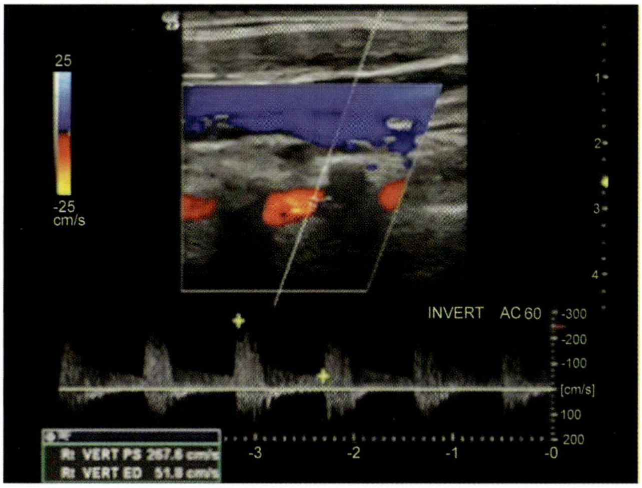

Fig. 9: High velocity in vertebral arteries of about 267.6 cm/s indicates stenosis.

sphygmomanometer cuff on ipsilateral arm and then inflate above the baseline systolic pressure for about 3–5 minutes and then deflate rapidly. On release of the cuff pressure, reactive hyperemia is induced leading to dilatation of distal vessels and a decrease in vascular resistance. Simultaneous Doppler recordings demonstrate corresponding changes in the waveforms, which usually show varying grades of flow reversal. Although, demonstrable changes in Doppler waveform patterns indicate significant SA stenosis. Failure to show these changes does not necessarily exclude the presence of hemodynamically subclavian narrowing.

VERTEBRAL ARTERY STENOSIS

Vertebral artery stenosis is usually diagnosed incidentally during routine carotid or VA Doppler study. Several noninvasive imaging modalities like duplex US, computed tomography (CT) scan, magnetic resonance imaging

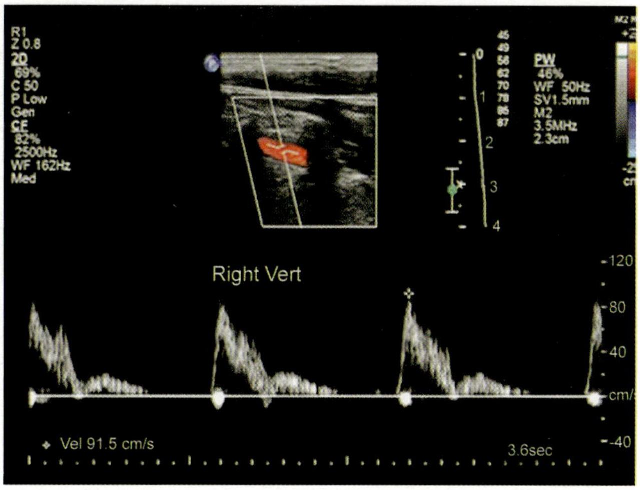

Fig. 10: A high resistance flow in vertebral artery showing low-diastolic flow. Diastolic flow almost nil in later part of diastole indicates high resistance in vertebral artery due to blockage near basilar artery.

(MRI) can detect VA stenosis. There are no widely accepted duplex criteria for the diagnosis of VA stenosis. Some authors have used a peak systolic velocity of more than 125 cm/s to categorize more than 50% diameter stenosis in VA (Fig. 9).[13,14] A significantly elevated diastolic velocity indicates a high-grade stenosis (more than 70%).

The usual location of VA stenosis is at its origin which could be difficult to interrogate.

Duplex imaging of VA is a reliable method to detect significant VA stenosis. In one prospective blinded study involving 158 patients, color Doppler was found to have sensitivity and specificity of 71% and 99%, respectively in detecting VA stenosis of more than 70% reduction in luminal diameter when compared with digital subtraction angiography as the reference standard.[15,16,17]

A high-resistance Doppler spectral pattern (high systolic velocity and low or absent diastolic velocity) as shown in Figure 10, indicates obstruction at the basal artery (if seen bilaterally) or just proximal to the basilar artery (if seen ipsilaterally).[18]

VERTEBRAL ARTERY VENOUS FISTULA

Vertebral artery venous (VAV) fistula is a rare condition which could be congenital or traumatic due to blunt trauma or internal jugular vein catheterization. This could present as an intractable tinnitus or pulsatile bruit. However these fistulas may be asymptomatic and may be detected incidentally. VAV fistula is readily diagnosed using color Doppler technique. Color flow mapping reveals continuous turbulent flow in the region of VA and vertebral vein and Doppler spectral waveform reveals a high velocity continuous pattern of flow. Surgical ligation or endovascular

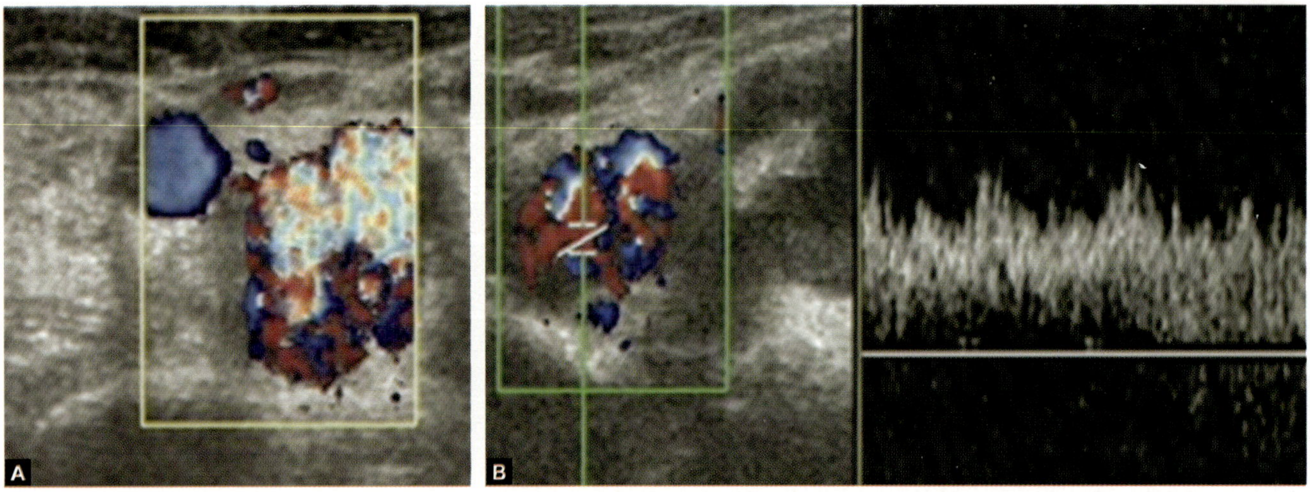

Figs. 11A and B: (A) Color Doppler ultrasound image shows high-grade vascularity in vertebral artery and vertebral vein; (B) Pulse Doppler shows high-grade velocity, low-resistance, monophasic spectrum in the vascular structures indicating fistulous communication between vertebral artery and vein.

closure of the high-flow arteriovenous fistula is the treatment of choice for VAV fistula (Figs. 11A and B).[19-22]

REFERENCES

1. Cacciola F, Phalke U, Goel A. Vertebral artery in relationship to C1-C2 vertebrae: an anatomical study. Neurol India. 2004;52(2):178-84.
2. Sidhu PS. Ultrasound of the carotid and vertebral arteries. Br Med Bull. 2000;56(2):346-66.
3. Sternic NC, Pavlovic AM, Podgorac A, et al. Ultrasound diagnostics of carotid and vertebral arteries. Period Biol. 2012;114(3):303-11.
4. Bluth EI, Merritt CR, Sullivan MA, et al. Usefulness of duplex ultrasound in evaluating vertebral arteries. J Ultrasound Med. 1989;8(5):229-35.
5. Nemati M, Bavil AS, Taheri N, et al. Comparison of normal values of Duplex indices of vertebral arteries in young and elderly adults. Cardiovasc Ultrasound. 2009;7:2.
6. Seidel E, Eicke BM, Tettenborn B, et al. Reference values for vertebral artery flow volume by duplex sonography in young and elderly adults. Stroke. 1999;30(12):2692-6.
7. Horrow MM, Stassi J. Sonography of the vertebral arteries: a window to disease of the proximal great vessels. AJR Am J Roentgenol. 2001;177(1):53-9.
8. Osiro S, Zurada A, Gielecki J, et al. A review of subclavian steal syndrome with clinical correlation. Med Sci Monit. 2012:18(5):RA57-63.
9. Päivänsalo M, Heikkilä O, Tikkakoski T, et al. Duplex ultrasound in the subclavian steal syndrome. Acta Radiol. 1998;39(2):183-8.
10. Kliewer MA, Hertzberg BS, Kim DH, et al. Vertebral artery Doppler waveform changes indicating subclavian steal physiology. AJR Am J Roentgenol. 2000;174(3):815-9.
11. Chen SP, Hu YP. Waveform patterns and peak reversed velocity in vertebral arteries predict severe subclavian artery stenosis and occlusion. Ultrasound Med Biol. 2015;41(5):1328-33.
12. Rohren EM, Kliewer MA, Carroll BA, et al. A spectrum of Doppler waveforms in the carotid and vertebral arteries. AJR Am J Roentgenol. 2003;181(6):1695-704.
13. Yurdakul M, Tola M. Doppler criteria for identifying proximal vertebral artery stenosis of 50% or more. J Ultrasound Med. 2011;30(2):163-8.
14. Hua Y, Meng XF, Jia LY, et al. Color Doppler imaging evaluation of proximal vertebral artery stenosis. AJR Am J Roentgenol. 2009;193(5):1434-8.
15. Rozeman AD, Hund H, Westein M, et al. Duplex ultrasonography for the detection of vertebral artery stenosis: a comparison with CT angiography. Brain Behav. 2017;7(8):e00750.
16. Kizilkilic O, Hurcan C, Mihmanli I, et al. Color Doppler analysis of vertebral arteries correlative study with angiographic data. J Ultrasound Med. 2004;23(11):1483-91.
17. de Bray JM, Pasco A, Tranquart F, et al. Accuracy of color-Doppler in the quantification of proximal vertebral artery stenoses. Cerebrovasc Dis. 2001;11(4):335-40.
18. Kim ES, Thompson M, Nacion KM, et al. Radiologic importance of a high-resistive vertebral artery Doppler waveform on carotid duplex ultrasonography. J Ultrasound Med. 2010;29(8):1161-5.
19. Edwards MK, Christenson EN, Corliss BM, et al. Vertebral arteriovenous fistula: an unwelcome thrill. Case Rep Emerg Med. 2017;2017:8386459.
20. Jang HJ, Oh SY, Shim YS, et al. Endovascular treatment of symptomatic high-flow vertebral arteriovenous fistula as a complication after c1 screw insertion. J Korean Neurosurg Soc. 2014;56 (4):348-52.
21. Yeh CH, Chen YL, Wu YM, et al. Anatomically based approach for endovascular treatment of vertebra-vertebral arteriovenous fistula. Interv Neuroradiol. 2014;20(6):766-73.
22. Umesh B, Pramodbhai P, Laxmidas C, et al. MR findings of vertebral AVM. Internet J Radiol. 2012;14(1):1-10.

SECTION 22

Peripheral Arterial and Venous Disease

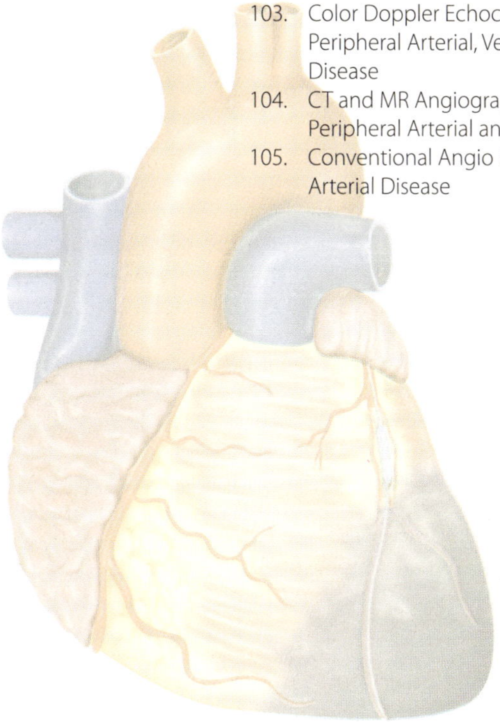

103

CHAPTER

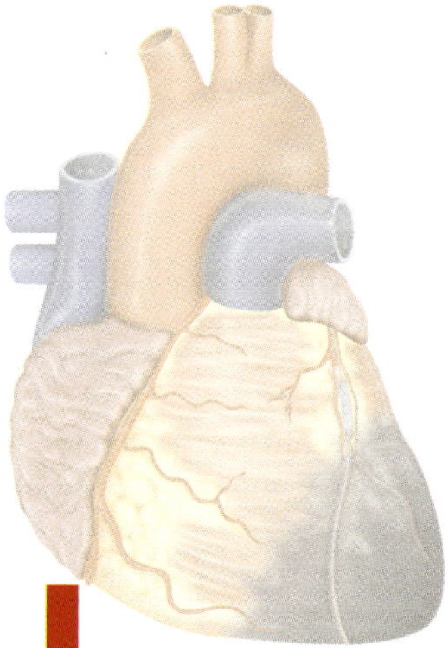

Color Doppler Echocardiographic Evaluation of Peripheral Arterial, Venous, and Carotid Artery Disease

Naveen Garg, KK Kapur, HK Chopra

INTRODUCTION

Doppler ultrasound (US) interrogation helps in analyzing peripheral vascular diseases (PVD) that include blockage, spasm, narrowing, or aneurysmal dilatation in arteries and incompetence, clots, or thrombus in venous system.[1,2] Moreover, this technique can be used to monitor disease progression, direct appropriate interventions and assess therapeutic response. The common causes of PVD are in Table 1.

VASCULAR ULTRASOUND AND TERMINOLOGY

Doppler US measures frequency shifts are provided by moving red blood cells in vessels.[3,4] The spectral velocity–time display is called velocity waveform. This waveform patterns depend on many factors.

- *Blood velocity*: A prominent Doppler waveform is obtained in proximal large vessels due to relatively high velocity as compared to distal vessels (Fig. 1).
  In the presence of significant luminal stenosis, higher velocities are obtained at the stenotic site or just beyond as compared to the flows in the relatively normal segment proximal to the stenotic region (Fig. 2). However, in near total occlusions or in long-segment tubular stenosis, this effect may not be observed, and significantly damped flow is observed at the end of the stenotic segment.
- *The angle of insonation*: A parallel alignment of Doppler beam in the direction of blood flow results in high-quality crisp and clear velocity waveforms. An angle correction higher than maximum of 60° usually results in significant overestimations of peak velocities.

TABLE 1: Common causes of PVD.

Hypertension	Sedentary lifestyle	Smoking/tobacco/drug abuse
Injuries	Diabetes	Inflammation or infections
Obesity	High cholesterol	Muscles or ligaments abnormalities
Emotional stress	Cold temperature	Operating on vibrating machinery/tools

(PVD: peripheral vascular diseases)

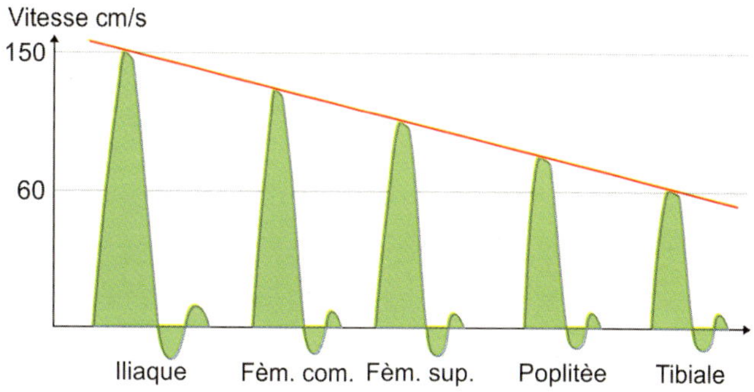

Fig. 1: Blood velocity tracing on Doppler. Large proximal arteries show higher velocities than distal ones.

- The angle of insonation should be less than 60° (Figs. 3A and B).

PULSED WAVE DOPPLER

In this mode, the Doppler interrogation of blood vessel is performed by placing a sample volume (<1.5 mm) usually in the center of its lumen, and the resulting spectral waveforms are analyzed. Color Doppler flow mapping facilitates appropriate placement of Doppler sample volume (Fig. 4).

COLOR FLOW MAPPING AND DOPPLER SCANNING

Doppler color flow mapping superimposed on two-dimensional (2D) image of blood vessel helps in establishing the direction of the blood flow. Brighter shades of color and aliasing indicate high velocities which could indicate either a stenotic lesion or a high flow state. A display of both Doppler spectral waveform together with color mapping is called duplex scanning (Fig. 4). The Nyquist limit (color scale) is usually set about 20–25 cm/s for the large and medium size vessels and about 10 cm/s for small distal vessels. By convention, red signals are taken moving toward the ultrasonic probe (transducer), whereas blue-colored signals are taken moving away from the probe (Figs. 5A and B).

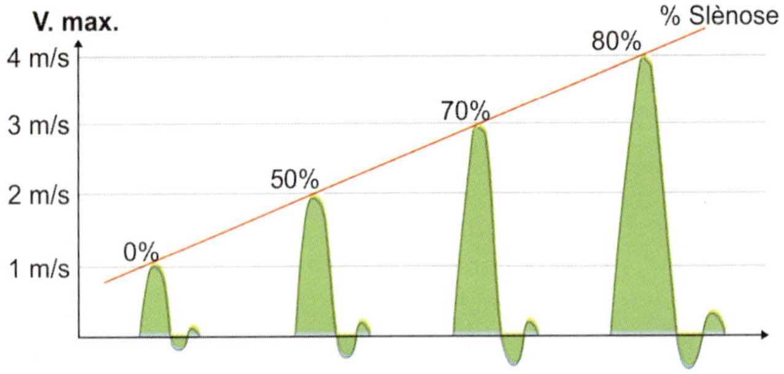

Fig. 2: Poststenotic waveform is larger than proximal waveform due to jet effect.

Gain Settings

The appropriate use of the gain control is essential for technical as well as interpretative accuracy of Doppler US. These gain settings apply to B-mode US, color flow mapping as well as to the spectral Doppler display.

For the B-mode US, an optimum gain is achieved when the vessel lumen appears as "jet black" contrasting well with the gray scale of vascular wall.

At appropriate color gain settings the spillover of color signals beyond the vessel wall boundary does not occur.

Adequate Doppler gain is seen as "crisp and clear" well-defined Doppler waveforms without the feathery overshoots of peak velocities.

Arterial Diseases

Duplex ultrasound (DUS) is widely used for the screening and diagnosis of vascular lesions.

Duplex ultrasound provides information regarding cardiovascular risk assessment. It readily detects intimal medial thickness (IMT) which is predictor of cardiovascular morbidity and mortality.[3-9]

Duplex ultrasound allows a complete evaluation of the different vascular beds and is often the first step in the clinical management. Novel additions, such as live three-dimensional (3-D) imaging, as well as the use of US contrast agents, could further enhance the performance of DUS. DUS of arteries facilitates the diagnosis of the following lesions—stenosis, thrombus, aneurysm, fistula, and collaterals.

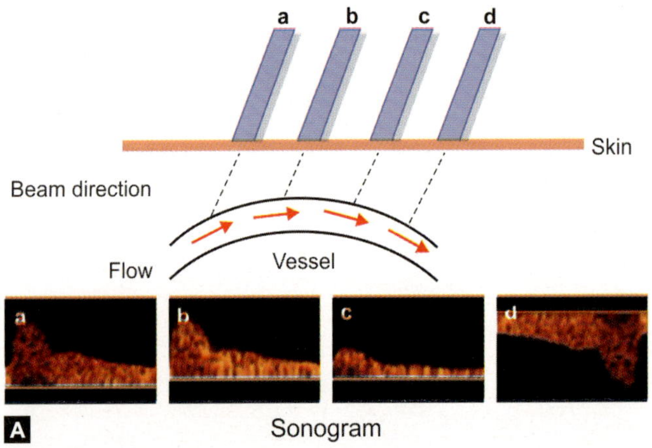

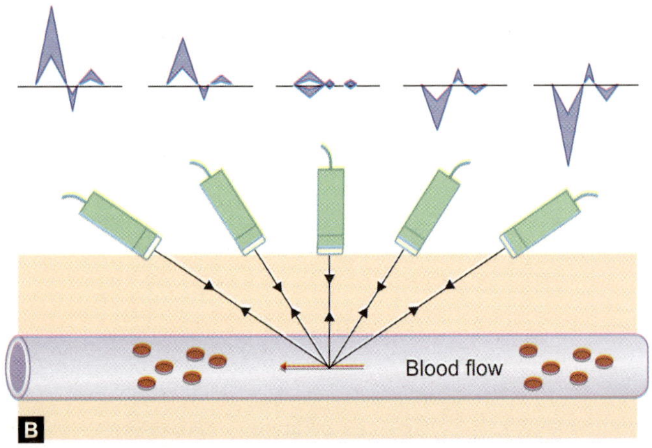

Figs. 3A and B: Importance of Doppler angle. When ultrasound beam is parallel to blood flow direction as in "a," the Doppler waveform is sharp and shows the highest velocity, whereas in "b" or "c" the ultrasound waves are not in parallel and thus shows damped flows. In "d" the flow is opposite to as in "a."

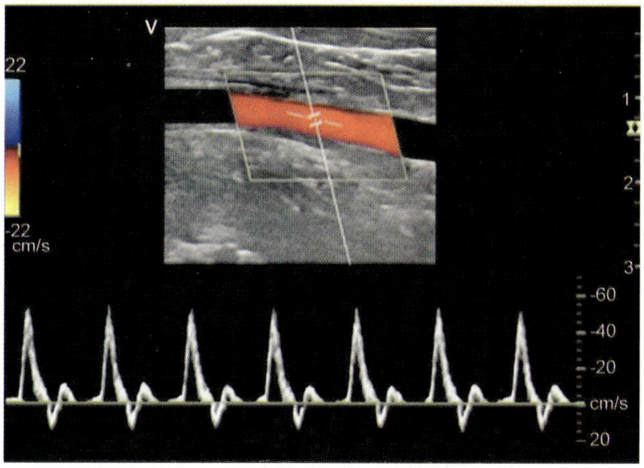

Fig. 4: Pulse wave Doppler.

Duplex scanning provides a combination of anatomic and physiologic information that is usually not obtained with other imaging modalities.

Arterial Waveforms

Doppler waveform patterns in the various arterial circulations show remarkable variations depending on the site, size, and distance from the heart. The spectral profile of these waveforms could also provide important clues to the various pathological conditions.[10,11] The different waveform profiles are as illustrated below:

Triphasic

A triphasic waveform with three components (Fig. 6)

1. Forward flow in systole
2. Reverse flow (late systole/early diastole due to elastic recoil)
3. Forward flow (late diastole)

This flow pattern is considered a reference pattern for a normal flow in high-resistance circulations (e.g. arteries of upper and lower limb). A thin spectrum with a "clear window" implies a nonturbulent flow.

Biphasic

This pattern of Doppler flow is also present in high-resistant arteries and could imply a minimal to mild disease. This is depicted as a forward flow in systole and a reverse flow in late systole/early diastole (Fig. 7).

Monophasic Flow

This pattern is found in low-resistant arteries (e.g. hepatic, renal, splenic, cerebral, gravid uterus, and umbilical artery circulations) and is depicted as a single phase with slow acceleration and deceleration. However, this pattern is also seen in limb arteries with advanced disease distal to the site of high-grade stenosis, near total occlusions, or distal to a total block. Good collateral flow to the arteries distal to the site of occlusions results in a more prominent monophasic waveform (Figs. 8A and B).

Criteria for Estimating Severity of Peripheral Arterial Narrowing

The degree of arterial narrowing can be estimated on B-mode US together with color flow mapping by direct computation, or it can also be assessed indirectly by using Doppler velocity ratios (Vrs) as shown here:

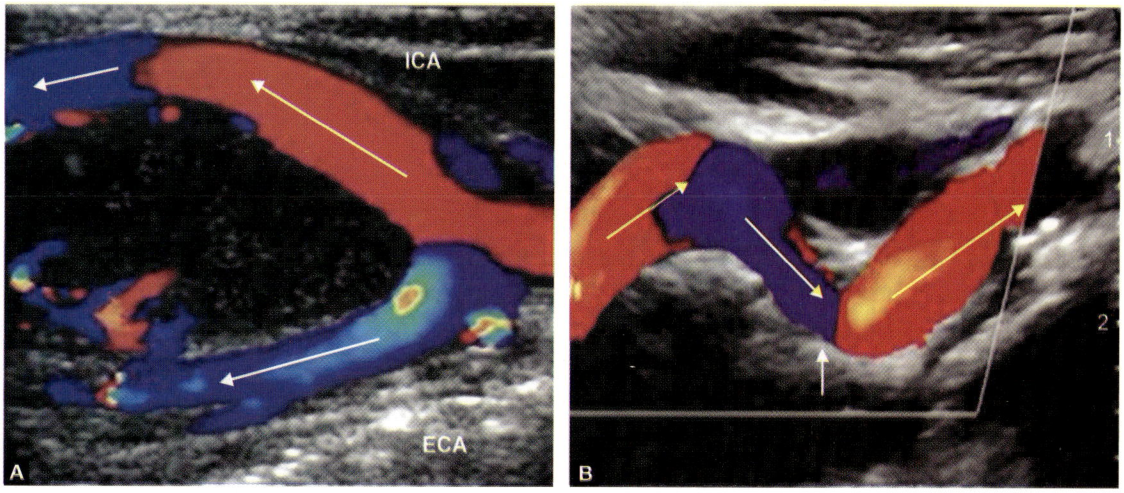

Figs. 5A and B: This figure depicts red and blue color of Doppler signals. (A) Arrows shows the direction of moving blood; (B) The blood is moving in tortuous artery and shows change in color as it flows away from the transducer. (ICA: internal carotid artery; ECA: external carotid artery)

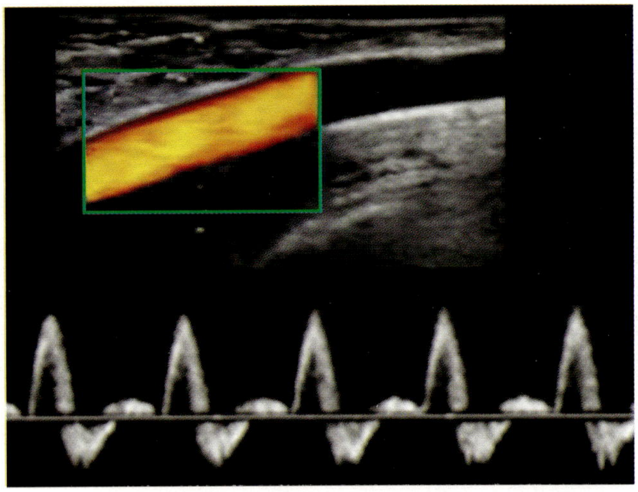

Fig. 6: Triphasic waveform.

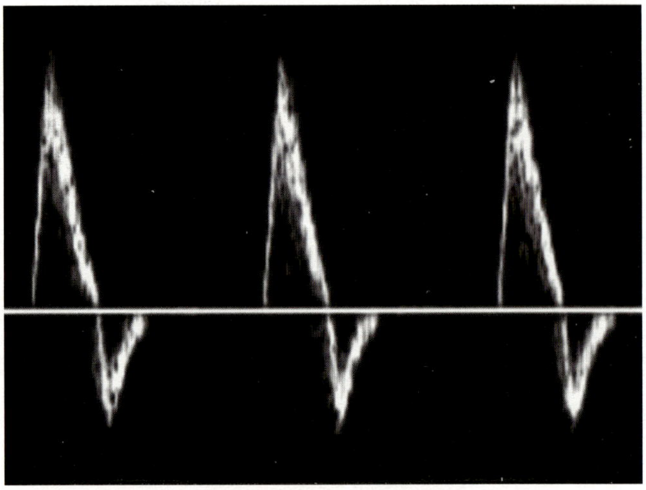

Fig. 7: Biphasic pattern.

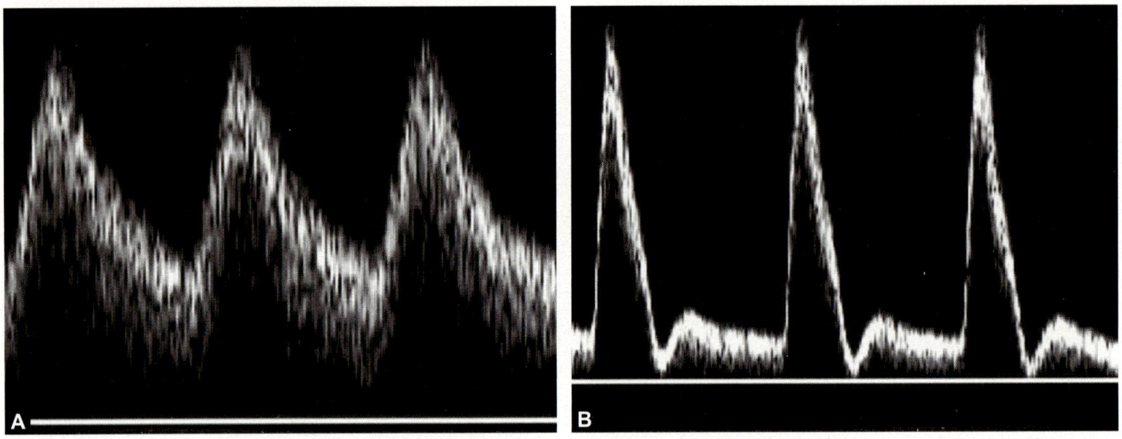

Figs. 8A and B: Monophasic arterial Doppler flow pattern.

- *Peak flow Vr*: It can be defined as the ratio of peak flow at the site of stenosis to the peak flow proximal to the stenosis. This gives some indication as to the percentage of the stenosis (Table 2 and Figs. 9A and B).

The shape of the Doppler waveform as assessed by the *time to peak flow velocity* also gives some indications about the degree of stenosis.

Doppler waveform of slanted pattern (long time to peak) implies significant stenosis and damped flows than of brisk pattern of undamped flow (Figs. 10A and B).

The overall assessment of severity of arterial narrowing is depicted in Table 3.

Limitations

Obesity and heavily calcified vessels may produce poor acoustic window that may limit the ability to analyze Doppler trace.

TABLE 2: Indications for the percentage of velocity ratio and stenosis.

Velocity ratio	*Percentage stenosis*
<1.5:1	Normal
1.5–2:1	25–50%
2–4:1	50–75%
4:1	>75%
No flow	Occluded

EQUIPMENT SELECTION

A good color Doppler machine with a dedicated vascular capability or combined equipment for echocardiography and vascular applications is essential for Doppler assessment of arterial circulation. A linear probe of 5–12 MHz is used to assess arteries of upper and lower extremities. However, interrogation of abdominal aorta and iliac arteries as well as edematous/bulky limbs is performed using a lower frequency (2–5 MHz) curvilinear (convex) probe.

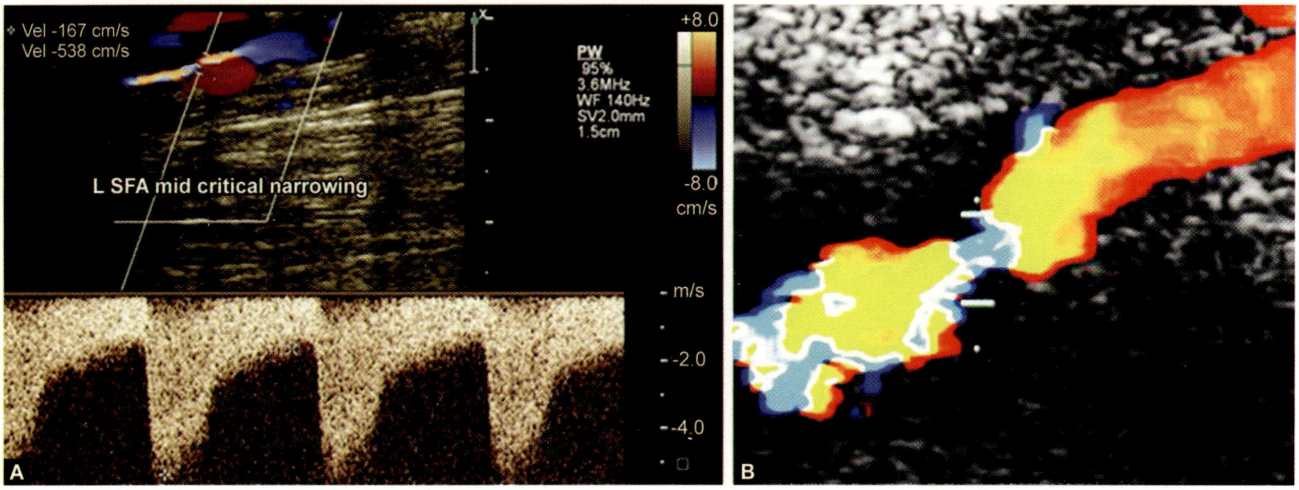

Figs. 9A and B: (A) Monophasic with marked spectral broadening indicating severe blockage. PSV is more than 100% increase (538 cm/s); (B) Color flow pattern showing stenosis. (PSV: peak systolic velocity)

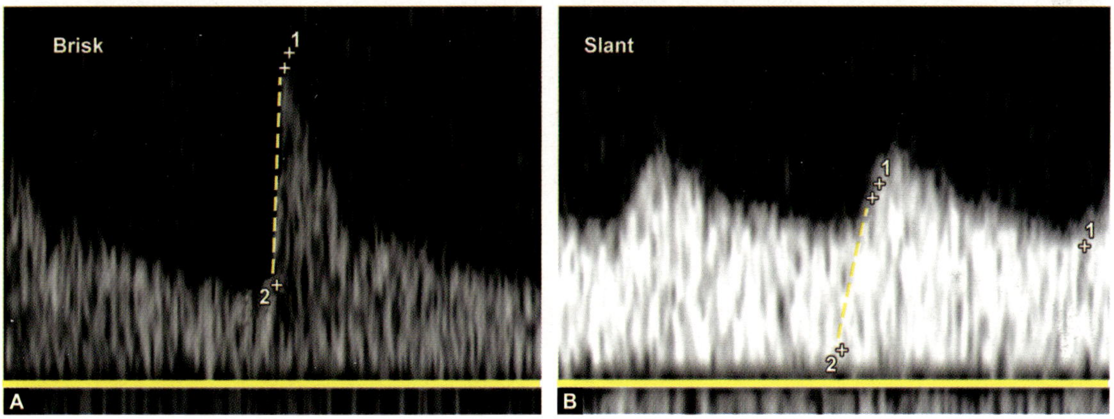

Figs. 10A and B: Slanted pattern is seen in damped flows due to occlusion.

Lower Limb

Anatomies of lower limb arteries are depicted in Figures 11A and B.

Duplex Scan Thigh

Duplex scan of the thigh begins below the inguinal crease in the middle. Pulsatile common femoral artery is lateral to femoral vein (FV) and may show the superficial femoral artery and the deep femoral artery are present alongside the FV, producing Mickey Mouse's sign in transverse imaging and Y-sign in longitudinal view (Figs. 12 to 14).[12-14]

Pseudoaneurysm: A pseudoaneurysm is defined as an arterial wall deficiency, which leads to the accumulation of oxygenated blood in a sac surrounding by soft tissue and compressed thrombus. Color imaging shows sac around the vessel, and Doppler waveform depicts "to-and-fro" pattern of blood movement (Figs. 15A and B).

TABLE 3: Assessment of severity of arterial narrowing.

Disease severity	*Spectral waveform*
1–19% diameter reduction	Triphasic pattern
20–49%	Triphasic with minimal reverse wave and prominent spectral broadening with increased PSV to more than 50–100%
50–99%	Monophasic waveform with extensive spectral broadening. PSV > 100% increase. Distal waveforms show damped flow
Total occlusion	No flow. Proximal waveform may show thump wave pattern (tardus-parvus wave)

(PSV: peak systolic velocity)

Criteria for the diagnosis of pseudoaneurysm includes:

- Extravascular arterial sac with flow
- A relatively narrow communication or rent between sac and artery

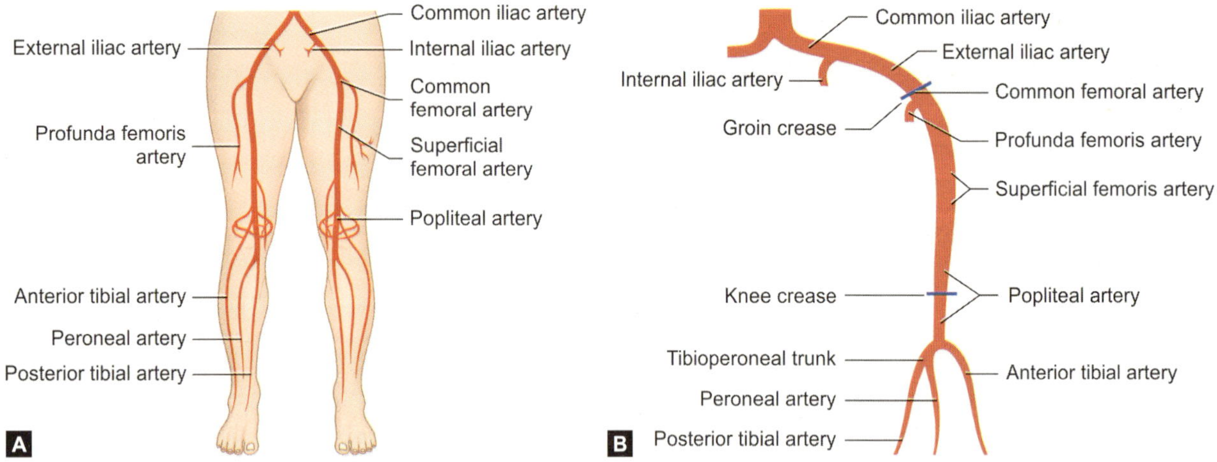

Figs. 11A and B: Basic anatomy of lower limb arteries.

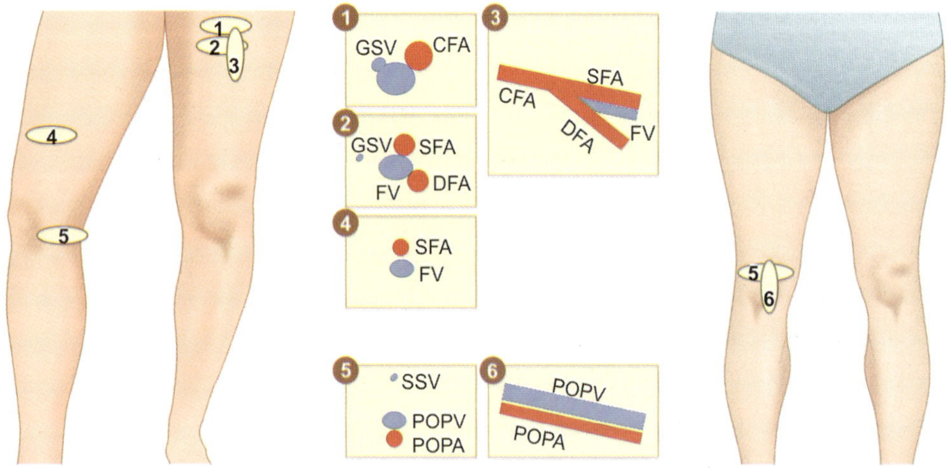

Fig. 12: It shows the areas of US scan for lower limb arteries as well corresponding pictorial views. (POPA: popliteal artery; POPV: popliteal vein; US: ultrasound; GSV: great saphenous vein; SSV: small saphenous vein; SFA: superficial femoral artery; DFA: deep femoral artery; FV: femoral vein; CFA: common femoral artery)

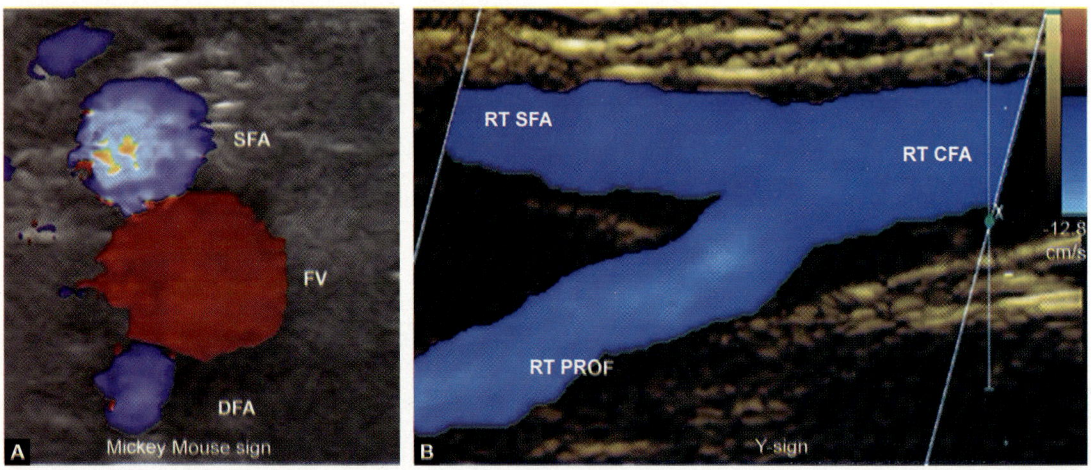

Figs. 13A and B: Ultrasonic imaging showing transverse view at inguinal region (Mickey Mouse sign) and longitudinal view (Y-sign) of femoral arteries. Usually a peak flow velocity in common femoral and SFA arteries below 55 cm/s could indicate a significant stenosis either proximal or distal to this site in a patient with a normal cardiac output.[12-14] It is better to compare Doppler patterns with normal (asymptomatic) leg. Figure 14 depicts the comparison of Doppler patterns in both the legs of a patient with claudication pain. (SFA: superficial femoral artery; FV: femoral vein; DFA: deep femoral artery)

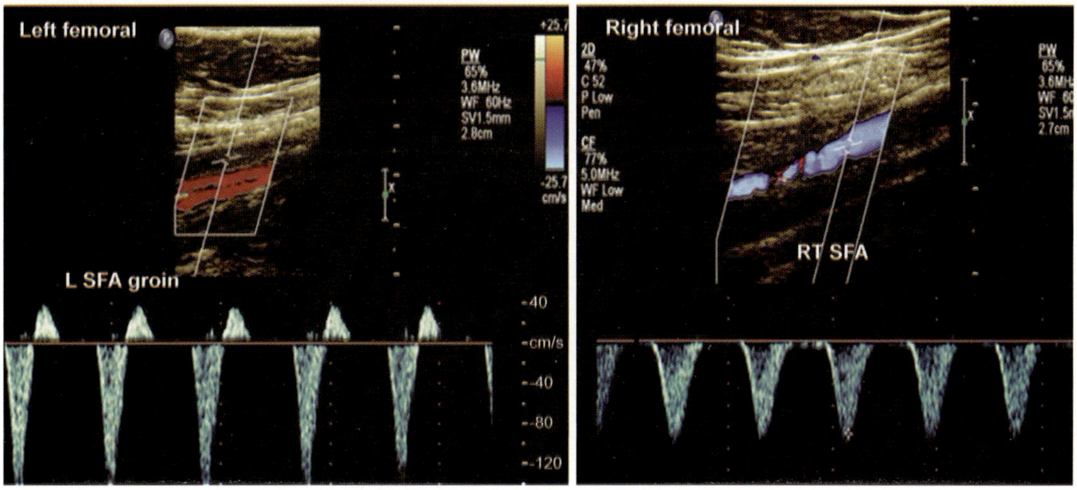

Fig. 14: Claudication pain in the right leg in a 66-year-old woman. Left femoral artery shows triphasic pattern, while right SFA is monophasic. (SFA: superficial femoral artery)

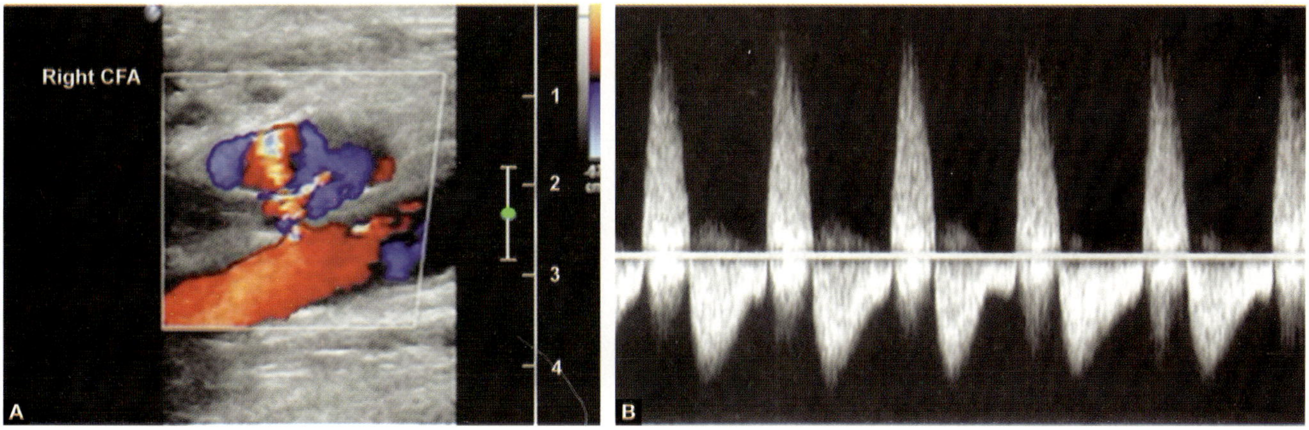

Figs. 15A and B: (A) Pseudoaneurysm sac; and (B) To-and-fro pattern. (CFA: common femoral artery)

- To-and-fro flow pattern between the native artery and the extravascular sac.

Infrapopliteal Doppler

The popliteal artery is seen in the middle of popliteal fossa. Posterior tibial artery is scanned from knee to medial malleolus on medial aspect of the lower leg, and anterior tibial artery is on anterolateral aspect. The peroneal artery is scanned along the lateral side of the posterior calf and is visualized alongside the fibular bone (Figs. 16 and 17A to C).

Case example: Right tibial artery shows damp flows due to obstruction at popliteal artery. After stent graft (endovascular procedure), triphasic patterns were restored in both popliteal as well as in tibial arteries (Figs. 18A to C).

Upper Limb (Fig. 19)[15-19]

Areas of interrogation Doppler are shown in Figures 20A and B.

Evaluations should be made bilaterally and is compared. In addition to the evaluation of arterial diseases of upper limb, color Doppler examination is frequently used to assess for surgically created arteriovenous fistulae (AVF), arteriovenous (AV) grafts. Interrogations of aortic arch as well as carotids and vertebral circulations may also be required for a complete evaluation of upper extremity arterial circulation.

Arteriovenous Fistula/Grafts

Arteriovenous fistulae and AV grafts are frequently created surgically to provide a suitable and stable access for hemodialysis.

The most preferred sites for AVF are the wrist and distal forearm (radiocephalic) and the elbow (brachiocephalic or brachiobasilic). The selection of the fistula site and prediction of its maturation, adequacy, and function can be easily and rapidly achieved by Duplex ultrasonography. Scanning of the artery is done by using B-mode and M-mode

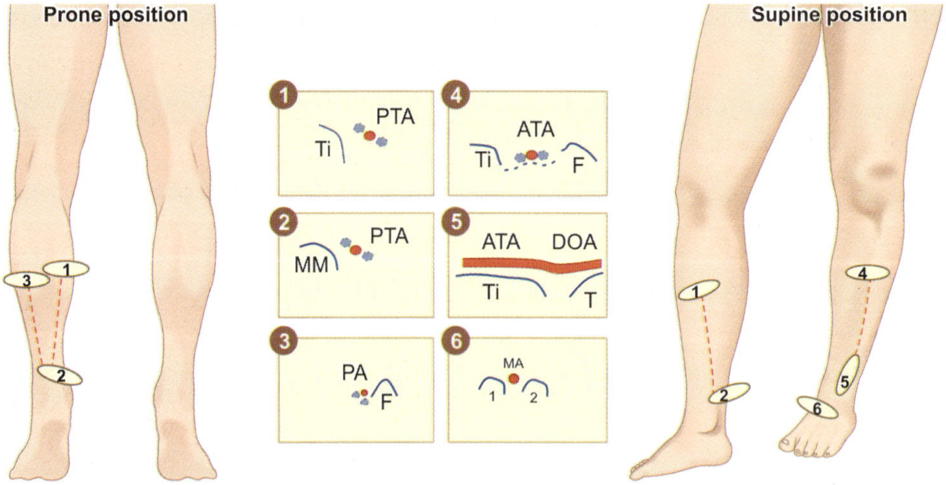

Fig. 16: Depicting the area of US scanning for infrapopliteal arteries with corresponding pictorial 2D views. (US: ultrasound; 2D: two-dimensional)

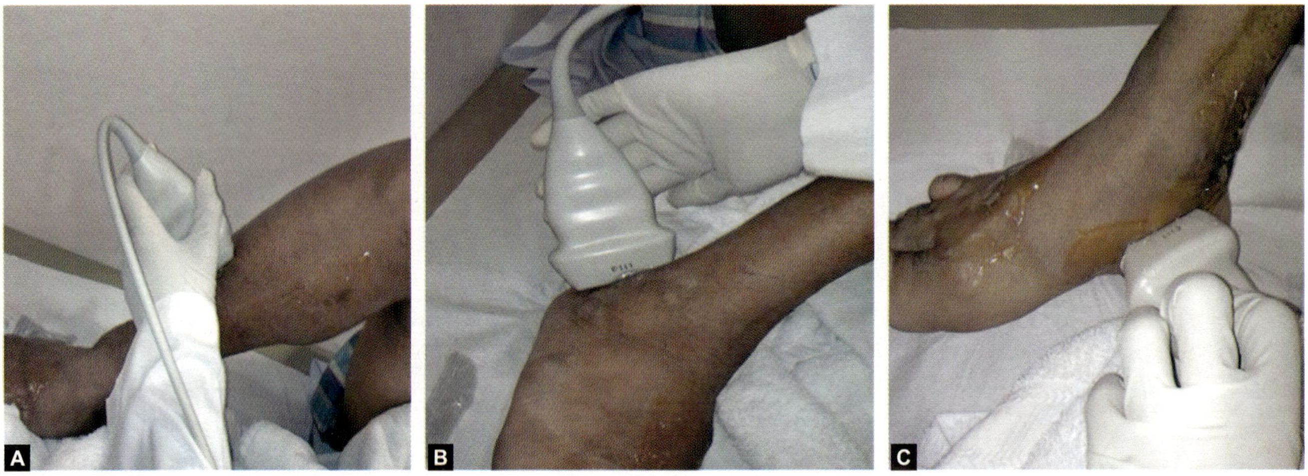

Figs. 17A to C: (A) US scan at the middle of lower limb for tibial arteries; (B) Posterior to lateral malleolus; and (C) Below medial malleolus.

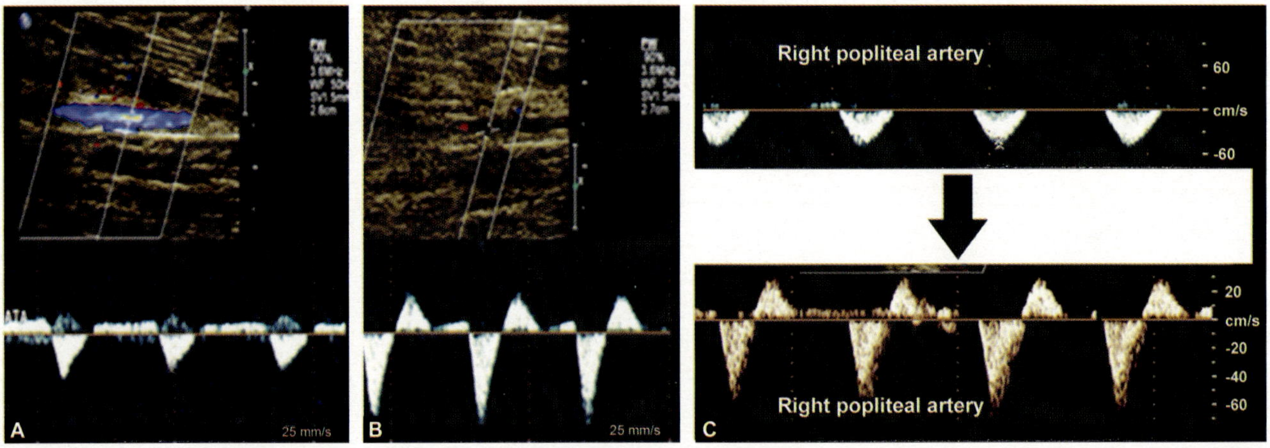

Figs. 18A to C: (A) Right tibial artery showing damp, monophasic flow; (B) After stent graft triphasic pattern was restored; and (C) Same with popliteal artery.

US and using both transverse as well as longitudinal projections.

The likelihood of AVF patency and survival increases with the diameter of the artery (>2.5 mm), and this is an important factor which determines the probability of success of the AVF.[20-22]

A normal superficial vein for the creation of good AVF (cephalic or basilic) should have a thin, regular wall, and a anechoic lumen; should be nontortuous for 8–10 cm of its length and diameter of more than 2 mm (distending more than 1 mm after 2 minutes of tourniquet application); and should also be superficial (less than 6 cm from skin surface).[23-28]

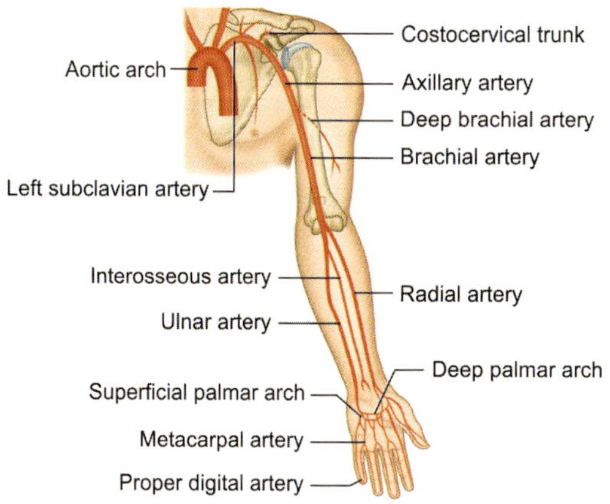

Fig. 19: Anatomy of upper limb arteries.[15-19]

Diagnosing Peripheral Arterial Disease with Doppler

Ankle-brachial index (ABI): ABI is measured in both arms as well as at the ankles by sphygmomanometer cuff occlusion and using the Doppler technique to detect flow signals after occlusion release. It is a ratio of systolic pressure at ankle to average of the systolic pressure in both the arms. Peripheral arterial disease (PAD) can then be semiquantitatively assessed as shown in Table 4.

Exercise ABI (Hyperemia study): The patient is allowed to walk on a treadmill at low grade for 5 minutes or until claudication symptoms develop. ABIs are then measured immediately after exercise and every minute until ABIs normalize to pre-exercise values.

A decrease in the ABI after exercise of greater than 0.2 indicates PAD (due to decrease in ankle systolic pressure). Moreover, a delayed return of ankle pressure to baseline (after 10–12 minutes), together with a change in arterial Doppler pattern (from triphasic or biphasic to monophasic), indicates a critical/multisegment disease.

Although ABI is a good screening test for the detection of significant PAD, its utility is limited in the presence of calcified peripheral arteries, increased arterial stiffness, as well as in arterial diseases involving upper extremities or aortic diseases of thoracic or abdominal aorta.[29-32]

Carotids

The anatomy and US technique for carotids have been described as in Figures 21A and B.

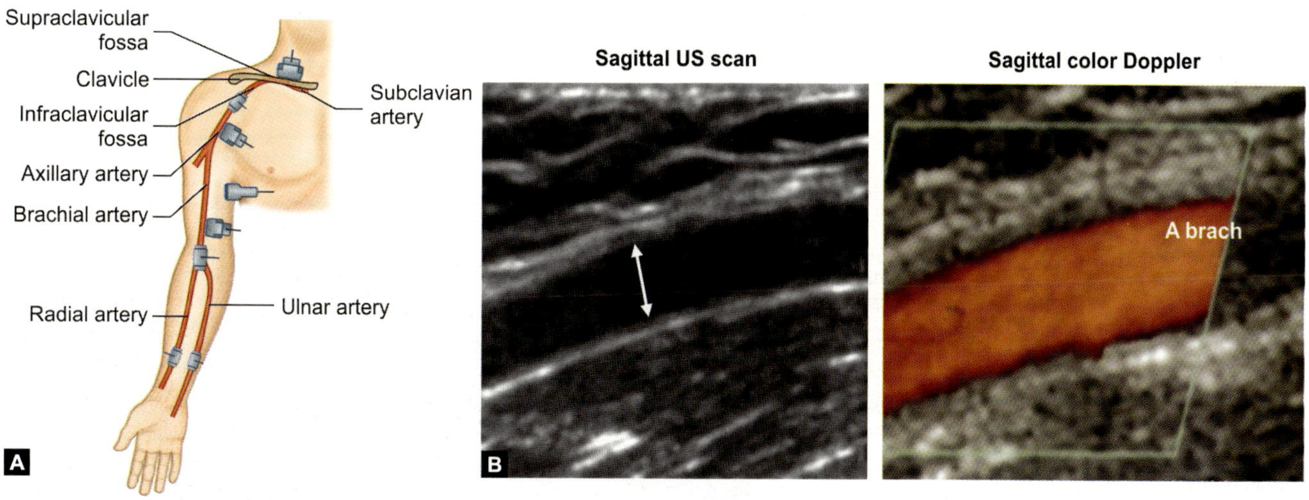

Figs. 20A and B: (A) Different segments of upper extremity artery for Doppler interrogation; and (B) Normal ultrasound of brachial artery in longitudinal view. Diameter is measured from intima-to-intima, color mode shows homogeneous color indicating normal laminar flow.

Imaging

A high-frequency linear array probe is of 7 MHz or higher frequency.[33,34] The difference between internal versus external carotid artery (ECA) on duplex examination has been depicted in Table 5.

Intimal medial thickness: It is known that an increase in IMT correlates with the risks for atherosclerotic diseases. The minimum unit of IMT measurement should be 0.1 mm (Fig. 22).

It is desirable to magnify the image for this measurement so that the error in measurement may be minimized.

Plaques

These can be defined as localized or diffuse elevated lesions, with a thickness at maximum point more than 1.5 mm. Plaques should be measured in both long and transverse imaging (Fig. 23).

Morphological characteristics of vulnerable plaques: The risk of cerebrovascular events depends not only on the severity of carotid luminal stenosis but also upon the vulnerability of the plaques. Plaques with high lipid core and thin fibrous cap tend to burst and produce thromboembolic events.[35-40] Vulnerability of plaques can be assessed sonographically under as follows:

- *Echogenicity*: Plaques with low echogenicity (predominantly echo lucent) are considered to be more vulnerable than plaques with high echogenicity.
- *Texture*: Heterogeneous plaques are considered more vulnerable than with homogeneous texture.
- *Surface*: Plaques with smooth, regular surface are less vulnerable than plaques with irregular surfaces. A significant breach in surface together with a concavity is considered ulceration.[37]

1. *Gray-scale median (GSM) analysis*: This is a novel computer-assisted technique. The frequency distribution of gray values of the pixels within the plaque is used as the measure of echogenicity. The GSM value is normalized between "0" (for blood and is denoted as "black") and 255 (for adventitia, denoted as "white"). The incidence of stroke is found to be more if GSM value for plaque is less than 50.[41]

TABLE 4: Assessment for peripheral arterial disease.

Ankle-brachial index	*Vessel disease*
0.9–1.4	Normal
0.7–0.89	Mild PAD
0.51–0.69	Moderate PAD
<0.5	Severe PAD
>1.4	Calcified or stiff arteries

(PAD: peripheral arterial disease)

TABLE 5: Internal versus external carotid artery on duplex examination.

Interal carotid artery	*External carotid artery*
Usually larger	Usually smaller
Usually lateral and posterior	Usually medial and anterior
Usually incorporates carotid bulb	Usually does not incorporate blub
Low-resistance spectral waveform	High-resistance spectral waveform at rest
No branches in the neck	Eight branches in the neck
Usually no oscillations in Doppler or temporal tap test	Visible and audible oscillations on Doppler signal waveform on temporal tap test

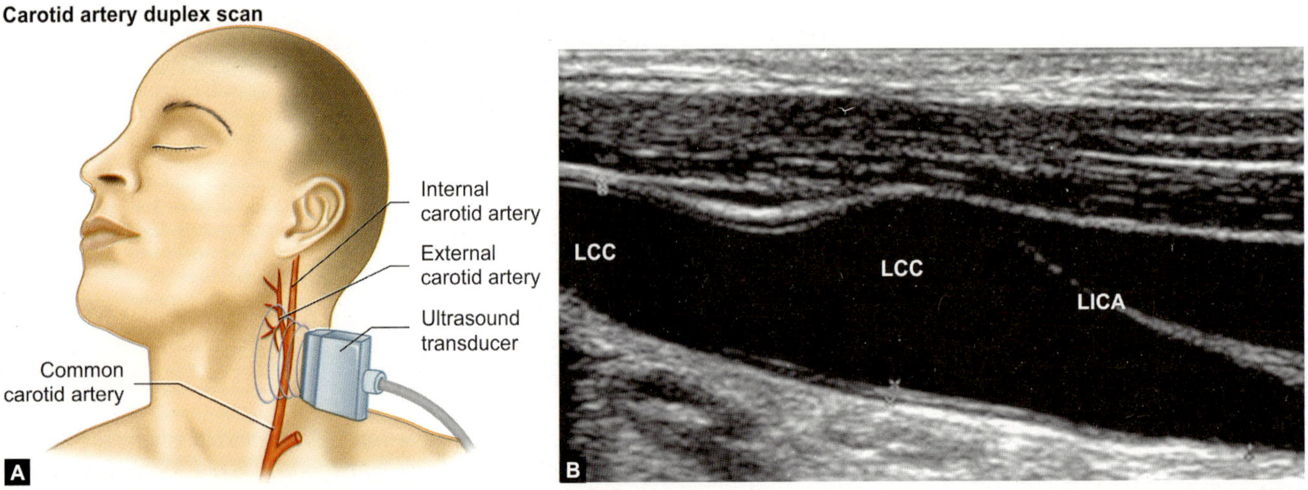

Figs. 21A and B: (A) Carotid anatomy and ultrasound position for its analysis; (B) 2D view of carotids. (LCB: left carotid bulb; LCC: left common carotid; LICA: left internal carotid artery; 2D: two-dimensional)

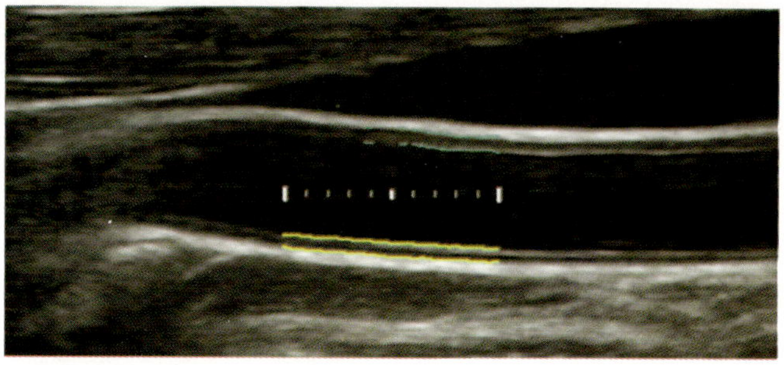

Fig. 22: Depicting the measurement of intimal medial thickness (IMT).

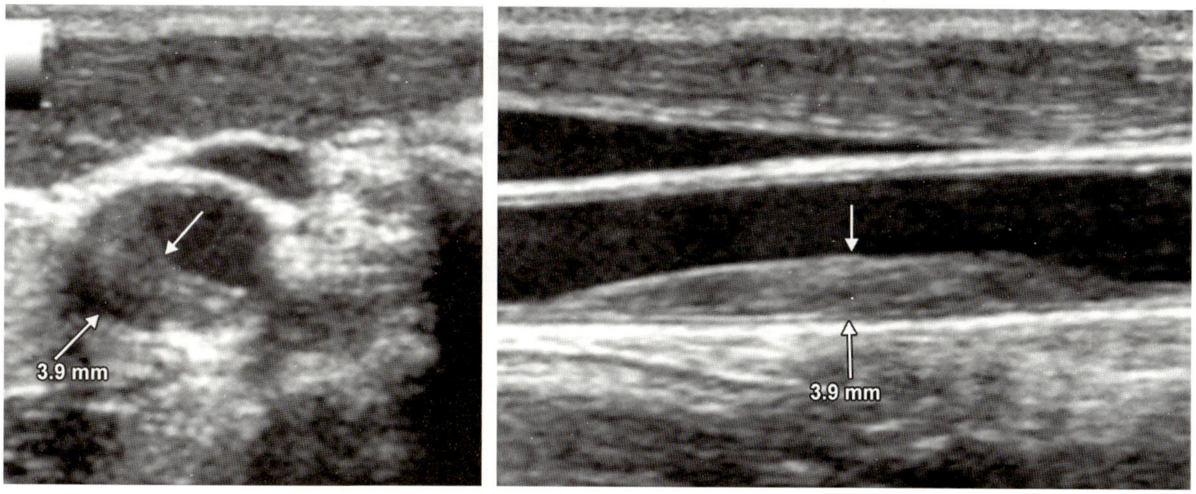

Fig. 23: Plaques in common carotids: (A) Short-axis veiw; and (B) long-axis veiw.

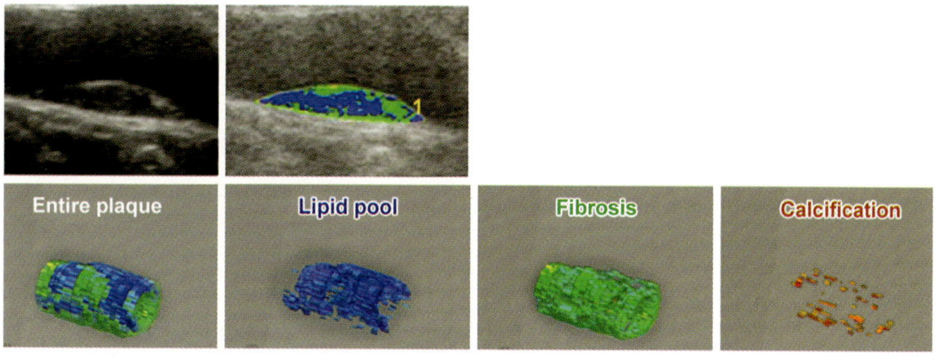

Fig. 24: Computerized-assisted color mapping of a plaque and its significance. (Red: calcification; Yellow: dense fibrosis; Green: fibrosis; Blue and purple: lipid pool)

2. *Integrated backscatter analysis*: This is a novel technique of color coding of plaques according to its composition,[42-45] as shown in Figure 24.

- *Three-dimensional analysis*: 3D US is superior to 2D as it allows better visualization of the plaque geometry and its surface features. 3D analysis of plaque volume has been demonstrated as a risk factor for cardiovascular disease.

The novel techniques are still under research and needs to be validated.

Indices of carotid stenosis:[46-48]

- *Carotid ratio*: The velocity in distal common carotid artery (CCA) measurement should be made within 2 cm of the bifurcation at a point where the vessel still has a uniform diameter, before its widening toward the bulb. Peak systolic velocity (PSV) at internal carotid artery (ICA) stenosis is taken. The degree of stenosis as measured with carotid ratio (Fig. 25) has been depicted in Table 6.

- *String sign*: It is seen on color Doppler at near total occlusion (Fig. 26).

Criteria of Stenosis Calculation

The NASCET (North American Symptomatic Carotid Endarterectomy Trial) and ECST (European Carotid Surgery Trial) had defined different methodology for calculating the stenotic percentage for the evaluation of risk for stroke and evaluating preventive strategies, such as carotid endarterectomy, carotid angioplasty or stenting.[49] The most commonly used index is NASCET (Fig. 27).

Precautions and pitfalls in carotid duplex:

- High and low cardiac output can affect PSV. In the setting of markedly abnormal cardiac output, the ICA/CCA PSV ratio should be the primary diagnostic criteria for ICA stenosis.
- Contralateral ICA occlusion may result in the overestimation of stenosis in the ipsilateral carotid artery, due to compensatory increase in PSV.
- A long-segment plaque with uniform or tapering stenosis often results in a nonturbulent damped flow pattern which could lead to the underestimation of the degree of stenosis.

SYNDROME OF TOTAL INTERNAL CAROTID ARTERY BLOCK

Total occlusion of the ICA could be fairly common occurrence and has an incident rate 6 per 100,000. It could be asymptomatic and detected incidentally during a routine Doppler interrogation of carotid arteries. However, it could also result in disabling strokes.[50,51]

The various criteria which could suggest a total occlusion are as follows (Fig. 28):

- Low-velocity high-resistance flows in ipsilateral CCA
- Extremely low velocity to-and-fro flow ("stump flow") in the carotid bulb just proximal to the block
- Nonvisualized flow in the identified ICA
- Occlusion of the ICA lumen artery by hypodense or hyperdense echogenicity
- Prominent flow in the ipsilateral ECA

$$Index = \frac{PSV_{ICA}}{PSV_{CCA}}$$

Fig. 25: Carotid ratio (index).

TABLE 6: Degree of stenosis as calculated from ratio.

Degree of stenosis	*Index*
<50%	<2
50–69	2–4
>70%	>4
Subtotal	Variable
Total	<1

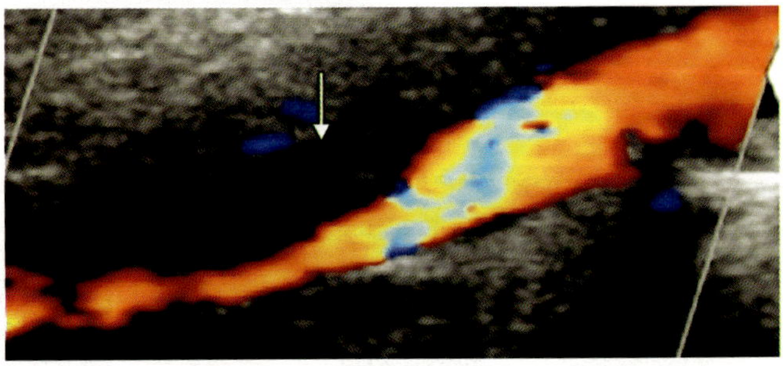

Fig. 26: String sign or trickle sign: Low velocity in subtotal occlusion.

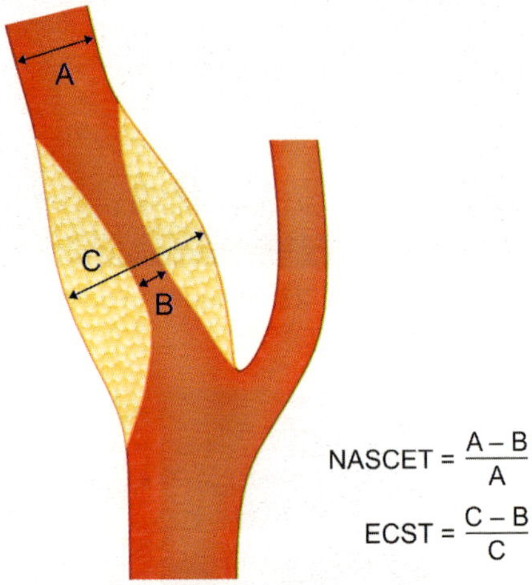

Fig. 27: Calculation of stenosis in internal carotid artery by both NASCET and ECST methods. (ECST: European Carotid Surgery Trial; NASCET: North American Symptomatic Carotid Endarterectomy Trial)

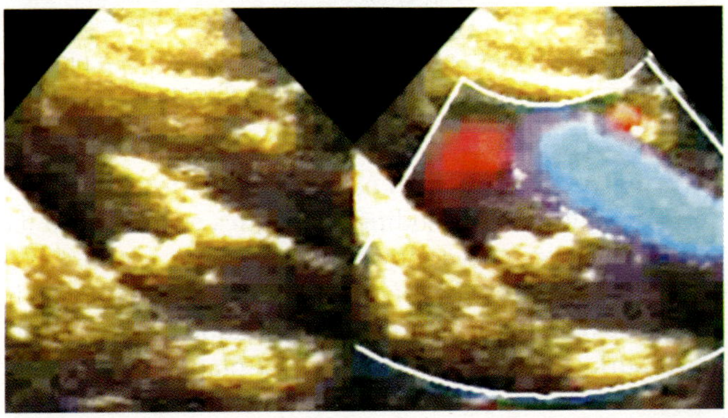

Fig. 28: Total occlusion of ICA. (ICA: internal carotid artery)

- Prominent flows in either of or both the vertebral arteries
- Prominent flows in contralateral CCA and ICA (if free of significant occlusive disease)

Doppler Ultrasound in Small Vessel Disease and Vasculitis

Raynaud's Disease/Phenomenon

Raynaud's phenomenon is characterized by the occurrence of discoloration of the fingers or toes in response to cold or emotional stress.[52-55] On Doppler US, patients with Raynaud's disease have smaller diameter of medium and small vessel arteries and a high-resistance flow in the arteries of the digits and the pulp.

Buerger's Disease or Thromboangiitis Obliterans

It is a segmental occlusive nonatherosclerotic inflammatory disease involving small-to-medium size of arteries and veins, characterized by thrombosis and recanalization of the affected vessels.[56-58]

Assessment of Pregangrenous Limb

Doppler US helps in the overall evaluation of a critically ischemic limb as regards to its viability as well as assessment of the adequacy of arterial perfusion. Owing to extremely low-flow state in the affected limb, arterial Doppler interrogation is technically challenging. However, visualization of venous flows on Doppler US indicates viability in the affected limb segment. Moreover, identification of good arterial collateral flow pattern could help in identifying a point distal to which the amputation can be performed.

Utility of Peripheral Arterial Doppler after Endovascular Surgery

The importance of peripheral Doppler study has been greatly enhanced after the introduction of interventional treatment modalities, such as stent grafts in the management of patients with thoracoabdominal aneurysms or aortoiliac occlusions.

In patients with aortoiliac disease treated with *stent grafts,* a Doppler evaluation involves interrogation of the graft as well as arterial flows distal to the graft in the affected limb. A stenosis or occlusion of stent graft can be readily evaluated by Doppler, and adequacy of distal flow can also be reliably assessed noninvasively.

In the management of patients with thoracoabdominal aneurysms by stent grafts, Doppler evaluation provides a good noninvasive method to assess the patency of the graft across the aneurysm sac as well as assessment of *endovascular leak* that could occur at the junction of stent graft with nonaneurysmal segments of the arteries.[59-62]

VENOUS DOPPLER

Duplex ultrasound scanning of peripheral veins has become a central diagnostic modality to detect reliably the anatomy and pathologies, such as deep vein thrombosis (DVT), varicose veins, or chronic venous insufficiency.[63,64]

A higher frequency probe of 12 MHz is needed for venous interrogation. For patients who have thick adipose tissue, a lower frequency probe of 5–7.5 MHz is appropriate. Examination of the abdominal vein (inferior vena cava and iliac) is best performed using 2.5–5-MHz convex probe. The probes of wide range of frequencies are available for optimal interrogation.[65-67]

LOWER LIMB VEINS

Superficial Veins

- Telangiectasia/Reticular veins
- Great saphenous vein (GSV)
- Small saphenous vein (SSV)
- Perforator veins

Telangiectasia/Reticular Veins

Leg telangiectasia is often associated with underlying venous disease even when no obvious visible varicose veins are present. DUS reveals incompetence of the superficial venous system without clinically apparent varicose veins, in about 23% of patients with telangiectasia (Fig. 29).

Great Saphenous Vein

The great saphenous vein (GSV) originates at the medial marginal vein of the dorsum of the foot, ascends medially upward to knee, and then to join the common FV below

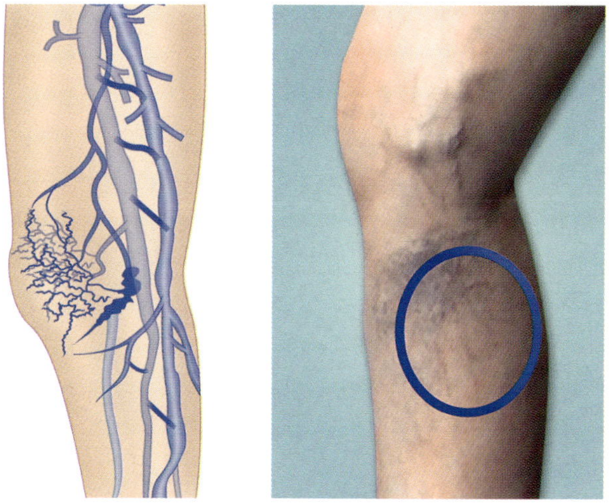

Fig. 29: Small superficial veins known as telangiectasia (outlined with circle).

inguinal ligament (Figs. 30A to C). The saphenofemoral junction is guarded by two valves, namely preterminal valve and terminal valve at the termination of GSV.

Imaging of Great Saphenous Vein and Saphenofemoral Junction: This should be performed both in supine and the erect position. In the transverse view, GSV and the surrounding superficial fascia give an "Egyptian eye" appearance (Figs. 31A to D).[68,69]

Small Saphenous Vein

The SSV arises from the dorsal pedal arch and ascends posterolaterally from behind the lateral malleolus. It courses along the midline of the calf and joins the popliteal vein about 4–6 cm proximal to popliteal crease at the junction of the lateral one-third and medial two-thirds. However, saphenopopliteal junction (SPJ) is present in only about half of the patients and when absent SSV usually joins the

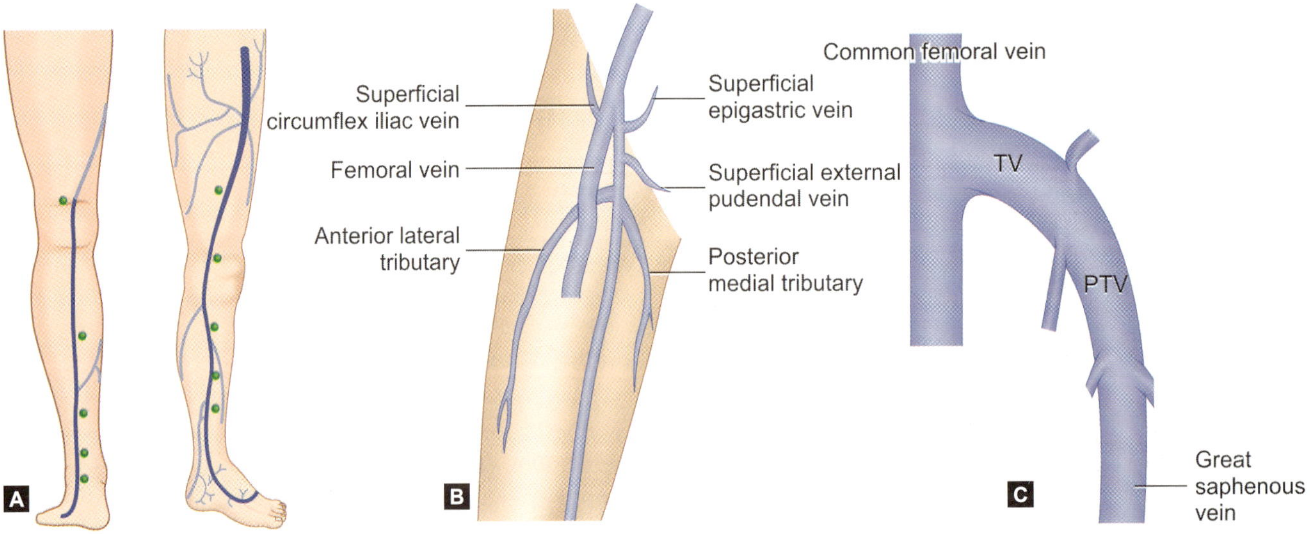

Figs. 30A to C: (A) Anatomical course of GSV; (B) It shows major tributaries of GSV before it merges with femoral vein; and (C) It shows two valves present near its merger with femoral vein, preterminal and terminal valves. (GSV: great saphenous vein)

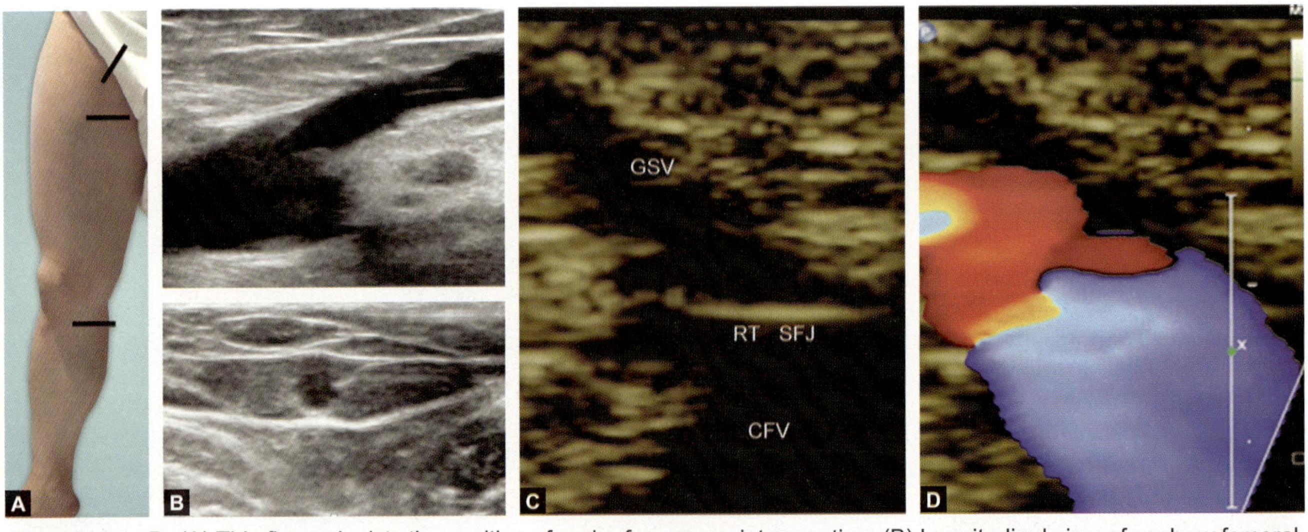

Figs. 31A to D: (A) This figure depicts the position of probe for venous interrogation; (B) Longitudinal view of saphenofemoral junction; (C) Transverse view depicting "Egyptian eye" appearance; and (D) Color mode of saphenofemoral junction.

terminal tributaries of the FV in the distal thigh. Venous reflux at SPJ (if present) or at the proximal SSV can be identified by Valsalva maneuver or coughing usually in the standing position (Figs. 32A to C).[70]

Perforator Veins

Perforator veins connect the superficial veins or their tributaries with the deep veins. Four groups of clinically important perforating veins have been identified as shown in Figure 33. These perforators are guided by valves which become incompetent causing perforator insufficiency usually as a result of the pathology in the superficial or deep venous system. The exact point at which perforator insufficiency should be marked as a guide to ligation or sclerotherapy.[71,72]

Assessment of Venous Competence

It should be performed in both standing and supine position, using Valsalva maneuver (performed either by blowing into a sphygmomanometer cuff, coughing, or abdominal strain). During this maneuver, normally, there is no retrograde flow. Venous incompetence is characterized by retrograde flow of more than 0.5 seconds. Inspiratory reflux also indicates significant venous incompetence (Figs. 34A to C).[73-76]

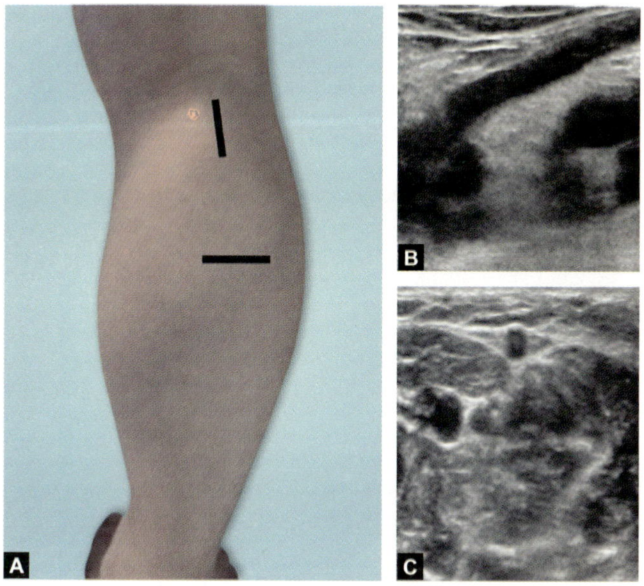

Figs. 32A to C: (A) Probe position for SSV. (B and C) Longitudinal as well transverse view of SSV at popliteal fossa. (SSV: small saphenous vein).

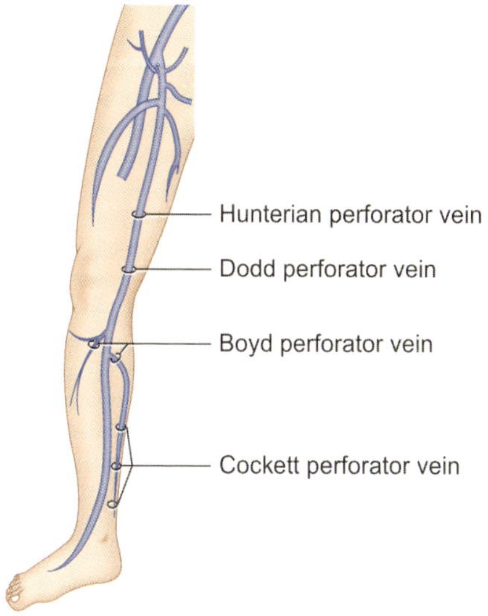

Fig. 33: Perforators of lower limb.

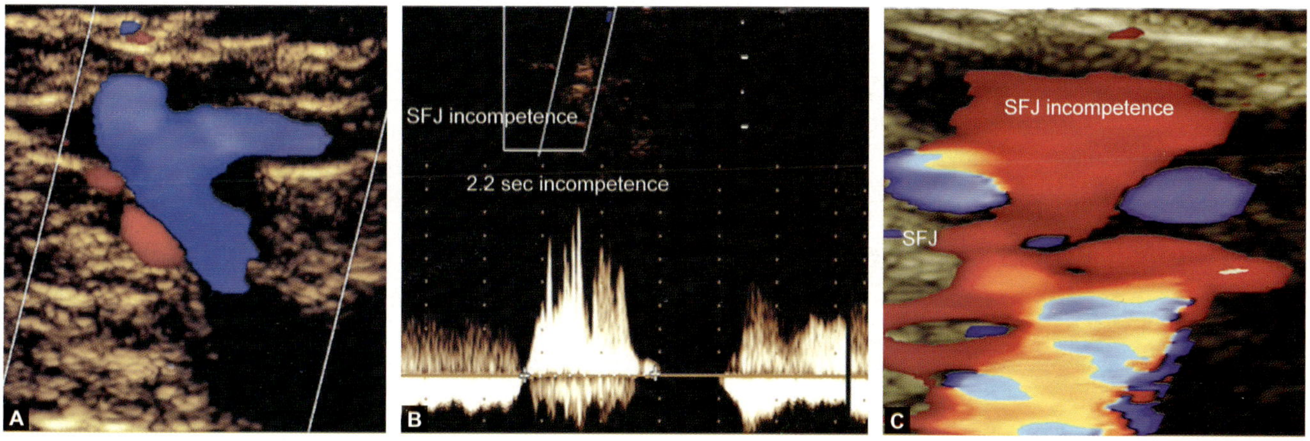

Figs. 34A to C: (A) Color mode of saphenofemoral junction (SFJ); (B) Back flow Doppler tracing of 2.2 s noticed after Valsalva maneuver; and (C) Color mode of back flow regurgitation.

TABLE 7: Difference between superficial and deep veins

Superficial veins	*Deep veins*
Not accompanied by artery	Always accompanied by artery
Extremely thin walled	Relatively thicker walls
Easily obliterated, so only minimal compression applied	Not so easily obliterated, but compressible
Relatively superficial at an average depth of 1.5–2.5 cm below skin surface	Relatively deeper at depths of 2.0–4 cm below skin surface

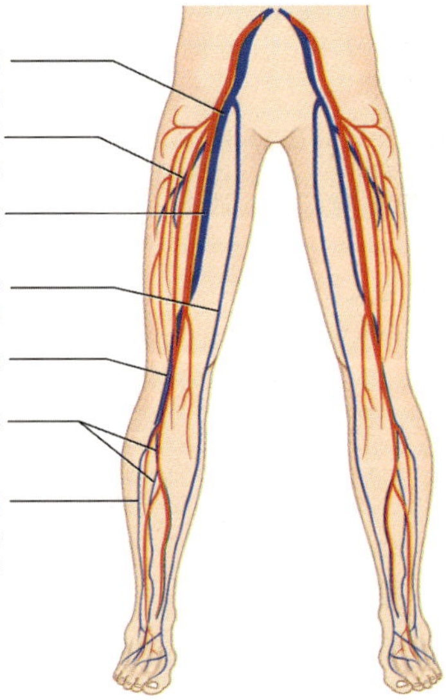

Fig. 35: Deep venous system of lower limbs.

Deep Veins

The deep veins are situated in the deep fascia along with the arteries. The difference between superficial and deep veins of lower limb is described in Table 7. The anatomy of deep veins is illustrated in Figure 35. Color Doppler of FV at inguinal region has been depicted in Figure 36, while the tributaries of the femoral, popliteal, and tibial veins are shown in Figure 35.

Deep Vein Thrombosis

The presence of clots in the deep venous system is the hallmark of DVT. The DVT could involve only a small segment or could be more extensive involving the part or whole of the venous system of lower limb.[77-81] The various signs of DVT on Doppler scan are as follows:

- Absent or reduced compressibility (this is a hallmark in the diagnosis of DVT as shown in Figure 37)
- Visualized thrombus of varying echogenicity
- Incomplete color fill-in
- Absent flow on color or spectral Doppler
- Impaired or absent augmentation of flow
- Lack of spontaneous flow
- Increased flow in collateral channels.

The presence of DVT in a patient has significant potential implications especially as regards to embolization to the pulmonary circulation.

Deep vein thrombosis could be acute, subacute, or chronic depending on the time duration after the episode of DVT depending upon recanalizing channels and venous collaterals.

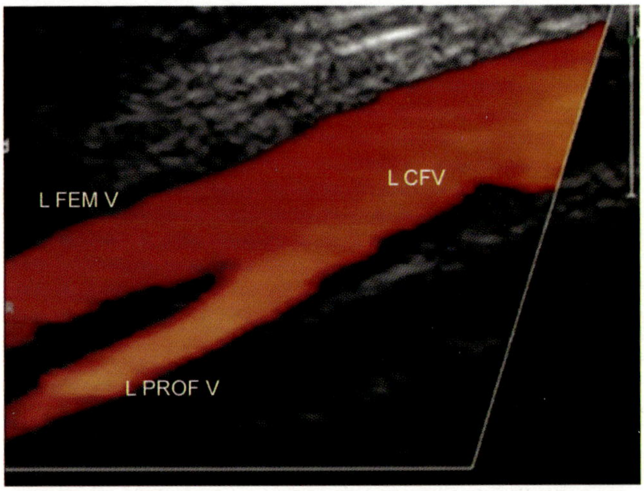

Fig. 36: Color mode of common femoral vein with its draining tributaries.

UPPER LIMB VEINS

Superficial Veins

The major superficial veins of the upper limb are shown in Figures 38A and B.

The interrogation of cephalic and basilic veins is usually performed for assessing their suitability for dialysis access (refer to section on AVF).[82-84]

Deep Veins

Upper limb deep vein thrombosis (UL-DVT) is about 5–10% of all cases of DVT with incidence increasing due to large use of intravenous catheter.

- The most common site of UL-DVT involves the axillary and subclavian veins, though brachial vein may also get involved. Internal jugular veins are also included in upper limb deep veins, though their proximity to central venous system. UL-DVT can be primary or secondary.
- *Primary UL-DVT* is less common and most typically is effort induced, known as *Paget-Schroetter syndrome (PSS)*, a venous form of thoracic outlet syndrome which classically occurs in young athletes.

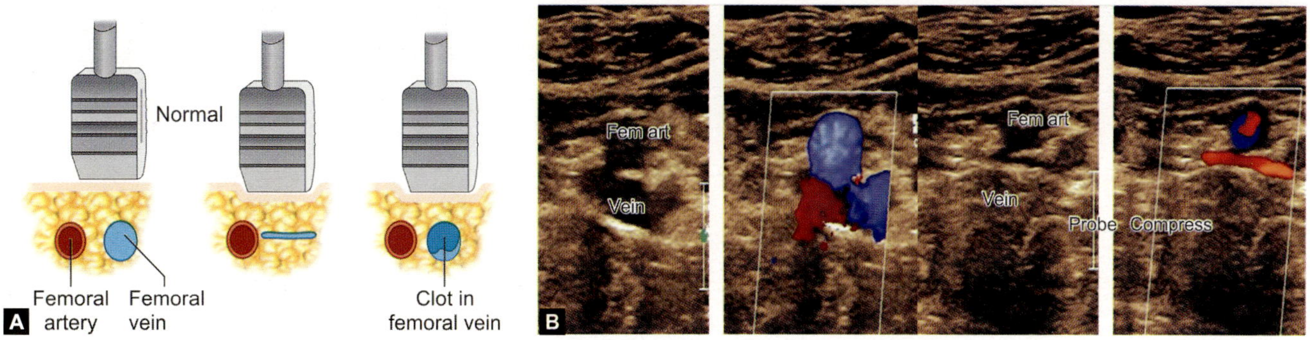

Figs. 37A and B: (A) When the pressure is applied on probe the veins tend to collapse, noncollapsibility of veins indicates pathology, such as thrombus; and (B) compressibility of vein with color Doppler.

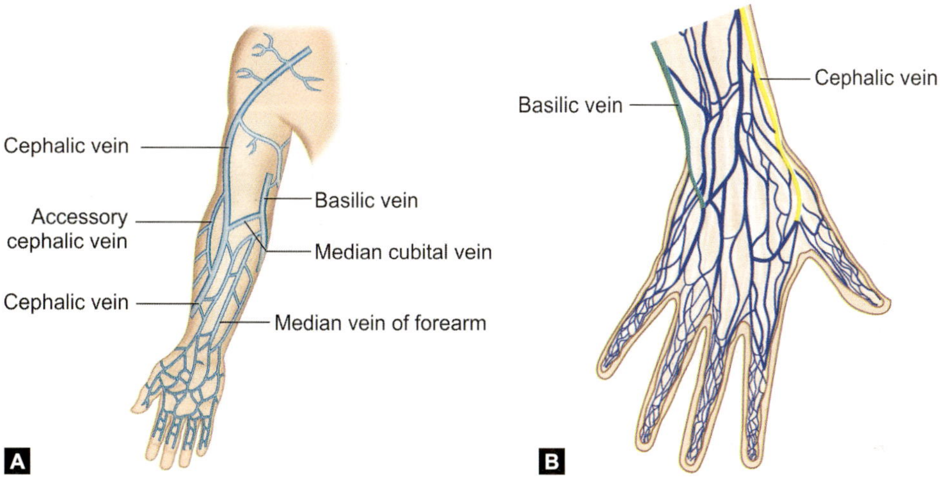

Figs. 38A and B: Venous system in upper limb.

- *Secondary UL-DVT* occurs due to indwelling devices, such as central venous catheters, pacemaker or defibrillator leads. Catheter-associated thrombosis is the most common etiology comprising 93% of all UL-DVT. Other factors include thrombophilia and malignancy.[82-84]
- Brachial veins are deep veins. These are paired veins which accompany the brachial artery on either side (Fig. 39).
- Doppler positions and 2D views are illustrated in Figures 40A to E and Jugular vein clot is shown in Figure 41.

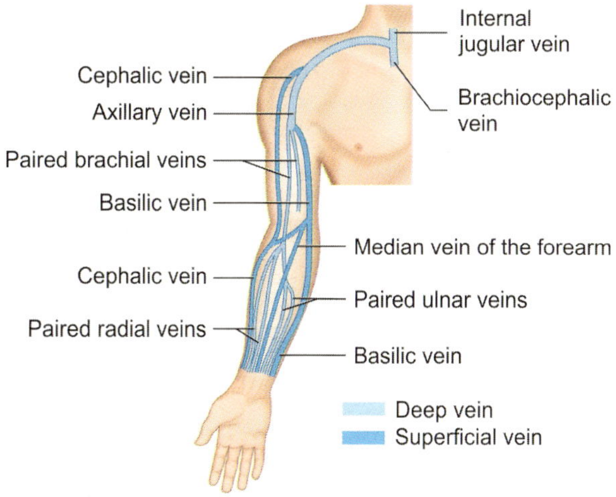

Fig. 39: Deep venous system of arm.

Diagnostic Accuracy of Venous Doppler

The diagnostic accuracy of US for lower limb DVT varies according to the technique used. Optimal sensitivity is attained by using duplex or triplex (duplex with compression) US for proximal limb is 96% and for distal limb is 71% and 75%, respectively, and specificity for both techniques is 94%, whereas compression US alone has sensitivity for proximal and distal limb is 94% and 57%, respectively, with specificity 98% in both parts of the limb.[85-88]

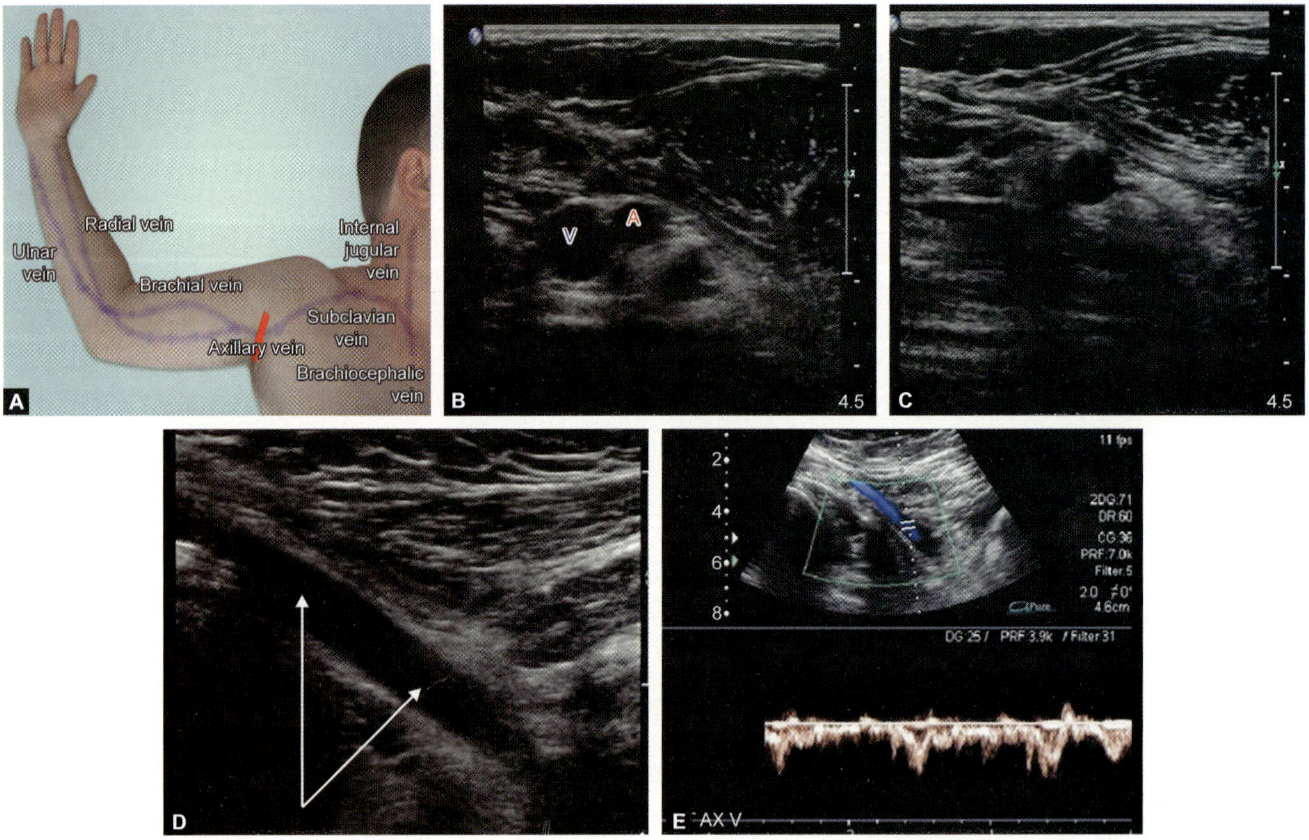

Figs. 40A to E: (A) Transducer position on arm for deep venous analysis (at axillary vein); (B and C) Compressibility of axillary vein; (D) Longitudinal view of axillary vein; and (E) Doppler of axillary vein. Note that pulsatile flow in axillary vein due to its proximity with heart.

Similarly for upper limb analysis, sensitivity for compression ultrasonography was 97% (90–100%), and for Doppler ultrasonography was 84% (72–97%).[89]

VENOUS COMPRESSION SYNDROMES

- *May-Thurner syndrome (MTS)* in which the left common iliac vein is compressed against the fifth lumbar vertebra by the right common iliac artery. The prevalence is about 20% of the population and predominantly present in females. It results in lower extremity venous outflow obstruction and can present as acute or chronic DVT with the symptoms of unilateral leg pain, edema, and/or varicosities. It should be considered when a standard venous Doppler US shows that the DVT extends proximally to the iliofemoral vein. At present, the use of endovascular techniques in the treatment of MTS is quite successful. Common endovascular treatment

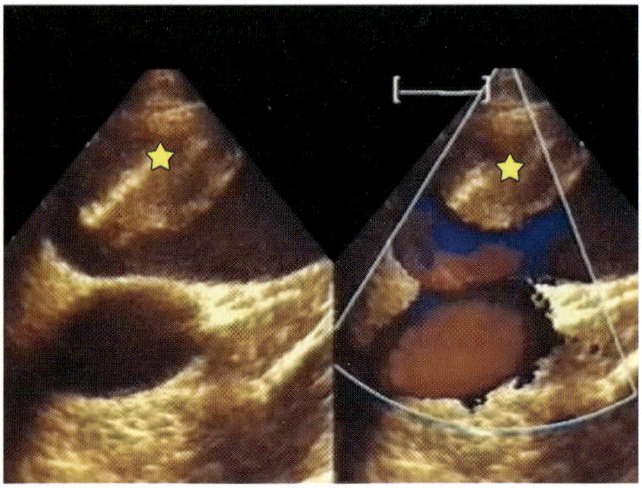

Fig. 41: Jugular vein clot. Star is placed on clot present in jugular vein.

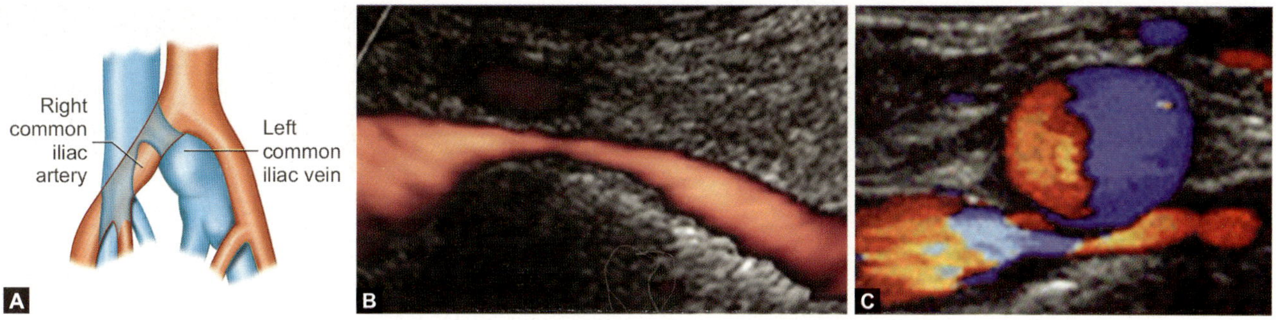

Figs. 42A to C: Skeptical diagram showing left common iliac vein is being compressed by the right common iliac artery; (B) Color power mode of left common iliac vein; and (C) Color mode showing artery (above) compressing vein (below).

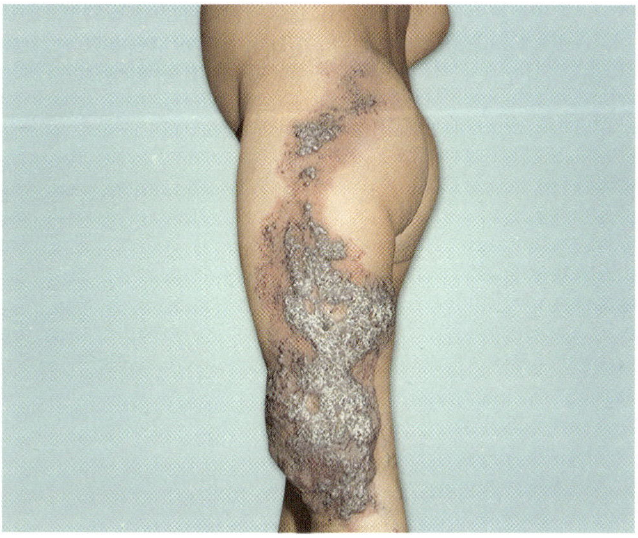

Fig. 43: Phlebectasic dysplasias in Klippel–Trenaunay syndrome (KTS).

options include catheter-directed thrombolysis, angioplasty, and ultimately stent placement (Figs. 42A to C).[90]

- *Klippel–Trenaunay syndrome* is a venous maldevelopment of the deep veins with or without the involvement of superficial venous system and is characterized by the presence of multiple skin hemangioma, asymmetric limb hypertrophy, and AVF (Fig. 43).[91]
- *Paget-Schroetter syndrome* is an uncommon cause of DVT of the subclavian vein, most commonly seen as a consequence of chronic compression of the subclavian vein at the level of the thoracic outlet (Figs. 44A to D). PSS is most commonly seen in the dominant arm of patients who are physically active and is provoked by excessive overhead activity. Venous thrombosis in the axillary and subclavian veins can be easily confirmed by US. US has a sensitivity of 78–100% and a specificity of 88–100% in the identification of acute DVT of the subclavian vein that extends into the axillary vein and sometimes even more distally (Figs. 44A to D).[92-95]

Utility of Doppler Technique in Venous Interventions for Varicose Veins

The treatment of incompetent GSV in patients with chronic venous insufficiency and varicose veins was traditionally performed by surgical ligation and/or stripping. However, the use of endovascular ablation technique (laser or radio frequency) has been a major breakthrough in the interventional management of these patients. The success of endovascular ablation of GSV can be analyzed with subsequent Doppler US. The possible complication of this technique includes thrombus extension into deep venous system (iliac-FVs), or there may be recanalization of ablated vein (Figs. 45A and B).[96,97]

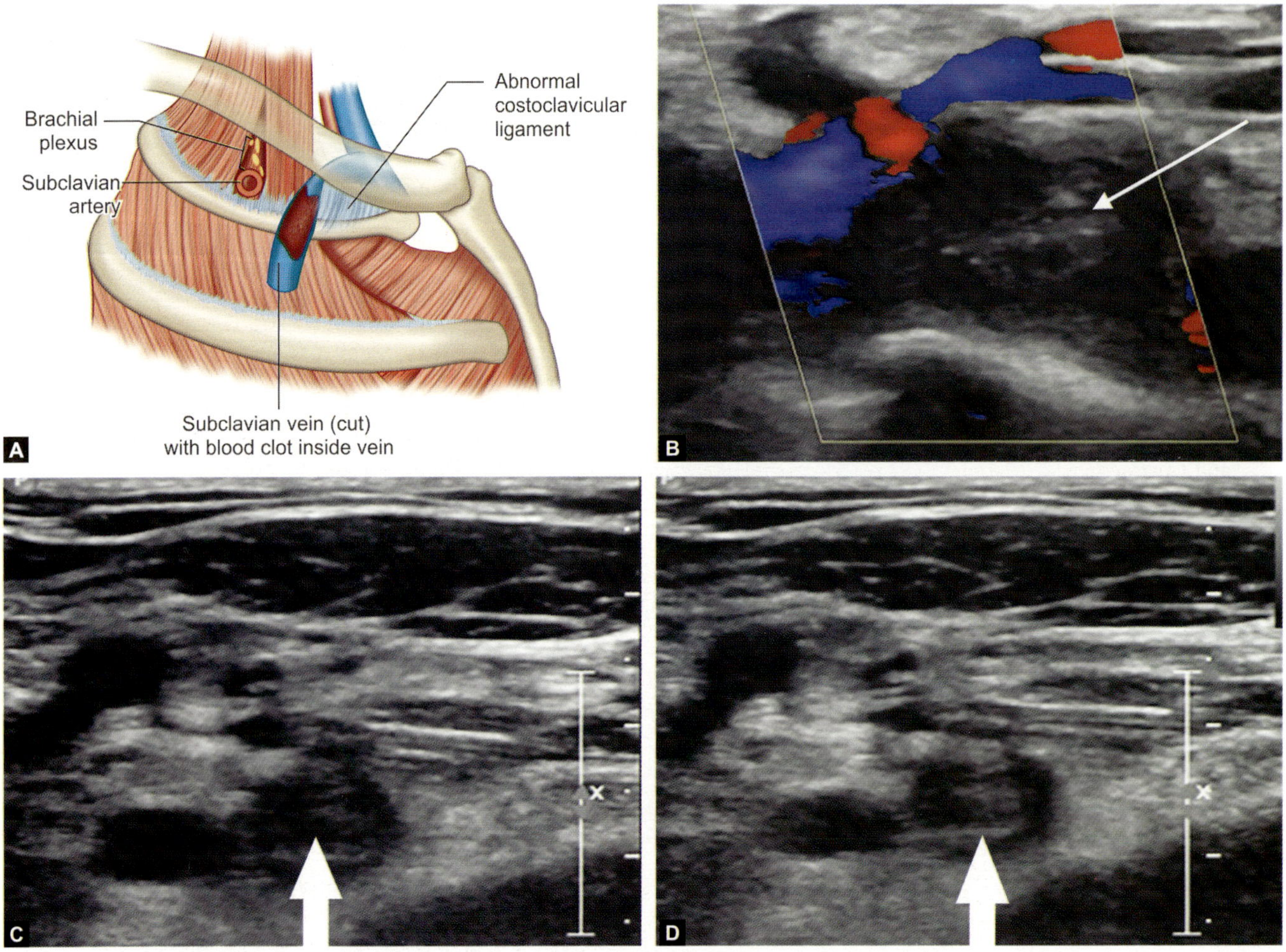

Figs. 44A to D: (A) Diagrammatic representation of PSS, showing compressed subclavian vein; (B) Ultrasound image showing thrombosed subclavian vein; (C and D) Compression test, vein being thrombosed did not get compressed. (PSS: Paget–Schroetter syndrome)

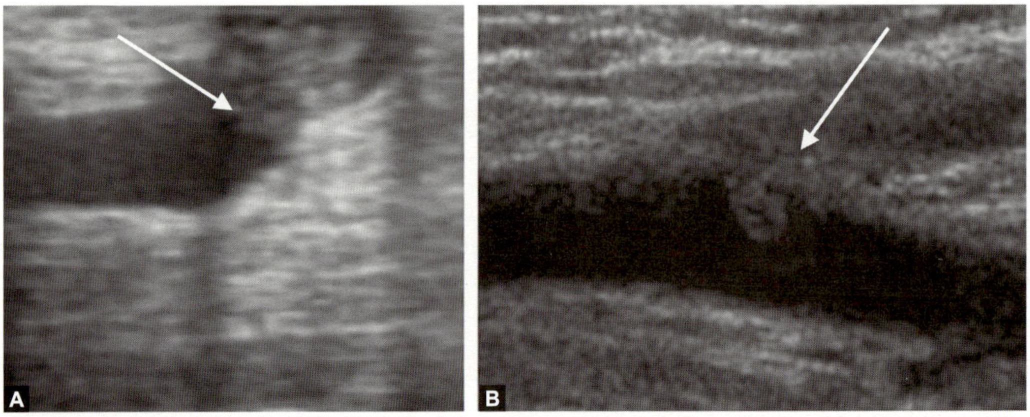

Figs. 45A and B: Extension of thrombus from GSV to deeper venous system. (GSV: great saphenous vein)

REFERENCES

1. Federman DG, Trent JT, Froelich CW, et al. Epidemiology of peripheral vascular disease: a predictor of systemic vascular disease. Ostomy Wound Manage. 1998;44:58-62.
2. Criqui MH, Aboyans V. Epidemiology of peripheral artery disease. Circ Res. 2015;116:1509-26.
3. Gerhard-Hermana M, Gardin JM, Jaff M, et al. Guidelines for noninvasive vascular laboratory testing: a report from the American Society of Echocardiography and the Society for Vascular Medicine and Biology. Vasc Med. 2006;11:183-200.
4. European Stroke Organisation, Tendera M, Aboyans V, et al. ESC Guidelines on the diagnosis and treatment of peripheral artery diseases: Document covering atherosclerotic disease of extracranial carotid and vertebral, mesenteric, renal, upper and lower extremity arteries: the Task Force on the Diagnosis and Treatment of Peripheral Artery Diseases of the European Society of Cardiology (ESC). Eur Heart J. 2011;32:2851-906.
5. Sacks D, Robinson ML, Marinelli DL, et al. Peripheral arterial Doppler ultrasonography: diagnostic criteria. J Ultrasound Med. 1992;11:95-103.
6. Morley RL, Sharma A, Horsch AD, et al. Peripheral artery disease. BMJ. 2018;360:j5842.
7. Sibley RC III, Reis SP, MacFarlane JJ, et al. Noninvasive physiologic vascular studies: a guide to diagnosing peripheral arterial disease. Radiographics. 2017;37:346-57.
8. Thoracic Key. (2016). Role of vascular ultrasonography in peripheral artery disease. https://thoracickey.com/role-of-vascular-ultrasonography-in-peripheral-artery-disease/ [Accessed October, 2018].
9. Ismail A, Saleh MK, Tabari AM, et al. Clinical and Doppler ultrasound evaluation of peripheral arterial diseases in Kano, North-Western Nigeria. Niger Postgrad Med J. 2015;22:217-22.
10. Scissons R, Comerota A. Confusion of peripheral arterial Doppler waveform terminology. JDMS. 2009;25:185-94.
11. Rohren EM, Kliewer MA, Carroll BA, et al. A spectrum of Doppler waveforms in the carotid and vertebral arteries. AJR Am J Roentgenol. 2003;181:1695-704.
12. Choudhary VA, Patil SS, Shah VR. Evaluation of peripheral arterial disease of lower extremity by doppler imaging. Int J Sci Stud. 2016;3:163-168
13. Verim S, Taşçı I. Doppler ultrasonography in lower extremity peripheral arterial disease. Turk Kardiyol Dern Ars. 2013;41:248-55.
14. Hwang JY. Doppler ultrasonography of the lower extremity arteries: anatomy and scanning guidelines. Ultrasonography. 2017;36:111-9.
15. Taneja K, Jain R, Sawhney S, et al. Occlusive arterial disease of the upper extremity: colour Doppler as a screening technique and for assessment of distal circulation. Australas Radiol. 1996;40:226-9.
16. Radiopaedia. (2018). Arterial supply of the upper limb. [online]. https://radiopaedia.org/articles/arterial-supply-of-the-upper-limb [Accessed October, 2018].
17. Salles-Cunha SX. Ultrasound imaging of upper extremity arteries: clinical applications. In: Noninvasive Vascular Diagnosis. London: Springer; 2007. pp. 325-33.
18. Toprak U, Hayretci M, Erhuner Z, et al. Dynamic Doppler evaluation of the hand arteries to distinguish between primary and secondary Raynaud phenomenon. AJR Am J Roentgenol. 2011;197:W175-80.
19. Tola M, Yurdakul M, Ökten S, et al. Diagnosis of arterial occlusive disease of the upper extremities: comparison of color duplex sonography and angiography. J Clin Ultrasound. 2003;31:407-11.
20. Malovrh M. Non-invasive evaluation of vessels by duplex sonography prior to construction of arteriovenous fistulas for haemodialysis. Nephrol Dial Transplant. 1998;13:125-9.
21. Zamboli P, Fiorini F, D'Amelio A et al. Color Doppler ultrasound and arteriovenous fistulas for hemodialysis. J Ultrasound. 2014;17:253-63.
22. Finlay DE, Longley DG, Foshager MC, et al. Duplex and color Doppler sonography of hemodialysis arteriovenous fistulas and grafts. Radiographics. 1993;13:983-9.
23. Silva MB Jr, Hobson RW, Pappas PJ, et al. A strategy for increasing use of autogenous hemodialysis access procedures: impact of preoperative noninvasive evaluation. J Vasc Surg. 1998;27:302-7.
24. Nalesso F, Garzotto F, Petrucci I, et al. Standardized protocol for hemodialysis vascular access assessment: the role of ultrasound and color Doppler. Blood Purif. 2018;45:260-9.
25. Chienga D, Patela B. Arteriovenous fistula as a rare early complication of transradial coronary angiography: with literature review on management strategies. J Med Cases. 2015;6:453-6.
26. Banerjee S. Fistula maturation and patency for successful dialysis. Dialysis Transplant. 2009;38:442.
27. Sarı F, Taşkapan H, Sığırcı A, et al. Evaluation of risk factors for arteriovenous fistula failure in patients undergoing hemodialysis. Erciyes Med J. 2016;38:12-9.
28. Da Fonseca Junior JH, Pitta GBB, Miranda Júnior F. Accuracy of Doppler ultrasonography in the evaluation of hemodialysis arteriovenous fistula maturity. Rev Col Bras Cir. 2015;42:138-42.
29. Sibley RC, Reis SP, MacFarlane JJ, et al. Noninvasive physiologic vascular studies: a guide to diagnosing peripheral arterial disease. Radiographics. 2017;37:346-57.
30. American Heart Association. Practice Guidelines: AHA Releases Recommendations on Ankle-Brachial Index Measurement and Interpretation. Am Fam Physician. 2013;88:866-7.
31. Takahashi I, Furukawa K, Ohishi W, et al. Comparison between oscillometric- and Doppler ABI in elderly individuals. Vasc Health Risk Manag. 2013;9:89-94.
32. Davies JH, Kenkre J, Williams EM. Current utility of the ankle-brachial index (ABI) in general practice: implications for its use in cardiovascular disease screening. BMC Fam Pract. 2014;15:69.
33. Oates CP, Naylor AR, Hartshorne T, et al. Joint recommendations for reporting carotid ultrasound investigations in the United Kingdom. Eur J Vasc Endovasc Surg. 2009;37:251-61.
34. Grant EG, Benson CB, Moneta GL, et al. Carotid artery stenosis: gray-scale and Doppler US diagnosis—society of radiologists in ultrasound consensus conference. Radiology. 2003;229:340-6.

35. Petersen C, Peçanha PB, Venneri L, et al. The impact of carotid plaque presence and morphology on mortality outcome in cardiological patients. Cardiovasc Ultrasound. 2006;4:16.
36. Casadei A, Floreani M, Catalini R, et al. Sonographic characteristics of carotid artery plaques: implications for follow-up planning?. J Ultrasound. 2012;15:151-7.
37. Muraki M, Mikami T, Yoshimoto T, et al. New criteria for the sonographic diagnosis of a plaque ulcer in the extracranial carotid artery. AJR Am J Roentgenol. 2012;198:1161-6.
38. Lukanova DV, Nikolov NK, Genova KZ, et al. The accuracy of noninvasive imaging techniques in diagnosis of carotid plaque morphology. Open Access Maced J Med Sci. 2015;3:224-30.
39. Ho SSY. Current status of carotid ultrasound in atherosclerosis. Quant Imaging Med Surg. 2016;6:285-96.
40. Park TH. Evaluation of carotid plaque using ultrasound imaging. J Cardiovasc Ultrasound. 2016;24:91-5.
41. Johri AM, Herr JE, Li TY, et al. Novel ultrasound methods to investigate carotid artery plaque vulnerability. J Am Soc Echocardiogr. 2017;30:139-48.
42. Bando M, Yamada H, Kusunose K, et al. Noninvasive quantitative tissue characterization of carotid plaques using color-coded mapping based on ultrasound integrated backscatter. JACC Cardiovasc Imaging. 2016;9:625-7.
43. Kawasaki M, Takatsu H, Noda T, et al. Noninvasive quantitative tissue characterization and two-dimensional color-coded map of human atherosclerotic lesions using ultrasound integrated backscatter: comparison between histology and integrated backscatter images. J Am Coll Cardiol. 2001;38:486-92.
44. Bando M, Yamada H, Kusunose K, et al. Comparison of carotid plaque tissue characteristics in patients with acute coronary syndrome or stable angina pectoris: assessment by iPlaque, transcutaneous carotid ultrasonography with integrated backscatter analysis. Cardiovasc Ultrasound. 2015;13:34.
45. Kawasaki M. An integrated backscatter ultrasound technique for the detection of coronary and carotid atherosclerotic lesions. Sensors. 2015;15:979-94.
46. Yoshida K, Miyamoto S. Evidence for management of carotid artery stenosis. Neurol Med Chir (Tokyo). 2015;55:230-40.
47. Fritz VU, Voll CL, Levien LJ. Internal carotid artery occlusion: clinical and therapeutic implications. Stroke. 1985;16:940-4.
48. Mozzini C, Roscia G, Casadei A, et al. Searching the perfect ultrasonic classification in assessing carotid artery stenosis: comparison and remarks upon the existing ultrasound criteria. J Ultrasound. 2016;19:83-90.
49. Saba L, Mallarini G. A comparison between NASCET and ECST methods in the study of carotids: evaluation using Multi-Detector-Row CT angiography. Eur J Radiol. 2010;76:42-7.
50. Giannoukas AD, Labropoulos N, Smith FC, et al. Management of the near total internal carotid artery occlusion. Eur J Vasc Endovasc Surg. 2005;29:250-5.
51. Zachrisson H, Berthelsen B, Blomstrand C, et al. High diastolic flow velocities in severe internal carotid artery stenosis: a sign of increased surgical risk? J Vasc Surg. 2000;31:477-83.
52. Toprak U, Hayretci M, Erhuner Z, et al. Dynamic Doppler evaluation of the hand arteries to distinguish between primary and secondary Raynaud phenomenon. AJR Am J Roentgenol. 2011;197:W175-80.
53. Chikui T, Izumi M, Eguchi K, et al. Doppler spectral waveform analysis of arteries of the hand in patients with Raynaud's phenomenon as compared with healthy subjects. AJR Am J Roentgenol. 1999;172:1605-9.
54. Schmidt WA. Role of ultrasound in the understanding and management of vasculitis. Ther Adv Musculoskelet Dis. 2014;6:39-47.
55. Lai K-L, Chen H-H, Lan JL, et al. Ultrasonography of large-vessel vasculitides. J Med Ultrasound. 2012;20:72-8.
56. Fujii Y, Soga J, Hidaka T, et al. Color Doppler flows of corkscrew collaterals in thromboangiitis obliterans (Buerger's disease) using color duplex ultrasonography. J Am Coll Cardiol. 2011;57:2539.
57. Yoshimuta T, Akutsu K, Okajima T, et al. Corkscrew collaterals in Buerger's disease. Can J Cardiol. 2009;25:365.
58. Busch K. Buerger's disease (thromboangiitis obliterans): clinical features and assessment by colour duplex ultrasound. Australas J Ultrasound Med. 2011;14:18-22.
59. Shah A, Stavropoulos SW. Imaging surveillance following endovascular aneurysm repair. Semin Intervent Radiol. 2009;26:10-6.
60. Filho DM, Trevisan FB, da Silva Silvestre JM, et al. Vascular ultrasonography for follow-up of endovascular repair of abdominal aorta aneurysms. J Vasc Bras. 2014;13:168-74.
61. Picel AC, Kansal N. Essentials of endovascular abdominal aortic aneurysm repair imaging: postprocedure surveillance and complications. AJR Am J Roentgenol. 2014;203:W358-72.
62. Wang PS, Verma R. Endoleak. Ultrasound Quarterly. 2017;33:96-7.
63. Monreal M, Ruiz J, Olazabal A, et al. Deep venous thrombosis and the risk of pulmonary embolism. A systematic study. Chest. 1992;102:677-81.
64. Eklof B, Rutherford RB, Bergan JJ, et al. Revision of the CEAP classification for chronic venous disorders: consensus statement. J Vasc Sur. 2004;40:1248-52.
65. Galeandro AI, Quistelli G, Scicchitano P, et al. Doppler ultrasound venous mapping of the lower limbs. Vasc Health Risk Manag. 2012;8:59-64.
66. Adam A, Yousef M, Wahab BA, et al. Duplex ultrasound for evaluation of deep venous blood flow in fractured lower extremities. Pol J Radiol. 2018;83:e47-53.
67. Khilnani NM. Duplex ultrasound evaluation of patients with chronic venous disease of the lower extremities. AJR Am J Roentgenol. 2014;202:633-42.
68. Coleridge-Smith P, Labropoulos N, Partsch H, et al. Duplex ultrasound investigation of the veins in chronic venous disease of the lower limbs—UIP consensus document. Part I. Basic principles. Eur J Vasc Endovasc Surg. 2006;31:83-92.
69. Lee DK, Ahn K-S, Kang CH, et al. Ultrasonography of the lower extremity veins: anatomy and basic approach. Ultrasonography. 2017;36:120-30.

70. Foley WD, Middleton WD, Lawson TL, et al. Color Doppler ultrasound imaging of lower-extremity venous disease. AJR Am J Roentgenol. 1989;152:371-6.
71. Liu CH, Wu CJ, Yu CY, et al. Evaluation of lower limb varicose vein by ultrasonic venous duplex examination. J Med Ultrasound. 2013;21:76-80.
72. De Maeseneer M, Pichot O, Cavezzi A, et al. Duplex ultrasound investigation of the veins of the lower limbs after treatment for varicose veins UIP consensus document. Eur J Vasc Endovasc Surg. 2011;42:89-102.
73. Robertson LA, Evans CJ, Lee AJ, et al. Incidence and risk factors for venous reflux in the general population: Edinburgh vein study. Eur J Vasc Endovasc Surg. 2014;48:208-14.
74. Magnusson M, Kälebo P, Lukes P, et al. Colour Doppler ultrasound in diagnosing venous insufficiency. A comparison to descending phlebography. Eur J Vasc Endovasc Surg. 1995;9:437-43.
75. Garcia R, Labropoulos N. Duplex ultrasound for the diagnosis of acute and chronic venous diseases. Surg Clin N Am. 2018;98:201-18.
76. Min RJ, Khilnani NM, Golia P. Duplex ultrasound evaluation of lower extremity venous insufficiency. J Vasc Interv Radiol. 2003;14:1233-41.
77. Markel A, Weich Y, Gaitini D, et al. Doppler ultrasound in the diagnosis of venous thrombosis. Angiology. 1995;46:65-73.
78. Mantoni M. Diagnosis of deep venous thrombosis by duplex sonography. Acta Radiologica. 1989;30:575-9.
79. Baker M, dela Cruz J. Deep venous thrombosis, ultrasound. 2017. [online]. https://www.ncbi.nlm.nih.gov/books/NBK470453/ [Accessed October, 2018].
80. Tanaka S, Nishigami K, Taniguchi N, et al. Criteria for ultrasound diagnosis of deep venous thrombosis of lower extremities. J Med Ultrason. 2008;35:33-6.
81. Karande GY, Hedgire SS, Sanchez Y, et al. Advanced imaging in acute and chronic deep vein thrombosis. Cardiovasc Diagn Ther. 2016;6:493-507.
82. Weber TM, Lockhart ME, Robbin ML Upper extremity venous Doppler ultrasound. Radiol Clin North Am. 2007;45:513-24.
83. Chin EE, Zimmerman PT, Grant EG. Sonographic evaluation of upper extremity deep venous thrombosis. J Ultrasound Med. 2005;24:829-38.
84. Czihal M, Hoffmann U. Upper extremity deep venous thrombosis. Vasc Med. 2011;16:191-202.
85. Goodacre S, Sampson F, Thomas S, et al. Systematic review and meta-analysis of the diagnostic accuracy of ultrasonography for deep vein thrombosis. BMC Med Imaging. 2005;5:6.
86. Lensing AWA, Doris CI, McGrath FP, et al. A comparison of compression ultrasound with color Doppler ultrasound for the diagnosis of symptomless postoperative deep vein thrombosis. Arch Intern Med. 1997;157:765-8.
87. Amin MA, Khan MZ, Khan MA, et al. Diagnosis of deep vein thrombosis in the leg by using colour coded duplex sonography. J Ayub Med Coll Abbottabad. 2001;13:22-3.
88. Naz R, Naz S, Mehboob M, et al. Diagnostic yield of color Doppler ultrasonography in deep vein thrombosis. J Coll Physicians Surg Pak. 2005;15:276-9.
89. Di Nisio M, Van Sluis GL, Bossuyt PM, et al. Accuracy of diagnostic tests for clinically suspected upper extremity deep vein thrombosis: a systematic review. J Thromb Haemost. 2010;8:684-92.
90. Galang LD, Tulsidas H. May-Thurner syndrome: an important differential diagnosis for DVT. Vasc Med Surg. 2016;4:2.
91. Radiopaedia. (2018). Klippel–Trénaunay–Weber syndrome. [online]. Available from https://radiopaedia.org/articles/klippel-tr-naunay-weber-syndrome [Accessed October, 2018].
92. Krishna K, Shah A, Garg A, et al. Paget-Schroetter syndrome. J Assoc Physicians India. 2007;55:371-3.
93. DeLisa LC, Hensley CP, Jackson S. Diagnosis of Paget-Schroetter syndrome/primary effort thrombosis in a recreational weight lifter. Phys Ther. 2017;97:13-9.
94. Alla VM, Natarajan N, Kaushik M, et al. Paget-Schroetter syndrome: review of pathogenesis and treatment of effort thrombosis. West J Emerg Med. 2010;11:358-62.
95. Svensson C, Lassvik C, Zachrisson H. Nutcracker syndrome, vascular imaging with ultrasound—a case report. Cardiovasc Pharm Open Access. 2018;7:235.
96. Shin JI, Park JM, Lee JS, et al. Effect of renal Doppler ultrasound on the detection of nutcracker syndrome in children with hematuria. Eur J Pediatr. 2007;166:399-404.
97. Salles-Cunha SX, Comerota AJ, Tzilinis A, et al. Ultrasound findings after radiofrequency ablation of the great saphenous vein: descriptive analysis. J Vasc Surg. 2004;40:1166-73.

104

CHAPTER

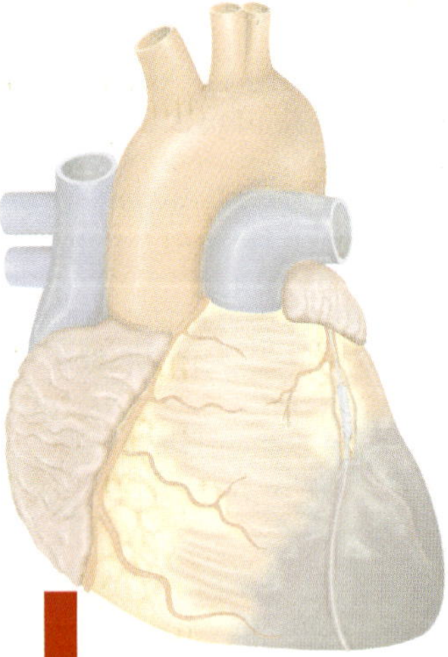

CT and MR Angiography Evaluation of Peripheral Arterial and Venous Disease

Chandrashekhara SH, Priya Jagia, Mumun Sinha

INTRODUCTION

Peripheral arterial disease (PAD) represents one of the most prevalent manifestations of systemic atherosclerosis with critical limb ischemia (CLI) being its most severe form and affecting 1–2% of the patients with PAD.[1] Its prompt recognition and early intervention whether surgical or endovascular aimed at improving the blood flow is of paramount importance both for alleviating symptoms and saving the affected limb. Clinical assessment of PAD entails comprehensive risk assessment which includes increasing age especially above or equal to 65 years; age 50–64 years with risk factors for atherosclerosis (e.g. diabetes mellitus, history of smoking, hyperlipidemia, hypertension) or family history; age less than 50 years with diabetes mellitus and one additional risk factor for atherosclerosis; individuals with known atherosclerotic disease in another vascular bed (e.g. coronary, carotid, subclavian, renal, mesenteric artery stenosis, or abdominal aortic aneurysm).[2] Patients at risk of PAD should undergo a complete medical history with review of symptoms, vascular examination with palpation of pulses and noninvasive blood pressure measurement at least once during initial assessment (Class of recommendation I). The assessment of symptomatic patients is much more comprehensive and encompassing multiple modalities including radiological investigations viz, duplex ultrasonography, computed tomography angiography (CTA) or magnetic resonance angiography (MRA) and digital subtraction angiography (DSA).

DIAGNOSTIC CRITERION

Diagnostic testing for the patient with suspected lower extremity PAD (claudication or CLI) begins with history and clinical examination. In patients with history or physical examination findings suggestive of PAD, the resting ankle-brachial index (ABI), with or without segmental pressures and waveforms, is recommended to establish the diagnosis with patients being put on guideline directed management and therapy in case of abnormal results.[2] The indications for imaging for anatomic assessment are as follows:

- Duplex ultrasound, CTA, or MRA of the lower extremities is useful to diagnose anatomic location and severity of stenosis for patients with symptomatic PAD in whom revascularization is considered (Class of recommendation I).
- Invasive angiography is useful for patients with CLI in whom revascularization is considered (Class of recommendation I).
- Invasive angiography is reasonable for patients with lifestyle-limiting claudication with an inadequate response to guideline-directed management and therapy (GDMT) for whom revascularization is considered (Class of recommendation IIa).

Invasive and noninvasive angiography (i.e. CTA, MRA) should never be performed for the anatomic assessment of patients with asymptomatic PAD. Though the gold standard for the assessment of PAD is DSA, it has the disadvantage of invasive nature, access site complication, ionizing radiation and use of iodinated contrast media.

In multidetector CT (MDCT) fine collimation is combined with rapid (arterial phase) contrast-enhanced (CE) imaging, and this has enabled evaluation of the lower limb vasculature. The overall diagnostic performance of 64-section CTA is equivalent to that of conventional DSA in the detection and treatment planning of PAD with sensitivity, specificity, and accuracy exceeding 98%.[3] However, it still exposes the patient to ionizing radiation and intravenous contrast agents.

DISCUSSION

Magnetic resonance angiography is the preferred modality for noninvasive comprehensive assessment of PAD as it has several advantages over CTA. Both the techniques are discussed here.

Computed Tomography Angiography

Computed tomography angiography is done after injecting 80–100 mL of nonionic iodinated contrast media with flow rate of 4–6 mL/s using dual channel power injector with saline chase followed after contrast injection for a better image quality with reduction of artifacts. Images are acquired from the aortic diaphragmatic hiatus unto the toes, for complete evaluation. For the assessment of visceral branches of aorta, patient is asked to breath-hold. Contrast transit time is calculated either by bolus tracking or by small test bolus. The scanning delay is chosen to be equal to contrast medium transit time (initiated as soon as contrast medium arrives in the aorta), or equal to predefined interval after the contrast medium transit time. In certain conditions like high-grade stenosis and aneurysms which delay the contrast transit time, it is possible (because of fast acquisitions) that the scanner outruns the bolus. In these conditions, it is better to plan a delayed phase short acquisition for better opacification of the distal vessels. Additionally, a biphasic injection of contrast media may be tried for optimum opacification of distal as well as proximal vessels. The overlying osseous structures may obscure the vessels, which may be overcome by the usage of advanced bone removal softwares, partial maximum intensity projections (MIP) excluding bone attenuation and dual energy CT technology. Also, the evaluation of axial source images is indispensable in the evaluation of vascular lesions. Vascular calcifications may obscure the vessel lumen. To avoid these, a window level of 200 Hounsfield units (HU) and width of 1,000 HU for the assessment of calcified vessels.[4] Image reconstruction using a sharp kernel (B46) may be helpful in calcified vessels and metallic stents.[5] As CT scan involves ionizing radiation, it recommended to use the appropriate KVp setting during acquisition.[6] The KVp may be reduced in thin and pediatric patients, which significantly decreases the radiation dose. New image domain-based iterative reconstruction (IR) algorithms, may reduce the noise and help in acquiring images with less radiation dose with same image quality. They may also increase the image sharpness and help in assessing small stents or calcified arteries.

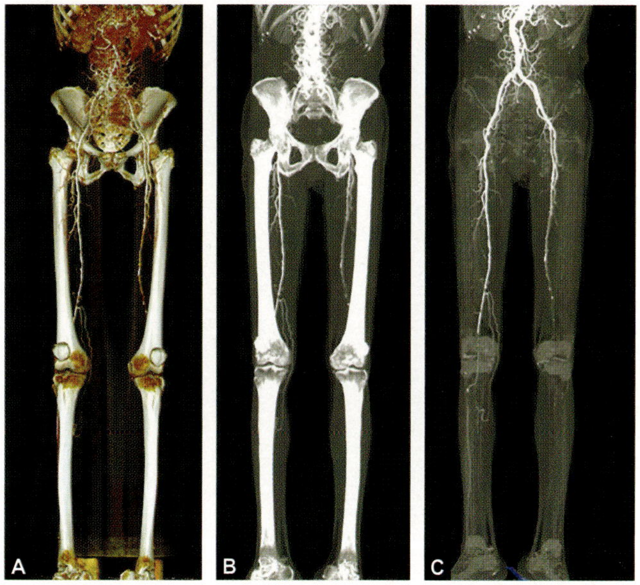

Figs. 1A to C: Contrast-enhanced computed tomography (CT) angiogram of 79-year-old male patient of bilateral claudication. Volume rendering technique (A), maximum intensity projections (B and C) reconstructions of CT angiogram demonstrating significant popliteal and infrapopliteal disease (occlusion of right popliteal artery and proximal trifurcation vessels with reformation of right anterior tibial artery; occlusion of left popliteal and infrapopliteal arteries).

Various postprocessing techniques are used in this setting (Figs. 1A to C). With multiplanar reformation (MPR) any section and orientation can be generated without loss of resolution from the base images because of isotropic data. These are important because they depict the lumen shape. Volume rendering (VR) generates images based on a threshold value. CT values above a threshold are displayed in various colors and at various enhancement levels.[7] In MIP, the highest CT value along any viewing ray from the desired direction is extracted and projected onto the image.[8] It generates an angiography like image. In curved planar reformation (CPR), a two-dimensional image is created by sampling CT volume data along an expected curved plane and a plane oriented along the long axis of the target vessel is usually used for vascular analysis. With these techniques in hand, there are no differences of treatment recommendations made on the basis of CT angiographic

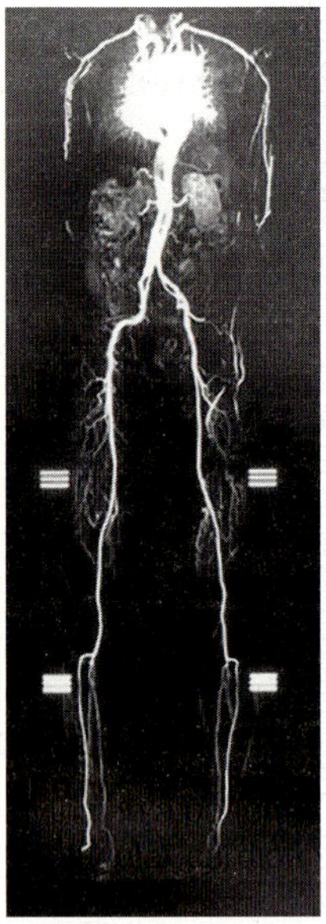

Fig. 2: Contrast magnetic resonance angiogram of 71-year-old male patient demonstrating entire peripheral arterial system.

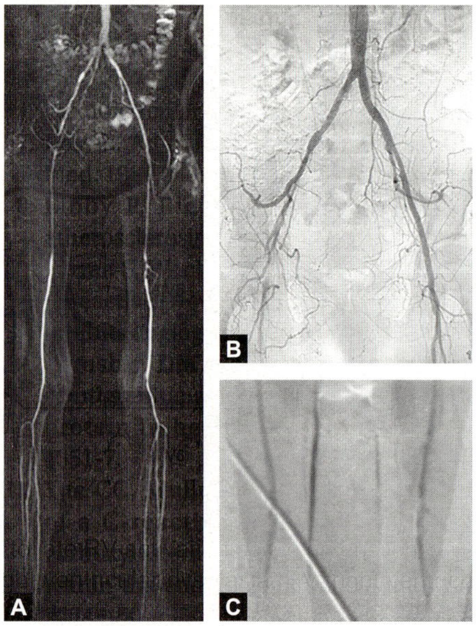

Figs. 3A to C: Magnetic resonance and digital subtraction angiography demonstrating right common femoral artery (CFA) occlusion with significant stenosis of left superficial FA. The vessels distal to stenosis and infrapopliteal arteries are better visualized with MRA.

findings and those made on the basis of DSA findings. Both investigations provide vascular surgeons and interventional radiologists equal and reliable information to plan their respective or combined procedures.

Magnetic Resonance Angiography

Magnetic resonance angiography has advantage of no radiation. Another benefit is the lower susceptibility to calcification relative to that of CT with clear depiction of vessels close to bones and vessels that are difficult to visualize with CTA, even with image postprocessing. CE MRA using gadolinium-based contrast agents is the technique of choice for the evaluation of peripheral angiogram with fast T1-weighted gradient echo low flip angle sequences or dynamic first pass imaging with fast field echo sequences to acquire angiogram images (Fig. 2).[9] Postprocessing reconstructions technique such as MIP and MPR may provide angiographic image. 3T MRA has better signal-to-noise ratio and spatial resolution in comparison to 1.5 T providing excellent angiographic images.[10] In fact, MRA is better than DSA to assess vessels distal to occlusion or significant stenosis as well as infrapopliteal arteries (Figs. 3A to C).

Multistation MRA is obtained using 0.2 mmol/kg body weight, in a bolus technique at aorto-iliac, femoropopliteal and infrapopliteal regions acquired in three to four stations (Figs. 4A to E). However, there may be venous contamination in infrapopliteal regions, especially in the case of CLI. Several techniques have been tried to avoid

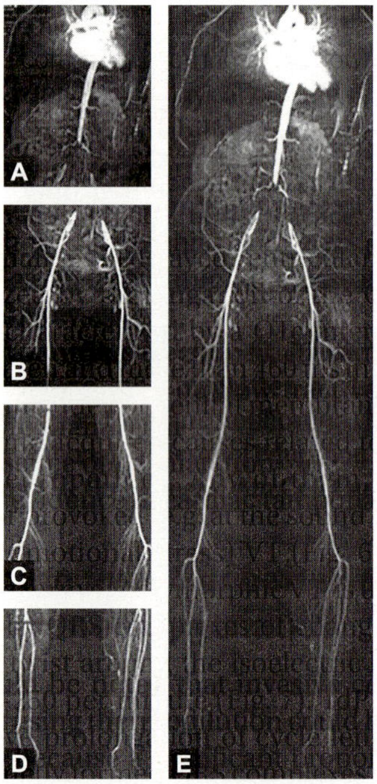

Figs. 4A to E: Contrast magnetic resonance angiogram (MRA) of 57-year-old male patient of bilateral claudication. MRA is acquired in four stations (A to D). Reconstructed MRA (E) demonstrating aorto-iliac occlusion.

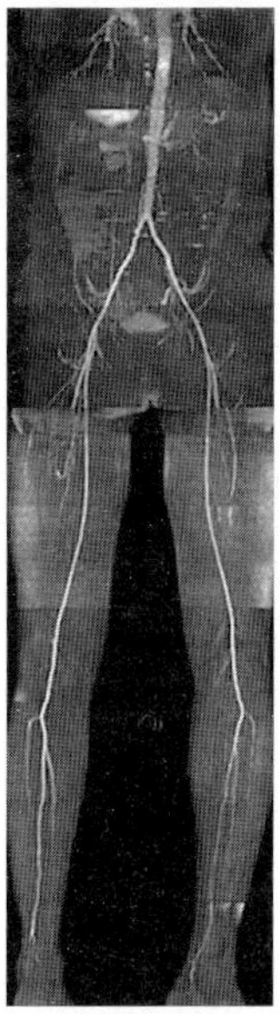

Fig. 5: Noncontrast magnetic resonance angiogram (MRA) of 57-year-old male patient of bilateral claudication. Noncontrast MRA showing significant disease with distal occlusion in bilateral anterior tibial arteries, significant disease involving right posterior tibial artery and left distal peroneal artery.

venous contamination in infrapopliteal region such as thigh compression cuffs, usage of foam pillow behind the knee to reduce venous return, acquiring the leg vessels first using separate contrast bolus.[11] New imaging sequences such as time-resolved MRA can provide the dynamic angiographic images of contrast flow from arterial to venous phases.

To avoid possible systemic complications, recent guidelines recommend assessment of renal function with estimated glomerular filtration rate (eGFR) before use of contrast materials and according to these guidelines, gadolinium should be used with caution in patients with an eGFR of less than 30 mL/min/1.73 m^2, including dialysis patients, to avoid nephrogenic systemic fibrosis.[12]

Magnetic resonance angiography can also be obtained with noncontrast techniques (Fig. 5). Time of flight imaging is a technique used for two-dimensional imaging of the peripheral and neck arteries and three-dimensional imaging of the intracranial arteries, but is limited by long imaging times, signal loss in turbulent and complex flows and susceptibility to field heterogeneities.[13]

Phase contrast imaging is used for hemodynamic rather than morphological imaging.[14] Electrocardiogram (ECG)-gated fast spin echo (FSE) MRA uses the flow void effect of fast arterial flow during systole. Imaging is based on subtracting systolic images (with flow voids) from diastolic images (which have high signal intensity due to slow flow) also effectively cancelling out background signals. Though, the imaging is complex and sensitive to motion, the imaging time is short, sensitive to slow flow and less susceptible to field heterogeneity and is used for imaging of peripheral arteries and aorta.[14]

Steady state free precession (SSFP) angiography, also known as balanced fast field echo (FFE), fast imaging with steady-state precession (TrueFISP), fast imaging employing steady state acquisition (FIESTA), and TrueSSFP, is a gradient-echo based sequence based on steady-state longitudinal and transverse magnetization. The image contrast is T2/T1-weighted, which gives blood high-signal intensity with little reliance on inflow.[15] Three-dimensional acquisition is used to produce angiographic images with a high signal-to-noise ratio of the aorta, renal and coronary territory. Limitations of this sequence are presence of high background signals and susceptibility to field heterogeneity.

Balanced SSFP with arterial spin labeling (ASL; a relatively complex imaging, susceptible to field heterogeneities, fast and complex flow) gives bright blood images with single acquisition by tagging the blood and provides excellent images with high signal-to-noise ratio and background suppression.[16]

The newest sequence is quiescent interval steady state (QISS). MRA use modified single shot two-dimensional balanced SSFP pulse sequence and has a sensitivity of 85–90% and specificity of 95–97% for the evaluation of PAD.[17]

THERAPEUTIC AND PROGNOSTIC IMPLICATIONS IN SPECIAL SITUATIONS

The choice of imaging modalities for acquiring angiographic images depend on imaging time, need to evaluate other anatomy such as renovascular disease, imaging of native disease or for follow-up after revascularization and patient factors (such as renal disease, diabetes, metallic stents). European Society of Cardiology (ESC), American Heart Association (AHA)/American College of Cardiology (ACC) and Inter-Society Consensus for the Management of Peripheral Arterial Disease (TASC II) have recommended guidelines for imaging modality to evaluate PAD.

The native vessel disease can be evaluated using duplex ultrasonography, CTA or MRA depending on the availability, cost and expertize. For patients with normal renal function who are not diabetic, PAD assessment can be done using either CTA or MRA. Various studies have demonstrated the sensitivities and specificities of CTA and MRA more than 95%.[18,19]

For arterial bypass grafts, Doppler ultrasonography (USG) used for the follow-up of the lower limb bypass graft with cross-sectional imaging done in case of inconclusive results or significant stenosis. Doppler study may detect graft stenosis and acute thrombosis.

For stent evaluation, CTA is better for assessment of stent restenosis, though beam hardening artifacts are real challenge (Figs. 6A to D). The metallic stents may deter the accurate assessment of stenosis by MRA due the artifacts and radiofrequency shielding. Usually recently available stents are magnetic resonance imaging (MRI) compatible. DSA is better for the evaluation of in-stent stenosis, when compared to CTA or MRA. Doppler USG can be used for the assessment of in-stent stenosis of peripheral arteries. Peak systolic velocity more than 275 cm/s and velocity ratio with the stent and disease-free vessel more than 3.5 may suggest significant stenosis of more than 80%.[20]

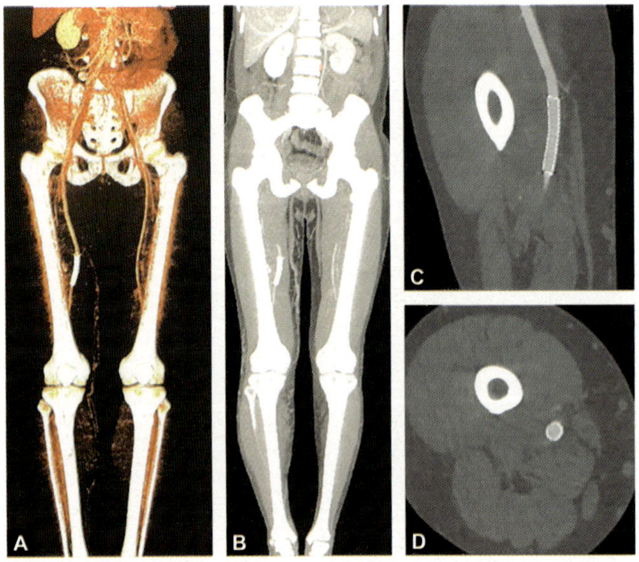

Figs. 6A to D: Post stent contrast-enhanced computed tomography (CT) angiogram of 32-year-old male patient of treated arteriovenous fistula. Volume rendered technique (A) and maximum intensity projection (B) showing the stent in the lower part of right superficial femoral artery. Axial CT sections with adjusted window settings (C and D) showing patent intra-stent segment.

Diabetic patients may have increased likelihood of vascular calcifications, which may hinder the proper assessment by Doppler USG and CTA. CE MRA would be better choice for assessment of calcified vessels calcifications. Noncontrast MRA can be used in case of advanced renal failure having an eGFR less than 30 mL/min/1.73 m^2.

In the evaluation of implanted metal devices, MRI may be contraindicated in patients with implanted pacemaker or defibrillator, ferromagnetic aneurysm clips, cochlear implant electrodes used in deep brain stimulation, metallic foreign bodies, ocular implants, etc. Some newer pacemakers are MRI compatible. Even MRI compatible stents or metallic implants may be difficult to assess due to artifacts generated by them. CTA also has challenges of beam hardening artifacts. Recent advances in CT hardware and software technologies enabled the adequate assessment of the vessels.

To summarize, characterization of PAD can be performed with noninvasive angiography using CTA or MRA as well as with duplex ultrasonography depending on patient specific characteristics. A comparison between the various imaging modalities is enlisted in the Table 1. The imaging algorithm for assessment of PAD is illustrated in Flowchart 1.

TABLE 1: Comparison between various imaging modalities in evaluating peripheral arterial disease.

Imaging modality	*Advantages*	*Disadvantages*
Doppler ultrasonography	Easy No radiation No contrast Can be done bedside Inexpensive	Operator dependent Difficult in evaluation of aorto-iliac lesions Difficult in assessing calcified vessels and multilevel stenosis Time consuming
CTA	Fast High spatial resolution Better for in-stent restenosis than MRA	Involves ionizing radiation Iodinated contrast Calcified plaques obscure the stenosis
MRA	No radiation Both contrast and noncontrast angiogram can be done Better for calcified stenotic lesions	Risk of nephrogenic systemic fibrosis In-stent restenosis difficult to assess
DSA	High temporal resolution Simultaneous treatment can be done	Involves ionizing radiation Iodinated contrast Provides 2D intraluminal image Risk of procedure related complications

(CTA: Computed tomography angiography; DSA: digital subtraction angiography; MRA: magnetic resonance angiography)

Flowchart 1: Imaging algorithm for evaluation of peripheral arterial disease.

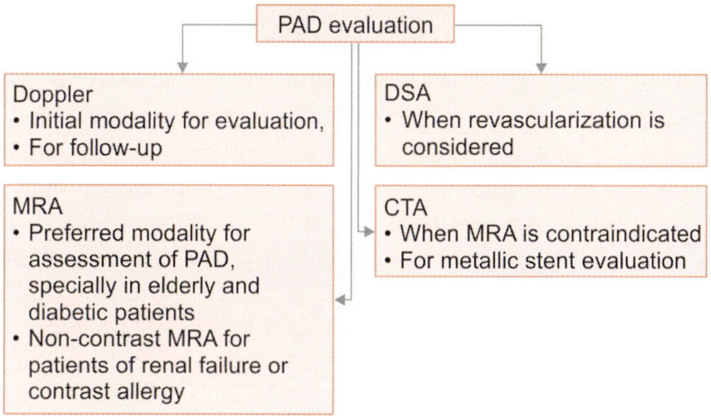

(CTA: computed tomography angiography; DSA: Digital subtraction angiography; MRA: Magnetic resonance angiography; PAD: Peripheral arterial disease)

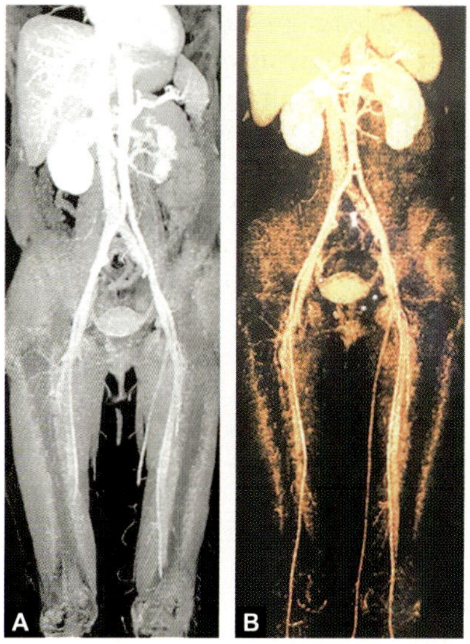

Figs. 7A and B: Computed tomography venogram with maximum intensity projections (A) and volume rendering technique (B) reconstructions demonstrating bilateral normal lower-limb deep veins and inferior vena cava.

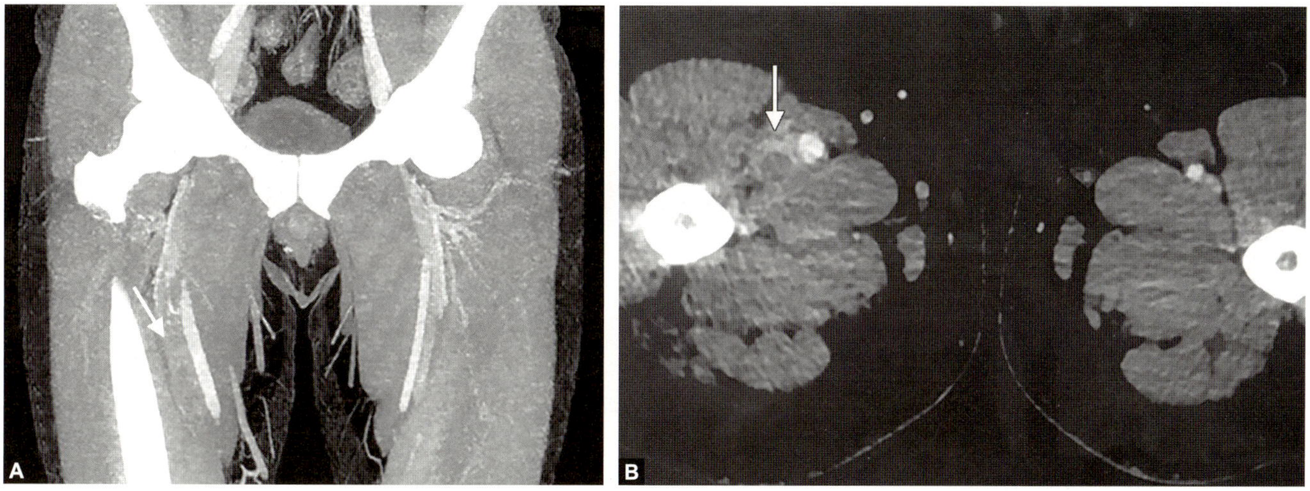

Figs. 8A and B: Computed tomography venogram in maximum intensity projections (A) and axial (B) images showing acute thrombosis involving superficial femoral vein (arrow).

CT AND MR VENOGRAPHY IN THE EVALUATION OF PERIPHERAL DEEP VENOUS SYSTEM

Computed tomography and MR venography techniques can assess venous thromboembolic disease in peripheral venous system. Though Doppler remains initial modality for evaluation of peripheral venous system, CT and MR venography has certain advantages, especially in the assessment of pelvic veins and inferior vena cava.

Computerized Tomography Venography

Lower-limb deep venous system can be best evaluated by Doppler study. CTA with venous phase imaging (CTA-CTV) will not only evaluate patients of pulmonary embolism, but also can assess inferior vena cava, pelvic veins, and lower-limb veins. CTA done using 80–100 mL contrast can be followed by delayed venous phase imaging (up to 4 minutes) of lower limbs up to upper calves (Figs. 7A and B). Deep vein thrombosis can be seen as hypodense filling defect, which may be surrounded by rim of hyperdense contrast medium (Figs. 8A and B). The prospective investigation of

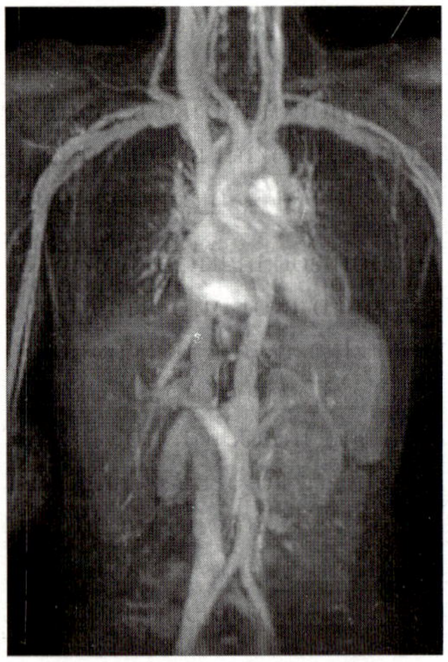

Fig. 9: Magnetic resonance imaging venogram with maximum intensity projections reconstructions demonstrating upper-limb deep veins and inferior vena cava.

pulmonary embolism diagnosis (PIOPED) II trial showed sensitivity and specificity of 83% and 96% respectively.[21] CTV may also demonstrate any thrombus in inferior vena cava and pelvic veins better than Doppler study.

Magnetic Resonance Venography

Magnetic resonance venography (MRV) can be performed either with contrast or noncontrast. Noncontrast MRV using time-of-flight venography (TOF-MRV) can evaluate the deep venous system. Thrombus may be seen as filling defect in the venous system. Meta-analysis by Abdalla et al. showed MRV has sensitivity of 93% and specificity of 96% diagnosing deep vein thrombosis.[22] It is more sensitive for the assessment of proximal veins in comparison to distal veins. It can evaluate pelvic veins or inferior vena cava similar to CTA, but without radiation and usage of iodinated contrast media (Fig. 9). It can be very helpful in the evaluation of pregnant patients for thrombosis. As the thrombus may show different signal intensities depended the age of the thrombus, MRV can differentiate acute from chronic thrombus. Though MRI is inferior to Doppler USG for evaluation of lower-limb deep vein thrombosis, it may better evaluate pelvic veins and inferior vena cava. Because of high cost and less availability, its use has not been picked up.

CONCLUSION

Recent advances in CTA and MRA have made these investigations excellent techniques for noninvasive evaluation of lower limb PAD. They can identify the site and morphology of the stenotic lesions, which may help in the management of these lesions. Though Doppler study is the initial modality for the assessment of peripheral arterial and venous disease, complete anatomical detail and morphology of the lesions are best assessed by CTA and MRA. CT and MR venography techniques can adequately evaluate peripheral venous system. Further developments in the hardware and software of these technologies may eliminate the few deficiencies of these modalities.

REFERENCES

1. Dua A, Lee CJ. Epidemiology of peripheral arterial disease and critical limb ischemia. Tech Vasc Interv Radiol. 2016;19(2):91-5.
2. Gerhard-Herman MD, Gornik HL, Barrett C, et al. 2016 AHA/ACC guideline on the management of patients with lower extremity peripheral artery disease: executive summary: a report of the American College of Cardiology/American Heart Association Task Force on Clinical Practice Guidelines. Circulation. 2017;135(12):e686-725.
3. Pollak AW, Norton P, Kramer CM. Multimodality imaging of lower extremity peripheral arterial disease: current role and future directions. Circ Cardiovasc Imaging. 2012;5(6):797-807.
4. Kock MCJM, Dijkshoorn ML, Pattynama PMT, et al. Multi-detector row computed tomography angiography of peripheral arterial disease. Eur Radiol. 2007;17(12):3208-22.
5. Suzuki S, Furui S, Kaminaga T, et al. Evaluation of coronary stents in vitro with CT angiography: effect of stent diameter, convolution kernel, and vessel orientation to the Z-axis. Circ J Off J Jpn Circ Soc. 2005;69(9):1124-31.
6. Schindera ST, Graca P, Patak MA, et al. Thoracoabdominal-aortoiliac multidetector-row CT angiography at 80 and 100 kVp: assessment of image quality and radiation dose. Invest Radiol. 2009;44(10):650-5.
7. Dalrymple NC, Prasad SR, Freckleton MW, et al. Informatics in radiology (infoRAD): introduction to the language of three-dimensional imaging with multidetector CT. Radiogr Rev Publ Radiol Soc N Am Inc. 2005;25(5):1409-28.
8. Napel S, Marks MP, Rubin GD, et al. CT angiography with spiral CT and maximum intensity projection. Radiology. 1992;185(2):607-10.
9. Watanabe Y, Dohke M, Okumura A, et al. Dynamic subtraction contrast-enhanced MR angiography: technique, clinical applications, and pitfalls. Radiogr Rev Publ Radiol Soc N Am Inc. 2000;20(1):135-52.
10. van den Bosch H, Westenberg JJ, Duijm LE, et al. 3T versus 1.5T MR angiography in peripheral arterial occlusive disease: an equivalence trial in comparison with digital subtraction angiography. J Cardiovasc Magn Reson. 2012;14(Suppl 1):P139.
11. Roditi G, Kusumawidjaja D. Magnetic resonance angiography and computed tomography angiography for peripheral arterial disease. Imaging. 2009;21:85-108.

12. Kribben A, Witzke O, Hillen U, et al. Nephrogenic systemic fibrosis: pathogenesis, diagnosis, and therapy. J Am Coll Cardiol. 2009;53(18):1621-8.
13. Kaufman JA, McCarter D, Geller SC, et al. Two-dimensional time-of-flight MR angiography of the lower extremities: artifacts and pitfalls. AJR Am J Roentgenol. 1998;171(1):129-35.
14. Miyazaki M, Lee VS. Nonenhanced MR angiography. Radiology. 2008;248(1):20-43.
15. Scheffler K, Lehnhardt S. Principles and applications of balanced SSFP techniques. Eur Radiol. 2003;13(11):2409-18.
16. van Laar PJ, van der Grond J, Hendrikse J. Brain perfusion territory imaging: methods and clinical applications of selective arterial spin-labeling MR imaging. Radiology. 2008;246(2):354-64.
17. Edelman R, Giri S, Dunkle E, et al. Quiescent-inflow single-shot (QISS) magnetic resonance angiography using a highly undersampled radial k-space trajectory. Magn Reson Med. 2013;70(6):1662-8.
18. Menke J, Larsen J. Meta-analysis: accuracy of contrast-enhanced magnetic resonance angiography for assessing steno-occlusions in peripheral arterial disease. Ann Intern Med. 2010;153(5):325-34.
19. Napoli A, Anzidei M, Zaccagna F, et al. Peripheral arterial occlusive disease: diagnostic performance and effect on therapeutic management of 64-section CT angiography. Radiology. 2011;261(3):976-86.
20. Baril DT, Rhee RY, Kim J, et al. Duplex criteria for determination of in-stent stenosis after angioplasty and stenting of the superficial femoral artery. J Vasc Surg. 2009;49(1):133-8.
21. Stein PD, Woodard PK, Weg JG, et al. Diagnostic pathways in acute pulmonary embolism: recommendations of the PIOPED II investigators. Am J Med. 2006;119(12):1048-55.
22. Abdalla G, Fawzi Matuk R, Venugopal V, et al. The diagnostic accuracy of magnetic resonance venography in the detection of deep venous thrombosis: a systematic review and meta-analysis. Clin Radiol. 2015;70(8):858-71.

105

CHAPTER

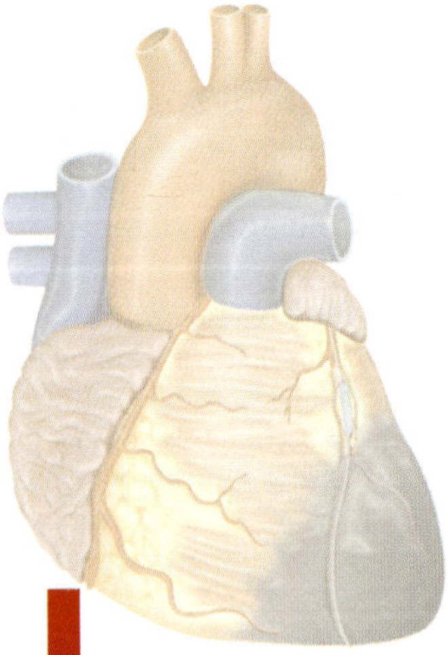

Conventional Angio Evaluation of Peripheral Arterial Disease

NN Khanna, Dyah W Anggrahini, Suparna Rao, Oladimeji Oluwaseye

INTRODUCTION

Peripheral vascular disease comprises the noncoronary arterial and venous disease. Most common cause of peripheral arterial disease (PAD) remains atherosclerosis, which can manifest as stenosis or aneurysm in various vascular beds. Recent 2017 European Society of Cardiology (ESC) Guidelines for the management of patients with PAD mentioned that it has a major decrement effect on functional capacity, quality of life, and limb amputation and has increased risk of death.[1,2] Peripheral venous disease (PVD) is a different type of disease. The most common cause of PVD is thrombosis and perivascular fibrosis.

The prevalence of both diseases has been increased in the past decades and will keep increasing considering the changes in lifestyle and disease pattern and better investigation methodologies. While awareness for coronary artery disease (CAD) has significantly increased, the awareness, diagnosis, and treatment of PAD and PVD remain underappreciated.[3]

A good imaging strategy is a must for diagnostic workup of the patients, to provide complete diagnostic information needed for diagnosis and further surgical or interventional management. Computed tomography (CT) angiography and MR angiography (MRA) are two sophisticated imaging other than conventional angiography or digital subtraction angiography (DSA). Both provide detailed information for the diagnosis and planning of the interventions.[4] Conventional catheter-based angiography/DSA is consistently more accurate than other imaging modalities, such as MR and CT angiography for below-the-knee lesions. In addition, it is the most universally accepted technology for guiding the percutaneous peripheral vascular intervention.[5] Therefore, this catheter-based angiography is considered as the gold standard reference for vascular imaging.

CONVENTIONAL ANGIOGRAPHY/ DIGITAL SUBTRACTION ANGIOGRAPHY

Imaging of peripheral vasculature is different from that of coronary vasculature. Several considerations should be taken into account when performing the peripheral angiography. It usually requires imaging of a large area, which in the absence of large field of view will require multiple injections. Thus, large image intensifier (36 cm) is recommended to accommodate large regions of interest. Cine angiography is usually done at a lower frame rate per second as the structures are not moving.

Most of the times, the best image acquisition will be obtained by performing DSA. Using DSA technique, a mask will be produced by making baseline background image just before injecting certain amount of dye to a digitally subtracted background.

Following contrast injection, subtraction of the image will allow enhancement and visualization of the vessel only by masking the non-vessel structures.[6]

Digital subtraction techniques reduce the dose of the contrast required. Good spatial and temporal resolution, combined with a large field of view, allows bolus chasing from the aorta to the feet. The peripheral arterial tree can be seen and mapped quickly with overlapping runs. Large numbers of collaterals can be anatomically visualized quickly and in one session.

INDICATIONS OF CONVENTIONAL ANGIOGRAPHY WITH DIGITAL SUBTRACTION ANGIOGRAPHY

The availability of more sophisticated noninvasive imaging technology has reduced the class recommendation of conventional angiography/DSA as a sole diagnostic approach for PAD or PVD. The general indication for angiography is to define the vascular anatomy, whenever a definite diagnosis is required and/or revascularization is planned. The 2017 ESC Guidelines, 2016 American College of Cardiology/American Heart Association (ACC/AHA) Guidelines, and 2018 American College of Chest Physician Guidelines recommend the following indications for DSA.[1,7]

Indications and Recommendations for Arterial Disease

- *Aortic arch, thoracic aorta, and its branches*: Angiography with/without DSA technique will be required for the aneurysm to specifically evaluate the anatomical abnormalities especially in the aortic arch when the exact location of these branches is necessary prior to the endovascular treatment.
- *Carotid disease*: In patients with transient ischemic attack or stroke, urgent imaging using a noninvasive modality is recommended. Intra-arterial DSA will be necessary for guiding carotid artery stenting but not carotid endarterectomy. DSA is rarely required for diagnostic purposes and is used only in highly selected situations with discordant noninvasive imaging.[4,8]
- *Abdominal aorta*: The indication for angiography in those with abdominal aortic aneurysm is to delineate the anatomy particularly if endovascular treatment is considered. It is usually not needed solely to define the anatomy in whom surgical treatment may be most beneficial. In the case of suspected mesenteric ischemia, angiography has ACC/AHA Class I indication.
- *Upper extremities*: Upper extremity claudication is one of the indications for evaluation by angiography for the presence of subclavian artery (SCA) stenosis. Subclavian and vertebral angiography is also very important in patients with angina after left internal mammary artery graft to left anterior descending or in vertebral or subclavian steal syndrome.[1]
- *Lower extremities*: In those with lower extremities artery disease, DSA is often required for guiding percutaneous peripheral interventional procedures or for checking the patency of distal bypass grafts. It is also often needed for below-the-knee arteries, especially in patients with critical limb ischemia, because of the limitation of all other imaging tools to detect ankle/pedal segments suitable for distal bypass. Several clinical conditions required for further diagnostic evaluation are:[1,7]
  - Peripheral occlusive disease with rest pain/gangrene (Fontaine III or IV)
  - Severe intermittent claudication (Fontaine IIb and selected IIa)
  - Critical limb ischemia (acute and chronic)
  - Femoropopliteal aneurysm
  - Thromboangiitis obliterans
  - Microembolism, e.g. blue toe syndrome
  - Arteriovenous malformation
  - Vascular trauma
  - Tumors of soft-tissue and bones
  - Follow-up evaluations after revascularization.
- *Renal*: Digital subtraction angiography remains the gold standard for the diagnosis of renal artery stenosis. Angiography is generally limited to visualization and quantification of the stenosis before vascular intervention. The major advantage of conventional angiography is the possibility to measure the pressure gradient across the lesions with moderate stenosis. The 2017 European Society of Cardiology guidelines recommendation mentioned that DSA may be considered to confirm a diagnosis of reactive attachment disorder when clinical suspicion is high and the results of noninvasive examinations are inconclusive (Class IIb). Several clinical conditions that may require angiography are:
  - Those with evidence of significant stenosis on noninvasive testing
  - Uncontrolled hypertension in patients younger than 30 years or older than 55 years
  - Refractory hypertension
  - Rising creatinine level (especially after the initiation of angiotensin-converting-enzyme inhibitor therapy).

IMAGING TECHNIQUES

Access Sites

Successful angiographic procedures require the correct choice of access site. If necessary, the noninvasive imaging studies, such as CT, MRA, or duplex ultrasound scanning, might be useful to determine the access site. Most common vascular sites are common femoral artery (CFA), brachial artery, and radial artery.[6]

Contrast Dose

An optimal contrast dose is necessary to obtain best result. Since peripheral artery and veins differ in size, length, and complexity of the branches, therefore, different dose and injection rate are necessary to define to get accurate images. The following table gives the injection rates and contrast volume for defining different vessels.[6]

Vessel type	*Injection rate (mL/s)*	*Contrast volume (mL)*
Aortoiliac	14–16	15–25
CFA-SFA-Popliteal	5–7	16–20
Run CFA-BTK	4	9–12
SFA	4–5	8–10
Run BTK	3–4	10–12
BTK	3–4	5–7
Pedal arteries	3–4	5–7

(BTK: Bruton's tyrosine kinase; CFA: common femoral artery; SFA: superficial femoral artery)

ANGIOGRAPHY PROCEDURE

Angiography for Aortic Arch and Thoracic Aorta

Conventional angiography is essential for the assessment for the type of aortic arch, although CT and MRA should be done prior to angiography. It may be necessary to selectively cannulate the arch vessels for interventional purposes. Four-vessel angiography is required before carotid or intracranial intervention (Figs. 1A and B). One should evaluate the diameter of the thoracic aorta, the presence of aneurysm or dissection and also evaluate aortic transection when there is blunt trauma to chest. For the evaluation of thoracic aortic dissection, conventional angiography has a sensitivity of 80% and specificity of 95%. If thoracic endovascular aortic repair will be performed, detailed coronary, brachiocephalic, visceral, and renal arteriography should be obtained.

The most common view for aortic arch and thoracic aorta evaluation is 30–40 left anterior oblique (LAO) projection. The injection of 30–40 mL of dye at 20–30 mL/s generally gives adequate opacification. Anteroposterior (AP) view and lateral images will be needed to evaluate in patients with coarctation of aorta. It gives information about anatomical details, including the relation with the origin of left SCA. Furthermore, the idea of collateral flows may be obtained. Selective angiography in lateral 90° views may also be used in the case of patent ductus arteriosus (PDA); and in some cases the extreme lateral of 120° LAO may be necessary to evaluate the angulation of the PDA tract.

Angiography for Carotid Studies

The default views used for evaluation of the carotid artery are AP and lateral. Patient is asked to do hyperextension of the neck. In selective cases, LAO or right anterior oblique (RAO) view may be needed to obtain better visualization of the stenotic vessel (Figs. 2A and B). In the case that LAO view is used, patient is advised to turn the head toward the contralateral side and vice versa for RAO view. Sometimes, rotational angiography, if available, should be used.[9]

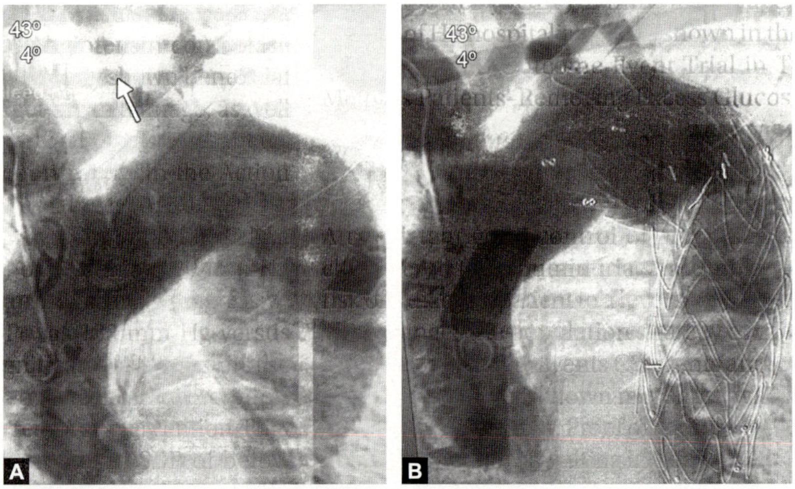

Figs. 1A and B: Angiography aortic arch and aorta also show the branches. Aneurysm of the descending thoracic aorta before stent graft placement (A) and after stent graft (B).

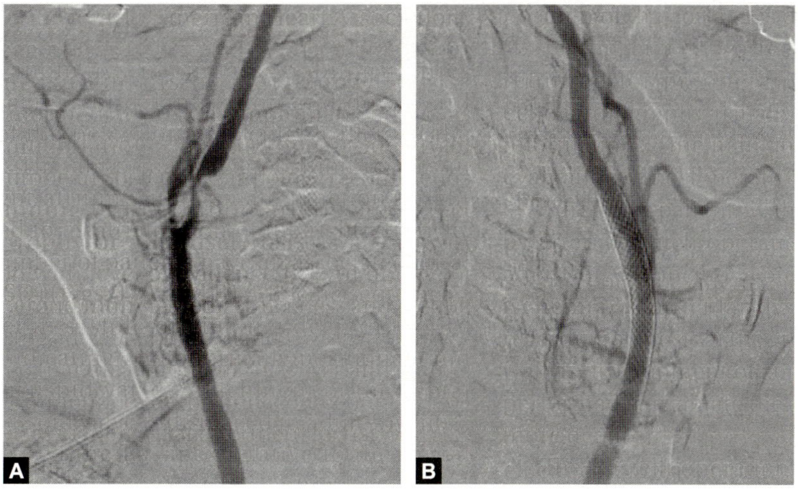

Figs. 2A and B: DSA visualization of right carotid artery showing 80% stenosis (A) and left carotid artery with implanted stent (B). (DSA: digital subtraction angiography)

Angiography for Abdominal Aorta

The best view to delineate the abdominal aorta is AP and lateral view. The celiac artery will be at the L1 level; the superior mesenteric artery (SMA) will be at L2 level; the renal artery at the L2-3 level just caudal to the SMA; and the inferior mesenteric artery at the L4 level. The 20–40 mL of the contrast using power injector at the rate of 15–30 mL/s at 1000 PSI will give adequate opacification (Figs. 3A to E).[10]

Angiography for Renal Artery

The most common approach for renal angiography is CFA with 5 or 6 F sheath. In case that there is tortuosity of the iliac artery, a long sheath may be used. Brachial approach or radial approach can be used when femoral artery is not assessable. DSA is done at 4 FPS with 30 mL iodinated contrast at the rate of 15 mL/s. The default view for evaluation of the renal artery is LAO 15–30°, which may be able to show osteal portion of both renal artery. AP view may be used, sometimes one may miss the osteal stenosis in both arteries and SMA after overlaps in the right renal artery shading the stenosis of the osteal.[9]

In borderline lesions, a translesional gradient should be measured. A systolic pressure gradient more than 20 mm Hg or a resting pressure ratio distal to the stenosis less than 0.90 is considered to be indicative of significant stenosis in symptomatic patients. Renal artery fractional flow reserve measured during maximum hyperemia induced by nitroglycerin (100–300 μg) or papaverine 20–30 mg is an alternative method to assess the stenosis severity (Figs. 4A and B).[11]

Angiography for Subclavian and Upper Extremities Arteries

When performing angiography of subclavian or upper extremities vessels, 5 mL to 10 mL of contrast with hand injection using DSA will give good visualization. Orthogonal oblique views are used for subclavian vessels and its branches. The right SCA is best viewed in LAO position while the left SCA in RAO. Patient's arm should be adducted to the neutral position during angiography.

Angiography for Lower Extremity Vessels

The iliofemoral arteries are the most common site for atheroesclerotic PAD. For angiography procedure, CFA, brachial, or radial approaches are common access sites using 4–6 F catheters.

For aortoiliac disease, the basic view is AP, but in this view, the internal iliac artery may overlap with [external iliac artery (EIA)] and the EIA stenosis may be missed. Modified 30° contralateral oblique view is used to visualize the contralateral common iliac bifurcation. Femoropopliteal lesion are usually long, multiple, and chronic total occlusions. The basic view is AP by which profunda femoral artery will overlie with superficial femoral artery. To overcome this, the ipsilateral 30° oblique view is recommended for visualizing the CFA bifurcation, e.g. RAO for right and LAO for left can be taken. Infragenicular lesion needs a DSA with injection as close to the arteries as possible (Figs. 5 and 6).[10]

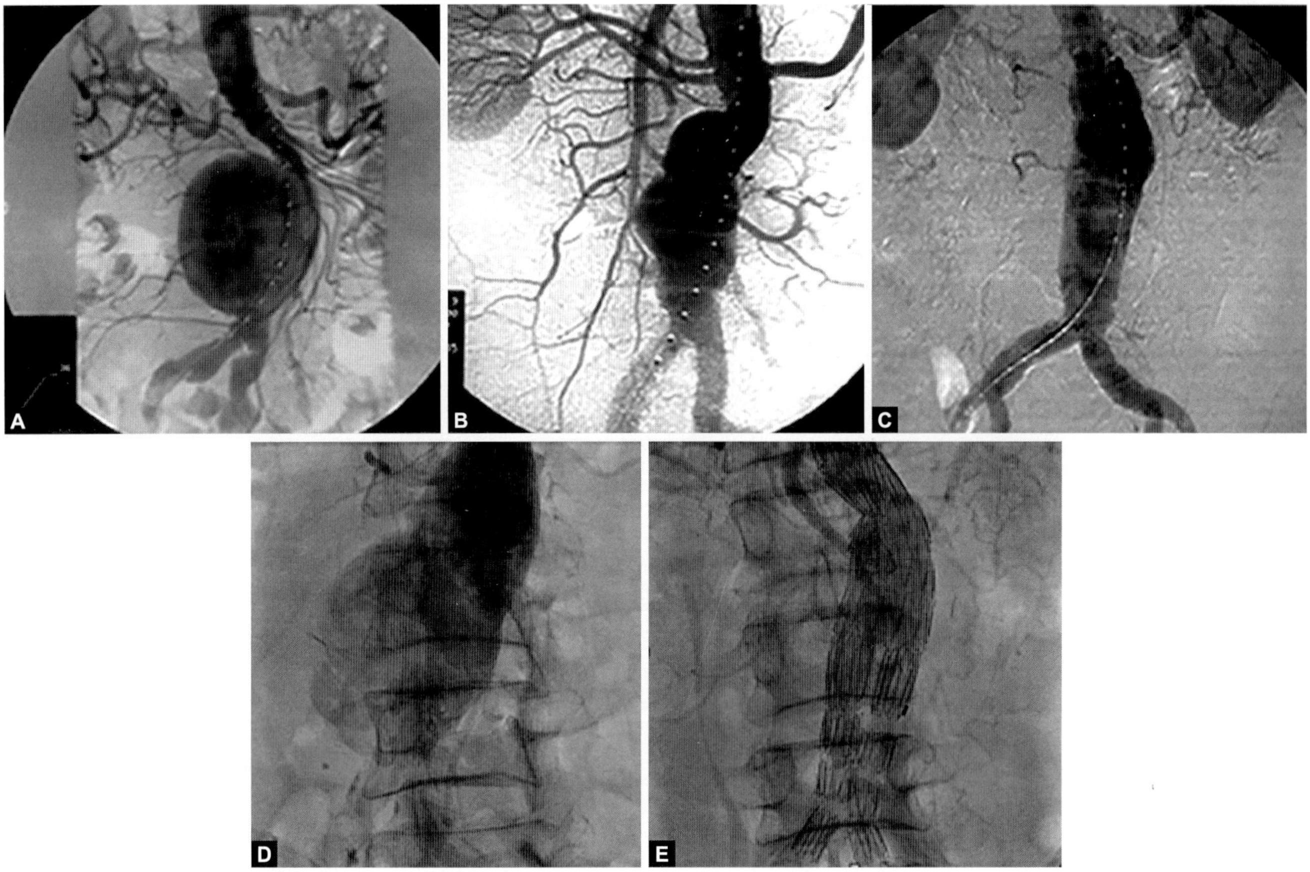

Figs. 3A to E: Several types of abdominal aortic aneurysm evaluated by contrast angiography to delineate the detail anatomy prior to intervention. (E) showed after stent graft implantation.

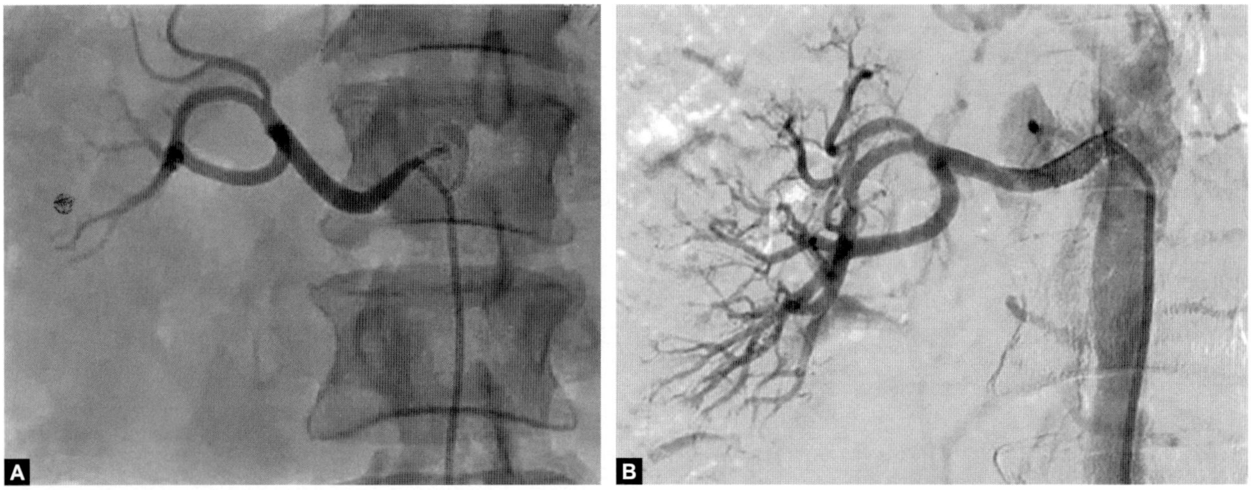

Figs. 4A and B: Renal angiography shows stenosis at the osteal of renal artery (A) and DSA evaluation after renal artery stenting (B). (DSA: digital subtraction angiography)

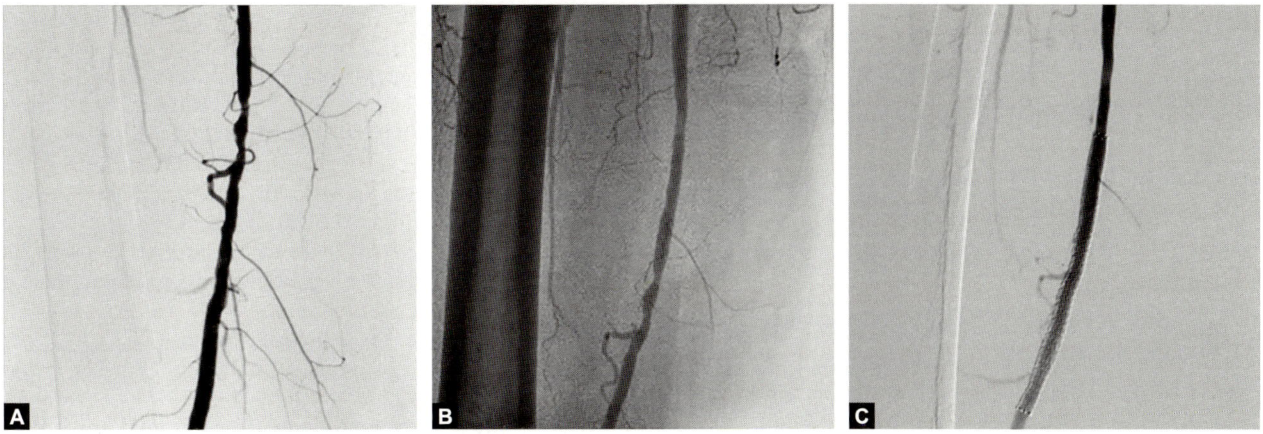

Figs. 5A to C: DSA and contrast angiography of SFA lesion (A) and the final result after stent implantation (B and C). (DSA: digital subtraction angiography; SFA: superficial femoral artery)

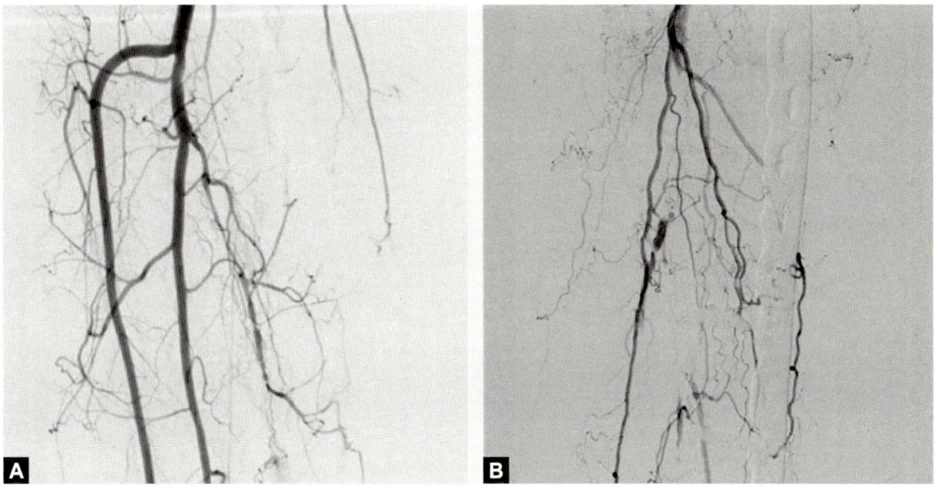

Figs. 6A and B: DSA of below-the-knee arteries showing normal vessel (A) and diffusely diseased (B). (DSA: digital subtraction angiography)

COMPLICATIONS AND LIMITATIONS

The main disadvantage of contrast angiography or DSA is the fact that it is an invasive procedure. Thus, complications, such as hematoma, perforation, dissection, arteriovenous fistula, or pseudoaneurysm, may occur. In addition, DSA involves ionizing radiation (for both patients and staff and the operator) nephrotoxicity of contrast. Contrast-related events including contrast-induced nephropathy may occur at the rate of 0.1% and increase in those with renal dysfunction, left ventricular dysfunction, and advance age.

GUIDELINE ALGORITHM/SUMMARY ILLUSTRATION

The algorithm for diagnosis and treatment of PVD is given in Flowchart 1.

Flowchart 1: An algorithmic approach for the diagnosis and treatment of PVD.

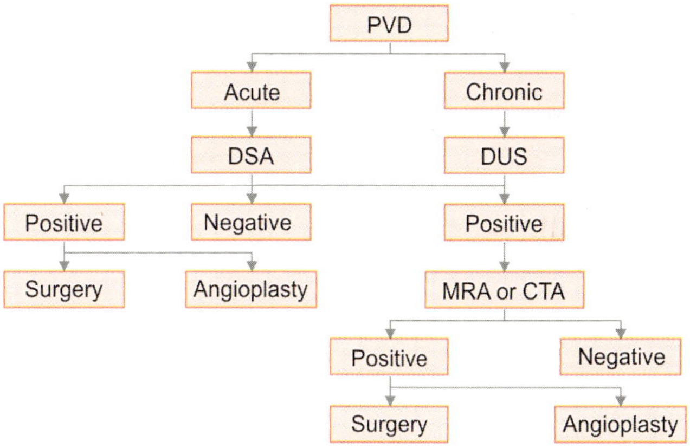

(PVD: peripheral venous disease; DSA: digital subtraction angiography; DUS: diagnostic ultrasonography; MRA: magnetic resonance angiography; CTA: computed tomography angiography)

CONCLUSION

Although a number of imaging technologies are available for evaluating arterial and venous diseases, conventional angiography still remains the gold standard for diagnosis and treatment of peripheral arterial and venous diseases and is essential before any interventional procedure.

REFERENCES

1. Victor A, Jean-Baptiste R, Marie-Louise B, et al. 2017 ESC guidelines on the diagnosis and treatment of peripheral arterial diseases, in collaboration with the European Society for Vascular Surgery (ESVS). Eur J Vasc Endovasc Surg. 2018;55:305-68.
2. Fowkes GR, Aboyans V, Fowkes FJI, et al. Peripheral artery disease: epidemiology and global perspectives. Nat Rev Cardiol. 2017;14:156-70.
3. Criqui M, Denenberg J, Langer R, et al. The epidemiology of peripheral arterial disease: importance of identifying the population at risk. Vasc Med. 1997;2:221-6.
4. Chilcote WA, Modic MT, Pavlicek WA, et al. Digital subtraction angiography of the carotid arteries: a comparative study in 100 patients. Radiology. 1981;139(2):287-95.
5. Collins R, Cranny G, Burch J, et al. A systematic review of duplex ultrasound, magnetic resonance angiography and computed tomography angiography for the diagnosis and assessment of symptomatic, lower limb peripheral arterial disease. Health Technol Assess. 2007;11(20):1-184.
6. Koci T, Mehringer C, Allgood M, et al. Peripheral angiography: optimal technique and current status in vascular imaging. Am J Card Imaging. 1993;7(2):73-91.
7. Gerhard-Herman MD, Gornik HL, Barrett C, et al. 2016 AHA/ACC guideline on the management of patients with lower extremity peripheral artery disease: a report of the American College of Cardiology/American Heart Association task force on clinical practice guidelines. J Am Coll Cardiol. 2017;69(11):e71-126.
8. Guidelines for percutaneous transluminal angioplasty. Standards of Practice Committee of the Society of Cardiovascular and Interventional Radiology. Radiology. 1990;177:619-26.
9. Krishnan M. Peripheral angiography: views and technique. J Indian Coll Cardiol 2016;6(Suppl. 1):114-7.
10. Pentecost M, Criqui M, Dorros G, et al. Guidelines for peripheral percutaneous transluminal angioplasty of the abdominal aorta and lower extremity vessels. Circulation. 1994;84:511-31.
11. Erwin PA, Shishehbor MH. Renal artery stenting: indications, techniques, and devices. Minerva Cardioangiol. 2013;61(2):188-99.

106

CHAPTER

Advanced Image-guided Peripheral Vascular Interventions

NN Khanna, Suparna Rao, Oladimeji Oluwaseye, Wulan Anggrahini

INTRODUCTION

Aging population increases the risk of patients for atherosclerotic disease involving all vascular beds, such as the coronary, cerebral, and peripheral circulation. Vascular diseases contribute to morbidity and mortality more than any other type of disease. Endovascular interventions have grown immensely over the past few decades. The technique has emerged as a first-line therapy in the management of peripheral vascular diseases (arterial and venous). Most of the vascular diseases (obstructive or nonobstructive) today are being treated by various endovascular techniques, which developed from the concept of serial dilatation with catheters and plain balloon angioplasty. Advances in the hardware, including catheter, sheath, wire, balloon and stent design, and the introduction of embolic protection devices and other novel technologies have led to new therapeutic options and improved clinical outcomes. Today, endovascular procedures are performed by variety of operators, including interventional cardiologists, radiologists, and vascular surgeons trained in endovascular techniques. The prerequisites for performing good vascular interventions are need of proper imaging, reduced contrast, reduced radiation, precision, and optimization of intervention. Cardiologists, radiologists, and vascular surgeons rely on imaging modalities for both diagnostic and procedural assistance when treating patients with peripheral arterial diseases (PAD). The role of imaging includes: (1) diagnosis of vascular disease (2) to provide road map for treatment (3) to follow-up after the treatment (4) for prognostication. Image accuracy in angiography is limited by vessel tortuosity, arterial wall motion artifacts, and overlying structures and vessels, which may lead to inaccurate interpretation of the diseased vessel.

COMPUTED TOMOGRAPHY ANGIOGRAPHY

Computed tomography angiography (CTA) has revolutionized vascular imaging in the recent years. Multi-detector computed tomography (MDCT) technology has rapidly evolved, which enables high-resolution imaging of the peripheral vasculature (Figs. 1 to 3). It is now possible to image the entire inflow and runoff vessels with a single acquisition by a single injection of intravenous contrast medium. Isotropic volumetric data sets acquired with MDCT angiography enable three-dimensional (3-D) reconstruction of vascular tree and many postprocessing methods. The advantages of peripheral vascular CTA are accurate localization of the pathological lesion, which helps in reliable procedure planning and vascular access planning.[1] It is also useful as a baseline study and to assess the disease progression and evaluation of the graft/stent. The major drawback of CTA is its potential radiation hazards; however, with the development of newer generation CT scanners, there has been a reduction in the radiation dose and shorter scan time. Adequate precautions should be taken prior to injection of contrast agents in patients with renal impairment. Other pitfalls of CTA include foreign objects such as metallic implants, stents, and clips causing artifactual pseudolesions.

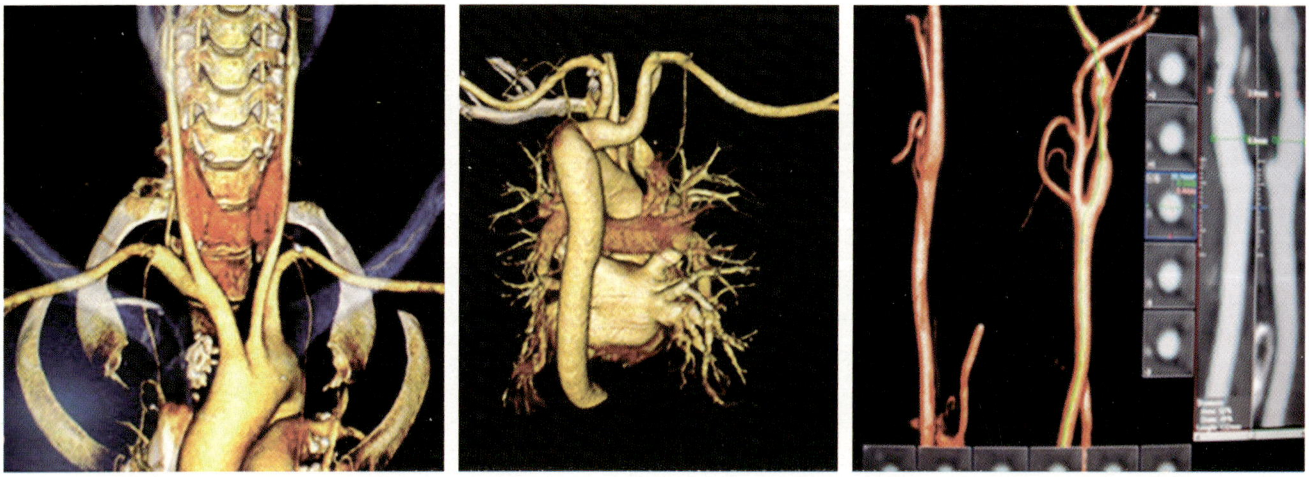

Fig. 1: Excellent depiction of vascular anatomy and pathological lesions involving major arch and neck vessels.[1]

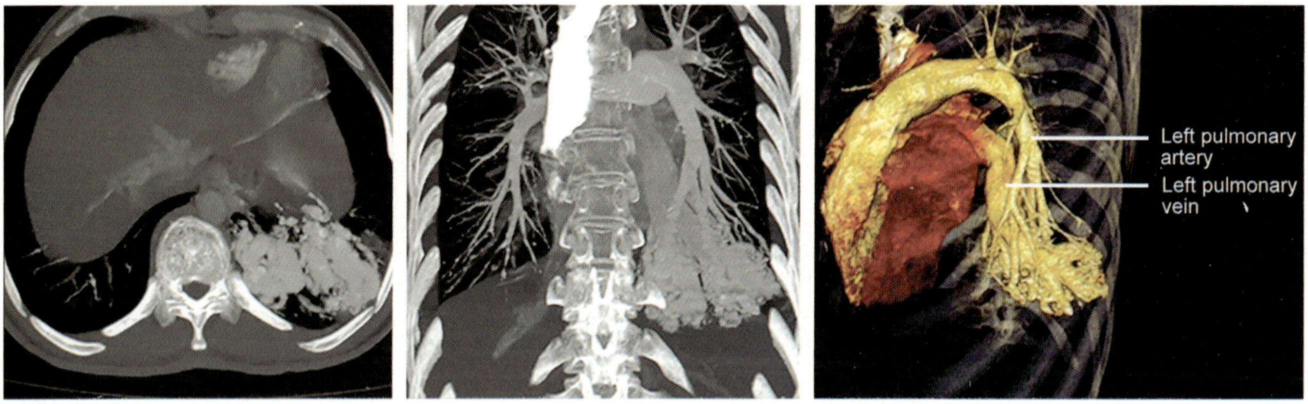

Fig. 2: Young man presented with exertional dyspnea and central cyanosis. Echocardiography revealed severe mitral stenosis with hyperdynamic pulmonary flow. Pulmonary CT angiogram revealed large AVM involving left lower lobe lung.[1] (CT: computed tomography; AVM: arteriovenous malformation)

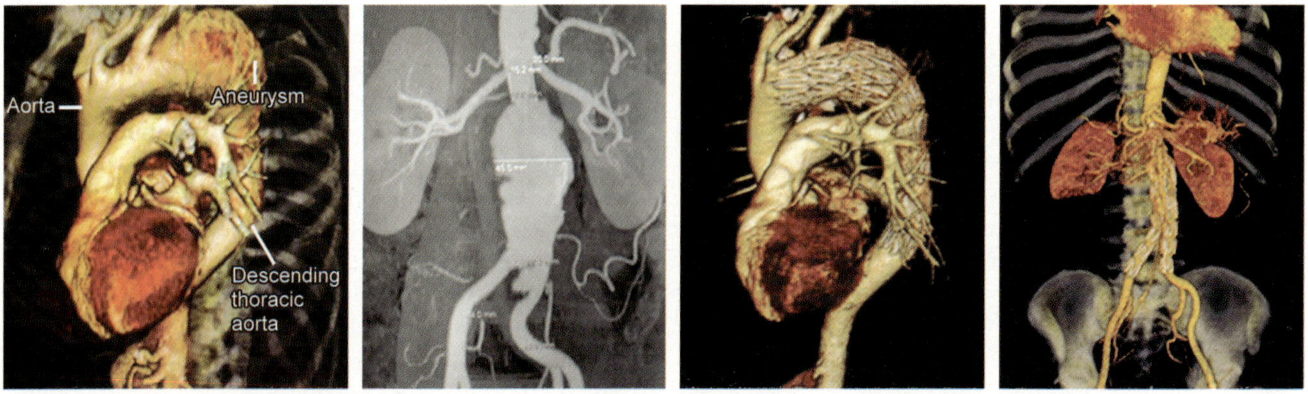

Fig. 3: Aortic aneurysms (arch and infrarenal aorta) status pre- and poststenting. Nice depiction of aneurysms as well as stents in prestenting and poststenting CT angiograms.[1] (CT: computed tomography)

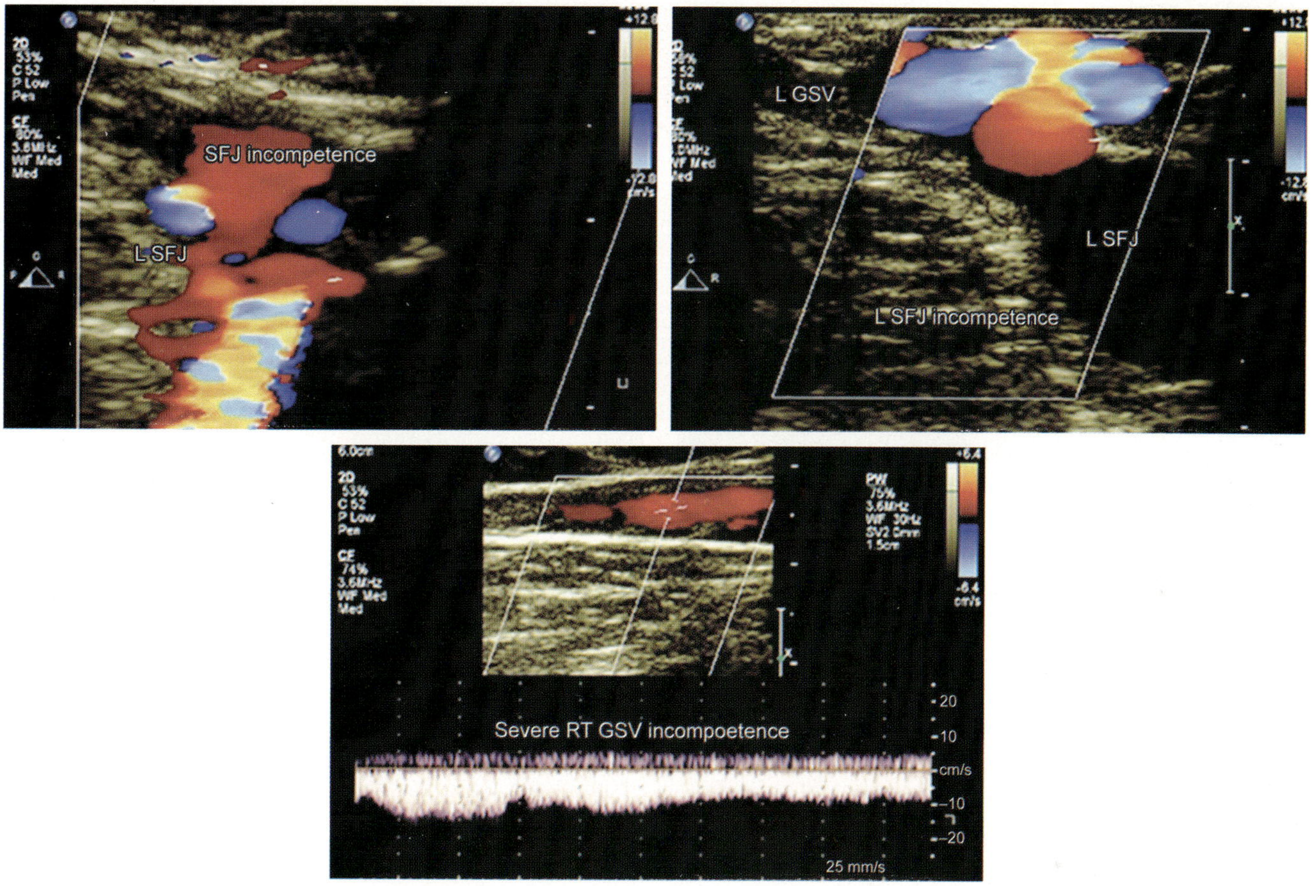

Fig. 4: Great saphenous valve (GSV) incompetence visualization for ultrasound-guided endovenous laser therapy. (L: left; R: right; SFJ: saphenofemoral junction)

Various advanced imaging modalities used for guiding peripheral vascular interventions (PVI) include the following:

- Duplex imaging
- Intravascular ultrasound (IVUS)
- CO_2 angiography
- Robotics
- Optical coherence tomography (OCT)
- Magnetic resonance imaging (MRI).

DUPLEX-GUIDED PERIPHERAL VASCULAR INTERVENTIONS

Because of the inherent disadvantages of contrast angiography, there have been attempts to do PVI under duplex guidance. The advantages of duplex are as follows:

- Better visualization of the peripheral vessels (arteries and veins) irrespective of the patency
- Possibility of up to five times magnification
- Precise measurements to the tune of 0.1 mm
- Imaging and characterization of arterial wall and the plaque
- Availability of real-time hemodynamic parameters, such as flow, velocity, and waveform

The various procedures, which are routinely being done using duplex guidance as the only imaging, are as follows:

- Endovenous laser therapy (Fig. 4)
- Foam sclerotherapy
- Radiofrequency ablation of varicose veins
- Thrombin injection of pseudoaneurysm
- Angioplasty for venous access [for stenosis and delayed maturation of arteriovenous (AV) fistula].

The newer and promising indications are as follows:

- Superficial femoral artery, popliteal, and tibial artery revascularization
- Bypass graft revascularization
- Subintimal angioplasties
- Duplex-assisted carotid angioplasty.

Duplex-guided Angioplasty for Femoral and Popliteal Arteries

This was first reported by Ahmadi et al.[2] and Ramaswami et al.[3] They demonstrated the safety and effectiveness of this procedure. However, the largest series of 360 cases was reported by Ascher.[4-8]

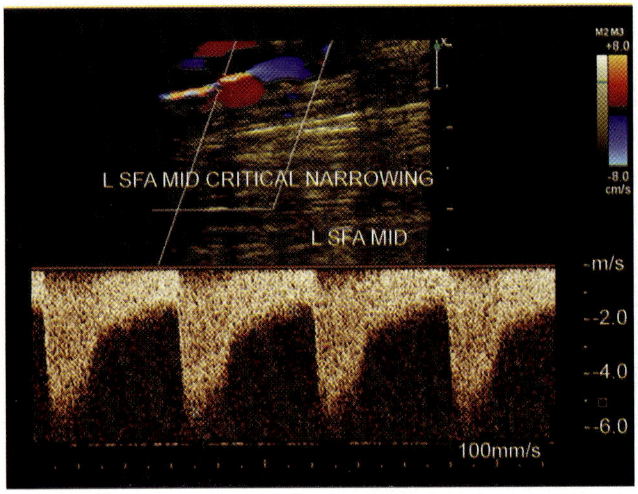

Fig. 5: Duplex scan showing critical stenosis of superficial femoral artery (SFA).

Technique

Baseline duplex ultrasound is first recorded (Fig. 5). The duplex is performed by a registered vascular technologist using linear 7–4 MHz probe with a foot length of 4 cm and additional specialized probes of frequency ranging from 15–7 MHz to 5–2 MHz. The prerequisite is to rule out stenosis in aortoiliac segment by demonstrating triphasic waveform in common femoral artery (CFA) and absence of biphasic and monophasic waveforms.

The severity and the length of stenosis/occlusion are measured and the skin marking is made. Access is gained in CFA from ultrasound-guided puncture. This avoids dissections and posterior wall punctures and reduces the bleeding complications. Usually, ipsilateral antegrade puncture is done. The advantages of antegrade puncture are easier manipulation of endovascular devices, and avoidance of difficult contralateral access because of tortuous anatomy, narrow bifurcation of aorta and aorto-iliac disease. The arteries in the thigh and calf which are usually 1–5 cm deep are assessed by 7–4 MHz linear probe, while superficial arteries (<1 cm deep) at level of ankle or feet are insonated by 15–7 MHz hockey stick probe. Ascher et al.[4-8] reported their experience of 360 femoropopliteal angioplasties where ipsilateral CFA approach was used in 91% cases. Contralateral CFA was used in 32 (9%) cases. Contralateral CFA access requires fluoroscopy and is used only when antegrade puncture is contraindicated because of high bifurcation or deep location (>3 cm from the skin). Both luminal and subluminal angioplasties are possible and the wire tracking can be easily visualized on real-time duplex scanning both for luminal and subintimal angioplasty (Figs. 6A to D).

The advantage of duplex over fluoroscopy in subintimal angioplasty is that it allows to identify the segment with least amount of calcification and thinnest intima media layer which is suitable for the entry. The guidewire entry in true lumen beyond the chronic total occlusion (CTO) in subintimal angioplasty technique is confirmed by color flow imaging in both longitudinal and transverse views. The lesions are dilated with adequate-sized balloons as determined by duplex, and the results are assessed after removing the balloon by using duplex, color and power images, and spectral analysis. Recoil leading to less than 30% diameter reduction with peak systolic velocity (PSV) ratio less than 2 is considered to be a good balloon angioplasty result. If PSV ratio is more than 2 or recoil is more than 30% diameter reduction, putting in a stent is warranted to maintain the patency. Stents were used in 68% cases in the series by Ascher.[4-8] Ascher et al. reported technical success in 95% (342/360 cases). It was 100% for TransAtlantic Inter-Society Consensus (TASC) A and B lesions, 96% for TASC C, and 74% for TASC D lesions. Hemodialysis was the only statistically significant predictive factor for technical failure of duplex-guided subintimal angioplasty. The 6-month patency rates for TASC A, B, C, and D lesions were 90%, 74%, 71%, and 64%, respectively, while 12-month patency rates for TASC A, B, C, and D lesions were 90%, 59%, 52%, and 46%, respectively. Limb salvage rates at 12 months were 90%. Adjunctive infrapopliteal angioplasty is always warranted to maintain good outflow and long-term patency of femoropopliteal angioplasty.

Duplex-guided Angioplasty of Infrainguinal Arterial Bypass Grafts

Duplex-guided angioplasty of infrainguinal arterial bypass grafts is feasible and done by the same technique as described above. It has an advantage of fluoroscopic-guided angioplasty in the form of direct visualization of access site and accurate entry and also additional guidance by hemodynamic information. Ascher et al.[4-8] reported 47 duplex-guided balloon angioplasty procedures for arterial bypass grafts being performed in both vein grafts (77%) and polytetrafluoroethylene grafts (23%).

Duplex-guided Angioplasty for Arteriovenous Access/Fistulas

Arteriovenous access/fistulas are predisposed for multiple stenosis or maturation failure. Their patency is directly related to the quality and survival of life in hemodialysis patients of end-stage renal disease (ESRD). The contrast

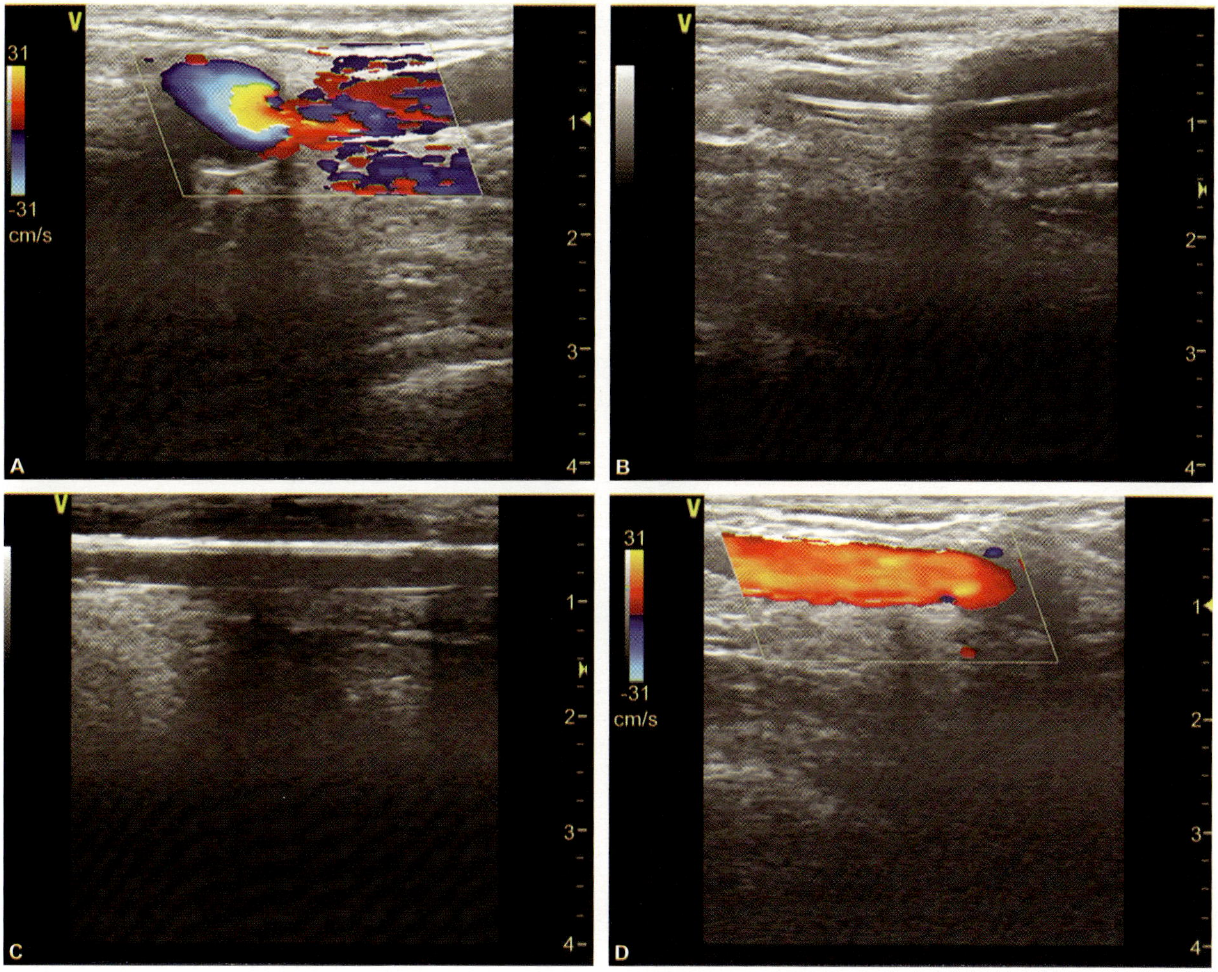

Figs. 6A to D: Duplex-guided angioplasty: (A) Baseline duplex; (B) Guidewire passage; (C) Balloon angioplasty; and (D) Final result.

administration becomes an important issue in patients with nonmaturation of AV fistulas in patients with borderline renal functions and also in patients of ESRD with AV fistulas having multiple stenosis and allergy to iodine contrast. Duplex ultrasound-guided angioplasties become especially useful in these patients (Fig. 7).

Technique

Real-time visualization of AV access (both inflow and outflow) is done by duplex ultrasound to delineate the level of stenosis or obstruction, and skin marking is done. Additional information, which is required, is the location of stenosis in relation to the anastomosis, diameter of the fistula, depth, and tortuosity. The procedure can be performed both in the operating room or outpatient clinic. Usually a 15–7-MHz transducer is used for insonation of superficial structures (<2-cm deep), and linear 7–4-MHz probe is used for deeper (>2 cm) and for measurements of very-high-flow velocities. Both inflow and outflow stenosis can be treated by ultrasound guidance, and the final results can be confirmed by color/power images and measurement of PSV ratios. Balloon angioplasty is done using adequate-sized, high-pressure, noncompliant balloons or cutting balloons.

Duplex-assisted Internal Carotid Artery Stenting

Although complete procedure of carotid artery stenting cannot be completely done under duplex image guidance and fluoroscopic guidance is essential, duplex does give additional benefits in terms of verification of hemodynamic success and identification of intrastent protrusion of plaque after carotid artery stenting (Fig. 8). Severe arterial calcification of carotids creates an acoustic shadow and limits the use of duplex scanning.

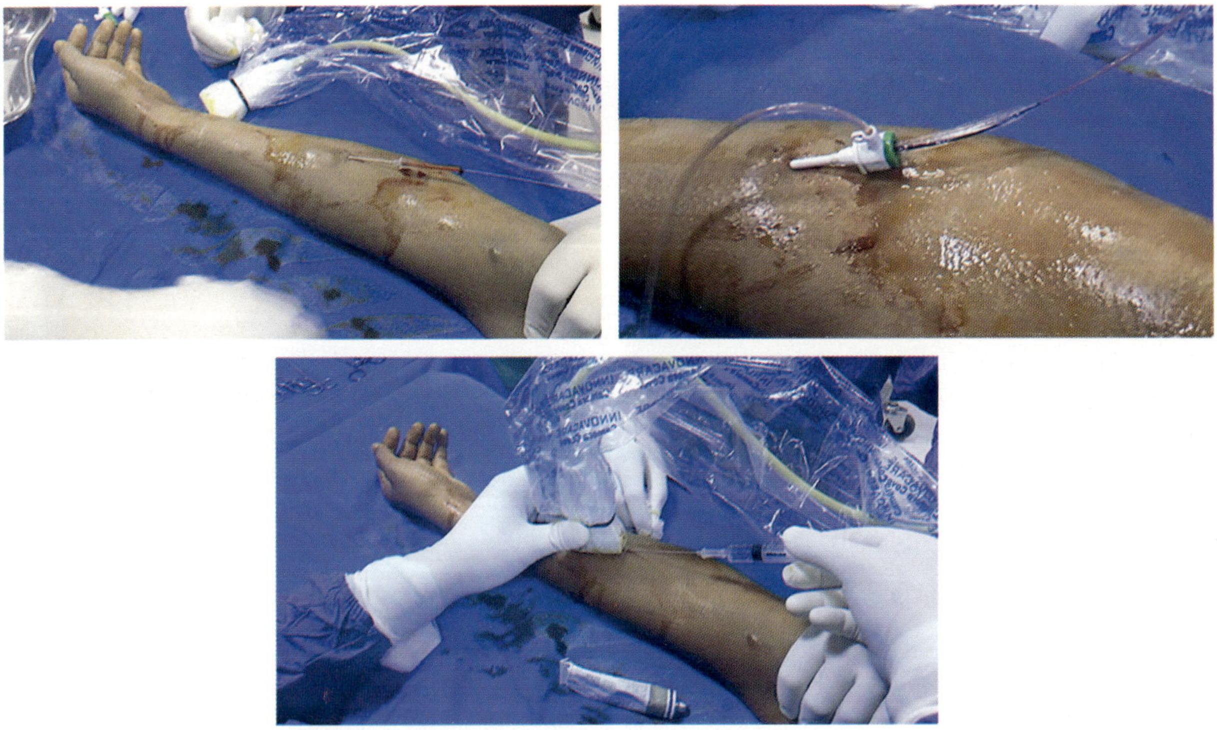

Fig. 7: Duplex-guided hemodialysis access angioplasty.

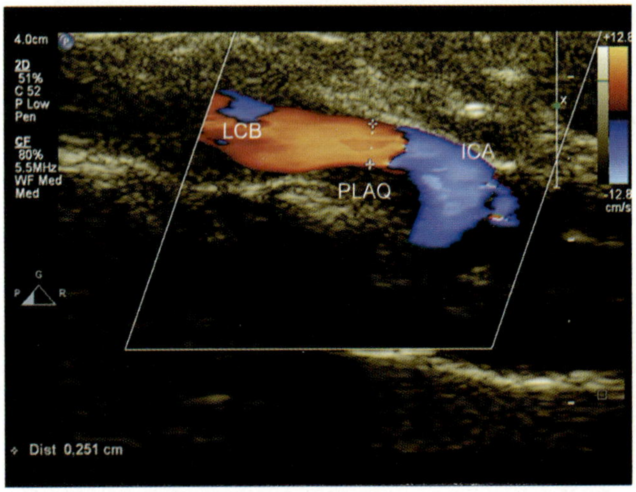

Fig. 8: Carotid artery stenosis and plaque visualized in carotid duplex scan.

ROLE OF INTRAVASCULAR ULTRASOUND IN PERIPHERAL VASCULAR INTERVENTIONS

The inability to objectively evaluate plaque burden, composition, morphology, and vessel wall architecture through conventional angiography in patients suffering from PAD may lead to inaccuracies in arterial dimensions and degrees of stenosis. IVUS has improved the outcomes in both diagnostic and interventional procedures by providing intraluminal cross-sectional images with higher image resolution than angiography. IVUS potentially improves outcomes in the peripheral vasculature and has been demonstrated with better patency of iliac stents (Figs. 9A to C).

Intravascular ultrasound, similar to angiography, uses a system of guidewires and catheters with a small ultrasound device on the distal end of the catheter. This device allows the operator to visualize the inner wall of blood vessels from inside the vessel itself. IVUS catheters capture cross-sectional images that enable 360° intraluminal visualization of peripheral vasculature. A revolving transducer is present on the catheter tip, which emits ultrasound waves during pullback of the probe. A gray scale is used to differentiate amplitudes of reflecting ultrasound waves from different tissue types. Calcified plaques appear white, as they reflect brightly impeding ultrasound waves, whereas thrombus is hypoechoic and reflects dark gray.[9] A higher image resolution and magnification is provided due to close proximity of the probe allowing for higher frequency ultrasound to be used. This enables more accurate assessment for detecting vessel diameter, visualizing edge dissection, stent expansion (optimization), calcification, and crossing CTO. IVUS can also stack consecutive images to create a 3-D image of the plaque. When these

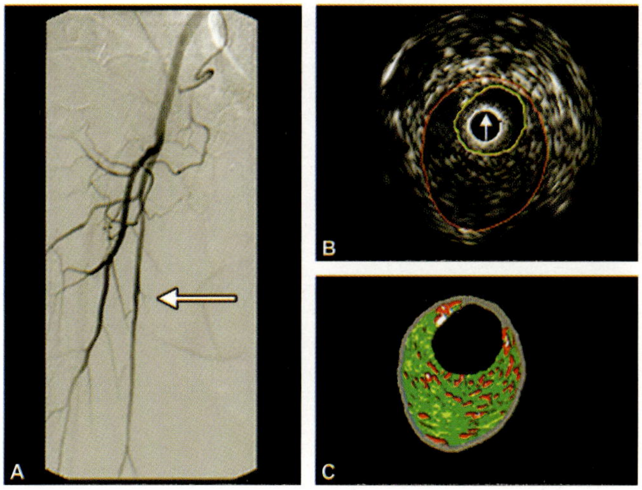

Figs. 9A to C: An example of angiographic and IVUS analysis. (A) The white arrow in the angiogram depicts the area for analysis—interpreted as 30% stenosis based on angiogram; (B) IVUS gray scale imaging through this area (yellow line—internal elastic lamina; red line—external elastic lamina); by IVUS this represents a 76% area stenosis; (C) Virtual histology analysis—dark and light green shades depict fibrous plaque; red areas represent necrotic plaque, and white areas denote calcium. (IVUS: intravascular ultrasound)
Courtesy: TJ Collins. JICC APVIC VII Special Supplement.

cross-sectional images are used with angiography, it increases the capability and accuracy of diagnostic and interventional procedures for patients with PAD.

Stenosis

Intravascular ultrasound correlates 95% with angiography in calculation of luminal diameters. It determines true vessel wall dimensions in both diseased and normal arteries. The accurate measurements and detection of any plaque burden, not identified by angiography, increase the accuracy when computing stenosis area.[10] Using true arterial dimensions to compute the maximal percent area stenosis, IVUS determined a 10% degree of stenosis was unaccounted for by angiography, most likely because luminal diameter measurements do not account for positive remodeling.[11]

Vessel Wall Morphology

Details of morphological characteristics of the vessel wall, plaque identification, and location of lesions are provided by the analysis of the high-resolution images captured by IVUS. Compared to angiography, IVUS images and their morphological analysis produce more detailed information regarding the location, eccentricity, and luminal cross-sectional area.[12] Details of vessel wall morphology are also helpful in determining plaque characteristics, branch vessel location in addition to the extent of disease involvement.

Calcified Plaques

Calcified plaques are identified as bright white locations on IVUS images, providing a better understanding of lesion morphology, shape, and location. The choice of atherectomy device to be used depends on the location of calcified plaque. High-speed rotational atherectomy is best suited for superficial plaques close to the lumen surface, whereas for deep calcified plaques in contact with the media, directional atherectomy may be more appropriate.[13] Hence, objective measurements on specific plaque morphologies using IVUS are more helpful than the subjective angiographic representation when selecting the appropriate therapy and predicting results of the different interventions.

Optimization of Stent Expansion

Intravascular ultrasound images provide accurate measurements enabling accurate stent sizing. It also enables more accurate stent positioning and expansion. Prior to stent deployment, IVUS can accurately assess the correct size to which a vessel should be dilated. In the case of incomplete apposition of the stent to the vessel wall, platelets, fibrin, and thrombus can accumulate between the stent and arterial wall, forming a lesion that may serve as the starting point for restenosis.[10] Stent oversizing or overexpansion severely increases the rates of ischemic complications, such as perforated or ruptured vessels. After implantation, IVUS can help in evaluation of stent placement, ensuring full stent expansion with complete stent-vessel wall apposition and no prolapsed plaque.

Limitations

The biggest limitation of IVUS is its implementation, due to associated costs of operation. Other limitations of IVUS are associated with its clinical applications. Since the procedure is operator dependent, it can cause inconsistent retraction rates of the transducer, resulting in incorrectly stacked images or poor image quality. To overcome this, now we have automated pullback for doing IVUS. Investment in IVUS also mandates additional time, equipment, and personnel.

CO_2 ANGIOGRAPHY-DIRECTED VASCULAR INTERVENTIONS

CO_2 angiography is an imaging modality employed in peripheral interventions. It allows visualization of vessels without the use of contrast. The method involves

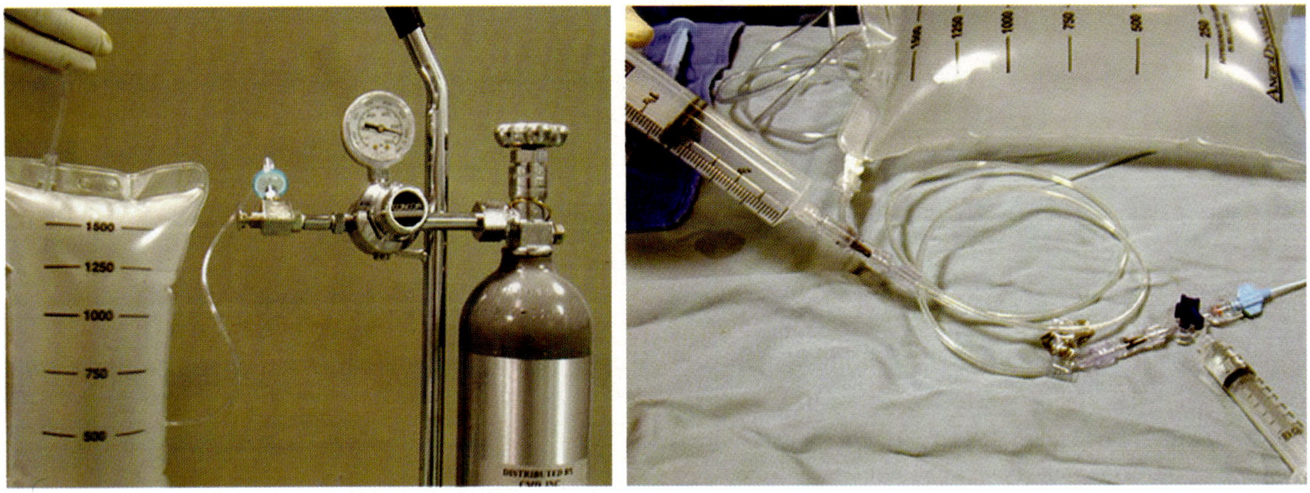

Fig. 10: Equipment of CO_2 angiography and intervention.

injection 10–15-mL from the CO_2 cylinder into the vascular system, and angiography is done with digital subtraction angiography (DSA) technique (Fig.10). The opacification is similar to the conventional DSA angiogram. It is of special use in patients at risk of contrast-induced nephropathy and borderline renal dysfunction and patients with contrast allergy.[14,15]

CO_2 can be used for all peripheral arterial interventions below the level of diaphragm and entire range of venous work except intracranial interventions (Fig. 11). CO_2 is a buoyant gas and works by the displacement of blood column. It stays in the vessel before getting dissolved, and because it is lighter than blood, the area of interest can be elevated or made nondependent to have better opacification.

The potential risk of CO_2 angiography is air contamination and contamination of other gases, which can lead to severe air embolism. Sometimes, excessive volume of CO_2 can result in air block of mesenteric arteries leading to abdominal pain and sometimes mesenteric infarction in extreme cases.

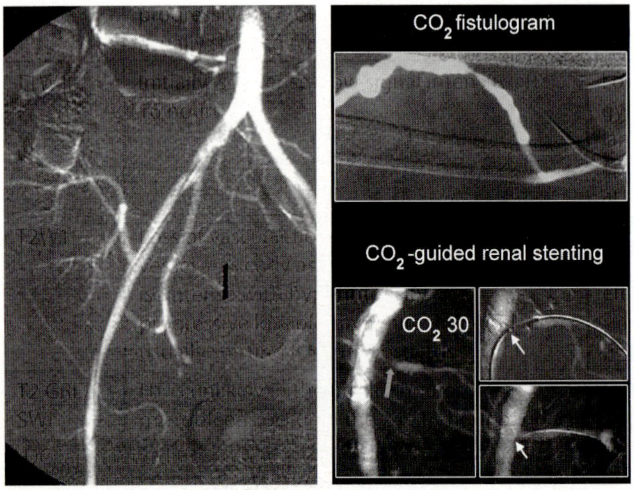

Fig. 11: CO_2 angiogram.

FUTURE TRENDS IN IMAGE-GUIDED PERIPHERAL VASCULAR INTERVENTIONS

Robotic Peripheral Vascular Interventions

Although PVI have been perfected to a large extent, there are some unmet needs in the form of the safety of cardiovascular interventionalists as regards to radiation hazards and prevention of orthopedic complications as a result of heavy lead aprons and ergonomically compromised position of interventionalist. To address this, robotic-assisted PVI is being developed.

Two robotic systems are currently in use—(1) CorPath system (Corindus Vascular Robotics, Waltham, Massachusetts) (Fig. 12) and (2) Hansen system (Hansen Medical, Mountain View, California). Hansen medical system uses proprietary catheters, which are robotically reshapable in vivo. On the other hand, CorPath system uses proprietary catheters and balloons. Both the systems have shown to improve physician ergonomics, reduced radiation exposure and improved accuracy of the procedure.

A recent study, Rheumatoid Arthritis Prevention of structural Damage trial (feasibility and safety of robotic PVI) by Mahmud et al., was published in *Journal of the American College of Cardiology Cardiovascular Interventions*.[16] The goal of this study was to evaluate the safety of CorPath robot-assisted PVI for treating PAD in femoropopliteal segment. This was a prospective single-arm trial with primary

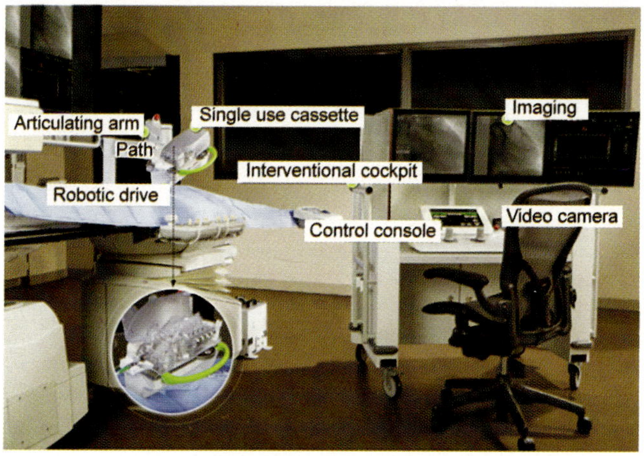

Fig. 12: CorPath Robotic system.[16]

endpoints being device technical success and safety. A total of 20 patients were enrolled (mean age 65.5 ± 9.3 years of age) with Rutherford II or III symptoms. A total of 29 lesions (lesion length—33.1 ± 15.5 mm) were treated. Device technical success, safety and clinical procedural success were 100%. Stents were required in 34.5% lesions, and fluoroscopy time was 7.1 ± 3.2 min. Contrast used compared favorably in studies with similar patient cohorts. There was no adverse event associated with the use of robotic system demonstrating its feasibility and safety in robot-assisted PVI.

Optical Coherence Tomography-guided Vascular Interventions

Optical coherence tomography is an innovative imaging modality with high resolution for effective assessment of atherosclerotic plaque and internal anatomy of the arteries. It was first introduced by Huang et al.[17] in 1991 and was originally designed for use in transparent tissues, such as cornea of the eye.[18] It can be used to identify thin cap plaques in carotids, which have high risk for rupture. It has excellent resolution in evaluating postinterventional dissections. OCT combines the principles of ultrasound with imaging performance of a microscope. It measures intensity of back reflected near infrared light to measure thickness of different biological tissues, which are similar to B-mode imaging, except that it uses light instead of sound. It provides significantly higher spatial resolution than that of any ultrasound technique. It is the only modality with the potential to characterize the nature of atherosclerotic plaque. It has an axial resolution of 10 μm, which is 10–20 times greater than ultrasound imaging. OCT finds special application in PVI, such as cutting balloon angioplasty, intravascular cryoablation, and atherectomy. Meissner et al. studied the potential role of OCT in posterior vitreous detachment and showed it to be comparable to that reported for coronary arteries.[19] The modern atherectomy devices have OCT guidance (optical atherectomy). In times to come, OCT technology is likely to advance and be a very useful armamentarium for OCT-guided PVI. Optical coherence tomography (OCT) generates high-resolution cross-sectional images of arterial structure and pathology. It can identify components of the vessel wall. Unlike IVUS, it is not limited by calcification.

Magnetic Resonance Angiography

Magnetic resonance (MR) angiography with and without gadolinium contrast gives an excellent delineation of peripheral vasculature and totally avoids the need of iodinated contrast and radiation. This is especially important in patients with borderline renal failure and contrast allergy. As of now, MRI is not used for guiding vascular interventions because of the lack of dedicated MRI compatible hardware. However, like MR-guided neurosurgical procedures, in future, MR compatible hardware for PVI are being developed. This will be a revolutionary change in the way vascular interventions would be done and would totally avoid the need of contrast and radiation protection and would be very convenient for the operators by preventing radiation hazards and orthopedic issues.

REFERENCES

1. Bera ML. Computed tomography angiogram in peripheral arterial disease: an overview. In: Khanna H (Ed). Handbook of Interventions for Structural Heart and Peripheral Vascular Disease. New Delhi: Jaypee Brothers Medical Publishers (P) Ltd; 2016.
2. Ahmadi R, Ugurluoglu A, Schillinger M, et al. Duplex ultrasound-guided femoropopliteal angioplasty; initial and 12-month results from a case controlled study. J Endovasc Ther. 2002;9(6):873-81.
3. Ramaswami G, Al-Kutoubi A, Nicolaides AN, et al. Angioplasty of lower limb arterial stenoses under ultrasound guidance: single-center experience. J Endovasc Surg. 1999;6(1):52-8.
4. Ascher E, Marks NA, Schutzer RW, et al. Duplex-guided balloon angioplasty and stenting for femoropopliteal arterial occlusive disease: an alternative in patients with renal insufficiency. J Vasc Surg. 2005;42(6):1108-13.
5. Ascher E, Marks NA, Hingorani AP, et al. Duplex-guided endovascular treatment for occlusive and stenotic lesions of the femoral-popliteal arterial segment: a comparative study in the first 253 cases. J Vasc Surg. 2006;44(6):1230-37.
6. Ascher E, Hingorani AP, Marks NA. Duplex-guided angioplasty of lower extremity arteries. Perspect Vasc Endovasc Ther. 2007;9(1):23-31.
7. Ascher E, Marks NA, Hingorani AP, et al. Duplex-guided balloon angioplasty and subintimal dissection of infrapopliteal arteries: early results with a new approach to

avoid radiation exposure and contrast material. J Vasc Surg. 2005;42(6):1114-21.
8. Marks NA, Hingorani AP, Ascher E. Duplex-guided balloon angioplasty of failing infrainguinal bypass grafts. Eur J Vasc Endovasc Surg. 2006;32(2):176-81.
9. Reid DB, Douglas M, Diethrich EB. The clinical value of three-dimensional intravascular ultrasound imaging. J Endovasc Surg. 1995;2:356-64.
10. Jacobson J, Maehara A, Mintz GS. Clinical applications of intravascular ultrasound in the implantation of drug-eluting stents. Cardiovasc Ther. 2012;10(5):543-7.
11. Arthurs ZM, Bishop PD, Feiten LE, et al. Evaluation of peripheral atherosclerosis: a comparative analysis of angiography and intravascular ultrasound. J Vasc Surg. 2010;51(4):933-9.
12. Tabbara M, White R, Cavaye D, et al. In vivo human comparison of intravascular ultrasonography and angiography. J Vasc Surg. 1991;14:496-504.
13. Scoccianti M, Verbin CS, Kopchok GE, et al. Intravascular ultrasound guidance for peripheral vascular interventions. J Endovasc Surg. 1994;1:71-80.
14. Caridi JG, Cho KJ, Fauria C, et al. (2014). Carbon dioxide digital subtraction angiography (CO2 DSA): a comprehensive user guide for all operators. [online]. Available from: http://www.vasculardiseasemanagement.com/content/carbondioxide-digital-subtraction-angiography-co2-dsa-comprehensive-user-guide-all> [Accessed October, 2018].
15. Nicolini A, Ferraresso M, Lovaria A, et al. Carbon dioxide as a valuable contrast agent for identifying iatrogenic arteriovenous fistulas in transplanted kidneys. Nephrol Dial Transplant. 2003;18(10):2189-92.
16. Mahmud E, Schmid F, Kalmar P, et al. Feasibility and safety of robotic peripheral vascular interventions: results of the RAPID trial. JACC Cardiovasc Interv. 2016;9(19):2058-64.
17. Huang D, Swanson EA, Lin CP, et al. Optical coherence tomography. Science. 1991;254:1178-81.
18. Swanson EA. In vivo retinal imaging by optical coherence tomography. Optics Lett. 1993;18:1864-6.
19. Meissner OA, Rieber J, Babaryka G, et al. Intravascular optical coherence tomography: comparison with histopathology in atherosclerotic peripheral artery specimens. J Vasc Interv Radiol. 2006;17:343-9.

107

CHAPTER

Color Doppler Evaluation of Erectile Dysfunction

Naveen Garg, KK Kapur

INTRODUCTION

Penile Doppler study (PDS) was first introduced in 1985, and since then, it has become a major tool to investigate the vasculogenic causes contributing to erectile dysfunction (ED). Erectile disease is an emerging menace and has been thought to be the precursor of cardiovascular events.[1] Montorsi et al. had shown that ED precedes coronary artery disease (CAD) about 39 months due to small-sized penile arteries. This study showed that a normal PDS excludes CAD with a 98% negative predictive value, while an abnormal PDS has a 30% positive predictive value.[2] El-Sakka and Morsy also demonstrated that 77% males having peak systolic velocity (PSV) of less than 25 cm/s during PDS were suffering from ischemic heart disease.[3] Similarly, Gazzaruso et al. demonstrated that diabetics with silent CAD had about eight times more ED than diabetics with no CAD.[4] The hemodynamic physiology of penile erection includes sudden rush of blood into the organ. Cavernosal arteries dilates and sinusoids get filled with incoming blood causing penis to get enlarge. This in turn squeezes the peripheral veins, and so blood gets trapped within the organ causing its erection (Fig. 1).

Penile Doppler study is a safe, accurate, and most cost-effective technique for diagnosing ED. Some of the techniques used in the past were highly invasive and

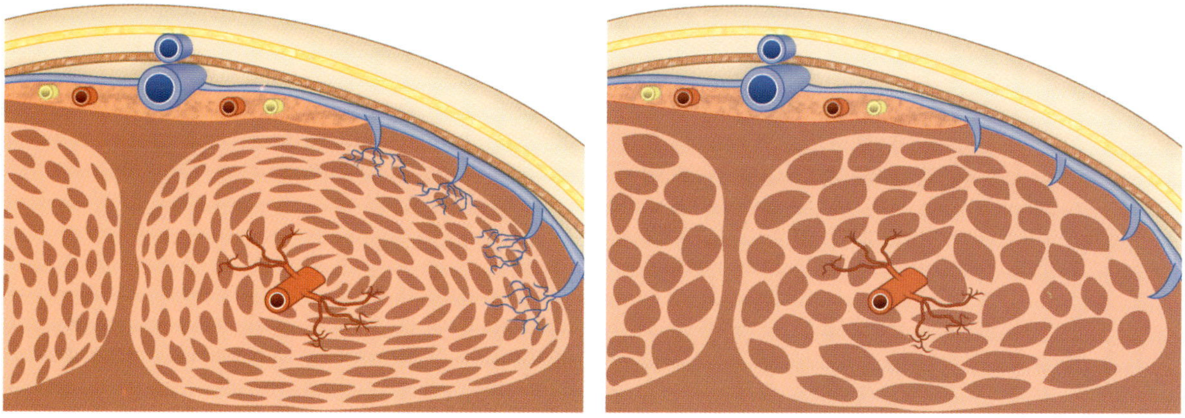

Fig. 1: Cavernosal changes during erection process. In flaccid state, cavernosal sinusoids are collapsed, while in arousal state, these are filled with blood, resulting in swollen cavernosa that blocks the draining veins and causes rigid and hard erection.

not suitable for routine clinical use. Some of the recent noninvasive techniques, such as penile magnetic resonance imaging and near-infrared spectrometry, are cumbersome and expensive and therefore are only used in research labs. The introduction of pharmacological duplex using cavernosal stimulants, such as Papaverine, Phentolamine, and Prostaglandins E1, has markedly changed the understanding of pathophysiology in vasculogenic causes of ED.[5-11]

VASOACTIVE SUBSTANCES

The PDS is usually done after injecting either Pepaverine or Alprostadil or Phentolamine. These can be used singly or mixed together as Bimix or Trimix. Their effects can be reversed by using vasoconstrictor, such as Phenylephrine 0.8–1.4 mg intracavernosaly. An additional short bust of dynamic exercise is usually helpful in alleviating the priapism. These vasoactive pharmacological agents are listed in Table 1.

Vascular evaluation and imaging are indicated:[12,13]

- Arterial/arteriolar arteriogenic dysfunction
- Venoocclusive disorder
- Peyronie's disease
- Priapism
- Penile trauma, fractures, hematoma
- Fistulas
- Assess the risk of cardiovascular disease
- Venous thrombosis

Preparation of Patients and Technique

A linear array probe of 5–11-MHz frequency is used for this test. A low Nyquist limit 10–15 cm/s, a low filter setting 50 Hz and low-pulse repetition frequency of 2–4 kHz is used for this procedure (Fig. 2).

With the patient in the supine position, his penis is positioned so as to "lie on his abdomen" (dorsal side is posterior). The ultrasonic probe is placed at the basal region with a sufficient amount of acoustic gel interface. Penile shaft is then imaged from basal region to glans both longitudinally and in cross-sectional view (transverse view) to know the anatomical variations in cavernosal muscles. The two corpora cavernosa are homogeneous and hypoechoic circular structures. The tunica albuginea is visualized as a linear hyperechoic structure covering the corpora cavernosa. The cavernosal artery can be visualized in the middle of each cavernosa as a pulsating echolucent lumen with echogenic borders. The corpus spongiosum is seen as compressed elliptical structure on the ventral aspect of the two cavernosa (on the probe side if placed ventrally and remote to the probe if placed dorsally. With imaging from right lateral aspect, the right cavernosa is visualized adjacent to the probe, and left cavernosa is deeper and vice versa). At the basal region, near proximal one-third of the penile shaft cavernosal artery is identified in longitudinal plane, and color-guided pulse study is performed. The diameter and the peak flow velocity of cavernosal artery are then measured and documented during this flaccid stage. Either Pepaverine or Alprostadil (Caverject) is injected into either of the cavernosa (preferably right side) using 28–30-gauge needle. The peak systolic and diastolic velocities as well as the cavernosal artery diameter is measured every 3–5 min up to 20 min. If the tumescence or erectile response is delayed, the patient is then advised a suggestive visual imaginary along with tactile self-stimulation. Interrogation of the superficial or deep dorsal veins does not provide any additional diagnostic information (Figs. 3A to D; Table 2).

TABLE 1: Pharmacological agents with their dosage as used in penile studies.

Agent	Dosage
• Papaverine	30–60 mg
• Phentolamine	1–2.5 mg
• PGE-1	2–25 µg
• Alprostadil	10–30 µg
• Chlorpromazine	6.25–12.5 µg

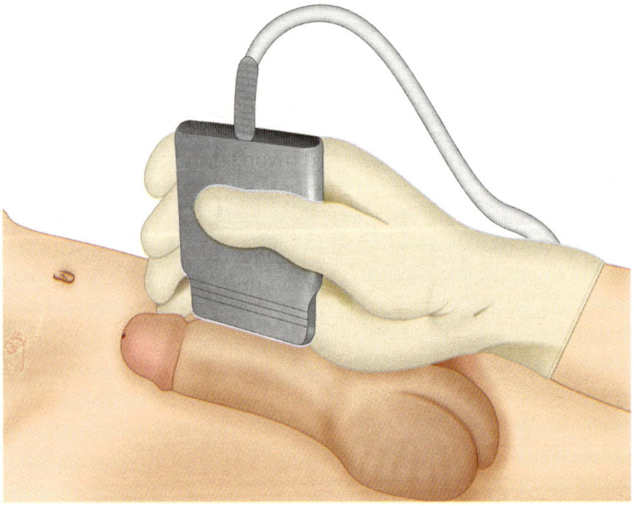

Fig. 2: Positioning of penis during PDS. (PDS: penile Doppler study)

Interpretations

The diameter of cavernosal artery varies normally 0.6–1 mm in its basal flaccid state of penis. The vasoactive stimulation or the sexual arousal increases its diameter by 75%. The basal peak velocity of cavernosal artery is about 6–10 cm/s in flaccid state which increases above 40 cm/s in aroused erect penis. The normal pattern of peak velocity shows an acceleration time of less than 100 ms with little or no diastolic flow after the first 10 min of injection of cavernosal

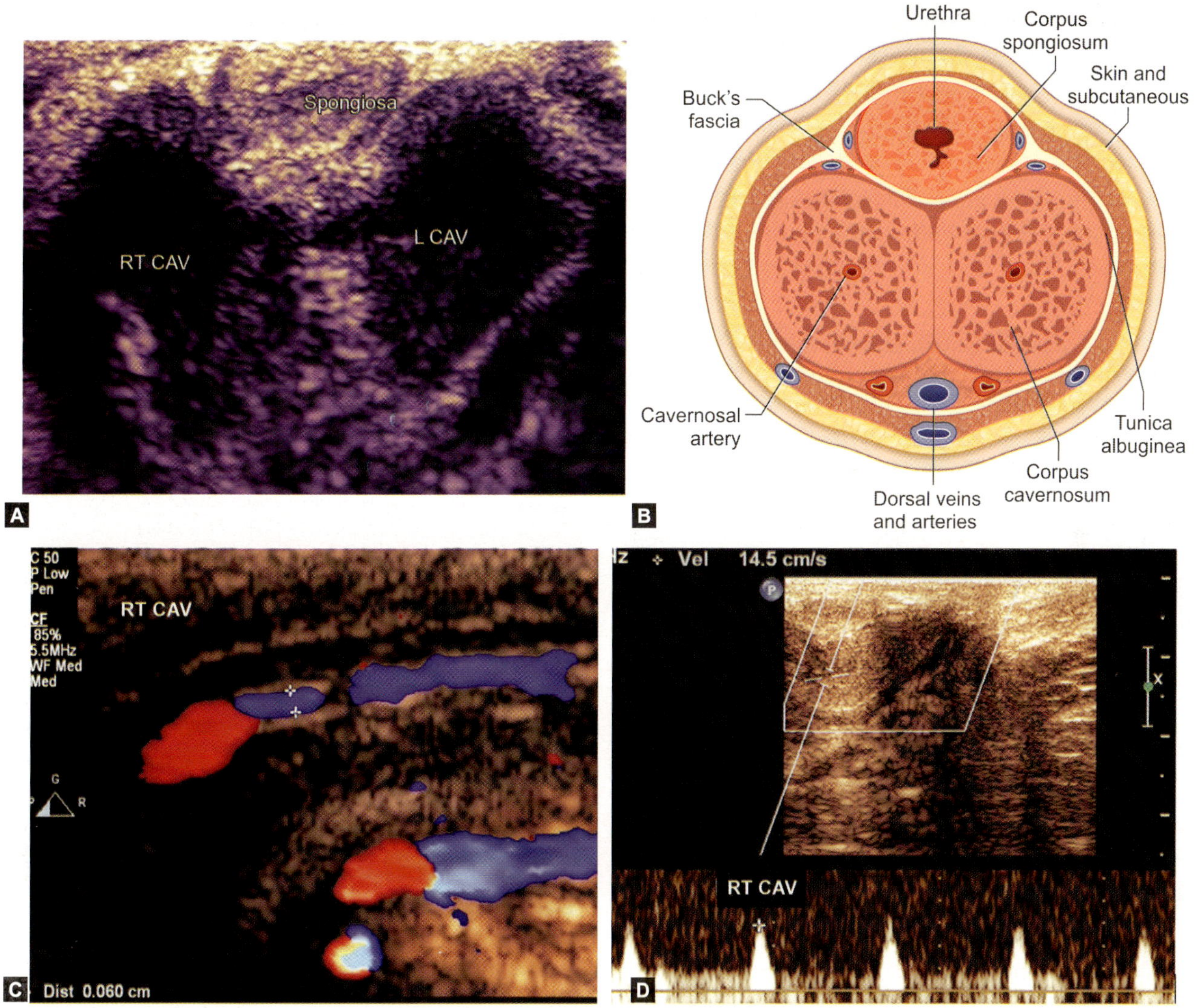

Figs. 3A to D: Part (A) showing ultrasonic image of penis (transverse view) with probe placed ventrally, depicting two cavernosa with cavernosal arteries and deep dorsal arteries. Shadow of corpous spongiosum can be appreciated. Part (B) shows the pictorial diagram of ultrasonic image; (C and D) Cavernosal artery in longitudinal plane. Size of artery is 0.060 cm with basal velocity 14.5 cm/s.

TABLE 2: Doppler flow profile.

Physiological stages	*Doppler pattren*
Latent	Rapid increase in systolic and diastolic velocities
Tumensence	Slow or no increase in systolic velocity. Decrease in diastoloc velocity
Full erection	End-diastolic velocity is zero
Rigid erection	Decrease in systolic velocity with the reversal of diastolic velocity
Detumensence	Decrease systolic velocity with the reapperance of diastolic velocities

stimulant.[14,15] This test is read as abnormal if there is any variation in the above-mentioned parameters. However, the most applied parameter is PSV. The PSV, if less than 25 cm/s after the injection of cavernosal stimulant, implies an arteriogenic etiology for ED with 92% of accuracy. A PSV above 35 cm/s is considered normal.[12,16] An end-diastolic antegrade velocity (EDV) of less than 5 cm/s is considered normal, whereas a value of above 10 cm/s is considered abnormal; however, this is interpreted in conjunction with resistive index (RI). This index semiquantifies the vascular resistance and is computed as

$$RI = \frac{PSV - EDV}{PSV}$$

The maximum value for RI is 1.0, and if this index is below 0.75, it implies failure of venoocclusive mechanism. RI more than 0.9 is consistent with a normal response to the cavernosal stimulant in approximately 90% of the patients.

A semiquantitative grading of erectile response of penis can be obtained using the Erection Hardness Score (EHS) as:

1. Flaccid
2. Tumescence without hardness
3. Tumescence with nonpenetrable hardness
4. Tumescence with penetrable hardness
5. Tumescence with complete hardness

Analysis

- The *normal* pattern is of high PSV with EHS 3 or 4. Such patients often are anxious and need psychotherapy (Fig. 4).
- *Arteriogenic* abnormalities are mostly due to atherosclerosis. The PSV is often less than 25 cm/s with low EHS (Fig. 5).
- *Myogenic* abnormalities are characterized by a decreased plasticity or malleability of cavernosal muscle which prevents a rigid erection. This leads to high PSV with low EHS (Figs. 6A and B).
- Since the erection is physiologically considered to occur via nitric oxide, produced by the endothelium, a less sustained erection even with normal PSV may be due to *endothelial dysfunction* (Fig. 7).
- *Peyronie's disease* is characterized by a prominent deformity or the extreme deviation of the penis during erectile phase. This gives an appearance of "bent penis."

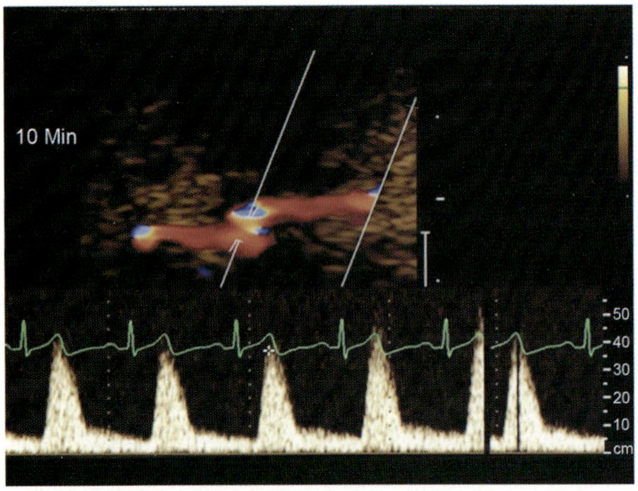

Fig. 4: A normal response of high PSV after 10 min of pharmacological stimulation with high EHS. (EHS: erection hardness score; PSV: peak systolic velocity)

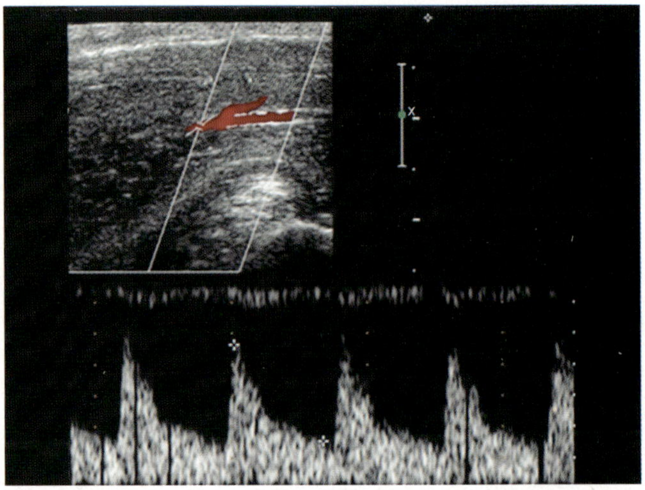

Fig. 5: Showing PSV 23.1 cm/s is consistent with arteriogenic etiology of ED. (ED: erectile dysfunction; PSV: peak systolic velocity)

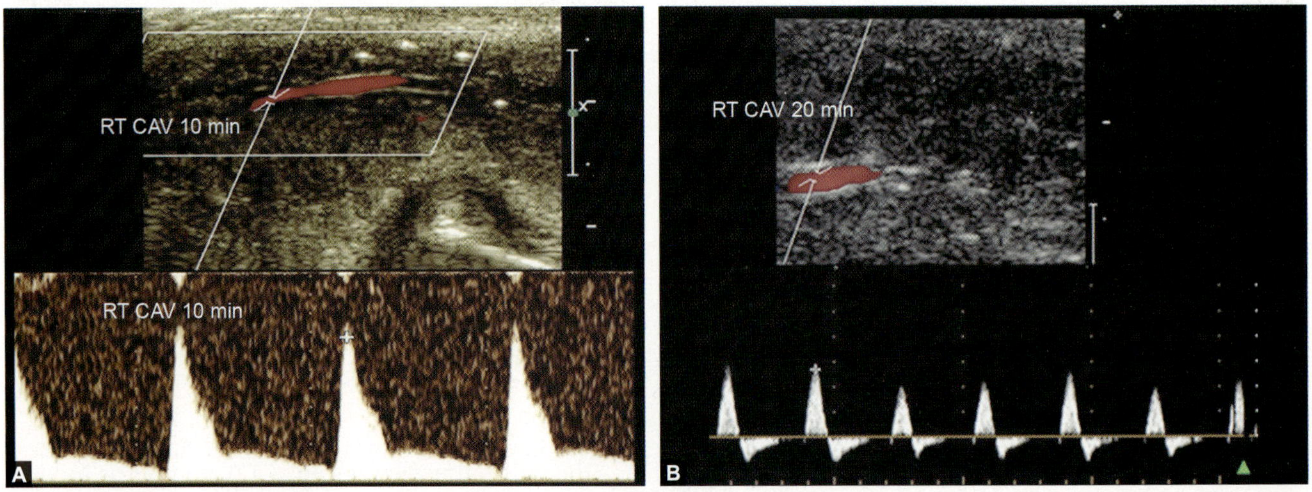

Figs. 6A and B: (A) A high PSV 38.6 cm/s with low end-diastolic velocity and low EHS. (B) Patient with good response after injection of 60 mg of Papaverine, PSV of 53.7 cm/s and a biphasic flow pattern. A low EHS of 2 in this patient implies a myogenic etiology. (EHS: erection hardness score; PSV: peak systolic velocity)

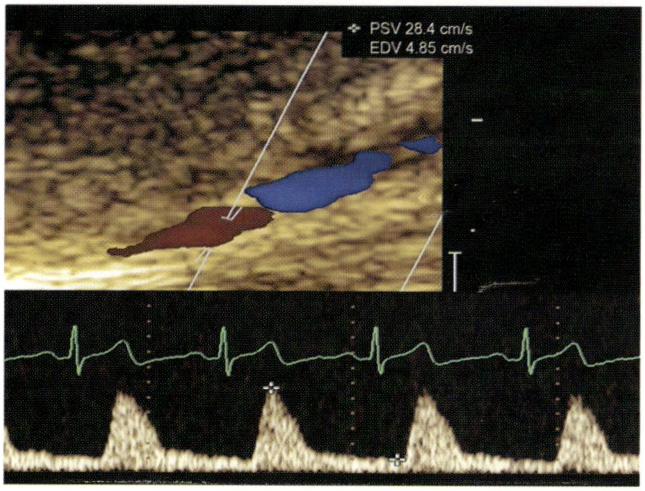

Fig. 7: Relatively high PSV with low EHS consistent with endothelial dysfunction. (EHS: erection hardness score; PSV: peak systolic velocity)

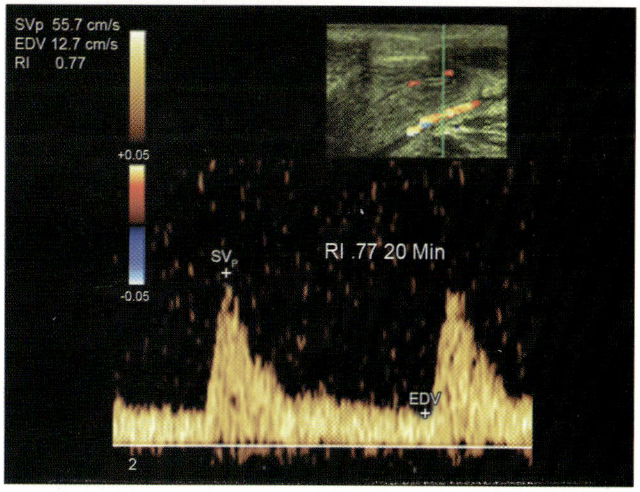

Fig. 9: This figure showing PSV 55.7 cm/s, EDV 12.7 cm/s, and RI 0.77 at 20 min highly suggestive of anatomical venous leak. (EDV: end-diastolic antegrade velocity; PSV: peak systolic velocity; RI: resistive index)

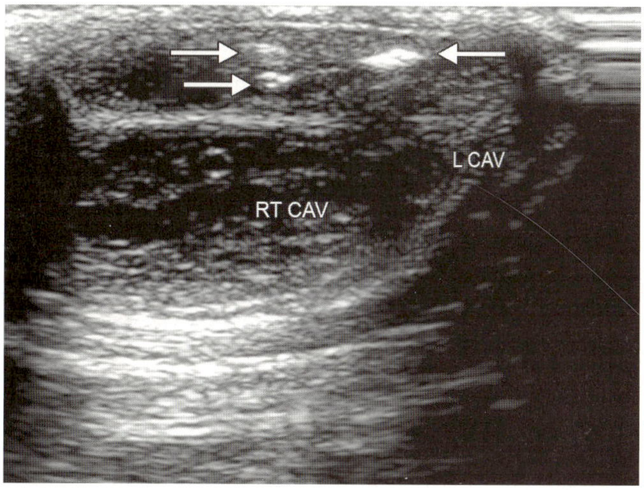

Fig. 8: This figure showing (arrows) calcified plaques.

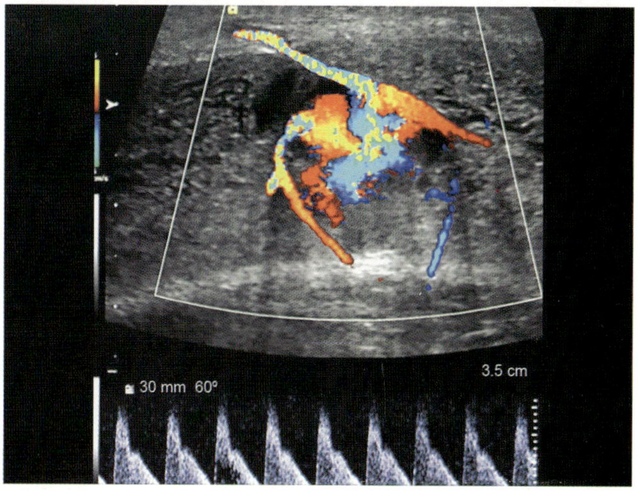

Fig. 10: This figure showing a large fistula between cavernosal artery and the venous sinusoids (turbulent flow). Spectral trace shows high PSV and high EDV indicating a low-resistance pattern seen in nonischemic priapism. (EDV: end-diastolic antegrade velocity; PSV: peak systolic velocity)

Sonographic findings include hyperechoic thickening of the tunica albuginea or plaques with or without calcification. Power Doppler may reveal hyperperfusion around the plaques as a sign of inflammation in the active state of the disease (Fig. 8).

- *Venous leak* phenomenon thought to occur when there is high PSV and high end-diastolic velocity. It implies the failure of venoocclusive mechanism, thus leading to increased outflow of blood and a nonsustained erection (Fig. 9).
- *Priapism*—This is a prolonged and sustained erection without arousal. It could be classified as low flow and high flow depending upon the PSV. The low-flow priapism is a medical emergency. Owing to venous occlusion, there is a complete absence of venous outflow; this leads to reduced arterial inflow. This leads to the deoxygenation of sinusoidal cavernosal blood causing intense discomfort and pain. On the other hand, in high-flow priapism, there is a definite presence of venous outflow. There is a corresponding increase in arterial flow which is shown on Doppler as high as detected by PSV. This causes a painless, nonischemic sustained erection (Fig. 10). High-flow priapism is commonly associated with fistulas usually near the glans.[12,17]
- *Penile fractures* are characterized by a breach in the continuity or integrity of tunica albuginea. This is readily

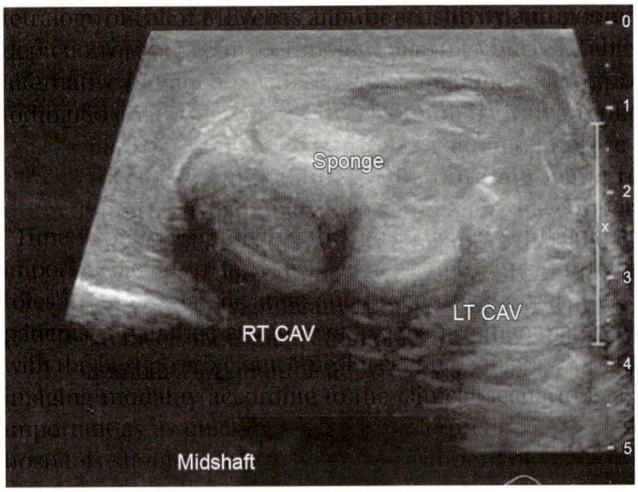

Fig. 11: Midshaft echogenic tunica albuginea overlying the left corpora cavernosa with an adjacent hematoma.

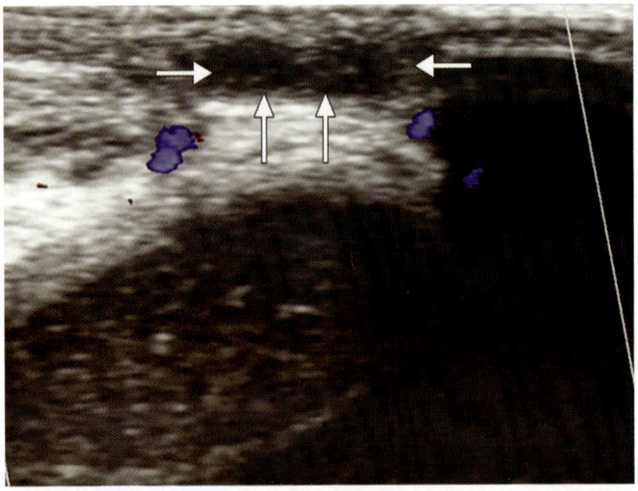

Fig. 12: Color Doppler ultrasound showing thrombosis of the superficial dorsal vein of the penis (arrows).
Source: Adapted from Polat H, Yucel MO, Gok A, et al. Penile Mondor's disease: primum non nocere! Urol J. 2015;12(2):2096-8.

imaged on Doppler ultrasound. A *penile hematoma* is a localized hypoechoic collection with/without a disruption in the continuity of tunica albuginea. Both these entities could be missed on clinical evaluation, color Doppler examination further helps in identifying the integrity of the cavernosal vasculature (Fig. 11).[18]

- *Penile Mondor's disease*—A rare disease manifested as thrombosis of deep dorsal veins. A Doppler interrogation of dorsal aspect of penis in its flaccid state could visualize a thrombus in the vein at this point (Fig. 12).[19]

Analysis of PDS can be summarized in Table 3.

TABLE 3: Analysis of penile Doppler study.

PSV cm/s at 20 min	*EDV cm/s (RI)*	*EHS*	*Interpretation*
<25			Atherosclerosis/ Arteriogenic
25–35		3 or less	Endothelial dysfunction
>35	<5	3 or 4	Normal
>35	<5	Less than 3	Myogenic
>35	>10 (<0.75)	Variable, nonsustained	Venous leak

(EDV: end-diastolic antegrade velocity; EHS: erection hardness score; PSV: peak systolic velocity; RI: resistive index)

Termination of Test

At the end of 20 min, after the injection of cavernosal stimulant and obtaining the complete data, the study is terminated. The penis is examined for any hematoma or discoloration at the injection site as well as for residual tumescence or priapism. He is advised to inform the treating physician for any sign of abnormal penile swelling or pain.

LIMITATIONS[20–23]

- Failure to achieve an adequate PSV and impaired EHS response does not always imply a vasculogenic etiology for the ED. This could be often due to excessive patient anxiety. Therefore it is imperative that the study should be performed in a relaxed atmosphere and at complete privacy.
- A normal penile artery Doppler study with normal EHS response does not always imply an absence of ED. Erectile problems in these patients could be due to the psychogenic stress factors. Therefore as in many other diagnostic procedures, interpretation of PDS should be made in conjunction with the overall clinical profile of the patient and not in isolation.
- Because the penile arteries are small and torturous, it may be technically difficult to measure their diameters accurately, especially in the flaccid state. Moreover, obtaining technically adequate flow may be challenging in flaccid state.
- Velocities in cavernosal arteries could vary widely along their length, with higher velocities at the basal region and lower near the glans. It is thus advisable to measure and interpret the velocities only at the basal segments. Moreover, the same segment of the artery should be interrogated during the course of PDS.

- Angle dependency is an important limitation of the Doppler technique. This problem could be resolved to large extent by appropriately aligning the ultrasound beam in the direction of the artery. Angle correction is often required; however, it should not exceed 60°, or else overcorrection results.
- While scheduling the PDS, patient should be advised to abstain from any sexual activity 24–48 hours prior to the test. A misdiagnosis of ED could be made if PDS is performed within a few hours of sexual activity which results in ejaculation. For example *semen analysis and PDS should not be scheduled on the same day.*[19-23]

REFERENCES

1. Golijanin D, Singer E, Davis R, et al. Doppler evaluation of erectile dysfunction—Part 1. Int J Impot Res. 2007;19(1):37-42.
2. Montorsi P, Ravagnani PM, Galli S, et al. Association between erectile dysfunction and coronary artery disease: a case report study. J Sex Med. 2005;2(4):575-82.
3. El-Sakka AI, Morsy AM. Screening for ischemic heart disease in patients with erectile dysfunction: role of penile Doppler ultrasonography. Urology. 2004;64(2):346-50.
4. Gazzaruso C, Giordanetti S, De Amici E, et al. Relationship between erectile dysfunction and silent myocardial ischemia in apparently uncomplicated type 2 diabetic patients. Circulation. 2004;110:22-6.
5. Gratzke C, Angulo J, Chitaley K, et al. Anatomy, physiology, and pathophysiology of erectile dysfunction. J Sex Med. 2010;7(1 Pt 2):445-75.
6. Hsu G, Hung YP, Tsai MH, et al. Penile veins are the principal component in erectile rigidity: a study of penile venous stripping on defrosted human cadavers. J Androl. 2012;33(6):1176-85.
7. Shamloul R, Ghanem HM, Salem A, et al. Correlation between penile duplex findings and stress electrocardiography in men with erectile dysfunction. Int J Impot Res. 2004;16(3):235-7.
8. Elhanbly S, Abdel-Gaber S, Fathy H, et al. Erectile dysfunction in smokers: a penile dynamic and vascular study. J Androl. 2004;25(6):991-5.
9. Muneer A, Kalsi J, Nazareth I, et al. Erectile dysfunction. BMJ. 2014;348:g129.
10. Hatzimouratidis K, Eardley I, Giuliano F, et al. Guidelines on male sexual dysfunction: erectile dysfunction and premature ejaculation. Eur Urol. 2014;57(5):804-14.
11. Padma-Nathan H. Diagnostic and treatment strategies for erectile dysfunction: the 'Process of Care' model. Int J Impot Res. 2000;12(4):S119-21.
12. Golijanin D, Singer E, Davis R, et al. Doppler evaluation of erectile dysfunction—Part 2. Int J Impot Res. 2007;19(1):43-8.
13. Quam JP, King BF, James EM, et al. Duplex and color Doppler sonographic evaluation of vasculogenic impotence. AJR Am J Roentgenol. 1989;153:1141-7.
14. Clifford A, Toppo JN. Role of penile color Doppler in the evaluation of erectile dysfunction. Indian J Radiol Imaging. 2006;16(4):891-6.
15. Fitzgerald SW, Erickson SJ, Foley WD, et al. Color Doppler sonography in the evaluation of erectile dysfunction. Radiographics. 1992;12(1):3-17.
16. Lee B, Sikka SC, Randrup ER, et al. Standardization of penile blood flow parameters in normal men using intracavernous prostaglandin E1 and visual sexual stimulation. J Urol. 1993;149(1):49-52.
17. Speel TG, van Langen H, Wijkstra H, et al. Penile duplex pharmaco-ultrasonography revisited: revalidation of the parameters of the cavernous arterial response. J Urol. 2003;169(1):216-20.
18. Gupta N, Goyal P, Sharma K, et al. Penile fracture: role of ultrasound. Transl Androl Urol. 2017;6(3):580-4.
19. Polat H, Yucel MO, Gok A, et al. Penile Mondor's disease: primum non nocere! Urol J. 2015;12(2):2096-8.
20. Slob AK, Cornelissen S, Dohle GR, et al. Brief report the limited practical value of color Doppler sonography in the differential diagnosis of men with erectile dysfunction. Int J Impot Res. 2002;14:201-3.
21. Gall H, Bähren W, Scherb W, et al. Diagnostic accuracy of Doppler ultrasound technique of the penile arteries in correlation to selective arteriography. Cardiovasc Intervent Radiol. 1988;11:225-31.
22. Lue TF, Hricak H, Marich KW, et al. Vasculogenic impotence evaluated by high-resolution ultrasonography and pulsed Doppler spectrum analysis. Radiology. 1985;155(3):777-81.
23. Golubinski AJ, Sikorski A. Usefulness of power Doppler ultrasonography in evaluating erectile dysfunction. BJU Int. 2002;89:779-82.

SECTION 23

Syncope

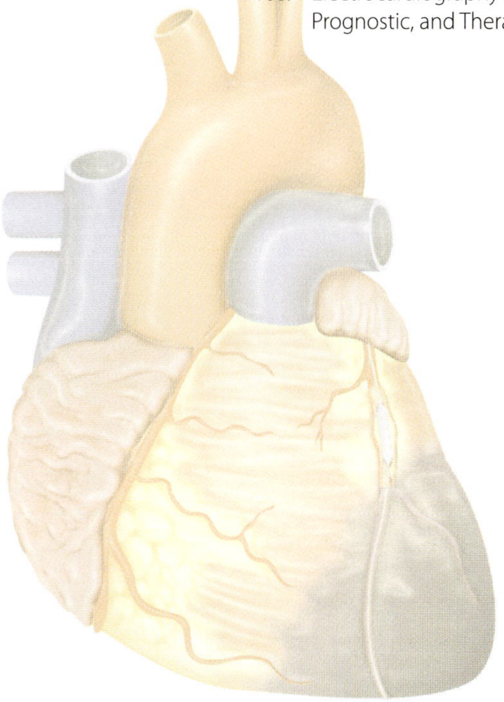

CHAPTER 108

Electrocardiography in Syncope: Diagnostic, Prognostic, and Therapeutic Implications

Vivek Kumar, Vanita Arora

INTRODUCTION

Syncope is transient loss of consciousness presumably as a result of transient cerebral hypoperfusion. It is an important clinical problem that accounts for 1% of hospital admissions and 3% of emergency department (ED) visits.[1] Although the cause of syncope is most common vascular, followed by cardiac causes, but on presentation, it is utmost important to consider several less common but potentially lethal causes of syncope in differential diagnosis. Here electrocardiography (EKG or ECG) becomes a vital tool. It is often challenging to reach a precise cause of the syncope as the syncope itself usually occurs sporadically and infrequently. So it is extremely difficult to evaluate a patient during an episode of syncope. A resting 12-lead EKG is useful (class I) in the initial evaluation of syncope.[2] ECG is widely available and inexpensive and can provide information about the potential and specific cause of the syncope episode (Box 1).[3] The ECG findings may suggest of, acute coronary syndrome, left ventricular hypertrophy (LVH), dysrhythmias, or conduction system problems (Box 2). It may demonstrate an underlying arrhythmogenic substrate for syncope or sudden cardiac death (SCD). Subsets of patients with Wolff-Parkinson-White (WPW) syndrome, Brugada syndrome, long QT syndrome (LQTS), hypertrophic cardiomyopathy (HCM), or arrhythmogenic right ventricular (RV) cardiomyopathy (ARVC) have characteristic ECG features, which can prompt the decision to pursue further evaluation.

CORONARY ARTERY DISEASE

Syncope associated with coronary ischemia can have many causes, including paroxysmal dysrhythmia [ventricular tachycardia (VT), atrial fibrillation (AF), reperfusion arrhythmia, etc.], left ventricular (LV) pump failure, and acute mitral regurgitation. Acute inferior wall myocardial infarction (MI) may present as syncope and complete heart block (Fig. 1). Left main lesion may present with syncope and subtle ST elevation in augmented vector right and V1 (Fig. 2). ECG diagnosis of ST-elevation myocardial infarction mandates time-defined intervention in the form of percutaneous coronary intervention or thrombolysis and has prognostic implications. In the setting of VT happening beyond first 24–48 hours of MI mandates consideration for automatic implantable cardioverter-defibrillator implantation for seasonal affective disorder prevention.[4]

OBSTRUCTIVE CARDIAC VALVE DISEASE AND OTHER ANATOMIC CAUSES OF SYNCOPE

In adult patients, severe aortic stenosis is an important cause of syncope and carries a grim prognosis if aortic valve replacement is not done. The classic ECG finding is of LVH, and others are left atrial enlargement, left axis deviation, and left bundle branch block (LBBB). The ECG does not correlate with the disease severity. The presence of LVH in ECG in a syncope patient should prompt to look for another important cause, i.e. HCM (Fig. 3). Apart from the above mentioned

BOX 1: Cardiac causes of syncope.

Anatomic:
- Obstructive cardiac valve disease
- Aortic dissection
- Atrial myxoma
- Pericardial disease, tamponade
- Hypertrophic obstructive cardiomyopathy
- Myocardial ischemia, infarction
- Pulmonary embolism
- Pulmonary hypertension

Arrhythmias:
- Bradyarrhythmia
  - Atrioventricular block
  - Sinus node dysfunction
- Tachyarrhythmia
  - Supraventricular tachycardia
    - Atrial fibrillation
    - Paroxysmal supraventricular tachycardia (AVNRT, AVRT, WPW)
  - Ventricular tachycardia
    - Structural heart disease
    - Inherited syndromes (ARVD, HCM, Brugada syndrome, long QT syndrome)
    - Drug-induced proarrhythmia
  - Implanted pacemaker or ICD malfunction

(ARVD: arrhythmogenic right ventricular dysplasia; AVNRT: atrioventricular nodal reentry tachycardia; AVRT: atrioventricular reentrant tachycardia; HCM: hypertrophic cardiomyopathy; ICD: implantable cardioverter-defibrillators; WPW: Wolff–Parkinson–White)

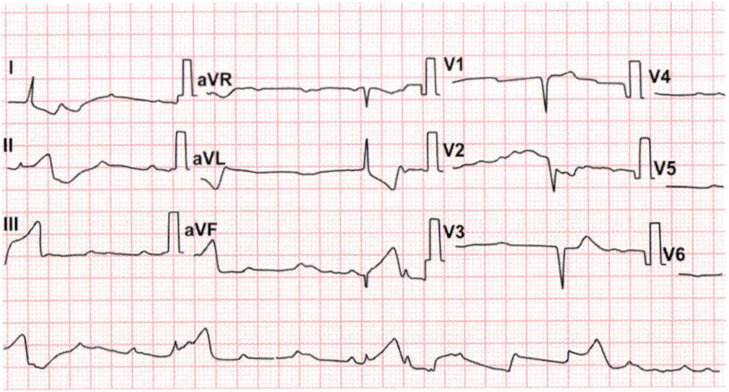

Fig. 1: CHB, ST elevation in II, III, and AVF, S/O of inferior wall myocardial infarction. (AVF: arteriovenous fistula; CHB: complete heart block)

features, characteristic deep and narrow Q wave may be present in precordial leads indicating severe septal hypertrophy. ECG is abnormal in most of the HCM patients. Normal ECG patterns are more commonly associated with mild LVH and a favorable clinical course, but do not exclude the possibility of future seasonal depression events.

Pulmonary embolism (PE) causes nonspecific symptoms and signs. Hence, clinical suspicion for PE is of paramount importance in guiding diagnostic testing. Syncope portends

BOX 2: Common electrocardiography findings in syncope.

- Paroxysmal or sustained dysrhythmia on monitoring in clinic
- Nonsinus rhythm of any sort
- Nonspecific intraventricular conduction delay (QRS > 100 ms without left or right bundle branch pattern)
- Left bundle branch block or left anterior or posterior hemiblock
- ECG signs of coronary ischemia
- Long QT syndrome QTc > 440–450 ms in men or > 460 ms in women
- Brugada sign—right bundle branch block and anterior ST elevation
- Left ventricular hypertrophy
- Pre-excitation syndromes (PR interval < 120 ms) with or without delta wave

(ECG: Electrocardiography)

a major life-threatening PE. The ECG may not be especially remarkable and may exhibit sinus tachycardia or slight ST-segment and T-wave abnormalities, or may even have an entirely normal appearance. The presence of $S_1Q_3T_3$ is the classic sign of right heart strain in PE specific but it is not very sensitive (Fig. 4).

BRADYARRHYTHMIA/ TACHYARRHYTHMIA

Patients with symptomatic bradycardia [sick sinus syndrome/atrioventricular (AV) block] often present with syncope. ECG may show features of conduction block at various levels depending on the underlying pathology. Patients with persistent, symptomatic bradycardia due to sinoatrial nodal or AV nodal pathology often need permanent pacemaker implantation (PPI). ECG in such patients often has high-degree AV block or sinus pauses and often heart rate less than 40 bpm. But at times, patient's ECG may be normal or having 1° heart block or various forms of bundle branch block. In such scenario, establishing the causal relation based on ECG becomes difficult, then Holter monitoring or electrophysiological study may be needed. PPI is definitely found to have morbidity benefit in such patients but mortality benefit remains doubtful.[5] VT or very rapid supraventricular tachycardia cause syncope more often than AF, atrial flutter, or multifocal atrial tachycardia do. Of course, any culprit dysrhythmia may have resolved by the time the patient presents to ED. It becomes very important to analyze the ECG thoroughly to look for condition that predispose to tachyarrhythmia. There may be evidence of ischemia, metabolic, or electrolyte abnormality.

SPECIFIC TACHYARRHYTHMIAS

There are several conditions, in healthy patients without structural heart disease, associated with inherent

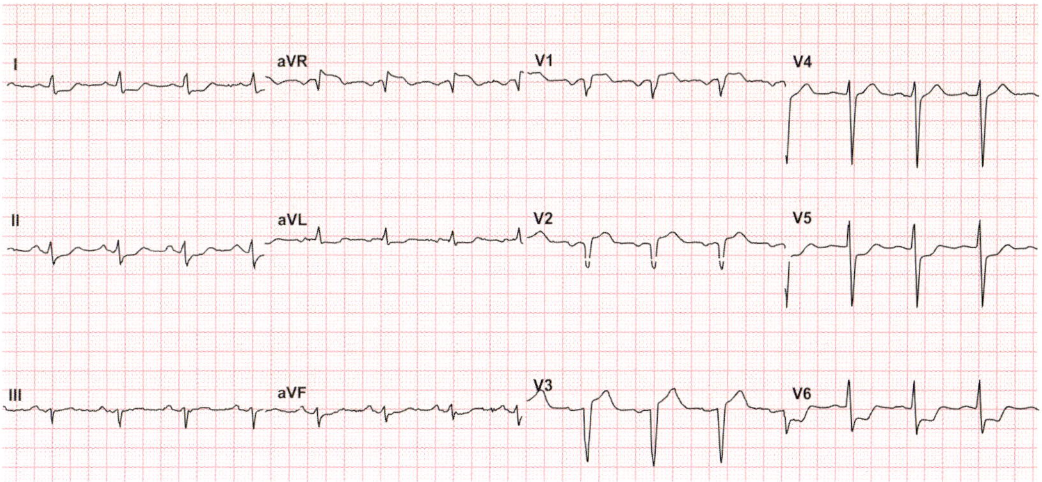

Fig. 2: Chest pain and syncope. ST elevation in aVR and V1, suggestive of LM lesion. (aVR: augmented vector right; LM: left main)

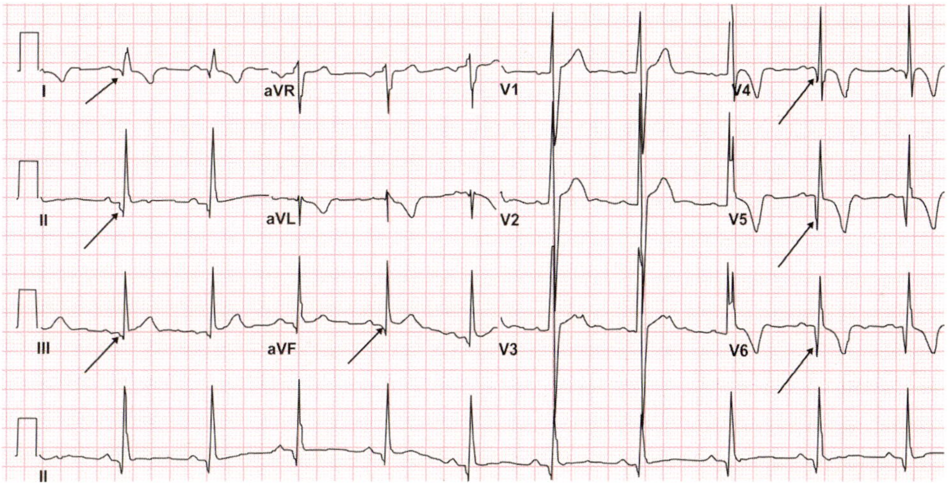

Fig. 3: Deep, narrow ("dagger-like") Q waves in the lateral (V5-6, I, aVL) and inferior (II, III, aVF) leads indicating asymmetrical septal hypertrophy. (aVF: augmented vector foot; aVL: augmented vector left)

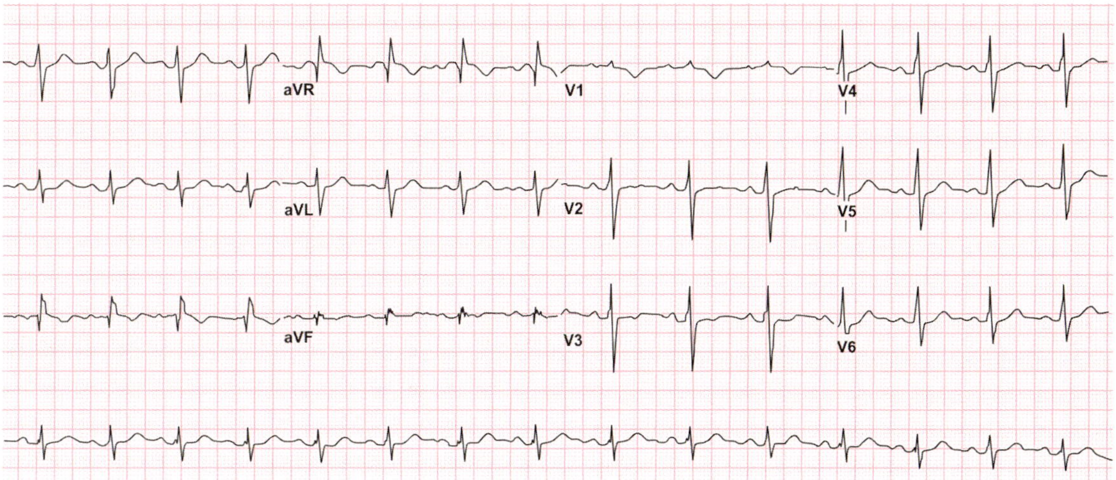

Fig. 4: Tracing shows an $S_1Q_3T_3$ (leads I and III) with an S wave in lead I, Q wave in lead III, and inverted T wave in lead III.

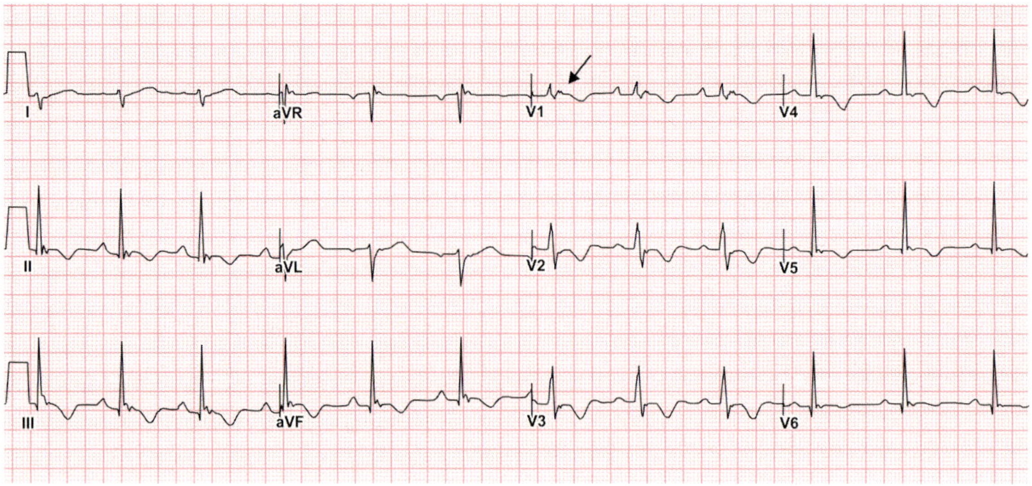

Fig. 5: Normal sinus rhythm in a patient ARVC/ARVD. The arrow in V1 point to late RV activation called an epsilon wave. (ARVC: arrhythmogenic right ventricular cardiomyopathy; ARVD: arrhythmogenic right ventricular dysplasia; RV: right ventricular)

predisposition to tachyarrhythmia and syncope. They are relatively rare but potentially lethal causes and require high degree of suspicion on presentation to reach a diagnosis. The knowledge of characteristic ECG features unique to these rare disorders is useful in making a diagnosis and timely planned intervention. As the occurrence of syncope portends higher risk, these patients need immediate, or at least extremely close, specialty follow-up.

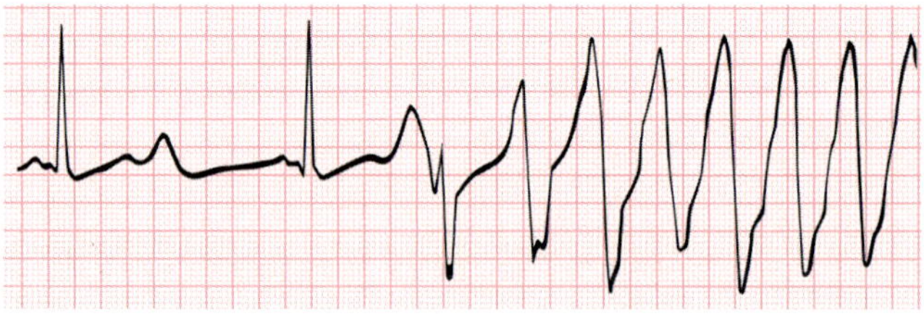

Fig. 6: The QTU interval in the sinus beats is at least 600 ms. Note the TU wave alternans in the first and second complexes. A late premature complex occurring in the downslope of the TU wave initiates an episode of VT. (VT: ventricular tachycardia)

ARRHYTHMOGENIC RIGHT VENTRICULAR CARDIOMYOPATHY (ARRHYTHMOGENIC RIGHT VENTRICULAR DYSPLASIA)

Arrhythmogenic RV cardiomyopathy/arrhythmogenic RV dysplasia is a heterogeneous inherited disease that results in fibrofatty infiltration of predominantly the right ventricle. Right-sided heart failure or asymptomatic RV enlargement can be present.[6] Patients with ARVC have VT that generally has an LBBB contour and can have several morphologies (including those consistent with outflow tract VT). The ECG during sinus rhythm can exhibit complete or incomplete right bundle branch block and T-wave inversions in V1–V3. A characteristic terminal notch in the QRS, called an epsilon wave, can be present as a result of slowed intraventricular conduction (Fig. 5). Because of the progressive nature of the disease and poor prognosis, particularly if the patient has poorly tolerated VT, implantable cardioverter-defibrillators (ICDs) are generally preferable to pharmacologic approaches.

LONG QT SYNDROME

Several abnormalities of delayed ventricular repolarization are characterized by prolongation of the QT interval on ECG. LQTS is characterized by a QTc interval more than 440–450 ms in men and more than 460 ms in women. These abnormalities include congenital membrane-ion-channel defects and some acquired causes related to medications, toxins, and neuropathies. Any of them may result in spontaneous or provoked (e.g. at the sound of a loud noise or physical or emotional stress) VT (Fig. 6). Torsades de pointes (TdP), a form of polymorphic VT, is unique to LQTS characterized by QRS complexes of changing amplitude that appear to twist around the isoelectric line and occur at rates of 200–250 per minute (Fig. 7). TdP can terminate with progressive prolongation of cycle length and larger and more distinctly formed QRS complexes and culminate in a return to the basal rhythm, a period of ventricular standstill, and a new attack of TdP or ventricular fibrillation (VF). Patients with congenital LQTS can initially have syncope, at times misdiagnosed as epilepsy, as a result of

TdP. Management is directed toward ameliorating reversible causes in acquired LQT and beta-blocker, with or without PPI/ICD in congenital LQTS.

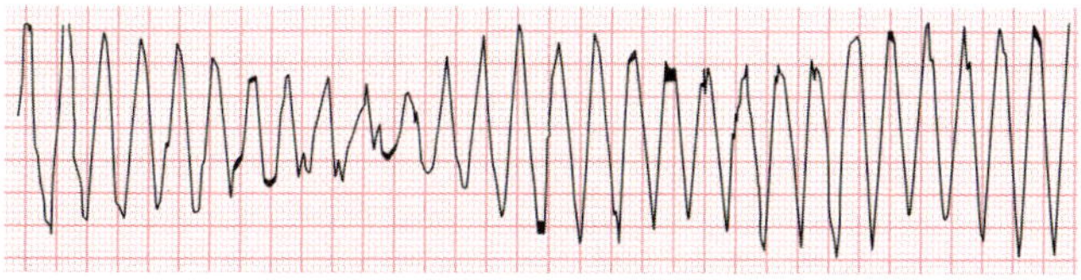

Fig. 7: Torsades de pointes.

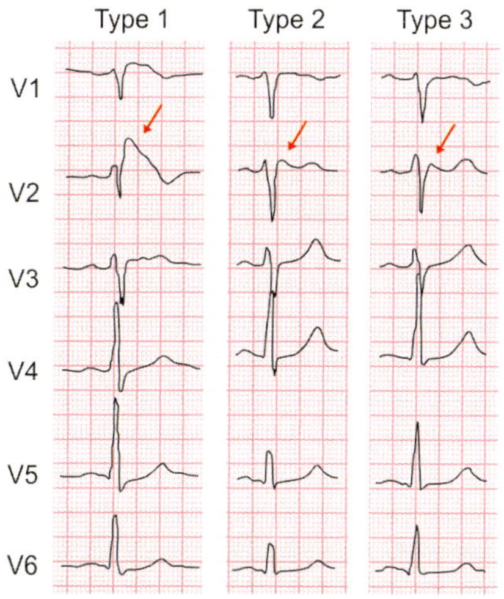

Fig. 8: Precordial leads of a patient with Brugada syndrome showing dynamic changes on the ECG. (ECG: electrocardiography)

BRUGADA SYNDROME

Brugada syndrome is an inherited channelopathy as a result of specific chromosomal mutation most frequently a defect in sodium membrane channel, often without evidence of structural heart disease. The defective channel predisposes to VT and fibrillation. The ECG hallmark of this disorder is a right bundle branch pattern with anterior ST-segment elevation in either a coved-downsloping or saddle-shaped pattern (Fig. 8). The ECG findings may be transient and are reported to be unmasked by fever or some medications. Type 1 pattern either occurring spontaneously or provoked by drug challenge with class I antiarrhythmic drug (AAD) (procainamide, flecainide, ajmaline) is diagnostic of Brugada syndrome.[7] Placing the right precordial leads in the second or third intercostal space ("high leads") can increase the sensitivity of detecting a type 1 pattern. ICD implantation is warranted in patients with Brugada syndrome with aborted SCD or spontaneous VT/VF (class I indication) or with a history of syncope (class IIa).[7] In patients with diagnosed or suspected Brugada syndrome, drugs that can provoke Brugada syndrome should be avoided.

VENTRICULAR PRE-EXCITATION SYNDROMES

Accessory pathway having antegrade conduction property manifest as ventricular pre-excitation syndrome and has the potential of very rapid conduction over the accessory pathway in the presence of AF, resulting in fast ventricular excitation likely to result in syncope and at times it may degenerate into VF (Fig. 9). If the resting ECG captures

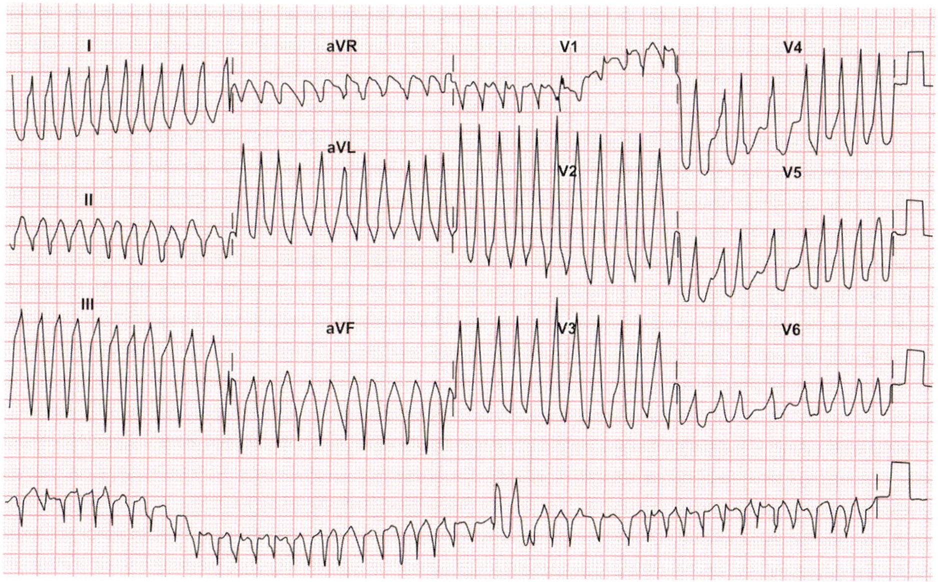

Fig. 9: Right posteroseptal accessory pathway with atrial fibrillation.

conduction of the AV impulses along the accessory pathway, the classic pattern of WPW syndrome will be apparent. This includes shortening of the PR interval to less than 120 ms, widening of the QRS complex, and a "delta wave," which describes a slurred upstroke of the initial part of the R wave. Patients with WPW will not have these findings if AV impulses are traveling along the normal conduction system at the time the ECG is performed.

CONCLUSION

Despite the benefit of identifying a likely cause or potential clue about the cause of syncope from the ECG, the prognostic value of an abnormal ECG in patients with syncope has been questioned.[8] However, a multicenter, prospective, observational study[9] concluded that the presence of AF, intraventricular conduction disturbances, voltage criteria for LVH, and ventricular pacing were associated with increased risk of death from all causes at 1 year. Though of limited sensitivity, ECG is inexpensive and is uniformly recommended in the evaluation of patients after syncope. Patients with ECG findings of obvious arrhythmia or the potential for arrhythmia, conduction disturbances, coronary ischemia, or cardiac outflow obstruction require further cardiac evaluation, including electrophysiology. Syncope is an uncommon occurrence but truly represent a chance to potentially save a life, if appropriate diagnosis and timely intervention is done.

REFERENCES

1. Sutton R, Benditt DG. Epidemiology and economic impact of cardiac syncope in western countries. Future Cardiol. 2012;8:467.
2. Shen WK, Sheldon RS, Benditt DG, et al. 2017 ACC/AHA/HRS guideline for the evaluation and management of patients with syncope: a report of the American College of Cardiology/American Heart Association task force on clinical practice guidelines and the Heart Rhythm Society. J Am Coll Cardiol. 2017;70:e39-110.
3. Zipes DP, Libby P, Bonow RO, et al. Braunwald's heart disease: A Textbook of Cardiovascular Medicine, Single Volume, 11th edition. Philadelphia: Elsevier; 2018. pp. e848-59.
4. O'Gara PT, Kushner FG, Ascheim DD, et al. 2013 ACCF/AHA guideline for the management of ST-elevation myocardial infarction: a report of the American College of Cardiology Foundation/American Heart Association Task Force on Practice Guidelines. J Am Coll Cardiol. 2013;61(4):e78-140.
5. Brunner M, Olschewski M, Geibel A, et al. Long-term survival after pacemaker implantation: prognostic importance of gender and baseline patient characteristics. Eur Heart J. 2004;25(1):88-95.
6. Haugaa KH, Haland TF, Leren IS, et al. Arrhythmogenic right ventricular cardiomyopathy, clinical manifestations, and diagnosis. Europace. 2016;18:965-72.
7. Priori SG, Blomström-Lundqvist C, Mazzanti A, et al. 2015 ESC guidelines for the management of patients with ventricular arrhythmias and the prevention of sudden cardiac death. The Task Force for the Management of Patients with Ventricular Arrhythmias and the Prevention of Sudden Cardiac Death of the European Society of Cardiology (ESC). Endorsed by: Association for European Paediatric and Congenital Cardiology (AEPC). Europace. 2015;17:1601-87.
8. Thiruganasambandamoorthy V, Hess EP, Turko E, et al. Defining abnormal electrocardiography in adult emergency department syncope patients: the Ottawa Electrocardiographic Criteria. CJEM. 2012;14:248-58.
9. Pérez-Rodon J, Martínez-Alday J, Baron-Esquivias G, et al. Prognostic value of the electrocardiogram in patients with syncope: data from the group for syncope study in the emergency room (GESINUR). Heart Rhythm. 2014;11:2035-44.

109

CHAPTER

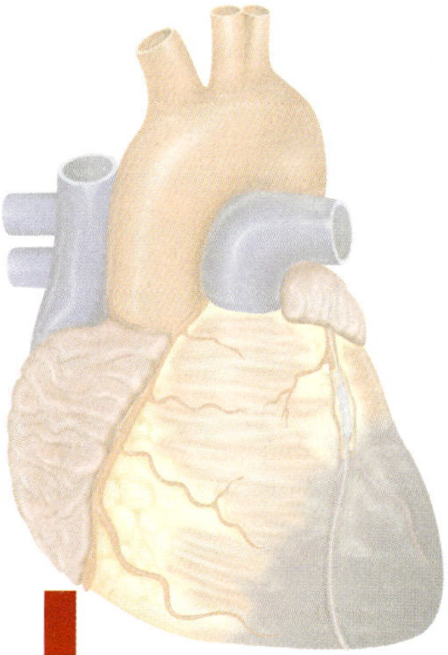

Cardiac Color Doppler Echo Evaluation in Syncope

Rajan J Manjuran, Sulthan R Salih

INTRODUCTION

Syncope is defined as a transient loss of consciousness (TLOC) with loss of postural tone due to global cerebral hypoperfusion, characterized by a rapid onset, short duration, and spontaneous complete recovery.[1] Syncope comes under a broad spectrum of disorders with TLOC. TLOC is defined as a state of real or apparent loss of consciousness with loss of awareness, characterized by amnesia for the period of unconsciousness, abnormal motor control, loss of responsiveness, and of short duration. TLOC can be traumatic and nontraumatic; nontraumatic is classified based on pathophysiology into cerebral hypoperfusion related (syncope), abnormal excessive neuronal discharge related (seizures), or psychogenic. Syncope is a fairly common disorder amounting to significant morbidity. Around 1% of all emergency department visits are due to syncope and are more common in the elderly.[2] The common causes of syncope are of noncardiac etiology. Cardiac syncope is mostly related to various bradyarrhythmias or tachyarrhythmias. Structural heart disease leading to syncope is among the least common of the cardiac causes. Initial evaluation of syncope mainly consists of history and physical examination, electrocardiogram (ECG), and postural blood pressure (BP) fluctuation to reach a diagnosis. If a diagnosis is not reached or is uncertain, it calls for further detailed evaluation especially in high-risk individuals. High-risk features in history are history of structural or coronary artery disease, new onset chest discomfort, dyspnea, abdominal pain or headache, exertional syncope, and syncope associated with palpitations. High-risk features of examination and investigations findings are systolic BP < 90 mm Hg, gastrointestinal bleed on rectal examination, bradycardia, undiagnosed murmur(s), and abnormal ECG. High-risk features on examination or investigations, recurrent episodes, severe coexisting disease, and syncope causing injury require further evaluation and admission if indicated. Further evaluation includes head-up tilt test (HUTT), tests of autonomic function, ECG monitoring, cardiac biomarkers, exercise stress testing, and echocardiography. These tests are ordered based on the observations in history, symptoms, and signs. Echocardiography is ordered if there is suspicion of underlying heart disease. The present article deals with the usefulness of electrocardiography in evaluating syncope patients.

CLASSIFICATION OF SYNCOPE

The central mechanism for syncope is cerebral hypoperfusion due to fall in systemic BP. This can be due to a low cardiac output or a fall in peripheral resistance or both. Syncope is classified based on pathophysiology into three categories; reflex (neurogenic) syncope, orthostatic hypotension (OH) induced syncope, and cardiac syncope. There is usually interplay between the primary mechanisms leading to considerable overlap.

Reflex syncope: It is a neurally mediated reaction triggered by special situations. Reflex syncope is further classified into vasovagal, situational, and carotid sinus hypersensitivity. Reflex syncope can be due to a vasodepressor reaction secondary to an inappropriate loss of sympathetically mediated vasoconstriction leading to a sudden dip in peripheral resistance, a cardioinhibitory reaction leading to a low cardiac output or a mixed reaction. This category comprises the most common cause of syncope.

Orthostatic hypotension: Upright position results in reduced venous return to heart, due to a drug action, failure of autonomic system to maintain vascular tone, or a volume depleted status. Most common causes are drugs, such as diuretics and vasodilators. Autonomic failure can be a primary neurologic disease or a secondary to another disease involving the autonomic system, such as diabetes mellitus or amyloidosis. Autonomic failure leads to an inappropriately low peripheral resistance whereas a volume depleted status leads to a low cardiac output.

Cardiac syncope: Cardiac syncope is either due an arrhythmia, a structural heart disease causing low output, or a disease of the great vessels, such as an embolism or acute aortic dissection. Arrhythmias, bradycardia or tachycardia, is more common than the structural disease of the heart or great vessels in causing syncope.

ROLE OF ECHOCARDIOGRAPHY IN SYNCOPE

The role of echocardiography depends upon the cause.

Reflex syncope: Echocardiography has no role in the diagnosis of reflex syncope. However, Goel et al.[3] observed reduced educed resting left ventricular (LV) strain in HUTT-positive patients. Further, Hensel et al.[4] found lower LV resting longitudinal strain rate in children with neurocardiogenic (vasovagal) syncope. This was pronounced in the children with HUTT positive. However, it is too early to include this investigation as part of syncope work up. A study by Cho KI et al.[5] reported correlation of syncope with epicardial fat thickness (EFT) as measured in parasternal long axis view on echocardiography. The study is concluded with positive correlation between EFT and HUTT. EFT was an independent predictor of HUTT positivity. EFT could be related to endocrine or paracrine functions and can mediate reflex syncope.

Orthostatic hypotension: Orthostatic hypotension is primarily not diagnosed by echocardiography. Patients with OH should undergo a drug chart review and tests of autonomic function. The volume depleted status can be checked by the use of inferior vena cava assessment of echocardiography.

Cardiac syncope: Cardiac syncope can be due to obstructive lesions, myocardial disease, or disease of the great vessels.

Obstructive lesions and structural heart disease: This is the category in which echocardiography is most useful. Left-sided obstructive lesions are uncommonly present with syncope. Echocardiography can accurately diagnose valvular aortic stenosis and tumors producing left ventricular outflow tract/right ventricular outflow tract (LVOT/RVOT) obstruction, such as rhabdomyomas or fibromas. Papillary fibroelastoma presenting as syncope has also been reported.[6] Left atrial myxoma prolapsing into the mitral valve apparatus can cause mitral valve obstruction and lead to syncope.[7,8] Similarly, cases of right atrial myxoma presenting as syncope have also been reported.[9-11] Ball valve thrombus obstructing the mitral or tricuspid orifices also present, such as myxomas.[12] Cardiac tamponade can be presented as syncope and diagnosed by echocardiography.[13] There has also been a case report of malignant pectus excavatum which caused compression on the right atrium and ventricle presenting with syncopal episodes.[14] LV dysfunction and heart failure are other causes that are diagnosed readily by echocardiography. Rare lesions which cause syncope-like cortriatriatum[15] and primary cardiac sarcoidosis[16] can also be detected in patients presenting as syncope.

Myocardial disease: Cardiomyopathies are associated with arrhythmia-related syncope.[17] A diagnosis of arrhythmia related to cardiomyopathy cannot be diagnosed by echocardiography. But the identification of a cardiomyopathy, such as hypertrophic cardiomyopathy, noncompaction, and arrhythmogenic right ventricular cardiomyopathy, can help in further evaluation of these patients. In addition, dynamic obstruction with LV outflow tract gradient more than or equal to 50 mm Hg in hypertrophic obstructive cardiomyopathy at rest or demonstrated in stress echocardiography is also predictive of the cause of syncope. Infiltrative cardiomyopathy of amyloidosis also can be presented with recurrent syncope although the syncope could be due to the associated polyneuropathy causing postural hypotension.[18,19]

Disease of the great vessels: Acute pulmonary embolism, both massive and submassive, can be presented with syncope and may not be readily diagnosed on initial evaluation.[20-22] Features suggestive of pulmonary embolism, such as dilated right heart, McConells sign, and mild-to-moderate pulmonary arterial hypertension, can be readily picked up on echocardiography. Acute aortic dissection is a great masquerade. Involvement of the common carotid artery in aortic dissection can be presented as syncope. Although transthoracic echocardiography is not the ideal investigation in suspected aortic dissection, it can detect the dissection flap in one fourth cases. Transesophageal echocardiography has much higher sensitivity.

YIELD OF ECHOCARDIOGRAPHY IN THE EVALUATION OF SYNCOPE

Over the years, a good number of studies have evaluated the positive yield of various tests in syncope to formulate an ideal plan of evaluation. The study by Recchia et al.[23] in 1995 used echocardiography for syncope evaluation in 64% of the cases in the study. Although 48% cases had some echocardiographic abnormality, most of these could not be related to syncope. LV dysfunction with heart failure had the diagnosis made from history and ECG even before the echocardiogram. The additional diagnostic yield for echocardiography was negligible. Sarasin et al. diagnosed LV dysfunction in 27% and there was 1.2% with aortic stenosis. But all these patients had an abnormal ECG and/or examination abnormality. Arrhythmia was diagnosed as the cause in half of the patients with LV dysfunction by Holter monitoring. Although echocardiography helped in risk stratifying in these patients, the ultimate diagnostic yield for echocardiography alone was very low. Ruwald et al.[24,25] studied unexplained syncope and the usefulness of diagnostic tests in 600 patients. Echocardiography could help in the diagnosis in one diagnostic cause in 4% patients. Mendu et al.[26] found that although 63% of echocardiograms had abnormal findings, only 2% revealed findings that were directly contributing to syncope. Chang et al.[27] could find diagnostic echocardiogram in none of the patients with normal physical examination and ECG; and in 6.5% with abnormal physical examination and/or ECG. Han et al.[28] reported 28% abnormal echocardiogram in patients with risk factors and 2% in patients without risk factors based on positive history, examination, biomarkers, and/or abnormal ECG. But the true yield of a cause of syncope by echocardiogram was not reported in this study and is likely to be lower than the above quoted values. Anderson et al.[29] reported abnormal echocardiogram in 7 of 323 patients (2.17%) of syncope and all of them had abnormal ECG. There was evidence of myocardial ischemia defined in three patients (0.9%) on stress echocardiography. The author suggested echocardiography as not useful or cost effective in evaluating syncope. A recent study[30] compared syncope in patients of structural heart disease and found that there was a significantly more readmission and shorter event-free interval in cardiac cause for syncope versus a vasovagal or OH group. It is clear from the above studies that echocardiography delineating a direct cause for syncope is rare (Fig. 1). But echocardiogram is shown to identify high-risk patients for syncope for whom another episode can be catastrophic and require measures to prevent such episodes. Majority of the authors do not recommend echocardiography among the first-line investigations for syncope.

RECOMMENDATIONS OF VARIOUS INTERNATIONAL BODIES ON USE OF ECHOCARDIOGRAPHY IN SYNCOPE

2011 Automotive Service Excellence Appropriate use Criteria for Echocardiography[31] strongly recommends (score 9/9) echocardiography in patients with positive cardiac history and syncope or presyncope. It also gives a moderate recommendation (score 7/9) for echocardiographic examination in syncope but not for presyncope (score 3/9) without a cardiac history. American College of Cardiology/American Heart Association/Heart Rhythm Society 2017 syncopeguidelines[32] gives a 2-A recommendation for the use of echocardiography in patients with syncope and suspected heart disease. It gives a class 3 (no benefit) recommendation for routine use of echocardiography in patients of syncope not suspected to have cardiac illness.

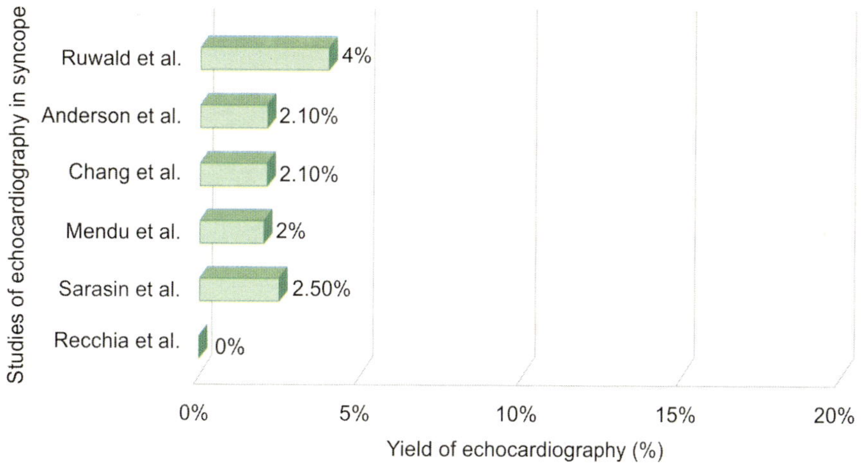

Fig. 1: Yield of echocardiography in syncope as reported in various studies.

European Society of Cardiology 2018 syncope guidelines[1] for the diagnosis and management of syncope give a 1-B recommendation for echocardiography in patients with structural heart disease for syncope evaluation. It also gives a 1-B recommendation for stress echocardiography testing in hypertrophic cardiomyopathy to look for dynamic LVOT gradient. But it does not recommend the use of echocardiography if there are no features of cardiac disease on history, physical examination, or ECG. If we are to accept the recommendations from world bodies, echocardiography is useful in diagnosing the cause of syncope only when history, examination, or ECG revealed abnormalities. In otherwise normal person with syncope, the yield from echocardiography examination is low.

RECOMMENDATIONS

From the above discussion it is clear that echocardiography is rarely diagnostic in patients with a negative history, physical examination, and ECG for cardiac disease. Even in patients with cardiac disease suggested by initial evaluation, the yield of echocardiography for a diagnostic cause for syncope is low. But echocardiography helps in the risk stratification of patients with structural heart disease. Also based on the case reports, there are cases of syncope with negative initial evaluation in which echocardiogram was diagnostic, such as the myxomas and the malignant pectus excavatum. Most guidelines and studies do not recommend a routine use of echocardiography as the cost of an echocardiogram is high in those countries. But in a country, such as India, where the cost of echocardiogram is low and is affordable to the majority of the patients, it is unwise not to use the available armamentaria for a complete evaluation. Also, missing a cause for cardiac syncope can be disastrous for the patient. Although the initial evaluation for syncope does not need an echocardiogram, it is recommended to use echocardiography in the detailed evaluation of patients with syncope.

REFERENCES

1. Brignole M, Moya A, de Lange FJ, et al. 2018 ESC Guidelines for the diagnosis and management of syncope. Eur Heart J. 2018;39:1883-1948.
2. Sun BC, Emond JA, Camargo CA. Characteristics and admission patterns of patients presenting with syncope to U.S. Emergency Departments, 1992-2000. Acad Emerg Med. 2004;11:1029-34.
3. Goel R, Caracciolo G, Wilansky S, et al. Effect of head-up tilt-table testing on left ventricular longitudinal strain in patients with neurocardiogenic syncope. Am J Cardiol. 2013;112:1252-7.
4. Hensel KO, Roskopf M, Abellan Schneyder F, et al. Novel functional advanced echocardiography for the assessment of myocardial mechanics in children with neurocardiogenic syncope—a blinded prospective speckle tracking head-up tilt-table challenge study. BMC Cardiovasc Disord. 2018;18:87.
5. Cho KI, Lee YS, Kim BK, et al. Epicardial fat thickness is correlated with vagal hyperactivity in patients with neurally-mediated syncope. J Cardiovasc Ultrasound. 2017;25:57-62.
6. De Portu G, Nickels LC, Flach E, et al. Fibroelastoma as a culprit of syncope. Case Rep Crit Care. 2013;2013:416168.
7. Rashidi N, Montazeri M, Montazeri M. Large left atrial myxoma causing mitral valve obstruction: a rare cause of syncope. J Cardiovasc Echogr. 2014;24:125-7.
8. Sinha AK, Singh BP. LA myxoma presenting as recurrent syncope. Indian Heart J. 2013;65:643.
9. Azevedo O, Almeida J, Nolasco T, et al. Massive right atrial myxoma presenting as syncope and exertional dyspnea: case report. Cardiovasc Ultrasound. 2010;8:23.
10. Babs Animashaun I, Akinseye OA, Akinseye LI, et al. Right atrial myxoma and syncope. Am J Case Rep. 2015;16:645-7.
11. Yazici M, Ozhan H, Tetik O, et al. Isolated large right atrial myxoma manifested by syncope. Texas Hear Inst J. 2004;31:324-5.
12. Miura K, Ikegami Y, Momiyama Y. Syncope due to a free-floating left atrial thrombus. Intern Med. 2017;56:3115-6.
13. Chen MC, Wu HH, Hsia CP. Syncope due to impending cardiac tamponade in Hashimoto's thyroiditis. Acta Cardiol Sin. 2014;30:253-5.
14. Crossland DS, Auldist AW, Davis AM. Malignant pectus excavatum. Heart. 2006;92:1511.
15. Eichholz JL, Hodroge SS, Crook JJ, et al. Cor triatriatum sinister in a 43-year-old man with syncope. Tex Heart Inst J. 2013;40:602-5.
16. Thangam M, Nathan S, Kar B, et al. Primary cardiac sarcoidosis with syncope and refractory atrial arrhythmia: a case report and review of the literature. Tex Heart Inst J. 2016;43:236-40.
17. Bhogal S, Ladia V, Sitwala P, et al. Isolated ventricular noncompaction cardiomyopathy presenting as recurrent syncope. Case Rep Med. 2016;2016:3742171.
18. Marin-Acevedo JA, Sanchez-Alvarez C, Alsaad AA, et al. Recurrent syncope, a clue in amyloid cardiomyopathy. Case Rep Med. 2018;2018:1864962.
19. Mugnai G, Cicoira M, Rossi A, et al. Syncope in cardiac amyloidosis and chronic ischemic heart disease: a case report. Exp Clin Cardiol. 2011;16:51-3.
20. Wang SY, Chen H, Di LG. Caution for acute submassive pulmonary embolism with syncope as initial symptom: a case report. J Thorac Dis. 2014;6:E212-6.
21. Demircan A, Aygencel G, Keles A, et al. Pulmonary embolism presenting as syncope: a case report. J Med Case Rep. 2009;3:7440.
22. Epstein D, Berger G, Barda N, et al. The incidence of acute pulmonary embolism following syncope in anticoagulant-naïve patients: a retrospective cohort study. PLoS One. 2018;13:e0193725.
23. Recchia D, Barzilai B. Echocardiography in the evaluation of patients with syncope. J Gen Intern Med. 1995;10:649-55.

24. Chung SY, Lin FC, Chua S, et al. Clinical profile and outcome of first acute myocardial infarction with ischemic mitral regurgitation. Chang Gung Med J. 2008;31:268-75.
25. Ruwald MH, Lock Hansen M, Lamberts M, et al. Unexplained syncope and diagnostic yield of tests in syncope according to the ICD-10 discharge diagnosis. J Clin Med Res. 2013;5:441-50.
26. Mendu ML, McAvay G, Lampert R, et al. Yield of diagnostic tests in evaluating syncopal episodes in older patients. Arch Intern Med. 2009;169:1299.
27. Chang N-L, Shah P, Bajaj S, et al. Diagnostic yield of echocardiography in syncope patients with normal ECG. Cardiol Res Pract. 2016;2016:1-7.
28. Han SK, Yeom SR, Lee SH, et al. Transthoracic echocardiogram in syncope patients with normal initial evaluation. Am J Emerg Med. 2017;35:281-4.
29. Anderson KL, Limkakeng A, Damuth E, et al. Cardiac evaluation for structural abnormalities may not be required in patients presenting with syncope and a normal ECG result in an observation unit setting. Ann Emerg Med. 2012;60:478-84.
30. Guimarães RB, Essebag V, Furlanetto M, et al. Structural heart disease as the cause of syncope. Braz J Med Biol Res. 2018;51:e6989.
31. Douglas PS, Garcia MJ, Haines DE, et al. ACCF/ASE/AHA/ASNC/HFSA/HRS/SCAI/SCCM/SCCT/SCMR 2011 appropriate use criteria for echocardiography. A report of the American College of Cardiology Foundation Appropriate Use Criteria Task Force, American Society of Echocardiography, American Heart Associa. J Am Soc Echocardiogr. 2011;24:229-67.
32. Shen WK, Sheldon RS, Benditt DG, et al. 2017 ACC/AHA/HRS guideline for the evaluation and management of patients with syncope: a report of the American College of Cardiology/American Heart Association Task Force on Clinical Practice Guidelines and the Heart Rhythm Society. Circulation. 2017;136:e60-122.

SECTION 24

Stroke

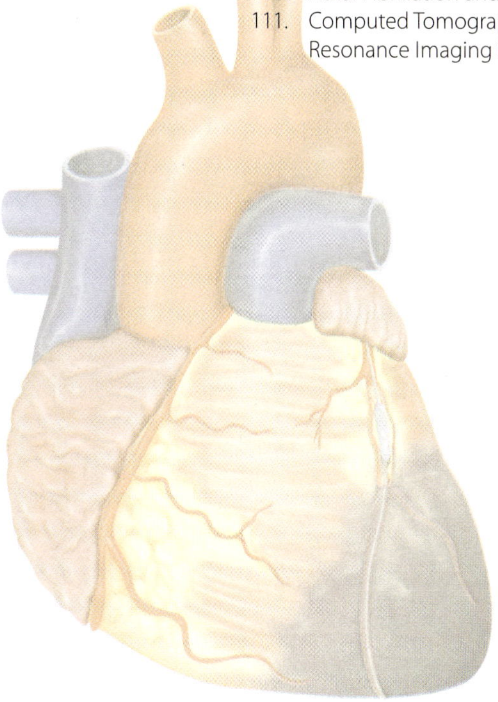

CHAPTER 110

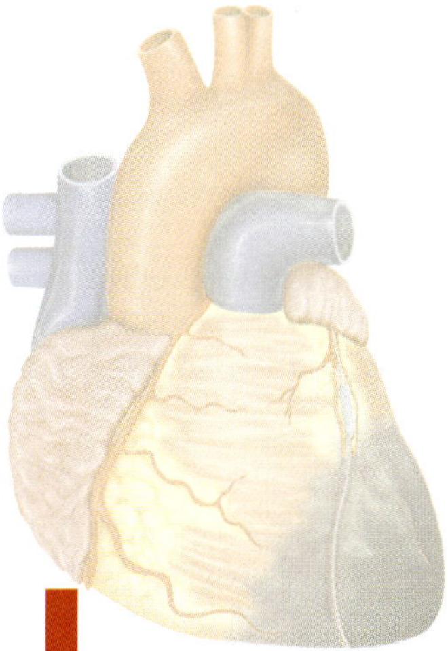

Atrial Fibrillation and Stroke

Himashu Agarwal, Chandril Chugh

INTRODUCTION

Stroke is defined by the World Health Organization as a clinical syndrome consisting of rapidly developing clinical signs of focal (or global in the case of coma) disturbance of cerebral function lasting more than 24 hours or leading to death with no apparent cause other than a vascular origin.[1] Stroke is classified broadly into three categories: ischemic stroke, hemorrhagic stroke, and subarachnoid hemorrhage. Ischemic stroke occurs due to blockage of blood vessel which limits the blood supply to the brain, whereas hemorrhagic stroke occurs due to the rupture of blood vessel leading spillage of blood in the intracranial cavity.[2] Depending on the site of blood spillage, the hemorrhagic stroke could be classified as intracerebral or subarachnoid hemorrhage. Approximately 60–80% of all strokes are ischemic and more common in cardiovascular patients as well. Atrial fibrillation (AF) is one of the most common causes of ischemic stroke. Up to 33 million people are affected by AF, and they are 3–5 times more likely to have a stroke.[3] AF is associated with larger ischemic strokes and longer transient ischemic attacks as compared to the patients with carotid artery disease. This is primarily due to the fact that larger emboli tend to form in the left atrial appendage which affects the larger brain blood vessels.[4,5] Although AF has been associated with cardioembolic strokes, there is conflicting evidence which points toward other mechanisms of stroke. About 10% of patients with lacunar strokes have associated AF, and large-vessel atherosclerosis is twice as common in patients with AF.[6,7]

MECHANISM OF STROKE IN ATRIAL FIBRILLATION

Atrial fibrillation is a rhythm abnormality; however, there are structural abnormalities associated with AF which predispose the patient to an ischemic stroke. AF is frequently associated with chamber dilatation, endothelial dysfunction, fibrosis, and impaired myocyte function. Data suggests that left atrial size,[8] premature ventricular contractions,[9] electrocardiographic evidence of left atrial dysfunction, and paroxysmal supraventricular tachycardia[10,11] are associated with additional risk of ischemic stroke. Stroke in AF thus cannot be attributed to only the rhythm, instead structural heart changes, systemic vascular, and hematological changes might play an equally important role. Aging and systemic factors cause atrial cardiopathy which increases the risk of arterial embolism. Atrial cardiopathy can progress to AF which further elevates the risk of clot formation due to impaired contractility. In prolonged AF, there is atrial remodeling which further increases the risk of thromboembolism. In parallel, systemic risk factors increase stroke risk via other mechanisms outside the atrium, such as large artery atherosclerosis, ventricular systolic dysfunction, and in situ cerebral small-vessel occlusion.[12]

Historical Perspective

Intravenous thrombolysis has for long been the only proven treatment available for ischemic stroke. It has to be given within 4.5 hours and is not particularly effective for large-vessel arterial occlusion.[13,14] A number of intra-arterial therapy trials have been published in the last two decades. Many of them failed to show significant difference as compared to routine care until recently. Initially the results of intra-arterial thrombolysis was published in Prolyse in Acute Cerebral Thromboembolism (PROACT) I and PROACT II.[15,16] The results were encouraging as they showed higher recanalization rates with prourokinase. However, prourokinase was never approved by Food and Drug Administration (FDA) for this indication due to lack of a confirmatory trial.

First-generation Thrombectomy Device

Mechanical embolus removal in cerebra ischemia (MERCI) retriever device was the first device approved by FDA for mechanical thrombectomy. MERCI trial was able to achieve recanalization in internal carotid artery (ICA), M1 middle cerebral artery (MCA), and M2 MCA in 46% cases [thrombolysis in myocardial infarction (TIMI) 2 or 3].[17] In subsequent Multi-MERCI trial, recanalization was achieved in 55% of the cases. Both single-arm trials treated patients within 8 hours of onset. Good clinical outcome [Modified Rankin Score (MRS) <2] was achieved in 28% and 36% cases, respectively, with not much improvement in mortality.[18] Nevertheless, patients with early recanalization had good outcomes which paved the way for further trials.

Second-generation Thrombectomy Devices

Penumbra aspiration device is a second-generation thrombectomy device which was studied under the Penumbra Pivotal Stroke Trial. Device showed high rates of recanalization (TIMI 2 or 3) in about 82% of cases. It was a nonrandomized trial with high rates of mortality and morbidity.[19]

Third-generation Thrombectomy Devices

The Solitaire and Trevo are third-generation thrombectomy devices. Better recanalization rates and clinical outcomes were reported with these retrievable stents.[20,21] Recent endovascular trials have shown promising results using these stentrievers, with higher rates of recanalization and better clinical outcomes.

PERFUSION CHANGES IN ISCHEMIC STROKE

As the intracranial vessel gets occluded, territory of brain supplied by that vessel tries to compensate for the compromised blood supply through leptomeningeal collaterals. Due to these collaterals region of brain at risk, it has three zones depending on cerebral blood flow (CBF):

1. *Core*: Irreversibly damaged region.
2. *Penumbra*: Region with low CBF, but salvageable if blood supply is restored.
3. *Region of benign oligemia*: Region with low CBF, but not at the risk of irreversible damage.

After the stroke, onset infarct core grows progressively and penumbra decreases. The rate of infarct core growth depends on the collaterals of individual patients.[22]

Patient Selection

Major breakthrough in acute stroke treatment with mechanical thrombectomy came from five successful trials published since 2015 [Multicenter Randomized Clinical Trial of Endovascular Treatment for Acute Ischemic Stroke in the Netherlands (MR CLEAN), Solitaire™ With the Intention For Thrombectomy as PRIMary Endovascular Treatment (SWIFT PRIME), Endovascular Treatment for Small Core and Proximal Occlusion Ischemic Stroke (ESCAPE), Emergency Neurological Deficits with Intra-arterial therapy (EXTEND IA), and REVASCAT].[20,23-26] One major difference from the previous negative trials (MERCI, Interventional Management of Stroke 3, SYNTHESIS) was more refined criteria for patient selection in later trials, such as:[27-30]

- Presence of significant neurological deficit [National Institutes of Health Stroke Scale (NIHSS)>6], which justifies the risk of endovascular intervention.
- Presence of small infarct core, identified by either noncontrast computed tomography (CT) (NCCT) [Alberta Stroke Program Early CT Score (ASPECTS) >6] or collateral score or diffusion-weighted imaging (DWI) or perfusion imaging.
- Presence of large-vessel occlusion (LVO) (ICA, M1 MCA, and proximal M2 MCA), for targeted thrombectomy.
- Treatment initiation within defined time window, which was variable in trials (Table 1).

To summarize, patients with significant neurological deficits (NIHSS > 6) with small infract core (ASPECT > 6) and a LVO (ICA, M1 MCA, and proximal M2 MCA), who present early (0–6 h), benefit most from the mechanical thrombectomy. The response to mechanical thrombectomy in young patients with large infarct core, who present very early, is still debatable and needs further research.[31]

Patients with Extended Time Window

Two recent trials, Data Analysis WorkbeNch (DAWN) and Endovascular Therapy Following Imaging Evaluation for Ischemic Stroke 3 (DEFUSE 3), showed the better outcomes in patients presenting beyond 6 hours' time window.[32,33]

TABLE 1

Trial	Baseline NIHSS median	Time window (h)	Median ASPECTS	Median time onset to groin access (min)	Retrievable stent %	Screening imaging modality
MR CLEAN	17	0–6	9	260	87	NCCT CTA/MRA/DSA
ESCAPE	16	0–12	9	211	73	NCCT/Multiphase CTA
EXTEND-IA	17	0–6	NA (median core <12 mL)	210	100	NCCT/CTA/CTP
SWIFT-PRIME	17	0–6	9	224	100	NCCT, CTA/MRA, CTP/MRP
REVASCAT	17	0–8	7	269	70	NCCT, CTA/MRA, CTP/MRP

(ASPECTS: Alberta Stroke Program Early Computed Tomography Score; CTA: computed tomography angiography; CTP: computed tomography perfusion; DSA: digital subtraction angiography; ESCAPE: Endovascular Treatment for Small Core and Proximal Occlusion Ischemic Stroke; EXTEND-1A: Endovascular Therapy for Ischemic Stroke with Perfusion-Imaging Selection; MRA: magnetic resonance angiography; MR CLEAN: Multicenter Randomized Clinical Trial of Endovascular Treatment for Acute Ischemic Stroke in the Netherlands; MRP: multiplanar reformation; NCCT: noncontrast computed tomography; NIHSS: National Institutes of Health Stroke Scale; SWIFT PRIME: Solitaire with the Intention for Thrombectomy as Primary Endovascular Treatment)

TABLE 2

Trial	Baseline NIHSS median	Time window (h)	Median ASPECTS	Selection criteria	Median time onset to groin access (h:min)	Screening imaging modality
DAWN	17	6–24	NA	Core: <31 and NIHSS > 10 Core 31–51 mL and NIHSS > 20	12:12	NCCT, CTA/MRA
DEFUSE 3	16	6–16	8	Core < 70 mL, ischemic tissue to core volume > 1.8	11:28	NCCT, CTA/MRA, CTP/MRP

(ASPECTS: Alberta Stroke Program Early Computed Tomography Score; CTA: computed tomography angiography; CTP: computed tomography perfusion; DAWN: Data Analysis WorkbeNch; DEFUSE 3: Endovascular Therapy Following Imaging Evaluation for Ischemic Stroke 3; MRA: magnetic resonance angiography; MRP: multiplanar reformation; NIHSS: National Institutes of Health Stroke Scale; NCCT: noncontrast computed tomography)

These trials used the same principle of small core, significant neurological deficits, and LVO (ICA and M1 MCA). However, they used specialized software to accurately identify volume of core either by DWI or CT perfusion imaging and identifying penumbra using NIHSS score discordance or by regional CBF (Table 2).

Imaging Modalities

Goal of imaging in acute ischemic stroke is to identify (Table 3):

- Core
- Penumbra
- Site of occlusion

Ideal imaging for acute ischemic stroke should be able to give quick and reliable results with minimal interobserver variability. NCCT scan is the primary imaging modality used in almost all the trials. It can be obtained quickly and is highly sensitive and specific to rule out hemorrhage. However, major drawback of NCCT is its low sensitivity for early ischemic changes. ASPECTS is used to decrease the interobserver variability.[34,35] However, results from major trials have proved that within 6 hours of the onset of NCCT with CT angiography is reliable to make treatment decision.[36] Diffusion is highly accurate to identify core,

TABLE 3

Goal	CT (level of evidence)	MRI (level of evidence)
Core	ASPECTS (level 2/class 2a) CTA—collateral score (level 2/class 3)	DWI (level 1/class 1)
Penumbra	CTP (level 3/class 2b)	PWI
Site of occlusion	CTA (level 1/class 1)	MRA

(ASPECTS: Alberta Stroke Program Early Computed Tomography Score; CT: computed tomography; DWI: diffusion-weighted imaging; CTA: computed tomography angiography; CTP: computed tomography perfusion; MRA: magnetic resonance angiography; MRI: magnetic resonance imaging; PWI: perfusion-weighted imaging) but is limited by time taken to obtain it.[37,38] Often the time is lost to scan patients for magnetic objects, availability of free machine in busy radiology department, ineligibility of patient due to pacemakers and other metallic implants.[39]

POSTERIOR CIRCULATION STROKE

There are no randomized trials available to define criteria for the selection of patients eligible for mechanical thrombectomy in posterior circulation stroke, though Basilar Artery International Cooperation Study trial is ongoing to see the efficacy of mechanical thrombectomy in basilar artery occlusion. Time window in basilar artery occlusion is not defined, it is known that brain stem is resilient to ischemia, which gives more time window in posterior circulation stroke in selected patients.[40,41] NCCT is less sensitive to pick acute brain stem strokes; therefore, in patients with suspected brain stem stroke, it is wiser to have diffusion imaging.

Procedural Considerations

There is enough evidence to suggest that general anesthesia in acute stroke patients is associated with bad outcomes. Reasons may be delay in initiation of procedure due to intubation, hemodynamic compromise, hypotension induced by induction can lead to expansion of infarct core, longer intensive care unit (ICU) stay. On the other hand, monitored anesthesia care or conscious sedation is associated with better outcomes, small infarct load, and shorter ICU stays. Exceptions are posterior fossa strokes that may often need general anesthesia. Conscious sedation should be the preferred approach; however, rapid intubation may be required if patient develops acute decompensation or hemodynamic compromise.[42-44]

TABLE 4

Trial	*MRS (0–2) at 90 days—EMT arm%*	*MRS (0–2) at 90 days—control arm%*
MR CLEAN	32.6	19.1
ESCAPE	53	29.3
SWIFT PRIME	60.2	35.5
EXTEND IA	71.4	40
REVASCAT	43.7	28.2
HERMES	46	26.5
DAWN	52	13
DEFUSE 3	41	15

(ASPECTS: Alberta Stroke Program Early Computed Tomography Score; DAWN: Data Analysis WorkbeNch; DEFUSE 3: Endovascular Therapy Following Imaging Evaluation for Ischemic Stroke 3; EMT: endovascular mechanical thrombectomy; ESCAPE: Endovascular Treatment for Small Core and Proximal Occlusion Ischemic Stroke; EXTEND-1A: Endovascular Therapy for Ischemic Stroke with Perfusion-Imaging Selection; HERMES: Highly Effective Reperfusion Evaluated in Multiple Endovascular Stroke Trials; MRS: modified rankin score; SWIFT PRIME: Solitaire with the Intention for Thrombectomy as Primary Endovascular Treatment)

Benefits of Mechanical Thrombectomy and Improvement in Disability

Seven successful trials (MR CLEAN, ESCAPE, EXTEND IA, SWIFT PRIME, REVASCAT, DEFUSE 3, and DAWN) of endovascular mechanical thrombectomy (EMT) and Highly Effective Reperfusion Evaluated in Multiple Endovascular Stroke Trials meta-analysis have proven beyond doubt that EMT in selected patients of acute ischemic stroke is associated with significant reduction in disability and mortality. Outcome measured from MRS at 90 days showed significant shift toward good MRS (0–2) in EMT arm as compared to control arm (Table 4).[20,23-26,32,33,45]

CONCLUSION

There is major paradigm shift in acute ischemic stroke care in last few years. Recent trials have shown significant reduction of disability in patients receiving EMT and are now the standard of care in selected patients of acute ischemic stroke with LVO. Ongoing research has improved the understanding of ischemic stroke. Improvement in imaging software with better understating of pathogenesis has allowed for precise patient selection. Continuous advances in hardware, especially thrombectomy devices, have allowed quick and safe thrombectomy. Now there is more focus on tissue window as oppose to time windows. Mechanical thrombectomy in patients with large infarct core at presentation needs further research, so as to become a standard of care.

REFERENCES

1. Hatano S. Experience from a multicentre stroke register: a preliminary report. Bull World Health Organ. 1976;54(5):541-53.
2. Caplan LR. Basic pathology, anatomy, and pathophysiology of stroke. In: Caplan's Stroke: A Clinical Approach, 4th edition. Philadelphia, PA: Elsevier Saunders; 2009. p. 22.
3. Chugh SS, Havmoeller R, Narayanan K, et al. Worldwide epidemiology of atrial fibrillation: a Global Burden of Disease 2010 Study. Circulation. 2014;129:837-47.
4. Harrison MJ, Marshall J. Atrial fibrillation, TIAs and completed strokes. Stroke 1984;15(3):441-2.
5. Chesebro JH, Fuster V, Halperin JL. Atrial fibrillation—risk marker for stroke. N Engl J Med. 1990;323:1556-8.
6. Lodder J, Bamford JM, Sandercock PA, et al. Are hypertension or cardiac embolism likely causes of lacunar infarction? Stroke. 1990;21:375-81.

7. Larsen BS, Kumarathurai P, Falkenberg J, et al. Excessive atrial ectopy and short atrial runs increase the risk of stroke beyond incident atrial fibrillation. J Am Coll Cardiol. 2015;66:232-41.
8. Kamel H, Elkind MS, Bhave PD, et al. Paroxysmal supraventricular tachycardia and the risk of ischemic stroke. Stroke. 2013;44:1550-4.
9. Kamel H, O'Neal WT, Okin PM, et al. Electrocardiographic left atrial abnormality and stroke subtype in the atherosclerosis risk in communities study. Ann Neurol. 2015;78:670-8.
10. Kamel H, Soliman EZ, Heckbert SR, et al. P-wave morphology and the risk of incident ischemic stroke in the Multi-Ethnic Study of Atherosclerosis. Stroke. 2014;45:2786-88.
11. Kamel H, Hunter M, Moon YP, et al. Electrocardiographic left atrial abnormality and risk of stroke: Northern Manhattan Study. Stroke. 2015;46:3208-12.
12. Kamel H, Okin PM, Elkind MS, et al. Atrial fibrillation and mechanisms of stroke: time for a new model. Stroke. 2016;47(3):895-900.
13. National Institute of Neurological Disorders and Stroke rt-PA Study Group. Tissue plasminogen activator for acute ischemic stroke. N Engl J Med. 1995;333:1581-7.
14. Hacke W, Kaste M, Bluhmki E, et al. Thrombolysis with alteplase 3 to 4.5 hours after acute ischemic stroke. N Engl J Med. 2008;359:1317-29.
15. Del Zoppo G, Higashida R, Furlan A, et al. PROACT: a phase II randomized trial of recombinant pro-urokinase by direct arterial delivery in acute middle cerebral artery stroke. Stroke. 1998;29:4-11.
16. Furlan A, Higashida R, Wechsler L, et al. Intra-arterial prourokinase for acute ischemic stroke. The PROACT II study: a randomized controlled trial. JAMA. 1999;282:2003-11.
17. Smith W, Sung G, Starkman S, et al. Safety and efficacy of mechanical embolectomy in acute ischemic stroke: results of the MERCI trial. Stroke. 2005;36:1432-8.
18. Smith W, Sunf G, Saver J, et al. Mechanical thrombectomy for acute ischemic stroke: final results of the multi MERCI trial. Stroke. 2008;39:1205-12.
19. The Penumbra Pivotal Stroke Trial Investigators. The penumbra pivotal stroke trial: safety and effectiveness of a new generation of mechanical devices for clot removal in intracranial large vessel occlusive disease. Stroke. 2009;40:2761-8.
20. Saver J, Goyal M, Bonafe A, et al. Stent-retriever thrombectomy after intravenous t-PA vs. t-PA alone in stroke (SWIFT-PRIME). N Engl J Med. 2015;372:2285-95.
21. Nogueira R, Lutsep H, Gupta R, et al. Trevo versus Merci retrievers for thrombectomy revascularisation of large vessel occlusions in acute ischaemic stroke (TREVO 2): a randomised trial. Lancet. 2012;380:1231-40.
22. Goyal M, Menon BK, Derdeyn CP. Perfusion imaging in acute ischemic stroke: let us improve the science before changing clinical practice. Radiology. 2013;266:16-21.
23. Berkhemer O, Beumer F, van den Berg L, et al. A randomized trial of intraarterial treatment for acute ischemic stroke (MR CLEAN). N Engl J Med. 2015;372:11-20.
24. Goyal M, Demchuk A, Menon B. Randomized assessment of rapid endovascular treatment of ischemic stroke (ESCAPE). N Engl J Med. 2015;372:1019-30.
25. Campbell B, Mitchell P, Kleinig T, et al. Endovascular therapy for ischemic stroke with perfusion-imaging selection (EXTEND-IA). N Engl J Med. 2015;372:1009-18.
26. Jovin T, Chamorro A, Cobo E, et al. Thrombectomy within 8 hours after symptom onset in ischemic stroke (REVASCAT). N Engl J Med. 2015;372:2296-306.
27. Kidwell CS, Jahan R, Gornbein J, et al. A trial of imaging selection and endovascular treatment for ischemic stroke. N Engl J Med. 2013;368:914-23.
28. Broderick JP, Palesch YY, Demchuk AM, et al. Endovascular therapy after intravenous t-PA versus t-PA alone for stroke. N Engl J Med. 2013;368:893-903.
29. Ciccone A, Valvassori L, Nichelatti M, et al. SYNTHESIS expansion investigators. Endovascular treatment for acute ischemic stroke. N Engl J Med. 2013;368:904-13.
30. Goyal M, Almekhlafi MA, Fan L, et al. Evaluation of interval times from onset to reperfusion in patients undergoing endovascular therapy in the Interventional Management of Stroke III trial. Circulation. 2014;130:265-72.
31. Gilgen MD, Klimek D, Liesirova KT, et al. Younger stroke patients with large pretreatment diffusion weighted imaging lesions may benefit from endovascular treatment. Stroke. 2015;46:2510-6.
32. Nogueira RG, Jadhav AP, Haussen DC, et al. Thrombectomy 6 to 24 hours after stroke with a mismatch between deficit and infarct. N Engl J Med. 2018;378:11-21.
33. Albers GW, Marks MP, Kemp S, et al. Thrombectomy for stroke at 6 to 16 hours with selection by perfusion imaging. N Engl J Med. 2018;378:708-18.
34. Yoo AJ, Zaidat OO, Chaudhry ZA, et al. Impact of pretreatment noncontrast CT Alberta Stroke Program Early CT Score on clinical outcome after intra-arterial stroke therapy. Stroke. 2014;45:746-51.
35. Gupta AC, Schaefer PW, Chaudhry ZA, et al. Interobserver reliability of baseline noncontrast CT Alberta Stroke Program Early CT Score for intra-arterial stroke treatment selection. AJNR Am J Neuroradiol. 2012;33:1046-9.
36. Menon BK, d'Esterre CD, Qazi EM, et al. Multiphase CT angiography: a new tool for the imaging triage of patients with acute ischemic stroke. Radiology. 2015;275:510-20.
37. Yoo AJ, Verduzco LA, Schaefer PW, et al. MRI-based selection for intra-arterial stroke therapy: value of pretreatment diffusion weighted imaging lesion volume in selecting patients with acute stroke who will benefit from early recanalization. Stroke. 2009;40:2046-54.
38. González RG, Copen WA, Schaefer PW, et al. The Massachusetts General Hospital acute stroke imaging algorithm: an experience and evidence based approach. J Neurointerv Surg. 2013;5(Suppl. 1):i7-12.
39. Hwang DY, Silva GS, Furie KL, et al. Comparative sensitivity of computed tomography vs. magnetic resonance imaging for detecting acute posterior fossa infarct. J Emerg Med. 2012;42(5):559-65.
40. Vergouwen MD, Algra A, Pfefferkorn T, et al. Time is brain(stem) in basilar artery occlusion. Stroke. 2012;43:3003-6.
41. Schonewille WJ, Wijman CA, Michel P, et al. Treatment and outcomes of acute basilar artery occlusion in the

Basilar Artery International Cooperation Study (BASICS): a prospective registry study. Lancet Neurol. 2009;8:724-30.
42. Abou-Chebl A, Lin R, Hussain MS, et al. Conscious sedation versus general anesthesia during endovascular therapy for acute anterior circulation stroke: preliminary results from a retrospective, multicenter study. Stroke. 2010;41:1175-9.
43. Jumaa MA, Zhang F, Ruiz-Ares G, et al. Comparison of safety and clinical and radiographic outcomes in endovascular acute stroke therapy for proximal middle cerebral artery occlusion with intubation and general anesthesia versus the nonintubated state. Stroke. 2010;41:1180-4.
44. van den Berg LA, Koelman DL, Berkhemer OA. Type of anesthesia and differences in clinical outcome after intra-arterial treatment for ischemic stroke. Stroke. 2015;46(5):1257-62.
45. Goyal M, Menon BK, van Zwam WH, et al. Endovascular thrombectomy after large-vessel ischaemic stroke: a meta-analysis of individual patient data from five randomised trials. Lancet. 2016;387:1723-31.

111

CHAPTER

Computed Tomography and Magnetic Resonance Imaging in Stroke

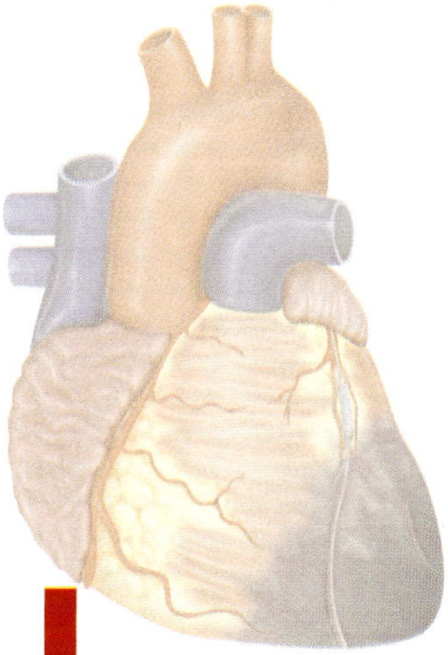

Vivek Lanka, Ajay Garg

INTRODUCTION

Twenty four centuries ago, when Greeks described a disease entity called "apoplexy" ("struck down by violence"), they had little understanding of brain anatomy and function. Over the years, as we grew wiser, we started calling it a "cerebrovascular accident" (CVA). Today, the WHO defines CVA as a clinical syndrome consisting of rapidly developing clinical signs of focal (or global in the case of coma) disturbance of cerebral function lasting more than 24 hours or leading to death with no apparent cause other than a vascular origin.[1] Pathologically, the process may be an ischemic or a hemorrhagic event.

ISCHEMIC STROKE

It is a CVA secondary to acute arterial occlusion and accounts for 80% of all strokes.[2] Ischemic brain parenchyma consists of a central core of infarcted tissue and a peripheral "penumbra" of hypoperfused tissue "at risk of infarction." The goals of imaging in acute ischemic stroke (AIS) are:

- Exclusion of hemorrhage [noncontrast computed tomography (NCCT)]
- Presence/absence of a large vessel occlusion (LVO) [computed tomography (CT) angiography]
- Estimation of volumes of infarcted and at risk tissues [CT perfusion (CTP)/magnetic resonance (MR) perfusion (MRP) ± MR diffusion].

The roles of various available imaging modalities are as follows:

Noncontrast Computed Tomography

It is often the first imaging modality used in CVA patients, because of its speed, widespread availability, and its accuracy in ruling out hemorrhage. AIS has some well-described early ischemic changes (EIC) in the hyperacute (0–6 hours) and acute (6–48 hours) phases on NCCT, which give a quick and approximate estimate of the infarct volume (Table 1) (Figs. 1A to D). It is often difficult to determine the true extent of these soft signs on NCCT images. Alberta Stroke Protocol Early CT Score (ASPECTS) is a 10-point semiquantitative topographic scoring system developed for determining the approximate volume of EICs on NCCT in patients with AIS involving the middle cerebral artery (MCA) territory.[3] The MCA territory is divided into 10 ASPECTS regions (Fig. 2): caudate (C), insular ribbon (I), posterior limb of internal capsule (IC), lentiform nucleus (L), anterior inferior frontal cortex (M1), anterior temporal cortex (lateral to the insular ribbon; M2), posterior temporal cortex (M3), anterior superior MCA cortex (ACA-MCA border zone; M4), posterior frontal cortex (M5), and parietal cortex (M6). The M4, M5, and M6 regions are the MCA territories immediately superior to the M1, M2, and M3 regions, respectively. For involvement of each of these regions, 1 point is subtracted from a total score of 10. Smaller scores represent larger areas of infarction. All slices should be inspected and each hemisphere should be scored separately.

Subacute phase (48 hours to 2 weeks) is marked by increase in hypoattenuation and mass effect. About 13–43%

TABLE 1: Early ischemic changes of acute ischemic stroke on NCCT (Fig. 1).

Sign	*Description*	*Confounders*
Hyperdense artery sign/MCA dot sign	Hyperdensity along the expected course of a thrombosed artery, most commonly MCA. High sensitivity (79%) and specificity (82%) for LVO	Polycythemia, dehydration, atherosclerosis—hyperdensity is usually symmetrical
Sulcal effacement and loss of gray–white differentiation ("loss of insular ribbon" in case of insula)	Loss of gray-white differentiation, with/without a hypodense cortex and poor definition of sulci	Asymmetric sections
Hypodensity/Poor definition of basal ganglia	Hypodensity in the basal ganglia, causing them to "merge" with the white matter	Other causes of basal ganglia hypodensities including hypoxia, hypoglycemia, viral encephalitis, etc.

(LVO: large vessel occlusions; MCA: middle cerebral artery; NCCT: noncontrast computed tomography).

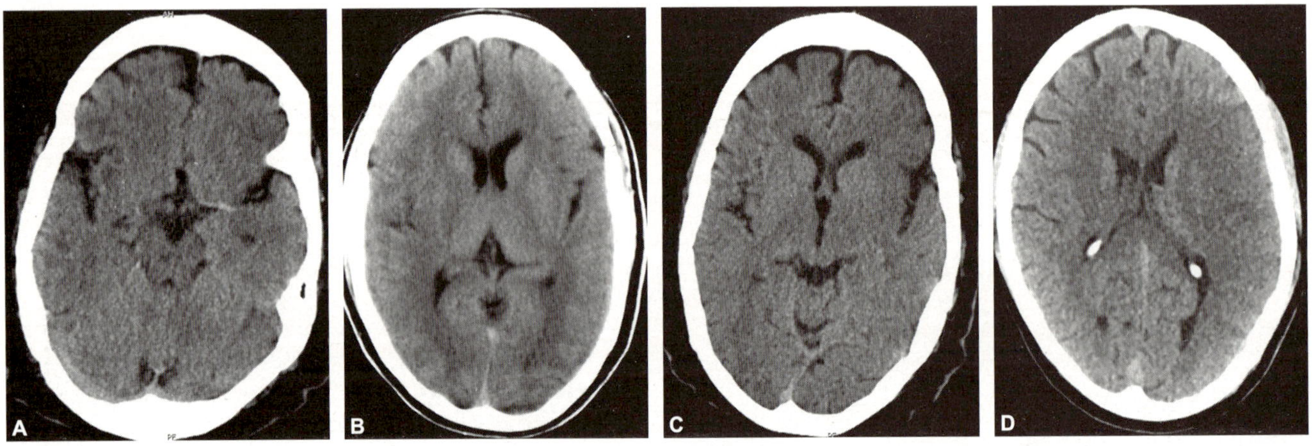

Figs. 1A to D: Common NCCT signs of AIS. NCCT axial sections of four different patients showing hyperdensity along the expected course of the left MCA ("Hyperdense artery" sign) (A); Loss of delineation of the left putamen, due to blurring of its gray-white matter interface and hypoattenuation (B); Hypodensity and loss of gray-white interface in the left insula ("Loss of insular ribbon" sign) (C); and Sulcal effacement and loss of gray-white matter interface in the superior part of the left MCA territory (D). (AIS: acute ischemic stroke; MCA: middle cerebral artery; NCCT: noncontrast computed tomography).

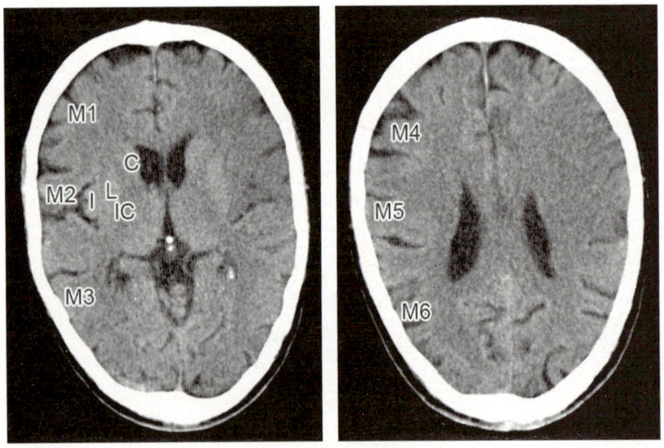

Fig. 2: Regional subdivisions of the MCA territory according to the ASPECTS. Two NCCT axial sections are shown showing the caudate (C), insular ribbon (I), posterior limb of internal capsule (IC), lentiform nucleus (L), anterior inferior frontal cortex (M1), anterior temporal cortex (lateral to the insular ribbon; M2), posterior temporal cortex (M3), anterior superior MCA cortex (ACA-MCA border zone; M4), posterior frontal cortex (M5), and the parietal cortex (M6). (ACA: anterior cerebral artery; ASPECTS: Alberta Stroke Protocol Early Computed Tomography Score; MCA: middle cerebral artery; NCCT: noncontrast computed tomography)

of infarcts may show internal hyperattenuating areas in varied morphological patterns suggestive of hemorrhagic transformation.[4] In the later part of the subacute phase, the decreasing mass effect and increasing attenuation of the infarcted cortex (attributable to lipid laden macrophages and capillary proliferation) result in poor contrast between the infarcted tissue and the surrounding normal parenchyma in about 50% of cases, the so-called CT fogging phenomenon.[5] When the diagnosis is in doubt, administration of iodinated contrast shows gyriform enhancement of the overlying cortex (cortical laminar necrosis), a phenomenon, which starts 2 days postictus, peaks at 2 weeks, and persists for 2 months.

Computed Tomography Angiography

Recently published American Heart Association guidelines for early management of stroke[6] as well as the results of the DAWN II (Data Analysis WorkbeNch II)[7] and DEFUSE III (Endovascular Therapy Following Imaging Evaluation for Ischemic Stroke III) trials[8] have emphasized the importance of early diagnosis of LVOs in AIS. A timely mechanical thrombectomy after careful patient selection in these patients shows a significant reduction in morbidity and mortality. Computed tomography angiography (CTA) is fast, widely available, and has a high diagnostic yield in diagnosing LVOs.[9,10] Other uses include:

- Road map for mechanical thrombectomy, including assessment of ease of vascular access across the aortic arch.
- Assessment for extracranial atherosclerotic/dissection-related occlusive vascular disease and the identification of candidates for interventions, such as carotid artery stenting and end-arterectomy[11] (Figs. 3A to F).
- Assessment of clot burden ("clot burden score") and collateral circulation (collateral scoring systems like), which predict the success of recanalization procedures and the overall prognosis.[12]

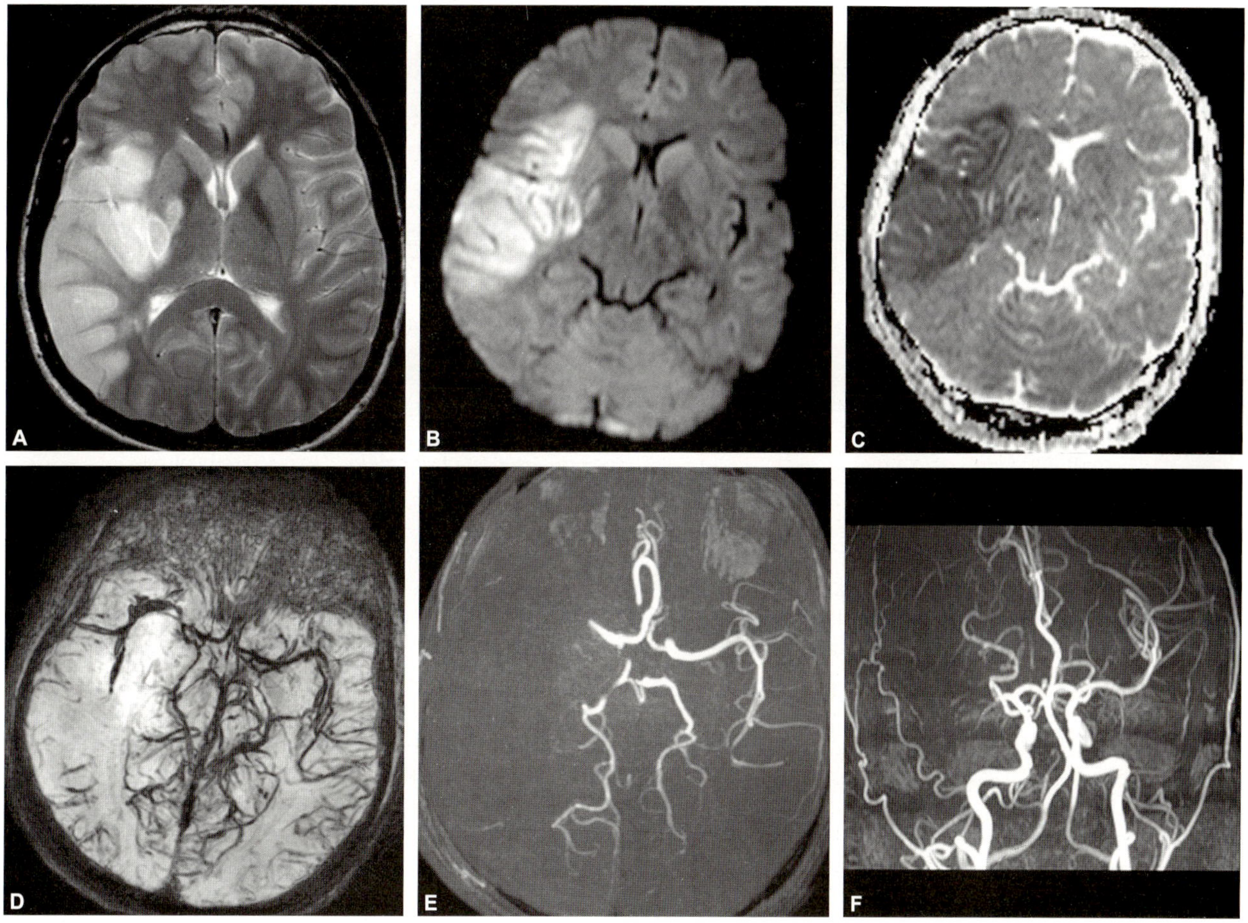

Figs. 3A to F: Appearance of an acute infarct on MRI. T2WI axial section shows hyperintensity and loss of gray-white differentiation in the right insula, posterior frontal, and anterior temporal lobes (conforming to the right MCA territory) (A). The lesion appears bright on DWI (B) and dark on ADC maps (C) suggestive of diffusion restriction. SWI shows blooming along the expected course of the right MCA suggestive of a thrombus (D) with a corresponding complete cutoff of the right M1 MCA seen on TOF-MRA images (E and F). (ADC: apparent diffusion coefficient; DWI: diffusion-weighted imaging; MCA: middle cerebral artery; MRI: magnetic resonance imaging; SWI: susceptibility-weighted imaging; T2WI: T2-weighted image; TOF-MRA: tetralogy of Fallot magnetic resonance angiography).

- Source images obtained during CTA compared with NCCT scans could be more sensitive in the detection of early irreversible ischemia and thus more accurate for the prediction of final infarct volume.[13]
- Information about vascular variants, which not only helps to guide catheter-directed therapies but also explains the nonpathological perfusion asymmetry that may be seen in perfusion studies.[14]

Computed Tomography Perfusion

Since its first description in animal models in the late 1970s, the "ischemic penumbra" has been a "hot cake" subject in stroke imaging. It is defined as "ischemic tissue potentially destined for infarction but is not irreversibly injured and is the target of any acute therapies."[15] One way to map it is by estimating the extent of reduction in tissue perfusion. In dynamic CTP, multiple CT acquisitions are done to monitor progressive attenuation changes after a bolus of contrast infusion. Pharmacokinetic modeling allows calculation of various parameters including cerebral blood flow (CBF), cerebral blood volume (CBV), mean transit time (MTT), and T_{max} (time to maximum residue function). Their color-coded maps are used to define the infarcted core and the penumbra. Areas showing increased MTT (>145% of normal contralateral parenchyma) and T_{max} (>6 seconds) represent the total hypoperfused brain while those showing reduced CBV (usually < 2 mL/100 g of tissue) represent the infarcted core.[8,16] The mismatch between CBV and MTT/T_{max} maps represents the penumbra, which is potentially salvageable with reperfusion. CBF is mildly reduced in the penumbra, while markedly reduced in the infarcted tissues (<20–30% that of normal contralateral parenchyma).[17] Although MRP was the initially studied modality, wider availability of CTP and the less time it takes when part of "stroke protocols", made it overtake MRP in the last few years. Its role in improving outcomes in AIS beyond 6 hours of onset was further highlighted in the recent DAWN II[7] and DEFUSE III trials.[8] Results of the DEFUSE III trial advocate endovascular management in patients with < 16 hours old strokes, core/penumbra volume ratio of 1.8, absolute penumbra volume of > 15 mL, and a core infarct volume of < 70 mL.

Magnetic Resonance Imaging, Magnetic Resonance Angiography, and Magnetic Resonance Perfusion

Salient imaging findings on standard MR imaging (MRI) sequences are summarized as follows in Table 2 (Figs. 4A to C).

TABLE 2: Sequence specific evolution of ischemic changes with time on standard MRI sequences.

Sequence	*Acute*	*Subacute*	*Chronic phase*
DWI	High signal on DWI and low signal on ADC (diffusion restriction) as early as within 15 minutes of ictus	Restriction peaks at 2–3 days and persists for 7–10 days. Pseudonormalization of signal on ADC at 1–2 weeks	Variable signal on DWI and usually high signal on ADC with associated volume loss
FLAIR	Loss of vascular flow void in the occluded vessel—as early as 0–2 hours. Initially isointense with hyperintensity and progressive loss of gray-white differentiation usually starting 6 hours postictus	High signal intensity, loss of gray-white differentiation and mass effect	Variable signal intensity (gliosis and cystic encephalomalacia) with volume loss
T1W1	Initially isointense. Low signal intensity after 16 hours	Low signal intensity. Cortical gyriform hyperintensity (cortical laminar necrosis) may start to appear after 3–5 days and peaks at 2 weeks	Low signal intensity with volume loss. Cortical gyriform hyperintensity (cortical laminar necrosis) may persist up to 2 months after which it disappears
T2W1	Loss of vascular flow void in the occluded vessel—as early as 0–2 hours. Initially isointense with hyperintensity and progressive loss of gray-white differentiation usually starting 8 hours postictus	High signal intensity, loss of gray-white differentiation and mass effect. "Fogging" phenomenon similar to that described on CT peaks at 2–3 weeks	High signal intensity with volume loss
T2 GRE/ SWI	HT is unlikely in the first 12 hours. Most microbleeds occur in the 24–48-hour period	Significant risk of HT exists up to 1 week, after which it is unlikely	Persistent hemosiderin deposits from an old bleed may be seen

(ADC: apparent diffusion coefficient; CT: computed tomography; DWI: Diffusion-weighted imaging; FLAIR: fluid attenuation inversion recovery; HT: hemorrhagic transformation; MRI: magnetic resonance imaging; T1WI: T1-weighted imaging; T2 GRE/SWI: T2-gradient echo/ susceptibility-weighted imaging; T2WI: T2-weighted imaging)

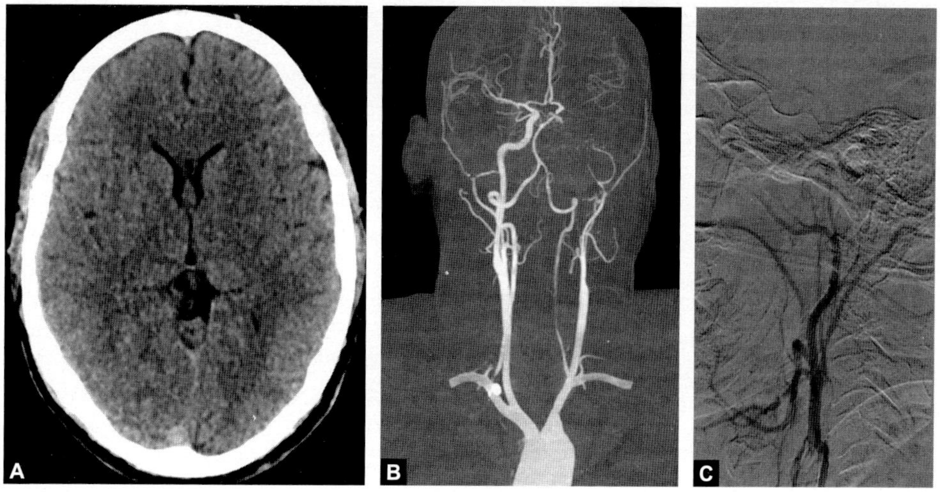

Figs. 4A to C: Infarct secondary to left ICA dissection. NCCT axial section shows poor delineation of the left putamen with loss of gray-white interface in the left MCA territory suggestive of an acute infarct (A). Reconstructed MIP of the CT angiogram of the same patient (B) and selective common carotid angiogram lateral view (C) of the same patient show tapering followed by complete cutoff of the left ICA at its origin suggestive of dissection. Left M2 and M3 MCA and the left ACA are seen to reform from collaterals. (ACA: anterior cerebral artery; CT: computed tomography; ICA: internal carotid artery; MCA: middle cerebral artery; MIP: maximum intensity projection; NCCT: noncontrast computed tomography).

Among all the available sequences, diffusion-weighted imaging (DWI) has the highest sensitivity and specificity to detect infarction in the acute and hyperacute stages and hence is the workhorse of AIS MRI. The lesions likely to be missed on DWI are usually lacunar infarcts in and around the basal ganglia and the brainstem. Diffusion-restricting parenchyma, in a patient with AIS, has been shown to accurately represent the irreversibly ischemic core.[18] Although there have been several reports of partial reversibility in the periphery of diffusion-restricting lesions,[19] they were confounded by the natural course of infarct volume loss and the transient normalization of diffusion with subsequent reappearance, which can occur in the first 24 hours postreperfusion.[17] At most centers, MRI is primarily used as a problem-solving modality in cases where a clinical diagnosis of AIS is equivocal (especially in posterior circulation stroke) or to time the infarct when the onset of ictus is uncertain. Many patients with uncertain time of stroke onset routinely get excluded from intravenous thrombolysis. Some authors have shown that an infarct, which shows restriction on DWI and is either partly or completely nonvisualized on the corresponding fluid-attenuated inversion recovery (FLAIR) images *(the DWI/FLAIR mismatch)*, is highly likely to be less than 4.5–6 hours old.[20-22] Studies using this "mismatch" to select uncertain stroke onset patients for thrombolysis have shown significant improvement in overall outcomes.[22,23] Although this approach may have a good specificity (78–100%) for selecting patients (especially for infarcts > 15 mL) who might be within the window period, it has poor sensitivity (56–62%) and may falsely exclude many patients from treatment.[22-25]

Dynamic susceptibility contrast (DSC) perfusion is the most commonly performed and the most well-studied MRP technique in stroke. It uses the T2* relaxation properties of a bolus of gadolinium contrast to generate time-dependent tissue concentration curves and follows similar principles as CTP (vide supra) to calculate perfusion parameters, such as CBF, CBV, MTT, and T_{max}. Unlike CTP, it provides whole-brain coverage and zero radiation exposure. However, like any other single compartmental model of perfusion assuming a nondiffusible tracer, it is prone to errors due to recirculation of contrast and leakage across the blood–brain barrier. Moreover, it is unreliable in the presence of hemorrhage, due to its unwanted T2* effects. It is commonly used in combination with DWI to map out the so-called *DWI//perfusion mismatch (PM)*. When the DWI lesion (which represents the ischemic core) is excluded from the total volume of hypoperfused parenchyma on MRP, the resultant "mismatch" forms an imaging surrogate for the ischemic penumbra.[26] The initial DWI lesion eventually grows to encompass nearly the entire hypoperfused volume if no reperfusion occurs. PM is known to mildly overestimate the penumbra, due to its inherent propensity to underestimate CBF and CBV in collateral perfused tissues (due to delay and dispersion of the arterial input function) as well as due to its inability to differentiate benign oligemia from ischemic perfusion.[26] Nevertheless, it has shown significant benefit in selecting patients for reperfusion therapies in several large clinical stroke trials, such as DEFUSE III, EXTEND

IA (Extending the Time for Thrombolysis in Emergency Neurological Deficits—Intra-Arterial), and SWIFT PRIME (Solitaire™ With the Intention For Thrombectomy as PRIMary Endovascular Treatment).[8,27,28]

Arterial spin labeling (ASL) perfusion labels blood protons in a proximal blood vessel with an excitation pulse and uses them as endogenous contrast material to be imaged at the slice of interest after a delay. Some recent stroke studies have demonstrated comparable estimates of penumbra between ASL and DSC perfusion.[29] ASL does not need contrast administration, allows repeated measurements, and offers absolute flow quantification (unlike relative quantification to normal contralateral parenchyma in DSC perfusion). However, it has lower signal-to-noise ratio compared to DSC and higher susceptibility to ASL-specific artifacts, such as vascular transit, and vessel-specific reduction in labeling efficiency in tortuous anatomy. *MR angiography (MRA)* is less popular than CTA in the setting of AIS, due to its inferior spatial resolution. However, it provides similar information as the latter in the case of LVOs, with no need for radiation.[30] MRA can be done with/without the use of intravenous contrast. Imaging protocol for AIS at our institution is summarized in Flowchart 1.

HEMORRHAGIC STROKE

It is a CVA secondary to an acute spontaneous intracranial bleed and accounts for 20% of all the strokes. Of this, about 15% are due to intracerebral hemorrhage (ICH) while the remaining 5% are due to subarachnoid hemorrhage (SAH).

Nontraumatic Intracerebral Hemorrhage

The goals of imaging in nontraumatic ICH are:

- Diagnosis of ICH
- Prognostication and assessment of risk of expansion
- Monitoring for mass effect and resulting complications
- Narrowing down the etiology for hemorrhage and guiding further investigation.

Computed Tomography

Sensitivity of NCCT for "clinically relevant" acute ICH is considered to be close to 100% and is the gold standard imaging modality for its detection. It is seen as a hyperdense space occupying lesion with surrounding edema and mass effect. Very rarely, a small isodense hematoma may result in a missed diagnosis, especially in cases with severe anemia.[31] NCCT helps in accurate volume estimation,

Flowchart 1: Imaging protocol for acute ischemic stroke. Protocol structured on the basis of guidelines issued by the AHA for early management of AIS in 2018.

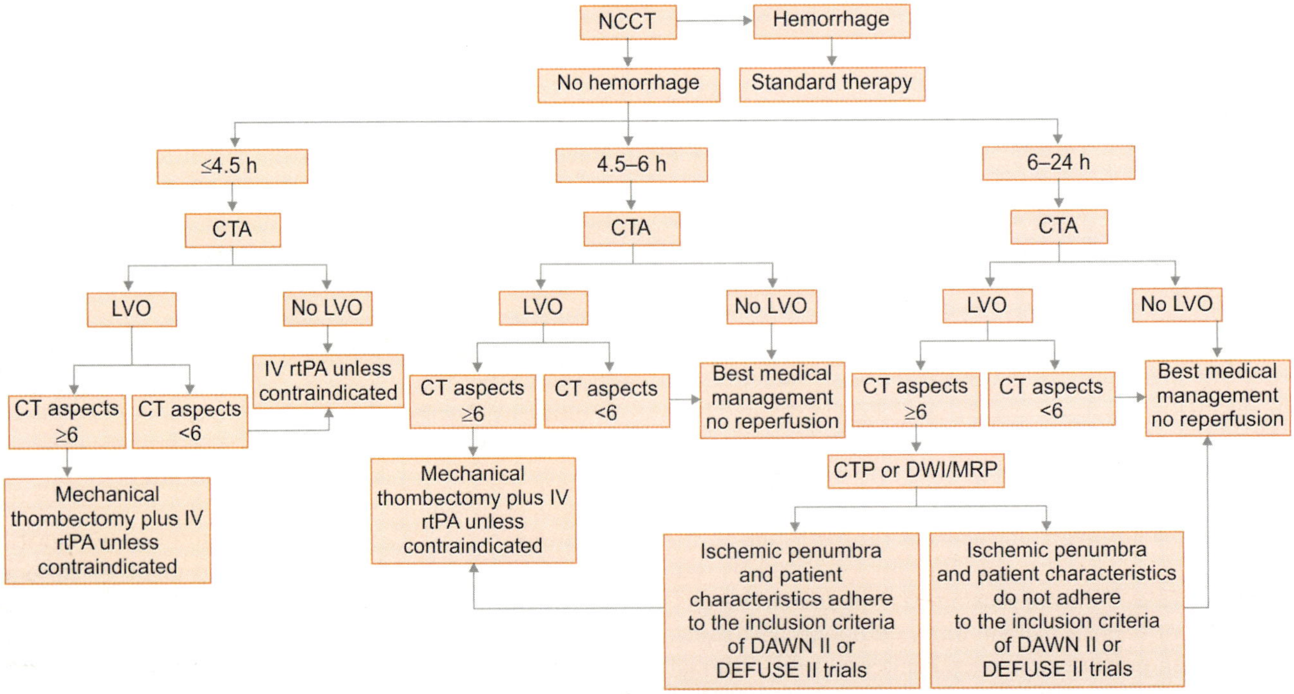

(AHA: American Heart Association; ASPECTS: Alberta Stroke Protocol Early Computed Tomography Score; AIS: acute ischemic stroke; CTA: computed tomographic angiography; CTP: computed tomographic perfusion; DWI: diffusion-weighted imaging; LVO: large vessel occlusion; MRP: magnetic resonance perfusion; NCCT: noncontrast computed tomography)

which in turn helps in initial prognostication as well as in monitoring for hematoma expansion.[32] In recent years, segmentation software and its derivative volumetry have superseded the traditional ellipsoid approximations. Volume overestimations are a common phenomenon with the latter.[33] Presence of isodense or hypodense areas within the hematoma (the "swirl sign") and contrast extravasation (the "spot sign") on CTA are predictive of significant hematoma expansion and mandate follow-up imaging at shorter intervals.[34] Cerebellar hematomas more than 3 cm in size need to be communicated to the surgeon immediately, as an early evacuation can be life-saving. Perihematoma edema usually peaks on the third day and lasts for about 5 days. Hematomas tend to become isodense between 1 week and 6 weeks, usually from periphery to center with progressive clot retraction and reduction in edema and mass effect. Fluid-fluid levels within a hematoma are rare, but fairly specific for an underlying coagulopathy.[35] However, this finding has been described in some large hypertensive bleeds, tumors, and vascular malformations as well.[35,36]

Magnetic Resonance Imaging

T2* gradient echo and susceptibility-weighted MRI are at least as sensitive as CT for acute ICH and are more sensitive for prior ICH.[37] Signal characteristics of a hematoma vary with time, depending on the varying molecular structure of its iron carrying proteins as well as its red cell membrane integrity.[38] These are summarized in Table 3 and help in approximate aging of the ICH. MRI also plays a vital role in diagnosing various secondary causes of ICH including vascular malformations, tumors, cerebral amyloid angiopathy (CAA), vasculitides and cerebral venous thrombosis (CVT) (see Table 4).

Etiology of Intracerebral Hemorrhage

Hypertension is usually the only identifiable etiology in most patients. MRI and vascular imaging help diagnose most other underlying micro- and macrovascular pathologies. However, selection of patients for further imaging is a subject of ongoing debate and varies widely among institutions. It has been shown that patients older than 55 years, with known hypertension (defined as previously diagnosed hypertension or electrocardiography changes of left ventricular hypertrophy plus a high blood pressure recording on admission) and a bleed in the thalamus, basal ganglia, or the posterior fossa have a very low probability of an underlying vascular pathology[39] (Figs. 5A to C). This subgroup does not need further imaging. All other scenarios need case-based selection of appropriate imaging modalities and their interpretation to arrive at the right diagnosis. Clues, which help to pick out some common etiologies of spontaneous ICH, are elucidated in Table 4.

Nontraumatic Subarachnoid Hemorrhage

Rupture of an intracranial saccular aneurysm (aneurysmal SAH/aSAH) is the most common cause of nontraumatic SAH, accounting for 85% of cases. Of the remaining 15%, 10% are due to perimesencephalic non-aSAH (an idiopathic bleed, confined to the perimesencephalic region attributed to venous causes) and the remaining 5% encompass a broad differential diagnosis including CAA, reversible cerebral vasoconstriction syndrome and other vasculitides, CVT, posterior reversible encephalopathy syndrome, arterial dissections, arteriovenous malformations, dural arteriovenous fistulas vascular tumors, such as hemangioblastomas, mycotic aneurysms, coagulopathy, and moyamoya disease.[40] On CT, SAH appears as a hyperdensity

TABLE 3: Temporal evolution of ICH on CT and MRI (1.5 T).

Approximate stage	*CT*	*Clinical biochemical forms*	*T1-weighted MRI*	*T2-weighted MRI*	*GRE MRI*
Hyperacute (<12 hours)	Hyperdense	OxyHb in RBCs	Isointense or mildly hyperintense	Hyperintense	Thin hypointense rim
Acute (12 hours to 2 days)	Hyperdense	DeOxyHb in RBCs	Isointense or hypointense	Hypointense	Hypointense rim that progresses to center
Early subacute (2–7 days)	Hyperdense	MethHb in RBCs	Hyperintense	Hypointense	Hypointense
Late subacute (8 days to 1 month)	Isodense	Extracellular MethHb	Hyperintense	Hyperintense	Hypointense
Chronic (>1 month)	Hypodense	Hemosiderin	Isointense or hypointense	Hypointense	Hypointense

(CT: computed tomography; DeOxyHb: deoxyhemoglobin; GRE: gradient echo; ICH: intracerebral hemorrhage; MethHb: methemoglobin; MRI: magnetic resonance imaging; OxyHb: oxyhemoglobin; RBCs: red blood cells)

TABLE 4: Pattern recognition clues to the etiology of ICH.

	Location	*Imaging*	*Comments*
Hypertension	External capsule/ putamen thalamus, pons	Acute hematoma with classical imaging findings	Suggest angiography unless all three criteria are met, i.e. age > 55 years, known hypertension and a deeply located bleed
Cavernoma	Pons—favorite location; abuts ventricular surface	"Popcorn"-like lesions on T2WI with hypointense rim (Figs. 6A to C)	May be associated with developmental venous anomalies—scan after intravenous contrast
Hemorrhagic transformation of infarct	Hemorrhage localized to cortex	Nonhemorrhagic component following a vascular territory	
Venous infarct	Hematoma in white matter or white matter-gray matter junction	Evidence of CVT, diffusion-variable. Disproportionate edema for the size of the hematoma (Figs. 7 and 8)	Parasagittal region if thrombosis is superficial; bithalamic if thrombosis is in deep venous system; posterior temporal lobe if vein of Labbe is involved
Cerebral amyloid angiopathy	Lobar bleed, spares basal ganglia	Multiple hemorrhages of different ages	Old age
Neoplasm	Anywhere in brain	Nonhemorrhagic component; heterogeneous; delayed evolution of signal changes; multiple stages of hematoma in the same lesion; absent, diminished or very irregular hypointense rim; persistent perihematoma edema and mass effect; inappropriate enhancement in acute lesion	
Aneurysm	Medial frontal lobe (ruptured anterior communicating artery or anterior cerebral artery aneurysm) or the temporal lobe (ruptured MCA aneurysm)	Associated parenchymal hematoma is not uncommon in patients with SAH due to saccular aneurysms	When ICH is immediately adjacent to the subarachnoid space at the base of the brain or basal interhemispheric fissure, vascular imaging should be strongly considered to exclude saccular aneurysm
Trauma	Orbitofrontal regions, anterior temporal lobes	Presence of fluid-blood level; evidence of head trauma-scalp hematoma, subdural/ extradural hematomas	
AVMs	Anywhere in brain	Suggestive but not sensitive imaging findings include dilated feeding and draining vessels on MR T2WI, CT angiography, or MR angiography, as well as patchy enhancement (Figs. 9A and B)	Young age

(AVMs: arteriovenous malformations; CT: computed tomography; CVT: cerebral venous thrombosis; ICH: intracerebral hemorrhage; MCA: middle cerebral artery; MR: magnetic resonance; SAH: subarachnoid hemorrhage; T2WI: T2-weighted imaging)

of the cerebrospinal fluid (CSF) within the sulcal spaces and/or the cisterns, with/without reflux into the ventricular system. It has decreasing attenuation and eventual disappearance with time. A modified Fisher grading system is used to grade the severity of SAH on NCCT with higher grades predicting poorer prognosis and greater risk of delayed cerebral ischemia.[41]

Common causes of false positives on NCCT include cerebral edema (venous engorgement and hypodense cortex), CVT (venous engorgement), beam-hardening artifacts in the posterior fossa and severe meningitis (iso- to hyperdense proteinaceous exudates). Sensitivity of NCCT for SAH depends on the amount of bleed as well as the time since ictus. The overall sensitivity is close to 100% in

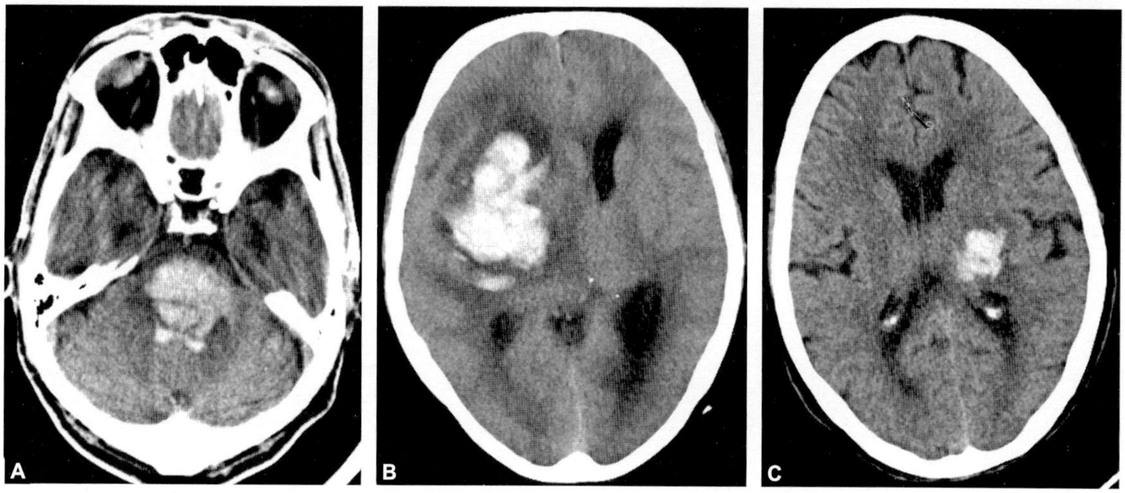

Figs. 5A to C: Common sites of hypertensive bleeding. NCCT axial sections of three different patients show hematoma formation in the pons (A), right gangliocapsular region (B), and the right thalamus (C). A patient who is a known hypertensive, over 55 years of age and has a bleeding in one or more of these sites has an extremely low probability of an underlying vascular pathology and a routine diagnostic DSA is redundant in such cases. (DSA: digital subtraction angiography; NCCT: noncontrast computed tomography)

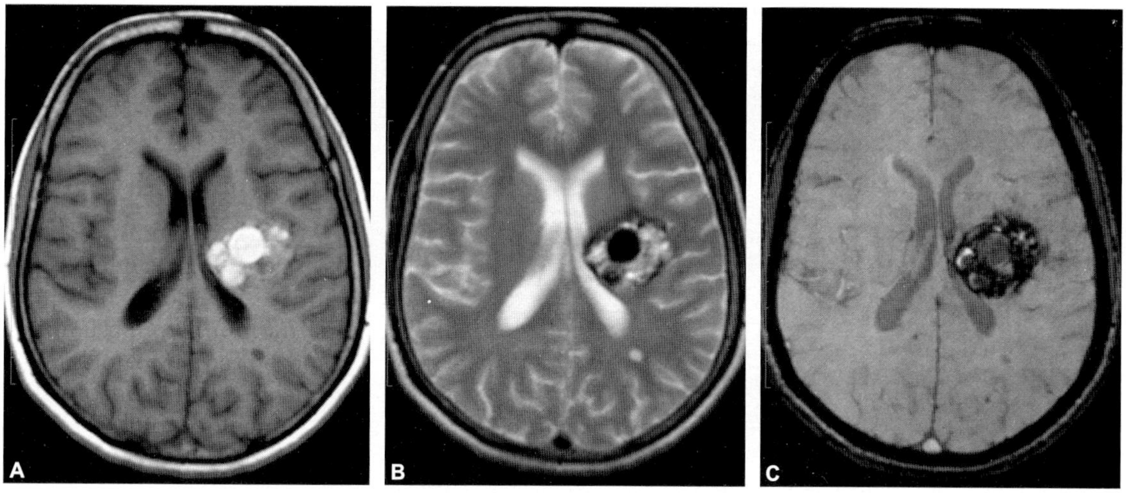

Figs. 6A to C: Appearance of a cavernoma with bleeding. MRI axial sections show a mass in the left corona radiata. On T1WI (A), it shows T1 hyperintense areas within it. On T2WI (B), the mass is "popcorn" like and has a T2 heterogeneous signal with markedly hypointense internal areas as well as a markedly hypointense rim surrounding it. These hypointense areas also show blooming on SWI (C) suggestive of blood products. (MRI: magnetic resonance imaging; SWI: susceptibility-weighted imaging; T1WI: T1-weighted image; T2WI: T2-weighted image)

the first 6 hours, 93% within the first 24 hours, 85% within 5 days, 60% within the first 1 week, and almost 0% at the end of 3 weeks.[42,43] Hence, within the first 6 hours, using thin section CT (1 mm), NCCT alone is sufficient to rule out SAH. Beyond 6 hours, using lumbar puncture (LP) for CT negative cases picks up nearly 100% of cases missed on CT.[43] In cases where LP is contraindicated or a less invasive alternative is sought, MRI detects additional cases to CT, especially in the subacute and chronic phases of SAH. T2 FLAIR is the most extensively studied MRI sequence for SAH detection, with sensitivity comparable to CT in the acute phase and better than CT in the subacute phase.[44] Common causes of false positivity on the FLAIR images include meningitis, hyperoxygenation therapy, and artifacts secondary to CSF flow and magnetic field inhomogeneities.

Diagnosis of an underlying aneurysm is paramount in a case of nontraumatic SAH (Figs. 10A and B) to prevent a rebleed. This has traditionally been done with digital

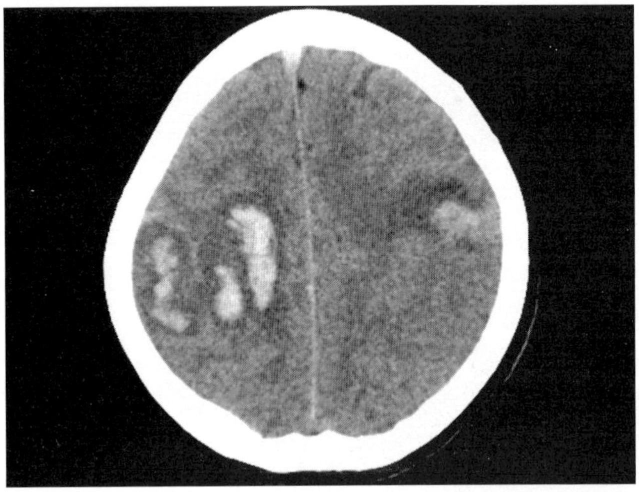

Fig. 7: NCCT appearance of a bleeding secondary to CVST. NCCT axial section shows bilateral parasagittal lobar bleedings along with a hyperdense superior sagittal sinus suggestive of thrombus formation. (NCCT: noncontrast computed tomography; CVST: cortical venous sinus thrombosis)

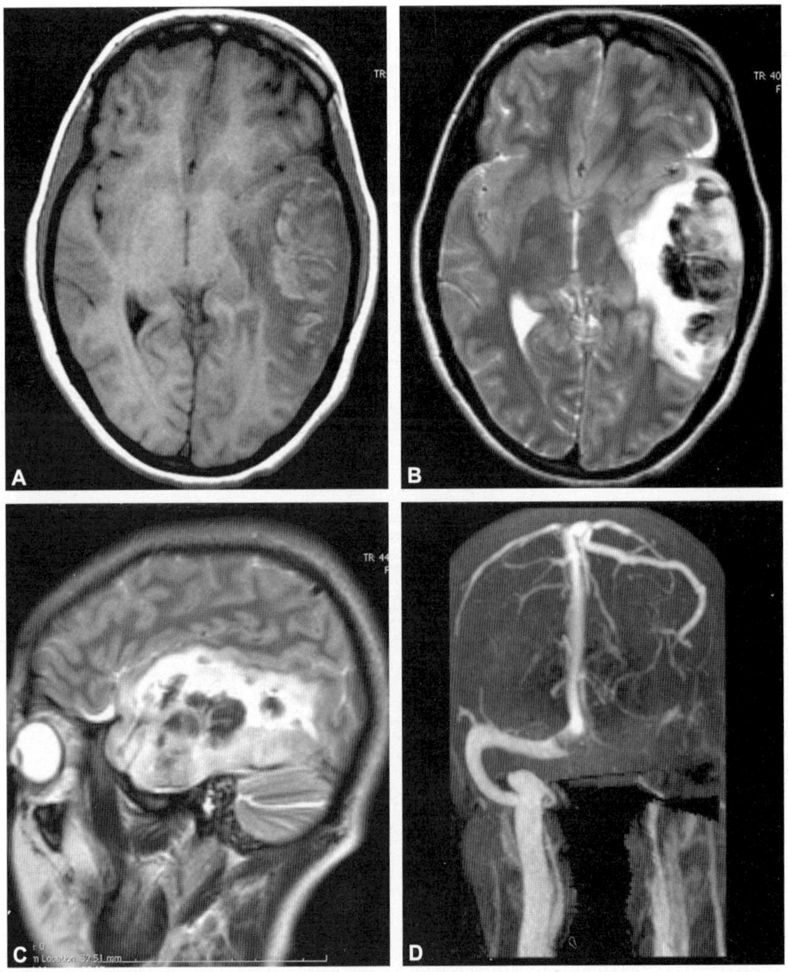

Figs. 8A to C: MRI appearance of a bleeding secondary to CVST. T1WI axial section (A) shows swelling of the left temporal lobe with T1 hyperintense areas within. T2WI axial (B) and sagittal (C) sections show a mass-like hemorrhagic lesion in the left temporal lobe with disproportionate amount of perilesional edema. Corresponding contrast-enhanced MR venogram MIP image (D) shows absence of contrast flow in the left transverse and sigmoid sinuses and a prominent ipsilateral superior superficial anastomotic vein. (CVST: cortical venous sinus thrombosis; MR: magnetic resonance; MRI: magnetic resonance imaging; MIP: macrophage inflammatory protein; T1WI: T1-weighted image; T2WI: T2-weighted image)

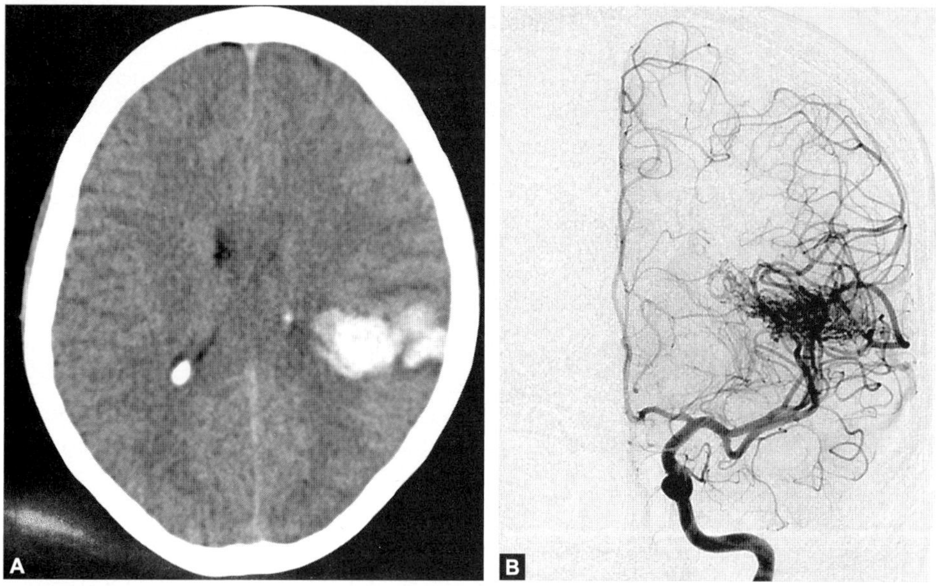

Figs. 9A and B: Intracerebral hemorrhage secondary to AVM. NCCT axial section (A) shows a left parietal lobar bleeding. Selective ICA angiogram AP view (B) shows a tangle of tortuous vessels deriving supply from left M3 MCA branches, suggestive of an AVM. Presence of a lobar bleeding in a young nonhypertensive patient should rise suspicion of an underlying vascular pathology and prompt a DSA. (AP: anterior-posterior; AVM: arteriovenous malformations; DSA: digital subtraction angiography; ICA: internal carotid artery; MCA: middle cerebral artery; NCCT: noncontrast computed tomography)

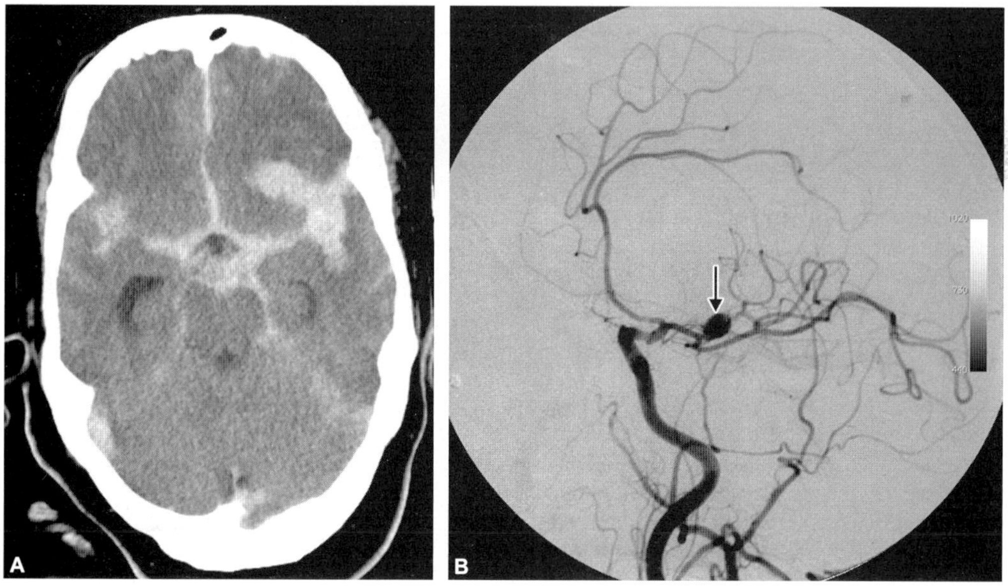

Figs. 10A and B: SAH secondary to an intracranial aneurysm. NCCT axial section (A) shows hyperdensity in the suprasellar cistern, bilateral ambient cisterns, anterior interhemispheric fissure, and the bilateral Sylvian fissures suggestive of SAH. The maximum thickness of the SAH is in the left Sylvian fissure (sentinel clot sign), pointing to the likely site of the aneurysm. Corresponding selective left ICA angiogram oblique view (B) shows a saccular narrow neck aneurysm at the left MCA bifurcation (arrow). (ICA: internal carotid artery; MCA: middle cerebral artery; NCCT: noncontrast computed tomography; SAH: subarachnoid hemorrhage)

subtraction angiography (DSA) and more recently with three-dimensional (3-D) rotational DSA (the current gold standard). Although CTA with new-generation scanners and near-perfect bone removal has achieved sensitivities comparable to DSA for aneurysms more than 3 mm,[43,45] most cases still need a 3-D rotational DSA for accurate depiction of neck and body morphology of these aneurysms, which in turn guides further management. High-resolution tetralogy of Fallot MRA has a lower sensitivity and poorer depiction of aneurysm morphology than CTA but is a viable alternative in patients with renal dysfunction or allergy to iodinated contrast media.[46]

CONCLUSION

"Time is brain" is probably the most clichéd yet the most important dictum in stroke management. Imaging plays central roles in timely classification and prognostication of stroke patients and in their assignment to a management pathway with the best possible outcome. Selection of an appropriate imaging modality according to the clinical scenario is as important as its quick and accurate interpretation. Hence, hospitals should strive toward establishment of standard operating procedures for managing stroke patients based on a thorough understanding in imaging.

REFERENCES

1. Hatano S. Experience from a multicentre stroke register: a preliminary report. Bull World Health Organ. 1976;54(5): 541-53.
2. Aguilar MI. Acute ischemic stroke and transient ischemic attack. In: Evidence-based Neurology: Management of Neurological Disorders. New Jersey, United States: Wiley-Blackwell; 2015. p. 53-66. [online]. Available from: https://onlinelibrary.wiley.com/doi/abs/10.1002/9781119067344.ch6 [Accessed October, 2018].
3. Prakkamakul S, Yoo AJ. ASPECTS CT in acute ischemia: review of current data. Top Magn Reson Imaging. 2017;26(3):103.
4. Zhang J, Yang Y, Sun H, et al. Hemorrhagic transformation after cerebral infarction: current concepts and challenges. Ann Transl Med. 2014;2(8):81.
5. Skriver EB, Olsen TS. Transient disappearance of cerebral infarcts on CT scan, the so-called fogging effect. Neuroradiology. 1981;22(2):61-5.
6. Powers WJ, Rabinstein AA, Ackerson T, et al. 2018 Guidelines for the early management of patients with acute ischemic stroke: a guideline for healthcare professionals from the American Heart Association/American Stroke Association. Stroke. 2018;49:e46-e110.
7. Nogueira RG, Jadhav AP, Haussen DC, et al. Thrombectomy 6 to 24 hours after stroke with a mismatch between deficit and infarct. N Engl J Med. 2018;378(1):11-21.
8. Albers GW, Marks MP, Kemp S, et al. Thrombectomy for stroke at 6 to 16 hours with selection by perfusion imaging. N Engl J Med. 2018;378(8):708-18.
9. Smith WS, Lev MH, English JD, et al. Significance of large vessel intracranial occlusion causing acute ischemic stroke and TIA. Stroke J Cereb Circ. 2009;40(12):3834-40.
10. Bash S, Villablanca JP, Jahan R, et al. Intracranial vascular stenosis and occlusive disease: evaluation with CT angiography, MR angiography, and digital subtraction angiography. Am J Neuroradiol. 2005;26(5):1012-21.
11. Abbott AL, Paraskevas KI, Kakkos SK, et al. Systematic review of guidelines for the management of asymptomatic and symptomatic carotid stenosis. Stroke. 2015;46:3288-301.
12. Puetz V, Dzialowski I, Hill MD, et al. Intracranial thrombus extent predicts clinical outcome, final infarct size and hemorrhagic transformation in ischemic stroke: the clot burden score. Int J Stroke. 2008;3(4):230-6.
13. Schramm P, Schellinger PD, Fiebach JB, et al. Comparison of CT and CT angiography source images with diffusion-weighted imaging in patients with acute stroke within 6 hours after onset. Stroke. 2002;33(10):2426-32.
14. Raghuram K, Hou BL, Roberts TD, et al. CT perfusion imaging pitfall related to fetal posterior cerebral artery. Am J Roentgenol. 2012;199(6):1371-4.
15. Fisher M, Ginsberg M. Current concepts of the ischemic penumbra: introduction. Stroke. 2004;35(11suppl 1):2657-8.
16. Lui YW, Tang ER, Allmendinger AM, et al. Evaluation of CT perfusion in the setting of cerebral ischemia: patterns and pitfalls. Am J Neuroradiol. 2010;31(9):1552-63.
17. Campbell BC, Parsons MW. Imaging selection for acute stroke intervention. Int J Stroke. 2018;13:554-67.
18. Baird AE, Benfield A, Schlaug G, et al. Enlargement of human cerebral ischemic lesion volumes measured by diffusion-weighted magnetic resonance imaging. Ann Neurol. 1997;41(5):581-9.
19. Kranz PG, Eastwood JD. Does diffusion-weighted imaging represent the ischemic core? An evidence-based systematic review. Am J Neuroradiol. 2009;30(6):1206-12.
20. Aoki J, Kimura K, Iguchi Y, et al. FLAIR can estimate the onset time in acute ischemic stroke patients. J Neurol Sci. 2010;293(1-2):39-44.
21. Thomalla G, Rossbach P, Rosenkranz M, et al. Negative fluid-attenuated inversion recovery imaging identifies acute ischemic stroke at 3 hours or less. Ann Neurol. 2009;65(6):724-32.
22. Thomalla G, Cheng B, Ebinger M, et al. DWI-FLAIR mismatch for the identification of patients with acute ischaemic stroke within 4·5 h of symptom onset (PRE-FLAIR): a multicentre observational study. Lancet Neurol. 2011;10(11):978-86.
23. Mourand I, Milhaud D, Arquizan C, et al. Favorable bridging therapy based on DWI-FLAIR mismatch in patients with unclear-onset stroke. Am J Neuroradiol. 2016;37(1):88-93.
24. Jeong JY, Han SK, Shin DH, et al. Diffusion-weighted imaging–fluid-attenuated inversion recovery mismatch is associated with better neurologic response to intravenous thrombolytic therapy in acute ischemic stroke patients. Clin Exp Emerg Med. 2015;2(1):31-7.
25. Odland A, Særvoll P, Advani R, et al. Are the current MRI criteria using the DWI-FLAIR mismatch concept for selection of patients with wake-up stroke to thrombolysis excluding too many patients? Scand J Trauma Resusc Emerg Med. 2015;23:22.
26. Chen F, Ni YC. Magnetic resonance diffusion-perfusion mismatch in acute ischemic stroke: an update. World J Radiol. 2012;4(3):63-74.
27. Campbell BCV, Mitchell PJ, Kleinig TJ, et al. Endovascular therapy for ischemic stroke with perfusion-imaging selection. N Engl J Med. 2015;372(11):1009-18.

28. Saver JL, Goyal M, Bonafe A, et al. Stent-retriever thrombectomy after intravenous t-PA vs. t-PA alone in stroke. N Engl J Med. 2015;372(24):2285-95.
29. Wang DJJ, Alger JR, Qiao JX, et al. The value of arterial spin-labeled perfusion imaging in acute ischemic stroke: comparison with dynamic susceptibility contrast-enhanced MRI. Stroke. 2012;43(4):1018-24.
30. Vymazal J, Rulseh AM, Keller J, et al. Comparison of CT and MR imaging in ischemic stroke. Insights Imaging. 2012;3(6):619-27.
31. Packard AS, Kase CS, Aly AS, et al. Computed tomography-negative intracerebral hemorrhage: case report and implications for management. Arch Neurol. 2003;60(8):1156-9.
32. Chang GY. Hematoma growth is a determinant of mortality and poor outcome after intracerebral hemorrhage. Neurology. 2018;66(8):1175-81.
33. Divani AA, Majidi S, Luo X, et al. The ABCs of accurate volumetric measurement of cerebral hematoma. Stroke. 2011;42(6):1569-74.
34. Ng D, Churilov L, Mitchell P, et al. The CT swirl sign is associated with hematoma expansion in intracerebral hemorrhage. Am J Neuroradiol. 2018;39(2):232-7.
35. Pfleger MJ, Hardee EP, Contant CF, et al. Sensitivity and specificity of fluid-blood levels for coagulopathy in acute intracerebral hematomas. AJNR Am J Neuroradiol. 1994;15(2):217-23.
36. Sawaya R, Rämö OJ, Shi ML, et al. Biological significance of tissue plasminogen activator content in brain tumors. J Neurosurg. 1991;74(3):480-6.
37. Hemphill JC, Greenberg SM, Anderson CS, et al. Guidelines for the management of spontaneous intracerebral hemorrhage: a guideline for healthcare professionals from the American Heart Association/American Stroke Association. Stroke. 2015;46(7):2032-60.
38. Saad AF, Chaudhari R, Fischbein NJ, et al. Intracranial hemorrhage imaging. Semin Ultrasound CT MRI. 2018;39(5):441-56.
39. Kamel H, Navi BB, Hemphill JC. A rule to identify patients who require magnetic resonance imaging after intracerebral hemorrhage. Neurocrit Care. 2013;18(1):59-63.
40. Marder CP, Narla V, Fink JR, et al. Subarachnoid hemorrhage: beyond aneurysms. Am J Roentgenol. 2013;202(1):25-37.
41. Frontera JA, Claassen J, Schmidt JM, et al. Prediction of symptomatic vasospasm after subarachnoid hemorrhage: the modified fisher scale. Neurosurgery. 2006;59(1):21-7.
42. van Gijn J, van Dongen KJ. The time course of aneurysmal haemorrhage on computed tomograms. Neuroradiology. 1982;23(3):153-6.
43. de Oliveira Manoel AL, Mansur A, Murphy A, et al. Aneurysmal subarachnoid haemorrhage from a neuro-imaging perspective. Crit Care. 2014;18(6):557.
44. Abdel Ghaffar MK, Eleya RZ, Nassef MA. Detection of acute small amount of subarachnoid hemorrhage: comparison between fluid-attenuated inversion recovery MR imaging and CT. Egypt J Radiol Nucl Med. 2014;45(3):833-9.
45. Chen W, Xing W, Peng Y, et al. Cerebral aneurysms: accuracy of 320-detector row nonsubtracted and subtracted volumetric CT angiography for diagnosis. Radiology. 2013;269(3):841-9.
46. Farahmand M, Farahangiz S, Yadollahi M. Diagnostic accuracy of magnetic resonance angiography for detection of intracranial aneurysms in patients with acute subarachnoid hemorrhage; a comparison to digital subtraction angiography. Bull Emerg Trauma. 2013;1(4):147-51.

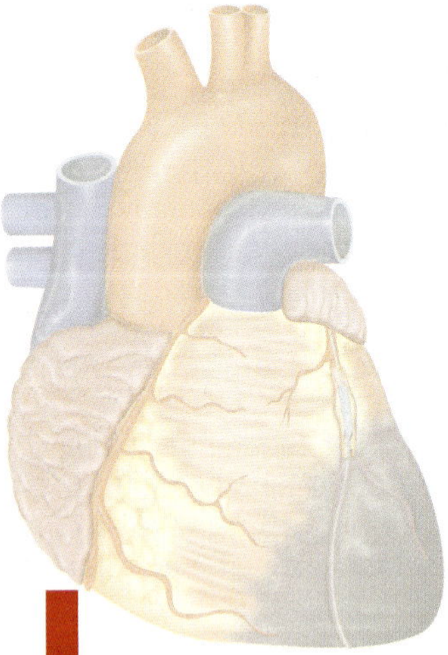

CHAPTER 112

Recent Advances in Neurointervention

Sanjeev Kumar, Tariq Matin

INTRODUCTION

The field of neurointerventional surgery has emerged in recent decades to provide safe and effective options for the treatment of intracranial aneurysms.

The first experience with cerebral angiography was reported by Portuguese doctor Egas Moniz at the University of Lisbon, in order to identify central nervous system (CNS) diseases, such as tumors or arteriovenous malformations (AVMs). He performed the first brain angiography in Lisbon in 1927 by injecting iodinated contrast medium into a carotid and using the X-rays to visualize the cerebral vessels.[1] In precomputed tomography (CT) and premagnetic resonance imaging era, it was the only tool to observe the structures within the skull and was also used to diagnose extravascular pathologies.

Subsequently, European radiologists further developed the angiographic technic by replacing the traumatic direct puncture with catheterization. In 1953, Swedish physician Sven Seldinger introduced the technique of arterial and venous catheterization, which is still in practice. In 1964, the Norwegian radiologist, Amudsen, was the first to perform a complete brain angiography with a transfemoral approach, as it is performed today. He then moved to San Francisco to teach the technique to American neuroradiologists. These two stages, at the basis of modern invasive vascular diagnostics, prepared the way for later therapeutic developments.

EVOLUTION OF NEUROCATHETERIZATION LABORATORY

X-ray based catheterization laboratory suites having subtraction and roadmap software are the workplace of all the neuroendovascular procedures. Tremendous developments have happened in the tube technology and image processing hardwares to obtain good-quality images while not trading with radiation dosages, which always has remained of concern both with the medical personnel and patients. In fact, newer machines have got radiation reduction programs which have served the purpose immensely.

Biplanar systems have increased the safety and feasibility of the more and more complex procedures. Add-on processing software, such as three-dimensional (3D) rotational angiogram, cone beam CT technology, perfusion and flow dynamics software, have aided a great deal with leaving nothing for imagination (Figs. 1 and 2).

ACCESS SYSTEM

For nearly all the neuroendovascular procedures, the access is taken from femoral artery. The success for the endovascular procedures depends upon the stable access below. Distal reach as far as possible have enabled us to accomplish procedures, which were unimaginable few years back.

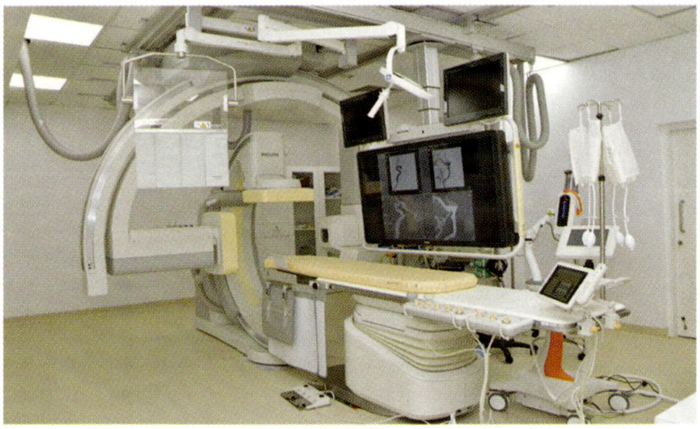

Fig. 1: The Biplane Neuro cath Lab. Philips Allura FD 20.

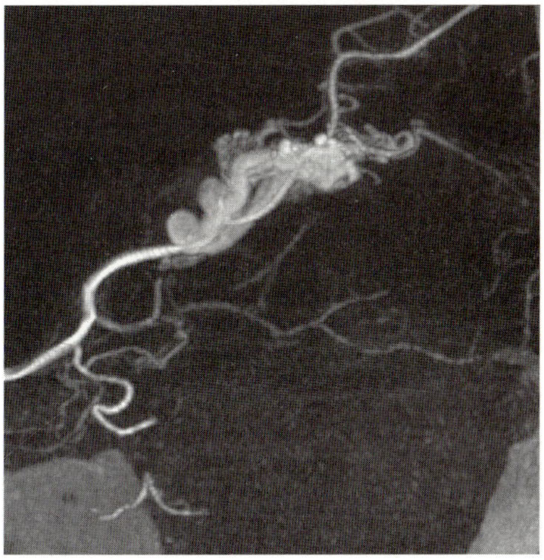

Fig. 2: Cone Beam CT angio showing site of ruptured leading to ICH.

Treatment of Cerebral Aneurysms

While the first endovascular treatment of an intracranial aneurysm was performed in 1939, it was not until the mid-1970s that Gerard Debrun, the father of interventional neuroradiology, developed a detachable latex balloon catheter for the treatment of carotid-cavernous fistulae and giant intracavernous aneurysms. This was followed by a report of 300 patients treated via an endovascular approach by Serbinenko using a modified version of Debrun's catheter.

By 1990, the invention of the Guglielmi detachable coils by Guido Guglielmi, an Italian neurosurgeon, was set to change intracranial aneurysm treatment.

International Subarachnoid Aneurysm Trial 1 and 2[2]

The International Subarachnoid Aneurysm Trial (ISAT) in 2005 compared endovascular with open surgical treatment of ruptured intracranial aneurysms and showed that endovascular coiling resulted in better independent survival at 1 year, with absolute risk reduction of 7.4% [95% confidence interval (3.6–11.2), p = 0.0001].

The results showed that the early survival advantage was maintained for up to 7 years and was significant in patients treated with endovascular technics (p = 0.03). The risk of epilepsy was substantially lower in patients allocated to the endovascular treatment group but the risk of late rebleeding was higher. This treatment effect continued for at least 7 years. The conclusion was that in patients with ruptured intracranial aneurysms suitable for both types of treatments, endovascular and microsurgery, endovascular therapy is more likely to result in independent survival at 1 year and at 84 months. Despite the fact that rebleeding has a higher incidence with endovascular therapy, the survival benefit continues for 7 years on the basis of data from ISAT 2 (Figs. 3A to E).

Barrows Trial[3]

The strongest criticism of the ISAT was the design of the study promoting cherry picking and influencing the outcome. To address the issue of the broader applicability of the ISAT results, the Barrow Ruptured Aneurysm Trial (BRAT) used a prospective intent-to-treat design that randomized all patients admitted with a diagnosis of subarachnoid hemorrhage. The 1-, 3- and 6-year results have been published. Although BRAT was statistically underpowered to detect small differences, these results suggest little difference in outcome between the two treatments for anterior circulation aneurysms. This was not the case for the posterior circulation aneurysms, where coil embolization appeared to provide a sustained advantage over clipping. Aneurysm obliteration rates in BRAT were significantly lower and retreatment rates significantly higher in the patients undergoing coiling than in those undergoing clipping.

However, despite the fact that retreatment rates were higher after coiling, no recurrent hemorrhages were known to have occurred in patients undergoing coiling in BRAT who were followed up for 6 years. Sufficient questions remain about the relative benefits of the two treatment modalities to warrant further well-designed randomized trials. The BRAT remains an ongoing trial with a final follow-up to occur 10 years after the enrollment (Fig. 4).

Evolution in Coil Technology (Figs. 5 A to W)[4]

The development of detachable coils is one of the most pivotal developments in neurointervention, providing a tool that could be used to treat a wide variety of hemorrhagic stroke. From the original Guglielmi detachable coil, a

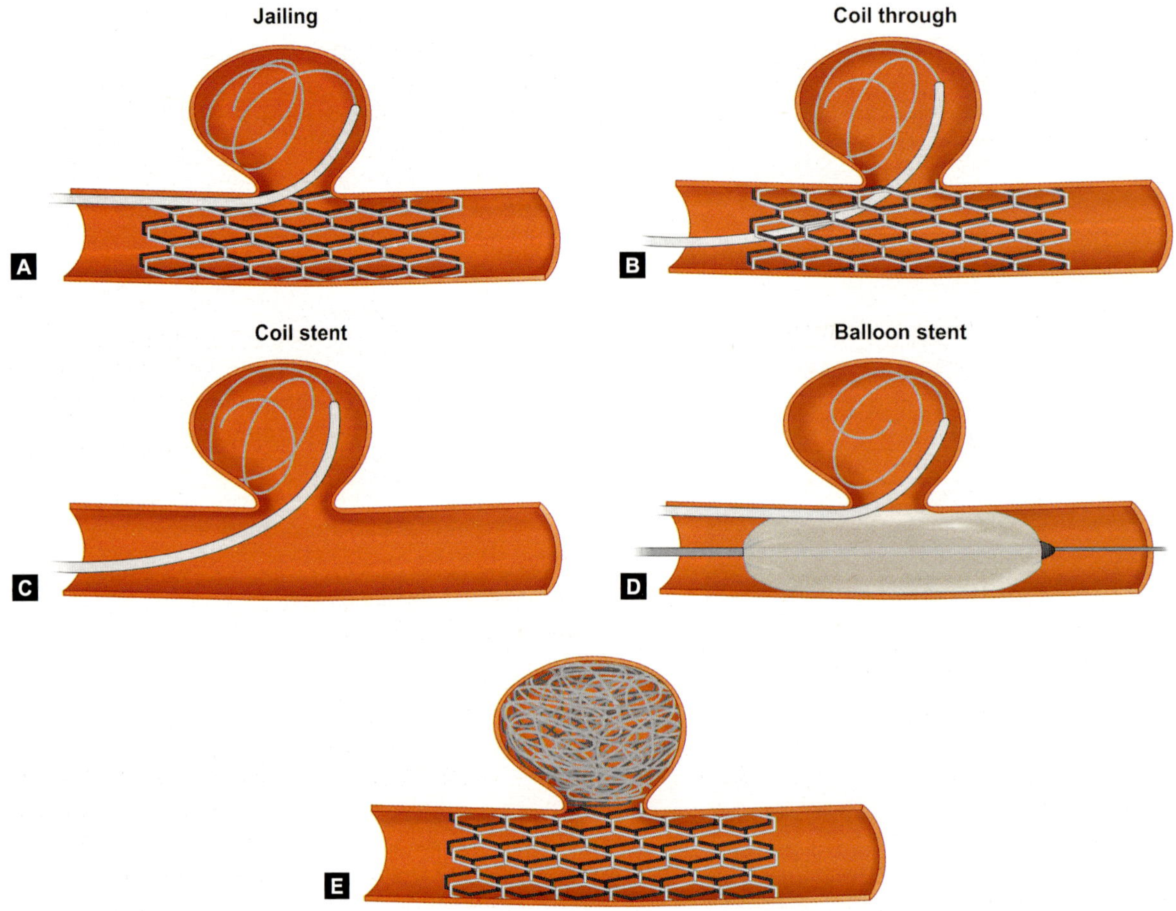

Figs. 3A to E: Coiling of aneurysm.

number of different coil designs and delivery designs have evolved.[5]

While it is likely that we do not yet fully understand the mechanism of coil function in aneurysms, case series histology reports have shown thrombus formation in the early phases after coil insertion. With later ingrowth of angiogenesis and scar formation, differing at the fundus, within and around the coil mass with demonstrable endothelialization.

Surgical experience with coiled aneurysms has anecdotally shown that coils are not irreversibly adherent to the aneurysm fundus during removal. Histopathologic analysis of bioactive and gel coils has also been performed. However, widespread histopathologic analysis of aneurysms has not been performed, and further insight into aneurysm pathophysiology and mechanisms of growth, recurrence, and progression is desirable.

The First Coil

The first commercially available detachable coil was relatively stiff by today's standards, helical, and most importantly, detachable. While the duration required for detachment ranged up to 45 min, the detachment mechanism allowed for controlled deployment, repositioning and removal. The helical morphology of the coil allowed the loops to

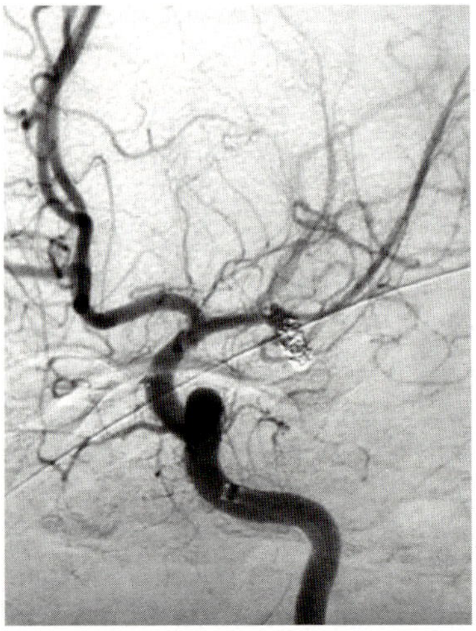

Fig. 4: Completely obliterated aneurysm with patent bifurcation.

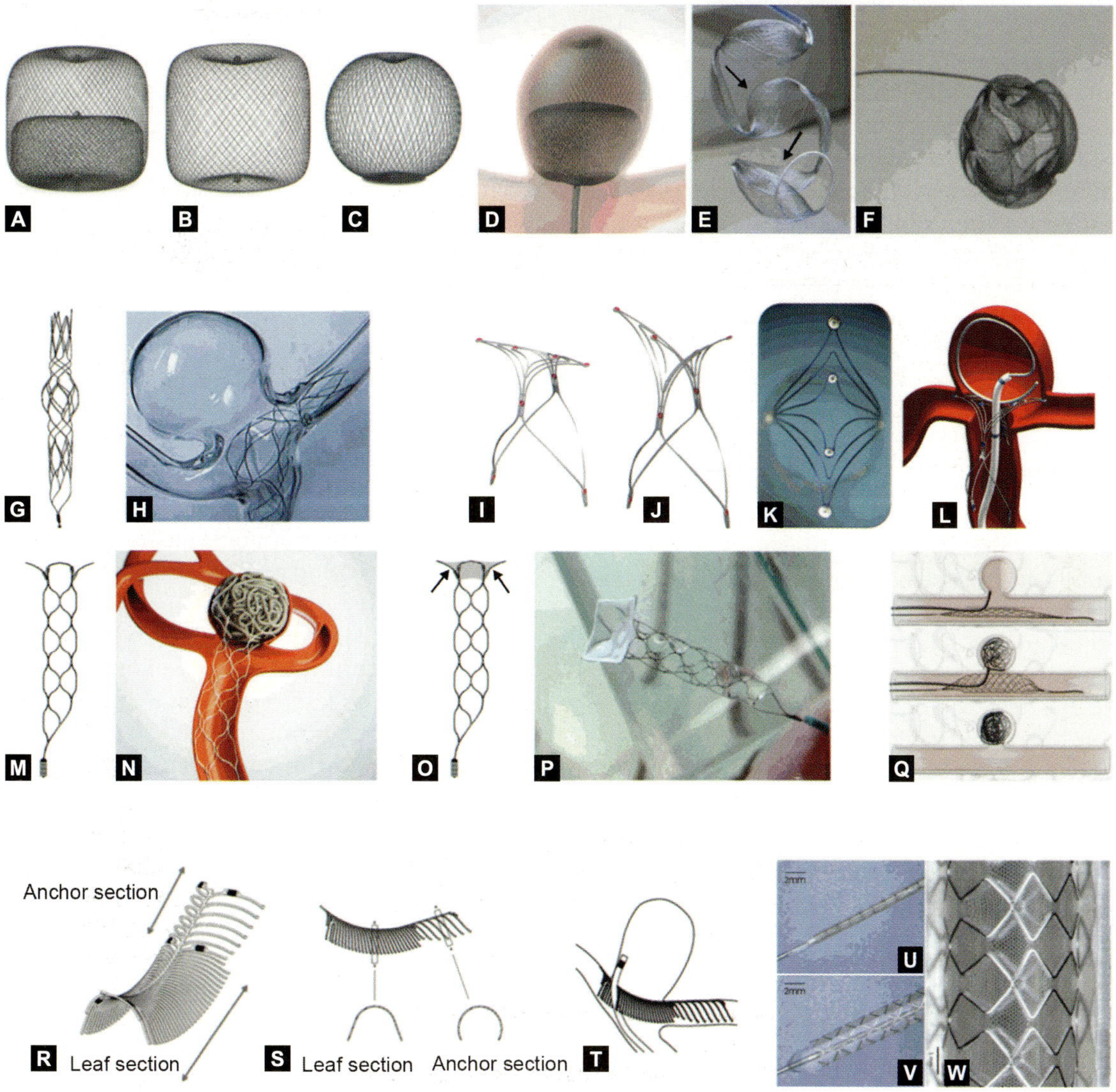

Figs. 5A to W: Development of new endovascular devices for aneurysm treatment.

approximate the periphery of the aneurysm at a given size. However, distribution of the two-dimensional design did not consistently allow for good neck coverage. Moreover, the initial cross-sectional diameter was small, and thus neck coverage in larger aneurysms was not reliable.

Three-Dimensional Coils

Target introduced a 3D coil with an intrinsic shape that would seek to retain a spherical overall configuration when fully deployed. These would become known as framing coils, which marked a major advance in the philosophy of aneurysm embolization. With a relatively robust frame bounding the neck and dome of an aneurysm, filling the frame with softer coils allowed the operator a greater "safety" margin in filling coil behavior as the frame would bound the outward movement of subsequent coils toward both the aneurysm dome and the parent vessel.

Finishing Coils

With both framing coils and two-dimensional helical filling coils, it was possible to fill much of most aneurysms. However, the irregular residual spaces in the coil mass were sometimes not spacious enough to allow for easy deployment of even small-sized helical coils. By introducing even softer coils (0.010-inch system) based around more filamentous core wires and less tightly wound secondary winds, coils better suited for filling in the small irregular residual space became available.

Stretch Resistance

The withdrawal of coils from the aneurysm sac would occasionally be complicated by the trapping or locking of the distal end of the coil within the coil mass. This effect would result in stretching and unwinding of the coil—and even fracture. Once the platinum coil unwinds, it is difficult or impossible to either advance the coil back into the aneurysm or withdraw the coil completely back into the microcatheter. The addition of a polymer filament in the center of the coil wind would resist stretching of the metallic coil, helping to maintain the desired physical characteristics of the implant. This feature became an essentially standard facet of coil design.

Material Choice

While platinum is now essentially the only primary material in clinical use, efforts were made to use other materials, such as nitinol and tungsten. The relative stiffness of these materials may have been an impediment to widespread acceptance and use. Platinum is an inert metal with material characteristics favorable for coil manufacturing. It is possible that new materials for coil embolization will be found in the future with benefits overexisting technologies.

Fibered Coils

Some coils, such as the VortX Coil (Stryker), or more recently, the Axium and polyglycolic acid (PGA)-fibered and nylon coils (ev3/Covidien) were designed with coils of polymer attached to the primary coil. The thinking behind the fibered coils was that the presence of the fibers might be useful in impeding blood flow and encouraging stasis and thrombosis. While these coil designs never became widely used or extensively studied, they remain an interesting concept.

Bioactive Coils

Since optimal aneurysm repair would result in endothelialization of the coil mass at the neck, the idea of a proinflammatory bioactive coil arose, ostensibly to accelerate the wound healing cascade and cellular ingrowth into the coil mass and at the neck. Early formulations of these coils included the original Matrix coil which was nearly 50% poly (lactic-co-glycolic) acid (PGLA) by volume, arranged at the outer surface of the coils.

The PGLA was reintroduced as a filament inside the secondary wind of the coil, thus limiting the degree of coil volume loss after PGLA dissolution. The Matrix 2 coil (Stryker) is of this design and was shown to be not inferior to bare platinum coils in the Matrix, and Platinum Science trial PGA21 is present in the Cerecyte22–24 coil series (Codman) and some of the fibered coils available from ev3/Covidien.

Packing Density and Hydrocoil

Packing density has been associated with a lower rate of recurrence by multiple authors, spurring the development of softer coils that can be placed to increase the volumetric fill from a coil during aneurysm embolization, with the most recent data from randomized controlled HELPS (HydroCoil Endovascular Aneurysm Occlusion and Packing Study) and GREAT trials.

Gel-platinum hybrid coils were introduced by Microvention, starting with nominal 0.018-inch system coils that swell to four times the volume once introduced into an aqueous milieu. While stiffer than equivalently sized coils during delivery, after delivery the coils would swell, increasing the volume of inserted coils, thus increasing the packing density of the coil mass. The initial acrylamide-based formulation was then extended to 0.012-inch system sizes and a 0.010-inch system. The hydrogel was wrapped by the secondary wind and provided a marked increase in coil volume.

The introduction of HydroSoft and HydroFrame coils reduced the amount of gel as well as changing the gel formulation. The later coils were constructed with gel inserted within the primary wind. With a lesser volume of gel, it softened the coils relative to earlier designs, also improving working time. For instance, the original Hydrocoil design had a limited working time and required heating in either steam or warm solution, whereas the new coils did not have such a limited working time.

Recent histopathologic data showed a reduced inflammatory response of gel-coated coils in comparison with bare platinum which is of uncertain effect. The HELPS trial showed a 7% reduction in recurrence rates in patients treated with hydrogel, but no statistically significant difference in outcomes compared with bare platinum coils. The role of gel in aneurysm coiling remains uncertain.

Remodeling Techniques[6]

Aneurysms with an unfavorable dome-to-neck ratio and wide-necked aneurysms with a favorable dome-to-neck ratio were exposed to the risk of coil protrusion or lower packing densities.

The balloon remodeling technique, as described by Moret et al., primarily offers temporary balloon inflation during coil delivery to achieve homogeneous packing density of wide-necked, complex-shaped cerebral aneurysms that otherwise would not be amenable to primary coiling without any coil protrusion into the parent artery. Despite the revolutionizing effect of the balloon remodeling technique on the era of wide-necked aneurysm treatment, low-compliant, over-the-wire balloons were limiting the applicability of the technique to sidewall

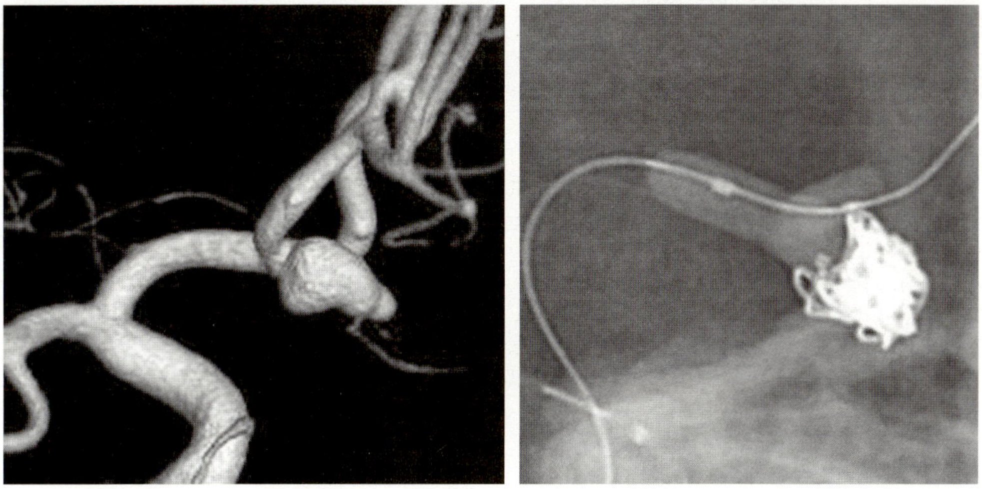

Fig. 6: Balloon remodelling technique for coiling broad necked a COM aneurysm.

aneurysms, while more compliant latex balloons glued to a flow-dependent microcatheter were providing less directionality, less stability, and less accurate balloon positioning across the aneurysm neck. In the subsequent years, a new, more compliant balloon microcatheter (HyperForm, ev3 Inc., Plymouth, MN) appeared on the market, offering trackability and accurate positioning over a specified 0.01-inch guidewire, along with the ability to adapt its shape to the anatomy of the arterial bifurcation by bulging into the aneurysm neck or the branches coming off the sac. From 0.010 wire to 0.012 wire and then 0.014 wire improved the trackability and navigability of the balloon to difficult arterial location (Fig. 6).

Double-Lumen Balloon

The Scepter balloon catheter (Scepter C™ or Scepter XC™, Microvention, Inc., Tustin, CA, USA) is a newly developed balloon catheter with a coaxial double lumen, which is compatible with any type of 0.014-inch micro-guidewire, and the other serves for balloon inflation.

STENTS[7]

The technique of stent-assisted coiling (SAC) in the clinical setting was first described in 1997. Soon after, the availability of new flexible, self-expanding intracranial stents allowed the increasing application of this technique and observation of its benefits (Fig. 7).[8]

Low-Profile Stents

Until recently, the deployment of self-expandable stents necessitated the catheterization of the parent artery with 0.021–0.027-inch microcatheters. Low-profile, self-expandable stents (BRAIDED LEO Baby and LVIS Jr NON BRAIDED ATLAS), deliverable through microcatheters with an internal diameter of 0.0165 inch, were developed in 2011. These low-profile stents allow easier catheterization and navigation in small-sized, delicate vessels and enable safer stent placement during the treatment of distal wide-neck aneurysms.

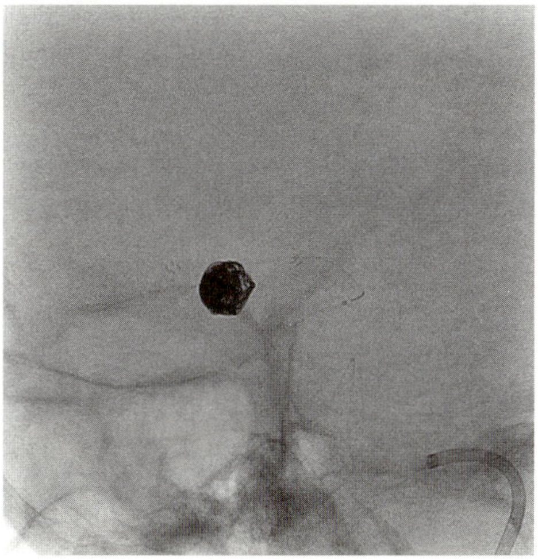

Fig. 7: Stent assisted coiling of broad neck aneurysm.

Baby stents are available with diameters of 2.0 mm and 2.5 mm and lengths of 12 mm, 18 mm, 25 mm, 30 mm, and 35 mm. These stents are labeled for deployment in arteries with diameters between 1.5 mm and 3.2 mm. Therefore, these are the only self-expandable stents that are labeled for deployment in arteries with diameters of less than 2 mm. Low-profile stents were successfully deployed in arteries with diameters as small as 1.3 mm. Furthermore, these stents could be deployed in branches having a diameter discrepancy of up to 60%.

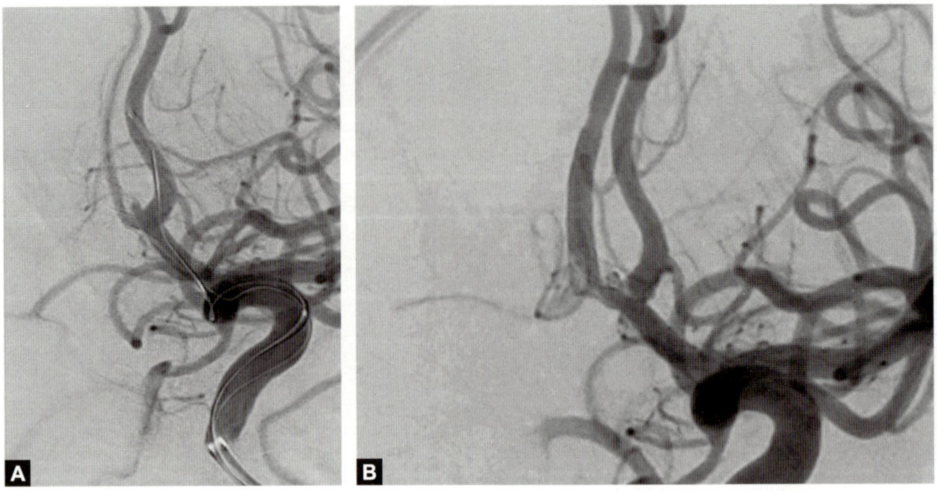

Figs. 8A and B: Baby Leo assisted coiling with shelfing technique.

These stents can be deployed in various configurations, such as X, Y, T, or half T to treat various complex aneurysms (Figs. 8A and B).

COMANECI

The Comaneci device represents a unique flexible mesh that allows for temporary neck bridging during embolization of the aneurysm while averting flow arrest. The Comaneci device is designed to bridge the neck of an aneurysm during coil embolization. It consists of a 183-cm length core wire with a diameter of 0.5 mm. The stent device is 32 mm in length but when fully expanded foreshortens to 20 mm with a 3-mm diameter (Fig. 9).

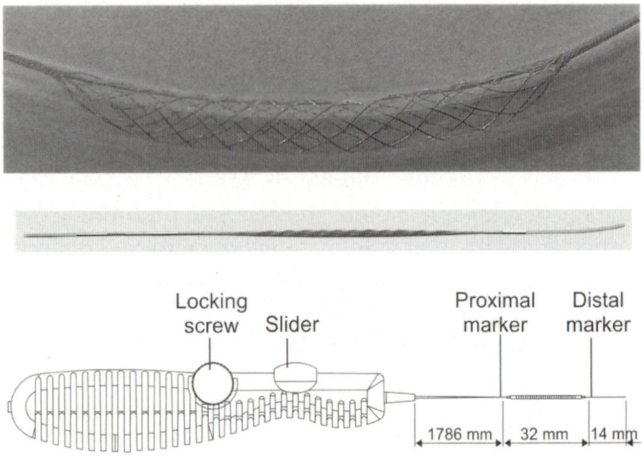

Fig. 9: Commaneci device.

BARREL

The Barrel vascular remodeling device is a self-expandable, laser-cut stent that has a bulged center section. It is designed as a single device for stent-assisted coil embolization of wide-necked bifurcation aneurysms to lower the metal-to-artery ratio and the inherent risk of thromboembolic complications due to multiple stents.

BIFURCATION DEVICE (FIG. 10)[9]

Intracranial bifurcation aneurysms are complex lesions for which current therapy, including simple coiling, balloon-assisted coiling or SAC, coil retention, or intrasaccular devices, is inadequate. These devices help in bridging the aneurysm neck, allow coil retention, disrupt flow away from the aneurysm, leave the main vessel and side branches unencumbered by intraluminal metal, and serve as a platform for endothelial growth across the neck, excluding the aneurysm from the circulation.

Flow Diverters (Figs. 11A to C)[10,11]

Flow diversion has become a well-accepted option for the treatment of cerebral aneurysms. The first clinical use of a flow diverter [pipeline embolization device (PED)] in North America was reported in 2008 and involved treatment of patients with fusiform vertebral artery aneurysms. Between the 1990s and 2008, the so-called intracranial stent underwent significant gain-of-function mutations to arrive at intracranial aneurysm occlusion via flow diversion. The flow diverter has become a separate entity from the stent, with a different purpose and set of indications.

Originally, the PED was indicated for wide-necked or fusiform aneurysms from the petrous segment to the clinoid segment of the internal carotid artery. Nowadays, however, flow diversion is being more broadly applied to small aneurysms, anterior cerebral artery aneurysms, M3–M4 aneurysms, recurrent aneurysms, dissecting aneurysms, ruptured aneurysms, and posterior circulation aneurysm.

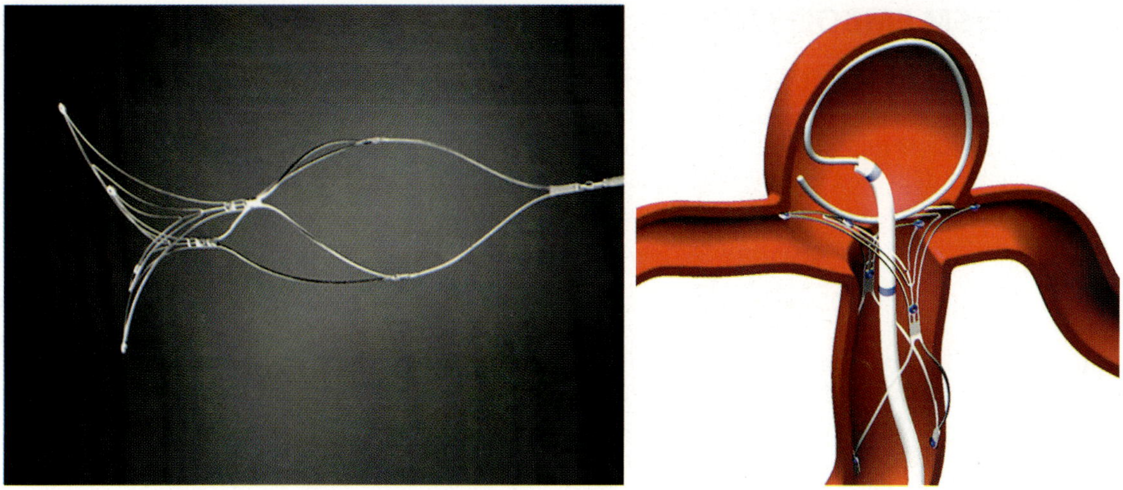

Fig. 10: Pulse rider.

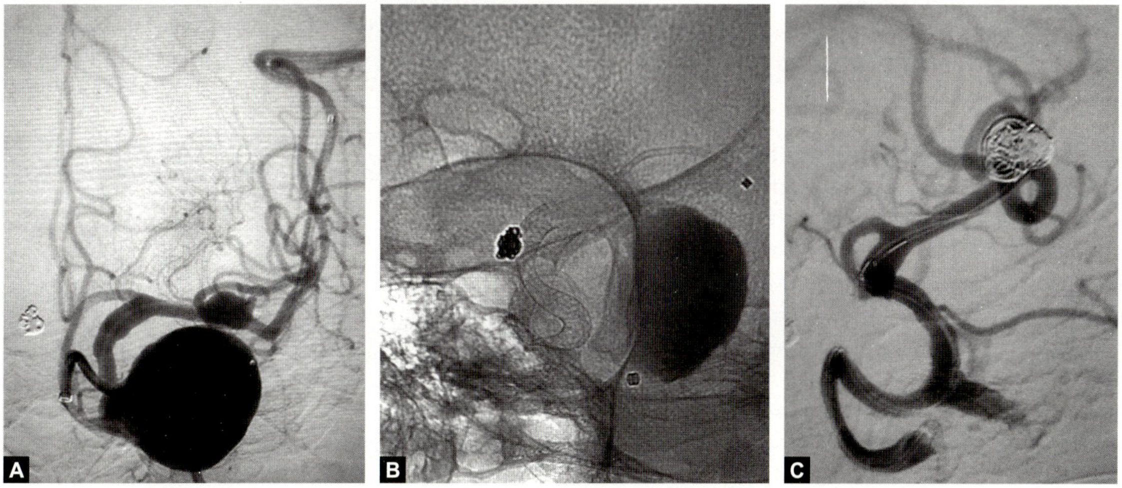

Figs. 11A to C: Case of giant ICA aneursym with dysplastic MCA bifurcation aneurysm treated in same session with flow diverter and a bifurcation device.

Multiple flow diverters are currently available: the PED (Medtronic), Surpass (Stryker), FRED (flow redirection endoluminal device, MicroVention), SILK (Balt Extrusion), and p64 (Phenox). A new generation of intraluminal support devices incorporates braided designs with 18–22% metal coverage and possible flow-modifying properties. These include: LVIS (low-profile visualized intraluminal support device, MicroVention), LVIS Jr. (MicroVention), and LVIS Blue (MicroVention). Incidentally, two overlapping LVIS devices have been reported to create a better flow diverting effect than a single PED.

Flow Disruptors

Intrasaccular devices, as a group, provide high metal coverage at the aneurysm neck, but unlike the endoluminal flow-diversion devices, these devices are placed within the aneurysm itself.

Woven EndoBridge

The Woven EndoBridge (WEB) device (Sequent Medical) is an endosaccular/intrasaccular flow diverter/disrupter composed of braided nitinol wires with proximal and distal platinum markers. The wire mesh spanning the aneurysm inflow provides 35–45% metal coverage.

The device has an inner and outer wire mesh, forming two compartments. The stent-like structure of the device provides adherence to the aneurysm wall. The device is deployed in a manner similar to available stents or coils and has an electrothermal detachment system.

The WEB device comes in two configurations: standard (SL, "single layer") and spherical (SLS, "SL sphere"). The WEB SL is available in a diameter range of 4–11 mm and a height range of 3–9 mm.

LUNA ANEURYSM EMBOLIZATION SYSTEM

The LUNA AES (aneurysm embolization system) is a self-expanding double-layer nitinol mesh with platinum markers. The device is delivered via a standard 0.027-inch microcatheter and takes an ovoid shape within the aneurysm.

Medina[12]

The Medina Embolic Device (Medtronic) is a 3D coil made from shape-set core wire with shape-set alloy outer filaments forming petals. The coil is deployed linearly through a microcatheter but assumes a spherical shape within the aneurysm, providing neck coverage with the petals and stable intrasaccular structure with its 3D shape. It is available in framing and filling styles.

ARTERIOVENOUS MALFORMATION

For AVM, therapeutic approach is multidisciplinary: a cure may be achieved by surgery, radiosurgery, neuro-interventional surgery, or a combination of the three. More specifically, the endovascular management for AVM may include interventions providing a reduction of AVM nidus dimension in a presurgical setting, reduction prior to radiosurgery, or elimination of certain, often associated, vascular anomalies, such as aneurysms, venous varices, and fistulae.

Supporting evidences on the behavior of AVMs managed conservatively performed through mere observation and radiological follow-up may be a viable option considering the risk of complications entailed with the treatment of these complex and unpredictable lesions. Even though the final goal of AVM therapy is the complete obliteration of its nidus, this is not always possible. An endovascular approach may be adopted in at least five possible scenarios: indeed an embolization may be performed either prior to surgery/radiosurgery, or to treat vascular anomalies with an AVM, as a curative therapy or in a palliation setting (i.e. mitigation of blood flow steal symptoms). Embolic agents are numerous, each with peculiar advantages and limitations. Among the most commonly used *n*-butyl cyanoacrylate, ethyl alcohol, polyvinyl alcohol/Embospheres, coils and, more recently, Onyx, are biocompatible polymers.

CONCLUSION

Endovascular neurosurgery is an exciting field. There has been tremendous amount of progress in its various aspects in the recent times. Advances in neurocatheterization laboratories/evolution of different coils/evolution of different technics in the case of wide-neck aneurysms have significantly broadened the horizon of its application in hitherto untreatable lesions of CNS.

In spite of these advances, it remains equally important to further explore the basic biological processes involved in these diseases through combined research in this field. A combined team work of neurosurgeons/intervention neuroradiologists/neurocritical care specialists is the need of the hour to offer the best possible management to the victims of the vascular diseases of CNS.

REFERENCES

1. Antunes JL. Egas Moniz and cerebral angiography. J Neurosurg. 1974;40:427-32.
2. International Subarachnoid Aneurysm Trial (ISAT) Collaborative Group. International Subarachnoid Aneurysm Trial (ISAT) of neurosurgical clipping versus endovascular coiling in 2143 patients with ruptured intracranial aneurysms: a randomised trial. Lancet. 2002;360:1267-74.
3. Spetzler RF, McDougall CG, Zabramski JM, et al. The Barrow Ruptured Aneurysm Trial: 6-year results. Neurosurgery. 2015;123(3):609-17.
4. Hui FK, Fiorella D, Masaryk TJ, et al. A history of detachable coils: 1987–2012. J Neurointerv Surg. 2014;6(2):134-8.
5. Guglielmi G. History of the genesis of detachable coils. J Neurosurg. 2009;111:1-8.
6. Moret J, Cognard C, Castaings L, et al. Reconstruction technique in the treatment of wide-neck intracranial aneurysms: long-term angiographic and clinical results-apropos of 56 cases. J Neuroradiol. 1997;24:30-44.
7. Chalouhi N, Jabbour P, Singhal S, et al. Stent assisted coiling of intracranial aneurysm: predictors of complications, recanalization and outcome in 508 cases. Stroke. 2013;44(5):1348-53.
8. Spiotta AM, Wheeler AM, Smithason S, et al. Comparison of techniques for stent assisted coil embolization of aneurysms. J NeuroInterv Surg. 2011;4(5):339–44.
9. Aguilar-Perez M, Kurre W, Fischer S, et al. Coil occlusion of wide-neck bifurcation aneurysms assisted by a novel intra- to extra-aneurysmatic neck-bridging device (pCONus): initial experience. AJNR Am J Neuroradiol. 2014;35:965-71.
10. Becske T, Kallmes DF, Saatci I, et al. Pipeline for uncoilable or failed aneurysms: results from a multicenter clinical trial. Radiology. 2013;267(3):858-68.
11. Nelson PK, Lylyk P, Szikora I, et al. The pipeline embolization device for the intracranial treatment of aneurysms trial. Am J Neuroradiol. 2011;32(1):34-40.
12. Jia ZY, Shi HB, Miyachi S, et al. Development of new endovascular devices for aneurysm treatment. J Stroke. 2018;20(1):46-56.

SECTION 25

Congenital Heart Disease

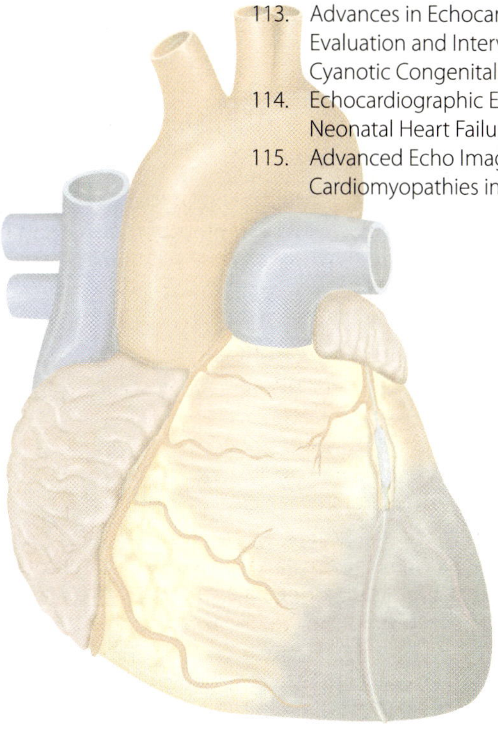

113

CHAPTER

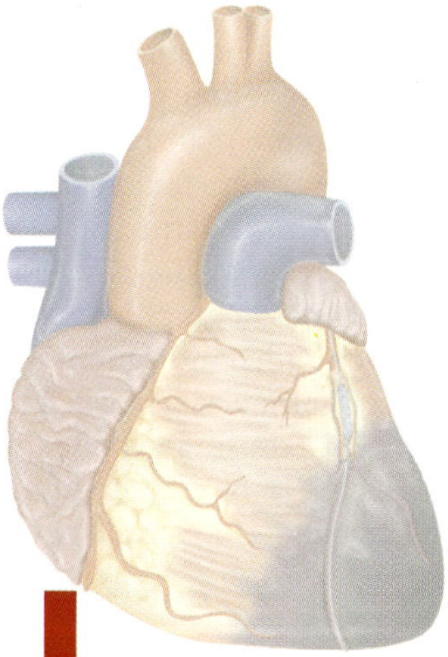

Advances in Echocardiographic Evaluation and Intervention of Cyanotic Congenital Heart Disease

Sakshi Sachdeva, S Ramakrishnan

INTRODUCTION

Worldwide incidence of congenital heart disease (CHD) is approximately 7–8 per 1,000 live births.[1] Of all the CHDs, cyanotic CHDs (CCHDs) constitute around 40%. Unlike the acyanotic CHDs, which may remain undiagnosed till the patient develops clinically significant symptoms, CCHDs are easily diagnosed and detected by an astute pediatrician or physician due to the presence of clinically apparent central cyanosis or due to low saturation of peripheral oxygen (SpO_2) values on pulse oximetry. Clinically, the CCHDs can be divided into three groups, i.e. reduced pulmonary blood flow, increased pulmonary blood flow, and transposition physiology. Table 1 shows a broad classification of CCHDs. Most of the CCHDs require surgical intervention for treatment or palliation. In all these diseases, echocardiogram is an indispensible tool for the diagnosis of the exact morphology and for decision-making about the management plan. In few conditions, percutaneous intervention may help to stabilize the acute phase and may help in temporizing the surgical intervention. In some conditions, percutaneous intervention may be the only required treatment. In the following sections, echocardiographic evaluation of CCHDs requiring percutaneous intervention is described.

TABLE 1: Classification of cyanotic congenital heart disease.

Increased pulmonary blood flow	*Reduced pulmonary blood flow*
Total anomalous pulmonary venous connection	Tetralogy of Fallot
Common atrium	DORV VSD PS
DORV without PS	Tricuspid atresia VSD PS
Tricuspid atresia without PS	TGA VSD PS
Single ventricle without PS	CTGA VSD PS
Truncus arteriosus	Single ventricle PS
Transposition of great arteries	AVSD PS
Hypoplastic left heart syndrome	Pulmonary atresia with VSD
	Pulmonary atresia with intact ventricular septum
	Ebstein anomaly

(CTGA: corrected transposition of the great arteries, DORV: double outlet right ventricle, PS: pulmonary stenosis, TGA: transposition of great arteries, VSD: ventricular septal defect)

TRANSPOSITION OF GREAT ARTERIES

Transposition of great arteries is the most common cyanotic congenital disease presenting with cyanosis at birth. Due to the presence of parallel systemic and pulmonary circulation, children need communication at interatrial, interventricular, or great artery level for having adequate intercirculatory mixing between oxygenated and deoxygenated blood. Hence, the neonates with poor intercirculatory mixing are early presenters with deep cyanosis. These include transposition of great arteries (TGA) and intact ventricular septum and restrictive patent foramen ovale (PFO) and small/absent patent ductus arteriosus (PDA). Figure 1 shows echocardiographic image of TGA and intact ventricular septum with small PFO.

Balloon Atrial Septostomy

Interatrial communication is the best site of intercirculatory mixing. Hence, for stabilization, these patients require percutaneous intervention in the form of balloon atrial septostomy (BAS).[2] In this procedure, interatrial communication is enlarged by tearing it with a Fogarty balloon. Figure 2 shows angiocardigraphic still image depicting the BAS procedure. The procedure is usually done through the femoral venous route. The balloon is parked across the PFO in the left atrium and inflated with diluted radiopaque contrast. Balloon position in the left atrium is confirmed by echocardiogram, and the balloon is pulled across the interatrial communication, tearing and enlarging it. Important precaution during the procedure is correct localization of balloon before pulling it as sometimes balloon may reach left atrial appendage or pulmonary vein or across the tricuspid valve into right ventricle. These locations of balloon can cause injury to pulmonary vein and appendage or damage to tricuspid apparatus, leading to hemopericardium or tricuspid regurgitation. Criteria for successful BAS include rise in SpO_2 more than 10%, wide interatrial communication with nonrestrictive bidirectional flow as assessed by echocardiogram. Postprocedure echocardiogram should be checked for pericardial effusion. Figure 3 shows postprocedure echocardiographic image with wide interatrial communication. Other indications for BAS in TGA include TGA with large ventricular septal defect (VSD) or large PDA, and small PFO causing significant pulmonary venous hypertension (PVH). In this situation, BAS is done for relieving PVH by enlarging atrial septal defect (ASD).

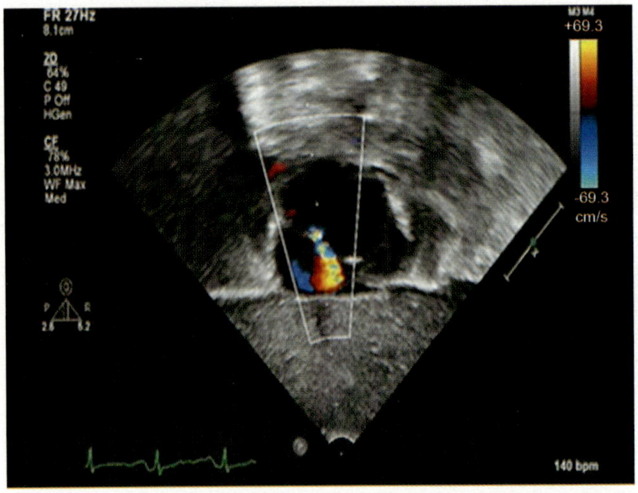

Fig. 1: Echocardiographic image from subcostal view, showing restrictive interatrial communication with narrow jet of flow from left atrium to right atrium.

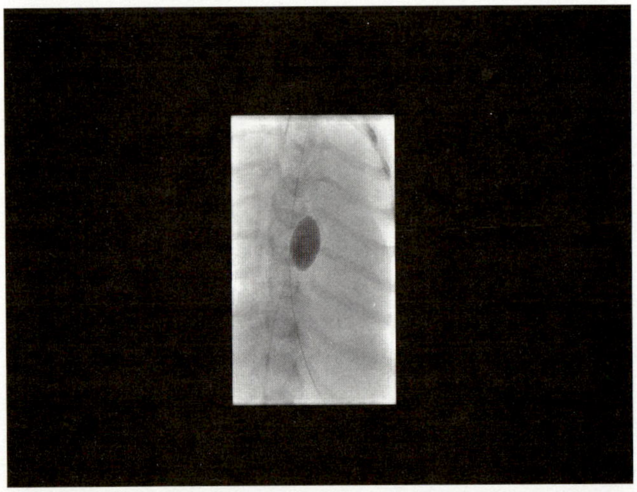

Fig. 2: Angiographic image showing balloon atrial septostomy being done with a Fogarty balloon. Balloon position is across the atrial septal defect into the left atrium.

Patent Ductus Arteriosus Stenting in Transposition of Great Arteries with Regressed Left Ventricle

In TGAs, the left ventricle (LV) supports the pulmonary circulation. After 4–6 weeks of life when neonatal pulmonary vascular resistance regresses and pulmonary pressures fall, LV loses its muscle mass and becomes "regressed". Table 2 gives criteria for a regressed LV. This regressed LV becomes ineffective to support systemic circulation if arterial switch operation is done. Hence, in the cases of TGA with regressed LV, LV needs to be trained to make it prepared to withstand systemic pressures postprocedure. This can be done surgically by putting a pulmonary atresia (PA) band and Blalock-Taussig (BT) shunt or interventionally by doing a PDA stenting. PDA stenting procedure details are described in the section on tetralogy of Fallot (TOF) subsequently. Figures 4 and 5 show echocardiographic images for the assessment of regressed and retrained LV. Figure 6 shows angiocardiographic image of PDA stent being deployed. Figures 7A to D show PDA stent flowing from left to right.[3]

CRITICAL PULMONARY STENOSIS

When the severity of pulmonary stenosis increases to such an extent that right ventricle is not able to sustain cardiac output to the pulmonary circulation, there starts a right-to-left shunt at the level of ASD/PFO, which leads to the appearance of cyanosis as the output decreases. Echocardiographic evaluation includes the assessment of severity of pulmonary stenosis by assessing the gradient across the pulmonary valve. Figures 8A to D show images for echocardiographic assessment of pulmonary stenosis. The size of pulmonary annulus is measured to decide the size of balloon required for pulmonary valve balloon dilation (PVBD). Atrial septal defect shows right-to-left shunt as seen in bicaval view.

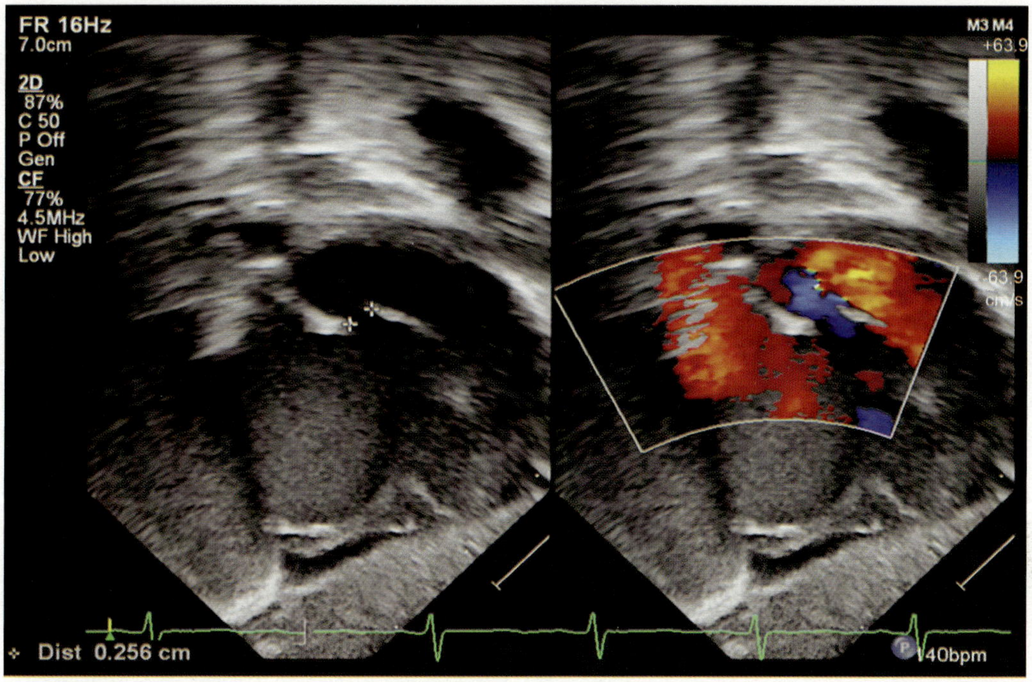

Fig. 3: Echocardiographic image post-balloon atrial septostomy, from subcostal view showing nonrestrictive interatrial communication with bidirectional flow.

TABLE 2: Criteria for a regressed and nonregressed left ventricle in transposition of great arteries with intact ventricular septum.

	Nonregressed	*Regressed*
Apical 4 chamber view	LV forms apex of heart	RV forms apex
Parasternal short axis	Spherical shape of LV	Crescent shape/squashed LV
LV sphericity index	≤ 2	≥3
M-mode	IVS motion synchronous with LV free wall	IVS motion with right ventricle free wall
LV posterior wall diastolic thickness	>4 mm >12 mm/m^2	< 4 mm <12 mm/m^2
LV mass index	>35 g/m^2	<35 g/m^2
LV end diastolic volume	>20 mL/m^2	<20 mL/m^2

(LV: left ventricle; RV: right ventricular; IVS: intact ventricular septum)

Pulmonary Valve Balloon Dilation

By doing right heart catheterization, right ventricular (RV) and pulmonary artery pressure is measured and the severity of pulmonary stenosis is assessed. RV angiogram is done in lateral view. Then, a balloon of size 100–120% of the annulus measured by echocardiogram is used to do PVBD. Postprocedure fall in gradient may not be significant, which is due to infundibular hypertrophy causing subvalvar dynamic RV outflow tract (RVOT) obstruction. Echocardiographic assessment can differentiate the predominant site of obstruction as infundibular or valvar. Severity of residual stenosis can be assessed and the severity of pulmonary regurgitation can be assessed. Shunting across ASD can become bidirectional or remain right to left for some time till the RV hypertrophy resolves.

TETRALOGY OF FALLOT

Tetralogy of Fallot is the most common CCHD beyond neonatal age. Morphologically, it comprises of four components: a large malaligned VSD, overriding of aorta, severe infundibular and valvar pulmonary stenosis, and RV hypertrophy. Important aspect of imaging TOF patients is to look for the size of pulmonary annulus and morphology and size of branch pulmonary arteries because the timing and type of surgery depends on these factors. But if a patient presents with cyanotic spells in early infancy and

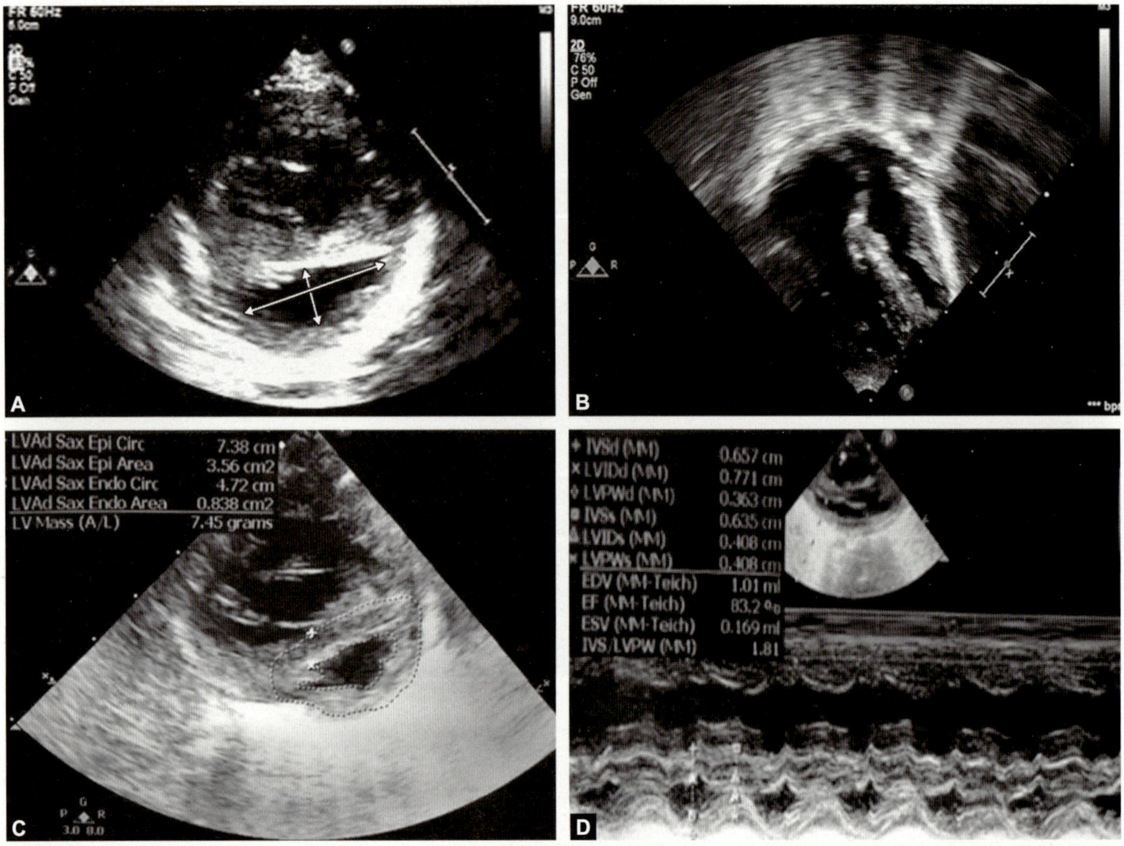

Figs. 4A to D: Echocardiographic panel of images of TGA with regressed LV. (A) Short axis view showing crescent-shaped LV with poor sphericity index; (B) Apical four chamber view with nonapex-forming LV; (C) LV mass assessment; (D) Low LV posterior wall thickness. (TGA: transposition of great arteries; LV: left ventricle)

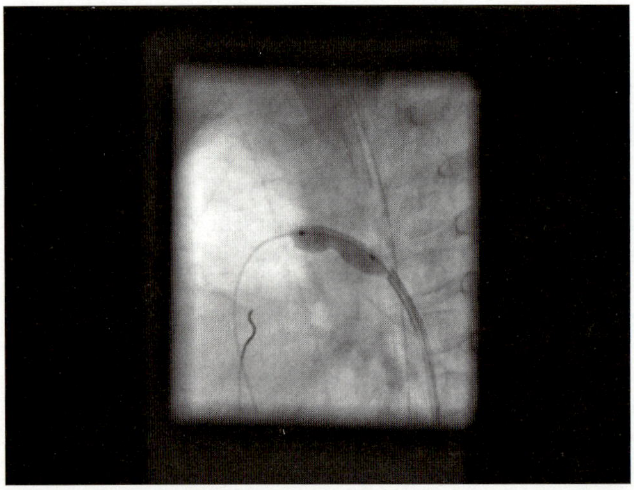

Fig. 5: Angiographic image showing patent ductus arteriosus stent being deployed in transposition of great arteries with regressed left ventricle.

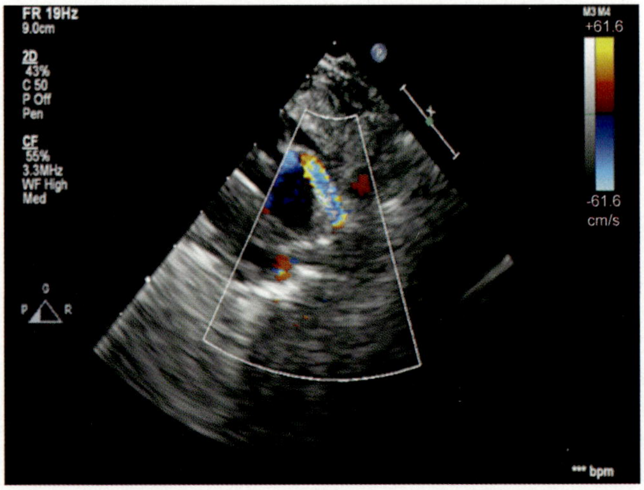

Fig. 6: Echocardiographic image showing well flowing patent ductus arteriosus stent in situ.

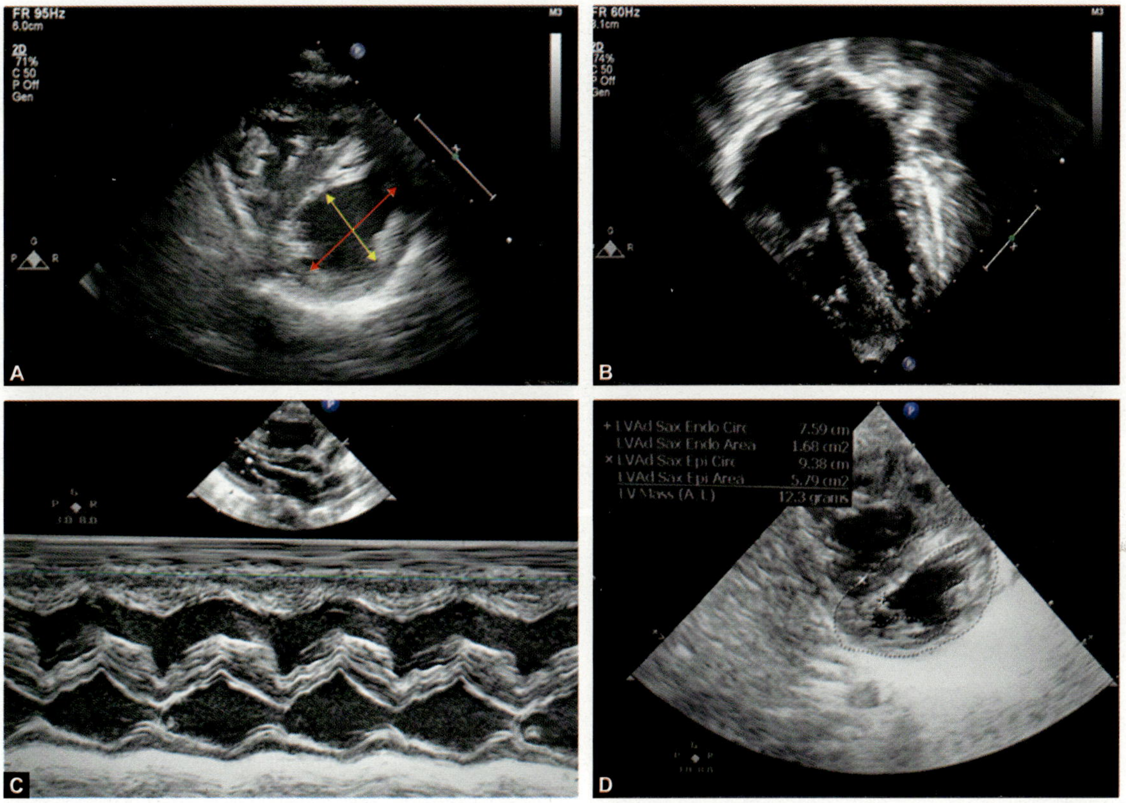

Figs. 7A to D: Echocardiographic panel of images of TGA with prepared LV. (A) Short axis view showing crescent-shaped LV with good sphericity index; (B) Apical four chamber view with apex forming LV; (C) Low LV posterior wall thickness; (D) LV mass assessment. (TGA: transposition of great arteries; LV: left ventricle).

total correction is not possible either due to sick condition of patient or due to small branch pulmonary arteries, BT shunt is the preferred mode of management. Interventional alternatives to BT shunt include PDA stenting, RVOT individually.

Patent Ductus Arteriosus Stenting

Patent ductus arteriosus is an unreliable source of pulmonary blood flow because it is a fetal structure and tends to restrict and close completely in postnatal life. Hence, ductal stenting is an option to establish reliable source of pulmonary blood flow in emergency situation, such as refractory spell, or electively as an alternative to BT shunt in situations where total correction is not possible at the time of presentation. Echocardiographic assessment prior to intervention should focus on ductus morphology; a long tortuous ductus is a difficult subset for stenting and will require a long stent with higher risk of stent thrombosis. Morphology of branch pulmonary arteries should be assessed thoroughly as nonconfluent PAs and those with ostial stenosis of one branch PA generally left pulmonary artery will lead to contralateral pulmonary edema after stent placement.[4-6]

Patent ductus arteriosus is imaged by arch and descending aortic angiogram, and its morphology is assessed and length measured to choose the length of stent. Coronary stenting hardware is utilized to cross the ductus. Coronary stent of 3.5-mm diameter is preferred in infants weighing up to 3 kg, and for higher weight infants, stent of size 4 mm is chosen. A stent is deployed using coronary balloon. Attention is given to the following facts:

- Prostaglandin injection should be kept standby in catheterization laboratory, as sudden ductal spasm while passing wire or balloon-stent assembly may precipitate spell in the patient.
- The length of stent chosen should be such that no part of ductus remains uncovered with stent; otherwise, it can go into spasm and occlude entire flow to the pulmonary arteries.
- Aortic end of stent should not project into arch or descending aorta.
- Pulmonary end of stent should just cover the PDA. It should not project into pulmonary artery

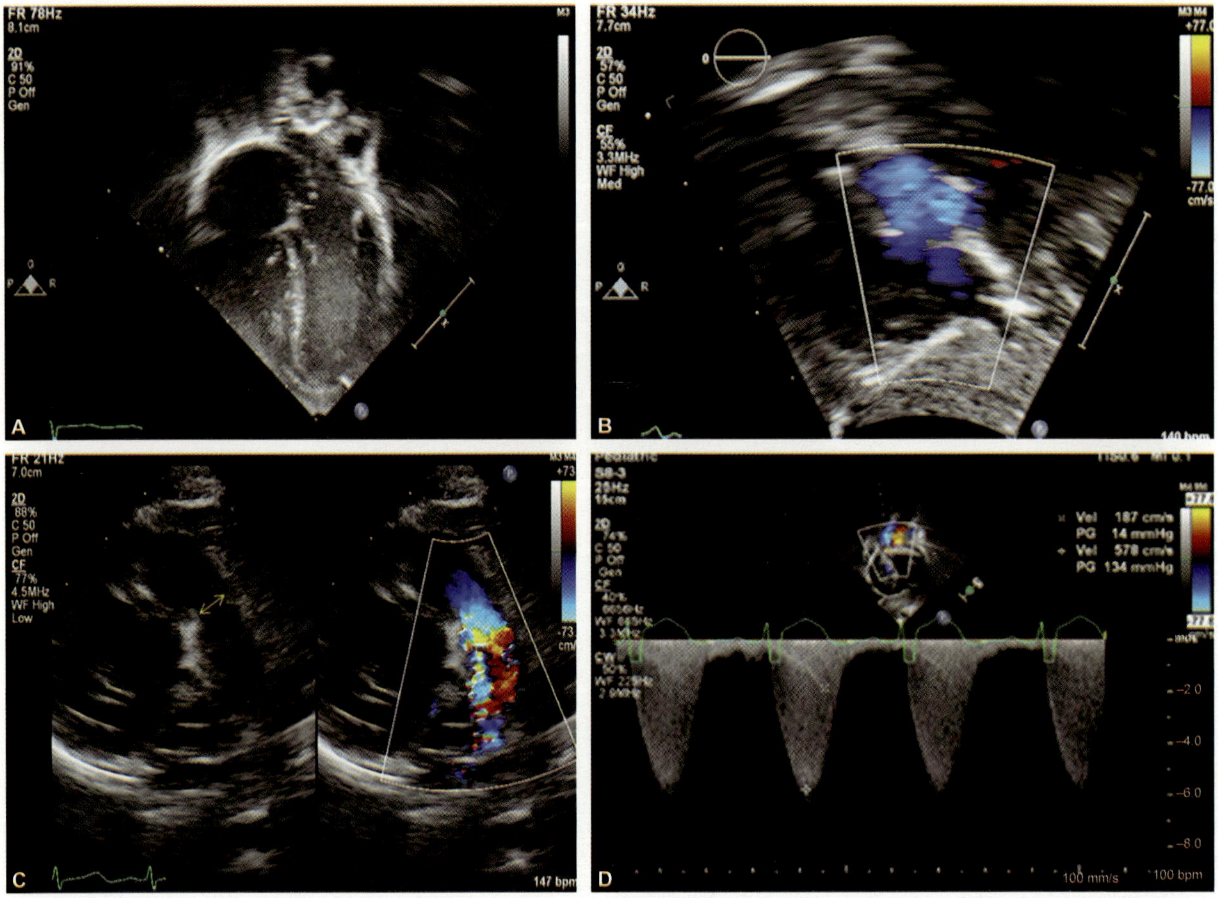

Figs. 8A to D: Echocardiographic panel of images showing the assessment of pulmonary stenosis. (A) Four chamber view showing IAS bulging toward left; (B) Subcostal view shows ASD shunting right to left; (C) Short axis view showing pulmonary annulus being measured, and narrow pulmonary outflow jet; (D) Doppler flow across pulmonary valve showing high gradient indicating severe pulmonary stenosis. (ASD: atrial septal defect; IAS: intact atrial septum)

branch; otherwise, unilateral pulmonary edema and contralateral oligemia may occur.

- Heparin infusion is initiated just after the control of vascular access site bleeding. Dual antiplatelet therapy is started after 24 hours to prevent stent thrombosis.

Right Ventricular Outflow Tract Stenting

Right ventricular outflow tract stenting is another option for palliation in patients with TOF presenting with spells in whom branch pulmonary arteries are hypoplastic and nonsuitable for total correction or BT shunt. Echocardiographic assessment prior to RVOT stent includes measurement of the length of stenotic infundibular segment to decide the length of stent needed. The diameter of stent generally varies from 5 mm to 7 mm. Site of obstruction should be clearly assessed as RVOT stenting is ineffective in patients with predominantly valvar stenosis and those having supravalvar stenosis.

Right ventricular angiogram is done to define RVOT anatomy. The length is measured in lateral view to choose the length of stent. The length of stent should be optimal to cover the entire infundibulum.

Apart from the technical details, precautions while RVOT stenting in laboratory include the following:

- Optimal stent length should be chosen.
- Small length of stent may lead to some parts of infundibulum remaining uncovered which may cause it to undergo spasm and lead to failure of procedure.
- Longer stent may project proximally and interfere with tricuspid valve mechanism leading to tricuspid regurgitation.
- Longer stent may project distally and encroach upon the pulmonary valve leading to its incompetence and pulmonary regurgitation.
- Laboratory should be pre-equipped to manage cyanotic spell, which may precipitate during procedure.

Pulmonary Valve Balloon Dilation

The occasional patient with TOF who has predominantly valvar stenosis, PVBD may be attempted in these subsets of patients. Preprocedure echo assessment includes assessing the predominant site of obstruction and pulmonary annulus diameter. If obstruction is at infundibular level predominantly, PVBD cannot be attempted. Any degree of supravalvar stenosis is a contraindication of PVBD in TOF. Pulmonary annulus diameter should be assessed accurately as the size of balloon required for procedure depends on its optimal assessment. Balloon-to-annulus ratio can be 100–120%. Postprocedure echocardiographic evaluation includes assessment of presence of residual obstruction and the level of obstruction, development of pulmonary regurgitation, and its severity assessment.

Tetralogy of Fallot with Pulmonary Atresia

In this situation, BT shunt is preferred option for palliation till total correction with conduit is feasible. But in certain cases, PDA stenting can be done. Assessment, procedure, and precautions are similar to PDA stenting as described in the previous section of TOF.

Pulmonary Atresia with Intact Ventricular Septum

Pulmonary atresia in absence of VSD has varying degrees of RV hypoplasia. Patient presents with cyanosis since birth, and some children have symptoms of heart failure specially right side failure in the early neonatal age. Echocardiographic assessment includes the evaluation of type of PA, i.e. membranous or muscular. Only membranous type of pulmonary atresia is amenable for percutaneous intervention. The next step in evaluation is the assessment of tricuspid valve morphology and degree of hypoplasia. Tricuspid valve annulus dimensions and *Z* score are measured. Value less than –3*Z* makes it less suitable for biventricular repair. Right ventricular size and morphology is the next important part of evaluation. Normal right ventricle has three parts; it is tripartite and is composed of inflow, trabecular, and outflow parts. In PA/intact ventricular septum (IVS), the right ventricle may have one or more parts undeveloped, i.e. it may be unipartite or bipartite. Such RV morphology may be unsuitable for biventricular repair. In addition, there may be a presence of coronary sinusoids in the right ventricle wall causing RV dependent coronary circulation (RVDCC). In this situation, coronary artery filling happens through blood flowing retrograde from ventricular cavity into main epicardial coronary arteries. The presence of RVDCC is a contraindication to pulmonary valve perforation. Figures 9A to D show echocardiographic images for PA with intact ventricular segment. In PA/IVS with tripartite right ventricle, tricuspid valve *Z* score more than –3*Z*, and absence of RVDCC, pulmonary valve perforation is carried out. In this procedure, the atretic pulmonary outflow is perforated using chronic total occlusion (CTO) coronary hardware and made patent. This perforation is followed by balloon dilation of pulmonary annulus.

Pulmonary Valve Perforation

In this procedure, first RV angiogram is done. Filling of coronary artery or presence of coronary sinusoids is an indicator of RVDCC. In this case, pulmonary valve perforation cannot be carried out, because coronary filling is dependent on high RV pressure, which if decompressed by pulmonary valve perforation may cause myocardial ischemia by reducing the coronary perfusion pressure and coronary blood flow. In such cases, either BT shunt or PDA stenting is done for future univentricular pathway. Once it is made sure that RVDCC is not present, the next step is to use CTO coronary wires with high tip load and perforate the pulmonary annular membrane.[7] Care must be taken to avoid perforating the RVOT. Echocardiographic assessment for the presence of pericardial effusion should be done during the procedure even at minor suspicion. Other options for perforation include the use of radiofrequency ablation wires. After perforating the membranous pulmonary annulus, coronary balloon is advanced over the wire and balloon dilation of pulmonary annulus is done (Figs. 10A and B). After this, the balloon size is upgraded to that of the size of pulmonary annulus, and PVBD is done to establish good antegrade flow. Postprocedure echocardiographic assessment (Figs. 11A and B) for the presence of effusion, quantum of antegrade flow, severity of pulmonary stenosis, and regurgitation should be done.

Tricuspid Atresia

This CCHD is suitable for univentricular pathway only. Biventricular repair is impossible due to atretic tricuspid valve and hypoplastic right ventricle. A series of percutaneous interventions are possible in cases of tricuspid atresia depending on the morphology.

Tricuspid Atresia with Restrictive Atrial Septal Defect

In tricuspid atresia, ASD has obligatory right-to-left shunt. Systemic venous return from superior vena cava and inferior vena cava should flow through ASD to left atrium and then to ventricle to reach the pulmonary arteries. Generally, ASD is nonrestrictive, but in some cases, it may be small. Restrictive ASD acts as obstruction to systemic venous return and such neonates present with severe cyanosis and symptoms of systemic venous congestion.

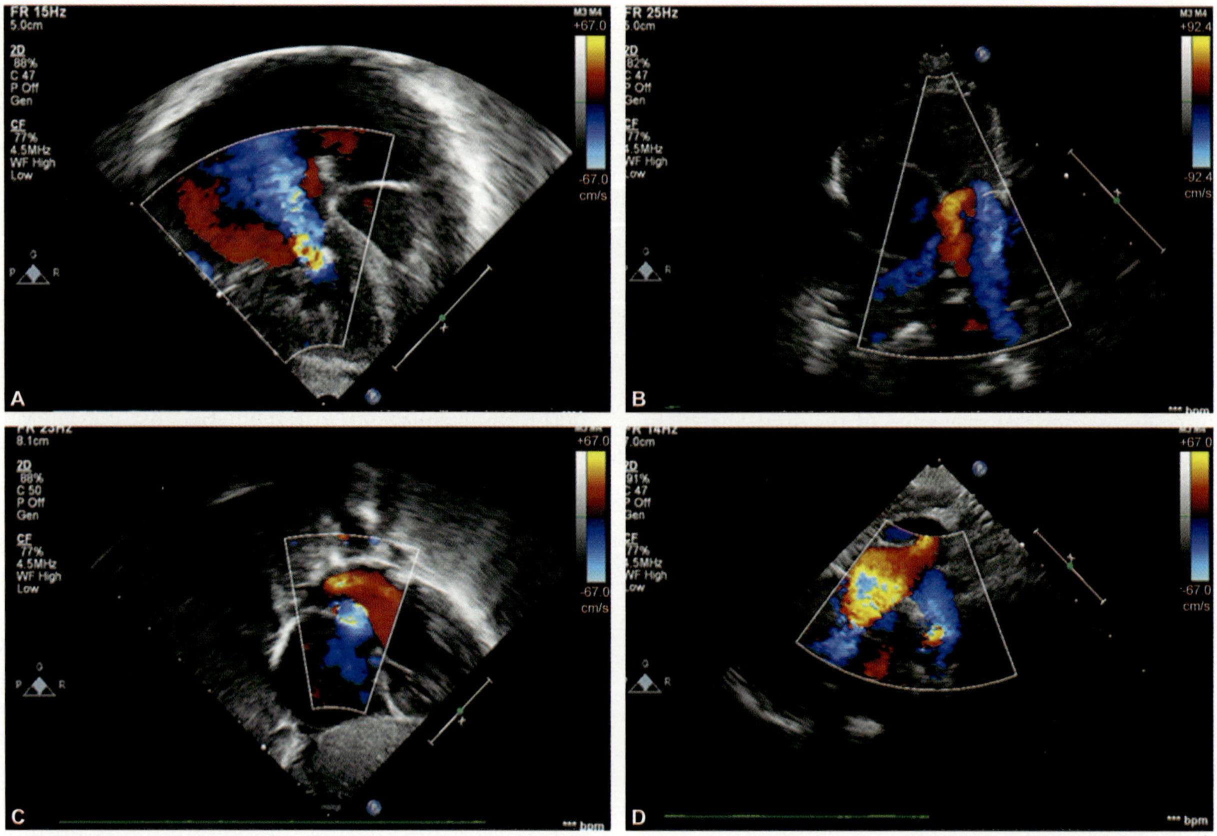

Figs. 9A to D: Echocardiographic panel of images showing assessment of pulmonary atresia with intact ventricular septum. (A) Apical four chamber view showing severe tricuspid regurgitation; (B) Parasternal short axis view showing good size main pulmonary artery and confluent branch pulmonary arteries with no antegrade flow and retrograde flow from PDA supplying pulmonary arteries; (C) Subcostal short axis view showing ASD with right-to-left shunt; (D) Suprasternal view showing PDA from descending thoracic aorta. (ASD: atrial septal defect; PDA: patent ductus arteriosus)

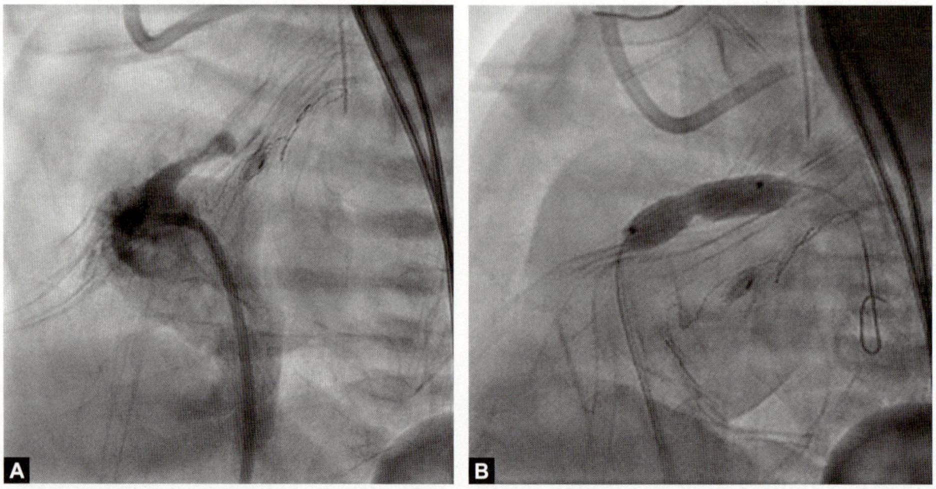

Figs. 10A and B: Angiocardiographic images showing pulmonary valve perforation followed by balloon dilation. (A) Right ventricular angiogram showing pulmonary atresia with no antegrade flow; (B) Pulmonary valve being balloon dilated after perforation.

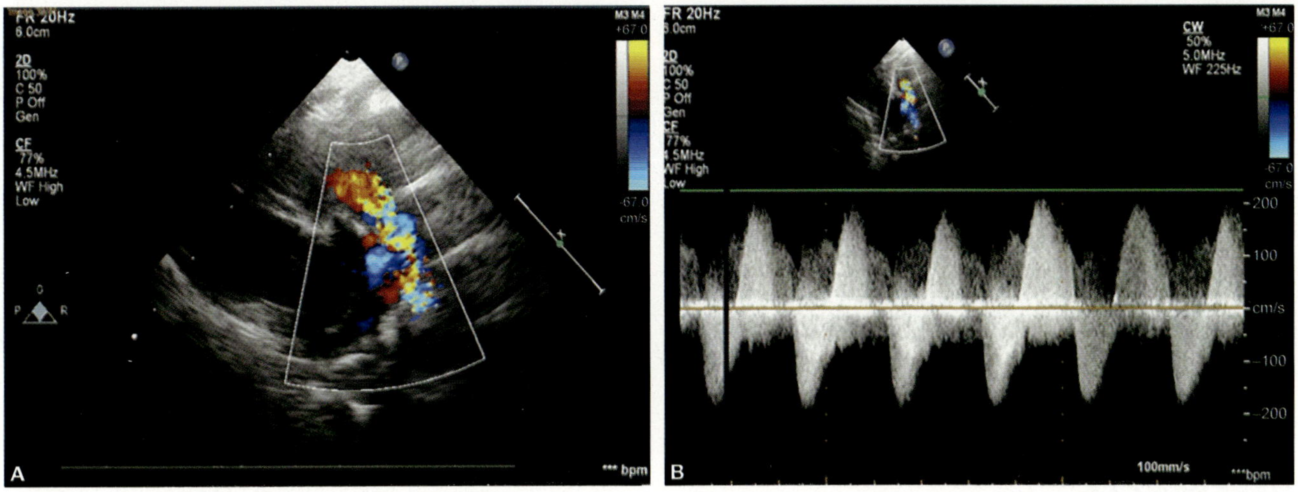

Figs. 11A and B: Echocardiographic images after pulmonary valve perforation and balloon dilation in a case of pulmonary atresia with intact ventricular septum without right ventricular dependent coronary circulation. (A) Parasternal short axis view showing pulmonary regurgitation through the perforated and dilated pulmonary valve; (B) Doppler signal across the pulmonary valve showing good antegrade flow and pulmonary regurgitation.

In these situations, BAS will improve cyanosis and relieve symptoms of right heart failure. The procedure is similar to that described for BAS in TGA.

Tricuspid Atresia with Pulmonary Atresia

Interventional PDA stenting may be done to improve saturation in this subset of patients. Assessment and procedure are similar to PDA stenting in TOF patients.

TOTAL ANOMALOUS PULMONARY VENOUS CONNECTION

Total anomalous pulmonary venous connection is a cyanotic congenial heart disease with admixture of systemic and pulmonary venous blood happening at the level of atrium. According to the site of drainage of pulmonary veins, total anomalous pulmonary venous connection (TAPVC) can be classified into supracardiac, cardiac, infracardiac, and mixed, if there is more than one site of pulmonary venous drainage. All the four pulmonary veins drain into a common pulmonary venous chamber which drains through ascending or descending vertical vein into supracardiac or infracardiac location.

Generally, TAPVC is nonobstructive and presents with features of congestive cardiac failure and mild cyanosis. If TAPVC is obstructive, infants present very early in life with severe cyanosis and respiratory distress due to PVH. Obstruction to pulmonary venous blood can be at any level, i.e. individual pulmonary vein level, common chamber to vertical vein junction, within the vertical vein, or at the level of interatrial communication. Some of these sites of obstruction can be handled by percutaneous interventions.

Total Anomalous Pulmonary Venous Connection with Obstruction at Interatrial Communication

Restrictive interatrial communication is the most common site of obstruction in TAPVC. BAS may be done in this situation to enlarge the interatrial communication and relieve the obstruction. Steps of procedure are same as those described in BAS for TGA. After the procedure, the right-to-left shunt through the ASD becomes nonrestrictive as assessed by echocardiography.

Total Anomalous Pulmonary Venous Connection with Obstruction at Vertical Vein Level

Inherent stenosis at vertical vein level makes these neonates sicker and makes them present early in life. Ideally, these neonates should undergo early surgery for TAPVC correction, but if the patients are very sick and unstable, palliation to tide over crisis can be done by percutaneous intervention in the form of vertical vein stenting. In this procedure, angiogram is done within the vertical vein to assess the length of stenotic segment. Then, a balloon mounted stent is advanced, and it is deployed across the stenotic segment to relieve the gradient. Postprocedure echo assessment includes residual gradient measurement and assessment of obstruction to individual pulmonary veins.[8,9]

CONCLUSION

Cyanotic congenital heart diseases are a group of disorders that invariably require surgical intervention for their palliation or treatment. Echocardiographic assessment is the mainstay of diagnosis in these disorders. Percutaneous intervention is generally limited to tiding over the crisis situation and preparing the patient for ultimate surgical intervention in a stable condition. The role of echocardiogram is important in the postoperative period to look for residual lesions.

REFERENCES

1. Saxena A, Mehta A, Sharma M, et al. Birth prevalence of congenital heart disease: a cross-sectional observational study from North India. Ann Pediatr Card. 2016;9:205-9.
2. Boehm W, Emmel M, Sreeram N. Balloon atrial septostomy: history and technique. Images Paediatr Cardiol. 2006;8(1):8-14.
3. Kothari SS, Ramakrishnan S, Senguttuvan NB, et al. Ductal recanalization and stenting for late presenters with TGA intact ventricular septum. Ann Pediatr Card. 2011;4(2):135-8.
4. Alwi M. Stenting the ductus arteriosus: case selection, technique and possible complications. Ann Pediatr Card. 2008;1(1):38-45.
5. Sluysmans T, Neven B, Rubay J, et al. Early balloon dilatation of the pulmonary valve in infants with tetralogy of Fallot. Risks Benefits Circ. 1995;91:1506-11.
6. Quandt D, Ramchandani B, Stickley J, et al. Stenting of the right ventricular outflow tract promotes better pulmonary arterial growth compared with modified Blalock-Taussig shunt palliation in tetralogy of Fallot-type lesions. JACC: Cardiovasc Interv. 2017;10(17):1774-84.
7. Patil NC, Saxena A, Gupta SK, et al. Perforating the atretic pulmonary valve with CTO hardware: technical aspects. Cathet Cardiovasc Interv. 2016;88:E145-50.
8. Ramakrishnan S, Kothari SS. Preoperative balloon dilatation of obstructed total anomalous pulmonary venous connection in a neonate. Cathet Cardiovasc Interv. 2004;61(1):128-30.
9. Lim WK, Leong MC, Samion H. Stenting of vertical vein in an infant with obstructed supracardiac total anomalous pulmonary venous drainage. Ann Pediatr Card. 2016;9:183-5.

114

CHAPTER

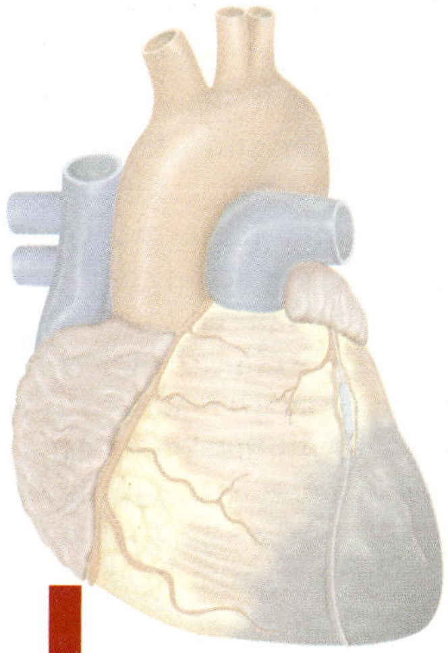

Echocardiographic Evaluation in Neonatal Heart Failure

Hala El Marsafaway

INTRODUCTION

Neonatal heart failure is characterized by many unique anatomic and physiologic features. Anatomically, the newborn myocardium is disorganized in its structure and has a lower density of contractile proteins. Also, decreased cellular transport, may play a role in the relatively impaired contractile and relaxation functions of the immature heart. Despite these differences, the Frank-Starling relationship in the neonatal heart is intact and functional as cardiac output can be augmented with increased ventricular filling, as well as higher heart rates and inotropy. The treatment of the clinical syndrome of heart failure in the neonate depends, on the underlying cause of heart failure. Understanding the developmental changes in myocardial structure and function will provide optimal care of the newborn in the setting of a failing myocardium.

NEONATAL CARDIOVASCULAR PHYSIOLOGY

Postnatal Circulation

At delivery, when the umbilical cord and placenta are divided, the systemic vascular resistance rises acutely. At the same time, the pulmonary vascular resistance begins to decrease. At the level of the ductus arteriosus, blood flow shifts from a fetal right-to-left circulation to a post-natal left-to-right shunt. Functionally, this usually occurs within 12 hour of birth in term infants and may occur later in preterm infants, leading to pulmonary overcirculation.[1] An increase in the partial pressure of oxygen in the blood acts as a stimulus for closure of the patent ductus arteriosus.[2,3] Other factors that may play a role in ductal closure include nitric oxide and bradykinins.[4,5] Shortly after birth the ductus venosus also closes. It is speculated that decreased umbilical-placental blood flow to the ductus venosus leads to contraction of the vessel. Constriction of a sphincter at the origin of the ductus venosus may also contribute to closure.[6] Inhibitors of prostaglandin synthesis (indomethacin) have been shown to cause constriction of the ductus venosus in the fetal lamb.[7] The closure of the foramen ovale is caused by the passive forces of increased blood return to the left heart. In the fetus, a high pulmonary vascular resistance limits blood flow to the lungs. Less than 10% of the combined venous return enters the left atrium by way of the pulmonary veins. After birth, as the pulmonary vascular resistance falls and shunting in the ductus arteriosus becomes left-to-right, blood flow to the left atrium through the pulmonary veins increases substantially. Left atrial pressure rises and the septum primum apposes the crista, resulting in closure of the foramen ovale. Pulmonary vascular resistance is high in the fetal lung but falls abruptly at birth.[8]

This rapid drop in pulmonary vascular resistance can be attributed to changes in both ventilation and oxygenation.[9,10] Although ventilation is the major component of the fall of pulmonary vascular resistance, improved oxygenation also plays a role. Increases in oxygen concentration cause a modest increase in pulmonary blood flow and decrease in mean pulmonary artery pressure.[10] This may be partly due to the fact that oxygen modulates the production of the vasoactive substances nitric oxide and prostacyclin.

Neonatal Myocardium

At birth, physiologic changes in pressure and volume loads on the heart require that the neonatal myocardium compensate rapidly. Left ventricular volume and mass increase in early postnatal life in response to the changes in workloads of the left and right ventricles.[11,12] Myocyte numbers increase during this transition period. This hyperplastic growth response may be modulated by locally released ventricular acidic fibroblast growth factor.[13] Because of the increased demands of a higher vascular resistance to which it is exposed, myocyte proliferation occurs more rapidly in the left ventricle than the right. Cell growth continues through the first several weeks or months of life but becomes senescent later in life.[14] After these first few weeks, myocycte hypertrophy accounts for most of the increase in ventricular mass that occurs after birth. The postnatal hypertrophic growth response is thought to be stimulated by a change in workload demands on the ventricles as well as circulating growth factors and catecholamines. Acidic fibroblast growth factor and transforming growth factors produced by the cardiac myocycte may mediate cellular proliferation and differentiation.[15] Rising concentrations of circulating catecholamines also stimulate hypertrophy of cultured neonatal myocytes.[16]

The neonatal myocycte is quite different structurally from the mature myocyte. The immature cardiac myocyte is rounded, relatively short, and quite disorganized intracellularly.

It changes into a slender and longer shape and takes on a more organized ultrastructural appearance as it matures. The myofibrils are contractile proteins that help to give the myocyte its shape and structural organization. In the mature cell, the myofibrils are densely concentrated and are aligned in parallel with the axis of the cell, organized into alternating rows of mitochondria. In the neonatal cardiomyocyte, however, the myofibrils are relatively less dense and are more likely to be situated along the periphery of the cell. The more central portion of the myocyte is made up of disorganized clumps of mitochondria and nuclei.[11,17,18] The mitochondria increase in number, relative volume, and cristae thickness as the cell matures.[19,20] As the mitochondria increase in volume and take on a more orderly relationship, the myocardium matures to utilize activated long chain fatty acids as its primary source of energy rather than carbohydrate.[21-23] The sarcomere is the contractile unit of cardiac muscle and is organized into overlapping strands of thick and think filaments (contractile proteins). The number of sarcomeres increases and their organizational structure is transformed during the first few months of life.[14] During development, several different isoforms of contractile proteins change their expression, and therefore the functional properties of the sarcomere.[24]

The cardiac myocyte plasma membrane, or sarcolemma, is made up of ion channels pumps that allow for trans-sarcolemmal transport of calcium and other ions. Age-dependent density and current properties of ion channels may impact on myocardial performance. In human atria, decreased calcium current density has been demonstrated in children when compared to adults.[25] Calcium ion current in the atria also inactivates more rapidly in infants and children compared to adults.[26] The sarcolemma is tightly associated with the sarcoplasmic reticulum, a tubular meshwork surrounding the myofibrils and responsible for the uptake and release of cytosolic calcium. The sarcoplasmic reticulum from fetal sheep contains a lower density of Ca^{2+} channels and decreased pump activity compared to maternal sheep.[27] These differences in composition and function of calcium transporters may contribute to decreased myocardial reserve and contractility in the immature myocardium. The extracellular matrix represents another unique feature of the neonatal myocardium. This complex of proteoglycans, glycoproteins, and collagen provides structural support and contributes to the active and passive properties of the myocyte.[28] The composition of the extracellular matrix changes over time. Laminin, a matrix protein found in the basal laminae and important for cell adhesion, is sparsely distributed in the embryonic myocardium and localized to discrete areas of the matrix related to the sarcolemma during fetal development.[29-31] Later, in the mature myocyte, islaminin is found throughout the basement membrane, closely associated with the Z discs of the sarcomere. This association suggests a possible mechanical contribution of the extracellular matrix to myocardial contraction and relaxation.[28]

Ventricular Contraction and Relaxation

During the first few weeks and months of life, the composition of the myocardium changes significantly and with that the functional capacity of the heart. The immature myocardium is less compliant, generates less contractile force, and is inefficiently shaped when compared to the mature heart. Developmental changes in the composition of the sarcolemma, contractile proteins, mitochondria, and extracellular matrix play important roles in the myocyte's ability to develop sarcomeric shortening and myocardial tension. A combination of a greater ratio of noncontractile elements to contractile elements in the neonatal heart and less organized and efficient myofibrils impact on myocardial contractility.[32] The neonatal heart is not capable of generating the same tension per unit cross-sectional area as the myocardium of adults.[33-37] Fetal myocardial contractility is reduced at all cardiac muscle lengths. Additionally, at any given tension, the velocity of shortening is diminished compared to the adult. The resting, or passive tension, is also higher in the fetus than the adult suggesting reduced compliance of these muscles.[38] Despite a relatively reduced ability to develop tension, the neonatal myocardial contractility can be augmented with inotropes.[39]

Although the neonatal myocardium has the capacity to augment contractility when exposed to inotropic agents, that capacity may be reduced compared to the older infant and child.[40] Higher baseline concentrations of catecholamines may limit the ability of the immature myocyte to further increase cardiac output. Circulating concentrations of norepinephrine are elevated at birth[41] and may cause a transient increase in myocardial contractility in the perinatal period. Pressure loads on the immature myocardium can also negatively impact on cardiac function. The fetal myocardium is very sensitive to afterload and has a limited capacity for improved cardiac performance in the presence of raised arterial pressure.[42] This limited capacity for improved function and high baseline levels of circulating catecholamines suggest that cardiac performance is normally near maximum in the fetus. Even so, cardiac output can be augmented to some degree with various manipulations including volume loading and catecholamines.

The increase in pressure and volume that occurs as blood enters the heart is determined by the compliance of the ventricular myocardium. The compliance of the newborn heart is relatively reduced compared to the adult. Ventricular filling is affected by several factors including the active and passive properties of myocardium, ventricular interdependence, and the pericardium. Developmental changes in the extracellular matrix and cytoskeleton as well as the decreased ability of the neonatal myocardium to sequester calcium from the cytosol [43,44] may also impact on the mechanical relaxation properties of the neonatal heart.

The newborn myocardium responds to volume loading differently than the adult myocardium. Higher pressures are achieved with a given volume load in the right ventricle compared to the left. In the neonate, left ventricular compliance is altered and becomes intermediate to that of the fetus and adult. At all ages the right ventricle is more compliant than the left.[45] The influence of ventricular interdependence also differs by age, with filling of one ventricle reducing the distensibility of the opposite ventricle, occurring most profoundly in the fetus and less so in the adult myocardium. Ventricular compliance Increases with maturation throughout many species.[33,38,46-49]

The Frank-Starling curve is operative and effective in the neonatal heart although shifted due to a limited capacity for developing active tension. Compared to more mature myocardium, little change in cardiac output is seen when the immature ventricle is volume loaded.[50,51]

This limited capacity for augmenting cardiac output with ventricular filling means that increasing heart rate becomes an important mechanism for increasing cardiac output in the neonate.[52] Naturally occurring heart rate changes associated with changes in venous return to the heart combine to produce a positive relationship between heart rate and left ventricular output.[53]

Sympathetic Activity

Afferent baroreceptor input to the brain signals low cardiac output states. Efferent sympathetic pathways are then activated, causing vasoconstriction of the renal and peripheral vasculature as well as the release of renin and angiotensin II and the nonosmotic release of arginine vasopressin. Baseline plasma concentrations of catecholamines are elevated in the neonate compared to the older child and adult.[41,54] Myocardial catecholamine concentrations, however, are higher in the adult than the fetus and neonate.[55] Several studies have demonstrated that cardiac sympathetic innervation is incomplete in the neonate but gradually matures postnatally.[38,54-56]

Developmental differences in the hemodynamic response to similar doses of exogenous catecholamines exists and is likely due in large part to differences in drug pharmacokinetics between the age groups.[57,58] Age-dependent differences in the clearance rates of sympathomimetic inotropes have been demonstrated.[59,60] Dopamine clearance rates decrease significantly with age, with rates in children under 2 years of age nearly twice as great as older children. Because they have a higher percentage of body water than adults, neonates and infants have a larger volume of distribution for water soluble drugs, including phosphodiesterase inhibitors[61-63] and digoxin.[63] Individual differences as hypoperfusion to vital organs, systemic inflammatory response syndrome, and differences in enzyme activity also may affect clearance.[58,64] Age-related variation in the hemodynamic response to exogenous catecholamines may also result from different responses to the adrenergic receptor. While the relative receptor density of beta-adrenergic receptor subtypes is similar in both neonatal and adult rats, a difference in response to receptor stimulation can be measured.[65] At low agonist concentrations, beta-2-adrenergic receptor activation improves contractile performance in the neonatal rat but has no effect on the adult rat myocardium. It is further affected by the relatively low concentration of the inhibitory (Gi) G protein isoform in the neonatal rat ventricular myocardium.[66] Prolonged stimulation of the b-adrenergic receptor normally leads to desensitization and down-regulation. The neonate is unique, however, in that desensitization does not occur with chronic stimulation of the agonist-occupied receptor. In fact, the opposite occurs—the receptor becomes sensitized and the response to stimulation is enhanced.[67-70]

ETIOLOGY OF HEART FAILURE

Neonatal heart failure can manifest in both acquired and congenital forms with etiologies as disparate as structural, metabolic, and environmental in origin.

Excessive Pulmonary Blood Flow

Heart failure is a clinical syndrome characterized by elevated filling pressures, compensatory activation of the neurohormonal system and progressive symptomatology, which typically occurs in situations of pulmonary overcirculation. Circulatory adaptive mechanisms are triggered in symptomatic pulmonary overcirculation to preserve cardiac output and end organ perfusion. The sympathetic nervous system is activated and plasma concentrations of norepinephrine increase, stimulating the renin–angiotensin–aldosterone system, causing peripheral vasoconstriction and increased heart rate. Plasma norepinephrine levels are elevated in infants and children with heart failure due to left-to-right shunting lesions,[71] and these concentrations normalize after surgical repair of the structural defects.[72] Likewise, plasma concentrations of arginine vasopressin, a neurohormone that causes peripheral vasoconstriction and free water retention, are also increased in children with heart failure due to shunting lesions as well as in situations of ventricular dysfunction.[73] Natriuretic peptides are secreted by the atria and ventricles in response to myocardial stretch due to pressure or volume loads on the heart. Plasma levels of atrial natriuretic peptide,[74] and B-type natriuretic peptide,[75] are elevated in children with congenital heart disease and correlate with Qp:Qs in patients with left-to-right intracardiac shunts.

In acyanotic cardiac lesions such as ventricular septal defect and complete atrioventricular canal defect, signs and symptoms of heart failure usually develop during the neonatal period, as the pulmonary vascular resistance falls. Signs such as tachypnea, retractions, grunting, and diaphoresis with feeding usually herald this change in physiology. Other acyanotic lesions also associated with large left-to-right shunting include the patent ductus arteriosus, aortopulmonary window, and systemic arteriovenous malformations. These "run off" lesions may manifest with signs of heart failure in the first few days (in premature infants) or weeks of life with bounding pulses in addition to signs of respiratory compromise. If left uncorrected, these defects can lead to pulmonary vascular disease over time.

Cyanotic cardiac defects can also be associated with pulmonary overcirculation and heart failure and include common arterial trunk, total anomalous pulmonary venous connection, tricuspid atresia (without obstructed pulmonary blood flow) and double outlet right ventricle (without obstructed pulmonary blood flow). In these lesions, an admixture of highly oxygen-saturated and less oxygen-saturated blood occurs at the atrial, ventricular or great arterial level and the mixed blood is then sent to the pulmonary and systemic circulations, taking the path of least resistance. Chest radiography may reveal increased pulmonary vascular markings despite low systemic arterial oxygen saturations. Classic signs of heart failure are also seen in infants with unrepaired or non-palliated forms of cyanotic pulmonary overcirculation and include cardiomegaly, hepatomegaly, tachypnea, and poor weight gain.

Children born with ductal-dependent systemic blood flow lesions such as hypoplastic left heart syndrome or a variant, thereof can develop signs of heart failure while being administered prostaglandin E1 and awaiting surgical palliation. As pulmonary vascular resistance falls, increased pulmonary blood flow may lead to heart failure of pulmonary overcirculation and low cardiac output syndrome. This progressive imbalance of Qp:Qs places an increased demand on the systemic right ventricle to maintain cardiac output while producing a falsely reassuring high systemic oxygen saturation. These newborns may develop pulmonary vascular congestion, poor perfusion, metabolic acidosis, and endorgan injury from inadequate systemic blood flow. Efforts to limit excessive pulmonary blood flow and increase pulmonary vascular resistance by either reducing alveolar PO_2 or increasing alveolar PCO_2 may improve cardiac output. Strategies such as intubation and administration of inspired CO_2,[76,77] reduction of minute ventilation, and adding nitrogen to the inspired gases to create a subambient FiO_2 concentration have been employed with variable success. Once a patient has been stabilized and acidosis has been corrected a more definitive therapy such as the Norwood procedure or Sano modification of stage 1 reconstruction is required.

Pressure Overload

Other forms of congenital heart disease can manifest with signs of heart failure in the early newborn period (first 3 days of life). Infants with critical aortic or pulmonary valvar stenosis may present with shock or cyanosis, respectively. Critical coarctation of the aorta or interrupted aortic arch may also present in the first few days of life as the ductus arteriosus closes. These left-sided obstructive lesions often coexist, and the clinical spectrum can vary between an isolated bicuspid aortic valve with minimal obstruction to hypoplastic left heart syndrome. The right ventricle generally will support the systemic circulation in the setting of a widely patent ductus arteriosus. When the ductus closes the right ventricle cannot adequately perfuse the systemic circulation resulting in a profound metabolic acidosis, and if untreated, multiorgan system failure and death. Initial stabilization of neonates with low cardiac output and hypotension with suspected heart disease may require volume resuscitation, correction of acidosis and initiation of inotropic support. Infusion of prostaglandin E1 should be started in an effort to maintain patency of the ductus arteriosus. Opening the ductus provides palliative blood flow to the systemic circulation in the presence of critical left-sided obstructive lesions such as critical aortic stenosis, coarctation, interrupted aortic arch, and hypoplastic left heart syndrome and allows for augmented pulmonary blood flow in the situation of critical pulmonary stenosis. The benefits of prostaglandin E1 in these clinical scenarios usually outweigh any risks or side effects (e.g. apnea, fever, peripheral vasodilation). If the patient is anemic, transfusion with packed red blood cells can improve oxygen delivery. Concurrent with starting prostaglandin should be intubation and control of ventilation as a key element of decreasing metabolic demand. Additionally, positive pressure ventilation can improve left ventricular dysfunction by decreasing left ventricular afterload.[78]

A more definitive intervention can be performed, once the patient has been stabilized and a diagnosis confirmed. In valvular aortic stenosis, the leaflets are usually dysplastic, thickened, doming in systole and the aortic valve is frequently bicommissural. Balloon valvuloplasty for either critical pulmonary or aortic valve stenosis can provide rapid hemodynamic relief. Balloon valvuloplasty may be the treatment of choice for infants with aortic stenosis and depressed left ventricular systolic function, avoiding surgical intervention in the newborn period. Balloon valvuloplasty has been associated with decreased residual gradient, higher degree of aortic insufficiency, and an increased need or reintervention as compared with surgical valvotomy.[79] Surgical repair of coarctation of the aorta or aortic arch hypoplasia is the preferred treatment for native coarctation of the aorta in the newborn period. Systemic hypertension is thought to be the etiology of dilated cardiomyopathy with depressed myocardial function in pediatric patients with neuroblastoma and Wilm's tumor. In neuroblastoma, high levels of circulating catecholamines cause peripheral vasoconstriction and raise the systemic vascular resistance. Additionally, norepinephrine is directly toxic to the myocardium and a protracted period of high concentrations can lead to myocyte drop out and apoptosis. Patients with Wilms tumor may have high circulating levels of renin which also increases systemic vascular resistance. Treatment of these tumors can lead to reverse remodeling of the myocardium and improved ventricular function. Other renal causes of systemic hypertension (e.g. renal artery stenosis, nephritis) in children may also lead to ventricular dysfunction and heart failure, but these diseases often manifest with ventricular hypertrophy initially.

Valvular Insufficiency

Pulmonary valvar insufficiency causing ventricular dysfunction or heart failure is usually a result of previous surgery or catheter-based interventions on the pulmonary valve. Congenital forms of pulmonary insufficiency are also recognized, such as absent pulmonary valve syndrome. Tricuspid regurgitation is an uncommon cause of heart failure in children. Clinically significant tricuspid regurgitation is most often seen in patients with Ebstein's anomaly, a congenital defect of the heart in which the annular attachments of the tricuspid valve are displaced towards the apex of the right ventricle. The ventricle becomes divided into an "atrialized" inlet portion and functional apical and infundibular portions. The tricuspid valve leaflets fail to coapt, causing severe tricuspid regurgitation and right atrial enlargement. Prograde pulmonary blood flow may be significantly compromised and right ventricular function may eventually deteriorate. Symptomatic patients diagnosed in the newborn or infant period usually have the most severe form of the disease and develop signs of heart failure early on. The mortality rate is high among patients who require surgical intervention at this age. Older individuals with less severe disease may develop symptoms of right heart failure including hepatomegaly, jugular venous distention, peripheral edema, and dyspnea with exertion. Atrial arrhythmias are also common in this cohort. Other causes of significant tricuspid regurgitation include endocarditis and tricuspid valvar dysplasia.

Functional tricuspid regurgitation, in the setting of a structurally normal valve, may occur secondary to pressure or volume loads on the right ventricle. A hypertensive right ventricle will eventually dilate, causing the annulus to stretch and the valve leaflets to fail to coapt properly resulting in tricuspid regurgitation. Elevated right ventricular pressures and subsequent valvar incompetence in the neonate are usually caused by persistent pulmonary hypertension, left atrial hypertension (e.g. mitral stenosis), or pulmonary valve stenosis. Correcting the underlying cause of right ventricular hypertension may reduce the degree of valvar regurgitation and ameliorate the clinical features of heart failure. A volume load on right ventricle can also lead to annular dilation and incompetence. Congenital defects such as total anomalous pulmonary venous return, cerebral or hepatic arteriovenous malformations, and absent pulmonary valve syndrome cause an increase in blood flow to the right heart producing progressive right ventricular dilation.

Other forms of valvar insufficiency causing heart failure in the newborn period are rare. Aortic insufficiency in the neonate usually occurs secondary to surgery or a catheter-based intervention. A dilated aortic root, as a result of neonatal Marfan syndrome, is frequently associated with aortic insufficiency and may cause left ventricular dilation and dysfunction. [80] The mitral valve may also be affected in Marfan syndrome, causing leaflet prolapsed and regurgitation. Congenital mitral regurgitation leading to heart failure in the neonate is rare and is usually associated with other cardiac defects or occurs secondary to dilated cardiomyopathy or infarction of the papillary muscles.

Ischemic Cardiomyopathy

Myocardial ischemia, as a result of anomalous origin of the coronary arteries, is an infrequent and potentially reversible cause congestive heart failure in the neonate and infant.

Anomalous origin of the left coronary artery from the pulmonary artery (ALCAPA) usually is an isolated malformation that occurs during embryogenesis. In the fetus, pulmonary artery pressure is relatively high and coronary artery perfusion is therefore adequate. Postnatally, as pulmonary vascular resistance falls, pulmonary arterial pressure decreases leading to diminished left coronary artery (LCA) perfusion. Blood flow to the left coronary artery is then dependent on retrograde filling from collateral vessels that originate from the higher pressure right coronary artery (RCA).[81] A small left-to-right shunt is created with oxygenated blood from the RCA coursing through collaterals to the LCA and ultimately draining into the pulmonary artery. This failure of antegrade perfusion through the LCA leads to myocardial ischemia that may cause subendocardial or transmural infarction and, eventually, the clinical syndrome of heart failure.

Most patients with ALCAPA develop signs of heart failure in the first few weeks or months of life. The earliest signs of heart failure include failure to thrive, tachypnea, wheezing, diaphoresis, and angina-like episodes that manifest as sudden inconsolability and pallor.[82] A gallop rhythm and blowing holosystolic murmur of mitral insufficiency may be appreciated on physical examination. Chest radiograph typically reveals cardiomegaly and prominent pulmonary vascular markings may be present. The electrocardiogram classically demonstrates ST segment elevation in the anterolateral leads and Q waves in leads I and aVL.

Although the signs and symptoms of heart failure in ALCAPA can be relieved with medicinal therapy, the goal should be to correct any hemodynamic derangements and stabilize the patient in preparation for surgery. Myocardial ischemia in ALCAPA is potentially reversible with surgical repair[83,84] and improved ventricular function is frequently observed after reimplantation of the coronary artery.[85]

TREATMENT OF HEART FAILURE IN THE NEONATE

The clinical spectrum of heart failure is broad in the newborn period, ranging from the hypoxemic infant with persistent pulmonary hypertension and fulminant right-sided heart failure to the hydropic infant with neonatal myocarditis and severely depressed left ventricular function, to the child with respiratory insufficiency caused by diastolic heart failure of hypertrophic cardiomyopathy. The care of these patients must be individualized as one aims to provide symptomatic relief, correct metabolic abnormalities, and reverse hemodynamic derangements. Treatment options for decompensated heart failure are limited and almost all are untested in children. Most of the data and insight relied upon for managing pediatric patients with advanced heart failure have been derived from studies and experience in adults, the majority of whom have an ischemic etiology for their LV dysfunction. There are no formal recommendations for the treatment of advanced heart failure in children, therefore we must respect the principle that we should first do no harm.

Intravenous diuretics (usually loop diuretics) are considered standard of care therapy for the initial treatment of decompensated heart failure in neonates and children and should be given without delay. Diuretic "resistance" may respond to the addition of thiazide diuretics such as metolazone or intravenous chlorothiazide. Another consideration is the use of a continuous infusion of a loop diuretic instead of scheduled intermittent dosing when patients fail to respond to diuretic therapy. Fluid restriction in neonates is rarely ever necessary. During intravenous diuretic therapy, a variety of side effects should be monitored including electrolyte disturbances, renal insufficiency, and hypotension. Because of immature renal secretory control in the neonate, urinary loss of potassium, magnesium and calcium can be profound. Newborns with decompensated heart failure and reduced blood pressure with normal or low systemic vascular resistance should be considered for inotropic therapy. Inotropic agents may be necessary to maintain circulatory function and improve end-organ function. Milrinone, sometimes referred to as an inodilator, is a phosphodiesterase inhibitor that acts by increasing cyclic adenosine monophosphate (cAMP), thereby providing inotropy with additional afterload reduction. Milrinone also reduces pulmonary vascular tone and is less likely to cause tachycardia like other inotropic agents. Although it can be proarrhythmic, milrinone is not typically associated with the sustained tachycardia, increased myocardial oxygen consumption, or elevated systemic vascular resistance that often occurs with the use of other inotropic agents. Few studies have evaluated the safety and efficacy of milrinone for the treatment of decompensated heart failure in adults, they have failed to show any clinical benefit when used for this indication.[86-88] A few studies have examined the cardiovascular effects of phosphodiesterase inhibitors in children.[89,90] In the PRIMACORP study, milrinone used in neonates in the immediate postoperative period reduced the risk of low cardiac output syndrome.[91] Dosing and utility of milrinone for the treatment of decompensated pediatric heart failure are not known. Previously, infusions should be started at a relatively low dose (0.1–0.3 μg/kg/min) and uptitrated to a maximum of approximately 0.75 μg/kg/min, depending on systemic blood pressure response.

In situations of hypotension an alternative to milrinone, are the sympathomimetic agents—dobutamine, dopamine and epinephrine. These agents stimulate adrenergic receptors in the myocardium and smooth muscle causing increased cAMP concentrations and enhanced inotropy and vascular resistance. They may also result in tachycardia, increased myocardial oxygen consumption and an increased incidence of arrhythmias.

Dobutamine is a sympathomimetic drug that stimulates β-adrenergic receptors in the myocardium and peripheral vasculature causing increased myocardial contractility and decreased peripheral and pulmonary vascular tone.[91,92]

Dobutamine is also known to increase heart rate, myocardial oxygen consumption and the incidence of atrial and ventricular arrhythmias. If dobutamine is to be used for the treatment of decompensated heart failure, it should be started at the lowest dose capable of achieving the desired effect and should be weaned or discontinued as soon as possible. Doses of 2.5–10 μg/kg/min are capable of increasing cardiac output, reducing systemic vascular resistance and improving stroke volume. Higher doses are unlikely to provide further improvement in hemodynamics and are more likely to be associated with adverse effects.

Dopamine is a sympathomimetic that stimulates β-adrenergic receptors, as well as α-adrenergic receptors and dopaminergic receptors on the peripheral vasculature. It acts predominantly on β_1 receptors in the myocardium causing increased contractility and heart rate at doses of 3 μg/kg/min and greater. The α-adrenergic receptor response is seen at doses of 5 μg/kg/min and higher, causing peripheral vasoconstriction and overwhelming any beta-2-induced vasodilation. The dopaminergic or renal effects occur at doses less than 3 μg/kg/min, augmenting renal blood flow. Whether this improves renal function or urine output in patients with heart failure remains controversial. Dopamine is a good choice for patients in low cardiac output when sustained pressor support is needed quickly. Common side effects of dopamine infusions include tachycardia, ventricular arrhythmias, hypertension, and headache.

In life-threatening situations or cardiogenic shock, an epinephrine infusion is indicated. Even low dose epinephrine boluses can sustain systemic pressure until a more reliable therapy can be initiated. Epinephrine stimulates both a and b receptors with pressor effects occurring at doses of 0.02 μg/kg/min or greater. Although epinephrine may increase blood pressure, heart rate, and contractility it also may cause ischemia, atrial or ventricular arrhythmias and increased myocardial oxygen consumption. When catecholamine-resistant hypotension is encountered, a vasopressin infusion may improve systemic vascular resistance. Vasopressin has not been studied in a controlled fashion for this indication in heart failure patients, but doses of 0.01–0.05 units/kg/hr for the purpose of treating hypotension in end-stage heart failure have been used. A calcium chloride infusion may also support blood pressure and provide increased contractility in emergency situations. Doses of 2.5–5.0 mg/kg/hr, have been used while monitoring ionized calcium concentrations.

CONCLUSION

The syndrome of heart failure in neonates differs in its etiology, physiology, and clinical manifestations when compared to older children and adults. Structural heart disease is the most common cause of heart failure in the newborn period, causing either pulmonary overcirculation, low cardiac output syndrome or both. Most anatomic defects that cause heart failure, fortunately, can be surgically palliated, if not repaired. Functionally, the neonatal myocardium generates less contractile force and exhibits less compliance than the more mature myocardium. Despite this difference, cardiac output in the neonate may be augmented with increased filling, higher heart rate, and inotropic stimulation. Treating heart failure in this population can be quite challenging.

REFERENCES

1. Rudolph AM, Drorbaugh JE, Auld PA, et al. Studies on the circulation in the neonatal period. The circulation in the respiratory distress syndrome. Pediatrics. 1961;27:551-66.

2. Clyman RI, Mauray F, Wong L. et al. The developmental response of the ductus arteriosus to oxygen. Biol Neonate. 1978;34:177-81.
3. Oberhansli-Weis I, Heymann MA, Rudolph AM, et al. The pattern and mechanism of response to oxygen by the ductus arteriosus and umbilical artery. Ped Res. 1972;6:693-700.
4. Clyman RI, Waleh N, Black SM, et al. Regulations of ductus arteriosus patency by nitric oxide in fetal lambs: the role of gestation, oxygen tension, and vasa vasorum. Ped Res. 1998;43:633-44.
5. Friedman WF, Printz MP, Kirkpatrick SE, et al. The vasoactivity of the fetal lamb ductus arteriosus studied in utero. Ped Res. 1983;17:331-337.
6. Meyer WW, Lind J. The ductus venosus and the mechanism of its closure. Arch Dis Child. 1966;41:597-605.
7. Adeagbo AS, Coceani F, Olley PM. The response of the lamb ductus venosus to prostaglandins and inhibitors of prostaglandin and thromboxane. Circ Res. 1982;51:580-6.
8. Heyman MA, Rudolph AM. Effects of congenital heart disease on fetal and neonatal circulations. Prog Cardiovasc Dis. 1972;15:115-43.
9. Cook CD, Drinker PA, Jacobson HN, et al. Control of pulmonary blood flow in the foetal and newly born lamb. J Physiol. 1963;169:10-29.
10. Teitel DF, Iwamoto HS, Rudolph AM. Changes in the pulmonary circulation during birth-related events. Ped Res. 1990;27:372-8.
11. Anversa P, Olivetti G, Loud AV. Morphometric study of early postnatal development in the left and right ventricular myocardium of the rat. Circ Res. 1998;46:495-502.
12. Korecky B, Rakusan K. Normal and hypertrophic growth of the rat heart: changes in cell dimension and number. Am J Physiol. 1978;234:H123.
13. Englemann GL, Dionne CA, Jaye MC. Acidic fibroblast growth factor and heart development. Role in myocyte proliferation and capillary angiogenesis. Circ Res. 1993;72:7-19.
14. Zak R. Development and proliferative capacity of cardiac muscle cells. Circ Res. 1993;35(Supp II):17-26.
15. Weiner HL, Swain JL. Acidic fibroblast growth factor mRNA is expressed by cardiac myocytes in culture and the protein is localized to the extracellular matrix. Proc Natl Acad USA. 1989;86:2683-7.
16. Simpson P. Stimulation of hypertrophy of cultured neonatal rat heart cells through an alpha 1-adrenergic receptor and induction of beating through an alpha 1- and beta 1-adrenergic receptor interaction. Evidence for independent regulation of growth and beating. Circ Res. 1985;56:884-94.
17. Nassar R, Reedy MC, Anderson PA. Developmental changes in the ultrastructure and sarcomere shortening of the isolated rabbit ventricular myocyte. Circ Res. 1987;61:465-83.
18. Sheridan DJ, Cullen MJ, Tynan MJ. Qualitative and quantitative observations on ultrastructural changes during postnatal development in the cat myocardium. J Mol Cell Cardiol. 1979;11:1173-81.
19. Hoerter J, Mazet F, Vassort G. Perinatal growth of the rabbit cardiac cell. Possible implications for the mechanism of relaxation. J Mol Cell Cardiol. 1981;13:725-40.
20. Olivetti G, Anversa P, Loud AV. Morphometric study of early postnatal development in the left and right ventricular myocardium of the rat. Tissue composition, capillary growth, and sarcoplasmic alterations. Circ Res. 1980;46:503-12.
21. Fisher DJ, Heymann MA, Rudolph AM. Myocardial oxygen and carbohydrate consumption in fetal lambs in utero and in adult sheep. Am J Phys. 1980;238:H399-H405.
22. Warshaw JB, Terry ML. Cellular energy metabolism during fetal development. II. Fatty acid oxidation by the developing heart. J Cell Biol. 1970;44:354-60.
23. Wittels B, Bressler R. Lipid metabolism in the newborn heart. J Clin Invest 1965;44:1639-46.
24. Swynghedauw B. Developmental and functional adaptation of contractile proteins in cardiac and skeletal muscles. Physiol Rev 1986;66:710-71.
25. Hatem SN, Sweeten T, Vetter V, et al. Evidence for presence of Ca^{2+} stores in neonatal human atrial myocytes. Am J Physiol. 1995;268:H1195-H1201.
26. Roca TP, Pigott JD, Clarkson CW, et al. L-type calcium current in pediatric and adult human atrial myocytes: evidence for developmental changes in channel inactivation. Pediatr Res. 1996;40:462-8.
27. Mahony L, Jones LR. Developmental changes in cardiac sarcoplasmic reticulum in sheep. J Biol Chem 1986;261:15257-65.
28. Anderson RH, Baker EJ, Macartney FJ, et al. Myocardium and development in paediatric cardiology, 2nd edition. London: Harcourt Publishers; 2002.
29. Kitten GT, Markwald RR, Bolender DL. Distribution of basement membrane antigens in cryopreserved early embryonic hearts. Anatom Record. 1978;217:379-90.
30. Little CD, Piquet DM, Davis LA, et al. Distribution of laminin, collagen type IV, collagen type I, and fibronectin in chicken cardiac jelly basement membrane. Anatom Record. 1989;224:417-25.
31. Price RL, Nakagawa M, Terracio L, et al. Ultrastructural localization of laminin on in vivo embryonic neonatal and adult rate cardiac myocytes and in early rat embryos raised in whole embryo culture. J Histochem and Cytochem. 1992;40:1373-81.
32. Legato MJ. Cellular mechanisms of normal growth in the mammalian heart. Qualitative and quantitative features of ventricular architecture in the dog from birth to five months of age. Circ Res. 1979;44:250-62.
33. Davies P, Dewar J, Tynan M. Post-natal developmental changes in the length-tension relationship of cat papillary muscles. J Physiol. 1975;253:95-102.
34. Friedman WF, Lesch M, Sonnenblick EH. Neonatal heart disease. New York: Grune and Stratton; 1973, pp. 21-49.
35. Hoerter J. Changes in the sensitivity to hypoxia and glucose deprivation in the isolated perfused rabbit heart during perinatal development. Pfluegers Arch. 1976;363:1-6.
36. Hopkins SF Jr. McCutcheon EP, Wekstein DR. Postnatal changes in rat ventricular function. Circ Res. 1973;32:685-91.
37. Park MK, Sheridan PH, Morgan WW, et al. Comparative inotropic response of newborn and adult rabbit papillary

muscles to isoproterenol and calcium. Dev Pharmacol Ther. 1980;1:70-82.

38. Friedman WF. The intrinsic physiologic properties of the developing heart. Prog Cardiovasc Dis. 1972;15:87-111.
39. Anderson PA, Manring A, Glick KL, et al Biophysics of the developing heart. A comparison of the left ventricular dynamics of the fetal and neonatal lamb heart. Am J Obstet Gynecol. 1982;143:195-203.
40. Teitel DF, Sidi DD, Chin T, et al. Developmental changes in myocardial contractile reserve in the lamb. Pediatr Res. 1985;19:948-55.
41. Eliot RJ, Lam R, Leake RD, et al. Plasma catecholamine concentrations in infants at birth and during the first 48 hours of life. J Pediatr. 1980;96:311-5.
42. Gilbert RD. Effects of afterload and baroreceptors on cardiac function in fetal sheep. J Dev Physiol. 1982;4:299-309.
43. Mahony L. Calcium homeostasis and control of contractility in the developing heart. Semin Perinatol. 1996;20:510-9.
44. Spotnitz WD, Spotnitz HM, Truccone NJ, et al. Relation of ultrastructure and function. Sarcomere dimensions, pressure-volume curves, and geometry of the intact left ventricle of the immature canine heart. Circ Res. 1979;44:679-91.
45. Romero T, Covell J, Friedman WF. A comparison of pressure-volume relations of the fetal, newborn, and adult heart. Am J Phys. 1972;222:1285-90.
46. Nakazawa M, Miyagawa S, Ohno T, et al. Developmental hemodynamic changes in rat embryos at 11 to 15 days of gestation: normal data of blood pressure and the effect of caffeine compared to data from chick embryo. Pedtr Res. 1988;23:200-5.
47. Reed KL, Sahn DJ, Scagnelli S et al. Doppler echocardiographic studies of diastolic function in the human fetal heart: changes during gestation. J Am Coll Cardiol. 1986;8:391-5.
48. Wladimiroff JW, Huisman TW, Stewart PA, et al. Normal fetal Doppler inferior vena cava, transtricuspid and umbilical artery flow velocity waveforms between 11 and 16 weeks' gestation. Am J Obstet Gynecol. 1992;166:921-4.
49. Hu N, Connuck DM, Keller BB, Clark EB. Diastolic filling characteristics in the stage 12 to 27 chick embryo ventricle. Pediatr Res. 1991;29:334-7.
50. Kirkpatrick SE, Pitlick PT, Naliboff J, et al. Frank-Starling relationship as an important determinant of fetal cardiac output. Am J Physiol. 1976;231:495-500.
51. Romero TE, Friedman WF. Limited left ventricular response to volume overload in the neonatal period: a comparative study with the adult animal. Pediatr Res. 1979;13:910-5.
52. Anderson PA, Killam AP, Mainwaring RD, et al. In utero right ventricular output in the fetal lamb: the effect of heart rate. J Physiol. 1987;387:297-16.
53. Anderson PA, Glick KL, Killam AP, et al. The effect of heart rate on in utero left ventricular output in the fetal sheep. J Physiol. 1986;372:557-73.
54. Geis WP, Tatooles CJ, Priola DV, et al. Factors influencing neurohormonal control of the heart in the newborn dog. Am J Physiol. 1975;228:1685-9.
55. Friedman WF, Pool PE, Jacobowitz D et al. Sympathetic innervation of the developing rabbit heart: Biochemical and histochemical comparisons of fetal, neonatal, and adult myocardium. Circ Res. 1968;23:25-32.
56. Lebowitz EA, Novich JS, Rudolph AM. Development of myocardial sympathetic innervations in the fetal lamb. Pediatr Res. 1992;6:887-93.
57. Erath HG Jr, Boerth RC, Graham TP Jr. Functional significance of reduced cardiac sympathetic innervation in the newborn dog. Am J Physiol. 1982;243:H20-6.
58. Booker PD. Pharmacological support for childrenn with myocardial dysfunction. Paediatr Anesth. 2002;12:5-25.
59. Allen E, Pettigrew A, Frank D, et al. Alterations in dopamine clearance and catechol-O-methyltransferase activity by dopamine infusions in children. Crit Care Med. 1997;25:181-89.
60. Nottemran DA, Greenwald BM, Moran F, et al. Dopamine clearance in critically ill infants and children: effect of age and organ system dysfuntion. Clin Pharmacol Ther. 1990;48:138-147.
61. Lawless S, Burckart G, Diven W, et al. Amrinone in neonates and infants after cardiac surgery. Crit Care Med. 1989;17:751-754.
62. Ramamoorthy C, Anderson GD, Williams GD, et al. Pharmacokinetics and side effects of milrinone in infants and children after open heart surgery. Anesth Analg. 1998;86:283-9.
63. Wettrell G. Distribution and elimination of digoxin in infants. Eur J Clin Pharmacol. 1977;11:329-335.
64. Schwartz PH, Eldadah MK, Newth CJ. The pharmacokinetics of dobutamine in pediatric intensive care. Drug Metab Dispos. 1991;19:614-9.
65. Kuznetsov V, Pak E, Robinson RB, et al. β_2-adrenergic receptor actions in neonatal and adult rat ventricular myocytes. Cir Res. 1995;76:40-52.
66. Bartel S, Karczewski P, Krause EG. G proteins, adenylyl cyclase and related phosphoproteins in the developing rat heart. Mol Cell Biochem. 1996;163/164:31-8.
67. Giannuzzi CE, Seidler FJ, Slotkin TA. Beta-adrenoceptor control of cardiac adenylyl cyclase during development: agonist pre-treatment in the neonate uniquely causes heterologous sensitization, not desensitization. Brain Res. 1995;694:271-8.
68. Zeiders JL, Seidler FJ, Iaccarino G, et al. Ontogeny of cardiac beta-adrenoceptor desensitization mechanisms: agonist treatment enhances receptor/G-protein transduction rather than eliciting ncoupling. J Mol Cell Cardiol. 1999;31:413-23.
69. Zeiders JL, Seidler FJ, Slotkin TA. Agonist-induced sensitization of β-adrenoceptor signaling in neonatal rat heart: expression and catalytic activity of adenylyl cyclase. J Pharmacol Exp Ther. 1999;291:503-10.
70. Auman JT, Seidler FJ, Slotkin TA. β-adrenoceptor control of G protein function in the neonate: Determinant of desensitization or sensitization. Am J Physiol Regul Integr Comp Physiol. 2002;283:1236-44.

71. Ross RD, Daniels SR, Schwartz DC, et al. Plasma norepinephrine levels in infants and children with congestive heart failure. Am J Cardiol. 1987;59:911-4.
72. Wu JR, Chang HR, Huang TY, et al. Reduction in lymphocyte beta-adrenegic receptor density in infants and children with heart failure secondary to congenital heart disease. Am J Cardiol. 1996;77:170-4.
73. Price JF, Towbin JA, Denfield SW, et al. Arginine vasopressin levels are elevated and correlate with functional status in infants and children with congestive heart failure. Circulation. 2004;109:2550-3.
74. Kikuchi K, Nishioka K, Ueda T, et al. Relationship between plasma atrial natriuretic polypeptide concentration and hemodynamic measurements in children with congenital heart disease. J Pediatr. 1987;111:335-42.
75. Kunii Y, Kamada M, Ohtsuki S, et al. Plasma brain natriuretic peptide and the evaluation of volume overload in infants and children with congenital heart disease. Acta Med Okayama. 2003;57:191-7.
76. Jobes DR, Nicholson SC, Steven JM, et al. Carbon dioxide prevents pulmonary overcirculation in hypoplastic left heart syndrome. Ann Thorac Surg 1992;54:150-1.
77. Tabbutt S, Ramamoorthy C, Montenegro LM, et al. Impact of inspired gas mixtures on preoperative infants with hypoplastic left heart syndrome during controlled ventilation. Circulation. 2001;104;I159-64.
78. Acosta B, DiBenedetto R, Rahimi A, et al. Hemodynamic effects of noninvasive bilevel positive airway pressure on patients with chronic congestive heart failure with systolic dysfunction. Chest. 2000;118:1004-9.
79. McCrindle BW, Blackstone EH, Williams WG, et al. Are outcomes of surgical versus transcatheter balloon valvotomy equivalent in neonatal critical aortic stenosis? Circulation. 2001;104(12 Supp 1):I152-8.
80. Morse PM, Rockenmacher S, Pyeritz RE, et al. Diagnosis and management of infantile Marfan syndrome. Pediatrics. 1990;86:888-95.
81. Case RB, Morrow AG, Stainsby W, Nestor JO. Anomalous origin of the left coronary artery: the physiologic defect and suggested surgical treatment. Circulation. 1958;17:1062-8.
82. Wesselhoeft H, Fawcett JS, Johnson AL. Anomalous origin of the left coronary artery from the pulmonary trunk: Its clinical spectrum, pathology, and pathophysiology, based on a review of 140 cases with seven further cases. Circulation. 1968;38:403-25.
83. Arciniegas E, Farooki ZQ, Hakimi M, et al. Management of anomalous left coronary artery from the pulmonary artery. Circulation. 1980;62:I180-9.
84. Kakou GM, Sidi D, Kachaner J, et al. Anomalous left coronary artery arising from the pulmonary artery in infancy: is early operation better? Br Heart J. 1988;60:522-6.
85. Carvalho JS, Redington AN, Oldershaw PJ, et al. Analysis of left ventricular wall movement before and after reimplantation of anomalous left coronary artery in infancy. Br Heart J. 1991;65:218-22.
86. Adams KF, Fonarow GC, Emerman CL, et al. In-hospital mortality in patients with acute decompensated heart failure requiring intravenous vasoactive medications: an analysis from the Acute Decompensated Heart Failure National Registry (ADHERE). J Am Coll Cardiol. 2005;46: 57-64.
87. Cuffe MS, Califf RM, Adams KF, et al. Short-term intravenous milrinone for acute exacerbation of chronic heart failure: a randomized controlled trial. JAMA. 2002;287:1541-7.
88. Felker MG, Benza RL, Chandler AB, et al. Heart failure etiology and response to milrinone in decompensated heart failure: results from the OPTIME-CHF study. J Am Coll Cardiol. 2003;41:997-1003.
89. Chang AC, Atz AM, Wernovsky G, et al. Milrinone: systemic and pulmonary emodynamic effects in neonates after cardiac surgery. Crit Care Med. 1995;23:1907-14.
90. Teshima H, Tobita K, Yamamura H, et al. Cardiovascular effects of a phosphodiesterase III inhibitor, amrinone, in infants: Noninvasive echocardiographic evaluation. Pediatr Int. 2002;44:259-263.
91. Hoffman TM, Wernovsky G, Atz AM, et al. Efficacy and safety of milrinone in preventing low cardiac output syndrome in infants and children after corrective surgery for congenital heart disease. Circulation. 2003;107:996-1002.
92. Leier CV, Webel J, Bush CA. The cardiovascular effects of the continuous infusion of dobutamine in patients with severe cardiac failure. Circulation. 1977;56:468-72.

115

CHAPTER

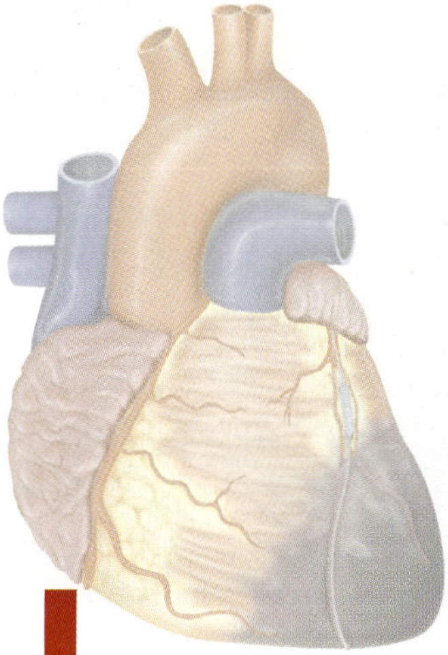

Advanced Echo Imaging in Cardiomyopathies in Children

Sonia A El-Saiedi, Hosam Ibrahim, Wael A Attia

INTRODUCTION

Patients with subclinical left ventricular (LV) dysfunction have an increased risk of developing symptomatic congestive heart failure (HF) leading to higher morbidity and mortality. Speckle-tracking echocardiography emerged recently to detect the understated changes in cardiac function and help in characterization and quantification of myocardial deformation.[1] Left ventricular ejection fraction (LVEF) over time proved its practicality and reliability but it is not enough to expose subtle or regional myocardial dysfunction. Two-dimensional speckle-tracking echocardiography (2D-STE) is a promising new imaging technique that can early detect imperceptible myocardial dysfunction prior to full blown decrease in LVEF.[2] Two-dimensional speckle-tracking echocardiography allows offline calculation of myocardial velocities and deformation parameters such as strain and strain rate (SR).[3] It also gives an impartial and quantitative evaluation of global and regional myocardial function independently from the angle and from cardiac movements.[4]

DIAGNOSTIC CRITERIA MEASURED BY TWO-DIMENSIONAL SPECKLE-TRACKING ECHOCARDIOGRAPHY

Longitudinal Strain

Longitudinal strain measures deformation of myocardium from the base to the apex. It is represented by negative trend curves (Fig. 1). Longitudinal strain analyses in four-chamber, two-chamber, and apical long-axis views give both regional and global strain values (global longitudinal strain). Global longitudinal strain lately has been authenticated as a quantitative index for global LV function (Figs. 1, 5, and 6).[5]

Radial Strain

Radial strain measures radial deformation of myocardium where the myocardium is deformed toward the center of the LV cavity, this will identify the LV thickening and thinning motions during the cardiac cycle. It is represented by positive curves (Fig. 2). Radial strain values are obtained by

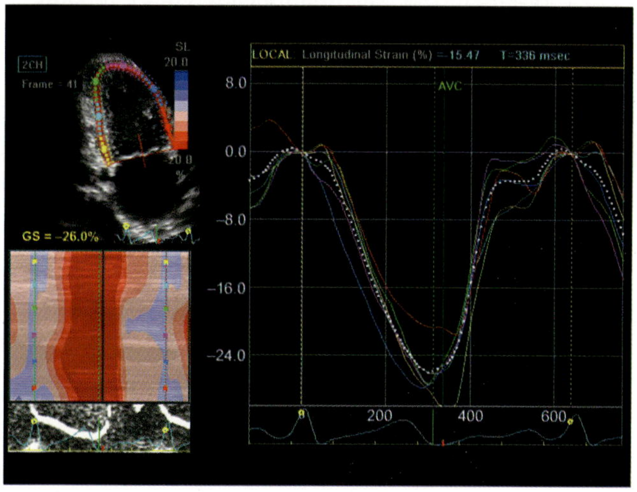

Fig. 1: Normal longitudinal strain.

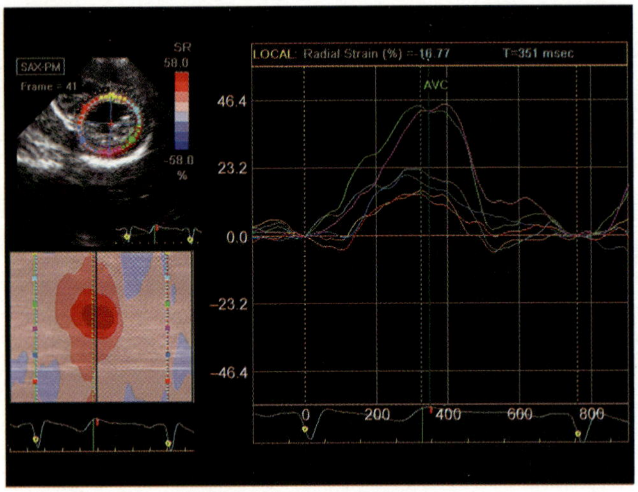

Fig. 2: Normal radial strain.

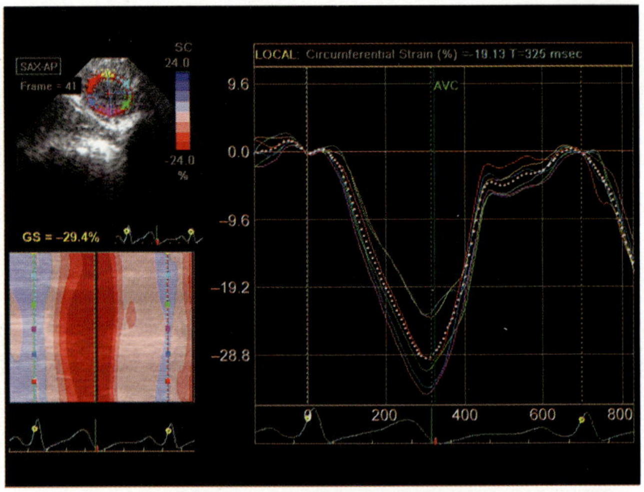

Fig. 3: Normal circumferential strain.

speckle-tracking echocardiographic analysis of basal, mid, and apical LV short-axis views.[6]

Circumferential Strain

Circumferential strain represents LV myocardial fiber shortening along the circular boundary evaluated on a short-axis view. Circumferential strain measurements are represented by negative curves (Fig. 3).[6]

Torsion

The LV spiral myocardial fibers are responsible for producing more than 60% of LVEF through LV torsional deformation, compared to the simple longitudinal or circumferential fibers whose shortening cannot produce LVEF more than 30%. The quantification of LV torsion by speckle-tracking echocardiography is made conceivable by analyzing the reciprocal rotation of the LV apex and base during systole (Fig. 4). Left ventricular torsion is then calculated as the net difference in mean rotation between the apical and basal levels.[7]

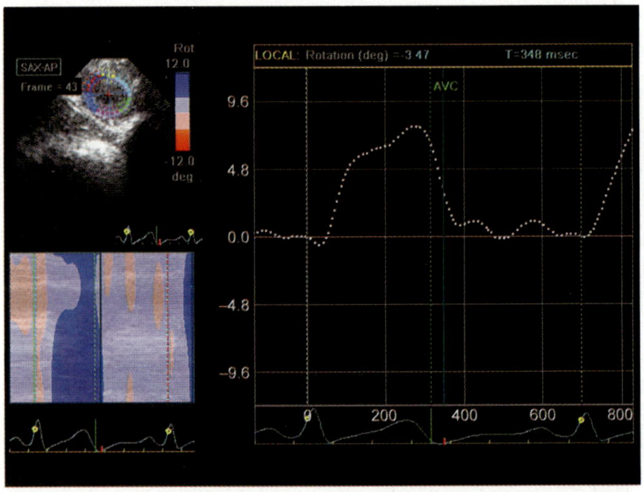

Fig. 4: Normal apical rotation.

THERAPEUTIC IMPLICATIONS OF SPECKLE TRACKING IN CARDIOMYOPATHY

Detection of Subclinical and Clinical Myocardial Dysfunction

Early detection of myocardial dysfunction by speckle tracking in subclinical stages has significant implications especially in patients receiving cardiotoxic medications, as reduction of LV function will be already a very late finding where significant myocardial damage has already happened. Several published studies reported the decrease of the different types of systolic strain (LV longitudinal, radial, and circumferential deformation) in cases of dilated cardiomyopathy (DCM) and hypertrophic cardiomyopathy (HCM)[8,9] confirmed by several limited studies from our own center.

Detection of Myocardial Fibrosis and Left Ventricular Reverse Remodeling

Myocardial fibrosis is associated with a poor prognosis, LV remodeling, and impaired response to treatment in patients with DCM. Myocardial fibrosis is detected with late gadolinium enhancement cardiovascular magnetic resonance imaging and ultrasonic myocardial tissue characterization by integrated backscatter in patients with DCM. These imaging modalities were found to be related with the LV longitudinal, radial, and circumferential deformation, while LV reverse remodeling was found to be correlated with circumferential deformation. Accordingly, 2D-STE can be used in assessment of LV dysfunction, prognosis, and response to treatment in cases of DCM and HF.[10]

Also, cardiac fibrosis index is closely related to myocardial torsion. Reversed apical systolic function can detect extensive fibrosis that may be an indicator for severe LV dyssynchrony and poor LV performance.[11]

Monitoring Response to Treatment

Global longitudinal strain can be used as an objective, quantitative parameter for monitoring response to therapies indicated for improving LV contractility in cases of cardiomyopathy.[10]

Role in Cardiac Resynchronization Therapy

The role of 2D-STE in the assessment of mechanical dyssynchrony is that radial strain estimated by STE has been shown to be a reliable measure of intraventricular mechanical dyssynchrony and a solid indicator of the response to cardiac resynchronization therapy (CRT) in patients with DCM when the time difference in peak septal wall-to-posterior wall strain is more than or equal to130 ms with sensitivity 89% and specificity 83% (*see* Fig. 4).[12] Time to peak radial strain can also help recognize the site of latest activation and thus help in directing us to the proper LV lead placement.[13] Dyssynchrony between the time of peak apical rotation and basal rotation has appeared to happen in HF and is improved with CRT. The standard deviation of times to peak longitudinal strain can as well be utilized to portray LV dyssynchrony with cutoff value more than37 ms (Fig. 5).[14]

Assessment of Left Ventricular Diastolic Function

Early diastolic SR, peak untwist velocity, and time to peak untwist velocity have all been used as indicators of LV diastolic function which are affected in cases of cardiomyopathy with variable outcomes.[15]

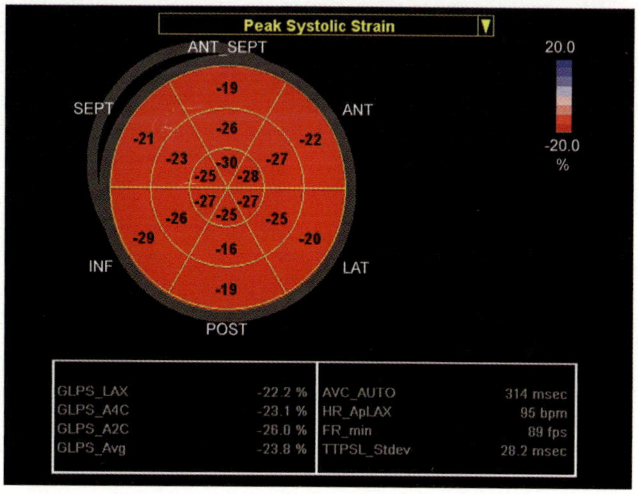

Fig. 5: Bull's eye of global longitudinal strain of normal child.

Assessment of Left Ventricular Rotation Patterns and Amplitude and Their Effect on Left Ventricular Function in Cardiomyopathy

Apical rotation pattern varies with increasing LV dilatation in patients of DCM with reduced amplitude of positive rotation (Fig. 6) than reversed apical rotation in severe conditions. Putting in mind that reversed basal rotation occurs only in 30% of cases of reversed rotation in cases of DCM (Fig. 7),[16] high LV outflow tract gradient in patients of HCM might be one of many factors in such condition that triggers deterioration of LV longitudinal strain and twist mechanics in patients with HCM.[9]

Left Atrial Function

Speckle-tracking echocardiography, being an angle-independent technique, allows as well evaluation of left atrial (LA) strain which can aid in determination of LA function in cases of cardiomyopathy. In these cases, the magnitude of LA dysfunction is strictly related to LV filling pressures.[17]

Assessment of Right Ventricular Function

Strain and SR imaging have been made available of late for the assessment of regional LV and right ventricular (RV) function which are altered in cases of DCM and HF as well as being used as a predictive for worse outcome. Right ventricular function significantly certainly influences the reaction to various HF remedies including CRT and might be a target in some cases.[18]

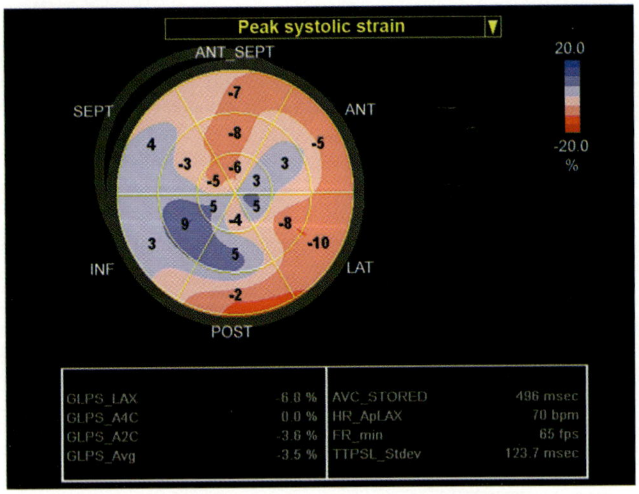

Fig. 6: Bull's eye of global longitudinal strain in a dilated cardiomyopathy patient.

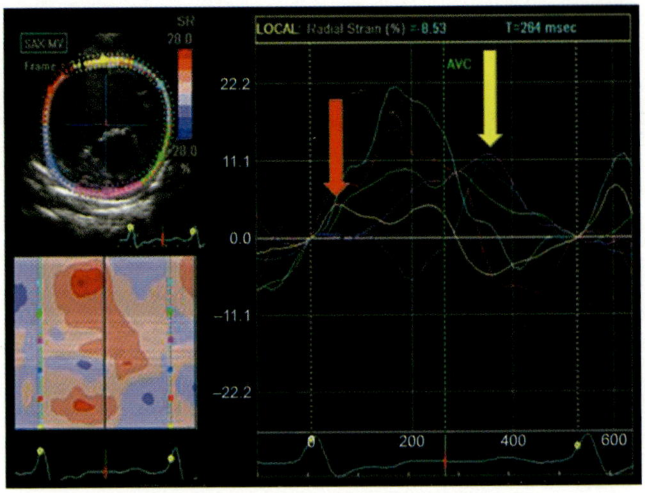

Fig. 7: Time to peak radial strain with significant anteroseptal to posterior delay denoting intraventricular dyssynchrony (yellow arrow represents posterior segment and red arrow represents anteroseptal segment).

The Prognostic Implications of Two-dimensional Speckle-tracking Echocardiography in Hypertrophic Cardiomyopathy

Decreased global longitudinal strain is correlated with more severe disease and points to an increased risk for major cardiac events, separate from other clinical and echocardiographic risk factors. Left ventricular dyssynchrony also seems promising as a risk factor for unexpected cardiac events. With respect to LA mechanics, LA reservoir, conduit, and contractile strain all of which may present significant predictors for atrial fibrillation, major cardiac events, and even sudden death.[19]

DISCUSSION

Myocardial fiber arrangement is complex and encompassed two primary arrangements (circumferential and longitudinal) that change smoothly from one direction to the other responsible for the heterogeneous, miscellaneous, and sophisticated fiber architecture. Thus, it is expected that myocardial regions must be electrically activated temporally for efficient pump function. Normally, electrical activation is initiated at the apical endocardium and propagates outward to the epicardium and simultaneously upward toward the base, resulting in a synchronized and energetically efficient mechanical contraction for optimal LV performance.[20] Hence, the need to discuss variable types of mechanical movements (circumferential, longitudinal, and torsion) and assessment of regional function by new modality, such as speckle tracking, and not only reliant on evaluation of global function by traditional echocardiography. The acceptance and fame of fractional shortening (FS) is due to the ease and rapidity with which it can be carried out. However, it is not free of constraints: (1) Regional motion of the septum and posterior wall are used as factors for global function. On the other hand, this assumes that there are no regional wall motion abnormalities. The measurement becomes inaccurate or impossible when regional septal hypokinesia or dyskinesia is present. This occurs in different circumstances, such as in the context of RV volume overload, which can be associated with dyskinetic (paradoxical) septal motion, similarly in bundle branch block or dyssynchrony accompanied with septal hypokinesia or dyskinesia. These conditions affect the measurement of %FS and overestimate the reduction in global systolic function. Conversely, when regional function is preserved in the septum and posterior wall but reduced in other regions, calculated %FS overestimates global LV function. (2) Another important restriction of %FS is its load dependency. The technique is affected largely by changes in both preload and afterload and does not solely reflect intrinsic myocardial function. Increased preload will increase left ventricular end-diastolic diameter and will therefore affect the measurement. Increased afterload will influence left ventricular end-systolic diameter as it may result in earlier closure of the aortic valve, thus resulting in a lower %FS. (3) A final important limitation is the dependency of the calculation on LV geometry. With volume loading, the shape of the LV ventricle becomes more spherical, affecting measurements and dimensional changes. When hypertrophy of the wall occurs, as in the context of HCM, endocardial dimensional changes are influenced by the effect of the thickened wall resulting in an overestimation of systolic function.[21] Using speckle tracking as a new approach for assessment of regional systolic function of different types of strain in cases of cardiomyopathy has become critical for improved prognosis and management of these patients. *Two different working groups* reported decrease of the different types of systolic strain (LV longitudinal, radial, and circumferential deformation) in the cases of DCM and HCM.[8,9]

Notomi and his colleagues assessed LV torsion and twisting velocities in individuals from 9 months to 49 years. He studied how the age influences basal rotation and he stated that 10–15 years is the switch age from counterclockwise to clockwise rotation. Accordingly, he proposed that counterclockwise basal rotation is dominant in infancy and gradually change to adult clockwise rotation at this age group. *Bogdan A* investigated LV rotation pattern in patients of DCM and as a result observed a change of apical rotation pattern with increasing LV dilatation in patients of DCM with reduced amplitude of positive rotation than reversed apical rotation in severe cases. *Udink ten Cate* noticed reversed basal rotation in 30% of cases of DCM. There is controversy in the literature whether children with DCM have LV dyssynchrony or not, and to what extent. Therefore, precise diagnosis and measurement of LV mechanical dyssynchrony in the pediatric population have to be made by using 2D speckle-tracking techniques.[22] *Friedberg in 2007* described intraventricular dyssynchrony by significant prolongation of standard deviation of time to peak longitudinal strain with cutoff value more than37 ms, while *Maurizio G and his co-authors* described intraventricular dyssynchrony by significant delay between peak septal wall-to-posterior wall radial strain more than or equal to130 ms with sensitivity 89% and specificity 83%.

Cardiac fibrosis index in patients of cardiomyopathy was commonly examined by different imaging techniques as cardiac MRI as it is associated with poor prognosis, serious complications, and poor response to treatment. It was found to be associated with reversed apical systolic rotation and circumferential deformation.[10] Finally, speckle-tracking techniques are expected to be a portion of the echocardiographic assessment of children with cardiomyopathy (Figs. 8 to 10).

LIMITATIONS OF TWO-DIMENSIONAL SPECKLE-TRACKING ECHOCARDIOGRAPHY

Image Quality

Even though 2D-STE is fairly robust, image quality is still an issue. Poor image quality can result of failure to analyze almost 6% of all LV segments in young healthy subjects.[23]

Correct Tracing of Myocardial Region of Interest

One of the major limitations is the exact detection of borders. Although speckle tracking is useful in delineating endocardium, yet manual correction of its contour is still needed. Furthermore, the evaluation of strain and SR

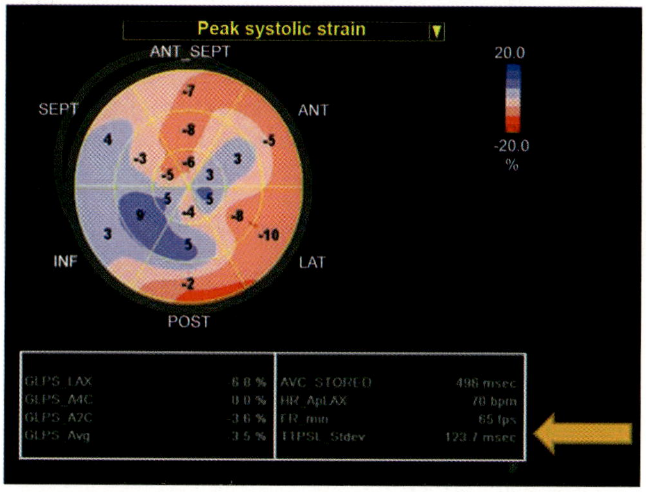

Fig. 8: Patient with dilated cardiomyopathy with significant delay of SD of time to peak longitudinal strain denoting intraventricular dyssynchrony.

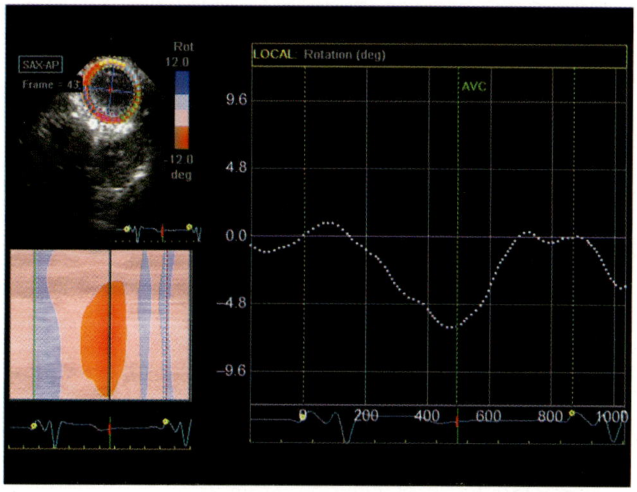

Fig. 9: Reversed apical rotation in patient of dilated cardiomyopathy.

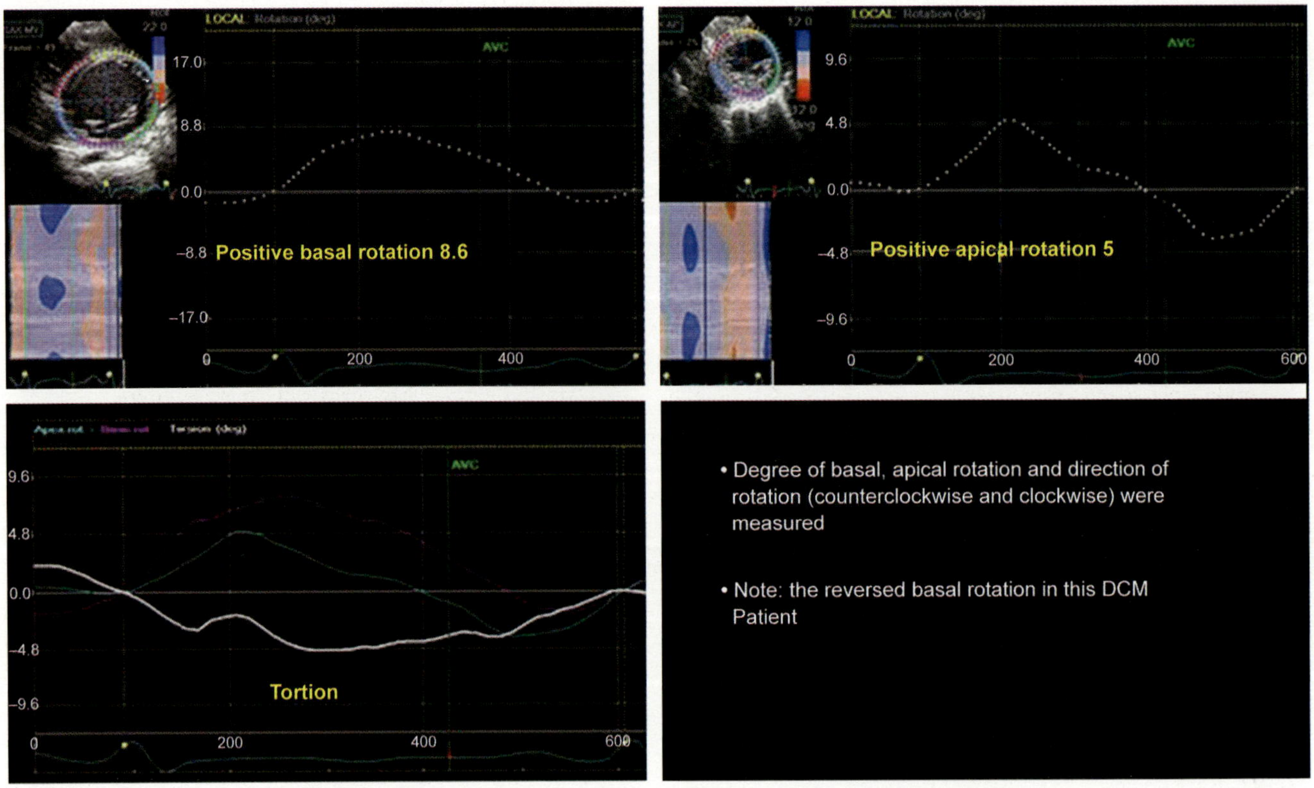

Fig. 10: Reversed basal rotation in patient of dilated cardiomyopathy.

requires delineating the epicardial borders. Most software versions assume a uniform thickness of the myocardium which is not true.[24-26]

Size of Left Ventricle

Large ventricles also represent a challenge as it may be difficult to image the entire myocardium, especially the apical segments.[3]

CONCLUSION

Two-dimensional speckle-tracking echocardiography is an emerging imaging technique that can be useful in early identification, prediction of outcome, and treatment in cardiomyopathic patients.

REFERENCES

1. Wang T, Evans J, Benjamin E, et al. Natural history of asymptomatic left ventricular systolic dysfunction in the community. Circulation. 2003;108:977-98.
2. Neilan T, Jassal D, Perez-Sanz T, et al. Tissue Doppler imaging predicts left ventricular dysfunction and mortality in a murine model of cardiac injury. Eur Heart J. 2006;27:1868-75.
3. Blessberger H, Binder T. 2D speckle tracking echocardiography: basic principles. Heart. 2010;96:716-22.
4. Geyer H, Caracciolo G, Abe H. Assessment of myocardial mechanics using speckle tracking echocardiography: fundamentals and clinical applications. J Am Soc Echocardiogr. 2010;23:351-69.
5. Brown J, Jenkins C, Marwick T. Use of myocardial strain to assess global left ventricular function: a comparison with cardiac magnetic resonance and 3-dimensional echocardiography. Am Heart J. 2009;157:102e1-5.
6. Saito K, Okura H, Watanabe N, et al. Comprehensive evaluation of left ventricular strain using speckle tracking echocardiography in normal adults: comparison of three-dimensional and two-dimensional approaches. J Am Soc Echocardiogr. 2009;22:1025-30.
7. Van Dalen B, Soliman O, Vletter W, et al. Age related changes in the biomechanics of left ventricular twist measured by speckle tracking echocardiography. Am J Physiol Heart Circ Physiol. 2008;295:1705-11.
8. Meluzin J, Spinarova L, Hude P, et al. Left ventricular mechanics in idiopathic dilated cardiomyopathy: systolic–diastolic coupling and torsion. J Am Soc Echocardiogr. 2009;22(5):486-93.
9. Tigen K, Sunbul M, Karaahmet T, et al. Left ventricular and atrial functions in hypertrophic cardiomyopathy patients with very high LVOT gradient: a speckle tracking

echocardiographic study. Echocardiography. 2014;31(7): 833-41.

10. Seong-Mi P, Yong-Hyun K, Chul-Min A, et al. Relationship between ultrasonic tissue characterization and myocardial deformation for prediction of left ventricular reverse remodelling in non-ischaemic dilated cardiomyopathy. Eur J Echocardiogr. 2011;12:887-94.
11. Karaahmet T, Gürel E, Tigen K, et al. The effect of myocardial fibrosis on left ventricular torsion and twist in patients with non-ischemic dilated cardiomyopathy. Cardiol J. 2013;20(3):276-86.
12. Galderisi M, Cattaneo F, Mondillo S. Doppler echocardiography and myocardial dyssynchrony: a practical update of old and new ultrasound technologies. Cardiovasc Ultrasound. 2007;5:28.
13. van der Hulst AE, Delgado V, Blom NA, et al. Cardiac resynchronization therapy in paediatric and congenital heart disease patients. Eur Heart J. 2011;32:2236-46.
14. Friedberg MK, Silverman NH, Dubin AM, et al. Mechanical dyssynchrony in children with systolic dysfunction secondary to cardiomyopathy: Doppler tissue and vector velocity imaging study. J Am Soc Echocardiogr. 2007;20:756-63.
15. Jin SM, Noh CL, Bae EJ, et al. Decreased left ventricular torsion and untwisting in children with dilated cardiomyopathy. J Korean Med Sci. 2007;22:633-40.
16. Udink ten Cate FEA, Lorenz SRW, Khalil M, et al. Does reversed apical or basal left ventricular rotation in children with dilated cardiomyopathy recover following medical therapy? A two-dimensional speckle tracking imaging study. Int J Cardiol. 2011;153(3):330-3.
17. Cameli M, Caputo M, Mondillo S, et al. Feasibility and reference values of left atrial longitudinal strain imaging by two-dimensional speckle tracking. Cardiovasc Ultrasound. 2009;22:299-305.
18. Guendouz S, Rappeneau S, Nahum J, et al. Prognostic significance and normal values of 2D strain to assess right ventricular systolic function in chronic heart failure. Circ J. 2012;76:127-36.
19. Zegkos T, Parcharidou D, Ntelios D, et al. The prognostic implications of two-dimensional speckle tracking echocardiography in hypertrophic cardiomyopathy: current and future. Perspectives. 2018;26(3):130-6.
20. Helm P, Beg MF, Miller MI, et al. Measuring and mapping cardiac fiber and laminar architecture using diffusion tensor MR imaging. Ann NY Acad Sci. 2005;1047:296-307.
21. Lai W, Mertens L, Ganame J, et al. Echocardiography in pediatric and congenital heart disease: from fetus to adult, 1st edition. US: Wiley-Blackwell; 2009. pp. 76-94.
22. Gorcsan J, Tanabe M, Bleeker GB, et al. Combined longitudinal and radial dyssynchrony predicts ventricular response after resynchronization therapy. J Am Coll Cardiol. 2007;15:1476-83.
23. Hurlburt H, Aurigemma G, Hill J, et al. Direct ultrasound measurement of longitudinal, circumferential, and radial strain using 2-dimensional strain imaging in normal adults. Echocardiography. 2007;24:723-31.
24. Mor-Avi V, Lang R, Badano L, et al. Current and evolving echocardiographic techniques for the quantitative evaluation of cardiac mechanics. J Am Soc Echocardiogr. 2011;24:277-313.
25. Notomi Y, Srinath G, Shiota T, et al. Maturational and adaptive modulation of left ventricular torsional biomechanics. Doppler tissue imaging observation from infancy to adulthood. Circulation. 2006;113:2534-41.
26. Bogdan AP, Carmen CB, Andreea C, et al. Left ventricular remodelling and torsional dynamics in dilated cardiomyopathy: reversed apical rotation as a marker of disease severity. Eur J Heart Fail. 2009;11:945-51.

CHAPTER 116

Cross-sectional Imaging in Congenital Heart Disease

Richa Kothari, Vimal Raj

INTRODUCTION

Major advances in the field of pediatric cardiology and cardiac surgery over the last several decades have led to a dramatic improvement in survival rates for most forms of congenital heart disease (CHD). Improvements in surgical and medical treatments have been accompanied by developments in diagnostic modalities. Imaging plays a major role in pre- and postoperative management of patients with CHD. Transthoracic echocardiography is reliable in diagnosing most CHDs in the pediatric and adult populations.[1,2] Additional imaging is required, if the necessary information is not achieved with echocardiography. Noninvasive imaging options include cardiac magnetic resonance (CMR), computed tomography (CT), and nuclear scintigraphy. Cardiac catheterization, though invasive, remains the gold standard for direct hemodynamic assessment.

DIFFERENT IMAGING MODALITIES

Radiographs provide a simple, cheap overview of the heart, mediastinum, pulmonary vessels, lungs, and thoracic skeleton. This remains the first imaging that patients get exposed to, as it gives a good overview and helps in making further clinical decisions. Classical description of pathological abnormalities in CHD is often not recognized.

Transthoracic echocardiography is the first-line imaging modality in CHD. It is widely available, inexpensive, portable, real time; has high temporal resolution; and is free from ionizing radiation. *Fetal echocardiography* is used with excellent diagnostic accuracy for most CHDs. With recent advances, about 30–50% of the severe CHD are diagnosed before birth.[3] In adolescents and adults, there is progressive degradation in the quality of echocardiographic images due to poor acoustic windows. In such patients, CMR plays an increasing role. *Transesophageal echocardiography* provides access to more posterior parts of the heart, particularly for visualization of the valves. However, it is invasive, generally requiring sedation or anesthesia, and has limited field of view. Multidetector computed tomography (*MDCT*) assessment of heart has excellent three-dimensional (3D) spatial resolution and allows for detailed evaluation of small blood vessels such as coronary arteries, pulmonary veins, collaterals, and distal pulmonary artery branches. Ultrafast scan times are making imaging of all patients possible, especially those who are unable to lie still or flat for long time. MDCT is an excellent tool to assess aberrant coronary anatomy and a good alternative to selective coronary catheter angiography in older patients referred for CHD surgery. A major disadvantage of MDCT, especially in children, is the exposure to ionizing radiation. This drawback is compounded when multiple follow-up studies are necessary. This is being addressed worldwide with the development of ultralow dose scan protocols reducing the overall radiation exposure of the patient. MDCT also requires the use of iodinated contrast agents and does not provide information on hemodynamics, flow rate, or velocity.

Cardiac magnetic resonance does not involve ionizing radiation and is therefore ideally suited and recommended for long-term CHD follow-up.[4] CMR provides anatomic assessment of cardiovascular anomalies before and after surgery, quantification of biventricular function, measurement of systemic and pulmonary blood flow, quantification of valve regurgitation, identification of myocardial ischemia, and fibrosis and tissue characterization. CMR is the reference standard for accurate and reproducible quantification of right ventricular (RV) and left ventricular (LV) volumes, mass, and function.[4] Limitations include availability, higher cost, artifacts from implants, and relative contraindication in patients with pacemakers or implantable cardioverter-defibrillators. MR-compatible devices are increasingly used and are desirable for CHD patients. However, predicting the impact of artifact noise on image quality is difficult. It is necessary to establish a strict policy of screening before CMR, such as other MR examinations, for the patient and all accompanying persons.[5] MR eliminates the use of iodinated contrast or exposure to radiation as compared to CT. In younger children, typically before school-age, a CMR examination usually requires sedation or general anesthesia. In these patients, appropriate monitoring by an expert team which is well equipped to deal with emergencies is necessary.

NUCLEAR SCINTIGRAPHY

Nuclear scintigraphy has been reserved for selected patients only, such as for myocardial stress perfusion imaging or differential pulmonary blood flow quantification when CMR is not available. Nuclear scintigraphy plays a limited role especially in the pediatric age group due to the risks associated with exposure to ionizing radiation and its relatively low spatial resolution.

CATHETERIZATION

Although used less for diagnosis since improved noninvasive approaches have become available, catheterization has role in the calculation of pulmonary resistance, coronary artery disease, and for percutaneous interventions using balloons, stents, occlusion devices, or implantable valves. Increasing use of MDCT/CMR can help in reducing procedure time and radiation exposure for catheterization by providing most of the anatomical data prior to procedure itself.

IMAGING IN SPECIFIC CONGENITAL HEART DISEASES

Tetralogy of Fallot

Tetralogy of Fallot (TOF) is the most common cyanotic congenital cardiac condition, accounting for 6–10% of all CHDs.[6,7] Tetralogy of Fallot has four components: subpulmonary infundibular stenosis, a ventricular septal defect (VSD), an aorta that overrides the VSD by less than 50% of its diameter, and RV hypertrophy. There can be varying levels of severity, and a morphological spectrum exists. Echocardiography is usually sufficient to define anatomy prior to surgery in most patients during infancy; however, those with complex pulmonary stenosis or atresia can be effectively assessed with MDCT/CMR.[8] CT orMR angiography can provide anatomical road map to aid in surgical repair by determining pulmonary vascular anatomy, source of pulmonary blood supply, origin and course of the coronaries, and other associated lesions, such as anomalies of the aortic arch.[9,10] Surgical repair can be accomplished through a variety of approaches depending on the severity of obstruction, presence, and sizes of the branch pulmonary arteries. Surgical approach may change if a coronary artery crosses the RV outflow tract (RVOT). The size of the pulmonary arteries is standardized using McGoon ratio (the ratio of sum of diameters of right and left pulmonary arteries just before their bifurcation and aortic diameter at the level of diaphragm). McGoon ratio above 1.2 is associated with acceptable postoperative outcome in TOF, and the ratio below 0.8 is inadequate for complete repair of pulmonary arteries.[11] Palliative surgery is used for infants with pulmonary arterial hypoplasia, which necessitates postponing definitive repair to allow for pulmonary arterial growth.[10] Modified Blalock-Taussig shunt (shunt between subclavian artery to pulmonary artery) is most commonly performed. When pulmonary arteries are adequate in size, definitive repair called intracardiac repair (ICR) is done. ICR consists of VSD closure and relief of RVOT obstruction. An adult who has undergone palliation earlier in life can be considered for ICR provided there is favorable pulmonary anatomy and hemodynamics. Relief of RVOT obstruction may include simple resection of infundibular stenosis, but if the pulmonary annulus is small, more extensive surgery, such as RV outflow patch augmentation or placement of a transannular patch, may be necessary. Occasionally, an extracardiac conduit must be placed from the RV to the pulmonary artery. Although prognosis for patients who have undergone ICR is favorable (early mortality rate—2%), residual defects, complications, and sequelae are common.[12-16] Key postoperative issues are summarized below[17]:

- Residual pulmonary regurgitation (PR)
- Right ventricular dilation and dysfunction from PR, possibly with associated tricuspid regurgitation (TR)
- Residual RVOT obstruction
- Branch pulmonary artery stenosis or hypoplasia
- Sustained ventricular tachycardia
- Sudden cardiac death

The most common problem encountered in the patient after repair is that of PR. Significant PR can lead to RV dysfunction and failure with systemic complications including arrhythmias and sudden death. The probability of adverse events has been shown to increase with RV enlargement or dysfunction.[18] Currently, the main treatment of severe PR in these patients is the replacement of the pulmonary valve. Pulmonary valve replacement has been shown to improve RV volumes, improve exercise tolerance, and stabilize QRS duration while reducing clinical arrhythmias.[19] Oosterhof et al. have reported that indexed RV end diastolic volume more than 160 mL/m^2 or RV end systolic volume more than 82 mL/m^2 in CMR prior to repair of significant PR is associated with decreased chances of normalization of RV volume.[20] CMR is the gold standard for quantification of RV size, shape, and function as well as for calculation of PR both volumetrically and by flow calculations with velocity-encoded imaging.[21] Right ventricular diastolic function can be assessed with tricuspid valve inflow volumetric curves using phase-contrast MRI (MR imaging).[22] Late gadolinium enhancement CMR can also be utilized to detect ventricular fibrosis, which has been shown to predict worse outcomes such as ventricular dysfunction, exercise intolerance, and clinical arrhythmia in repaired TOF patients.[23] Pulmonary stenosis following TOF repair can be well characterized by CMR, using cine imaging, flow mapping, and angiography (Figs. 1A to E). CMR has been shown to be sensitive and specific in

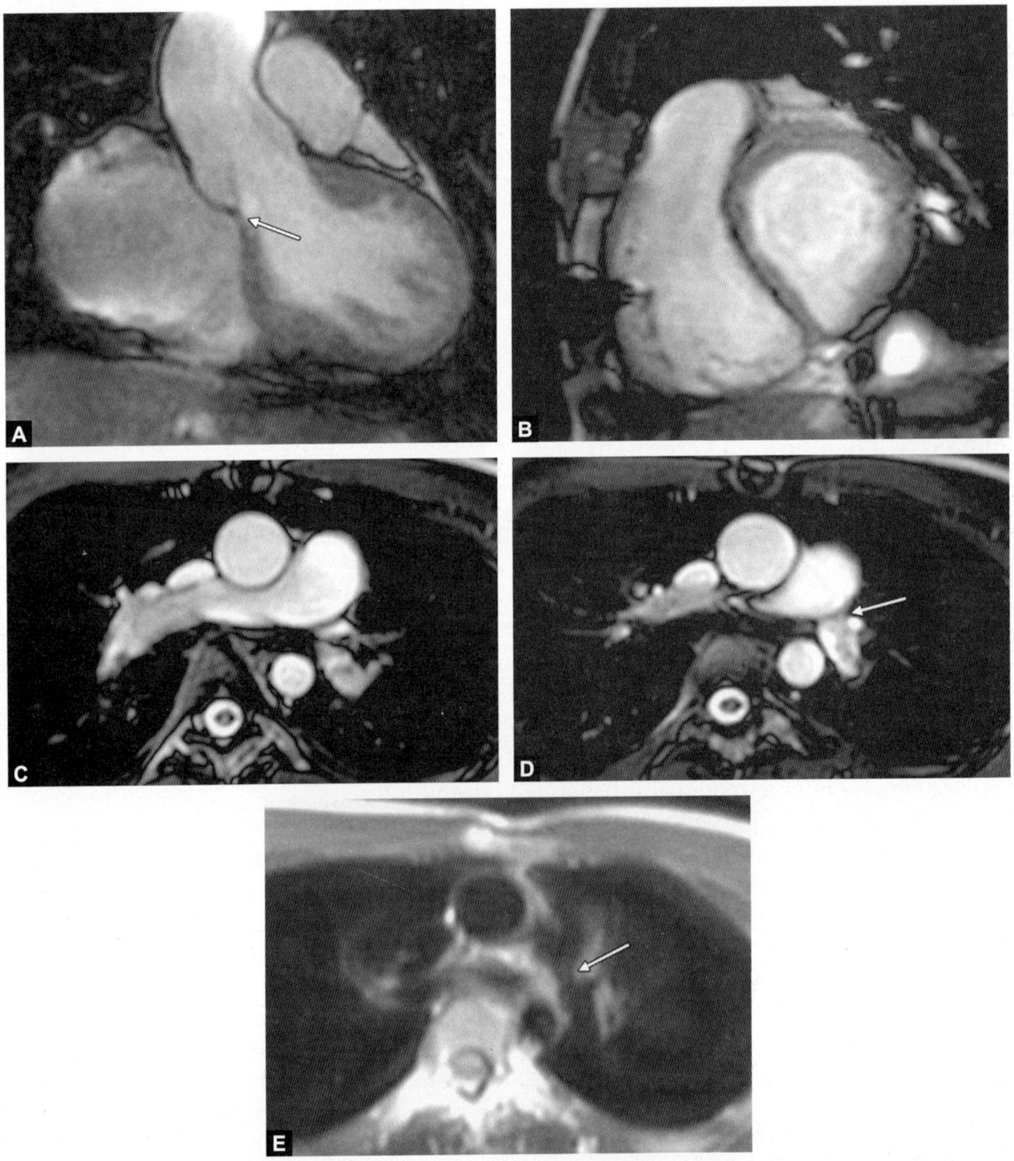

Figs. 1A to E: SSFP images of post-ICR case showing (A) intact VSD patch (arrow) in LVOT view, (B) repaired RVOT in RVOT view, (C) normal right pulmonary artery, and (D) mild left pulmonary artery ostial stenosis (arrow) with associated flow acceleration in axial view. (E) The mild left pulmonary artery ostial stenosis (arrow) can be well seen in the black blood axial images. (ICR: Intracardiac repair; LVOT: Left ventricular outflow tract; RVOT: Right ventricular outflow tract; SSFP: Steady-state free precession; VSD: Ventricular septal defect)

detecting branch pulmonary artery stenosis following TOF, especially 3D MR angiography. Contrast-enhanced MR angiography can depict the entire course of a postsurgical shunt and quantify its caliber, patency, and function.[24-26] Phase-contrast MRI is the best modality in demonstrating the relative volume of blood flow to each lung after TOF repair.[27]

TRANSPOSITION OF GREAT ARTERIES

There are two types of CHD with ventriculoarterial (VA) discordance resulting in a systemic RV: dextro-transposition of the great arteries (D-TGA) and congenitally corrected TGA [CC-TGA or levo-TGA (L-TGA)].

Dextro-transposition of the great arteries is more common, with an incidence of 4–8% in the population.[28] Survival of patients with D-TGA is dependent on sufficient mixing of oxygen saturated and depleted blood on the atrial level. This mixing is augmented by additional shunt connections that increase pulmonary vascular perfusion and thereby left atrial pressure (i.e. VSD, patent ductus arteriosus). Most patients will have had one or more operations in childhood. Mustard/Senning atrial baffle procedure (atrial switch operation) was developed first and is more commonly seen in older D-TGA survivors. Patients with D-TGA are nowadays corrected by arterial switch operation (ASO). The Mustard/Senning procedure consists of a superior vena cava baffle and inferior vena cava (IVC) baffle that meet together and redirect systemic venous blood through the mitral valve into subpulmonic LV; a pulmonary venous baffle is created to direct oxygenated blood through the tricuspid valve to the subaortic RV.[17,29] Characteristic problems encountered after repair include baffle obstruction, baffle leaks, subpulmonary/pulmonary stenosis, arrhythmias, long-term failure of the systemic RV and systemic TR. Systemic baffle obstruction has the potential to cause superior vena cava syndrome or, less commonly, hepatic congestion if the IVC limb is obstructed. The need for reoperation is not uncommon.[30] All of these complications have a major impact on morbidity and mortality. Early and frequent monitoring with serial imaging modalities is therefore crucial. Baffle leaks or obstructions can be very well depicted by CT. The systemic RV and subpulmonary LV function, baffle leaks, or obstructions can be detected by CMR using cine imaging and flow maps. The ASO procedure is the present-day surgical standard of care for repair of D-TGA. It offers patients a significantly better quality of life and long-term health status than the Mustard/Senning procedure, as the LV is reestablished as the systemic ventricle.[31] The ASO involves reposition of the great arteries to their corresponding ventricle (Lecompte maneuver) (Figs. 2A to C), accompanied by excision and reimplantation of the coronary arteries, early in life.[32] The characteristic long-term problems following this procedure include coronary insufficiency, coronary artery stenosis or occlusion, myocardial ischemia, ventricular dysfunction and arrhythmias, stenosis at the great arterial anastomotic sites, pulmonary hypertension, branch pulmonary arterial stenosis, and neoaortic or PR. The most common complication is residual or recurrent RVOT obstruction, which typically occurs at the suture line of the pulmonary arterial anastomosis.[33] CMR is an important imaging modality in patients who have undergone an ASO, similar to those who have undergone an atrial switch.

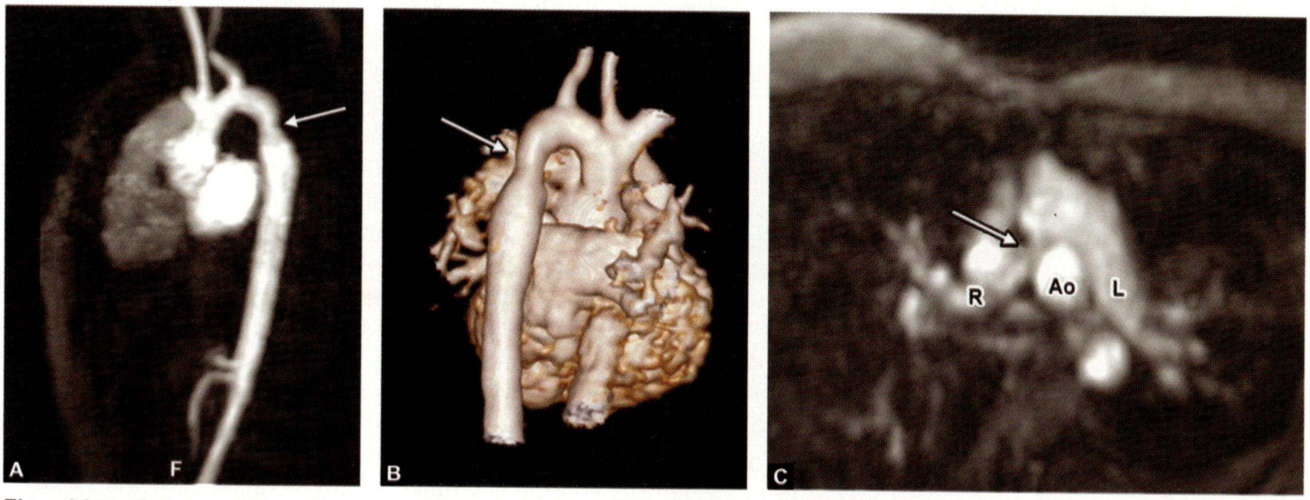

Figs. 2A to C: In a patient with transposition of great arteries who underwent arterial switch operation, magnetic resonance angiography images in (A) sagittal oblique multiplanar reconstruction plane and (B) 3D volume rendered images from MR angiography showing moderate coarctation of aorta (arrow). (C) The Lecompte maneuver with pulmonary artery anterior to ascending aorta and right (R) and left (L) pulmonary artery passing on either side of ascending aorta. The right pulmonary artery is uniformly small compared to the left and also shows moderate proximal narrowing (arrow).

Studies have shown that branch pulmonary artery stenosis is detected more accurately by CMR as compared with echocardiography.[34] Cardiac CT is usually a third-line imaging modality but may be the most useful, particularly when there is possible coronary artery ostial stenosis. CT should be considered for supplemental imaging after echocardiography in patients whose MRI is contraindicated (pacemaker, foreign body artifact, size to fit in scanner, critically ill condition, etc.).[32]

Congenitally corrected transposition of the great arteries or L-TGA is a complex anomaly with variable phenotype. Congenitally corrected TGA patients may be first recognized in adulthood, as the physiology can be asymptomatic before this time and discordance can go unrecognized with imaging if other defects are not present.[35] There are atrioventricular (AV) discordance and VA discordance.[36] Although "congenitally corrected," this physiology still results in a systemic RV, and the tricuspid valve functioning as the systemic AV valve. Systemic RV failure is the most significant cause of morbidity and mortality in these patients.[37] CMR remains the standard of care to assess systemic RV function. The onset of symptoms related to systemic RV dysfunction or development of systemic AV valve regurgitation is an indication for surgery, and patients may be referred for early systemic AV valve replacement.[38]

COARCTATION OF AORTA

Coarctation of aorta is congenital narrowing of aorta, usually at site of ductus insertion. There may also be several associated cardiac defects including bicuspid aortic valve, subaortic stenosis, VSD, and varying degrees of arch hypoplasia. 3D MRI or CT angiography identifies the precise location and anatomy of the coarctation (Figs. 3A and B) and caliber of entire aorta, as well as collateral vessels[39] and allows decision-making on the most appropriate treatment technique, i.e. cardiac surgery or catheter-guided intervention.[40-43] The sensitivity of CMR to detect vascular abnormalities is as good as that of conventional catheter angiography, so that cardiac catheterization can be reserved for selected cases and for catheter-guided interventions.[40] CT angiography is a sound alternative particularly when associated airway anomalies are suspected and/or when the clinical scenario is that of a young and sick infant or neonate who may require anesthesia for CMR examination.

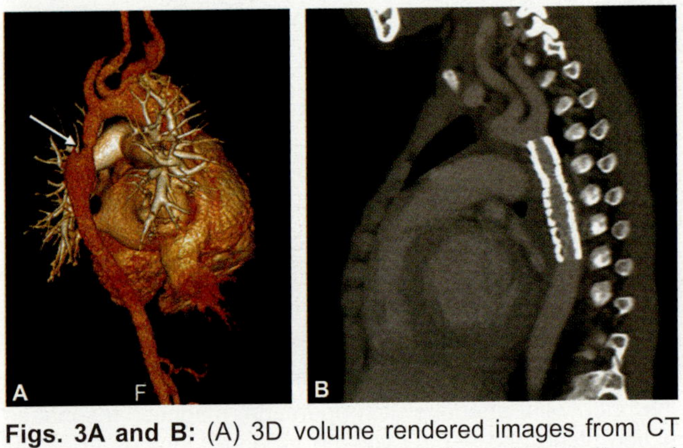

Figs. 3A and B: (A) 3D volume rendered images from CT angiography showing severe coarctation of aorta (arrow) with poststenotic dilatation. (B) Sagittal oblique multiplanar reconstruction from CT of same patient poststenting.

Hemodynamic assessment can be performed with a velocity-encoded phase-contrast cine sequence using high velocity encoding typically of at least 200 cm/s[44] in CMR. MR angiography may also be useful to quantify collateral flow. Flow measurements are usually performed in a perpendicular plane through the ascending aorta, proximal descending aorta (immediately distal to the stenosis), and at the level of the diaphragm. An increase in flow between the distal aortic arch and the descending aorta at the level of the diaphragm is indicative for significant collateral circulation. CMR is an excellent tool to evaluate LV function and associated defects, such as aortic valve malformation. New imaging techniques such as four-dimensional flow measurements can be used to evaluate hemodynamic indicators such as vortex formation, vascular strain, and collateral vessel flow. CT or CMR can be performed for follow-up after surgical correction or catheter intervention, when residual or recurrent stenoses and/or aneurysms need to be ruled out.[45-47] In the follow-up of poststenting patients, stent associated stenosis can be estimated using MR angiography and phase-contrast flow mapping.[48,49] Also, depending on the material of the stent used, there are limitations for the assessment of in-stent stenosis and morphology using CMR, which may necessitate the alternative use of CT.[50-52]

SHUNTS

Two of the most common types of shunts are atrial septal defect (ASD) and VSD. There are several types of *ASD* that are categorized according to the location of the defect: secundum ASD, primum ASD, sinus venosus ASD, and coronary sinus septal defect. Blood is shunted across the defect from the left atrium into the right atrium, resulting in greater right atrium and RV blood volume, ultimately leading to RV volume overload and pulmonary overcirculation. CMR provides an additional noninvasive imaging modality, if findings by echocardiography are uncertain. Direct visualization of the defect and pulmonary veins is possible, RV volume and function can be quantified, and estimate of shunt size can also be obtained.[53-55] *Ventricular septal defect* is the most common congenital heart defect at birth,[56] although the incidence is much lower in older children and adults because of the frequency of spontaneous closure.[57,58]

Moderate-to-large defects can lead to LV volume overload and pulmonary arterial hypertension. MRI or CT may be useful to assess pulmonary artery, pulmonary venous, and aortic anatomy, if there are coexisting lesions and to confirm the anatomy of unusual VSDs such as inlet or apical defects not well seen by echocardiography. CMR can provide a noninvasive assessment of left-to-right shunting (Qp/Qs), a measurement that is utilized in determining intervention plans. Closure is indicated when the Qp/Qs ratio is 2.0 or greater.[17] Similar to an ASD, closure is not recommended with severe irreversible pulmonary hypertension. The basic morphology of *atrioventricular septal defect* includes a large and central defect that may extend to variable degrees above and below the AV valve. There is a common AV valve annulus that stretches across both ventricles. The AV valve may be misaligned with respect to the ventricles, in association with hypoplasia of the right or left ventricle.[17] CMR will be useful to evaluate venous and arterial anatomy when associated lesions are suspected.

In *anomalous pulmonary venous connection*, it is important to detail the course and connection of each pulmonary vein, diagnose or rule out the presence of pulmonary venous obstruction and describe associated lesions.[59,60] CT is an excellent modality to define the pulmonary venous anatomy. CMR is an established modality for the noninvasive assessment of shunt location, flow direction, and magnitude.[61] It also quantifies the degree of Qp/Qs which is part of the comprehensive hemodynamic evaluation in many patients with CHD and often a determinant factor for surgery. Extracardiac shunts, such as major aortopulmonary collaterals are readily delineated by CT/MR angiography.[62,63]

COMPLEX CONGENITAL HEART DISEASE

Complex CHD frequently consists of a combination of situs anomalies, abnormal AV and/or VA connections, and/or additional defects, including septal defects, ventricular looping anomalies, and malformations of the outflow tracts. In addition, malformations of the extracardiac thoracic vessels and tracheobronchial anomalies may also be present (Figs. 4 and 5).[64] CT can be extremely useful

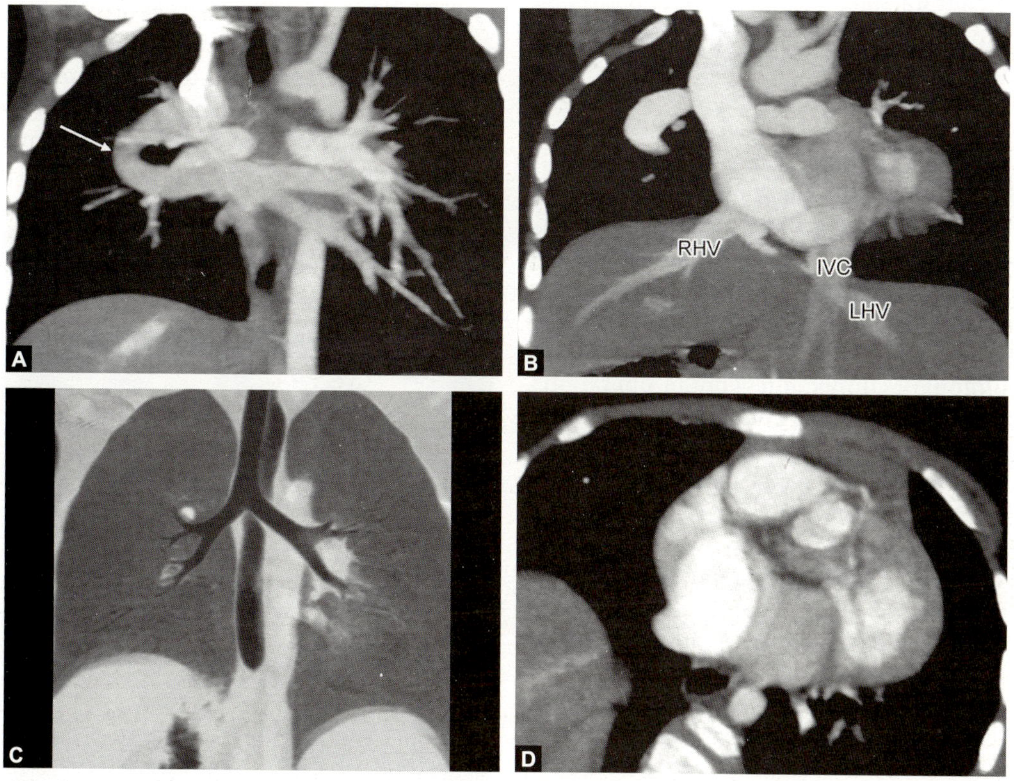

Figs. 4A to D: CT of a child with heterotaxy syndrome with right isomerism (A) coronal oblique multiplanar reconstruction image shows all pulmonary veins forming a common channel (arrow) with an intrapulmonary course draining into right superior vena cava to right-sided atrium—total anomalous pulmonary venous drainage. (B) Coronal oblique multiplanar reconstruction image shows right superior vena cava, RHV and middle hepatic veins draining into right-sided atrium, LHV, IVC draining into left-sided atrium. Midline liver can be appreciated. (C) Minimum intensity projection images show bilateral right bronchial morphology. (D) Axial oblique multiplanar reconstruction image shows left main coronary artery (arrow) crossing pulmonary infundibulum and then bifurcating into left anterior descending and circumflex arteries. (CT: Computed tomography; IVC: Inferior vena cava; LHV: Left hepatic vein; RHV: Right hepatic vein)

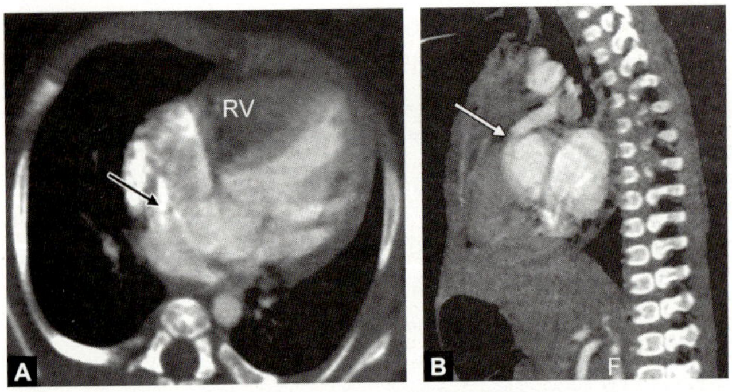

Figs. 5A and B: CT of a 4-month-old child (A) reconstructed image in the horizontal long axis showing tricuspid atresia with hypoplastic right ventricle. Atrial septal defect can be appreciated (black arrow) and (B) sagittal oblique multiplanar reconstruction image showing pulmonary atresia (white arrow).

for imaging systemic and pulmonary arterial and venous anatomy and intracardiac complex anatomy. Dedicated CMR examinations provide a comprehensive picture of complex CHD, including anatomy and hemodynamics including determining ventricular volumes, ejection fraction, regurgitant fraction, and degree of hypertrophy. Planning and performing imaging in these patients require thorough expertise in congenital malformations to avoid misinterpretation or incomplete results. While performing CMR in complex CHD, views in axial, coronal, and sagittal orientations at the beginning help to facilitate orientation within the thorax. The abdomen is included in the scout images to determine anatomy of the upper abdominal organs.[65] Surgical management of these patients usually involves various modifications or a series of staged procedures allowing systemic venous return to enter pulmonary circulation directly such as a total cavopulmonary connection (Fontan operation). Prior to the creation of any such connection, imaging of the ascending aorta and aortic arch, pulmonary arteries, and of the systemic and pulmonary veins are mandatory.[66] Ventricular size and function, valve function, and the subaortic outflow tract are also studied. After completion of the Fontan circulation, CMR is recommended for serial follow-up of systolic and diastolic ventricular function, ventricular geometry, and serial quantification of valvular incompetence.[66-68] Useful information provided by CMR during follow-up includes identifying obstructions, baffle leaks, thrombus formation, and collateral flow.

CORONARY ASSESSMENT/ANOMALIES

Congenital anomalous origin of the coronary arteries may occur in 1–1.2% of all coronary angiograms performed, with 0.5% of them having the highest risk lesions of the left main or left anterior descending branch artery arising from the opposite sinus of Valsalva.[69] Coronary anomalies account for approximately 15% of the sudden cardiac deaths in athletes (potentially due to torsion or slit-like compression of the proximal coronary artery, exercise-induced compression, vasospasm, or ischemic or scar-induced ventricular arrhythmia).[70,71] In patients younger than 50 years, coronary CT or CMR is recommended for more definitive definition of coronary origin and course in patients suspected of having anomalous coronary origins.

Coronary abnormalities associated with CHD include single coronary artery, coronary cameral fistula (Fig. 6), accessory left anterior descending coronary artery, and anomalous coronary artery from the pulmonary artery. The most common and important abnormality in TOF patients is the left anterior descending coronary artery arising from the right coronary artery and crossing the RV outflow.[17] Coronary artery origin and course should be delineated before any surgical or interventional procedure, because the potential exists for damage to anomalous coronary arteries to occur during cardiac exposure, surgery on the RVOT, and stenting of RV outflow. Electrocardiography-gated multidetector CT is an established noninvasive alternative for catheter angiography because of its ease of use, generally availability, and fast acquisition times compared with CMR. However, important limitations in children remain radiation exposure and fast heart rate.[72] MR coronary artery imaging of the proximal and mid regions of the major epicardial coronary artery by using noncontrast 3D whole heart sequence can be performed in infants and children[73-75] (Fig. 7). As the patient's growth increases and heart rate

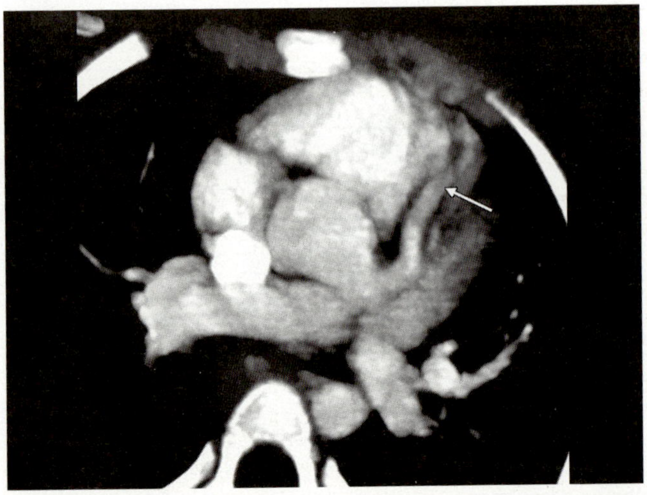

Fig. 6: CT of a child with coronary cameral fistula—axial oblique reconstructed image shows dilated left main coronary artery arising from left coronary cusp. It gives rise to a dilated left descending artery (arrow) which is seen draining into the right ventricle.

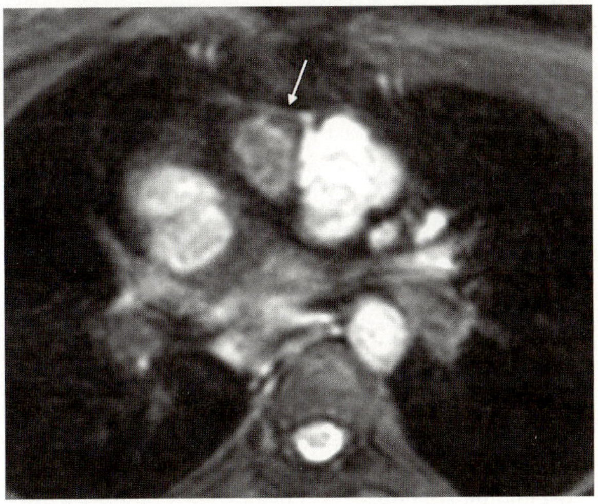

Fig. 7: Axial oblique multiplanar reconstruction image of noncontrast 3D whole heart sequence shows a case of transposition of great arteries with right coronary artery (arrow) seen crossing pulmonary infundibulum.

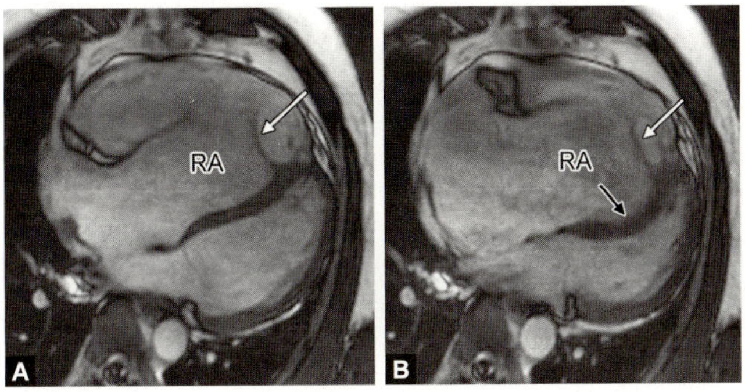

Figs. 8A and B: Steady-state free precession images in a case of Ebstein's anomaly showing apically displaced tricuspid valve (white arrow) with atrialized right atrium in four-chamber view in diastole (A) and systole (B). Also seen is leftward bowing of interventricular septum (black arrow) in systole.

decreases, image quality improves. This technique can be used to detect an anomalous origin and proximal course of the coronary artery.[76]

EBSTEIN'S ANOMALY

Ebstein's anomaly is a rare congenital malformation that accounts for approximately 1% of all congenital defects.[77-79] Ebstein's anomaly is a combination of an atrialized portion of the RV, tricuspid valve dysplasia with displacement of the septal origin of the valve toward the apex of more than 25 mm and RV dysfunction (Figs. 8A and B). CMR is reliably used for verifying the initial diagnosis and follow-up of RV function.[80] RV volume is also an important parameter in deciding future management.

CONCLUSION

Imaging is fundamental to the lifelong care of CHD patients. Cross-sectional imaging with CMR or CT provides complementary and invaluable information on cardiac and vascular anatomy and other intrathoracic structures. Furthermore, CMR provides quantification of cardiac function and vascular flow. To realize their full potential and to avoid pitfalls, however, echocardiography, MRI, and CT of CHD require appropriate training and experience.

REFERENCES

1. Dorfman AL, Levine JC, Colan SD, et al. Accuracy of echocardiography in low birth weight infants with congenital heart disease. Pediatrics. 2005;115:102-7.
2. Tworetzky W, McElhinney DB, Brook MM, et al. Echocardiographic diagnosis alone for the complete repair of major congenital heart defects. J Am Coll Cardiol. 1999;33:228-33.
3. Chew C, Halliday JL, Riley MM, et al. Population-based study of antenatal detection of congenital heart disease by ultrasound examination. Ultrasound Obstet Gynecol. 2007;29:619-24.
4. Kilner PJ, Geva T, Kaemmerer H, et al. Recommendations for cardiovascular magnetic resonance in adults with congenital heart disease from the respective working groups of the European Society of Cardiology. Eur Heart J. 2010;31:794-805.
5. Shellock FG, Spinazzi A. MRI safety update 2008: part 2, screening patients for MRI. AJR Am J Roentgenol. 2008;191:1140-9.
6. Helbing WA, de Roos A. Clinical applications of cardiac magnetic resonance imaging after repair of tetralogy of Fallot. Pediatr Cardiol. 2000;21:70-9.
7. Nadas AS. Tetralogy of Fallot. In: Fyler DC (Ed). Nadas' Pediatric Cardiology. Philadelphia, PA: Hanley & Belfus; 1992.
8. Powell AJ, Chung T, Landzberg MJ, et al. Accuracy of MRI evaluation of pulmonary blood supply in patients with complex pulmonary stenosis or atresia. Int J Card Imaging. 2000;16:169-74.
9. Norton K, Tong C, Glass R, et al. Cardiac MR imaging assessment following tetralogy of Fallot repair. Radiographics. 2006;26:197-211.
10. Babu-Narayan S, Chung N, Shore D, et al. Tetralogy of Fallot and common arterial trunk. In: Crawford M, DiMarco J, Paulus W (Eds). Cardiology, 3rd edition. US: Elsevier Ltd.; 2010. pp. 1471-84.
11. Balaguru D, Dilawar M. Pulmonary atresia with ventricular septal defect: systematic review. Heart Views. 2007;8:52-61.
12. Nollert G, Fischlein T, Bouterwek S, et al. Long-term survival in patients with repair of tetralogy of Fallot: 36-year follow-up of 490 survivors of the first year after surgical repair. J Am Coll Cardiol. 1997;30:1374-83.
13. Murphy JG, Gersh BJ, Mair DD, et al. Long-term outcome in patients undergoing surgical repair of tetralogy of Fallot. N Engl J Med. 1993;329:593-9.

14. Gatzoulis MA, Balaji S, Webber SA, et al. Risk factors for arrhythmia and sudden cardiac death late after repair of tetralogy of Fallot: a multicentre study. Lancet. 2000;356: 975-81.
15. Bacha EA, Scheule AM, Zurakowski D, et al. Long-term results after early primary repair of tetralogy of Fallot. J Thorac Cardiovasc Surg. 2001;122:154-61.
16. Lillehei CW, Varco RL, Cohen M, et al. The first open heart corrections of tetralogy of Fallot: a 26–31 year follow-up of 106 patients. Ann Surg. 1986;204:490-502.
17. Warnes CA, Williams RG, Bashore TM, et al. ACC/AHA 2008 guidelines for the management of adults with congenital heart disease: a report of the American College of Cardiology/ American Heart Association Task Force on Practice Guidelines (Writing Committee to Develop Guidelines for the Management of Adults with Congenital Heart Disease). Circulation. 2008;118:e714-833.
18. Knauth AL, Gauvreau K, Powell AJ, et al. Ventricular size and function assessed by cardiac MRI predict major adverse clinical outcomes late after tetralogy of Fallot repair. Heart. 2008;94:211-6.
19. Therrien J, Siu SC, Harris L, et al. Impact of pulmonary valve replacement on arrhythmia propensity late after repair of tetralogy of Fallot. Circulation. 2001;103:2489-94.
20. Oosterhof T, van Straten A, Vliegen HW, et al. Preoperative thresholds for pulmonary valve replacement in patients with corrected tetralogy of Fallot using cardiovascular magnetic resonance. Circulation. 2007;116:545-51.
21. Davlouros PA, Kilner PJ, Hornung TS, et al. Right ventricular function in adults with repaired tetralogy of Fallot assessed with cardiovascular magnetic resonance imaging: detrimental role of right ventricular outflow aneurysms or akinesia and adverse right-to-left ventricular interaction. J Am Coll Cardiol. 2002;40:2044-52.
22. Helbing MDWA, Niezen MDRA, Le Cessie MS, et al. Right ventricular diastolic function in children with pulmonary regurgitation after repair of tetralogy of Fallot: volumetric evaluation by magnetic resonance velocity mapping. J Am Coll Cardiol. 1996;28:1827-35.
23. Babu-Narayan SV, Kilner PJ, Li W, et al. Ventricular fibrosis suggested by cardiovascular magnetic resonance in adults with repaired tetralogy of Fallot and its relationship to adverse markers of clinical outcome. Circulation. 2006;113:405-13.
24. Greenberg SB, Crisci KL, Koenig P, et al. Magnetic resonance imaging compared with echocardiography in the evaluation of pulmonary artery abnormalities in children with tetralogy of Fallot following palliative and corrective surgery. Pediatr Radiol. 1997;27:932-5.
25. Ichida F, Hashimoto I, Tsubata S, et al. Evaluation of pulmonary blood supply by multiplanar cine magnetic resonance imaging in patients with pulmonary atresia and severe pulmonary stenosis. Int J Card Imaging. 1999;15: 473-81.
26. Kondo C, Takada K, Yokoyama U, et al. Comparison of three-dimensional contrast-enhanced magnetic resonance angiography and axial radiographic angiography for diagnosing congenital stenoses in small pulmonary arteries. Am J Cardiol. 2001;87:420-4.
27. Sridharan S, Derrick G, Deanfield J, et al. Assessment of differential branch pulmonary blood flow: a comparative study of phase contrast magnetic resonance imaging and radionuclide lung perfusion imaging. Heart. 2006;92:963-8.
28. Hoffman JI, Kaplan S. The incidence of congenital heart disease. J Am Coll Cardiol. 2002;39:1890-900.
29. Dearani JA, Connolly HM, Martinez R, et al. Caring for adults with congenital cardiac disease: successes and challenges for 2007 and beyond. Cardiol Young. 2007;17(Suppl. 2):87-96.
30. Oechslin E, Jenni R. 40 Years after the first atrial switch procedure in patients with transposition of the great arteries: long-term results in Toronto and Zurich. Thorac Cardiovasc Surg. 2000;48:233-7.
31. Culbert EL, Ashburn DA, Cullen-Dean G, et al. Quality of life of children after repair of transposition of the great arteries. Circulation. 2003;108:857-62.
32. Cohen MS, Eidem BW, Cetta F, et al. Multimodality imaging guidelines of patients with transposition of the great arteries: a report from the American Society of Echocardiography Developed in Collaboration with the Society for Cardiovascular Magnetic Resonance and the Society of Cardiovascular Computed Tomography. J Am Soc Echocardiogr. 2016;29:571-621.
33. Angeli E, Raisky O, Bonnet D, et al. Late reoperations after neonatal arterial switch operation for transposition of the great arteries. Eur J Cardiothorac Surg. 2008;34:32-6.
34. Weiss F, Habermann CR, Lilje C, et al. MRI of pulmonary arteries in follow-up after arterial-switch-operation (ASO) for transposition of great arteries (D-TGA). Rofo. 2005;177:849-55.
35. Beauchesne LM, Warnes CA, Connolly HM, et al. Outcome of the unoperated adult who presents with congenitally corrected transposition of the great arteries. J Am Coll Cardiol. 2002;40:285-90.
36. Warnes CA. Congenitally corrected transposition: the uncorrected misnomer. J Am Coll Cardiol. 1996;27:1244-5.
37. Connelly MS, Liu PP, Williams WG, et al. Congenitally corrected transposition of the great arteries in the adult: functional status and complications. J Am Coll Cardiol. 1996;27:1238-43.
38. van Son JA, Danielson GK, Huhta JC, et al. Late results of systemic atrioventricular valve replacement in corrected transposition. J Thorac Cardiovasc Surg. 1995;109:642-52.
39. Nielsen JC, Powell AJ, Gauvreau K, et al. Magnetic resonance imaging predictors of coarctation severity. Circulation. 2005;111:622-8.
40. Kaiser T, Kellenberger CJ, Albisetti M, et al. Normal values for aortic diameters in children and adolescents—assessment in vivo by contrast-enhanced CMR-angiography. J Cardiovasc Magn Reson. 2008;10:56.
41. Konen E, Merchant N, Provost Y, et al. Coarctation of the aorta before and after correction: the role of cardiovascular MRI. AJR Am J Roentgenol. 2004;182:1333-9.

42. Riquelme C, Laissy JP, Menegazzo D, et al. MR imaging of coarctation of the aorta and its postoperative complications in adults: assessment with spin-echo and cine-MR imaging. Magn Reson Imaging. 1999;17:37-46.
43. Prince MR, Narasimham DL, Jacoby WT, et al. Three-dimensional gadolinium-enhanced MR angiography of the thoracic aorta. AJR Am J Roentgenol. 1996;166:1387-97.
44. Oshinski JN, Parks WJ, Markou CP, et al. Improved measurement of pressure gradients in aortic coarctation by magnetic resonance imaging. J Am Coll Cardiol. 1996;28:1818-26.
45. Eichhorn JG, Krissak R, Rudiger HJ, et al. Compliance of the normal-sized aorta in adolescents with Marfan syndrome: comparison of MR measurements of aortic distensibility and pulse wave velocity. Rofo. 2007;179:841-6.
46. Kellenberger C. Aortic arch malformations. Pediatr Radiol. 2010;40:876-84.
47. Greil GF, Kramer U, Dammann F, et al. Diagnosis of vascular rings and slings using an interleaved 3D double-slab FISP MR angiography technique. Pediatr Radiol. 2005;35:396-401.
48. Nordmeyer J, Gaudin R, Tann OR, et al. MRI may be sufficient for noninvasive assessment of great vessel stents: an in vitro comparison of MRI, CT, and conventional angiography. AJR Am J Roentgenol. 2010;195:865-71.
49. Rasche V, Oberhuber A, Trumpp S, et al. MRI assessment of thoracic stent grafts after emergency implantation in multi trauma patients: a feasibility study. Eur Radiol. 2011;21:1397-405.
50. Sridharan S, Yates R, Taylor AM. Optimizing imaging after coarctation stenting: the clinical utility of multidetector computer tomography. Catheter Cardiovasc Interv. 2005;66:420-3.
51. Thanopoulos BV, Douskou M, Giannakoulas G. Multislice computed tomography after stent implantation for aortic coarctation. Eur Heart J. 2010;31:2270.
52. Iezzi R, Dattesi R, Pirro F, et al. CT angiography in stent-graft sizing: impact of using inner vs. outer wall measurements of aortic neck diameters. J Endovasc Ther. 2011;18:280-8.
53. Hundley WG, Li HF, Lange RA, et al. Assessment of left-to-right intracardiac shunting by velocity-encoded, phase-difference magnetic resonance imaging. A comparison with oximetric and indicator dilution techniques. Circulation. 1995;91:2955-60.
54. Holmvang G, Palacios IF, Vlahakes GJ, et al. Imaging and sizing of atrial septal defects by magnetic resonance. Circulation. 1995;92:3473-80.
55. Taylor AM, Stables RH, Poole-Wilson PA, et al. Definitive clinical assessment of atrial septal defect by magnetic resonance imaging. J Cardiovasc Magn Reson. 1999;1:43-7.
56. Hoffman JI, Kaplan S. The incidence of congenital heart disease. J Am Coll Cardiol. 2002;39:1890-900.
57. Du ZD, Roguin N, Wu XJ. Spontaneous closure of muscular ventricular septal defect identified by echocardiography in neonates. Cardiol Young. 1998;8:500-5.
58. Kidd L, Driscoll DJ, Gersony WM, et al. Second natural history study of congenital heart defects. Results of treatment of patients with ventricular septal defects. Circulation. 1993;87:I38-51.
59. Roman KS, Kellenberger CJ, Macgowan CK, et al. How is pulmonary arterial blood flow affected by pulmonary venous obstruction in children? A phase-contrast magnetic resonance study. Pediatr Radiol. 2005;35:580-6.
60. Riesenkampff EM, Schmitt B, Schnackenburg B, et al. Partial anomalous pulmonary venous drainage in young pediatric patients: the role of magnetic resonance imaging. Pediatr Cardiol. 2009;30:458-64.
61. Beerbaum P, Korperich H, Barth P, et al. Noninvasive quantification of left-to-right shunt in pediatric patients: phase-contrast cine magnetic resonance imaging compared with invasive oximetry. Circulation. 2001;103:2476-82.
62. Valsangiacomo ER, Hornberger LK, Barrea C, et al. Partial and total anomalous pulmonary venous connection in the fetus: two-dimensional and Doppler echocardiographic findings. Ultrasound Obstet Gynecol. 2003;22:257-63.
63. Valente A, Sena L, Powell A, et al. Cardiac magnetic resonance imaging evaluation of sinus venosus defects: comparison to surgical findings. Pediatr Cardiol. 2007;28:51-6.
64. Valsangiacomo Buechel ER, Grosse-Wortmann L, Fratz S, et al. Indications for cardiovascular magnetic resonance in children with congenital and acquired heart disease: an expert consensus paper of the Imaging Working Group of the AEPC and the Cardiovascular Magnetic Resonance Section of the EACVI. Eur Heart J Cardiovasc Imaging. 2015;16:281-97.
65. Geva T, Vick GWIII, Wendt RE, et al. Role of spin echo and cine magnetic resonance imaging in presurgical planning of heterotaxy syndrome. Comparison with echocardiography and catheterization. Circulation. 1994;90:348-56.
66. Fogel MA. Cardiac magnetic resonance of single ventricles. J Cardiovasc Magn Reson. 2006;8:661-70.
67. Fogel MA, Weinberg PM, Chin AJ, et al. Late ventricular geometry and performance changes of functional single ventricle throughout staged Fontan reconstruction assessed by magnetic resonance imaging. J Am Coll Cardiol. 1996;28:212-21.
68. Robbers-Visser D, Kapusta L, van Osch-Gevers L, et al. Clinical outcome 5 to 18 years after the Fontan operation performed on children younger than 5 years. J Thorac Cardiovasc Surg. 2009;138:89-95.
69. Angelini P. Coronary artery anomalies: an entity in search of an identity. Circulation. 2007;115:1296-305.
70. Angelini P, Velasco JA, Flamm S. Coronary anomalies: incidence, pathophysiology, and clinical relevance. Circulation. 2002;105:2449-54.
71. Maron BJ, Shirani J, Poliac LC, et al. Sudden death in young competitive athletes. Clinical, demographic, and pathological profiles. JAMA. 1996;276:199-204.
72. Brenner DJ, Hall EJ. Computed tomography—an increasing source of radiation exposure. N Engl J Med. 2007;357:2277-84.
73. Greil GF, Desai MY, Fenchel M, et al. Reproducibility of free-breathing cardiovascular magnetic resonance coronary angiography. J Cardiovasc Magn Reson. 2007;9:49-56.

74. Piccini D, Monney P, Sierro C, et al. Respiratory self-navigated postcontrast whole-heart coronary MR angiography: initial experience in patients. Radiology. 2014;270:378-86.
75. Tangcharoen T, Bell A, Hegde S, et al. Detection of coronary artery anomalies in infants and young children with congenital heart disease by using MR imaging. Radiology. 2011;259:240-7.
76. Beerbaum P, Sarikouch S, Laser KT, et al. Coronary anomalies assessed by whole-heart isotropic 3D magnetic resonance imaging for cardiac morphology in congenital heart disease. J Magn Reson Imaging. 2009;29:320-7.
77. Brickner ME, Hillis LD, Lange RA. Congenital heart disease in adults. Second of two parts. N Engl J Med. 2000;342:334-42.
78. Perloff JK, Hart EM, Greaves SM, et al. Proximal pulmonary arterial and intrapulmonary radiologic features of Eisenmenger syndrome and primary pulmonary hypertension. Am J Cardiol. 2003;92:182-7.
79. Perloff JK. Clinical recognition of congenital heart disease, 5th edition. Philadelphia, PA: Saunders; 2003.
80. Yalonetsky S, Tobler D, Greutmann M, et al. Cardiac magnetic resonance imaging and the assessment of Ebstein anomaly in adults. Am J Cardiol. 2011;107:767-73.

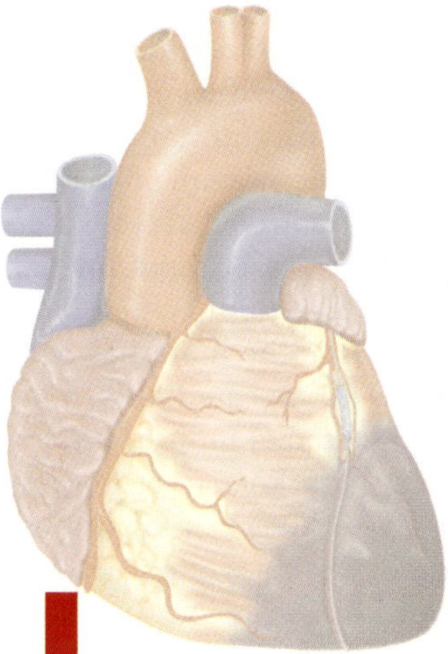

117

CHAPTER

Role of Cardiac MRI in Evaluation of Congenital Heart Disease

Richa Kothari, Vimal Raj

INTRODUCTION

Imaging of congenital heart disease (CHD) has been a domain of plain chest radiographs (CXRs), cardiac catheterization, and echocardiography. Recent years have seen the rise of magnetic resonance imaging (MRI) and computed tomography (CT) as imaging modalities for CHD. Both of these modalities provide a noninvasive method of assessing the anatomy of the cardiovascular system in any imaging plane. Compared to CT, MRI has the advantage of providing functional data without any exposure to ionizing radiation. Therefore, MRI has become the source of important insights into individualized pathophysiologic changes in CHD for both morphologic and functional aspects.[1,2] It has become the standard of reference for providing an accurate and reproducible measurement of right ventricular (RV) volume and function.[3] MRI is excellent in the diagnosis and follow-up of CHD due to its ability to deliver detailed three-dimensional (3D) imaging of complex anatomy in a noninvasive manner before as well as after surgical interventions.[4]

PATIENT PREPARATION

Cardiac MRI (CMR) examinations may last from 20 minutes to 60 minutes, depending on the clinical scenario. Patients are expected to remain still in the scanner during the procedure to obtain high-quality images by minimize motion artifact. For all patients, MR-compatible electrocardiographic (ECG) leads are placed on the anterior chest wall and for ECG gating. In patients with dextrocardia, ECG leads are best placed on the right half of the chest (Figs. 1A and B). A flat "body coil" is placed on top of the patient (either over a frame or directly on the patient) to acquire the images. In older children, parents are provided with a detailed description of the CMR examination and asked to discuss it with their child in an age-appropriate manner in advance to increase the likelihood of a successful study. Images can be acquired during breath-hold if the child is cooperative; otherwise, imaging can be performed during normal respiration (free breathing).

Sedation

Young children (usually less than 6 to 8 years) and cognitively impaired older patients typically require some form of sedation. Multiple factors should be taken into account when deciding whether a patient should have an examination with sedation including the length of the anticipated examination protocol, developmental maturity, the patient's experience with prior procedures, the parents opinion of their child's capability to cooperate with the examination, the risks of sedation, and the benefits of the diagnostic information.[5] The preferences and availability of sedation and/or general anesthesia (GA) differ from center to center. When sedation or GA is used, appropriate monitoring of the patient and presence of an expert team which is versed in the administration of drugs and equipped to deal with emergencies are mandatory. Each study is tailored so as to keep time of anesthesia as minimum as possible. Newer advances in technology have improved "free-breathing" protocols, thereby reducing the requirement of GA with majority of the studies being performed under mild sedation. Distraction techniques with a monitor playing cartoon movies within the scanner room are also very useful in improving patient experience and reducing the requirement of sedation.

Safety

Prior to bringing the patient into the scanner room, the patient's history and safety screening form should be reviewed to identify implanted devices which may be hazardous in the CMR environment or produce image artifact. For patients who may have undergone a cardiac procedure and have an incomplete or unreliable history, a CXR is obtained to assist screening. The most important step to reduce potential risks of CMR scanning is to establish a strict policy of screening before CMR for the patient and all accompanying persons, including parents and medical personnel.[6] This is particularly important to avoid the so-called missile effect caused by ferromagnetic objects drawn rapidly into the scanner by massive magnetic forces.[7] Following safety screening, physiological monitoring devices, and hearing protection (for both awake and sedated patients) are put in place. A high-quality ECG signal is essential for optimum data quality in cardiac-gated sequences. Common contraindications for CMR, like claustrophobia, must be respected. CMR is generally contraindicated in patients after non-MRI compatible pacemaker or implantable cardioverter-defibrillator implantation. However, several implantable electrodes, generators, and mechanical prosthetic valves of the newer generations are MRI conditional; performing CMR examinations with these devices is safe and yields high-quality images.[8] In case of doubt, information about product safety is available on dedicated websites (e.g. www.mrisafety.com). The presence of epicardial pacemaker leads is a relative contraindication for CMR because of potential heating of the leads. Gadolinium-based contrast agents (GBCAs) are generally safe. Major adverse events are very rare and consist of allergic reactions and nephrogenic systemic fibrosis (NSF).[8] Nephrogenic systemic fibrosis is an exceedingly rarely reported generalized disease. Risk is increased in patients with severely decreased renal function and a glomerular filtration rate below 30 mL/min. More recently, deposition of gadolinium in the brain has been reported in patients who underwent repeated MRI (more than five times) for various (noncardiac) indications; the clinical significance of this finding is not known yet. In many CHD cases, there is no need to give GBCAs, especially those on follow-up. If administration of GBCAs is required, such as for angiography (Figs. 2A and B), perfusion studies, or late gadolinium enhancement, the use of nonlinear, cyclic GBCAs is preferred, as for this group of contrast agents, NSF and brain deposition are significantly lower. In patients with a glomerular filtration rate below 30 mL/min, the use of a cyclic GBCA should be carefully weighed against the potential risks and, if possible, avoided, while some linear GBCAs are contraindicated.[8] In pregnant females, CMR should be preferred to radioactive imaging modalities. The use of GBCA in pregnancy should be avoided as they cross the blood–placenta barrier and their effects on the fetus are not known.[8] The main advantages of CMR are the lack of ionizing radiation and its noninvasiveness. Particularly, the use of radiation-free modalities is very important in children as they may require multiple follow-up studies. CT scan has the advantages of being faster with good isotropic spatial resolution. Patients in whom MRI is contraindicated and those with a high risk for sedation/GA, CT imaging of the chest can be performed. Disadvantages of CT include exposure to radiation and iodinated contrast media.

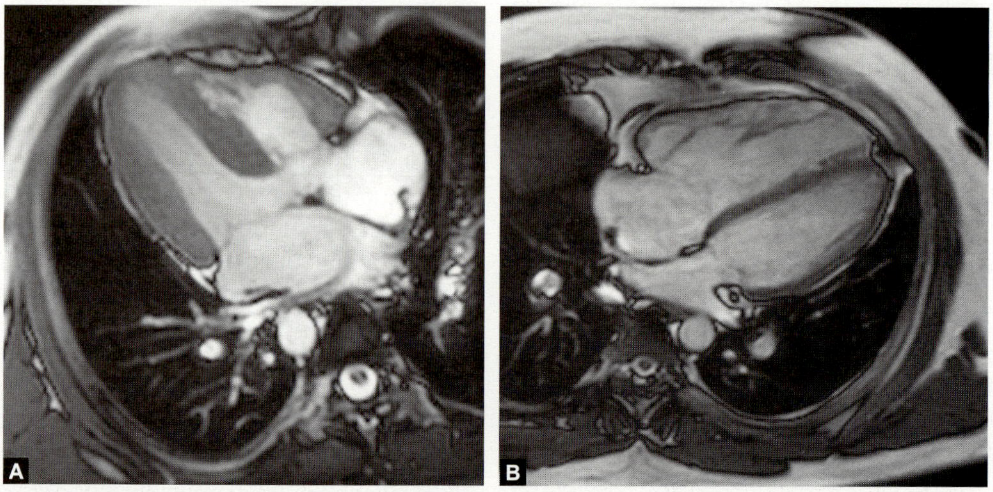

Figs. 1A and B: Orientation of the heart determines placement of the leads on the chest: (A) dextrocardia and (B) levocardia.

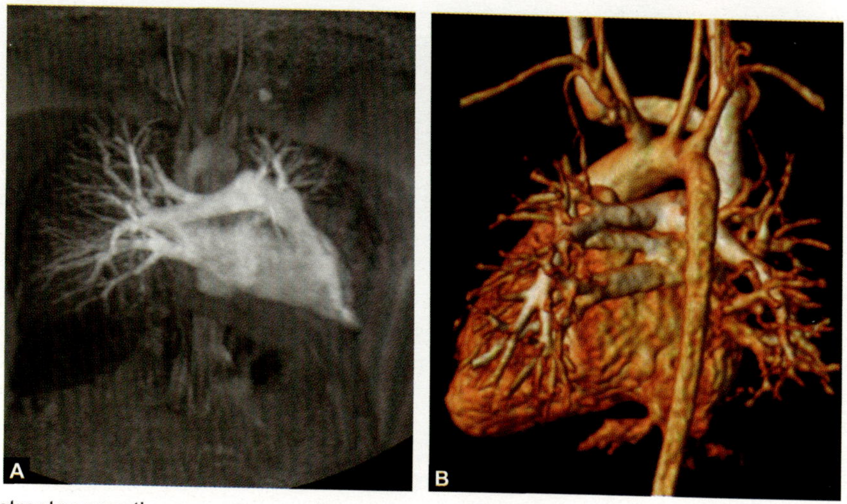

Figs. 2A and B: Contrast magnetic resonance angiography showing (A) maximum-intensity projection image of pulmonary angiography and (B) a 3D volume-rendered image of aortography.

Protocol

With advances in technology, various imaging sequences have become widely available that allow detailed anatomic and functional assessment of CHD.[2,9,10] High spatial resolution can be achieved by using thin slices, a small field of view and a large matrix. Static and cine imaging is generally performed with a section thickness of 3–5 mm in children.

Cardiac magnetic resonance imaging protocol (Table 1):

- Localizers.
- Black-blood spin-echo sequences provide a good overview of the anatomy and can be helpful in directing additional sequences. These are noncine images and are of high resolution (Figs. 3A and B).

TABLE 1: Magnetic resonance imaging sequences in routine cardiac MRI.

CMR protocol
• Localizers • Black-blood axial spin-echo sequence covering entire chest • Axial cine SSFP acquisition of entire heart with no slice gap • Additional cine stacks may be acquired in coronal, sagittal, or an oblique plane, if needed • Dedicated cine SSFP acquisition in two-, four-, and three-chamber views • Cine SSFP LVOT view • Cine SSFP RVOT view • Phase-contrast imaging of MPA and aorta • Gadolinium-enhanced MR angiography for thoracic vasculature with 3D reformats • 3D whole heart sequence

(3D: Three-dimensional; CMR: cardiac MRI; LVOT: left ventricular outflow tract; MPA: main pulmonary artery; MR: magnetic resonance; RVOT: RV outflow tract; SSFP: steady-state free precession)

- Cine images are acquired using steady-state free precession (SSFP) sequence. The entire heart is covered in an axial plane with no slice gap. These sequences provide most of the diagnostic information. Ventricular volumes and function can be calculated from these and any shunts can be diagnosed.
- Additional cine images may be acquired in coronal, sagittal, or an oblique plane in case of complicated anatomy.
- Dedicated cine SSFP acquisition in two-, four-, and three-chamber views.
- Cine SSFP left ventricular (LV) outflow tract (LVOT) view. It further gives the information of LVOT angulation for ventricular septal defect (VSD) routability and better visualization of VSD patch postoperatively.
- Cine SSFP RV outflow tract (RVOT) view. It provides visualization and extent of akinesis or aneurysmal infundibulum. It allows direct visualization of pulmonary regurgitation (PR) and stenosis.[11]
- Phase-contrast imaging of main pulmonary artery and aorta is vital for the assessment of blood flow characteristics, including the direction and magnitude of flow, and hence, the detection and quantification of any valvular, vessel, or conduit stenosis or regurgitation. It allows calculation of pulmonary-to-systemic-flow ratio (Qp and Qs).
- Gadolinium-enhanced MR angiography is used when detailed anatomic information relating to the thoracic vasculature is needed. 3D imaging data sets can be displayed in any orientation with maximum-intensity projection reformatted images or as an overview of the anatomy with 3D volume-rendered images.

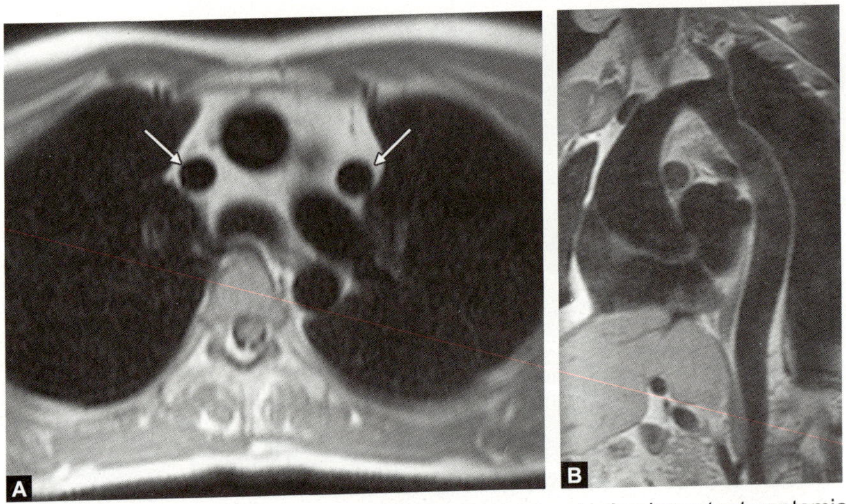

Figs. 3A and B: (A) Axial and (B) oblique sagittal black-blood images demonstrating important anatomical abnormalities, such as double superior vena cava (white arrow) and mild coarctation of aorta in proximal descending aorta.

Preoperative Assessment

Preoperative assessment is usually accomplished by two-dimensional echocardiography. In addition, cross-sectional imaging using CT or MR angiography can provide anatomical details to aid in surgical repair by determining pulmonary vascular anatomy (specifically size and branching pattern of the pulmonary arteries), origin, and course of the coronaries and other associated lesions, such as anomalies of the aortic arch.[11,12] It is especially useful in complex CHD.

Postoperative Assessment

Cardiac magnetic resonance imaging provides excellent anatomic and functional details with a large field of view, excellent in-plane spatial resolution, and good temporal resolution. In follow-up of postoperative patients, it provides precise measurements of LV and RV volumes and function, PR fraction, anatomy of pulmonary arteries. It is also useful in ascertaining the integrity of the VSD patch. Serial objective follow-up is also possible in patients without exposure to ionizing radiation or intravenous contrast.

CLINICAL APPLICATIONS

Left Heart Obstructive Defects

Left ventricular outflow tract obstruction syndromes include subaortic stenosis, valvular aortic stenosis (AS), supra-AS, and aortic coarctation.[13] Obstruction can occur singly or at multiple levels, as an isolated lesion or in combination with septal defects or conotruncal anomalies.

Subaortic stenosis refers to a discrete fibrous ring or fibromuscular narrowing and is distinct from genetic hypertrophic cardiomyopathy with dynamic LVOT obstruction. Subaortic stenosis is usually a solitary congenital defect but may be superimposed on other congenital heart defects (e.g. VSD) or acquired under certain circumstances (e.g. after VSD patch repair).[14] Cine SSFP three-chamber and LVOT views would demonstrate dark systolic jets compatible with flow acceleration. Subvalvular stenosis can be differentiated from valvular AS based on the origin of the jet in LVOT view rather than aortic valve cusps (Figs. 4A and B). The diastolic phase would show the anatomy of the thin ridge/thick membrane. Associated LV hypertrophy can also be quantified and assessed for

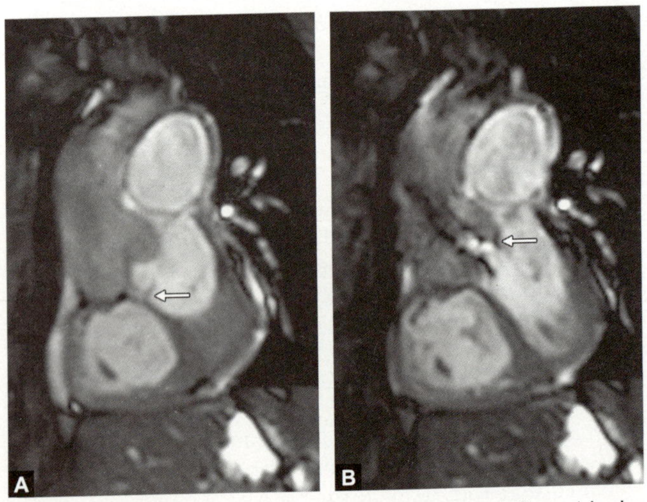

Figs. 4A and B: Steady-state free precession left ventricular outflow tract view: (A) flow acceleration jet can be seen in systole originating in subvalvular region (arrow) proximal to the valve cusps. (B) An eccentric 2-mm-thick membrane (arrow) is seen as the cause of the subvalvular stenosis in diastole.

myocardial fibrosis. Bicuspid aortic valve (BAV) is the most common cause of *valvular stenosis* in the young. BAV abnormalities arise from abnormal cusp formation during valve genesis, commonly with fusion between two cusps, forming one smaller and one larger cusp. Variants range from a nearly trileaflet aortic valve with cusp inequality to a unicuspid and dysplastic valve. A BAV can be predominately obstructive or regurgitant, depending on the degree of commissural fusion[14] (Figs. 5A and B). Additional cine views along the aortic valve in thin slices of 3–4 mm help to evaluate the aortic valve area. Cine SSFP three-chamber and LVOT views would demonstrate dark systolic jets compatible with flow acceleration at the level of the valve. Phase-contrast imaging along the aortic valve gives pressure gradient across valve; however, CMR underestimates the gradient compared to catheter based studies.

Supraaortic stenosis is a fixed obstruction that arises just above the sinus of Valsalva (Figs. 6A to C) and extends a variable distance along the aorta. It is commonly associated with varying degrees of hypoplasia of the aortic arch. Determination of arch dimension is important in planning the surgical management of these patients. CMR can easily demonstrate the area, length of stenosis, and the arch anatomy.

Discrete *coarctation of the aorta* consists of short-segment narrowing in the region of ligamentum arteriosum

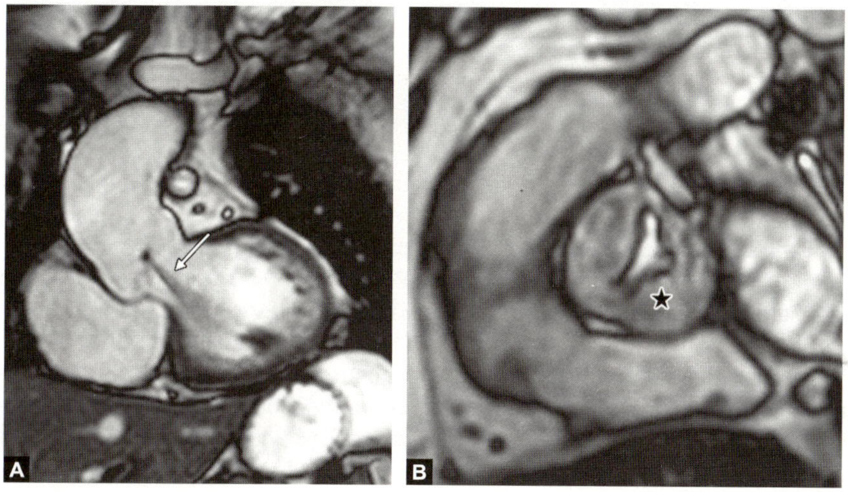

Figs. 5A and B: Steady-state free precession left ventricular outflow tract view: (A) moderate aortic regurgitation jet (arrow) and (B) dedicated crosscut view of the aortic valve showing a bicuspid aortic valve (star).

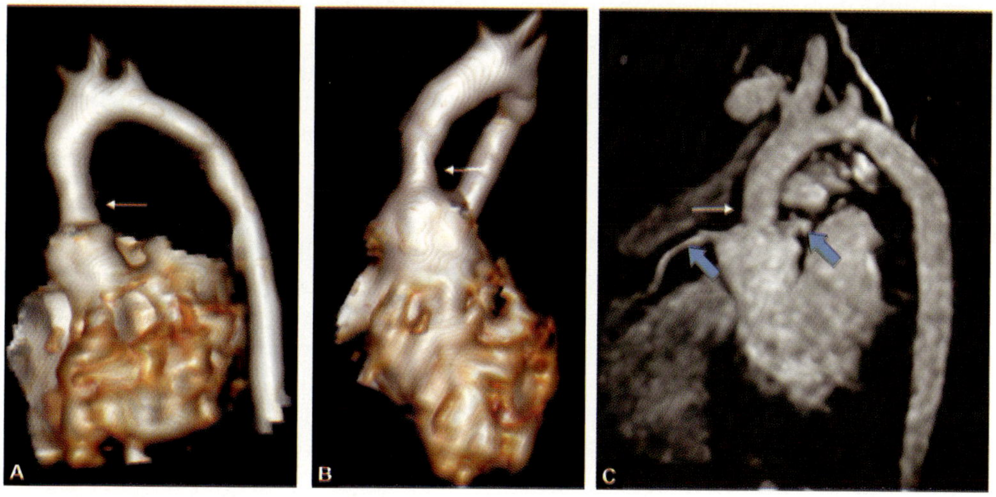

Figs. 6A to C: 3D volume rendered images from magnetic resonance angiography showing supravalvular aortic stenosis (arrow) as seen from (A) front and (B) side. (C) Sagittal oblique multiplanar reconstruction from 3D noncontrast whole heart sequence showing supravalvular aortic stenosis (white arrow) in another patient. The coronaries (blue arrows) can be seen arising from aorta below the level of stenosis.

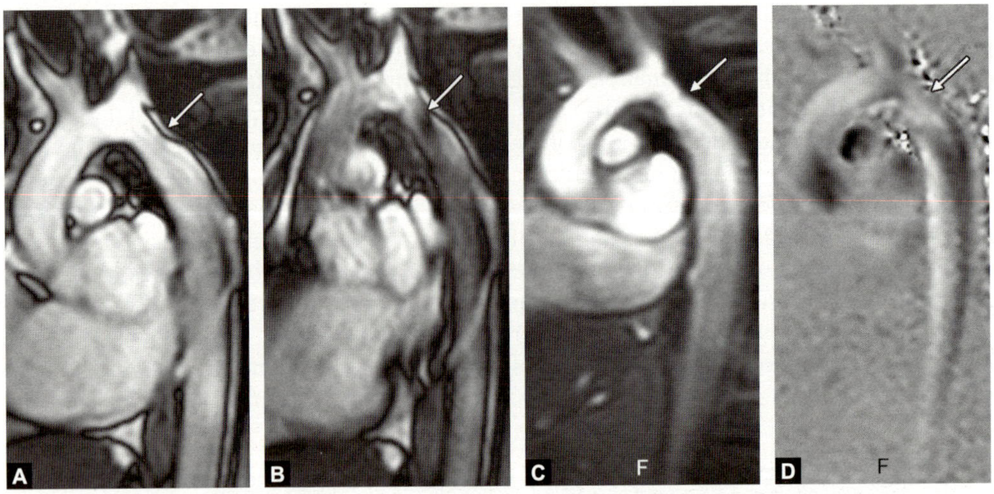

Figs. 7A to D: Cine steady-state free precession sequence along the aorta shows mild coarctation (arrow) just beyond the left subclavian artery origin in diastole (A) with flow acceleration across it in systole (B). In-plane phase-contrast images (C and D) of same patient.

adjacent to the origin of the left subclavian artery (Figs. 7A to D). Anatomical determination of the severity of stenosis and its relationship with the left subclavian artery is very important in management of these patients. Pressure gradients across the obstruction can be calculated on CMR. The presence of abundant collaterals may also reduce the gradient across the coarctation and mask the severity of the obstruction.[14] Phase-contrast imaging may also be useful to quantify collateral flow. 3D MRI or CT angiography identifies the precise location and anatomy of the coarctation and entire aorta, as well as collateral vessels.[15]

Cardiac magnetic resonance imaging is a sensitive modality for the identification of left heart obstructive defects. It is well suited for the evaluation of the clinical significance of the stenosis as well as the precise location of the gradient, detection, and quantification of aortic insufficiency, quantitative and qualitative evaluation of LV hypertrophy, and ventricular function.

Right Heart Obstructive Defects

Congenital obstruction can be at, below, or above the pulmonary valve. Infundibular stenosis is a crucial component of tetralogy of Fallot (TOF).[16] Supravalvular pulmonary stenosis (PS) or pulmonary arterial stenosis is caused by narrowing of the main pulmonary trunk, the pulmonary arterial bifurcation, or the primary and/or intrapulmonary branches. Sub-infundibular stenosis or double-chambered right ventricle is a rare form of outflow obstruction that results in the RV being divided into a high-pressure inlet portion and a low-pressure outlet portion by a thick muscle bundle, the hypertrophied septoparietal trabeculation, an anomalous apical shelf, or an abnormal moderator band.[17,18] The sequelae from surgical intervention may also result in stenosis, at times requiring reintervention. Postoperatively, there may be valvular or conduit stenosis and regurgitation of implanted bioprosthetic pulmonary valves placed during childhood. The role of MRI or CT in uncomplicated valvular PS is confirmatory and to assess the degree and location of stenosis. Cardiac magnetic resonance imaging provides excellent imaging of the main, branch, and peripheral pulmonary arteries without the requirement of contrast administration. It is also useful in confirming the presence and quantifying the amount of PR or tricuspid regurgitation (TR). MRI is the most useful imaging modality for defining the anatomy in double-chambered right ventricle and in follow-up of these patients.[19] In patients with any RV pulmonary artery conduit or bioprosthetic valve placed in the RVOT, it may help define lesion severity and may demonstrate conduit adherence to the sternum.

Tetralogy of Fallot

Tetralogy of Fallot is the most common cyanotic CHD. CMR has become a prominent diagnostic and monitoring tool for both pre- and postoperative assessments of TOF.[20-22] Preoperative CMR shows the pulmonary and coronary vascular anatomy which helps determine the surgical approach. The size of the pulmonary arteries are standardized using McGoon's ratio, which is the ratio of sum of diameters of distal right and left pulmonary arteries and aortic diameter at the level of diaphragm. McGoon's ratio above 1.2 is associated with acceptable postoperative outcome in TOF, and definite intracardiac repair (ICR) may be done. The ratio below 0.8 is inadequate for complete repair of pulmonary arteries and palliative surgery like Blalock-Taussig shunt may be done to allow for pulmonary arterial growth.[23] Coronary artery that crosses anterior to the surface of the RVOT may alter the surgical approach (Figs. 8A to D). PR is the most common sequel following ICR. It is present in nearly all TOF patients undergoing ICR. PR can be accurately quantified with phase-contrast imaging (Figs. 9A to D). Also, CMR is very useful in quantifying the secondary effects of PR on RV size and function. This can be measured and serially monitored and with no exposure to radiation or iodinated contrast. CMR quantification of PR fraction, RV dilatation, and ejection fraction plays a critical role in decision of timing of pulmonary valve replacement.[24] RV dilation more than 150–160 mL/m^2 with decreased RV function is now regarded an important cutoff parameter for the timing of pulmonary valve replacement.[25] CMR helps delineate the level and severity of lesions in residual PS (Figs. 10A to C) or conduit obstruction, especially MR angiography. Tricuspid regurgitation may develop as a consequence of progressive RV dilatation due to free PR. Residual VSD can be demonstrated in the cine LVOT view and also shunt quantification done using phase-contrast imaging avoiding invasive catheterization.

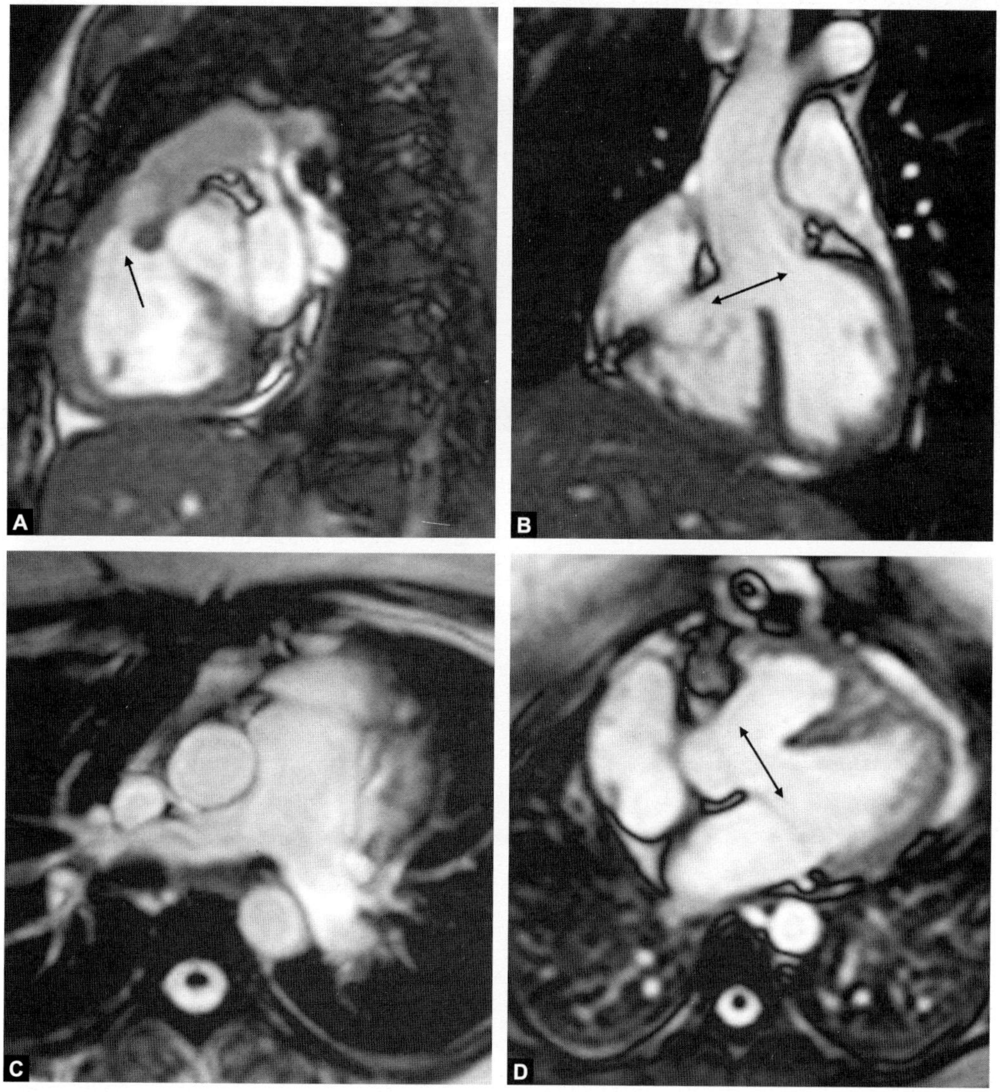

Figs. 8A to D: Steady-state free precession images in (A) RVOT, (B) LVOT, and (C and D) axial planes in a patient with TOF. There is severe RVOT narrowing (single black arrow) with subaortic VSD (double black arrow) and good size confluent branch pulmonary arteries. (LVOT: left ventricular outflow tract; RVOT: RV outflow tract; VSD: ventricular septal defect)

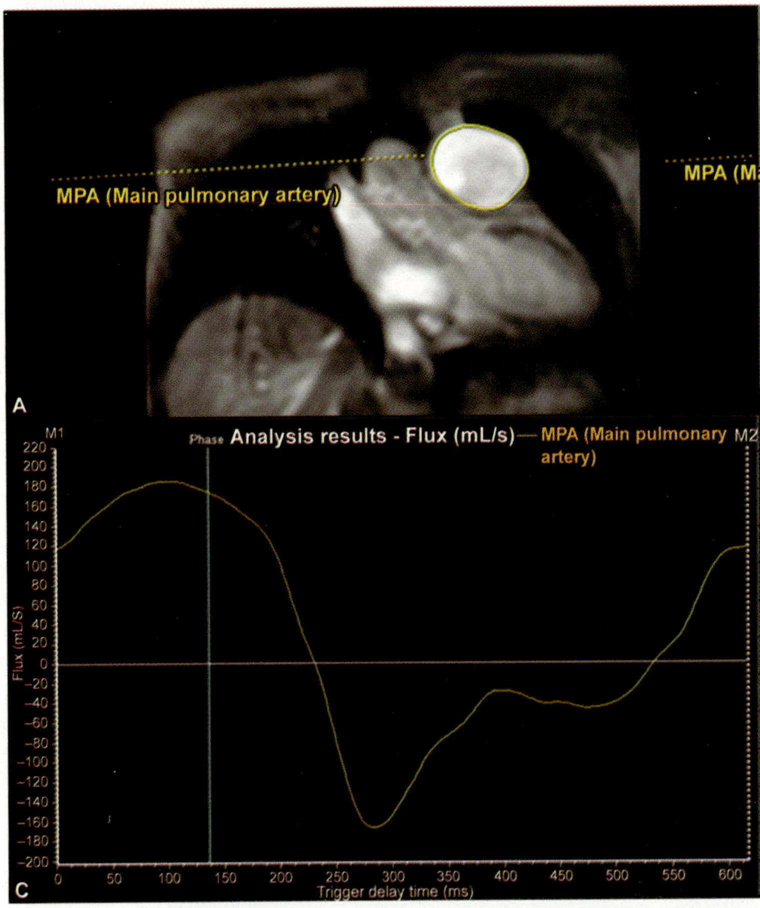

D

Analysis results	MPM (Main pulmonary artery)
Stroke volume	19.70 mL
Forward flow vol	40.42 mL
Backward flow vol	20.72 mL
Regurgitant fract	51.25 %
Abs. stroke volume	61.14 mL
Mean flux	31.86 mL/s
Stroke distance	1.65 cm
Mean velocity	2.67 cm/s
Peak velociity	64.48 cm/s
Peak pressure gradient	1.66 mm Hg (k=4)
Heart rate	97 bpm

Figs. 9A to D: Phase-contrast images through (A and B) main pulmonary artery and (C) analysis graph—positive peak in the graph denotes forward flow and trough denotes regurgitation—showing free PR (~51%) as seen in results table (D) in a post-ICR patient. (ICR: intracardiac repair; PR: pulmonary regurgitation)

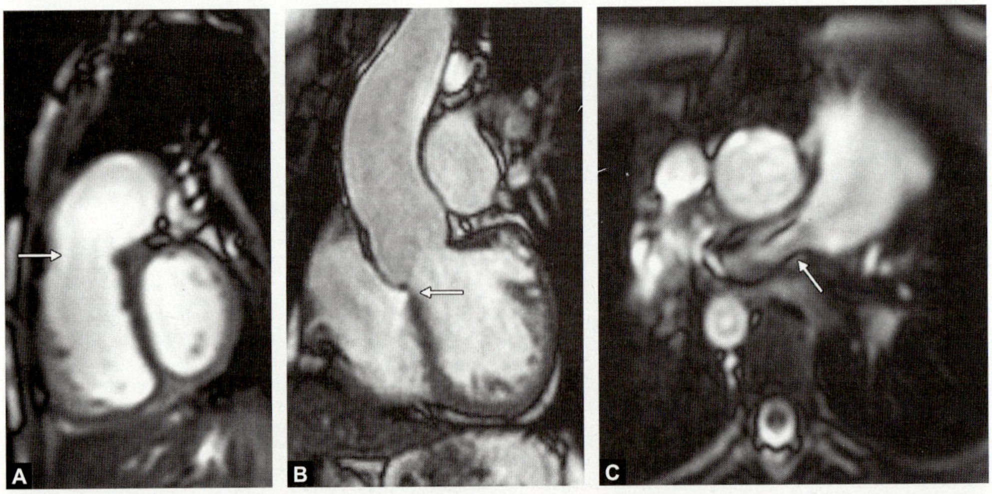

Figs. 10A to C: Steady-state free precession images of post-ICR case showing (A) repaired capacious RVOT (arrow) in RVOT view, (B) intact VSD patch (arrow) in LVOT view, and (C) mild-RPA ostial stenosis (arrow) with associated flow acceleration in axial view. (ICR: intracardiac repair; LVOT: left ventricular outflow tract; RPA: right pulmonary artery; RVOT: RV outflow tract; VSD: ventricular septal defect)

Ebstein's Anomaly

The Ebstein's anomaly encompasses abnormalities with varying degrees of delamination and downward displacement of the posterior and septal leaflets of the tricuspid valve. The abnormal valve position results in an enlarged right atrium with a small, functional right ventricle referred to as atrialization of the right ventricle. A substantial number of patients have an associated atrial septal defect (ASD) (Figs. 11A and B).[26] In cine sequences, a regurgitant jet in systole originating deep in the RV cavity is seen, indicating an abnormally positioned and incompetent tricuspid valve. Attachment of the septal leaflet of the tricuspid valve is displaced in adults by more than 20 mm toward the RV apex relative to the mitral insertion point.[27] Bowing of the interventricular septum may be seen (Figs. 11A and B). Echocardiography remains the mainstay of valve function imaging, owing to higher temporal resolution, but CMR can help provide an accurate assessment of right atrial and RV size and, most important, can provide reproducible RV function measurements.[28] It also allows calculation of potential RV volume and function after corrective valve reimplantation.

ABNORMAL CONNECTIONS

Transposition of Great Arteries

Transposition of the great arteries (TGA) is the second most common cyanotic CHD after TOF. As the name suggests, each great artery arises from the wrong ventricle. In TGA, there is atrioventricular (AV) concordance with ventriculoarterial (VA) discordance. Depending on the position of the aorta, it is divided into dextro (D) and levo (L) or congenitally corrected (CC) TGA. CMR is seldom required for preoperative assessment of D-TGA, as echocardiography usually provides adequate diagnostic information.[29] The main indication for CMR in TGA is the evaluation of postoperative complications.

Surgically, patients with D-TGA are nowadays corrected by arterial switch operation (ASO). Long-term concerns after the ASO include coronary insufficiency, myocardial ischemia, ventricular dysfunction, arrhythmias, issues regarding stenosis at the great arterial anastomotic sites, as well as development of aortic or PR. Periodic CMR can be performed to evaluate the anatomy and hemodynamics in more detail.

The Rastelli operation may be done in patients with combination of D-TGA, PS, and VSD. Postoperative complications include RVOT or pulmonary conduit obstruction (Figs. 12A and B), superimposed RV failure, and TR. These can be well assessed with CMR. Additional important features include assessment of PR, residual or baffle-margin VSD, and development of pulmonary arterial hypertension. Senning and Mustard procedures (atrial switch operation) are no longer routinely done. In older D-TGA survivors, radiological imaging with CMR can be used to further assess atrial baffle patency and coronary anatomy. MR angiography is excellent for the evaluation of the extracardiac great arteries and veins. Cine and 3D imaging is used for the evaluation of the venous pathways for baffle leaks or obstruction, and assessing systemic RV systolic function and tricuspid valve function. Congenitally corrected TGA (L-TGA) consists of AV and VA discordance—the right atrium connects to the morphological left ventricle,

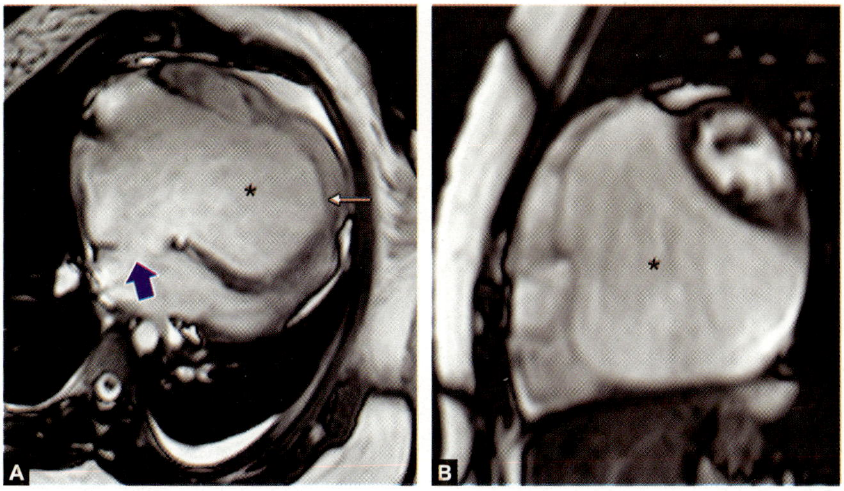

Figs. 11A and B: Steady-state free precession images in a case of Ebstein's anomaly showing (A) apically displaced tricuspid valve (white arrow) with atrialized right ventricle (*) and atrial septal defect (blue arrow) in four-chamber view, (B) straightening of interventricular septum in short axis view.

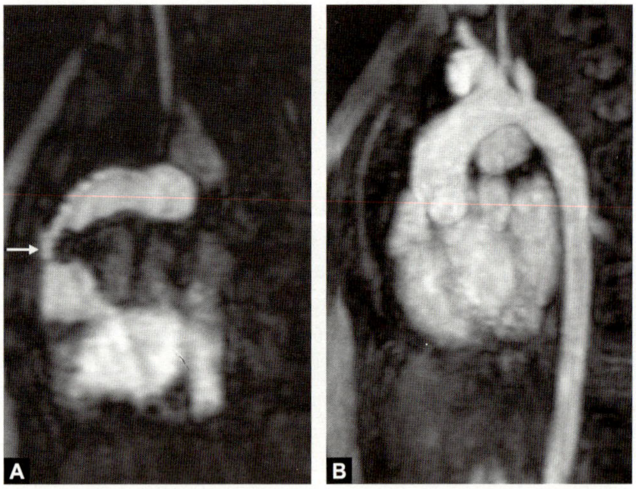

Figs. 12A and B: In a case of post–Rastelli procedure, MR angiography images in (A) sagittal oblique multiplanar reconstruction plane showing severe right ventricle outflow tract conduit obstruction (arrow), (B) maximum-intensity projection images in sagittal oblique view showing aortic arch.

which gives rise to the pulmonary artery, and the left atrium connects to the morphological right ventricle, which gives rise to the aorta (Figs. 13A and B).[30] The morphological right ventricle therefore functions as the systemic ventricle, whereas the morphological left ventricle functions as the pulmonary ventricle. The reference standard for assessing systemic ventricle function is generally accepted as being CMR. Surgical intervention in the adult often consists of systemic AV valve (morphologically tricuspid) replacement alone and ideally should be performed before the systemic ventricle ejection fraction has deteriorated below 45%.[31]

Single Ventricle Syndromes

Single ventricle syndromes include a spectrum of disorders characterized by an anatomic or functional single ventricle, with a variable-sized rudimentary ventricle that results in mixing of oxygenated and deoxygenated blood. The relationship of the atrium can be situs solitus, inversus, or ambiguous. The AV valves of the univentricle can be made up of two separate valves (double-inlet left or right ventricle) or one patent valve and one atretic valve (referred to as a common AV valve) (Figs. 14A and B). The VA connections are also variable, often being discordant (transposed) in single ventricle morphology. The most common conditions in this category are double-inlet left ventricle and tricuspid atresia.[26] Multistage procedures such as partial cavopulmonary (bidirectional Glenn shunt) and atriopulmonary (Fontan) anastomoses are done. CMR is very helpful in imaging the anatomy, identifying the stenosis at the anastomotic sites, and assessing ventricular function and valve patency. The assessment of systemic ventricular dysfunction and/or significant AV valve regurgitation can be accurately done by CMR. Pulmonary artery or Fontan circuit stenosis can be demonstrated by cine images and MR angiography.

Intra- and Extracardiac Shunts

Ventricular septal defects and ASDs are some of the most commonly encountered congenital cardiac malformations in clinical practice. CMR can help to determine the site, size, number of defects, degree of shunting, and ventricular function and help identify any associated valvular dysfunction. The degree of shunting with either an

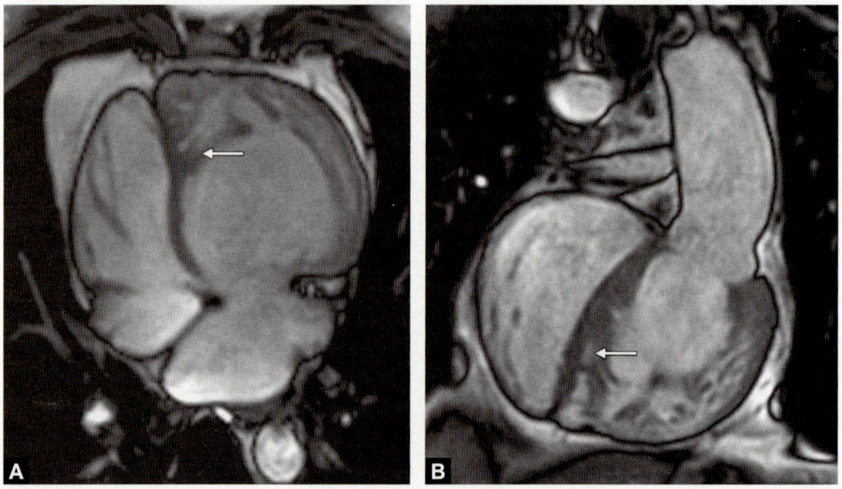

Figs. 13A and B: Steady-state free precession images (A) in four-chamber view showing right atrium draining into morphological left ventricle and left atrium draining into hypertrophied morphological right ventricle (arrow denotes moderator band) and (B) coronal plane showing aorta arising from morphological right ventricle, thus making it systemic ventricle.

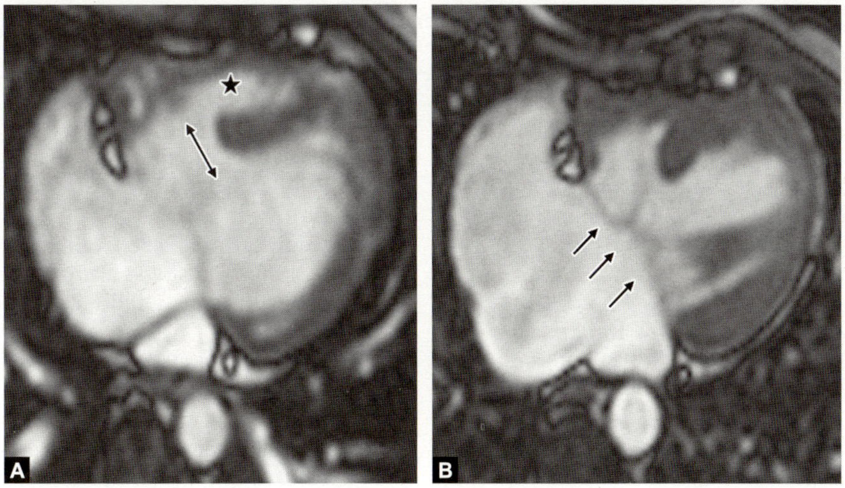

Figs. 14A and B: Steady-state free precession axial images at different planes showing hypoplastic right ventricle (star) with a large VSD (double black arrow) and a common AV valve (multiple arrows). (AV: Atrioventricular; SSFP: Steady-state free precession; VSD: Ventricular septal defect)

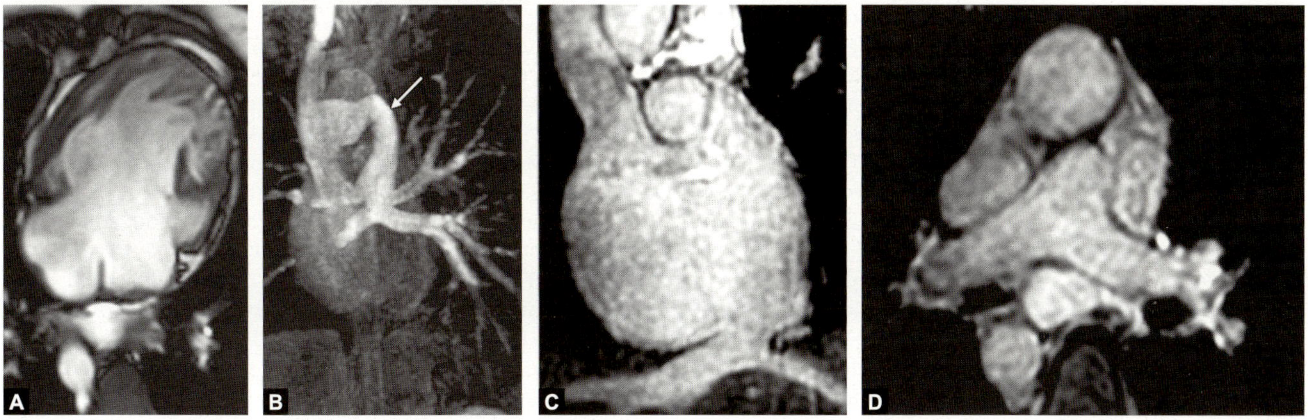

Figs. 15A to D: (A) Steady-state free precession axial image shows single ventricle morphology with large AV septal defect. (B) Oblique maximum-intensity projection images of MR angiography show all pulmonary veins forming a common channel (arrow) and draining into RSVC to right-sided atrium—total anomalous pulmonary venous drainage. Noncontrast 3D whole heart sequence (C) coronal multiplanar reconstruction image shows RSVC draining into right-sided atrium, hepatic veins, IVC draining into left-sided atrium and (D) axial image shows confluent pulmonary arteries. (AV: atrioventricular; IVC: inferior caval vein; MR: magnetic resonance; RSVC: right superior vena cava; SSFP: steady-state free precession)

intra- or extracardiac shunt is calculated by comparing flow measurements obtained in phase-contrast studies within the pulmonary trunk and ascending aorta, which reflect the pulmonary-to-systemic-flow ratio (Qp and Qs).[32] Total and partial anomalous pulmonary venous return can be diagnosed by CMR. Anatomic details and vessel aberrancy can also be shown by MR angiography and dedicated 3D multiplanar reconstructions (Figs. 15A to D) can be performed to help in surgical planning. The magnitude of the shunt volume can be assessed by phase-contrast studies.[33-35]

CONCLUSION

Cardiac magnetic resonance imaging has a central role in the diagnosis, evaluation, and serial monitoring of CHD patients by helping to assess cardiovascular anatomy, function and identifying complications related to previous corrective surgery. It is noninvasive; performed as an outpatient procedure; and obviates the use of ionizing radiation, arterial puncture, and iodinated contrast media.

REFERENCES

1. Ntsinjana HN, Hughes ML, Taylor AM. The role of cardiovascular magnetic resonance in pediatric congenital heart disease. J Cardiovasc Magn Reson. 2011;13:51.
2. Powell AJ, Geva T. Blood flow measurement by magnetic resonance imaging in congenital heart disease. Pediatr Cardiol. 2000;21: 47-58.
3. Grothues F, Moon JC, Bellenger NG, et al. Inter-study reproducibility of right ventricular volumes, function, and

mass with cardiovascular magnetic resonance. Am Heart J. 2004;147:218-23.

4. Riesenkampff E, Rietdorf U, Wolf I, et al. The practical clinical value of three-dimensional models of complex congenitally malformed hearts. J Thorac Cardiovasc Surg. 2009;138:571-80.
5. Fratz S, Chung T, Greil G, et al. Guidelines and protocols for cardiovascular magnetic resonance in children and adults with congenital heart disease: SCMR expert consensus on congenital heart disease. J Cardiovasc Magn Reson. 2013;15:51.
6. Shellock FG, Spinazzi A. MRI safety update 2008: part 2, screening patients for MRI. AJR Am J Roentgenol. 2008;191:1140-9.
7. Chaljub G, Kramer LA, Johnson RFI, et al. Projectile cylinder accidents resulting from the presence of ferromagnetic nitrous oxide or oxygen tanks in the MR suite. AJR Am J Roentgenol. 2001;177:27-30.
8. Rutz T, Wustmann K, Prsa M, et al. Cardiac magnetic resonance imaging in congenital heart disease. Cardiovasc Med. 2016;19(6):176-84.
9. Chung T. Assessment of cardiovascular anatomy in patients with congenital heart disease by magnetic resonance imaging. Pediatr Cardiol. 2000;21(1):18-26.
10. Fogel MA. Assessment of cardiac function by magnetic resonance imaging. Pediatr Cardiol. 2000;21(1):59-69.
11. Babu-Narayan S, Chung N, Shore D, et al. Tetralogy of Fallot and common arterial trunk. In: Crawford M, DiMarco J, Paulus W (Eds). Cardiology. 3rd edition. Elsevier Ltd.; 2010. p. 1471-84.
12. Norton K, Tong C, Glass R, et al. Cardiac MR imaging assessment following tetralogy of Fallot repair. Radiographics. 2006;26:197-211.
13. Aboulhosn J, Child JS. Left ventricular outflow obstruction: subaortic stenosis, bicuspid aortic valve, supravalvar aortic stenosis, and coarctation of the aorta. Circulation. 2006;114:2412-22.
14. Warnes CA, Williams RG, Bashore TM, et al. ACC/AHA 2008 guidelines for the management of adults with congenital heart disease: a report of the American College of Cardiology/American Heart Association Task Force on Practice Guidelines (Writing Committee to Develop Guidelines for the Management of Adults With Congenital Heart Disease). Circulation. 2008;118:e714-833.
15. Nielsen JC, Powell AJ, Gauvreau K, et al. Magnetic resonance imaging predictors of coarctation severity. Circulation. 2005;111:622-8.
16. Anderson RH, Weinberg PM. The clinical anatomy of transposition. Cardiol Young. 2005;15(Suppl. 1):76-87.
17. Freedom RM, Li J, Yoo SJ. Late complications following the Fontan operation. In: Gatzoulis MA, Webb GD, Daubeney PE (Eds). Diagnosis and management of adult congenital heart disease. London: Churchill Livingston; 2003. pp. 85-91.
18. Freedom RM, Yoo SJ. The divided right ventricle. In: The natural and modified history of congenital heart disease. Elmsford, NY: Futura; 2004. pp. 232-5.
19. Ibrahim T, Dennig K, Schwaiger M, et al. Images in cardiovascular medicine. Assessment of double chamber right ventricle by magnetic resonance imaging. Circulation. 2002;105:2692-3.
20. Boechat MI, Ratib O, Williams PL, et al. Cardiac MR imaging and MR angiography for assessment of complex tetralogy of Fallot and pulmonary atresia. Radiographics. 2005;25:1535-46.
21. Gatzoulis MA, Balaji S, Webber SA, et al. Risk factors for arrhythmia and sudden cardiac death late after repair of tetralogy of Fallot: a multicentre study. Lancet. 2000;356:975-81.
22. Dorfman AL, Geva T. Magnetic resonance imaging evaluation of congenital heart disease: conotruncal anomalies. J Cardiovasc Magn Reson. 2006;8:645-59.
23. Balaguru D, Dilawar M. Pulmonary atresia with ventricular septal defect: systematic review. Heart Views. 2007;8:52-61.
24. Geva T. Repaired tetralogy of Fallot: the roles of cardiovascular magnetic resonance in evaluating pathophysiology and for pulmonary valve replacement decision support. J Cardiovasc Magn Reson. 2011;13:9.
25. Oosterhof T, van Straten A, Vliegen HW, et al. Preoperative thresholds for pulmonary valve replacement in patients with corrected tetralogy of Fallot using cardiovascular magnetic resonance. Circulation. 2007;116:545-51.
26. Babar J, Jones R, Hudsmith L, et al. Application of MR imaging in assessment and follow-up of congenital heart disease in adults. Radiographics. 2010;30:e40.
27. Hartnell G, Meier RA. MR angiography of congenital heart disease in adults. Radiographics. 1995;15:781-94.
28. Choi YH, Park JH, Choe YH, et al. MR imaging of Ebstein's anomaly of the tricuspid valve. Am J Roentgenol. 1994;163:539-43.
29. Blume ED, Altmann K, Mayer JE, et al. Evolution of risk factors influencing early mortality of the arterial switch operation. J Am Coll Cardiol. 1999,33:1702-09.
30. Allwork SP, Bentall HH, Becker AE, et al. Congenitally corrected transposition of the great arteries: morphologic study of 32 cases. Am J Cardiol. 1976;38:910-23.
31. van Son JA, Danielson GK, Huhta JC, et al. Late results of systemic atrioventricular valve replacement in corrected transposition. J Thorac Cardiovasc Surg. 1995;109:642-52.
32. Wang ZJ, Reddy GP, Gotway MB, et al. Cardiovascular shunts: MR imaging evaluation. Radiographics. 2003;23:S181-94.
33. Riesenkampff EM, Schmitt B, Schnackenburg B, et al. Partial anomalous pulmonary venous drainage in young pediatric patients: the role of magnetic resonance imaging. Pediatr Cardiol. 2009;30:458-64.
34. Dellegrottaglie S, Pedrotti P, Pedretti S, et al. Atrial septal defect combined with partial anomalous pulmonary venous return: complete anatomic and functional characterization by cardiac magnetic resonance. J Cardiovasc Med (Hagerstown). 2008;9:1184-86.
35. Beerbaum P, Parish V, Bell A, et al. Atypical atrial septal defects in children: noninvasive evaluation by cardiac MRI. Pediatr Radiol. 2008;38:1188-94.

SECTION 26

Echo in Extracorporeal Membrane Oxygenation

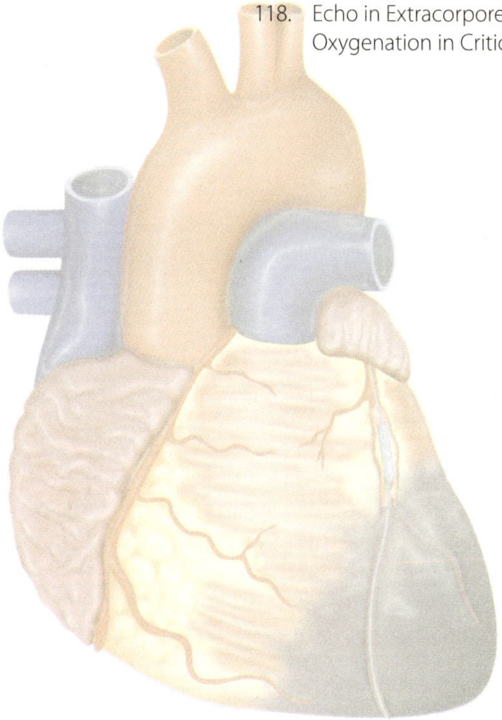

118

CHAPTER

Echo in Extracorporeal Membrane Oxygenation in Critical Care

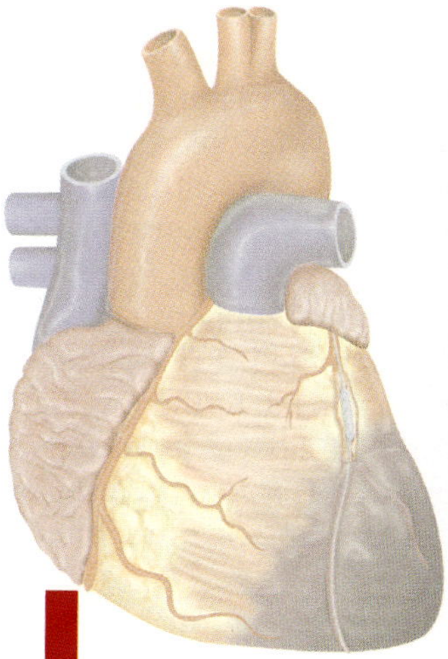

Poonam Malhotra

INTRODUCTION

In this era of using imaging as a diagnostic modality for a better prognosis, a lifesaving procedure, such as extracorporeal membrane oxygenation (ECMO), too needs good imaging modality for success.[1] The placement of cannulas and the right patient selection for ECMO, all requires echocardiography. Combes et al.,[2] Douflé et al.,[3] and Platts et al.[4] have all in recent literature elaborated on the judicious advantages of echocardiography for a successful ECMO run, particularly in a busy emergency department, where ECMO is put following an arrest with chest compression on and cannula placement is a problem. It is particularly useful for the detection of cardiac complications that may arise during ECMO (Fig. 1). It helps in many ways during the ECMO run, as shown in Box 1.

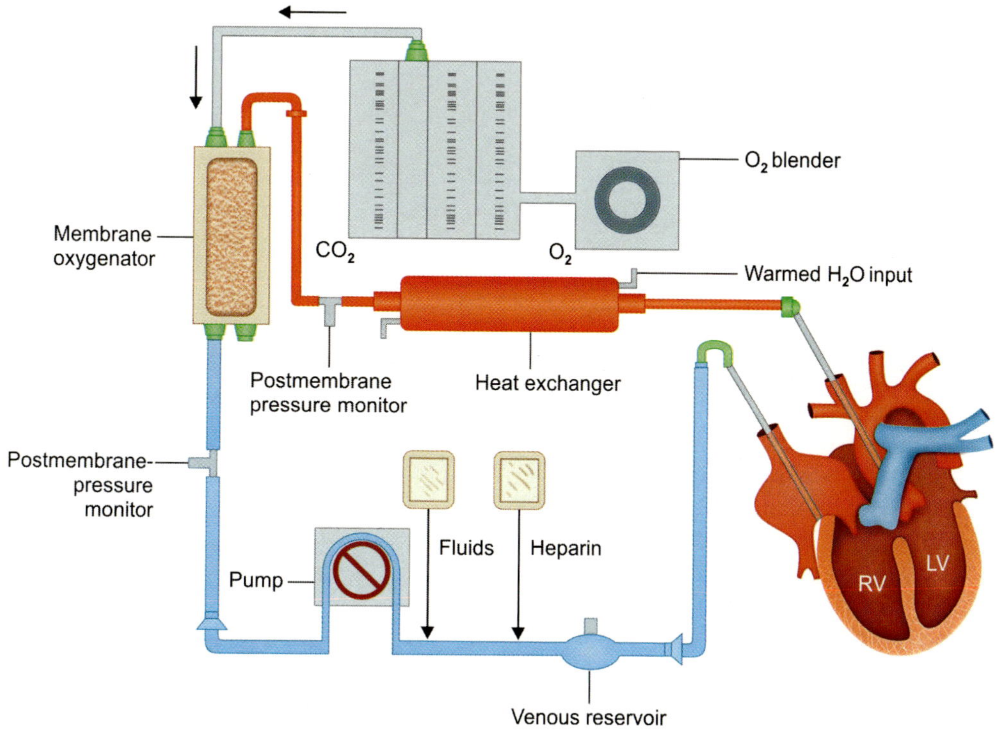

Fig. 1: The ECMO system. (ECMO: extracorporeal membrane oxygenation)

BOX 1: Echocardiographic monitoring on extracorporeal membrane oxygenation.

- Patient selection for ECMO
- Monitoring during support
- Insertion and correct placement of cannulas
- Detecting complications during ECMO
- Decision-making: Cardiac recovery, weaning from ECMO, bridge to transplant/VAD, etc.

(ECMO: extracorporeal membrane oxygenation; VAD: ventricular assist device)

CRITICAL CARE ECHOCARDIOGRAPHY DURING EXTRACORPOREAL MEMBRANE OXYGENATION

Critical care echocardiography (CCE) is performed and interpreted by the intensivist at the bedside to help in the diagnostic work-up and to guide therapy for patients with acute circulatory and respiratory failure on ECMO. Due to the statement of educational standards, the validation of echocardiography against alternative hemodynamic monitoring tools, and continuous technological improvement, CCE is increasingly being considered as an unparalleled technique to hemodynamically assess critically ill patients on ECMO.[5]

THE ROLE AND IMPACT OF EXTRACORPOREAL MEMBRANE OXYGENATION IN CRITICAL CARE

The use of ECMO has been exponentially increasing over the last decade and is now considered a mainstream lifesaving treatment modality in critical care medicine. However, the need for physician education, training, and experience remains imperative. Although ECMO has traditionally been used in end-stage lung disease and circulatory collapse, it is being adopted for use in right heart failure, as a bridge to heart and lung transplantation, and as rescue therapy for both sepsis and postorgan transplantation.

The use of cardiopulmonary bypass (CPB) technologies, such as ECMO, allows for more aggressive lung rest strategies and cardiovascular support than could be provided otherwise. Depending on the choice of cannulation techniques, ECMO can deliver purely respiratory support, respiratory support with right ventricular support, and full cardiopulmonary support. Today, with careful patient selection, ECMO is used as a rescue therapy to allow for recovery or bridge to transplant for hypoxic respiratory failure and severe refractory cardiogenic shock. The following review discusses the role and impact of ECMO in critical care delivery as well as the challenges and experience at our own institution.[6]

TYPES OF EXTRACORPOREAL MEMBRANE OXYGENATION

Both venovenous (VV) and venoarterial (VA)-ECMO can be used in patients with acute respiratory failure, and ECMO can be used for both hypoxemia and hypercarbia (Figs. 2 and 3A and B). Since the Conventional Ventilatory Support versus Extracorporeal Membrane Oxygenation for Severe Adult Respiratory Failure (CESAR) trial supporting ECMO for acute respiratory distress syndrome (ARDS) patients, three multiple studies have been done to further evaluate the outcomes of ECMO use in ARDS because questions remained as to whether or not ECMO should be used as rescue therapy or more proactively as protective mechanical support.

Extracorporeal membrane oxygenation has been successfully used for lung rest in patients with inhalation injuries and traumatic lung injuries. Outcomes in patients with severe traumatic lung injury treated with ECMO appear to be better than those in patients treated with conventional modalities.[7]

OVERVIEW OF EXTRACORPOREAL MEMBRANE OXYGENATION

The two main configurations of ECMO currently used are VV-ECMO, for respiratory support, and VA-ECMO, for cardiorespiratory support (Fig. 1). VV-ECMO does not directly provide cardiac support; however, resolution of severe hypoxemia and hypercapnia will decrease the pulmonary vascular resistance, reducing the right

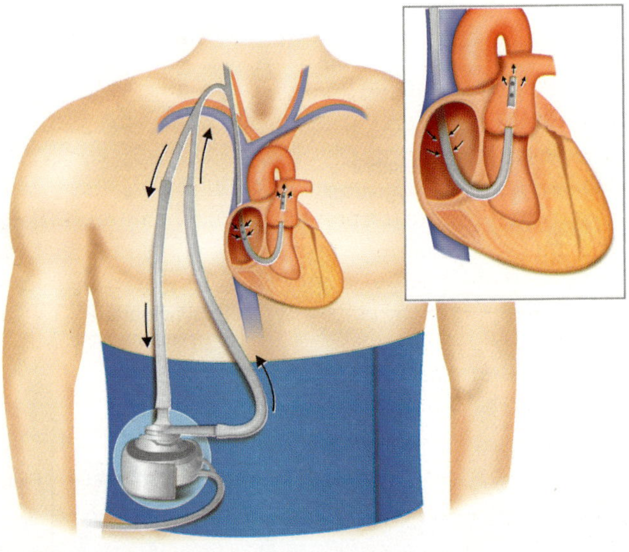

Fig. 2: The PROTEK Duo venovenous cannula (Cardiac Assist, Inc.) provides venous drainage and reinfusion of blood through an internal jugular vein while on ECMO support. (ECMO: extracorporeal membrane oxygenation)

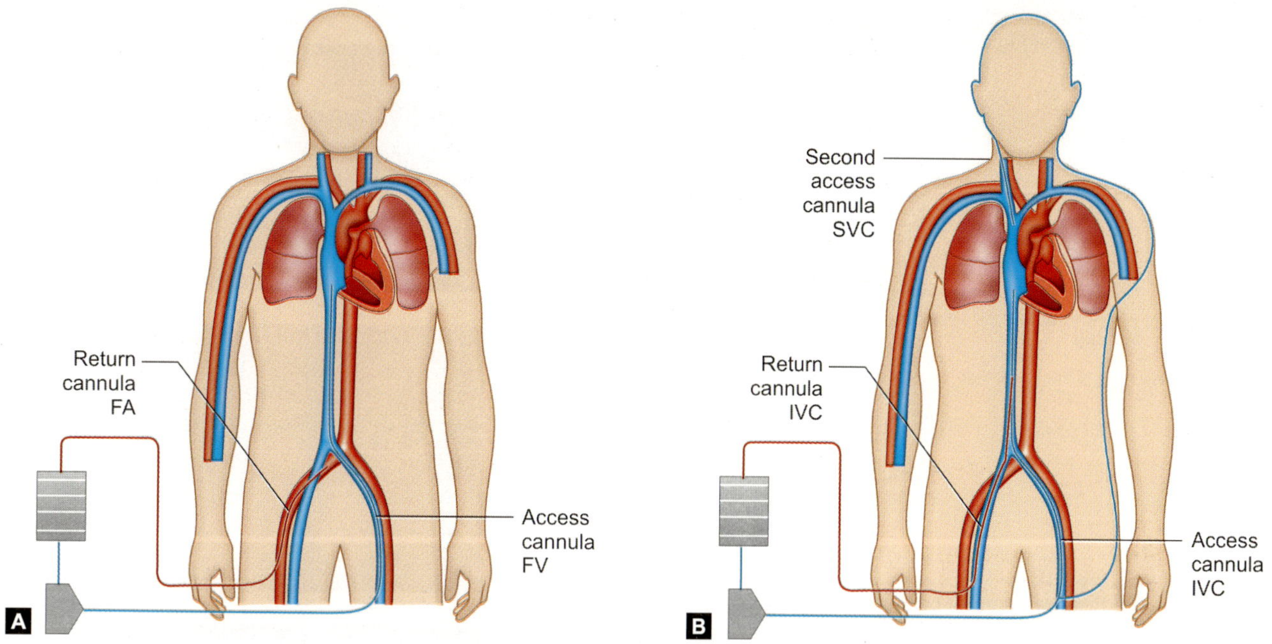

Figs. 3A and B: (A) VA-ECMO; and (B) VV-ECMO. (ECMO: extracorporeal membrane oxygenation; FA: femoral artery; FV: femoral vein; IVC: inferior vena cava; SVC: superior vena cava; VA: venoarterial; VV: venovenous)

ventricle (RV) afterload, and improving RV function.[8] This should augment left ventricle (LV) filling. In addition, the institution of VV-ECMO usually results in the reduction of airway pressures, which also decreases RV afterload. In patients with cardiorespiratory compromise, VA-ECMO is the modality of choice and provides full cardiopulmonary support (Figs. 4A to C).

VENOARTERIAL EXTRACORPOREAL MEMBRANE OXYGENATION

In VA-ECMO, drainage cannula is commonly placed in the inferior vena cava (IVC) or right atrium (RA). This can be done either via a sternotomy or percutaneously by inserting the cannula via the internal jugular or the femoral vein. Blood is returned to the patient through a cannula inserted in either the ascending aorta (central ECMO, inserted surgically) or the femoral artery (peripheral ECMO, either surgically or percutaneously inserted). Central ECMO is a preferred option when used immediately after CPB as the location of the cannulae is similar to the one used during surgery (Figs. 5A to C).

PRE-EXTRACORPOREAL MEMBRANE OXYGENATION ASSESSMENT

Even with predominant respiratory failure the choice of ECMO modality that would best benefit the patient is not always straightforward. Institution of VV-ECMO leads to the resolution of hypoxemia and hypercapnia, with lower airway pressures required, resulting in decreased pulmonary vascular resistance. This may reverse the hemodynamic instability associated with RV dysfunction. However, the causes of RV failure may not be immediately reversible, and it may be difficult to ascertain what proportion of the hemodynamic instability can be ascribed to the underlying metabolic disturbances. The presence of significant concomitant LV dysfunction warrants the use of VA-ECMO, and echocardiography plays a crucial role in assessing the degree of residual LV contractility.

ROLE OF ECHOCARDIOGRAPHY

Echocardiography helps in identifying or excluding new reversible pathology, which could be the actual cause of patient hemodynamic deterioration (cardiac tamponade/ undiagnosed valvular lesions, and LV dysfunction); thus avoiding the need for ECMO support. It also helps in providing information regarding contraindications, for example ECMO is not to be put for an aortic dissection. Identification of significant aortic regurgitation (AR) is a relative contraindication in VA-ECMO; in which, the LV afterload is increased, leading to further increase in the AR. It also provides information as regards to aortic atherosclerosis, thus guiding the intensivist in deciding the cannulation sites (central vs peripheral) or the technique (surgical vs percutaneous). Echocardiography also helps in evaluating the right heart morphology for any structural abnormality, which could impede the positioning of venous cannula for VV-ECMO or VA-ECMO. Chest X-ray is the most

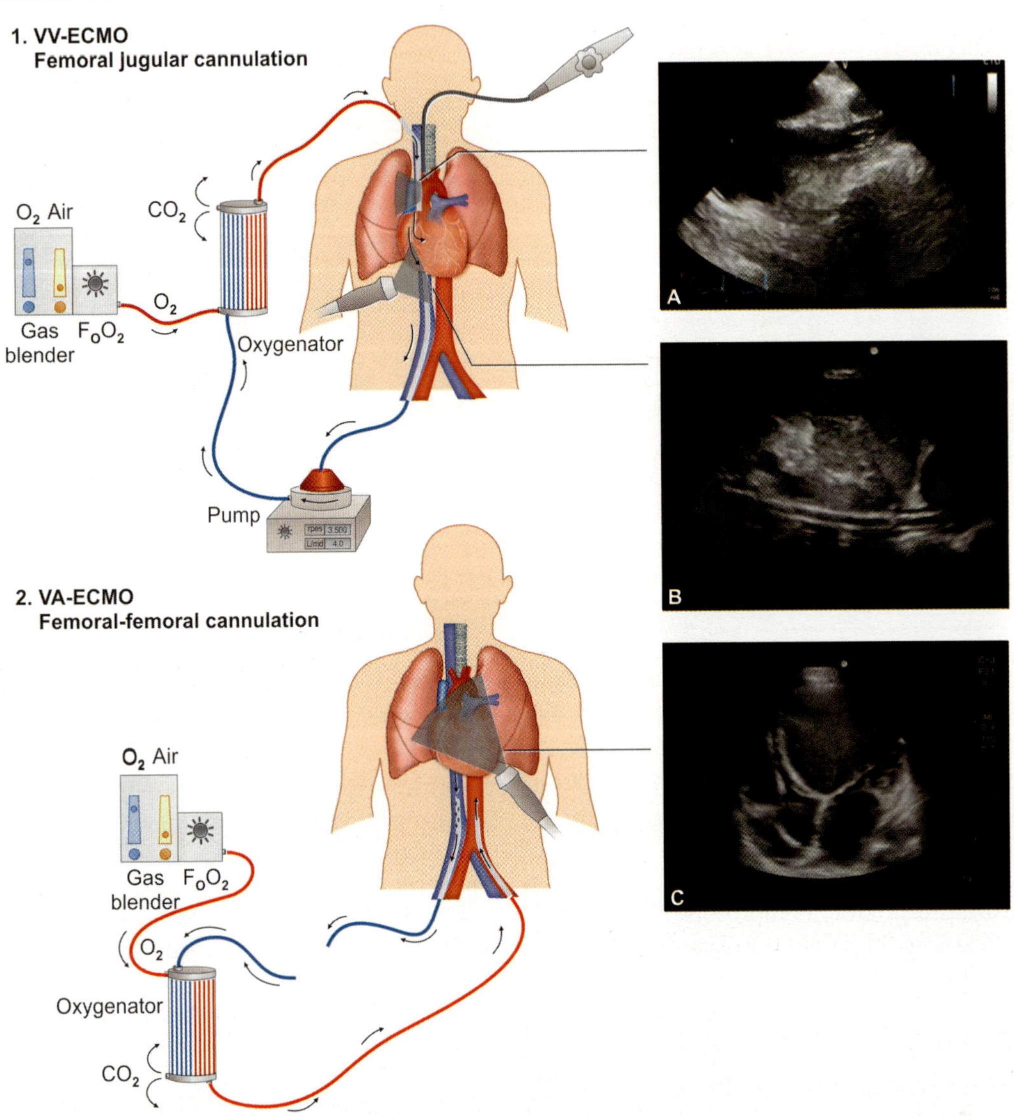

Figs. 4A to C: VV- and VA-ECMO configurations and corresponding echocardiographic views. This diagram shows the most common ECMO configurations in our center. (1) Bicannulation VV-ECMO (femoro-jugular cannulation) with the drainage cannula in the femoral vein and the reinjection in the SVC, via the jugular vein. (A) Midesophageal view showing the SVC and reinjection cannula within it (transesophageal echocardiography); (B) IVC subcostal view. The drainage cannula is visualized within the IVC in long axis (transthoracic echocardiography). (2) Femoro-femoral VA-ECMO cannulation. The drainage cannula is located in the IVC, and the reinjection cannula is in the iliac artery/distal descending aorta; and (C) Transthoracic apical four-chamber of a patient with a dilated cardiomyopathy. The cannulae are not visualized on this view but note the presence of an automatic implantable cardioverter-defibrillator within the right ventricle. (ECMO: extracorporeal membrane oxygenation; IVC: inferior vena cava; SVC: superior vena cava; VA: venoarterial; VV: venovenous)

common modality used, so far during ECMO run to observe the positions of the return and access cannulas (Fig. 6).[9]

ECHOCARDIOGRAPHY BEFORE EXTRACORPOREAL MEMBRANE OXYGENATION COMMENCEMENT: SELECTION OF PATIENTS

Echocardiography helps in identifying or excluding new reversible pathology which could be the actual cause of patient hemodynamic deterioration (cardiac tamponade/undiagnosed valvular lesions and left ventricular dysfunction); thus avoiding the need for ECMO support. It also helps in providing information regarding contraindications, for example aortic dissection. Identification of significant AR is relative contraindication in VA-ECMO; in which, the LV afterload is increased, leading to further increase in the AR. It also provides information as regards to aortic atherosclerosis, thus guiding the cannulation sites (central vs peripheral) or the technique (surgical vs percutaneous). Echocardiography also helps

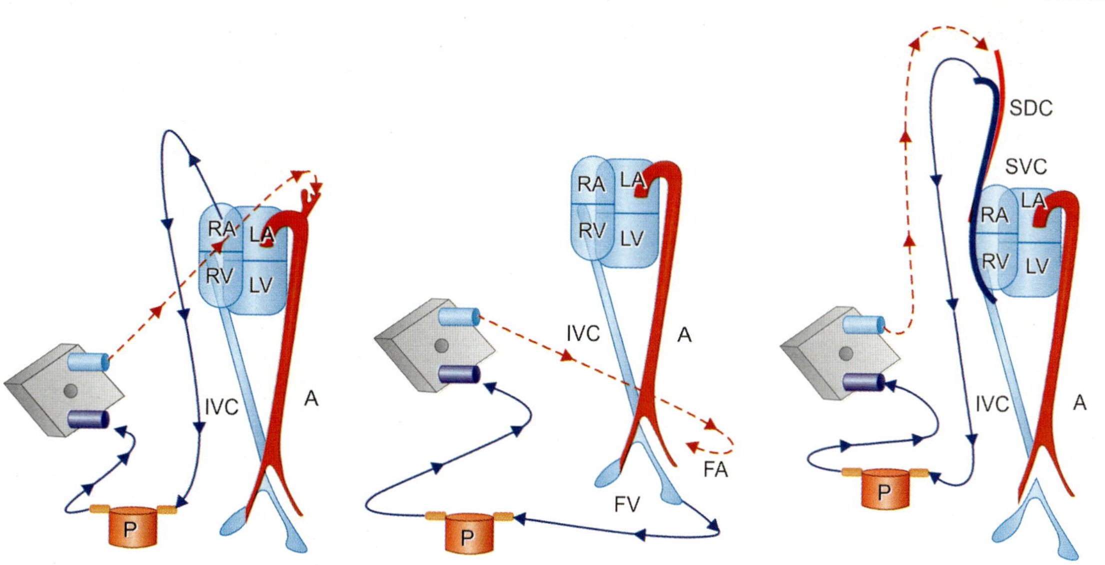

Figs. 5A to C: Dotted red arrow: Oxygenated blood. Solid blue arrows: Deoxygenated blood. (A) VA central ECMO: the two-stage venous cannula drains the blood from the RA and IVC toward a centrifugal pump "P" which pushes the blood into the oxygenator "O" with an integrated heat exchanger; the circuit is completed with a returning cannula placed into the ascending aorta "A"; (B) VA peripheral ECMO: the drainage cannula leaves the FV run through the circuit and return into the FA; and (C) VV-ECMO: SDC venous cannulation strategy. One chamber has the distal orifice in the IVC and another orifice in the SVC, together they drain the blood into the pump/oxygenator which returns through an outflow exit orifice into the RA. (ECMO: extracorporeal membrane oxygenation; FA: femoral artery; FV: femoral vein; IVC: inferior vena cava; LA: left atrium; LV: left ventricle; RA: right atrium; RV: right ventricle; SDC: single–dual chamber; SVC: superior vena cava; VA: venoarterial; VV: venovenous)

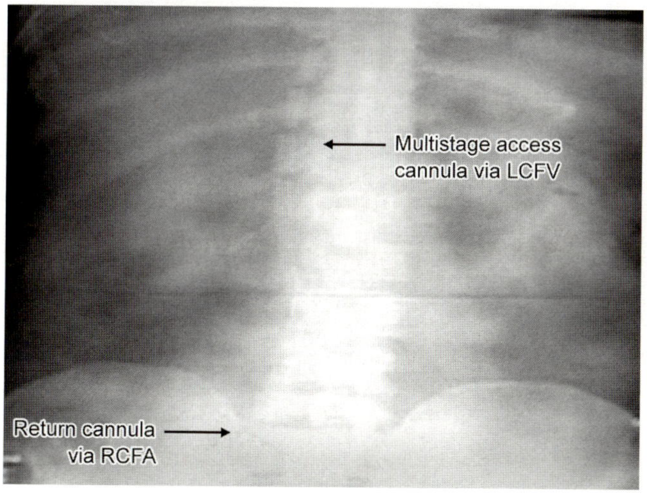

Fig. 6: Chest X-ray on day 2 of extracorporeal membrane oxygenation run (arrow).

in evaluating the right heart morphology for any structural abnormality which could impede the positioning of venous cannula for VV-ECMO or VA-ECMO. These abnormalities include prominent patent foramen ovale, ASD, atrial septal aneurysm, tricuspid stenosis, as well as pacemaker or automatic implantable cardioverter-defibrillator leads in the RA. Assessment of right ventricular and left ventricular functions enables decision-making as regards to VV-ECMO or VA-ECMO in patients with fulminant pneumonia with or without septic cardiomyopathy.[9]

Patient Selection and Pre-extracorporeal Membrane Oxygenation Assessment

Although imperfect, the objective assessment of the LV includes the measurement of its size along with global and regional function. The presence of thin walls usually indicates a chronic process. Similarly, a dilated left atrium (LA) will be in keeping with chronically elevated left atrial and ventricular diastolic pressures. The global function can be assessed by the modified Simpson's method, to give an estimate of ejection fraction (EF).[10] The consideration for VA-ECMO implies severely decreased systolic function, with an EF $< 20\%$, with or without wall-motion abnormalities.

Pre-extracorporeal life support (ECLS), a transthoracic echocardiography (TTE), or transesophageal echocardiography (TEE) study is useful to detect certain important pathologies. The initiation of VA-ECMO increases the LV afterload and the severity of any preexisting AR will worsen, leading to increasing LV dilatation, pulmonary edema, and risk of subendocardial ischemia secondary to increased myocardial oxygen consumption and wall stress.[11-14] The presence of significant mitral regurgitation may be associated with increased pulmonary edema. It is important to determine the etiology of any significant mitral regurgitation to exclude pathology that may be amenable to surgical intervention.

EXTRACORPOREAL MEMBRANE OXYGENATION COMPLICATIONS

- Bleeding (Cyklokapron/Novo 7)
- Heparin-induced thrombocytopenia (Rx with argatroban)
- Thromboembolism
- *Cannulation-related*: Limb ischemia, vessel perforation, and arterial dissection
- Hemolysis
- Gastrointestinal tract perforation, ulceration due to changes in splanchnic perfusion
- *Venoarterial extracorporeal membrane oxygenation*: Pulmonary hemorrhage, pulmonary infarction, arterial thrombosis, coronary, and cerebral hypoxia (Fig. 7).

ECHOCARDIOGRAPHY DURING EXTRACORPOREAL MEMBRANE OXYGENATION INITIATION AND CANNULATION

General Principles

Cannulation for ECLS is always an urgent or emergency operation. The indications are acute, severe cardiac,

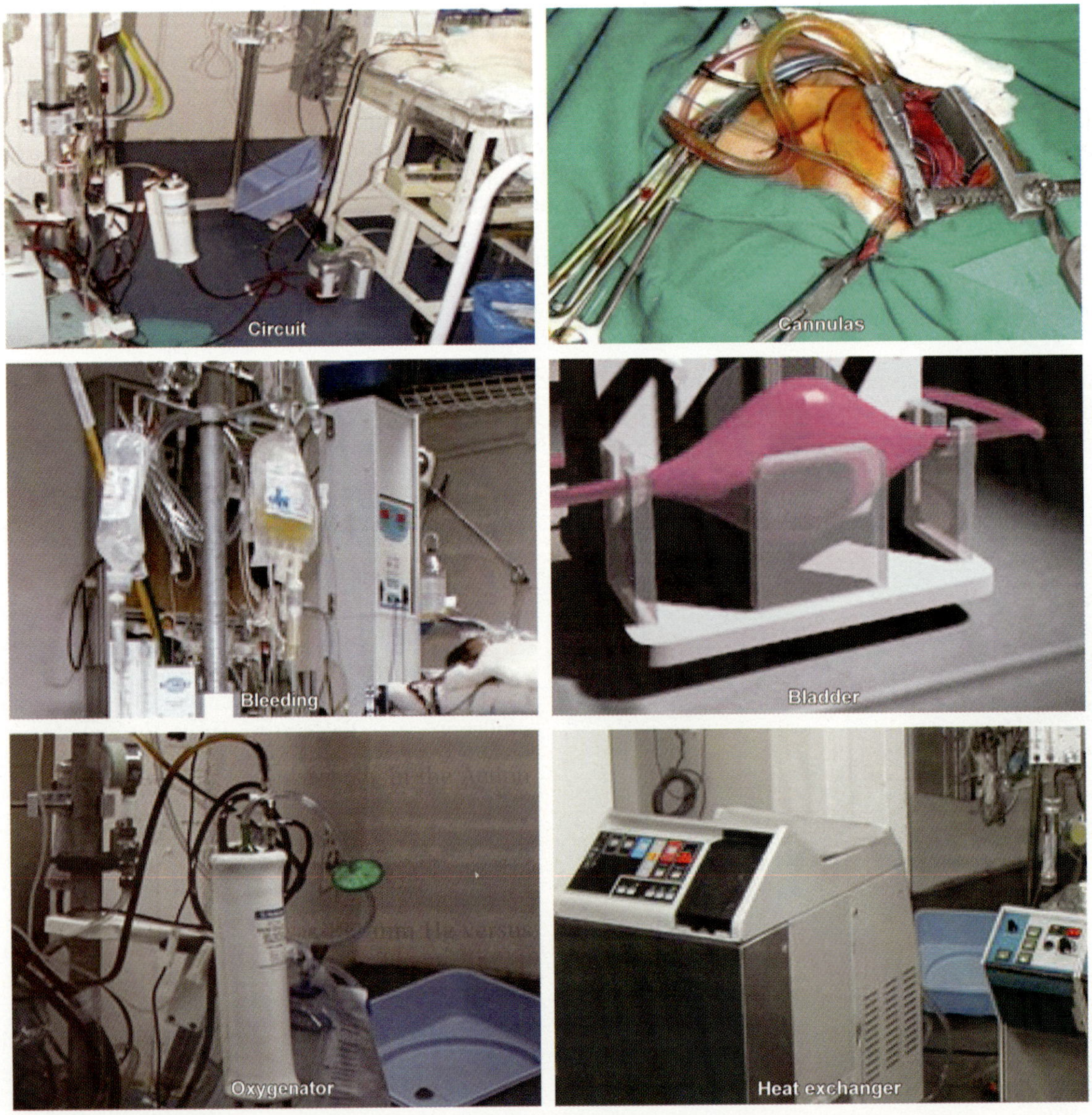

Fig. 7: Complications of ECMO. (ECMO: extracorporeal membrane oxygenation)

respiratory, or liver failure in which, organ recovery or replacement can be expected within 2–4 weeks of time. Cannulation is either VV (for pulmonary or liver support) or VA (for cardiac or cardiac and respiratory support). The size (resistance) of the venous drainage catheter limits the extracorporeal blood flow; the size (resistance) of the blood return (arterial) catheter determines the ECLS system pressure at any given flow (Fig. 8).

Echocardiography has a crucial role during ECMO cannulation as it guides the correct placement of the ECMO cannulas. TTE may not have the adequate spatial resolution to guide ECMO cannulation and therefore, TEE. There should be a direct communication between the operator and the echocardiologist as to the site of the indented cannula insertion. For example, in VV-ECMO when one cannula is used for access and one to return the blood—this position of the access cannula tip is in the proximal IVC, just before the entry into the RA. On the other hand, the optimal position for the return cannula is in the mid-RA but well clear from the interatrial septum (IAS) and the tricuspid valve (TV); this is apparent in Figure 9.

If the access cannula is placed more proximally than the return cannula or if the two cannulas are too close together, recirculation will occur resulting in very little oxygenated blood passing into the pulmonary and systemic circulation. Incorrect cannula positioning requires reoperation or manipulation and to achieve an appropriate location and this could increase the risk for bleeding and infection and can delay the delivery of ECMO support. The abnormal sites include the IAS through a patent foramen ovale and then into the LA. Abnormal sites also include coronary sinus and across the tricuspid subvalvular apparatus. Malpositioning of the cannula could also result vascular or cardiac injury and inadequate flows.

ECHOCARDIOGRAPHIC FEATURES OF RIGHT VENTRICLE FAILURE

Echocardiographic features of RV dysfunction include RV chamber dilatation, flattening of the interventricular septum, creating a D-shaped LV with an eccentricity index greater than 1; RA and TV annular dilation, with significant tricuspid regurgitation (TR); and RV contribution to the apex of the heart, typically visualized in the TTE or TEE four-chamber view. Objective measurements of RV systolic function include the tricuspid annular plane systolic excursion; the tricuspid annular systolic peak velocity (S'), using tissue Doppler imaging; and fractional area change. McConnell's sign, severe basal and mid-RV hypokinesia with apical hyperkinesia, is the indicative of acute onset pulmonary hypertension.[10,15]

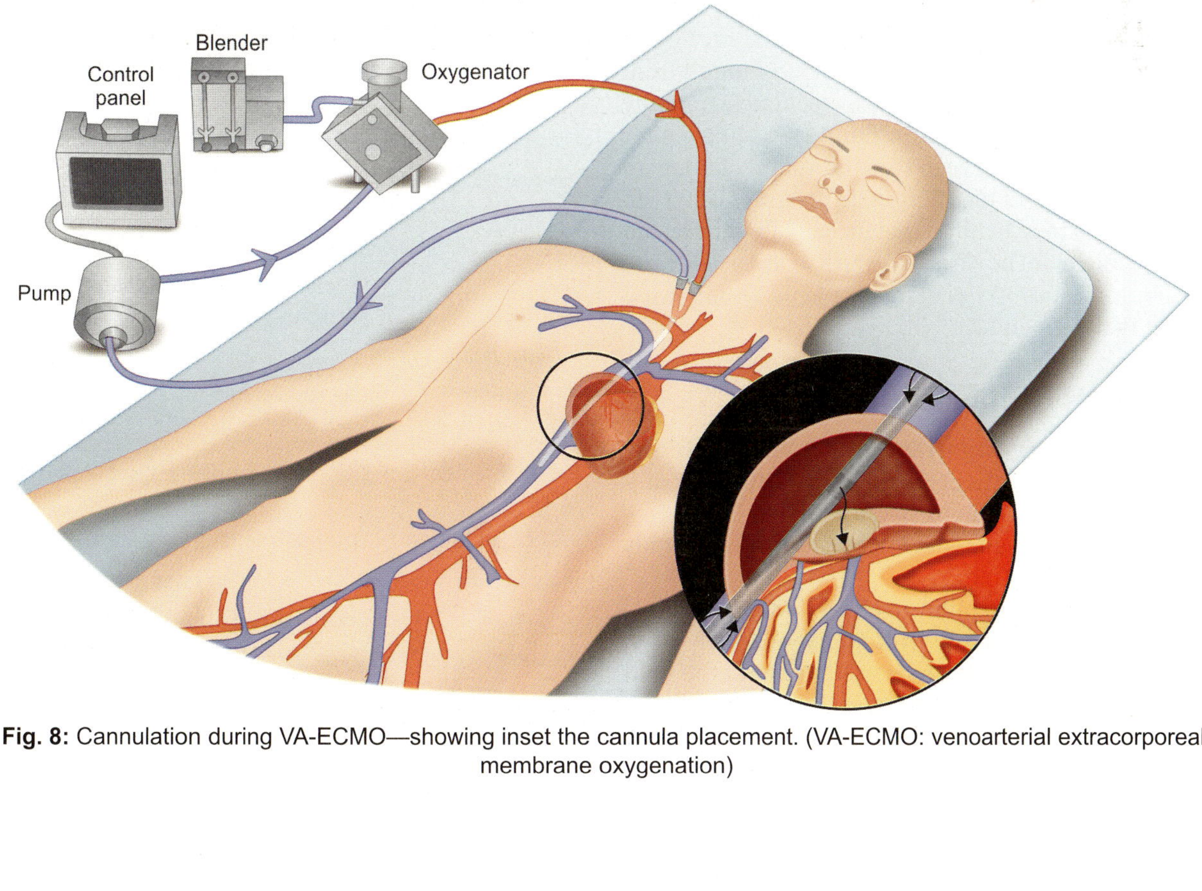

Fig. 8: Cannulation during VA-ECMO—showing inset the cannula placement. (VA-ECMO: venoarterial extracorporeal membrane oxygenation)

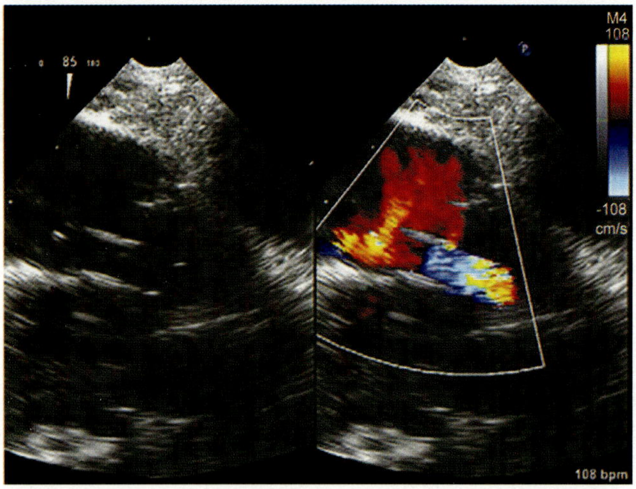

Fig. 9: 2D TEE of a VV-ECMO returns cannula in right atrium. (2D TEE: two-dimensional transesophageal echocardiography; VV-ECMO: venovenous extracorporeal membrane oxygenation)

The RV systolic pressure can be estimated using the simplified Bernoulli's equation, by measuring the peak velocity of the TR jet. Increased pulmonary artery (PA) pressure can also be estimated by pulse-wave Doppler interrogation of the PA systolic flow. The presence of a biphasic waveform and a PA acceleration time (time from the onset of systole to time to peak pressure) shorter than 100 ms are indicative of increased pulmonary pressure.[16] These numbers will serve as a reference as the TR is not considered to be accurate once the patient is on ECMO support. Indeed, drainage and reinjection of blood from and into the RA make it impossible to accurately quantify TR. The drainage of blood from the RA will likely alter the pressure gradient between RV and RA, precluding an accurate assessment of the RV systolic pressure. However, it is important to bear in mind that in acute RV failure, the PA pressure might not be elevated if the RV cannot generate a sufficient pressure in the setting of acutely increased afterload (Tables 1A and B).

RIGHT VENTRICLE (FIG. 10)

- The RV plays an important role in the morbidity and mortality of patients presenting with signs and symptoms of cardiopulmonary disease.
  - Systematic assessment of right heart not uniformly carried out:
    - Enormous attention given to left heart
    - Lack of familiarity with ultrasonography (u/s) techniques that can be used to assess the right heart
    - Scarcity of u/s studies providing normal reference values.

TABLE 1A: Parameters to be assessed prior to extracorporeal membrane oxygenation initiation.

Left ventricle	
Morphology	Size, wall thickness
Systolic function	Ejection fraction (Simpson's method) or FAC
	Wall-motion abnormalities
	S wave at mitral annulus
	Velocity time integral in LVOT
Diastolic function	E/A ratio (transmitral flow)
	E/e′ ratio at mitral annulus
Left atrium	Size and volume
Valvular assessment	Diagnosis and quantification of potential aortic/mitral regurgitation/stenosis

(A: atrial; E: early; FAC: fractional area change; LVOT: left ventricular outflow tract)

TABLE 1B: Parameters to be assessed prior to extracorporeal membrane oxygenation initiation.

Right ventricle	
Morphology	RV end-diastolic area/LV end-diastolic area
	Triangular shape vs rounded shape of apex
	RV wall thickness
	McConnell's sign
Systolic function	TAPSE, tissue Doppler at tricuspid annulus, S wave
	Fractional area of change
	Pulse-wave Doppler through pulmonary valve (acceleration time/biphasic pattern)
Diastolic function	E/A transtricuspid flow
Interventricular septum	Presence of paradoxical septum
	Eccentricity index
Tricuspid regurgitation	Estimation of right ventricular systolic pressure
Valvular pathology	
Right atrium	Size and volume
Other	
Patent foramen ovale	Color flow Doppler ± bubble study
IVC/SVC (if TEE)	Size and respiratory variation
Right atrium	Dilated coronary sinus
	Chiari network
Vascular	Thrombosis/Stenosis/Aortic dissection/ Severe atheroma

(A: atrial; E: early; IVC: inferior vena cava; LV: left ventricle; RV: right ventricle; SVC: superior vena cava; TAPSE: tricuspid annular plane systolic excursion; TEE: transesophageal echocardiography)

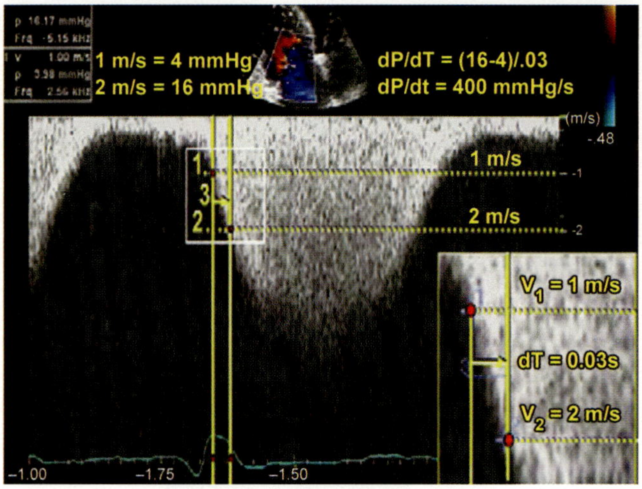

Fig. 10

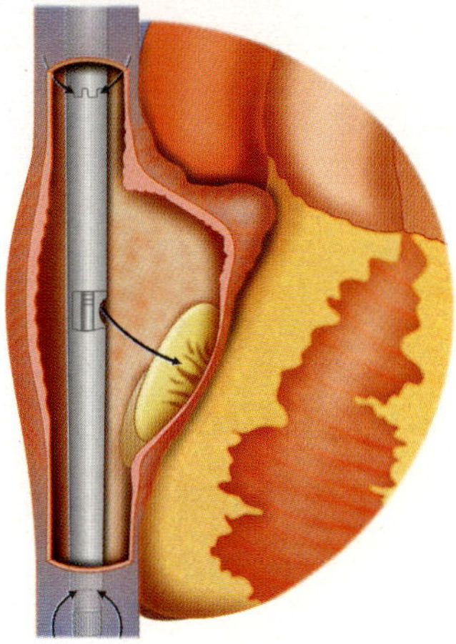

Fig. 11: Avalon cannula.

CANNULATION

The Avalon Elite® (Maquet, Rastatt, Germany) bicaval dual-lumen cannula is designed to drain blood from both the IVC and superior vena cava (SVC), and return oxygenated blood into the RA, with the flow directed toward the TV (Fig. 9). Its advantages are single-site cannulation and a decreased propensity for recirculation. Echocardiography provides excellent views of the appropriate position of the different portions of the cannula. Correct positioning of the cannula tip in the IVC must be confirmed to avoid cannulation of one of the hepatic veins. The utilization of color flow Doppler can demonstrate the direction of the returned blood toward the TV, and not the IAS or into the hepatic veins (Figs. 11 and 12).

Avalon Cannula

It consists of two lumens:

- One lumen allows the deoxygenated:
  - Blood to drain from the IVC and the SVC.
- The second lumen allows the oxygenated:
  - Blood to return directed toward the TV
  - Reduces the recirculation seen with the traditional VV setup.

ECHOCARDIOGRAPHY AND MONITORING EXTRACORPOREAL MEMBRANE OXYGENATION RESPONSE

After initiation of ECMO support, severe hemodynamic alterations take place which are dependent on the type of ECMO and cannulation location in ECMO circuit. During the peripheral VA-ECMO, LV preload usually decreases because of decreased pulmonary blood flow, but LV afterload increases because of the pressurized return of blood via the arterial return cannula.

In the cases of severe LV dysfunction associated with severe mitral regurgitation, the LV becomes more enlarged and the aortic valve may not open because of markedly reduced cardiac output. This can lead to stasis and thrombosis in the ascending aorta, the LV cavity, and pulmonary veins. In this situation, a left venting procedure or percutaneous balloon atrial septostomy has been found to be useful. TEE is an ideal procedure for guiding the septostomy catheter and balloon inflation (Figs. 12A and B).

Failure of the aortic valve to open during peripheral VA-ECMO support poses a critical problem. To tide over this situation, anticoagulation is increased and afterload is decreased, while native LV output is optimized using inodilators to facilitate aortic valve opening. In this setting, changing the ECMO circuit to VAD should be considered.

The hemodynamics in VV-ECMO is less complicated and more beneficial to the patient. In this mode, the blood is taken from and return to the right heart with no significant change to the RV preload and no adverse effects on left heart hemodynamics. VV-ECMO also increased mixed venous oxygen saturation, and this leads to decrease pulmonary vascular resistance and thus a lower RV afterload. The increased oxygenation of the LV indirectly improves the LV function and increases oxygen delivery to the coronary artery circulation.

Most of the studies on ECMO-induced changes in hemodynamics have been carried out in the pediatric populations. Martin and Short in 1988 evaluated echocardiographic hemodynamic parameters before and during VA-ECMO support on cardiac performance in 19 patients with postpartum hemorrhage. Both the LV and RV stroke volumes decreased by 50% at ECMO initiations

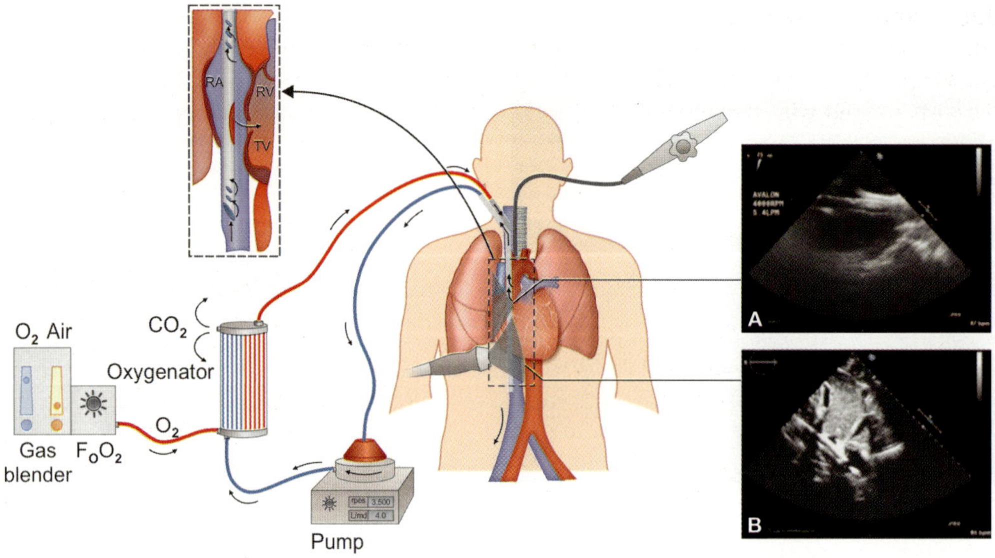

Figs. 12A and B: Bicaval dual-lumen cannula for VV-ECMO (Avalon Elite®) and corresponding echocardiographic views. This picture depicts a bicaval dual-lumen cannula, inserted via the internal jugular vein. The drainage holes are located in the superior vena cava and IVC, and the reinjection hole is facing the TV. (A) Midesophageal bicaval view showing the cannula within the RA (transesophageal echocardiography); and (B) Transthoracic subcostal view showing the cannula in the RA; the tip of the cannula is located in the IVC. The reinjection hole is visible, oriented toward the tricuspid valve. (IVC: inferior vena cava; RA: right atrium; RV: right ventricle; TV: tricuspid valve; VV-ECMO: venovenous extracorporeal membrane oxygenation)

but returned to baseline levels at 72 hours with parallel changes in the LV and RV cardiac output.[17] PA systolic pressure decreased between 48 hours and 72 hours of VA-ECMO support and was normal after ECMO. Striper et al. in 1993 prospectively evaluated 15 infants requiring VV-ECMO. There was considerable improvement in the PA mean pressure and peak velocities and time to peak velocity in patients on ECMO. There was no deterioration in cardiac function measured by aortic flow velocities, LV dimensions, LV fractional shortening, and LV EF. The improved delivery of mixed venous oxygenated blood via VV-ECMO to the left heart and coronary arteries along with the absence of increased afterload seen in VA-ECMO may account for favorable cardiac performance in the setting of VV-ECMO. In another study by Balasubramaniam et al. in 2007, cardiac function in 10 adult patients requiring VV-ECMO for severe acute respiratory failure was assessed using echocardiography. This was performed before ECMO and after the cessation of ECMO. There were no significant changes in LV fractional shortening, EF, or peak aortic velocity.[18]

In ARDS as well as in sepsis, there is increased pulmonary vascular resistance and decreased RV function due to significant hypoxemia-echocardiography is useful in documenting the effects of improved oxygenation and acid-base status on the adequacy of RV function when VV-ECMO is used.

ECHOCARDIOGRAPHY DURING PATIENT'S RECOVERY AND WEANING OF SUPPORT

Echocardiography plays an important role in the assessment of recovery and suitability for weaning from ECMO support. The level of recovery and likelihood of weaning ECMO support are based on multitude of clinical hemodynamic and echocardiographic parameters. The echocardiographic variables that determine the cessation of ECMO support are as follows:

- Left ventricle ejection fraction more than 35–40%
- Left ventricular outflow tract velocity time integral of more than 10 cm
- Absence of LV dilatation
- No evidence of cardiac tamponade.

Weaning from Venoarterial-extracorporeal Membrane Oxygenation

It should be noted that invasive computation of cardiac output using thermodilution could be misleading from VA-ECMO because a significant proportion of the circulatory blood flow actually bypasses the PA. During weaning VA-ECMO flows are reduced in 0.5–1.0 L/min increments, during which clinical hemodynamic and echocardiographic parameters (stroke volume, ventricular dimensions, ventricular volume, and EF) are monitored. In a study by Konishi et al. in 1999, Doppler evaluation of flow in descending aorta was used to evaluate the cardiac recovery after viral myocarditis treated with peripheral VA-ECMO, based on adequacy of cardiac output generated by the native heart (Fig. 13).

Weaning from Venoarterial-extracorporeal Membrane Oxygenation

Weaning from VV-ECMO relies primarily on the assessment on the oxygenation and pulmonary compliance, during which the gas flow through the ECMO circuit is gradually reduced, and conventional lung protective ventilation is resumed. However the ECMO circuit blood flow is not reduced; therefore, echocardiography is usually not required for weaning from VV-ECMO.

CONCLUSION

Despite various challenges, ECMO is a vital lifesaving modality in patients with respiratory and cardiorespiratory failure. New frontiers are demonstrating the benefit of ECMO in right heart failure and as a bridge and rescue modality in lung and heart transplant, and it has recently been used for patients in cardiogenic shock due to severe sepsis. We are witnessing more and more institutions adapting its use despite the challenges of cost and staff training. Although the institutional learning curve may take a few years, significant reductions in mortality can be achieved in high-risk patients who may otherwise not survive.

Critical care echocardiography offers a wide range of modalities and hemodynamic parameters to best help the front-line intensivist in adjusting acute therapy individually in patients with cardiopulmonary compromise, irrespective of their level of competence (basic, advanced, or expert). Recently proposed echocardiography-based management strategies and newly available technologies need further validation in large cohorts of critically ill patients. The best has yet to come.

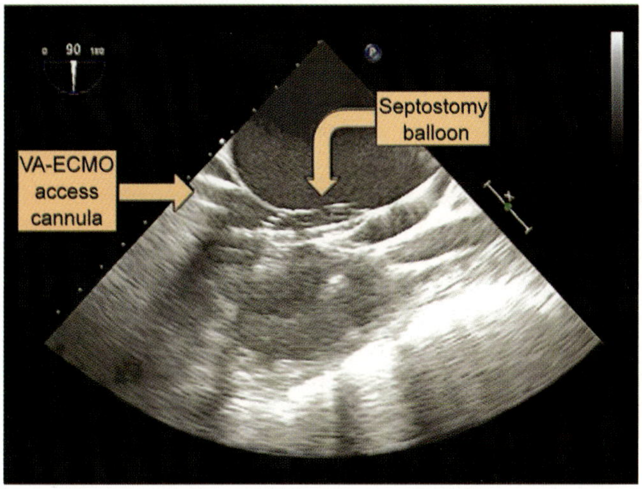

Fig. 13: Septostomy balloon.

REFERENCES

1. Kapoor PM. Echocardiography in extracorporeal membrane oxygenation. Ann Card Anaesth. 2017;20(Suppl 1):S1-3.
2. Combes A, Brodie D, Bartlett R, et al. Position paper for the organization of extracorporeal membrane oxygenation programs for acute respiratory failure in adult patients. Am J Respir Crit Care Med. 2014;190:488-96.
3. Douflé G, Roscoe A, Billia F, et al. Echocardiography for adult patients supported with extracorporeal membrane oxygenation. Crit Care. 2015;19:326.
4. Platts DG, Sedgwick JF, Burstow DJ, et al. The role of echocardiography in the management of patients supported by extracorporeal membrane oxygenation. J Am Soc Echocardiogr. 2012;25:131-41.
5. Vignon P. What is new in critical care echocardiography?. Crit Care. 2018;22:40.
6. Ratnani I, Tuazon D, Zainab A, et al. The role and impact of extracorporeal membrane oxygenation in critical care. Methodist Debakey Cardiovasc J. 2018;14(2):110-9.
7. Cordell-Smith JA, Roberts N, Peek GJ, et al. Traumatic lung injury treated by extracorporeal membrane oxygenation (ECMO). Injury. 2006;371:29-32.
8. Miranda DR, van Thiel R, Brodie D, et al. Right ventricular unloading after initiation of VV ECMO. Am J Respir Crit Care Med. 2015;191:346-7.
9. Kapur K. Echocardiographic imaging of patients on extracorporeal membrane oxygenation. In: Kapur K (Ed). Manual of ECMO in ICU book, 1st edition. New Delhi: Jaypee Brothers Medical Publishers (P) Ltd; 2014. pp. 165-71.
10. Lang RM, Badano LP, Mor-Avi V, et al. Recommendations for cardiac chamber quantification by echocardiography in adults: an update from the American Society of Echocardiography and the European Association of Cardiovascular Imaging. J Am Soc Echocardiogr. 2015;28:1-39.
11. Mills SA, Hansen K, Vinten-Johansen J, et al. Enhanced functional recovery with venting during cardioplegic arrest in chronically damaged hearts. Ann Thoracic Surg. 1985;40:566-73.
12. Kanter KR, Schaff HV, Gott VL, et al. Reduced oxygen consumption with effective left ventricular venting during postischemic reperfusion. Circulation. 1982;66:I50-4.
13. Lucas SK, Schaff HV, Flaherty JT, et al. The harmful effects of ventricular distention during postischemic reperfusion. Ann Thoracic Surg. 1981;32:486-94.
14. Martin GR, Short BL. Doppler echocardiographic evaluation of cardiac performance in infants on prolonged ECMO. Am J Cardiol. 1988;62:929-34.
15. Rudski LG, Lai WW, Afilalo J, et al. Guidelines for the echocardiographic assessment of the right heart in adults: a report from the American Society of Echocardiography

endorsed by the European Association of Echocardiography, a registered branch of the European Society of Cardiology, and the Canadian Society of Echocardiography. J Am Soc Echocardiogr. 2010;23:685-713.
16. Arkles JS, Opotowsky AR, Ojeda J, et al. Shape of the right ventricular Doppler envelope predicts hemodynamics and right heart function in pulmonary hypertension. Am J Respir Crit Care Med. 2011;183:268-76.
17. Martin GR, Short BL. Doppler echocardiographic evaluation of cardiac performance in infants on prolonged extracorporeal membrane oxygenation. Am J Cardiol. 1988;62:929-34.
18. Balasubramanian SK, Tiruvoipati R, Amin M, et al. Factors influencing the outcome of paediatric cardiac surgical patients during extracorporeal circulatory support. J Cardiovasc Surg. 2007;2:4.

SECTION 27

Shock

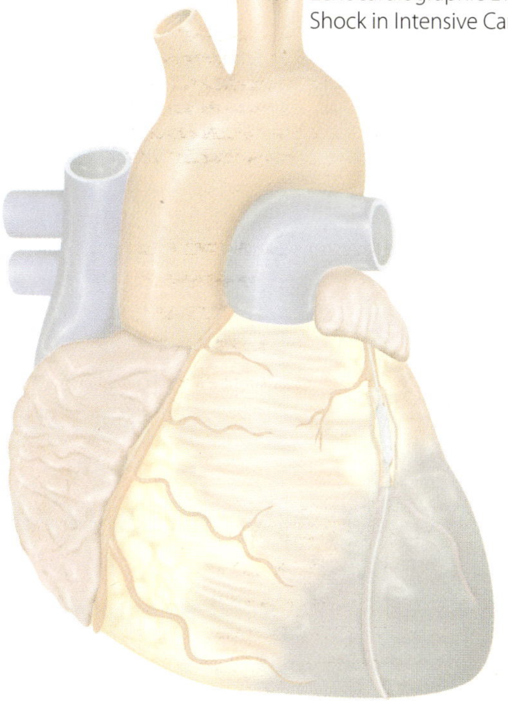

CHAPTER 119

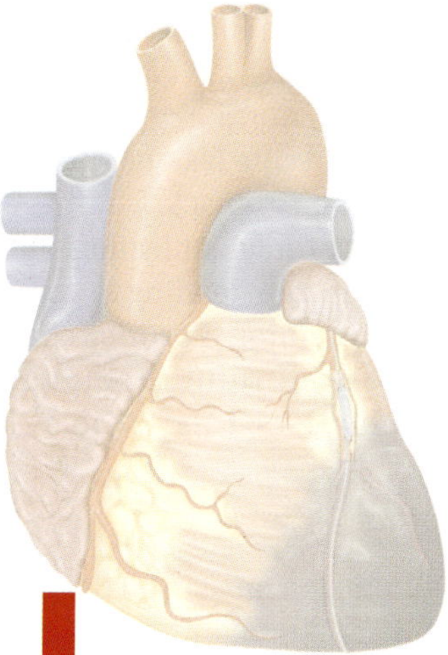

Echocardiographic Evaluation of Shock in Intensive Care Unit

Rekha Mishra, Rakesh Bachloo, Shashwat Mishra

INTRODUCTION

Echocardiography is an invaluable tool in the management of patients with shock. Its versatility lies in the fact that it is noninvasive, cost-effective, portable, yields immediate effect, and can be done repeatedly for ongoing monitoring of the patient. The main goal of the echocardiography should be to rapidly identify and differentiate the cause of hemodynamic instability. It is recommended as the modality of first choice in consensus guidelines.[1] Up to one-third of the patients admitted to the intensive care unit (ICU) are in shock,[2] and early recognition of the condition is vital, if subsequent tissue injuries are to be avoided. It is associated with high mortality and adverse outcomes in nontraumatic patients in the emergency department.[3]

DEFINITION OF SHOCK

Shock is defined as a life-threatening, generalized form of acute circulatory failure associated with inadequate oxygen utilization by the cells.[1] The presentation of shock can vary with different causes of shocks and the degree of physiological abnormalities.

Shock can be classified into four different categories according to the underlying mechanisms, either alone or in combination (Table 1).

DIAGNOSTIC CRITERION

Cardiogenic Shock

Cardiogenic shock is the leading cause of death in acute myocardial infarction (MI), with mortality rates as high as 70–90% in the absence of aggressive management and early revascularization. The clinical definition of cardiogenic shock is decreased cardiac output (CO) and evidence of tissue hypoxia in the presence of adequate intravascular volume. Hemodynamic criteria for cardiogenic shock are sustained hypotension (systolic blood pressure <90 mm Hg for ≥30 minutes) and a reduced cardiac index (<2.2 L/min/m^2) in the presence of normal or elevated pulmonary capillary wedge pressure (PCWP) (>15 mm Hg) or right ventricular end-diastolic pressure (>10 mm Hg).[4] Although coronary artery pathology is the major underlying cause of cardiogenic shock, but other pathologies, such as acute valvular heart diseases, dissection of aorta, sepsis resulting in severe cardiac failure, are encountered, and echocardiography is the only bedside tool that can accurately diagnose the underlying pathology. A rapid cardiac assessment by echocardiography, using just two-dimensional (2D) and M-mode echocardiography, demonstrates major underlying abnormality in the acute scenario, followed by a more detailed advanced echocardiographic assessment.[5] The overall left ventricular (LV) size and systolic function including ejection

TABLE 1: Diagnostic criterion.

1.	Cardiogenic shock (Pump function failure)
2.	Hypovolemic shock (inadequate circulating volume)
3.	Obstructive shock (Obstruction to blood flow)
4.	Distributive shock (loss of vascular tone)

fraction, fractional shortening (FS), regional wall motion abnormalities, myocardial thickness, interventricular septal thickness and motion, right ventricular size and function, intravascular volume status, pericardial or pleural effusion, presence of intramural mass, and aorta can be identified.[6] Additional hemodynamic status, such as LV end-diastolic pressure and pulmonary artery pressures, can be determined using spectral Doppler and tissue Doppler imaging (TDI).

Left Ventricular Systolic Function

Echocardiography is used to assess LV systolic function by demonstrating systolic excursion as well as systolic thickening of the myocardium. The most common cause of cardiogenic shock results from marked reduction in systolic contractility. Left ventricular systolic function can traditionally be assessed by LV ejection fraction (LVEF) and FS. Left ventricular ejection fraction can be estimated by modified Simpson biplane method; the endocardial borders of the LV are traced in systole and diastole from two different views (i.e. apical 4C and 2C views) to calculate the volume change between systole and diastole [(LVEDV – LVESV)/LVEDV × 100%]. In an emergency situation, subjective evaluation or "eyeballing" is often used in suboptimal images of the LV where endocardial delineation is not clear, which is reasonably accurate by an experienced echocardiographer. The size of the LV and left atrial (LA) may provide clue to the duration of LV systolic dysfunction, with dilatation indicating a degree of chronicity. Fractional shortening of the LV can be assessed in M-mode by placing a cursor near the tip of the mitral leaflets in long-axis view which shows the change in LV diameter during the cardiac cycle [FS = (LVEDD – LVESD)/LVEDD × 100%]. Other advanced parameters with the help of pulse Doppler and TDI can be used to quantify the LV systolic dysfunction more accurately. Using pulse wave Doppler, the LV outflow tract (LVOT) velocity–time integral (VTI) can be measured and can be used as a surrogate for the stroke volume (SV).[7] A value above 18 cm implies an adequate SV. Using TDI, the myocardial systolic velocity S', measured from an average of readings from multiple segments, correlates with LVEF. In a study involving four basal segments, an S' more than 7.5 correlated with an LVEF more than 50% with a sensitivity of 79% and specificity of 88%.[8] Gulati et al., using an average of six basal segments, found an S' more than 5.4 to have LVEF of more than 50% with sensitivity of 88% and specificity of 97%.[9] A number of comorbidities contribute to a systemic inflammatory state leading to coronary microvascular endothelial dysfunction and exacerbate cardiac failure by worsening diastolic function with preserved ejection fraction.[10]

Valvular Pathology and Other Complications

Echocardiography helps in delineating the etiology as well as the severity of acute as well as pre-existing valvular lesions, such as degenerative aortic stenosis, aortic regurgitation (AR), and mitral regurgitation (MR). Acute lesions such as the peri-infarction rupture of a papillary muscle leading to a severe MR, perforation or rupture of valvular leaflets due to infective endocarditis, aortic dissection leading to acute severe AR would need immediate attention. Postinfarction ventricular septal defects, free-wall rupture, though uncommon, are usually catastrophic (Figs. 1 and 2; Table 2).

Hypovolemic Shock

Assessment of intravascular volume is a must in all types of circulatory failure. The size of the heart chambers reflects the intravascular volume and heart function based on the volume–pressure relationship of a compliant heart chamber, in the absence of a pre-existing or concurrent diseases, such as MI or cardiomyopathies.[11] Obliteration of the LV cavity at end-systole, the so-called kissing walls and hyperdynamic LV would be seen in severe hypovolemia.[12] In contrast, LV would be dilated in presence of volume overload. Also fixed bowing of the atrial septum into the right atrium throughout the cardiac cycle suggests elevated LA pressures, and further fluid administration is not required. A LV end-diastolic area (LVEDA) of less than 10 cm^2 or a LVEDA index (LVEDA/body surface area) of less than 5.5 cm^2/m^2 indicates significant hypovolemia, whereas an LVEDA of more than 20 cm^2 indicates volume overload.[13] However, these parameters should be used cautiously as in certain conditions, such as marked concentric LV hypertrophy and constrictive pericarditis, where LVEDA may be small; dilated LV in case of pre-existing dilated or ischemic cardiomyopathy. In severe right ventricle (RV) dysfunction, LV can be small due to underfilling.

Current guidelines recommend the use of inferior vena cava (IVC) diameter, its respiratory variation and percentage of diameter alteration as a useful parameter to assess right atrial (RA) pressure (RAP).[14] The IVC diameter should be measured within 1–2 cm from the caval–RA junction in the subcostal view.[15] M-mode tracing of the size of the IVC throughout the respiratory cycle in the longitudinal axis can be obtained at this point. The IVC collapses on inspiration but distends on expiration due to the changes in intrathoracic pressure in the patients with spontaneous breathing, whereas the reverse occurs in the patients on mechanical ventilation. The American Society of Echocardiography suggested the cut-off value of 2.1 cm and use of IVC collapsibility index (CI), which equals [IVCmax – IVCmin]/IVCmax[16] (Table 3).

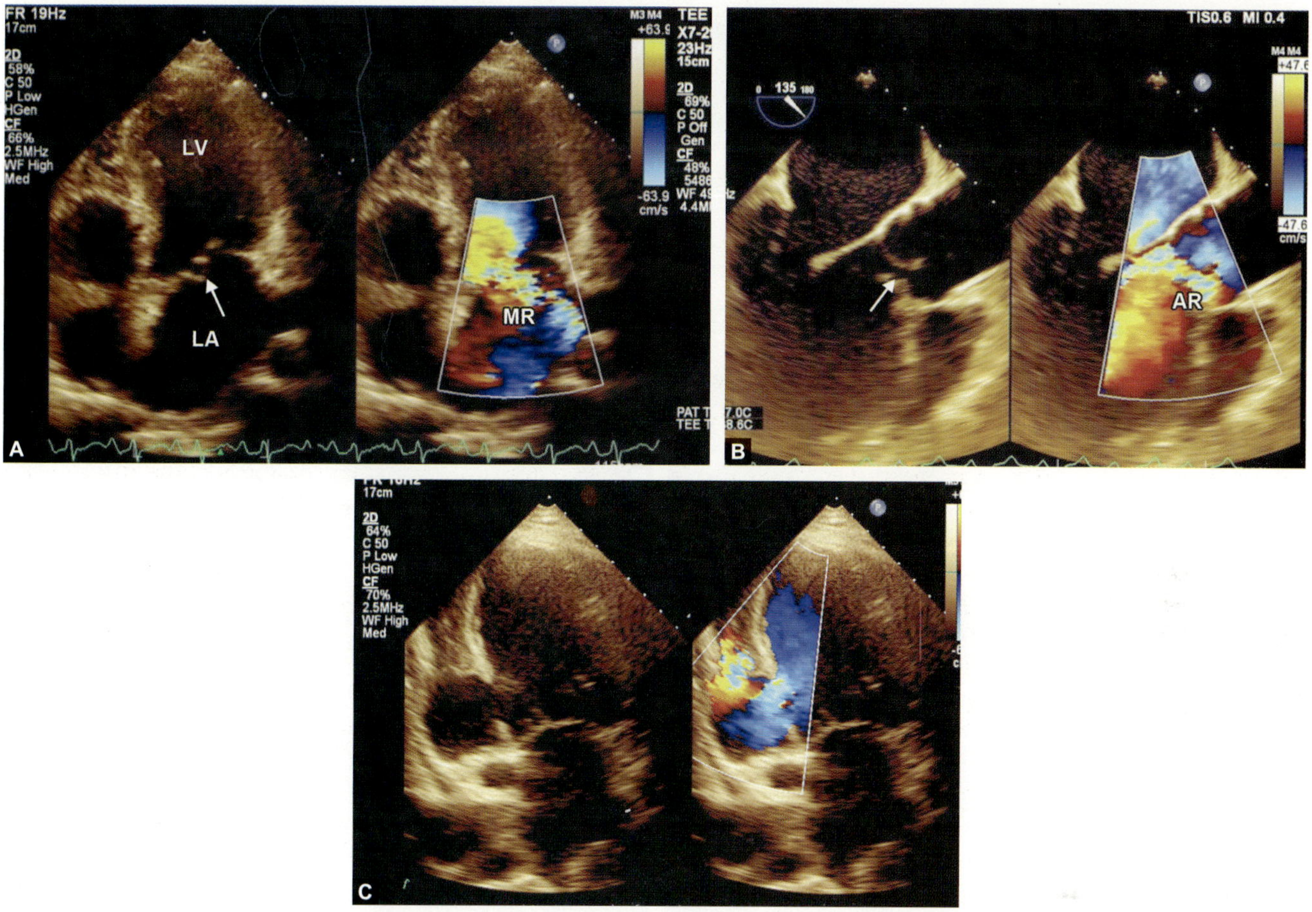

Figs. 1A to C: (A) Transthoracic echocardiography showing a large infero-VSD postinferior wall myocardial infarction. Color flow imaging shows a shunt from left to right ventricle via the VSD. (B) TEE demonstrating longitudinal view with flail right coronary cusp (white arrow) and color flow imaging shows severe aortic regurgitation directed toward anterior mitral leaflet. (C) Apical 4-C view of a patient with infective endocarditis leading to perforation (white arrow) of anterior mitral leaflet. Color Doppler demonstrating severe mitral regurgitation directed posterolaterally.(TEE: Transesophageal echocardiography; VSD: Ventricular septal defect)

IVC diameter less than 2.1 cm that collapses more than 50% with inspiration would correlate with RA pressure of 3 mm Hg (range, 0–5 mm Hg), while an IVC diameter more than 2.1 cm that collapses less than 50% with inspiration suggests a high RAP of 15 mm Hg (range, 10–20 mm Hg). In conditions where the IVC diameter and collapse do not fit in this paradigm, an intermediate value of 8 mm Hg (range, 5–10 mm Hg) may be used. For practical purposes, when the diameter is less than 10 mm, the patient is likely to respond to fluid, but when it is more than 20 mm, it is unlikely. In the collapse of more than 50% between the diameters of 10 mm and 20 mm, the trial of fluid should be done. The dynamic inspiratory change of more than 50% is more important than the IVC size. However, it should not be used in patients on mechanical ventilation as the IVC is commonly dilated and may not collapse. With the cutoff of 40%, the IVC CI would give a sensitivity of 70%, specificity of 80%, positive predictive value of 72%, and negative predictive value of 83%.[17] In the patient on fully supported positive pressure ventilation, the distensibility index (DI) is a good guide to fluid responsiveness. The DI is calculated as the ratio of $(IVC_{max} - IVC_{min})/IVC_{min}$ with a threshold of 18% discriminating between fluid responders and nonresponders with 90% sensitivity and specificity.[18]

In case uncertainty persists about the intravascular fluid status, more advanced techniques using Doppler-like SV and CO and dynamic measures, such as passive leg raising should be applied. Fluid responders are defined as more than or equal to 15% increase in CO or SV after fluid administration.[19] Other secondary indices of elevated RA pressure are restrictive right-sided diastolic filling pattern, tricuspid E/E′ of more than 6 and diastolic flow predominance in hepatic venous (HV) flow (at low or normal RA pressures, there is systolic predominance in hepatic vein flow). Nagueh et al. used HV systolic filling fraction (HVFF = VsVTI/VdVTI) less than 55%, which showed a sensitivity

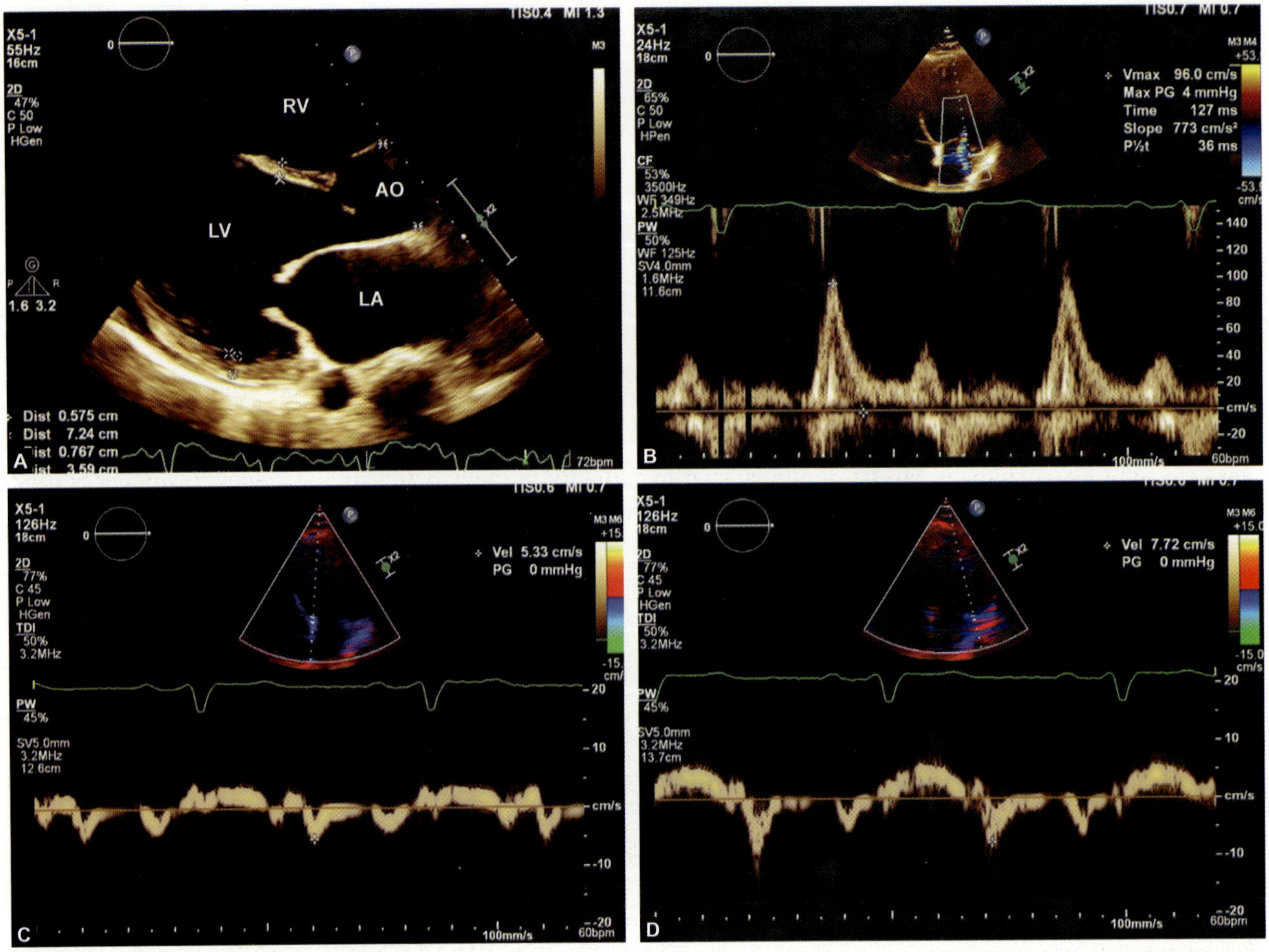

Figs. 2A to D: (A) Parasternal long-axis view shows ischemic cardiomyopathy with dilated LV and LA, a kinetic and scarred interventricular septum. (B) Mitral inflow shows restrictive filling pattern with E/A of >2 and deceleration time of 127 ms. (C) and (D) Septal and lateral annular tissue Doppler velocities with average velocity of 6.5 cm/s and E/e′ of 14.4 indicative of high LV filling pressure. (LA: Left atrial; LV: Left ventricular)

TABLE 2: Echocardiographic parameters in evaluation of cardiac function.

2-D and M-Mode	*Echo Doppler*
• Size, thickness, and configuration of chambers	• Evaluation of stroke volume and cardiac output
• Global systolic function—EF and FS	• Evaluation of regurgitation and valve stenosis
• Global and regional systolic function of LV and RV	• Evaluation of diastolic function
• Assessment of valvular function and anatomy	• Estimation of pulmonary artery pressure
• Detection and assessment of pericardial effusion	

(2D: Two-dimensional; EF: Ejection fraction; FS: Fractional shortening; LV: Left ventricular; RV: Right ventricle)

TABLE 3: Correlation between IVC diameter, CI and CVP

IVC Diameter (cm)	*% collapse on inspiration*	*CVP (mm Hg)*
<2.1	>50%	3 (0–5)
>2.1	>50%	8 (5–10)
>2.1	<50%	15 (10–20)
>2.1 cm with dilated hepatic veins	None	>20

(CVP: Central venous pressure; IVC: Inferior vena cava diameter)

and specificity of 86% and 90%, respectively, for diagnosing RAP more than 8 mm Hg.[20] (VsVTI : systolic HV VTI; VdVTI : diastolic HV VTI). Another formula has been used in mechanically ventilated patients which incorporates the tricuspid inflow and TDI of the tricuspid annulus: $1.62 \times E/e' + 2.13 = RAP$ (r = 0.7).[21] This was assessed in recent cardiac surgery (Figs. 3A to D; Table 4).

Obstructive Shock

Obstructive shock is a form of shock associated with resistance to blood flow through the cardiopulmonary circulation. The specific pathological diagnoses are acute pulmonary embolism, cardiac tamponade, dynamic outflow obstruction, type A dissection of aorta, tension pneumothorax, rarely constrictive pericarditis, and a cardiac tumor.

Acute Pulmonary Embolism

Classical right heart changes can be demonstrated by echocardiography in massive pulmonary embolism which includes acute RV dysfunction associated with dilatation, paradoxical motion of interventricular septum, D-shaped LV in parasternal short-axis view, elevated pulmonary artery pressure with high resistant flow in pulmonary artery, decreased CO, and rarely intracavitary emboli. The IVC may be distended with minimal or no respiratory variation. Dilatation of the RV is assessed in the apical 4-C view with basal diameter of more than 4 cm and RV/LV area ratio more than 0.6; an RV/LV ratio of 0.6–1.0 indicates moderate RV dilatation; gross dilatation is seen with a ratio of more than 1.0.[22,23] McConnell sign which is defined as mid RV free-wall akinesia with sparing of the apex may occasionally be seen.[24] It is thought to be specific but not very sensitive sign for acute pulmonary embolism (sensitivity 77%; specificity 96%). This sign is believed to be caused by tethering of the RV to the hyperdynamic LV apex.[25] Doppler is used to estimate pulmonary artery systolic pressure using a

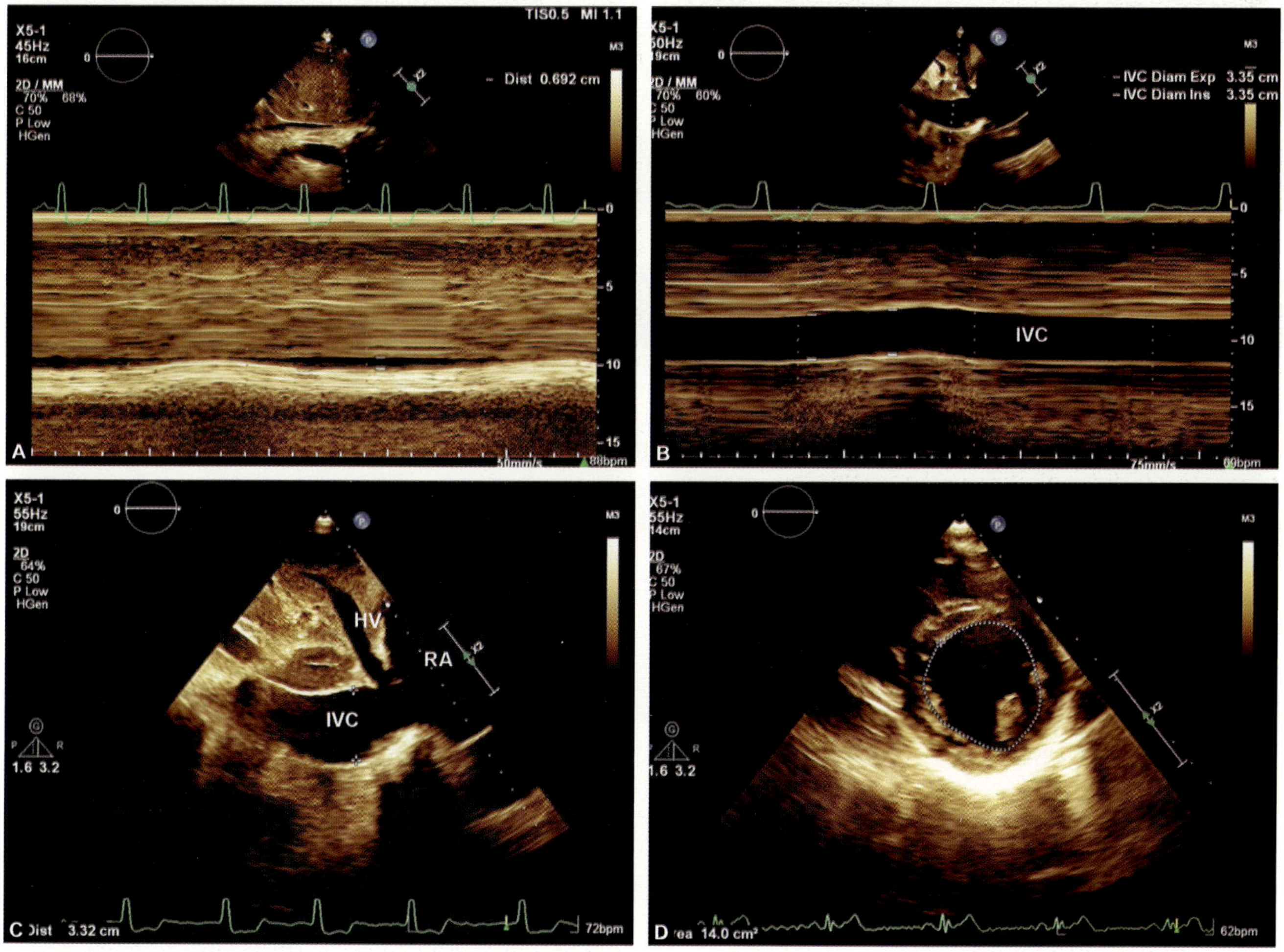

Figs. 3A to D: (A) 2D-guided M-mode of IVC showing markedly reduced luminal diameter with total inspiratory collapse consistent with hypovolemia. (B) M-mode echocardiography showing markedly dilated IVC with no respiratory variation s/o increased RA pressure. (C) Subcostal view showing markedly dilated IVC with prominent hepatic vein. (D) LVEDA measurement in short-axis view at the level of papillary muscle level. (IVC: Inferior vena cava; LVDA: Left ventricular end-diastolic area; RA: Right atrial)

TABLE 4: Limitation of right atrial pressure evaluation by Echo.

1.	Low respiratory compliance
2.	Mechanically ventilated patients
3.	Trained athletes
4.	Prominent Eustachian valve
5.	Narrowing of the IVC-RA junction
6.	Web or tissue present in the IVC

(IVC: Inferior vena cava; RA: Right atrial)

tricuspid regurgitation (TR) jet. The acceleration time of the pulmonary ejection signal (PAcT) is often used in case of absence of a reliable TR jet.[26] PAcT of 70–90 ms indicates a pulmonary artery systolic pressure of more than 70 mm Hg. The presence of mid systolic notch in PAcT also indicates severe pulmonary hypertension (Figs. 4A and B).

Cardiac Tamponade

One of the most common causes of obstructive shock is cardiac tamponade and echocardiography is the investigation of choice. When the intrapericardial pressure exceeds the right heart filling pressure (diastole), impaired filling of the chambers results in tamponade. The echocardiography not only helps in the diagnosis but also in establishing the qualitative size of effusion, its distribution, to some extend the nature of the effusion, and differentiating it from a pericardial fat pad or a pleural effusion. It also assists with urgent pericardiocentesis.

The 2D echocardiography findings of the atrial systolic collapse, diastolic collapse of RV, and dilated IVC with minimal or no respiratory variation establish the presence of tamponade and need for rapid drainage.[27] Brief RA collapse is sensitive but not specific, whereas RA collapse that exceeds one third of the cardiac cycle is nearly 100%

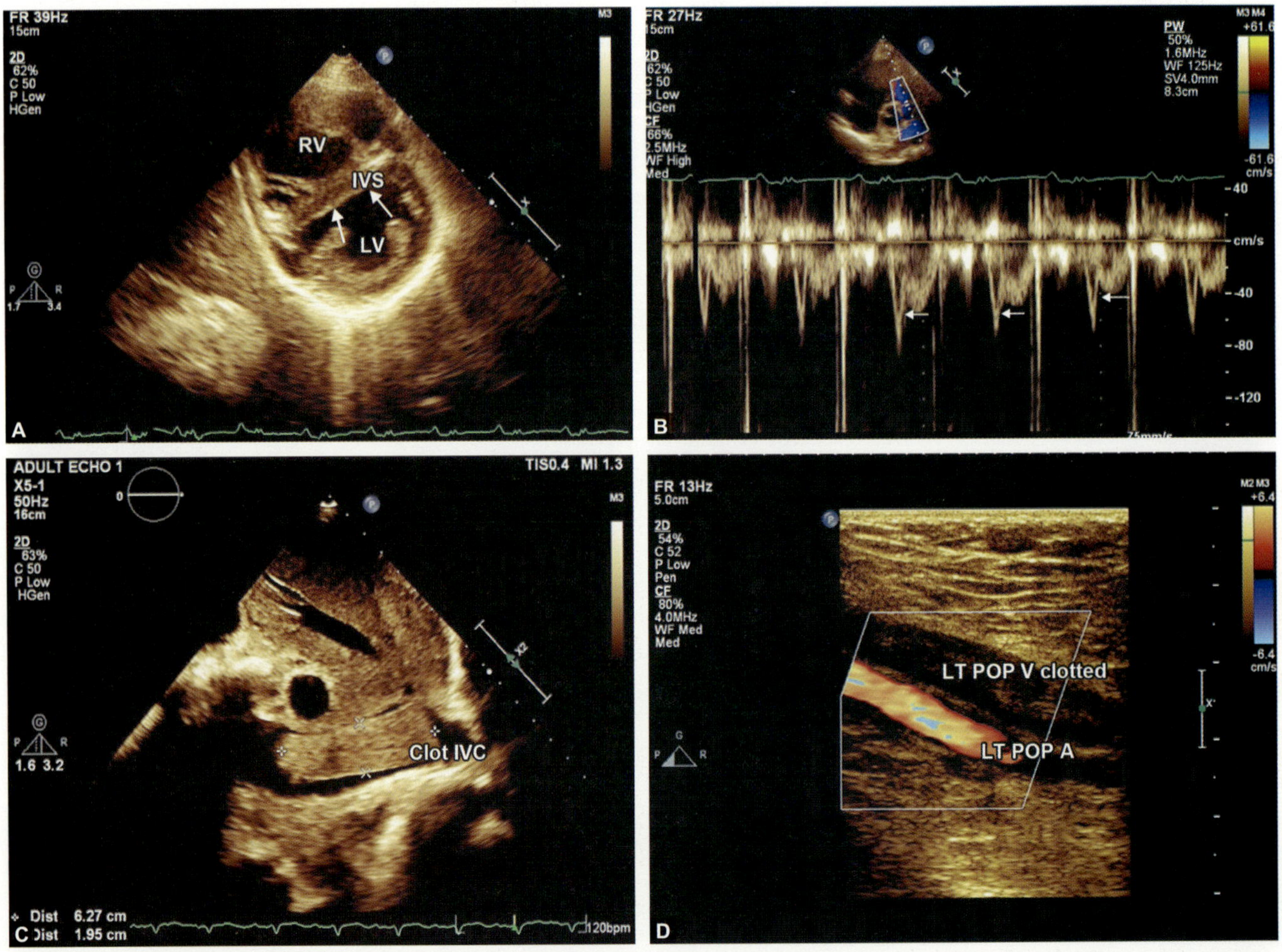

Figs. 4A to D: (A) Short-axis view demonstrating flattening of IVS with D-shaped LV cavity and enlarged RV s/o pulmonary hypertension. (B) Pulse wave Doppler of pulmonary flow with a notch consistent with high resistant flow. (C) Subcostal view shows a large clot in IVC close to RA junction. (D) Venous Doppler of lower limb demonstrating deep vein thrombosis of left popliteal vein. (IVC: Inferior vena cava; IVS: Interventricular septum; LV: Left ventricular; RA: Right atrial; RV: Right ventricle)

sensitive and specific for clinical cardiac tamponade.[28] When the effusion is massive, the heart swings freely in the pericardial space.

Added diagnostic support can be derived by Doppler assessment of mitral and tricuspid inflow pattern. Normally there is respiratory variation in tricuspid and mitral inflow with increase of tricuspid flow during inspiration (<25%) and reciprocal changes occurring in mitral flow; mitral inflow increases during expiration (<15%), whereas with tamponade the variation is much greater (Figs. 5A and B).

Dynamic Left Ventricular Outflow Tract Obstruction

Hypertrophic cardiomyopathy (HCM) with hypertrophy of the basal septum is the most common cause of dynamic LVOT obstruction (LVOTO). The LVOTO has been associated with systolic anterior motion (SAM) of the mitral valve, which is observed in 30–60% of patients with HCM. However, it is clear now that dynamic LVOTO is not associated only with HCM. It is one of the more common causes of unexplained hypotension seen in ICU.[29,30] Dynamic LVOTO can also be seen in elderly patients in a structurally normal heart without wall hypertrophy.[31] Factors which make the critically ill patients more susceptible, apart from age, includes hypertensive hypertrophy, hypovolemia, tachycardia, treatment with inotropes, sepsis and vasodilatation, and general anesthesia.[32] It is also seen in postoperative patients, both cardiac as well as noncardiac surgery, and it can be life threatening.[33] Rarely, LVOTO is seen in acute anterior wall MI or Takotsubo cardiomyopathy when the basal segments of LV are hypercontractile. Echocardiography is the modality of choice to diagnose this transient LVOTO. The 2D echocardiography reveals hypercontractile LV, SAM of anterior mitral leaflet (better appreciated by M-mode). Color Doppler reveals narrow turbulent flow in LVOT with continuous wave Doppler showing late peaking high-velocity flow of the so-called dagger-shaped LVOT gradient. Color Doppler also shows significant MR due to disrupted mitral coaptation. These hemodynamic features lead to reduction in SV and CO. Once the presence of SAM/LVOTO is confirmed, treatment includes reestablishing adequate intravascular volume, reducing heart rate (HR) to enhance diastolic filling time and ceasing inotropes (Figs. 6A and B).[34]

Aortic Dissection

Aortic dissection is a potentially fatal vascular emergency. The sensitivity and specificity of transthoracic echocardiography (TTE) for type A dissection are 78–90% and 87–96%, respectively.[35,36] The pathognomic echocardiographic feature of aortic dissection is the presence of intimal flap which appears as a thin linear echogenic structure, separating the true and false lumens within the aorta. The entire aorta should be thoroughly scanned including abdominal aorta to rule out distal aortic dissection. With the availability of echocardiography, the associated complications can also be detected, e.g. AR, aneurysms of the aortic root, pericardial effusion, cardiac tamponade, pleural effusion, myocardial ischemia. Regional wall motion abnormality may be detected secondary to ostial occlusion by intimal flap, usually involving the right coronary artery (Figs. 7A and B).[37]

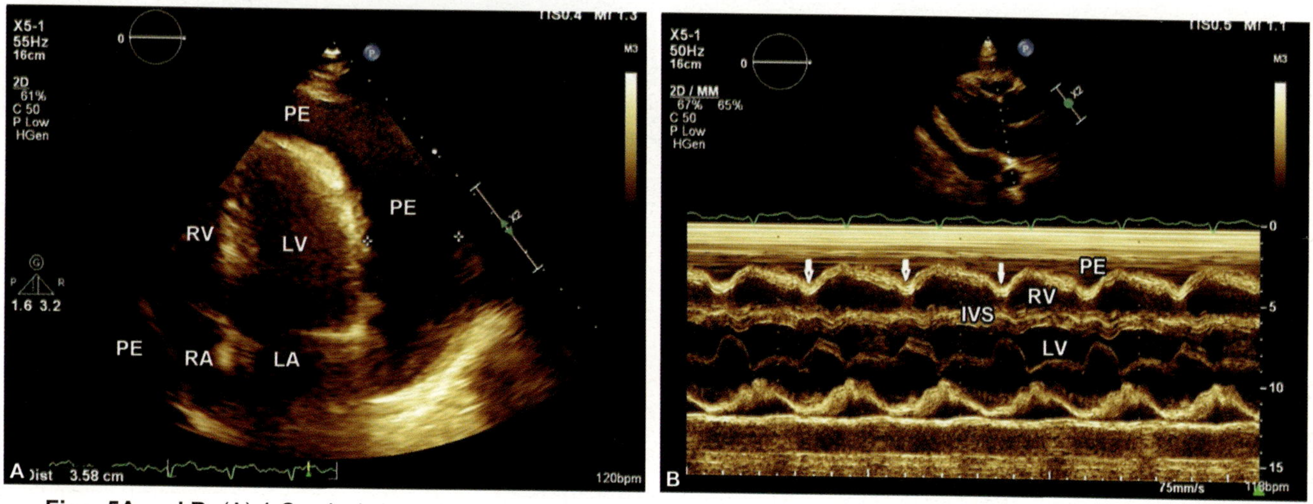

Figs. 5A and B: (A) 4-C apical view of a patient with large pericardial effusion circumferentially. (B) 2D-guided M-mode echocardiography showing early diastolic collapse of right ventricle (white arrows) consistent with cardiac tamponade.

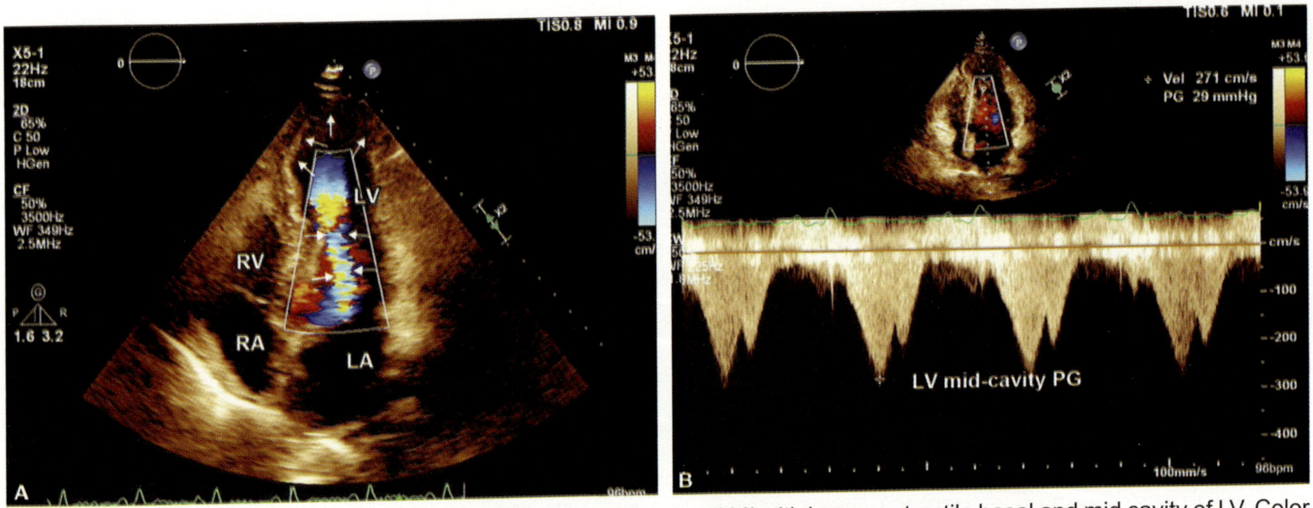

Figs. 6A and B: (A) Apical 4-C view of a patient with acute anterior wall MI with hypercontractile basal and mid cavity of LV. Color Doppler reveals a narrow mosaic flow in basal and mid cavity, suggesting turbulent flow characteristic of cavitary obstruction. (B) Continuous wave Doppler spectrum across LV cavity demonstrating "dagger-shaped" spectrum with peak instantaneous pressure gradient of 29 mm Hg. (LV: Left ventricular; MI: Myocardial infarction)

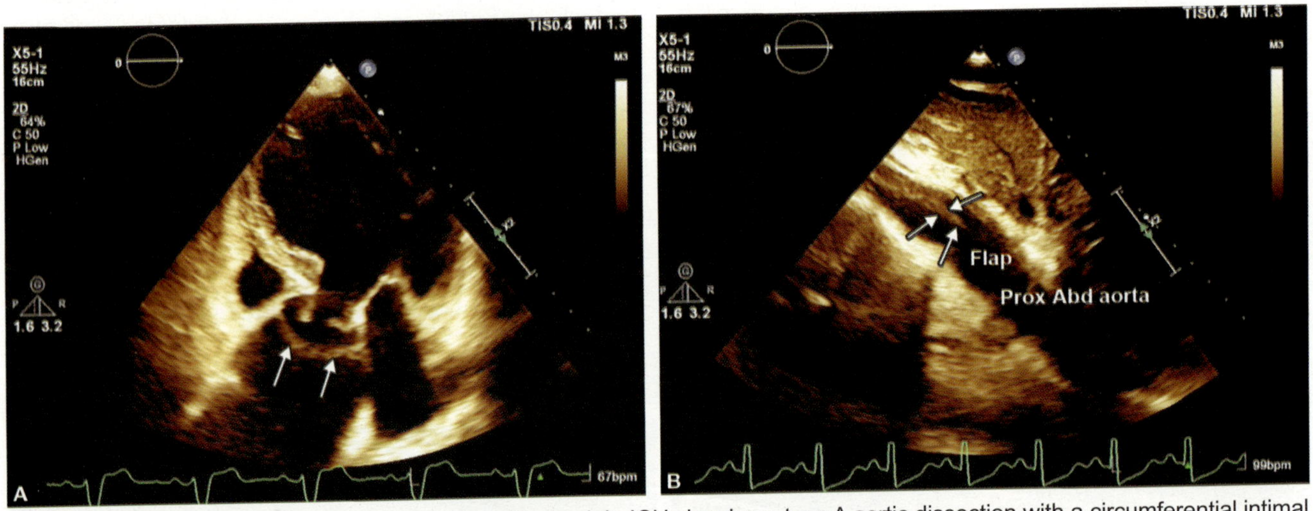

Figs. 7A and B: (A) Apical 5-C view of a patient with shock in ICU showing a type A aortic dissection with a circumferential intimal flap close to the aortic leaflets, also ascending aorta is aneurysmally dilated. (B) Intimal flap is extending into abdominal aorta.

Tension Pneumothorax

Lung ultrasound is nowadays considered as an effective technique for the diagnosis of pneumothorax at bedside.[38] Sensitivity of a lung ultrasound in the diagnosis of pneumothorax is higher than that of a conventional chest X-ray. Ultrasound diagnosis of pneumothorax relies on the recognition of four sonographic artifact signs: the lung sliding sign, the B-lines or comet-tail artifacts, the lung point, and the lung pulse.[39] Absence of sliding line, B-lines, and lung pulse in an unstable patient is enough to conclude the diagnosis of pneumothorax. Additionally, if lung point is not detected, tension pneumothorax is the diagnosis and should move on to an immediate lifesaving invasive treatment.[40] Other conditions, such as inferior or superior vena cava compression or thrombosis, intracardiac tumors or clot, aortic stenosis, can also lead to obstructive shock. As a result of the low CO, the patient may have tachycardia with the signs of tissue hypoperfusion and will have an increase in the systemic vascular resistance (SVR) to compensate.

Distributive Shock

Distributive shock results from excessive vasodilatation and the impaired distribution of blood flow. Septic shock (SS) is the most common cause of cardiovascular failure in critical care and is the most frequent cause of mortality in ICUs.[41]

Septic shock is one of the most complex hemodynamic failure syndromes, as it may involve derangement of all the three mainstays of cardiovascular homeostasis—absolute or relative reduction in central blood volume, peripheral vasodilatation, and myocardial failure may coexist and variably overlap in different phases of SS's course.[42] Echocardiography plays a key role in the critical septic patient management as an ideal monitoring tool. It not only excludes cardiac causes for sepsis but also guides in recognition of the dominant features of the failing cardiovascular system with subsequent appropriate management.[43,44] In the early stage, though LV dysfunction is present, it is masked by severely reduced afterload due to vasodilatation in sepsis.[42,45] Thus, LV is hyperdynamic with normal LVEDA, but a small LV end-systolic area (LVESA) in sharp contrast to hypovolemia where both LVEDA as well as LVESA are small. The IVC would be smaller in this phase. After this initial hyperdynamic stage, myocardial depression occurs in around 60% of the patients.[46] Once the afterload is restored by vasopressors and fluid therapy, LV myocardial dysfunction is unmasked. Left ventricular would be normal sized or dilated with global/segmental hypokinesia. Inferior vena cava would be distended with or without minimal respiratory variation having a similar profile as in cardiogenic shock (Figs. 8A and B; Table 5).

Hemodynamic Evaluation by Echocardiography

The use of echocardiography in the ICU for patients in shock allows the accurate measurement of several hemodynamics, such as SV, CO, central venous pressure (CVP), intracavitary pressures, SVR, myocardial contractility, and biventricular interactions (Box 1). This basic hemodynamic assessment allows differentiation of the four major categories of circulatory shock and enables proper and immediate hemodynamic support.

Stroke volume can be measured by using pulse wave Doppler and calculating the VTI of blood flow with the sample volume placed at the level of aortic annulus at 5-C view, multiplying with cross-sectional area (CSA) of LVOT derived from parasternal long-axis view

$$[CSA = (\pi(LVOT\ diameter/2)]2$$

(where SV = VTI × CSA and CO = SV × HR). Systemic vascular resistance, expressed in Woods units, can be calculated using the equation:

SVR = mean arterial pressure – RAP/CO; another equation that can be used by Doppler echocardiography is MR velocity/LVOT VTI. Mitral regurgitation velocity/LVOT VTI more than 0.27 has 70% sensitivity and 77% specificity for identifying SVR more than 14 Woods units.[47] The LV filling pressure is equal to PCWP in the absence of mitral stenosis and any pulmonary veno-occlusive disease. According to the latest guidelines from American Society of Echocardiography and European Association of Cardiovascular Imaging, only four variables need to be evaluated in determining the diastolic function, if LV systolic is preserved.[48] These four variables and their abnormal variables are:

1. Annular e' velocity (septal e' velocity <7.0 cm/s, lateral e' < 10 cm/s)
2. An average E/e' ratio of more than 14
3. LA maximum volume index more than or equal to 34 mL/m^2
4. Peak TR velocity of more than 2.8 m/s.

At times only the medial or lateral e' velocity is available, and in these circumstances, a medial E/e' ratio more than 15 or a lateral E/e' more than 13 is considered abnormal.

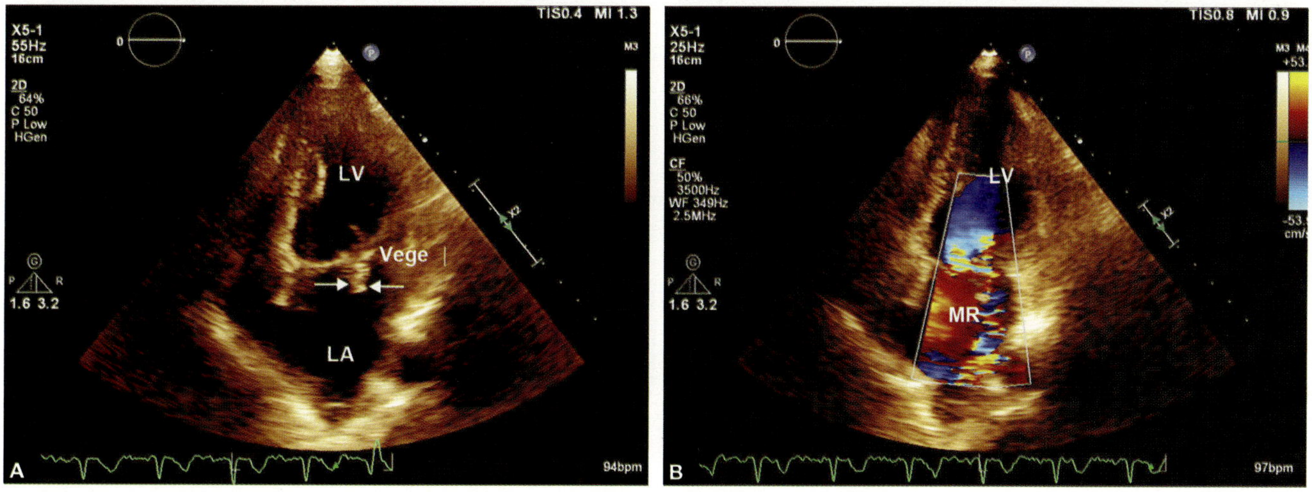

Figs. 8A and B: (A) Apical 4-C view of a patient with septic shock showing a vegetation attached to posterior mitral leaflet. (B) Color-guided Doppler demonstrating a highly eccentric jet of severe mitral regurgitation (MR).

TABLE 5: Cardiac abnormalities in severe sepsis.

- Left ventricular dilatation
- LV systolic dysfunction
  - Global
  - Segmental
- LV diastolic dysfunction
- RV systolic or diastolic dysfunction
- Valvular lesions
  - Functional
  - Endocarditis

BOX 1: Targets of the echocardiographic hemodynamic assessment.

- Left ventricle and right ventricle systolic function
- Volume status, volume responsiveness
- Stroke volume, cardiac output
- Left ventricle filling pressure
- Systemic arterial resistances

In patients with reduced LV systolic function, transmitral inflow pattern is the first variable to be assessed. If the ratio of mitral E/A is less than 0.8 and mitral E wave velocity is less than 50 cm/s then usually the LV filling pressure/PCWP is normal. If E/A is more than 2.0 then it indicates significantly increased PCWP (Figs. 9A and B). In case of indeterminate values, the three other parameters to be evaluated are:[49]

1. Average E/e' more than 14
2. TR velocity more than 2.8 cm/s
3. LA volume index more than or equal to 34 mL/m^2

The routine use of echocardiography to determine the four parameters (CVP, PCWP, SV, and CO) helps the intensivist to ensure the optimum balance of fluids, inotropes, and vasoconstrictors (Table 6).

Limitations of Echocardiography in the Intensive Care Unit

- Echocardiography is operator dependent, hence can lead to subjectivity and operator variability. Also it does not provide continuous monitoring. Repeated scanning causes a significant burden on resources
- Suboptimal windows are present due to positioning of the patients, mechanical ventilations, chest tubes, surgical dressings, etc. therefore may not be possible to acquire all the echocardiographic views. In patients with chronic obstructive pulmonary disease or obese patients, TTE can be challenging
- Cardiac function can be overestimated when patients receive mechanical or inotropic support. Also pre-existing cardiac disease may cause interpretation difficult. For example, LVEDA is not predictive of fluid responsiveness in dilated LV due to cardiac disease
- Measurement errors are one of the major limitations for hemodynamic assessment. For example, for estimation of SV and CO, LVOT diameter if not taken accurately can lead to doubling the error and for Doppler measurement; poor angle alignment will lead to underestimation of the velocity of flow
- Finally, if not properly decontaminated, the echocardiography probe can be a source of transmission of infection in the ICU.

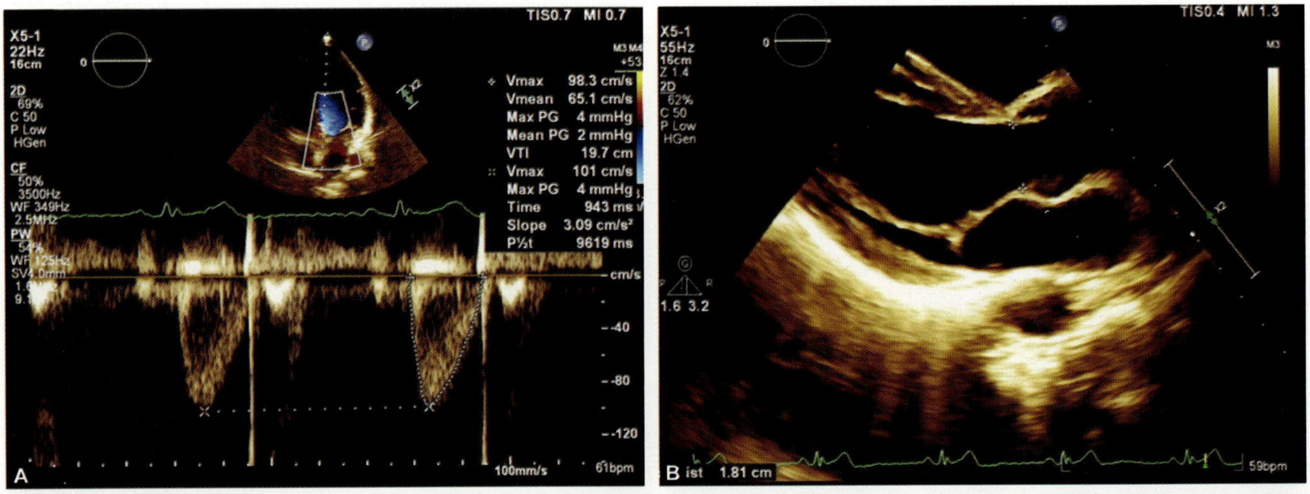

Figs. 9A and B: Measurement of stroke volume and cardiac output. (A) LVOT diameter is measured in zoomed parasternal long-axis view at the level of aortic annulus during systole perpendicular to the anterior aortic wall. (B) Measurement of LVOT VTI from the apical 5-C view using pulse wave Doppler with sample volume placed at the center of the aortic annulus. VTI is the area under the velocity curve. Interval between two VTI spectrums is the heart rate. (LVOT: Left ventricular outflow tract; VTI: Velocity time integral)

TABLE 6: Hemodynamics of shock.

	CVP	PCWP	Cardiac output	SVR
Hypovolemic	↓	↓	↑	↑
	↑			
Cardiogenic	↑	↑	↓	↑
Septic	↓	↓	↑	↓
Obstructive	↑ or ↓	↑	↓	↑

(CVP: central venous pressure; PCPW: pulmonary capillary wedge pressure; SVR: systemic vascular resistance; ↑-Increased, ↓-Decreased)

CONCLUSION

Echocardiography has become an indispensable tool in ICU in recent years. In properly trained hands, it provides valuable information on the pathology and physiology of circulatory system to differentiate between different types of shock and guide-specific management.

REFERENCES

1. Cecconi M, De Backer A, Antonelli M, et al. Consensus on circulatory shock and hemodynamic monitoring. Task force of the European Society of Intensive Care Medicine. Intensive Care Med. 2014;40:1795-815.
2. Sakr Y, Reinhart K, Vincent JL, et al. Does dopamine administration in shock influence outcome? Results of the Sepsis Occurrence in Acutely Ill Patients (SOAP) Study. Crit Care Med. 2006;34:589-97.
3. Jones AE, Aborn LS, Kline JA. Severity of emergency department hypotension predicts adverse hospital outcome. Shock. 2004;22(5):410-4.
4. Ren X (Mike), Ooi HH, Brandler ES, et al. (2017). Cardiogenic shock: practice essentials, background, pathophysiology. Available from https://emedicine.medscape.com/article/152191-overview [Accessed October 2018].
5. McLean AS, Huang SH. Critical Care Ultrasound Manual, 1st edition. Australia: Elsevier; 2012.
6. Mok KL. Make it simple: enhanced shock management by focussed cardiac ultrasound. J Intensive Care. 2016 4:51.
7. Dalen H, Thorstensen A, Vattan LJ, et al. Reference values and distribution of conventional echocardiography Doppler measures and longitudinal tissue doppler velocities in a population free from cardiovascular disease. Circ Cardiovasc Imaging. 2010;3:614-22.
8. Alam M, Wardell J, Andersson E, et al. Effects of first myocardial infarction on left ventricular systolic and diastolic function determined by pulsed wave Doppler tissue imaging. J Am Soc Echocardiogr. 2000;13:343.
9. Gulati VK, Katz WE, Follansbee WP, Gorcsan J. Mitral annular descent velocity by tissue Doppler echocardiography as an index of global left ventricular function. Am J Cardiol. 1996;77:979-84.
10. Paulus WJ, Tschope C. A novel paradigm for heart failure with preserved ejection fraction: comorbidities drive myocardial dysfunction and remodelling through microvascular endothelial inflammation. J Am Coll Cardiol. 2013;62:263-71.
11. Cheung AT, Savino JS, Weiss SJ, et al. Echocardiographic and hemodynamic indexes of left ventricular preload in patients with normal and abnormal ventricular function. Anesthiology. 1994;81:376-87.
12. Leung JM, Levine EH. Left ventricular end-systolic cavity obliteration as an estimate of intraoperative hypovolemia. Anesthesiology. 1994;81:1102-9.
13. Vermeiren G, Malbrain M, Walpot J. Cardiac ultrasonography in the critical care setting: a practical approach to assess cardiac function and preload for the "non-cardiologist". Anesthesiol Intensive Ther. 2015;47s89-104.
14. Kicher BJ, Himelman RB, Schiller NB. Noninvasive estimation of right atrial pressure with 2-dimensional and Doppler echocardiography :a simultaneous catheterization and echocardiographic study. Am J Cardiol. 1990;66(4):493-6.
15. Wallace DJ, Allison M, Stone MB. Inferior vena cava percentage collapse during respiration is affected by the sampling location : an ultrasound study in healthy volunteers. Acad Emerg Med. 2010:1796-9.
16. Lawrence G. Rudski, Lai WW, et al. Guidelines for the echocardiographic assessment of the right heart in adults: a report from the American Society of Echocardiography endorsed by the European Association of Echocardiography, a registered branch of the European Society of Cardiology, and the Canadian Society of Echocardiography. J Am Soc Echocardiogr. 2010;23(7):685.
17. Muller L, Bobbia X, Toumi M et al. Respiratory variations of inferior vena cava diameter to predict fluid responsiveness in spontaneously breathing patients with acute circulatory failure: need for a cautious use. Crit Care. 2012;16(5):R188.
18. Barbier C, Loubieres Y, Schmit C, et al. Respiratory changes in inferior vena cava diameter are helpful in predicting fluid responsiveness in ventilated septic patients. Intensive Care Med. 2004;30:1740-6.
19. Marik PE, Monnet X, Teboul JL. Haemodynamic parameters to guide fluid therapy. Ann Int Care. 2011;1:1.
20. Nagueh SF, Kopelen HA, Zoghbi WA. Relation of mean right atrial pressure to echocardiographic and Doppler parameters of right atrial and right ventricular function. Circulation. 1996;93(6):1160-9.
21. Sade LE, Gulmez O, Eroglu S, et al. Noninvasive estimation of right ventricular filling pressure by ratio of early tricuspid inflow to annular diastolic velocity in patients with and without recent cardiac surgery. J Am Soc Echocardiogr. 2007;20(8):982-8.
22. Jardin F, Duboung O, Boundarias JP. Echocardiographic pattern of acute cor pulmonale. Chest. 1997;111:209-17.
23. Beaulieu Y. Bedside echocardiography in the assessment of the critically ill. Crit Care Med. 2007;35(5 Suppl.):S235-49.
24. McConnell MV, Solomon SD, Rayan ME, et al. Regional right ventricular dysfunction detected by echocardiography in acute pulmonary embolism. Am J Cardiol. 1996;78:469-73.

25. Lopez-Candales A, Edelman K, Candales MD. Right ventricular apical contractility in acute pulmonary embolism: the McConnell sign revisited. Echocardiography. 2010;27:614-20.
26. Tossavainen E, Soderberg S, Gronlund C, et al. Pulmonary artery acceleration time in identifying pulmonary hypertension patients with raised pulmonary vascular resistance. Eur Heart J (Cardiovasc Imag). 2013;14:890-7.
27. Ristic AD, Imazio M, Adler y, et al. Triage strategy for urgent management of cardiac tamponade: a position statement of the European Society of Cardiology Working Group of Myocardial and Pericardial Disease. Eur Heart J. 2014;35:2279-84.
28. Gillam LD, Guyer DE, Gibson TS, et al. Hydrodynamic compression of the right atrium: a new echocardiographic sign of cardiac tamponade. Circulation. 1983;68(2):294-301.
29. Luckner G, Margreiter J, Jochberger S, et al. Systolic anterior motion of the mitral valve with left ventricular outflow tract obstruction: three cases of acute perioperative hypotension in noncardiac surgery. Anesth Analg. 2005;100:1594-8.
30. Luckie M, Khattar RS. Systolic anterior motion of the mitral valve-beyond hypertrophic cardiomyopathy. Heart. 2008:1383-5.
31. Yang JH, Park SW, Kim HJ, et al. Dynamic left ventricular outflow tract obstruction without basal septal hypertrophy, caused by catecholamine therapy and volume depletion. Korean J Intern Med. 2008;23(2):106-9.
32. Roldan FJ, Vargas-Barron J, Espinola-Zavaleta N, et al. Severe dynamic obstruction of the left ventricular outflow tract induced by dobutamine. Echocardiography. 2000;17:37-40.
33. Sobczyk D. Dynamic left ventricular outflow tract obstruction: underestimated cause of hypotension and hemodynamic instability. J Ultrason. 2014;14(59):421-7.
34. Ibrahim M, Rao C, Ashrafian H, et al. Modern management of systolic anterior motion of the mitral valve. Eur J Cardiothorac Surg. 2012;41:1260-70.
35. Nienaber CA, Von Kodolitsch Y, Nicolas V, et al. The diagnosis of thoracic aortic dissection by noninvasive imaging procedures. N Engl J Med. 1993;328:1-9.
36. Evangelista A, Flachskamp FA, Erbel R, et al. Echocardiography in aortic diseases: EAE recommendations for clinical practice. Eur J Echocardiogr. 2010;11:645-58.
37. Spittell PC, Spittell Jr JA, Joyce JW, et al. Clinical features and differential diagnosis of aortic dissection: experience with 236 cases (1980 through 1990). Mayo Clin Proc. 1993;68:642-51.
38. Volpicelli G, Elbarbary M, Blaivas M, et al. International Liaison Committee on Lung Ultrasound for International Consensus Conference on Lung Ultrasound. International evidence-based recommendations for point-of-care lung ultrasound. Intensive Care Med. 2012;38(4):577-91.
39. Volpicelli G. Sonographic diagnosis of pneumothorax. Intensive Care Med. 2011;37(2):224-32.
40. Volpicelli G, Boero E, Stefanone V, et al. Unusual new signs of pneumothorax at lung ultrasound. Crit Ultrasound J. 2013;5:10.
41. Brun-Buisson C, Doyon F, Carlet J, et al. Incidence, risk factors, and outcome of severe sepsis and septic shock in adults. A multicenter prospective study in intensive care units: French ICU Group for Severe Sepsis. JAMA. 1995;274(12):968-74.
42. Via G, Price S, Storti E. Echocardiography in the sepsis syndromes. Crit Ultrasound J. 2011;3(2):71-85.
43. Zanotti Cavazzoni SL, Dellinger RP. Hemodynamic optimization of sepsis-induced hypoperfusion. Crit Care. 2006;10(Suppl. 6):S2.
44. Dellinger RP, Levy MM, Carlet JM, et al. Surviving Sepsis Campaign: international guidelines for management of severe sepsis and septic shock. Intensive Care Med. 2008;36:296-327.
45. Repesse X, Charron C, Viellard-Baron CV. Evaluation of left ventricular systolic function revisited in septic shock. Crit Care. 2013;17(4):64.
46. Viellard-Baron A, Caille V, Charron C, et al. The actual incidence of global left ventricular hypokinesia in adult septic shock. Crit Care Med. 2008;36:1701-6.
47. Abbas AE, Fortuin FD, Patel B, et al. Noninvasive measurement of systemic vascular resistance using Doppler echocardiography. J Am Soc Echocardiogr. 2004;17:834-8.
48. Nagueh SF, Smiseth OA, Appleton CP, et al. Recommendations for the evaluation of left ventricular diastolic function by echocardiography: an update from American Society of Echocardiography and the European Association of Cardiovascular Imaging. J Am Soc Echocardiogr. 2016:19:277-314.
49. Dokainish H, Nguyen JS, Bobek J, et al. Assessment of the American Society of Echocardiography: European Society of Echocardiography Guidelines for Diastolic Function in Patients with Depressed Ejection Fraction: an echocardiography and invasive hemodynamic study. Eur J Echocardiogr. 2011;12:857-64.

SECTION 28

Epidemiological

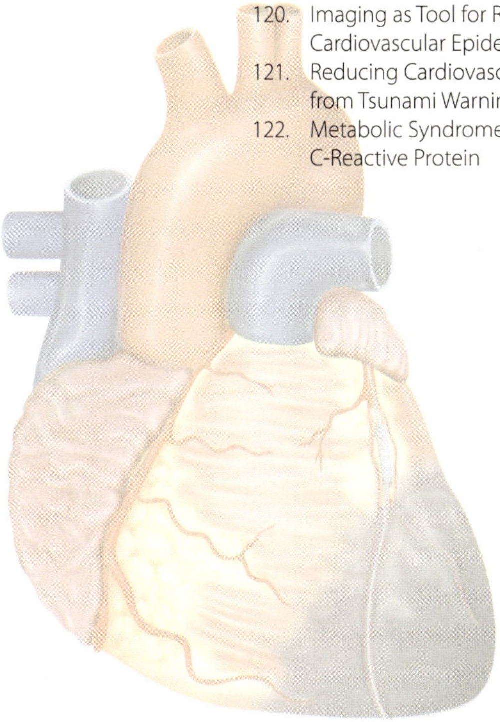

120

CHAPTER

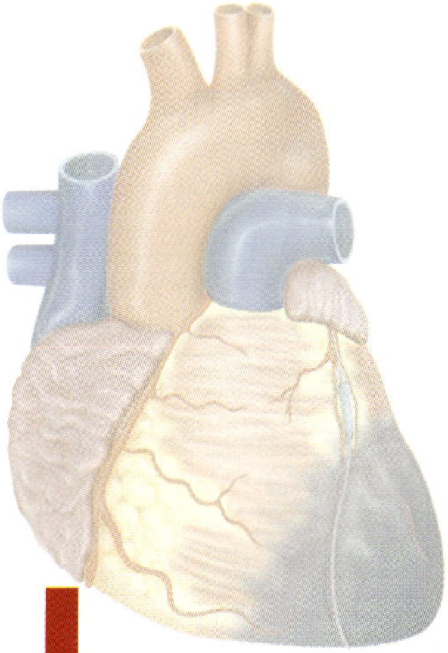

Imaging as Tool for Risk Prediction in Cardiovascular Epidemiology

Suman Singhal, Rajeev Gupta

INTRODUCTION

Coronary artery disease (CAD) or ischemic heart disease (IHD) is epidemic in India and has rapidly evolved to achieve the dubious distinction of principal cause of death in the country.[1] Global Burden of Diseases Study has reported that IHD mortality rates in India are more than twice the rates in North America and Western Europe. The Million Death Study has reported that IHD deaths have increased in India by more than 20% in the last 15 years (years 2000–2016).[1] Coronary heart disease (CHD) in Indians is characterized by premature occurrence, widespread atherosclerosis, and high mortality. It is extremely important to predict its occurrence, so we can employ preventive strategies with emphasis on risk stratification and primary prevention in asymptomatic patients to decrease the IHD-related mortality and morbidity in the country. Tools for identifying individuals at increased risk are important because effective preventive treatments are available.

A number of clinical risk prediction tools are available (Table 1) and have been recently reviewed.[2] These risk prediction tools have been more validated than others and may be better for risk prediction in selected populations.[3] On comparison of eight risk prediction tools (two variants of Framingham risk score, Assessing Cardiovascular Risk to Scottish Intercollegiate Guidelines Network, Systematic Coronary Risk Evaluation, Prospective Cardiovascular Münster, QRISK-1, QRISK-2, and Reynold risk score) in 56 studies, it was concluded that only for 18% comparisons exceeded 5% relative difference.[2] This suggests that most of the risk tools provide similar information. It has been observed that most of the risk prediction models have not been externally validated, especially in the Indian populations, making them of unknown value for practitioners, policy makers, and guideline developers in our country; most developed models are inadequately reported to allow external validation or implementation in clinical practice, and rather than developing new models, researchers should make better use of available evidence by validating, making head-to-head comparisons, and tailoring the promising existing models.[2] On the other hand, multiple imaging modalities are continuously emerging as coronary risk prediction tools over last few years and their

TABLE 1: Commonly used clinical risk prediction tools in coronary artery disease.

Region/country	*Tool eponym*
North America	Framingham, old, and new Reynold ACC/AHA Pooled Cohort Equation
Europe	SCORE QRISK-1, QRISK-2 PROCAM ASSIGN
International	WHO INTERHEART GLOBORISK-2

(AHA/ACC: American Heart Association/American College of Cardiology; ASSIGN: Assessing cardiovascular risk to Scottish intercollegiate guidelines network; PROCAM: Prospective Cardiovascular Münster; SCORE: Systematic coronary risk evaluation)

role in risk stratification is being studied and justified. In this review article, we discuss the current status of various imaging modalities in risk stratification of CHD based on commonly assed technologies listed in Table 2.

CAROTID INTIMA MEDIA THICKNESS

Common carotid intima media thickness (CIMT) is a noninvasive ultrasound measurement between the intimal luminal and the medial–adventitial interfaces of the carotid artery wall represented as a characteristic double-line density on B mode ultrasound image (Fig. 1). It is measured in supine position with neck extended and head turned to the contralateral side of examination, allowing maximal access to the great arteries of the neck.[4,5] The common carotid artery (CCA) far-wall IMT measurement represents the true biological thickness of the vessel wall,[6] whereas the near-wall IMT measurement has systematic measurement error because of the echogenicity of the adventitial layer masking the adventitial–medial boundary, as well as being affected by gain settings. The development of automated edge-tracking software in ultrasound machines has further improved the reproducibility of CIMT measurements.[6]

TABLE 2: Imaging-based coronary risk prediction tools.

Imaging modality	*Risk assessment technologies*
Ultrasonographic imaging	Common CIMT Carotid plaques Plaques in femoral arteries, aorta
CT scan	EBCT coronary calcium imaging Coronary artery calcium scoring MDCT, CTCA
MR imaging	MR coronary angiography
Plaque imaging	Coronary CT angiography CMRI IVUS
Novel techniques	OCT NIRS Thermography
Nuclear imaging	SPECT PET

(CAD: coronary artery disease; CIMT: carotid intima media thickness; CMRI: cardiac magnetic resonance imaging; CT: computed tomographic; CTCA: computed tomographic coronary angiography; EBCT: electron beam computed tomographic; IVUS: intravascular ultrasound; MDCT: multidetector computed tomography; MR: magnetic resonance; NIRS: near-infrared spectroscopy; OCT: optical coherent tomography; PET: positron emission tomography; SPECT: single photon emission cardiac tomography)

There is no common consensus regarding cutoff value of abnormal CIMT and varies from IMT greater than the 75th percentile,[7,8] IMT that is more than 1 standard deviation from the mean or IMT at the upper quartile or IMT at the upper tertile, or an absolute IMT value of more than or equal to 0.9 mm or more than or equal to 1.0 mm.[9] American Society of Echocardiography consensus statement recommends the use of CIMT greater than the 75th percentile for age, ethnicity, and sex as being abnormal.[7]

Risk prediction: Various studies have shown an association between CIMT and future CAD events. Initially, the Kuoppio Ischaemic Heart Disease study demonstrated an association of CIMT with future coronary events. In this study, every 0.1-mm increment of IMT was associated with an 11% increased risk of myocardial infarction during follow-up.[10] Subsequently, several other large clinical studies, including the Atherosclerosis Risk in Communities study,[9] Cardiovascular Health Study,[11] and Carotid Atherosclerosis Progression Study,[12] showed that CIMT can be used to assess incident CAD risk. Plaque presence seemed to have a more profound effect on improving the risk prediction.

Limitations: The major limitation of CIMT-based risk assessment is that there is little or no additional prognostic value found by adding CIMT to a traditional risk factor score, such as the Framingham Risk Score.[13-15] The contradictory results regarding the value of CIMT in CAD risk prediction are due to various discrepancies in its measurement, whether plaque to be included or excluded, and is also shown in conflicting results from two meta-analyses.[16,17] Another limitation when using CIMT for risk prediction is the significant influence of age on CIMT as it increases with age.

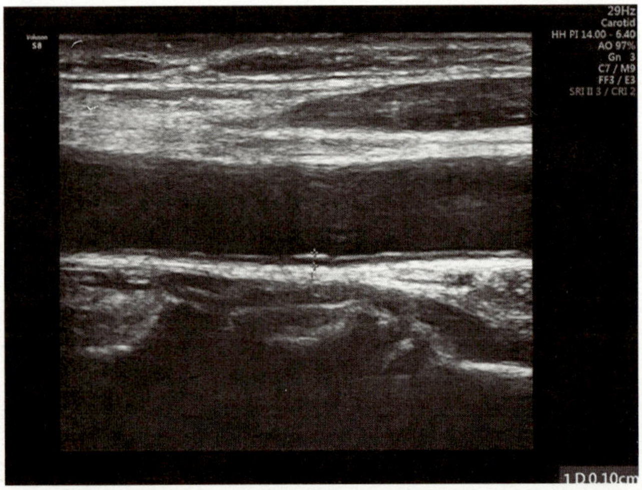

Fig. 1: Carotid intima media thickness with automatic edge enhancement.

Recommendations: The 2010 American Heart Association/American College of Cardiology (AHA/ACC) guidelines recommend measurements of CIMT for CHD risk assessment in intermediate-risk asymptomatic adults as Class IIB recommendation.[18] The European Society of Hypertension/European Society of Cardiology recommends ultrasound scanning of the carotid arteries to detect vascular hypertrophy or atherosclerosis as a class IIA recommendation with level of evidence B.[19] An update of the Mannheim Carotid Intima-Media Thickness and Plaque Consensus from the advisory board of the *Watching the Risk* symposium stated that measurements of CIMT and plaque presence are recommended for the initial detection of CAD risk in asymptomatic patients if at intermediate risk or if risk factors were present.[20]

However, in 2013, the AHA/ACC guidelines recommend against the use of CIMT for individual risk prediction in clinical practice.[21] These varying guideline recommendations are probably caused by differences in study design, specifically discrepancies regarding CIMT measurements, such as measuring the common or internal segment and whether plaques are included or excluded in analyses, as seen in review by Naqvi and Lee.[22] Recent studies with better imaging techniques which are able to image internal carotid artery (ICA)-IMT found that ICA-IMT is associated with higher relative risk of incident CAD compared with CCA-IMT,[23] and inclusion of plaque in measurement of CIMT is better for risk prediction[22] (Fig. 2). In Multiethnic Study of Atherosclerosis (MESA), it has been postulated that combined CIMT and ICA-IMT percentile score offers incremental value to Framingham CHD risk factors and coronary artery calcium (CAC) score for predicting incident coronary artery events.[24]

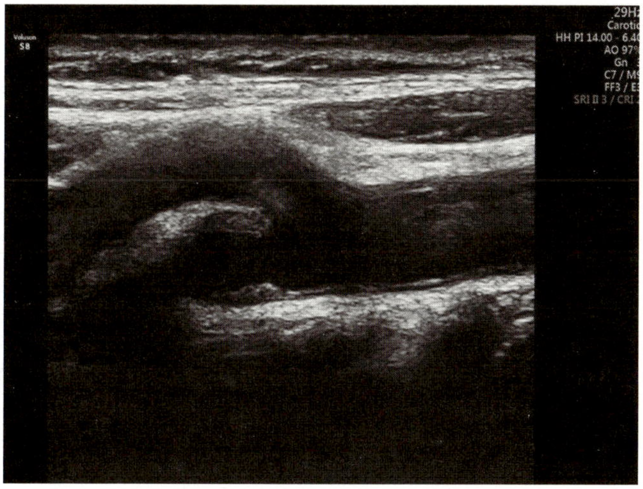

Fig. 2: Mixed eccentric plaque in common carotid artery bulb with normal intima media thickness.

CORONARY ARTERY CALCIUM SCORE

Initially electron beam computed tomography (EBCT) was used to estimate CAC score and ample scientific literature is being based on this technique. Later multidetector computed tomography (MDCT) became the modality of choice for CAC evaluation; EBCT is now practically obsolete.

Coronary artery calcium score: Calcification is identified as areas of hyperattenuation of at least 1 mm^2 with more than 130 Hounsfield units (HU) or more than or equal to 3 adjacent pixels.[25] The determination of the CAC score by MDCT is based on axial slices, with a thickness of 3 mm, without overlapping or gaps, limited to the cardiac region, acquired prospectively in synchrony with the electrocardiogram at a predetermined moment in the R-R interval, usually in the mid/late diastole, without the use of intravenous contrast medium.[26] The radiation dose is usually low, typically less than or equal to 1.5 mSv,[27] which is the highest effective dose recommended for use in image acquisition, according to the Society of Cardiovascular Computed Tomography.[27] The main methods for CAC score quantification are the Agatston method,[25] calcium volume score,[28] and relative calcium mass score.[29] Agatston method, first described by Agatston and Janowitz in 1991, is used as a reference for most population databases and publications involving risk stratification and is therefore most often used in clinical practice. The Agatston method uses the weighted sum of lesions with a density above 130 HU, multiplying the area of calcium by a factor related to maximum plaque attenuation: 130–199 HU, factor 1; 200–299 HU, factor 2; 300–399 HU, factor 3; and more than or equal to 400 HU, factor 4. The slice thickness and the interval must follow the standard protocols to reduce the noise variation and for reproducibility of calcium score (Fig. 3).

Calcium volume score: It has proven to be the most robust and reproducible method[30] and is calculated by multiplying the number of voxels with calcification by the volume of each voxel, including all voxels with an attenuation more than 130 HU. However, this method is particularly sensitive to the partial volume (especially in plaques with high attenuation) and subject to variability between tests, depending on the position of the plaque in the axial slice acquired.

Relative calcium mass score: It is calculated by multiplying the mean attenuation of the calcified plaque by the plaque volume in each image, thus reducing the variation caused by the partial volume. The absolute calcium mass score uses a correction factor based on the attenuation of water.[30]

Risk stratification: CAC score adds value to the Framingham risk score and to other risk assessment methods, providing a substantial increase in the accuracy of the risk

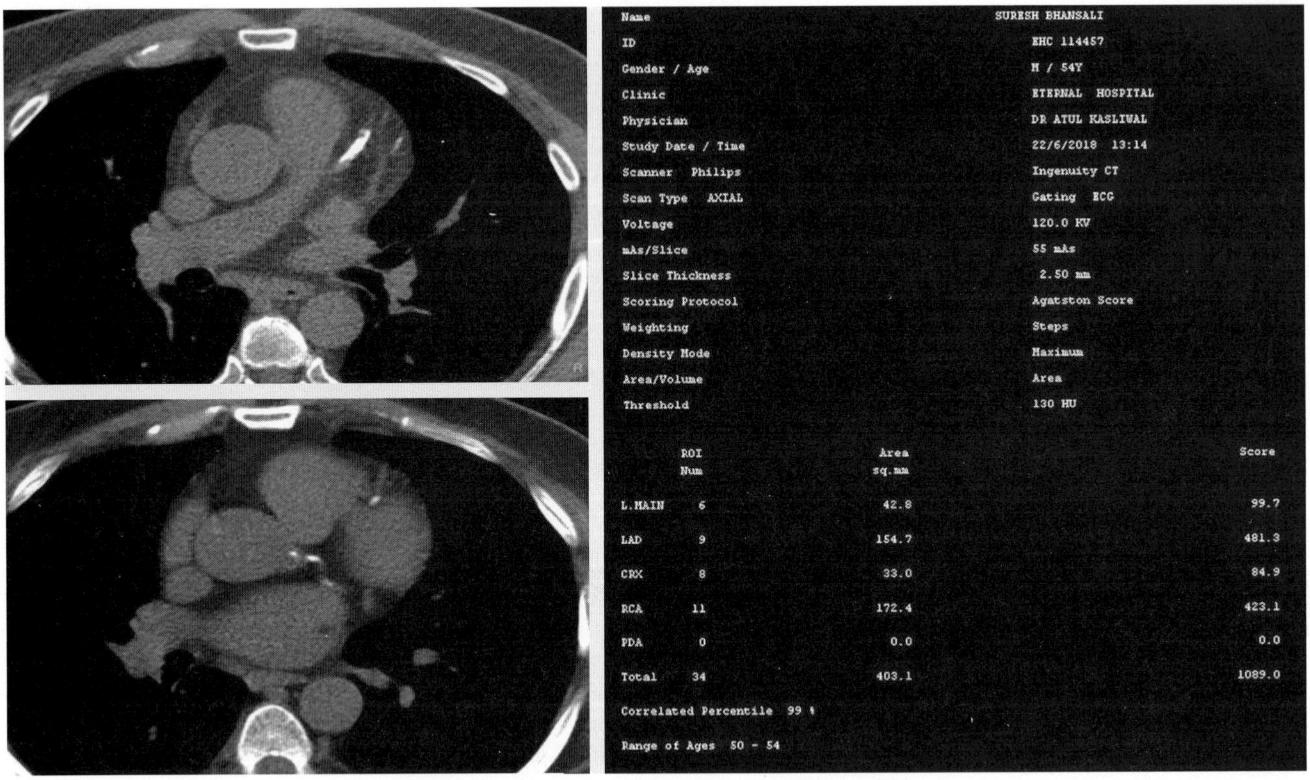

Fig. 3: Coronary calcium score (Agatston score).

stratification.[26,31] The incidence of cardiovascular events reported for patients classified as being at intermediate risk by the Framingham risk score and with an elevated CAC score is equal to or greater than that reported for patients classified as being at high risk by the Framingham risk score and with a low CAC score.[26] The CAC score is also an independent predictor of the risk of major cardiovascular events, with demonstrated superiority over the Framingham risk score, C-reactive protein level, and CIMT.[32,33]

Asymptomatic patients: The use of CAC score is indicated in intermediate-risk group and not in high-risk group as aggressive preventive measures will already be indicated in high-risk asymptomatic patients. Within the low-risk group, a subgroup is identified with a significant long-term risk of a cardiovascular event, for which preventive measures should be adopted. Recent evidence has shown that a family history of premature CAD (in a male first-degree relative <55 years of age or female first-degree relative <65 years of age) is an independent risk factor and is associated with increased atherosclerotic burden.[26] Recommendations for the use of the CAC score in asymptomatic patients, according to the main published guidelines, are summarized in Table 3. The 2010 ACC/AHA guidelines[18] on risk stratification of asymptomatic adults were more favorable for the use of CAC score offering a IIA recommendation for intermediate group patients; however, the 2013 ACC/AHA guidelines[34] give a IIB recommendation implying that a risk-based treatment decision is uncertain and clinical judgment is required. The interpretation methods for CAC score can be classified in two ways—one using absolute values and other based on percentiles adjusted for gender, age, and ethnicity—as shown in Table 4. Clinical interpretation is also shown.[33,35] Both classification systems provide valuable prognostic information.

Coronary artery calcium in guiding treatment: Preliminary retrospective studies and prospective cohort studies have suggested that statin use slows the progression of the CAC score. The consensus statements issued till date do not indicate that the CAC score should be determined as a method of monitoring therapeutic interventions. Various studies have demonstrated the utility of CAC scores in guiding the clinical management of CAD in asymptomatic patients. Although not in the high-risk group, the data by Nasir et al.[36] from MESA study provides reassurance that withholding statins in those with a CAC score of 0 may likely be safe. In addition, the CAC score could be an important tool to avoid statin overtreatment if conventional scores overestimate risk. Studies have shown that a follow-up examination of patients with a CAC score of 0 would not be needed until 4 or 5 years after the initial examination.[37,38]

TABLE 3: Use of coronary artery calcium score in asymptomatic persons.

Guidelines	*Low risk*	*Low risk + diabetes*	*Low risk + family history of premature CAD**	*Intermediate risk*	*High risk*
ACC/SCCT/ACR 2010	Inappropriate	–	Appropriate	Appropriate	Uncertain
ACR 2010	Inappropriate	–	Maybe	Appropriate	Inappropriate
ACC/AHA 2010[18]	IIB	–	–	IIA	–
ESC 2014[19]	–	–	–	IIA	–
ADA 2014	–	IIA	IIA	I	III
SBC/CBR[41]	III	–	–	–	–
ACC/AHA 2013[34]	–	–	–	IIB	–

(ACC: American College of Cardiology; ACR: American College of Roentgenology; ADA: American Diabetes Association; AHA: American Heart Association; CBR: Community-based rehabilitation; ESC: European Society of Cardiology; SBC: Brazilian Society of Cardiology; SCCT: Society of Cardiac Computed Tomography)
*If, after risk assessment, the treatment based on the decision is uncertain, evaluation with the CAC score can be considered in order to define the most appropriate therapeutic strategy.

TABLE 4: Degree of coronary artery calcification by absolute coronary artery calcium score and coronary artery calcium scores adjusted for gender, age, and ethnicity, with clinical interpretation.

Degree of CAC	*Absolute CAC score (Agatston)*	*Sex-adjusted CAC score (Agatston)*	*Clinical interpretation*
Absent	0	0	Very low risk of future coronary events
Discrete	1–100	≤75	Low risk of future coronary events; low probability of myocardial ischemia
Moderate	101–400	76–90	Increased risk of future coronary events (aggravating factor); consider reclassifying the individual as high risk
Accentuated	>400	>90	Increased probability of myocardial ischemia

(CAC: coronary artery calcium)

Symptomatic patients: In symptomatic patients, the use of the CAC score alone is limited, and pretest probability should always be given more weightage. The 2007 ACC Foundation/AHA consensus[39] suggested that the CAC score can be used as a filter before the indication for coronary angiography or for hospitalization of patients with chest pain, especially those with atypical symptoms. The consensus published by The National Institute for Health and Clinical Excellence recommends that the CAC score be applied in patients with chest pain who are classified as being at low-to-intermediate risk. If the CAC score is 0, no other examination would be indicated; if the score is between 1 and 400, the consensus recommends coronary angiography, and if the score is more than 400, coronary angiography would be indicated.[40] Despite the small number of studies involving symptomatic patients, there is evidence that the risk of cardiovascular events is lower in individuals with a CAC score of 0. However, more studies are needed in order to determine the true role of the CAC score, along with other diagnostic methods, such as coronary computed tomography angiography (CCTA) and stress myocardial perfusion imaging, in symptomatic patients.

Diabetes: The presence of any degree of CAC in patients with diabetes mellitus translates to a higher risk of all-cause mortality than in patients without diabetes. Various international guidelines have shown that screening for silent ischemia is not warranted in patients with diabetes and a CAC score less than 100, although it is recommended in those with a CAC score more than 400.[41] Despite the higher cardiovascular risk and higher prevalence of ischemia on functional tests, there is no evidence so far that routine screening for silent ischemia reduces mortality in this group of patients.

MULTIDETECTOR COMPUTED TOMOGRAPHY CORONARY ANGIOGRAPHY

Multidetector computed tomographic coronary angiography or CCTA is a useful first-line diagnostic test for appropriately selected patients with symptoms of angina and a low-to-moderate pretest probability of CAD. Multidetector computed tomography CA, due to its high negative predictive value, improved spatial and temporal resolution, prospective gating with low-radiation protocols, helps to exclude CAD when the clinical diagnosis is doubtful[42] and is considered as gatekeeper to cardiac catheterization laboratory. It is often performed in conjunction with CAC score as a risk stratification tool.[43] Current guidelines do not support the use of CCTA over clinical risk ± CAC scores in asymptomatic patients;[44] however, there is significant additional diagnostic benefit when CCTA is added to standard care for patients with suspected angina and might lead to changes in management that improve long-term survival.[45] It has also been shown to be superior to noninvasive functional testing for detection of angiographically significant coronary stenosis in patients with CAC less than 400.[46,47]

MAGNETIC RESONANCE CORONARY ANGIOGRAPHY

Magnetic resonance (MR) coronary angiography (MRA) at 1.5 T can identify coronary stenosis more than 50% with reasonable certainty[48,49] and identify left main stem and three-vessel CAD in 94% patients.[50] Significant improved diagnostic accuracy has been reported with 3 T contrast-enhanced whole-heart MRA when compared with gold standard X-ray angiography in a single center.[51] Absence of significant stenosis on coronary MRA has also been associated with a low risk of subsequent cardiac events when monitored over 2 years.[52] Though MRI has superior soft tissue differentiation, better temporal resolution, and no radiation, its routine clinical use as a first-line screening tool for atherosclerosis is not recommended owing to increased signal-to-noise ratio, longer can times, difficult image acquisition, high cost, and limited availability. Integration of coronary MRA with other MR functionalities in future can potentially provide a comprehensive evaluation of coronary anatomy, ventricular wall motion, myocardial perfusion, viability, and help in risk assessment.

PLAQUE IMAGING

"Vulnerable plaque" is an atheromatous plaque in wall of an artery that is particularly unstable thrombosis-prone with a high probability of undergoing rapid progression and rupture, thus becoming culprit plaque.[53] Narula et al.[54] compared 105 stable plaques, 88 thin-cap fibroatheromas (TCFA), and 102 ruptured plaques with respect to features of plaque morphology: fibrous cap thickness, percent luminal stenosis, plaque area, necrotic core area, macrophage area, and calcification. Fibrous cap thickness was the best discriminator of plaque type, measuring less than 54 μm in ruptured plaques, 54–84 μm in most TCFA, and more than 84 μm in the stable plaques. Upon exclusion of cap thickness, the best discriminators of TCFA were macrophage infiltration and necrotic core. Thin-cap fibroatheromas less than 65 μm has close resemblance to ruptured plaque but lacks luminal thrombosis and is, therefore, regarded as the most likely precursor lesion to the plaque rupture. Identification of the "vulnerable plaque" can be achieved both invasively and noninvasively. The noninvasive modalities to visualize atherosclerosis are CT coronary angiography (CTCA)/CAC score and MRI. They are used in low-intermediate-risk population, often in primary prevention setting, to facilitate further risk stratification and identify those who may benefit from invasive treatment in addition to medical management. Intravascular ultrasound (IVUS), optical coherence tomography (OCT), near-infrared spectroscopy (NIRS), angioscopy, thermography are all being used for invasive plaque imaging in the high-risk group.[55]

Computed tomographic coronary angiography for plaque imaging: Depending on the attenuation values plaque can be identified as calcified, mixed, and soft plaques by CTCA (*see* Fig. 3). The submillimeter spatial resolution of CTCA enables the assessment of plaque characteristics, including identification of the vulnerable plaques. Motoyama et al. targeted positive remodeling (defined as diameter of plaque 10% larger than reference vessel) and low attenuation plaque (<30 HU) as potential predictors of acute coronary syndromes (ACS). Patients with both factors had a 22.2% chance of developing acute syndromes versus 3.7% for only one of the above and 0.5% chance if a plaque had none of the above features. Positive remodeling and/or low attenuation plaques independently predicted acute coronary events with hazard ratios of 22.8 (95% CI, 6.9–75.2, $p < 0.001$).[56] The napkin-ring sign describes a low attenuation plaque surrounded by a rim of higher attenuation and helps in the prediction of ACS (Fig. 4). Since CTCA has an ability to document significant stenosis and characterize high-risk plaque, it has incremental prognostic value over and above a CAC score, though the magnitude of this benefit varies across studies. Currently, a CTCA should be reserved for low-to-intermediate risk symptomatic patients for whom coronary angiography is not deemed appropriate.

Cardiac magnetic resonance (CMR) imaging: CMR has been mainly used as a functional tool rather than an anatomical tool. There has been restrained utilization of the CMR due to its spatial resolution (1–1.5 mm) and longer acquisition times. Using knowledge from carotid plaques (where plaque hemorrhage and lipid-rich necrotic cores manifest as high

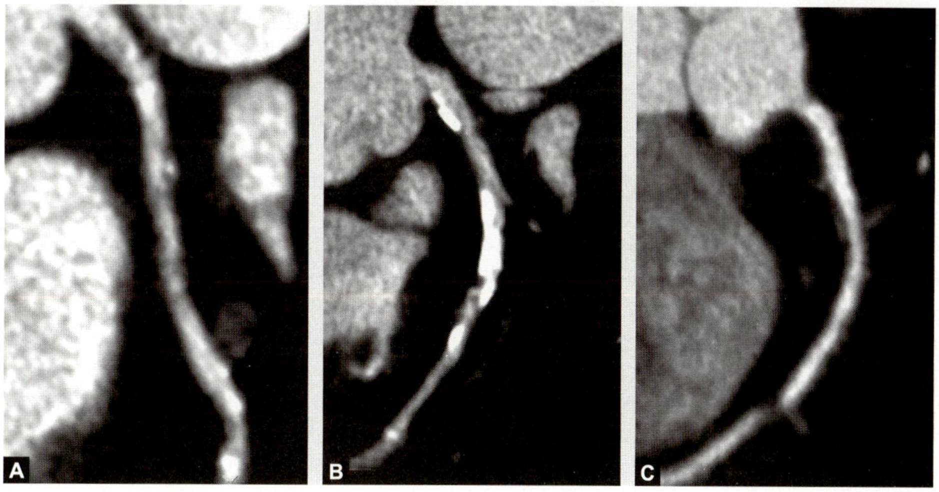

Figs. 4A to C: Curved reformat of coronary vessels showing plaques: (A) Eccentric mixed plaque; (B) Multiple dense calcific plaques; and (C) Eccentric and concentric soft plaques.

signal intensity on T-1 weighted sequence), high-intensity plaques and plaques with plaque to myocardium signal intensity ratio more than or equal to 1.4 independently predicted coronary events.[57] Further prognostic studies with large cohorts are required before CTCA is dethroned as the primary noninvasive imaging modality for visualizing coronary atherosclerosis.

Intravascular ultrasound for plaque imaging: Over the decades, IVUS has been used as a primary invasive tool for coronary plaque assessment, utilizing its superiority over coronary luminography (i.e. coronary angiography). With an axial resolution of 150–250 µm and a lateral resolution of 250 µm, vulnerability has been identified by IVUS. In addition to conventional gray scale IVUS, a new generation of IVUS is available: virtual histology (VH)-IVUS and intravascular ultrasound radiofrequency (IVUS-RF). Given the inherent limitations placed on IVUS by its spatial resolution, a necrotic core more than 10% without evident overlying fibrous tissue and a plaque volume of more than 40% is required as a surrogate for TCFA detection.[58,59] IVUS elastography and palpography have also been used to characterize the stress strain relationship in coronary arteries and plaques. Three-dimensional IVUS assessment of local shear stress has recently been shown to be feasible and might prove to be a useful approach to identify vulnerable plaques and potential sites of upcoming rupture.

Although RF-IVUS–determined TCFA were independent predictors of subsequent ischemic events in the PROSPECT and VIVA (VH-IVUS in Vulnerable Atherosclerosis).[60,61] Because the axial resolution of RF-IVUS is insufficient to accurately measure fibrous cap thickness, RF-IVUS defines TCFA on the basis of the presence of a necrotic core abutting the lumen, without evident overlying fibrous tissue, and plaque volume of more than or equal to 40% on at least three consecutive images. There are significant prognostic data supporting the use of IVUS; furthermore, direct relationships among atherosclerotic burden, progression, and adverse cardiovascular events have been documented. The strength of IVUS is to facilitate real-time decision-making. In a meta-analysis of three randomized controlled trials and 14 observational studies, it was reported that IVUS-guided revascularization resulted in more stents, longer stents, and larger stents—reflecting true assessment of atherosclerotic disease burden and vessel and plaque size.[60] Virtual histology-intravascular ultrasound has also been used to follow-up effect of statin therapy on plaque characteristics, offering not only initial prognostic information, but data on how the vulnerable characteristics of a plaque can be modified by therapy.[61]

OPTICAL COHERENCE TOMOGRAPHY

Optical coherent tomography (OCT) has been used initially in ophthalmology and is now clinically available in cardiology. Compared with IVUS, OCT offers more precise assessment of coronary plaques, utilizing a 10-time greater resolution than that of IVUS (a spatial resolution of 10 µm axially and 20–40 µm laterally). OCT enables the visualization of several important plaque features assisting in determining plaque vulnerability: TCFA, plaque rupture, plaque erosion, lipid core, microcalcification, and neovascularization. Though OCT is superior in regards to assessment of fibrous cap thickness and endothelial assessment, it is unable to give us vessel dimensions, plaque area, or "necrotic core" area, due to limited penetration. There is limited data on the long-term predictive value of OCT for TCFA lesions as it is a younger technology and is more for clinical research and trials. OCT has been used to follow TCFA and demonstrated an increase in the fibrous cap thickness of patients who were treated with lipid lowering therapy.[62]

NEAR-INFRARED SPECTROSCOPY

Near-infrared light can penetrate arterial tissue and the reflected spectral pattern is used to assess the lipid content of arterial walls. Near-infrared spectroscopy (NIRS)—defined lipid-rich plaque has been assessed in various settings.[63] A large lipid core is an essential component of the NIRS-identified vulnerable plaque similar to IVUS and OCT and lipid core burden index (LCBI) is assessed. NIRS can be used to assess coronary lesions not apparent on angiography, such as ulcerated plaques with a recanalized lumen following treatment or identifying culprit vessel in the context of an infarct with multivessel disease. In stable coronary disease, a high LCBI and lipid chemogram can be used to assess vulnerability of a lesion. Oemrawsingh et al. showed that an LCBI value greater than the median of 43 was associated with a four-fold increase in major adverse cardiac events at 12-month follow-up in a prospective study.[64]

THERMOGRAPHY

Intracoronary thermography (ICT) is a catheter-based technique based on the assumption that plaque inflammation and neoangiogenesis produces heat that can be measured at the surface of the plaque with a dedicated catheter.[65] It has ability to identify potential vulnerable and culprit plaques. ICT is able to detect thermal heterogeneity, which has been positively correlated to vulnerable plaque morphology and characteristics such as positive remodeling.[66-68] ICT has several important limitations and is yet to be validated in large prospective trials, but may be used in the future to detect vulnerable or culprit plaques and thus can be used to direct local and/or systemic therapy in patients with CAD.

NUCLEAR IMAGING (SINGLE PHOTON EMISSION CARDIAC TOMOGRAPHY AND POSITRON EMISSION TOMOGRAPHY)

^{18}F-fluorodeoxyglucose (FDG)-positron emission tomography (PET) is noninvasive imaging modality for assessing plaque vulnerability, particularly plaque inflammation. FDG is taken up by macrophages and can be imaged with PET to identify areas of inflammation and vulnerability to rupture.[69] Key limitations of FDG-PET include low specificity of FDG uptake (intense tracer uptake in adjacent myocardium and its poor resolution as compared with MRI or CT). To compensate for this, PET has been coupled with MRI or CT in PET/MRI or PET/CT scanners and, in theory, can provide integrated measurement of factors, including stenosis severity, markers of hemodynamic significance, myocardial viability, plaque burden, and composition. Although nuclear imaging is currently the leading modality for the detection of vulnerable atherosclerotic plaques, repeated radiation exposure limits its widespread use for the longitudinal monitoring of patients with atherosclerotic risk factors, many of whom are women of childbearing age.[70] Thus, future studies should probably concentrate not only on demonstrating the diagnostic accuracy of these techniques but also on investigating their risk/benefit ratio.

CONCLUSION

Cardiovascular epidemiology has traditionally relied on clinical risk assessment tools for prediction of hard cardiovascular events such as ACS, stroke, and mortality (*see* Table 1). These risk scores have not been prospectively evaluated in Indian populations, but positive predictive value of these scores is low. Imaging modalities (*see* Table 2) are potentially useful, especially in the low- and intermediate-risk persons with no symptoms. CIMT and other ultrasound-based techniques are low-cost enterprises and could be a potential game changer. However, prospective studies within India are needed to confirm their importance. Other technologies, which include CT-, MRI-, and isotope-based technologies, are useful but are expensive, especially in India. Gene-based risk prediction tools are being developed and low cost of such technologies could be a game changer.[71] It is important to evaluate all these technologies using scientific and economic tools for use in the common clinical practice.

REFERENCES

1. Gupta R, Xavier D. Hypertension: the most important non-communicable disease risk factor in India. Indian Heart J. 2018;70(4):565-72.
2. Chopra HK, Gupta R. Coronary risk assessment and risk stratification in India. In: Deb PK (Ed). CSI Textbook of Cardiology: The Indian Perspective. New Delhi: Jaypee Brothers Medical Publishers (P) Ltd; 2018. pp. 377-85.
3. Conroy RM, Pyorala K, Fitzgerald AP, et al. Estimation of ten-year risk of fatal cardiovascular disease in Europe: the SCORE project. Eur Heart J. 2003;24:987-1003.
4. Pignoli P, Tremoli E, Poli A, et al. Intimal plus medial thickness of the arterial wall: a direct measurement with ultrasound imaging. Circulation. 1986;74:1399-406.
5. Wikstrand J. Methodological considerations of ultrasound measurement of carotid artery intima media thickness and lumen diameter. Clin Physiol Funct Imaging. 2007;27:341-5.

6. Kanters SD, Algra A, van Leeuwen MS, et al. Reproducibility of in vivo carotid intima media thickness measurements: a review. Stroke. 1997;28:665-71.
7. Stein JH, Korcarz CE, Hurst RT, et al. Use of carotid ultrasound to identify subclinical vascular disease and evaluate cardiovascular disease risk: a consensus statement from the American Society of Echocardiography Carotid Intima-Media Thickness Task Force. Endorsed by the Society for Vascular Medicine. J Am Soc Echocardiogr. 2008;21:93-111, 189-190.
8. Ali YS, Rembold KE, Weaver B, et al. Prediction of major adverse cardiovascular events by age normalized carotid intimal medial thickness. Atherosclerosis. 2006;187:186-90.
9. Chambless LE, Heiss G, Folsom AR, et al. Association of coronary heart disease incidence with carotid arterial wall thickness and major risk factors: the Atherosclerosis Risk in Communities (ARIC) Study, 1987-1993. Am J Epidemiol. 1997;146:483-94.
10. Salonen JT, Salonen R. Ultrasonographically assessed carotid morphology and the risk of coronary heart disease. Arterioscler Thromb. 1991;11:1245-9.
11. O'Leary DH, Polak JF, Kronmal RA, et al. Distribution and correlates of sonographically detected carotid artery disease in the Cardiovascular Health Study. The CHS Collaborative Research Group. Stroke. 1992;23:1752-60.
12. Lorenz MW, Schaefer C, Steinmetz H, Sitzer M. Is carotid intima media thickness useful for individual prediction of cardiovascular risk? Ten-year results from the Carotid Atherosclerosis Progression Study (CAPS). Eur Heart J. 2010;31:2041-8.
13. Lau KK, Chan YH, Yiu KH, et al. Incremental predictive value of vascular assessments combined with the Framingham Risk Score for prediction of coronary events in subjects of low-intermediate risk. Postgrad Med J. 2008;84:153-7.
14. Yeboah J, McClelland RL, Polonsky TS, et al. Comparison of novel risk markers for improvement in cardiovascular risk assessment in intermediate-risk individuals. JAMA. 2012;308:788-95.
15. Simon A, Megnien JL, Chironi G, et al. The value of carotid intima-media thickness for predicting cardiovascular risk. Arterioscler Thromb Vasc Biol. 2010;30:182-5.
16. Lorenz MW, Markus HS, Bots ML, et al. Prediction of clinical cardiovascular events with carotid intima-media thickness: a systematic review and meta-analysis. Circulation. 2007;115:459-67.
17. Den Ruijter HM, Peters SA, Anderson TJ, et al. Common carotid intima media thickness measurements in cardiovascular risk prediction: a meta analysis. JAMA. 2012;308: 796-803.
18. Greenland P, Alpert JS, Beller GA, et al.; American College of Cardiology Foundation and American Heart Association. 2010 ACCF/AHA guideline for assessment of cardiovascular risk in asymptomatic adults: a report of the American College of Cardiology Foundation/American Heart Association Task Force on Practice Guidelines. J Am Coll Cardiol. 2010;56:e50-103.
19. Mancia G, Fagard R, Jaarsma T, et al. Task Force for the management of arterial hypertension of the European Society of Hypertension and the European Society of Cardiology. 2013 ESH/ESC practice guidelines for the management of arterial hypertension. Blood Press. 2014;23:3-16.
20. Touboul PJ, Hennerici MG, Meairs S, et al. Mannheim carotid intima-media thickness and plaque consensus (2004-2006-2011). An update on behalf of the advisory board of the 3rd, 4th and 5th *Watching The Risk* Symposia, at the 13th, 15th and 20th European Stroke Conferences, Mannheim, Germany, 2004, Brussels, Belgium, 2006, and Hamburg, Germany, 2011. Cerebrovasc Dis. 2012;34:290-6.
21. Goff DC, Bennett G, Coady S, et al. American College of Cardiology/American Heart Association Task Force on Practice Guidelines. 2013 ACC/AHA guideline on the assessment of cardiovascular risk: a report of the American College of Cardiology/American Heart Association Task Force on Practice Guidelines. J Am Coll Cardiol. 2014;63:2935-59.
22. Naqvi TZ, Lee MS. Carotid intima-media thickness and plaque in cardiovascular risk assessment. JACC Cardiovasc Imaging. 2014;7:1025-38.
23. O'Leary DH, Polak JF, Kronmal RA, et al. Carotid artery intima and media thickness as a risk factor for myocardial infarction and stroke in older adults. Cardiovascular Health Study Collaborative Research Group. N Engl J Med. 1999;340:14-22.
24. Joseph F, Polak S, Szklo M, et al. Carotid intima-media thickness score, positive coronary artery calcium score, and incident coronary heart disease: the Multi-Ethnic Study of Atherosclerosis. J Am Heart Assoc. 2017;6:e004612.
25. Agatston AS, Janowitz WR, Hildner FJ, et al. Quantification of coronary artery calcium using ultrafast computed tomography. J Am Coll Cardiol. 1990;15:827-32.
26. Nasir K, Clouse M. Role of non-enhanced multidetector CT coronary artery calcium testing in asymptomatic and symptomatic individuals. Radiology. 2012;264:637-49.
27. Budoff MJ, Achenbach S, Blumenthal RS, et al. Assessment of coronary artery disease by cardiac computed tomography: a scientific statement from the American Heart Association Committee on Cardiovascular Imaging and Intervention, Council on Cardiovascular Radiology and Intervention, and Committee on Cardiac Imaging, Council on Clinical Cardiology. Circulation. 2006;114:1761-91.
28. Hong C, Bae KT, Pilgram TK, et al. Coronary artery calcium measurement with multi-detector row CT: in vitro assessment of effect of radiation dose. Radiology. 2002;225:901-6.
29. Yoon HC, Greaser LE, Mather R, et al. Coronary artery calcium: alternate methods for accurate and reproducible quantitation. Acad Radiol. 1997;4:666-73.
30. McCollough CH, Ulzheimer S, Halliburton SS, et al. Coronary artery calcium: a multi-institutional, multi-manufacturer international standard for quantification at cardiac CT. Radiology. 2007;243:527-38.
31. Greenland P, LaBree L, Azen SP, et al. Coronary artery calcium score combined with Framingham score for risk prediction in asymptomatic individuals. JAMA. 2004;291:210-5.
32. Arad Y, Goodman KJ, Roth M, et al. Coronary calcification, coronary disease risk factors, C-reactive protein, and

atherosclerotic cardiovascular disease events: the St. Francis Heart Study. J Am Coll Cardiol. 2005;46:158-65.
33. Budoff MJ, Nasir K, McClelland RL, et al. Coronary calcium predicts events better with absolute calcium scores than age-sex-race/ethnicity percentiles: MESA (Multi-Ethnic Study of Atherosclerosis). J Am Coll Cardiol. 2009;53:345-52.
34. Goff DC Jr, Lloyd-Jones DM, Bennett G, et al. 2013 ACC/AHA guideline on the assessment of cardiovascular risk: a report of the American College of Cardiology/American Heart Association Task Force on Practice Guidelines. Circulation. 2014;129(Suppl. 2):S49-73.
35. Neves PO, Andrade J, Monção H. Coronary artery calcium score: current status. Radiol Bras. 2017;50:182-9.
36. Nasir K, Bittencourt MS, Blaha MJ, et al. Implications of coronary artery calcium testing among statin candidates according to American College of Cardiology/American Heart Association cholesterol management guidelines: MESA (Multi-Ethnic Study of Atherosclerosis). J Am Coll Cardiol. 2015;66:1657-68.
37. Miedema MD, Duprez DA, Misialek JR, et al. Use of coronary artery calcium testing to guide aspirin utilization for primary prevention: estimates from the multi-ethnic study of atherosclerosis. Circ Cardiovasc Qual Outcomes. 2014;7:453-60.
38. Blaha MJ, Budoff MJ, Defilippis AP, et al. Associations between C-reactive protein, coronary artery calcium, and cardiovascular events: implications for the JUPITER population from MESA, a population-based cohort study. Lancet. 2011;378:684-92.
39. Greenland P, Bonow RO, Brundage BH, et al. ACCF/AHA 2007 clinical expert consensus document on coronary artery calcium scoring by computed tomography in global cardiovascular risk assessment and in evaluation of patients with chest pain. J Am Coll Cardiol. 2007;49:378-402.
40. Skinner JS, Smeeth L, Kendall JM, et al. NICE guidance. Chest pain of recent onset: assessment and diagnosis of recent onset chest pain or discomfort of suspected cardiac origin. Heart. 2010;96:974-8.
41. Sara L, Szarf G, Tachibana A, et al. II Diretriz de Ressonância Magnética e Tomografia Computadorizada Cardiovascular da Sociedade Brasileira de Cardiologia e do Colégio Brasileiro de Radiologia. Arq Bras Cardiol. 2014;103:1-86.
42. Shaw LJ, Hausleiter J, Achenbach S, et al.; CONFIRM Registry Investigators. Coronary computed tomographic angiography as a gatekeeper to invasive diagnostic and surgical procedures: results from the multicenter CONFIRM (Coronary CT Angiography Evaluation for Clinical Outcomes: an International Multicenter) registry. J Am Coll Cardiol. 2012;60:2103-14.
43. Editorial. Coronary artery calcium scanning: past, present, and future. JACC Cardiovasc Imaging. 2015;8:579-96.
44. Cho I, Chang HJ, Sung JM, et al.; CONFIRM Investigators. Coronary computed tomographic angiography and risk of all-cause mortality and nonfatal myocardial infarction in subjects without chest pain syndrome from the CONFIRM Registry (coronary CT angiography evaluation for clinical outcomes: an international multicenter registry). Circulation. 2012;126:304-13.
45. SCOT-HEART Investigators. CT coronary angiography in patients with suspected angina due to coronar4 heart disease (SCOT-HEART): an open-label, parallel-group, multicentre trial. Lancet. 2015;385:2383-91.
46. Neglia D, Rovai D, Caselli C, et al.; EVINCI Study Investigators. Detection of significant coronary artery disease by noninvasive anatomical and functional imaging. Circ Cardiovasc Imaging. 2015;8:e002179.
47. Arbab-Zadeh A, Di Carli MF, Cerci R, et al. Accuracy of computed tomographic angiography and single-photon emission computed tomography-acquired myocardial perfusion imaging for the diagnosis of coronary artery disease. Circ Cardiovasc Imaging. 2015;8:e003533.
48. Sakuma H, Ichikawa Y, et al. Detection of coronary artery stenosis with whole-heart coronary magnetic resonance angiography. J Am Coll Cardiol. 2006;48:1946-50.
49. Kato S, Kitagawa K, Ishida N, et al. Assessment of coronary artery disease using magnetic resonance coronary angiography: a national multicenter trial. J Am Coll Cardiol. 2010;56:983-91.
50. Kim WY, Danias PG, Stuber M, et al. Coronary magnetic resonance angiography for the detection of coronary stenoses. N Engl J Med. 2001;345:1863-9.
51. Yang Q, Li K, Liu X, et al. 3.0T whole-heart coronary magnetic resonance angiography performed with 32-channel cardiac coils: a single-center experience. Circ Cardiovasc Imaging. 2012;5:573-9.
52. Yoon YE, Kitagawa K, Kato S, et al. Prognostic value of coronary magnetic resonance angiography for prediction of cardiac events in patients with suspected coronary artery disease. J Am Coll Cardiol. 2012;60:2316-22.
53. Naghavi M, Libby P, Falk E, et al. From vulnerable plaque to vulnerable patient: a call for new definitions and risk assessment strategies: Part I. Circulation. 2003;108:1664-72.
54. Narula J, Nakano M, Virmani R, et al. Histopathologic characteristics of atherosclerotic coronary disease and implications of the findings for the invasive and noninvasive detection of vulnerable plaques. J Am Coll Cardiol. 2013;61:1041-51.
55. Pathan F, Negishi K. Prediction of cardiovascular outcomes by imaging coronary atherosclerosis. Cardiovasc Diagn Ther. 2016;6:322-39.
56. Motoyama S, Sarai M, Harigaya H, et al. Computed tomographic angiography characteristics of atherosclerotic plaques subsequently resulting in acute coronary syndrome. J Am Coll Cardiol. 2009;54:49-57.
57. Noguchi T, Kawasaki T, Tanaka A, et al. High-intensity signals in coronary plaques on non-contrast T1-weighted magnetic resonance imaging as a novel determinant of coronary events. J Am Coll Cardiol. 2014;63:989-99.
58. Suh WM, Seto AH, Margey RJP, et al. Intravascular detection of the vulnerable plaque. Circ Cardiovasc Imag. 2011;4:169-78.
59. Nozue T, Yamamoto S, Tohyama S, et al. Statin treatment for coronary artery plaque composition based on intravascular ultrasound radiofrequency data analysis. Am Heart J. 2012;163:191-9.

60. Stone GW, Maehara A, Lansky AJ, et al. A prospective natural history study of coronary atherosclerosis. N Engl J Med. 2011;364:226-35.
61. Calvert PA, Obaid DR, O'Sullivan M, et al. Association between IVUS findings and adverse outcomes in patients with coronary artery disease: the VIVA (VH-IVUS in Vulnerable Atherosclerosis) study. J Am Coll Cardiol Imag. 2011;4:894-901.
62. Hattori K, Ozaki Y, Ismail TF, et al. Impact of statin therapy on plaque characteristics as assessed by serial OCT and grayscale and integrated backscatter IVUS. JACC Cardiovasc Imag. 2012;5:169-77.
63. Erlinge D. Near-infrared spectroscopy for intracoronary detection of lipid-rich plaques to understand atherosclerotic plaque biology in man and guide clinical therapy. J Intern Med. 2015;278:110-25.
64. Oemrawsingh RM, Cheng JM, Garcia-Garcia HM, et al. Near-infrared spectroscopy predicts cardiovascular outcome in patients with coronary artery disease. J Am Coll Cardiol. 2014;64:2510-8.
65. Madjid M, Willerson JT, Casscells SW. Intracoronary thermography for detection of high-risk vulnerable plaques. J Am Coll Cardiol. 2006;47:C80-5.
66. Stefanadis C, Diamantopoulos L, Vlachopoulos C, et al. Thermal heterogeneity within human atherosclerotic coronary arteries detected in vivo: a new method of detection by application of a special thermography catheter. Circulation. 1999;99:1965-71.
67. Toutouzas K, Synetos A, Stefanadi E, et al. Correlation between morphologic characteristics and local temperature differences in culprit lesions of patients with symptomatic coronary artery disease. J Am Coll Cardiol. 2007;49:2264-71.
68. Wainstein M, Costa M, Ribeiro J. Vulnerable plaque detection by temperature heterogeneity measured with a guidewire system: clinical, intravascular ultrasound and histopathologic correlates. J Invasive Cardiol. 2007;19:49-54.
69. Figueroa AL, Subramanian SS, Curry R, et al. Distribution of inflammation within carotid atherosclerotic plaques with high-risk morphological features: a comparison between positron emission tomography activity, plaque morphology, and histopathology. Circ Cardiovasc Imag. 2012;5:69-77.
70. Davies JR, Rudd JHF, Narula J. Radionuclide imaging for the detection of inflammation in vulnerable plaques. J Am Coll Cardiol. 2006;47:C57-68.
71. Khera AV, Kathiresan S. Genetics of coronary artery disease: discovery, biology and clinical translation. Nat Rev Genet. 2017; 18:331-44.

121

CHAPTER

Reducing Cardiovascular Risk in Diabetes from Tsunami Warning to Zebra Line

Tiny Nair

INTRODUCTION

It is estimated that roughly 380 million people suffer from diabetes mellitus worldwide. This number is likely to escalate to around 500 million by 2025 and 600 million by the year 2035. India is likely to be the epicenter of this huge diabetic epidemic with roughly 100 million diabetic by 2025. Addition of a substantial number of patients with impaired fasting glucose and impaired glucose tolerance adds up to the enormity and complexity of the problem.[1,2] Most people with diabetes tend to develop micro- and macrovascular disease over a period of time. While good glycemic control has showed to reduce microvascular complications, such as retinopathy and neuropathy, it seems to have lesser effect on progression of macrovascular disease manifested by the entire spectrum of atherosclerotic cardiovascular (CV) disease (ASCVD): from ischemic heart disease, acute coronary syndrome, heart failure (HF), cerebrovascular accident, and peripheral occlusive vascular disease (POVD). It is estimated that POVD is the most common vascular disease, HF being the second common. Framingham study shows that HF is 2.5 times more common in diabetic men compared to nondiabetic, while it is 5 times more common for a diabetic lady to have HF compared to nondiabetic.[3,4] The reduction of microvascular disease with good control of diabetes is in sharp contrast to the lack of effect on macrovascular complications (ASCVD) is important not just for brainstorming academic sessions but to decide on the optimal strategy, in formulating guidelines for risk reduction at the community level. Data show that the wheel of concept has turned a full 360° from a general high-risk warning to a focused risk stratification for ASCVD in diabetes.

THE SCARE

The patients of diabetes not only have a higher incidence of ASCVD but also higher mortality, younger age of onset of ASCVD, and a higher incidence of associated comorbidities. It is estimated that ASCVD occurs in patients of type 2 diabetes approximately 14.6 years earlier compared to nondiabetic patients. Also the disease tends to be more severe and diffuse in distribution. The spectrum of ASCVD in diabetes ranges from chronic stable angina to ischemic acute cardiac syndromes and finally HF with progressive decline in the systolic function. Haffner et al. in 1998[5] showed that the risk of CV event rate in a diabetic patient is very high and is equivalent to a person who already had a myocardial infarction (MI) in the past. This concept of diabetes being equivalent to CV disease inculcated a sense of fear of impending an unavoidable CV event in the mind of the physician and a sense of hopelessness in the mind of the patient. Coupled with the data showing that reduction of blood sugar has very little to do with control of ASCVD and vascular events, such as MI and stroke, development of ASCVD and CV events tended to be equated as a part of progression of natural history of type 2 diabetes. Subsequent studies failed to confirm this notion. Meta-analysis[6] published in 2009 showed that the risk of future events in an uncomplicated diabetes patient was 30% lower than that of a person who had a previous MI. This indicated that the so-called risk is not homogeneous and that there is likelihood of at least some subgroup of patients who have a much less risk and much less aggressive course of macrovascular disease and CV events.

THE TARGETS: AIRWAY, BREATHING, AND CIRCULATION AND BEYOND

Hyperglycemia or A1c

Type 2 diabetes is diagnosed when the fasting blood sugar is more than 126 mg%, postprandial blood sugar is more than 200 g%, and glycated hemoglobin (HbA1c) is more than 6.5%. It is estimated that for every 1% increase in HbA1c the risk of CV events increases by 11–16%. Overall, relationship between blood sugar levels and CV event rates seem to be weak, nonlinear, and follows a J shape. The correlation between macrovascular disease and HbA1c is linear only when the duration of diabetes is longer than 4 years. The emerging risk factor collaboration group data also show similar results.[7,8] The concept of insulin resistance follows the same line of relationship between CV events and hyperinsulinemia. Insulin resistance and a higher circulating levels of serum insulin and C-peptide levels tend to correlate with increased incidence of ASCVD and CV events. In clinical scenario, the benefit of reduction of MI and stroke in patients of diabetes on treatment with pioglitazone (an agent that reduces insulin resistance) confirms this assumption.

Blood Pressure

Elevated blood pressure (BP) is an important risk factor in presence of diabetes, contributing to development of ASCVD. Cardiovascular events and mortality of atherosclerotic vascular disease have a strong linear correlation with systolic BP (SBP).[9]

Cholesterol Elevation (Dyslipidemia)

Up to two thirds of patients with diabetes have abnormal lipid profile. It is characterized by elevated triglycerides, low high-density lipoproteins, and high apolipoprotein (Apo) B levels. It is also associated with modestly increased low-density lipoprotein (LDL) levels, LDL being more atherogenic with more abundant small dense LDL. Abnormal lipid profile in presence of diabetes increases the risk of ASCVD and hastens its progression. Also CV events tend to be higher in diabetic patients with abnormal lipid profile. The relationship between CV mortality and elevated LDL in diabetes tends to be linear and strong. Treatments with statins have shown to improve outcome.

Inflammatory Markers (High-Sensitivity C-Reactive Protein)

High-sensitivity C-reactive protein (HsCRP) is a biomarker indicative of vascular inflammation. Elevated HsCRP when combined with standard risk score tend to predict CV risk better. Further stratification of risk between low (less than 1 mg/L), intermediate (1–3 mg/L), and high (more than 3 mg/L) can further help in stratifying risk.[10]

Lipoprotein (a)

Lipoprotein (a) (LPA) is an LDL particle with Apo LPA that helps in risk stratification of diabetes. A high level of LPA, more than 30 mg/dL predicts high CV risk.[11]

Imaging

Estimation of coronary artery calcium (CAC) level score gives us a rough idea of the status of degree of coronary atherosclerosis. The Early Identification of Subclinical Atherosclerosis by Noninvasive Imaging Research study examined CAC score among 2,100 patients and showed that addition of CAC score to standard risk predictions increases the predictability.[12]

Carotid Intima Media Thickness

Carotid intima media thickness (CIMT) is an ultrasound measurement of extent of carotid atherosclerotic disease. This indirectly shows overall atherosclerosis and endothelial dysfunction. Large studies have showed that addition of CIMT to traditional risk factors only modestly improves risk prediction.[13]

STRATEGY OF RISK REDUCTION

Overall, it seems that macrovascular complications are more strongly dependent on optimal control of BP and lipid levels along with lifestyle management (weight control, active lifestyle, and smoking avoidance) compared to strict glucose control alone. This is a major "concept shift" in management strategy.

In STENO II trial,[14] the strategy of targeting multiple risk factors (aggressive management) was compared to standard management of diabetes. Intensive multiple risk management of glycemia, BP, lipids, and microalbuminuria (intensive; n = 80) was compared to a standard therapy (conventional; n = 80), over a mean period of 7.8 years resulted in a significant 53% of reduction of the primary composite end point of CV death, nonfatal MI, nonfatal stroke, revascularization, and amputation. This clearly showed that the strategy of "multipronged" intensive therapy, targeting risk factors is better than standard sugar control.

LIPID LOWERING IN DIABETES

There is a total shift of goal in lipid lowering therapy from a "target number" to "target risk" approach. In this strategy, the total risk of a patient is assessed and therapy started. Patients with established ASCVD, known diabetes, those with very high lipid levels, and those with more than 7.5% risk score are considered candidates for statin therapy. It is estimated that lowering of 40 mg% (1 mmol) of LDL cholesterol with statins reduced coronary heart disease mortality by about 20%. In the Collaborative Atorvastatin Diabetes Study trial, the patients of type 2 diabetes with a mean LDL of 110 mg% benefited by 37% reduction of primary composite end points on being treated with 10 mg of atorvastatin compared to placebo. The slightly elevated risk of new-onset diabetes with statins (9% increase in relative risk with all statins across the board) does not reduce the efficacy and benefit of statins in CV prevention of ASCVD or CV events. Today evidence-based medicine dictates that every type 2 diabetic patient should be prescribed a statin unless contraindicated.

BLOOD PRESSURE CONTROL IN DIABETES

It is estimated that roughly about 30% of adult population worldwide has elevated BP. The prevalence of hypertension in diabetes goes up to as high as 57.3%. Presence of hypertension significantly increases the risk of CV events in diabetes. Since renin–angiotensin system axis is closely implicated in the genesis and progression of hypertension in diabetes, an angiotensin convertase enzyme inhibitor or angiotensin receptor blocker (ARB) is considered as a drug of choice in this situation. Angiotensin convertase enzyme inhibitors and ARBs have clearly shown beneficial in lowering BP, prevention of target organ damage, as well as prevent CV events. The "target" BP goals in diabetes had been the subject of lot of controversy. In the Action to Control Cardiovascular Risk in Diabetes (ACCORD)-BP study,[15] patients were randomized to an SBP of less than 140 mm Hg (standard therapy) or less than 120 mm Hg (aggressive therapy). On less than 120 mm Hg (aggressive therapy), the mean attained BP was 133 mm Hg versus 119.3 mm Hg. There was no significant difference in the primary composite outcome between these two groups. In contrast, the Systolic Blood Pressure Intervention Trial (SPRINT)[16,17] randomized patients to an SBP of below 140 mm Hg (standard treatment) or below 120 mm Hg (intensive treatment). The group assigned to intensive treatment had a significantly reduced CV event rate compared to standard therapy.

A meta-analysis,[18] which included three trials including ACCORD and SPRINT, showed that reduction of BP less than 130/80 mm Hg resulted in a 35% decrease in the risk of stroke and a trend for mortality reduction (compared to BP target of 140/85 mm Hg).

DRAWING THE SAFE ZONE (ZEBRA LINE)

In a cohort study published in New England Journal of Medicine 2018, Rawshani et al.[19] from the Department of Molecular and Clinical Medicine, University of Gothenburg, Sweden analyzed the Swedish National Diabetes database of 271,174 type 2 diabetic patient data and matched them with data of 1,355,870 controls. They computed the effect of presence (or absence) of five risk factors—HbA1c, elevated LDL cholesterol, elevated BP, albuminuria, and smoking on the primary outcome. The primary outcomes analyzed were a combination of death, acute MI, stroke, and HF hospitalization. After median follow-up of 5.7 years, the effect of these five risk parameters contributing to the primary outcome was assessed. Among those patients with diabetes who had all five variables within the target range, the hazard ratio for death (1.06), acute MI (0.84), stroke (0.95) was not higher than nondiabetic patients. The risk for hospitalization for HF was consistently high in patients with diabetes even with control risk factors. They also found that an HbA1c level outside the target range was the strongest predictor of stroke and acute MI. Presence of smoking was the strongest prediction of death.

The only parameter that remained unchanged was HF hospitalization. Introduction of sodium-glucose cotransporter (SGLT)-2 inhibitors have clearly shown benefit of HF hospitalization as shown in the Empagliflozin Cardiovascular Outcome Event Trial in Type 2 Diabetes Mellitus Patients–Removing Excess Glucose study.[20]

CONCLUSION

A consistent good control of blood sugar (HbA1c), LDL cholesterol, BP, albuminuria, and smoking can reduce CV risk of a diabetic patient to a level same that of a nondiabetic. This changes the population strategy of trying to search for a magic drug that prevents CV events and ASCVD to simply implementing well-known measures, which are simple but difficult to implement. Proof of addition of SGLT-2 inhibitors to diabetic therapy resulting in a consistent improvement in HF hospitalization seems to overcome the only remaining problem that is not yet overcome.

REFERENCES

1. Guariguata L, Whiting DR, Hambleton I, et al. Global estimates of diabetes prevalence for 2013 and projections for 2035. Diabetes Res Clin Pract. 2014;103:137-49.
2. Tancredi M, Rosengren A, Svensson AM, et al. Excess mortality among persons with type 2 diabetes. N Engl J Med. 2015;373:1720-32.
3. Kannel WB, McGee DL. Diabetes and cardiovascular disease. The Framingham study. JAMA. 1979;241:2035-8.
4. Shah AD, Langenberg C, Rapsomaniki E, et al. Type 2 diabetes and incidence of cardiovascular diseases: a cohort study in 19 million people. Lancet Diabetes Endocrinol. 2015;3:105-13.
5. Haffner SM, Lehto S, Rönnemaa T, et al. Mortality from coronary heart disease in subjects with type 2 diabetes and in nondiabetic subjects with and without prior myocardial infarction. N Engl J Med. 1998;339:229-34.
6. Bulugahapitiya U, Siyambalapitiya S, Sithole J, et al. Is diabetes a coronary risk equivalent? Systematic review and meta-analysis. Diabet Med. 2009;26:142-8.
7. Stratton IM, Adler AI, Neil HA, et al. Association of glycaemia with macrovascular and microvascular complications of type 2 diabetes (UKPDS 35): prospective observational study. BMJ. 2000;321:405-12.
8. Seshasai SR, Kaptoge S, Thompson A, et al. Diabetes mellitus, fasting glucose, and risk of cause-specific death. N Engl J Med. 2011;364:829-41.
9. Cushman WC, Evans GW, Byington RP, et al. Effects of intensive blood-pressure control in type 2 diabetes mellitus. N Engl J Med. 2010;362:1575-85.
10. Ridker PM, Silvertown JD. Inflammation, C-reactive protein, and atherothrombosis. J Periodontol. 2008;79(Suppl.): 1544-51.
11. Hernandez C, Francisco G, Chacon P, et al. Lipoprotein(a) as a risk factor for cardiovascular mortality in type 2 diabetic patients: a 10-year follow-up study. Diabetes Care. 2005;28:931-3.
12. Malik S, Budoff MJ, Katz R, et al. Impact of subclinical atherosclerosis on cardiovascular disease events in individuals with metabolic syndrome and diabetes: the multi-ethnic study of atherosclerosis. Diabetes Care. 2011;34:2285-90.
13. Nambi V, Chambless L, Folsom AR, et al. Carotid intima-media thickness and presence or absence of plaque improves prediction of coronary heart disease risk: the ARIC (Atherosclerosis Risk In Communities) study. J Am Coll Cardiol. 2010;55:1600-7.
14. Gaede P, Vedel P, Larsen N, et al. Multifactorial intervention and cardiovascular disease in patients with type 2 diabetes. N Engl J Med. 2003;348:383-93.
15. Ginsberg SN, Elam MB, Lovato LC, et al.; for the ACCORD Study Group. Effect of combination lipid therapy for type 2 diabetes mellitus. N Engl J Med. 2010;362:1563-74.
16. Wright JT, Jr., Williamson JD, Whelton PK, et al. A randomized trial of intensive versus standard blood-pressure control. N Engl J Med. 2015;373:2103-16.
17. Perkovic V, Rodgers A. Redefining blood-pressure targets—SPRINT starts the marathon. N Engl J Med. 2015;373:2175-8.
18. McBrien K, Rabi DM, Campbell N, et al. Intensive and standard blood pressure targets in patients with type 2 diabetes mellitus: systematic review and meta-analysis. Arch Intern Med. 2012;172:1296-303.
19. Rawshani A, Rawshani A, Franzen S, et al. Risk factors, mortality and cardiovascular outcomes in patients with type 2 diabetes. N Engl J Med. 2018;379:633-44.
20. Zinman B, Wanner C, Lachin JM, et al. EMPA-REG OUTCOME investigators. Empagliflozin, cardio-vascular outcomes, and mortality in type 2 diabetes. N Engl J Med. 2015;373:2117-28.

122

CHAPTER

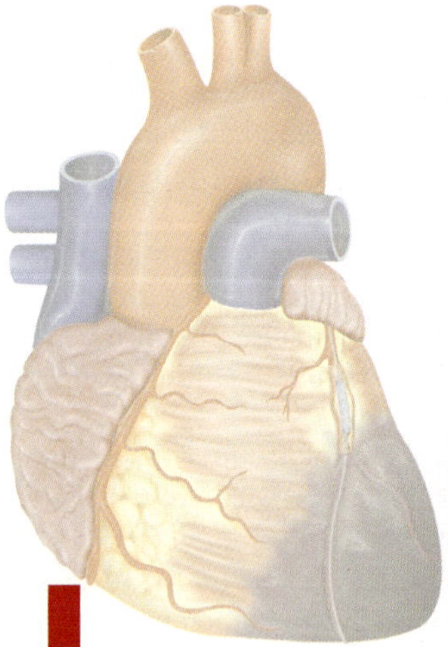

Metabolic Syndrome and C-Reactive Protein

SN Pathak, Rajesh Meena, HK Chopra

INTRODUCTION

Metabolic syndrome (MetS) is a clinical condition characterized by the co-occurrence of abdominal obesity, impaired glucose tolerance, dyslipidemia, and hypertension, associated with a high risk of coronary heart disease (CHD) and mortality.

The National Cholesterol Education Program's Adult Treatment Panel III (ATP III) report identified the following components of the MetS, which relate to cardiovascular (CV) disease (CVD): (1) abdominal obesity, (2) dyslipidemia, (3) hypertension, (4) insulin resistance, (5) proinflammatory state, and (6) prothrombotic state. These components of the MetS are classified into underlying, major, and emerging risk factors. According to ATP III, underlying risk factors for CVD are abdominal obesity, physical inactivity, and an atherogenic diet. The major risk factors are cigarette smoking, raised blood pressure, high low-density lipoprotein (LDL) cholesterol, low high-density lipoprotein cholesterol, family history of premature CHD, and aging. The emerging risk factors include elevated triglycerides, small LDL particles, insulin resistance, glucose intolerance, proinflammatory state, and prothrombotic state.[1]

C-REACTIVE PROTEIN

C-reactive protein (CRP) is considered to be a major inflammatory cytokine that functions as a nonspecific defense mechanism in response to tissue injury or infection. Synthesized mainly in the liver, CRP activity is stimulated by other cytokines, especially interleukin (IL)-6, IL-1β, and tumor necrosis factor-α. CRP binds to a variety of molecules, particularly liposomes and lipoproteins, such as LDL and very LDL cholesterol, and is a powerful activator of the classic complement system. Accumulating evidence suggests that CRP, which is also found within macrophages of atheromatous plaques, is causally or mechanistically related to atherothrombosis. Higher values of high-sensitivity CRP (hs-CRP) are associated with MetS and its components and provide additional prognostic information on future development of CV events in them (Fig. 1).

C-reactive protein has become the subject of avid interest in recent years, but the history of CRP began more than seven decades ago and has been one of discovery and continuing dispute. In 1930, Tillet and Francis[2] observed a substance in the serum of people with pneumococcal infections that formed a precipitate when mixed with the C-polysaccharide coat of *Streptococcus pneumoniae*. This

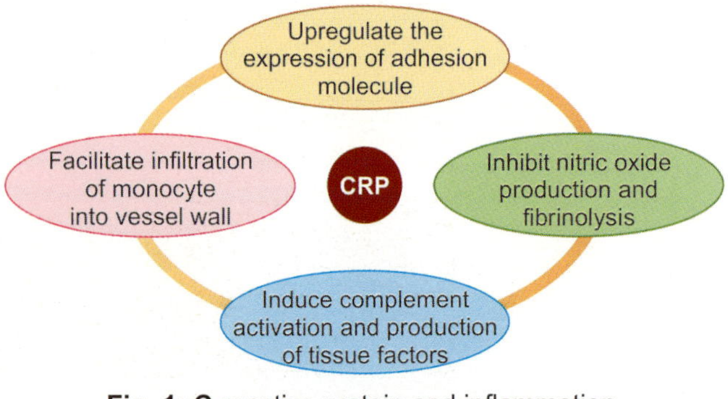

Fig. 1: C-reactive protein and inflammation.
Source: Egypt Heart J. 2015;67:89-97.

"C-reactive" activity was absent from the sera of healthy individuals. MacLeod and Avery[3] subsequently found this substance to be a protein and coined the term "acute phase" to characterize the serum of patients with various acute infections. Lofstrom[4] found a similar acute-phase response in acute and chronic inflammatory conditions, and CRP became recognized as a nonspecific acute-phase protein. In healthy individuals, CRP levels are only minimal. Under acute conditions, levels of CRP in the circulation increase during the first 6–8 hours and reach a peak value after approximately 48 hours.[5]

C-reactive protein is an effective clinical marker because of its analytical stability, reproducible results, and commercial availability of high-sensitivity assays with good precision. Recent studies suggest that CRP may have direct proinflammatory effects and contributes to the initiation and progression of atherosclerotic lesions. Functionally, CRP activates circulating monocytes and induces their recruitment to the arterial wall. It also mediates LDL uptake by macrophages and induces expression of cell-adhesion molecules and tissue factor. Latest epidemiological studies have supported the significance of CRP level in predicting future CV risk. Low-grade inflammation is characteristic of the MetS. CRP, the best characterized biomarker of inflammation, is also an independent predictor of future CV events. MetS is associated with an up to five times increased risk of type 2 diabetes mellitus and an approximately twofold increased risk of CVD.[6]

C-REACTIVE PROTEIN CAN PREDICT CARDIOVASCULAR EVENT

A progressive rise in CRP can reflect augmented stages of vascular inflammation. A wealth of data suggests that chronic inflammation is a major factor that drives the progression of atherosclerosis and atherothrombosis.[7,8] Elevated CRP levels are associated with diminished expression of endothelial nitric oxide (NO) synthase, which may attenuate production of NO, promote oxidative modification of LDL, and induce expression of plasminogen activator inhibitor-1 (Fig. 2).[9]

C-REACTIVE PROTEIN IN CLINICAL PRACTICE

C-reactive protein is among the most rapidly acting acute-phase proteins and has a prolonged elimination half-life of ~19 hours.[10] Concentrations of CRP usually appear to rise rapidly in proportion to the degree and severity of inflammatory stimuli.[11] However, thus far, diurnal levels appear to be stable, and CRP concentrations are similarly distributed among men and women, except for women on hormone replacement therapy.[12] These properties of CRP would appear to render this analyte ideal to detect the occurrence of various inflammatory, infectious, and other acute pathological processes. However, elevations of CRP may be uncommon in the absence of traditional risk factors for CHD.[13] CRP elevations may therefore be attributable to and already accounted for by traditional risk factors. A recent meta-analysis of studies of CRP and other circulating markers of inflammation in CHD risk prediction concluded that CRP may be a somewhat moderate predictor of CHD risk.[14] The Centers for Disease Control and Prevention and the American Heart Association have published combined evidence-based guidelines for the optimal use of CRP in clinical practice.[15] These guidelines confirm that, although hs-CRP measurement may be useful as an independent marker of prognosis for recurrent events, this analyte

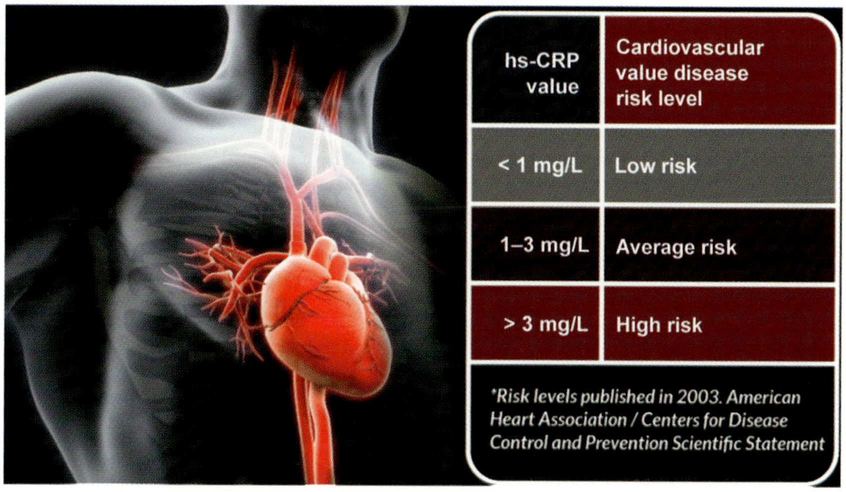

Fig. 2

Source: Danesh J, Wheeler JG, Hirschfield GM, et al. C-reactive protein and other circulating markers of inflammation in the prediction of coronary heart disease. N Engl J Med. 2004;350(14):1387-97.

should not be used at present for routine screening, and application of secondary prevention measures should not be influenced by hs-CRP determination. However, in intermediate-risk patients without known CHD but with 10-year risk for CHD of 10–20%, the guidelines suggest that measurement of hs-CRP may be considered an independent marker of CHD risk and may be useful, at the discretion of the physician, to help determine optimal treatment. Patients are categorized according to hs-CRP level as follows: less than 1 mg/L = low risk, 1.0–3.0 mg/L = average risk, and more than 3.0 mg/L = high risk. The report of the ATP III panel of the National Cholesterol Education Program also addressed the clinical use of CRP. This report does not recommend routine measurement of CRP for the purpose of modifying LDL cholesterol goals in primary prevention. However, because CRP may have predictive power beyond the classical lipid risk factors, this report indicates that some investigators consider lowering LDL cholesterol more aggressively in adults with elevated levels of CRP than may otherwise be indicated by an evaluation solely of the major risk factors. The 2004 update to the ATP III guidelines also suggests that CRP measurements may be useful as a guide to treatment targets. Thus a patient with an hs-CRP more than 3 mg/L would be allocated to the moderately high-risk category for CVD, even with unremarkable lipid levels.[16] Whichever guidelines are used, CRP as a nonspecific marker of inflammation must always be interpreted under the clinical conditions of the patient undergoing assessment.

REFERENCES

1. Int J Clin Biochem Res. 2015;2(3):162-5.
2. Tillet WS, Francis T. Serological reaction in pneumonia with a non-protein somatic fraction of pneumococcus. J Exp Med. 1930;52:561-71.
3. MacLeod CM, Avery OT. The occurrence during acute infections of a protein not normally present in the blood. II. Isolation and properties of the reactive protein. J Exp Med. 1943;73:183-91.
4. Lofstrom G. Comparison between the reaction of acute phase serum with pneumococcus C-polysaccaride and with pneumococcus type 27. Br J Exp Pathol. 1944;25:21-6.
5. Falk E. Why do plaques rupture? Circulation. 1992;86(6 Suppl.):III30-42.
6. Grundy SM. Pre-diabetes, metabolic syndrome, and cardiovascular risk. J Am Coll Cardiol. 2012;59(7):635-43.
7. Ross R. Atherosclerosis: an inflammatory disease. N Engl J Med. 1999;340:115-26.
8. Libby P, Ridker PM, Maseri A. Inflammation and atherosclerosis. Circulation. 2002;105:1135-43.
9. Verma S, Wang CH, Li SH, et al. A self-fulfilling prophecy: C-reactive protein attenuates nitric oxide production and inhibits angiogenesis. Circulation. 2002;106:913-9.
10. Vigushin DM, Pepys MB, Hawkins PN. Metabolic and scintigraphic studies of radioiodinated human C-reactive protein in health and disease. J Clin Invest. 1993;91:1351-7.
11. Yue CC, Muller-Greven J, Dailey P, et al. Identification of a C-reactive protein binding site in two hepatic carboxylesterases capable of retaining C-reactive protein within the endoplasmic reticulum. J Biol Chem. 1996;271:22245-50.
12. Ledue TB, Rifai N. Preanalytic and analytic sources of variations in C-reactive protein measurement: implications for cardiovascular disease risk assessment. Clin Chem. 2003;49:1258-71.
13. Miller M, Zhan M, Havas S. High attributable risk of elevated C-reactive protein level to conventional coronary heart disease risk factors: the Third National Health and Nutrition Examination Survey. Arch Intern Med. 2005;165:2063-8.
14. Danesh J, Wheeler JG, Hirschfield GM, et al. C-reactive protein and other circulating markers of inflammation in the prediction of coronary heart disease. N Engl J Med. 2004;350:1387-97.
15. Pearson TA, Mensah GA, Alexander RW, et al. Markers of inflammation and cardiovascular disease: application to clinical and public health practice. A statement for healthcare professionals from the Centers for Disease Control and Prevention and the American Heart Association. Circulation. 2003;107:499-511.
16. Grundy SM, Cleeman JI, Bairey Merz CN, et al.; for the Coordinating Committee of the National Cholesterol Education Program. Implications of recent clinical trials for the National Cholesterol Education Program Adult Treatment Panel III Guidelines. J Am Coll Cardiol. 2004;44:720-32.

123

CHAPTER

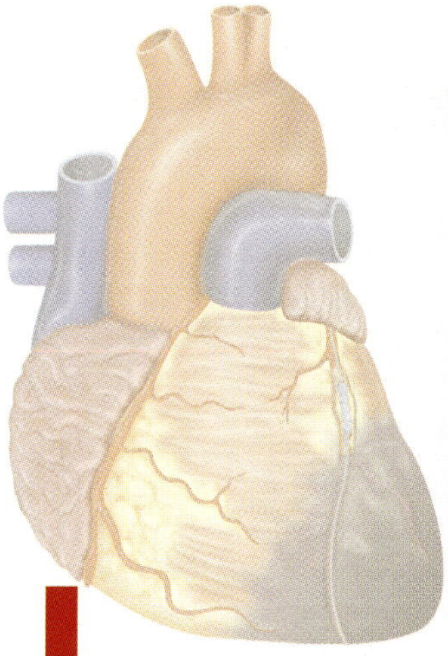

Biomarker B-type Natriuretic Peptide Imaging in Heart Failure

Srikant Sharma, HK Chopra, M Srihari Babu, Surabhi Awasthi, Nisarg Patel

INTRODUCTION

B-type natriuretic peptide (BNP) is a protein hormone, one among the nine natriuretic peptides (seven are atrial in origin). Atrial NP (ANP) is produced from muscle cells of atria, BNP is produced from ventricles, C-type NP produced from blood vessels, and dynamic nuclear polarization is formed in blood plasma. They reduce adrenaline, angiotensin, and aldosterone leading to decreased heart rate and vasodilation. They are natural defense designed to protect heart from stress. PreproBNP is a 134-amino-acid-preprohormone from which ProBNP is formed, which thereafter is cleaved by corin into N-terminal (NT) ProBNP and *biological active 32-amino acid polypeptide BNP.* Once released, BNP binds and activates NP receptor (NPR)-A (atrial natriuretic factor receptor) and to a lesser extent NPR-B and NPR-C receptors. Binding of NP induces a conformational change in the receptor that causes receptor dimerization and activation. This causes the conversion of guanosine triphosphate (GTP) to cyclic guanosine 3′–5′ cyclic monophosphate (GMP) and raises intracellular cyclic GMP, which *activates a cyclic GMP-dependent kinase Protein Kinase G.* These lead to actions, such as *natriuresis, vasodilatation, increase glomerular filtration rate (GFR), increase renal blood flow, enhancement of ventricular relaxation, antifibroblastic, antiproliferative, antithrombotic, suppression of renin-angiotensin-aldosterone system (RAAS), and sympathetic nervous system.*[1] Natriuretic peptide receptor-C functions mainly as a clearance receptor by binding and sequestering BNP from the circulation. Neutral endopeptidase also known as neprilysin is the enzyme that metabolizes NP, less than or equal to 5% is excreted via kidney. N-terminal ProBNP relies solely on kidney for excretion (Fig. 1).

There are *three volume-regulating systems*, two salt-saving systems—the RAAS and renal sympathetic system (RSS)—and the third is salt-excreting NP, a hormone system. When the vascular space contracts, the RASS and RSS are turned on; when the atria expands, NP are turned on. B-type natriuretic peptide *inhibits cardiac hypertrophy* and remodeling. Although hypertension can cause cardiac hypertrophy, the level of hypertrophy in NPR-A-deficient mice is significantly greater than others with similar hypertension, suggesting that NPR-A elicits a local growth inhibitory signal in heart. Knowles et al. (2001) showed that NPR-A knockout mice have enlarged heart even when they are treated effectively with antihypertensive drugs since birth. B-type natriuretic peptide and NT-ProBNP are detected by specific assays, biochemically, or by mass spectrometry. B-type natriuretic peptide half-life is 20 minutes; hence, it reflects current ventricular status (NT-ProBNP half-life is 1–2 hours). The biological half-life of BNP is longer than ANP, and that of NT-ProBNP is even longer, making these peptides better targets for diagnostic. B-type natriuretic peptide and NT-ProBNP, both peptides, show similar accuracy in three studies,[2,3] and BNP was superior to NT-ProBNP in one study. This study exclusively enrolled patients above the age of 65 years;[4] therefore, BNP seems to have an advantage in elderly patients.

Physiologic effects: NP has following functions in different organs:

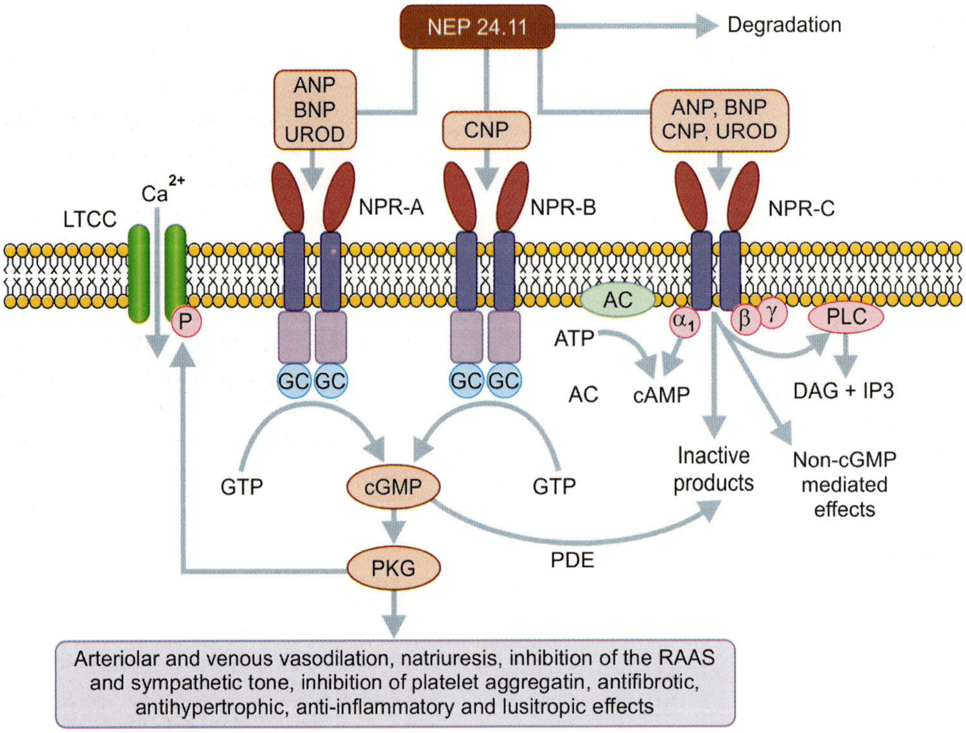

ANP: atrial natriuretic peptide; BNP: B-type natriuretic peptide; CNP: C-type natriuretic peptide; cGMP: cyclic guanosine monophospate; DAG: diacilglicerol; GC: guanylylcyclase-A; GMP: guanosine monophosphate; GTP: guanosine triphosphate; IP3: inositol 1, 4, 5-trifosfato; LTCC: L-type calcium channel; NEP: neprilysin (neutral endopeptidase); NPR: natriuretic peptide receptor; PDE: phosphodiesterase; PKG: protein kinase G; PLC: phospholypase C; RAAS: renin-angiotensin-aldosterone system; UROD: Urodilatine

Fig. 1

- *Renal*: It dilates afferent and constricts efferent arteriole and relaxes mesangial cells, leading to increase GFR, resulting in greater filtration of sodium and water. In vasa recta, flow increases, and due to lower osmolarity of medullary interstitium, less tubular reabsorption leads to increased excretion of sodium and water and decreased sodium reabsorption of distal convoluted tubule and collecting duct, via GMP-dependent phosphorylation of epithelial sodium channel. Natriuretic effect is affected by dopamine, and dopamine receptor D1 activity inhibits renin secretion, thereby inhibiting RAAS. This inhibits renal sympathetic nervous system.
- *Adrenal*: It decreases aldosterone secretion by zona glomerulosa of adrenal cortex.
- *Vascular*: It relaxes vascular smooth muscles of arterioles and venules by membrane receptor-mediated elevation of cyclic guanosine monophosphate (cGMP). Catecholamines inhibition promotes uterine spiral artery remodeling, which prevents pregnancy-induced hypertension.
- *Cardiac*: It inhibits maladaptive cardiac hypertrophy.
- *Adipose tissue*: It increases the release of free fatty acid from adipose tissue, increases intracellular cGMP levels that induce the phosphorylation of a hormone-sensitive lipase and perilipin A via the activation of a cGMP-dependent protein kinase-I, and does not modulate cyclic adenosine monophosphate production or protein kinase A activity.

HISTORY OF NPs

Kisch (1956) found that atrial cells contained highly developed Golgi networks, similar to secretary cells. Henry et al. (1956) revealed that balloon distension of the atria correlated with increased urination of dogs. De bold et al. (1981) showed that atrial extracts contain a potent blood pressure–decreasing component that stimulates renal sodium and water excretion. This was the first NP discovery. Thereafter, several names were given to this peptide as atrial natriuretic factor, atriopeptin, cardionatrin, and cardiodilantin. The second member discovered in this family was BNP, originally called brain NP, because it was purified and sequenced from porcine brain (Sudoh et al., 1988). Subsequently, Mukoyama et al. (1991) found that BNP was more concentrated in cardiac ventricles of heart failure (HF) patients, rather than in normal subjects (BNP as low as 1 fmol/mL). The gene-encoding human BNP, NP precursor B (Gene ID 4879), is located on chromosome 1 at 1p36. The current indication for BNP measurements in HF from American College of Cardiology (ACC)/American Heart Association (AHA) guidelines, for diagnosis (acute and ambulatory) and prognosis (acute and ambulatory), is I-A class-level of evidence.

HEART FAILURE AND B-TYPE NATRIURETIC PEPTIDE

The ACC foundation/AHA guidelines define HF as *a complex clinical syndrome that results from any structural or functional impairment of ventricular filling or ejection of blood.* Four clinical stages of development of HF have been recognized. Stage A occurs in individuals at risk but without structural heart disease or HF symptoms. Stage B includes evidence of structural heart disease without HF symptoms. Stage C is associated with HF, and Stage D includes severe end-stage HF. Heart failure with Stages C and D are associated with increased blood levels of BNP,[5-8] with the onset of pulmonary edema, and rise in plasma levels of cGMP.

Comparison between HF with reduced ejection fraction (EF) and HF with preserved EF: In comparison with reduced EF HF, population with preserved HF were older, female, presented higher serum NT-ProBNP levels at hospitalization, had longer length of hospital stay, showed lower proportion of presenting pulmonary edema, but with accurate and equal predictive ability for in-hospital mortality in both groups.[9]

Heightened release of BNP is a direct consequence of mechanical stretch of atrial muscle.[10] It may be that changes in atrial dimensions rather than atrial pressure stimulate NP release. Hence, NP is also increased in atrial fibrillation, supraventricular tachycardia, and after pericardiocentesis.

Diagnostic Implications

Advanced HF can be diagnosed from clinical grounds, electrocardiography, chest X-ray, and echocardiogram (ECHO). But mild HF diagnosis is difficult to diagnose as it may mimic lung disease, kidney disease, or liver disease. In this situation, symptoms are nonspecific, and typical findings of HF are present in <50% of patients.[11,12] Heart failure is usually diagnosed in persons with known heart disease who presents with nonspecific symptoms (breathlessness, ankle swelling) and signs (basal lung crepitation). Thereafter, left ventricular (LV) EF (LVEF) by ECHO is measured. Few patients, such as elderly, females, have preserved EF HF (diastolic HF). To diagnose these in patients is sometime difficult. B-type natriuretic peptide increases when cardiac myocytes are strained; therefore, BNP is an effective method for detecting HF with or without systolic dysfunction. A recent European Society of Cardiology Guideline[13] suggested stagewise approach to ambulatory suspicious HF patients with initial BNP levels and was followed by ECHO in patients with elevated values of BNP. B-type natriuretic peptide monitoring in HF also correlates with pulmonary capillary wedge pressure.[14] Original studies by Troughton et al.,[15] Maisel et al.,[16] Januzzi et al.,[17] and others demonstrated that NPs are extremely useful in the diagnosis of HF. Normal level of NT-ProBNP, as per *Cleveland clinic's reference range*, is <125 pg/mL for patients aged 0–74 years; and <450 pg/mL for patient's aged >75 years. B-type natriuretic peptide of <100 pg/mL rules out of HF. B-type natriuretic peptide levels >450 pg/mL for <50 years, >900 pg/mL in 50–75 years, and >1,200 pg/mL in >75 years support HF diagnosis in 90% of time. Normal BNP excludes HF by 98%. Between normal and HF zone is the gray zone.

In other large validating study, BNP and NT-ProBNP levels, as in Boxes 1 and 2, were found to be diagnostic with high accuracy.

In patients with kidney disease with *GFR of<60 mL/min, 200–225 pg/mL* is the appropriate cutoff value to rule out HF.[18,19] In patients with severe *obesity with body mass index (BMI) more than 35, BNP cutoff value of 60 pg/mL* to rule out, and 200 pg/mL to rule in HF is the cause of dyspnea.[20,21] In *intensive care unit, BNP lower cutoff of 150 pg/mL* to rule out HF as the cause of respiratory failure, and 600 pg/mL as a reasonable higher cutoff value to rule in HF.[22-24]

B-type natriuretic peptide–increased levels in noncardiac cases are: Increased age, female gender, and genotype. A single-nucleotide polymorphism in the promoter region

BOX 1: Interpretation of BNP levels in patients with acute dyspnea.

Always in conjunction with other clinical information

<100 pg/mL	100–400 pg/mL	>400 pg/mL
↓	↓	↓
No HF	Clinical evaluation	HF
	↓ No HF ↓↓↓ HF	↓
		→ Diuretics Nitrates

(*Source*: Maisel et al.)

BOX 2: Interpretation of NT-pro BNP levels in patients with acute dyspnea.

Always in conjunction with other clinical information

<300 pg/mL	Age <50	>450 pg/mL
↓	50–75	>900 pg/mL
No HF	>75	>1800 pg/mL
		↓
		HF

(*Source:* Wright et al.)

of the *BNP gene* (rs 198389; also referred to as T-381C) *was associated with 30% higher BNP* levels per C allele.[13,25-29] B-type natriuretic peptide also increases in lung disease, advanced liver disease, overactive thyroid, cortisol excess, brain hemorrhage, certain tumors, chronic hypoxia, renal failure (reduced clearance),[30] pulmonary embolism, and pulmonary hypertension.[31-33]

B-type natriuretic peptide–increased levels in cardiac cases are: Acute coronary syndrome, valvular heart disease (aortic stenosis, mitral regurgitation), and high blood pressure with LV hypertrophy; atrial fibrillations are also the causes of high BNP. B-type natriuretic peptides are also high in diastolic dysfunction, hypertrophic cardiomyopathy, or associated systolic dysfunction. B-type natriuretic peptide also correlated with ECHO finding includes LV mass index, end diastolic volume, and isometric relaxation time.

Decreased BNP level is seen in obesity and in the use of angiotensin-converting enzyme (ACE) inhibitors, diuretics, and beta blockers.

In the setting of acute HF, the contribution of these above factors is small compared to the impact of cardiac overload so that *even single, unadjusted BNP values can provide very good diagnostic yield.* In the setting of asymptomatic disease, however, the contribution of these other factors is more relevant, and adjusting may significantly improve test characteristics (Table 1).[29,34]

The diagnosis of HF with BNP, in patients with dyspnea in either *urgent care or ambulatory setting,* is among the strongest indication, with *class I level of evidence, as per ACC/AHA guidelines.*

Guidelines by European Society of Cardiology indicate that evidence supports the use of NPs, for the *diagnosis, staging, making hospitalization/discharge decisions, and identifying patients at risk* of clinical events. The evidence for their use in monitoring and adjusting drug therapy is less clearly established.[35]

A study "Breathing Not Properly" trial evaluated 1,586 *emergency dyspneic patients* and demonstrated that BNP threshold of 100 pg/mL could distinguish between a diagnosis of HF and other causes of dyspnea, with high degree of accuracy.[16] Similar data from PRIDE (ProBNP investigation of Dyspnea in the Emergency department) study support the accuracy of NT-ProBNP for diagnosis in the same setting,[17] although age-specific threshold (NT-ProBNP > 450 pg/mL for patients <50 years of age and more than 900 pg/mL for >50 years of age) has been proposed. Interpretation of results must take in consideration, e.g. decrease levels in obesity and increased levels in chronic kidney disease, aging, acute pulmonary emboli, acute coronary syndrome, genotype preponderance, etc.

TABLE 1: Indication of natriuretic peptide measurement in HF.

Indications	*ACC/AHA recommendation class level of evidence*
Diagnosis in patients with dyspnea (acute)	I-A
Diagnosis in patients with dyspnea (ambulatory)	I-A
Prognosis in patients with known HF (acute)	I-A
Prognosis in patients with known HF (ambulatory)	I-A
Achieving guideline-directed medical therapy (ambulatory)	IIa-B
Natriuretic peptide guided therapy for chronic HF	IIb-B

Class I: Conditions for which there is evidence and/or general agreement that a given procedure or treatment is useful and effective; Class IIa: Weight of evidence/opinion is in favor of usefulness/efficacy; Class IIb: Usefulness/efficacy is less well established by evidence/opinion. Level of Evidence: A: Recommendation on the basis of evidence from multiple randomized trials or meta-analyses; Level of Evidence; B: Recommendation on the basis of evidence from a single randomized trial or nonrandomized studies.

(ACC/AHA: American College of Cardiology/American Heart Association; HF: heart failure)

B-Type Natriuretic Peptide in Risk Population

Wang et al. showed in the Framingham Offspring study that in *asymptomatic individuals,* BNP elevations well below levels used in the diagnosis of acute HF were associated with increased risk of death, first cardiovascular event, HF, atrial fibrillation, and stroke or transient ischemic attack, after adjustment for cardiovascular risk factors.[36] There is an increasing interest in using BNP measurement to target at *risk population,* without HF, for preventing strategy. Two randomized clinical trials, PONTIAC (NT-ProBNP Guide of Primary Prevention of Cardiovascular Events in Diabetic Patients)[37] and STOP-HF (Screening to Prevent HF),[38] have demonstrated improvement in clinical outcome; with a strategy of using BNP to identify high-risk patients for more aggressive HF prevention strategy. Hence, BNP screening in specific populations at higher risk, e.g. patients with coronary artery disease, hypertension, diabetes, or elderly, may be cost effective. McKie et al. confirm in a *general population* of Olmsted County, MN, that higher BNP and NT-ProBNP levels are associated with increased mortality even after adjusting for risk factors and echocardiographic parameters including systolic and diastolic dysfunction, LV hypertrophy, and left atrial enlargement.[39] There was a small number of subjects with BNP levels in the highest tertile without risk factors or echocardiographic abnormalities; these individuals did not show higher mortality. This could be explained by the impact of genetic contribution. In *asymptomatic patients,* the relative risk of death during the *4–5 years of follow-up* approximately doubled in patients with BNP value higher than in relatively low cutoff levels.[36,40] B-type natriuretic peptide levels average 12 pg/mL in patient who turned out to have healthy coronary arteries, but they averaged 16, 19, and 39 pg/mL, respectively, in patients who had blockages in one, two, or three of their *coronary arteries.* Patients who are admitted for acute coronary syndrome, high BNP level, predicted a high risk of mortality during the next 2 years. B-type natriuretic peptide levels in *mitral insufficiency* are correlated with mortality and the onset of congestive HF, regardless of the degree of regurgitation present on ECHO, suggesting that BNP is a reflection of atrial and ventricular consequences. B-type natriuretic peptide is also correlated with symptoms and echocardiographic severity of mitral stenosis.[33] Increased levels of NT-ProBNP were associated with *increased Trop-I, peak creatine kinase-MB, and low LVEF.*[41] Henriksen et al.[42] showed that BNP correlated with *severity of hepatic cirrhosis* and with heart dysfunction.[43] A study on *liver transplant patients* determines that higher BNP levels (>391 pg/mL) immediately post-transplant (on day 1) appeared to be an early marker for heart dysfunction related to liver cirrhosis.[44]

Prognostic Implications

Prognostic studies have shown that BNP levels measured after treatment were more predictive for the risk of death or cardiovascular events than those initiated at first presentation.[45,46] The BNPs are among the most powerful prognostic markers in all forms of clinical HF, including HF with reduced EF,[47] with preserved EF,[48] and acute HF.[49] In acute setting, both elevations of the initial value at the time of presentation[49] and changes with therapy (value at hospital discharge) are strong predictors of short-[50] and long-term outcomes.[51] The persistence higher than 5,000 pg/mL NT-ProBNP levels long after decongestion portends poor outcomes regardless of relative changes, as per PROTECT (ProBNP Outpatient Tailored Chronic HF Trial).[52] For chronic cases, in the data from Valsartan Heart Failure Trial (Val-HeFT), both baseline values and changes over 3 months in BNP and NT-ProBNP have been shown to be among the most powerful predictors of future outcome.[53] Miller et al. investigated whether baseline cardiac troponin T and BNP as well as changes over time were predictive of outcome (death, cardiac transplantation, hospitalization) in *stable HF* patients in an *outpatient setting.* Both elevated baseline troponin and elevated BNP were associated with worse outcomes. An increase in troponin overtime increased risk, while a decrease reduces risk. In contrast, a change from normal to elevated BNP indicated an increase in risk, but, once elevated, this increased risk persisted regardless of subsequent changes. B-type natriuretic peptide reduction more than 80% was associated with risk reduction, while an increase from below to above 500 pg/mL was associated with an increased risk. The Acute Decompensated Heart Failure National Registry (ADHERE) study which included over 48,000 patients indicated as prognosticators of mortality values over 430 pg/mL.[54] B-type natriuretic peptide–elevated levels in HF patients are associated with increased risk of death and cardiac events, as evidenced by 19 studies.[55] *B-type natriuretic peptide increase of 100 pg/mL causes a 35% increase in risk of death.* Moreover, BNP is potentially more useful than traditional predictors of mortality (e.g. age, etiology, ischemic, LVEF, New York Heart Association (NYHA) class, and *s*-creatinine level).[55]

The measurement of BNP or NT-ProBNP prior to discharge can reliably identify those patients at higher risk. There is consistent evidence from two independent studies that we should try to achieve *predischarge BNP* levels below 350–400 pg/mL.[56,57] If this level is not achieved at the time of planned discharge, intensification of acute HF therapy with uptitration of drugs is warranted. Patients of acute HF with a predischarge BNP levels of 350–700 pg/mL had a five times increased mortality or readmission for HF risk as compared to patient with predischarge BNP below 350 pg/mL. Once the predischarge BNP was above 700 pg/mL, mortality or readmission for HF risk increased by a factor 15 and reached at a rate of 90%.[57] Similar results were reported for NT-ProBNP.[58]

In *acute HF in hospitalized patients*, Logeart et al. evaluated predictors of postdischarge outcomes, by BNP levels. In multivariate analysis, only predischarge BNP levels remained significant. Further analysis showed BNP level of 350 ng/L best discriminated between patients with and without event, and that the range from 350 ng/L to 700 ng/L represented an intermediate risk. B-type natriuretic peptide may help in identifying people with *risk of stroke and atrial fibrillation.* Moreover, it can play a role in predicting the stroke mortality. Admission BNP is an independent powerful marker of early and late cardiac mortality in patients with *acute chest pain* without ST-segment elevation. In the Val-HeFT, subjects with the largest proportion of reduction of BNP levels at *4 months* after randomization experienced the best outcomes, whereas those with the greatest increase in BNP levels experienced the highest event rates.[59] Among patients *hospitalized with decompensated HF*, both the *predischarged BNP* levels and the *relative changes in BNP* levels during hospital treatment are strong predictors of the risk for death or hospital readmission at 6 months.[50,56,60] Study published from Taiwan (January 2011 to December 2013, with 269 patients) hypothesized that NT-ProBNP may provide better predictive power for *in-hospital mortality* among patients with HF, when serum NT-ProBNP levels were above 8,100 mg/dL.[9]

Treatment Implications

If cardiac overload negatively impacts prognosis, and BNP reflects cardiac overload, then reductions in BNP would be expected to indicate an improved prognosis. If this were so, BNP could be used to help assess the efficacy of therapeutic intervention in normal clinical practice as well as in clinical trials. The prognostic importance of NP levels and their potential for modulation with treatment have fueled interest in the use of serial NP measurements to guide HF therapy. The fundamental premise is an alluring one: that patients with high biomarker levels (therefore high risk for advance outcomes) should receive more intensive disease-modifying therapy, and those with low or normal biomarker levels (low risk) should receive less intensive treatment. A number of randomized controlled trials of NP-guided treatment were done.[15,61-68] The overall *results are mixed*, with the largest studies showing no clear evidence of benefit, but recent positive trials resurrecting enthusiasm for this approach, although some have leveraged meta-analytic technique to infer mortality benefit from the biomarker-guided approach.[69] Clinical approach of NP-guided therapy is generally tested by two approaches—one, a uniform strategy in which treatment for all patients is adjusted to target a *single absolute level of BNP* or NT-ProBNP, or two, an *individual strategy* in which different targets are defined for different patients based on the measured baseline value (Tables 2 and 3).

The trials that have demonstrated benefit for NP-guided therapy have not been those with the most stringent NP targets, arguing against the notion that more aggressive efforts to reduce NP levels are necessarily better. Although many therapies with proven benefit in HF patients reduce circulating NP concentrations, it is not clear that ideal NP levels are achievable in every patient. High-circulating NP levels may become harder to modulate with conventional treatment for the elderly or those with more advanced HF. However, the absolute reduction in NP levels from baseline is modest in most studies, leaving many patients well above the established targets at the end of the follow-up. The lower the set targets are, the less likely patients are to achieve

TABLE 2: Trials of natriuretic peptide-guided management using an individualized natriuretic peptide target.

	n	*Inclusion criteria*	*Mean age years*	*Target for NP-guided arm*	*Primary end point*	*Favors NP guided treatment*
Starbrite	130	HF hospitalization LVEF ≤35% NYHA III-IV	59	BNP <2 hospital discharge	Hospitalization free survival	No
Prima	345	HF hospitalization NT-Pro BNP≥ 1,700 on admission, NT-pro BNP drop >10% (>850 pg/mL) before discharge	72	Lowest NT-pro BNP at discharge and subsequent 2 weeks follow-up	No. of days alive outside hospital	No
Signal-HF	252	LVEF <50%, NYHA II-IV, elevated NT-Pro BNP (men >800 pg/mL, women >1,000 pg/mL)	77	50% reduction from baseline NT- pro BNP	Days alive, days out of hospital, and qualigy of life (KCCQ)	No

BNP: B-type natriuretic peptide; HF: heart failure; KCCQ: Kansas City Cardiomyopathy Questionnaire; LVEF: left ventricular ejection fiaction; NP: natriuretic peptide; NT-Pro BNP, N-terminal B-type natriuretic peptide; NYHA: New York Heart Association; PRIMA: can Pro-brain-natriuretic peptide guided therapy of chronic heart failure improve heart failure morbidity and mortality? SIGNAL-HF: Swedish intervention study-guidelines and NT-ProBNP analysis in heart failure; and STARBRITE: strategies for tailoring advanced heart failure regimes in the outpatient setting; Brain natriuretic peptide versus the clinical congestion score.

TABLE 3: Trials of natriuretic peptide-guided management using a fixed natriuretic peptide target.

	n	*Inclusion criteria*	*Mean age years*	*Target for NP-guided arm*	*Primary end point (s)*	*Favors NP-guided treatment*
Troughton et al.	69	HF hospitalization LVEF <40% NYHA III-IV	70	NT-ProBNP <200 pmo/L (1,700 pg/mL)	Cardiovascular death of HF hospitalization	Yes
STARS-BNP	20	Stable outpatient, optimal background therapy, LVEF <45% NYHA-II-III	65	BNP <100 pg/mL	Unplanned HF hospitalization or death	Yes
TIME-CHF	499	Age ≥ 60, LVEF ≤ 45%, NYHA II-IV, HF hospitalization with last year, NT-ProBNP > 2 × upper limit of normal	78	NT-proBNP <400 pg/mL if < 75 year of age or < 800 pg/mL if ≥ 75 year of age	Hospitalization free survival and quality of life	No
BATTLESCA RRED	364	Symptomatic HF with preserved or reduced LVEF HF hospitalization within 2 weeks, NT-ProBNP > 400 pg/mL	76	NT-ProBNP <150 pmo/L (1,300 pg/mL)	Total mortality and death of HF hospitalization	No
PROTECT	151	Hospital admission emergency room visit or outpatient therapy for HF within 6 month LVEF <40% NYHA II-IV	63	NT ProBNP ≤ 1,000 pg/mL	Total cardiovascular events	Yes
Berger et al.	278	HF hospitalization, NYHA III-IV on admission LVEF <40% or CTR >0.5	71	NT-ProBNP <2,200 pg/mL	Days of HF hospitalization time to death of HF hospitalization	Yes

BATTLESCARRED indicates NT-ProBNP assisted treatment to lessen serial cardia readmissions and death BNP: B-type natriuretic peptide; CTR: cardiothoracic ratio; HF: heart failure; LVEF: left ventricular ejection fraction; NP: natriuretic peptide; MT-ProBNP, N-terminal B-type natriuretic peptide; NYHA: New York Heart Association; PROTECT: use of NT-ProBNP testing to guide heart failure therapy in the outpatient setting; STARS-BNP: systolic heart failure treatment supported by BNP, and TIME-CHF: trial of untesified vs standard medical therapy in elderly patients with congestive heart failure.

them. Trials applying more liberal thresholds, particularly those using individual NP targets, tend to report greater success in achieving the set goals but have failed to show relative benefit to the NP-guided approach. Because high NP levels frequently direct intensification of therapy even in patients who may be clinically *asymptomatic*, the NP-guided therapy is typically associated with a relative increase in the use of ACE inhibitors, beta blockers, angiotensin receptor blockers, and spironolactone over standard, symptom-guided care; therefore, the minimization of diuretic dosing in all HF patients with reduced EF has been noticed. There is little evidence that the benefit of HF therapy varies according to HF severity or NP levels. Excessive reliance on NP levels to assess volume status might prompt inappropriate dose escalation of loop diuretics among patients without significant congestion and increase the rate of hypotension, renal dysfunction, and other adverse events. Aggressive medication titration to manage high NP values may also be poorly tolerated in the elderly or those with significant renal dysfunction. In addition, for nearly 50% of patients with HF with *preserved EF* for whom there is little evidence-based treatment, it is unclear how elevated NP levels should influence clinicians to adapt their approach. In the Prevention of Events with Angiotensin Converting Enzyme Inhibition (PEACE) trial, ACE inhibition with trandolapril compared to placebo in patients with *established coronary artery* disease and an LVEF > 40% did not improve the primary endpoint, (which was death from cardiovascular causes, myocardial infarction, or coronary revascularization), but it reduced the number of patients requiring hospitalization due to HF. B-type natriuretic peptide correlates well with *pulmonary capillary wedge pressure*,[14] hence, may be a tool for monitoring treatment response. Troughton et al., in patients with symptomatic chronic HF with low EF (<40%), BNP-guided management at *6 months*, 27% of patients in BNP group and 53% of patients in clinical group had experienced the first cardiovascular event.[15] This finding has recently been confirmed by a French multicenter study (STARS-BNP).[70] Study by Berger et al. favored NP-guided therapy, in which, patients with

BNP levels >2,200 pg/mL were deliberately triaged to HF specialist for more intensive management, and the remainder were managed by primary-care physicians-/nurse-led multidisciplinary team.[60]

The TIME-CHF [Trial of Intensified (BNP guided) versus Standard (symptom guided) Medical Therapy in Elderly Patients with Congestive HF] trial was designed to assess BNP-guided therapy both in younger (60–74 years) and older (>75 years) HF patients. Mortality was reduced with BNP guidance in the younger group, but not in the older group. The older patient group was on average not only older but also more symptomatic, had worse renal function, more comorbidities, a higher proportion of females and patients with coronary artery disease, and higher NT-ProBNP values compared to the younger group. In other words, the lack of benefits seen in older patients does not disprove the concept of hormone-guided treatment approach but rather questions the efficacy of the treatment. In addition, the age interaction suggested in TIME-CHF and BNP-Assisted Treatment to LEssen Serial CARdiac REadmissions and Death (BATTLE SCARRED) studies and the positive results of the PROTECT trial reserve the possibility that there may be a role for BNP-targeted treatment in younger patients with reduced EF. However, with normal BNP levels and those with advanced age, preserved EF and significant medical comorbidities, who make up the majority of the HF burden, will continue to rely on the clinical decision of physicians. Studies as Val-HeFT[71,72] and Carvedilol Prospective Randomized Cumulative Survival (COPERNICUS)[73] indicated that *chronic treatment* with beta blockers and blockers of RAAS led to the reduction of BNP in plasma and improved the prognosis, which was possibly a reflection of the improvement in cardiac function secondary to treatment.[33] Treatment, which proves beneficial in HF patients with reduced EF, includes ACE inhibitors,[74] ARB[75] spironolactone,[76] beta blockers,[77] and cardiac resynchronization therapy[78] that appear to decrease BNP levels in parallel with improvements in cardiac remodeling and clinical outcomes. The concept of existing *chronic HF* therapy to target a specific NP level has been tested and reviewed.[79] Analysis of these pooled studies indicates a 20–25% reduction in mortality with NP-guided therapy. Generalization has been limited by small size study, heterogeneity inclusion criteria, BNP cut points and results.[69,80] Hence, important question remains: Should there be individualized target NP values, e.g. considering age, sex, renal function, BMI, and genotype? Due to this uncertainty, *ACC/AHA guidelines recommend the use of serial BNP measurements to guide titration of therapy in chronic HF that is class level of evidence IIb-B*. Risk stratification by BNP levels may be important to identify a subset of patients who benefit from more intensive treatment. In addition, the BNP-targeted treatment is suggestive more in younger patients with reduced EF.

CONCLUSION

B-type natriuretic peptide is a noble NP, by receptor dimerization, it causes the conversion of GTP to cyclic GMP-activating protein kinase G leading to natriuresis, vasodilation, increased GFR, enhanced ventricular relaxation, antiproliferative, antifibrotic, antithrombotic, and inhibition of RAAS and RSS. Heightened release of BNP is a direct consequence of atrial muscles stretch (dimensions), rather than pressure. B-type natriuretic peptide, in acute/ambulatory dyspneic patients, is an effective diagnostic marker of HF cases (ACC/AHA class level of evidence I-A). B-type natriuretic peptide more than 400 pg/mL supports HF diagnosis, whereas <100 excludes HF diagnosis (in conjunction with other clinical information). B-type natriuretic peptide levels are used in prognosis in patients with acute and ambulatory known HF (ACC/AHA class level of evidence I-A). B-type natriuretic peptides are prognostic markers in clinical acute HF and HF with reduced EF and preserved EF. They are predictors of short- and long-term outcomes. High BNP levels in risky asymptomatic individuals were associated with increased risk of death, first cardiovascular event, HF, atrial fibrillation, and transient ischemic attack. Moreover, screening BNP in specific population at higher risk may be cost effective. There may be a role of BNP-targeted treatment in younger patients with reduced EF. But probably due to its variability in different age, sex, renal function, BMI and genotype: ACC/AHA guidelines recommendation for BNP guideline directed therapy in ambulatory, and BNP-guided therapy for chronic HF, is respectably class level of evidence are IIa-B and IIb-B. Risk stratification by BNP levels may be important to identify a subset of patients who benefit from more intensive treatment.

REFERENCES

1. Sharma S, Chhabra S. ARNI in heart failure with cardiodiabetes: the way forward. In: Cardiodiabetes Update: A Textbook of Cardiology. New Delhi: Jaypee Brothers Medical Publishers (P) Ltd.; 2018. pp. 505-13.
2. Maisel A, Mueller C, Adams K, Jr, et al. State of the art: using natriuretic peptide levels in clinical practice. Eur J Heart Fail. 2008;10(9):824-39.
3. Clerico A, Fontana M, Zyw L, et al. Comparison of the diagnostic accuracy of brain natriuretic peptide (BNP) and the N-terminal part of the propeptide of BNP immunoassays in chronic and acute heart failure: a systematic review. Clin Chem. 2007;53(5):813-22.
4. Ray P, Arthaud M, Birolleau S, et al. Comparison of brain natriuretic peptide and pro brain natriuretic peptide in the

diagnosis of cardiogenic pulmonary edema in patients aged 65 and older. J Am Geriatr Soc. 2005;53:643-8.

5. Boerrigter G, Costello-Boerrigter LC, Burnett JC. Natriuretic peptides in the diagnosis and management of chronic heart failure. Heart Fail Clin. 2009;5:501-14.
6. Kim HN, Januzzi JL. Natriuretic peptide testing in heart failure. Circulation. 2011;123:2015-9.
7. Roberts E, Ludman AJ, Dworzynski K, et al.; NICE Guideline Development Group for Acute Heart Failure. The diagnostic accuracy of the natriuretic peptides in heart failure: systematic review and diagnostic meta-analysis in the acute care setting. BMJ. 2015;350:h910.
8. Gottlieb SS, Kukin ML, Ahern D, et al. Prognostic importance of atrial natriuretic peptide in patients with chronic heart failure. J Am Coll Cardiol. 1989;13:1534-9.
9. Huang YT, Tseng YT, Chu TW, et al. N-terminal pro b-type natriuretic peptide (NT-pro-BNP)-based score can predict in-hospital mortality in patients with heart failure. Sci Rep. 2016;6:29590.
10. Agnoletti G, Rodella A, Ferrari R, et al. Release of atrial natriuretic peptide-like immunoreactive material during stretching of the rat atrium in vitro. J Mol Cell Cardiol. 1987;19:217-20.
11. Redfield MM, Jacobsen SJ, Burnett JC, Jr, et al. Burden of systolic and diastolic ventricular dysfunction in the community: appreciating the scope of the heart failure epidemic. JAMA. 2003;289(2):194-202.
12. McDonagh TA, Morrison CE, Lawrence A, et al. Symptomatic and asymptomatic left-ventricular systolic dysfunction in an urban population. Lancet. 1997;350(9081):829-33.
13. Meirhaeghe A, Sandhu MS, McCarthy MI, et al. Association between the T-381C polymorphism of the brain natriuretic peptide gene and risk of type 2 diabetes in human populations. Hum Mol Genet. 2007;16(11):1343-50.
14. Kazanegra R, Cheng V, Garcia A, et al. A rapid test for B-type natriuretic peptide correlates with falling wedge pressures in patients treated for decompensated heart failure: a pilot study. J Card Fail. 2001;7:21-9.
15. Troughton RW, Frampton CM, Yandle TG, et al. Treatment of heart failure guided by plasma aminoterminal brain natriuretic peptide (N-BNP) concentrations. Lancet. 2000;355:1126-30.
16. Maisel AS, Krishnaswamy P, Nowak RM, et al.; Breathing Not Properly Multinational Study Investigators. Rapid measurement of B-type natriuretic peptide in the emergency diagnosis of heart failure. N Engl J Med. 2002;347:161-7.
17. Januzzi JL, Jr, Camargo CA, Anwaruddin S, et al. The N-terminal Pro-BNP investigation of dyspnea in the emergency department (PRIDE) study. Am J Cardiol. 2005;95:948-54.
18. McCullough PA, Duc P, Omland T, et al. B-type natriuretic peptide and renal function in the diagnosis of heart failure: an analysis from the breathing not properly multinational study. Am J Kidney Dis. 2003;41:571-5.
19. Mueller C, Laule Kilian K, Scholer A, et al. B-type natriuretic peptide for acute dyspnea in patients with kidney disease: insights from a randomized comparison. Kidney Int. 2005;67:278-84.
20. Wang TJ, Larson MG, Levy D, et al. Impact of obesity on plasma natriuretic peptide levels. Circulation. 2004;109: 594-600.
21. McCord J, Mundy BJ, Hudson MP, et al. Relationship between obesity and B-type natriuretic peptide levels. Arch Intern Med. 2004;164:2247-52.
22. McLean AS, Tang B, Nalos M, et al. Increased B-type natriuretic peptide (BNP) level is a strong predictor for cardiac dysfunction in intensive care unit patients. Anaesth Intensive Care. 2003;31:21-7.
23. McLean AS, Huang SJ, Nalos M, et al. The confounding effects of age, gender, serum creatinine, and electrolyte concentrations on plasma B-type natriuretic peptide concentrations in critically ill patients. Crit Care Med. 2003;31:2611-8.
24. Silver MA, Maisel A, Yancy CW, et al. BNP consensus panel 2004: a clinical approach for the diagnostic, prognostic, screening, treatment monitoring, and therapeutic roles of natriuretic peptides in cardiovascular diseases. Congest Heart Fail. 2004;10(Suppl. 3):10-1.
25. Wang TJ, Larson MG, Levy D, et al. Heritability and genetic linkage of plasma natriuretic peptide levels. Circulation. 2003;108(1):13-6.
26. Lanfear DE, Stolker JM, Marsh S, et al. Genetic variation in the B-type natriuretic peptide pathway affects BNP levels. Cardiovasc Drugs Ther. 2007;21(1):55-62.
27. Costello-Boerrigter LC, Boerrigter G, Ameenuddin S, et al. The B-type natriuretic peptide T-381C polymorphism is associated with increased BNP plasma immunoreactivity and higher prevalence of type 2 diabetes mellitus and atrial fibrillation. Eur Heart J. 2008;29(Abstract Suppl.):766.
28. Redfield MM, Rodeheffer RJ, Jacobsen SJ, et al. Plasma brain natriuretic peptide concentration: impact of age and gender. J Am Coll Cardiol. 2002;40(5):976-82.
29. Costello-Boerrigter LC, Boerrigter G, Redfield MM, et al. Amino-terminal pro-B-type natriuretic peptide and B-type natriuretic peptide in the general community: determinants and detection of left ventricular dysfunction. J Am Coll Cardiol. 2006;47(2):345-53.
30. Siebenhofer A, Ng LL, Plank J, et al. Plasma N-terminal pro-brain natriuretic peptide in type 1 diabetic patients with and without diabetic nephropathy. Diabet Med. 2003;20:535-9.
31. Kucher N, Goldhaber SZ. Cardiac biomarkers for risk stratification of patients with acute pulmonary embolism. Circulation. 2003;108:2191-4.
32. Pruszczyk P, Kostrubiec M, Bochowicz A, et al. N-terminal pro-brain natriuretic peptide in patients with acute pulmonary embolism. Eur Respir J. 2003;22:649-53.
33. Burke MA, Cotts WG. Interpretation of B-type natriuretic peptide in cardiac disease and other comorbid conditions. Heart Fail Rev. 2007;12:23-36.
34. Redfield MM, Rodeheffer RJ, Jacobsen SJ, et al. Plasma brain natriuretic peptide to detect preclinical ventricular systolic or diastolic dysfunction: a community-based study. Circulation. 2004;109(25):3176-81.

35. Dickstein K, Cohen-Solal A, Filippatos G, et al. ESC Guidelines for the diagnosis and treatment of acute and chronic heart failure 2008: the Task Force for the Diagnosis and Treatment of Acute and Chronic Heart Failure 2008 of the European Society of Cardiology. Developed in collaboration with the Heart Failure Association of the ESC (HFA) and endorsed by the European Society of Intensive Care Medicine (ESICM). Eur Heart J. 2008;29(19):2388-442.
36. Wang TJ, Larson MG, Levy D, et al. Plasma natriuretic peptide levels and the risk of cardiovascular events and death. N Engl J Med. 2004;350:655-63.
37. Huelsmann M, Neuhold S, Resl M, et al. PONTIAC (NT-proBNP Selected PreventiOn of cardiac events in a population of dIabetic patients without A history of Cardiac disease): a prospective randomized controlled trial. J Am Coll Cardiol. 2013;62:1365-72.
38. Ledwidge M, Gallagher J, Conlon C, et al. Natriuretic peptide-based screening and collaborative care for heart failure: the STOP-HF randomized trial. JAMA. 2013;310:66-74.
39. McKie PM, Rodeheffer RJ, Cataliotti A, et al. Amino-terminal pro-B-type natriuretic peptide and B-type natriuretic peptide: biomarkers for mortality in a large community-based cohort free of heart failure. Hypertension. 2006;47(5):874-80. (PMC free article).
40. McDonagh TA, Cunningham AD, Morrison CE, et al. Left ventricular dysfunction, natriuretic peptides, and mortality in an urban population. Heart. 2001;86:21-6.
41. Castro LR, Alencar MC, Barbosa MM, et al. NT-proBNP levels in patients with non-ST-segment elevation acute coronary syndrome. Arq Bras Cardiol. 2011;97(6):456-61.
42. Henriksen JH, Goetze JP, Fuglsang S, et al. Increased circulating pro brain natriuretic peptide (proBNP) and brain natriuretic peptide (BNP) in patients with cirrhosis: relation to cardiovascular dysfunction and severity of disease. Gut. 2003;52(10):1511-7.
43. Kneiseler G, Herzer K, Marggraf G. Die Interaktion zwischen Leber und Herz. Z Herz-, Thorax- Gefäßchirurgie. 2010;24(6):334-40.
44. Gallinat A, Neumann T, Kaiser G, et al. Brain natriuretic peptide (BNP): an early marker of cardiac dysfunction after liver transplantation?. Liver Outcomes Suppl. Transplant. 2010;90(2S):1739.
45. Anand IS, Fisher LD, Chiang YT, et al.; For the Bal-HeFT Investigators. Changes in brain natriuretic peptide and norepinephrine over time and mortality and morbidity in the Valsartan Heart Failure Trial (Val-HeFT). Circulation. 2003;107:1278-83.
46. Wijeysundera HC, Hansen MS, Stanton E, et al., For the PRAISE II Investigators. Neurohormones and oxidative stress in nonischemic cardiomyopathy: relationship to survival and the effect of treatment with amlodipine. Am Heart J. 2003;146:291-7.
47. Anand IS, Fisher LD, Chiang YT, et al. The Val-HeFT Investigators Changes in brain natriuretic peptide and norepinephrine over time and mortality and morbidity in the Valsartan Heart Failure Trial (Val-HeFT). Circulation. 2003;107:1278-83.
48. Anand IS, Rector TS, Cleland JG, et al. Prognostic value of baseline plasma amino-terminal pro-brain natriuretic peptide and its interactions with irbesartan treatment effects in patients with heart failure and preserved ejection fraction: findings from the I-PRESERVE trial. Circ Heart Fail. 2011;4:569-77.
49. Fonarow GC, Peacock WF, Phillips CO, et al.; The ADHERE Scientific Advisory Committee and Investigators. Admission B-type natriuretic peptide levels and in-hospital mortality in acute decompensated heart failure. J Am Coll Cardiol. 2007;49:1943-50.
50. Bettencourt P, Azevedo A, Pimenta J, et al. N-terminal-pro-brain natriuretic peptide predicts outcome after hospital discharge in heart failure patients. Circulation. 2004;110:2168-74.
51. Kociol RD, Horton JR, Fonarow GC, et al. Admission, discharge, or change in B-type natriuretic peptide and long-term outcomes: data from Organized Program to Initiate Lifesaving Treatment in Hospitalized Patients with Heart Failure (OPTIMIZE-HF) linked to Medicare claims. Circ Heart Fail. 2011;4:628-36.
52. Gaggin HK, Truong QA, Rehman SU, et al. Characterization and prediction of natriuretic peptide "nonresponse" during heart failure management: results from the ProBNP Outpatient Tailored Chronic Heart Failure (PROTECT) and the NT-proBNP-Assisted Treatment to Lessen Serial Cardiac Readmissions and Death (BATTLESCARRED) study. Congest Heart Fail. 2013;19:135-42.
53. Masson S, Latini R, Anand IS, et al. The Val-HeFT Investigators Prognostic value of changes in N-terminal pro-brain natriuretic peptide in Val-HeFT (Valsartan Heart Failure Trial). J Am Coll Cardiol. 2008;52:997-1003.
54. Fonarow GC, Peacock WF, Phillips CO, et al.; ADHERE Scientific Advisory Committee and Investigators. Admission B-type natriuretic peptide levels and in-hospital mortality in acute decompensated heart failure. J Am Coll Cardiol. 2007;49:1943-50.
55. Doust JA, Pietrzak E, Dobson A, et al. How well does B-type natriuretic peptide predict death and cardiac events in patients with heart failure: systematic review. BMJ. 2005;330:625.
56. Logeart D, Thabut G, Jourdain P, et al. Predischarge B-type natriuretic peptide assay for identifying patients at high risk of readmission after decompensated heart failure. J Am Coll Cardiol. 2004;43:635-41.
57. Verdiani V, Nozzoli C, Bacci F, et al. Pre-discharge B-type natriuretic peptide predicts early recurrence of decompensated heart failure in patients admitted to a general medical unit. Eur J Heart Fail. 2005;7:566-71.
58. Bettencourt P, Azevedo A, Pimenta J, et al. N-Terminal-Pro-Brain natriuretic peptide predicts outcome after hospital discharge in heart failure patients. Circulation. 2004;110:2168-74.
59. Anand IS, Fisher LD, Chiang YT, et al.; Val-HeFT Investigators. Changes in brain natriuretic peptide and norepinephrine over time and mortality and morbidity in the Valsartan Heart Failure Trial (Val-HeFT). Circulation. 2003;107:1278-83.

60a. O'Connor CM, Hasselblad V, Mehta RH, et al. Triage after hospitalization with advanced heart failure: the ESCAPE (Evaluation Study of Congestive Heart Failure and Pulmonary Artery Catheterization Effectiveness) risk model and discharge score. J Am Coll Cardiol. 2010;55:872-8.
60b. Berger R, Moertl D, Peter S, et al. N-terminal pro-B-type natriuretic peptide-guided, intensive patient management in addition to multidisciplinary care in chronic heart failure a 3-arm, prospective, randomized pilot study. J Am Coll Cardiol. 2010;55:645-53.
61. Jourdain P, Jondeau G, Funck F, et al. Plasma brain natriuretic peptide-guided therapy to improve outcome in heart failure: the STARS-BNP Multicenter Study. J Am Coll Cardiol. 2007;49:1733-9.
62. Shah MR, Califf RM, Nohria A, et al. The STARBRITE trial: a randomized, pilot study of B-type natriuretic peptide-guided therapy in patients with advanced heart failure. J Card Fail. 2011;17:613-21.
63. Pfisterer M, Buser P, Rickli H, et al.; TIME-CHF Investigators. BNP-guided vs symptom-guided heart failure therapy: the Trial of Intensified vs Standard Medical Therapy in Elderly Patients with Congestive Heart Failure (TIME-CHF) randomized trial. JAMA. 2009;301:383-92.
64. Lainchbury JG, Troughton RW, Strangman KM, et al. N-terminal pro-B-type natriuretic peptide-guided treatment for chronic heart failure: results from the BATTLESCARRED (NT-proBNP-Assisted Treatment to Lessen Serial Cardiac Readmissions and Death) trial. J Am Coll Cardiol. 2009;55:53-60.
65. Eurlings LW, van Pol PE, Kok WE, et al. Management of chronic heart failure guided by individual N-terminal pro-B-type natriuretic peptide targets: results of the PRIMA (Can PRo-brain-natriuretic peptide guided therapy of chronic heart failure IMprove heart fAilure morbidity and mortality?) study. J Am Coll Cardiol. 2010;56:2090-100.
66. Januzzi JL, Rehman SU, Mohammed AA, et al. Use of amino-terminal pro-B-type natriuretic peptide to guide outpatient therapy of patients with chronic left ventricular systolic dysfunction. J Am Coll Cardiol. 2011;58:1881-9.
67. Berger R, Moertl D, Peter S, et al. N-terminal pro-B-type natriuretic peptide-guided, intensive patient management in addition to multidisciplinary care in chronic heart failure a 3-arm, prospective, randomized pilot study. J Am Coll Cardiol. 2010;55:645-53.
68. Persson H, Erntell H, Eriksson B, et al. Improved pharmacological therapy of chronic heart failure in primary care: a randomized Study of NT-proBNP Guided Management of Heart Failure—SIGNAL-HF (Swedish Intervention study—Guidelines and NT-proBNP AnaLysis in Heart Failure). Eur J Heart Fail. 2011;12:1300-08.
69. Felker GM, Hasselblad V, Hernandez AF, et al. Biomarker-guided therapy in chronic heart failure: a meta-analysis of randomized controlled trials. Am Heart J. 2009;158:422-30.
70. Jourdain P, Funck F, Gueffet P, et al. Benefit of BNP plasma levels for optimising therapy: the systolic heart failure treatment supported by BNP multicenter trial (STARS-BNP). J Am Coll Cardiol. 2005;45:1001-151. (abstract).
71. Latini R, Masson S, Anand I, et al. The comparative prognostic value of plasma neurohormones at baseline in patients with heart failure enrolled in Val-HeFT. Eur Heart J. 2004;25:292-9.
72. Masson S, Latini R, Arnand IS, et al. Prognostic value of changes in N-terminal proBNP in Val-HeFT. J Am Coll Cardiol. 2008;52:997-1003.
73. Hartmann F, Packer M, Coats A, et al. Prognostic impact of plasma N-terminal pro-brain natriuretic peptide in severe chronic congestive heart failure: a substudy of the Carvedilol Prospective Randomized Cumulative Survival (COPERNICUS) trial. Circulation. 2004;110:1780-6.
74. Motwani JG, McAlpine H, Kennedy N, et al. Plasma brain natriuretic peptide as an indicator for angiotensin-converting-enzyme inhibition after myocardial infarction. Lancet. 1993;341:1109-13.
75. Latini R, Masson S, Anand I, et al.; Valsartan Heart Failure Trial Investigators. Effects of valsartan on circulating brain natriuretic peptide and norepinephrine in symptomatic chronic heart failure: the Valsartan Heart Failure Trial (Val-HeFT). Circulation. 2002;106:2454-8.
76. Tsutamoto T, Wada A, Maeda K, et al. Effect of spironolactone on plasma brain natriuretic peptide and left ventricular remodeling in patients with congestive heart failure. J Am Coll Cardiol. 2001;37:1228-33.
77. Stanek B, Frey B, Hülsmann M, et al. Prognostic evaluation of neurohumoral plasma levels before and during beta-blocker therapy in advanced left ventricular dysfunction. J Am Coll Cardiol. 2001;38:436-42.
78. Cleland JG, Daubert JC, Erdmann E, et al.; Cardiac Resynchronization-Heart Failure (CARE-HF) Study Investigators. The effect of cardiac resynchronization on morbidity and mortality in heart failure. N Engl J Med. 2005;352:1539-49.
79. Troughton R, Felker GM, Januzzi JL, Jr. Natriuretic peptide-guided heart failure management. Eur Heart J. 2014;35:16-24.
80. Troughton RW, Frampton CM, Brunner-La Rocca HP, et al. Effect of B-type natriuretic peptide-guided treatment of chronic heart failure on total mortality and hospitalization: an individual patient meta-analysis. Eur Heart J. 2014;35:1559-67.

124

CHAPTER

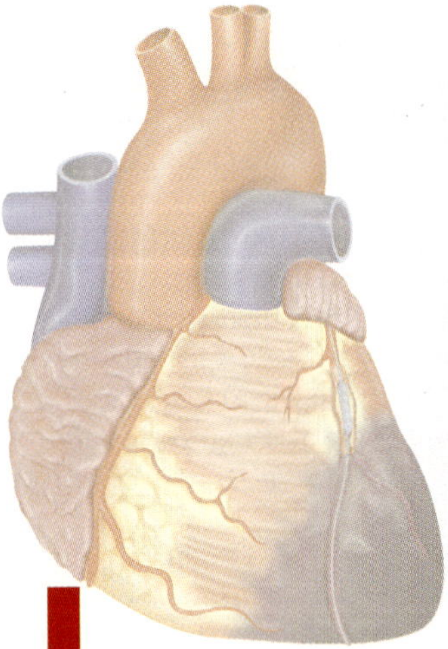

Neuroimaging in Meditation

Subash Khushu, Richa Trivedi, Kushal Madan, SC Manchanda

INTRODUCTION

Meditation is an essential component of yoga and can be defined as a practice where an individual uses a technique, such as focusing their mind on a particular object, thought, or activity, to achieve a mentally clear and emotionally calm state. Meditative practices have been shown to be beneficial in a wide variety of cognitive and health-related functions, including self-regulation, attention, interoceptive awareness, somatosensory processing, stress, anxiety, depression, immune functions, chronic pain, sleep, and heart-related disorders.[1-9] Mental stress has emerged as an important risk factor for the causation of cardiovascular disease, hypertension, diabetes mellitus, and metabolic syndrome.[10] The mechanism of reduction of stress by meditation has been the subject of interest for quite a long time. It appears that meditation can alter the structure and function of brain which could contribute to the beneficial effect of meditation. Several neuroimaging techniques, especially functional magnetic resonance imaging (fMRI), have been utilized to study the alterations in the brain activity during meditation.

NEUROIMAGING IN MEDITATION

Neuroimaging has evolved as a great tool to explore changes at the functional and structural level of the brain. Analysis of brain images has developed their indispensable importance for diagnosis or prognosis of any disorder or inflammation caused by pathogens in the human brain. Particularly, the architecture of functional networks was deciphered with neuroimaging. The scientific bases of mindfulness are attention, body awareness, emotion regulation, changes in self-perspective, and the neural modulation of brain areas, including the posterior cingulate cortex (PCC), anterior cingulate cortex (ACC), medial prefrontal cortex (MPFC), temporoparietal junction (TPJ), insula, amygdale, and hippocampus.[11] Meditation is a method to train brain networks. It is able to change its architecture.[12] The effects of meditation on brain structure and functions have received increasing attention in neuroimaging studies, and the numbers of published studies are growing steadily. The change in neuroarchitecture can be seen as altered cortical thickness,[13] gray matter (GM) volume, and white matter properties at macro/micro level.[14] Resting state[15,16] and task-based fMRI experiments[17] show functional changes in neural network as well. Based on imaging modalities and techniques, studies can be divided broadly into two groups: (1) structural brain modification in meditators and (2) neurofunctional modifications after meditation training.

Structural Brain Modification in Meditators

Fox et al. reported a systematic review and meta-analysis of morphometric neuroimaging studies in meditation practitioners.[18] Eight brain regions were consistently altered in meditators. The majority of studies investigated the effects of meditation on GM regions. They utilized voxel-based morphometry and demonstrated increased regional GM volumes and thicker cortical areas in meditators compared with nonmeditators. Lazar et al. reported thicker prefrontal cortex as well as a thicker anterior insula in meditators.[13]

A study found larger GM density in the right hippocampus and orbitofrontal cortex.[19] Higher GM matter concentration was detected in meditators in the right anterior insula, left inferior temporal gyrus, and right hippocampus.[20] After 8 weeks of mindfulness meditation practice, Hölzel et al. also found increased GM concentration within the left hippocampus, the TPJ, the PCC, and the cerebellum.[11] In the human brain, neurons communicate via dendrites locally but extend their axonal process for farthest signal conduction. These axons can connect to many different regions in brain. Axons reaching out to the same region form a huge bundle called white matter. Human brain has many white matter tracts which have distinct and collective functional importance to brain activity. These tracts can run in different orientation, such as anterior–posterior which runs between frontal to the temporal or occipital lobe. Rostral–caudal tracts run for corticosubcortical integration. For interhemispheric connectivity, major white matter tract is corpus callosum (CC), which connects left and right hemispheres. These white matter tracts transmit the information among neurons and resemble the functionality of a shielded electric wire. Exclusive to vertebrates, oligodendrocytes synthesize lipid substance called myelin which provides ensheathing to axonal processes. White matter is involved in learning, processing and transfer of information, neurological, cognitive, and psychological disorders.[21]

Diffusion tensor imaging (DTI) enables to visualize structural changes, especially in white matter regions in the health and disease.[22] It noninvasively characterizes properties of soft tissue on a microstructural scale. It works by sensitizing the MRI signals to the diffusion of water molecules by adding "diffusion-encoding gradients" to a standard MRI pulse sequence.[23] Water molecules exhibit random motion called as Brownian movement or diffusion. It is primarily caused by random changes in temperature. Diffusion is termed isotropic if the motion is equal in all directions. However, water diffuses asymmetrically in the white matter along the restricted pathways of axonal processes. This diffusion is restricted perpendicular to the long axis of the axons. This preferential diffusion along one axis is known as anisotropy; it may be used to define the direction of the axons in a particular voxel.[24] The data from the tensor model at the level of each individual voxel and subsequently in a region can be summarized and visualized in three different ways: mean diffusivity (MD), degree of anisotropy, and the main direction of diffusivity (Figs. 1 and 2). To define microstructural and macrostructural properties of white matter, these diffusivity measures can be calculated. Due to its sensitivity to microstructural tissue properties, DTI can explore anatomy and structure of axonal fibers in vivo. The measurement of diffusion and

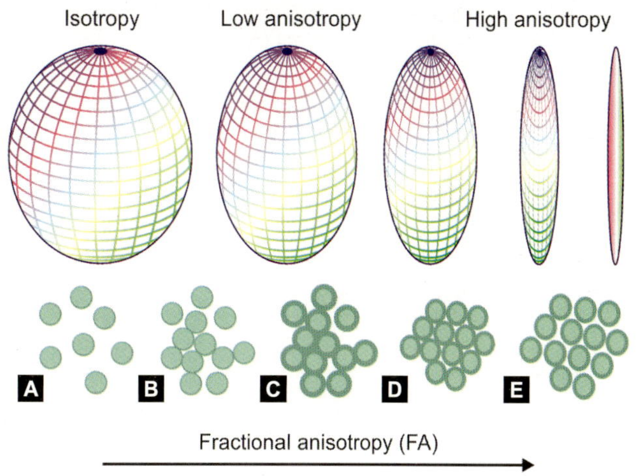

Figs. 1A to E: Description of fractional anisotropy.
Courtesy: Nagy Z, Lindström K, Westerberg H, et al. Diffusion tensor imaging on teenagers, born at term with moderate hypoxic-ischemic encephalopathy. Pediatr Res. 2005;58:936-40.

tissue fiber orientation made DTI widely used clinical tool in white matter abnormalities related to myelination levels and axonal injuries.[25,26] Anisotropy estimates the axonal organization of the brain. Diffused water should move more easily along the axonal bundles rather than perpendicular to these bundles because there are fewer obstacles to prevent movement along the fibers. So, higher anisotropy, suggesting a higher density of fibers oriented in one direction.[27] Practicing music,[28] video gaming,[29] and meditation[30,31] lead to changes in fractional anisotropy (FA) and diffusivity values. Expertise in Baduk game brings increased FA in white matter tracts associated with attention, working memory, and problem-solving.[32] Reasoning training led to decreased diffusivity in the frontal white matter and left frontal and right parietal cortices.[33] Experience-induced neuroplasticity suggests the relationship between behavior and underlying cortical structures.[34] These experiences include learning music, sports, meditation, or any cognitive training. Meditation involves information flow between brain parts associated in emotion and attention types.[35,36] Diffusion tensor imaging enables to visualize structural changes in the healthy human brain caused by any such training.[22] Music training leads to changes in FA and diffusivity values. Kang et al. in the year 2012 have shown significantly different FA values in cuneus, precuneus, and occipital regions (majority of) in comparison with controls in meditators with an average of 40 months of training period.[37] Short-term meditation practice increases FA in anterior corona radiate connecting to ACC and genu of CC.[14,38] Ceko et al. reported increased FA and axial diffusivity in pain-related regions, which confirms higher tolerance of pain in long-term meditators.[39]

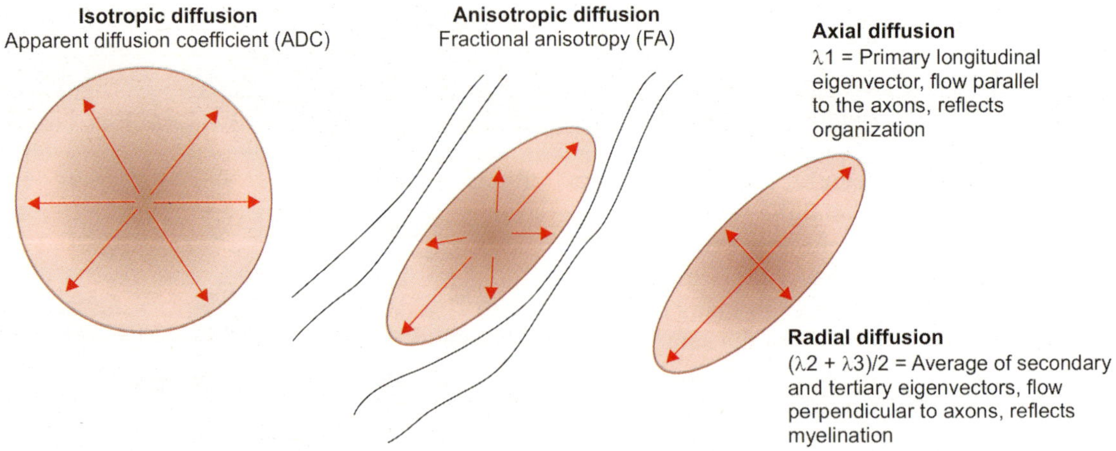

Fig. 2: Diffusion tensor imaging diagram showing radial diffusion, axial diffusion, and apparent diffusion coefficient as related to fractional anisotropy.
Courtesy: Karlsgodt KH, Rosser T, Lutkenhoff ES, et al. Alterations in white matter microstructure in neurofibromatosis-1. PLoS ONE. 2012;7(10):e47854.

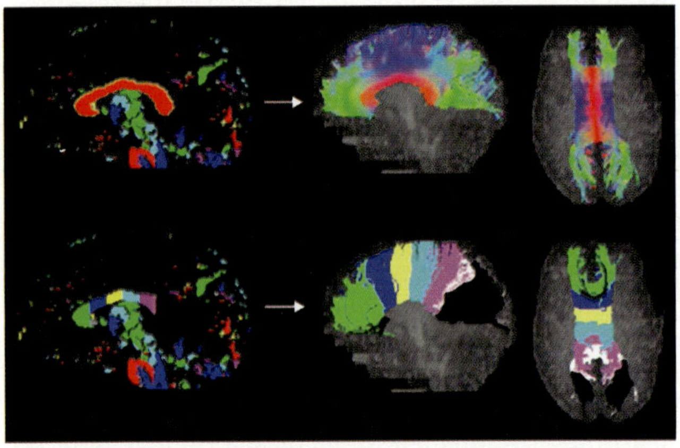

Fig. 3: Segmentation of corpus callosum based on cortical–callosal relationship.
Courtesy: Sharma et al.[42]

Enhanced FA was found in discrete meditators with thicker callosal regions,[12] and significant larger FA values were found in long-term meditators in many fiber tracts,[19] including superior longitudinal fasciculus (SLF) and uncinated fasciculus (UNC). Both SLF and UNC are known to play an important role in emotion regulation and emotion response control.[40,41] In one recent Indian study[42] on long-term Raj yoga meditators, high FA values with low MD in whole as well as different segments of CC were observed compared with age-matched controls (Fig. 3). Moreover, the experience of meditation was correlated with FA values of CC tracts. Findings may suggest Raj yoga meditation to bring potential changes in myelination of CC segments.

Neurofunctional Modifications in Meditators

Functional MRI is an indirect measure of brain activity. It observes neural activity in the real time when scans are taken in a repeated manner over trials of any task. Distinct brain areas work in the synchronous or non-synchronized manner in order to accomplish a mental task. This functional synchrony activates a network of these brain regions which is visualized in blood oxygenated level-dependent (BOLD) activation. MRI studies have shown that due to short- or long-term meditation practice, brain areas comprising the prefrontal cortex, ACC,[43] the basal ganglia,[44] the hippocampus, the pre- and postcentral gyri as well as the dorsolateral prefrontal and parietal cortices[45] activate or deactivate. Davidson et al. reported enhancement in the activation of specific brain areas in long-term meditatiors. They also reported that long-term meditation promotes attention and sustainability.[46] Meditation modulates plasticity in neural circuits which commonly process attention.[47] The fMRI studies have shown a reduction of neural responses in widespread brain regions. It can be linked to conceptual processing suggesting enhanced neural efficiency.[17,48] Studies are available[49] reporting how meditation experience modulates brain networks involved in the development of cognitive skills and cognitive actions. Meditation practitioners were subjected to fMRI scan during meditation task of focused attention on breathing. It revealed that repeated engagement of relevant brain networks over time induces neuroplastic changes and also mediates positive outcomes in cognitive, behavioral, and

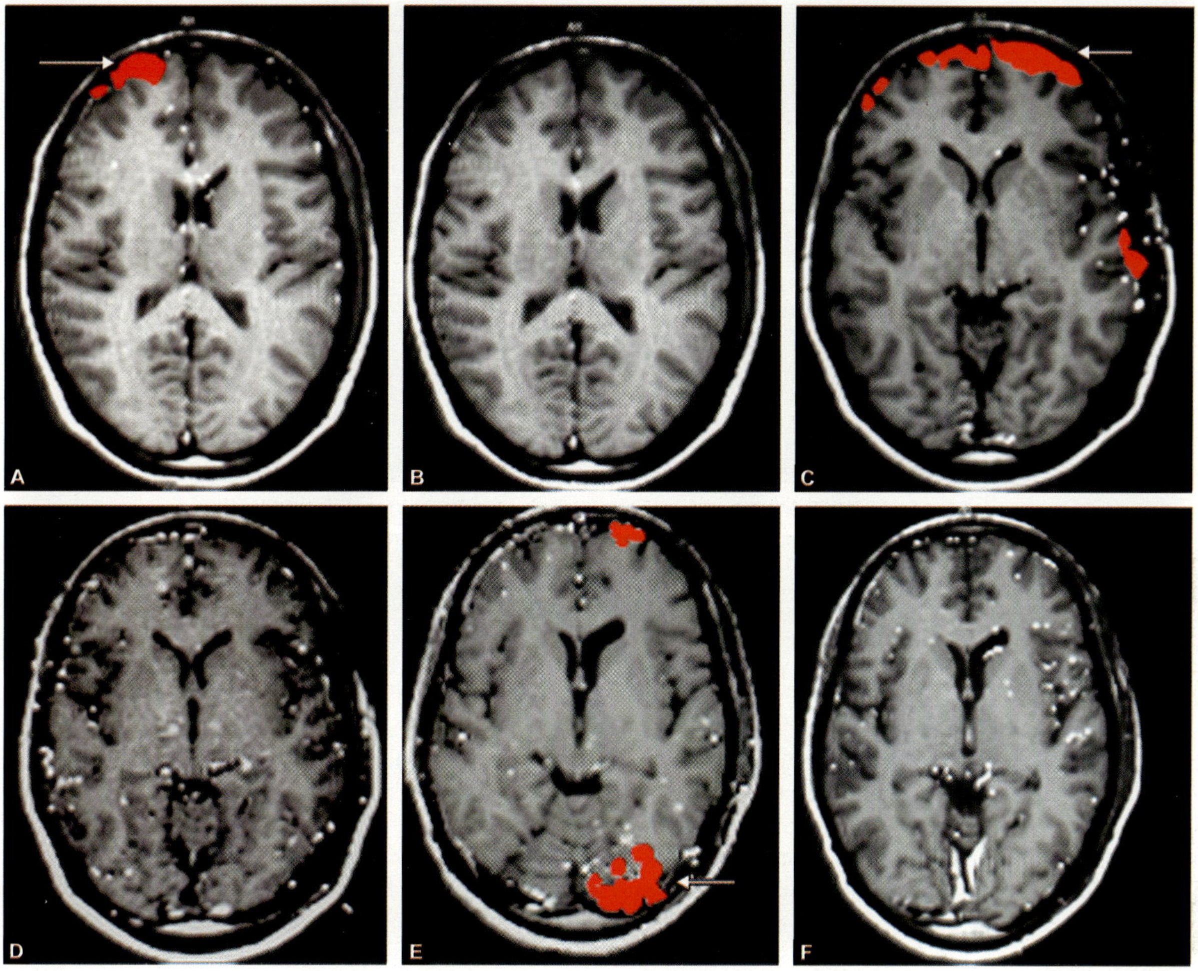

Figs. 4A to F: The neural activation maps during meditation (A, C, and E) and baseline (B, D, and F) states in subjects with 3–5 years of experience (A and B), experience ranging from 5 years to 15 years (C and D), and beyond 15 years (E and F). *Courtesy:* Khushu et al.[52]

emotional domains. The effects of long-term meditation have been studied with respect to physiological and cognitive changes. Studies have shown trait-related changes with mindfulness meditation, Vipassana, Zen meditation, transcendental meditation, and Sahaja yoga.[50] An fMRI-based experiment on Tibetan long-term meditators with extensive practice of meditation (10,000–54,000 hours) has shown expertise-related changes in the brain networks.[51] In a study by Khushu et al. frontal lobe activation was observed in the meditators. Moreover, the activation of left occipital lobe was observed in subjects having meditation practice of more than 15 years. The results of our study were explained in terms of directed attention and visual imagery[52] (Figs. 4A to F). Resting-state functional connectivity analyzes neural activity which is intrinsically generated by the brain (Fig. 5). This phenomenon was attempted to observe in fMRI scans of 35 meditators in comparison with 33 control subjects.[53] Increased activation of default mode network (DMN) in the MPFC was found in meditators. Earlier studies have suggested that increased activity of DMN is associated with the internalized attention (detached from external stimuli).[54] The results of this study concluded that long-term meditation provides functional changes in regions associated with internalized attention and also indicate induction in brain plasticity by meditation. Dickenson et al.[55] used fMRI to explore the basic mechanism of mindfulness and expected an increased BOLD signal in DMN and attention regulatory networks. In their study, a brief task of focused breathing and mind-wandering was given to perform during fMRI scan, followed by some set of questions. An interaction between focused breathing on brain activation and trait mindfulness scale was expected to be seen. However, results provided evidence on reduced DMN activation while subjects were engaged in mindfulness

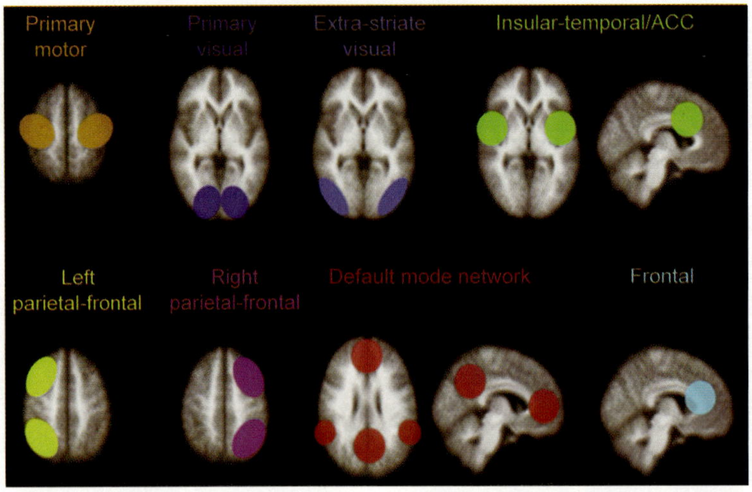

Fig. 5: Most consistent reported resting-state networks across different studies. The figure illustrates resting-state networks reported by the different studies.
Courtesy: Van Den Heuvel and Pol (2010).

after a very simple and brief induction with little prior training. Overall, in control subjects, attention networks were found to be engaged during task but moderated due to meditation practice. Default mode network activations were seen by Brewer et al. using functional connectivity MRI (fcMRI) analysis in 12 meditators and 13 control subjects.[15] The results of fcMRI analysis revealed stronger activations in the posterior cingulate, dorsal anterior cingulate, and dorsolateral prefrontal cortices during baseline and meditation and also found a positive association with meditation expertise. Reduced mind-wandering was found in expert meditators in comparison to naïve controls. Lutz et al. hypothesized positive correlation of the BOLD signal with changes in heart rate (HR) during compassion, as a function of compassion meditation.[22] In a study, 10 expert Buddhist meditators and 13 control subjects were randomly presented to affective sounds from a database of international affective digital sounds in headphones during MR scan. Subjects were asked to meditate during sounds. Change in HR was positively correlated with the BOLD signals collected from right middle insula and somatosensory regions, right inferior parietal lobule (IPL), and premotor regions [Brodmann area 6 (BA6)], as well as right TPJs. Right middle insula showed a significant association with HR across state and group. The strong correlation of HR was found with large cluster, including right somatosensory cortex and right IPL along with parahippocampal/fusiform gyrus/occipital gyrus. This strong association suggested enhanced brain activation related to other's emotions due to compassion in expert meditators. Meditators with an average experience of around 40 months showed heightened activation of the DMN in the MPFC. Studies suggested activation of brain areas responsible for internalized attention (i.e. MPFC) in meditators while they were not practicing meditation. Internalized attention may relate to the increased sense of stimuli and can provide usefulness while managing multimodal stress.[53] Kozasa et al.[17] have reported effects of meditation on fMRI adapted Stroop Word-Color Task with respect to brain activation pattern. No significant difference was observed between the meditators and controls; however, accuracy was found to be reduced during incongruent trials. Right medial frontal, middle temporal, precentral and postcentral gyri, and the lentiform nucleus during the incongruent conditions were found to be highly activated in control group. Results suggested that long-term practice of meditation may increase efficiency of the executive attentional network and facilitated neural pathways involved in identification of task-related stimuli. Froeliger et al.[56] have demonstrated effects of yoga meditation practice on affective and cognitive processing as well as interaction of emotions in cognitive processing. They recruited Hatha yoga meditation practitioners and controls (meditation naïve) and affective Stroop task with pictures from International Affective Picture System database was performed on them. No significant difference was observed in reaction time or accuracy in the task performance. Results of brain activation pattern revealed right dorsolateral prefrontal cortex activations during negative emotions in controls. Regions responsible for inhibitory control (i.e. ventrolateral prefrontal cortex) were activated in meditators, while emotionally irrelevant distractor stimuli were presented in cognitive task. In controls, decrease in positive affect was correlated with increased amygdala activation. Findings suggested that meditators were able to process emotions without effortful cognitive control. This ability in meditators might have developed due to mindful awareness and virtue of acceptance and can prevent suppression while in the process of emotion regulation. Attention subtypes are most practiced cognitive abilities by any type of meditators. In our resting-state MRI study, we observed four networks which showed difference on group analysis between long-term meditators and controls. These networks included lateral visual, sensorimotor, posterior DMN, and frontal medial cortex. Lateral visual, including precentral gyrus, postcentral gyrus, superior parietal lobule, supramarginal gyrus at both anterior and posterior division, superior parietal lobule, and this network, was found to be more active in control subjects as compared to long-term memory.

CONCLUSION

Efforts to image the energy field (aura) around objects or people with the help of machines or specific techniques has been going on for past many decades. In 1939, Russian scientist, Semyon Kirlian, and his wife, Valentina, developed Kirlian photography which was believed to capture that aura around objects. They believed that their images showed a life force or energy field that reflected the emotional and physical states of their living subjects. They thought that these images could be used to diagnose illnesses in the earlier stages. Konstantin Korotkov developed a technique similar to Kirlian photography called "gas discharge visualization" (Figs. 6A and B). However, the results were inconclusive. Harry Oldfield, a UK biologist, developed an energy field imaging system, polycontrast interference photography, which is an energy field video imaging process. The instrument was used by the researchers trying to understand how a person's biofield is a telltale sign of their future health. However, this needs further confirmation.

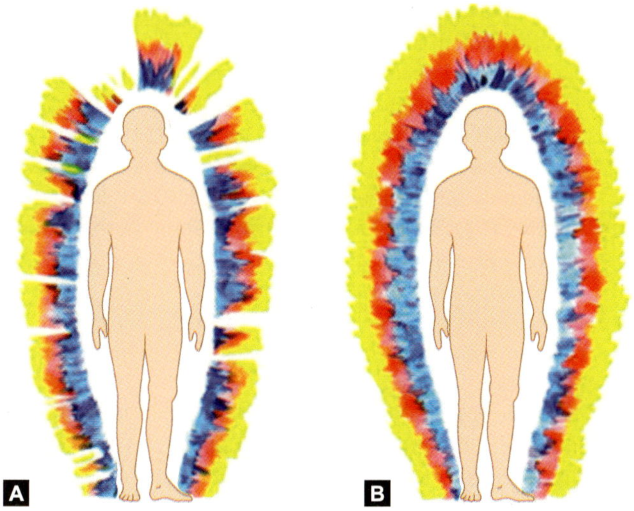

Figs. 6A and B: Gas discharge visualization. Kirlian photography of (A) unhealthy and (B) healthy person.

REFERENCES

1. Jha AP, Krompinger J, Baime MJ. Mindfulness training modifies subsystems of attention. Cogn Affect Behav Neurosci. 2007;7(2):109-19.
2. Farb NA, Segal ZV, Anderson AK. Mindfulness meditation training alters cortical representations of interoceptive attention. Soc Cogn Affect Neurosci. 2013;8(1):15-26.
3. Kerr CE, Sacchet MD, Lazar SW, et al. Mindfulness starts with the body: somatosensory attention and top-down modulation of cortical alpha rhythms in mindfulness meditation. Front Hum Neurosci. 2013;7:12.
4. Tang YY, Posner MI, Rothbart MK. Meditation improves self-regulation over the life span. Ann NY Acad Sci. 2014;1307: 104-11.
5. Infante JR, Peran F, Rayo JI, et al. Levels of immune cells in transcendental meditation practitioners. Int J Yoga. 2014;7(2):147-51.
6. Jain S, Shapiro SL, Swanick S, et al. A randomized controlled trial of mindfulness meditation versus relaxation training: effects on distress, positive states of mind, rumination, and distraction. Ann Behav Med. 2007;33(1):11-21.
7. la Cour P, Petersen M. Effects of mindfulness meditation on chronic pain: a randomized controlled trial. Pain Med. 2015;16(4):641-52.
8. Nagendra RP, Maruthai N, Kutty BM. Meditation and its regulatory role on sleep. Front Neurol. 2012;3:54.
9. Manchanda SC, Madan K. Yoga and meditation in cardiovascular disease. Clin Res Cardiol. 2014;103(9):675-80.
10. Innes KE, Bourguignon C, Taylor AG. Risk indices associated with the insulin resistance syndrome, cardiovascular disease, and possible protection with yoga: a systematic review. J Am Board Fam Pract. 2005;18(6):491-519.
11. Hölzel BK, Carmody J, Vangel M, et al. Mindfulness practice leads to increases in regional brain gray matter density. Psychiatry Res. 2011;191(1):36-43.
12. Luders E, Kurth F, Mayer EA, et al. The unique brain anatomy of meditation practitioners: alterations in cortical gyrification. Front Hum Neurosci. 2012;6:34.
13. Lazar SW, Kerr CE, Wasserman RH, et al. Meditation experience is associated with increased cortical thickness. Neuroreport. 2005;16(17):1893.
14. Tang YY, Lu Q, Fan M, et al. Mechanisms of white matter changes induced by meditation. Proc Natl Acad Sci USA. 2012;109(26):10570-4.
15. Brewer JA, Worhunsky PD, Gray JR, et al. Meditation experience is associated with differences in default mode network activity and connectivity. Proc Natl Acad Sci USA. 2011;108(50):20254-9.

16. Taylor VA, Daneault V, Grant J, et al. Impact of meditation training on the default mode network during a restful state. Soc Cogn Affect Neurosci. 2013;8(1):4-14.
17. Kozasa EH, Sato JR, Lacerda SS, et al. Meditation training increases brain efficiency in an attention task. Neuroimage. 2012;59(1):745-9.
18. Fox KC, Nijeboer S, Dixon ML, et al. Is meditation associated with altered brain structure? A systematic review and meta-analysis of morphometric neuroimaging in meditation practitioners. Neurosci Biobehav Revi. 2014;43:48-73.
19. Luders E, Toga AW, Lepore N, et al. The underlying anatomical correlates of long-term meditation: larger hippocampal and frontal volumes of gray matter. Neuroimage. 2009;45(3): 672-78.
20. Hölzel BK, Ott U, Gard T, et al. Investigation of mindfulness meditation practitioners with voxel-based morphometry. Soc Cogn Affect Neurosci. 2008;3(1):55-61.
21. Fields RD. White matter in learning, cognition and psychiatric disorders. Trends Neurosci. 2008;31:361-70.
22. Scholz J, Klein MC, Behrens TE, et al. Training induces changes in white-matter architecture. Nat Neurosci. 2009;12(11):1370.
23. Jones DK, Leemans A. Diffusion tensor imaging. In: Modo M, Bulte JWM (Eds). Magnetic resonance neuroimaging. US: Humana Press; 2011. pp. 127-44.
24. Moseley ME, Cohen Y, Kucharczyk J, et al. Diffusion-weighted MR imaging of anisotropic water diffusion in cat central nervous system. Radiology. 1990;176:439-45.
25. Song SK, Sun SW, Ramsbottom MJ, et al. Dysmyelination revealed through MRI as increased radial (but unchanged axial) diffusion of water. Neuroimage. 2002;17:1429-36.
26. Gupta RK, Trivedi R, Awasthi R, et al. Understanding changes in DTI metrics in patients with different stages of neurocysticercosis. Magn Reson Imaging. 2012;30:104-11.
27. Mori S, Zhang J. Principles of diffusion tensor imaging and its applications to basic neuroscience research. Neuron. 2006;51:527-39.
28. Imfeld A, Oechslin MS, Meyer M, et al. White matter plasticity in the corticospinal tract of musicians: a diffusion tensor imaging study. Neuroimage. 2009;46(3):600-7.
29. Zhang Y, Du G, Yang Y, et al. Higher integrity of the motor and visual pathways in long-term video game players. Front Hum Neurosci. 2015;9:98.
30. Posner MI., Tang YY, Lynch G. Mechanisms of white matter change induced by meditation training. Front Psychol. 2014;5:1220.
31. Luders E, Clark K, Narr KL, et al. Enhanced brain connectivity in long-term meditation practitioners. Neuroimage. 2011;57(4):1308-16.
32. Lee B, Park JY, Jung WH, et al. White matter neuroplastic changes in long-term trained players of the game of "Baduk" 1 (GO): a voxel-based diffusion-tensor imaging study. Neuroimage. 2010;52(1):9-19.
33. Mackey AP, Whitaker KJ, Bunge SA. Experience-dependent plasticity in white matter microstructure: reasoning training alters structural connectivity. Front Neuroanat. 2012;6:32.
34. Driemeyer J, Boyke J, Gaser C, et al. Changes in gray matter induced by learning—revisited. PLoS One. 2008;3(7):e2669.
35. Pagnoni G, Cekic M. Age effects on gray matter volume and attentional performance in Zen meditation. Neurobiol Aging. 2007;28:1623-7.
36. Lutz A, Slagter HA, Dunne JD, et al. Attention regulation and monitoring in meditation. Trends Cogn Sci. 2008;12(4):163-9.
37. Kang DH, Jo HJ, Jung WH, et al. The effect of meditation on brain structure: cortical thickness mapping and diffusion tensor imaging. Soc Cogn Affect Neurosci. 2012;8(1):27-33.
38. Tang YY, Lu Q, Geng X, et al. Short-term meditation induces white matter changes in the anterior cingulate. Proc Natl Acad Sci USA. 2010;107:15649-52.
39. Ceko M, Bushnell MC, Gracely RH. Neurobiology underlying fibromyalgia symptoms. Pain Res Treat. 2012;2012:585419.
40. Quirk GJ, Beer JS. Prefrontal involvement in the regulation of emotion: convergence of rat and human studies. Curr Opin Neurobiol. 2006;16:723-7.
41. Davidson RJ, Jackson DC, Kalin NH. Emotion, plasticity, context, and regulation: perspectives from affective neuroscience. Psychol Bull. 2000;126:890-909.
42. Sharma K, Trivedi R, Chandra S, et al. Enhanced white matter integrity in corpus callosum of long-term Brahmakumaris Rajayoga meditators. Brain Connect. 2018;8:49-55.
43. Hölzel BK, Ott U, Hempel H, et al. Differential engagement of anterior cingulate and adjacent medial frontal cortex in adept meditators and non-meditators. Neurosci Lett. 2007;421:16-21.
44. Ritskes R, Ritskes-Hoitinga M, Stødkilde-Jørgensen H, et al. MRI scanning during Zen meditation: the picture of enlightenment?. Constructivism Hum Sci. 2003;8:85-9.
45. Lazar SW, Bush G, Gollub RL, et al. Functional brain mapping of the relaxation response and meditation. Neuroreport. 2000;11:1581-5.
46. Davidson RJ, Kabat-Zinn J, Schumacher J, et al. Alterations in brain and immune function produced by mindfulness meditation. Psychosom Med. 2003;65:564-70.
47. Davidson RJ, Lutz A. Buddha's brain: neuroplasticity and meditation. IEEE Signal Process Mag. 2008;25:176-4.
48. Pagnoni G, Cekic M, Guo Y. "Thinking about not-thinking": neural correlates of conceptual processing during Zen meditation. PLoS One. 2008;3(9):e3083.
49. Hasenkamp W, Barsalou LW. Effects of meditation experience on functional connectivity of distributed brain networks. Front Hum Neurosci. 2012;6:38.
50. Cahn BR, Polich J. Meditation states and traits: EEG, ERP, and neuroimaging studies. Psychol Bull. 2006;132:180.
51. Brefczynski-Lewis JA, Lutz A, Schaefer HS, et al. Neural correlates of attentional expertise in long-term meditation practitioners. Proc Natl Acad Sci USA. 2007;104:11483-8.

52. Khushu S, Kumaran SS, Telles S, et al. Functional mapping of human brain during meditation: an fMRI study. Biomedicine. 2005;25(2):40-7.
53. Jang JH, Jung WH, Kang DH, et al. Increased default mode network connectivity associated with meditation. Neurosci Lett. 2011;487(3):358-62.
54. Buckner RL, Andrews-Hanna JR, Schacter DL. The brain's default network: anatomy, function, and relevance to disease. Ann NY Acad Sci. 2008;1124:1-38.
55. Dickenson J, Berkman ET, Arch J, et al. Neural correlates of focused attention during a brief mindfulness induction. Soc Cogn Affect Neurosci. 2013;8(1):40-7.
56. Froeliger B, Garland EL, McClernon FJ. Yoga meditation practitioners exhibit greater gray matter volume and fewer reported cognitive failures: results of a preliminary voxel-based morphometric analysis. Evid Based Complement Alternat Med. 2012;2012:821307.

125

CHAPTER

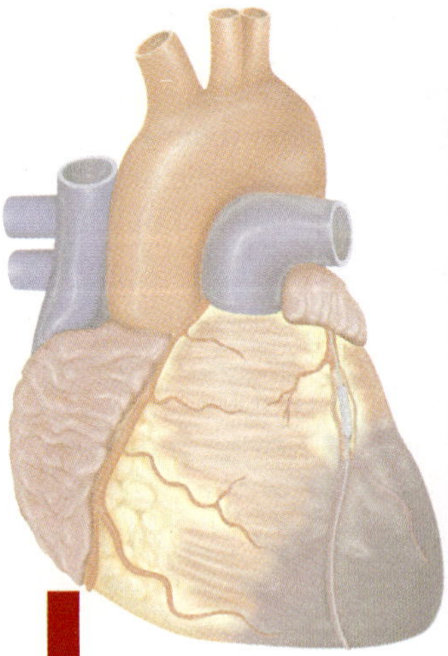

Multimodality Imaging and Telemedicine in Cardiology

P Krishnam Raju, SG Prasad

INTRODUCTION

The advent of newer communication technologies with higher bandwidths, the exponential increase in the noninvasive and minimally invasive imaging technologies having the ability of providing detailed information about the overall functioning and structure of the heart and the vasculature, and the flexibility of integrating various imaging modalities adhering to imaging protocols have enabled specialists to assimilate all relevant data and transmit the same in a systematic manner to facilitate diagnosing even from distant locations. The merging of science and innovation in our dynamic advanced time has brought about the improvement of inventive digital gadgets that permit simple and exact portrayal in well-being and disease. In today's medical arena, imaging technologies are beginning to play a very important role in diagnosing and suggesting an appropriate course of treatment. One of the distinct advantages that arise from imaging diagnostics is that there is already a set proprietary format, namely digital imaging and communications in medicine (DICOM) involved in the acquisition and storage formulated by the American College of Radiology and National Engineers Manufacturing Association which makes interoperability with various application software simpler. The best of experienced specialists with knowledge are often concentrated in specialty centers in cities, and the number is very low compared to the number of patients seeking their advice. In this context, telemedicine can now be an effective tool in facilitating transmission and viewing of these images along with relevant clinical information over network by specialists sitting anywhere in the world to get the best of opinions. With advances in the imaging technology in providing high sensitivity and spatial resolution, quantitative molecular imaging for understanding the physiology at cellular and molecular levels is now one of the areas where active research is happening which can lead to a new unique platform in diagnostic imaging. Any increase in the resolution of images at the molecular level can bring about a significant advance to the outcome of research. Imaging is fast emerging as the frontline diagnostic investigation for evaluation or identification of diseases. Imaging technologies have brought about a change in clinical approach to the management of diseases significantly.[1] This leads us to the need of having an integrated platform which helps in integrating multimodality imaging devices through one interface and providing the relevant images easily. Picture archiving and communication system (PACS) is more often associated with radiology, but with increasing imaging investigations in cardiology, they have started using this technology more effectively. Unlike radiology where PACS finds maximum utilization since most of the modalities are not dependent on radiologists for performing the test, cardiology have been conservative in the utilization of this technology. However, many cardiology departments have started implementing PACS, and they typically begin from the catheterization (XA) laboratory before integrating other modalities. The dynamic nature of images in cardiac imaging and the associated file size for these play an important role in designing an imaging system for retrieving and archiving.

Picture archiving and communication system essentially is an image management system. They consist of image display systems, archiving systems, networks, and interfaces, presenting one unified system to the user. Radiology has been actively using the PACS platform since the 1980s and changing film-based environment to a filmless environment. The success and acceptance of the DICOM standard in radiology have led to other health-care specialties adopting the standard and thereby moving into a shared electronic digital world. Seeing the success in radiology and also the increase in image-based investigations in cardiology, cardiac imaging equipment started adhering to DICOM standards which led to a PACS specifically designed for cardiology. Since cardiology studies are dynamic (in motion), huge numbers of images and a vast amount of data are generated per study (a single study can range from 200 MB to 1 GB). It has been observed that there is a 20% increase every year on the cardiology studies being done.[2]

As all advances made in communication technology, especially bandwidth, are not available at all locations, it is important that the telemedicine technology caters to the actual needs of the communities by having the appropriate technology. Different specialties need different requirements, such as cardiology basic investigations use still images which can be transmitted over low bandwidths than orthopedics wherein higher resolution of images are required.[3] Live consultations provided through telemedicine require high bandwidth to ensure good quality as also having continuous education programs being transmitted through the same ICT (information and communication technology) platform. As telemedicine is slowing finding itself more usage than before, it is necessary that not too many restrictions and over use of technology become a deterrent. For example, telecardiology has moved beyond the transmission of simple electrocardiograms (ECGs) or echocardiographic images to include interactive video for patient consultation and remote diagnosis for cardiac problems. Such growth and exploration of new ways to utilize electronic imaging technology can be beneficial to patients. Newer applications must further have the flexibility to explore ways that this technology can continue to grow and improve health-care delivery. Mobile smart phone technologies and accessibility of them everywhere has made them very useful and convenient tools to deliver good and prompt health-care diagnostics, follow-up, and treatment. New technologies, such as cloud computing, storage, retrieval, block chain technology, and balloon-based internet connectivity, are making health care accessible and useful even in remote areas, hilly regions, islands, and desert areas as well. Electronic health records are making it possible to share patient data within the hospital system among different departments and between different health facilities across cities and continents. Patient outcomes and cost effectiveness of these new technologies are yet to be worked out and proven.

PICTURE ARCHIVING AND COMMUNICATION SYSTEM ARCHITECTURE

Picture archiving and communication system is an ensemble health-care technology which comprises various modules for acquisition of medical images from multiple modalities, reliable storage of these images along with easy and convenient access when needed.[4] Picture archiving and communication system acquires the images of DICOM format which is the industry standard in medical imaging (Table 1).

TABLE 1: Advantages and disadvantages of film-based system and PACS.

Film-based system	*PACS*
Advantages • Initial investment is low • No extra training is required • Film-based X-rays cannot be altered **Disadvantages** • Requires additional infrastructure, such as dark room for processing films and is a manual-based consuming time • If the quality of film is bad, then patient needs to undergo repeated examination, leading to more exposure to radiation • Expensive in the long run	**Advantages** • Increased availability of images • Increased processing, no lost film, multiple copies of the same image can be generated • Image manipulation to overcome under or over exposure • Increased accessibility, speed, and quality of reporting • Cost effective in the long run **Disadvantages** • Initial investment is high • Needs training for proper maintenance • Possibility of alteration exposes digital radiography to fraudulent use and legal issues • In the case of PACS system failure, it is not possible to view the radiological investigations

(PACS: picture archiving communication system)

Picture archiving and communication system has enabled many hospitals to streamline their way of operation in terms of storage, viewing, accessing critical patient data, and ability to share images to specialists in a seamless manner. They provide viewing of high-resolution images, thereby facilitating in the process of diagnosis. With proper design for storage of data, both online as well as offline, retrieval of images become independent on the location of the storage (Fig. 1). Essentially, PACS architecture consists of the following three modules:

- Acquisition
- Storage
- Viewing.

Acquisition System

Today, virtually all imaging equipment are fully DICOM compliant. Each imaging modality is configured to send images to a server which hosts a DICOM gateway service that permits the handshake between the imaging modality and the server. Thus, images can be stored on a network or a workstation in the DICOM format. Earlier, these images were transmitted over telephone line with bandwidths being as low as 2,400 bps.[5] The availability of high bandwidths even at distant locations has made centers connect directly over internet for transmitting images to the PACS server.

Storage System

All the images received by the DICOM gateway service are archived in the storage server. There are compression algorithms which are lossy and lossless based that help in reducing the file size with varying degree of loss in the quality of image. It must be noted that imaging investigations related to cardiology generally consume more storage as the size of the study tend to be high ranging anywhere from 200 MB to 1.5 GB. Accordingly, the storage and the compression techniques to be adopted need to be planned well to ensure optimal storage consumption. Another important aspect that needs to be looked into is the time taken for retrieval of images. Obviously, if the size of the study is large and the number of images more, the time taken to retrieve becomes longer. Hence, compression techniques and methodologies of streaming data to software applications play an important role.

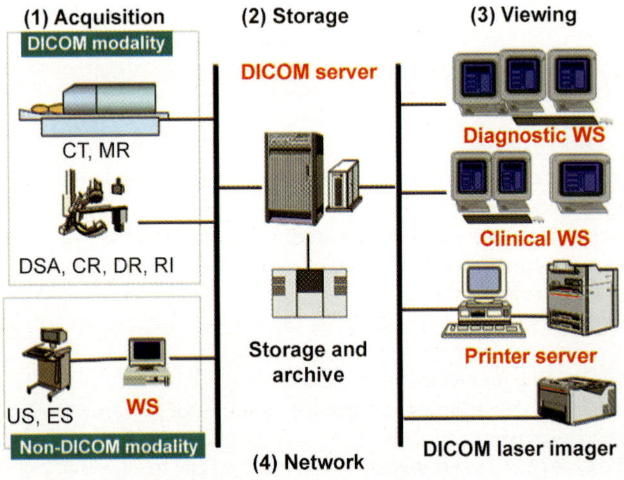

Fig. 1: PACS architecture.

Viewing System

This module forms the front end of any PACS solution. The acquisition and storage modules are back-end operations which happen seamlessly once each imaging modality is configured to the DICOM gateway service in the server. The viewing segment enables retrieving images from the server and displaying them on the viewer. All functionalities that assist in image manipulation, such as gray shade control, zoom, measurements, volume rendering, and reconstruction, are part of this module which assist the radiologists/cardiologists to work around with images and give an opinion. This module also enables in providing templates for various studies, thereby facilitating the efficiency in terms of turnaround time for reporting.

In fact, it is the PACS architecture and application that permits transmission of images across network for getting specialists' opinions or second opinion. More and more hospitals are adopting to higher utilization of PACS as it gives them the flexibility to view and report cases from anywhere provided they have the due credentials to access the PACS servers.

APPLICATION OF IMAGING TECHNOLOGY IN CARDIOLOGY

There are varied clinical presentations, such as chest pain, dyspnea, syncope, palpitations, which are the first signs to raise doubts of a cardiovascular problem. Based on the clinical history and general examination, cardiologists generally recommend a list of investigations that include blood chemistry and diagnostic tests which have been listed below. Cardiac imaging investigations may also be required to monitor patients with known pathology in many cardiovascular diseases such as interval monitoring of aortic stenosis, heart failure, cardiac devices, etc. The basic choice of cardiac imaging modality essentially is dependent on the disease being investigated, individual patient characteristics, and the accessibility of tests. The advantage of imaging diagnostics is because of the availability of these images in the digital format, the transmission of these images to relevant select specialists has become lot more easier than before. The two most common scenarios in the clinical side that require cardiac imaging are dyspnea and coronary artery disease. Imaging is also indicated in the diagnosis of cardiomyopathy, structural, and congenital heart disease.[6]

Electrocardiogram

The 12-lead ECG is one of the basic diagnostic tests that is commonly suggested in the assessment of cardiovascular disease (Box 1). The use of standardized terminology is recommended to allow the application of ECG diagnoses across many different hospital systems and countries.[7] Today, we have ECG machines, which are portable and ones that give the option of giving a single lead or 3 lead or the standard 12-lead ECG. These devices are coming with interfaces that can be integrated to applications, thereby facilitating getting them in a digital format. The biggest advantage of this is that ECGs can now be transmitted to cardiologists who can view the ECG on their mobiles. One of the most important factors for management of ST-elevation myocardial infarction (STEMI) is to facilitate prehospital diagnosis leading to early reperfusion in patients. Electrocardiography is the gold standard for the diagnosis of STEMI in both prehospital and hospital settings. Prehospital transmission of ECGs through telemedicine has revolutionized the management of STEMI by ensuring that health-care professionals can decide a plan of care before the patient reaches the hospital. The transmission of ECG has been in practice for quite some time and with Internet of Things (IoT)-based medical devices, the portability concerns and the ease of capture have more or less become less of an issue. The typical size of an ECG ranges from 100 kB to 300 kB suggesting a low bandwidth requirement for transmission. The ability to transmit a patient's ECG is a good example of the benefits telecardiology can bring, and it has impacted greatly on the treatment of acute heart attacks.

X-ray (Computed Radiography/Digital Radiography)

Chest X-ray is another common investigation that is recommended in the assessment of cardiovascular disease after the ECG (Box 2). While being one of the most common investigations, reading of a chest X-ray requires a lot of experience as the imaging is based on interpreting shadows generated by radiation exposure. More often, findings are misinterpreted and, therefore, the option of using the ICT platform to get opinions from experienced professionals always helps even within the hospital. Today, most hospitals and diagnostics centers have computed radiography machines which provide the digital format (DICOM), enabling easy transmission of images over the network. A lossless X-ray image size is about 10–15 MB, but using acceptable lossless compression techniques, the sizes can be reduced to 4–5 MB. It is important to note that a normal chest X-ray however does not exclude other cardiac problems. Specific cardiac conditions, such as valvular heart problems, congenital heart diseases, or pulmonary arterial hypertension, may not be comprehensively confirmed with this investigation.[6]

Echocardiography

Echocardiography (ECHO) is fast being considered as the mainstream cardiac imaging modality and the availability of portable machines have made this modality an ideal tool to be used in the Telemedicine platform (Box 3). As echocardiographic images are dynamic in nature, the data associated is much more than those with still images. Image compression algorithms are used to compress to

BOX 1: Assessment by ECG.

- Cardiac rhythm
- Detection of myocardial ischemia and infarction
- Conduction system abnormalities
- Preexcitation
- Long QT syndromes
- Atrial abnormalities
- Ventricular hypertrophy
- Pericarditis

BOX 2: Assessment by X-ray.

- Size of heart
- Pulmonary markings or pleural effusion that may be indicative of pulmonary congestion secondary to cardiac failure
- Pulmonary hypertension
- Pericardial effusion
- Pulmonary pathology, such as infection, malignancy, or fibrosis

BOX 3: Assessment by echocardiography.

- Size and shape of the heart and the size, thickness, and wall motion abnormalities
- Heart's systolic/diastolic functioning
- Functionality of the heart valves
- Stenotic valves or regurgitation
- Tumor or infectious growth around heart valves
- Infective endocarditis
- Congenital heart defects
- Pericardial/myocardial disease

enable quicker transmission which can affect the quality of images. With the modern ECHO machines adhering to DICOM protocol, integration of this modality to the PACS platform has become possible. Patients with cardiac failure and valvular problems are often recommended to undergo ECHO investigation to suggest a course of treatment. Septal defects which are congenital and the presence of pulmonary arterial hypertension can be identified on ECHO (Box 4).

Cardiac-computed Tomography Angiography

The multislice computed tomography (CT), gated by ECG, is now considered as a cost effective diagnostic test for the evaluation of coronary arteries and helps in the assessment of heart structure along with coronary circulation. The latest advances over the last decade in CT technology have not only results in enhancing image quality but also in achieving the same with lower radiation dosage. The speed of acquisition has increased tremendously allowing the imaging of the heart with minimal involuntary motion that can affect the image quality.[8] Cardiac-computed tomography angiography (CCTA) as a diagnostic option has found widespread application for patients having suspected coronary artery disease. It has also been found as an effective test to evaluate the coronary grafts for patients who have undergone coronary bypass surgery. For patients at an intermediate level of risk of cardiovascular events, quantifying the coronary artery calcification using the CCTA is now emerging to be reliable measure. Based on the age-specific quartiles, a calcium score is given based on the degree of calcification present. Significantly, elevated scores are at greater risk of myocardial infarction according to a multiple, large observational studies that have been carried out. A low calcium score is indicative of the absence of significant coronary stenosis, thereby suggesting a favorable cardiac prognosis.

Cardiac Magnetic Resonance Imaging

Cardiac magnetic resonance imaging (MRI) is now being used as a good diagnostic measure for assessing the heart structure and vasculature, and it helps in the assessment of various heart diseases, including congenital (Box 5). As this imaging technology does not use ionizing radiation, the diagnostic quality of images is better for certain cardiac conditions. Consequently, this is a safer and preferred investigation for patients having complex congenital diseases requiring multiple scans than CT, decreasing the risk of radiation exposure. Electrocardiogram-gated MRI produces the needed imaging of the heart with higher temporal resolution. The severity of aortic regurgitation and measurement of the associated volumes can be evaluated which is helpful in planning the management for patient suffering with diseased aortic valve with associated aortopathy and detecting the presence of aortic coarctation.

Catheterization

The older and the most reliable investigation for evaluating any cardiac disease is coronary angiography (Box 6). Critical information related to the heart and the blood vessels surrounding it are obtained which gives us a fair picture of heart function both in terms of the valves and blood flow of the arteries surrounding it. Most XA laboratories are DICOM compliant which facilitates seamless integration to the PACS platform. Once images are there in the digital format, transmission of the same to specialists anywhere is very much possible. PACS software today also provide the option of converting DICOM images to other digital formats, such as Audio Video Interleave and Moving Picture Experts Group (MPEG), which reduces the files size of the images without much loss in the quality of image. This option is exercised more when specialists do not have access to DICOM viewers and need to see images on an emergency basis for an opinion. The MPEG format permits angiography sequences sent through mail or even on WhatsApp for a quick look on the cardiologists' smartphones.

BOX 4: Assessment by cardiac CT.

- Anatomic origin and course of the coronary arteries
- Coronary artery disease and calcium scoring
- Evaluation of thoracic aorta, aortic valve, bypass grafts, left atrium, and various structural cardiac abnormalities
- Coronary venous system for cardiac electrophysiology procedures
- Calcium scoring

BOX 5: Assessment by cardiac MRI.

- Anatomy and function of the heart chambers, valves, size, and blood flow through major vessels, and surrounding structures, such as the pericardium
- Diagnosing a variety of cardiovascular disorders, such as tumors, infections, and inflammatory conditions
- Myocardial pathologies
- Evaluating the effects of coronary artery disease such as ischemia of heart muscle, scarring within the heart muscle after a heart attack and for the assessment of myocardial viability

BOX 6: Assessment by catheterization (XA).

- Coronary artery disease
- Valvular heart disease
- Congenital heart disease

Positron Emission Tomography

Positron emission tomography (PET) is fast finding its applications in cardiac imaging. The last decade has witnessed extensive application of PET techniques to assess myocardial viability and has provided valuable information important in analyzing the risk:benefit ratio for several therapeutic measures (Box 7). Positron emission tomography helps us to understand the physiological and pathophysiological mechanisms of myocardial metabolism, receptor physiology, and blood flow. This technique involves the induction of radiotracer which mixes with the blood and the gamma detector circling the heart picks up the signals from the tracer and digital images are constructed from these signals. The scan gives an indication of the blood flowing across the arteries. This technique helps in documenting the exact percentage of coronary artery stenosis as a basis for therapeutic planning and the identification of viable myocardium in patients after myocardial infarction. This form of diagnostic imaging has traditionally been perceived as cost-prohibitive in comparison to general nuclear medicine cardiac stress testing using single photon emission CT. However, due to significant gains in access to scanners, related to the widely accepted role of PET/CT in clinical oncology, cardiac PET is likely to become more widely available, particularly given various clinical and technical advantages that might make this a potential test of choice in the diagnosis of coronary artery and other heart diseases.[9]

Internet of Things Devices

The health-care landscape is dramatically changing, and in the face of such a rapid evolution, many organizations are seeking ways to keep pace and remain contemporary. Continuity in patient care and adopting better efficiencies in patient management with the use of technology now need to have real-time intelligence regarding aspects, such as patient history, point of care diagnostics, medications, and supply of inventory. Although the concept of IoT is not new, a lot of attention is currently being placed because of the wide range of clinical applications that can be designed with this technology. These devices can communicate directly through Bluetooth or Wi-Fi to applications hosted in systems or laptops or portable devices, such as mobiles or tablets. This helps us in monitoring patient data which may be ECG or blood-glucose levels or blood pressure in a systematic and comprehensive way. A large portion of these measures require interaction with a specialist as a follow-up. This makes an opening for more intelligent gadgets to convey more important information, decreasing the requirement for direct patient–doctor collaboration.

BOX 7: Assessment by PET.

- Infective endocarditis
- Granulomatous myocardial disease
- Aortitis
- Pacemaker infections
- Assessment of ischemic heart disease for ischemia and myocardial viability

OUR EXPERIENCE

Cooperative for assistance and relief everywhere (CARE) has been actively using the PACS system for over 8 years. The PACS application has been developed in-house and integrated with open-source viewer tailor made to our requirement and has undergone several iterations in the design based on clinical inputs from team of cardiologists and radiologists (Table 2). All imaging modalities are seamlessly integrated over the DICOM network to the PACS server, and a viewing module has been provided for all doctors and other clinical staff for viewing all studies. The viewer has all the features of a typical stand-alone modality workstation, wherein the viewer can perform many post processing tasks, such as gray shade leveling, calculation of area and volume of images, Hounsfield unit, and converting DICOM images to various other picture or video file formats. Integration of PACS solution with open-source advanced viewer so that all advanced features, such as scout lines, maximum intensity projection, and multiplanar reconstructions, are available for users of the application. This solution is also integrated with a reporting module with the option of macro-based templates to ensure reporting in an efficient manner and ensuring that reports are in a structured manner. This component makes PACS suitable for telecardiology or teleradiology applications (Fig. 2).

Cooperative for assistance and relief everywhere (CARE) has three of its centers at Banjara, Nampally, and Hitech City Centre that perform cardiac CT and cardiac MR. Cardiologists assigned on these modalities report on these cases by viewing images through PACS irrespective of

TABLE 2: Number of cardiac CT and MR at CARE.

Sl. No	Location	Modality	Number
1	Banjara (6 years)	Cardiac CT	4841
		Cardiac MR	1864
2	Nampally (3 years)	Cardiac MR	390
3	Hitech City (2 years)	Cardiac CT	289
		Cardiac MR	128

their place of work within the CARE network. It also gives the flexibility of getting opinion from other cardiologists/radiologists as every specialist having the PACS application with appropriate credentials can view the images. We have a good repository of images over the last 5 years in our server and maintain a library of all interesting cases which are often discussed in our in-house weekly academic programs. Echocardiography and XA laboratory are also integrated to the PACS and can be viewed from any of the CARE locations.

Case Examples

The important case examples are given in Figures 3 to 6.

- Cardiac magnetic resonance imaging (Figs. 3 and 4)
- Cardiac-computed tomography angiogram (Fig. 5).
- *CARE, Mahabubnagar:* An ECG was taken for all the patients for whom an ECHO investigation was suggested. A paramedic who was resident of Mahabubnagar town about 100 km away from the hub center was trained at our hub center for a duration of 1 month on providing the echocardiographic views (Fig. 6). As part of the process of telemedicine, the specialist would first have a face-to-face interaction with the patient to understand the condition and complaints of the patient all of which were recorded through the application software.[10] A two-way interactive video conferencing (VC) system was provided for the live interaction, and the output of the echocardiographic machine was given as an input to the VC which enabled all echocardiographic images to be streamed live as the case was being done. The paramedic provided the necessary views through the established ICT platform for the specialist at the hub center to diagnose. The report was generated online and post completion of the test the specialist would again explain to patient the findings and advice accordingly for further course of action.
- *Case example:* Coronary heart disease with large patent ductus arteriosus and atrial septal aneurysm (Fig. 7)
- *Case example:* Dilated left ventricle with noncompaction of left ventricle apex (Fig. 8)
- *Case example:* Fetal echocardiography (Fig. 9).

Electrocardiogram Reporting from Rural Centers

As a part of our rural initiative, CARE conducts a rural health program covering 124 villages in the East and West Godavari districts of Andhra Pradesh and about 10 villages from the Ranga Reddy district of Telangana (Fig. 10). The program involves conducting consultations via telemedicine network and performs routine blood investigations and ECG. Electrocardiograms from these villages are transmitted to the hub center at Hyderabad through Telemedicine application. Cardiologists access images and report the same. The ICT platform has indeed made it easy for people at distant locations to get specialists' opinions on the ECG.

Patient Remote Monitoring System

CARE foundation in collaboration with VIOS Medical devices clinically validated the sensors for capturing vital information, namely ECG, oxygen saturation (SpO_2) with the gold standard (standard bed side monitors) (Fig. 11).

More than 500 patients have availed the benefit of this technology at CARE Hitech Hospitals, Hyderabad, thereby reducing their stay at the ICU and maintaining same standards of monitoring at rooms through IoT sensors.

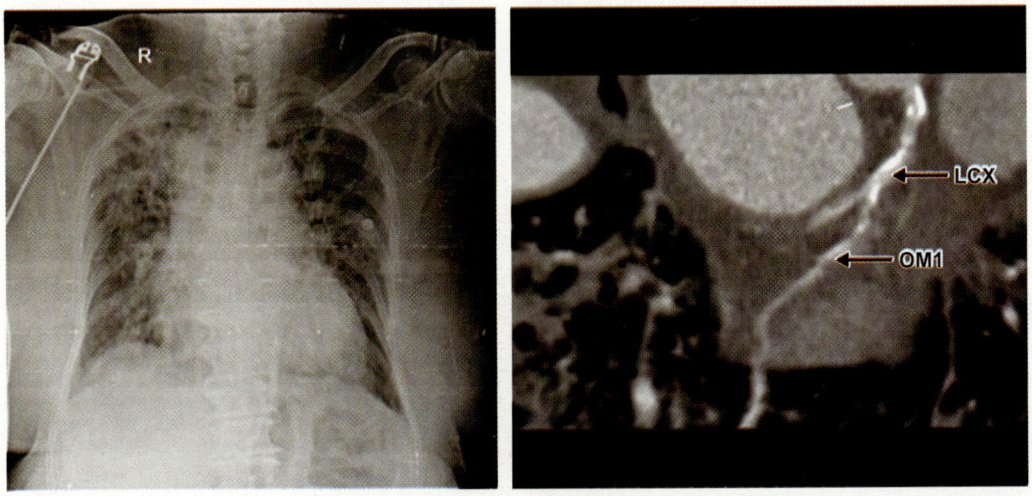

Fig. 2: Cardiac PACS viewer.

This technology has also opened up the doors for providing monitoring patients discharged from hospitals to their homes ensuring continuity of care. Patients having chronic ailments, such as congestive heart failure who need regular monitoring but not necessarily hospitalization all the time, are best suited to use these devices.

Second Opinion

The PACS platform provides an ideal solution to share images to both patients as well as other clinicians for getting a second opinion. Typically, the request is most for coronary angiograms, wherein patients like to get a

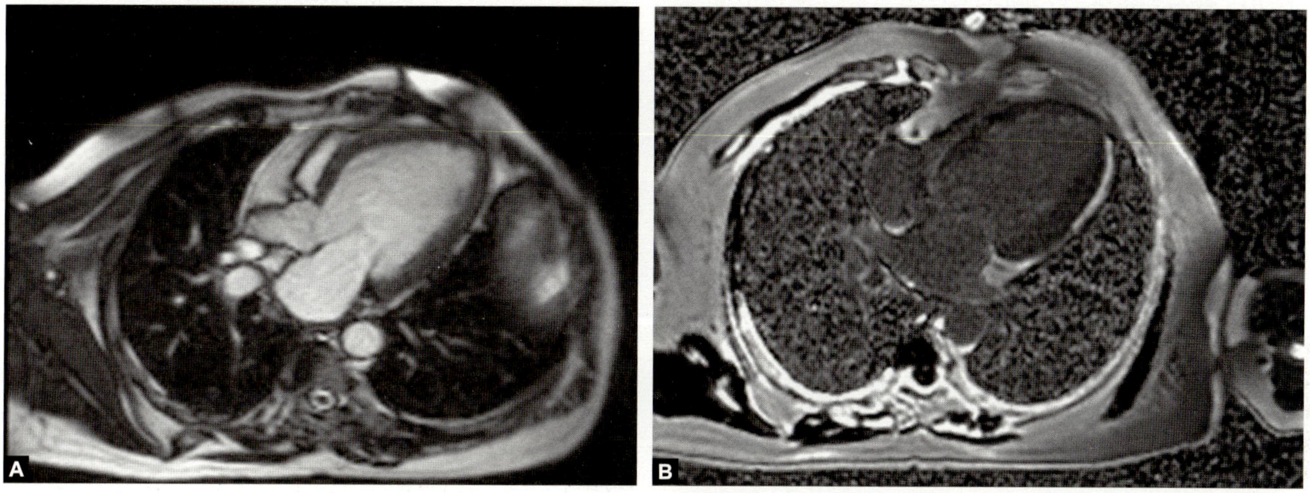

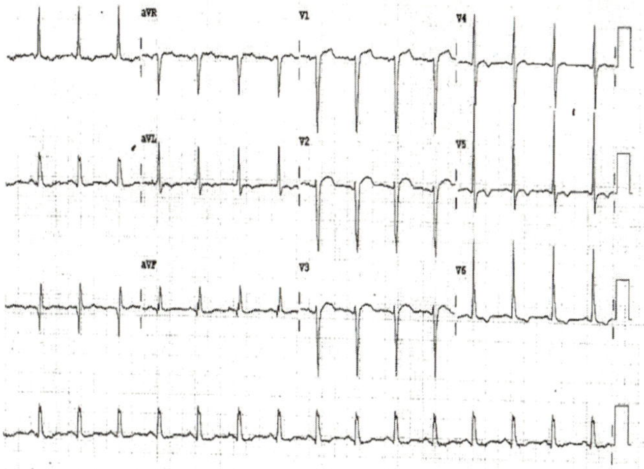

Study suggestive of dilated cardiomyopathy 2° to left bundle branch block (LBBB) with underlying hibernating ischemic heart disease (IHD)

- Dilated left ventricle (LV)/left atrial (LA)
- Regional wall motion abnormalities (RWMA) in left anterior descending (LAD) and right coronary artery (RCA) territory
- Abnormal septal motion suggestive of left bundle branch block
- Severe LV dysfunction
- 0–25% subendocardial scar in mid LAD territory (partially viable)
- 25–50% subendocardial scar in distal LAD territory (partially viable)
- 25–50% subendocardial scar in RCA territory (partially viable)
- Significant viable myocardium in LAD and RCA territory
- Normal right ventricular (RV) size and function
- Mild MR/no LV thrombus/no pericardial effusion

Figs. 3A and B: Cardiac MRI showing dilated cardiomyopathy.

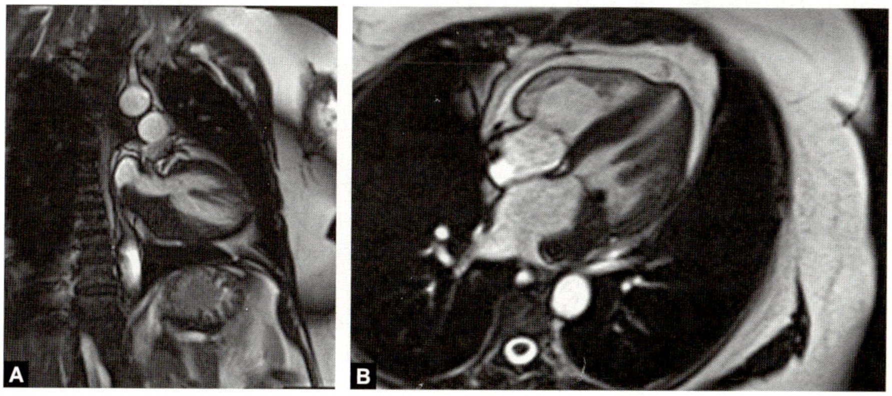

Study suggestive of Calcified LA thrombus

- Normal LV size/Dilated LA
- No RWMA
- Good LV function
- Normal RV size and function
- Homogenous calcified LA mass extending into the basal LV cavity
- No evidence of malignant behavior of the mass
- Mild MR/ No LV thrombus/No pericardial effusion

Figs. 4A and B: Cardiac MRI showing calcified LA thrombus.

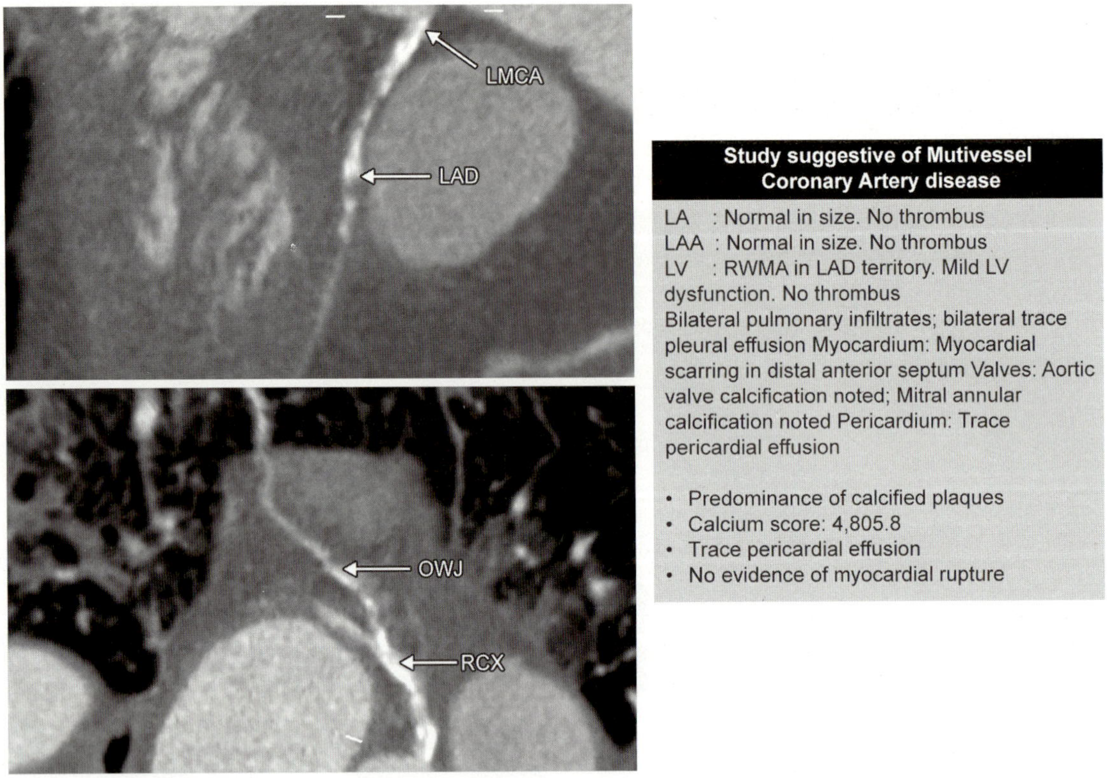

Fig. 5: Cardiac CTA showing multivessel CAD.

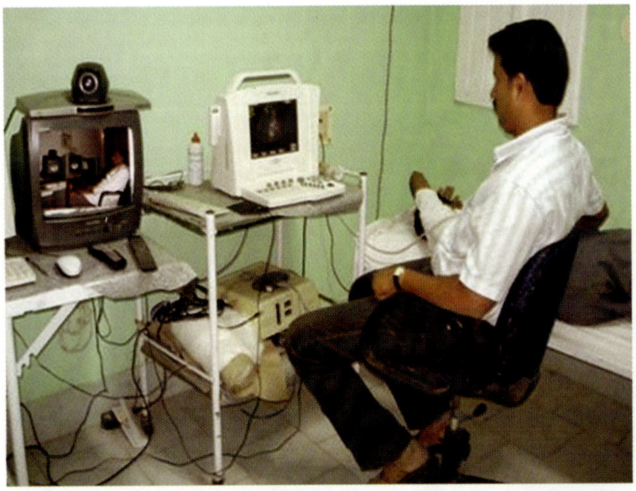

Fig. 6

second opinion on the kind of procedure that needs to be undertaken after the coronary angiogram is performed. One issue that is prevalent is that CDs are provided to patients upon request, and it is left to them to possibly get the second opinion. Our PACS solution provides the feature of ensuring that all angiography sequences are converted into MPEG format, maintaining a specific resolution for viewing. The advantage with this is that these sequences can be sent to respective emails making them accessible to specialists on their mobiles, tablets, or laptops/computers, making it convenient for them to get advice and in also maintaining a transparent system for getting the best for the patients.

ROLE OF ARTIFICIAL INTELLIGENCE IN CARDIOLOGY

The continuous development in communication technologies and increase of IoT-based medical devices have led to an outburst in the kind of data emerging. The good side of this is that the bandwidth to do analytics with this data is now available which can help us in developing algorithms based on pattern recognitions on the data and assist in predictive analysis. As decision-making is not easy and rather complex in medicine, algorithms that are developed based on the availability of reliable and objective facts can assist the concerned specialist in making well-informed diagnosis. Artificial intelligence (AI) is generally defined as the assemblage of items (algorithms, robotics,

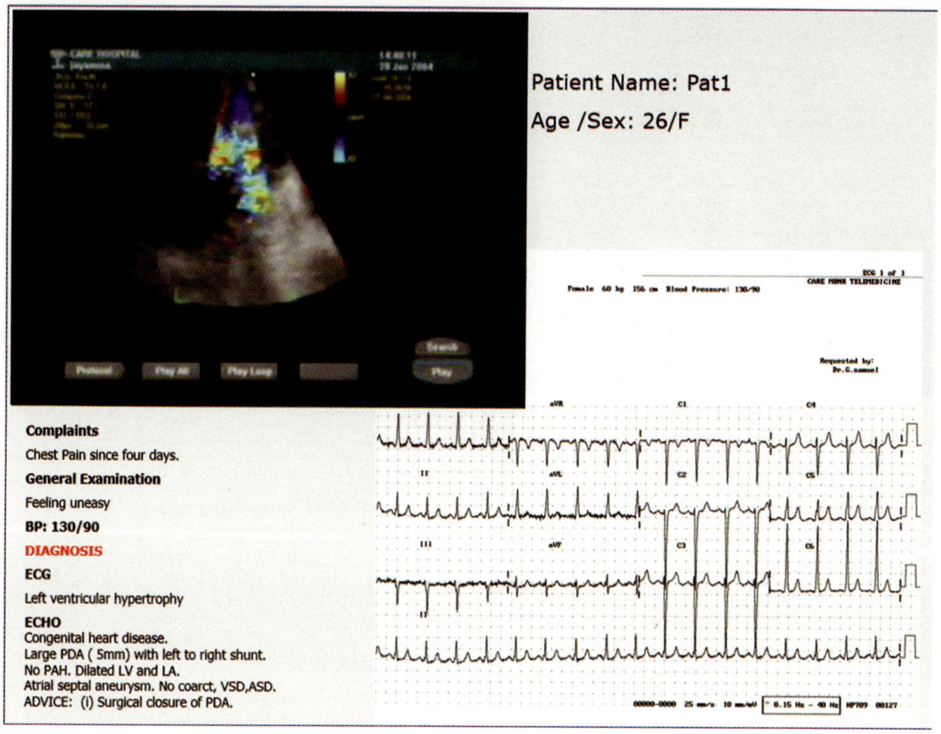

Fig. 7: CHD with large PDA and atrial septal aneurysm.

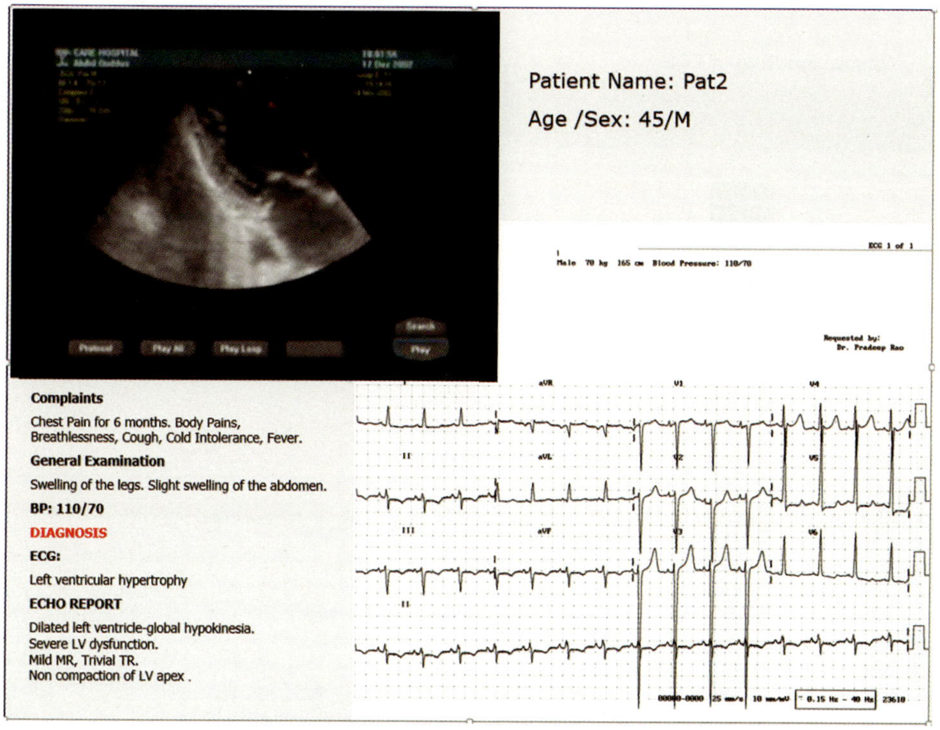

Fig. 8: Dilated LV with non-compaction of LV apex.

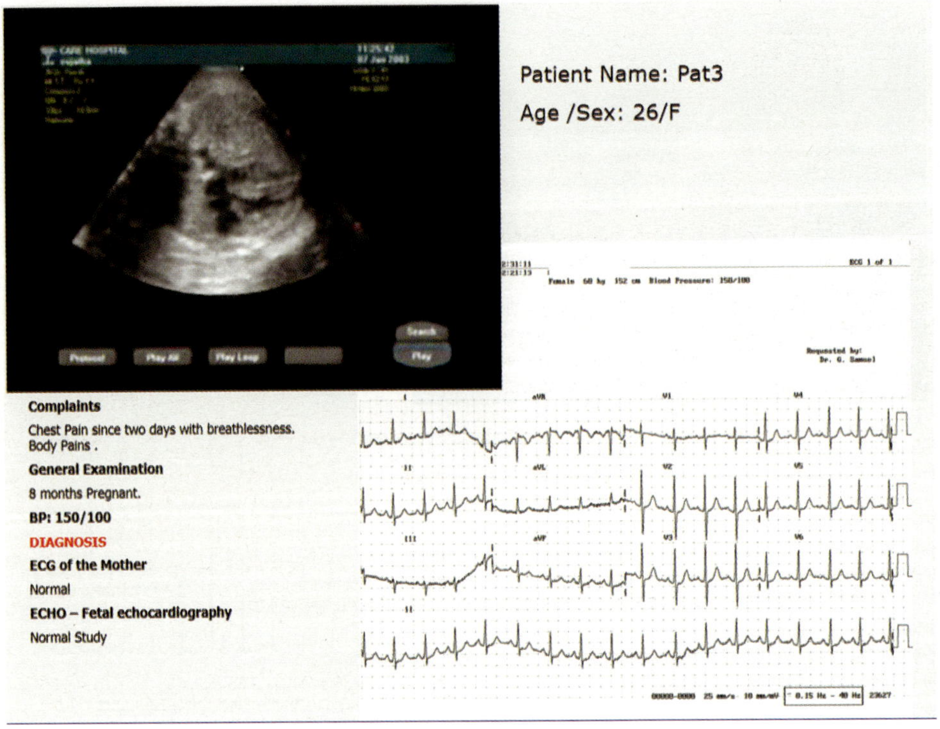

Fig. 9: Fetal echocardiography.

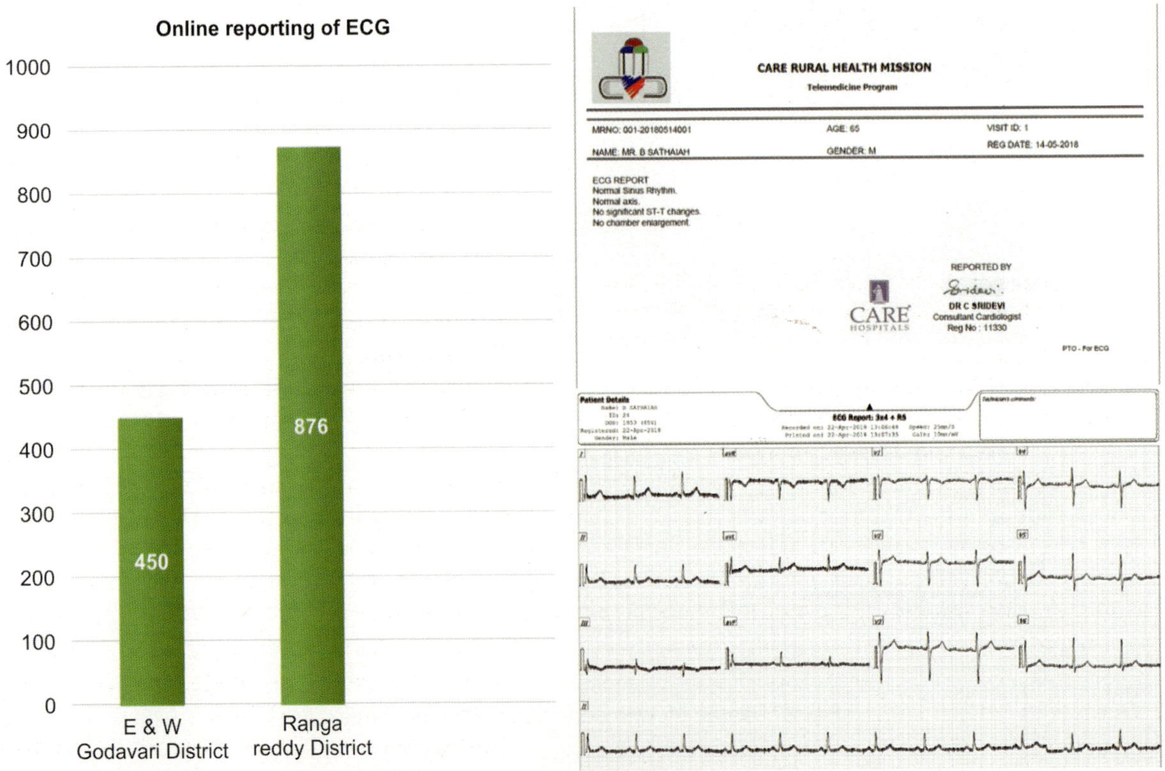

Fig. 10: Online reporting of ECG by CARE.

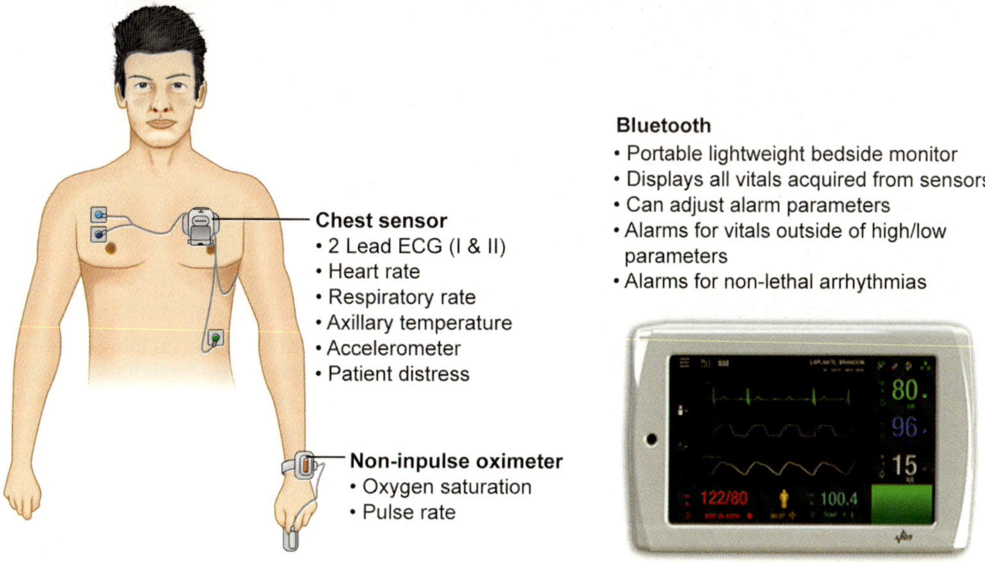

Fig. 11: Patient remote monitoring system.

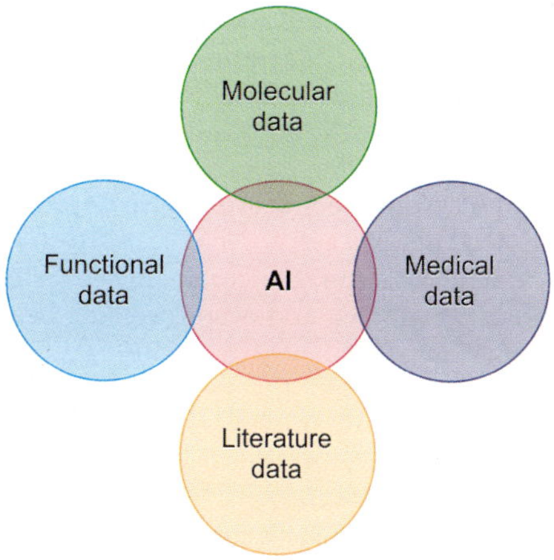

Fig. 12: Four areas of big data sources in cardiovascular biomedicine. (AI: artificial intelligence)

and neural networks) and an application software which is developed with the kind of intelligence comparable to those of a human being, and whose database is constantly updated to permit the software to acquire the learning with minimal human interference.[11]

Artificial intelligence can play a specific role in cardiology by using techniques, such as machine learning, deep learning, and cognitive thinking. Machine learning is focused on building automated clinical decision systems (such as readmission and mortality score systems) that help doctors make more accurate predictions, rather than simple estimated score systems. Deep learning mimics the functionality of the brain through multiple layers of neural network that create training datasets to automatically generate predictions based on the input data. This technique is very powerful with relation to image recognition and can potentially be used in cardiovascular imaging. Cognitive computing is self-learning systems which adopts the techniques of machine learning and pattern recognition to simulate the functioning of a human thought. The kind of big data available in cardiology can be broadly classified as shown in the Figure 12.

In cardiovascular biomedicine, there are four areas of big data sources which are important (Fig. 12):

1. Functional data which includes patient demographics as well as imaging data that includes ECG, ECHO, vital monitoring data and from and other, hemodynamics, and imaging data.
2. Molecular data is associated data that comes from genomics/proteomics acquired in large trials or the clinical setting.
3. Medical data which includes the complete patient medical record, including patient electronic medical records along with physician's notes and other information on disease, treatment, outcomes, and epidemiology that may be mined for association studies and predictive modeling on prognosis and drug responses leading to precision medicine.
4. Literature data that is assimilated information on all kinds of research going on and the outcomes of the research work which can be easily mined and structured by deep learning algorithms.

The use of AI is evolving increasingly in cardiology, and there are already excellent examples in several areas. Using a sophisticated learning system to electrocardiographic interpretation, Li et al. achieved that electrocardiographic patterns were automatically recognized with an accuracy of 88% for the classification of abnormal rhythms.[12] One of the studies conducted used a machine learning and data-mining system to evaluate and classify patients with heart failure and found that although the system was superior to conventional methods for predicting heart failure with preserved ejection fraction, there were no advantages over the traditional logistic regression.[13]

We are currently working with the data generated from the patient remote monitoring system to develop:

- Predictive algorithms for atrial fibrillation detection.
- Derive the blood pressure from ECG and photoplethysmography based on the pulse wave transit time.

CONCLUSION

Cardiac imaging is becoming an integral part for cardiac disease diagnosis and more so for monitoring patients. The minimally invasive nature involved in acquisition of images has made it more convenient from the patient's perspective, and the advances made in the spatial and temporal resolution obtained give clinicians a fairly good perspective to make their diagnosis. The availability of the images in a digital format (DICOM) and the PACS system has further made viewing of these images from anywhere, irrespective of the location of the specialist to seek medical advice whether it is the first or second opinion. The lossless compression algorithms help in reducing the associated file sizes proportionately without compromising on the quality of the image and thereby reducing the time needed for retrieval of images from the server and the bandwidth requirements. With the advances made in communication technology and the availability of 3G/4G, bandwidth availability even in distant locations is posing less of a challenge than a couple of years ago. The numerous amount of data that is being generated from all this has now opened up the doors for the development of algorithms that help in the design of a clinical decision support system as well as in predictive analysis. We, however, need to take a cautious approach in the application of AI in medicine though the initial trends have been encouraging. Artificial intelligence should more be considered as a tool to assist clinicians in making their diagnosis and have a 360° view of all data before making their diagnosis.

REFERENCES

1. Di Carli MF, Geva T, Davidoff R. The future of cardiovascular imaging. Circulation. 2016;133:2640-61.
2. Diagnostic Imaging. Cardiology PACS basics: with large studies and growing volume, cardiology can benefit from PACS. [online] Available from http://www.diagnosticimaging.com/pacs-and-informatics/cardiology-pacs-basics-large-studies-and-growing-volume-cardiology-can-benefit-pacs. [Accessed October, 2018].
3. Taylor JM, Picciano LD. Color imaging in telemedicine. Current trends and future needs. In: Color and imaging conference, 3rd color and imaging conference final program and proceedings. Oxford: Igneta Connect; 2017. pp. 181-5.
4. Heckman K, Schultz TJ. PACS: a guide to the digital revolution. New York: Springer; 1999. pp. 249-67.
5. Burute N, Jankharia B. Teleradiology: the Indian perspective. Indian J Radiol Imaging. 2009;19:16-8.
6. Stokes MB, Roberts-Thomson R. The role of cardiac imaging in clinical practice. Aust Prescr. 2017;40(4):151-5.
7. Mason JW, Hancock EW, Gettes LS, et al. Recommendations for the standardization and interpretation of the electrocardiogram: Part II: Electrocardiography diagnostic statement list a scientific statement from the American Heart Association Electrocardiography and Arrhythmias Committee, Council on Clinical Cardiology; the American College of Cardiology Foundation; and the Heart Rhythm Society Endorsed by the International Society for Computerized Electrocardiology. J Am Coll Cardiol. 2007;49(10):1128-35.
8. DeVane MS. Heart smart a cardiologist's 5-step plan for detecting, preventing, and even reversing heart disease. Hoboken: Wiley; 2006.
9. Nandalur K, Dwamena B, Choudhri A, et al. Diagnostic performance of positron emission tomography in the detection of coronary artery disease: a meta-analysis. Acad Radiol. 2008;15(4):444-51.
10. Raju KP, Prasad SG. Telemedicine and tele-echocardiography in India. J Indian Acad Echocardiogr Cardiovasc Imaging. 2017;1:109-18.
11. Forsting M. Hot topics: will machine learning change medicine? J Nucl Med. 2017;58(3):357-8.
12. Li Q, Rajagopalan C, Clifford GD. A machine learning approach to multi-level ECG signal quality classification. Comput Methods Programs Biomed. 2014;117(3):435-47.
13. Austin PC, Tu JV, Ho JE, et al. Using methods from the data-mining and machine-learning literature for disease classification and prediction: a case study examining classification of heart failure subtypes. J Clin Epidemiol. 2013;66(4):398-407.

126

CHAPTER

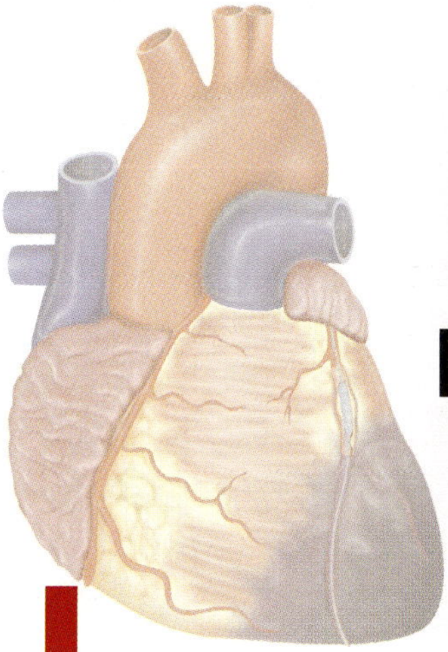

Echocardiography in Noncardiac Surgery

Yatin Mehta, Dheeraj Arora

INTRODUCTION

Echocardiography has been introduced in clinical practice since 1980s, and intraoperative transesophageal echocardiography (TEE) was introduced in operating rooms in later years. Its clinical usage has been steadily increased over the years, particularly in cardiac surgery, and also proved to be beneficial. Intraoperative TEE has been reported as beneficial in 40%–80% of patients with a change in medical therapy.[1] Based on the advantage in cardiac surgery, its role in noncardiac surgery is also gaining popularity.

APPROACHES

There are two approaches for perioperative echocardiography either by transthoracic echocardiography (TTE) or TEE. TTE has been used as a clinical guide for treatment and follow-up in patient with cardiovascular diseases as well as in critical care units to diagnose and follow the treatment. However, it may not be used intraoperatively when surgical site overlaps with the site of placement of standard ultrasound probe. TEE may solve this problem by providing new window to the heart and provides real-time information about cardiac anatomy and functioning with a posteriorly placed probe. Moreover, it can provide better quality images without any obstruction by the related structures.

GUIDELINES AND STANDARD VIEWS

Guidelines for perioperative echocardiography were written to standardize its usage and help in surgical decision-making. Most of the previous guidelines, including American Society of Anesthesiologists (ASA)/Society of Cardiovascular Anesthesiologists (SCA), one were for the use of echocardiography, are relevant to cardiac surgery. Practice guidelines were introduced in 1996, followed by comprehensive guidelines in 1999 and for quality improvement in 2006.[2-4] However, one of the most common category I indications for the use of intraoperative TEE during noncardiac surgery is the role of "rescue TEE" for the evaluation of acute persistent and life-threatening hemodynamic disturbances not responding to the treatment. Recent guidelines of ASA/SCA suggest the use of perioperative transesophageal echocardiography (PTE) in patients where the nature of the planned surgery or the patient's known or suspected cardiovascular pathology might result in severe hemodynamic, pulmonary, or neurologic compromise in addition to as a rescue tool. The goals of a basic PTE examination in a patient with hemodynamic instability include early diagnosis of the etiology of hypotension despite the use of inotropic and vasoactive support and guidance of therapeutic interventions to treat the underlying cause.[5] The guidelines also suggested that for basic PTE examination, at least 11 views should be practiced. These views can provide necessary information for diagnosing the general etiology of hemodynamic instability in surgical patients[5] (Fig. 1). If any abnormality or pathology is suspected then comprehensive examination should be performed. Basic views are as follows: (1) Midesophageal (ME) four chamber, (2) ME two chamber, (3) ME long-axis (LAX), (4) ME ascending aortic LAX, (5) ME ascending aortic short-axis (SAX) (6) ME right

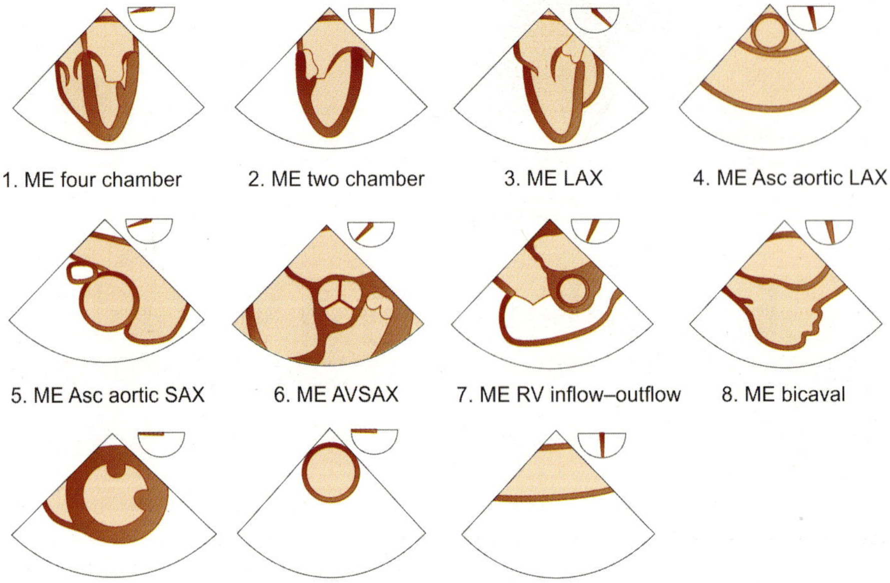

Fig. 1: 11 basic views for PTE examination. (Asc: ascending; Desc: descending; AV: aortic valve; LAX: long-axis; ME: midesophageal; PTE: perioperative transesophageal echocardiography; RV: right ventricular; SAX: short axis; TG: transgastric)

ventricular (RV) inflow-outflow, (7) ME aortic valve (AV) SAX, (8) ME bicaval, (9) Transgastric (TG) midpapillary SAX, (10) Descending aortic SAX, and (11) Descending aortic LAX.

CLINICAL USAGE OF ECHOCARDIOGRAPHY IN NONCARDIAC SURGERY

Hypovolemia

Hypovolemia is one of the common causes of hemodynamic instability in the perioperative period. Echocardiography, particularly TEE, is useful to diagnose hypovolemia by "eyeballing" or by measuring left ventricle (LV) end-diastolic diameter and LV end-diastolic area (LVEDA). In an emergency situation, TEE probe can be placed quickly and provides real-time assessment of LV cavity size. "Eyeballing" or direct visual assessment is done in TG midpapillary SAX view used to measure volume status by measuring the degree of approximation of papillary muscles. "Kissing sign," i.e. approximation of papillary muscles, denotes hypovolemia (Fig. 2). Major bleeding during surgical procedure may cause decrease in LVEDA, filling pressures, and LV end-diastolic wall stress. Transesophageal echocardiography is useful in predicting LV preload by measuring LVEDA (Fig. 3).[5] Hypovolemia is suspected if LVEDA of less than 10 cm^2 or a LVEDA index (LVEDA/body surface area) is less than 5.5 cm^2/m^2 and volume overload is suspected if LVEDA is more than 20 cm^2. Moreover, positive correlation has been found between central venous pressure and inferior vena cava (IVC) diameter in anesthetized patients.[6]

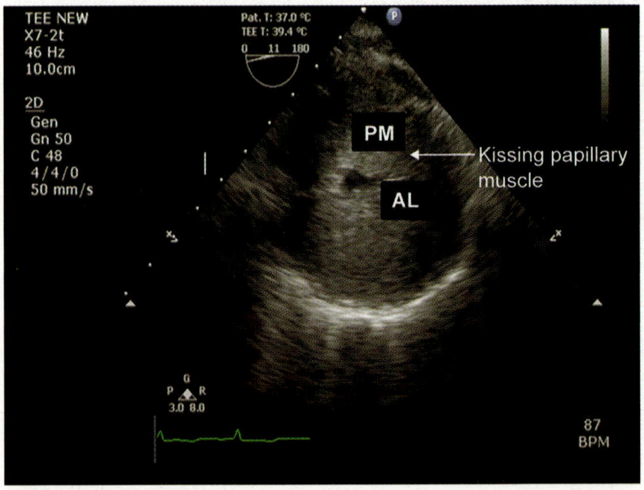

Fig. 2: TGSAX view showing "kissing sign", i.e. approximation of papillary muscles. (AL: anterolateral; PM: posteromedial papillary muscles; TGSAX: transgastric short-axis)

Perioperative Ischemia Monitoring

Qualitative assessment of LV function is an important indication of perioperative echocardiography. "Eyeballing" or direct visual assessment of LV and RV functions can be done easily, and quantitative methods can also be used in selected group of patients. Perioperative echocardiography is useful in detecting new regional wall motion abnormalities (RWMAs) and also helps in the detection of complications, such as congestive heart failure,

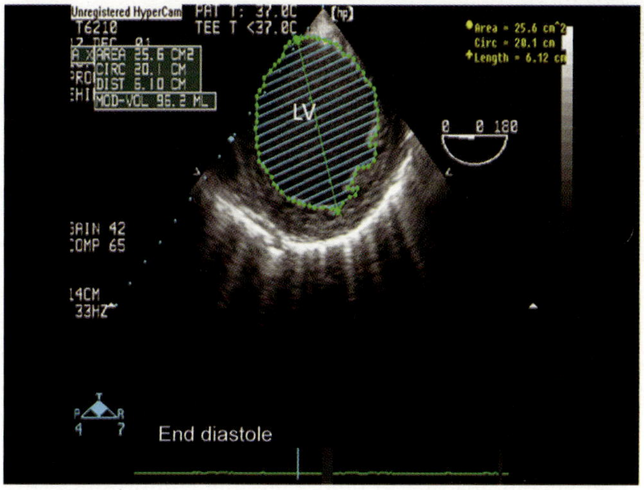

Fig. 3: TGSAX view showing LVEDA. (LV: left ventricle; LVEDA: left ventricular end-diastolic area; TGSAX: transgastric short-axis)

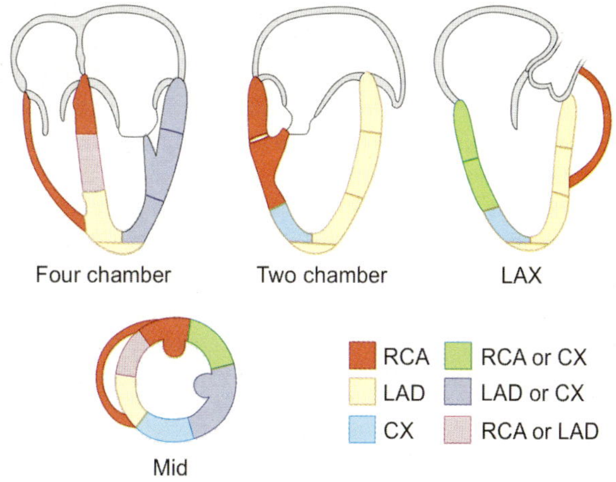

Fig. 6: Coronary distribution of the left ventricle in various TEE views. (CX: circumflex artery; LAD: left anterior descending; LAX: long-axis; RCA: right coronary artery; TEE: transesophageal echocardiography)

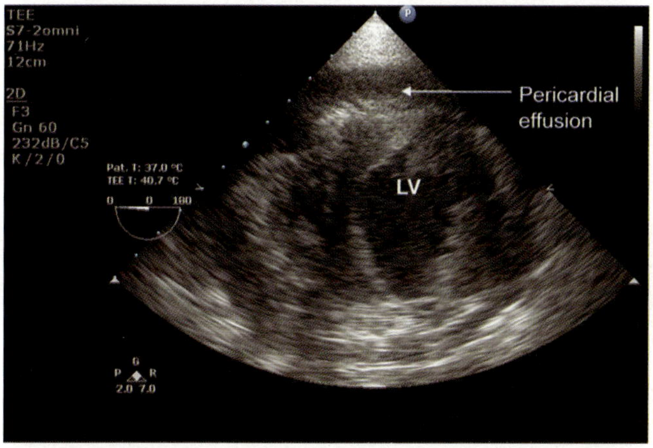

Fig. 4: TGSAX view showing pericardial effusion. (LV: left ventricle; TGSAX: transgastric short-axis)

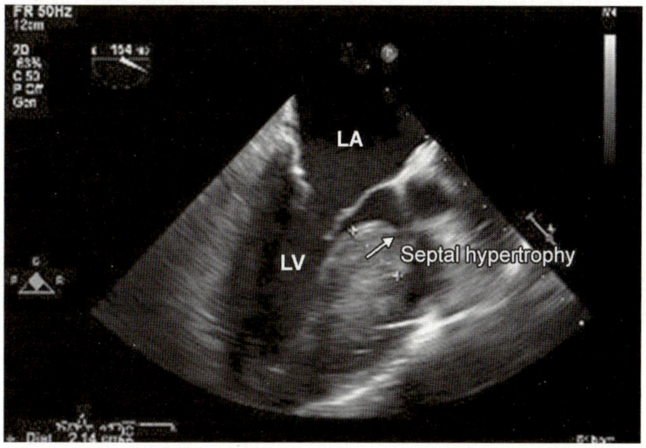

Fig. 7: ME long-axis view LVOT obstruction. (LA: left atrium; LVOT: left ventricular outflow tract; ME: midesophageal; LV: left ventricle)

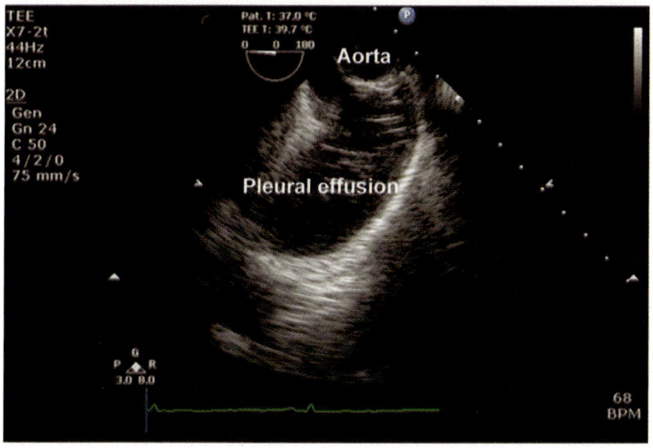

Fig. 5: Transesophageal echocardiography view showing pleural effusion.

valvular regurgitation, septal defects, thrombi, pericardial effusions, and ventricular free-wall rupture (Figs. 4 to 6). Regional wall motion abnormalities can be quantified by 17-segment wall motion score by TEE using the ME four-chamber, ME two-chamber, ME LAX views, and by six midpapillary segments from the TG midpapillary SAX (Fig. 7).[7] However, RWMA may be overestimated as it might be due to other conditions, such as myocardial stunning, hibernation, and tethering as well as changes in loading conditions. Therefore, it is not clear that routine TEE is either cost effective or more beneficial than electrocardiogram monitoring with ST-segment analysis in patients undergoing noncardiac surgery.[8] TEE may be a good diagnostic tool for the initial assessment of myocardial ischemia or myocardial infarction-related complications for high-risk patients undergoing noncardiac surgery.

Vascular Surgery

Clamping of aorta during aortic reconstruction may lead to new RWMA that may not be related to myocardial ischemia. It has a reported incidence of 55% during aortic cross-clamping primarily during supraceliac clamping (92%).[9] The RWMA occurred during vascular surgery is usually transient, and prompt diagnosis and treatment can be done if echocardiography monitoring is done. Most of patients undergoing vascular surgery have associated comorbidities, particularly hypertension, coronary artery disease, or diabetes mellitus. Thus perioperative echocardiography, particularly TEE, will be beneficial in these patients.

Transplantation

Transesophageal echocardiography has now been used quite frequently in patients undergoing liver and lung transplantation. During liver transplantation, TEE monitoring has shown to impact overall perioperative care in 11% of patients with new findings in more than 50% of patients and also improved hemodynamic management. Although there is risk of bleeding due to coagulopathy and esophageal varices, however, the reported incidence is only 1–2%.[10] The advantages of PTE in liver transplantation are that it gives real-time assessment of cardiac function and cardiac output measurement is not affected by temperature changes. Moreover, ventricular dysfunction (systolic and diastolic) and new RWMA during clamping and unclamping of IVC or portal vein, any evidence of embolism/shunting during reperfusion and LV outflow tract obstruction (Fig. 7) can be easily diagnosed. It is useful during all the phases (prehepatic, anhepatic, and reperfusion) of liver transplantation. Contrast TEE also helps in detection of intrapulmonary shunt in patients of liver disease. Injection of agitated saline through a peripheral vein and presence of microbubbles in the left heart chambers four to six beats after initial appearance of contrast in the right side of the heart is an indicator of intracardiac shunt (ICS).

During lung transplantation, echocardiography, especially TEE, has been used to assess pulmonary hypertension, ventricular function, and surgical repair. Moreover, any evidence of pulmonary artery (PA) thrombosis (Fig. 8) can also be assessed. Use of echocardiography resulted in a major impact on patient management in 11% of patients.[11] Authors have recommended the use of TEE in patients undergoing lung transplantation for early detection of PA thrombosis.[12]

Neurosurgery

Craniotomy, especially in sitting position and transsphenoidal resection, may cause venous air embolism (VAE) that may be small with little clinical significance or massive that may lead to paradoxical embolism across a patent foramen ovale leading to hemodynamic instability. TEE is a sensitive monitor to detect air bubbles intraoperatively and is an important tool to prevent VAE.[5] It is more sensitive than precordial Doppler and may even detect hemodynamically insignificant bubbles (Fig. 9). Therefore preoperative echocardiographic evaluation should also be done to rule out any ICS in patients scheduled for surgery in sitting or semisitting positions.[13]

Orthopedic Surgery

Total hip replacement surgery may lead to fat embolism that can cause increase in PA pressure, new RWMA, and hypotension, leading to hemodynamic compromise. The incidence varies from 0.6% to 10% with mortality of 0.02%. It has also been observed in knee replacement also after tourniquet release. TEE may be useful in elderly patients

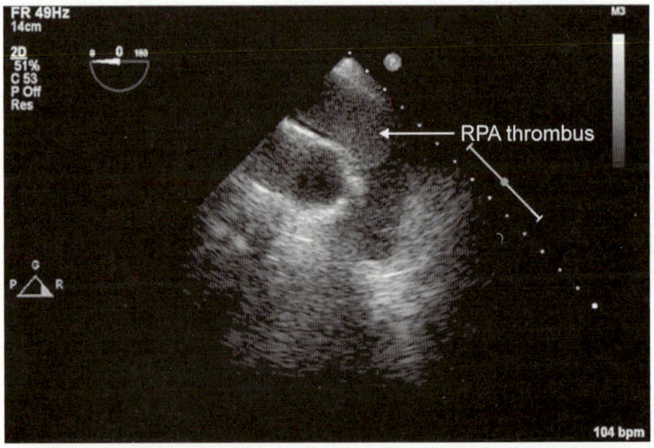

Fig. 8: Transesophageal echocardiography view showing thrombus in right pulmonary artery (RPA).

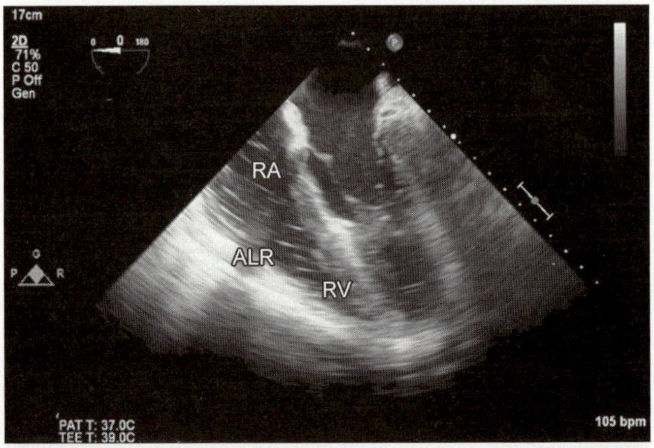

Fig. 9: Midesophageal four-chamber view showing air in the right side of heart.

and those with significant cardiovascular and pulmonary comorbidity undergoing orthopedic surgery.[14] We have also used echocardiography in patient undergoing simultaneous cardiac and noncardiac surgery.[15]

Obstetric Surgery

Echocardiography is useful in high-risk obstetrical patients with cardiac disease. It has been used in patients with valvular heart disease, congenital heart disease, and cardiomyopathies undergoing cesarean section. In patients with pregnancy-induced hypertension, pulmonary embolism, and peripartum cardiomyopathy, it is used to assess the hemodynamic profile.[16] Therefore, its use is recommended only for high-risk subgroups.

Oncosurgery

Echocardiography is helpful in inserting peripherally inserted central catheter line is correctly positioned in patients receiving concurrent chemotherapy or total parenteral nutrition. Chemotherapeutic agents, such as adriamycin, cause cardiotoxicity that may lead to LV dysfunction. Echocardiographic monitoring should be done in this subset of patients undergoing surgery.

Laparoscopic Surgery

Pneumoperitoneum by insufflation of carbon dioxide during laparoscopic surgery leads to increase in abdominal pressure that may affect myocardial pressure–volume relationship. It may cause abnormal myocardial compliance leading to abnormal intracardiac pressures.[17] Moreover, it decreases the venous return, increases vascular resistance that may lead to hemodynamic instability in susceptible patients. Echocardiography should be used electively in high-risk patients and geriatric population with comorbidities, morbidly obese patients undergoing bariatric surgery, or may be used as a rescue technique in the case of hemodynamic instability. Authors have reported use of rescue TEE in the case of hemodynamic instability due to carbon dioxide paradoxical embolism.[18]

Intraoperative Cardiac Arrest in Noncardiac Surgery

Transesophageal echocardiography has been considered useful in cardiac arrest scenario in operating rooms. It is useful in establishing cause of arrest. Authors have found definitive diagnosis of the underlying pathology in 19 out of 22 patients with intraoperative cardiac arrest with the use of TEE.[19] TEE is more reliable than TTE in diagnosing the etiology. Finally, an audit of anesthesiologist performed echocardiography was published that showed greater impact on the perioperative management of the patients. Various actions, such as cancelation of the procedure, diagnosis of newer pathologies, and change in the hemodynamic management, were done.[20,21]

CONCLUSION

Echocardiography, especially TEE, is a useful tool for hemodynamic monitoring in cardiac and noncardiac surgery. TEE being semi-invasive and noninterference in the surgical field has an edge over TTE in the intraoperative period. It should be used without delay in patients undergoing noncardiac surgery having hemodynamic compromise not responding to the standard treatment. Nowadays with the easy availability of the equipment and training facilities, anesthesiologist should train themselves in echocardiography.

REFERENCES

1. Denault AY, Couture P, McKenty S, et al. Perioperative use of transesophageal echocardiography by anesthesiologists: impact in non-cardiac surgery and in the intensive care unit. Can J Anesth. 2002;40:287-93.
2. Practice guidelines for perioperative transesophageal echocardiography. A report by the American Society of Anesthesiologists and the Society of Cardiovascular Anesthesiologists Task Force on Transesophageal Echocardiography. Anesthesiology. 1996;84:986-1006.
3. Shanewise JS, Cheung AT, Aronson S, et al. ASE/SCA guidelines for performing a comprehensive intraoperative multiplane transesophageal echocardiography examination: recommendations of the American Society of Echocardiography Council for Intraoperative Echocardiography and the Society of Cardiovascular Anesthesiologists Task Force for Certification in Perioperative Transesophageal Echocardiography. Anesth Analg. 1999;89:870-84.
4. Mathew JP, Glas K, Troianos CA, et al. American Society of Echocardiography/Society of Cardiovascular Anesthesiologists recommendations and guidelines for continuous quality improvement in perioperative echocardiography. J Am Soc Echocardiogr. 2006;19:1303-13.
5. Reeves ST, Finley AC, Skubas NJ, et al. Basic Perioperative Transesophageal Echocardiography Examination: A consensus statement of the American Society of Echocardiography and the Society of Cardiovascular Anesthesiologists. J Am Soc Echocardiogr. 2013;26(5):443-56.
6. Arthur ME, Landolfo C, Wade M, et al. Inferior vena cava diameter (IVCD) measured with transesophageal echocardiography (TEE) can be used to derive the central venous pressure (CVP) in anesthetized mechanically ventilated patients. Echocardiography. 2009;26(2):140-9.

7. Lang RM, Bierig M, Devereux RB, et al. Recommendations for chamber quantification: a report from the American Society of Echocardiography's Guidelines and Standards Committee and the Chamber Quantification Writing Group, developed in conjunction with the European Association of Echocardiography, a branch of the European Society of Cardiology. J Am Soc Echocardiogr. 2005;18:1440-63.
8. Benson MJ, Cahalan MK. Cost-benefit analysis of transesophageal echocardiography in cardiac surgery. Echocardiography. 1995;12:171-83.
9. Roizen MF, Beaupre PN, Alpert RA, et al. Monitoring with two-dimensional transesophageal echocardiography: comparison of myocardial function in patients undergoing supraceliac, suprarenal-infraceliac, or infrarenal aortic occlusion. J Vasc Surg. 1984;1:300-5.
10. Prah GN, Lisman SR, Maslow AD, et al. Transesophageal echocardiography reveals an unusual cause of hemodynamic collapse during orthotopic liver transplantation: two case reports. Transplantation. 1995;59:921-5.
11. Michel-Cherqui M, Brusset A, Liu N, et al. Intraoperative transesophageal echocardiographic assessment of vascular anastamoses in lung transplantation: a report on 11 cases. Chest. 1997;111:1229-35.
12. Aleem Siddique A, Bose AK, Özalp F, et al. Vascular anastomotic complications in lung transplantation: a single institution's experience. Interact Cardiovasc Thorac Surg. 2013;17(4):625-31.
13. Mammoto T, Hayashi Y, Ohnishi Y, et al. Incidence of venous and paradoxical air embolism in neurosurgical patients in the sitting position: detection by transesophageal echocardiography. Acta Anaesthesiol Scand. 1998;42:643-7.
14. Koessler MJ, Fabiani R, Hamer H, et al. The clinical relevance of embolic events detected by transesophageal echocardiography during cemented total hip arthroplasty: a randomized clinical trial. Anesth Analg. 2001;92:49-55.
15. Mehta Y, Sujatha P, Rajgopal A, et al. Off pump CABG along with hip and knee replacement: anaesthetic management—a case report. J Anaesthesiol Clin Pharm. 2005;21:445-47.
16. Belfort MA, Rokey R, Saade GR, et al. Rapid echocardiographic assessment of left and right heart hemodynamics in critically ill obstetric patients. Am J Obstet Gynecol. 1994;171:884-92.
17. Andersson L, Lindberg G, Bringman S, et al. Pneumoperitoneum versus abdominal wall lift: effects on central hemodynamics and intrathoracic pressure during laparoscopic cholecystectomy. Acta Anaesthesiol Scand. 2003;47(7):838-46.
18. Patel JH, Szymanski T, Metzler EC, et al. Rescue transesophageal echocardiography for the diagnosis and management of paradoxical carbon dioxide embolism with hemodynamic compromise during laparoscopic surgery. J Cardiothorac Vasc Anesth. 2013;27(3):e23-4.
19. Memtsoudis SG, Rosenberger P, Loffler M, et al. The usefulness of transesophageal echocardiography during intraoperative cardiac arrest in noncardiac surgery. Anesth Analg. 2006;102(6):1653-7.
20. Canty DJ, Royse CF. Audit of anaesthetist-performed echocardiography on perioperative management decisions for non-cardiac surgery. Br J Anaesth. 2009;103:352-8.
21. Pietri LD, Mocchegiani F, Leuzzi C, et al. Transesophageal echocardiography during liver transplantation. World J Hepatol. 2015;7(23):2432-48.

SECTION 29

Metabolic: Nutritional Imaging

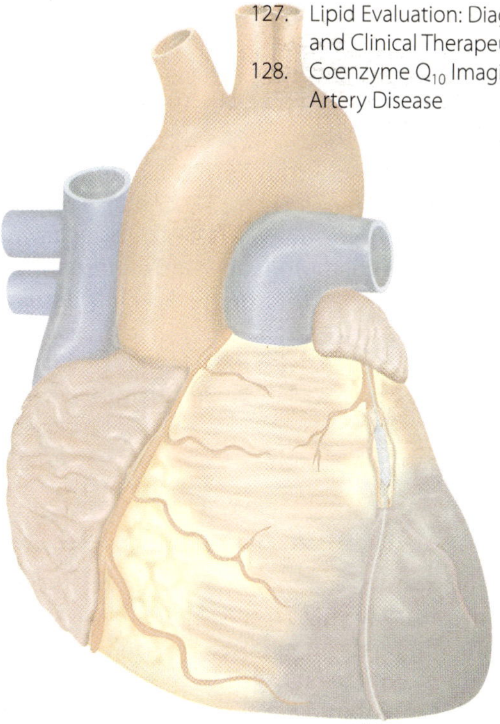

127
CHAPTER

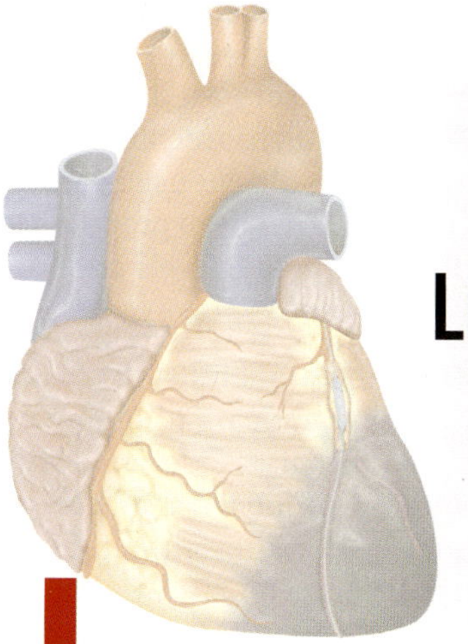

Lipid Evaluation: Diagnostic, Prognostic, and Clinical Therapeutic Implications

JPS Sawhney, Prashant Wankhade, Simran Sawhney

INTRODUCTION

The burden of atherosclerotic cardiovascular (CV) disease (CVD) (ASCVD) worldwide is alarmingly high. Developing countries bear special consideration regarding ASCVD problems. Indians are at high risk of developing ASCVD as well as they usually get the disease at an early age, have a more severe form of the disease and have poorer outcome as compared to the Western populations.[1] Developing countries in addition have poor access to health care, and the treatment of ASCVD remains expensive. Therefore, prevention of ASCVD needs to take priority on all fronts, including personal level, healthcare providers, and governmental agencies. There are modifiable and nonmodifiable risk factors for ASCVD. Of modifiable risk factors, dyslipidemia has the highest population attributable risk for myocardial infarction (MI), both because of its high prevalence and also because of its direct pathogenic association with atherosclerosis.[2] Effective management of dyslipidemia constitutes one of the most important healthcare targets for ASCVD prevention. The distribution and interplay of concomitant CV risk factors and genetic susceptibility also plays role in manifestation of disease. Along with this, population awareness, socioeconomic conditions, and cultural beliefs are also important factors for the prevention and management of ASCVD. Lipid metabolism can be altered in different ways, leading to changes in its various components and their functions. These alterations in lipids and its interaction with other CV risk factors may affect the development of atherosclerosis. Dyslipidemias can be secondary to other diseases or to the interaction between genetic predisposition and environmental factors. Elevation of low-density lipoprotein-cholesterol (LDL-C) can be modified by lifestyle changes and drug therapies and hence has received particular attention. There are also evidences showing reduction in LDL-C can prevent CVD. Therefore, the LDL-C levels continue to constitute the primary targets of therapy. In addition to the elevation of LDL-C levels, some other types of dyslipidemias also appear to predispose to premature CVD. Atherogenic lipid triad consisting of increased very LDL (VLDL) remnants manifested as increased small dense LDL particles, reduced high-density lipoprotein-cholesterol (HDL-C), and mildly elevated triglycerides (TGs) levels is more common than others.[1] However, there is limited evidence on the effectiveness and safety of intervening in this pattern to reduce CVD risk; therefore, this pattern or its components should be regarded as optional targets of prevention of ASCVD.

DIAGNOSIS

Fasting versus nonfasting lipid evaluation: Serum lipid profile has become routine part of CV risk prediction. The test consists of four basic components: total cholesterol (TC), HDL-C, LDL-C, and TG. Most of the guidelines in the past including National Institute for Health and Care Excellence (NICE) [National Cholesterol Education Program (NCEP)] and European guidelines recommend doing the test on 12–14 hours fasting blood samples.[3,4] Lipid profile in fasting is advised due to two main reasons, i.e. postprandial TG remain elevated for several hours and most reference values for serum lipids are established on fasting blood samples.[5] National Cholesterol Education Program[3] and European guidelines[4] also recommend doing lipid profile in fasting blood specimen for assessment of CV risk. Fasting state is essential for TG estimation as it remains high for several hours after meal, highest levels 4–5 hours postprandially.[6] This postprandial lipemia is also affected by various factors like ethnicity, alcohol consumption, and menopausal status.[7] Total cholesterol and HDL-C are not much different in fasting and nonfasting specimens so guidelines allow their evaluation even in nonfasting states. Non-HDL-C (TC – HDL-C) may also be used in the nonfasting state.[3] The Friedewald equation is used for calculation of LDL-C (LDL-C = TC – HDL-C – [TG/5]). So if nonfasting TG value is used in this equation, the LDL-C levels will be underestimated. Direct LDL-C estimation can solve this problem up to some extent as this can be done in nonfasting specimen. But this method of direct LDL-C measurement has few drawbacks. It sometimes underestimates of LDL-C[8,9] are costly and studies have shown the lack of association of nonfasting direct LDL-C with CVD in women.[9] During the last few years, efforts have been made to simplify blood sampling by replacing fasting lipid profile with nonfasting, as it has been found that lipids, lipoproteins, and apolipoproteins were not much different in fasting than nonfasting state with the exception of TG.[10] Thus, fasting sample is preferred if CVD risk assessment is based on TC, LDL-C, or non-HDL-C, whereas HDL-C, TG, TC/HDL-C ratio, and apolipoprotein A-1 can be used in nonfasting states.[7] The interesting fact is that nonfasting TG levels may be even better predictor of CV risk as compared to fasting TG, but cutoff levels of nonfasting TG for CV risk have not yet been defined.[11]

Other factors may also affect the levels of these lipid components, such as,[12-16]

- Change from an upright to a supine position can reduce the cholesterol levels by 10% and TG by 12% due to dilutional effect.[12]
- Application of tourniquet for longer period (2–5 minutes) can increase cholesterol from 5% to 15%.[13]
- Cholesterol levels are slightly higher in winter than in summer and the opposite is true in case of TG.[14]
- Various disease conditions can affect the levels of these lipid components, like nephrotic syndrome increase TC, LDL-C, and VLDL cholesterol, whereas hypothyroidism increases LDL-C and TC. Infection and inflammation may decrease TC and HDL-C and cause increase the TG levels.[15,16]

Lipids also get altered following MI which may persist for several weeks.[17,18] That is why it is better to do lipid profile within 24 hours after MI. In patients admitted with acute illness, individual components of the lipid profile vary significantly during and after hospital stay, whereas the ratio of TC to HDL-C has shown to remain relatively stable.[19] A joint consensus statement from the European Federation of Clinical Chemistry and Laboratory Medicine and European Atherosclerosis Society (EAS) has recommended that nonfasting blood samples should be used for the assessment of plasma lipid profiles. It has been proposed to repeat fasting lipid profile if nonfasting TG levels are more than 440 mg/dL.[20]

Lipoprotein a [Lp(a)]: A large meta-analysis of 126,634 participants and 1.3 million person-years of follow-up has shown that Lp(a) level >24 mg/dL is associated with increased risk of MI.[21] The EAS proposed Lp(a) levels of <50 mg/dL as an optimal level representing 20% of the population with higher levels. The 2016 Canadian Cardiovascular Society Guidelines for the Management of Dyslipidemia consider Lp(a) > 30 mg/dL to be a risk factor. Canadian Cardiovascular Society guidelines also suggest measuring Lp(a) to inform decision-making, especially in patients at intermediate risk and those with a family history of premature coronary artery disease (CAD) and in younger patients who may not meet treatment risk criteria.[22]

Familial hypercholesterolemia (FH): This autosomal dominant disorder causes severe elevations in TC and LDL-C levels.[23] They usually presents with premature ASCVD or at times found to have high LDL-C levels in the absence of secondary causes of hypercholesterolemia. Definitive diagnosis can be made only with genetic studies. Familial hypercholesterolemia is typically caused by mutations in LDL-receptor, apolipoprotein B, and proprotein convertase subtilisin/kexin type 9 (*PCSK9*) genes in 60–80% of patients; 20–40% patients have unknown genetic mutations. Various clinical and laboratory based criteria have been proposed to ease the diagnosis of FH which include Make Early Diagnosis to Prevent Early Death, Simon Broome criteria, Dutch Lipid Clinic Network Score, etc.

Dutch Lipid Clinic Network Score includes components like family history, clinical history, physical examination, and LDL-C levels[24] (Table 1).

Based on this scoring system, FH can be diagnose as definite (>8), probable (6–8), possible (3–5), or unlikely (<3). Sensitivity and specificity of these criteria for diagnosis of definite FH is 41.5% and 87.9%, respectively. Though these patients are at very high risk of developing ASCVD, most of them remain undiagnosed, untreated, or inadequately treated. Early diagnosis and treatment of these patients with FH can reduce the risk significantly (≈80%).[25] Cascade screening has been recommended for first- and second-degree and if possible for third-degree relatives.[26] In most families, cascade screening is best performed with TC or LDL-C analysis, but if the causative mutation is known,

TABLE 1: Dutch Lipid Clinic Network Score for diagnosis of familial hypercholesterolemia.

Criteria	*Score*
Family history	
First-degree relative with known premature coronary and/or vascular disease (men aged <55 years, women aged <60 years) OR First-degree relative with known LDL-C above the 95th percentile for age and gender	1
First-degree relative with tendinous xanthomata and/or arcus cornealis OR Children aged <18 years with LDL-C above 95th percentile for age and gender	2
Clinical history	
Patients with premature coronary artery disease (men aged <55 years, women aged <60 years)	2
Patients with premature cerebral or peripheral vascular disease (men aged <55 years, women aged <60 years)	1
Physical examination	
Tendinous xanthomata	6
Arcus cornealis before 45 years of age	4
Investigation (LDL-C)	
≥330 mg/dL	8
250–329 mg/dL	5
190–249 mg/dL	3
155–189 mg/dL	1
DNA analysis	
Genetic test results confirming functional mutation in *LDL-R, Apo-B*, or *PCSK9* gene	8

(Apo-B: apolipoprotein B; LDL-C: low-density lipoprotein-cholesterol; DNA: deoxyribonucleic acid; LDL-R: low-density lipoprotein-receptor; PCSK9: proprotein convertase subtilisin/kexin type 9)

genetic testing is recommended since affected individuals may present with TC below the clinical diagnostic criteria.[27]

PROGNOSTIC AND CLINICAL IMPLICATIONS

American College of Cardiology/American Heart Association (ACC/AHA) recommendations: ACC/AHA has proposed ASCVD risk algorithm for management of dyslipidemia. Recommendations of ACC/AHA for dyslipidemia management have been shown in Table 2.[28]

European Society of Cardiology (ESC)/EAS recommendations: ESC/EAS has proposed principles of risk assessment as follows:[27]

- Those automatically at very high or high total CV risk and need active management of all risk factors
  - Known CVD
  - Type 2 diabetes mellitus (DM) or type 1 DM with microalbuminuria
  - Very high levels of individual risk factors
  - Chronic kidney disease.
- For all the other people, the use of a risk estimation system such as Systematic Coronary Risk Estimation is recommended to estimate total CV risk as many people have several risk factors, which in combination, may result in high levels of total CV risk. Recommendations by ESC/EAS have been shown in Table 3.

Statins has been considered first-line therapy for management of dyslipidemia. Atorvastatin, rosuvastatin, and pitavastatin are more potent amongst the family. Use of fenofibrates should be considered in high CV risk patients with TG levels >200 mg/dL despite of statin therapy.[27] If TG is not controlled by statins or fibrates, addition of n-3 fatty acids may be considered, and these combinations are safe and well tolerated.[27]

In case unable to achieve desired lipid goals, addition of ezetimibe and PCSK9 inhibitor should be considered. The Improved Reduction of Outcomes: Vytorin Efficacy International Trial,[29] which compared simvastatin only with simvastatin plus ezetimibe combination in patients with acute coronary syndrome (ACS), has shown more reduction in LDL-C in combination group compared to simvastatin monotherapy. The median time-weighted average LDL-C level during the study was 53.7 mg/dL in the combination group. This laboratory data were reflected in clinical outcomes in the form of reduction in composite of CV death, nonfatal MI, unstable angina (USA) requiring

TABLE 2: American College of Cardiology/American Heart Association recommendations for lipid management.

Age group	*Risk*	*Treatment goal*	*Intervention*
Adults ≥21 years old	Known ASCVD	≥50% reduction in LDL-C	High-intensity* statin therapy except age more than 75 years and statin-associated adverse events
	LDL-C >190 mg/dL	≥50% reduction in LDL-C	
	≥7.5% 10 years ASCVD risk with LDL-C levels 70–180 mg/dL	30–50% reduction in LDL-C	Moderate† intensity statins
40–75 years old	Diabetes	30–50% reduction in LDL-C	
	LDL-C levels 70–189 mg/dL	30–50% reduction in LDL-C	

(ASCVD: atherosclerotic cardiovascular disease; LDL-C: low-density lipoprotein-cholesterol)

**High-intensity statin therapy*: Atorvastatin 40–80 mg QD or rosuvastatin 20–40 mg QD.

†*Moderate intensity statin therapy*: Atorvastatin 20–40 mg QD or rosuvastatin 10–20 mg QD.

TABLE 3: European Society of Cardiology/European Atherosclerosis Society (ESC/EAS) recommendations for lipid management.

Risk group	*Patient population*	*Goal*	*Recommendations*
Very high CV risk	• Known CV disease, stroke or TIA, PAD • Diabetes with target organ damage such as proteinuria or with a major risk factor such as smoking, hypertension or dyslipidemia • Severe CKD (GFR <30 mL/min/1.73 m^2) • SCORE level >10%	LDL-C <70 mg/dL or a reduction of at least 50% if the baseline LDL-C is between 70 mg/dL and 135 mg/dL	I-B
High CV risk	• SCORE level >5% to <10% • Markedly elevated single risk factor • Most other people with diabetes (some young people with type 1 DM may be at low or moderate risk) • Moderate CKD (GFR 30–59 mL/min/1.73 m^2)	LDL-C <100 mg/dL or a reduction of at least 50% if the baseline LDL-C is between 100 mg/dL and 200 mg/dL	I-B
Moderate CV risk	• SCORE level >1% to <5%	LDL-C <115 mg/dL	IIa-C

(CKD: chronic kidney disease; CV: cardiovascular; DM: diabetes mellitus; GFR: glomerular filtration rate; LDL-C: low-density lipoprotein-cholesterol; SCORE: systematic coronary risk estimation; TIA: transient ischemic attack; PAD: peripheral arterial disease)

rehospitalization, coronary revascularization (≥30 days after randomization), or nonfatal stroke.

Further Cardiovascular Outcomes Research with PCSK9 Inhibition in Subjects with Elevated Risk (FOURIER) trial established that evolocumab prevents CV events on the background statin therapy.[30] The FOURIER trial was a randomized trial involving 27,564 stable CAD patients from 49 countries. At 48-week follow-up, compared to placebo evolocumab caused 59% reduction in LDL-C from a median baseline value of 92–30 mg/dL. Trial concluded that evolocumab significantly reduced the risk of CV death, MI, stroke, hospitalization for USA, or coronary revascularization.

Another PCSK9 inhibitor alirocumab was tested for efficacy in reducing LDL-C and Lp(a) levels in patients with heterozygous FH on maximally tolerated lipid-lowering therapy. In phase 3 studies ODYSSEY FH I and FH II, patients were randomized to receive alirocumab 75 mg every 2 weeks with dose uptitration to 150 mg every 2 weeks if LDL-C levels remained above 70 mg/dL or placebo. After 24 weeks, alirocumab treatment led to a 49% reduction in LDL-C levels, with 40% of patients requiring the 150-mg dose.[31]

First evidence of survival benefit from PCSK9 inhibitors came from ODYSSEY outcomes trial in which patients (n = 18,924) received every other week injections of alirocumab. Drug was titrated between 75 mg and 150 mg to keep the LDL-C between 25 mg/dL and 50 mg/dL, but more than 15 mg/dL. At 4 months, LDL-C reduction in alirocumab versus placebo was 37.6 mg/dL versus 93.3 mg/dL, i.e. 62.7% reduction, and at 48 months, it was 53.3 mg/dL versus 101.4 mg/dL, i.e. 54.7% reduction. Those with baseline LDL-C ≥ 100 mg/dL appeared to derive the highest benefit. Trial showed that use of alirocumab reduces all-cause mortality and MI among patients presented with ACS who were already on maximum tolerated statin therapy.[32]

These findings in above-mentioned recent trials have shown that patients with ASCVD benefit from lowering of LDL-C levels below current targets.

American Association of Clinical Endocrinologists/American College of Endocrinology (AACE/ACE) recommendations: AACE/ACE advocates the use of Framingham risk score to assess the CV risk and advice LDL-C levels of <55 mg/dL in extreme risk group.[33] AACE/ACE has recommended LDL-C levels below 55 mg/dL in extreme risk population (Table 4).

TABLE 4: American Association of Clinical Endocrinologists/American College of Endocrinology (AACE/ACE) recommendations for lipid management.

Risk category	Risk factors/10-year risk	Treatment goals		
		LDL-C (mg/dL)	Non-HDL-C (mg/dL)	Apo-B (mg/dL)
Extreme risk	• Progressive ASCVD including unstable angina in patients after achieving an LDL-C <70 mg/dL • Established clinical CVD in patients with diabetes, CKD 3/4, or HeFH • History of premature ASCVD (<55 years in male and <65 years in females)	<55	<80	<70
Very high risk	• Established or recent hospitalization for ACS, coronary, carotid, or peripheral vascular disease, 10-year risk >20% • Diabetes or CKD 3/4 with 1 or more risk factor(s) • HeFH	<70	<100	<80
High risk	• ≥2 risk factors and 10-year risk 10–20% • Diabetes or CKD 3/4 with no other risk factors	<100	<130	<90
Moderate risk	≤2 risk factors and 10-year risk <10%	<100	<130	<90
Low risk	0 risk factors	<130	<160	NR

(ACS: acute coronary syndrome; Apo-B: apolipoprotein B; ASCVD: atherosclerotic cardiovascular disease; CKD: chronic kidney disease; CVD: cardiovascular disease; HeFH: heterozygous familial hypercholesterolemia, NR: not recommended; LDL-C: low-density lipoprotein-cholesterol; HDL-C: high-density lipoprotein-cholesterol)

Therapies directed against Lp(a): It must be emphasized that there are no approved medications to specifically lower Lp(a). Currently drugs used to lower Lp(a) levels are limited to niacin, with PCSK9 inhibitors, mipomersen, and estrogen in more limited populations. Apheresis performed to lower Lp(a) has suggested reduction in CV risk, but these studies have their own limitations in the form of absence of control group.[34,35]

Atherothrombosis Intervention in Metabolic Syndrome with low HDL/HIGH Triglycerides trial showed no additional CV benefit when niacin was added to excellent LDL-C control. Niacin reduced mean Lp(a) level from 13.5 mg/dL to 11 mg/dL (19% reduction).[36] Niacin did not reduce the event rate even in the subgroup of patients in fourth quartile of Lp(a) (approximately >50 mg/dL), despite achieving a mean Lp(a) reduction of 39%. This analysis was underpowered, with around 700 patients and an event rate of around 16%.

In HERS (Heart and Estrogen/Progestin Replacement Study), estrogen with progestin lowered Lp(a) by approximately 15–20%. In post hoc analysis, postmenopausal women with elevated Lp(a) in the fourth quartile (55–236 mg/dL) had the most benefit.[37] Mipomersen and PCSK9 inhibitors may reduce Lp(a) by 20–30%, but currently indicated for rare patient populations only.[38,39] Thus till date, Lp(a) hypothesis has not been tested with any currently available therapy.

FOLLOW-UP

There is limited evidence regarding the test to monitor lipids, its interval, and safety evaluation. Recommendations from most guidelines are consensus based. Response to therapy can be assessed at 6–8 weeks from initiation of statin therapy, but it is not true for fibrates and lifestyle which may take longer.[40]

National Institute for Health and Care Excellence guidelines recommend measurement of TC, HDL-C, and non-HDL-C at 3 months after starting high-intensity statin therapy with an aim of greater than 40% reduction in non-HDL-C. If this goal is not achieved then one should assess adherence to therapy, and subsequent dose, diet, and lifestyle optimization should be considered.[26]

European Society of Cardiology guidelines recommend at least two measurements of lipid profiles with an interval of 1–12 weeks before starting lipid-lowering therapy except in conditions such as ACS. After starting lipid-lowering therapy, lipids should be assessed after 8 ± 4 weeks and should be reassessed 8 ± 4 weeks after adjusting the dosage. Once target lipid levels achieved, lipid testing should be done annually unless there is adherence problem or any another specific reason.[27]

Range of studies has shown that regular lipid monitoring has positive effect on sustaining lifestyle changes and treatment adherence. The reason behind this is not clear, whether it is critical monitoring or additional effect of education, regular contact, and adherence assessment.[41]

Safety Assessments

National Institute for Health and Care Excellence guidelines recommend against the routine measurement of creatine kinase (CK) levels in asymptomatic people whereas advocates for the measurement of liver transaminase enzymes [alanine aminotransferase (ALT) or aspartate aminotransferase] within 3 months of treatment initiation and at 12 months, but not again unless indicated clinically.[26]

European Society of Cardiology guidelines recommend liver enzyme (ALT) measurement at baseline, 8 weeks after starting lipid-lowering therapy or any dose increments and thereafter annually if levels are <3 times upper limit of normal (ULN). If liver enzymes are raised, but <3 times ULN, continue therapy and recheck levels after 4–6 weeks and if levels are >3 times the ULN, stop statins or reduce dose and recheck levels after 4–6 weeks. Creatine kinase levels should be measured at baselines and if found >5 times ULN, do not start statins. It is advised to check CK levels if patient develops myalgia. Routine checkup of CK is not recommended. If CK levels are elevated >5 times ULN, stop treatment, evaluate renal functions, and measure CK levels every 2 weeks. If CK levels are persistently elevated then one should consider secondary cause for the same. If CK levels are raised but <5 times ULN and if there are no symptoms of muscle pain then one can continue statins with close observation for development of symptoms. Symptomatic patient with raised CK levels with values <5 times ULN, regular monitoring of symptoms and CK has been advised.[27]

Statin Intolerance/Statin-associated Muscle Symptoms

Statin intolerance has been defined as a clinical syndrome characterized by inability to use statins for long-term reduction of lipids and/or CV risk because of significant symptoms and/or biomarker abnormalities that can be temporally attributed to the initiation or dose escalation of statins and is not attributable to established predispositions such as drug–drug interactions and untreated hypothyroidism; if appropriate, drug withdrawal and rechallenge can strengthen this association. Intolerance can be "complete", i.e. intolerant to any statin at any dose or "partial", i.e. intolerant to some statins at some doses.[42]

European Society of Cardiology/European Atherosclerosis Society preferred to use term statin-associated muscle symptoms instead of statin intolerance. If there is evidence of rhabdomyolysis or CK ≥4 times ULN, statins should be withheld for 6 weeks to allow statin washout until normalization of CK. After 6 weeks of statin abstinence, another efficacious statin with either low dose or alternate day or once/twice a week therapy should be considered. If patient is symptomatic with CK levels <4 times ULN withhold statins for 2–4 weeks. If symptoms improved then second statin at usual dose should be considered, and if symptoms persist then statin rechallenge should be tried. If symptoms recur, another efficacious statin with either low dose or alternate day or once/twice a week therapy should be advise. In case of intolerable symptoms or unable to achieve desired lipid goals consider ezetimibe, bile acid sequestrants, PCSK9 inhibitor, or their combinations.[27]

CONCLUSION

Thus, LDL-C remains the most important target for lipid-lowering therapy, and recent trial has shown that lesser the better. Strict fasting lipid evaluation is no longer recommended. Statins remain the first choice lipid-lowering agent.

REFERENCES

1. Iyengar SS, Puri R, Narasingan SN, et al. Lipid association of India expert consensus statement on management of dyslipidemia in Indians 2016: Part 1. J Assoc Physicians India. 2016;64(3):7-52.
2. Yusuf S, Hawken S, Ounpuu S, et al. Effect of potentially modifiable risk factors associated with myocardial infarction in 52 countries (the INTERHEART study): case-control study. Lancet. 2004;364:937-52.
3. National Cholesterol Education Program (NCEP) Expert Panel on Detection, Evaluation, and Treatment of High Blood Cholesterol in Adults (Adult Treatment Panel III). Third report of the National Cholesterol Education Program (NCEP) expert panel on detection, evaluation and treatment of high blood cholesterol in adults (adult treatment panel III) final report. Circulation. 2002;106:3143-421.
4. De Backer G, Ambrosioni E, Borch-Johnson K, et al. European guidelines on cardiovascular disease and prevention in clinical practice. Atherosclerosis. 2003;171:145-55.
5. Campose H, Khoo C, Sacks FM. Diurnal and acute pattern of postprandial apolipoprotein B-48 in VLDL, IDL and LDL from normolipidemic human. Atherosclerosis. 2005;181:345-51.
6. Nordestgaard BG, Benn M, Schnohr P, et al. Nonfasting triglycerides and risk of myocardial infarction, ischemic heart disease and death in men and women. JAMA. 2007;298:299-308.
7. Ridker PM. Fasting versus nonfasting triglycerides and prediction of cardiovascular risk: do we need to revisit the oral triglyceride tolerance test? Clin Chem. 2008;54:11-3.
8. Sahu S, Chawla R, Uppal B. Comparison of two methods of estimation of low density lipoprotein cholesterol, the direct versus Friedewald estimation. Indian J Clin Biochem. 2005;20:54-61.
9. Mora S, Rifai N, Buring JE, et al. Comparison of LDL cholesterol concentration by Friedewald calculation and direct measurement in relation to cardiovascular events in 27,331 women. Clin Chem. 2009;55:888-94.
10. Nordestgaard BG, Langsted A, Freiberg JJ. Nonfasting hyperlipidemia and cardiovascular disease. Curr Drug Targets. 2009;10:54-61.
11. Bansal S, Buring JE, Rifai N, et al. Fasting compared with nonfasting triglycerides and risk of cardiovascular events in women. JAMA. 2007;298:309-16.

12. Narayana S. Pre and post analytical errors in lipid determination. Indian J Clin Biochem. 1996;11:12-6.
13. Young DS. Biological variability. In: Brown SS, Mitchell FL, Young DS (Eds). Chemical Diagnosis of Disease. New York, NY: Elsevier; 1979. pp. 1-113.
14. Narayanan S. Physiological variables in blood sampling. Mitt Klin Chem. 1993;24:130-4.
15. Joven J, Villabona C, Vilella E. Abnormalities of lipoprotein metabolism in patients with nephrotic syndrome. N Engl J Med. 1990;323:579-84.
16. Alvarez C, Ramos A. Lipids, lipoproteins and apolipoproteins in serum during infection. Clin Chem. 1986;32:142-5.
17. Ryder REJ, Hayes TM, Mulligan JP, et al. How soon after myocardial infarction should plasma lipid values be assessed? Br Med J. 1984;289:1651-3.
18. Nigam PK, Narain VS, Hasan M. Serum lipid profile in patients with acute myocardial infarction. Indian J Clin Biochem. 2004;19:67-70.
19. Nawaz H, Comerford BP, Njike VY, et al. Repeated serum lipid measurements during the perihospitalization period. Am J Cardiol. 2006;98:1379-82.
20. Nordestgaard BG, Langsted A, Mora S, et al. Fasting is not routinely required for determination of a lipid profile: clinical and laboratory implications including flagging at desirable concentration cut-points—a joint consensus statement from the European Atherosclerosis Society and European Federation of Clinical Chemistry and Laboratory Medicine. Eur Heart J. 2016;37(25):1944-58.
21. Emerging Risk Factors Collaboration. Lipoprotein(a) concentration and the risk of coronary heart disease, stroke, and nonvascular mortality. JAMA. 2009;302:412-23.
22. Anderson TJ, Grégoire J, Pearson GJ, et al. Canadian Cardiovascular Society guidelines for the management of dyslipidemia for the prevention of cardiovascular disease in the adult. Can J Cardiol. 2016;32:1263-82.
23. Illingworth DR, Duell PB, Connor WE. Disorders of lipid metabolism. In: Felig P, Baxter JD, Frohman LA (Eds). Endocrinology and metabolism. New York, McGraw Hill; 1995. pp. 1315-403.
24. Nordestgaard BG, Chapman MJ, Humphries SE, et al. Familial hypercholesterolaemia is underdiagnosed and undertreated in the general population: guidance for clinicians to prevent coronary heart disease: consensus statement of the European Atherosclerosis Society. Eur Heart J. 2013;34:3478-90.
25. Knowles JW, Rader DJ, Khoury MJ. Cascade screening for familial hypercholesterolemia and the use of genetic testing. JAMA. 2017;318(4):381-2.
26. NICE. Cardiovascular disease: risk assessment and reduction, including lipid modification. <https://www.nice.org.uk/guidance/cg181/chapter/1-recommendations>; 2014 July [updated September 2016].
27. Gueyffier F, Krstačić G, Lettino M, et al. The Task Force for the management of dyslipidaemias of the European Society of Cardiology (ESC) and European Atherosclerosis Society (EAS). Eur Heart J. 2016;37:2999-3058.
28. Stone NJ, Robinson JG, Lichtenstein AH, et al; American College of Cardiology/American Heart Association Task Force on Practice Guidelines. 2013 ACC/AHA guideline on the treatment of blood cholesterol to reduce atherosclerotic cardiovascular risk in adults: a report of the American College of Cardiology/American Heart Association Task Force on Practice Guidelines. Circulation. 2014;129(25 Suppl. 2):S1-45.
29. Cannon CP, Blazing MA, Giugliano RP, et al. Ezetimibe added to statin therapy after acute coronary syndromes. N Engl J Med. 2015;372:2387-97.
30. Sabatine MS, Giugliano RP, Keech AC, et al. Evolocumab and clinical outcomes in patients with cardiovascular disease. N Engl J Med. 2017;376:1713-22.
31. Kastelein JJ, Ginsberg HN, Langslet G, et al. ODYSSEY FH I and FH II: 78 week results with alirocumab treatment in 735 patients with heterozygous familial hypercholesterolaemia. Eur Heart J. 2015;36(43):2996-3003.
32. Gabriel P. Evaluation of cardiovascular outcomes after an acute coronary syndrome during treatment with alirocumab—ODYSSEY outcomes. <https://www.acc.org/latest-in-cardiology/clinical-trials/2018/03/09/08/02/odyssey-outcomes>; March 2018.
33. Jellinger PS, Handelsman Y, Rosenblit PD, et al. American Association of Clinical Endocrinologists and American College of Endocrinology Guidelines for Management of Dyslipidemia and Prevention of Cardiovascular Disease. Endocr Pract. 2017;23(Suppl. 2):1-87.
34. Moriarty PM, Hemphill L. Lipoprotein apheresis. Endocrinol Metab Clin North Am. 2016;45:39-54.
35. Roeseler E, Julius U, Heigl F, et al. Lipoprotein apheresis for lipoprotein(a)-associated cardiovascular disease: prospective 5 years of follow-up and apolipoprotein(a) characterization. Arterioscler Thromb Vasc Biol. 2016;36:2019-27.
36. Nordestgaard BG, Chapman MJ, Ray K, et al. Lipoprotein(a) as a cardiovascular risk factor: current status. Eur Heart J. 2010;31:2844-53.
37. Shlipak MG, Simon JA, Vittinghoff E, et al. Estrogen and progestin, lipoprotein(a), and the risk of recurrent coronary heart disease events after menopause. JAMA. 2000;283:1845-52.
38. Duell PB, Santos RD, Kirwan BA, et al. Long-term mipomersen treatment is associated with a reduction in cardiovascular events in patients with familial hypercholesterolemia. J Clin Lipidol. 2016;10:1011-21.
39. Hossne NA, Cruz E, Buffolo E, et al. Long-term and sustained therapeutic results of a specific promonocyte cell formulation in refractory angina: ReACT (Refractory Angina Cell Therapy) clinical update and cost-effective analysis. Cell Transplant. 2015;24:955-70.
40. Reiner Z, Catapano AL, De Backer G, et al. The Task Force for the management of dyslipidaemias of the European Society of Cardiology (ESC) and the European Atherosclerosis Society (EAS). Eur Heart J. 2011;32:1769-818.
41. Coodley GO, Jorgensen M, Kirschenbaum J, et al. Lowering LDL cholesterol in adults: a prospective, community-based practice initiative. Am J Med. 2008;121:604-10.
42. Banach M, Rizzo M, Toth PP, et al. Statin intolerance—an attempt at a unified definition—position paper from an International Lipid Expert Panel. Arch Med Sci. 2015;11:1-23.

128

CHAPTER

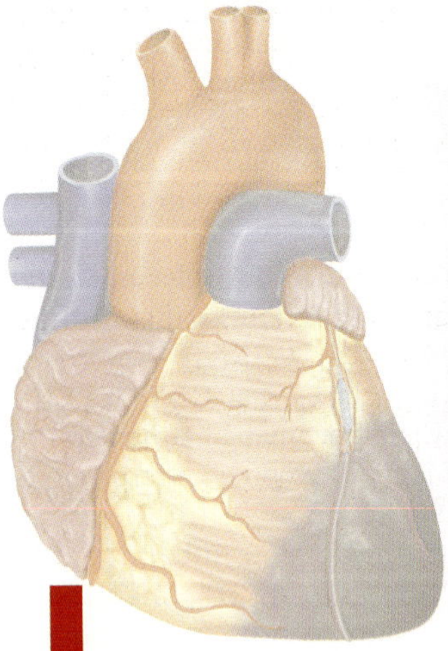

Coenzyme Q_{10} Imaging and Coronary Artery Disease

Pawan K Sharma, HK Chopra

INTRODUCTION

Coenzyme Q_{10} (CoQ_{10}) was first isolated from beef heart mitochondria in 1957.[1] Deficiency of CoQ_{10} in human heart disease was documented in 1972.[2] CoQ_{10} is a provitamin present in every cell of the body and is found in aerobic microorganisms, plant, and animals. It is structurally similar to vitamin K. Normal blood levels of CoQ_{10} are 0.7–1.0 µg/mL.[3] Natural production of CoQ_{10} drops during aging, especially the concentration significantly decreases in the heart.[4] CoQ_{10} occurs in organ meats, such as heart, liver, kidney, beef, and other food sources, such as soybean oil, sardines, and peanuts.[5] The CoQ_{10} is also synthesized in the body cells, especially within the liver. CoQ_{10} is the coenzyme for at least three mitochondria enzymes (complexes I, II, and III). It exists in three oxidation states[1]; the fully reduced ubiquinol form ($CoQ_{10}H_2$),[2] the radical semiquinone intermediate ($CoQ_{10}H$), and[3] fully oxidized ubiquinone form (CoQ_{10}). It plays a key role in producing the mitochondria enzyme phosphate—adenosine triphosphate—upon which all cellular functions depend.[6] CoQ_{10} also functions as a powerful antioxidant by inhibiting the function of free radicals, which have damaging effects on the body.[7,8]

BIOLOGICAL ACTIVITIES OF COENZYME Q_{10}

Coenzyme Q_{10} is insoluble in water and very slightly soluble in alcohol. It should be protected from light.[3] It is slowly absorbed with peak blood levels occurring 5–10 hours after oral administration. The CoQ_{10} is fat soluble, and its absorption is dependent on the presence of postprandial lipids in the gastrointestinal tract.[9] In the mitochondria, CoQ_{10} continually transports protons and electrons from one bioenergy enzyme to another. Cells in the body continuously generate energy to support their functions, and this process depends on each cell having adequate amount of CoQ_{10}.[10,11] CoQ_{10} also plays an important role in the transport of protons across lysosomal membranes to maintain the optimal power of hydrogen.[11,12] In isolated mitochondria, CoQ_{10} can protect membrane proteins and deoxyribonucleic acid from the oxidative damage that occurs during lipid peroxidation.[13] The effects and mechanisms of action of CoQ_{10} may include stabilization of Ca-dependent slow channels, inhibition of intracellular phospholipases, prostaglandin metabolism, free radical scavenging, and direct membrane stabilization (Box 1).[9]

BOX 1: Biological effects of coenzyme Q_{10}.

- Transport of protons and electrons from one bioenergy enzyme to another
- Transport of protons across lysosomal membranes to maintain the optimal pH
- Protect membrane proteins and DNA from the oxidative damage due to lipid peroxidation (antioxidant effect)
- Stabilization of Ca-dependent slow channels
- Inhibition of intracellular phospholipases, prostaglandin metabolism, free radical scavenging, and direct membrane stabilization

(DNA: Deoxyribonucleic acid; pH: Power of hydrogen)

Deficiency of Coenzyme Q_{10}

There are no specific symptoms of CoQ_{10} deficiency that have been reported in general population.[14] At present, there are no specific dietary intake recommendations for CoQ_{10} from the Institute of Medicine.[15] Primary CoQ_{10} deficiency is a rare, autosomal recessive disorder caused by genetic defects in CoQ_{10} biosynthesis. The resultant low levels of CoQ_{10} severely compromise neuronal and muscular function. Oral CoQ_{10} supplementation improves neurological and muscular symptoms in some patients with primary CoQ_{10} deficiency.[16] Decreased levels of CoQ_{10} have been observed in diabetes, cancer, and congestive heart failure patients. The 3-hydroxy-3-methyl-glutaryl-coenzyme A reductase inhibitors (statins) decrease the plasma level of CoQ_{10}. It is not clear whether statin therapy affects CoQ_{10} concentrations in the body tissues.[17-19] It, therefore, remains unclear whether this has clinical or symptomatic implications.

ROLE IN CARDIOVASCULAR DISEASES

Coenzyme Q_{10} is known to be highly concentrated in heart muscle cells due to high-energy requirements of myocardial cells. It has shown promise in the treatment of chronic heart failure, mitral valve prolapse, and improved stress-induced cardiac dysfunction.[20,21]

CONGESTIVE HEART FAILURE

From 1985 to 1993, Langsjoen et al. treated 424 patients with various cardiovascular diseases, including ischemic cardiomyopathy, dilated cardiomyopathy, primary diastolic dysfunction, hypertension, mitral valve prolapse, and valvular heart disease, by adding CoQ_{10} to their medical regimens. Of the 424 patients, 58% improved by one New York Heart Association (NYHA) class, 28% by two classes, and 1.2% by three classes. A statistically significant improvement in myocardial function was noted using the echocardiographic parameters. Before treatment with CoQ_{10}, most patients were taking from one to five cardiac medications. During this study, overall medication requirements dropped considerably: 43% of patients were able to stop taking between one and three cardiovascular drugs as a result of CoQ_{10} therapy. Only 6% of the patients required the addition of one drug.[22] It was postulated that the improved diastolic function lowered the blood pressure leading to a decrease in the high catecholamine state of hypertensive disease. It is also possible that the lowering of blood viscosity and effects on vascular endothelium may favorably influence hypertension.[22] A meta-analysis of 10 randomized controlled trials found that CoQ_{10} supplementation (99–200 mg/day for 1–6 months) in heart failure patients resulted in a significant 3.7% improvement in left ventricular ejection fraction, and this effect was stronger in patients not taking angiotensin-converting enzyme inhibitors.[23] A study involving 236 patients with heart failure found that lower plasma CoQ_{10} levels were associated with an increased risk of mortality.[24] A large study of 1,191 heart failure patients found that plasma CoQ_{10} level was a biomarker of advanced heart disease and not an independent predictor of clinical outcomes in heart failure patients.[25] The Q-SYMBIO trial showed that long-term CoQ_{10} treatment of patients with chronic heart failure is safe, improves symptoms, and reduces major adverse cardiovascular events.[26]

HYPERTENSION

In a crossover, placebo-controlled, randomized study to evaluate antihypertensive effect of CoQ_{10} in patients with essential hypertension; 18 patients were randomly assigned to either group A (treatment with 100 mg of CoQ_{10} daily) or group B (placebo). After 10 weeks, treatment was stopped for 2 weeks, then each patient in group A was switched to group B and vice versa. Treatment with CoQ_{10} indicated a statistically significant decrease in both systolic blood pressure ($P < 0.001$) and diastolic blood pressure ($P < 0.001$) that confirms the antihypertensive effect of the drug.[27] In a study by Langsjoen et al., 109 patients with symptomatic essential hypertension were observed after adding an average oral dose of 225 mg/day of CoQ_{10} to their existing antihypertensive regimen. There was a gradual improvement in functional status and a decrease in antihypertensive drug therapy within 1–6 months. The NYHA functional class improved from a mean of 2.40 to 1.36 ($P < 0.001$), and 51% of patients stopped using one to three antihypertensive drugs at an average of 4.4 months after starting CoQ_{10}.[28]

In a trial, addition of 120 mg/day of CoQ_{10} to conventional medical therapy for 8 weeks in patients with hypertension and coronary artery disease decreased systolic blood pressure by an average of 12 mm Hg and diastolic blood pressure by an average of 6 mm Hg, in comparison to a placebo containing B-complex vitamins.[29] In patients with isolated systolic hypertension, supplementation with both CoQ_{10} (120 mg/day) and vitamin E (300 IU/day) for 12 weeks resulted in an average decrease of 17 mm Hg in systolic blood pressure compared with 300 IU/day of vitamin E alone.[30] In a meta-analysis of clinical trials, including 362 hypertensive patients using 100–120 mg/day of CoQ_{10}, the systolic blood pressure was found reduced by 11–17 mm Hg and diastolic blood pressure by 8–10 mm Hg.[31]

MYOCARDIAL INFARCTION AND CARDIAC SURGERY

Pretreatment of animals with CoQ_{10} has been found to decrease myocardial damage due to ischemia-reperfusion.[32] Three placebo-controlled trials found that CoQ_{10} pretreatment with 100–300 mg/day for 7–14 days prior to surgery provided some benefit in short-term outcome measures after coronary artery bypass grafting (CABG) surgery.[33,34] In another placebo-controlled trial, preoperative CoQ_{10} supplementation with 600 mg was used 12 hours prior to surgery and did not show any benefit.[35] These trials suggest that preoperative CoQ_{10} treatment may need to commence at least 1 week prior to CABG surgery in order to get any benefit. Although the results are promising, these trials have included relatively few people and have only examined outcomes shortly after CABG surgery.

ANGINA PECTORIS

Five small placebo-controlled studies have examined the effect of oral CoQ10 supplementation (60–600 mg/day) in addition to conventional medical therapy in patients with chronic stable angina.[36] In most of the studies, CoQ_{10} supplementation improved exercise tolerance and reduced or delayed electrocardiographic changes associated with myocardial ischemia compared to placebo. However, only two of the studies found significant decrease in symptom frequency and nitroglycerine consumption with CoQ_{10} supplementation. At present, there is only limited evidence suggesting that CoQ_{10} supplementation would be a useful adjunct to conventional angina therapy.

VASCULAR ENDOTHELIAL FUNCTION

A placebo-controlled trial showed that CoQ_{10} supplementation with 200 mg/day for 12 weeks improved endothelium-dependent vasodilation in diabetic patients with abnormal serum lipid profiles, although it did not restore vasodilation to level seen in nondiabetic individuals.[37] Another placebo-controlled study in 23 type 2 diabetics taking statins found that 200 mg/day of CoQ_{10} for 12 weeks improved flow-mediated dilation, but not nitrate-mediated dilation, of the brachial artery.[38] However, a placebo-controlled trial in 80 type 2 diabetics found that this supplementation protocol did not improve endothelial function.[39] A meta-analysis of five randomized controlled trials, including 194 subjects, found that CoQ_{10} supplementation of 150–300 mg/day for 4–12 weeks resulted in a clinically significant 1.7% increase in flow-dependent endothelial-mediated dilation.[40] Large-scale studies are needed to further elucidate the therapeutic role of CoQ_{10} in endothelial dysfunction (Box 2).

BOX 2: Potential role of coenzyme Q_{10} in cardiovascular conditions.

CHF:
- Improve myocardial function
- Reduction in number of medications taken by patient
- Improvement in diastolic function leading to reduction of blood pressure
- Improvement in vascular endothelium
- Lowering of blood viscosity
- Improvement of symptoms and reduction in NYHA class

Hypertension:
- Reduction of both systolic and diastolic blood pressure
- Improvement in functional class
- Decrease in number of antihypertensive medications used

Myocardial infarction and cardiac surgery:
- Pretreatment with CoQ_{10} may decrease myocardial damage
- Benefit in short-term outcome after CABG
- Preoperative CoQ_{10} supplementation may be beneficial but large randomized trials are needed

Angina pectoris:
- May improve exercise tolerance in chronic stable angina
- May reduce or delay ECG changes in chronic stable angina
- Reduction in nitroglycerine consumption
- Large randomized trial lacking

Vascular endothelial function:
- CoQ_{10} supplementation improved endothelium-dependent vasodilation in diabetics
- Large-scale studies needed to further assess therapeutic role of CoQ_{10}

(CABG: Coronary artery bypass grafting; CHF: Congestive heart failure; CoQ_{10}: Coenzyme Q_{10}; ECG: Electrocardiography; NYHA: New York Heart Association)

POTENTIAL ROLE IN OTHER DISEASES

Diabetes Mellitus

Reduced plasma levels of CoQ_{10} have been found in diabetic patients than healthy controls when normalized to plasma cholesterol levels.[41,42] However, CoQ_{10} supplementation has not decreased insulin requirement in type 1 diabetics,[43] not shown any improvement in glycemic control in type 1 or 2 diabetics, and did not improve serum lipid profiles in type 2 diabetics.[39,44] Since CoQ_{10} supplementation did not influence glycemic control, it has been concluded that CoQ_{10} supplements could be used safely in diabetic patients as an adjunct therapy for cardiovascular disease.

Use with Doxorubicin and Cancer

In a placebo-controlled trial in mice, 100 mg/day of CoQ_{10} was given for 3–5 days prior to doxorubicin treatment. In two separate protocols the control group had only 36% and 42% survival rates. Pretreatment with CoQ_{10} groups had 80% and 86% survival rates, respectively. The differences are significant ($P < 0.05$). This reduction in acute toxicity of doxorubicin may be due to the effect of CoQ_{10} on the inhibition of CoQ_{10}-dependent enzymes in cardiac and other tissues that can be caused by doxorubicin.[45]

Cancer patients have been noted to show CoQ_{10} deficiency.[46,47] In an 18-month study of 32 patients, aged 32–81 years with "high-risk" breast cancer due to the disease's spread to axillary lymph nodes, nutritional therapy was added to surgical and therapeutic treatments. Patients were given 90 mg per os CoQ_{10}, antioxidants vitamin C 2,850 mg, vitamin E 2,500 IU, beta-carotene 32.5 IU, selenium 387 µg and secondary vitamins and minerals, fatty acids (omega 3 and omega 6). None of the patients had further metastasis and none died during the study. Of the 32 patients, 6 showed partial tumor regression.[48] However, large, controlled clinical trials are needed to determine the effects of CoQ_{10} supplementation in cancer patients.

ACQUIRED IMMUNODEFICIENCY SYNDROME

In 1991, Folkers et al. reported that two patients with acquired immunodeficiency syndrome (AIDS)-related complex had survived 4–5 years without any symptoms of adenopathy or infection after continuous treatment with CoQ_{10}. They found that 14 ordinary subjects responded to CoQ_{10} with increases in T4/T8 ratios and an increase in the blood levels of CoQ_{10}.[46]

Muscular Dystrophy

In 1995, 12 patients aged 7–69 years with muscular dystrophy were enrolled in a double-blind trial. The CoQ_{10} blood level of the control group was low, ranging from 0.5 µg/mL to 0.84 µg/mL. Patients were treated for 3 months with 100 mg of CoQ_{10} daily with a matching placebo in a double-blind trial. Improvement in physical performance was noted. Although the dosage 100 mg for 3 months was effective and safe, the authors believe that the dosage was too low and recommend using CoQ_{10} indefinitely in patients suffering from muscle dystrophy.[49]

Parkinson Disease

Decreased activity of complex I of the mitochondrial electron transport chain and oxidative stress in the substantia nigra are thought to play a role in Parkinson disease. CoQ_{10} as an electron acceptor for complex I and antioxidant effect may have a useful role. However, a phase III clinical trial of CoQ_{10} (1,200–2,400 mg/day) and vitamin E (1,200 IU/day) supplementation was terminated because it was felt that it is unlikely to show any benefit in treating patients with Parkinson disease.[50]

Pregnancy

The plasma CoQ_{10} levels rise during each trimester of normal pregnancy. However, there is a correlation between a low CoQ_{10} level and spontaneous abortion. A statistically significant difference ($P = 0.007$) was also found between the plasma CoQ_{10} value that was lower in spontaneous contractile activity, mainly in the third trimester, as compared with normal pregnancy. An increase in plasma CoQ_{10} level was related to decreased contractile activity of the uterine muscle.[51]

Periodontal Disease

Deficiency of CoQ_{10} has been noted in diseased gingiva but not in healthy gingiva. Oral administration of CoQ_{10} to patients with periodontal disease was effective in reducing gingival inflammation, as well as reducing periodontal pocket of depth and tooth mobility. No improvement was noted in the placebo group.

Topical application of CoQ_{10} dissolved in soybean oil (85 mg/mL) to affected areas (periodontal pockets) reduces bleeding and depth of pockets.[52]

Athletic Performance

Several placebo-controlled trials have examined the effects of 100–150 mg/day of CoQ_{10} supplementation for 3–8 weeks on physical performance in trained and untrained men. Most found no significant differences between groups taking CoQ_{10} and groups taking placebos with respect to the measures of aerobic exercise performance (Box 3).[53-56]

SIDE EFFECTS OF COENZYME Q_{10}

No serious side effects have been noted with CoQ_{10}. Less than 1% has epigastric discomfort, diarrhea, nausea, or appetite suppression. Side effects diminish when the dosage is decreased.[9] The adverse effects may be minimized if daily doses higher than 100 mg are divided into two or three daily doses. High dose (>100 mg) in the evening may cause mild insomnia in some individuals. Mild increase in serum transaminases can be seen in patients taking 300 mg/day for extended periods, but no hepatic toxicity has been observed.[9]

PHARMACOLOGY OF COENZYME Q_{10}

Coenzyme Q_{10} is available in capsules, gel, and toothpaste forms. Lipid vehicles, such as vegetable oil and vitamin E, yield higher absorption rate than the purified coenzyme alone. The half-life is about 34 hours. The elimination is primarily via the biliary tract, with up to 60% of oral

BOX 3: Potential role of coenzyme Q_{10} in noncardiac conditions.

Diabetes mellitus:
- Not shown any improvement in glycemic control in type 1 or 2 diabetics
- Did not decrease insulin requirement in type 1 diabetics
- No improvement in lipid profile in type 2 diabetics
- CoQ_{10} supplement can be safely used in diabetics as an adjunct therapy for cardiovascular disease

Cancer/doxorubicin use:
- Reduces the toxicity/side effects of doxorubicin
- Reduction in metastasis and mortality, especially in breast cancer
- May have beneficial effect in tumor regression
- Large, controlled clinical trials needed

AIDS:
- May have survival benefit
- Improvement of symptoms
- Increased T4/T8 ratio
- Large randomized trials needed

Muscular dystrophy:
- Improved physical performance
- Large randomized trials needed

Parkinson disease:
- Not much benefit seen

Pregnancy:
- May have beneficial effect in spontaneous abortion

Periodontal disease:
- Reduced gingival inflammation
- Reduces bleeding and depth of periodontal pockets

Athletic performance:
- No improvement in athletic performance

(AIDS: Acquired immunodeficiency syndrome; CoQ_{10}: Coenzyme Q_{10})

doses recoverable in the feces.[57] It is fat soluble, and absorption is significantly improved when taken with a meal containing some fat or even butter, in combination with soybean or vegetable oil. The recommended dose for health maintenance is 30 mg. A dose of 30–60 mg/day has been used to prevent deficiency. Therapeutic dose of CoQ_{10} ranges from 200 mg to 400 mg daily. Reported doses are 75–600 mg daily for cardiovascular disease; 30–60 mg/day have been used to prevent deficiency; and 100–200 mg/day to treat chronic heart disease. Treatment of cardiovascular disease requires elevated blood levels of 2–3 μg/mL, or even higher (Box 4).[27]

DRUG INTERACTIONS

Warfarin

Concomitant use of warfarin and CoQ_{10} supplements has been reported to decrease the anticoagulant effect of warfarin in at least four cases.[58] If warfarin and CoQ_{10} are to be used concomitantly, prothrombin time/international normalized ratio should be monitored closely, especially in the first 2 weeks.

BOX 4: Properties of coenzyme Q_{10}.

- Lipid soluble
- Half-life 34 hours
- Elimination: Biliary tract
- Disease prevention dose: 30–60 mg/day
- Dose to treat chronic heart disease: 100–200 mg/day
- Structurally similar to vitamin K. Monitor PT/INR closely if patients taking warfarin and CoQ_{10} concomitantly
- CoQ_{10} may protect against adverse effects of clonidine, diazoxide, hydralazine, hydrochlorothiazide, and methyldopa
- More research needed to determine if CoQ_{10} is beneficial for patients taking statins

(CoQ_{10}: Coenzyme Q_{10}; INR: International normalized ratio; PT: Prothrombin time)

3-Hydroxy-3-Methyl-Glutaryl-Coenzyme A Reductase Inhibitors (Statins)

Three-hydroxy-3-methyl-glutaryl-coenzyme A reductase inhibitors block CoQ_{10} biosynthesis, lowering blood levels by 20% to 30% because of the partially shared biosynthetic pathway of CoQ_{10} and cholesterol.[59] Since very few studies have examined CoQ_{10} content in target organs, it is not clear whether statin therapy affects CoQ_{10} concentration in body tissues.[17-19] More research is needed to determine whether CoQ_{10} supplementation is beneficial for those taking statins.

Gemfibrozil

Gemfibrozil lowers endogenous levels of CoQ_{10}.[60]

Other Drugs

Beta-blockers can inhibit CoQ_{10}-dependent enzymes. CoQ_{10} may protect against the adverse effects of clonidine, diazoxide, hydralazine, hydrochlorothiazide, and methyldopa.[61]

CONCLUSION

Coenzyme Q_{10} appears to be well tolerated and is relatively inexpensive. There is some evidence of potential benefit of CoQ_{10} in the treatment of congestive heart failure and other cardiovascular conditions. However, there is not enough evidence to support its benefit in cancer, periodontal disease, AIDS, or premature contractions in pregnancy. Numerous small studies on CoQ_{10} have shown potential benefits in various diseases, but large, randomized trials are needed to evaluate the relationship of CoQ_{10} to meaningful end points in important health areas.

REFERENCES

1. Crane FL, Hatefi Y, Lester EI, et al. Isolation of a quinone from beef heart mitochondria. Biochim Biophys Acta. 1957;25:220-1.
2. Littarru GP, Ho L, Folkers K. Deficiency of coenzyme Q10 in human heart disease: parts I and II. Internat J Vit Nutr Res. 1972;42(2):291,(3):413.
3. Allen LV. Coenzyme Q10 high strength capsules. US Pharm. 1999;24(5):96-9.
4. Marincola R. Neurobiology and quantified pharmaco EEG of coenzyme Q10. J Orthomolecular Med. 1997;12(2):87-95.
5. Challem J. Coenzyme Q10: It may just be the miracle vitamin of the 1990s. The Nutrition Reporter; December 4, 1996.
6. Silverman H, Romano J, Elmer G (Eds). The vitamin book, New York, NY: Bantam Books; 1993.
7. Weber C, Jakobsen TS, Mortensen SA, et al. Antioxidative effect of dietary coenzyme Q10 in human blood plasma. Internat J Vit Nutr Res. 1994;64:311-5.
8. Folkers K, Osterborg A, Nylander M, et al. Activities of vitamin Q10 in animal models and a serious deficiency in patients with cancer. Biochem Biophys Res Commu. 1997;234(2):296-9.
9. Pepping J. Alternative therapies: coenzyme Q10. Am J Health Syst Pharm. 1999;56(6):519-21.
10. Bliznakov EG. From sharks to coenzyme Q10. Adv Exp Med Biol. 1976;73:441-50.
11. Crane FL. Biochemical functions of coenzyme Q10. J Am Coll Nutr. 2001;20(6):591-8.
12. Nohl H, Gille L. The role of coenzyme Q in lysosomes, In Kagan VE, Quinn PJ (Eds). Coenzyme Q: molecular mechanisms in health and disease, Boca Raton, FL: CRC Press; 2001. pp. 99-106.
13. Ernster L, Dallner G. Biochemical, physiological and medical aspects of ubiquinone function. Biochim Biophys Acta. 1995;1271(1):195-204.
14. Overvad K, Diamant B, Holm L, et al. Coenzyme Q10 in health and disease. Eur J Clin Nutr. 1999;53(10):764-70.
15. Weber C. Dietary intake and absorption of coenzyme Q. In: Kagan VE, Quinn PJ (Eds). Coenzyme Q: molecular mechanisms in health disease. Boca Raton, FL: CRC Press; 2001. pp. 209-15.
16. Rustin P, Munnich A, Rotig A. Mitochondrial respiratory chain dysfunction caused by coenzyme Q deficiency. Methods Enzymol. 2004;382:81-8.
17. Laaksonen R, Jokelainen K, Laakso J, et al. The effect of simvastatin treatment on natural antioxidants in low-density lipoproteins and high-energy phosphates and ubiquinone in skeletal muscle. Am J Cardiol. 1996;77(10):851-4.
18. Elmberger PG, Kalen A, Lund E, et al. Effects of pravastatin and cholestyramine on products of the mevalonate pathway in familial hypercholesterolemia. J Lipid Res. 1991;32(6):935-40.
19. Laaksonen R, Jokelainen K, Sahi T, et al. Decreases in serum ubiquinone concentrations do not result in reduced levels in muscle tissue during short term simvastatin treatment in humans. Clin Pharmacol Ther. 1995;57(1):62-6.
20. Langsjoen P, Vadhanavikit S, Folker K. Response of patients in class III and IV of cardiomyopathy to therapy in a blind and crossover trial with coenzyme Q10. Proc Natl Acad Sci USA. 1985;82:4240-4.
21. Judy W, Hall J, Toth P, et al. Double blind-double crossover study of coenzyme CoQ10 in heart failure. In: Folkers K, Yamamura Y (Eds). Biomedical and clinical aspects of coenzyme Q. Amsterdam, The Netherlands: Elsevier Science; 1986.
22. Langsjoen H, Langsjoen P, Willis R, et al. Usefulness of coenzyme Q10 in clinical cardiology: a long-term study. Mol Aspects Med. 1994;15(Suppl.):S2165-75.
23. Sander S, Coleman CI, Patel AA, et al. The impact of coenzyme Q10 on systolic function in patients with chronic heart failure. J Card Fail. 2006;12:464-72.
24. Molyneux SL, Florkowski CM, George PM, et al. Coenzyme Q10: an independent predictor of mortality in chronic heart failure. J Am Coll Cardiol. 2008;52:1435-41.
25. McMurray JJ, Dunselman P, Wedel H, et al. Coenzyme Q10, rosuvastatin, and clinical outcomes in heart failure: a pre-specified substudy of CORONA (controlled rosuvastatin multinational study in heart failure). J Am Coll Cardiol. 2010;56:1196-204.
26. Mortensen SA, Rosenfeldt F, Kumar A, et al. The effect of coenzyme Q10 on morbidity and mortality in chronic heart failure. Results from Q-SYMBIO: a randomized double-blind trial. JACC Heart Fail. 2014;2:641-9.
27. Digiesi V, Cantini F, Brodeck B. Effect of coenzyme Q10 on essential arterial hypertension. Curr Ther Res. 1990;47:841-5.
28. Langsjoen P, Willis R, Folkers K. Treatment of essential hypertension with coenzyme Q10. Mol Aspects Med. 1994;15(Suppl.):S265-72.
29. ingh RB, Niaz MA, Rastogi SS, et al. Effect of hydrosoluble coenzyme Q10 on blood pressure and insulin resistance in hypertensive patients with coronary artery disease. J Hum Hypertens. 1999;13(3):203-8.
30. Burke BE, Neuenschwander R, Olson RD. Randomized, double-blind, placebo-controlled trial of coenzyme Q10 in isolated systolic hypertension. South Med J. 2001;94(11):1112-7.
31. Rosenfeldt FL, Haas SJ, Krum H, et al. Coenzyme Q10 in the treatment of hypertension: a meta-analysis of the clinical trials. J Hum Hypertens. 2007;21:297-306.
32. Lonnrot K, Tolvanen JP, Porsti I, et al. Coenzyme Q10 supplementation and recovery from ischemia in senescent rat myocardium. Life Sci. 1999;64(5):315-23.
33. Rosenfeldt FL, Pepe S, Linnane A, et al. The effects of ageing on the response to cardiac surgery: protective strategies for the ageing myocardium. Biogerontology. 2002;3(1-2):37-40.
34. Langsjoen PH, Langsjoen AM. Overview of the use of CoQ10 in cardiovascular disease. Biofactors. 1999;9(2-4):273-84.
35. Taggart DP, Jenkins M, Hooper J, et al. Effects of short-term supplementation with coenzyme Q10 on myocardial protection during cardiac operations. Ann Thorac Surg. 1996;61(3):829-33.
36. Tran MT, Mitchell TM, Kennedy DT, et al. Role of coenzyme Q10 in chronic heart failure, angina and hypertension. Pharmacotherapy. 2001;21(7):797-806.

37. Watts GF, Playford DA, Croft KD, et al. Coenzyme Q10 improves endothelial dysfunction of the brachial artery in Type II diabetes mellitus. Diabetologia. 2002;45(3):420-6.
38. Hamilton SJ, Chew GT, Watts GF. Coenzyme Q10 improves endothelial dysfunction in statin-treated type 2 diabetic patients. Diabetes Care. 2009;32:810-2.
39. Lim SC, Lekshminarayanan R, Goh SK, et al. The effect of coenzyme Q10 on microcirculatory endothelial function of subjects with type 2 diabetes mellitus. Atherosclerosis. 2008;196:966-9.
40. Gao L, Mao Q, Cao J, et al. Effects of coenzyme Q10 on vascular endothelial function in humans: a meta-analysis of randomized controlled trials. Atherosclerosis. 2011;221(2):311-6.
41. McDonnell MG, Archbold GP. Plasma ubiquinol/cholesterol ratios in patients with hyperlipidaemia, those with diabetes mellitus and in patients requiring dialysis. Clin Chim Acta. 1996;253(1-2):117-26.
42. Lim SC, Tan HH, Goh SK, et al. Oxidative burden in prediabetic and diabetic individuals: evidence from plasma coenzyme Q10. Diabet Med. 2006;23:1344-9.
43. Henriksen JE, Andersen CB, Hother-Nielsen O, et al. Impact of ubiquinone (coenzyme Q10) treatment on glycaemic control, insulin requirement and well-being in patients with Type I diabetes mellitus. Diabet Med. 1999;16(4):312-8.
44. Eriksson JG, Forsen TJ, Mortensen SA, et al. The effect of coenzyme Q10 administration on metabolic control in patients with type 2 diabetes mellitus. Biofactors. 1999;9(2-4):315-8.
45. Combs A, Choe J, Truong D, et al. Reduction by coenzyme Q10 of the acute toxicity of Adriamycin in mice. Res Commun Chem Pathol Pharmacol. 1977;18:565-8.
46. Folkers K, Hanioka T, Xia LJ, et al. Coenzyme Q10 increases T4/T8 ratios of lymphocytes in ordinary subjects and relevance to patients having the AIDS related complex Biochem Biophys Res Commun. 1991;176(2):786-91.
47. Folkers K, Morita M, McRee J Jr. The activities of coenzyme Q10 and vitamin B6 for immune responses. Biochem Biophys Res Commun. 1993;193(1):88-92.
48. Lockwood K, Moesgaard S, Hanioka T, et al. Apparent partial remission of breast cancer in "high risk" patients supplemented with nutritional antioxidants, essential fatty acids and coenzyme Q10. Mol Aspects Med. 1994;15(Suppl.):S231-40.
49. Folkers K, Simonsen R. Two successful double blind trials with coenzyme Q10 (vitamin Q 10) on muscular dystrophies and neurogenic atrophies. Biochem Biophys Acta. 1995;1271(1)281-6.
50. National Institute of Health. Effects of coenzyme Q10 in Parkinson disease (QE3). ClinicalTrials.gov. <http://www.clinicaltrials.gov/ct2/show/NCT00740714?>.
51. Nola G, Littarru G, De Santis M, et al. Coenzyme Q10 in pregnancy. Fetal Diagn Ther. 1996;11(4):264-70.
52. Wilkinson E, Arnold R, Folkers K. Treatment of periodontal and other soft tissue diseases of the oral cavity with coenzyme Q. In: Folkers K, Yamamura Y (Eds). Biomedical and clinical aspects of coenzyme Q, vol. 1. Amsterdam, The Netherlands: Elsevier/North Holland Biomedical; 1977.
53. Laaksonen R, Fogelholm M, Himberg JJ, et al. Ubiquinone supplementation and exercise capacity in trained young and older men. Eur J Appl Physiol Occup Physiol. 1995;72(1-2):95-100.
54. Malm C, Svensson M, Ekblom B, et al. Effects of ubiquinone-10 supplementation and high intensity training on physical performance in humans. Acta Physiol Scand. 1997;161(3):379-84.
55. Weston SB, Zhou S, Weatherby RP, et al. Does exogenous coenzyme Q10 affect aerobic capacity in endurance athletes? Int J Sport Nutr. 1997;7(3):197-206.
56. Porter DA, Costill DL, Zachwieja JJ, et al. The effect of oral coenzyme Q10 on the exercise tolerance of middle-aged, untrained men. Int J Sports Med. 1995;16(7):421-7.
57. Micromedex. Ubidecarenone drug monograph. Englewood, CO: Micromedex; May 1995 [updated March 1998].
58. Heck AM, DeWitt BA, Lukes AL. Potential interactions between alternative therapies and warfarin. Am J Health Syst Pharm. 2000;57(13):1221-7. quiz 1228–1230.
59. Mortensen S, Leh A, Agner E, et al. Dose related decrease of serum coenzyme Q10 during treatment with HMG-CoA reductase inhibitors. Mol Aspects Med. 1997;18(Suppl.):S137-44.
60. Aberg F, Appelkvist E, Broijersen A, et al. Gemfibrozil-induced decrease in serum ubiquinone and alpha and gamma-tocopherol levels in men with combined hyperlipidemia. Eur J Clin Invest. 1998;28:235-42.
61. Kishi T, Watanabe T, Folkers K. Bioenergetics in clinical medicine XV. Inhibition of coenzyme Q10 enzymes by clinically used adrenergic blockers of B receptors. Res Commun Chem Pathol Pharmacol. 1977;17(1):157-64.

129

CHAPTER

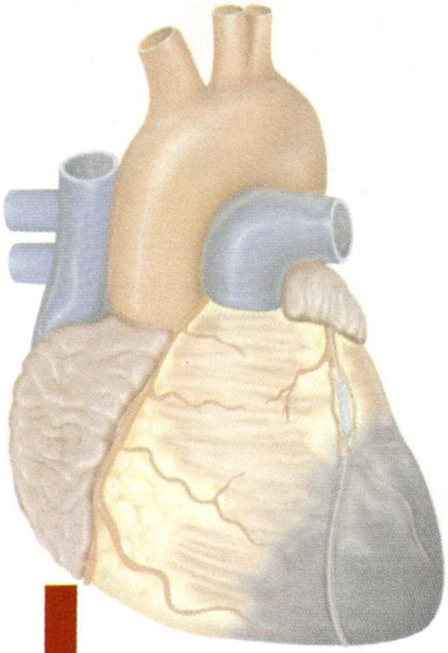

Myocardial Molecular Imaging of Fatty Acid Metabolism Using BMIPP

Pawan K Sharma, HK Chopra, Srikant Sharma

INTRODUCTION

The two major sources of energy in the myocardium are fatty acids and glucose. Fatty acids are the primary source of energy for heart muscle under normal conditions of blood flow and oxygen delivery. Alterations in myocardial fatty acid utilization may indicate ischemic myocardium.[1] Under hypoxic or ischemic conditions, oxidation of fatty acids is greatly suppressed, whereas glucose metabolism, requiring less oxygen consumption, plays a major role in residual oxidative metabolism. Therefore, under ischemic conditions, the source of energy in the myocardium shifts from fatty acid to glucose.[2] Decreased fatty acid metabolism is also observed in myocardial necrosis. Thus, alteration of fatty acid oxidation is considered to be a sensitive marker of ischemia and myocardial damage. Conversely, persistence of glucose utilization is regarded as a suitable marker of myocardial viability in the dysfunctional myocardium. The fatty acid analog iodine 123 15-(*p*-iodophenyl)-3-(*R*,*S*) methylpentadecanoic acid facilitates metabolic imaging of the diseased myocardium because 60–70% of the energy requirement of the normal myocardium under aerobic conditions is derived from the metabolism of free fatty acids.[3] Japan is the first country to approve BMIPP for clinical use in 1993. Single photon emission computed tomography (SPECT) with BMIPP, which does not require any kind of stress, detects abnormal metabolic findings in various cardiac conditions such as unstable angina, acute myocardial infarction (AMI), vasospastic angina, and cardiomyopathies.[4]

ISCHEMIC MEMORY OR METABOLIC STUNNING

Ischemia results in reduction of fatty acid utilization and there is shift from fatty acid to glucose utilization during ischemic conditions. In addition, such metabolic shift may persist shortly after recovery of ischemia with restoration of perfusion. Thus, BMIPP uptake remains affected for a longer time in ischemic myocardium, mainly due to persistent suppression of fatty acid metabolism after severe ischemia. This metabolic alteration as a result of prior ischemia is called *ischemic memory or metabolic stunning*.[1,5,6] Persistent fatty acid metabolic abnormality has been observed up to 30 hours after the transient stress-induced ischemic episode on the treadmill.[7]

PRINCIPLE OF IODINE 123 15-(*p*-IODOPHENYL)-3-(*R*,*S*) METHYLPENTADECANOIC ACID IMAGING AND TECHNIQUE

Iodine 123 15-(*p*-iodophenyl)-3-(*R*,*S*) methylpentadecanoic acid is distributed both in mitochondria and in cytosol and is incorporated into the triglyceride pool. Because of its rapid, high myocardial uptake with a low background and retention in the myocardium for a long period of time, it is a suitable agent for SPECT imaging.[8] Under ischemic conditions, beta-oxidation of fatty acid in the mitochondria is reduced and back-diffusion and early wash out of nonmetabolized BMIPP occur. Due to this abnormal metabolic pathway, there is reduced myocardial uptake of BMIPP which is detected by SPECT.[9,10] BMIPP uptake is similar to thallium and an overnight fast is required before myocardial metabolic imaging is performed. There is no requirement for any stress exercise or pharmacologic stress agent and 111–148 MBq (3–4 mCi) I-123 BMIPP is administered intravenously. The imaging scans are obtained 20–30 minutes after the injection. This may provide information about both perfusion and metabolic function of the myocardium and ameliorate the use of extra-perfusion tracer, e.g. Tl-201 or tetrofosmin. The earlier image acquisition reflects myocardial perfusion and may mask pure metabolic imaging.[11] Greater BMIPP uptake than thallium perfusion is observed in the septal and inferior regions in normal subjects, probably due to the greater photon attenuation of Tl-201 in these areas. The rotation of the gamma camera and acquisition time are similar to those with myocardial perfusion imaging. Although a multipurpose or low-energy high-resolution collimator can be used for I-123 BMIPP imaging, a multipurpose collimator yields better quality SPECT image. No attenuation or scatter correction is usually used.

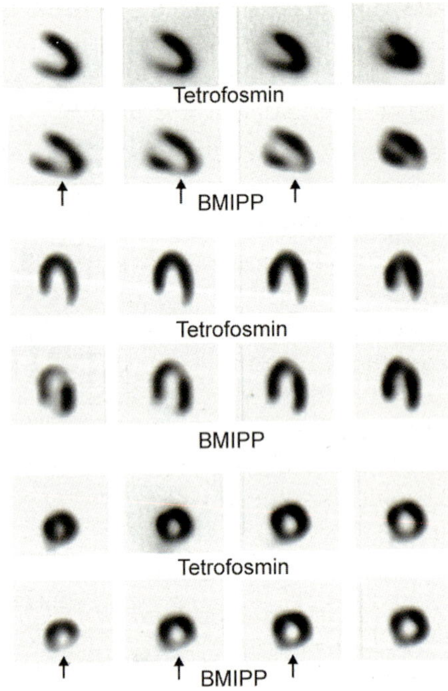

Fig. 1: Tetrofosmin and BMIPP SPECT images at rest in a patient with unstable angina. Myocardial perfusion SPECT on admission showed only mild perfusion abnormalities in the inferior region, but BMIPP SPECT taken next day showed significant reduction in the inferior region (arrows). (BMIPP: Iodine 123 15-(*p*-iodophenyl)-3-(*R,S*) methylpentadecanoic acid; SPECT: Single photon emission computed tomography).

CORONARY ARTERY DISEASE ASSESSMENT USING IODINE 123 15-(*p*-IODOPHENYL)-3-(*R,S*) METHYLPENTADECANOIC ACID IMAGING AND TECHNIQUE

Triaging acute chest pain in the emergency room: Elevated levels of cardiac troponins are present in AMI and are also seen in other conditions in the absence of acute coronary syndrome (ACS). For this reason, a resting perfusion-metabolism study via fatty acid imaging may potentially be a useful diagnostic tool in differentiating cardiac enzyme elevations due to ACS from other etiologies. The principle of ischemic memory imaging of BMIPP can be useful in triaging patients in the emergency room with acute chest pain with no evidence of acute myocardial infarction (MI). Using BMIPP metabolic imaging in 111 patients with acute chest pain whose symptoms had resolved 1–5 days previously, a sensitivity of 74% and specificity of 92% in the detection of coronary artery stenosis and spasm have been noted whereas Tc-99m tetrofosmin imaging at rest had a lower sensitivity of 38% (Fig. 1).[12]

Although Tc-99m sestamibi myocardial imaging at rest can also be used to evaluate patients with acute chest pain in the emergency room, imaging should be performed within 2–6 hours after chest pain is relieved.[13,14] It was, therefore, concluded that BMIPP metabolic imaging can be useful in stratifying patient risk long after chest pain has been resolved. Large-scale studies are needed to establish any definite conclusion.

Acute myocardial infarction: In acute chest pain and unstable angina, reduced uptake of myocardial BMIPP is the hallmark of diagnosis. But the BMIPP imaging alone in AMI is insufficient. Reduced uptake of myocardial BMIPP is caused by ischemic memory and myocardial necrosis, both of which usually coexist in the myocardium of AMI. Thus, abnormal findings on BMIPP imaging in AMI imply a combination of necrosis due to MI and ischemic memory. To clarify the diagnostic value of BMIPP imaging in AMI, this tracer is usually combined with perfusion tracers such as Tl-201 or Tc-99m-labeled agents.[4,15] BMIPP and perfusion imaging in patients with AMI show three different correlations between myocardial perfusion and fatty acid metabolism:

1. If the reduction of myocardial uptake of the two tracers (defects in perfusion and BMIPP scan) is similar, the segment is defined as *matching*. A matched defect with severely reduced uptake of the two tracers is considered to indicate nonviable scar tissue;

2. Lower BMIPP uptake relative to perfusion (perfusion-metabolism *mismatch*) implicates a metabolically damaged often dysynergic, but viable myocardium (stunned or hibernating myocardium);
3. Equivalently, *normal uptake* of the radiotracer in perfusion and BMIPP scan represents a completely salvaged myocardium.

These three imaging features contribute to the prediction of an ischemia-related myocardial injury, postinterventional functional recovery of the myocardium, and patients who have myocardium at ischemic risk.[16] The BMIPP imaging has also been found to be useful in many studies to evaluate the benefit of reperfusion therapy for AMI in the acute phase. In a study using I-123 BMIPP and Tc-99m sestamibi SPECT in 18 post-AMI patients, in most of whom thrombolytic therapy was performed. It was shown[17] that the analysis based on mismatched and matched uptake abnormalities of the two tracers had a sensitivity of 82% and specificity of 90% regarding improvement of wall motion 6 months after MI whereas dobutamine stress echo showed a sensitivity of 80% and specificity of 63%. In another study[18] involving patients with large AMIs treated only by percutaneous coronary intervention, the combination of I-123 BMIPP and Tc-99m tetrofosmin imaging had a sensitivity of 61% and specificity of 83% in predicting functional improvement after 6 months. Mismatched pattern in a dysfunctional myocardium before revascularization is associated with fewer hard events after successful revascularization.[19] This suggests that the mismatched myocardium before revascularization represents a hibernating or stunned but viable myocardium. Successful revascularization of such a myocardium may, therefore, confer survival benefit. Patients with matched myocardium suggesting scarred myocardium may not benefit from revascularization. The BMIPP imaging may therefore be useful for the planning of revascularization to determine which patients benefit from revascularization. Large, prospective randomized trials are needed to confirm this. In another[20] multicenter study involving 159 patients who were treated for AMI by only percutaneous coronary intervention, during a 34.5-month follow-up, 36 of these patients had major adverse cardiac events. Again, a greater extent of BMIPP uptake abnormality and mismatched defects between I-123 BMIPP and Tl-201 was closely and independently associated with major adverse cardiac events. The prediction of future cardiac events with these scintigraphic parameters was independent of clinical and angiographic parameters. Of note, mismatched defects were present at the initial evaluation in all six patients who subsequently died suddenly. These results demonstrated that the greater the BMIPP myocardial uptake abnormality, the worse the long-term prognosis of AMI patients, which might be explained by the prognostic influence of the amount of the area at risk.[21]

Unstable angina: Among patients with suspected ACS excluded for prior MI, the presence of reduced uptake on the BMIPP imaging was significantly associated with future cardiovascular events, whereas the negative test provided greater assurance with a negative predictive value of 98.9% for hard events over 3.5 years.[22] This meta-analysis demonstrated that negative BMIPP imaging gave 98.9% assurance that patient will not develop cardiac death or MI over 3.5 years. The repeated nature of chest pain in unstable angina allows BMIPP metabolic imaging to reveal "ischemic memory." Suzuki et al.[23] evaluated 28 patients with unstable angina and documented coronary artery disease (CAD) on coronary angiography compared with 12 control subjects. The BMIPP imaging at rest had a sensitivity of 89% and specificity of 100% in detecting patients, whereas Tl-201 perfusion imaging at rest had a lower sensitivity of 54%. Other studies also reported sensitivities of 71–100% and specificities of 83–100% using BMIPP for the diagnosis of patients with unstable angina.[11,24-26] Although these studies with BMIPP imaging showed acceptable diagnostic accuracy, the number of involved patients is very limited; therefore, a large-scale clinical study is necessary to confirm these promising observations.

Chronic stable angina: The prognostic value of BMIPP metabolic imaging was evaluated in patients with known or suspected CAD, excluding those with previous MI, and followed for a period of 3.9 years.[27] Kaplan-Meir survival estimates revealed an event-free survival rate of 92% at 3 years in patients with a BMIPP defect score of less than 5 but 80% in those with a defect score of 5 or more. Furthermore, patients with normal BMIPP myocardial imaging results had excellent outcomes, with a survival rate of 99% without any significant event at 1 year, 98% at 3 years, and 96% at 5 years. In addition, diabetic patients with a BMIPP defect score of 5 or more had a subsequent event rate of 41%, whereas nondiabetic patients with a defect score of less than 5 had an event rate of only 4%. These results suggested that BMIPP metabolic imaging is an independent predictor for subsequent cardiac events in patients with known or suspected CAD and that the combination of BMIPP with clinical factors such as diabetes mellitus further stratified the risk of patients.

Vasospastic angina: Provocative testing with the use of ergonovine or acetylcholine to visualize coronary spasm during diagnostic catheterization is usually necessary (Fig. 2). BMIPP metabolic imaging is promising because BMIPP can detect ischemic memory caused by recent vasospastic episodes. Using BMIPP metabolic imaging

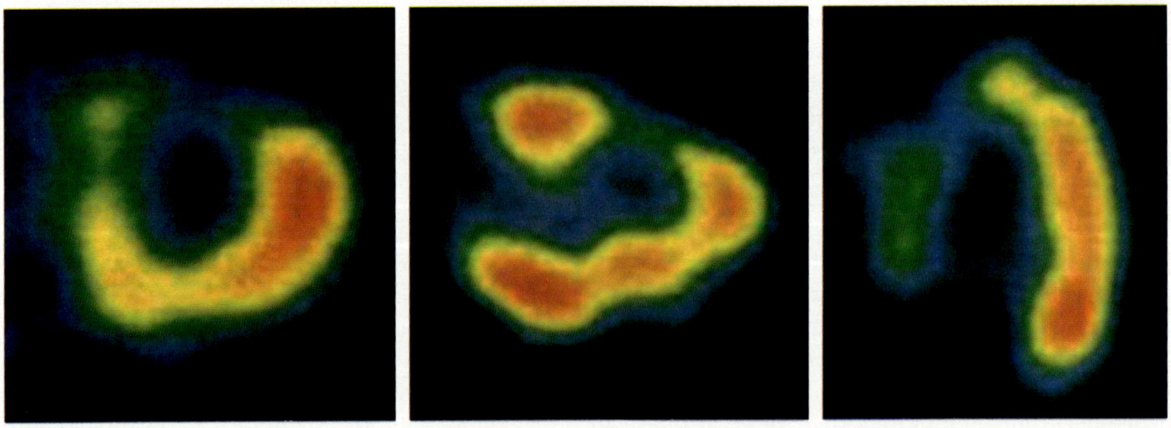

Fig. 2: BMIPP SPECT images showing reduced uptake in anteroseptal, anterolateral, and septal regions. The coronary angiogram showed acetylcholine-induced spasm of coronary arteries. (BMIPP: Iodine 123 15-(*p*-iodophenyl)-3-(*R*,*S*) methylpentadecanoic acid; SPECT: Single photon emission computed tomography).

without any provocative testing, Nakajima et al.[28] reported a sensitivity of 78% in 32 patients with angiographically documented vasospastic angina whereas a lower sensitivity of 31% was observed by using perfusion tracers (either Tl-201 or Tc-99m sestamibi).

CARDIOMYOPATHY ASSESSMENT USING IODINE 123 15-(*P*-IODOPHENYL)-3-(*R,S*) METHYLPENTADECANOIC ACID IMAGING AND TECHNIQUE

Hypertrophic Cardiomyopathy

The Tl-201 uptake is heterogeneous in a hypertrophied septal region, and BMIPP uptake is significantly decreased in the anteroseptal, posteroseptal, and the apical regions, indicating a perfusion-metabolism mismatch.[29-31] The extent of gadolinium-delayed hyperenhancement on magnetic resonance imaging or BMIPP defect are associated with progressive ventricular dilatation and are markers of sudden death.[30,32,33] The BMIPP imaging may therefore have a clinical role in the risk stratification of patients with hypertrophic cardiomyopathy.

Dilated Cardiomyopathy

In dilated cardiomyopathy (DCM), poor responders to beta-blocker therapy have decreased BMIPP uptake probably due to a severely injured myocardium. The patients who respond well to beta-blocker therapy have a relatively preserved BMIPP uptake. The BMIPP imaging, therefore, has a prognostic value in predicting response to therapy in DCM.[34] Studies have also suggested that the extent of BMIPP defects correlate with the severity of hemodynamic deterioration and histopathological changes as assessed by endomyocardial biopsy specimens[35] and that myocardial uptake of BMIPP could predict the response of DCM patients to beta-blocker therapy.[36] Further studies are needed to clarify the clinical usefulness of the BMIPP imaging in patients with DCM and those with heart failure.

Takotsubo Cardiomyopathy (Transient Apical Ballooning)

Patients with Takotsubo cardiomyopathy show normal perfusion with Tl-201 myocardial imaging, whereas a large area with reduced myocardial uptake of BMIPP is seen in the acute phase. The prognosis of Takotsubo cardiomyopathy is generally good and the BMIPP imaging shows improvement on follow-up. These findings may suggest that the transient left ventricular (LV) dysfunction may essentially be a stunned myocardium.[37]

Iodine 123 15-(*p*-Iodophenyl)-3-(*R,S*) Methylpentadecanoic Acid in Chronic Kidney Disease

Patients with end-stage renal disease (ESRD) have significant cardiovascular risk factors and have high prevalence of obstructive CAD. This results in higher incidence of cardiac death in ESRD patients on hemodialysis when compared with the general population.[38-40] The BMIPP imaging can be useful for the detection of CAD in hemodialysis patients.[41] High prevalence of BMIPP abnormalities and coronary angiography confirmed coronary stenosis on those showing BMIPP abnormalities. The BMIPP imaging showed high sensitivity (98%) and intermediate specificity (66%) for identifying stenosis in major coronary arteries. The relatively low specificity may possibly be due to small-vessel disease detected by BMIPP but not by coronary angiography. In a prospective study of 375 asymptomatic hemodialysis patients, severe BMIPP defect identified high risk for cardiac death on the follow-up study.[42] There are no definite studies showing the value of BMIPP imaging for general population of chronic kidney disease (CKD) without hemodialysis.

ASSESSMENT OF MYOCARDIAL VIABILITY

The size and severity of BMIPP defect areas in the subacute phase of infarction correlates with the areas at risk calculated by perfusion imaging on admission in the acute phase of MI. The difference in the areas between the perfusion and BMIPP abnormalities in the subacute phase of MI after revascularization correlates with the amount of salvaged myocardium as noted on the perfusion studies before and shortly after revascularization treatment in patients after AMI[6] (Fig. 3). The persistent abnormalities in the regional function after revascularization in AMI may be related to the delayed recovery of altered metabolism.

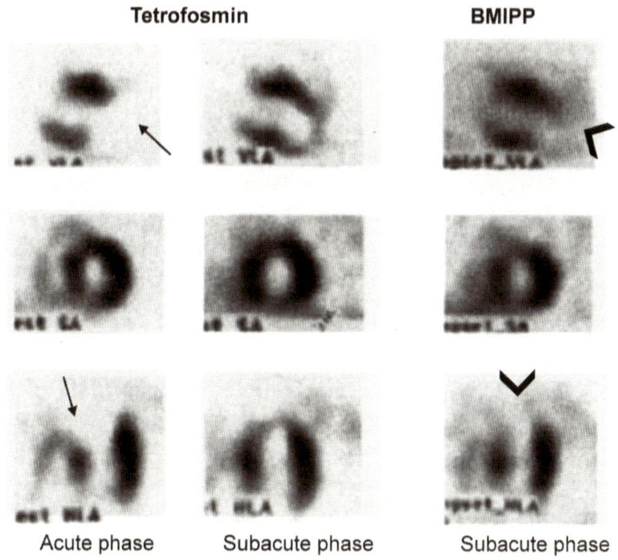

Fig. 3: Sequential tetrofosmin images and BMIPP images after AMI with successful PTCA. Perfusion defect (arrows) observed in the acute phase (left) significantly improved in the subacute phase (middle) (1 week). The BMIPP images taken in the subacute phase (right) showed reduced uptake (arrowheads), corresponding to the perfusion abnormalities in the acute phase, indicating delayed recovery of metabolic alteration after PTCA. (AMI: acute myocardial infarction; BMIPP: iodine 123 15-(*p*-iodophenyl)-3-(*R,S*) methylpentadecanoic acid; PTCA: percutaneous transluminal coronary angioplasty; SPECT: single photon emission computed tomography).

Such stunned myocardium can be identified as an area of less BMIPP uptake compared with perfusion. Thus, BMIPP may reflect prior severe ischemia after recovery of perfusion (i.e. ischemic memory).[1,6] The areas with less BMIPP uptake than perfusion are more likely to improve regional function, whereas those with similar defect of both BMIPP and perfusion are least likely to improve function. Thus, combined imaging with BMIPP and perfusion may be used for myocardial viability assessment. Further studies are needed to confirm the potential value of BMIPP imaging in combination with perfusion studies for assessing myocardial viability.

RISK STRATIFICATION

In a study involving 167 consecutive patients with angina followed for a period of 4 years, BMIPP defect score at rest, stress perfusion score, diabetes, and LV ejection fraction (LVEF) were found to be independent prognostic factors.[43] No hard event (cardiac death, nonfatal MI) was observed with normal BMIPP uptake, whereas two patients with nearly normal stress perfusion with abnormal BMIPP uptake had hard events. These data indicate that BMIPP imaging is an important prognostic indicator independent of stress myocardial imaging in patients with angina without prior MI. More clinical experience is required to confirm the prognostic value of the BMIPP imaging at rest in patients with suspected CAD.

Fractional anisotropy (FA) imaging is potentially useful in the determination of the risk spectrum for sudden cardiac death and can help in patient selection for an implantable cardioverter-defibrillator (ICD), particularly in the controversial early period after AMI. The Valsartan in Acute Myocardial Infarction Trial demonstrated that the risk of sudden death is highest in the first 30 days after MI among patients with LV dysfunction or heart failure (or both).[44] Thus, the ability of FA imaging to predict LV recovery early after MI may play a role in the early implementation of strategies to prevent sudden death in high-risk patients. The Defibrillator in Acute Myocardial Infarction Trial findings did not support the use of early ICD therapy in a high-risk population after MI suggesting an overreliance on LVEF as a risk stratification tool.[45] Metabolic assessment through FA imaging may add incremental value to risk stratification over measurement of LVEF alone, given that the metabolic consequences of severe ischemia may trigger ventricular fibrillation in AMI.[46]

CONCLUSION

Iodine 123 15-(*p*-iodophenyl)-3-(*R,S*) methylpentadecanoic acid plays an important role for identifying ischemia at rest, based on the unique capability to represent persistent metabolic alteration after recovery of ischemia, the so-called ischemic memory. Since it does not require any stress imaging, it can be very useful in triaging patients presenting to the emergency room who cannot or should not be exercising such as those with unstable angina, AMI, vasospastic angina, cardiomyopathies. It is a useful agent for ischemic imaging in patients whose chest pain has resolved 1–5 days earlier and present late for evaluation. Since BMIPP abnormalities may represent severe ischemia or jeopardized myocardium, it may permit risk stratification in CAD patients, particularly for those with CKD and on hemodialysis.

REFERENCES

1. Tamaki N, Morita K, Kuge Y, et al. The role of fatty acids in cardiac imaging. J Nucl Med. 2000;41:1525-34.
2. Liedke AJ. Alterations of carbohydrate and lipid metabolism in the acutely ischemic heart. Prog Cardiovasc Dis. 1981;23:321-36.
3. Neely JR, Rovetto MJ, Oram JF. Myocardial utilization of carbohydrate and lipids. Prog Cardiovasc Dis. 1972;15:289-329.
4. Tamaki N, Kusakabe K, Kubo A, et al. Guidelines for clinical use of cardiac nuclear medicine (JCS 2005) [In Japanese]. Circ J. 2005;65(Suppl. IV):1125-202.
5. Tamaki N, Morita K, Kawai Y. The Japanese experience with metabolic imaging in the clinical setting. J Nucl Cardiol. 2007;14:S145-52.
6. Kawai Y, Tsukamoto E, Nozaki Y, et al. Use of 123 I-BMIPP single-photon emission tomography to estimate areas at risk following successful revascularization in patients with acute myocardial infarction. Eur J Nucl Med. 1998;25:1390-5.
7. Dilsizian V, Bateman TM, Bergmann SR, et al. Metabolic imaging with beta-methyl-*p*-[^{123}I]-iodophenyl-pentadecanoic acid (BMIPP) identifies ischemic memory following demand ischemia. Circulation. 2005;112:2169-74.
8. Knapp FF Jr, Kropp J. Iodine-123 labeled fatty acids for myocardial SPECT: current status and future perspective. Eur J Nucl Med. 1995;22:361-81.
9. Nohara R, Okuda K, Ogino M, et al. Evaluation of myocardial viability with iodine-123-BMIPP in a canine model. J Nucl Med. 1996;37:1403-7.
10. Hosokawa R, Nohara R, Fujibayashi Y, et al. Myocardial kinetics of iodine-123-BMIPP in canine for clinical SPECT. J Nucl Med. 1997;38:1857-63.
11. Kobayashi H, Kusakabe K, Momose M, et al. Evaluation of myocardial perfusion and fatty acid uptake using a single injection of iodine-123-BMIPP in patients with acute coronary syndrome. J Nucl Med. 1998;39:1117-22.
12. Kawai Y, Tsukamoto E, Nozaki Y, et al. Significance of reduced uptake of iodinated fatty acid analogue for the evaluation of patients with acute chest pain. J Am Coll Cardiol. 2001;38:1888-94.
13. Udelson JE, Beshansky JR, Ballin DS, et al. Myocardial perfusion imaging for evaluation and triage of patients with suspected acute cardiac ischemia. A randomized controlled trial. JAMA. 2002;288:2693-700.
14. Klocke FJ, Baird MG, Lorell BH, et al. ACC/AHA/ASNC guidelines for the clinical use of cardiac radionuclide imaging. J Am Coll Cardiol. 2003;42:1318-33.
15. Torizuka K, Yonekura Y, Nishimura T, et al. Phase 3 study of beta-methyl-*p*-(^{123}I)-iodophenyl-pentadecanoic acid, a myocardial imaging agent for evaluating fatty acid metabolism: a multi-center trial [in Japanese]. Kakuikaku. 1992;29:413-33.
16. Nakata T, Hashimoto A, Eguchi M. Cardiac BMIPP imaging in acute myocardial infarction. Int J Card Imaging. 1999;15:21-6.
17. Franken PR, Dendale P, De Geeter F, et al. Prediction of functional outcome after myocardial infarction using BMIPP and sestamibi scintigraphy. J Nucl Med. 1996;37:718-22.
18. Seki H, Toyama T, Higuchi K, et al. Prediction of functional improvement of ischemic myocardium with 123 I-BMIPP SPECT and 99mTc-tetrofosmin SPECT imaging. Circ J. 2005;69:311-9.
19. Fukuzawa S, Ozawa S, Shimada K, et al. Prognostic values of perfusion-metabolic mismatch in Tl-201 and BMIPP scintigraphic imaging in patients with chronic coronary artery disease and left ventricular dysfunction undergoing revascularization. Ann Nucl Med. 2002;16:109-15.
20. Nanasato M, Hirayama H, Ando A, et al. Incremental predictive value of myocardial scintigraphy with 123 I-BMIPP in patients with acute myocardial infarction treated with primary percutaneous coronary intervention. Eur J Nucl Med Mol Imaging. 2004;31:1512-21.
21. Christian TF, Schwartz RS, Gibbons RJ. Determinants of infarct size in reperfusion therapy for acute myocardial infarction. Circulation. 1992;86:81-90.
22. Inaba Y, Bergmann SR. Prognostic value of myocardial metabolic imaging with BMIPP in the spectrum of coronary artery disease: a systemic review. J Nucl Cardiol. 2010;17:61-70.
23. Suzuki A, Takada Y, Nagasaka M, et al. Comparison of resting beta-methyl-iodophenylpentadecanoic acid (BMIPP) and thallium-201 tomography using quantitative polar maps in patients with unstable angina. Jpn Circ J. 1997;61:133-8.
24. Tateno M, Tamaki N, Yukihiro M, et al. Assessment of fatty acid uptake in ischemic heart disease without myocardial infarction. J Nucl Med. 1996;37:1981-5.
25. Takeishi Y, Fujiwara S, Atsumi H, et al. Iodine-123-BMIPP imaging in unstable angina: a guide for interventional strategy. J Nucl Med. 1997;38:1407-11.
26. Yamabe H, Abe H, Yokoyama M, et al. Resting 123 I-BMIPP scintigraphy in diagnosis of effort angina pectoris with reference to subsets of the disease. Ann Nucl Med. 1998;12:139-44.
27. Chikamori T, Fujita H, Nanasato M, et al. Prognostic value of I-123 15-(*p*-iodophenyl)-3-(*R*,*S*) methylpentadecanoic acid myocardial imaging in patients with known or suspected coronary artery disease. J Nucl Cardiol. 2005;12:172-8.

28. Nakajima K, Shimizu K, Taki J, et al. Utility of iodine-123-BMIPP in the diagnosis and follow-up of vasospastic angina. J Nucl Med. 1995;36:1934-40.
29. Kurata C, Tawarahara K, Taguchi T, et al. Myocardial emission computed tomography with iodine-123-labeled beta-methyl-branched fatty acid in patients with hypertrophic cardiomyopathy. J Nucl Med. 1992;33:6-13.
30. Ohtsuki K, Sugihara H, Kuribayashi T, et al. Impairment of BMIPP accumulation at junction of ventricular septum and left and right ventricular free walls in hypertrophic cardiomyopathy. J Nucl Med. 1999;40:2007-13.
31. Tadamura E, Kudoh T, Hattori N, et al. Impairment of BMIPP uptake precedes abnormalities in oxygen and glucose metabolism in hypertrophic cardiomyopathy. J Nucl Med. 1998;39:390-6.
32. Nishimura T, Nagata S, Uehara T, et al. Prognosis of hypertrophic cardiomyopathy: assessment by 123 I-BMIPP (beta-methyl-*p*-(123 I) iodophenyl pentadecanoic acid) myocardial single photon emission computed tomography. Ann Nucl Med. 1996;10:71-8.
33. Moon JCC, McKenna WJ, McCrohon JA, et al. Toward clinical risk assessment in hypertrophic cardiomyopathy with gadolinium cardiovascular magnetic resonance. J Am Coll Cardiol. 2003;41:1561-7.
34. Yoshinaga K, Tahara M, Torii H, et al. Predicting the effects on patients with dilated cardiomyopathy of beta-blocker therapy, by using iodine-123 15-(*p*-iodophenyl)-3-*R,S*-methylpentadecanoic acid (BMIPP) myocardial scintigraphy. Ann Nucl Med. 1998;12:341-7.
35. Yazaki Y, Isobe M, Takahashi W, et al. Assessment of myocardial fatty acid metabolic abnormalities in patients with idiopathic dilated cardiomyopathy using 123 I BMIPP SPECT: correlation with clinicopathological findings and clinical course. Heart. 1999;81:153-9.
36. Ito T, Hoshida S, Nishio M, et al. Relationship between evaluation by quantitative fatty acid myocardial scintigraphy and response to beta-blockade therapy in patients with dilated cardiomyopathy. Eur J Nucl Med. 2001;28:1811-6.
37. Kurisu S, Inoue I, Kawagoe K, et al. Myocardial perfusion and fatty acid metabolism in patients with tako-tsubo-like left ventricular dysfunction. J Am Coll Cardiol. 2003;41:743-8.
38. Rostand SG, Rutsky EA. Ischemic heart disease in chronic renal failure: management considerations. Semin Dial. 1989;2:98-101.
39. Ansell D, Roderick P, Hodsman A, et al. UK Renal Registry 11th annual report (December 2008): Chapter 7 Survival and causes of death of UK adult patients on renal replacement therapy in 2007: national and centre-specific analyses. Nephron Clin Pract. 2009;111:c113-39.
40. Foley RN, Parfrey PS, Sarnak MJ. Epidemiology of cardiovascular disease in chronic renal disease. J Am Soc Nephrol. 1998;9:S16-23.
41. Nishimura M, Hashimoto T, Kobayashi H, et al. Myocardial scintigraphy using a fatty acid analogue detects coronary artery disease in hemodialysis patients. Kidney Int. 2004;66:811-29.
42. Nishimura M, Tsukamoto K, Hasebe N, et al. Prediction of cardiac death in hemodialysis patients by myocardial fatty acid imaging. J Am Coll Cardiol 2008;51:139-45.
43. Matsuki T, Tamaki N, Nakata T, et al. Prognostic value of fatty acid imaging in patients with angina pectoris without prior myocardial infarction: comparison with stress thallium imaging. Eur J Nucl Med Mol Imaging. 2004;31:1512-21.
44. Solomon SD, Zelenkofske S, McMurray JJV, et al. Valsartan in Acute Myocardial Infarction Trial (VALIANT) Investigators. Sudden death in patients with myocardial infarction and left ventricular dysfunction, heart failure, or both. N Engl J Med. 2004;325:2581-8.
45. Hohnloser SH, Kuck KH, Dorian P, et al. Prophylactic use of an implantable cardioverter-defibrillator after acute myocardial infarction. N Engl J Med. 2004;351:2481-8.
46. Buxton AE. Sudden death after myocardial infarction—who needs prophylaxis, and when?. N Engl J Med. 2004;325:2638-40.

130

CHAPTER

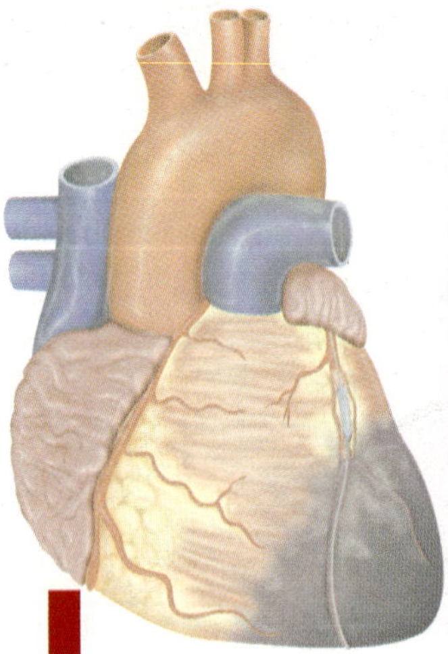

Homocysteine Imaging and Coronary Artery Disease

GS Sainani, Rajesh Sainani

INTRODUCTION

Homocysteine is a sulfur-containing amino acid derived from the breakdown of dietary methionine. It has now been recognized as a coronary risk factor. Several laboratory experiments have shown the relationship between hyperhomocysteinemia, endothelial cell dysfunction, platelet activation, and smooth muscle cell proliferation. Homocysteine metabolism is significantly influenced by life style choices and nutritional status. *Women seem to have lower levels than men.*[1]

Homocysteine regulates vascular tone and permeability through nitric oxide (NO). It also influences coagulation cascading through thrombomodulin-protein C and heparin sulfate antithrombin III interactions. Endothelium has fibrinolytic functions and it also influences composition of the subendothelial matrix and smooth muscle cell proliferation. These normal functions of endothelium are disturbed by elevated homocysteine levels. Anderson et al.[2] and Wall et al.[3] have reported that homocysteine is rapidly auto-oxidized, releasing hydrogen peroxides as a byproduct. Nitric oxide is formed from L-arginine by NO synthase. *Nitric oxide has various antithrombotic properties.*[4] It inhibits platelet adhesion and aggregation and it interacts with homocysteine forming *S*-nitrosothiols or *S*-nitrosohomocysteine which has *vasodilatory and antiplatelet actions.*[5]

Tawakol et al.[6] and Woo et al.[7] reported that hyperhomocysteinemia is associated with endothelial cell dysfunction. Tawakol et al.[6] studied endothelial-dependent vasodilation in arteries of hyperhomocysteinemia patients and controls and reported that endothelial-dependent vasodilation was significantly impaired in patients with hyperhomocysteinemia indicating that NO levels were reduced in these patients. One may conclude that elevated homocysteine results in *endothelial cytotoxicity.*[8] Stamler et al.[5] have reported that the raised homocysteine impair generation of NO by cultured endothelial cells. There is an increase in circulating markers of endothelial damage (*Von-Willebrand factor and thrombomodulin*) in patients with hyperhomocysteinemia and vascular disease and decrease after normalization of homocysteine with folate and vitamin B6 treatment.[8] Flow-mediated dilatation of brachial artery is significantly impaired in hyperhomocysteinemia.

Hyperhomocysteinemia causes oxidative stress and leads to oxidation of low-density lipoprotein (LDL) through generation of *superoxide anion radical.*[9] Oxidized LDL is taken up by intimal macrophages to form foam cells which is the beginning of developing atheromatous plaque. Heineckle et al.[10] have reported that homocysteine increases the formation of highly atherogenic oxycholesterol, and it promotes atherosclerosis by inducing proliferation of *vascular smooth muscle cells.*[11] According to Dey,[12] experimental and human studies show that homocysteine-induced atherosclerosis is characterized by platelet accumulation and platelet-rich thrombus formation in sites of endothelial injury. Majors et al.[13] have reported that homocysteine increases the mitogenic response of platelet derived growth factor on vascular smooth muscle cell, possibly by disturbing the activity of antioxidant enzyme. Fryer et al.[14] have reported that hyperhomocysteinemia may promote coagulation through the tissue factor pathway.

Kumbarsar et al.[15] have reported that patients with hyperhomocysteinemia have higher rate of restenosis of coronary artery after angioplasty.

Selhub et al.[16] conducted a study on 1,041 persons in the age group (members of Framingham Heart Study) where they with the help of color Doppler found that 43% of the men and 34% of the women showed more than 25% carotid artery stenosis. Plasma folate, pyridoxine, and dietary folate intake were inversely associated with the degree of carotid artery stenosis after adjusting for other risk factors.

A case-control study reported from London and Dublin,[17] involving 21,520 men (35–64 years old) who had no evidence of ischemic heart disease (IHD) at the baseline of study, showed that on mean follow-up of 8.7 years, 229 men died of IHD. The investigators[17] also enrolled 1,126 age-matched controls with no evidence of IHD. On comparison, homocysteine was found higher in cases than controls. In their case-control study of 21,626 patients reported by Arnesen et al.,[18] 123 subjects developed IHD within a mean follow-up of 4 years. Matched for age and sex, control cases were selected. The homocysteine levels in IHD cases were significantly higher.

US Physicians Health Study[19] elaborated on the development of IHD episodes [both fatal and nonfatal myocardial infarction (MI)] in their cohort of 14, 1,916 US male physicians. These were compared with 271 controls. They found an association between IHD and homocysteine in the upper 5% of homocysteine distribution compared with lower 90%. A positive relationship between homocysteine and risk of MI was reported in a large prospective community study from Norway. But Folson et al.[20] reported significant correlation of hyperhomocysteinemia with incidence of coronary artery disease (CAD) only in women.

Nygard et al.[21] in a secondary prospective study in which 587 CAD cases (angiographically documented) were followed up for a median period of 4.6 years reported that 64 patients died during that period. They found a strong graded correlation between raised homocysteine and mortality.

Graham et al.[22] have reported a large multicenter European trial of several hundred patients and controls (*the COMAC study*) in which elevated homocysteine was independently associated with a risk of CAD. However, in a study of 7,425 Finnish men and women who were followed for 9 years, no relationship was found between homocysteine and CAD. Chacko[23] studied CAD patients and 53 controls and concluded that homocysteine is not a major risk factor for CAD in Asian Indians. *Multiple Risk Factor Intervention Trial, atherosclerosis in communities,* and the *Finnish population study*[24] did not support any relation of plasma homocysteine levels to CVD. In contrast, Chambers et al.[25] and Deepa et al.[26] have confirmed that hyperhomocysteinemia is a CAD risk factor among immigrant Indians and Indians living in India. Anand et al.[27] have reported a population study from Canada in which they enrolled a thousand persons from three ethnic groups (South Asians, Chinese, and Europeans). Here, they correlated homocysteine levels with clinical features of cardiovascular disease (CVD) and carotid intimal medial thickness as measured on Doppler study. The South Asians had significant hyperhomocysteinemia than their Chinese and European counterparts; however, this did not confirm an independent association of hyperhomocysteinemia with CVD. The studies (population based by Anand et al.[27] in Canada and case-control study by Chambers et al. in the United Kingdom)[25] revealed that Indians tend to have a higher homocysteine levels compared to Chinese and European persons. This is probably attributable to low intake of vitamin B_{12} and folic acid by Indians and overcooking of vegetables by Indian community that destroys vitamins.

Gallagher PM et al.[28] studied homocysteine and risk of premature coronary heart disease as an evidence for a common gene mutation. Plasma homocysteine levels are modulated by nutritional and genetic factors, among which there is the role of enzyme *methylenetetrahydrofolate reductase (MTHFR)*. A common defective (thermolabile) variant of this enzyme is causally associated with elevated plasma homocysteine, which itself is an independent risk factor for coronary heart disease. The authors examined the hypothesis that the allele (T) that codes for the thermolabile defect increases the risk of coronary heart disease. They studied 111 patients with clinical and objective investigational evidence of coronary heart disease and 105 control subjects. The frequencies of the thermolabile defect (T) in patients and control subjects were measured, and the prevalence of elevated plasma total homocysteine according to genotype was assessed. The frequency of the defective allele was higher in patients than in the control subjects. Plasma total homocysteine levels were significantly associated with disease status, a relationship that matched the strength of the association between disease and homozygous inheritance of the defective enzyme.

Ridkar PM et al.[29] studied homocysteine and CVD among postmenopausal women. Women with elevated homocysteine levels tended to have high prevalence of CVD. The authors studied to determine whether elevated homocysteine levels in healthy postmenopausal women could predict the risk of developing CVD. They carried out a prospective nested care-control study with mean 3-year follow-up. The women's health study an ongoing US primary prevention trial was initiated in 1993. From total cohort of 23,263 postmenopausal women with no history of CVD or cancer at baseline, 122 women who subsequently experienced cardiovascular events were defined as cases and 244 age and smoking status-matched women who remained free of disease during the follow-up were defined as controls.

Amongst 122 cases, there were 85 events of MI or stroke and 37 coronary revascularizations. These subjects had significantly higher baseline homocysteine levels than controls. They concluded that among healthy postmenopausal women, elevated levels of homocysteine moderately increased the risk of future CVD.[30,31]

Foody JM et al.[32] studied atherosclerosis, lipoproteins, and homocysteine in young men and women. A biochemical link between homocysteine and lipoprotein(a) related to fibrin binding has been proposed. This hypothesis has not been specially examined in human beings. The authors thought to determine in a clinical setting whether their risk factors would interact to increase CAD risk. The authors performed a cross-sectional analysis of 750 men and 403 women referred to preventive *cardiology clinic at the Cleveland Clinic Foundation* in whom baseline homocysteine (Hcy) and Lp(a) data were available. Logistic regression after adjusting for standard cardiovascular risk factors was used to estimate the relative risks of CAD in patients with an Lp(a) > 30 mg/dL and Hcy > 17 mmol/L. Neither isolated high Hcy nor isolated Lp(a) appeared to be associated with CAD in women. However, strong evidence of an association was seen when both the risk factors were present.

Moreover, this increased risk showed evidence of an interactive effect beyond that attributed to either additive or multiplicative effect of Hcy and Lp(a) > 30 ($P = 0.03$). In contrast, both the elevated Hcy and Lp(a) showed evidence of being interdependent risk factors for CAD in men. The presence of both the risk factors in men did not appear to confer additional risk consistent with prior studies, Hcy level and Lp(a) are risk factors either independently or in concert for CAD in this clinical population. More significantly, the authors found evidence that when both risk factors were present in women, the associated risk was greater than what would be expected, if the two risk factors were simply acting independently. These clinical findings provide insights into the potential roles of both Hcy and Lp(a) in the pathogenesis of atherosclerosis.

Wald DS et al.[33] have reported from meta-analysis evidence of causality between homocysteine and CVDs. The objective was to assess whether the association of serum homocysteine concentration with ischemic heart disease, deep vein thrombosis and pulmonary embolism, and stroke are causal and, if so, to quantify the effect of homocysteine reduction in preventing them.

The meta-analyses of the above three diseases using: (1) 72 studies in which the prevalence of a mutation in the MTHFR gene (which increases homocysteine) was determined in cases ($n = 16,849$) and controls and (2) 20 prospective studies (3,820 participants) of serum homocysteine and disease risk were included. The authors found that there was significant association between homocysteine and the three diseases. The odds ratios for a 5-µmol/L increase in serum homocysteine were, for ischemic heart disease, 1.42 (95% confidence interval 1.11–1.84) in the genetic studies and 1.32 (1.19–1.45) in the prospective studies; for deep vein thrombosis with or without pulmonary embolism, 1.60 (1.15–2.22) in the genetic studies (there were no prospective studies); and, for stroke, 1.65 (0.66–4.13) in the genetic studies and 1.59 (1.29–1.96) in the prospective studies.

The authors concluded that the genetic studies and the prospective studies do not share the same potential sources of error, but both yield similar highly significant results—strong evidence that the association between homocysteine and CVD is causal. On this basis, lowering homocysteine concentrations by 3 µmol/L from current levels (achievable by increasing folic acid intake) would reduce the risk of ischemic heart disease by 16% (11–20%), deep vein thrombosis by 25% (8% to 38%), and stroke by 24% (15–33%).

Kazemi MB et al.[34] studied homocysteine levels and CAD. They aimed to assess the relationship between hyperhomocysteinemia and CAD in an Iranian population. In the case-control study, 197 persons (male: 123) who were scheduled for coronary angiography were selected. Blood samples were collected in fasting state before coronary angiography. Data about age, sex, and risk factors (e.g. hypertension, diabetes mellitus, smoking, hyperlipidemia, obesity) were obtained from prepared questionnaires. Homocysteine levels were measured by ELISA method. Homocysteine level above 15 mmol/L was considered high. Coronary angiography reports and homocysteine were analyzed by independent *simple test*.

In comparison with normal coronary angiography reports (32.5%), patients with abnormal coronary angiography reports (67.5%) had elevated homocysteine ($P = 0.001$), about 28.1% of the patients with normal coronary angiography reports had hyperhomocysteinemia. After further evaluation, linear correlations were detected between number of involved vessels and homocysteine ($P = 0.000$). Multiple linear regression analysis of data detected that in persons without any other risk factors, the relationship was stronger and more meaningful ($P = 0.000$). It is seen from these data that hyperhomocysteinemia is related to CAD as an independent risk factor. In persons without any other risk factors, a linear correlation between homocysteine levels and numbers of coronary artery involvement was present. If this equation is confirmed prospectively, one can predict the number of diseased coronary arteries.

Ankrah A et al.[35] studied association between plasma homocysteine and myocardial single photon emission-computed tomography (SPECT) abnormalities in patients referred for suspected myocardial ischemia. The authors in the study investigated the association of levels of homocysteine levels and quantitative indices of myocardial perfusion SPECT imaging in patients referred for myocardial ischemia.

Quantitative myocardial perfusion SPECT indices were obtained for 120 patients. Stress myocardial perfusion imaging was carried out. Plasma homocysteine was estimated in fasting state. Of the 120 persons (mean age 56 years, 53% males), 33% had elevated homocysteine levels. The plasma homocysteine levels were then compared with the results of imaging and other known factors. After adjusting for traditional risk factors of CAD, patients with elevated homocysteine levels had a significantly higher mean summed score (summed stress score) (34 hours 6.9, $P = 0.02$) than patients with normal homocysteine level. This was true with normal homocysteine level. This was true for both the single and multivessel disease. Also, patients with elevated homocysteine levels had higher stress end-systolic volume (137 mL vs 105 mL, $P = 0.03$) and lower post-stress left ventricular ejection fraction (54% vs 64%, $P = 0.02$).

Patients with elevated homocysteine levels also had significantly lower mean body mass index (26.6 kg/m^2 vs 30.6 kg/m^2, $P = 0.002$). There was a significant relationship between the total number of known risk factors in a patient with CAD and the proportion of patients presenting elevated plasma homocysteine levels ($P = 0.03$).

Also, the extent of infarct as measured by summed rest score was more closely correlated with elevated level than with the degree of ischemia. The authors concluded that there was a correlation between plasma homocysteine level and the presence and extent of myocardial perfusion abnormalities in patients with established CAD, in particular those with multiple risk factors and multivessel infarction. Bozkurt et al.[36] carried out a study on plasma homocysteine level and the angiographic extent of CAD. In this study, 156 consecutive patients presenting with CAD (group 1) and control group (group 2) of 35 age-matched persons with normal coronary angiography were enrolled. Blood samples for homocysteine were obtained on admission. Plasma homocysteine concentration was measured with high-performance liquid chromatography with fluorescence detection. Radiographs from coronary angiography were viewed and scored using *Sullivan method* to assess the atherosclerotic involvement of CAD. There were significant elevations in homocysteine level in group 1 compared to group 2. All scores (demonstrated angiographic extension of CAD) correlated significantly with plasma homocysteine levels; however, the *Sullivan* extent score correlated more closely than both the stenosis score and vessel score.

Schaffer A et al.[37] reported from a large prospective cohort study the relationship between homocysteine and CAD. Hyperhomocysteinemia is associated with increased thrombogenicity, oxidative stress status, and endothelial dysfunction. The authors investigated the association of Hcy with the prevalence and extent of CAD in a large consecutive cohort of patients undergoing coronary angiography. They studied a total of 3,056 consecutive patients undergoing coronary angiography at the *Azienda Ospedaliera "Maggiore della Carità," Novara, Italy*. Fasting samples were collected for homocysteine levels assessment. Coronary disease was defined for at least one vessel stenosis > 50% as evaluated by quantitative coronary angiography. The study population was divided according to Hcy tertiles (<13.3, 13.3–18.2, > 18.2 nmol/mL). High plasmatic level of homocysteine was related with age ($P < 0.001$), male gender ($P < 0.001$), hypertension ($P < 0.001$), renal failure ($P < 0.001$), family history of CAD ($P < 0.001$), previous cerebrovascular accident ($P < 0.001$), previous MI ($P = 0.002$), previous coronary artery bypass grafting ($P = 0.003$), and ejection fraction ($P < 0.001$), and higher significant relationship was found between Hcy levels and the extent of CAD. The authors concluded that high levels of plasmatic Hcy are independently associated with CAD.

Ranjith R et al.[38] studied clinical correlation between plasma homocysteine level and CAD in Indian patients.

CONCLUSION

The aim of this study was to evaluate correlation between plasma homocysteine and CAD in Indian patients. This study included 150 patients, 100 subjects in study group with angiographically diagnosed CAD and 50 subjects in the control group with a normal coronary angiogram. In the study group, patients were divided into three subgroups, viz. CAD only, CAD with hypertension, and CAD with type 2 diabetes mellitus. Plasma homocysteine, lipid profile, and other risk factors were compared. The results showed that the mean homocysteine levels were significantly higher than control group. Furthermore, no significant correlation was found between plasma homocysteine and lipid components in different groups of patients. They concluded that the study demonstrated that increased levels of homocysteine are independently related to CAD.

REFERENCES

1. Tucker KL, Selhub J, Wilson PW, et al. Dietary intake pattern relates to plasma folate and homocysteine concentration in the Framingham Heart Study. J Nutr. 1996;126:3025-31.
2. Anderson A, Lindgren A, Hultberg B, et al. Effect of thiol oxidation and thiol export from erythrocytes on determination of redox status of homocysteine and other thiols in plasma from healthy subjects and patients with cerebral infarction. Clin Chem. 1995;41:361-6.
3. Wall RT, Harlan JM, Harker LA, et al. Homocysteine-induced endothelial cell injury in vitro: a model for the study of vascular injury. Thromb Res. 1980;18:113-21.

4. Wu KK, Thiagarajan P. Role of endothelium in thrombosis and hemostasis. Annu Rev Med. 1996;47:315-31.
5. Stamler JS, Osborne JA, Jaraki O, et al. Adverse vascular effects of homocysteine are modulated by endothelium-derived relaxing factor and related oxides of nitrogen. J Clin Invest. 1993;91:308-18.
6. Tawakol A, Omland T, Gerhand M, et al. Hyperhomocysteinemia is associated with impaired endothelium-dependent vasodilatation in humans. Circulation. 1997;95:1119-21.
7. Woo KS, Chook P, Lolin YI, et al. Hyperhomocyst(e)inemia is a risk factor for arterial endothelial dysfunction in humans. Circulation. 1997;96:2542-4.
8. Van den Berg M, Boers GH, Franken DG, et al. Hyperhomocysteinaemia and endothelial dysfunction in young patients with peripheral arterial occlusive disease. Eur J Clin Invest. 1995;25:176-81.
9. Loscalzo J. The oxidant stress of hyperhomocysteinemia. J Clin Invest. 1966;98:5-7.
10. Heineckle JW, Kawarmura M. Suzuki L, et al. Oxidation of low density lipoprotein by thiols: superoxide-dependent and -independent mechanisms. J Lipid Res. 1993;34:2051-61.
11. Tsi JC, Wang H, Perrella MA, et al. Induction of cyclin A gene expression by homocysteine in vascular smooth muscle cell. J Clin Invest. 1996;97:146-53.
12. Dey SC. Homocysteine; a new risk factor in atherosclerotic vascular disease. Cardiol. Today. 2000;4:323-5.
13. Majors A, Ehrhart LA, Pezacka EH. Homocysteine as a risk factor for vascular disease: Enhanced collagen production and accumulation by smooth muscle cells. Arterioscler Thromb Vasc Biol. 1997;17:2074-81.
14. Fryer RH, Wilson BD, Gubler DB, et al. Homocysteine, a risk factor for premature vascular disease and thrombosis, induces tissue factor activity in endothelial cells. Arterioscler Thromb. 1993;13:1327-33.
15. Kumbarsar SD, Dincer I, Ertas F, et al. Hyperhomocysteinemia and restenosis. J Cardiovasc Risk. 2001;8:9-13.
16. Selhub J, Jacques PE, Bostom AG, et al. Association between plasma homocyteine concentrations and extracranial carotid artery stenosis. N Engl J Med. 1995;332:286-91.
17. Wald NJ, Watt HC, Law MR, et al. Homocysteine and ischaemic heart disease: results of a prospective study with implications on prevention. Arch Intern Med. 1998;158:862-7.
18. Arnesen E, Refsum H, Bona KH, et al. Serum total homocysteine and coronary heart disease. Int J Epidemiol. 1995;24:704-9.
19. Stampfer MJ, Malinow MR, Willett WC, et al. A prospective study of plasma homocyteine and risk of myocardial infarction in US physicians. JAMA. 1992;268:877-81.
20. Folson AR, Nieto FJ, McGovern PG, et al. Prospective study of coronary heart disease incidence in relation to fasting total homocysteine, and B vitamins: the Atherosclerosis Risk in Communities (ARIC) study. Circulation. 1998;98;204-10.
21. Nygard O, Nordrehaug JE, Refsum H, et al. Plasma homocysteine level and mortality in patients with coronary artery disease. New Engl J Med. 1997;337:230-36.
22. Graham IM, Daly LE, Refsum HM, et al. Plasma homocysteine as a risk factor for vascular disease. The European Concerted Action Project. JAMA. 1997;277:1775-81.
23. Chacko KA. Plasma homocysteine levels in patients with coronary heart disease. Indian Heart J. 1998;50:295-9.
24. Alftman G, Pekkanen J, Jauhiainen M, et al. Relation of serum homocysteine and lipoprotein(a) concentration to atherosclerotic disease in a prospective Finnish population based study. Atherosclerosis. 1994;106:9-19.
25. Chambers JC, Obeid OA, Refsum H, et al. Plasma homocysteine concentrations and risk of coronary heart disease in UK Indian Asian and European men. Lancet. 2000;355:523-7.
26. Deepa R, Velmurugan K, Saravanan G, et al. Absence of association between serum homocysteine levels and coronary artery disease in South Indian males. Indian Heart J. 2001;53:44-7.
27. Anand SS, Yusuf S, Vuksan V, et al. Differences in risk factors, atherosclerosis and cardiovascular disease between ethnic groups in Canada: the Study of Health Assessment and Risk Ethnic groups (SHARE). Indian Heart J. 2000;356:279-84.
28. Gallagher PM, Meleady R, Shields DC, et al. Homocysteine and risk of premature coronary heart disease. Evidence for a common gene mutation. Circulation. 1996,94:2154-58.
29. Ridkar PM, Manson JE, Buring JE, et al. Homocysteine and risk of cardiovascular disease among postmenopausal women. JAMA. 1999;281(19):1817-21.
30. McCully KS. Vascular pathology of homocysteinemia: implications for the pathogenesis of arteriosclerosis. Am J Pathol. 1969;56:111-28.
31. Welch GN, Loscalzo J. Mechanisms of disease: homocysteine and atherothrombosis. N Engl J Med. 1998;338:1042-50.
32. Foody JM, Milberg JA, Robinson K, et al. Homocysteine and lipoprotein(a) interact to increase CAD risk in young men and women. Arterioscler Thromb Vasc Biol. 2000;20:493-9.
33. Wald DS. Homocysteine and cardiovascular diseases: evidence of causality from a meta-analysis. BMJ. 2002; 325:1202.
34. Kazemi MB, Eshraghian K, Omrani GR, et al. Homocysteine level and coronary artery disease. Angiology. 2006;47(1):9-14.
35. Ankrah A, Buscombe J, Sathekge MM. Association between plasma homocysteine and myocardial SPECT abnormalities in patients referred for suspected myocardial ischemia. Cardiovasc J Afr. 2012;23(6):313-7.
36. Bozkurt E, Keles S, Acikel M, et al. Plasma homocysteine level and the angiographic extent of coronary artery disease. Angiology. 2004;55(3):265-70.
37. Schaffer A, Verdoia M, Cassetti E, et al. Relationship between homocysteine and coronary artery disease. Results from a large prospective cohort study. Thromb Res. 2014;134(2):288-93.
38. Ranjith R, Devika P. Clinical correlation between plasma homocysteine level and coronary artery disease in Indian patients. WJCD. 2017;07:477-85.

SECTION 30

Cardiac Space-occupying Lesion

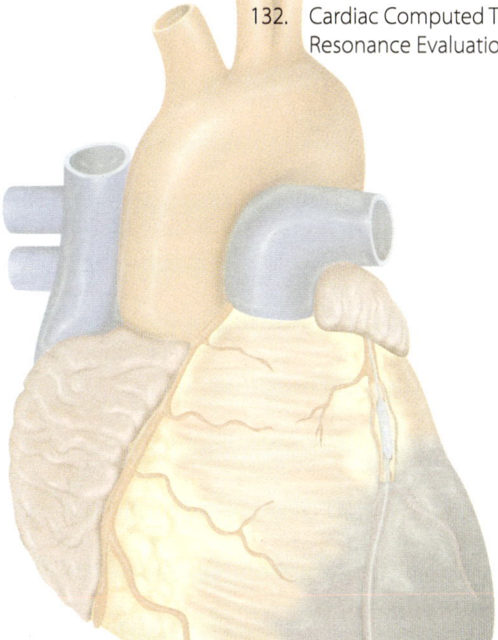

131

CHAPTER

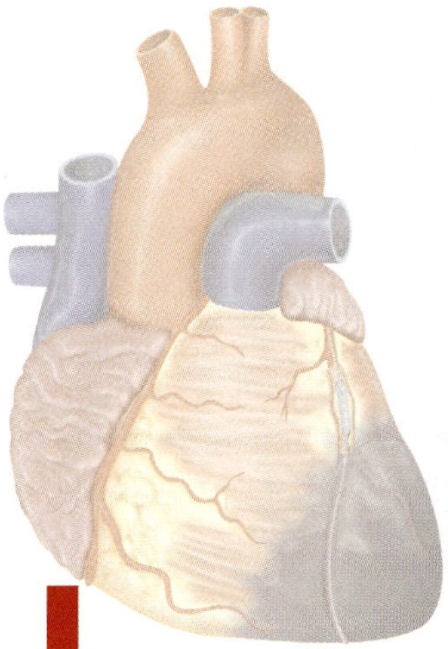

Cardiac Tumors

George Koshy, Mathew Iype, KM Krishnamoorthy

INTRODUCTION

Primary cardiac tumors are rare with a necropsy incidence of 0.05%.[1] However, secondary deposits are far more common and are seen in 1% of postmortem examinations.[1] Cardiac tumors were merely a curiosity till the 1950s, as effective diagnostic modalities and treatment was not available. Surgical management became a reality with the advent of cardiopulmonary bypass. Moreover, diagnostic modalities, such as echocardiography, computed tomography (CT), and magnetic resonance imaging (MRI), became widely available making precise preoperative diagnosis fairly easy. Atrial myxomas are the most common primary cardiac tumor in adults accounting for 75% of all cases. Rhabdomyoma is the most common cardiac tumor in children. About 25% of all cardiac tumors are malignant; the majority of which are angiosarcomas or rhabdomyosarcomas.[2] Primary cardiac tumors are diverse in clinical presentation, and hence, the diagnosis is frequently challenging. The symptoms associated with most primary cardiac tumors are very often nonspecific. Many cases are found incidentally during evaluation of an unrelated medical condition. The symptoms of cardiac tumors, especially myxomas, can mimic those associated with collagen vascular disease, malignancy, and infective endocarditis.

CLINICAL PRESENTATIONS

The symptoms and clinical findings of the cardiac tumors depend on their location, size, mobility, and friability. The clinical features can be broadly considered under the following headings:

- *Embolic phenomenon*: This is particularly common with myxomas. The tumor itself or adherent thrombi can embolize. Both systemic as well as pulmonary embolism can occur depending on the location of the tumor. Histopathological examination of the retrieved embolic material can help in the diagnosis. Multiple small emboli can mimic vasculitis or endocarditis. The brain is the most common site of involvement for systemic emboli, and the involvement of both hemispheres and multiple regions is not uncommon.[3] Right-sided tumors embolize to the lungs and can result in pulmonary hypertension and right heart failure.
- *Cardiac manifestations*: Atrial tumors, once they are large enough, usually lead to the obstruction of atrioventricular (AV) flow and behave like AV valve stenosis. They can also interfere with valve closure leading to AV valve regurgitation. Mechanical trauma over a long span of time can cause valve damage. Left atrial (LA) myxomas very often mimic mitral valve disease. Gradually progressive exertional dyspnea is common. Syncope and worsening of breathlessness related to particular postures, if present, are characteristic features. Ventricular tumors, though less common, can produce outflow tract obstruction leading to breathlessness, angina, or syncope.
- *Arrhythmias*: Conduction abnormalities and arrhythmias can occur depending on the location of the tumor. Intramyocardial and intracavity tumors may both

produce arrhythmias. The mechanisms include direct infiltration of the conduction tissue and irritation of the myocardium itself. Sudden cardiac death can occur both due to arrhythmias and conduction abnormalities as well as due to valvular obstruction.

- *Metastasis*: Infrequently, symptoms secondary to the metastatic disease may represent the initial clinical manifestation of the malignant primary cardiac tumor. The common sites of metastases include lung, brain, and bone. The diagnosis of cardiac tumors was extremely difficult before the advent of echocardiography. Now multiimaging modalities have transformed the clinical scenario.
- *Echocardiography*: Transthoracic and transesophageal as well as three-dimensional (3D) imaging modalities have made the diagnosis simple and precise in most of the cases. Cardiac CT and MRI can provide additional information in selected cases.

BENIGN CARDIAC TUMORS

Myxomas

Atrial myxoma is the most common primary cardiac tumor. Approximate incidence is 1 per 100,000 per year. Occurring more commonly in women, myxomas are usually diagnosed between the ages of 50 years and 70 years. It is a benign gelatinous growth composed of primitive connective tissue cells and stroma resembling mesenchyme. The exact cell of origin is not known. It can arise from the endocardial surfaces of all cardiac chambers and infrequently from the cardiac valves. About 75% myxomas arise from the endocardial surface of the left atrium and approximately 15% from the right atrium. Ventricular myxomas are uncommon. The commonest site of attachment is the interatrial septum near the fossa ovalis. Less frequent sites of attachment include posterior and anterior walls of the left atrium and the atrial appendage. Ventricular myxomas tend to be sessile and may be confused with thrombi. Valvular myxomas are usually smaller. Tricuspid valve is more often involved than the mitral valve. Myxomas are solitary in more than 90% of cases. *Syndrome myxomas*: "Syndrome myxoma" should be suspected in patients younger than 40 years who present with multiple cardiac myxomas.[4] These can include biatrial, ventricular, and recurrent myxomas. Multiple acronyms have been proposed for such syndromes. These include LAMB (lentigines, atrial myxoma, mucocutaneous myxoma, and blue nevus) and NAME (nevus, atrial myxoma, myxoid neurofibromata, and ephelides). Familial myxomas with a genetic background are collectively described as Carney complex.[5] If diagnosed, all first-degree relatives should be screened for the condition by echocardiography.

Clinical features: Symptoms include breathlessness, fever, weight loss, syncope, hemoptysis, and sometimes sudden death. Light headedness or syncope as well as worsening breathlessness can be related to particular postures. This is commoner with highly mobile LA myxomas. Echocardiographic evaluation of patients with transient ischemic attacks or stroke may lead to a diagnosis of LA myxoma. Anemia and raised acute-phase reactants are frequently present. The clinical findings of LA myxoma simulate mitral valve disease with loud first heart sound and mid-diastolic murmur with presystolic accentuation.[6] The characteristic "tumor plop" may be audible in diastole in some patients. This can be confused with the opening snap of mitral stenosis. Pansystolic murmur indicative of mitral regurgitation may also be audible. The murmur can sometimes show postural changes related to the mobility of the tumor.

Echocardiography: Transthoracic echocardiography (TTE) shows a pedunculated mass attached to interatrial septum in the left atrium. When the attachment to the interatrial septum is by a long stalk, the tumor tends to be highly mobile and prolapsing into the left ventricle in diastole. When the tumor is sessile, the movement is limited. They may contain areas of hemorrhage and calcification. Echo-free spaces within the tumor usually indicate areas of hemorrhage and necrosis.[7] Bright echo spots can signify calcification. Identification of hypoechoic spaces indicative of hemorrhage and necrosis helps in differentiating myxoma from thrombus or vegetations. Doppler interrogation can detect and quantify mitral regurgitation which usually disappears after the tumor has been surgically removed. Transmitral diastolic gradient due to mitral inflow obstruction can also be measured by Doppler. The M-mode tracing will simulate mitral stenosis with reduced EF slope but the valve per se is not significantly thickened. An echo-free clear space can be identified in early diastole between the DE excursion of the anterior mitral leaflet and the thick echoes of the prolapsing LA myxomas.

The 3D studies can accurately measure the size of the tumor, which very often is under estimated in a TTE examination. The site of attachment is also better made out in 3D studies. Transesophageal echocardiography (TEE) confirms the diagnosis in majority of cases. Multiple views including unconventional imaging planes are helpful for full characterization of the tumor. TEE can provide additional information, such as the site of attachment and the presence of lobulations and calcification. Additional small tumors which may be missed in the TTE can also be picked up. In TTE the site of attachment is usually best visualized in the apical or subcostal four-chamber view biatrial location of myxomas, which is not uncommon in the familial variety (Figs. 1 to 7).

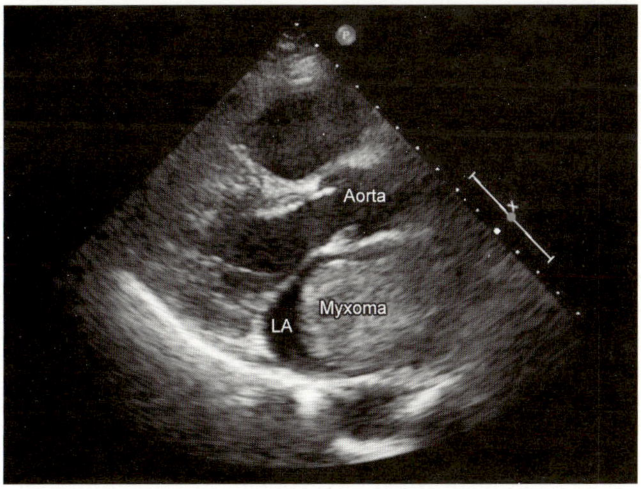

Fig. 1: A large myxoma in LA. (LA: left atrium)

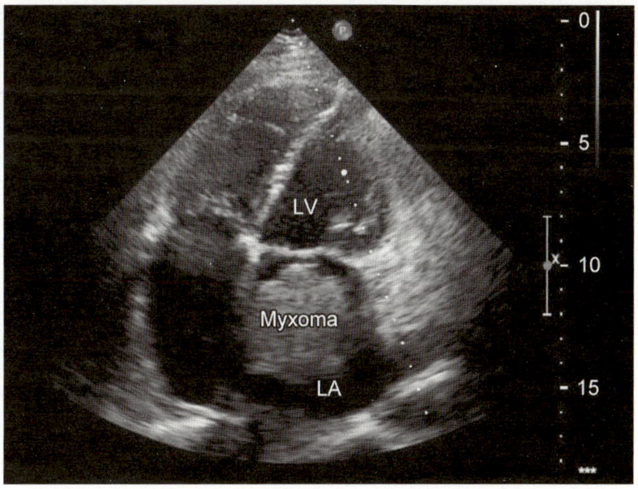

Fig. 2: A polypoidal myxoma in LA. (LV: left ventricle; LA: left atrium)

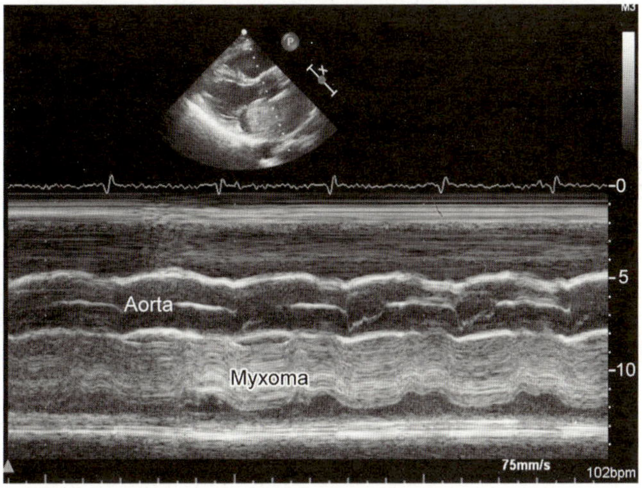

Fig. 3: M-mode across the left atrium showing myxoma.

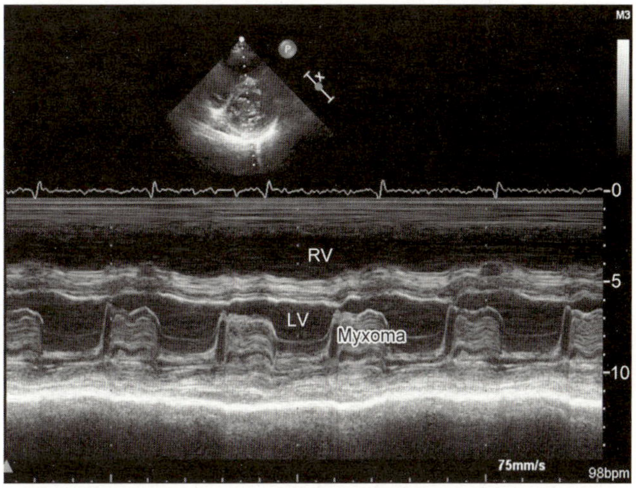

Fig. 4: M-mode across the mitral valve shows myxoma prolapsing through the valve. (LV: left ventricle; RV: right ventricle)

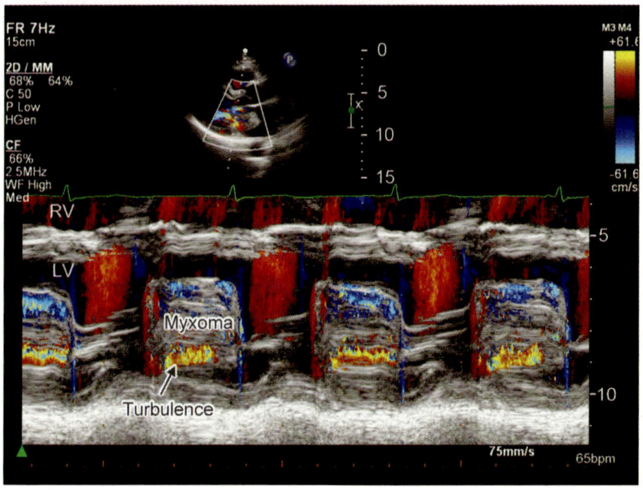

Fig. 5: Color M-mode across the mitral valve shows mitral valve obstruction. (LV: left ventricle; RV: right ventricle)

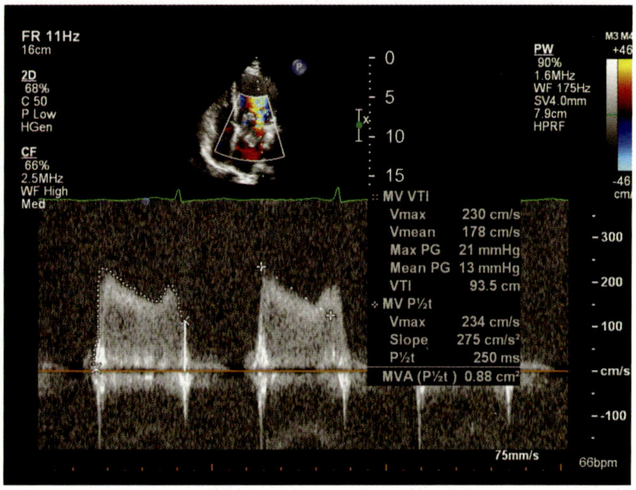

Fig. 6: Pulse-wave Doppler showing gradient across mitral valve in a patient with left atrial myxoma.

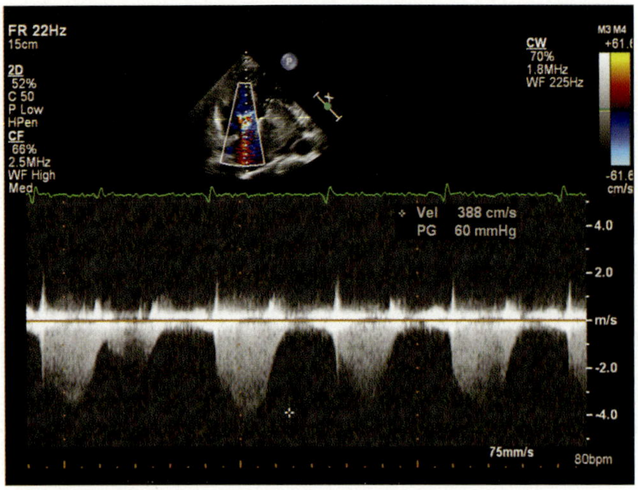

Fig. 7: Estimation of right ventricular systolic pressure from the tricuspid regurgitation signal in a patient with left atrial myxoma.

Echocardiographic classification of myxomas:[8]

- *Classification by size*: Myxomas are classified into large (largest diameter >5 cm, 54%) and small (largest diameter < 5 cm, 46%).
- *Classification by shape*: Myxomas are classified into polypoid (soft and irregular shape with mobile surface, 57%) and round types (solid and round shape with nonmobile surface, 43%).
- *Classification by the site of origin*: Myxomas could be divided into typical (attached to the interatrial septum in the left side, 71%) and atypical locations (attachment to sites other than the left side of the interatrial septum, 29%).

Differential diagnosis: Myxomas should be differentiated from atrial thrombi, vegetations, and other tumor-like structures. The characteristic appearance, motion, and site of origin are usually helpful. The clinical context is important. Vegetations occur in relation to the valve and tend to be smaller and with intrinsic mobility. When left-sided valves are involved, usually underlying structural heart disease can be picked up, and valve disruption may be sometimes evident, especially on TEE. Atrial thrombi are usually seen in the LA appendage in nonvalvular atrial fibrillation. In mitral stenosis, the thrombi can be seen anywhere in the left atrium. Ventricular thrombi usually occur in relation to an abnormally contracting segment of the myocardium or in the background of left ventricular (LV) dysfunction. Thrombi are often laminated, immobile, and tend to have broad-base attachment. Differentiation is more difficult when myxomas occur in unusual locations, such as valves and in relation to ventricular endothelium.

Right atrial myxomas can be visualized in apical four-chamber and subcostal views. They have a globular shape and well-defined borders in TEE. They should be differentiated from normal congenital variants, such as Chiari network, persistent eustachian valve, and lipomatous hypertrophy of the interatrial septum. Rarely, they occur in the ventricles, producing both inflow and outflow obstruction.

Rhabdomyomas

They are the commonest primary cardiac neoplasm in children. Cardiac rhabdomyoma is often associated with tuberous sclerosis.[9] Rhabdomyomas tend to be multiple and commonly involve the ventricles. Both ventricles are equally involved. Interventricular septum as well as the ventricular free wall can be involved. Symptoms may result from myocardial involvement or arrhythmias due to involvement of the conduction system. Obstruction to ventricular inflow as well as outflow can occur depending on the location and intracavitary extension of the tumor. Echocardiographically, these tumors appear as multiple, homogeneous, well-circumscribed, echogenic ventricular masses. Intracavitary extension may be seen in half of the cases, whereas the remaining half tends to be completely intramural. One important feature that is useful in differentiating rhabdomyoma from other cardiac tumors is the presence of multiple nodular masses. Doppler studies can determine the degree of outflow or inflow gradients as well as the presence of any regurgitant lesions. Spontaneous regression of the tumor is common, and hence, treatment is often conservative. But those with severe outflow obstruction may require surgical intervention.

Fibromas

They are low-grade tumors mostly occurring in children. This is the second most common primary cardiac neoplasm after rhabdomyomas.[10] Fibromas are characteristically found in the ventricular myocardium. They can present with obstructive symptoms, arrhythmias, and sometimes sudden cardiac death. Heart failure can also occur. Approximately half of cardiac fibromas are entirely asymptomatic and are detected incidentally because of the calcification in the chest X-ray or on CT scan of the chest. Echocardiographic appearance is usually as a solitary distinct, well-demarcated, highly echogenic mass within the myocardium. Calcification is common. It can be differentiated from rhabdomyomas by the fact that rhabdomyomas are frequently multicentric, without calcification and commonly associated with tuberous sclerosis. Surgical excision is the recommended treatment but may not be possible in all cases. Because of the potential for recurrence, follow-up echocardiographic evaluation is recommended.

Papillary Fibroelastomas

This accounts for only approximately 5% of all tumors of the heart but is the commonest tumor arising from the valve.[11] Males are more commonly affected, and usually patients are in their sixth or seventh decades but are often asymptomatic during life and are incidentally detected during autopsy. The real incidence may be higher as it is often asymptomatic. They are located on the ventricular aspect of the aortic valves and in relation to the atrial aspect of the mitral valves. Right-sided valves are less frequently involved. Despite their location in close proximity to the valve, significant valvular dysfunction is uncommon since these tumors are small measuring less than 1 cm. Because of its location in the LV outflow tract and the friable nature, systemic embolization is common. It can embolize to coronary and cerebral arteries. Acute coronary syndrome and transient ischemic attacks or stroke can be the initial presentation.

Echocardiographic appearance is characteristic. They are generally small, mobile, pedunculated, and echodense masses attached to valves. They have a speckled interior with stippling near the edges.[12] Transesophageal echocardiography is more sensitive and specific for the detection of these tumors. The finger-like projections on the surface and the mobility produce a fluttering appearance to the tumor surface which is better made out in TEE. Papillary fibroelastoma has to be distinguished from Lambl excrescences, valvular myxoma, and vegetations. Treatment is by surgical excision (Fig. 8).

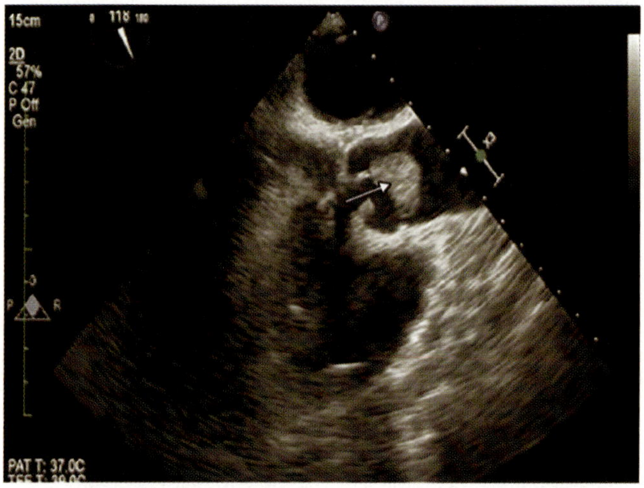

Fig. 8: TEE of papillary fibroelastoma attached to the aortic valve. (TEE: transesophageal echocardiography)

Source: Reprinted with permission from Saleh et al. Cardiac papillary fibroelastoma: single institution experience with 14 surgical patients. Tex Heart Inst J. 2016;43:148-51. © 2016 by the Texas Heart Institute, Houston.

Lipomas

They can occur at all ages, and both sexes are equally affected. They may occur anywhere in the heart but LV is the commonest site. About 25% are completely intramural. They can occur in relation to the interatrial septum as well as pericardium, subendocardium, and subepicardium. Subepicardial tumors are large, often pedunculated, whereas subendocardial lipomas tend to be smaller and sessile. They are usually asymptomatic, but arrhythmias and conduction abnormalities can occur. Obstructive symptoms and heart failure are less common. Echocardiographically, they are well circumscribed, broad based, and immobile. Lipomas are differentiated from myxomas by their location, higher echodensity, and lesser mobility. Lipomas involving the atrial septum must be differentiated from lipomatous hypertrophy of the interatrial septum.[13] The latter is mostly a benign condition usually found in obese patients. Globular thickening of the interatrial septum with central sparing gives a characteristic "dumb bell" shape to the interatrial septum, best seen in the subcostal view.

Cardiac Hemangiomas

They are the commonest benign vascular tumors of the heart. They are usually solitary but can be multiple. Though any site of the heart can get involved; epicardial involvement is commoner. It is very often associated with pericardial effusion. They can be intramural or intracavitary. Intracavitary tumors can present with obstructive symptoms or heart failure. Echocardiographic examination reveals nonpedunculated, nonhomogeneous masses with echo-free areas within the mass because of the presence of vascular channels. Right heart involvement with pericardial effusion should alert one about the possibility of the tumor being hemangioma.

PRIMARY MALIGNANT CARDIAC TUMORS

Approximately 25% of all cardiac tumors are malignant, and of these, 75% are sarcomas. However, a tumor present only on the right side of the heart has an almost 50% chance of being a malignant primary cardiac tumor.[14] Rapid increase in the size of a mass, local invasion, and hemorrhagic pericardial effusion are the signs of malignancy. A pericardial mass is more likely to be malignant than nonmalignant. All primary malignant tumors of the heart have a poor prognosis. The 5-year survival of cardiac sarcoma is only 11%.[15]

Angiosarcoma

Angiosarcoma is the commonest primary malignant cardiac neoplasm in an adult. It accounts for one third of primary cardiac neoplasms. They are common in the middle ages. Males are more affected than females. They occur more frequently in the right atria. Recurrent pericardial effusions and tricuspid valve involvement is common. Complications of angiosarcoma include superior venacaval syndrome, right heart failure, pulmonary embolism, and cardiac tamponade. Echocardiographically, they are seen as bulky, lobulated, and mobile mass with a broad base with or without extension to the pericardium. It has a heterogeneous appearance with the areas of necrosis or hemorrhage. In contrast to myxomas, they do not have a stalk. Treatment is generally not very effective. Surgery is usually ineffective. Chemotherapy or radiation does not generally provide long-lasting symptomatic relief.

Rhabdomyosarcoma

They are the commonest primary sarcoma of the heart in children. The tumor arises from embryonic cells in the septum. Males are slightly more commonly affected. It can originate from any cardiac chamber.[16] Echocardiographically, they appear as dense, multilobular, pedunculated mass with irregular borders. These tumors can occur in multiple sites within the heart and can cause obstruction at multiple levels. They are very aggressive tumors, and pericardial involvement is common at the time of initial diagnosis. These tumors have a dismal prognosis, and survival is usually less than 1 year.

Fibrosarcomas

They are primarily fibroblastic in origin. It can involve any cardiac chamber. Typical echocardiographic finding is that of mobile, heterogeneous mass in the left atrium. Pericardial effusion is common. Prognosis is generally poor.

Leiomyosarcomas

These are rare tumors found in the left atrium. Spindle-shaped cells are found on histology. Presenting symptoms include rapidly progressive dyspnea. Echocardiographically, they present as mass located in the left atrium (posterior wall) and invade pulmonary veins or mitral valve. They can present as multiple intracavitary nodules. They are highly aggressive tumors. Hemopericardium and cardiac tamponade are common. Arrhythmias and sudden cardiac death have also been described. Overall prognosis is very poor.

Lymphoma

Cardiac lymphomas are less common than sarcomas. It occurs mainly in immune-compromised patients, such as HIV patients and posttransplant.[17] Echocardiographically, they can appear as circumscribed, nodular homogenous masses in the myocardium. Pericardial effusion and tamponade are important complications.

Malignant Mesothelioma

Malignant mesotheliomas account for half of the primary pericardial tumors. Echocardiography typically reveals a pericardial effusion and a tumor encasing the heart. The mass around the heart can be confused with constrictive pericarditis.[18] Treatment is palliative surgery and radiation (Table 1).

SECONDARY MALIGNANT CARDIAC TUMORS (METASTASIS)

Secondaries from a malignancy elsewhere are more common than primary malignant tumors. These can involve the heart either by direct extension from adjacent structures, such as liver and breast, or metastatic spread via blood. The tumors which most commonly metastasize to heart are carcinomas of lung and breast and hematological malignancies. The tumors which have the highest potential to metastasize to heart are melanoma (usually pericardial metastasis).[19] But melanoma as such is a rare tumor. Secondaries in the heart most commonly involve the pericardium and epicardium so that pericardial effusion is the common finding. Confirmation of the tumor requires pericardial fluid study for malignant cells and rarely pericardial biopsy. However, it should be kept in mind that in the case of malignancy, in addition to secondary deposits, radiation pericarditis and idiopathic pericarditis are not the

TABLE 1: Differentiation between malignant and benign tumors.

Benign	*Malignant*
Left-sided chambers more involved	Right-sided chambers more often involved
Narrow pedicle favors benign nature	Broad attachment favors malignant nature
Chamber walls unaltered	Chamber walls may be replaced by tumor infiltration
No pericardial effusion	Pericardial effusion is common
No pericardial mass	Pericardial mass favors malignant tumor
Slow increase in size	Rapid increase in size

infrequent causes of pericardial effusion. It can present as intramyocardial masses on echocardiography.

Normal Variants and Other Masses

Chiari network is an embryological remnant related to the right valve of the sinus venosus, located in the right atrium appearing as a web-like structure with thread-like components. It is present in 2% of the population and should not be confused with other mobile structures in the right atrium. Eustachian valve is an embryologic remnant of the valve of the inferior vena cava. It appears as a mobile, linear echodense structure on echocardiography. Thebesian valve or the valve of the coronary sinus can sometimes be very prominent and may be mistaken for a right atrial mass. Echocardiographically, usually it appears as echodense crescentic fold that resembles bands or threads. Prominent crista terminalis can also be confused with right atrial mass. Prominent moderator band in the right ventricle can also be a source of confusion. Usually it is identified as linear echodense structure traversing the RV cavity at midventricular level, connecting the free wall to the interventricular septum. It is best seen in the apical four-chamber view and subcostal views. "Coumadin ridge" is a prominent muscular structure formed between the LA appendage and the atrial insertion of the left upper pulmonary vein. It can be confused with LA appendage thrombus. Prominent pectinate muscles in the LA appendage in TEE may also be confused with small thrombi. Thrombi and vegetations are sometimes difficult to differentiate from cardiac tumors. But in the clinical context, echocardiographic features and the associated findings usually help in the differentiation.

Thrombus

The most common location for thrombi in the atrium is the LA appendage. But in the presence of mitral stenosis, spontaneous echo contrast is very often detected echocardiographically indicating sluggish flow and thrombi can form in other areas also. In nonvalvular atrial fibrillation, thrombi are usually confined to LA appendage. Transesophageal echocardiography is far superior to TTE in detecting and characterizing LA appendage thrombi. Left atrial appendage emptying velocities are usually reduced in the presence of appendage thrombus. Left ventricular thrombi are generally located in relation to the apex in the setting of poor systolic function. With an anterior wall myocardial infarction, the thrombus is usually seen in relation to a dyskinetic segment, akinetic segment, or ventricular aneurysm. It is very unusual to find thrombus in relation to a normally contracting segment. Thrombus should be visualized at least in two echocardiographic views, and they should be differentiated from the normal variants, such as moderator band, accessory papillary muscles, false tendons, and aberrant trabeculae. Left ventricular thrombus can be lying flat or may be protruding into the cavity. It may be homogeneously echogenic or have a heterogeneous texture with central lucency. Thrombi can be mobile when the risk of embolization tends to be higher (Fig. 9).

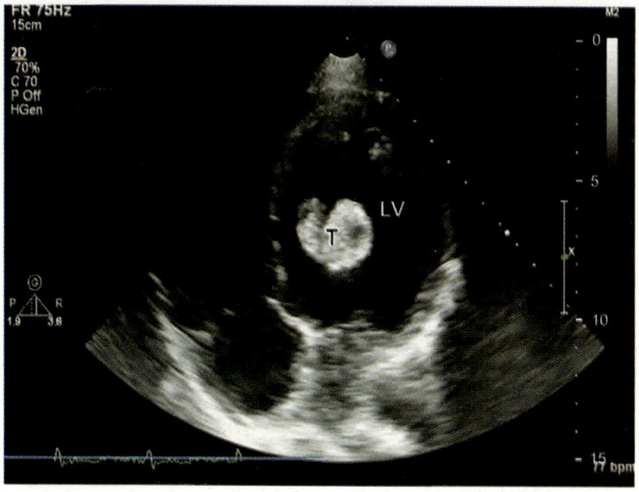

Fig. 9: Bilobed T in the LV. (LV: left ventricle; T: thrombus)

Vegetations

The clinical context is important in suspecting and making an accurate diagnosis. Echocardiographic criteria for the diagnosis of infective endocarditis are vegetations and abscesses. Vegetations are the pathological hallmark of infective endocarditis. The underlying structural heart disease can be diagnosed by echo Doppler studies. Vegetations appear as oscillating or nonoscillating mass attached to valves and other endocardial structures or on implanted intracardiac devices, such as pacemaker leads. The presence of intrinsic mobility is especially useful. Transesophageal echocardiography has better sensitivity (85–90%) as well as specificity compared to TTE (75%) for accurate diagnosis. This is especially so for the diagnosis of prosthetic valve endocarditis. Transesophageal echocardiography is mandatory in the assessment of prosthetic valve infective endocarditis. It has better sensitivity and specificity for the detection of vegetations, abscesses, and perivalvular lesions in these patients (Fig. 10).

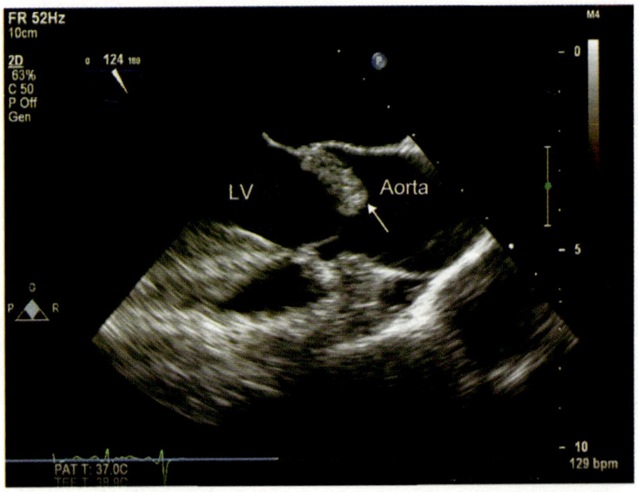

Fig. 10: Vegetation (arrow) attached to the aortic valve; LV. (LV: left ventricle)

VIDEO LEGENDS

Video 1: A large myxoma in left atrium.

Video 2: A myxoma in left atrium; smaller compared to Video 1, but producing mitral inflow obstruction.

Video 3: Parasternal long axis view of myxoma attached to anterior mitral leaflet and prolapsing to left ventricular outflow tract.

Video 4: Parasternal short axis view of myxoma shown in Video 3.

Video 5: Myxoma in right atrium producing tricuspid inlet obstruction.

Video 6: A sweep of four-chamber view showing multiple rhabdomyomas in the ventricular septum, apex, and lateral wall of ventricle.

Video 7: Myxosarcoma in left atrium prolapsing into left ventricle. Note the bulky, mobile, heterogeneous mass with the areas of echolucency suggestive of necrosis.

Video 8: Lymphoma in right ventricular outflow tract, producing turbulence in outflow tract.

Video 9: Thickening in free wall and septum due to secondaries from an unknown site.

Video 10: A small thrombus in the left atrial appendage.

REFERENCES

1. Lam KY, Dickens P, Chan AC. Tumors of the heart. A 20-year experience with a review of 12,485 consecutive autopsies. Arch Pathol Lab Med. 1993;117:1027-31.
2. Shapiro LM. Cardiac tumours: diagnosis and management. Heart. 2001;85:218-22.
3. Lee VH, Connolly HM, Brown RD, Jr. Central nervous system manifestations of cardiac myxoma. Arch Neurol. 2007;64:1115-20.
4. Vidaillet HJ Jr, Seward JB, Fyke FE 3rd, et al. 'Syndrome myxoma': a subset of patients with cardiac myxoma associated with pigmented skin lesions and peripheral and endocrine neoplasms. Br Heart J. 1987;57:247-55.
5. Casey M, Mah C, Merliss AD, et al. Identification of a novel genetic locus for familial cardiac myxomas and Carney complex. Circulation. 1998;98:2560-6.
6. Gonzalez-Juanatey C, Regueiro-Abel M, Lopez-Agreda H, et al. Giant left atrial myxoma mimicking severe mitral valve stenosis. Int J Cardiol. 2007;4:102.
7. Ragland MM, Tak T. The role of echocardiography in diagnosing space-occupying lesions of the heart. Clin Med Res. 2006;4(1):22-32.
8. Yu L, Gu T, Shi E. Echocardiographic findings and clinical correlation with cardiac myxoma. JACC Cardiovasc Imaging. 2016;9(5):618-21.
9. Beghetti M, Gow RM, Haney I, et al. Pediatric primary benign cardiac tumors: a 15-year review. Am Heart J. 1997;134:1107-14.
10. Elbardissi AW, Dearani JA, Daly RC, et al. Survival after resection of primary cardiac tumors: a 48-year experience. Circulation. 2008;118(Suppl. 14):S7-15.
11. Bossert T, Gummert JF, Battellini R, et al. Surgical experience with 77 primary cardiac tumors. Interact Cardiovasc Thorac Surg. 2005;4(4):311-5.
12. Klarich KW, Enriquez-Sarano M, Gura GM, et al. Papillary fibroelastoma: echocardiographic characteristics for diagnosis and pathologic correlation. J Am Coll Cardiol. 1997;30(3):784-90.
13. Basu S, Morshuis W, Heijmen R, et al. Lipomatous hypertrophy of the interatrial septum. Cardiovasc Surg. 1994;2:229-31.
14. Meng Q, Qian Y, Lai H, et al. Echocardiographic and pathologic characteristics of primary cardiac tumors: a study of 149 cases. Int J Cardiol. 2002;84:69-75.
15. Oliveira GH, Al-Kindi SG, Hoimes C, et al. Characteristics and survival of malignant cardiac tumors. A 40-year analysis of >500 patients. Circulation. 2015;132:2395-402.
16. McAllister HA, Hall RJ, Cooley DA. Tumors of the heart and pericardium. Curr Probl Cardiol. 1999;24:57-116.
17. Miguel CE, Bestetti RB. Primary cardiac lymphoma. Int J Cardiol. 2011;149:358-63.
18. Grebenc ML, Rosado de Christenson ML, Burke AP, et al. Primary cardiac and pericardial neoplasms: radiologic-pathologic correlation. Radiographics. 2000;20:1073-103.
19. Reynen K, Kockeritz U, Strasser RH. Metastases to the heart. Ann Oncol. 2004;15:375-81.

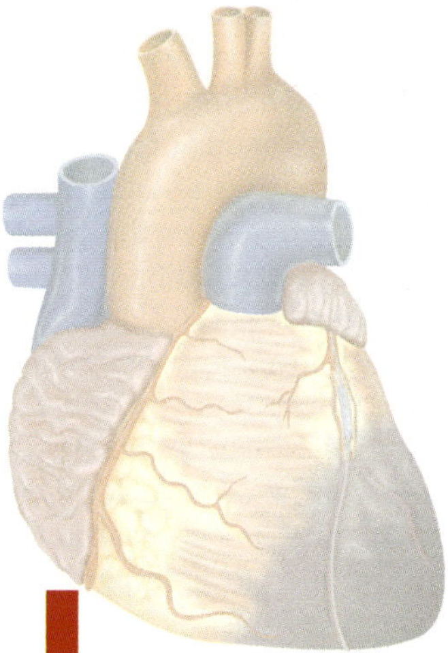

132 CHAPTER

Cardiac Computed Tomography and Magnetic Resonance Evaluation of Cardiac Masses

S Singhal, R Singhal

INTRODUCTION

Cardiac masses are uncommon with an estimated prevalence of 0.001–0.28% at autopsy.[1] They can be broadly classified as either neoplastic or nonneoplastic. Neoplastic cardiac masses are composed of primary benign tumors, primary malignant tumors, or metastatic tumors. Primary cardiac tumors are exceedingly rare with prevalence of 0.001–0.03% in an autopsy series, while metastatic tumors to the heart are reported to be 20–40 times more common.[2] Primary cardiac tumors originating in the heart are benign in approximately 75%, with myxoma accounting for at least half of total cases.[1,2] The remaining 25% are malignant with sarcoma comprising the majority of cases.[3] Nonneoplastic cardiac masses, such as thrombi, pericardial cysts, and prominent anatomic structures, can often mimic cardiac tumors. The evaluation of cardiac masses may therefore pose a diagnostic challenge. Multimodality imaging plays essential role in the diagnosis and treatment strategies of cardiac masses. Cardiac computed tomography (CT) and magnetic resonance (MR) are often utilized synergistically with echocardiography in the evaluation and management of cardiac masses. Echocardiography remains the first-line imaging modality for cardiac mass evaluation due to multitudes of reasons, such as its widespread availability, lack of iodinated contrast material or radiation exposure, and its dynamic assessment of cardiac masses in relation to the surrounding chambers, valves, and pericardium; however, it is limited by poor acoustic windows, particularly in obese patients and those with chronic lung disease, poor soft-tissue characterization, and due to limited evaluation of extracardiac structures.[4] This chapter provides an overview of cardiac masses, noninvasive imaging approach toward them including imaging characteristics of commonly encountered masses.

IMAGING APPROACH TO CARDIAC MASSES

Noninvasive imaging (cardiac MR and cardiac CT) plays a critical role in the diagnosis and surgical planning of cardiac masses. Typical locations of common cardiac masses are illustrated (Fig. 1).

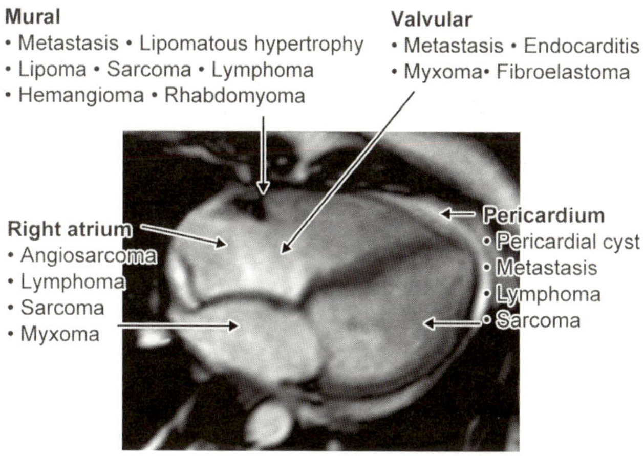

Fig. 1

Cardiac Magnetic Resonance

It is the preferred imaging modality for cardiac masses because of its superior soft-tissue characterization, high temporal resolution, multiplanar imaging capabilities, and unrestricted field of view.[5] As MR does not require the use of ionizing radiation, it is the modality of choice, along with echocardiography, for pediatric patients with cardiac masses. The goals of the cardiac magnetic resonance imaging (MRI) sequences selected are to define the extent and nature of the mass by its T1, T2, and T2* effects; to use cine sequences to determine mobility of the mass; to determine the presence and extent of compromise of valvular and cardiac function secondary to the mass; and to determine enhancement pattern of the mass. First-pass perfusion imaging allows assessment of mass vascularity, whereas late gadolinium enhancement imaging demonstrates the presence of extracellular matrix and is typically absent in the setting of thrombus. Box 1 summarizes indicators of malignancy on cardiac MR.

Limitations: Cardiac MR is dependent on patient cooperation to obtain quality images and is specifically contraindicated in patients with claustrophobia and implanted magnetic devices. MR may also be limited for evaluating small mobile masses (e.g. papillary fibroelastoma or valvular vegetations) due to limitations in spatial resolution and it also does not provide detailed assessment of coronary arteries in cases where the assessment of coronary artery disease (CAD) prior to surgery is an important clinical question.

Cardiac Computed Tomography

It is an effective, alternate imaging modality to assess cardiac masses, particularly in patients with known contra-indications to MR or in patients with inadequate images from other noninvasive methods. Cardiac CT is a fast imaging technique with electrocardiographic (ECG) gating that provides high-quality images with superior spatial resolution. Gated cardiac CT minimizes motion-related artifacts and allows a more precise delineation of the lesion margins. Compared to other cardiac imaging modalities, CT is optimal for the evaluation of calcified masses, the global assessment of chest and lung tissue, corresponding vascular structures, and exclusion of obstructive CAD. Computed tomography can provide anatomic information, functional assessment, and tissue characterization. There are specific CT protocols to assess cardiac masses and to acquire high-quality images. For example, right atrial or right ventricle masses may require a right heart contrast injection protocol with multiphasic contrast administration to obtain optimal images. In addition, low-dose, noncontrast, and delayed CT imaging may be helpful in distinguishing intracardiac thrombus from tumor and to detect calcifications. The differential diagnosis for cardiac masses on cardiac CT is based on several key aspects. They include size, quantity, location (cardiac chamber, pericardial involvement, extracardiac structures), morphology (attachment, margin appearance, infiltration), tissue characteristics (calcification, fat attenuation, vascularity), and clinical correlation (known malignancy or infection, presence of a catheter, associated syndromes). Cardiac CT is also useful to detect metastases in suspected malignancies especially coupled with 18-fluorodeoxyglucose positron emission tomography. Table 1 describes cardiac CT differentiating features between benign versus malignant tumors.

Limitations: Significant disadvantages with CT include radiation exposure, small risk of contrast-induced nephropathy, and lower soft tissue and temporal resolutions as compared with cardiac MR imaging. *Taking the discussion further, we are now highlighting the characteristic features of commonly encountered and selected cardiac masses on cardiac MR and CT.*

BOX 1: Indicators of malignancy using cardiac MRI.

Tumor characteristics:
- Large size—especially if >5 cm
- Irregular, ill-defined margins
- Direct invasion through tissue planes
- Most cardiac tumors involving the right heart are suspicious for malignancy
- Pericardial or pleural involvement
- Multiple lesions

Tissue characteristics:
- Tissue heterogeneity on T1- and T2-weighted images (hemorrhage and necrosis within mass)
- Hemorrhagic pericardial effusion (high signal intensity on T1-weighted images)
- Contrast enhancement
- High T1-weighted with low T2-weighted signal intensity is suggestive of metastatic malignant melanoma

CHARACTERISTICS FINDINGS OF VARIOUS NEOPLASMS BASED ON COMPUTED TOMOGRAPHY AND MAGNETIC RESONANCE IMAGING

Benign Neoplasms

Myxomas

Myxomas are the most common primary cardiac tumor, 25–50% of cases. It typically affects middle-aged adults, 30–60 years of age, with higher prevalence in women.[6] About 60–75% of cases are located in the left atrium attached to the fossa ovalis by a thin stalk, though less common

TABLE 1: Cardiac computed tomography (CT) features of benign and malignant tumors.

Feature	*Benign*	*Malignant*
Size/number	Small (<5 cm), single lesion	Large (>5 cm), multiple lesions
Location	Left >> right	Right >> left
Morphology	Intracameral	Intramural
Attachment	Narrow stalk, pedunculated	Usually broad based
Enhancement	Absent to minimal	Moderate, intense
Margin	Smooth, well-defined	Irregular, ill-defined
Invasion	None	Intra/extracardiac infiltration
Metastasis	None	May be present
Pericardial effusion	None	May be present
Calcification	Rare (except for small foci in fibroma, myxoma, or teratoma)	Large foci in osteosarcoma

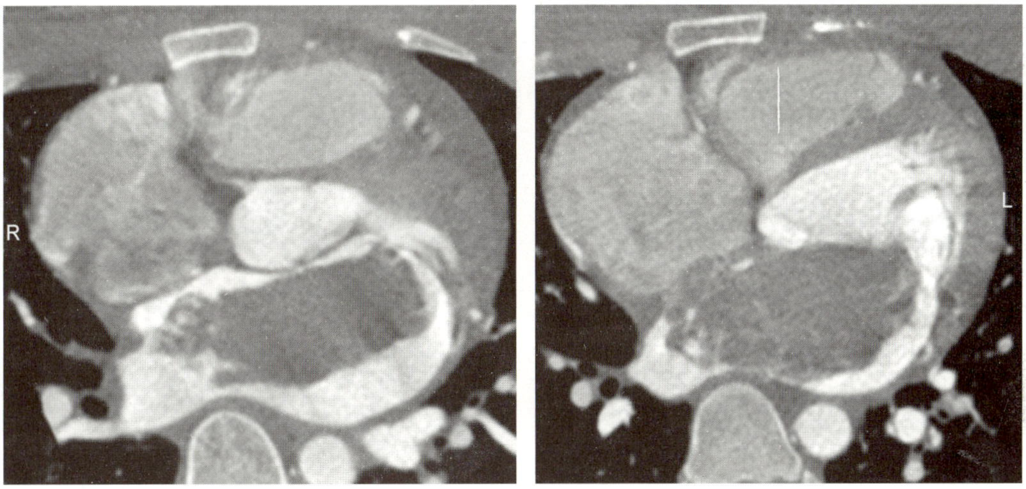

Fig. 2

locations include the right atrium (15–20%), inferior vena cava, ventricles, and the valve leaflets.[7] On cardiac CT, approximately two thirds of myxomas are ovoid with a smooth or lobular shape, with the remainder villous in appearance. On noncontrast CT, they typically appear hypodense, consistent with blood, and may demonstrate calcifications more often in the right atrial location. On contrast-enhanced cardiac CT, they appear as intracavitary filling defects with heterogeneous contrast enhancement, with variable intensity depending on their chronicity and whether necrosis or hemorrhage is present (Fig. 2). On mobile ECG-gated imaging, myxomas may prolapse across the atrioventricular valves causing outflow tract obstruction. At MRI, the vast majority of myxomas will demonstrate heterogeneous signal intensity. Myxomatous tissue is hypointense relative to myocardium on T1-weighted (T1W) images and has high signal intensity on T2-weighted (T2W) images due to the high extracellular water content; areas of fibrous tissue will be hypointense on both T1- and T2W images. Areas of acute hemorrhage within myxomas will be hypointense on both T1- and T2W images, whereas older areas of hemorrhage with localized methemoglobin formation will be hyperintense on both T1- and T2W images.[8-11] Myxomas generally show a heterogeneous pattern on enhancement following gadolinium contrast material.[6,7,11,12] On steady-state free precession images, myxomas will be hyperintense relative to myocardium but hypointense relative to the blood pool (Fig. 3).

The *main differential diagnoses* for myxoma include atrial thrombus or papillary fibroelastoma. It can be difficult to differentiate thrombus from a myxoma on MR images because both may have a heterogeneous appearance with areas of calcification; however, myxomas are more likely to arise anteriorly from the interatrial septum, whereas thrombus is more likely located posteriorly in the left atrium. In addition, myxomas will enhance with gadolinium

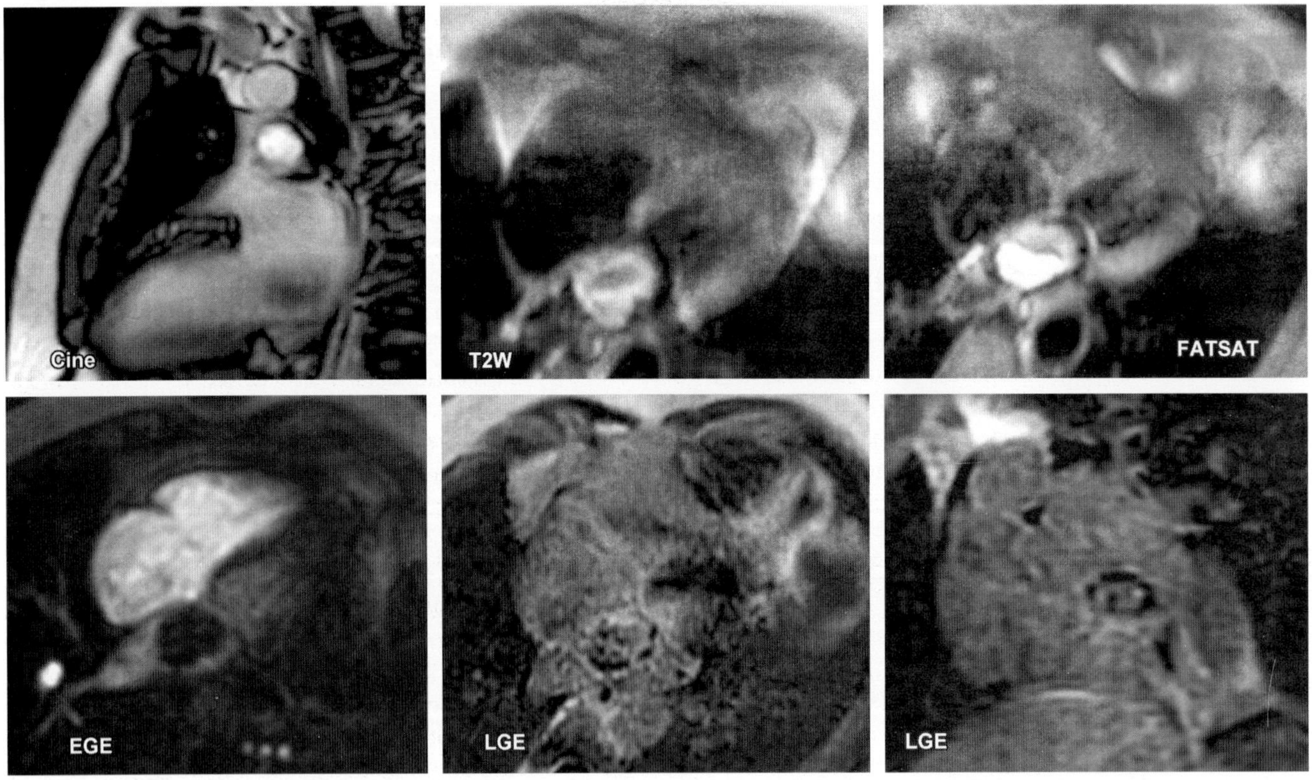

Fig. 3

contrast material, whereas thrombus, in most cases, does not.[13,14] Papillary fibroelastomas tend to be much smaller and demonstrate different signal intensity characteristics.

Lipoma

Lipoma is the second most common primary benign slow growing tumor (10%).[6] Lipomas commonly occur in middle-aged and older adults. Lipomas are encapsulated, well-circumscribed tumors consisting of mature adipocytes that can occur anywhere in the heart. Approximately 50% arise in the epicardial or midmyocardial layers, while the other half are subendocardial, where they create filling defects with a homogenous appearance of fat attenuation (density < –50 HU).

Lipomas have specific MRI characteristics, with homogeneous high signal intensity on T1W images, slightly less high signal intensity on T2W images, and signal suppression on fat-saturated images. The signal intensity is similar to that of adjacent subcutaneous or mediastinal fat. They do not enhance after contrast administration.

The *main differential diagnosis* is lipomatous infiltration of the interatrial septum characterized by deposit of fat in the atrial septum exceeding 2 cm in transverse diameter. On imaging, it again will demonstrate the well-described high signal intensity characteristics of fat with sparing of the fossa ovalis and a consequent dumbbell shape.[15]

Papillary Fibroelastoma

It is the most common neoplasm of the cardiac valves and papillary muscles.[16] The tumor occurs in any age with highest prevalence at 70–79 years, equally common in men and women.[17] The aortic valve is the most common site, followed by the mitral valve.[18] The majority are small and asymptomatic, may present with transient ischemic attack and stroke with mitral valve tumors, or sudden cardiac death and myocardial infarction with aortic valve tumors.[19] Valvular insufficiency is not a feature as these are located away from the free edge of the leaflet.[20]

Fibroelastomas are typically diagnosed by echocardiography, where they are seen as small mobile masses attached to the valve. These are difficult to identify on cardiac CT due to their small size, pronounced mobility and lack of calcification. If visible on cardiac CT, papillary fibroelastomas appear hypodense with irregular borders attached by a thin stalk. Electrocardiographic-gated CT angiography reveals a nodular lesion attached to the valve, away from the valvular free edge.[21] On MR images, fibroelastomas are of intermediate signal on both T1- and T2W images and are well demonstrated on cine MR images.[19]

Rhabdomyomas

Rhabdomyomas are the most common in children, particularly in infants, 50% are associated with tuberous sclerosis.[22,23] Most are asymptomatic and discovered incidentally, some patients may present with signs of heart failure or cardiac arrhythmias.[22]

Computed tomography may demonstrate myocardial thickening with spotty calcifications or a solid homogeneous mass.[24] Magnetic resonance images typically show a homogeneous mass within or attached to the ventricular myocardium, isointense on T1W images, mildly hyperintense on T2W images, and with enhancement after intravenous gadolinium administration.[18]

Fibroma

These constitutes second most common primary cardiac tumor in infants and children. About one third of fibromas occur before the age of 1 year.[2] Clinical picture varies from asymptomatic to heart failure, arrhythmias, and sudden death, likely due to involvement of the cardiac conduction system.[2]

Computed tomography demonstrates a heterogeneous mural mass with enhancement after intravenous contrast administration; calcifications are visible in about 25% of cases.[2] On MR images, typically seen as intramyocardial lesions involving the ventricular septum or free wall, with well-defined borders, heterogeneous signal on T1- and T2W images, and strong enhancement after intravenous gadolinium administration, with or without a hypoenhancing core correlating with fibrous tissue.[18]

Hemangiomas

Hemangiomas are vascular tumors that can affect a wide age group, 5–10% of benign tumors.[1] They can occur in any chamber.

Computed tomography images may demonstrate a heterogeneous mass with foci of calcifications and avid enhancement after intravenous contrast administration.[21] At MRI, they will be heterogeneously isointense or hypointense on T1W images and usually hyperintense on T2W images and may show heterogeneous appearance with low-signal-intensity areas on T2W images. An inhomogeneous hyperintense enhancement pattern has been reported after administration of gadolinium contrast material.[25-27]

Paragangliomas

Cardiac paragangliomas are very rare. They arise from the neuroendocrine cells in the normal cardiac ganglia and from visceral paraganglia in the left atrium, most frequently in the posterior wall or the left atrial roof, or from the interatrial septum or paraganglia along the coronary arteries. Patients are usually younger with mean age 40 years at diagnosis.[28,29]

On CT images, they appear as circumscribed, heterogeneous, low-attenuation masses that enhance avidly after contrast administration.[6] At MRI, paragangliomas exhibit isointensity on T1W images, bright hyperintensity on T2W images, and intense enhancement with contrast administration.[21,30] Central necrosis and hemorrhage may be present, as well as internal calcifications[27] (Fig. 4).

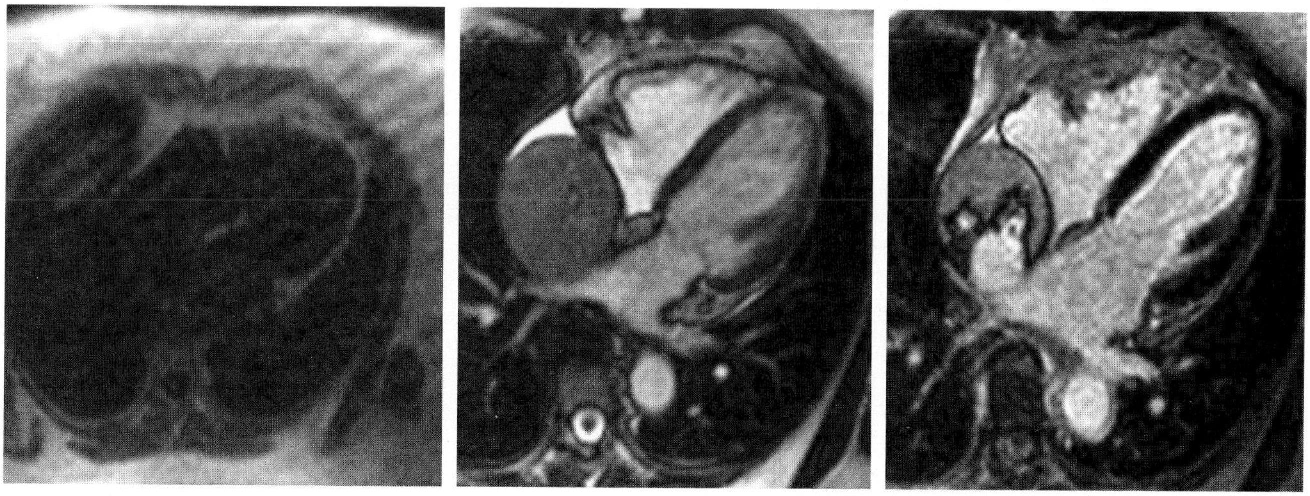

Fig. 4

Malignant Neoplasms

Metastases

Cardiac metastases are 20–40 times more frequent than primary tumors.[30,31] The most common primary sites are the lung, breast, and hematologic malignancies. The pericardium and epicardium are involved in 65–70% by direct invasion and the myocardium in 30%.

Imaging presentation varies with the primary origin of the tumor, and appearances and enhancing patterns identical to the primary lesion are clues for diagnosis. The presence of metastases involving other organs is also an indirect sign. In general, cardiac metastases are low-attenuation masses with heterogeneous enhancement on CT images, hypointense on T1W images, and hyperintense on T2W MR images. The exception is malignant melanoma, which demonstrates hyperintensity on T1W images.[30,32,33] Malignant pericardial effusion frequently occurs; exudative or hemorrhagic effusions exhibit high signal on T1W images, which can be differentiated from other pericardial effusions.[30,32]

Angiosarcoma

This is the most common primary cardiac malignancy of adulthood, 9% of primary cardiac tumors.[30] It is more common in men and occurs over a wide age range.[34] About 80% involve the right atrial free wall and may extend to the pericardium.[21,30,35] Right atrial perforation and cardiac tamponade may occur.[36]

On CT, they present as low-attenuation lesions that enhance heterogeneously after intravenous contrast administration.[21] There are two main morphologic appearances: focal nodules with cauliflower appearance protruding into a cardiac chamber and diffusely infiltrative masses extending along the epicardial surface.[30] Magnetic resonance images may demonstrate hemorrhage as hyperintense foci on T1W images. Areas of central necrosis and hemorrhage are characteristic findings and result in heterogeneous signal intensity on T2W images.[30-33,37] Intravenous contrast administration usually demonstrates avid enhancement.[21] In cases of pericardial infiltration, a "sunray appearance" may be seen with a sheet-like pericardial thickening and pericardial effusion.[34] Angiosarcomas metastasize in 66–89% of patients, most often to the lungs, liver, and brain.

Rhabdomyosarcomas

These are the most common primary cardiac malignancy in children, rarely in adults.[32] These tumors may occur in any chamber but involve the valves more often. Clinical symptoms depend on the location of the tumor, but congestive heart failure is a common presentation.[32]

On CT images, rhabdomyosarcomas typically appear as low-attenuation, bulky, infiltrative masses with central necrosis.[6] On MR images, the tumors exhibit heterogeneous signal intensity on both T1- and T2W images. Contrast enhancement of the solid, nonnecrotic portions is usually seen.[32]

Lymphoma

Primary cardiac lymphomas are extremely rare, with secondary lymphoma much more common.[32] In primary cardiac lymphomas, the most common is the diffuse large B-cell type[38] and usually occurs around 60 years and in men. They involve the right side of the heart and infrequently involve the valves.[1]

On CT images, lymphomas appear as thick myocardial or pericardial masses that are hypodense or isodense relative to the myocardium, with heterogeneous enhancement after intravenous contrast administration[39] (Fig. 5). On MR images, lymphomas typically exhibit low signal intensity on T1W images and high signal on T2W images.[40]

NONTUMORAL MASSES

Several mass-like lesions in the heart can mimic tumors.

Crista terminalis is a normal anatomical structure that may sometimes be mistaken for a tumor.[33]

Thrombi are also common and can usually be distinguished from tumors such as myxomas by shape and location.[41] Thrombi are usually smaller than myxomas, do not enhance, and are typically located in the left atrial appendage or posterior wall; myxomas tend to be attached at the fossa ovalis. In addition, thrombi do not prolapse through the cardiac valves as myxomas might[42] (Fig. 6). Table 2 highlights characteristics of thrombus on cardiac MR depending on the age.

Pericardial cysts can be identified by their well-demarcated appearance with water density on CT, low signal on T1W images, high signal on T2W images, and lack of contrast enhancement.[30]

Caseous necroses of the mitral valve are a rare variant of mitral annular calcification and typically involve the posterior mitral annulus at the atrioventricular groove. In the early phases, the mass is hyperintense on both T1- and T2W images.[30]

Valvular vegetations occur in the setting of infective endocarditis and can be identified as low-attenuation masses involving the valvular leaflet free edge, for which cardiac CT is both highly sensitive (97%) and specific (88%).[33]

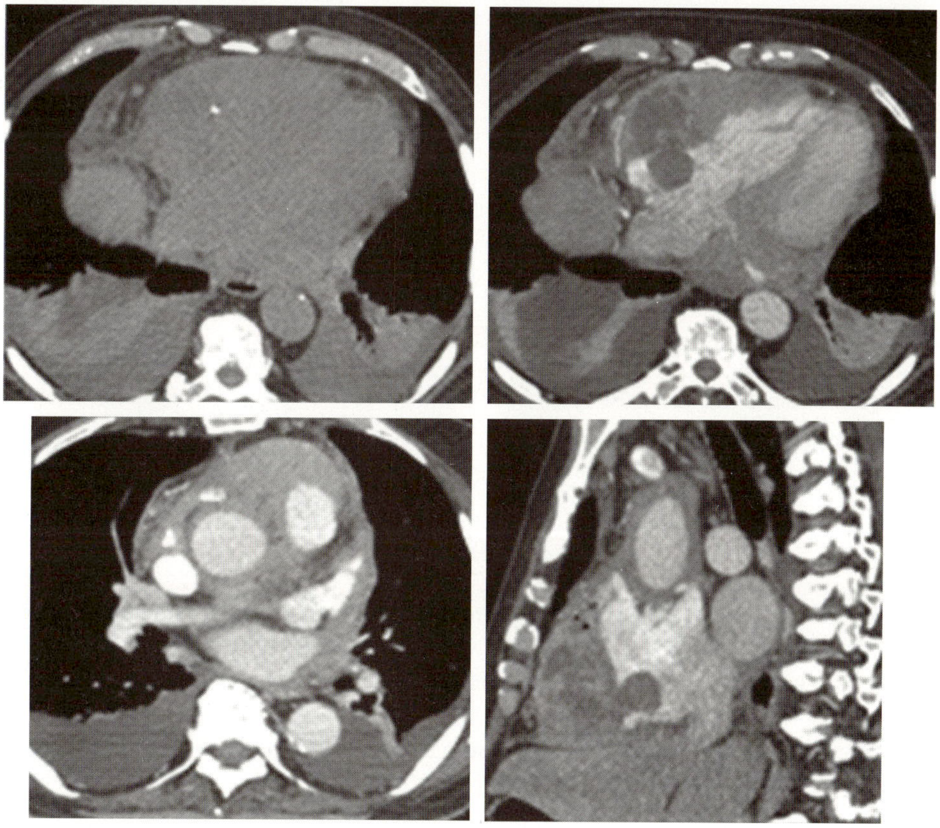

Fig. 5

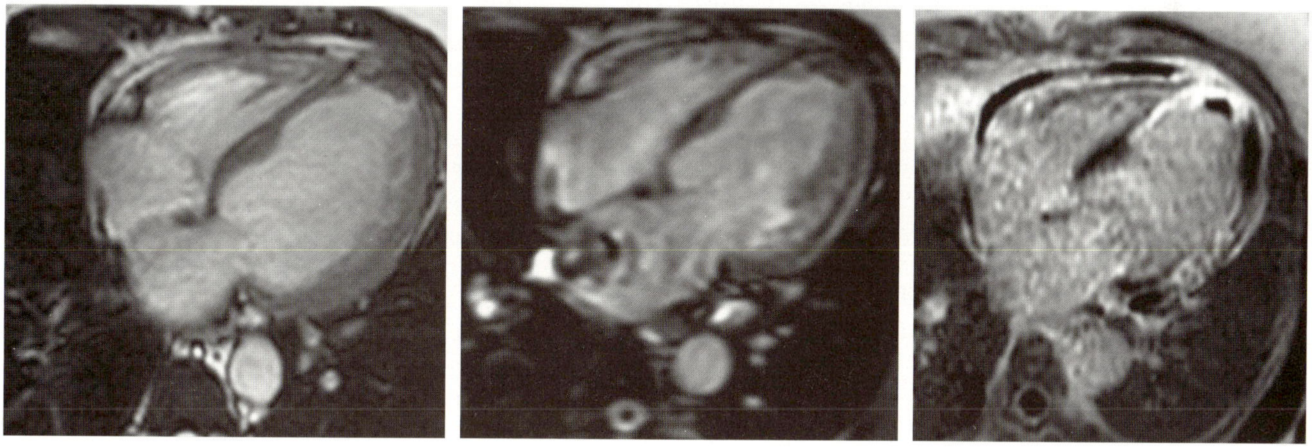

Fig. 6

TABLE 2: Cardiac MR imaging signal intensity characteristics for thrombus.

Age of thrombus	*T1W signal intensity*	*T2W signal intensity*	*EGE imaging*	*LGE imaging*
Acute	High	High	No uptake	No uptake
Subacute	High	Low	No uptake	No uptake
Chronic	Low	Low	No uptake	No uptake*

(EGE: early gadolinium enhancement; LGE: late gadolinium enhancement; MR: magnetic resonance; T1W: T1-weighted; T2W: T2-weighted)

*Organized chronic thrombus may show peripheral enhancement on LGE images owing to fibrous content.

TABLE 3: Recommendations for the use of noninvasive imaging to evaluate suspected cardiac and pericardial masses.

2006 Appropriate use criteria for cardiac MRI	
• Evaluation of cardiac mass (suspected tumor or thrombus)	Appropriate
• Evaluation of pericardial mass	Appropriate
2010 Appropriate use criteria for cardiac CT	
• Initial evaluation of cardiac mass (suspected tumor or thrombus)	Inappropriate
• Evaluation of cardiac mass (suspected tumor or thrombus) when inadequate images from other noninvasive methods	Appropriate
• Evaluation of pericardial anatomy	Appropriate
2013 Expert consensus for pericardial disease imaging	
• "Echocardiography is the initial imaging test to assess pericardial masses"	
• "CT and/or MRI should be done for better tissue characterization of the mass and detection of metastasis (if malignancy is suspected)"	

(MRI: magnetic resonance imaging; CT: computed tomography)

TABLE 4: Imaging features of cardiac masses.

Tumor	*Patient age at presentation*	*Most common location*	*CT features*	*MR imaging features*
Myxomas	30–60 years	Interatrial septum, left atrium > right	Heterogeneous, low attenuation	Heterogeneous, bright on T2WI, heterogeneous enhancement
Lipoma	Variable	Pericardial space or any cardiac chamber	Homogeneous fat attenuation	Homogeneous fat signal intensity: no enhancement
Papillary fibroelastomas	Middle-aged, elderly	Cardiac valves, especially aortic valve	Not seen usually	Not seen usually
Fibroma	Children, especially <1 years	Ventricles	Myocardial thickening, spotty calcifications, solid enhancing mass	Homogeneous mass, isointense to myocardium on T1WI, mildly hyperintense on T2W images
Hemangioma	Variable	Anywhere	Heterogeneous mass with calcifications, avid enhancement	Intermediate signal on T1WI, very bright on T2WI, marked enhancement
Paraganglioma	Young adults	Left atrium, coronary arteries, aortic root	Low attenuation, strong enhancement calcification rare: hemorrhage or necrosis common	Isointense on heterogeneous on T1WI, very bright on T2WI, marked enhancement
Metastasis	Variable	Epicardium or pericardium >myocardium >endocardium or intraluminal	Usually low attenuation, with heterogeneous enhancement	Usually hypointense on T1WI and hyperintense on T2WI except melanoma, heterogeneous enhancement
Angiosarcoma	Variable	Right atrium	Low-attenuation mass with heterogeneous avid enhancement	Hemorrhage hyperintense on T1WI, central necrosis, heterogeneous enhancement, "sunray appearance"
Rhabdomyo-sarcoma	Children	Any chamber or valves	Low attenuation, bulky infiltrative mass, central necrosis	Heterogeneous signal intensity on T1WI and T2WI, enhancement of nonnecrotic portions
Lymphoma	Around 60 years	Right heart	Hypodense or isodense, heterogeneous enhancement	Hypointense on T1WI, hyperintense on T2WI

(CT: computed tomography; MR: magnetic resonance; T1WI: T1-weighted images; T2WI: T2-weighted images)

Appropriateness criteria for cardiac MR[43] and cardiac CT[44] and an Expert Consensus statement for pericardial disease imaging[45] provide specific guidance on the approach to cardiac masses (Tables 3 and 4).

CONCLUSION

Cardiac tumors are rare, though may pose diagnostic and therapeutic challenge. Noninvasive cardiac imaging in form of cardiac CT and MR constitutes mainstay of diagnostic workshop for these masses, be it benign or malignant over and above echocardiography for various reasons discussed so far. Since it is important to accurately distinguish cardiac masses in order to provide optimal management cardiac CT by virtue of its high spatial and contrast resolution, fast acquisition times, capability to identify calcification and fat, having specific advantages in defining the cardiovascular extent of the mass and excluding CAD prior to surgical intervention, cardiac CT can provide best possible information. Also, the multiplanar assessment of the anatomy, tissue characteristics, and functional impact of a cardiac or juxtacardiac mass afforded by cardiac MRI allow early differentiation between benign and malignant tumors. This may enable rapid aggressive treatment of benign processes via surgical resection. Magnetic resonance imaging of malignant tumors may lead to complete diagnosis which may help in guiding more measured approach, appropriate in the majority of cases to the context of palliative treatment. With the increasing availability of an interest in gated cardiac MRI, imaging of suspected masses may form an infrequent but important tool for evaluating cardiac masses.

REFERENCES

1. Burke A, Virmani R. Tumors of the heart and great vessels. Fascicle 16, 3rd Series. In: Burke A, Virmani R (Eds). Atlas of tumor pathology. Washington, DC: Armed Forces Institute of Pathology; 1996. pp. 1-98.
2. Grebenc ML, Rosado-de-Christenson ML, Burke AP, et al. Primary cardiac and pericardial neoplasms: radiologic-pathologic correlation. Radiographics. 2000;20:1073-103.
3. Best AK, Dobson RL, Ahmad AR. Best cases from the AFIP: cardiac angiosarcoma. Radiographics. 2003;23:S141-5.
4. Buckley O, Madan R, Kwong R, et al. Cardiac masses, Part 1: Imaging strategies and technical considerations. Am J Roentgenol. 2011;197:W837-41.
5. O'Donnell DH, Abbara S, Chaithiraphan V, et al. Cardiac tumors: optimal cardiac MR sequences and spectrum of imaging appearances. Am J Roentgenol. 2009;193:377-87.
6. Araoz PA, Mulvagh SL, Tazelaar HD, et al. CT and MR imaging of benign primary cardiac neoplasms with echocardiographic correlation. Radiographics. 2000;20:1303-19.
7. Grebenc ML, Rosado-De-Christenson ML, Green CE, et al. Cardiac myxoma: imaging features in 83 patients. Radiographics. 2002;22:673-89.
8. Rubin JI, Gomori JM, Grossman RI, et al. High field MR imaging of extra-cranial hematomas. AJR Am J Roentgenol. 1987;148:813-7.
9. De Roos A, Weijers E, Van Duinen S, et al. Calcified right atrial myxoma demonstrated by magnetic resonance imaging. Chest. 1989;95:478-9.
10. Masui T, Takahashi M, Miura K, et al. Cardiac myxoma: identification of intratumoral hemorrhage and calcification on MR images. AJR Am J Roentgenol. 1995;164:850-2.
11. Matsuoka H, Hamada M, Honda T, et al. Morphologic and histologic characterization of cardiac myxomas by magnetic resonance imaging. Angiology. 1996;47:693-8.
12. Semelka RC, Shoenut JP, Wilson ME, et al. Cardiac masses: signal intensity features on spin-echo, gradient-echo, gadolinium enhanced spin-echo, and TurboFLASH images. J Magn Reson Imaging. 1992;2:415-20.
13. Funari M, Fujita N, Peck WW, et al. Cardiac tumors: assessment with Gd-DTPA enhanced MR imaging. J Comput Assist Tomogr. 1991;15:953-8.
14. Gomes AS, Lois JF, Child JS, et al. Cardiac tumors and thrombus: evaluation with MR imaging. AJR Am J Roentgenol. 1987;149:895-9.
15. Heyer CM, Kagel T, Lemburg SP, et al. Lipomatous hypertrophy of the interatrial septum: a prospective study of incidence, imaging findings, and clinical symptoms. Chest. 2003;124:2068-73.
16. Edwards FH, Hale D, Cohen A, et al. Primary cardiac valve tumors. Ann Thorac Surg. 1991;52:1127-31.
17. Gowda RM, Khan IA, Nair CK, et al. Cardiac papillary fibroelastoma: a comprehensive analysis of 725 cases. Am Heart J. 2003;146:404-10.
18. Beroukhim RS, Prakash A, Buechel ER, et al. Characterization of cardiac tumors in children by cardiovascular magnetic resonance imaging: a multicenter experience. J Am Coll Cardiol. 2011;58:1044-54.
19. Lembcke A, Meyer R, Kivelitz D, et al. Images in cardiovascular medicine. Papillary fibroelastoma of the aortic valve: appearance in 64-slice spiral computed tomography, magnetic resonance imaging, and echocardiography. Circulation. 2007;115:e3-6.
20. Klarich KW, Enriquez-Sarano M, Gura GM, et al. Papillary fibroelastoma: echocardiographic characteristics for diagnosis and pathologic correlation. J Am Coll Cardiol. 1997;30:784-90.
21. Plein S, Ridgway JP, Jones TR, et al. Coronary artery disease: assessment with a comprehensive MR imaging protocol—initial results. Radiology. 2002;225:300-7.
22. Webb DW, Thomas RD, Osborne JP. Cardiac rhabdomyomas and their association with tuberous sclerosis. Arch Dis Child. 1993;68:367-70.
23. Beghetti M, Gow RM, Haney I, et al. Pediatric primary benign cardiac tumors: a 15-year review. Am Heart J 1997;134:1107-14.
24. Kim EY, Choe YH, Sung K, et al. Multidetector CT and MR imaging of cardiac tumors. Korean J Radiol. 2009;10:164-75.
25. Brodwater B, Erasmus J, McAdams HP, et al. Pericardial hemangioma. J Comput Assist Tomogr. 1996;20:954-6.
26. Oshima H, Hara M, Kono T, et al. Cardiac hemangioma of the left atrial appendage: CT and MR findings. J Thorac Imaging. 2003;18:204-6.

27. Lo LJ, Nucho RC, Allen JW, et al. Left atrial cardiac hemangioma associated with shortness of breath and palpitations. Ann Thorac Surg. 2002;73:979-81.
28. Semionov A, Sayegh K. Multimodality imaging of a cardiac paraganglioma. Radiol Case Rep. 2016;11:277-81.
29. Wang JG, Han J, Jiang T, Li YJ. Cardiac paragangliomas. J Card Surg. 2015;30:55-60.
30. Motwani M, Kidambi A, Herzog BA, et al. MR imaging of cardiac tumors and masses: a review of methods and clinical applications. Radiology. 2013;268:26-43.
31. Shelton DK, Caputo G. Cardiac imaging in acquired diseases. In: Brant WE, Helms CA (Eds). Fundamentals of diagnostic radiology, 4th edition. Philadelphia, PA: Lippincott Williams and Wilkins; 2012. pp. 612-3.
32. Sparrow PJ, Kurian JB, Jones TR, et al. MR imaging of cardiac tumors. Radiographics. 2005;25:1255-76.
33. Kassop D, Donovan MS, Cheezum MK, et al. Cardiac masses on cardiac CT: a review. Curr Cardiovasc Imaging Rep. 2014;7:9281.
34. Burazor I, Aviel-Ronen S, Imazio M, et al. Primary malignancies of the heart and pericardium. Clin Cardiol. 2014;37:582-8.
35. Burke A. Primary malignant cardiac tumors. Semin Diagn Pathol. 2008;25:39-46.
36. Sakaguchi M, Minato N, Katayama Y, et al. Cardiac angiosarcoma with right atrial perforation and cardiac tamponade. Ann Thorac Cardiovasc Surg. 2006;12:145-8.
37. Yahata S, Endo T, Honma H, et al. Sunray appearance on enhanced magnetic resonance image of cardiac angiosarcoma with pericardial obliteration. Am Heart J. 1994;127:468-71.
38. O'Sullivan PJ, Gladish GW. Cardiac tumors. Semin Roentgenol. 2008;43:223-33.
39. Dorsay TA, Ho VB, Rovira MJ, et al. Primary cardiac lymphoma: CT and MR findings. J Comput Assist Tomogr. 1993;17:978-81.
40. Tada H, Asazuma K, Ohya E, et al. Images in cardiovascular medicine. Primary cardiac B-cell lymphoma. Circulation. 1998;97:220-1.
41. Tatli S, Lipton MJ. CT for intracardiac thrombi and tumors. Int J Cardiovasc Imaging. 2005;21:115-31.
42. Scheffel H, Baumueller S, Stolzmann P, et al. Atrial myxomas and thrombi: comparison of imaging features on CT. AJR Am J Roentgenol. 2009;192:639-45.
43. Hendel RC, Patel MR, Kramer CM, et al. ACCF/ACR/SCCT/SCMR/ASNC/NASCI/SCAI/SIR 2006 appropriateness criteria for cardiac computed tomography and cardiac magnetic resonance imaging: a report of the American College of Cardiology Foundation Quality Strategic Directions Committee Appropriateness Criteria Working Group, American College of Radiology, Society of Cardiovascular Computed Tomography, Society for Cardiovascular Magnetic Resonance, American Society of Nuclear Cardiology, North American Society for Cardiac Imaging, Society for Cardiovascular Angiography and Interventions, and Society of Interventional Radiology. J Am Coll Cardiol. 2006;48:1475-97.
44. Taylor AJ, Cerqueira M, Hodgson JM, et al. ACCF/SCCT/ACR/AHA/ASE/ASNC/NASCI/SCAI/SCMR 2010 appropriate use criteria for cardiac computed tomography. A Report of the American College of Cardiology Foundation Appropriate Use Criteria Task Force, the Society of Cardiovascular Computed Tomography, the American College of Radiology, the American Heart Association, the American Society of Echocardiography, the American Society of Nuclear Cardiology, the North American Society for Cardiovascular Imaging, the Society for Cardiovascular Angiography and Interventions, and the Society for Cardiovascular Magnetic Resonance. J Cardiovasc Comput Tomogr. 2010;4:407.e1-33.
45. Klein AL, Abbara S, Agler DA, et al. American Society of Echocardiography clinical recommendations for multimodality cardiovascular imaging of patients with pericardial disease. J Am Soc Echocardiogr. 2013;26:965-1012.

SECTION 31

Intraoperative Echocardiography in Operation Theater

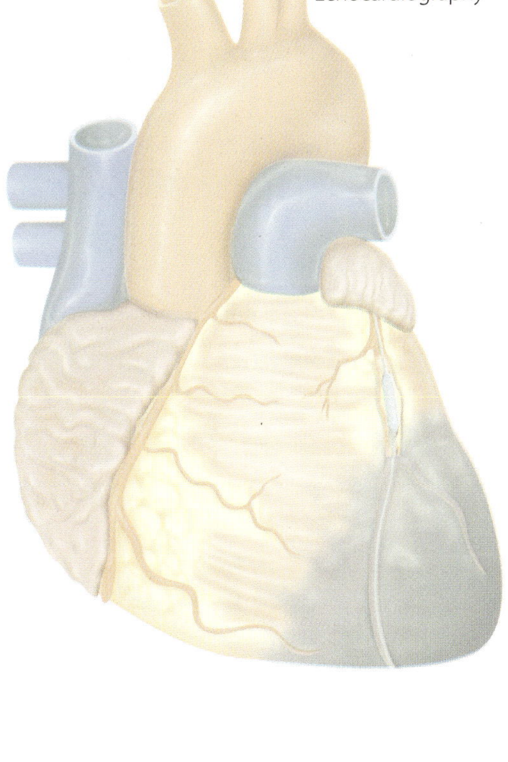

CHAPTER 133

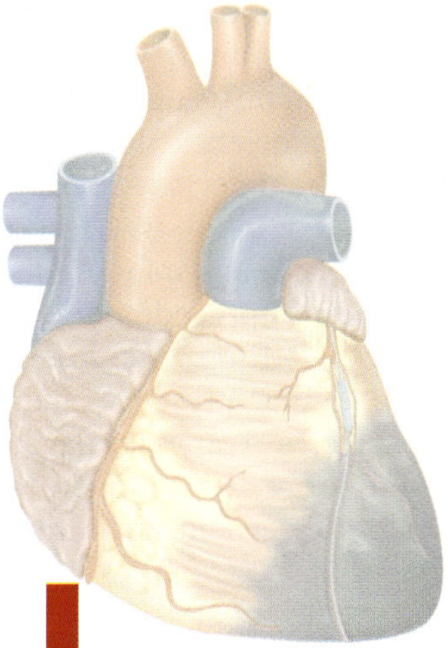

Intraoperative Transesophageal Echocardiography

Prateek Sharma, Ashley Pender, Roshini Malaney, Smadar Kort

INTRODUCTION

Advances in imaging quality, safety, and ability to obtain images in real time make transesophageal echocardiogram (TEE) the imaging modality of choice in both cardiac and noncardiac surgery. The utility of intraoperative TEE (IOTEE) is recognized and the procedure remains safe in cardiac and thoracic surgeries where studies have demonstrated new information is found in 9.2–11.4% of cases (resulting in changes in surgical decision-making in 5.8–9.2% of the cases).[1-4] As such, IOTEE is recommended in all open valvular procedures as well as thoracic aortic surgical procedures and should be considered in coronary artery bypass graft (CABG) surgeries. For patients undergoing noncardiac surgery, intraoperative TEE can be used in any patient with a diagnosed or potential cardiac pathology that could result in a surgical complication or instability and is also recommended during high-risk surgeries, such as lung transplantation and any major abdominal or thoracic procedure.[5,6] Intraoperative TEE can facilitate placement of central venous catheters, selection of anesthetic agents, confirmation of diagnosis, and exclusion of new pathology or defects and use of preoperative inotropic support by demonstrating ventricular systolic function and size.[7] Comprehensive assessment of the aorta should be performed as part of every IOTEE, as the presence of atherosclerotic plaques in the aorta poses a major risk for perioperative stroke and systemic embolization.[8] In this chapter, we discuss the role of IOTEE in many of its potential settings.

VALVE SURGERY

A comprehensive IOTEE assessment is tailored to the valve(s) of interest, including the measurement of valve area, mechanism of dysfunction, and quantification of regurgitation or stenosis.[1] Three-dimensional (3D) echocardiography complements two-dimensional (2D) echocardiography, allowing for improved topographical and spatial evaluation and should be included in the assessment of each valve. Furthermore, IOTEE helps to monitor for intraoperative complications, volume status, and global ventricular function. Owing to the posterior location of the mitral valve, ideal IOTEE views for thorough assessment of valvular function, leaflets, chordae, annulus, and papillary muscles include the four-chamber view, long-axis view, as well as the two-chamber and transgastric short-axis views. Proper sizing of the annuloplasty ring is dependent on the annulus measurement, and leaflets should be carefully evaluated with 2D and 3D imaging for restrictive or excessive motion and for clefts or perforations. Postintervention IOTEE should assess adequacy of repair and rule out potential complications of surgery. This includes exclusion of significant regurgitation, stenosis, systolic anterior motion (SAM) of the mitral valve, left ventricular (LV) dysfunction (mediated by circumflex artery compromise or increased afterload), and right ventricular (RV) dysfunction (mediated by right coronary artery air embolism or increased pulmonary vascular resistance).[9] Intraoperative TEE assessment of the aortic valve consists of the valve structure and function, identification of congenital or acquired lesions, assessment of volume status, and determination of prosthesis size when aortic valve replacement is performed.[10] Careful attention should be paid to the leaflets and their associated motion, aortic root, leaflet destruction, LV function, LV size, and LV outflow tract (LVOT). Ideal IOTEE views for aortic valve visualization are the midesophageal long-axis (at 120° with high TEE probe position), short-axis, and four-chamber views (at 0° with anterior angulation).[11] Postintervention assessment is to ensure adequate deairing and survey for complications. Potential complications include prosthetic valve dysfunction, SAM of the mitral valve/LVOT obstruction, wall-motion abnormalities (predominately mediated by coronary obstruction or air embolization).[12]

The tricuspid valve can be visualized with IOTEE in the midesophageal four-chamber and transgastric apical views. Given limited transducer positions with IOTEE, TTE provides more accurate assessment of the tricuspid regurgitant jet.[11] Three-dimensional TEE in the right atrial and RV views allow for simultaneous visualization of all three leaflets. The posterior leaflet is located inferiorly in the RV view, and the septal leaflet is located inferiorly in the right atrial view.[13] Intraoperative TEE can facilitate visualization of the pulmonic valve. Ideal views are the high esophageal position at 0° and the long-axis plane at 90°.[11] Three-dimensional TEE from the pulmonary artery allows for all three leaflets to be visualized with the anterior leaflet located superiorly.[14]

Congenital Heart Disease

The spectrum of diseases recognized as congenital heart disease includes shunts, obstructions to flow, regurgitant valves, or a combination of the above.[15] By utilizing biplane the horizontal and vertical planes allow for better visualization of pulmonary venous connections, atrial baffle function, atrioventricular anatomy and function, LVOT lesions, great artery positional relationships, systemic and pulmonary venous connections, atrial situs, venosus atrial septal defects (ASDs), the ventricular septum, and outflow tracts. It is also essential for complete assessment of complex RV outflow tract (RVOT) anatomy, ventriculoarterial alignment, and the sizing of all aortic segments in coarctation of the aorta.[16] It is important to differentiate between subtypes of ASDs. From the midesophageal level, the full length of septum is best seen at 0° along with the mitral and tricuspid valves and pulmonary venous return to the left atrium. The cleft associated with a primum ASD can also be assessed at 0° with a medially directed mitral regurgitant jet and the appearance of a split anterior leaflet. Alternatively, superior sinus venosus ASDs are best seen at 90°. The advent of 3D TEE has improved the visualization of patent foramen ovales and ASDs along with their surrounding tissue rim and nearby structures. As the interatrial septum is a complex, dynamic, and 3D anatomic structure, limitations exist in its evaluation using any single form of 2D echocardiography.[17] While ventricular septal defects are able to be seen at 0°, the defects to confirm tetralogy of Fallot are better viewed at in the RVOT view 60–90° where the pulmonary hypoplasia and infundibular obstruction can be assessed.[17] The postprocedure IOTEE assessment includes cardiac function, presence of intracardiac air, hemodynamics, and the presence of any potential residual anatomical defects. Transesophageal echocardiograms done immediately after congenital heart surgeries prior to chest closure have been shown to contribute to improved outcomes (Figs. 1 and 2).[7]

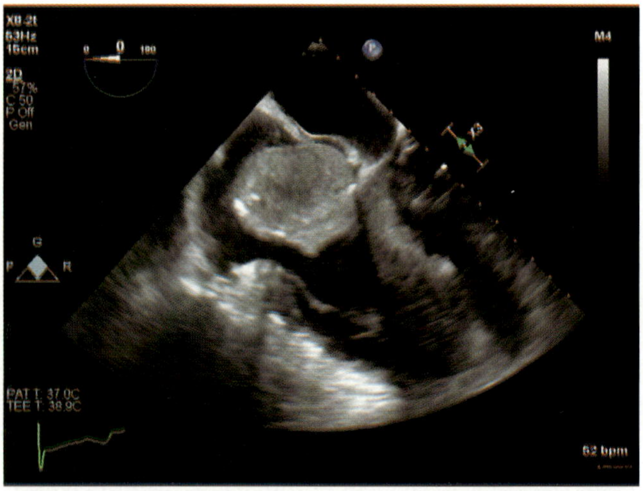

Fig. 1: Right atrial myxoma as seen from ME four-chamber view intraoperatively. (ME: midesophageal)

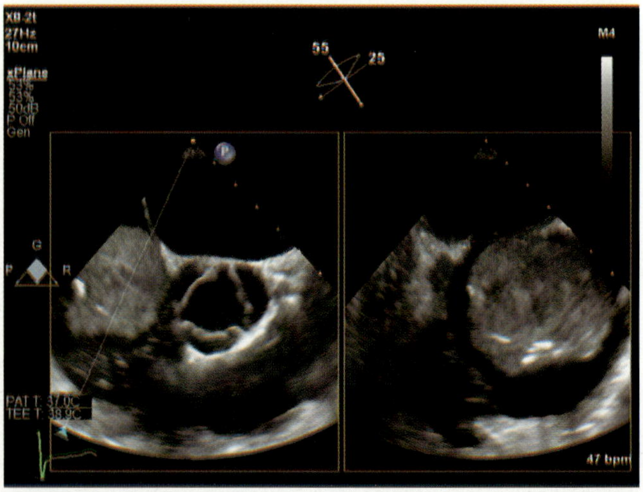

Fig. 2: Right atrial myxoma as visualized from ME biplane to evaluate for involvement of proximal structures. (ME: midesophageal)

Tumors

Although uncommon, when found, symptomatic cardiac masses and tumors should be surgically removed due to potential for embolic events, arrhythmia, discomfort/chest pain, malignant functional changes to involved chambers and valves, and heart failure.[18] Although many masses are found preoperatively, some may be found intraoperatively, which highlights the importance of a comprehensive intraoperative study.[19,20]

The primary cardiac tumors, although less common than secondary tumors, are more often amenable to surgical resection.[21] Intraoperative TEE is recommended for all open-heart and thoracic surgeries and is especially useful in the cases involving cardiac masses.[21,22] The most common primary cardiac tumor, cardiac myxoma, is a benign tumor mostly found in the left atrium and less frequently in the right atrium, where malignant tumors, such as sarcomas, are more commonly found.[23-25] Intraoperative TEE should be compared to all prior echocardiographic imaging to assess for new anatomical, mechanical, or valvular changes that may affect the surgical and anesthetic approach.[26] Intraoperative TEE can be especially helpful in evaluating masses that impinge on the right ventricle in the event of right-sided heart failure or suboptimal views in a transthoracic study.[13] It should also be utilized prior to the completion of a case to ensure complete removal of the mass and no significant remnants or physiological sequelae that would require further surgical intervention (e.g. significant valvular regurgitation or obstruction) (Figs. 3 to 11).[27,28]

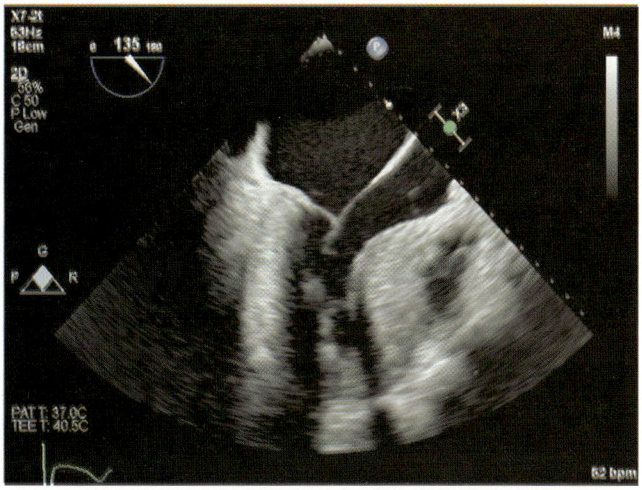

Fig. 3: Premyectomy ME two chamber of patient with HOCM. (HOCM: hypertrophic obstructive cardiomyopathy; ME: midesophageal)

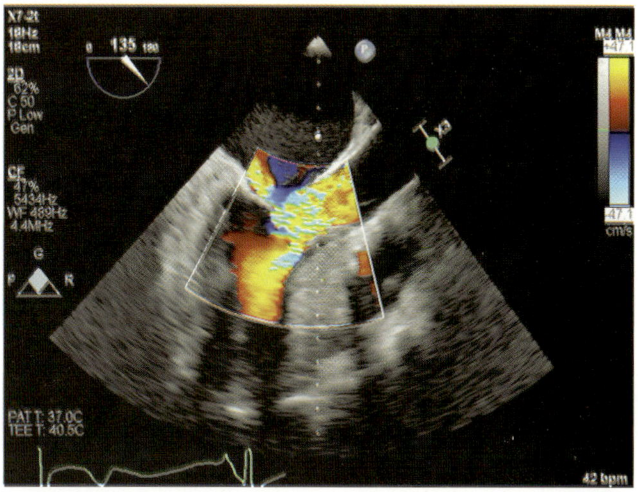

Fig. 5: Premyectomy of patient with HOCM with color flow Doppler. (HOCM: hypertrophic obstructive cardiomyopathy)

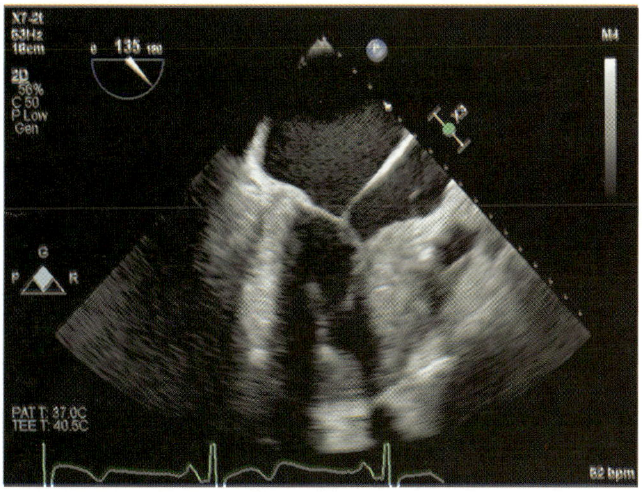

Fig. 4: Premyectomy ME two-chamber view of patient with HOCM highlighting SAM. (HOCM: hypertrophic obstructive cardiomyopathy; ME: midesophageal; SAM: systolic anterior motion)

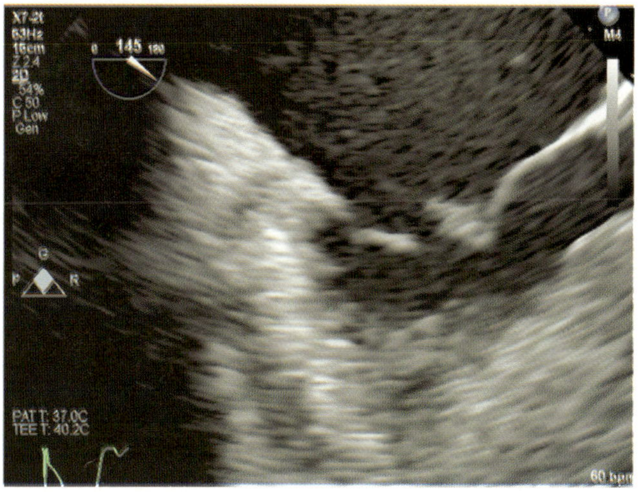

Fig. 6: Immediately postmyectomy of patient with HOCM demonstrating flail A1 segment. (HOCM: hypertrophic obstructive cardiomyopathy)

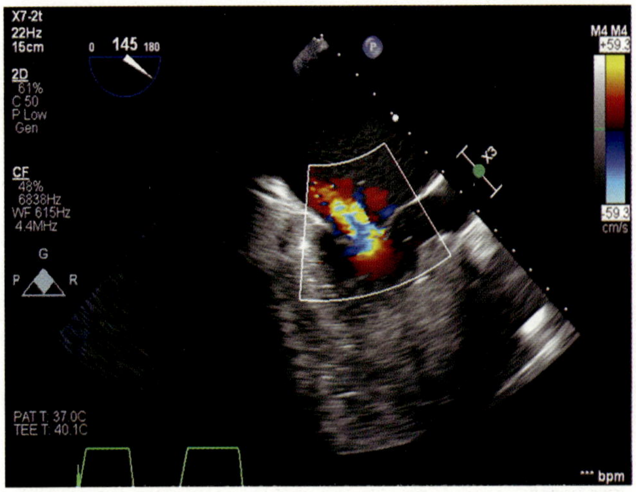

Fig. 7: Immediately postmyectomy of patient with HOCM demonstrating flail A1 segment and severe MR on color Doppler. (HOCM: hypertrophic obstructive cardiomyopathy; MR: mitral regurgitation)

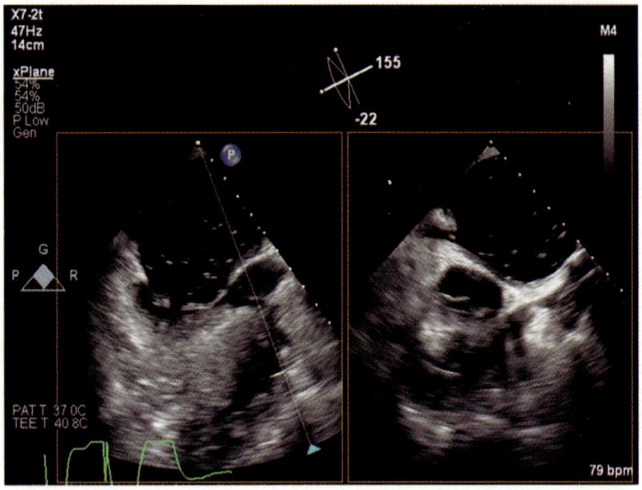

Fig. 9: Immediately postmyectomy of a patient with HOCM demonstrating right coronary cusp prolapse that resulted in severe aortic insufficiency. (HOCM: hypertrophic obstructive cardiomyopathy)

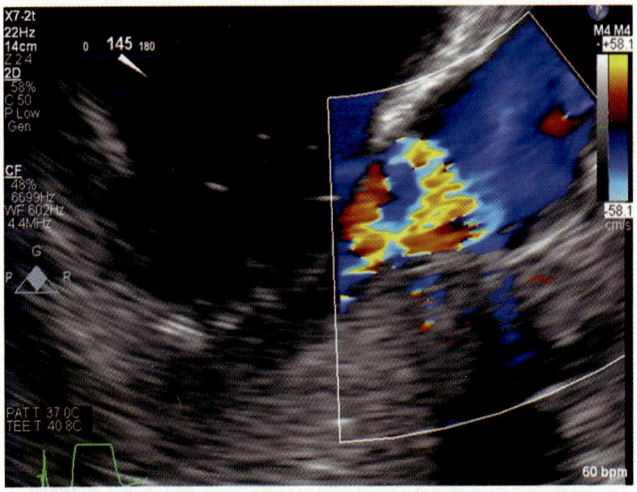

Fig. 8: Immediately postmyectomy of a patient with HOCM demonstrating severe AI on color flow Doppler secondary to right coronary cusp prolapse. (AI: aortic insufficiency; HOCM: hypertrophic obstructive cardiomyopathy)

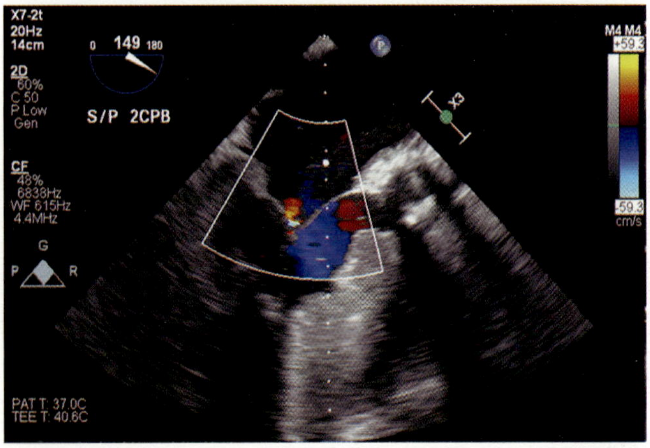

Fig. 10: Patient with HOCM who developed severe MR and severe AI after myectomy status postmitral valve repair and aortic valve replacement with color flow Doppler. (AI: aortic insufficiency; HOCM: hypertrophic obstructive cardiomyopathy; MR: mitral regurgitation)

Hypertrophic Obstructive Cardiomyopathy

Symptomatic hypertrophic cardiomyopathy that is refractory to medical management with demonstrated LVOT obstruction on echocardiographic studies is an indication for invasive management, such as surgical myectomy.[29] Surgical myectomy thins the septum, improving the LVOT, and reduces SAM of the mitral leaflet.[2,3] Prior to myectomy, imaging focused on systolic function and diastolic function, wall-motion abnormalities, the LVOT, and the mitral and subvalvular apparatus (including chordae and papillary muscles). The most recent American College of Cardiology/American Heart Association guidelines recommend IOTEE for intraoperative guidance of surgical myectomy (IB).[29] The transesophageal long-axis and four-chamber views allow the evaluation of the ventricular septum, the contact point between the anterior mitral leaflet and the basal septum, and to ensure no concomitant mitral or subvalvular pathology is present (e.g. the presence of a nonposteriorly directed mitral regurgitant jet or anomalous papillary muscle insertion). Defining these parameters is extremely important for the surgical team, especially to help prevent damage to nearby structures (e.g. bundle of His). The transgastric long-axis view should also be utilized to measure LVOT gradients with continuous-wave Doppler and the short-axis view to better elucidate concentric hypertrophy that may not be

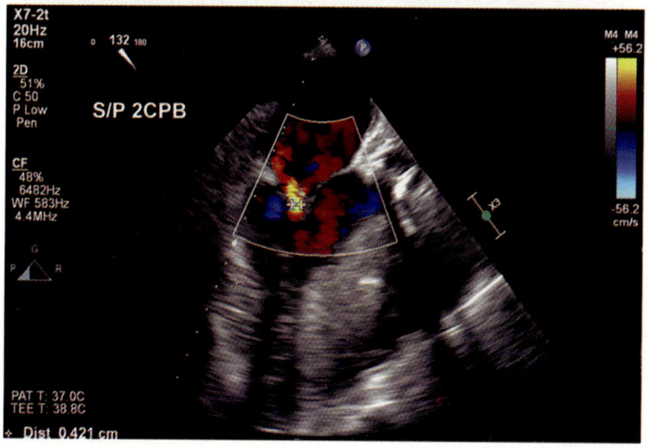

Fig. 11: Patient with HOCM who developed severe MR and severe AI after myectomy status postmitral valve repair and aortic valve replacement with color flow Doppler. (AI: aortic insufficiency; HOCM: hypertrophic obstructive cardiomyopathy; MR: mitral regurgitation)

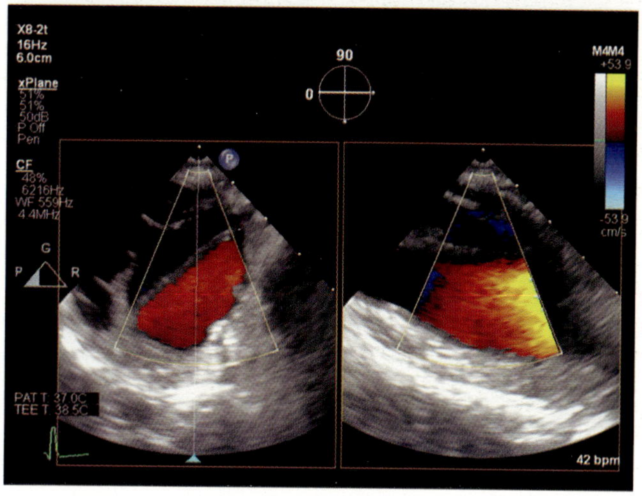

Fig. 13: Aortic dissection (ascending extending to descending) with color flow Doppler differentiating planes.

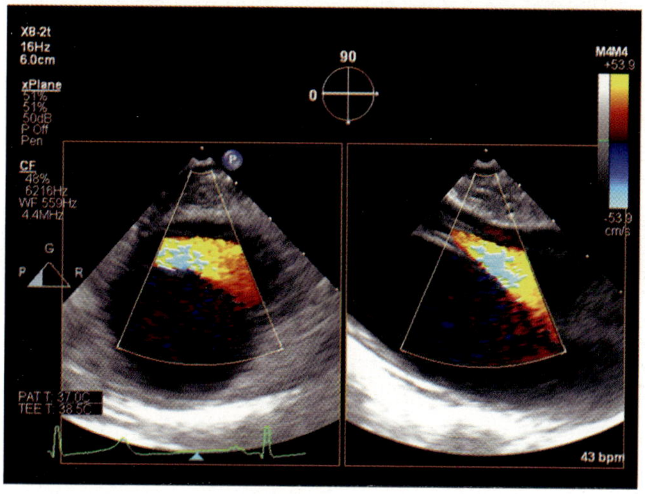

Fig. 12: Aortic dissection (ascending extending to descending) with color flow Doppler differentiating planes.

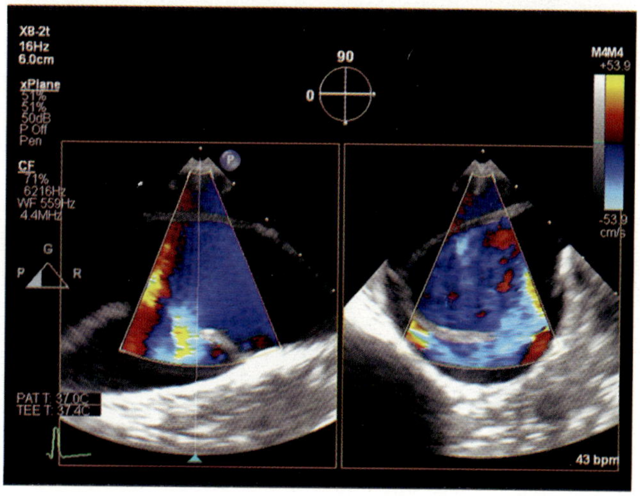

Fig. 14: Aortic dissection (ascending extending to descending) with color flow Doppler differentiating planes.

as well defined from other views.[16-29] At the completion of the resection, all views should be repeated not only to evaluate the LVOT gradient and SAM but also for any new aortic and mitral valve abnormalities (e.g. changes in mitral annulus can result in pathological regurgitation), damage to the interventricular septum or free wall, or abnormalities involving the subvalvular apparatus (Figs. 12 to 17).[2,4,30]

Aortic Dissection and Aortic Atheromas

Acute aortic dissection is the most common life-threatening disorder affecting the aorta.[8] The immediate mortality rate in aortic dissection is as high as 1% per hour over the first several hours, making early diagnosis and treatment critical for survival.[31] TEE is the first choice of imaging modalities to diagnose a suspected aortic dissection with a sensitivity of 86–100%, specificity 90–100%, and negative predictive value 86–100% in diagnosing an aortic dissection.[32-34] The mid and upper esophageal views in the long and short axis allow the best visualization of the aorta. The use of color flow Doppler allows delineation of the true and false lumen. The aortic valve must be evaluated along with the degree of aortic insufficiency to determine the need for replacement, especially in a Type I dissection. Other complications, such as the presence of a pericardial effusion or hemopericardium, branch vessel involvement, wall-motion abnormalities, and signs of rupture should also be excluded.[8] Postoperative IOTEE should be performed

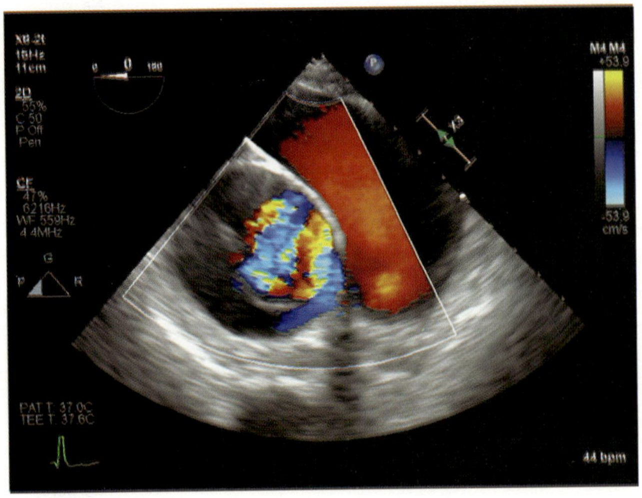

Fig. 15: Aortic dissection (ascending extending to descending) with color flow Doppler differentiating planes.

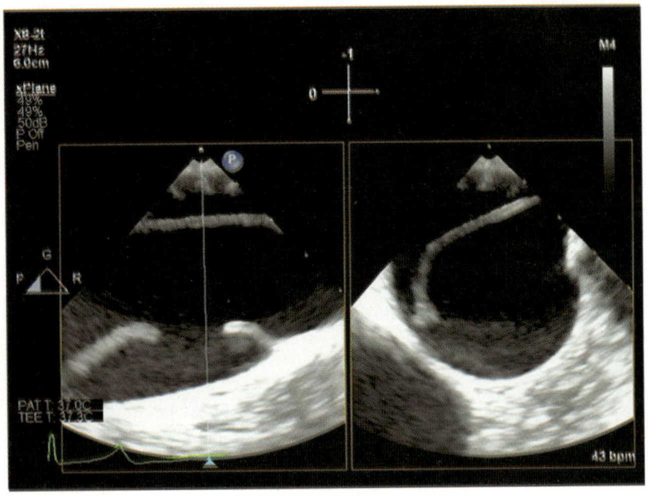

Fig. 17: Aortic dissection (ascending extending to descending) with true and false lumens visible.

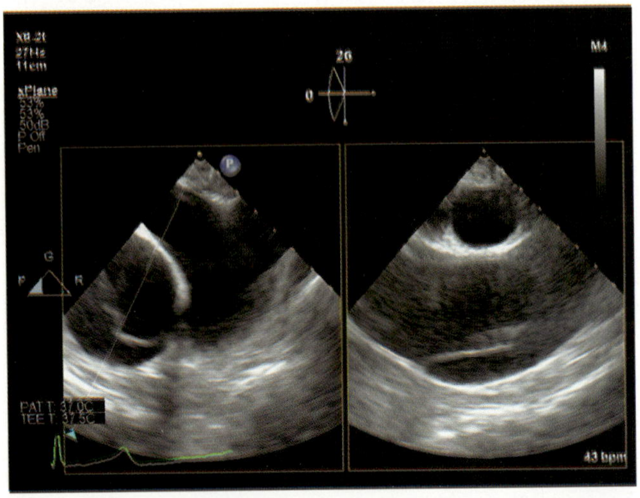

Fig. 16: Aortic dissection (ascending extending to descending) with true and false lumens visible.

to exclude residual aortic insufficiency; assess native or repaired valve function, the integrity of the aortic graft, tube connection to true lumen, and coronary artery attachment to graft tube; and exclude the presence of periaortic hemorrhage. The main limitation of TEE lies in the diagnosis of a Type II dissection and extension of dissection in the proximal portion of the ascending aorta. Positioning of the trachea, linear artifact, and reverberation artifact from the anterior wall of the left atrium can sometimes make the diagnosis of dissection challenging to make.[32]

Transesophageal echocardiogram is recommended prior to all cardiac and thoracic procedures to assess any aortic wall pathology, such as atheromas, aortic plaque complexity, and thrombus formation.[35] Intraoperative TEE can be performed after the induction of anesthesia and prior to sternotomy, and the information obtained used for planning the surgery, and deciding on the safest site of aortic clamping.[36] The assessment of the aorta is so critical that if a TEE cannot be safely performed, a periaortic ultrasound exam should be done instead.

Left Ventricular Assist Devices

Left ventricular assist devices (LVAD) provide mechanical circulatory support in patients with advanced heart failure. TEE plays an integral role in the success of the device from patient selection to long-term follow-up.

A comprehensive TEE is essential to detect atypical or undesirable findings just prior to LVAD placement. Valvular function and other findings must be reassessed due to the possibility of new or missed diagnoses, hemodynamic changes, and progression of disease that could have occurred between the surgery and prior study. Valvular assessment includes the degree of aortic, tricuspid, and pulmonic regurgitation; the presence of mitral valve stenosis; and evaluation of any prosthetic valve, if present.[37] It is recommended that aortic valve regurgitation be assessed while blood pressure is augmented with vasopressor support in order to accurately view the severity of regurgitation that the initial TEE may have underappreciated due to low mean arterial pressures and systemic vascular resistance.[38] Right ventricular function should also be determined, as poor function would indicate the need for biventricular mechanical circulatory support during LVAD placement.[37] Other components to be evaluated are the degree of mitral stenosis, pulmonary regurgitation, prosthetic valve function, presence of a pericardial effusion or vegetations, and the aorta for disease.[38] Intracardiac thrombi must be excluded.[32,39,40]

The presence of a patent foramen ovale or any other type of intracardiac shunt should also be reassessed at the time of surgery as an LVAD has a significant reducing effect on left-sided pressures and can present as new right-to-left shunt associated with hypoxemia.[38] During implantation, inflow and outflow cannula placement should be confirmed visually making sure the inflow cannula is not angled toward the septum or lateral wall.[38] Measurements on TEE can be used to aid in determining initial pump speed.[32] High velocities in the inflow cannula while using Doppler could indicate device thrombus or the cannula being against the ventricular wall. Color Doppler should be used to examine the aortic valve for new or worsening regurgitation and the outflow cannula anastomosis for kinking.[39] The aortic valve should be closely examined to note the function and degree of aortic regurgitation and can be done in M-mode.[37] Chamber size should decrease due to decompression by the device.[40] Other things to note specifically that may require prompt intervention are RV systolic function, RV size, septal shift, and increase in the amount of tricuspid insufficiency.[39]

Transesophageal echocardiogram in the postsurgical patient with an LVAD should evaluate placement and hemodynamics. TEE guidance is essential due to the risk of air trapping on the left side of the heart during coring of the LV apex which is a required step for both the Heartmate II and the Heartware ventricular assist device systems.[40] The left atrium, left ventricle, including the LV apex and inflow cannula, aortic root, ascending aorta, outflow graft-to-ascending aorta anastomosis, and transverse and descending aorta should all be directly visualized to rule out air.[40] Other complications to exclude are presence of a pericardial effusion or hematoma. Hemodynamic assessment using TEE includes determination of LVAD output and total cardiac output; pump speed and degree of offloading on the left ventricle by the LVAD.[37]

Cardiac Emergencies and Surgical Complications

Focused and emergent IOTEE should be considered during surgical emergencies and consists of high yield views—midesophageal four-chamber view (to evaluate biatrial size/filling and function, mitral and tricuspid valves, the LVOT, global RV and LV size/filling and function), the midesophageal long-axis view (to evaluate the aortic valve, the mitral valve, LVOT, RVOT, and portions of the anteroseptal and inferolateral LV walls), and the transgastric LV short-axis view (to evaluate global biventricular size/filling and function, for pericardial effusion, and LV regional wall-motion abnormalities).[21,22,41,42] The midesophageal short axis should also be utilized if the possibility of aortic pathology needs to be ruled out.[21,22,41] Intraoperative TEE during cardiac and noncardiac surgical emergencies should evaluate for volume status, thrombus, presence of air in the left side of the heart (postpump and emboli), global function and size, regional wall-motion abnormalities, wall integrity, valvular abnormalities, foreign objects (including loose suture material), and aortic pathology. The midesophageal short axis should be utilized to evaluate the main pulmonary artery and bifurcation if there is suspicion for pulmonary embolism. Intraoperative TEE in the emergency setting is also useful to guide placement of invasive catheters and support devices.

Myocardial infarction (MI) may present with a variety of complications including regional wall-motion dysfunction, heart failure, shock, valvular dysfunction secondary to ischemic injury to papillary muscles or chordae, aneurysm, pseudoaneurysm, septal or free-wall rupture, pericardial effusion, or pericarditis.[43] Intraoperative TEE can be considered in patients undergoing noncardiac surgery with changes suggestive of myocardial ischemia or infarction (i.e. hemodynamic changes or electrocardiography abnormalities). For patients who have perioperative MI in the context of CABG surgery, IOTEE, especially after coming off-pump or after graft anastomosis is complete, should be utilized to evaluate for sustained wall-motion abnormalities to identify areas of continued ischemia and quality of bypass anastomosis. Complete evaluation of all 16 segments will require midesophageal (four-chamber, two-chamber, and long-axis) and transgastric (mid and basal) views. Color flow Doppler, and ultrasound contrast agents, should be utilized if aneurysmal areas are identified, in order to detect mural thrombus in the post-MI setting. Color flow Doppler is valuable in all post-MI patients with hemodynamic compromise to evaluate for atrial and ventricular septal defects, free-wall rupture, and valvular dysfunction (e.g. to evaluate for ischemia-mediated papillary muscle rupture and subsequent acute mitral regurgitation or ischemia-mediated RV dysfunction and concomitant tricuspid regurgitation).[43,44] In the event of suspected pericardial effusion or tamponade the midesophageal four-chamber and bicaval views allow for evaluation of effusion size and right atrial and ventricular dysfunction. Intraoperative TEE, when used in conjunction with electrocardiographic monitoring and available hemodynamic data, can help diagnosis complications of MI and to guide therapy of potential complications.

DISCUSSION

The use of TEE in the perioperative setting allows for a comprehensive assessment of the cardiac anatomy pre- and postprocedure, including complete characterization of defects and hemodynamic evaluation. Intraoperative TEE facilitates real-time monitoring, evaluation, and decision-making for the entire surgical team and should be utilized in cardiac, thoracic, and selected surgical cases to help improve patient outcomes.

REFERENCES

1. Hahn RT, Abraham T, Adams MS, et al. Guidelines for performing a comprehensive transesophageal echocardiographic examination: recommendations from the American Society of Echocardiography and the Society of Cardiovascular Anesthesiologists. J Am Soc Echocardiogr. 2013;26(9):921-64.
2. Kihara C, Murata K, Wada Y, et al. Impact of intraoperative transesophageal echocardiography in cardiac and thoracic aortic surgery: experience in 1011 cases. J Cardiol. 2009;54:282-8.
3. Eltzschig HK, Rosenberger P, Loffler M, et al. Impact of intraoperative transesophageal echocardiography on surgical decisions in 12,566 patients undergoing cardiac surgery. Ann Thorac Surg. 2008;85:845-52.
4. Tresandí BD, Oyola JC, Gómez I, et al. Impact of intraoperative transesophageal echocardiography in cardiovascular and thoracic surgery: 4AP6-6. EJA. 2011;28:55.
5. American Society of Anesthesiologists and Society of Cardiovascular Anesthesiologists Task Force on Transesophageal Echocardiography. Practice guidelines for perioperative transesophageal echocardiography. An Updated Report by the American Society of Anesthesiologists and the Society of Cardiovascular Anesthesiologists Task Force on Transesophageal Echocardiography. Anesthesiology. 2010;112(5):1084-96.
6. Fayad A, Shillcutt SK. Perioperative transesophageal echocardiography for non-cardiac surgery. Can J Anaesth. 2018;65(4):381-98.
7. Ayres NA, Miller-Hance W, Fyfe DA, et al. Indications and guidelines for performance of transesophageal echocardiography in the patient with pediatric acquired or congenital heart disease. A report from the task force of the Pediatric Council of the American Society of Echocardiography. J Am Soc Echocardiogr. 2005;18:91-8.
8. Hagan PG, Nienaber CA, Isselbacher EM, et al. International Registry of Acute Aortic Dissection (IRAD): new insights from an old disease. JAMA. 2000;283:897-903.
9. Sidebotham DA, Allen SJ, Gerber IL, et al. Intraoperative transesophageal echocardiography for surgical repair of mitral regurgitation. J Am Soc Echocardiogr. 2014;27(4):345-66.
10. Michelena HI, Abel MD, Suri RM, et al. Intraoperative echocardiography in valvular heart disease: an evidence-based appraisal. Mayo Clin Proc. 2010;85(7):646-55.
11. Otto CM. Textbook of Clinical Echocardiography, 5th edition. Philadelphia, PA: Elsevier Health Sciences; 2013.
12. Qizilbash B, Couture P, Denault D. Impact of perioperative transesophageal echocardiography in aortic valve replacement. Semin Cardiothorac Vasc Anesth. 2007;11(4):288-300.
13. Luxford J, Bassin L, D'Ambra M. Echocardiography of the tricuspid valve: acknowledgements. Ann Cardiothorac Surg. 2017;6(3):223.
14. Vegas A. Three-dimensional transesophageal echocardiography: principles and clinical applications. Ann Card Anaesth. 2016;19(Suppl. 1):S35.
15. Rouine-Rapp K, Miller Hance WC. Transesophageal echocardiography for congenital heart disease in the adult. In: Perrino A, Reeves ST (Eds). A Practical Approach to Transesophageal Echocardiography, 2nd edition. Philadelphia: Lippincott Williams and Wilkins; 2008. pp. 387-9.
16. Marelli AJ, Child JS, Perloff JK. Transesophageal echocardiography in congenital heart disease in the adult. Cardio Clin. 1993;11(3):505-20.
17. Navaratham M, Punn R, Tracy TA. Imaging congenital heart disease in the perioperative period using transesophageal echocardiography. J Perioper Echocardiogr. 2014;2(1):10-28.
18. Shapiro LM. Cardiac tumours: diagnosis and management. Heart. 2001;85:218.
19. McAllister HA, Hall RJ, Cooley DA. Tumors of the heart and pericardium. Curr Probl Cardiol. 1999;24:59-116.
20. Walpot J, Shivalkar B, Rodrigus I, et al. Atrial myxomas grow faster than we think. Echocardiography. 2010;27:E128-31.
21. Deegan CA, Griffin MJ. Clinical utility of intraoperative 2D and 3D transesophageal echocardiography in the assessment of a left atrial mass during pneumonectomy. J Cardiothorac Vasc Anesth. 2011;25:833-5.
22. Dujardin KS, Click RL, Oh JK. The role of intraoperative transesophageal echocardiography in patients undergoing cardiac mass removal. J Am Soc Echocardiogr. 2000;13:1080-3.
23. Gersh BJ, Maron BJ, Bonow RO, et al. ACCF/AHA guideline for the diagnosis and treatment of hypertrophic cardiomyopathy: executive summary: a report of the American College of Cardiology Foundation/American Heart Association Task Force on Practice Guidelines. Circulation. 2011;124:2761-96.
24. Smedira NG, Lytle BW, Lever HM, et al. Current effectiveness and risks of isolated septal myectomy for hypertrophic obstructive cardiomyopathy. Ann Thorac Surg. 2008;85:127-33.
25. Grigg LE, Wigle ED, Williams WG, et al. Transesophageal Doppler echocardiography in obstructive hypertrophic cardiomyopathy: clarification of pathophysiology and importance in intraoperative decision making. J Am Coll Cardiol. 1992;20:42-52.
26. Iacovoni A, Spirito P, Simon C, et al. A contemporary European experience with surgical septal myectomy in hypertrophic cardiomyopathy. Eur Heart J. 2012;33:2080-7.
27. Nagueh SF, Bierig SM, Budoff MJ, et al. American Society of Echocardiography clinical recommendations for multimodality cardiovascular imaging of patients with hypertrophic cardiomyopathy: endorsed by the American Society of Nuclear Cardiology, Society for Cardiovascular Magnetic Resonance, and Society of Cardiovascular Computed Tomography. J Am Soc Echocardiogr. 2011;24:473-98.
28. Marwick TH, Stewart WJ, Lever HM, et al. Benefits of intraoperative echocardiography in the surgical management of hypertrophic cardiomyopathy. J Am Coll Cardiol. 1992;20:1066-72.

29. Minakata K, Dearani JA, Nishimura RA, et al. Extended septal myectomy for hypertrophic obstructive cardiomyopathy with anomalous mitral papillary muscles or chordae. J Thorac Cardiovasc Surg. 2004;127:481-9.
30. Brandt RR, Oh JK, Abel MD, et al. Role of emergency intraoperative transesophageal echocardiography. J Am Soc Echocardiogr. 1998;11:972-7.
31. Braverman, Allen C. Acute aortic dissection: a clinician update. Circulation. 2010;122:184-8.
32. Evangelista A, González-Alujas MT, García del Castillo H, et al. Ecocardiografía transesofágicaa en el diagnóstico de la disección aórtica. Rev Esp Cardiol. 1993;46:805-9.
33. Chirrillo F, Cavallini C, Longhini C, et al. Comparative diagnostic value of transesophageal echocardiography and retrograde aortography in the evaluation of thoracic aortic dissection. Am J Cardiol. 1994;74:590-5.
34. Keren A, Kim CB, Hu BS, et al. Accuracy of biplane and multiplane transesophageal echocardiography in diagnosis of typical acute aortic dissection and intramural hematoma. J Am Coll Cardiol. 1996;28:627-36.
35. Jansen Klomp WW, Brandon Bravo Bruinsma GJ, van't Hof AW, et al. Imaging techniques for diagnosis of thoracic aortic atherosclerosis. Int J Vasc Med. 2016;2016:4726094.
36. Vaduganathan, P, Ewton A, Nagueh SF, et al. Pathologic correlates of aortic plaques, thrombi and mobile "aortic debris" imaged in vivo with transesophageal echocardiography. J Am Coll Cardiol. 1997;30:357-63.
37. Stainback RF, Estep JD, Agler DA, et al. Echocardiography in the management of patients with left ventricular assist devices: recommendations from the American Society of Echocardiography. J Am Soc Echocardiogr. 2015;28:853-909.
38. Flores AS, Essandoh M, Yerington GC, et al. Echocardiographic assessment for ventricular assist device placement. J Thorac Dis. 2015;7(12):2139-50.
39. Cohen DG, Thomas JD, Freed BH, et al. Echocardiography and continuous-flow left ventricular assist devices: evidence and limitations. JACC Heart Fail. 2015;3(7):554-64.
40. Ammar, KA, Umland MM, Kramer C, et al. The ABCs of left ventricular assist device echocardiography: a systematic approach. Eur Heart J Cardiovasc Imaging. 2012;13:885-99.
41. Reeves ST, Finley AC, Skubas NJ, et al. Special article: basic perioperative transesophageal echocardiography examination: a consensus statement of the American Society of Echocardiography and the Society of Cardiovascular Anesthesiologists. Anesth Analg. 2013;117:543-58.
42. Shillcutt SK, Markin NW, Montzingo CR, et al. Use of rapid "rescue" perioperative echocardiography to improve outcomes after hemodynamic instability in noncardiac surgical patients. J Cardiothorac Vasc Anesth. 2012;26:362-70.
43. White HD, Chew DP. Acute myocardial infarction. Lancet. 2008;372:570-84.
44. Katsnelson Y, Raman J, Katsnelson F, et al. Current state of intraoperative echocardiography. Echocardiography. 2003;20:771-80.

134

CHAPTER

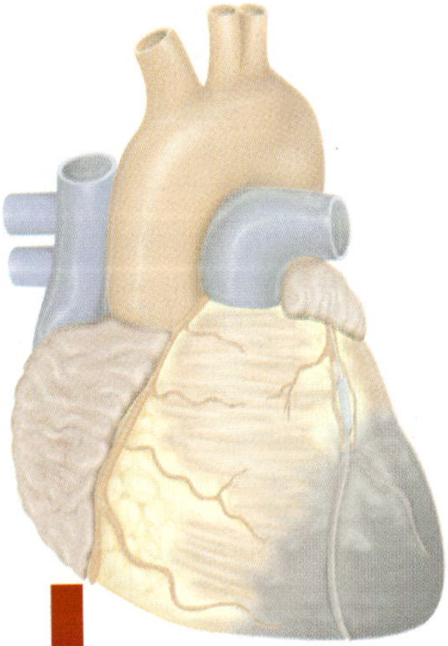

Echocardiographic Imaging in Operation Theater

Naman Shastri

INTRODUCTION

The introduction of transesophageal echocardiography (TEE) in the operating room (OR) represented a great advancement in cardiovascular monitoring and is routinely used in several cardiac surgery centers. Intraoperative echocardiography is used for diagnosis, to guide the surgical procedure, to assess immediate results, to detect complications, and to monitor left ventricular function. The usage has increased not only to the cardiac surgical operation theater but also to the noncardiac surgery very regularly in recent years. Obtaining real-time information allows the surgeon to correct inadequate repairs and prevent or treat surgical complications before the patient leaves the operating room, therefore reducing the need of reoperations.

IMPORTANT ROLE IN MODERN CARDIAC SURGERY

Several reports have shown the positive impact of using this technique in defining surgical strategy, assessment of operative results, and orientation of anesthetic management.[1] Minhaj et al.,[2] through a prospective clinical investigation of 283 patients undergoing cardiac surgeries, observed that the routine use of TEE revealed new pathologic findings (previously unidentified) in one in every three patients, and in 25% of the cases, it led to a change in surgical approach. So, intraoperative echocardiography is not only particularly useful in valvular disease but is also routinely used during aortic surgery, hypertrophic cardiomyopathy, off-pump bypass, maze procedure, congenital heart disease, etc. Intraoperative echocardiography gives an excellent opportunity for the interaction between the cardiologist or anesthesiologists and the surgeon that translate in better patient care.

Indications for intraoperative echocardiography (Table 1) are accepted worldwide and now all major centers follow those indications.

ECHOCARDIOGRAPHIC TECHNIQUE IN OPERATION THEATER

There are two basic modalities of intraoperative echocardiography: (1) epicardial and (2) transesophageal. Transesophageal echocardiography is the most commonly used technique because cardiologists and anesthesiologists are more familiar with this technique and also because it does not interfere with the operative field and offer excellent visualization of posterior structures. Epicardial echocardiography is used more often in the evaluation of atherosclerosis of the ascending aorta or in the cases where it is not possible to introduce the TEE probe (i.e. esophageal pathology). It requires placing a high-frequency probe in the surface of the heart, therefore interfering with the surgical field and also increasing the potential for contamination. It is of critical importance to understand that the hemodynamic conditions in the OR are very different with preload and afterload affected by anesthesia and volume status. This may affect the degree of regurgitant lesion and often is necessary to increase the blood pressure

TABLE 1: Summary of indications for intraoperative echocardiography.

Class I	*Classes IIa and IIb*	*Class III*
Acute hemodynamic instability of unknown etiology	Risk of myocardial ischemia/infarction/ hemodynamic changes	Catheter placement (IABP, PAC)
Valvular repair	Valvular exchange/Maze surgery	
Congenital cardiopathies that require surgeries with ECC	Aneurysms and cardiac tumors/thrombi/ foreign body	Repair of other cardiomyopathies
Repair of hypertrophic cardiomyopathy	Detection of air embolism/Evaluation of myocardial perfusion	Surgical repair of noncomplicated ostio secundum IAC
Endocarditis Ross surgery	Evaluation of aortic atheromatous plaques Evaluation of pericardiectomy/pulmonary embolectomy	Monitoring of embolism in orthopedic surgeries
Aortic aneurysms and dissections with suspicion of aortic insufficiency	Aortic aneurysms and dissections without suspicion of aortic insufficiency	
Evaluation for pericardia! procedures (pericardia! window)	Cardiac trauma	
Implantation of circulatory assistance devices	Heart transplants	

ECC: extracorporeal circulation; IABP: intra-aortic balloon pump; PAC: pulmonary artery catheter.
Revista Brasileira de Anestesiologia Vol. 61 , N24, July-August, 2011

with the use of vasopressors. Possibly, the most important aspect in the use of intraoperative echocardiography is the interaction between the cardiologist, anesthesiologist, and the surgeon. The surgeon expects instant feedback of the echocardiography findings, but he/she must recognize that in many instances, it is necessary to use multiple views for optimal assessment of the lesions.

CARE FOR PROBE INSERTION IN OPERATION ROOM

Once the decision of using intraoperative TEE is made, it is possible to proceed with inserting the probe into the digestive tract shortly after tracheal intubation and correct fixation of the endotracheal tube. However, to provide better image quality, gastric contents should be aspirated with a gastric tube. Other care should also be taken before insertion of the TEE probe to achieve better safety: the probe should be inspected for structural integrity and cleanliness, controls should be unlocked, and a bit blocker should not be forgotten in order to avoid dental damage and injuries to the tongue or mouth gum. The probe should be lubricated with a hydrosoluble gel before insertion. Sometimes, decision is taken to inert the probe during the surgery when there is no practice to inert the probe at the time of induction of anesthesia. The probe should be gently introduced through the posterior oropharynx, without perception of greater resistance, being careful to position the transducer elements anteriorly. Occasionally, a lower jaw traction maneuver is necessary and, in the cases of greater difficulty and resistance, insertion may require the aid of a laryngoscope. In some cases, a hyperinflated tracheal tube balloon can hinder its passage; particularly, in the case of pediatric cardiac surgery, utmost care is necessary to inert and remove the probe to avoid accidental extubation or accidental migration of the tube in bronchus.

Patient Interactions

An explanation of the echocardiographic procedure including the indications, risks, and benefits should be provided to every patient and/or legal guardian whenever possible (i.e. elective procedures). It is also recommended that informed consent, in which the specific risks and benefits to the patient from the procedure are discussed with the patient before the examination, is obtained and documented in the patient's chart, either separately or as a part of the general anesthetic consent.

Performance and Interpretation Time

No minimal time has been established to perform a comprehensive evaluation; however, initial study time may last 10–45 minutes, including time for discussion between cardiologists, surgeons, and anesthesiologists. A verbal report must be provided throughout and, in particular, at the completion of the initial examination to both the surgical and anesthesia care teams.

Comprehensive versus Limited Perioperative Examination

A limited intraoperative TEE examination may also be warranted after a request to determine the cause of acute hemodynamic compromise, such as during an intraoperative cardiac arrest.

VALVULAR HEART DISEASE

The assessment of valvular heart disease constitutes the classical indication of the use of intraoperative echocardiography. This allows exquisite definition of the anatomy of the mitral and aortic valves, presence and severity of stenosis or regurgitation, mechanism of the regurgitant lesions, and associated abnormalities.

MITRAL VALVE DISEASE AND INTERPRETATION

Indications for Mitral Valve Repair and Timing of Intervention

The American College of Cardiology/American Heart Association Task Force on Practice Guidelines in Valvular Heart Disease recommends that patients with functional class II symptoms or higher and severe mitral regurgitation (MR) and asymptomatic patients with severe MR and echocardiographic evidence of left ventricular (LV) dysfunction (LV end-systolic dimension ≥45 mm, ejection fraction ≤0.60) undergo repair. When a successful repair is probable, the weight of evidence favors surgical intervention in asymptomatic patients with severe MR and normal LV function.[3] There are currently no widely accepted criteria for establishing which patients should undergo mitral valve (MV) repair. The feasibility of repair depends on the anatomic lesions of the valve and the skill of the surgeon. The advantages of mitral repair over mitral replacement include the preservation of LV function through preservation of the chordal attachments, low rates of thromboembolism, the lack of a requirement for anticoagulants (beyond aspirin), and excellent durability. Given the excellent long-term results of modern mitral repair techniques, the threshold for surgical intervention has been appreciably lowered. With the development of standardized techniques for MV reconstruction, Deloche et al.[4] demonstrated that MV repair was feasible in 95% of the patients with degenerative valve disease, 70% with rheumatic valve disease, and 75% with ischemic valve disease. The long-term results after MV repair were excellent, with very low rates of thromboembolism, reoperation, and valve-related mortality. Echocardiographic follow-up analysis revealed no or mild MR in 92% of the patients.

ASSESSMENT OF THE PATIENT FOR MITRAL VALVE REPAIR

What We Should be Looking in Preoperative Echocardiography Findings!

Preoperative transthoracic echocardiographic (TTE) imaging often provides satisfactory information regarding the degree of MR or mitral stenosis (MS), annular size, involvement of anterior or posterior leaflets, chordal and papillary muscle structural integrity, and overall LV size and LV systolic function. In the absence of satisfactory TTE images, TEE provides improved visualization of MV pathology. Figure 1 shows a standard view to asses MV by TEE.

To evaluate the MV apparatus with two-dimensional (2D) TEE, the standard views shown in Figure 1 are necessary.

Intraoperative Transesophageal Echocardiographic Evaluation of Mitral Valve

A detailed intraoperative TEE evaluation of the mitral apparatus is critical for planning surgery, assessing results, and predicting the long-term durability of the MV repair. Along with the MV assessment, a complete evaluation of the heart and great vessels by intraoperative TEE is critical because incidental findings [severe atherosclerotic aortic disease, undiagnosed aortic insufficiency, regional wall motion abnormalities suggestive of ischemia, left atrial (LA) thrombus, intracardiac masses] often significantly affect surgical planning.

For evaluation of MR, commonly Carpentier classification of leaflet motion is used worldwide (Fig. 2).

Assessment of Structural Analysis of Mitral Valve

In the prerepair period, TEE should evaluate (1) the MV apparatus, (2) the function of the MV leaflets and pathological segments, (3) the severity of MR under general anesthesia, (4) the potential risk factors for the surgical repair, and (5) the correct placement of the cannulas used for cardiopulmonary bypass (CPB). The assessment of mitral repair must include the degree of MR or MS, the specific location of prolapsing or flail leaflet segments, areas of tethering and restriction, and areas of normal leaflet function. Leaflets should also be assessed for perforations, calcifications, excessive length, thickened appearance, and mobility. Annular calcification (the most common posteriorly) should be noted. The subvalvular apparatus is assessed for chordal thickening and for papillary muscle

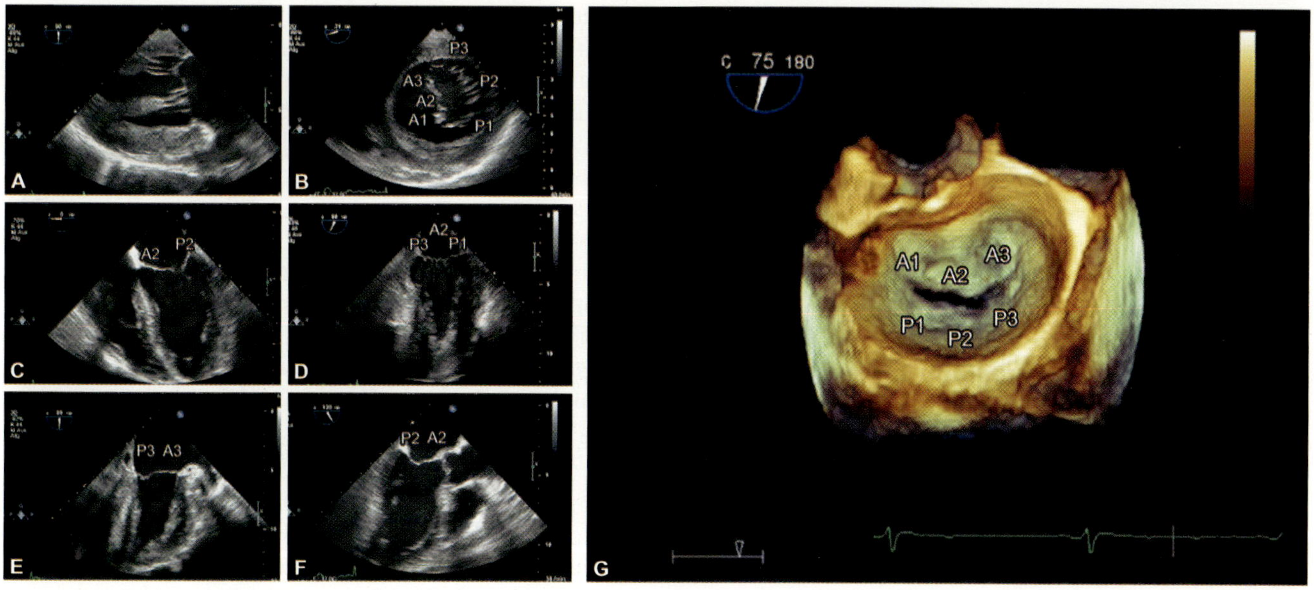

Figs. 1A to G: Standard view to assess mitral valve by TEE. (A) Transgastric two chamber; (B) Transgastric basal short axis; (C) ME four chamber; (D) Bicommissural view; (E) ME two chamber; and (F) ME long axis; (G) 3D en face view of mitral valve by 3D echocardiography. (3D: three-dimensional; ME: midesophageal; TEE: transesophageal echocardiography)
Source: Revista Brasieira de Anestesiologia Vol 61, No. 4, July-August, 2011

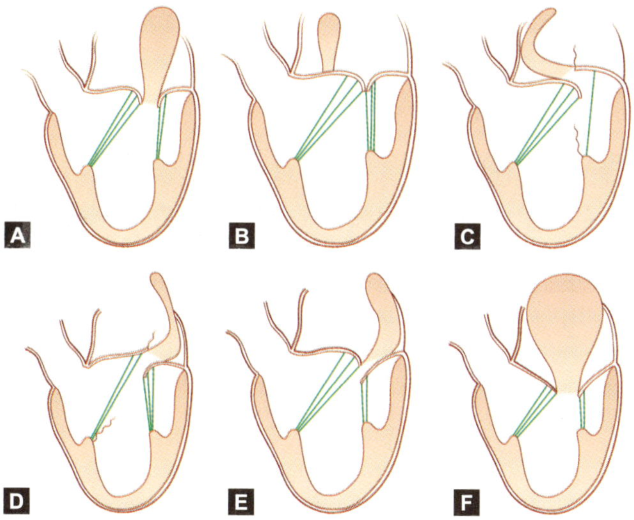

Figs. 2A to F: Carpentier classification of leaflet motion. (A) Type I, normal leaflet motion, depicted here with annular dilation and central MR jet; (B) Type I, normal leaflet motion with leaflet perforation; (C) Type II, flail of posterior leaflet, depicted here secondary to ruptured marginal chordae. The MR jet is directed anteriorly; (D) Type II, flail of anterior leaflet, depicted here secondary to ruptured marginal chordae. The MR jet is directed posteriorly; (E) Type III, restricted leaflet motion. The posterior leaflet and also anterior leaflet many times like in rheumatic pathology are depicted here as restricted, causing a "relative prolapse" of the anterior leaflet. The MR jet is directed posteriorly; and (F) Types I and III, restricted leaflet motion, depicted here in a dilated failing heart. Annular dilation (type I) and leaflet restriction secondary to downward displacement of the papillary muscle heads (type III) commonly coexist in this condition (ischemic MR). (MR: mitral regurgitant)

and ventricular wall function. Robust secondary chordae, which may be suitable for transposition to prolapsed leaflets, can often be identified by TEE.

So, basically we are looking for the MV structural indices and they measured in the length, such as anterior and posterior leaflet height, length of the mitral annulus, and coaptation area and height. *Because the goal of the intraoperative TEE examination before repair is to evaluate the function of the MV, it is critical to evaluate the valve in a hemodynamic state comparable to that of the awake, ambulatory patient. The use of inotropes or vasopressors may be necessary to achieve this end.* The secondary effects of the valvular disease, including LA enlargement with or without thrombus, and the size and function of the left and right ventricles should be discussed with the surgeon.

Isolated Anterior Leaflet Prolapse: "Respect, Less Resect"

Resection is not a reliable approach for the larger anterior leaflet, except for repair of a very small, focal prolapsing area by a triangular resection. The prolapsing anterior leaflet can be repaired by means of chordal transfer, artificial chordal replacement, or chordal-shortening techniques. Chordal transfer involves transferring robust chords either from a secondary position on the anterior leaflet or from an adjacent posterior leaflet edge (the latter requiring a quadrangular resection, as described earlier). Artificial chords (Gore-Tex) can be placed from the papillary muscle head to the leaflet edge. A major challenge is adjusting the length of the chords, often by judging adjacent, nonprolapsing leaflet segments.

Isolated P2 Prolapse

The P2 segment is resected from scallop to scallop in a quadrangular fashion. Intact chordae are detached from the papillary muscles (a robust, intact chord may be preserved to repair another prolapsing segment). The annulus is plicated with a horizontal mattress suture, and direct approximation of the leaflet edges is undertaken.

Bileaflet Prolapse

In the cases of prolapse of both the anterior and posterior leaflets, a systematic approach combining quadrangular resection with chordal transposition, shortening, or replacement is required. If there is a dominant posterior prolapse with a myxomatous, prolapsing anterior leaflet, isolated quadrangular resection with ring annuloplasty can be satisfactory.

Papillary Muscle Rupture

The posteromedial papillary muscle is most often affected (75% of the cases) because the coronary circulation to the inferior wall is not redundant. A single ruptured papillary head can be reimplanted in adjacent endocardium. In the cases with extensive necrosis of the papillary muscle and adjacent myocardium, an MV replacement with preservation of the remaining intact chords should be carried out.

Potential Risk Factors for Surgical Repair

Secondary SAM (systolic anterior motion of mitral leaflets) is a complication virtually unique to MV repair. The postoperative incidence is reported to range between 1% and 16%. Systolic anterior motion can be diagnosed as minor chordal protrusion in the left ventricular outflow tract (LVOT) to life-threatening LVOT obstruction with MR. In the mechanism of SAM/LVOT obstruction (LVOTO), it is multifactorial, the major cause being excess mitral leaflet tissue (as in the "floppy MV" of myxomatous disease). Anteriorly displaced papillary muscles, a nondilated LV, and a narrow mitral-aortic angle have also been proposed as contributing factors. The incidence of SAM/LVOTO after MV repair has been shown to increase in patients with a more anterior position of the leaflet coaptation point. This may be the consequence of a relatively large posterior leaflet, shifting coaptation closer to the base of the anterior leaflet and causing both the anterior displacement of the coaptation line and an increase in the amount of slack leaflet tissue in the outflow tract. An elongated anterior leaflet may cause a similar increase in the amount of slack leaflet available to obstruct LV outflow.

Preoperative TEE [midesophageal (ME) aortic valve short-axis view] structural and geometric factors like the anterior-to-posterior-leaflet-height ratio (<1.4), the absolute height of the posterior leaflet (>1.5 cm), and the minimum distance from the coaptation point to the septum (C-Sept, <2.5 cm) can be used as predictors of LVOT obstruction and SAM.[5] Distortion of the circumflex artery, due to sutures necessary to fix the annuloplasty ring during MV repair, occurs in up to 1.8% of the patients. With TEE, it is possible to visualize the circumflex artery in most of the patients undergoing MV repair.[6] The comparison between pre- and postoperative assessment of the circumflex artery helps to identify patients with compromised circumflex artery as early as possible after MV repair and should therefore be a part of the routine examination.[7]

Repair of Ischemic Mitral Regurgitation

Although mitral repair is demonstrably superior to replacement for nonischemic MR, the issue remains unresolved for ischemic MR because of the heterogeneity of this patient population. For example, Duarte et al.[8] reported very good 10-year survival in patients with 3+ MR treated with coronary artery bypass grafting alone, whereas Cohn et al.[9] reported better survival with replacement (with chordal preservation) than with repair.

Special Situations

Rheumatic Pathology

Mitral leaflet tissue can display varying degrees of thickening and calcium deposition that cause the MV leaflets to appear "enhanced", or echo-bright. The standard ME views (four-chamber, commissural, two-chamber, and long-axis) assist in evaluating the extent of disease. The chordal tendons can display varying degrees of thickening and contracture. The transgastric (TG) long-axis imaging plane provides the best information with regard to the extent of subvalvular involvement in the rheumatic process. The characteristic 2D echocardiographic findings associated with rheumatic MS are represented in rheumatic heart disease, which results in varying degrees of restricted mitral leaflet motion. In 2D TEE, restricted leaflet motion is characterized by decreased leaflet excursion and by diastolic "doming" of the anterior mitral leaflet. The appearance of "doming" is the result of fusion of the anterior and posterior leaflets along the medial and lateral commissures. The leaflets are restricted or abnormally stenotic at the tips, which demonstrate the characteristic "doming" or "hockey stick" deformity of the anterior mitral leaflet in diastole.

Because of the low-flow state, LA spontaneous echocardiography contrast or thrombus formation may be present. Left atrial spontaneous echocardiography contrast is useful in identifying those patients with MS who are at increased risk for thromboembolic events.

Transesophageal echocardiography (TEE) is more sensitive than transthoracic echocardiography in detecting LA spontaneous echocardiography contrast. Echocardiography cardiographer can discuss with surgeon to occlude the LA appendage by transfixing it.

Degenerative Pathology (Fig. 3)

Specifically, a distinction between Barlow disease and fibroelastic deficiency should be sought by the echocardiographer. Although both cause leaflet prolapse, there are key distinguishing features between these two degenerative diseases. Barlow disease is typically diagnosed in young adulthood, and patients are often under long follow-up before developing an indication for surgery, often during the fourth or fifth decade of life. The most common lesions are chordal elongation, tall leaflets with excess tissue, and very large annular size (Fig. 3B). Calcification can occur in the annulus or anterior papillary muscle. Billowing of the leaflet (in which the body of the leaflet rises above the annular plane due to excess tissue and elongation of intermediary chords) should be differentiated from prolapse of the margin (i.e. flail), with the latter used to differentiate single from bileaflet involvement (Fig. 3B).

The timing of the regurgitant jet can help differentiate the lesions in Barlow disease (if the regurgitant jet occurs in mid-to-late systole, it is usually due to chordal elongation as opposed to chordal rupture, which tends to cause holosystolic regurgitation). In contrast, fibroelastic deficiency results from a connective tissue deficiency rather than an excess of myxomatous tissue. Leaflets are generally thin and translucent, and chordae are thin, sparse, and deficient. Patients most commonly present in the sixth decade of life with relatively short histories of MV disease and severe holosystolic type II regurgitation that results from a ruptured chord or chords, usually involving a single segment of the valve (Fig. 3A). Although the affected segment may demonstrate myxomatous changes in the chronic setting, the remainder of the valve is small with normal leaflet height. Figure 2 illustrates the distinction (lesion and dysfunction) between these two forms of degenerative disease.

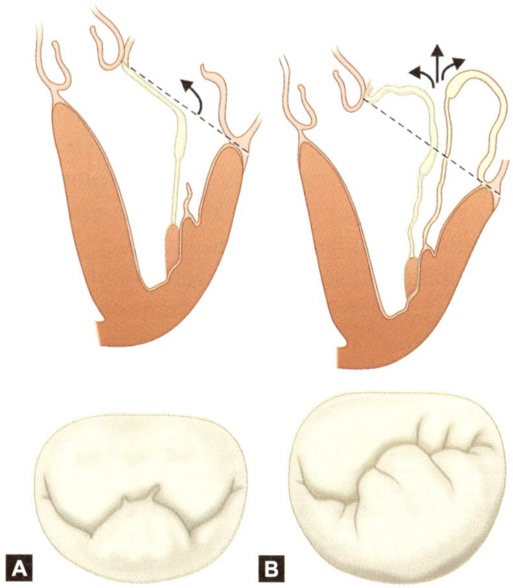

Figs. 3A and B: Degenerative pathology of mitral valve. (A) Fibroelastic disease; and (B) Myxomatous degeneration.

Postdegenerative Mitral Valve Repair (Fig. 3)

The depth of coaptation should be documented and be at least 5 mm in a 2D long-axis view to ensure the adequacy of coaptation. It is important to perform a segmental assessment to rule out regurgitation along any aspect of the coaptation surface, including the commissures. If a residual leak is identified, the lesions responsible and the residual dysfunction should be sought. Common causes of a residual leak include uncorrected segmental prolapse or restriction, a residual-restricted leaflet indentation, an incorrectly sized or positioned ring that distorts the coaptation zone, a perforation of the leaflet from an annuloplasty suture, or a defect in a leaflet closure line. Any significant degree of MV regurgitation (other than trivial to mild regurgitation) should prompt a return to CPB and valve reexploration to correct residual or new defects. This strategy is imperative to avoid a heightened risk of reoperation in the patient early during follow-up, as there is a correlation between residual MR and early reoperation. It is becoming increasingly clear that multisegment disease with excess tissue, typical of Barlow disease, is most appropriately referred to "mitral superspecialists" to optimize the repair rate in this most complex subgroup of degenerative MV regurgitation. Many patients receive unnecessary valve replacements because the echocardiogram has not been considered in surgical referral and operative planning. Given that current national repair rates generally approximate less than 60% of the operated patients, despite the guideline recommendations for valve reconstruction in all degenerative valves when feasible. By systematic documentation of segmental echocardiographic findings, it is easy to predict whether the repair would be simple or one that requires specialized surgical techniques. For example, whereas an isolated P2 prolapse secondary to a chordal rupture from fibroelastic deficiency can be repaired with high probability by most cardiac surgeons, a posterior leaflet prolapse with tall leaflets secondary to Barlow disease can only be consistently repaired in an MV reference center.

Possibility of repair by European Association of Echocardiography recommendations for the assessment of valvular regurgitation is listed in Table 2.

TABLE 2: Possibility of repair by European Association of Echocardiography recommendations for the assessment of valvular regurgitation.

Etiology	*Dysfunction*	*Calcification*	*Mitral annulus dilatation*	*Probability of repair*
Degenerative	II: Localized prolapse (P2 and/or A2)	No/localized	Mild/moderate	Feasible
Ischemic/functional	I or IIIb	No	Moderate	Feasible
Barlow	II: Extensive prolapse (≥3 scallops, posterior commissure)	Localized (annulus)	Moderate	Difficult
Rheumatic	IIIa but pliable anterior leaflet	Localized	Moderate	Difficult
Severe Barlow	II: Extensive prolapse (≥3 scallops, anterior commissure)	Extensive (annulus + leaflets)	Severe	Unlikely
Endocarditis	II: Prolapse but destructive lesions	No	No/mild	Unlikely
Rheumatic	IIIa but stiff anterior leaflet	Extensive (annulus + leaflets)	Moderate/severe	Unlikely
Ischemic/functional	IIIb but severe valvular deformation	No	No or severe	Unlikely

Evaluation of Repair in Operation Theater

Intraoperative TEE is mandatory for all MV repairs. It permits evaluation of immediate functional results: residual MR, reoperation factors, SAM, and other complications such as LV dysfunction, circumflex injury, aortic cusp stitch, or atrial septal defect. Residual MR is an unacceptable result except for mild and central regurgitation due to leaflet irregularities. Beyond severity, the objective of the echocardiography is to determine the precise mechanism and particularly to identify leaflet jet and segmental analysis; real-time 3D color TEE has a clear superiority over 2D analysis for this purpose. Immediately following MV repair, there are several important aspects of the MV anatomy, which must be addressed by the imager. Of course, the most critical aspect of postoperative valve analysis is to confirm the absence of significant residual MR. The depth of coaptation should be documented and be at least 5 mm in a 2D long-axis view to ensure the adequacy of coaptation.

It is important to perform a segmental assessment to rule out residual regurgitation along any aspect of the coaptation surface, including the commissures. If a residual leak is identified, the lesions responsible (such as a leaflet cleft or perforation) and the residual dysfunction (such as leaflet restriction or prolapse) should be sought and reported in a segmental fashion. Common causes of a residual leak include uncorrected segmental prolapse or restriction, a residual-restricted leaflet indentation, an incorrectly sized or positioned ring that distorts the zone of coaptation, leaflet perforation of the leaflet from an annuloplasty suture, or a defect in a leaflet closure line. Any significant degree of MV regurgitation (other than trivial to mild regurgitation) should usually prompt a return to CPB and subsequent valve reexploration to correct residual or new defects. This strategy is imperative to avoid a heightened risk of reoperation in the patient early during the follow-up, as there is a correlation between residual MR and early reoperation. Systolic anterior motion of the anterior mitral leaflet is a phenomenon almost unique to MV repair, resulting from a mismatch of annular septolateral dimension and the residual combined leaflet height. Typically, the margin of the anterior leaflet is displaced into the outflow tract, causing both a significant outflow tract gradient as well as varying degrees of mitral insufficiency. The best echocardiographic view to interrogate this is the ME long-axis view. In some circumstances, volume loading and increasing the ventricular afterload reposition the anterior leaflet minimizing the outflow tract gradient and valve regurgitation. If such maneuvers are not successful, valve reexploration, with the placement of a larger ring, leaflet height shortening, or even valve replacement, is required.

AORTIC VALVE PATHOLOGY AND EVALUATION FOR REPAIR IN OPERATION THEATER (FIG. 4)

Because of the oblique orientation of the aortic valve, a multiplanar assessment of the valve is helpful in order to correctly align the valve plane with the ultrasonic beam. With TTE, this requires imaging from multiple echocardiography windows, the preferred views being the parasternal long-axis and short-axis views. With TEE, one should combine the ME aortic valve long-axis and short-axis views, the TG, and the deep TG long-axis views to obtain a complete assessment of aortic valve morphology and analysis of the mechanism of aortic regurgitation (AR). It should be noted that from both the TTE parasternal view and the TEE ME view, only the coaptation between the right coronary cusp anteriorly and either the non- or left coronary cusp (depending on probe rotation) posteriorly can be measured. Clockwise rotation with TEE identifies coaptation between the right coronary and the noncoronary cusps, whereas counterclockwise rotation permits evaluation of coaptation between right and left coronary cusps. Normal values for length of apposition are more than 4–5 mm and for coaptation height is 4–10 mm (which normally projects into the middle of the sinuses of Valsalva). In this view, color-flow imaging enables not only the analysis of the origin but most importantly the orientation of the regurgitant jet. Midesophageal long-axis TEE view shows the aortic valve and root in end-diastole. Measurements are made at the level of the aortic annulus,[1] the sinuses of Valsalva,[2] and the sinotubular junction.[3] The length of cusp apposition (Fig. 4A) at the effective height (Fig. 4B) can also be measured.

Assessment of Aortic Regurgitation Severity during Surgery

The color jet area and length are unsatisfactory measures of the severity of AR because of their load-dependence and are not recommended. They are nonetheless helpful in the identification of the mechanisms of AR; for example, eccentric jets being often associated with aortic cusp prolapse or perforation. The diameter and the cross-sectional areas of the color-flow jet at its origin are better indices of AR severity. The maximum color jet diameter (width) is measured in diastole immediately below the aortic valve (at the junction of the LVOT and aortic annulus) in the parasternal long-axis view. The jet width is reasonably proportional to the size of the regurgitant orifice. Yet, if the orifice is irregular, as in bicuspid valves, the color jet width is less related to the degree of regurgitation. The accuracy of this method can be improved by dividing the jet width by the LVOT diameter. The cross-sectional areas of the jet from the parasternal short-axis view and its ratio to the LVOT area are also indicators of AR severity. Although these measurements suffer from a high interobserver variability, a jet-width ratio more than 65% is a strong argument for severe AR.

The functional classification of AR and management is given in Table 3.

Echocardiographic Prediction of "Repairability"

Unless severely calcified, most types 1 and 2 AR lesions are considered as "repairable", i.e. amenable to some form of conservative surgery, including valve sparing surgery, cusp repair, or a combination thereof. In moderately calcified valves (grade 3), the localization of the calcifications is taken into account. Whenever these calcifications are confined to the free margins, aortic repair is considered to be feasible. By contrast, when the calcifications

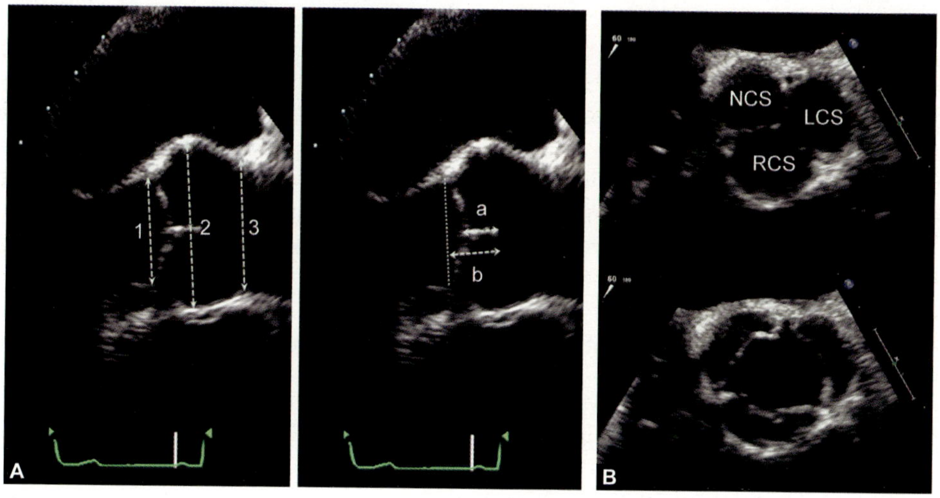

Figs. 4A and B: Normal values for length of apposition is more than 4–5 mm and for coaptation height is 4–10 mm (which normally projects into the middle of the sinuses of Valsalva).
(NCS: non-coronary sinus; LCS: left coronary sinus; RCS: right coronary sinus)

TABLE 3: Aortic regurgitation lesions and management (EL Khaury G,op.card 2005).

	Type I Normal cusp motion with FAA dilatation or cusp perforation				*Type II Cusp prolapse*	*Type III Cusp restriction*
AI class	*Ia*	*Ib*	*Ic*	*Id*		
Mechanism	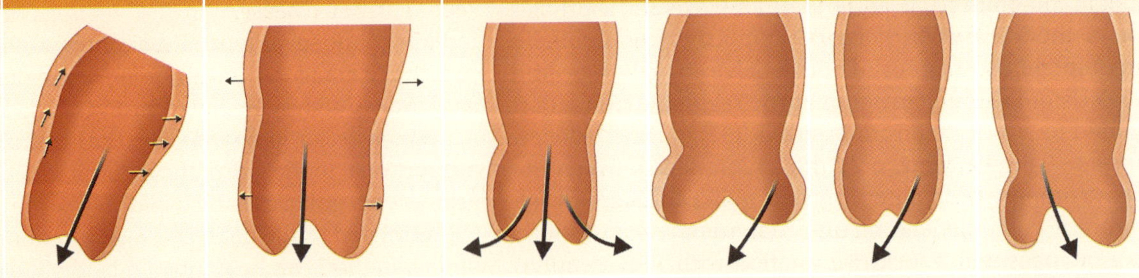					
Repair techniques (primary)	STJ remodeling *Ascending aortic graft*	Aortic valve *sparing: or remodeling with SCA*	SCA	Patch repair *Autologous or bovine pericardium*	Prolapse repair *Plication Triangular resection Free margin Resuspension Patch*	Leaflet repair *Shaving Decalciffication Patch*
(Secondary)	SCA		STJ annuloplasty	SCA	SCA	SCA

(STJ: sinotubular junction; SCA: subcommissural aortic annuloplasty)

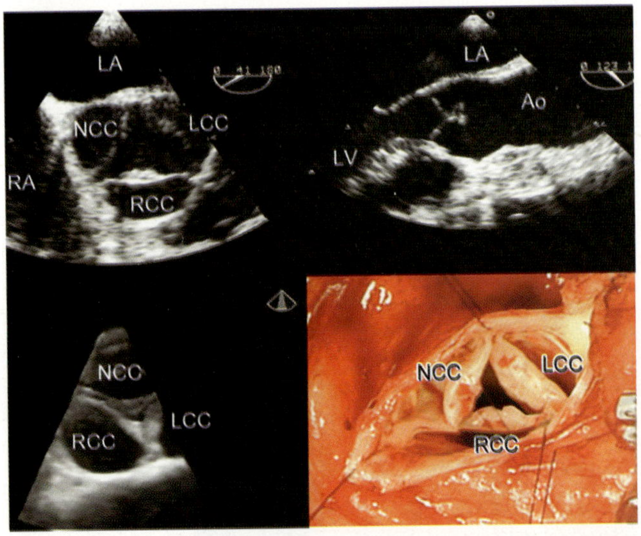

Fig. 5: Calcifications involved the body of the cusp, the valve is considered as nonrepairable.
(LA: left artery; LCC: left coronary cusp; LV: left rentricle; AO: aorta; NCC: non-coronary cusp; RCC: right coronary cusp)

involved the body of the cusp, the valve is considered as nonrepairable (Fig. 5). Finally, type 3 lesions are considered as nonrepairable.

As with any valve repair procedure, one of the primary roles of TEE is the immediate evaluation of the quality of valve repair. The expected postoperative result is an aortic valve that opens well and is competent without any residual insufficiency.

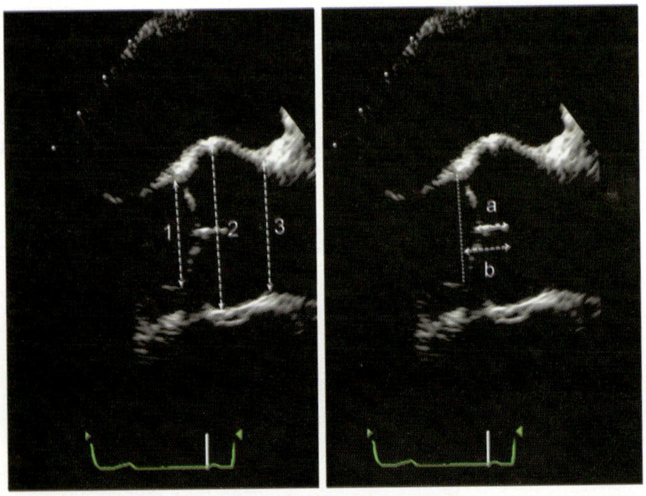

Fig. 6: Coaptation is less than 4 mm, it is associated with a 30–40% chance of recurrent severe AR. (AR: aortic regurgitation)

Algorithm for Assessing Aortic Valve Repair (Fig. 6)

This is based on a retrospective analysis of intraoperative echocardiographic data, incorporating functional and morphological features measured immediately after weaning from cardiopulmonary bypass. First, the level of cusp coaptation should occur above the aortic annulus. If cusp coaptation occurs below the aortic annulus, the risk of recurrent AR is more than 70%. Ideally, the height of coaptation should be more than 9 mm and reach the middle of the sinus of Valsalva. Second, the presence of any residual AR should be evaluated. If there is no residual AR and if coaptation is above the aortic annulus, recurrent AR is very unlikely. Finally, in patients with coaptation above the aortic annulus but who have residual AR, the length of cusp apposition should be measured. If this is less than 4 mm, it is associated with a 30–40% chance of recurrent severe AR in the follow-up.

TRICUSPID REGURGITATION

Pathophysiology of Tricuspid Regurgitation (Fig. 7)

The normal tricuspid regurgitation (TR) diameter, as measured by echocardiography in the four-chamber view between the base of the septal and the base of the lateral TV leaflets, is 2.8–0.5 cm. In addition, annular dilation and not pulmonary hypertension, RV dilation, or tricuspid tenting is the best determinant of functional TR. Reduced tricuspid annular shortening, encountered in patients with severe tricuspid annular dilation and RV dysfunction, also determines TR severity. Interestingly, in patients with chronic pulmonary thromboembolic hypertension in whom TR resolved after pulmonary thromboendarterectomy and

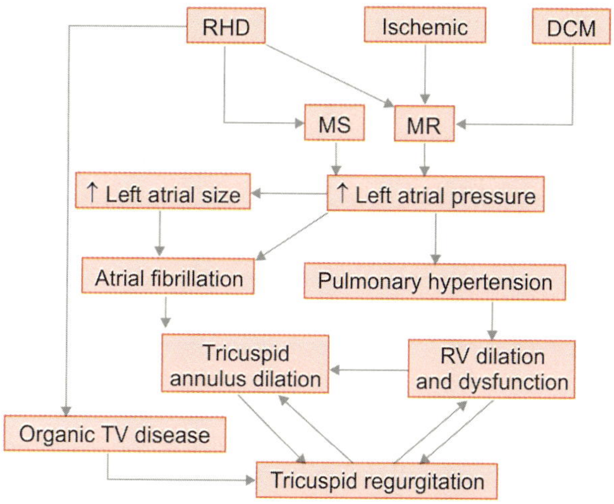

Fig. 7: Pathophysiology of TR. (TR: tricuspid regurgitation; RHD: rheumatic heart disease; DCM: dilated cardiomyopathy; MR: mitral regurgitation; MS: mitral stenosis; RV: right ventricular; TV: tricuspid valve)

in patients who had successful mitral balloon valvotomy, there was no change in TA diameter after the resolution of pulmonary hypertension. This implies that TA dilation might be irreversible and might explain the mechanism of late TR in MV disease.

Midesophageal four-chamber view (Fig. 8) indicates the position of the tricuspid annulus in diastole (Fig. 8A) and systole (Fig. 8B). These form the basis of calculation of the tricuspid annular plane systolic excursion ratio.

Infective Endocarditis and Intraoperative Echocardiography (Fig. 9)

Transesophageal echocardiography enhances the sensitivity of TTE to about 85–90% for the diagnosis of vegetations, while more than 90% specificity has been reported for both the TTE and TEE. The second major echocardiographic criterion for endocarditis is the presence of a perivalvular abscess. The infectious process may rapidly extend to form or worsen abscess and/or fistulous tracts or to involve other valves. Thus, a prepump TEE in the operative room allows a final evaluation of valvular and perivalvular lesions. This exam may provide new data on the extent of the infectious process and valve reparability and therefore confirm or modify the operative plan.

Prosthetic Valve Evaluation

Normal Backflow Patterns

A small amount of regurgitation is normally observed in all mechanical prosthetic valves and in approximately 10% of the bioprosthetic valves. *Closure backflow* is the reversal of flow required for closure of the valve. In contrast, *leakage backflow* occurs after the closure of mechanical valves and originates from the hinges and the regions of coaptation between the occluders and the valve ring. Physiologic regurgitation jets are small and short in duration. The leakage backflow patterns for each valve type are unique and distinct from pathologic regurgitation.

Paravalvular Regurgitation in Operation Theater

Paravalvular regurgitant jets imaged with color Doppler flow originate outside the sewing ring, characteristically track along the walls of the receiving chamber (Fig. 9), and usually produce zones of flow acceleration adjacent to the site of regurgitation in the chamber proximal to the prosthetic valve. Dehiscence of part of the sewing ring may destabilize the prosthetic valve, producing a "rocking" motion of the entire prosthesis and a visible separation of the native and prosthetic valve annulus on 2D imaging (Fig. 10).

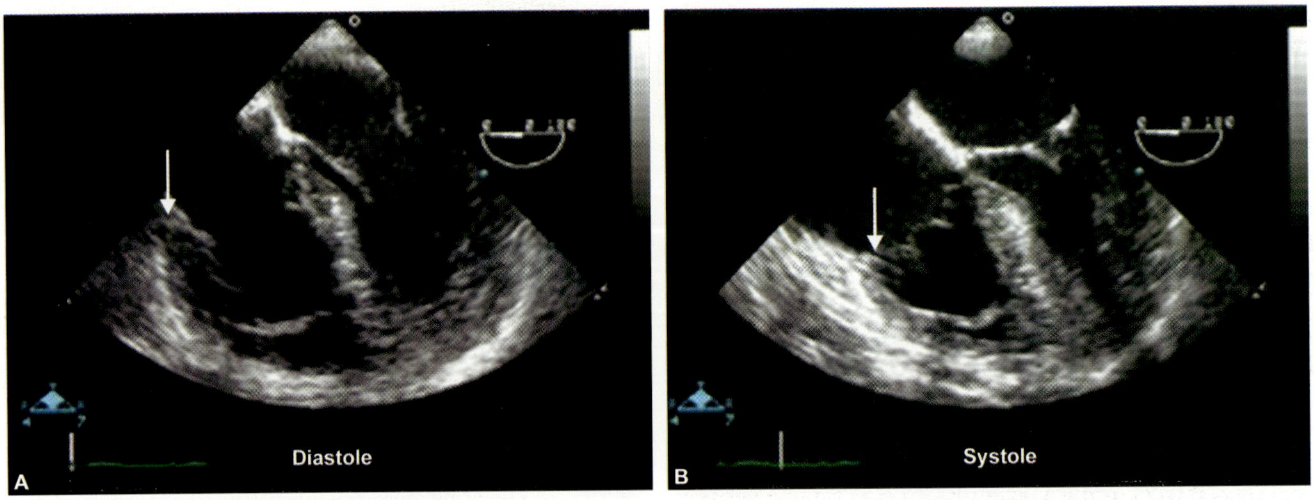

Figs. 8A and B: Midesophageal four-chamber view for measuring annulus dilatation.

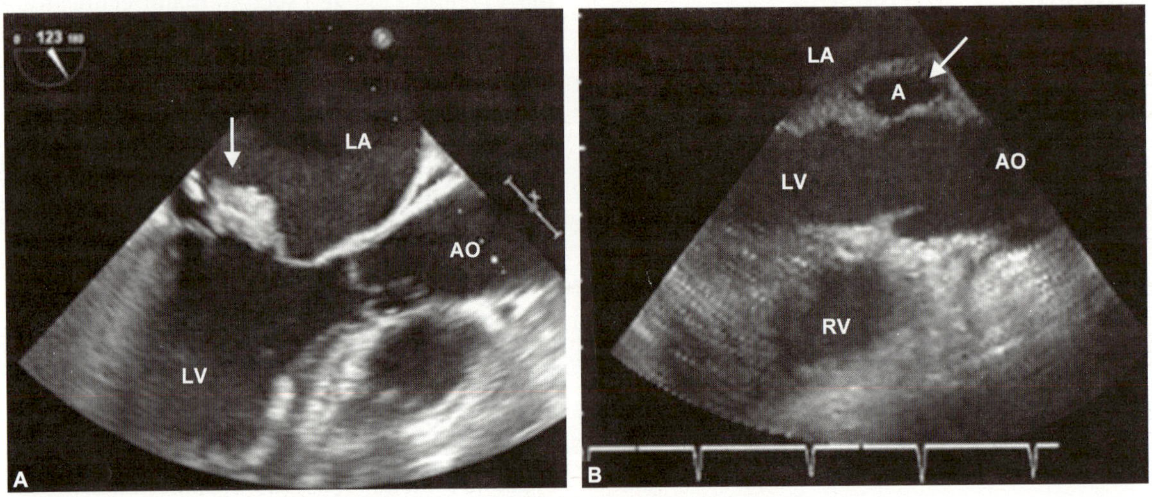

Figs. 9A and B: Vegetation seen on anterior mitral leaflet.

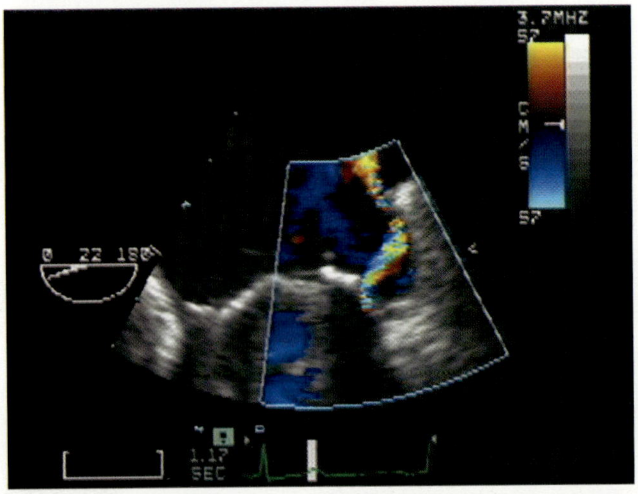

Fig. 10: Color Doppler flow originate outside the sewing ring.

PATHOLOGY OF AORTA AND ROLE OF TEE IN OT FOR ACUTE AORTIC SYNDROME

Intimal Tear Location

Two-dimensional echocardiography does not permit visualization of the intimal tear in the proximal part of the arch. In these cases, color Doppler may be helpful by showing a turbulent jet directed toward the false lumen. Using pulsed Doppler, it can be verified that the flow velocity at the tear is usually below 1.5 m/s and the flow goes from the true to the false lumen in systole. In diastole, the velocity is lower and the flow usually goes from the false to the true lumen.

Arterial branch involvement: Diagnosis of involvement of the main arterial vessels of the aorta is important as it may explain some of the symptoms or visceral complications.

The right brachiocephalic trunk is one of the arterial branches most frequently affected. Transesophageal echocardiography is not a good technique for assessing supra-aortic branch involvement. Usually, multiplanar probes, sensitivity, specificity, and accuracy in the diagnosis of supra-aortic trunks were 60%, 85%, and 78%, respectively. Transthoracic echocardiographic visualized the carotid artery and left subclavian artery in 92% of the cases and the right brachiocephalic trunk in 62%. Involvement of coronary arteries in dissection has been considered to be 10–15%, with the right coronary artery being the most frequently affected TEE permits assessment of the most proximal segment of the coronary arteries; thus, it can be verified whether the coronary ostium originates in the false lumen.

MINIMALLY INVASIVE CARDIAC SURGERY AND ECHOCARDIOGRAPHY IN OPERATION THEATER

Minimally invasive cardiac surgery (MICS) is gaining the popularity in cardiac surgery. Minimal incision and minimal anatomic disruption of the body tissues give better cosmetic results and provide psychological comfort to the patients. Patients are always afraid of the consequences of the surgery. Minimally invasive cardiac surgery reduces the duration of convalescence and allows patients to resume activities earlier and thus may reduce the fear of surgery.

Normally, following are the reasons for TEE evaluation during the MICS:

- Evaluation of cardiac pathology to see the possibilities of MICS
- Placing the cannula under small incision for both the venous drainage and arterial return
- Inserting coronary sinus cannula for ensuring infusion of proper cardioplegic solution
- Postsurgical procedure evaluation of the result.

"WANING-OFF CARDIOPULMONARY BYPASS" WITH THE HELP OF TRANSESOPHAGEAL ECHOCARDIOGRAPHY

Transesophageal echocardiography can be utilized to stabilize patient while discontinuing Cardiopulmonary bypass (CPB) at the time of cardiac surgery. General used flowchart for management is shown in Flowchart 1.

Flowchart 1: Flowchart of managing difficult separation from CPB. (CPB: cardiopulmonary bypass)

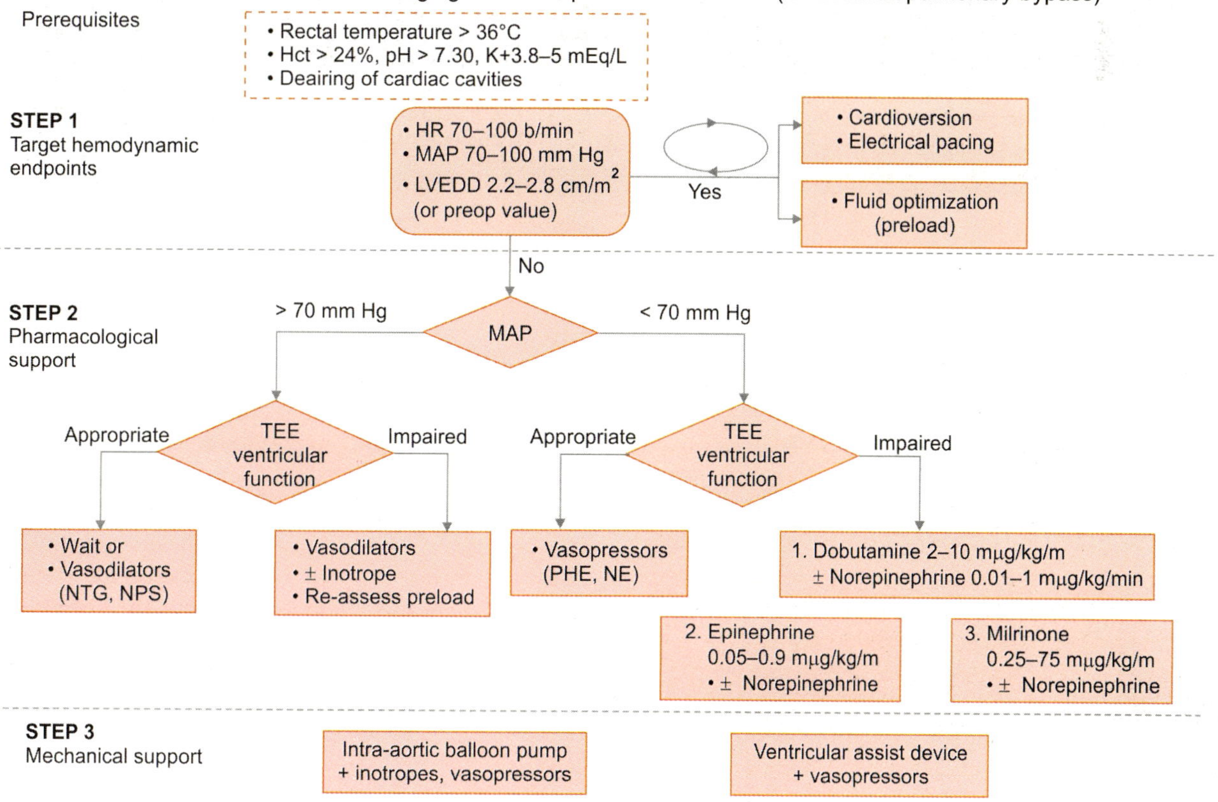

HCT: hematocrit; HR: heart rate, MAP: mean arterial pressure, LVEDD: left ventricular end-diastolic diameter, TEE: transesophageal echocardiography, NTG: nitroglycerine, NPS: nitroprussiate, PHE: phenylephrine

EPICARDIAL ECHOCARDIOGRAPHY IN OPERATION THEATER

More than a decade before the introduction of TEE, epicardial echocardiography was already in use as a diagnostic imaging modality to assist cardiac surgeons, anesthesiologists, and cardiologists with clinical decision-making.

Compared to TEE, epicardial echocardiography and epiaortic ultrasonography are unique in requiring a collaborative effort with the cardiac surgeon to either allow the echocardiographer to guide them in obtaining images or alternatively permit the echocardiographer to have direct access to the epicardial or epiaortic surface within the operative field. In addition, experience in epicardial echocardiography is considered an important component of advanced, rather than basic, perioperative echocardiographic training. Despite its overwhelming popularity and favorable influence on perioperative clinical decision-making and outcomes, the TEE approach to a comprehensive echocardiographic examination has some limitations. Transesophageal echocardiographic imaging of the distal ascending aorta and aortic arch may be impaired by the interposition of the trachea and main bronchi.

In addition, a TEE probe may occasionally be difficult or impossible to advance into the esophagus or in patients with significant gastroesophageal pathology.

REFERENCES

1. Eltzschig HK, Rosenberger P, Loffler M, et al. Impact of intraoperative transesophageal echocardiography on surgical decisions in 12,566 patients undergoing cardiac surgery. Ann Thorac Surg. 2008;85:845-52.
2. Minhaj M, Patel K, Muzic D, et al. The effect of routine intraoperative transesophageal echocardiography on surgical management. J Cardiothorac Vasc Anesth. 2007;21:800-4.
3. Bonow RO, Carabello B, De Leon AC, et al. ACC/AHA guidelines for the management of patients with valvular heart disease: executive summary. A report of the American College of Cardiology/American Heart Association Task Force on Practice Guidelines (Committee on Management of Patients with Valvular Heart Disease). J Heart Valve Dis. 1998;7:672-707.
4. Deloche A, Jebara VA, Relland JY, et al. Valve repair with Carpentier techniques. J Thorac Cardiovasc Surg. 1990;99:990-1002.
5. Maslow AD, Regan MM, Haering JM, et al. Echocardiographic predictors of left ventricular outflow tract obstruction and systolic anterior motion of the mitral valve after mitral valve reconstruction for myxomatous valve disease. J Am Coll Cardiol. 1999;34:2096-104.
6. Aybek T, Risteski P, Miskovic A, et al. Seven years' experience with suture annuloplasty for mitral valve repair. J Thorac Cardiovasc Surg. 2006;131:99-106.
7. Ender J, Gummert J, Fassl J, et al. Ligation or distortion of the right circumflex artery during minimal invasive mitral valve repair detected by transesophageal echocardiography. J Am Soc Echocardiogr. 2008;21:408.e4-5.
8. Duarte IG, Shen Y, MacDonald MJ, et al. Treatment of moderate mitral regurgitation and coronary disease by coronary bypass alone: late results. Ann Thorac Surg. 1999;68:426-30.
9. Cohn LH, Rizzo RJ, Adams DH, et al. The effect of pathophysiology on the surgical treatment of ischemic mitral regurgitation: operative and late risks of repair versus replacement. Eur J Cardiothorac Surg. 1995;9:568-74.

SECTION 32

Surgery and Imaging

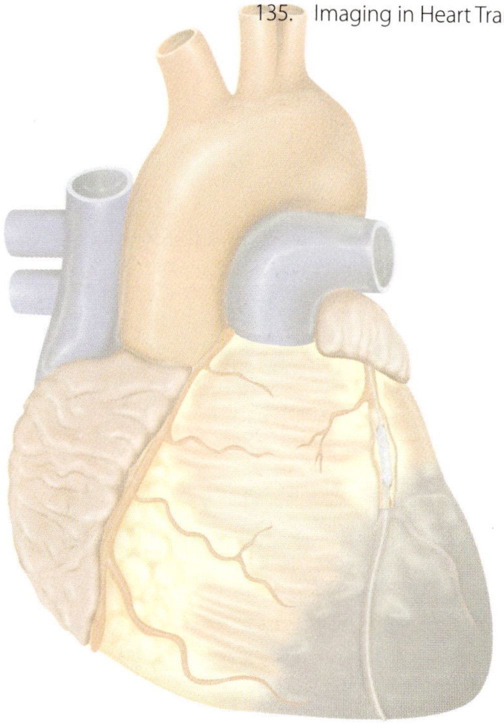

135

CHAPTER

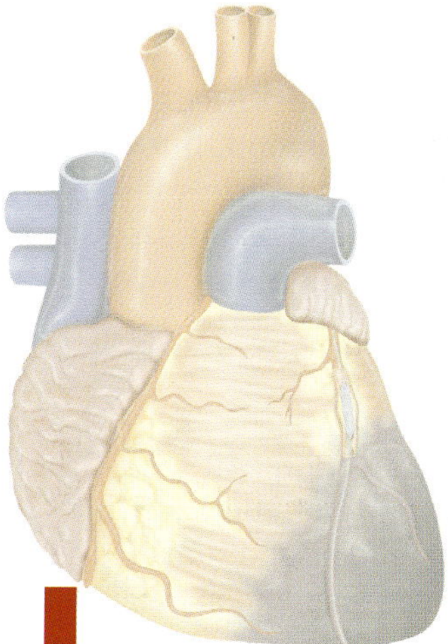

Imaging in Heart Transplant

Kewal Krishan, Reena Anand, Rajneesh Malhotra

INTRODUCTION

Heart failure (HF) is a complex clinical syndrome that can result from any structural or functional cardiac disorder that impairs the ability of the ventricle to fill with or eject blood. The cardinal manifestations of HF are dyspnea and fatigue, which may limit exercise tolerance, and fluid retention. Despite widespread use of evidence-based therapies, the morbidity and mortality of HF are still high. It remains the most common hospital discharge diagnosis for patients older than 65 years. The gold standard treatment for end-stage HF is heart transplant (HT). The alternative treatment is ventricular assist device (VAD) placement. The field of cardiac imaging and the management of patients with severe HF have advanced substantially during the past 10 years. Cardiac transplantation offers the best long-term survival with high quality of life for the patients with end-stage HF. However, acute cardiac rejection and cardiac allograft vasculopathy (CAV) can occur after cardiac transplantation and these problems necessitate regular surveillance. The short-term success of mechanical circulatory support devices, such as VADs, in improving survival and quality of life has led to a dramatic growth of the patient population with these devices. The development of optimal imaging techniques and algorithms to evaluate these advanced HF patients is evolving and multimodality noninvasive imaging approaches, and invasive techniques are commonly employed. So Imaging is playing great role in preoperative assessment, postoperative care, and follow-up.

PREOPERATIVE IMAGING

Chest Radiograph

To screen for contraindications to transplantation such as active infection or neoplasm, primarily pulmonary infection, and lung cancer, because either disease may progress in the post-transplant patient because of immunosuppression.

Computed Tomography

To identify conditions that might make transplantation more difficult or increase the chances of surgical complications, such as mediastinal fibrosis or adhesions from previous coronary artery bypass surgery. Anatomic variants or diseases of the thoracic great vessels, such as thoracic aorta aneurysms or dissection, and anomalies of the aorta, pulmonary artery, or vena cava should be identified, because the aorta, pulmonary artery, and cava will serve as anastomotic sites between the donor and recipient.

Cardiac Magnetic Resonance Imaging

Noninvasive and reproducible assessment of cardiac anatomy, deformation and function, perfusion, viability, and if required metabolism and tissue characterization without radiation exposure for the patients.

Evaluation of cardiac magnetic resonance imaging (CMR) parameters is useful for the prediction of outcomes in HT recipients. In this regard, myocardial scar assessed by late gadolinium enhancement and right ventricular end-diastolic volume index were independently associated with cardiac death and hospitalization due to cardiac symptoms.

Coronary Angiography

Coronary angiography (CA) is not routinely used in the workup of cardiac transplant donors or recipients but is used when there is suspected coronary artery disease.

POSTOPERATIVE IMAGING

It is usually done as routine investigations or to rule out any disease process. Common complications of cardiac transplantation include infection, rejection, accelerated coronary artery atherosclerosis, and lymphoproliferative disease.

Complication Directly Related to Cardiac Transplant

1. Infection—most common—pneumonia (aspergillus, CMV, *Pseudomonas*)
2. Acute allograft rejection—cardiomegaly may be demonstrated on chest X-ray but is neither specific nor sensitive
3. Accelerated graft atherosclerosis—CA and intracoronary sonography are methods currently used
4. Malignancy—prevalence is 100 times greater than that to general population. Most frequently observed is squamous cell carcinomas of skin, adenoma of lung and GIT, Kaposi's sarcoma, and acute leukemia and lymphoma.

Complications Related to Cardiothoracic Surgery

1. Chest wall and mediastinal complications
   a. *Acute mediastinitis*:
      i. Mediastinal widening, pneumomediastinum, obliteration of fat planes, localized fluid collections, and abscess formation
2. Aortic dissection and pseudoaneursym
3. Thromboembolism.

Following imaging are usually done after cardiac transplant other than routine chest X-ray:

- Echocardiography
- CT
- MRI

Techniques of echocardiography, CT, MRI, and nuclear cardiology have all progressed rapidly in recent years. There is thus a knowledge gap for cardiologists, radiologists, and clinicians, especially regarding the surveillance for CAV and ideal imaging approaches for patients with transplant. The purpose of this chapter is to provide an overview of different noninvasive imaging modalities used to evaluate the patients after cardiac transplantation. It focuses on the role of echocardiography, CT, and nuclear imaging in surveillance for CAV and rejection and on the assessment of ventricular structure and function and myocardial remodeling.

Role of Echocardiography

Close surveillance for acute rejection (AR) and CAV is essential for graft and patient survival.[1] Because CAV can arise and progress without symptoms and subclinical ARs can facilitate CAV development, standard surveillance of AR and CAV is based on routine endomyocardial biopsies (EMBs) and CAs performed at predefined time intervals. These invasive screening tests can be quite distressing for patients, yet they cannot identify all subclinical ARs or coronary stenoses prior to a clinical event. Additional close-meshed noninvasive surveillance strategies are therefore mandatory.

After the introduction of Doppler tissue-imaging (DTI) and strain-imaging for myocardial wall motion and deformation analysis, echocardiography became more promising for post-transplant patient surveillance because these techniques that allow quantification of minor myocardial dysfunction not detectable by standard echocardiography appeared particularly suited for early detection of subclinical AR and CAV.[2] The chapter summarizes the knowledge and clinical experience on the usefulness of echocardiography including DTI and strain-imaging for AR and CAV surveillance.

Computed Tomography Scan

Since the first successful cardiac transplantation performed in 1967, over one lac such operations have been recorded by the Registry of the International Society for Heart and Lung Transplantation. Cardiac transplantation is the currently accepted treatment for end-stage cardiomyopathy and has 1- and 5-year survival rates of 79% and 63%, respectively. Improvements in immunosuppression techniques and the widespread use of EMB to diagnose rejection account for most of the improvement in early survival rates. Infection and rejection remain significant causes of morbidity and death despite improvements in immunosuppression techniques with the most common complications of cardiac transplantation being infection, rejection, accelerated coronary artery atherosclerosis, and post-transplantation lymphoproliferative disease.

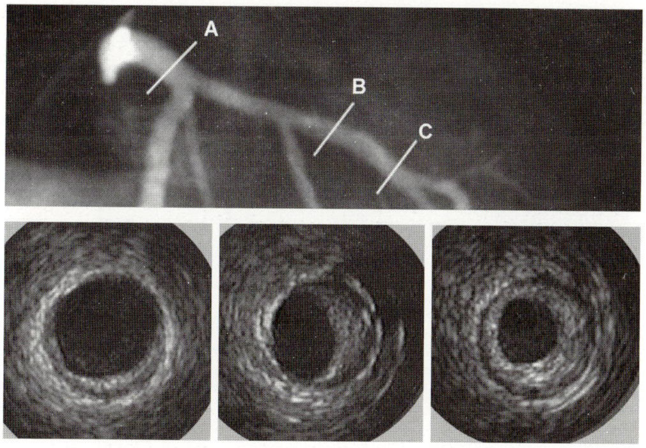

Fig. 1: CT and intravascular ultrasound of cardiac allograft vasculopathy imaging. (CT: computed tomography)

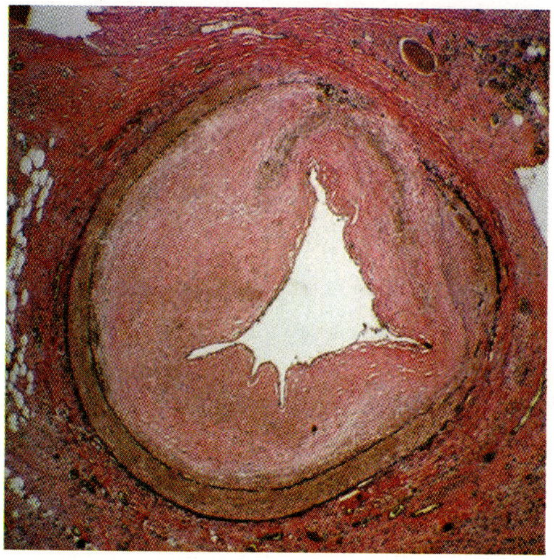

Fig. 2: Microscopic view of cardiac allograft vasculopathy.

With the emergence of heart transplantation as the ultimate treatment for end-stage HF, new diagnostic challenges have arisen. Computed tomography helps detect infectious, hemorrhagic, and cerebral complications in the early postoperative phase and allows accurate assessment of infectious, neoplastic, and allograft coronary disease in later postoperative years. The CT is now the diagnostic modality of choice for many transplant-related complications because it allows accurate assessment of some of the most daunting sequelae and may thus help improve patient treatment after heart transplantation.

Role of Magnetic Resonance Imaging

Cardiovascular imaging can contribute to noninvasively detecting and to evaluating both acute and chronic allograft rejection after heart transplantation, in particular, cardiovascular MRI (CMRI), and how CMRI can assess

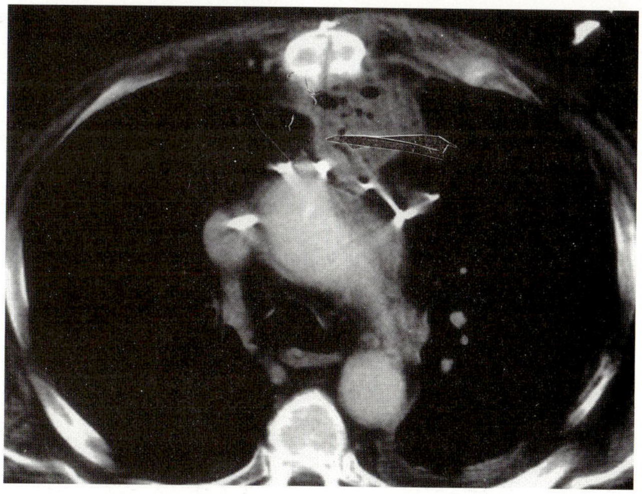

Fig. 3: CT chest showing mediastinal abscess after heart transplant. (CT: computed tomography)

both immune cell infiltration at the rejecting organ, and the cardiac dysfunctions resulting from allograft rejection. Current standard practices for monitoring rejection after heart transplantation are relying on invasive procedures: EMB (for AR surveillance; and CA or intravascular ultrasound[3] for chronic rejection diagnosis. These procedures need to be repeated over the life of the HT patients. They are not only invasive and costly, but the accuracy is less than ideal (due to a limited number of myocardial zones that can be biopsied). Although widely used, EMB is invasive, associated with finite risks of morbidity and mortality, and is prone to sampling errors due to limited sample sizes and locations available, especially in pediatric patients. In addition, the interpretation of EMB can be subjective, resulting in erroneous diagnosis and inability to predict the onset of rejection.

Up to now, most of the clinical applications for detecting cardiac allograft rejection with CMRI are mainly detecting manifestation of the rejection in the tissue or organ levels, viewing allograft rejection as one of the pathological states of the heart.[4] Reduced ejection fraction prolonged T_2, altered T_1, hyperenhancement with delayed enhancement (DE), and elevated Gd-based contrast agent uptake have been found to be associated with cardiac allograft rejection, probably due to edema, necrosis, and fibrosis resulting from rejection.[5] Decreased myocardial perfusion and changes in myocardial perfusion reserve have been found in transplant patients suffering from CAV. Combinations of multiparameter CMRI, accessing cine, T_1/T_2, perfusion, and DE together, can make a good diagnosis of compromised heart conditions with rejection in one CMRI session. In addition, ^{31}P MR chemical shift imaging has also been found to change in a small cohort of CAV patients. Simultaneous cellular and functional MRI provides potential noninvasive

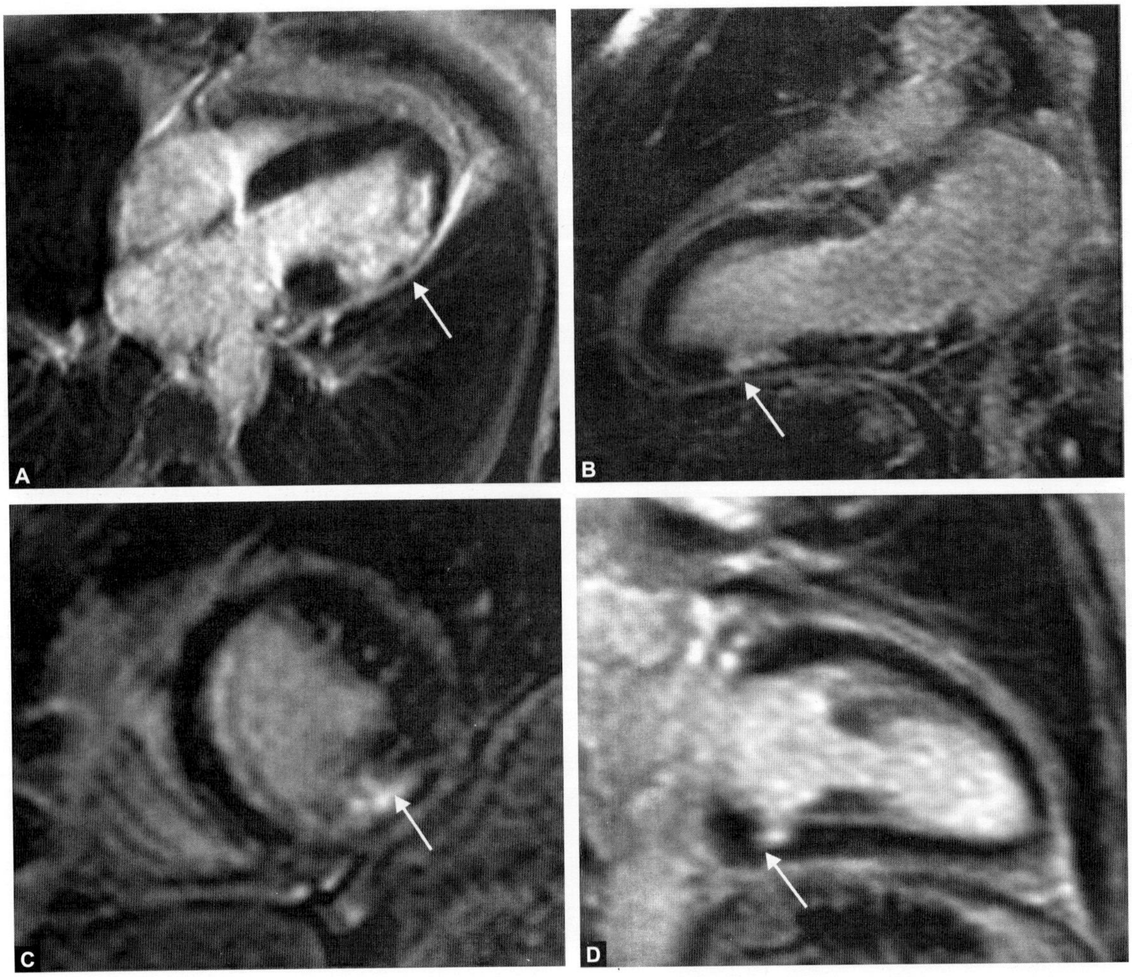

Fig. 4: MRI images of transplanted heart with allograft dysfunction. (MR: magnetic resonance)

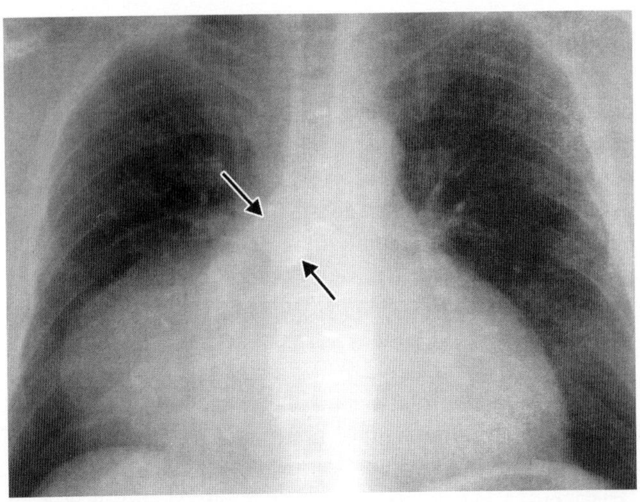

Fig. 5: Chest X-ray of heterotopic heart transplant.

and early detection of rejection before irreversible tissue damage has taken place. *In vivo* cellular MRI for macrophages and lymphocytes provides whole-volume perspective of graft rejection.

In addition, gadolinium use in patients with acute or chronic severe renal insufficiency (estimated glomerular filtration rate <30 mL/min) carries a significant risk for the development of nephrogenic systemic fibrosis. Because of these drawbacks and the lack of widespread availability, the role of CMR in evaluation of ACR is still evolving.

Heterotopic Cardiac Transplant

Heterotopic cardiac transplantation is reserved for patients who have high pulmonary vascular resistance, who receive a small donor organ, or who have acute or potentially reversible myocardial dysfunction.[6] In heterotopic cardiac transplantation, the donor heart is placed in the right thoracic cavity and connected to the recipient's heart in such a manner that the native right ventricle provides the majority of right-side cardiac output and the donor left ventricle provides the bulk of left-side cardiac output. Disadvantages of this procedure include angina, arrhythmias, and risk of thromboembolism from the recipient's native heart. Long-term therapy with anticoagulants is required to prevent potential systemic embolization.

At chest radiography, the heterotopic donor heart is located in the right hemithorax, lateral to patient's native heart. The patient may appear to have a markedly enlarged heart, if the heterotopic nature of the transplanted organ is not known. Substantial atelectasis in the right lower lobe may occur from the position of the heterotopic heart.

Thus, before and after HT, there are many imaging modalities, which play vital role in detecting, understanding, managing, and preventing the problems related to transplant. Thus, these modalities have helped in improving the survival of these patients.

REFERENCES

1. Wu HA, Kolias TJ. Cardiac transplantation: pretransplant and posttransplant evaluation. In: Otto CM (Ed). The practice of clinical echocardiography, 4th edition. Philadelphia, PA: WB Saunders Company; 2012. pp. 585-96.
2. Mehra MR, Uber PA, Uber WE, et al. Anything but a biopsy: noninvasive monitoring for cardiac allograft rejection. Curr Opin Cardiol. 2002;17:131-6.
3. Raichlin E, Bae JH, Kushwaha SS, et al. Inflammatory burden of cardiac allograft coronary atherosclerotic plaque is associated with early recurrent cellular rejection and predicts a higher risk of vasculopathy progression. J Am Coll Cardiol. 2009;53:1279-86.
4. McGiffin DC, Kirklin JK, Naftel DC, et al. Competing outcomes after heart transplantation: a comparison of eras and outcomes. J Heart Lung Transplant. 1997;16:190-8.
5. Bocchi EA, Mocelin AO, de Moraes AV, et al. Comparison between two strategies for rejection detection after heart transplantation: routine endomyocardial biopsy versus gallium-67 cardiac imaging. Transplant Proc. 1997;29:586-8.
6. Adey CK, Schwartz M, Nath PH, et al. Heterotopic heart transplantation: a radiographic review. RadioGraphics. 1987;7:151-60.

136

CHAPTER

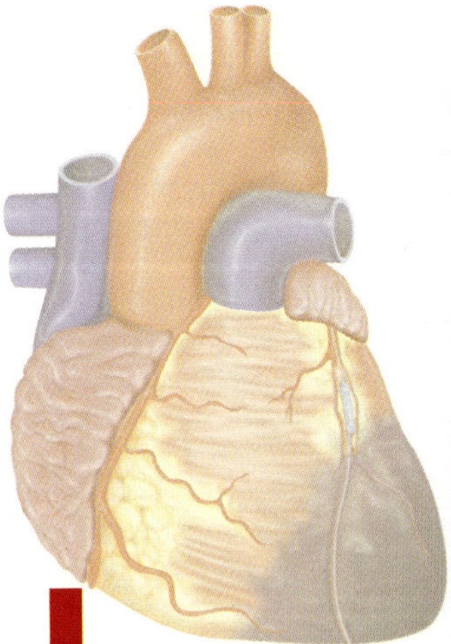

Intraoperative Graft Imaging

OP Yadava

INTRODUCTION

Despite coronary artery bypass graft (CABG) surgery being the commonest cardiac operation and the one most studied and scrutinized, intraoperative graft patency validation is still rarely performed and is an exception rather than a rule. Although failure of the Saphenous vein (SV) graft is well appreciated, with 3–12% failing even before the patient leaves the hospital, the fact that even the arterial grafts can fail early is not that well appreciated. Predischarge and radial arteries may fail in 3–4% patients and internal mammary artery (IMA) in 1.25%.[1,2] In the PREVENT IV study, 1-year failure rate of the IMA to left anterior descending coronary artery was 8.6%[3] and that of SV graft around 20%.[4] Besides anastomosis related issues, early graft failure could be due to competitive flow, kinking, twisting, oversizing, or tension due to undersizing of the length. Early graft failure may lead to perioperative myocardial infarction in up to 9% of patients[5] beside leading to higher morbidity and mortality in the longer run.[6] In the PREVENT IV trial, early events of perioperative infarct or death were 13.9% in patients with at least one occluded graft versus 0.9% in patients with patent grafts.[7]

Therefore, it is not only desirable, but infact mandatory, that some form of intraoperative graft validation should be done before the patient leaves the operating theater so that the grafts can be revised if the need be. Even European guidelines recommend intraoperative graft validation. The 2010 European Guidelines state, "Graft flow measurement, related to graft type, vessel size, degree of stenosis, quality of anastomosis, and outflow area, is useful at the end of surgery. Flow less than 20 mL/min and pulsatility index (PI) more than 5 predict technically inadequate grafts, mandating graft revision before leaving the operating theater."[8] The 2014 Guidelines are a bit more lucid and elaborate, "Graft flow measurement may be useful in confirming or excluding a technical graft problem indicated by hemodynamic instability or inability to wean the patient from cardiopulmonary bypass, new regional wall motion abnormalities on transesophageal echocardiography, or ventricular arrhythmias. It has also been shown to reduce the rate of adverse events and graft failure, although interpretation can be challenging in sequential grafts and T-grafts."[9] However, American guidelines have not yet mandated intraoperative graft validation and Michael Mack from Baylor, Texas bemoans, "Coronary artery bypass grafting is the only major vascular procedure currently performed that does not routinely undergo an assessment of patency at the end of the procedure."[10] Just finger palpation or a pulsatile feel in the graft, besides being very subjective, is not a proof positive sign of graft patency, nor does it pick partially obstructed grafts. Therefore, more definitive methods are resorted to assess bypass grafts. Various techniques used for intraoperative graft validation have been summarized by Balacumaraswami and Taggart[4] (Table 1).

TABLE 1: Different techniques for intraoperative graft patency assessment.[4]

Technique	Year	Reference Article	Patients (n)	Strengths	Limitations	Current Use
Conventional angiography	1998	Elbeery and colleagues (16)	50	Precise definition of graft patency	Invasive, requires contrast, rarely available in operating room	–
Electromagnetic flowmetry	1994	Louagie and colleagues (18)	262	Ease of use, noninvasive	Motion artifacts, interference	–
Transit- time flowmetry	1994	Canver and Dame (19)	63	Accurate graft flow value	Inability to define degree of stenosis	+
Thermal angiography	1995	Falk and colleagues (20)	370	No contrast or radiation	No clarity with increasing depth	–
Doppler velocity measurements	2000	Lin and colleagues (21)	35	Ease of use, noninvasive	Flow values affected by angle of insonation	–
Epicardial color Doppler scanning	2002	Haaverstad and colleagues (22)	23	Noninvasive	Imprecise definition of all coronary territories	–
Intraoperative fluorescence imaging	2003	2003 Taggart and colleagues (23)	84	Real- time "angiographic" images	Semiquantitative	+

CINE ANGIOGRAPHY

Intraoperative cine angiography in a hybrid lab is the gold standard for graft validation. Anastomoses are graded by Fitzgibbon grading system as follows:
Grade A—excellent
Grade B—fair but with clinically significant stenosis, and
Grade O—occluded

However, because of its relative nonavailability, the costs, the nephrotoxicity of the dye, radiation exposure, interuser variability especially for moderate degree of stenosis (50–70%),[11] and the invasive nature with a potential for anastomotic disruption, this is not a practical and pragmatic option. Some of the more well established techniques used in contemporary clinical practice are:

Transit Time Flowmetry

In this, the coronary conduit is placed in to a probe between two ultrasonic transducers on one side and a reflector on the opposite side. Ultrasonic signals are transmitted from the two transducers in a countervailing direction and are reflected by the reflector. The signals are received by the opposite transducers, which now act as receivers (Fig. 1). The velocity of the blood, and therefore the total blood flow volume, in the graft is calculated from the time delay (transit time) that occurs between the two signals.[13,14]

$$T2 - T1 \propto Q$$

(directly proportional)

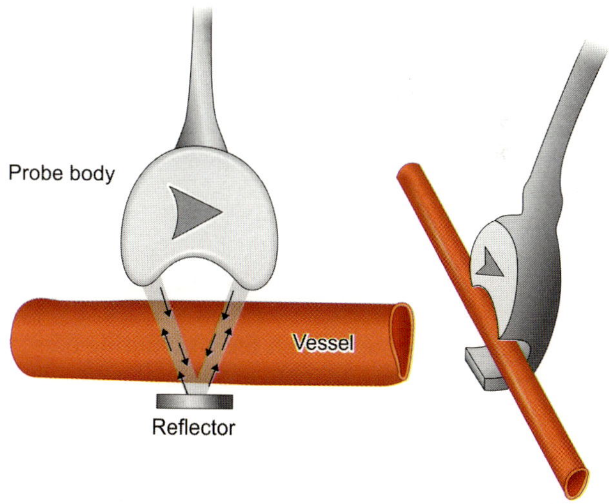

Fig. 1: Transit time flowmetry technique. The transducers in the transit time flowmeter are upstream and downstream of each other, and both act as a transmitter and a receiver.[12]

Four important variables are provided by the flowmeter:

1. Mean graft flow (MGF) is measured in mL/min; it is displayed as a color-coded waveform with red color depicting systolic and blue wave diastolic flow (Fig. 2).
2. Pulsatility index

$$PI = \frac{Q_{Mas} - Q_{Min}}{Q_{Mean}} \text{ where}$$

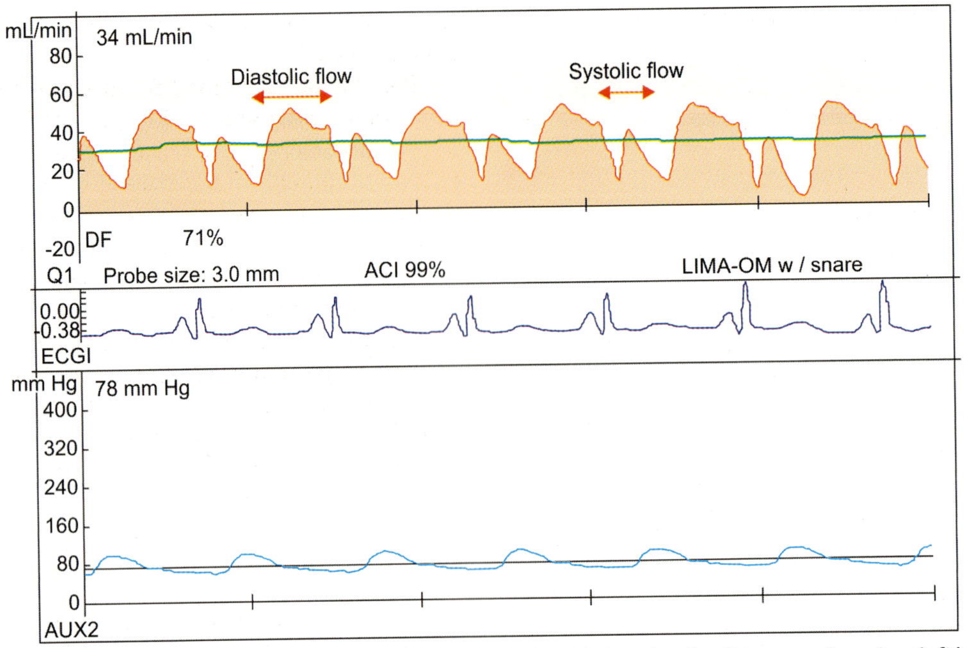

Fig. 2: Transit time flowmetry (TTFM) display (Medistim AS, Oslo, Norway) showing the flow waveform in a left internal mammary artery (LIMA) graft to obtuse marginal (OM) branch of circumflex artery with an MGF of 34 mL/min, PI of 1.5, and diastolic flow (DF) of 71%. The acoustic coupling index (ACI), which indicates the degree of contact, is 99%. Simultaneous electrocardiogram (ECG) and mean arterial pressure (78 mm Hg) are displayed on the auxiliary option (AUX 2).[4]

Q_{Max}—peak systolic flow
Q_{Min}—peak diastolic flow
Q_{Mean}—peak mean flow
This provides information on flow pattern and resistance (Fig. 2)

3. Diastolic filling percentage (DFP)

$$DFP = \frac{Q_{diastolic}}{Q_{systolic} + Q_{diastolic}}$$

It measures the flow through the graft during diastole and should ideally be more than 50% of the MGF.[14]

4. Backward flow percentage (BFP)
BFP expresses the percentage backward flow of the blood across the anastomosis and is influenced by competitive flow as also the severity of the distal native coronary stenosis.[15]

The MGF and PI are the two most frequently monitored parameters, and according to the ESC/EACTS guidelines, the recommended cutoff is 20 mL/min for MGF and <520 mL/min for the PI.[8] However, there is no universal agreement (Table 2) with Di Giammarco suggesting an MGF cutoff value of ≤15 mL/min[16] and Amin et al. recommending MGF values of 40 mL/min for venous graft and 20 mL/min for arterial grafts.[14] Similarly, PI should ideally be <3, with the gray zone between 3 and 5, and definitive evidence of association of graft failure with PI > 5. A BFP of 3% or greater is associated with graft failure, and thus, 3% or less cutoff is advocated. The DFP has not been shown to be predictive of graft patency. However, since the predominant flow in bypass graft should be diastolic, the DFP is recommended to be >50%.[12]

Depending on the cutoff parameters used, the sensitivity and specificity of TTFM have been reported at 96.2% and 76.9% respectively.[17] The TTFM can also be used for predicting mid and long-term results. Tokuda et al. found that a lower MGF and a higher BFP were predictors for mid-term graft failure.[18] Similarly, Kieser et al. found that a PI of more than 5 was associated with higher MACE of 17% versus 5% (p 0.005) and even higher mortality of 32% versus 12% (p 0.011).[19]

The TTFM, compared to its predecessor—the electromagnetic flowmetry of Grondin,[20] is not affected by the hematocrit, or the vessel caliber and does not need any calibration.[21] However, TTFM has a major limitation that it cannot locate the site of the obstruction and the MGF can be influenced by hemodynamic state of the patient. Further, the interpretation of the results is difficult because of nonstandardization of cutoff points. Also, the fact that with low sensitivity, TTFM may give false-positive results and thereby increase the incidence of unnecessary graft revisions has been stressed upon by Balacumaraswami et al.[22] and Di Giammarco et al.[21]

To increase the diagnostic yield of TTFM, Di Giammarco et al. recommend the addition of high-resolution epicardial

TABLE 2: Reported cutoffs for TTFM parameters in different experiences.[21]

Author	Cutoff values	Sensitivity	Specificity
Kim et al. (2005)	MGF < 15 mL/min	96%	77%
	PI > 3 (LCA) or PI > 5(RCA) PI>5		
Di Giammarco et al. (2006)	MGF ≤ 15 mL/min PI ≥ 3	94%	61%
	MGF ≤ 15 mL/min PI ≥ 5.1 (LCA)	26%	98%
Tokuda et al. (2007)	MGF ≤ 20 mL/min PI ≥ 4.7 (RCA)	60%	98%
Kieser et al. (2010)	PI > 5	nr	nr

(MGF: Mean graft flow; PI: Pulsatility index; LCA: Left coronary artery; RCA: Right coronary artery; nr: not reported)

ultrasonography,[23] as it increases the positive predictive value of TTFM from 10% to a whopping 100%.

Fluorescence Coronary Angiography

Indocyanine fluorescence imaging (IFI) is based on the property of indocyanine green (ICG) dye of emitting a fluorescence when stimulated by LASER energy at a wave length of 806 nm. This fluorescence is captured by a camera and the images collated. Safety of LASER use and ICG dye has been adequately demonstrated.[4] The ICG is injected into the central line for off-pump CABG or through the ascending aorta for on-pump CABG and the LASER source is positioned over the heart and is activated just prior to the first ICG bolus injection.[12] Taggart et al. found the images to be of quality similar to that of cine angiography.[24]

Indocyanine fluorescence imaging has been compared directly with cine angiography by Desai et al. in 106 patients.[25] Cine angiography detected 8.2% of the grafts to have ≥50% stenosis. Indocyanine fluorescence imaging detected 83.3% of these abnormal grafts, while TTFM succeeded in only 25.0% giving a sensitivity and specificity for detecting a 50% stenosis of 83.3% and 100% for IFI and 25.0% and 98.4% for TTFM, respectively (p 0.011). A graft revision rate of 1.4–5% has been reported by various authors based on IFI validation.[12,24,26] Takahashi et al. had to revise 1.2% of their grafts intraoperatively based on SPY ICG imaging.[26] All revised grafts were demonstrated to be patent in a follow-up angiography using 64-slice multidetector computerized tomography. Using the same system, Kawashima et al. had to revise 4.5% of their anastomoses in 10% of cases. However, in 2.8% cases, the grafts which were demonstrated to be patent on intraoperative SPY imaging were subsequently revealed to be occluded by postoperative angiography.[27]

The IFI has a major limitation in that it takes 3–4 minutes for each graft to be evaluated.[24] With a limited penetration depth of 1 mm, pedicled conduits may be poor candidates vis-a-vis skeletonized conduits for IFI use. Even heart may have to be displaced to ensure a direct "line of sight" to visualize the anastomosis so that kinking of graft in physiological position may be missed. It is also a semiqualitative assessment and gives very limited information on competitive flow and distal coronary bed.[28] Kawashima et al. sum up succinctly, "Although neither technology can constantly identify more minor, nonocclusive abnormalities, the intraoperative fluorescence imaging technique seems to be more sensitive and less susceptible to false-positive images."[27]

Thermal Coronary Angiography

This technique uses injection of solutions at different temperatures into the bypass graft and the temperature differential between the graft and the epicardial surface is then tracked by an infrared camera. Iwahashi et al.[29] were able to pick up 3.7% of the grafts as blocked and revised them. Ferguson et al. have developed a multi spectral physiologic visualization technology called I Certainty TM but the data are limited.[30]

High-resolution Epicardial Ultrasonography

Introduced in 1980s by Sahn et al., the technique of HR-ECUS did not find wide acceptance due to the limitation of the large size of the transducer. However, with the commercial launch of the smaller sized probes with frequencies ranging from 8 MHz to 18 MHz by Medistim, the use of HR-ECUS has been extended beyond graft patency to choosing even the site of anastomosis, both distally and proximally to aorta. Even HR-ECUS guided CABG sans coronary angiography has been reported in literature.[31] ECUS-derived two-dimensional longitudinal and cross-sectional images of the anastomosis can quantify anastomotic stenosis as diameter reduction or percentage area reduction, respectively. HR-ECUS has been validated against cine coronary angiography by Budde et al.[32] It may even predict long-term patency of anastomoses.[33] Development of automated stenosis quantification, especially using cross-sectional area, will further refine the technology and reduce human interface.

CONCLUSION

Much as we may wish otherwise, postmyocardial revascularization ischemia due to primary graft failure is not only a stark reality, but infact a common place event. However, it can be prevented to a large extent by intraoperative graft validation which should be made a mandatory quality metric to be monitored in every case.[34] As it stands today, transit time flowmetry is the most prevalent mode of intraoperative graft imaging and validation of CABG.

REFERENCES

1. Fitzgibbon GM, Kafka HP, Leach AJ, et al. Coronary bypass graft fate and patient outcome: angiographic follow-up of 5,065 grafts related to survival and reoperation in 1,388 patients during 25 years. J Am Coll Cardiol. 1996;28:616-26.
2. Goldman S, Copeland J, Mortiz T, et al. Starting aspirin therapy after operation. Effects on early graft patency. Department of Veterans Affairs Cooperative Study Group. Circulation. 1991;84:520-6.
3. Harskamp RE, Alexander JH, Ferguson B, et al. Frequency and predictors of Internal Mammary Artery Graft failure and subsequent clinical outcomes: insights from the PREVENT IV Trial. Circulation. 2016;133(2):133-8.
4. Balacumaraswami L, Taggart DP. Intraoperative imaging techniques to assess coronary artery bypass graft patency. Ann Thorac Surg. 2007;83:2251-7.
5. Taggart DP. Biochemical assessment of myocardial injury after cardiac surgery: effects of a platelet activating factor antagonist, bilateral internal thoracic artery grafts, and coronary endarterectomy. J Thorac Cardiovasc Surg. 2000;120:651-9.
6. Yusuf S, Zucker D, Peduzzi P, et al. Effect of coronary artery bypass graft surgery on survival: overview of 10-year results from randomised trials by the Coronary Artery Bypass Graft Surgery Trialists Collaboration. Lancet. 1994;344:563-70.
7. Alexander JH, Hafley G, Harrington RA et al. Efficacy and safety of edifoligide, an e2f transcription factor decoy, for prevention of vein graft failure following coronary artery bypass graft surgery: PREVENT IV: a randomized controlled trial. JAMA. 2005;294:2446-54.
8. The Task Force on Myocardial Revascularization of the European Society of Cardiology (ESC) and the European Association for Cardio-Thoracic Surgery (EACTS) 2010 guidelines on myocardial revascularization. Eur J Cardiothorac Surg. 2010;38:S1-52.
9. The Task Force on Myocardial Revascularization of the European Society of Cardiology (ESC) and the European Association for Cardio-Thoracic Surgery (EACTS) 2014 ESC/EACTS Guidelines on myocardial revascularization. Eur J Cardiothorac Surg. 2014;46(4):517-92.
10. Mack MJ. Intraoperative coronary graft assessment. Curr Opin Cardiol. 2008;23:568-72.
11. Beauman GJ, Vogel RA. Accuracy of individual and panel visual interpretations of coronary arteriograms; implications for clinical decisions. J Am Coll Cardiol. 1990;16(1):108-13.
12. Ohmes LB, Franco AD, Di Giammarco G, et al. Techniques for intraoperative graft assessment in coronary artery bypass surgery. J Thorac Dis. 2017;9(Suppl. 4):S327-32.
13. Niclauss L. Techniques and standards in intraoperative graft verification by transit time flow measurement after coronary artery bypass graft surgery: a critical review. Eur J Cardiothorac Surg. 2017;51:26-33.
14. Amin S, Pinho-Gomes AC, Taggart DP. Relationship of intraoperative transit time flowmetry findings to angiographic graft patency at follow-up. Ann Thorac Surg. 2016;101:1996-2006.
15. Honda K, Okamura Y, Nishimura Y, et al. Graft flow assessment using a transit time flow meter in fractional flow reserve-guided coronary artery bypass surgery. J Thorac Cardiovasc Surg. 2015;149:1622-8.
16. Di Giammarco G, Pano M, Cirmeni S, et al. Predictive value of intraoperative transit-time flow measurement for short-term graft patency in coronary surgery. J Thorac Cardiovasc Surg. 2006;132:468-74.
17. Kim KB, Kang CH, Lim C. Prediction of graft flow impairment by intraoperative transit time flow measurement in off-pump coronary artery bypass using arterial grafts. Ann Thorac Surg. 2005;80:594-8.
18. Tokuda Y, Song MH, Oshima H, et al. Predicting midterm coronary artery bypass graft failure by intraoperative transit time flow measurement. Ann Thorac Surg. 2008;86:532-6.
19. Kieser TM, Rose S, Kowalewski R, et al. Transit-time flow predicts outcomes in coronary artery bypass graft patients: a series of 1000 consecutive arterial grafts. Eur J Cardiothorac Surg. 2010;38:155-62.
20. Grondin CM, Castonguay YR, Lepage G, et al. Aortocoronary bypass grafts: early postoperative angiographic evaluation and reexploration for stenosis or thrombosis of the vein graft. Arch Surg. 1971;103(5):535-8.
21. Di Giammarco G, Marinelli D. Intraoperative graft assessment and imaging of native coronary arteries. Ind J Thorac Cardiovasc Surg. 2018. Accepted for Pub, In Press.
22. Balacumaraswami L, Abu-Omar Y, Choudhary B, et al. A comparison of transit-time flowmetry and intraoperative fluorescence imaging for assessing coronary artery bypass graft patency. J Thorac Cardiovasc Surg. 2005;130:315-20.
23. Di Giammarco G, Canosa C, Foschi M, et al. Intraoperative graft verification in coronary surgery: increased diagnostic accuracy adding high-resolution epicardial ultrasonography to transit-time flow measurement. Eur J Cardiothorac Surg. 2014;45:e41-5.
24. Taggart DP, Choudhary B, Anastasiadis K, et al. Preliminary experience with a novel intraoperative fluorescence imaging technique to evaluate the patency of bypass grafts in total arterial revascularization. Ann Thorac Surg. 2003;75:870-3.
25. Desai ND, Miwa S, Kodama D, et al. A randomized comparison of intraoperative indocyanine green angiography and transit-time flow measurement to detect technical errors in coronary bypass grafts. J Thorac Cardiovasc Surg. 2006;132:585-94.
26. Takahashi M, Ishikawa T, Higashidani K, et al. SPY: an innovative intraoperative imaging system to evaluate graft patency during off-pump coronary artery bypass grafting. Interact Cardiovasc Thorac Surg. 2004;3:479-83.
27. Kawashima T, Naraoka S, Kakizaki T. Intraoperative graft assessment using fluorescent imaging system (SPY). Kyobu Geka. 2009;62(7):519-22; discussion522-6.

28. Leacche M, Balaguer JM, Byrne JG. Intraoperative grafts assessment. Semin Thorac Cardiovasc Surg. 2009;21:207-12.
29. Iwahashi H, Tashiro T, Morishige N, et al. New method of thermal coronary angiography for intraoperative patency control in off-pump and on-pump coronary artery bypass grafting. Ann Thorac Surg. 2007;84:1504-07.
30. Ferguson TB Jr, Chen C, Kim S, et al. Noninvasive quantification of blood flow in epicardial coronary arteries, coronary artery bypass grafts, and anastomoses. Innovations (Phila). 2017;12:50-9.
31. Di Giammarco G, Marinelli D, Foschi M, et al. Intraoperative imaging to detect coronary stenosis in no-angiography patients. Asian Cardiovasc Thorac Ann. 2017;25(6):446-9.
32. Budde RPJ, Meijer R, Dessing TC. Detection of construction errors in ex vivo-coronary artery anastomoses by 13 MHz epicardial ultrasonography. J Thorac Cardiovasc Surg. 2005;129(5):1078-83.
33. Tjomsland O, Wiseth R, Wahba A et al. Intraoperative colour Doppler ultrasound assessment of anastomoses of the left internal mammary artery to the left anterior descending coronary artery during off pump coronary artery bypass surgery correlates with angiographic evaluation at the 8 month follow-up. Heart Surg Forum, Carden Jennings. 2003;6:375-9.
34. Kieser TM, Taggart DP. Current status of the intraoperative graft assessment: should it be standard of care for Coronary Artery Bypass Graft Surgery? J Card Surg. 2018;33(5):219-28.

SECTION 33

Echo Oncology

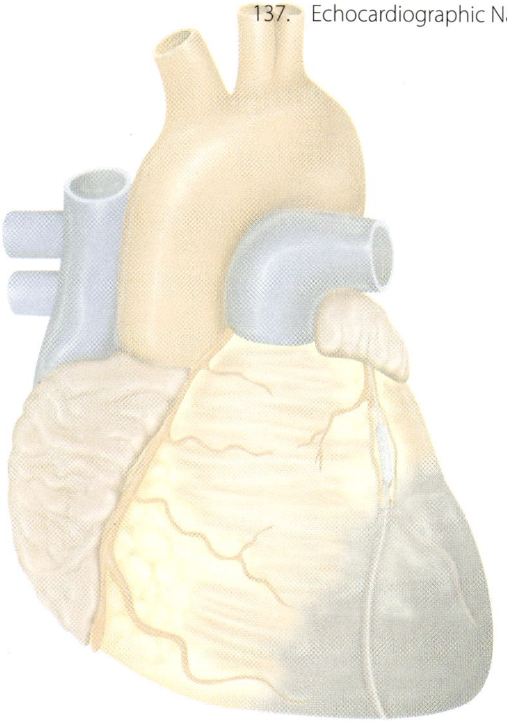

137

CHAPTER

Echocardiographic Navigation Cardio-oncology

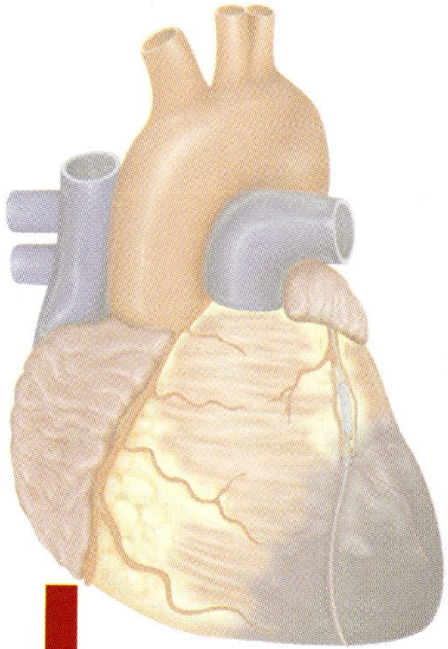

Madhu Mary Minz, Manish Bansal, Ravi R Kasliwal, HK Chopra

INTRODUCTION

Past few years have seen great advancements in the treatment of cancers which have led to increased survival of cancer patients. Unfortunately, these achievements have been partially offset by the side effects of these drugs which are associated with substantially morbidity and even mortality. The most dreaded among these side effects/complications is the chemotherapy-related cardiac dysfunction (CTRCD) which can lead to premature morbidity and mortality in cancer patients. The cardiotoxicity can be due to direct effect of cancer drugs on cardiac structure or ventricular function or can be due to acceleration of cardiac disease in presence of known risk factors, such as hypertension, diabetes mellitus, dyslipidemia, obesity, smoker, family history of cardiac disease, or sedentary life style. Chemotherapy and radiation therapy can put the cancer patients at a risk of a gamut of cardiovascular complications, such as cardiac failure, coronary artery disease, hypertension, arrhythmias, thromboembolism, pericardial disease, valvular heart disease, and peripheral heart disease.

CHEMOTHERAPY-RELATED CARDIAC DYSFUNCTION

Chemotherapy-related cardiac dysfunction is defined as a drop in left ventricular (LV) ejection fraction (LVEF) of >5% in symptomatic patients or >10 percentage points in asymptomatic patients, to a value <53% confirmed on two echocardiographic examinations at least 2–3 weeks apart.[1] Two types of CTRCD have been described:

1. *Type I*: This is dose-related, reversible toxicity which is due to structural changes in the myocardium. This form of toxicity is commonly seen with the anthracycline group of drugs, such as doxorubicin, daunorubicin, epirubicin, and idarubicin. Patients who have received >250–300 mg/m^2 of doxorubicin or equivalent are at higher risk of developing CTRCD.[2] Alkylating agents, mitoxantrone, mitomycin, and antimicrotubule agents are also known to cause type I cardiotoxicity (Table 1).
2. *Type II*: This form of cardiotoxicity is not dose related and is reversible as it does not cause any ultrastructural abnormalities in the myocytes. Type II cardiotoxicity is typically seen with monoclonal antibody-based agents (e.g. trastuzumab), tyrosine kinase inhibitors, etc. (Table 2).

The mechanism of action of anthracycline is related to deoxyribonucleic acid damage leading to death of dividing cancer cells and cardiotoxicity is due to free radical formation caused by its metabolism. In a meta-analysis, 6% patient receiving anthracycline presented with clinically relevant cardiotoxicity and 18% had subclinical cardiotoxicity.[3] Trastuzumab is an inhibitor of the HER2 receptor and is used in breast and gastric cancers. Sunitinib is a tyrosine kinase inhibitor used in renal cell cancer and cardiotoxicity is caused by mitochondrial injury and cardiomyocyte apoptosis.

TABLE 1: Cardiovascular toxicity of commonly used cancer therapies.

Class of drugs	*Agents*	*Cardiac side effects*
Anthracycline agents	Doxorubicin, daunorubicin, epirubicin, idarubicin, and mitoxantrone	LV dysfunction, CHF, and myopericarditis
Alkylating agents	Cyclophosphamide, ifosfamide, cisplatin, busulfan, and mitomycin	CHF, arrhythmias, hypertension, myopericarditis, and thromboembolism
Antiangiogenic antibodies	Bevacizumab	Hypertension, myocardial ischemia
Antimetabolites	5-Fluorouracil, capecitabine, cytarabine, methotrexate, and fludarabine	CHF, arrhythmias, coronary vasospasm, myocardial ischemia, and myopericarditis
Antimicrotubule agents	Docetaxel, paclitaxel, etoposide, teniposide, vincristine, and vinblastine	CHF, myocardial ischemia, QT prolongation, bradycardia, hypotension, and myocardial ischemia
TKI	Imatinib, dasatinib, erlotinib, lapatinib, lenvatinib, nilotinib, pazopanib, ponatinib, sorafenib, vandetanib, and sunitinib	CHF, QT prolongation, hypertension, myocardial ischemia, and thromboembolism
Miscellaneous	Bleomycin	Myopericarditis
	Interferons	Hypertension, hypotension, myocardial ischemia
	Interleukin-2	Arrhythmias, hypotension, and myocardial ischemia
	Tretinoin	CHF, hypotension
	Arsenic trioxide	QT prolongation

(CHF: Congestive heart failure; LV: Left ventricular; TKI: Tyrosine kinase inhibitors)

TABLE 2: Types of cancer chemotherapy-related left ventricular dysfunction.

Features	*Type I cardiotoxicity*	*Type II cardiotoxicity*
Causative chemotherapeutic agents	• Anthracycline (doxorubicin, epirubicin) • Alkylating agents (cyclophosphamide) • Mitoxantrone, mitomycin • Antimicrotubule (docetaxel, pacitaxel)	• Monoclonal antibody-based tyrosine kinase inhibitors (trastuzumab, bevacizumab) • Small molecule tyrosine kinase inhibitors (sunitinib, lapatinib)
Related to dose	Yes, cumulative	Not related to dose
Reversibility	Nonreversible, permanent damage May recur in months or years	Reversible; recovery can be near normal after stopping treatment
Structural change	Myofibrillar disarray, vacuolar swelling, necrosis	No ultrastructural changes
Rechallenge with same agent	High probability of recurrent dysfunction	Safe

HOW TO DIAGNOSE CARDIOTOXICITY?

Early detection of risk factors and recognition of symptoms of cardiotoxicity in patients receiving cancer chemotherapy are important to diagnose cardiotoxicity at an early stage so as to start cardioprotective medications or to modify/stop the cancer chemotherapy. Patients are assessed at baseline to elicit history of hypertension, diabetes mellitus, dyslipidemia, obesity, smoking, family history of cardiac disease, or sedentary life style which puts them at a higher than usual risk to develop cardiotoxicity. Importance of clinical examination to identify signs of heart failure, such as S3 gallop, tachycardia, or both, is imperative (Table 3).

BIOMARKERS

The use of biomarkers to identify early myocardial damage to predict the development of heart failure in apparently asymptomatic patients is becoming increasingly important. Cardiac troponin (cTn) and brain natriuretic peptide (BNP) are the two most commonly used biomarkers for this purpose. Cardiac troponin gets released due to cardiomyocyte damage whereas BNP is a measurement of elevation in LV filling pressure and wall stress. Other biomarker of inflammation [high sensitivity C-reactive protein (hs-CRP), interleukin-6, myeloperoxidase, etc.], markers of endothelial dysfunction (plasminogen activator

TABLE 3: A proposed risk assessment scoring for patients receiving potentially cardiotoxic chemotherapy.[25]

Medication-related risk	*Patient-related risk factors*
High (risk score 4): Anthracyclines, cyclophosphamide, trastuzumab, and ifosfamide	• Cardiomyopathy, heart failure • Coronary artery disease/peripheral artery disease • Hypertension • Diabetes mellitus • Prior anthracycline exposure • Prior radiotherapy • Age <15 years or >65 years • Female gender
Intermediate risk (risk score 2): Docetaxel, sunitinib, sorafenib, and pertuzumab	
Low risk (risk score 1): Bevacizumab, imatinib, lapatinib, and dasatinib	
Rare (risk score 0): Etoposide	
Interpretation	
• Total score is calculated by addition of medication-related risk score plus number of patient-related risk factors • Total score: 0—very low risk; 1–2—low risk; 3–4—intermediate risk; 5–6—high risk; >6—very high risk	

inhibitor, tissue plasminogen activator, etc.), and markers of myocardial ischemia (fatty acid binding protein, glycogen phosphorylase binding protein) have also been studied.[4]

Cardiac Troponins

Cardiac troponins are released from cardiomyocytes due to ischemia, inflammation, oxidative stress, or apoptosis. In several studies, cardiac troponin-I (cTnI) was found to be high in patients receiving high-dose chemotherapy and correlated well with adverse cardiac events.[4] cTnI elevation is seen in one-third patients—this proportion increases with cumulative dose:

- In patients with cTnI level >0.5 ng/mL, 33%, 27%, and 25% of increases occur right after, at 12 hours, and 24 hours after dose and such rise predicts a fall in LVEF after 1 month.
- Patients with cTnI > 0.5 ng/mL have a significant reduction in LVEF for 3–7 months, compared to patients with cTnI < 0.5 ng/mL who show a transient decrease in LVEF at 3 months followed by complete recovery at 7 months.
- High cardiac troponin-T levels during the first 90 days after chemotherapy predict cardiotoxicity at 4 years of follow-up.

N-Terminal Pro–Brain Natriuretic Peptide

Correlation between NT pro-BNP level and the cumulative dose has been seen in several studies.

- High NT pro-BNP levels during the first 90 days after therapy predict cardiotoxicity at 4 years of follow-up.
- Brain natriuretic peptide >51.3 ng/mL has an 83% sensitivity and 90% specificity for detection of cardiotoxicity.[4]
- With BNP > 100 pg/mL, heart failure is most common.[5]

In a cohort of 52 patients treated with chemotherapy, persistently elevated NT pro-BNP levels (defined as >88 ng/mL in males <50 years), >227 ng/L in males >50 years, >153 ng/L in females <50 years, and >334 ng/L in females >50 years) were noticed in 33% of the patients and this was associated with systolic and diastolic dysfunction in contrast to patients with transient elevation (36% of patients) or no elevation (31% of patients) who showed no significant effect during 12 months of follow-up.[4]

High Sensitivity C-Reactive Protein

High sensitivity C-reactive protein is a nonspecific marker of inflammation. A correlation between hs-CRP level and LV mass, wall thickness, and dimension has been demonstrated in patients with lymphoblastic leukemia after exposure to anthracycline.[4]

Cardiovascular Imaging

Cardiovascular imaging including echocardiography, magnetic resonance imaging, and radionuclide imaging plays a crucial role in the evaluation and management of patients receiving potentially cardiotoxic cancer chemotherapy. Imaging is very helpful in early diagnosis and prevention of heart failure in these patients. Of all the different imaging modalities, echocardiography is the most suited for this purpose owing to its wider availability, lower cost, noninvasive nature, safety, and repeatability.

ROLE OF ECHOCARDIOGRAPHY IN EARLY DIAGNOSIS AND FOLLOW-UP OF CANCER PATIENTS

Echocardiography is the most commonly used test for baseline assessment and serial follow-up of patients on chemotherapy. It provides a vast amount of information as described below.

Assessment of Left Ventricular Systolic Function

Left ventricular ejection fraction is the most commonly used parameter to assess LV systolic function and to diagnose the development of LV systolic dysfunction. As mentioned above, CTRCD is diagnosed when there is a decrease in LVEF of >10 percentage points to a value <53%, confirmed on two examinations at least 2–3 weeks apart.[1] Ejection fraction is determined by biplane Simpson method of disks in accordance with the current guidelines from the American Society of Echocardiography[6] or relevant societies. This is done by manually tracing the LV endocardial border in the apical four-chamber and two-chamber views at end-diastole and end-systole. Left ventricular ejection fraction in the range of 53–73% is considered normal. If endocardial borders are not well defined, ultrasonic contrast should be used to improve accuracy and reproducibility. Three-dimensional (3D) echocardiography has a temporal variability of 6% in LVEF and is considered the most accurate method for measurement of LVEF.[7] Compared with other echocardiographic techniques, 3D measurement has the least intraobserver, interobserver, and test–retest variability and correlates best with cardiac MRI. For estimation of LVEF by 3D echocardiography, a full-volume dataset of left ventricle is acquired which can be cropped in any orientation. Processing of this dataset allows estimation of LVEF without any geometric assumptions or mathematical approximations. Regardless of the modality used for estimation of LVEF, vital parameters, such as heart rate, blood pressure, etc., should be mentioned during each echocardiography study to indicate the hydration status of the patient.

Myocardial Strain

Earlier, tissue Doppler imaging (TDI) (more appropriately tissue velocity imaging) was developed to provide an objective myocardial contractile function. While it generated a lot of interest initially, it subsequently fell out of favor because of its angle dependence and the inability unable to differentiate translational movement or tethering effect from actual myocardial contraction. Strain imaging overcomes many of the limitations inherent in tissue velocity imaging. Consequently, strain imaging has rapidly evolved as an important technique to quantitatively estimate global or regional myocardial mechanical/contractile function and can detect early, subclinical LV dysfunction even before LVEF starts to decrease. Strain is a measurement of deformation and calculates fractional change in length of the myocardial segment. Strain rate is the rate at which deformation occurs. Deformation is expressed along longitudinal, radial, and circumferential coordinates. Strain imaging can be performed using either TDI or speckle tracking. Tissue Doppler-based strain is not much used because of the issues related to angle-dependent, and speckle-tracking echocardiography (STE) is the current modality of choice for myocardial strain imaging. Speckle-tracking echocardiography is a gray-scale-based, angle-independent technique which works by tracking frame-by-frame motion of acoustic speckles within a gray-scale image of myocardium. From the data thus gathered, the automated software calculates strain for each myocardial segment, which can be averaged to provide global strain (Fig. 1). Apical four-chamber, two-chamber, and three-chamber views are used for estimating longitudinal strain whereas short-axis views at base, mid, and apex of the left ventricle are used for deriving radial and circumferential strain.[8] Numerous studies have shown that reduction in global longitudinal strain (GLS) is an independent predictor of future development of cardiotoxicity and is able to detect ensuing LV systolic dysfunction even when LVEF is within the normal range also[1,9-19] (Fig. 2). Negishi et al. studied 81 women receiving trastuzumab, 37 of whom received anthracycline as well.[15] Conventional echocardiographic indices along with strain and strain rate were measured at baseline, 6 months, and 12 months. They concluded that GLS was an independent early predictor of later reduction in LVEF. A relative reduction of 11% in GLS from baseline is a sensitive marker for myocardial damage and CTRCD. In another study by Sawaya et al., 81 women with newly diagnosed HER2-positive breast cancer treated with anthracycline followed by trastuzumab were studied for 15 months using LVEF, peak systolic longitudinal radial, and circumferential myocardial strain.[12] They concluded that strain imaging was useful in prediction of subsequent cardiotoxicity and also helped to guide treatment to avoid cardiac side effects. Observational studies have also shown that the patients who are exposed to cardioprotective therapies, such as beta-blockers and angiotensin-converting enzyme inhibitor (ACE-I) while they are on cancer chemotherapy, are at lower risk of developing cardiotoxicity.[20-23] Moreover, among those who develop reduction in GLS, the abnormalities in myocardial strain seem to normalize once they are put on these therapies. However, no randomized study has so far been published to inform the utility of strain-guided management of the patients receiving cancer chemotherapy. SUCCOUR (Strain sUrveillance of Chemotherapy for improving Cardiovascular Outcomes)

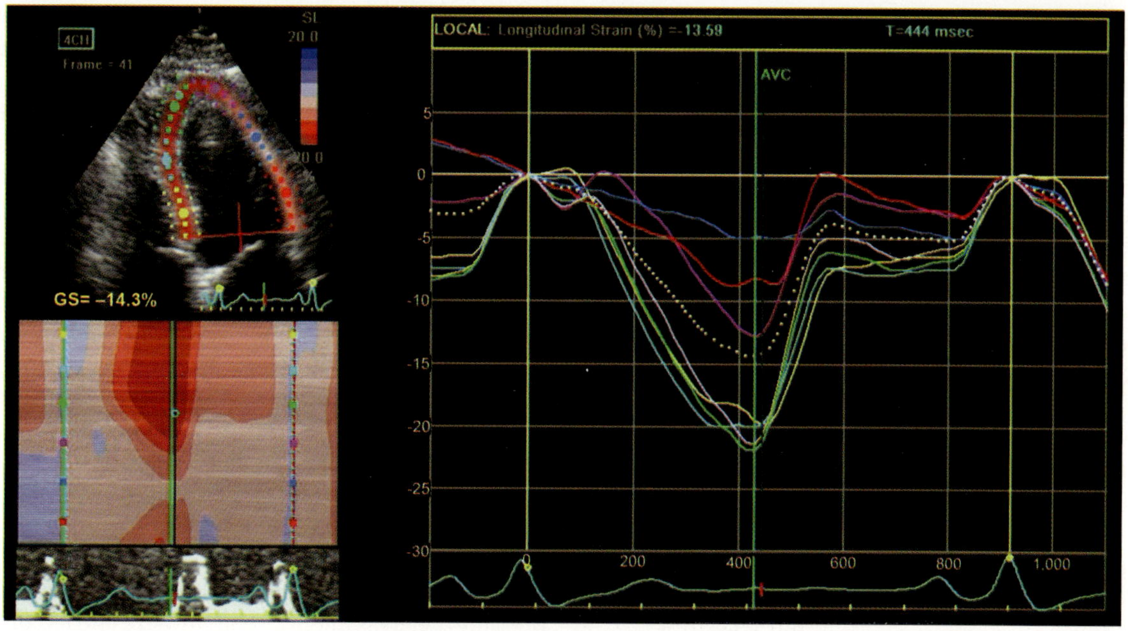

Fig. 1: Measurement of longitudinal strain by speckle-tracking echocardiography. Colored traced represent segmental strain whereas dotter white trace is average of all the six segments. (GS: Global strain)

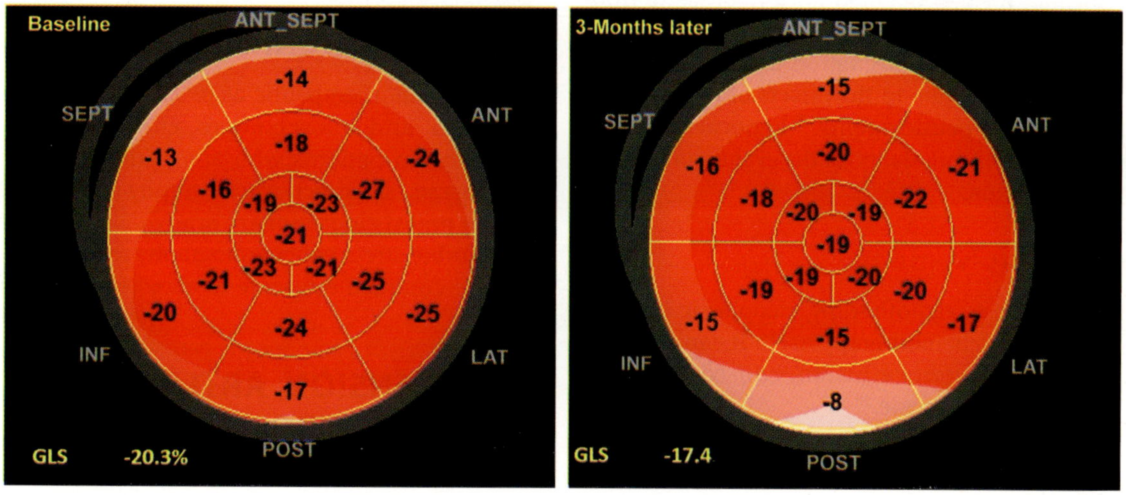

Fig. 2: Global longitudinal strain in a patient receiving trastuzumab for breast cancer. The strain was −20.3% at baseline but dropped to −17.4% at 3 months, representing a 14% relative reduction from the baseline. However, there was no reduction in left ventricular ejection fraction.
(Ant: Anterior; ant_sept: Anterior septum; GLS: Global longitudinal strain; inf: Inferior; lat: Lateral; post: Posterior; sept: Septum)

is the first, international, multicentric randomized study currently underway to address this very important question.[24] Nonetheless, based on the available data, all the current guidelines recommend measuring GLS in patients who are receiving potentially cardiotoxic drugs for early recognition of cardiotoxicity. A relative reduction in GLS ≤ 15% is considered to unequivocally represent subclinical LV systolic dysfunction.[1] However, the management approach once subclinical LV systolic dysfunction is diagnosed remains uncertain. While the American Society of Echocardiography makes no firm recommendation on this issue,[1] several investigators have suggested management protocols incorporating use of cardioprotective therapy based on strain measurement.[25] At this point, it is imperative to recognize some of the important limitations of strain imaging. First, STE is highly dependent on the image quality and the expertise of the examiner, though the interobserver variability for GLS is much lower than that for LVEF.[26] Second, the strain measurements vary according to the analysis software used for this purpose, which limits its cross-platform comparability. However, this intervendor variability has now decreased considerably due to the ongoing efforts of an industry–academia joint task force that has been looking in to this aspect.[27,28]

Assessment of Left Ventricular Diastolic Function

This includes evaluation of mitral inflow pattern and measurement of early diastolic mitral annulus velocity (e′) by tissue Doppler. This gives an indication of LV filling pressures. Left atrial volume estimation, pulmonary artery systolic pressure estimated from tricuspid regurgitation jet, and pulmonary vein flow pattern can provide additional information.

Valve Abnormality

Valve abnormalities can occur due to neoplastic infiltration, nonbacterial thrombotic endocarditis, infective endocarditis, functional regurgitation due to ventricular dysfunction, as well as due to the effects of radiotherapy or some chemotherapeutic agents.[29] Echocardiography remains the most useful modality for the evaluation of valve structure and function.

Pericardial Involvement

This can occur due to radiotherapy, neoplastic involvement, or the cancer chemotherapy itself. It can manifest as pericarditis, pericardial effusion, constrictive pericarditis, or cardiac tamponade.[29]

Right Heart Assessment

Chemotherapeutic agents, such as anthracycline, have been shown to cause a decrease in right ventricular (RV) systolic and diastolic functions in a short period. Some tissue Doppler indices have been shown to be markedly reduced even after the first dose of therapy, along with RV fractional area change (RVFAC) and tricuspid annular plane systolic excursion.[30] Although RV dysfunction is not considered in the diagnosis of cardiotoxicity, concomitant RV dysfunction may be a marker of more significant cardiac injury and a potential risk for persistent LV dysfunction during follow-up.[31] The right ventricle is divided anatomically into inflow and outflow tract and because of its crescentic structure, echocardiographic assessment is difficult. Hence, M-mode, 2D, Doppler, and myocardial strain are all used to evaluate the right heart.

Right ventricular size in parasternal, short-axis, and four-chamber views is measured. Right ventricular end diastolic area and end systolic area are measured to calculate RVFAC. Tricuspid annular plane systolic excursion, which is the systolic excursion of tricuspid annulus and a measure of RV systolic function, is derived using M-mode. Tricuspid annular systolic velocity measured using TDI is another measure of RV systolic function. It is derived by placing the pulsed-Doppler sample volume at lateral tricuspid annulus in the apical four-chamber view. Recently, the importance of RV strain obtained by STE has been established in many studies. In a study, RV dysfunction could be diagnosed in 10% of patients by using RVFAC and in 40% patients with strain analysis.[32] Several hemodynamic parameters can also be derived. Pulmonary artery systolic pressure and pulmonary acceleration time provide information about RV systolic pressure, whereas inferior vena cava size and its collapsibility with respiration are helpful in assessing RV diastolic pressure (which is equivalent to right atrial pressure in the absence of tricuspid inflow obstruction).[33]

STRESS ECHOCARDIOGRAPHY

Certain chemotherapeutic agents, such as 5-fluorouracil, sorafenib, and bevacizumab, can cause myocardial ischemia.[2] In patients who are going to receive one of these agents, stress echocardiography may be required to exclude preexisting coronary artery disease. Additionally, dobutamine stress echocardiography may be indicated to evaluate contractile reserve to allow early recognition of CTRCD.[34]

HYPERTENSION, ARTERIAL THROMBOEMBOLISM, PULMONARY HYPERTENSION

Hypertension and arterial thromboembolism are common side effects of drugs, such as bevacizumab, sunitinib, and cisplatin, whereas tyrosine kinase inhibitors, such as dasatinib, can cause pulmonary hypertension.[2,35] Echocardiography can be used to evaluate the heart in the above conditions so that treatment can be started at the right time.

ECHOCARDIOGRAPHIC MONITORING PROTOCOL

Different organizations have proposed different protocols for monitoring and decision-making in patients receiving

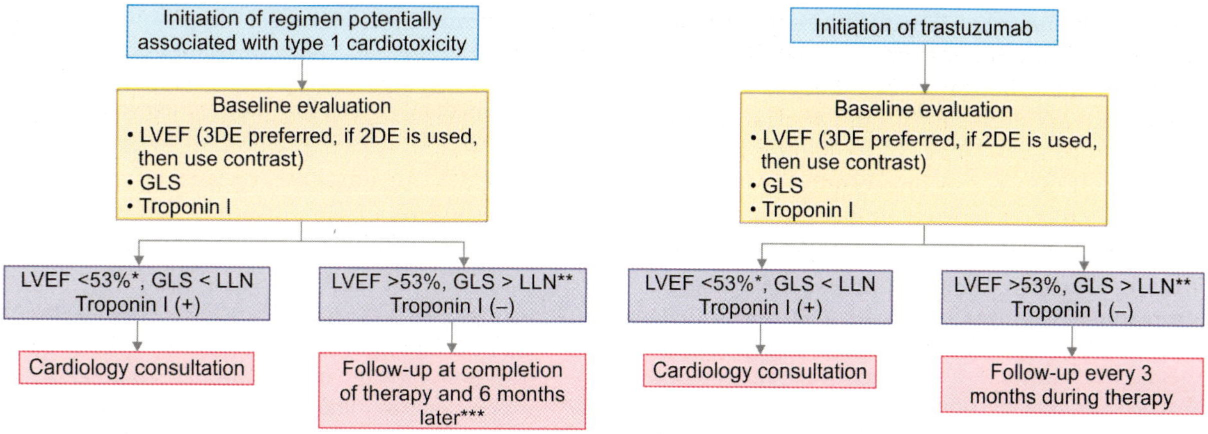

Fig. 3: Monitoring protocol in patients receiving potentially cardiotoxic chemotherapy, as recommended by the American Society of Echocardiography cardiotoxicity[1]: (A) protocol for regimen potentially associated with type 1 cardiotoxicity and (B) protocol for trastuzumab.
(2DE: Two-dimensional echocardiography; 3DE: Three-dimensional echocardiography; GLS: Global longitudinal strain; LLN: Lower limit of normal; LVEF: Left ventricular ejection fraction) *Consider confirmation with cardiac magnetic resonance imaging. **For the reference ranges, please refer the guideline document.[1] ***If the cumulative dose is more than 240 mg/m^2 (or equivalent), recommend measurement of LVEF, GLS, and troponin prior to each additional 50 mg/m^2 dose.

potentially cardiotoxic chemotherapy. The European Society of Medical Oncology published its recommendations in 2012, which are based only on LVEF.[36] In 2014, the American Society of Echocardiography published a guideline describing separate monitoring protocol for subjects receiving agents associated with types I and II cardiotoxicity[1] (Fig. 3). However, management approach in the case of LV systolic dysfunction (subclinical or overt) was not provided. In a recent review, Herrmann et al. have proposed a comprehensive strategy for risk assessment of patients based on medication-related risk and patient-related risk.[25] The subsequent monitoring and management approach is tailored according to the estimated risk, as described below.

Monitoring Protocol

- *Very high risk for cardiotoxicity*:
  Transthoracic echo with strain at baseline and before every cycle, at the end, 3–6 months, and every year, along with electrocardiogram (ECG) and cTn
- *High risk for cardiotoxicity*:
  Transthoracic echo with strain every three cycles, end of therapy, 3–6 months, and 1 year after chemotherapy
  Optional—ECG, cTn
- *Intermediate risk for cardiotoxicity*:
  Transthoracic with strain midterm, end, and 3–6 months after chemotherapy
  Optional—ECG, cTn midterm of chemotherapy
- *Low risk of cardiotoxicity*:
  Optional—Transthoracic with strain and/or ECG, cTn at the end of chemotherapy
- *Very low cardiotoxicity risk*:
  None

Management Protocol

The following protocol has been recommended for the use of cardioprotective agents.[25] These agents may be initiated prophylactically before the initiation of chemotherapy or can be added later, during or after chemotherapy, if there is any evidence of LV systolic dysfunction.

- *Very high risk for cardiotoxicity*:
  Initiate ACE-I/angiotensin receptor blocker (ARB), carvedilol, and statins, starting at lowest dose and start chemotherapy in 1 week from initiation to allow steady-state, up-titrate as tolerated
- *High risk for cardiotoxicity*:
  Initiate ACE-I/ARB, carvedilol, and/or statins
- *Intermediate risk for cardiotoxicity*:
  Discuss risk and benefit of medications
- *Low risk of cardiotoxicity*:
  None, monitoring only
- *Very low cardiotoxicity risk*:
  None, monitoring only

REFERENCES

1. Plana JC, Galderisi M, Barac A, et al. Expert consensus for multimodality imaging evaluation of adult patients during and after cancer therapy: a report from the American Society of Echocardiography and the European Association of Cardiovascular Imaging. J Am Soc Echocardiogr. 2014;27: 911-39.

2. Zamorano JL, Lancellotti P, Rodriguez Munoz D, et al. ESC Position Paper on cancer treatments and cardiovascular toxicity developed under the auspices of the ESC Committee for Practice Guidelines: the Task Force for cancer treatments and cardiovascular toxicity of the European Society of Cardiology (ESC). Eur Heart J. 2016;37:2768-801.
3. Lotrionte M, Biondi-Zoccai G, Abbate A, et al. Review and meta-analysis of incidence and clinical predictors of anthracycline cardiotoxicity. Am J Cardiol. 2013;112:1980-4.
4. Henri C, Heinonen T, Tardif JC. The role of biomarkers in decreasing risk of cardiac toxicity after cancer therapy. Biomark Cancer. 2016;8:39-45.
5. Sandri MT, Salvatici M, Cardinale D, et al. N-terminal pro-B-type natriuretic peptide after high-dose chemotherapy: a marker predictive of cardiac dysfunction? Clin Chem. 2005;51:1405-10.
6. Lang RM, Badano LP, Mor-Avi V, et al. Recommendations for cardiac chamber quantification by echocardiography in adults: an update from the American Society of Echocardiography and the European Association of Cardiovascular Imaging. J Am Soc Echocardiogr. 2015;28:1-39.e14.
7. Thavendiranathan P, Grant AD, Negishi T, et al. Reproducibility of echocardiographic techniques for sequential assessment of left ventricular ejection fraction and volumes: application to patients undergoing cancer chemotherapy. J Am Coll Cardiol. 2013;61:77-84.
8. Bansal M, Kasliwal RR. How do I do it? Speckle-tracking echocardiography. Indian Heart J. 2013;65:117-23.
9. Cheung YF, Hong WJ, Chan GC, et al. Left ventricular myocardial deformation and mechanical dyssynchrony in children with normal ventricular shortening fraction after anthracycline therapy. Heart. 2010;96:1137-41.
10. Hare JL, Brown JK, Leano R, et al. Use of myocardial deformation imaging to detect preclinical myocardial dysfunction before conventional measures in patients undergoing breast cancer treatment with trastuzumab. Am Heart J. 2009;158:294-301.
11. Stoodley PW, Richards DA, Hui R, et al. Two-dimensional myocardial strain imaging detects changes in left ventricular systolic function immediately after anthracycline chemotherapy. Eur J Echocardiogr. 2011;12:945-52.
12. Sawaya H, Sebag IA, Plana JC, et al. Assessment of echocardiography and biomarkers for the extended prediction of cardiotoxicity in patients treated with anthracyclines, taxanes, and trastuzumab. Circ Cardiovasc Imaging. 2012;5:596-603.
13. Poterucha JT, Kutty S, Lindquist RK, et al. Changes in left ventricular longitudinal strain with anthracycline chemotherapy in adolescents precede subsequent decreased left ventricular ejection fraction. J Am Soc Echocardiogr. 2012;25:733-40.
14. Jurcut R, Wildiers H, Ganame J, et al. Strain rate imaging detects early cardiac effects of pegylated liposomal doxorubicin as adjuvant therapy in elderly patients with breast cancer. J Am Soc Echocardiogr. 2008;21:1283-9.
15. Negishi K, Negishi T, Hare JL, et al. Independent and incremental value of deformation indices for prediction of trastuzumab-induced cardiotoxicity. J Am Soc Echocardiogr. 2013;26:493-8.
16. Ganame J, Claus P, Uyttebroeck A, et al. Myocardial dysfunction late after low-dose anthracycline treatment in asymptomatic pediatric patients. J Am Soc Echocardiogr. 2007;20:1351-8.
17. Sawaya H, Sebag IA, Plana JC, et al. Early detection and prediction of cardiotoxicity in chemotherapy-treated patients. Am J Cardiol. 2011;107:1375-80.
18. Tsai HR, Gjesdal O, Wethal T, et al. Left ventricular function assessed by two-dimensional speckle tracking echocardiography in long-term survivors of Hodgkin's lymphoma treated by mediastinal radiotherapy with or without anthracycline therapy. Am J Cardiol. 2011;107:472-7.
19. Thavendiranathan P, Poulin F, Lim KD, et al. Use of myocardial strain imaging by echocardiography for the early detection of cardiotoxicity in patients during and after cancer chemotherapy: a systematic review. J Am Coll Cardiol. 2014;63:2751-68.
20. Seicean S, Seicean A, Alan N, et al. Cardioprotective effect of beta-adrenoceptor blockade in patients with breast cancer undergoing chemotherapy: follow-up study of heart failure. Circ Heart Fail. 2013;6:420-6.
21. Bosch X, Rovira M, Sitges M, et al. Enalapril and carvedilol for preventing chemotherapy-induced left ventricular systolic dysfunction in patients with malignant hemopathies: the OVERCOME trial (preventiOn of left Ventricular dysfunction with Enalapril and caRvedilol in patients submitted to intensive ChemOtherapy for the treatment of Malignant hEmopathies). J Am Coll Cardiol. 2013;61:2355-62.
22. Cardinale D, Colombo A, Sandri MT, et al. Prevention of high-dose chemotherapy-induced cardiotoxicity in high-risk patients by angiotensin-converting enzyme inhibition. Circulation. 2006;114:2474-81.
23. Seicean S, Seicean A, Plana JC, et al. Effect of statin therapy on the risk for incident heart failure in patients with breast cancer receiving anthracycline chemotherapy: an observational clinical cohort study. J Am Coll Cardiol. 2012;60:2384-90.
24. Negishi T, Thavendiranathan P, Negishi K, et al.; SUCCOUR Investigators. Rationale and design of the strain surveillance of chemotherapy for improving cardiovascular outcomes (SUCCOUR) trial. JACC Cardiovasc Imaging. 2018.
25. Herrmann J, Lerman A, Sandhu NP, et al. Evaluation and management of patients with heart disease and cancer: cardio-oncology. Mayo Clin Proc. 2014;89:1287-306.
26. Farsalinos KE, Daraban AM, Unlu S, et al. Head-to-head comparison of global longitudinal strain measurements among nine different vendors: the EACVI/ASE Inter-Vendor Comparison Study. J Am Soc Echocardiogr. 2015;28:1171-81, e2.
27. Voigt JU, Pedrizzetti G, Lysyansky P, et al. Definitions for a common standard for 2D speckle tracking echocardiography: consensus document of the EACVI/ASE/Industry Task Force to Standardize Deformation Imaging. J Am Soc Echocardiogr. 2015;28:183-93.

28. Yang H, Marwick TH, Fukuda N, et al. Improvement in strain concordance between two major vendors after the strain standardization initiative. J Am Soc Echocardiogr. 2015;28:642-8.e7.
29. Lancellotti P, Nkomo VT, Badano LP, et al. Expert consensus for multi-modality imaging evaluation of cardiovascular complications of radiotherapy in adults: a report from the European Association of Cardiovascular Imaging and the American Society of Echocardiography. J Am Soc Echocardiogr. 2013;26:1013-32.
30. Boczar KE, Aseyev O, Sulpher J, et al. Right heart function deteriorates in breast cancer patients undergoing anthracycline-based chemotherapy. Echo Res Pract. 2016;3: 79-84.
31. Calleja A, Poulin F, Khorolsky C, et al. Right ventricular dysfunction in patients experiencing cardiotoxicity during breast cancer therapy. J Oncol. 2015;2015:609194.
32. Dutta T, Aronow WS. Echocardiographic evaluation of the right ventricle: clinical implications. Clin Cardiol. 2017;40:542-8.
33. Tanindi A, Demirci U, Tacoy G, et al. Assessment of right ventricular functions during cancer chemotherapy. Eur J Echocardiogr. 2011;12:834-40.
34. Civelli M, Cardinale D, Martinoni A, et al. Early reduction in left ventricular contractile reserve detected by dobutamine stress echo predicts high-dose chemotherapy-induced cardiac toxicity. Int J Cardiol. 2006;111:120-6.
35. Navi BB, Reiner AS, Kamel H, et al. Risk of arterial thromboembolism in patients with cancer. J Am Coll Cardiol. 2017;70:926-38.
36. Curigliano G, Cardinale D, Suter T, et al. Cardiovascular toxicity induced by chemotherapy, targeted agents and radiotherapy: ESMO Clinical Practice Guidelines. Ann Oncol. 2012;23(Suppl. 7):vii155-66.

SECTION 34

Ethical and Legal Issues

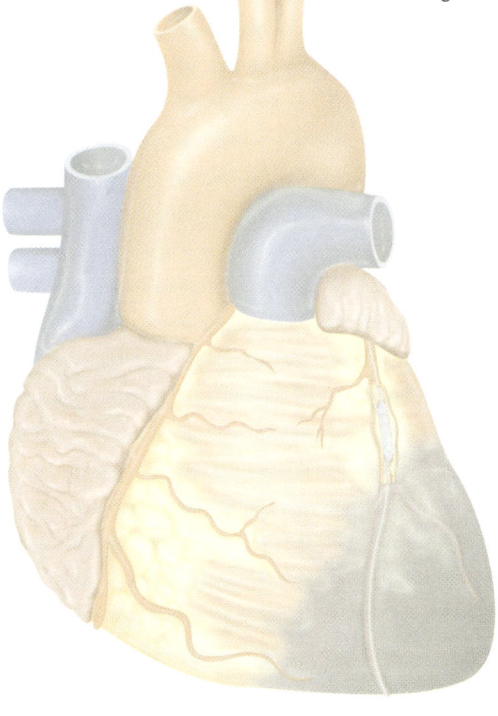

138

CHAPTER

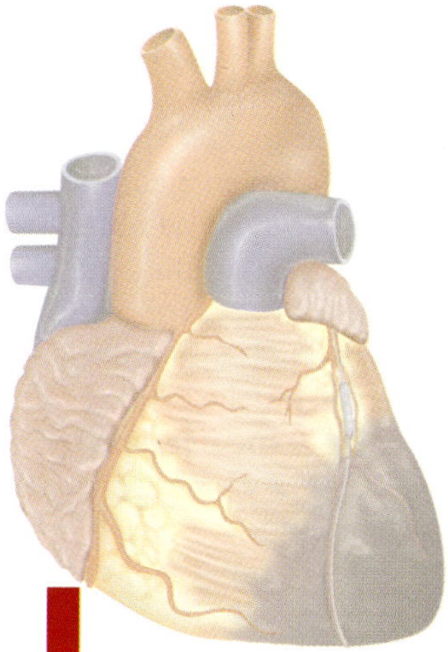

Ethical and Legal Issues in Cardiovascular Imaging

KK Aggarwal

INTRODUCTION

Diagnostics including diagnostic imaging form an important part of delivery of health care. Several billion diagnostic imaging studies and procedures are done annually; of these, one third are cardiovascular procedures.[1] While diagnostic advances have facilitated better management of patients, delivery of health care is increasingly becoming more technology dependent. This, in turn, has led to several ethical and legal issues in the use of imaging modalities in the management of cardiovascular diseases. Issues such as privacy and confidentiality, informed consent have become especially pertinent due to a gradual but perceptible shift in doctor–patient relationship, from paternalism to patient-centered, wherein the patient is a more fully informed and active participant.[2] Patients have the right to refuse treatment; this also implies the right to refuse examination.[3] Few judgements related to informed consent and privacy have drastically altered the ethical and legal scenario in the practice of medicine. The judgement of the Supreme Court of India in *Samira Kohli vs Dr Prabha Manchanda*, the Supreme Court of Pennsylvania in *Shinal vs Toms,* and the United Kingdom Supreme Court in *Montgomery vs Lanarkshire Health Board* and *Dr Bawa-Garba vs General Medical Council* is notable judgement in this regard. The gist of all these judgements is that consent is no longer simply a formality; it is now a legal necessity. In a historic judgement last year, the Supreme Court of India declared right to privacy as a fundamental "inviolable." Cardiologists in India should also know about the various provisions of the Pre-conception and Prenatal Diagnostic Techniques (Prohibition of Sex Selection) (PCPNDT) Act and the latest amendments because violation of any of the provisions therein is liable to criminal prosecution.

INFORMED CONSENT

The meaning of the term consent as defined in *Oxford English dictionary* is "permission for something to happen or agreement to do something."

Oxford Law Dictionary defines the term consent as "Deliberate or implied affirmation; compliance with a course of proposed action. Consent is essential in a number of circumstances. For example, contracts and marriages are invalid unless both parties give their consent. Consent must be given freely, without duress or deception, and with sufficient legal competence to give it."

Section 13 of the Indian Contract Act, 1872, defines the term consent as "Two or more persons are said to consent when they agree upon the same thing in the same sense." Thus, an agreement upon the same thing in the same sense is known as true consent or *consensus ad idem* and is at the root of every contract.

The tone of these definitions indicates that while the general meaning of consent is permission, the law regards consent as a contract, i.e. an agreement enforceable by law.[4]

Consent for the purpose of medical treatment means grant of permission by the patient for an act to be carried out by the doctor, such as a diagnostic, surgical, or therapeutic procedure. The relationship between a doctor and his patient is of an implied contract, i.e. a patient enters a doctor's clinic and sits in the examination chair; his consent is implied for examination, diagnosis, and consultation. This is the case almost always, except where a written informed consent is obtained because no formal contract is usually written when a patient visits a doctor. In medical profession, consent plays a remarkable legitimate role, especially in the field of medical negligence. It is important for the doctor, radiologist, imaging specialist, healthcare staff, etc. to obtain express or written consent from the patient in all major diagnostic procedures, general anesthesia, surgical operations, intimate examinations, examination for determining age, potency, and virginity, and in medicolegal cases. The said express or written consent has to be informed consent also.

Informed consent is nondelegable. This means that the treating doctor has the responsibility to obtain informed consent due to his/her advanced knowledge, training, and consequently expertise. He/she cannot delegate it to a junior doctor or nurse. This was also the position of the Supreme Court of Pennsylvania in *Shinal vs Toms*, which has held that "the duty to obtain informed consent belongs solely to the physician and that it is non-delegable [...] a physician may not delegate to others his or her obligation to provide sufficient information in order to obtain a patient's informed consent. Informed consent requires direct communication between physician and patient and contemplates a back-and-forth, face-to-face exchange, which might include questions that the patient feels the physician must answer personally before the patient feels informed and becomes willing to consent. The duty to obtain the patient's informed consent belongs solely to the physician."

Informed consent means voluntary agreement made by a well-advised and mentally competent patient to be treated or randomized into a research study. Blanket consent given at the time of admission may be invalid. A separate consent for the specific procedure and for anesthesia before conducting the procedure may be taken. A signed informed written consent form by itself does not constitute valid consent, though it is an evidence of consent given by the patient or his guardian. A valid consent has three essential components:

- *Voluntary:* The patient gives consent voluntarily without any coercion; he/she is free from extreme duress and is not intoxicated or under the influence of medication and the doctor has not coerced the patient into giving consent.
- *Competent:* The patient or the spouse/guardian of the patient has the capacity and competence to give consent, i.e. he/she must be major, i.e. 18 years and older and also, must be of sound mind. Competence is typically challenged only when a patient disagrees with the doctor's recommended treatment or refuses treatment altogether. If an individual understands the information presented regarding treatment, he/she is competent to either give consent to or refuse treatment.

When patient lacks the competence to make a decision about treatment, substitute decision maker(s) must be sought. Also, since consent obtained from an incompetent patient is invalid, substituted consent must be obtained. If doctors do not take substituted consent, they may be subject to claims of having treated the person without informed consent. A person is unable to make a decision and is incompetent to give consent, if he/she cannot:

- Understand the information about the decision to be made.
- Retain that information in their mind.
- Use or weigh that information as part of the decision-making process.
- Communicate their decision (by talking, using sign language, or any other means).

Adequate information: The patient must be provided full disclosure of information regarding the material risks, benefits of proposed treatment, alternatives, and consequences of no treatment so that the patient can make an informed choice. All information must be explained in comprehensible nonmedical terms, preferably in local language.

Several international conventions and declarations such as the *Nuremberg Code of 1947* and the *Declaration of Helsinki* adopted by the World Medical Association in 1964 have ratified the importance of obtaining consent from patients before investigations and treatment.

Article 6 of UNESCO's *Universal Declaration on Bioethics and Human Rights on consent* also says, "Any preventive, diagnostic, and therapeutic medical intervention is only to be carried out with the prior, free, and informed consent of the person concerned, based on adequate information. The consent should, where appropriate, be express and may be withdrawn by the person concerned at any time and for any reason without disadvantage or prejudice."

In India, the patient has a legal right to autonomy and self-determination enshrined within *Article 21* of the Constitution of India, 1950, which provides for protection of life and personal liberty by stating "No person shall be deprived of his life or personal liberty except according to procedure established by law." The patient can refuse treatment except in an emergency situation where the doctor need not get consent for treatment. *Clause 7.16 of the MCI Code of Ethics Regulations, 2002* places the responsibility of obtaining consent from the patient or his guardian, in case of a minor, before performing operation, upon the doctor. Failure to obtain consent is a professional misconduct rendering the doctor for disciplinary action.

The landmark judgement of Supreme Court in the case of *Samira Kohli vs Dr Prabha Manchanda & Anr, AIR 2008 SC 1385* has elaborated on different aspects of informed consent.

"32. We may now summarize the principles relating to consent as follows:

- A doctor has to seek and secure the consent of the patient before commencing a 'treatment' (the term 'treatment' includes surgery also). The consent so obtained should be real and valid, which means that: the patient should have the capacity and competence to consent; his consent should be voluntary, and his consent should be on the basis of adequate information concerning the nature of the treatment procedure, so that he knows what is consenting to.
- The 'adequate information' to be furnished by the doctor (or a member of his team) who treats the patient should enable the patient to make a balanced judgment as to whether he should submit himself to the particular treatment as to whether he should submit himself to the particular treatment or not. This means that the Doctor should disclose: (a) nature and procedure of the treatment and its purpose, benefits, and effect; (b) alternatives if any available; (c) an outline of the substantial risks; and (d) adverse consequences of refusing treatment. *But there is no need to explain remote or theoretical risks involved, which may frighten or confuse a patient and result in refusal of consent for the necessary treatment. Similarly, there is no need to explain the remote or theoretical risks of refusal to take treatment which may persuade a patient to undergo a fanciful or unnecessary treatment.* A balance should be achieved between the need for disclosing necessary and adequate information and at the same time avoid the possibility of the patient being deterred from agreeing to a necessary treatment or offering to undergo an unnecessary treatment.
- *Consent given only for a diagnostic procedure, cannot be considered as consent for therapeutic treatment.* Consent given for a specific treatment procedure will not be valid for conducting some other treatment procedure. The fact that the unauthorized additional surgery is beneficial to the patient, or that it would save considerable time and expense to the patient, or would relieve the patient from pain and suffering in future, are not grounds of defence in an action in tort for negligence or assault and battery. *The only exception to this rule* is where the additional procedure though unauthorized is necessary in order to save the life or preserve the health of the patient, and it would be unreasonable to delay such unauthorized procedure until patient regains consciousness and takes a decision.
- There can be a common consent for diagnostic and operative procedures where they are contemplated. There can also be a common consent for a particular surgical procedure and an additional or further procedure that may become necessary during the course of surgery.
- The nature and extent of information to be furnished by the doctor to the patient to secure the consent need not be of the stringent and high degree mentioned in Canterbury but should be of the extent which is accepted as normal and proper by a body of medical men skilled and experienced in the particular field. It will depend upon the physical and mental condition of the patient, the nature of treatment, and the risk and consequences attached to the treatment."

Contrary to what the Supreme Court of India has held in the *Samira Kohli vs Dr Manchanda* case as mentioned above in 32(ii), the UK Supreme Court in 2015 in the case of *Montgomery v Lanarkshire Health Board* changed the law on informed consent and disclosure of information regarding risks in the United Kingdom. When counseling the patients about the benefits and risks of various treatment options, doctors in the United Kingdom are now required to ensure that "the patient is aware of any material risks involved in any recommended treatment, and of any reasonable alternative or variant treatments." The doctor has to inform the patient of all possible risks, even though rare, and let the patient take a decision. The test of materiality would be whether "a reasonable person in the patient's position would be likely to attach significance to the risk, or the doctor is or should reasonably be aware that the particular patient would be likely to attach significance to it."

In the case of *Dr Hadiza Bawa-Garba vs GMC*, wherein a 6-year-old boy with Down syndrome died, the UK Supreme Court sentenced Dr Bawa-Garba to 2 years of imprisonment after she was found guilty of manslaughter and convicted for gross negligence. Her name was also subsequently erased from the Medical Register following action taken by the GMC. Delay in getting and reading the chest X-ray report was one among a series of errors she was held responsible for. The patient was examined at 10:30 AM when chest X-ray along with other blood tests were ordered, but the chest X-ray was available around 12:30 PM and it was reviewed at 3 PM (she was not informed before then that it was available). Not doing so may be potentially fatal to the patient as happened in this case. The X-ray showed that the patient had pneumonia, but the antibiotic was further delayed for another hour by 4 PM. The patient died of streptococcal sepsis. The lesson to be learnt here is that once any imaging study has been ordered, the treating doctor should be persistent in follow-up to avoid any delay in diagnosis. To err is human is no longer true in the United Kingdom.

The *National Consumer Disputes Redressal Commission* (NCDRC) has also ruled on consent in its various judgements.

"[...] Consent is not a one-off event of signatures on paper and not a submission of the patient to a particular treatment but rather a process of communication. It is then perceived as a proactive process empowering the patient to consciously decide on what s/he considers best. Thus, consent is a process of communication requiring the fulfilment of certain established elements, like competence, sufficient disclosure, understanding and volunteering [...]" (*C. Jayapal Reddy versus G. S. Rao, Managing Director, Yashoda Group of Hospitals, 2014 (1) CPJ 271*). "[...] It should not be presumed that a patient may not/need not know the procedure or is incapable of understanding the medical terms and, therefore, there is no use in explaining them. There cannot be a presumption that all patients are ignorant about their anatomy or the adverse effects or benefits of surgery, and, in any case, those days are over. Hence, properly informed written consent before operation is the necessity [...]"(*Saroj Chandhoke versus Sir Ganga Ram Hospital, 2007 (3) CPJ 189*).

A medical practitioner therefore cannot examine, treat, or operate upon the patient without the patient's consent, except by committing a trespass or assault.

WHEN IS CONSENT NOT NECESSARY?

Consent of a patient is not necessary in case of a medical emergency, when the doctor and medical practitioner can operate, examine, and treat the patient without his/her consent and the doctor and medical practitioner is protected by the defense of medical necessity of obtaining consent from the patient.

- In "*Samira Kohli vs Dr Prabha Manchanda, AIR 2008 SC 1385,*" the three-judge Constitution Bench of Hon'ble Supreme Court of India has held that: "[...] The doctor, therefore, is required to communicate all inherent and potential hazards of the proposed treatment, the alternatives to that treatment, if any, and the likely effect if the patient remained untreated. This stringent standard of disclosure was subjected to only two exceptions: (i) *where there was a genuine emergency*, e.g. the patient was unconscious; and (ii) *where the information would be harmful to the patient*, e.g. where it might cause psychological damage, or where the patient would become so emotionally distraught as to prevent a rational decision."
- The Hon'ble Madras High Court in the matter of "*Arun Balakrishnan Iyer vs Soni Hospital, AIR 2003 Madras 389*" has held that "22. When the doctor opines, in good faith, that emergency steps need to be taken in the interest of the patient, but fails to take such steps, he would be failing in his duty; and such failure would be a wrongful omission. Therefore, unless the patient proves that there was no such emergency or that those acts were not done bonafide, the doctor or surgeon cannot be found fault with."

Consent of a patient is also not necessary if in the course of one operation, there is a medical emergency requiring a medical procedure. In such a situation, the doctor can operate on the patient without his/her consent and is protected by the defense of medical necessity. In *Samira Kohli vs Dr Prabha Manchanda & Anr,* the Apex Court said, "What is relevant and of importance is the inviolable nature of the patient's right in regard to his body and his right to decide whether he should undergo the particular treatment or surgery or not. Therefore at the risk of repetition, we may add that unless the unauthorized additional or further procedure is necessary in order to save the life or preserve the health of the patient and it would be unreasonable (as contrasted from being merely inconvenient) to delay the further procedure until the patient regains consciousness and takes a decision, a doctor cannot perform such procedure without the consent of the patient."

In *Pravat Kumar Mukherjee vs Ruby General Hospital & Ors, 2005 (2) CPJ 35,* the NCDRC has held that "Considering the aforesaid law, it is apparent that: emergency treatment was required to be given to the deceased who was brought in a seriously injured condition; there was no question of waiting for the consent of the patient or a passerby who brought the patient to the hospital, and was not necessary to wait for consent to be given for treatment [...] Consent is implicit in such cases when patient is brought to the hospital for treatment, and a surgeon who fails to perform an emergency operation must prove that the patient refused to undergo the operation not only at the initial stage but even after the patient was informed about the dangerous consequences of not undergoing the operation."

Besides these general aspects, informed consent also has significant implications in cardiovascular imaging, particularly when an imaging modality that uses ionizing procedure is being considered as a diagnostic procedure.

Exposure to radiation during an imaging procedure, either radiological or nuclear medicine, is associated with a low but definite future risk of cancer. Patients, however, are mostly ignorant of the radiological dose they are exposed to and the risk of cancer consequent to that dose.[5] Radiation exposure is much higher in a CT scan compared to a plain film X-ray because of the larger radiation doses in the CT scan.[6]

Ironically, doctors are also not able to calculate the radiological doses at times even with years of experience behind them.[5] In a survey conducted in a tertiary care referral center of adult-pediatric cardiology center of excellence, the risk of fatal cancer associated with a stress myocardial perfusion scintigraphy procedure was erroneously estimated as "zero" or "less than 1 in 10 million" or "less than 1 in 1 million" by 95 physicians. Only 5% could give the right answer, i.e. more than 1 in 10,000 tests.[7] Few doctors cannot differentiate between "green" (nonionizing) and "red" (ionizing) imaging techniques or they have "imaging daltonism" as shown in a questionnaire study published in the BMJ, which assessed the knowledge of radiation exposure among doctors. Five percent doctors were unaware that ultrasound did not use ionizing radiation; likewise, 8% doctors were unaware that magnetic resonance imaging (MRI) did not use ionizing radiation.[8]

It has been suggested that a radiological dose may be communicated as multiples of a chest X-ray. Radiological dose in a thallium scan is equivalent to more than 1,000 chest X-rays; in a multislice CT scan, the radiological dose is more than 500 chest X-rays.[9]

Before taking informed consent for the diagnostic imaging procedure, the cardiologist has a responsibility to not only inform the patient of all the associated risks with the procedure recommended, but also the availability of alternative diagnostic modalities that do not use ionizing radiation such as echocardiography or cardiac MRI.[10] In a position paper published in the June 2016 issue of the *Journal of Radiological Protection*, the European Society of Cardiology (ESC) has recommended inclusion of the following information on the radiological consent form: type of imaging modality, effective dose (mSv) including the effective dose expressed as the number of chest X-rays, and the risk of cancer.[11]

PRE-CONCEPTION AND PRENATAL DIAGNOSTIC TECHNIQUES (PROHIBITION OF SEX SELECTION) ACT

The PCPNDT Act provides for the prohibition of sex selection, before or after conception, and for regulation of prenatal diagnostic techniques for the purposes of detecting genetic abnormalities or metabolic disorders or chromosomal abnormalities or certain congenital malformations or sex feticide and for matters connected therewith or incidental thereto. PCPNDT Act extends to whole of India except the State of Jammu and Kashmir. It came into force on 01.01.1996 vide S.O. 990(E) dated December 20, 1995 published in Gazette of India.

The Act was amended in the year 2003 vide Amendment Act 4 of 2003, keeping in view the emerging technologies for selection of sex before and after conception and problems faced in the working of implementation of the act and certain directions of Hon'ble Supreme Court after a PIL was filed in May 2000 by Centre For Enquiry Into Health (CEHAT) and Ors, a nongovernmental organization on slow implementation of the Act. These amendments have come into operation with effect from February 14, 2003.

The few basic requirements of the Act are as follows:

- Written consent of the pregnant woman and prohibition of communicating the sex of fetus under Section 5 of the Act
- Maintenance of records as provided under Section 29 of the Act
- Creating awareness among the public at large by placing the board of prohibition on sex determination

A look at the basic requirement of the Act shows the simplicity of the Act, but noncompliance of the Act in any manner, be it the smallest of an error brings wrath upon the errant. The Act penalizes all the errant, either involved in sex determination or nonmaintenance of records. It would not be out of place to therefore state that the most effective precautionary measures are to maintain records scrupulously, fill the Form-F as provided in the Act, accurately and correctly, and submit the records to the Appropriate Authority within the stipulated time.

Sex determination is prohibited under the PCPNDT Act. As per provisions of *Section 6 of PCPNDT Act*, the genetic counseling centers or genetic laboratory or genetic clinic are prohibited from conducting or cause to be conducting in its center, laboratory, or clinic prenatal diagnostic techniques including ultrasonography for the purposes of determining the sex of the fetus. Also, no person is allowed is conduct or cause to be conducted any prenatal diagnostic techniques including ultrasonography for the purposes of determining sex of the fetus or cause or allow to cause selection of sex before or after conception.

Under PCPNDT Act, it is mandatory for the genetic counseling centers, genetic laboratories, or genetic clinics to get themselves registered under the said Act. Not doing so would prohibit them from the following under *Section 3 of PCPNDT Act*:

- Conducting or associating with or helping in conducting activities relating to prenatal techniques
- Employing or cause to be employed or take services of any person whether on honorary basis or on payment who does not possess the qualifications as may be prescribed

All centers including the one using the ultrasound machine or imaging machine or scanner or any other equipment capable of detecting sex of fetus are compulsorily required to get registered under the PCPNDT Act, without which they cannot function or operate.

Further, as per the provisions of *Section 3B of PCPNDT Act* and *Rule 3A of PCPNDT Rules*, nobody can sell any ultrasound machine or imaging machine or scanner or any other equipment capable of detecting sex of the fetus to any genetic counseling center, genetic laboratory, genetic clinic, or any other person who is not registered under the PCPNDT Act.

Section 18 of the PCPNDT Act makes it mandatory for all genetic counseling centers, genetic laboratories, genetic clinics including all clinics, laboratories, or center having ultrasound or imaging machine or scanner or any other technology capable of undertaking determination of sex of fetus and sex selection or render services to any of them to get themselves registered under the said Act. Registration can be canceled or suspended by the Appropriate Authority either *suo moto* or on complaint after issuing a show cause notice to the said center or clinic thereby asking as to why its registration should not be canceled or suspended.

If after giving a reasonable opportunity of being heard to the Genetic Counseling Centre or Genetic Laboratory or Genetic Clinic, the Appropriate Authority is of the opinion that the said Centre or Clinic has breached the provisions of the PCPNDT Act/Rules, then the Appropriate Authority can suspend the registration for such period as it may think fit. The Appropriate Authority shall communicate with reasons as to why the registration has been rejected to the applicant in Form C (*Rule 6 of the PCPNDT Rules*).

The Genetic Counseling Centre or Genetic Laboratory or Genetic Clinic whose registration has been canceled or suspended can prefer an appeal within a period of 30 days from the date of the receipt of the order of suspension or cancellation of registration as passed by the Appropriate Authority before the Central Government if the appeal is against the order of Central Appropriate Authority, or the State Government, if the appeal is against the order of State Appropriate Authority.

COMPLIANCES UNDER THE PRE-CONCEPTION AND PRENATAL DIAGNOSTIC TECHNIQUES (PROHIBITION OF SEX SELECTION) ACT AND RULES

- *Display of Certificate of Registration*: It is compulsory for all the registered Genetic Counseling Centre, Genetic Laboratory, or Genetic Clinic to display the certificate of registration under the PCPNDT Act in a conspicuous place at its place of business. One copy of the certificate of registration has to be displayed by the registered mobile medical unit inside the vehicle at conspicuous place (*Rule 6 of the PCPNDT Rules*).
- *Maintenance of records*: Section 29 of the PCPNDT Act requires that all records, charts, forms, reports, consent letters, and all the documents be maintained and preserved for a period of 2 years. However, if any criminal or other proceedings are instituted against any Genetic Counseling Centre or Genetic Laboratory or Genetic Clinic, then the records have to be preserved till the final disposal of such proceedings.

It is mandatory that all such records are made available for inspection to the Appropriate Authority or to any other person authorized by the Appropriate Authority.

- Records to be maintained:
  - By every Genetic Counseling Centre in respect of each woman counseled is specified in Form D (*Rule 9(2) of PCPNDT Rules*).
  - By every Genetic Laboratory in respect of each man or woman subjected to any prenatal diagnostic technique is specified in Form E (*Rule 9(3) of PCPNDT Rules*).
  - By ever Genetic Clinic including a mobile Genetic Clinic in respect of each man or woman subjected to any prenatal diagnostic technique is specified in Form-F (*Rule 9(4) of PCPNDT Rules*).
- If records are maintained on computer or in electronic form, then the printed copy of the record shall be taken and preserved after authentication by a person responsible for such record.
- A complete report in respect of all pre-conception or pregnancy-related procedures, techniques, and tests conducted by the Genetic Counseling Centre, Genetic Laboratory, Genetic Clinic, Ultrasound Clinic or Imaging Centre in respect of a month by 5th day of the following month to the Appropriate Authority.
- *Intimation of changes in employees, place, or equipment*: Every Genetic Counseling Centre, Genetic Laboratory, Genetic Clinic, Ultrasound Clinic, or Imaging Centre shall intimate every change in the employees, place, address, and equipment at least 30 days in advance of the expected date of such change and seek re-issuance of the certificate of registration from the Appropriate Authority (*Rule 13 of PCPNDT Rules*).
- Public Notice: Every Genetic Counseling Centre, Genetic Laboratory, Genetic Clinic, Ultrasound Clinic, or Imaging Centre shall prominently display on its premises a notice in English and in local language for the information of the public that the disclosure of sex of the fetus is prohibited under law (*Rule 17(1) of PCPNDT Rules*).

- *Copy of PCPNDT Act and Rules*: Every Genetic Counseling Centre, Genetic Laboratory, Genetic Clinic, Ultrasound Clinic, or Imaging Centre has to keep at least one copy of the PCPNDT Act and Rules in its premises and has to make available the same to its client on demand (*Rule 17(2) of the PCPNDT Rules*).

PUNISHMENT UNDER THE PRE-CONCEPTION AND PRENATAL DIAGNOSTIC TECHNIQUES (PROHIBITION OF SEX SELECTION) ACT

- Prohibition of advertisement relating to pre-conception and prenatal determination of sex and in case of contravention, the person shall be punished with imprisonment for a term, which may extend to 3 years, and with fine, which may extend to ₹10,000/- (*Section 22 of PCPNDT Act*).
- Any medical geneticist, gynecologist, registered medical practitioner, or any person who owns a Genetic Counseling Centre, Genetic Laboratory, or a Genetic Clinic or is employed in any such Center, Laboratory, or Clinic and renders his professional or technical services to or at such Center, Laboratory, or Clinic whether on honorary basis or otherwise and contravenes any of the provisions of PCPNDT Act and Rules, then the said person shall be punishable with imprisonment, which may extend to 3 years, and with fine, which may extend to ₹10,000/- and on subsequent conviction, with imprisonment, which may extend to 5 years, and with fine, which may extend to ₹50,000/-. Also, the name of the registered medical practitioner shall be reported with the State Medical Council for taking appropriate action, including suspension of registration till the final disposal of the case and on conviction for removal of his name from the medical register (*Section 23 of the PCPNDT Act*).
- Penalty for contravention of the provisions of the PCPNDT Act or Rules for which no specific punishment is provided is imprisonment for a term, which may extend to 3 months, or with fine, which may extend to ₹1,000/- or with both and in case of subsequent contravention with an additional fine, which may extend to ₹500/- for every day during which such contravention continues after conviction for the first contravention (*Section 25 of PCPNDT Act*).
- In case of offenses by the company, then the person who was in charge and responsible for the conduct of the business of the company shall be proceeded against and punished accordingly unless he proves that the offense was committed without his knowledge or that he had exercised all due diligence to prevent the commission of the said offense (*Section 26 of PCPNDT Act*).
- Every offense under PCPNDT Act is cognizable, nonbailable, and noncompoundable (*Section 27 of PCPNDT Act*).

In the matter of *Voluntary Health Association of Punjab V. UOI & Ors* Writ Petition (C) No. 349/2006 dated 08.11.2016, the Hon'ble Supreme Court of India has issued directions as contained in para 33 of the said judgement. The court has observed that there is decrease in the sex ratio which is a sign of calamity and not be allowed to happen. However, the Supreme Court declined to interfere and grant any relief to Indian Medical Association (IMA) for striking down the provisions of the Act and the rules on the ground of their misuse by the authorities. The Supreme Court has observed that in all such cases of misuse of the provisions of the Act/Rules, the concerned person always has legal remedies available in law, and the Writ petition filed on behalf of IMA was dismissed.

Directions as para 33 are as follows:

a. All the States and the Union Territories in India shall maintain a centralized database of civil registration records from all registration units so that information can be made available from the website regarding the number of boys and girls being born.
b. The information that shall be displayed on the website shall contain the birth information for each District, Municipality, Corporation or Gram Panchayat so that a visual comparison of boys and girls born can be immediately seen.
c. The statutory authorities if not constituted as envisaged under the Act shall be constituted forthwith and the competent authorities shall take steps for the reconstitution of the statutory bodies so that they can become immediately functional after expiry of the term. That apart, they shall meet regularly so that the provisions of the Act can be implemented in reality and the effectiveness of the legislation is felt and realized in the society.
d. The provisions contained in Sections 22 and 23 shall be strictly adhered to. Section 23(2) shall be duly complied with and it shall be reported by the authorities so that the State Medical Council takes necessary action after the intimation is given under the said provision. The Appropriate Authorities who have been appointed under Sections 17(1) and 17(2) shall be imparted periodical training to carry out the functions as required under various provisions of the Act.
e. If there has been violation of any of the provisions of the Act or the Rules, proper action has to be taken

by the authorities under the Act so that the legally inapposite acts are immediately curbed.

f. The Courts which deal with the complaints under the Act shall be fast tracked and the concerned High Courts shall issue appropriate directions in that regard.
g. The judicial officers who are to deal with these cases under the Act shall be periodically imparted training in the Judicial Academies or Training Institutes, as the case may be, so that they can be sensitive and develop the requisite sensitivity as projected in the objects and reasons of the Act and its various provisions and in view of the need of the society.
h. The Director of Prosecution or, if the said post is not there, the Legal Remembrancer or the Law Secretary shall take stock of things with regard to the lodging of prosecution so that the purpose of the Act is sub served.
i. The Courts that deal with the complaints under the Act shall deal with the matters in promptitude and submit the quarterly report to the High Courts through the concerned Sessions and District Judge.
j. The learned Chief Justices of each of the High Courts in the country are requested to constitute a Committee of three Judges that can periodically oversee the progress of the cases.
k. The awareness campaigns with regard to the provisions of the Act as well as the social awareness shall be undertaken as per the direction No 9.8 in the order dated March 4, 2013 passed in Voluntary Health Association of Punjab (supra).
l. The State Legal Services Authorities of the States shall give emphasis on this campaign during the spread of legal aid and involve the para-legal volunteers.
m. The Union of India and the States shall see to it that appropriate directions are issued to the authorities of All India Radio and Doordarshan functioning in various States to give wide publicity pertaining to the saving of the girl child and the grave dangers the society shall face because of female foeticide.
n. All the appropriate authorities including the States and districts notified under the Act shall submit quarterly progress report to the Government of India through the State Government and maintain Form H for keeping the information of all registrations readily available as per subrule 6 of Rule 18A of the Rules.
o. The States and Union Territories shall implement the Pre-conception and Prenatal Diagnostic Techniques (Prohibition of Sex Selection) (Six Months Training) Rules, 2014 forthwith considering that the training provided therein is imperative for realising the objects and purpose of this Act.
p. As the Union of India and some States framed incentive schemes for the girl child, the States that have not framed such schemes may introduce such schemes."

THE ISSUE RELATING TO "SILENT OBSERVER" AND INFORMATION TO BE SUPPLIED IN "FORM-F" TO BE SUBMITTED ONLINE

In respect to the above issue the Hon'ble Division Bench Bombay High Court passed judgement on 26.08.2011 in writ petition No. 797/11 titled *"Radiological & Imaging Association/State chapter Jalna V. UOI &Ors"* had upheld the circular dated 14.01.2011 issued by the state authorities in Kolhapur, Maharashtra, to submit online Form-F with all relevant information within 24 hours and to install silent observer embodied on the ultrasound machine and to keep the ultrasonography slides stored in the silent observer.

The contention raised by the petitioners regarding invasion of privacy rights was turned down and rejected on the ground that the images stored in the silent observer are not transmitted online to any server except the appropriate authority only has access to them. Silent observer is an electronic device attached to a sonography machine and in case the appropriate authority requires to check the sonographies that have taken place through a particular machine, the appropriate authority/authorized officer will go to the site where the ultrasound machine is installed and take out the silent observer and can actually see the sonographies/images on a computer by entering the name and password under the control of the Collector. The court further gave directions to the appropriate authority not to allow access to such data stored in a silent observer to a nonmedical officer except the Collector himself or any senior officer not below the rank of Deputy Collector.

THE CONTROVERSY REGARDING THE AMENDMENTS MADE IN PRE-CONCEPTION AND PRENATAL DIAGNOSTIC TECHNIQUES (PROHIBITION OF SEX SELECTION) RULES, 1996 IN THE YEAR 2014 THEREBY AMENDING RULE 3(3)(1)(B) AND FURTHER INTRODUCING PRE-CONCEPTION AND PRENATAL DIAGNOSTIC TECHNIQUES (PROHIBITION OF SEX SELECTION) (6 MONTHS TRAINING) RULES, 2014

This controversy has been set at rest in the judgement of Hon'ble Delhi High Court, New Delhi, dated 17.02.2016 in W.P. (C) No. 6968/2011 titled *"Indian Radiological & Imaging Association V. UOI & Anr."* with WP (C) No. 2721/2014 titled *"Indian Medical Association V. UOI"* & W.P. (C) No. 3184/2014 titled *"Sonological Society of India V. UOI & Anr"* thereby striking down part of Section2 (p) of the Act and declaring illegal the rule 3(3)(1)(b) and other connecting provisions being contrary to the provisions of Indian Medical Council Act, 1954.

The Court held that Section 2(p) of the PCPNDT Act defining a Sonologist or Imaging Specialist is bad to the extent it includes persons possessing a postgraduate qualification in ultrasonography or imaging techniques. Also, it has been held that if the person seeking registration (a) makes a declaration in the form to be prescribed by the Central Supervisory Board to the effect that the said machine or equipment is not intended for conducting prenatal diagnostic procedures; (b) gives an undertaking to not use or allow the use of the same for prenatal diagnostic procedures; and (c) has a "silent observer" or any other equipment installed on the ultrasound machines, as may be prescribed by the Central Supervisory Board, capable of storing images of each sonography tests done therewith, such person would be exempt from complying with the provisions of the Act and the Rules with respect to Genetic Clinics, Genetic Laboratory, or Genetic Counseling Centre.

The matter titled as "Indian Radiological and Imaging Association versus UOI &Anr., SLP (C) 11046/2016" and "Union of India versus Indian Radiological & Imaging Association & Others, SLP (C) No. 16657/2016" were listed for hearing on 14.03.2018 in which the Hon'ble Supreme Court of India has vide order dated 14.03.2018 stayed the judgement of the Delhi High Court during the pendency of these proceedings. The Hon'ble Supreme Court has further held that the judgement of the High Court squarely impinges upon the directions issued by this Court in Voluntary Health Association of Punjab.

Thus, the Hon'ble Supreme Court has vide order dated 14.03.2018 has directed that the judgement of this Court in Voluntary Health Association of Punjab shall be strictly enforced by all states and union territories untrammeled by any order of any High Court or any other court.

The above-mentioned matters titled as "Indian Radiological and Imaging Association versus UOI &Anr., SLP (C) 11046/2016" and "Union of India versus Indian Radiological & Imaging Association & Others, SLP (C) No. 16657/2016" are pending adjudication before the Hon'ble Court and the same are likely to be listed on 05.10.2018.

Sex determination is also a professional misconduct as per Regulation 7.6 of the MCI Code of Ethics Regulations, 2002, which states as follows: "On no account sex determination test shall be undertaken with the intent to terminate the life of a female fetus developing in her mother's womb, unless there are other absolute indications for termination of pregnancy as specified in the Medical Termination of Pregnancy Act, 1971. Any act of termination of pregnancy of normal female fetus amounting to female feticide shall be regarded as professional misconduct on the part of the physician leading to penal erasure besides rendering him liable to criminal proceedings as per the provisions of this Act."

"Performing or enabling unqualified person to perform an abortion or any illegal operation for which there is no medical, surgical, or psychological indication (7.9)."

BENEFICENCE AND NONMALEFICENCE

Primum non nocere, i.e. "first (above all) do no harm" is the cardinal principle that guides the ethics of practice of medicine. From it is derived the principle of nonmaleficence (do no harm) and its natural corollary, the principle of beneficence (do good).

Beneficence and nonmaleficence along with patient autonomy and justice constitute the four guiding tenets of medical ethics and have been identified as most important for ethical decision-making in medical practice.

World Medical Association, in its Medical Ethics Manual, has stated that:

"Beneficence—literally, 'doing good.' Physicians are expected to act in the best interests of their patients.

Non-maleficence—literally, not doing wrong. Physicians and medical researchers are to avoid inflicting harm on patients and research subjects"

UNESCO addresses ethical issues related to medicine, life sciences, and associated technologies as applied to human beings, taking into account their social, legal, and environmental dimensions in various articles of its Universal Declaration on Bioethics and Human Rights. The relevant articles of the said Declaration are reproduced here under:

- "*Article 4—Benefit and harm*: In applying and advancing scientific knowledge, medical practice and associated technologies, direct and indirect benefits to patients, research participants, and other affected individuals should be maximized and any possible harm to such individuals should be minimized.
- *Article 5—Autonomy and individual responsibility*: The autonomy of persons to make decisions, while taking responsibility for those decisions and respecting the autonomy of others, is to be respected. For persons who are not capable of exercising autonomy, special measures are to be taken to protect their rights and interests.
- *Article 8—Respect for human vulnerability and personal integrity*: In applying and advancing scientific knowledge, medical practice and associated

technologies, human vulnerability should be taken into account. Individuals and groups of special vulnerability should be protected and the personal integrity of such individuals respected.

- *Article 10—Equality, justice and equity*: The fundamental equality of all human beings in dignity and rights is to be respected so that they are treated justly and equitably.
- *Article 11—Non-discrimination and non-stigmatization*: No individual or group should be discriminated against or stigmatized on any grounds, in violation of human dignity, human rights, and fundamental freedoms."

International Ethical Guidelines for Biomedical Research Involving Human Subjects prepared by the Council for International Organizations of Medical Sciences (CIOMS) in collaboration with the World Health Organization (WHO) provides the general ethical principles as follows:

"*General ethical principles. All research involving human subjects should be conducted in accordance with three basic ethical principles, namely respect for persons, beneficence and justice...*

Respect for persons incorporates at least two fundamental ethical considerations, namely:

a. *Respect for autonomy, which requires that those who are capable of deliberation about their personal choices should be treated with respect for their capacity for self-determination; and*
b. *Protection of persons with impaired or diminished autonomy, which requires that those who are dependent or vulnerable be afforded security against harm or abuse.*

Beneficence refers to the ethical obligation to maximize benefits and to minimize harms... Beneficence further proscribes the deliberate infliction of harm on persons; this aspect of beneficence is sometimes expressed as a separate principle, nonmaleficence (do no harm).

Justice refers to the ethical obligation to treat each person in accordance with what is morally right and proper, to give each person what is due to him or her...

'Vulnerability' refers to a substantial incapacity to protect one's own interests owing to such impediments as lack of capability to give informed consent, lack of alternative means of obtaining medical care or other expensive necessities or being a junior or subordinate member of a hierarchical group. Accordingly, special provision must be made for the protection of the rights and welfare of vulnerable persons."

In an article "Obligation of non-maleficence: moral dilemma in physician–patient relationship" published in JMBR June 2005, Peter F Omonzejele has written "The principles and rules of medical ethics are derived from the Hippocratic oath and various declarations (Declaration of Geneva as amended in Sydney 1968, Declaration of Tokyo 1975, Declaration of Oslo 1970, Declaration of Helsinki 1975, etc.) regulating medical practice. Despite the Hippocratic Oath and various declarations, a certain aspect (non-maleficence) of the oath and declaration is sometimes breached in what seems to be in the 'interest' of patients in circumstances that constitute moral dilemmas... The physician–patient relationship is fiduciary. The patient believes and trusts that the physician would apply his professional expertise in his/her (the patient's) interest and benefit. Even more importantly, the patient believes that his/her physicians (based on the principle of non-maleficence) would do nothing to harm him/her. The principle of non-maleficence runs through from the Hippocratic Oath to current versions and amendments of medical ethics. Non-maleficence in general, and medical non-maleficence in particular, recommends that one ought not to inflict evil or harm."

The doctor has a duty to maintain good medical practice, as directed in the MCI Code of Ethics regulations. Further elaborating on this, the Code of conduct says

"*... Who-so-ever chooses his profession, assumes the obligation to conduct himself in accordance with its ideals. A physician should be an upright man, instructed in the art of healings. He shall keep himself pure in character and be diligent in caring for the sick; he should be modest, sober, patient, prompt in discharging his duty without anxiety; conducting himself with propriety in his profession and in all the actions of his life (1.1.2).*"

"The Principal objective of the medical profession is to render service to humanity with full respect for the dignity of profession and man. Physicians should merit the confidence of patients entrusted to their care, rendering to each a full measure of service and devotion. Physicians should try continuously to improve medical knowledge and skills and should make available to their patients and colleagues the benefits of their professional attainments. The physician should practice methods of healing founded on scientific basis and should not associate professionally with anyone who violates this principle. The honoured ideals of the medical profession imply that the responsibilities of the physician extend not only to individuals but also to society (1.2.1)."

CONFIDENTIALITY AND PRIVACY

The terms privacy and confidentiality have often been considered as synonyms. But, the two are not the same, and it is important to know the difference between the two.

Privacy is the right of a person (patient) to keep his health information, including any other personal information, private, and undisclosed. Doctors are often privy to private information shared by the patients during the course of history taking and treatment.

However, confidentiality is what we, as doctors (or other concerned persons) do with the information that has been entrusted to us. Confidentiality implies the duty of everyone entrusted with any information to keep that information private.

Privacy and confidentiality have also been included among the important principles of bioethics defined by UNESCO under its Universal Declaration on Bioethics and Human Right in Article 9, which is reproduced hereunder: "The privacy of the persons concerned and the confidentiality of their personal information should be respected. To the greatest extent possible, such information should not be used or disclosed for purposes other than those for which it was collected or consented to, consistent with international law, in particular international human rights law."

Protecting the privacy of patient information is the ethical duty of the doctor as also mandated in the MCI Code of Ethics Regulations. According to Regulation 2.2, "Patience and delicacy should characterize the physician. Confidences concerning individual or domestic life entrusted by patients to a physician and defects in the disposition or character of patients observed during medical attendance should never be revealed unless their revelation is required by the laws of the State. Sometimes, however, a physician must determine whether his duty to society requires him to employ knowledge, obtained through confidence as a physician, to protect a healthy person against a communicable disease to which he is about to be exposed. In such instance, the physician should act as he would wish another to act toward one of his own family in like circumstances.

The following acts of commission or omission on the part of the physician shall constitute professional misconduct rendering him/her liable for disciplinary action:

7.14: The registered medical practitioner shall not disclose the secrets of a patient that have been learnt in the exercise of his/her profession except—(1) in a court of law under orders of the Presiding Judge, (2) in circumstances where there is a serious and identified risk to a specific person and/or community, and (3) notifiable diseases. In case of communicable/notifiable diseases, concerned public health authorities should be informed immediately.

7.17: A registered medical practitioner shall not publish photographs or case reports of his/her patients without their permission, in any medical or other journal in a manner by which their identity could be made out. If the identity is not to be disclosed, the consent is not needed."

As per the Electronic Health Record Standards for India 2016, "the term 'privacy' shall mean that only those person or person(s) including organizations duly authorized by the patient may view the recorded data or part thereof. The term 'security' shall mean that all recorded personally identifiable data will at all times be protected from any unauthorized access, particularly during transport (e.g. from healthcare provider to provider, healthcare provider to patient, etc.)."

USE OF SOCIAL MEDIA

Social media has become a very important mode of communication in any sphere of life, including medicine. It allows direct, faster, and almost instant sharing of information to a worldwide audience. Social media have proven to be a valuable learning tool not only for students but also for practicing doctors, by improving communication and allowing sharing of data and at times to seek an opinion in a difficult or complicated case or engage in discussion on the same. But this has also made patient information more vulnerable to breach of privacy and confidentiality. The healthcare sector is covered under the Information Technology (IT) Act, 2000, which has provisions relating to data protection and penalties and compensation for damage to computer, computer system, failure to protect data, failure to furnish information return, etc. and residuary penalty. Sharing of patient videos on social media like WhatsApp is a criminal offense punishable under the IT Act.

- As per *Section 43 of the IT Act, 2000* if any person without taking permission from the owner or any other person who may be in charge of a computer, computer system, or computer network accesses or secures access to such Computer; downloads, copies, or extracts any data or information from such Computer or helps any person in gaining access to such Computer, such person can be held liable to pay compensation up to ₹1 Crore to the person so affected. Furthermore, if any of these acts, as prescribed under Section 43 of the Act, is done with the dishonest or fraudulent intention, such person may have to face imprisonment for a term which may extend to 3 years or pay fine up to ₹5 lakh or both.
- *Section 43-A of the IT Act* provides even greater penal consequences for negligence in implementing and maintaining reasonable security practices and procedures in relation to sensitive personal data or information by a body corporate. Compensation for the violation of Section 43-A can even extent to the tune of ₹5 Crores.
- Similarly, *Section 72-A of the IT Act* deals with personal information and provides punishment for disclosure of information in breach of lawful contract or without the

information provider's consent. It is to be noted that even data which are outsourced to India get protection under these section.

Information relating to health of an individual is considered as sensitive personal data or information as per Rule 3 of "The Information Technology (Reasonable Security and Practices and Procedures and Sensitive Personal Data or Information) Rules, 2011." Information relating to password, financial information, such as Bank account or credit card or debit card or other payment instrument details, sexual orientation, and biometric information is also included under sensitive personal data or information.

Rule 6. Disclosure of information. Disclosure of sensitive personal data or information by body corporate to any third party shall require prior permission from the provider of such information, who has provided such information under lawful contract or otherwise, unless such disclosure has been agreed to in the contract between the body corporate and provider of information, or where the disclosure is necessary for compliance of a legal obligation.

Rule 7. Transfer of information. A body corporate or any person on its behalf may transfer sensitive personal data or information including any information, to any other body corporate or a person in India, or located in any other country, that ensures the same level of data protection that is adhered to by the body corporate as provided for under these Rules. The transfer may be allowed only if it is necessary for the performance of the lawful contract between the body corporate or any person on its behalf and provider of information or where such person has consented to data transfer.

In a historic judgement delivered on August 24, 2017, in the matter of *Justice KS Puttaswamy (Retd.) and Anr vs Union of India and Ors,* the nine-judge constitutional bench headed by Chief Justice of India ruled that privacy is a fundamental right and said, "The right to privacy is protected as an intrinsic part of the right to life and personal liberty under Article 21 and as a part of the freedoms guaranteed by Part III of the Constitution."

Following this judgement, doctors have a duty to respect the right to privacy of a patient not because it is prescribed by the MCI Ethics Code or any other regulatory body, privacy is now a fundamental "inviolable" right under the Constitution of India.

The patient is the supreme consent giver, and no action pertaining to his/her health information can be taken without consent from the patient. Any protected health information can be shared only after patient consent and that too only with the authorized person. Divulging this information to any unauthorized person without consent of the patient is breach of privacy and confidentiality.

The Central Government is now formulating a new legislation known as "*Digital Information Security in Health Care Act (DISHA)*" with the purpose to provide for establishment of National and State eHealth Authorities and Health Information Exchanges; to standardize and regulate the processes related to collection, storing, transmission, and use of digital health data; and to ensure reliability, data privacy, confidentiality, and security of digital health data and such other matters related and incidental thereto. The said DISHA is under consideration and has not been enacted till date.

MEDICAL RECORDS

Doctors are required to maintain medical records of their inpatients for a period of 3 years as stipulated in Regulation 1.3.1 of the MCI Code of Ethics Regulations. All documents must be issued within 72 hours if requested for either by the patients/authorized attendant or legal authorities involved (1.3.2). Failure to comply with the above regulations is professional misconduct liable for disciplinary action.

Regulation 1.3.4 says, "Efforts shall be made to computerize medical records for quick retrieval."

Ownership of medical records must be understood very clearly. While hospitals or healthcare establishments own the physical (or electronic) records, they are only "held in trust by them on behalf of the patient." The information or data contained in the records are owned by the patient. This information is protected health information.

According to the Electronic Health Record Standards for India 2016, Protected Health Information (PHI) would refer to any individually identifiable information whether oral or recorded in any form or medium that (1) is created, or received by a stakeholder and (2) relates to past, present, or future physical or mental health conditions of an individual; the provision of health care to the individual; or past, present, or future payment for health care to an individual.

Electronic Protected Health Information (ePHI) would refer to any PHI that is created, stored, transmitted, or received electronically. The healthcare provider has the ownership of the medium of storage or transmission of such electronic medical records.

ERRORS IN DIAGNOSIS

Imaging technology has undergone significant advances, yet it is still prone to errors in interpretation given its dependency on human perception.[12]

Broadly, two types of errors can be defined in radiology: perceptual errors (failure to see or detect the abnormality) and cognitive errors, where the doctor can see the abnormality but is not able to understand or appreciate its significance due to lack of knowledge or inadequate clinical information, leading to errors in diagnosis. Technical or physical limitations of the imaging modality may also cause a diagnosis to be missed in some cases.[13] Failure to diagnose is the most frequent cause of litigations.[14]

Medical opinion may differ with regard to course of action to be taken by a doctor treating a patient, but as long as a doctor acts in a manner, which is acceptable to the medical profession and the court finds that he has attended on the patient with due care, skill, and diligence and if the patient still does not survive or suffers a permanent ailment, it would be difficult to hold the doctor to be guilty of negligence.

It is now well established that where the doctors have two options and they exercise one, it cannot be described as negligence, unless the other party is able to show that the option exercised by the doctor was palpably wrong.

An error of judgement may or may not be negligent; it depends on nature of the error. If it is one that would not have been made by a reasonably competent professional man professing to have the standard and type of skill that he holds himself out as having and acting with ordinary care, then it is negligence. If, however, it is an error that such a man, acting with ordinary care might have made, then it is not negligence.

PROFESSIONAL COMPETENCY

Imaging modalities like echocardiography require advanced professional training and technical expertise. Despite technical advances, it has been described as "largely an operator-dependent technique."[15]

Patients are now becoming more aware about issues like competency and quality in imaging modalities.

The American Society of Echocardiography has defined minimum standards for the cardiac sonographer in a position chapter, which is reproduced hereunder[16]:

Principle I—To promote patient well-being, professionals shall:

- Provide information about the procedure and the reason it is being done. Respond to patient's concerns and questions.
- Respect the patient's self-determination and the right to refuse the procedure.
- Recognize the patient's individuality and provide care in a nonjudgemental and nondiscriminatory manner.
- Promote the privacy, dignity, and comfort of the patient and his or her family.
- Protect the confidentiality of acquired patient information.
- Strive to ensure patient safety.

Principle II—To promote the highest level of competent practice, professionals shall:

- Obtain the appropriate education and skills to ensure competence.
- Practice according to published and recognized standards.
- Work to achieve and maintain appropriate credentials.
- Acknowledge personal limits and not practice beyond capability and skills.
- Perform only those procedures that are medically indicated, restricting practice to validated and appropriate tests. For research studies, follow established research protocol, obtaining (and documenting) informed patient consent as needed.
- Ensure the completeness of examinations and the timely communication of important information.
- Strive for excellence and continued competence through continuing education.
- Perform ongoing quality assurance.
- Not compromise patient care by the use of substances that may alter judgement or skill.

Principle III—To promote professional Integrity and public trust, the professional shall

- Be truthful and promote honesty in interactions with patients, colleagues, and the public.
- Accurately represent their level of competence, education, and certification.
- Avoid situations that may constitute a conflict of interest.
- Maintain appropriate personal boundaries with patients including avoidance of inappropriate conduct, be it verbal or nonverbal.
- Promote cooperative relationships within the profession and with other members of the healthcare community.
- Avoid situations that exploit others for financial gain or misrepresent information to obtain reimbursement.
- Promote equitable access to care."

REFERENCES

1. Kaul P, Medvedev S, Hohmann SF, et al. Ionizing radiation exposure to patients admitted with acute myocardial infarction in the United States. Circulation. 2010;122(21):2160-9.
2. Terry PB. Informed consent in clinical medicine. Chest. 2007;131(2):563-8.
3. Lane AN. Medical imaging and consent: when is an X-ray assault? J Med Radiat Sci. 2016;63(2):133-7.

4. Singh SS, Jayaram N. Medico-legal issues in radiology: Indian context. J Med Soc. 2015;29:129-34.
5. Bedetti G, Loré C. Radiological informed consent in cardiovascular imaging: towards the medico-legal perfect storm? Cardiovasc Ultrasound. 2007;5:35.
6. Brenner DJ, Hall EJ. Computed tomography: an increasing source of radiation exposure. N Engl J Med. 2007;357(22):2277-84.
7. Correia MJ, Hellies A, Andreassi MG, et al. Lack of radiological awareness among physicians working in a tertiary-care cardiological centre. Int J Cardiol. 2005;103(3):307-11.
8. Shiralkar S, Rennie A, Snow M, et al. Doctors' knowledge of radiation exposure: questionnaire study. BMJ. 2003;327(7411):371-2.
9. Picano E, Lombardi M, Neglia D, et al. Sustainability of medical imaging in cardiology. Recenti Prog Med. 2006;97(11):652-62.
10. Paterick TE, Jan MF, Paterick ZR, et al. Cardiac imaging modalities with ionizing radiation: the role of informed consent. JACC Cardiovasc Imaging. 2012;5(6):634-40.
11. Carpeggiani C, Picano E. The radiology informed consent form: recommendations from the European Society of Cardiology position paper. J Radiol Prot. 2016;36(2):S175-86.
12. Waite S, Scott J, Gale B, et al. Interpretive error in radiology. AJR Am J Roentgenol. 2017;208(4):739-49.
13. Bruno MA, Walker EA, Abujudeh HH. Understanding and confronting our mistakes: the epidemiology of error in radiology and strategies for error reduction. Radiographics. 2015;35(6):1668-76.
14. Pinto A, Brunese L. Spectrum of diagnostic errors in radiology. World J Radiol. 2010;2(10):377-83.
15. Popescu BA, Andrade MJ, Badano LP, et al; European Association of Echocardiography. European Association of Echocardiography recommendations for training, competence, and quality improvement in echocardiography. Eur J Echocardiogr. 2009;10(8):893-905.
16. Bierig SM, Ehler D, Knoll ML, et al. American Society of Echocardiography minimum standards for the cardiac sonographer: a position paper. J Am Soc Echocardiogr. 2006;19(5):471-4.

SECTION 35

Future Directions

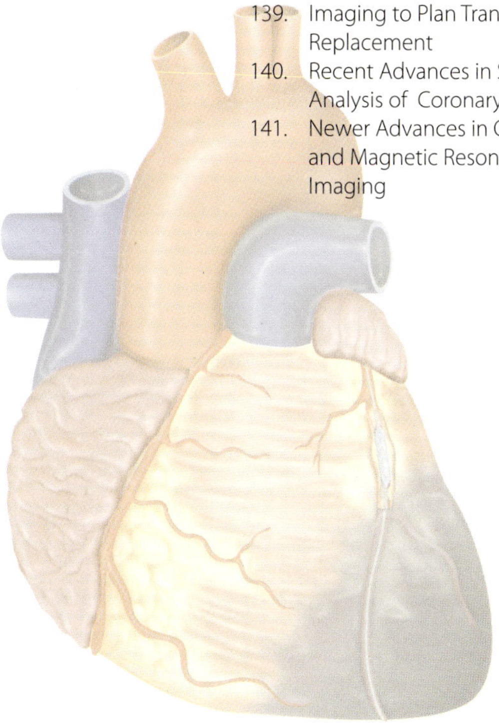

139

CHAPTER

Imaging to Plan Transcatheter Aortic Valve Replacement

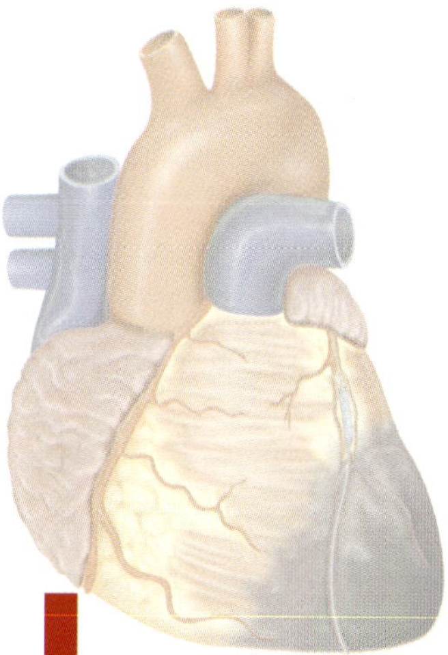

Anil Dhall, Nagendra Chouhan, Karan Chopra, Prashant Bharadwaj

INTRODUCTION

Echocardiography for aortic stenosis (AS) plays a pivotal role in diagnosis, prognostication, planning, execution, and follow-up of appropriate therapy. Updated recommendations focusing on a stepwise approach to evaluating AS have recently been published by the European Association of Cardiovascular Imaging and the American Society of Echocardiography. Technical considerations, sources of error in measurement of peak velocity, mean aortic valve gradient and aortic valve area (AVA) by continuity equation, application of flow status using indexed left ventricular (LV) stroke volume to distinguish patients with low gradients and a low calculated AVA, use of low-dose dobutamine stress echocardiography (DSE) in patients with low ejection fraction (EF) and application of the new classification scheme, and review of algorithm use for echocardiographic evaluation of severe AS have been discussed in these reviews. Echocardiography helps calculate the mean and peak instantaneous gradient across the valve area and also calculates the AVA using the continuity equation. Peak velocity requires parallel alignment of the ultrasound beam and therefore needs multiple views as flow in calcified valves may be eccentric. It is influenced by loading conditions and hemodynamic status. The mean gradient correlates well with invasive data and better reflects the pressure difference during systole. Aortic valve area using continuity equation is relatively independent of flow but requires due diligence to correct dimensions being used for calculations. Some inherent shape assumptions can cause miscalculations. Direct measurement of the LV outflow tract (LVOT) area by three-dimensional (3D) echocardiography or transesophageal echocardiography (TEE) has demonstrated better concordance of AVA with peak velocity and mean aortic gradients and may be increasingly adopted as technology improves (Table 1).

Grading AS relies on a complex hemodynamic framework as the transvalvular gradient is flow dependent. Severe AS is defined as an AVA <1.0 cm^2 or indexed valve area <0.6 cm^2/m^2 and is usually characterized by measures such as a peak velocity across the aortic valve on echocardiography of >4.0 m/s and a mean gradient of >40 mm Hg (Figs. 1 and 2).

In the cases where peak velocity and mean gradient are <4 m/s or 40 mm Hg, respectively, AVA is calculated. Left ventricular stroke volume index (LVSVi) can be calculated by multiplying the LVOT velocity time integral by the LVOT cross-sectional area, then dividing that number by the patient's body surface area. If the LVSVi is ≥35 mL/m^2 indicating normal flow, then most likely there is moderate or even mild AS. If LVSVi is <35 mL/m^2, then flow is reduced and low-flow low-gradient (LFLG) severe AS is present as long as measurement errors have been ruled out (Fig. 3).

In the setting of abnormal LV function (EF < 50%), severe AS can exist outside of these parameters. Low-flow low-gradient AS is defined as a low-flow state [EF < 50%, stroke volume index (SVI) <35 mL/m^2], AVA < 1.0 cm^2, with mean gradients that are <40 mm Hg on transthoracic echocardiographic (TTE) evaluation. In these cases, LFLG AS can be further distinguished by DSE. This group represents 5–15% of all patients with AS.

TABLE 1: Advantages and disadvantages of three criteria for echocardiographic assessment of AS severity (adapted from guidelines Baumgartner et al).

	Formula/method	*Cut-off for severe*	*Advantages*	*Limitations*
As jet velocity (m/s)	Direct measurement	4.0	Direct	Correct measurement requires parallel alignment of ultrasound beam, flow dependent
Mean gradient (mm Hg)	$\Delta P = \Sigma \frac{4v^2}{N}$	4.0	Units comparable to invasive measurements	Accurate pressure gradients depend on accurate velocity data, flow dependent
Continuity equation valve area (cm^2)	$AVA = \frac{CSA_{LVOT} \times VTI_{LVOT}}{VTI_{AV}}$	<1.0	Measures effective orifice area, relatively flow independent	Measurement error more likely

(AS = aortic stenosis; AV = aortic valve; AVA = aortic valve area; CSA = cross-sectional area; LVOT = left ventricular outflow tract; n = number of instantaneous measurements; P = pressure; V = velocity; VTI = velocity time integral)

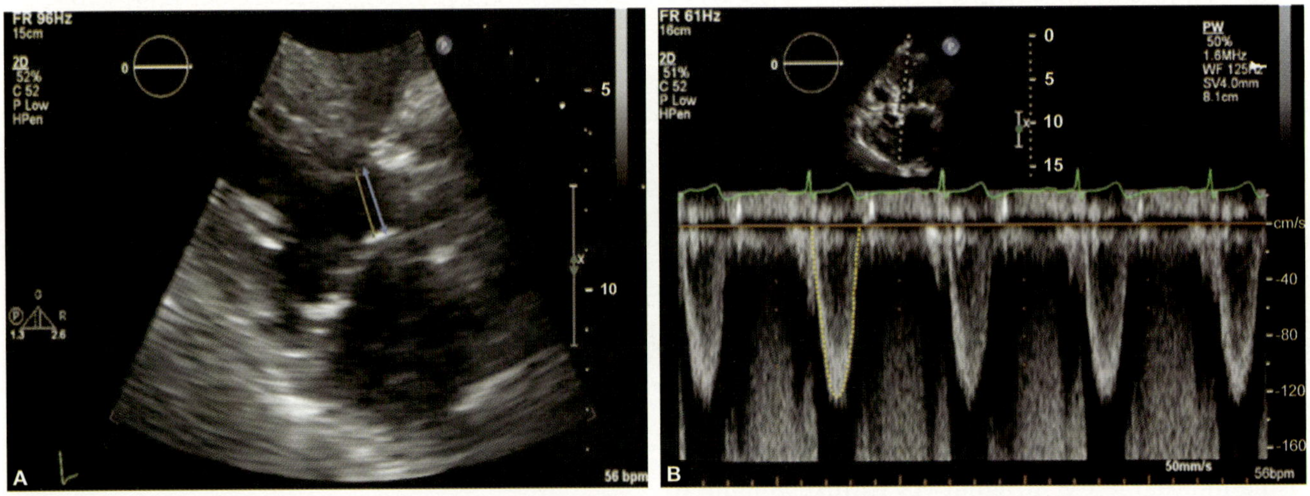

Fig. 1: Measurement of LVOT and LVOT VTI. (A) The LVOT should be measured from inner edge of the septal endocardium to the inner edge of the anterior mitral leaflet in midsystole; (B) The LVOT VTI should be a smooth velocity curve with a narrow band of velocities throughout systole and is highly dependent on sample volume positioning. (LVOT: left ventricular outflow tract; LVOT VTI: left ventricular outflow tract velocity time integral)

Paradoxical LFLG (PLFLG) AS is a separate clinical entity that occurs in patients with a normal LVEF (>50%), but abnormal SVI (SVI < 35 mL/m^2), an AVA < 1.0 cm^2 with a mean gradient across the aortic valve of <40 mm Hg and elevated valvuloarterial impedance. It is most often diagnosed in elderly patients with LV hypertrophy, small LV cavity, and possibly LV diastolic dysfunction. Paradoxical LFLG AS represents 10–25% of all patients with AS.

A new clinical entity has recently been described, normal-flow, low-gradient AS. This is defined as an AVA <1.0 cm^2 or indexed valve area <0.6 cm^2/m^2 in the presence of normal LVEF (>50%) and normal systolic flow (SVI > 35 mL/m^2) but with a mean gradient across the aortic valve of <40 mm Hg. This clinical syndrome has been less thoroughly studied than LFLG and PLFLG AS, and thus recommendations for management are less clear (Fig. 4).

After correctly measured peak velocity and mean gradient have been determined to be <4 m/s and <40 mm Hg, respectively, and AVA is calculated to be <1.0 cm^2, LVSVi of <35 mL/m^2 is required to make a diagnosis of LFLG AS, whether the LVEF is preserved or reduced. If the LVEF is <50%, a DSE should be performed to assess for LV contractile reserve and to exclude pseudosevere AS. Patients with pseudosevere AS show an increase in AVA

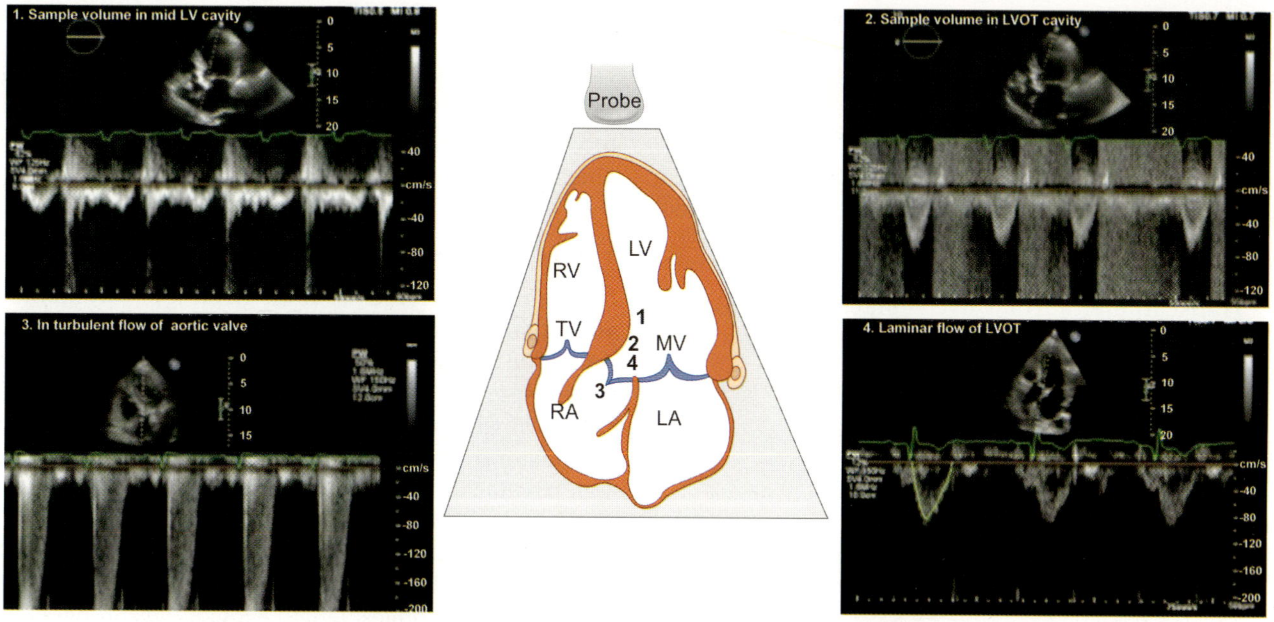

Fig. 2: Stepwise approach to obtaining a laminar LVOT flow. (LVOT: left ventricular outflow tract)

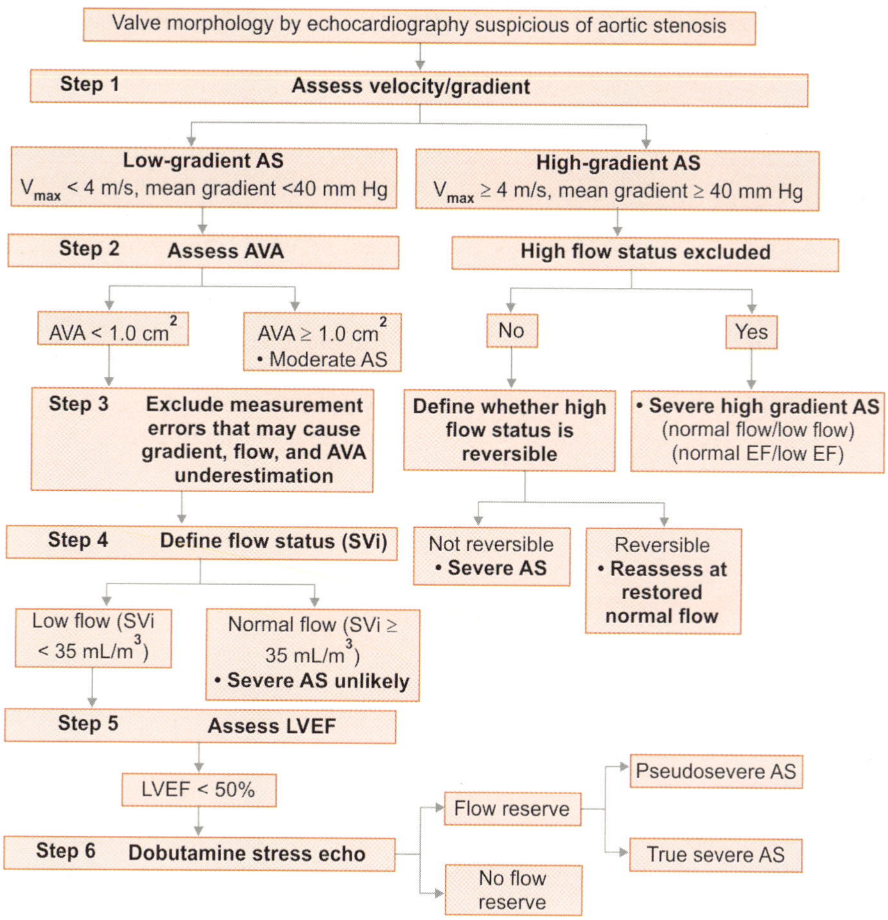

Fig. 3: AS grading algorithm using an integrated, stepwise approach. (AS: aortic stenosis; AVA: aortic valve area; LVEF: left ventricular ejection fraction; SVi: stroke volume indexed; V_{max}: peak aortic valve velocity)

and little increase in gradient in response to increased flow which does not represent significant AS, and the reason for low gradients and low flow is due to poor LV contractile function. Low-flow low-gradient AS with preserved LVEF is characterized by a hypertrophied LV with a small LV cavity. Low stroke volumes (hence low flow) are present due to small LV cavitary volumes. In Severe High-gradient Aortic Stenosis, we need to rule out concomitant high-output states such as anemia or thyrotoxicosis.

Transcatheter aortic valve replacement (TAVR) is now a well-established alternative to surgical aortic valve replacement, offering the opportunity of treatment of severe AS to those at prohibitive surgical risk. Performed without direct visualization of the valve, TAVR is reliant on noninvasive imaging both to guide implant selection and to create a virtual roadmap of the truncal vasculature which acts as the access pathway.

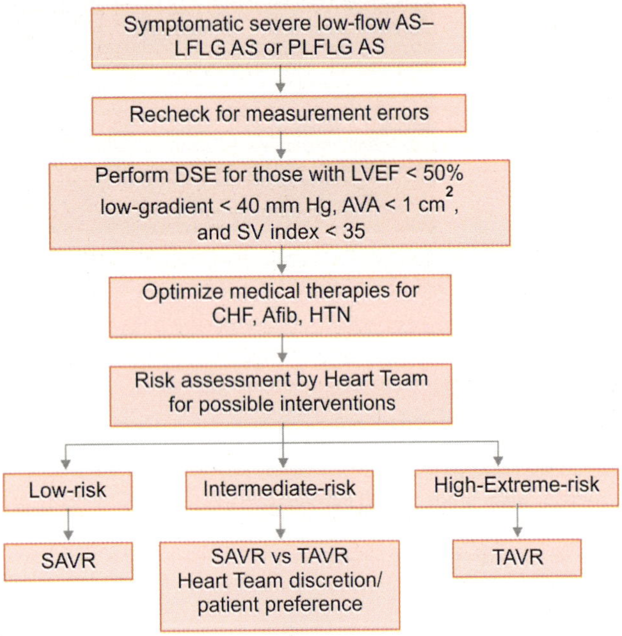

Fig. 4

(LFLG: low-flow low-gradient; AS: aortic stenosis; PLFLG: paradoxical low-flow low-gradient; LVEF: left ventricular ejection fraction; DSE: dobutamine stress echocardiography; TAVR: transcatheter aortic valve replacement; SAVR: surgical aortic valve replacement)

THE AORTIC ANNULUS

The annulus referred to in all TAVR measurements is not actually an anatomic one but rather a virtual entity composed of a ring formed by the basal hinge points of the valve cusps[1] (Fig. 4). Therefore, this is essentially a geometric best-fit of what an anatomic annulus would look like in this position and is actually ovoid in most cases rather than circular.[2] This has implications for its measurement, particularly diameters obtained by two-dimensional (2D) echocardiography, as the sagittal plane that is used to obtain the LVOT diameter represents the smallest cross section with the longest length lying in the coronal plane. Indeed, in progressively severe AS, the annulus becomes increasingly elliptical as a result of remodeling in the LVOT,[3] making the use of 2D echocardiography outdated in this area with almost unavoidable underestimation of annular size.

In addition to accounting for its elliptical profile, it is important to be aware of the change in annular measurements that occur across the cardiac cycle. Transesophageal echocardiography measurements are obtained during midsystole when the annulus is at its largest and most circular. This is the preferred time point to size the annulus, as TAVR implants predominantly assume a circular shape after deployment.[4] Conversely, multidetector computed tomography (MDCT) measurements size the annular area at any point in the cardiac cycle depending on where the optimal image is obtained (Fig. 5).

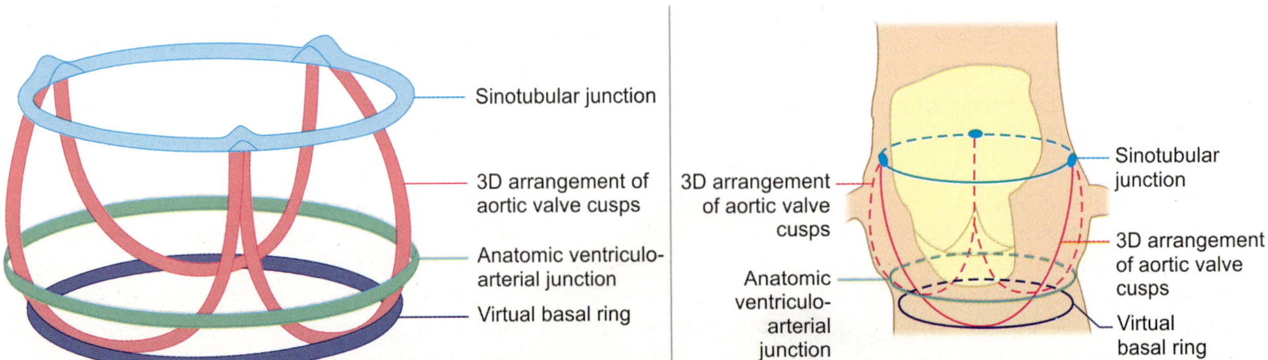

Fig. 5: Graphical depiction of the aortic annulus. The virtual ring formed by the basal hinge points of the valve cusps is the measured annulus in TAVR sizing.

The best correlation appears to be between systolic TEE and diastolic MDCT measurements,[5] whereas comparative systolic measures returned MDCT oversizing by approximately 0.28 mm^2. It must be noted, however, that discrepant time point sizing between modalities has not been proven to be a source of significant error in device selection.[6]

Perimeter or Area

The anatomy, the elliptical profile, and the potential to geometrical change during the cardiac cycle impact the annular sizing. Recent sizing charts are based on 3D area-derived measurements. While good correlation has been demonstrated between area and perimeter measures with seemingly equal predictive power for paravalvular regurgitation,[2,7] there are logical advantages in adopting the latter. As the annulus becomes progressively oval, area measurements are subject to potentially greater error as the area reduces in size disproportionately to the perimeter leading to potential underestimation of the true annular dimensions, an important potential source of unintentional under sizing.[8] A recent review suggested that perimeter sizing is a more robust measure, being less susceptible to inappropriate underestimation in the context of annular elongation.[9]

Among the major manufacturers, the self-expanding valves largely rely on perimeter measurement, while the balloon mounted valves use the area.

Preprocedural Imaging

Accurate sizing of the intended aortic implant is central to the success of TAVR. There are inherent technical issues with the use of 2D TEE, with limited ability either to account for the elliptical annulus or to identify the left main stem (LMS) origin which lies in the coronal plane. 3D TEE on the other hand is not subject to these limitations and can measure the distance from annulus to LMS origin as well as determine the length of the left coronary cusp which has the potential to occlude the ostium following valve deployment. The use of 2D imaging has been largely superseded by 3D (Fig. 6).

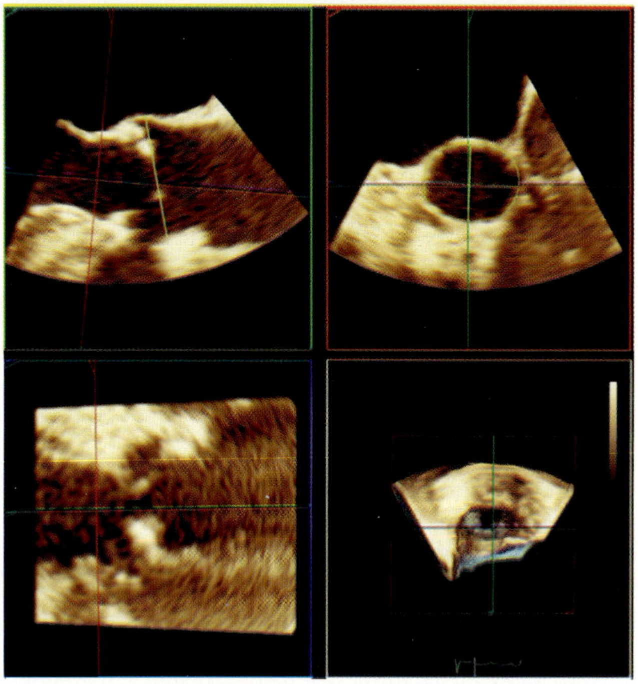

Fig. 6: Example of 3D TEE annular sizing. The yellow lines measure the annulus and sinus of Valsalva dimensions. Upper left panel = sagittal view; upper right panel = transverse view; bottom left panel = coronal view.

Multidetector computed tomography has evolved as a now well-validated tool, often cited as the gold standard in annular measurements. However, MDCT and 3D TEE have been shown to perform similarly in annular sizing. Several studies report good correlation between modalities with both methods having equivalence in predicting moderate or severe paravalvular regurgitation, an important potential complication of transcatheter heart valve (THV) implantation.[10-12] In a recent small retrospective study,[13] TEE, MDCT, and magnetic resonance imaging (MRI) all performed comparatively well with surgical device sizing, while a larger trial demonstrated good concordance in measurements for both area and perimeter between the three modalities.[7]

In spite of this, there has been concern that 3D TEE tends to undersize relative to MDCT with figures between 9% and 12% quoted for the degree of discrepancy.[14-16] Prosthesis sizing is of critical importance in TAVR; if the device is undersized, there is a risk of significant paravalvular leak (PVL) or device embolization. However, if the valve is oversized, the implant may disrupt the aortic root leading to rupture or, more frequently, bundle branch block or complete heart block due to impingement on the neighboring conduction system. Therefore, while intentional under or oversizing is a recognized strategy for limiting complications, unintentional (erroneous) prosthesis–annular mismatch can result in significant harm. The modality that is most widely used now worldwide to perform preprocedural sizing of the annulus is MDCT, and the most recent American College of Cardiology expert consensus statement on TAVR[17] advises that TEE is unnecessarily invasive in the high-risk, frail TAVR population and should not be used routinely pre-TAVR. Because patients with renal insufficiency may have a contraindication to contrast required for MDCT, and those with esophageal pathology may not be candidates for TEE, it is important to have both MDCT and 3D TEE imaging available within a TAVR center.

Beyond Annular Sizing

The sizing of the annulus is only one aspect of the imaging requirement of TAVR. Other preprocedural characteristics which require evaluation are:

- Left ventricular dysfunction, systolic or diastolic
- Mitral valve disease [secondary mitral regurgitation (MR) likely to improve postprocedure while primary MR typically does not[17]]
- Pulmonary hypertension
- Tricuspid regurgitation (preprocedural tricuspid annular diameter as predictive of significant tricuspid regurgitation at 1 year[18])
- Left ventricular outflow tract calcification (significant asymmetrical calcium deposition in the LVOT can result in PVL postprocedurally due to incomplete apposition of the valve struts against the surrounding wall and is also a risk factor for postprocedural ventricular septal defect)
- Low-gradient AS (present in up to 40% of AS patients[19] and known to carry a poorer TAVR outcome[20])

Low-gradient Aortic Stenosis

Low-gradient AS is of three types[19,20] (Table 2):

1. LFLG
2. PLFLG
3. Normal-flow low-gradient

Paradoxical LFLG AS is often seen in those with a small LV cavity resulting in a reduction in stroke volume despite the preserved EF, while the latter category of normal-flow low-gradient is thought secondary to elevated afterload such as systemic hypertension, driving down the gradient across the valve. Stress echocardiography is unrivalled for valve interrogation in LFLG AS, and it is only when it is unfeasible for a patient to undergo stress testing that assessment by other means should be considered. In these scenarios, MDCT has been gaining traction for the estimation of the degree of aortic valve calcification as a pseudomarker of low-gradient disease when stress testing is not feasible. The aortic valve calcium score derived by MDCT correlates strongly with the severity of stenosis, rate of progression, and clinical outcomes.[21] Less impressive has been the use of MRI velocity encoded flow imaging which will consistently underestimate aortic velocities and is therefore not useful in this setting.[17]

The judicious use of stress echocardiography in the evaluation of discrepancies between the visual appearance of the valve and the Doppler estimation of severity is of enormous importance in identifying those who may still benefit from TAVR in spite of low resting gradients. Overall, in the functional assessment of valvular heart disease and in the identification of potentially important adverse predictors of outcome, echocardiography remains an indispensable tool in the selection of appropriate patients for TAVR quite apart from its use in the sizing arena.

Vascular Access Planning

It is important to assess the aorta and the peripheral arterial system that may be used during TAVR, and MDCT is ideal for this purpose. The rate of complications related to vascular access during TAVR has been reported as anything between 6.3% and 30.7%.[22] Multidetector computed tomography offers a virtual roadmap of the truncal vasculature allowing identification of vessel size, tortuosity, calcification, and minimal lumen (Figs. 8A and B). Such information allows the planning of access routes with a view to minimizing vascular complications. Significant tortuosity in the iliofemoral system increases the risk of trauma with the catheter system used during TAVR. Eccentric calcification is associated with easier access

TABLE 2: Subtypes of aortic stenoses.

Type of Aortic Stenosis	*Mean gradient (mm Hg)*	*LVEF (%)*	*LV stroke volume index (mL/m²)*	*Assessment of contractile reserve*	*Elevated computed tomography AV calcium score*
Normal-flow high-gradient	≥40	≥50	>35	–	+
Normal flow and gradient, low EF	≥40	<50	>35	–	+
Classical low-flow, low-gradient	<40	<50	≤35	+	+
Paradoxical low-flow, low-gradient	<40	≥50	≤35	+/–	+
Pseudoaortic stenosis	<40	<50	≤35	–	–

(AV = aortic valve; EF = ejection fraction; LV = left ventricular)

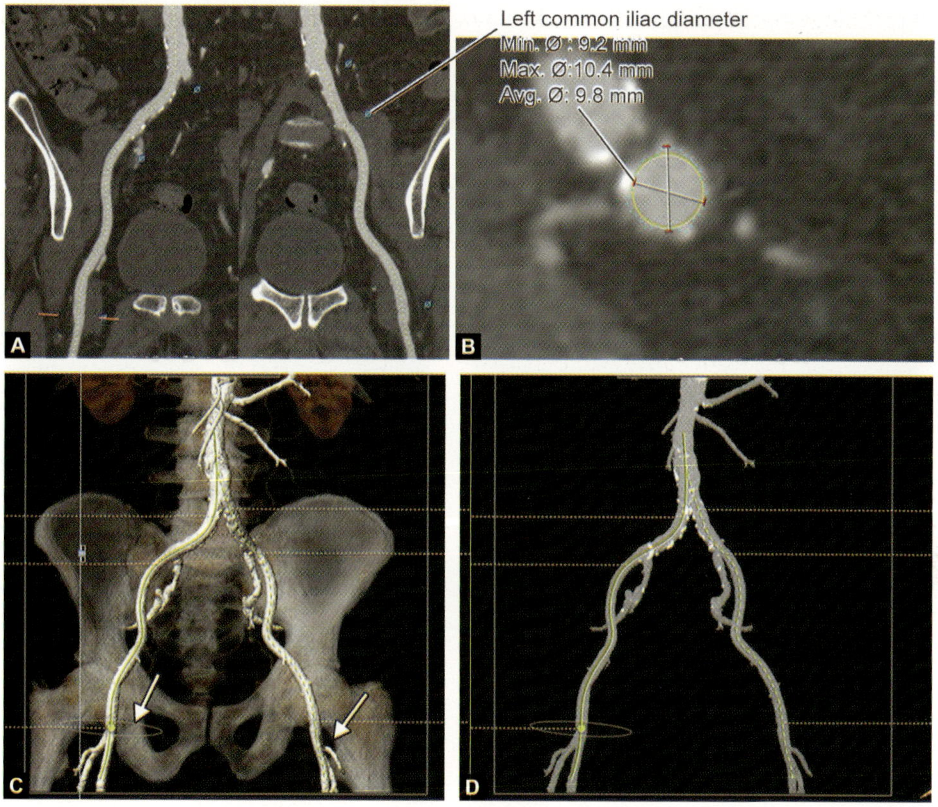

Figs. 7A to D:

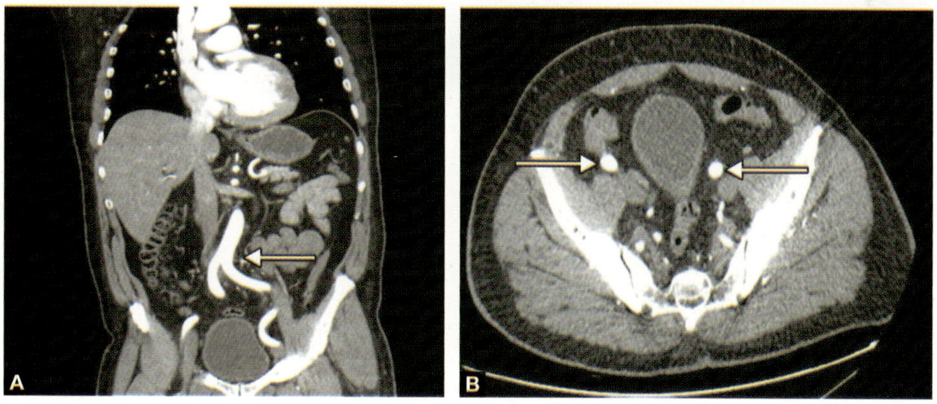

Figs. 8A and B: Coronal (A) and axial (B) views of the truncal vasculature. The arrows point to the aortofemoral bifurcation in the coronal image and the left and right femoral arteries in the axial image.

than vessels with circumferential calcification. Therefore, it is universally recommended to obtain vascular planning via MDCT pre-TAVR, with current MDCT scanners.

MULTIDETECTOR COMPUTED TOMOGRAPHY AND CORONARY ANGIOGRAPHY

While computed tomography (CT) coronary angiography (CTCA) might allow detection of significant stenosis in proximal or mid-vessel segments, the specificity and positive predictive values are limited (73% and 72%, respectively).[23] A recent study found diagnostic quality CTCA only in the LMS in a majority of patients and nondiagnostic CTCA rates ranging between 25% and 72% depending on the arterial segment analyzed.[24] This study concluded that CTCA did not provide adequate diagnostic information to exclude severe coronary artery disease, primarily as a result of the extensive calcification present in the TAVR population. However, there is agreement that MDCT is useful in the evaluation of coronary bypass grafts.[25]

Certainly, for the routine inspection of the native coronary system pre-TAVR, it seems that beam hardening artifact from extensive calcification will limit the applicability of the technique.

Case Planning

In any given case, we need to know:

- Calcification
- Valve anatomy
- Annulus sizing
- Coronary height
- Angle of implantation
- Sinuses size
- Ascending aorta
- Access site.

Valve Anatomy and Calcification

See Figure 9.

Annulus

See Figure 10.

Calcification

See Figure 11.

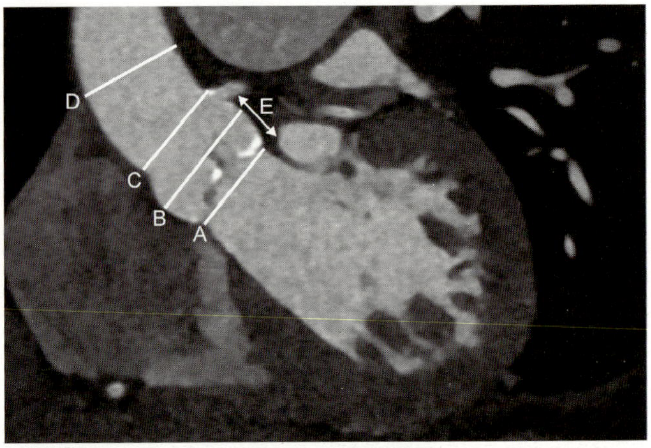

Fig. 9: Overview of standard measurements on cardiac CT for TAVR assessment on coronal-oblique multiplanar reformations along the axis of the aortic root. A: Diameter of the AA; B: Sinus of Valsalva; C: Sinotubular junction; D: Ascending aorta; E: Distance between AA and left coronary artery ostium.

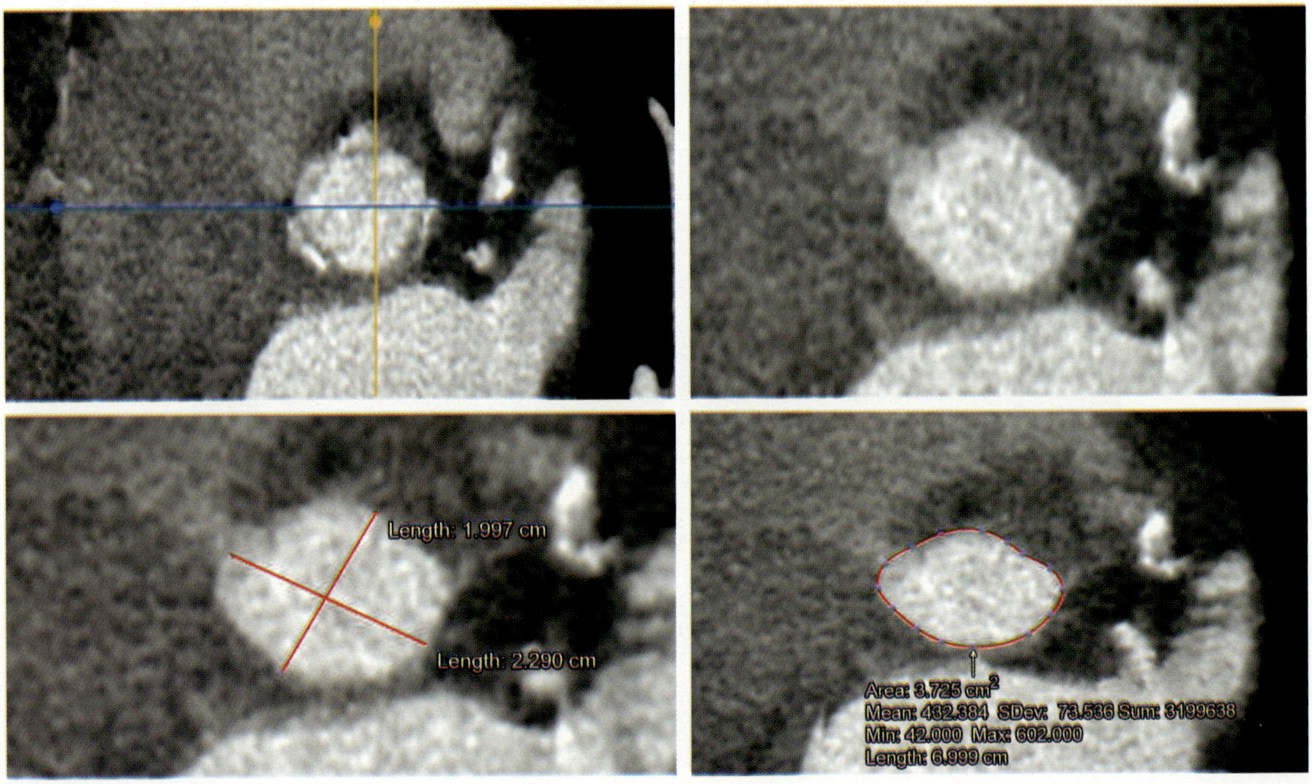

Fig. 10

Left Ventricular Outflow Tract

See Figure 12.

Left Ventricular Outflow Tract Calcification Grading

See Figures 13A to C.

Coronary Ostial Height

See Figures 14 and 15.

Mechanisms of occlusion are:
- Embolization
- Compression by the valve cage or valve skirt
- Aortic dissection
- Displacement of native leaflet against the ostium.

There is a higher risk of coronary occlusion if:
- The distance between the annulus and ostium is <10 mm
- Long leaflet
- Heavily calcified leaflet
- Shallow sinus
- Narrow sinotubular junction
- Balloon-expandable valve.

Sinus of Valsalva Size

See Figure 16.

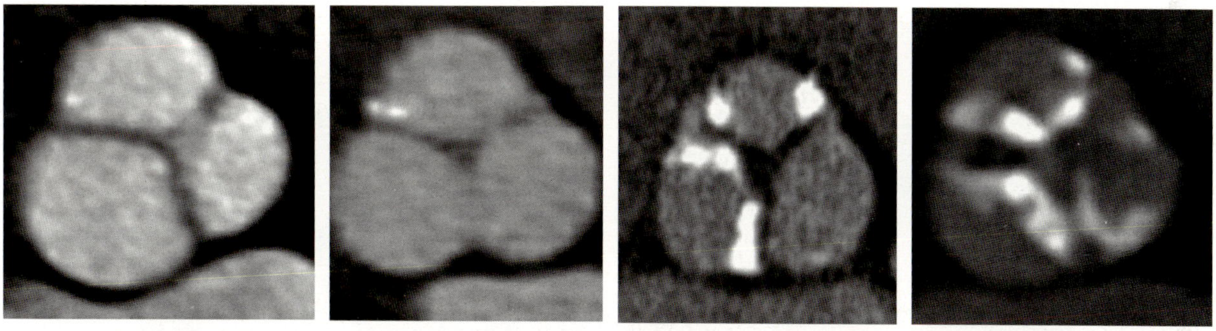

Bicuspid morphology with fused leaflets with no calcification (grade 1)

Trileaflet morphology with small isolated spots of mild calcification (grade 2)

Trileaflet valve with multiple, large spots of moderate calcification (grade 3)

Trileaflet valve with extensive calcification of all cusps (grade 4)

Fig. 11

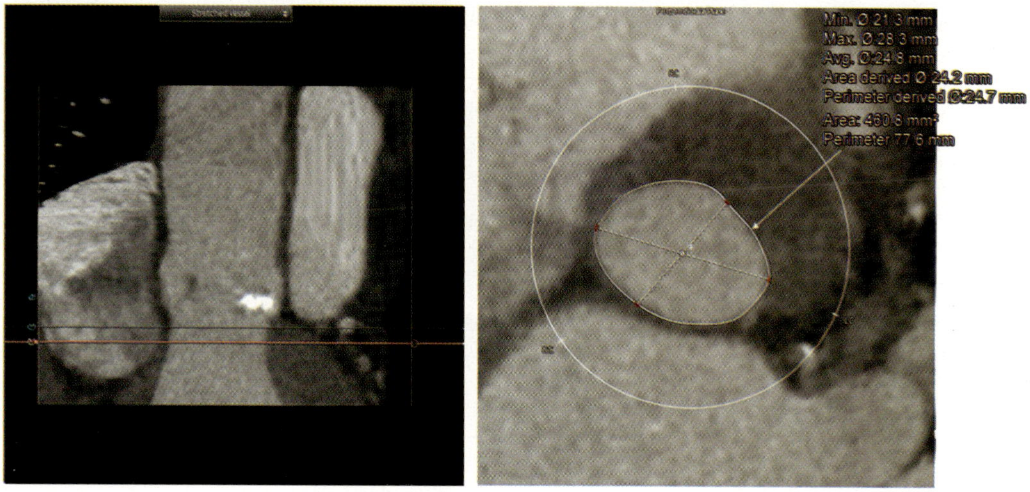

Fig. 12

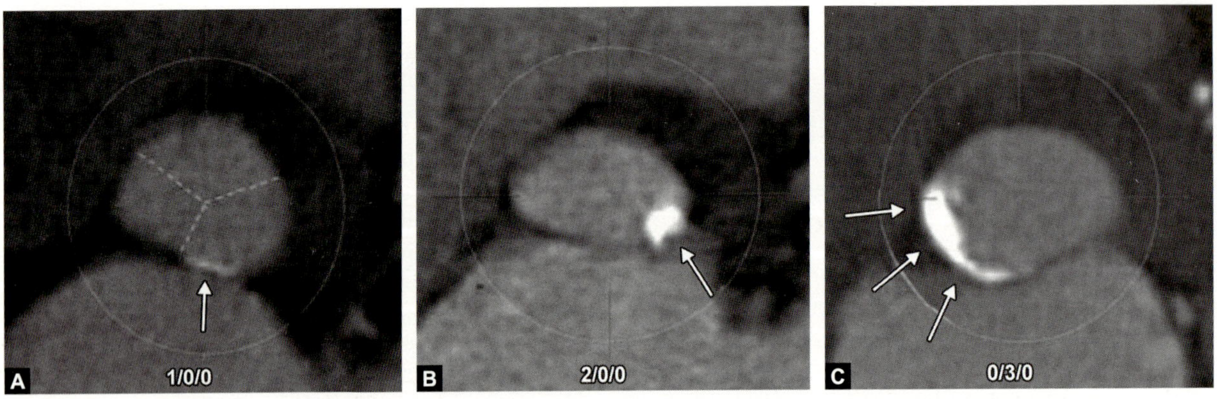

Grade 0	No calcification
Grade 1 (mild)	Small, non-protruding calcification
Grade 2 (moderate)	Protruding (>1 mm) or extensive (>50% of cusp sector) calcification
Grade 3 (severe)	Protruding (>1 mm) or extensive (>50% of cusp sector) calcification

Figs. 13A to C

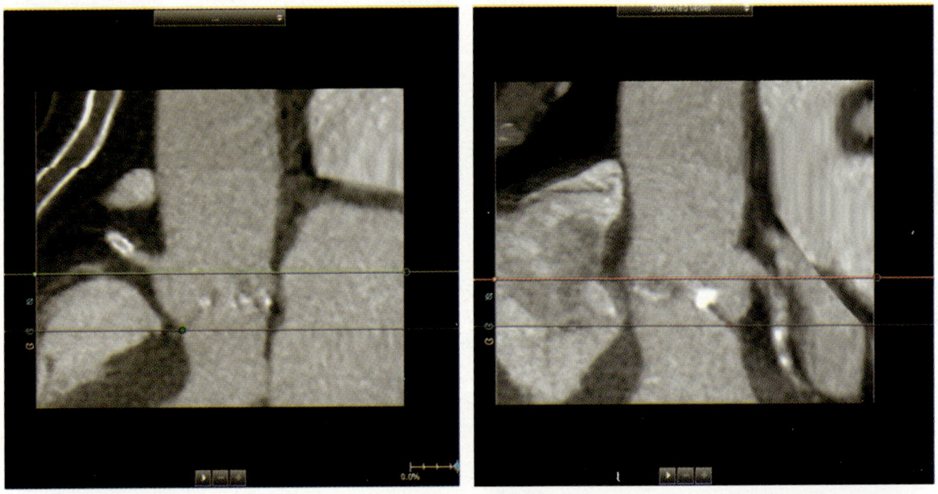

Fig. 14

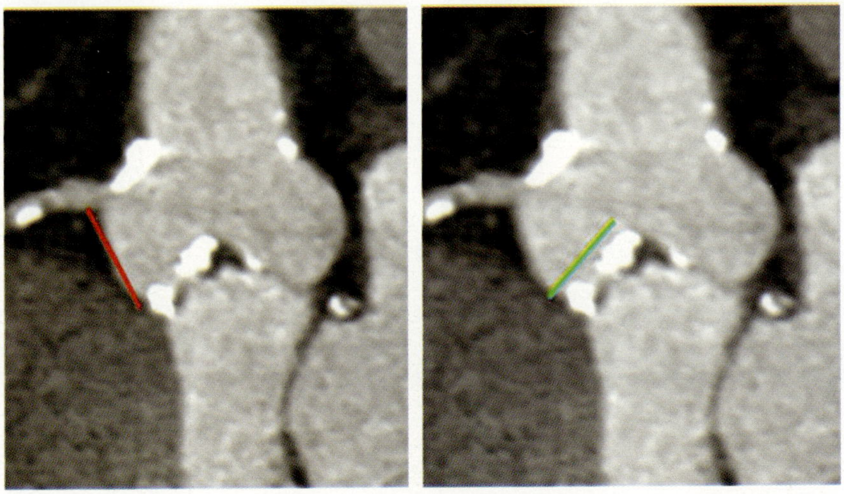

Fig. 15

Sinus of Valsalva Height

See Figure 17.

Horizontality of Aorta

See Figure 18.

Ascending Aorta

See Figure 19.

Challenging Transcatheter Aortic Valve Replacement Situations

This would include:
- Bicuspid aortic valve
- Valve-in-valve (VIV) procedures
- TAVR for pure aortic regurgitation.

Bicuspid Aortic Valve (Fig. 20)

Classification of bicuspid aortic valves is as shown:
- Transcatheter aortic valve replacement in bicuspid aortic valves has more annular rupture and paravalvular leaks; CT-based patient-specific planning is essential
- The incidence of PVL is increased compared to tricuspid aortic valve cohorts undergoing TAVR, particularly with self-expandable device. Aortic injury should be considered in TAVR with balloon-expandable device
- Annulus-based sizing for bicuspid aortic valve seems efficient for >80% of the patients
- Implantable cardioverter defibrillator–based sizing for tapered configurations

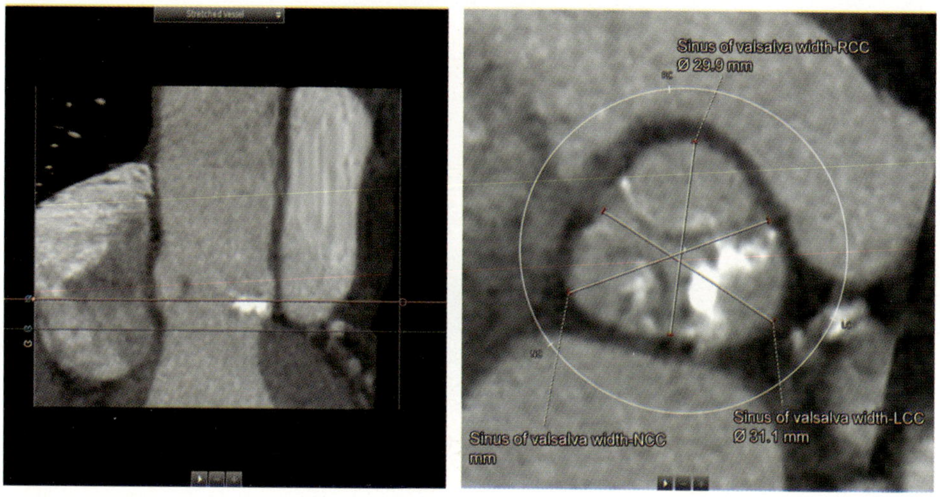

Fig. 16

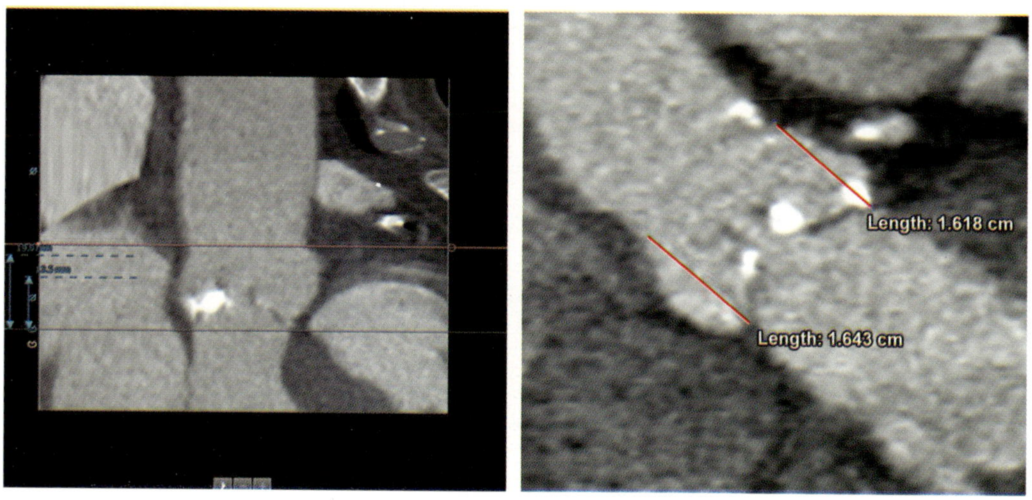

Fig. 17

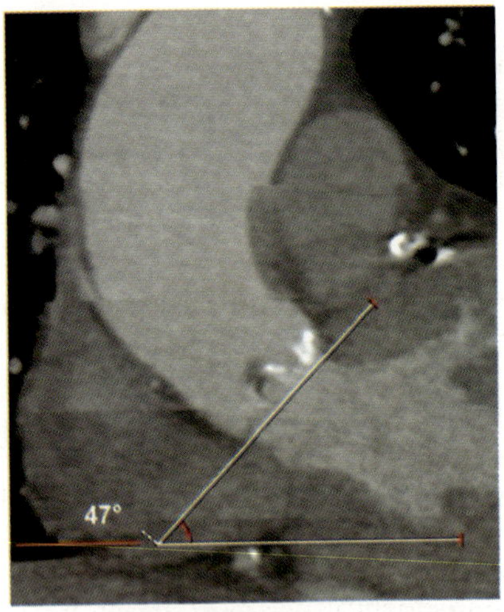

Fig. 18

- Contemporary oversizing is minimal
- Calcium distribution plays a role
- Ascending aorta dimension and peripheral vasculature may finally dictate the type of THV
- Unfavorable features are more elliptical valves, asymmetric and bulky calcium distribution, and lower coronary heights.

Pure Aortic Regurgitation

- *Limitations in TAVR with native aortic valve regurgitation (NAVR)*:
  - Absent cusp and leaflet calcification
  - Missing landmarks
  - Inadequate valve control
  - Risk of embolization or migration of the THV
  - Residual regurgitation and need for second THV

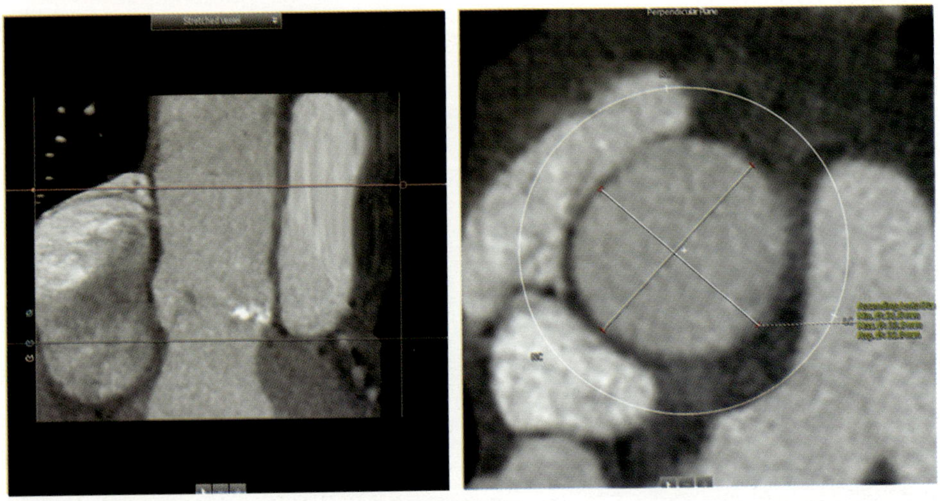

Fig. 19

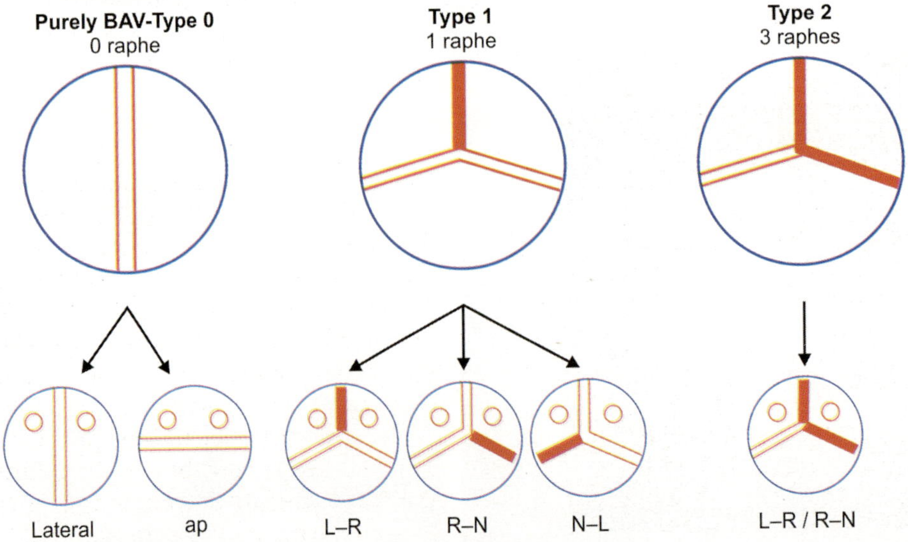

Fig. 20

- *Coronary occlusion has different pathophysiology with NAVR*:
  - Risk of coronary occlusion not higher in aortic insufficiency versus AS, although case literature smaller
  - However, unlike restricted leaflet mobility with AS, leaflets with AI are very mobile
  - Sinus of Valsalva and coronary heights are not sufficient in pre-CT evaluation, especially considering the mobile and elongated leaflets
  - Measurement of aortic valve leaflet lengths instrumental in preoperative evaluation
  - Calcium on valve helps in TAVRs (Fig. 21).

Valve-in-valve

The previously deployed surgical valves as well as the index procedure need to be carefully studied with careful analysis of the valve architecture and design. This information should be confirmed with the manufacturer and also using an app.

There are several potential risk factors for coronary occlusion during VIV interventions:

- *Anatomic factors*:
  - Narrow sinotubular junction/low sinus height
  - Narrow sinuses of Valsalva
  - Previous root repair (e.g. root graft and coronary reimplantation)
  - Low-lying coronary ostia
- *Bioprosthetic valve factors*:
  - Supra-annular position versus intra-annular
  - High leaflet profile
  - Internal stent frame (e.g. MitroFlow, Trifecta)
  - No stent frame (homograft, stentless valves)
  - Bulky leaflets
  - Transcatheter valve factors
  - Extended sealing cuff
  - High implantation.

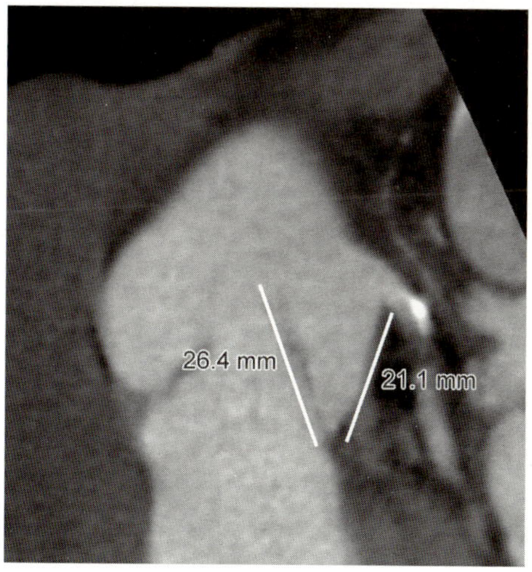

Fig. 21

Distortion of anatomy, tilting of the surgical prosthesis, and lower coronary height need to be kept in mind to analyze and predict the proximity of the coronary ostia to the anticipated final position of the displaced bioprosthetic leaflets after THV implantation (Figs. 22 and 23).

Valve Fracture

- Valve-in-valve TAVR in small surgical bioprostheses is associated with an increased incidence of PPM and higher mortality
- Most bioprosthetic valves can be fractured with a high-pressure balloon inflation
- Bioprosthetic valve fracture (BVF) results in lower residual valve gradients and larger valve effective orifice area after VIV TAVR
- Longer term data are needed to determine which patients are most likely to benefit from BVF in conjunction with VIV TAVR
- Trifecta and Hancock II valves do not fracture
- Older generation Carpentier-Edwards valves may not fracture—they do appear to stretch considerably though
- Concern for coronary artery/Sinotubular junction obstruction
  - Assess virtual THV to coronary distance
  - Coronary protection, BASILICA procedure if appropriate
- Small sinotubular junction, LVOT
  - Ensure that the aorta can accommodate the balloon used to perform fracture
  - Assess calcium burden
  - Smaller balloons can be used, but higher pressure may be needed.

Periprocedural Imaging

The shift away from general anesthesia has led to fewer patients having TEE-guided TAVR, but this did not have a detrimental impact on outcomes, as reported in the French registries.[26] This is likely in part a result of increasing operator experience. When TEE is used during implantation, it offers real-time diagnosis of complications such as tamponade, coronary occlusion, aortic dissection, aortic regurgitation, and mitral regurgitation.[22]

EchoNavigator technology provides fusion imaging of TEE and fluoroscopy in real time during TAVR, guiding the implanter to the most appropriate deployment position. This makes zero contrast TAVR procedures possible, which can be advantageous in patients with renal

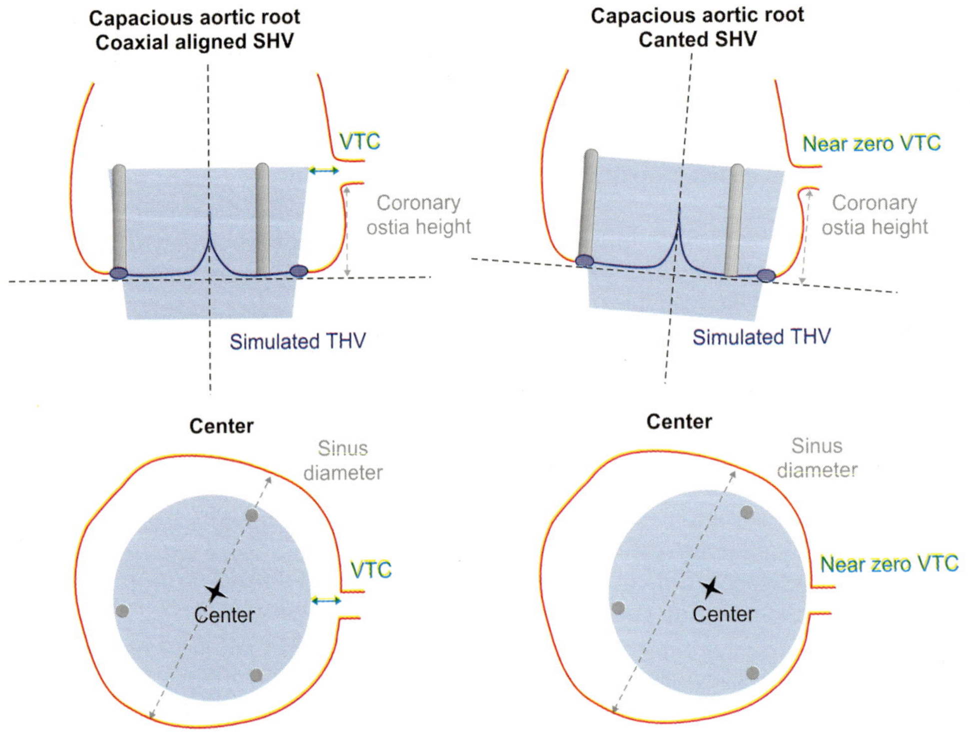

Fig. 22

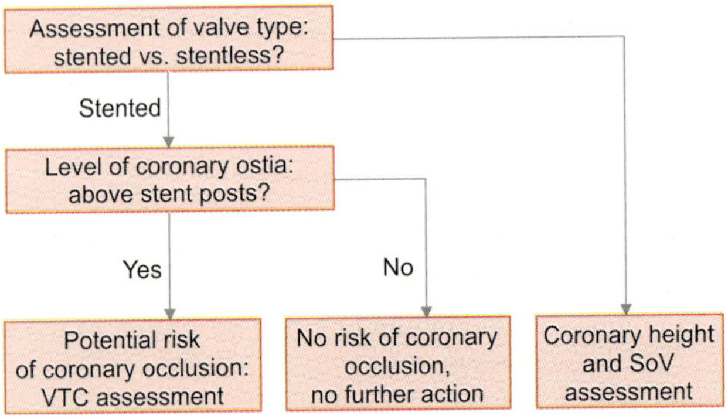

Fig. 23

impairment. However, in spite of the advantages offered by periprocedural TEE, it is gradually being used less with many centers increasingly relying on TTE to detect periprocedure complications and assess aortic regurgitation postimplant.

Multidetector computed tomography (MDCT) has not been adopted into the periprocedural domain despite having shown promise as a contrast sparing tool by predicting fluoroscopic views. The feasibility of CT fusion imaging has been established in interventional procedures such as TAVR, PVL closure, and in pulmonary vein anatomy for ablation studies.[27] The idea is to fuse or overlay reconstructed CT images onto fluoroscopic imaging in order to overcome the limitations common to all 2D modalities. This is not, however, a straightforward or timely process. MDCT does not presently play a significant role in periprocedural TAVR imaging.

Predictors of Permanent Pacemaker Implantation

Several predictors of permanent pacemaker implantation after TAVR have been consistently identified. The most important is history of right bundle branch block (RBBB) with an odds ratio of 3.7–8 according to different studies. Besides advanced age, the predictors can be differentiated in three groups:

1. *Electrocardiography*—RBBB, left anterior fascicular block, QRS duration.
2. *Anatomic*—Degree of annulus calcification and location, LV end-diastolic dimension LVEDd.
3. *Procedural*—Depth of implantation, degree of oversizing, balloon aortic valvuloplasty, or use of Medtronic CoreValve valve. The depth of implantation of CoreValve 6 mm below the annulus showed to be a very strong predictor when combined with presence of RBBB.

Paravalvular leak

Efforts to recognize patients at a higher risk of PVL based on multi-imaging analysis have shown predictors of significant PVL to include:

- Valve undersizing
- Device malpositioning
- Incomplete valve contact to the native aortic annulus, most often due to extensive and/or eccentric annular calcification.

Different anatomic and patient characteristics need to be considered before postdilatation. There should be a higher threshold to postdilate patients with anatomic risk for aortovalvar injury or coronary obstruction, unless moderate or worse PVL is noted. This holds true especially if the patient was initially deemed inoperable. On the other hand, a younger less comorbid patient should be treated aggressively, aiming for a perfect result, or tolerating up to mild PVL. The role of echocardiography is crucial in determining the risk of aortic injury while postdilatating and may guide to a more conservative or aggressive inflation, by identifying menacing calcific lesions deforming the aortic wall.

When repeated postdilatations are insufficient or generate an unaffordable risk, a second line of treatment is represented by retrograde transcatheter PVL closure with plug devices or the use of a second transcatheter valve. The decision depends on the morphology and localization of the PVL, as well as the type of valve used.

Given the association with mortality, the industry has focused on modifying valve systems to decrease the rate of PVL. The Edwards Sapien 3 was innovated with an outer sealing skirt of polyethylene terephthalate and modified its frame design to achieve better circularity. Medtronic has improved the radial force of its Evolut R valve and expanded its larger valve size to treat a broader group of patients, by reducing undersizing. Evolut Pro system is the new optional platform of the Medtronic valve, which has a thin pericardial sealing skirt that showed excellent results with absence of moderate or severe PVL in a small preapproval clinical study.

Follow-up of Transcatheter Aortic Valve Replacement

Bioprosthetic valves can degenerate and require to be followed-up. Clinical management depends on the stage of valve degeneration and dysfunction. It thus still remains uncertain whether transcatheter valves will be as durable as surgical valves. The type of tissue and anticalcifying processes used in transcatheter valves are similar to those of new generations of surgical valves. There are several factors specific to transcatheter aortic valve implantation (TAVI) that may limit the durability of transcatheter valves:

- The design of the bioprosthesis stent and the type of anchoring of the leaflets to the stent are very different
- The delivery of the transcatheter valves through an arterial access requires to crimp the valve over a balloon and then expand it with balloon inflation (balloon-expandable) or to crimp and load the valve within the catheter delivery system (self-expanding). Crimping is associated with significant alteration in structural morphology of collagen fibers and impairment of leaflet mechanical properties. The impact of these valve tissue alterations caused by crimping, loading, delivery, expansion, and postdilatation on valvular long-term durability remains unknown
- Due to the elliptical shape of the native aortic annulus and the frequent presence of bulky calcifications, the deployment of the stent is often noncircular and irregular. This increases stresses and abnormal flows
- Oversizing of the transcatheter valve relative to the native annulus size is recommended to reduce the risk of paravalvular regurgitation following TAVI. However, this strategy may result in incomplete expansion of the transcatheter valves and thus some degree of valve leaflet—stent orifice mismatch. This may, in turn, cause pin-wheeling motion of leaflets during closure with ensuing increased mechanical stress.

Reaccessing the Coronaries

We need to understand the device as well as its original deployment position to be able to reaccess the coronaries.

- For self-expanding valves, we obtain 6-7F access from femoral or left radial. An initial nonselective angiogram is performed. Selective access is facilitated by using J-wire to enter diamond in front/adjacent to ostia (angled stiff glide wire is also useful for entering diamond or tracking the catheter). For self-expanding transcatheter aortic valve, reduce catheter size by 0.5 mm and leave wire in coronary while retracting guide.
- *For LCA access*:
  - Use FL3.0/3.5 guide
  - *Second line guide*: Ikari right 1.0/1.5
  - If difficulty with coronary engagement, rail guide toward the ostium using
    - Coronary guidewire ±
    - Balloon support ±
    - Guide extension catheter

- *For RCA access*:
  - Use FR4 guide
  - *Second line guide*: Ikari Right 1.5, AR2 (wide sinuses), MP
  - If skirt is high, use Ikari Right or MP guide to enter diamond from above coronary ostia and rail guide toward ostium using
    - Coronary guidewire ±
    - Balloon support ±
    - Guide extension catheter
- For Balloon mounted valves, we obtain 6-7F access from femoral or left radial.
- Use standard diagnostic catheters to engage coronary arteries LCA JL4/JL3.5 RCA - JR4.
- Use standard guide catheters to engage coronary arteries LCA - VL3.5/EBU 3.5/FL4—RCA- FR4/IM (Figs. 24 to 27).

CONCLUSION

The development of TAVR has not only resulted in implantable AVR technology but has also given birth to new approaches to guide and image percutaneous procedures. These include real-time guidance pre-acquired roadmaps and intense planning. The available imaging modalities have each been evaluated and optimized to help predict accurately both the size of the intended implant and potential obstacles to procedural success. Transesophageal echocardiography and MDCT have been shown to be equitable in sizing the annulus appropriately. However, as many TAVR patients have potentially confounding structural or functional heart disease, it is likely that such patients may require both MDCT and TEE for optimal TAVR assessment and placement.

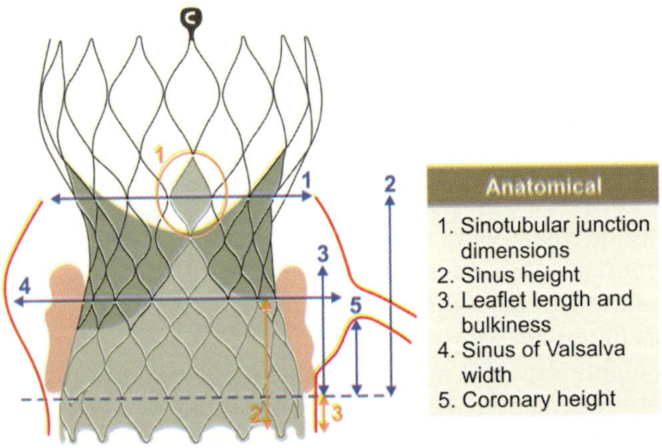

Fig. 24

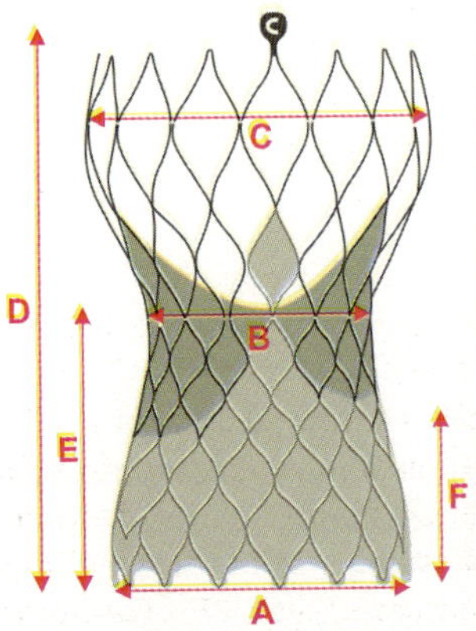

	23 mm Evolut R / PRO	26 mm Evolut R / PRO	29 mm Evolut R / PRO	34 mm Evolut R
A. Inflow diameter	23 mm	26 mm	29 mm	34 mm
B. Waist diameter	20 mm	22 mm	23 mm	24 mm
C. Outflow diameter	34 mm	32 mm	34 mm	38 mm
D. Frame height	45 mm	45 mm	45 mm	46 mm
E. Commissure height	26 mm	26 mm	26 mm	26 mm
F. Skirt height	13 mm	13 mm	13 mm	14 mm

Fig. 25: Repositionable self-expanding valves with and without an external pericardial wrap: features and dimensions.

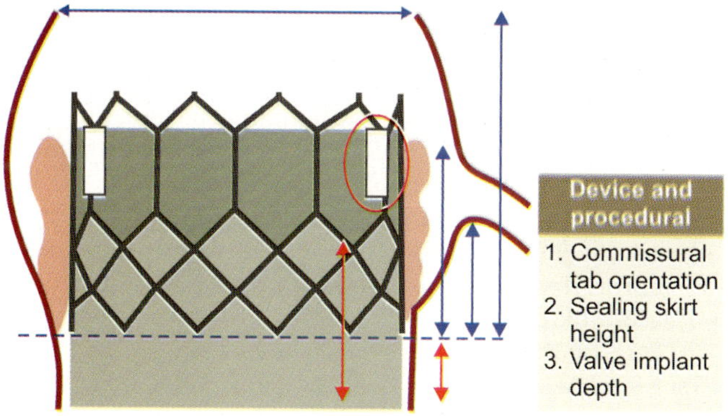

Fig. 26

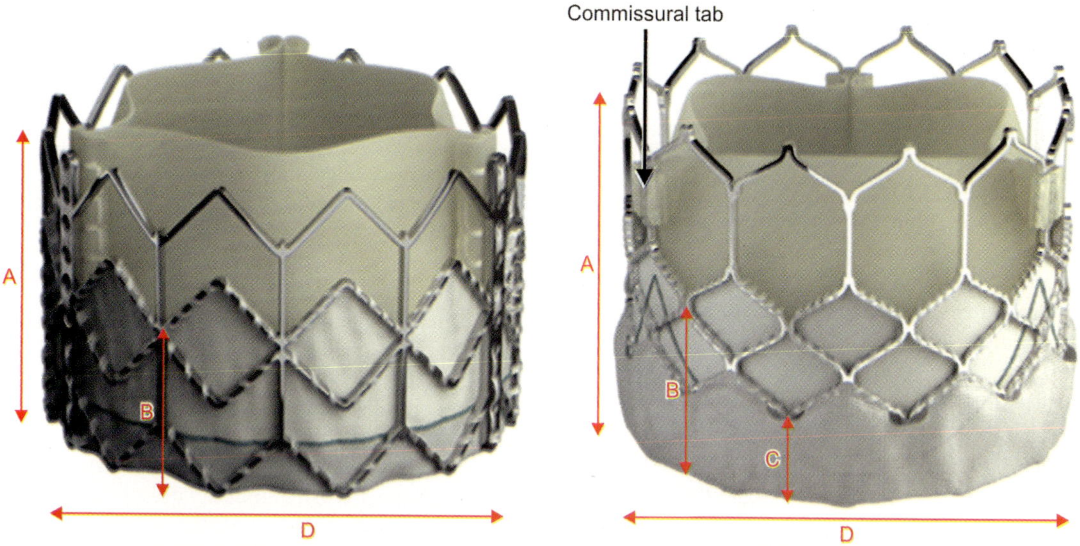

	23 mm Sapien XT	26 mm Sapien XT	29 mm Sapien XT	20 mm Sapien 3	23 mm Sapien 3	26 mm Sapien 3	29 mm Sapien 3
A. Frame height	14 mm	17 mm	19 mm	15.5 mm	18 mm	20 mm	22.5 mm
B. Inner skirt height	6.7 mm	8.7 mm	11.6 mm	7.9 mm	9.3 mm	10.2 mm	11.6 mm
C. Outer skirt height	N/A	N/A	N/A	5.2 mm	6.6 mm	7.0 mm	8.1 mm
D. Valve diameter	23 mm	26 mm	29 mm	20 mm	23 mm	26 mm	29 mm

Fig. 27

REFERENCES

1. Kasel AM, Cassese S, Bleiziffer S, et al. Standardized imaging for aortic annular sizing: implications for transcatheter valve selection. JACC Cardiovasc Imaging. 2013;6(2):249-62.
2. Khalique OK, Kodali SK, Paradis JM, et al. Aortic annular sizing using a novel 3-dimensional echocardiographic method: use and comparison with cardiac computed tomography. Circ Cardiovasc Imaging. 2014;7(1):155-63.
3. Mehrotra P, Flynn AW, Jansen K, et al. Differential left ventricular outflow tract remodeling and dynamics in aortic stenosis. J Am Soc Echocardiogr. 2015;28(11):1259-66.
4. Ng ACT, Delgado V, van der Kley F, et al. Comparison of aortic root dimensions and geometries before and after transcatheter aortic valve implantation by 2- and 3-dimensional transesophageal echocardiography and multislice computed tomography. Circ: Cardiovasc Imaging. 2010;3(1):94-102.

5. Guez D, Boroumand G, Ruggiero NJ, et al. Automated and manual measurements of the aortic annulus with ECG-gated cardiac CT angiography prior to transcatheter aortic valve replacement: comparison with 3D-transesophageal echocardiography. Acad Radiol. 2017;24(5):587-93.
6. Kim WK, Meyer A, Möllmann H, et al. Cyclic changes in area- and perimeter derived effective dimensions of the aortic annulus measured with multislice computed tomography and comparison with metric intraoperative sizing. Clin Res Cardiol. 2016;105(7):622-9.
7. Stortecky S, Heg D, Gloekler S, et al. Accuracy and reproducibility of aortic annulus sizing using a dedicated three-dimensional computed tomography reconstruction tool in patients evaluated for transcatheter aortic valve replacement. EuroIntervention. 2014;10(3):339-46.
8. Hamdan A, Guetta V, Konen E, et al. Deformation dynamics and mechanical properties of the aortic annulus by 4-dimensional computed tomography: insights into the functional anatomy of the aortic valve complex and implications for transcatheter aortic valve therapy. J Am Coll Cardiol. 2012;59(2):119-27.
9. Papachristidis A, Papitsas M, Roper D, et al. Three-dimensional measurement of aortic annulus dimensions using area or circumference for transcatheter aortic valve replacement valve sizing: does it make a difference? J Am Soc Echocardiogr. 2017;30(9):871-8.
10. Willson AB, Webb JG, TM LB, et al. 3-Dimensional aortic annular assessment by multidetector computed tomography predicts moderate or severe paravalvular regurgitation after transcatheter aortic valve replacement: a multicenter retrospective analysis. J Am Coll Cardiol. 2012;59(14):1287-94.
11. Gripari P, Ewe SH, Fusini L, et al. Intraoperative 2D and 3D transoesophageal echocardiographic predictors of aortic regurgitation after transcatheter aortic valve implantation. Heart. 2012;98(16):1229-36.
12. Buzzatti N, Maisano F, Latib A, et al. Computed tomography-based evaluation of aortic annulus, prosthesis size and impact on early residual aortic regurgitation after transcatheter aortic valve implantation. Eur J Cardiothorac Surg. 2013;43(1):43-51.
13. Faletti R, Gatti M, Salizzoni S, et al. Cardiovascular magnetic resonance as a reliable alternative to cardiovascular computed tomography and transesophageal echocardiography for aortic annulus valve sizing. Int J Cardiovasc Imaging. 2016;32(8):1255-63.
14. Tsang W, Bateman MG, Weinert L, et al. Accuracy of aortic annular measurements obtained from three-dimensional echocardiography, CT and MRI: human in vitro and in vivo studies. Heart. 2012;98(15):1146-52.
15. Wang H, Hanna JM, Ganapathi A, et al. Comparison of aortic annulus size by transesophageal echocardiography and computed tomography angiography with direct surgical measurement. Am J Cardiol. 2015;115(11):1568-73.
16. Jilaihawi H, Doctor N, Kashif M, et al. Aortic annular sizing for transcatheter aortic valve replacement using cross-sectional 3-dimensional transesophageal echocardiography. J Am Coll Cardiol. 2013;61(9):908-16.
17. Otto CM, Kumbhani DJ, Alexander KP, et al. ACC expert consensus decision pathway for transcatheter aortic valve replacement in the management of adults with aortic stenosis. J Am Coll Cardiol. 2017;69(10):1313-46.
18. Dumont C, Galli E, Oger E, et al. Pre- and postoperative tricuspid regurgitation in patients with severe symptomatic aortic stenosis: importance of pre-operative tricuspid annulus diameter. Eur Heart J Cardiovasc Imaging. 2018;19(3):319-28.
19. Clavel MA, Burwash IG, Pibarot P. Cardiac imaging for assessing low-gradient severe aortic stenosis. JACC Cardiovasc Imaging. 2017;10(2):185-202.
20. Kataoka A, Watanabe Y, Kozuma K, et al.; OCEAN-TAVI Investigators. Prognostic impact of low-flow severe aortic stenosis in small-body patients undergoing TAVR: the OCEAN-TAVI Registry. JACC Cardiovasc Imaging. 2018;11(5):659-69.
21. Clavel M-A, Malouf J, Messika-Zeitoun D, et al. Aortic valve area calculation in aortic stenosis by CT and Doppler echocardiography. JACC Cardiovasc Imaging. 2015;8(3):248-57.
22. Bloomfield GS, Gillam LD, Hahn RT, et al. A practical guide to multimodality imaging of transcatheter aortic valve replacement. JACC Cardiovasc Imaging. 2012;5(4):441-55.
23. Hamdan A, Wellnhofer E, Konen E, et al. Coronary CT angiography for the detection of coronary artery stenosis in patients referred for transcatheter aortic valve replacement. J Cardiovasc Comput Tomogr. 2015;9(1):31-41.
24. Chava S, Gentchos G, Abernethy A, et al. Routine CT angiography to detect severe coronary artery disease prior to transcatheter aortic valve replacement. J Thromb Thrombolysis. 2017;44(2):154-60
25. Park H-B, Heo R, ó Hartaigh B, et al. Atherosclerotic plaque characteristics by CT angiography identify coronary lesions that cause ischemia. A direct comparison to fractional flow reserve. JACC Cardiovasc Imaging. 2015;8(1):1-10.
26. Auffret V, Lefevre T, Van Belle E, et al. Temporal trends in transcatheter aortic valve replacement in France. J Am Coll Cardiol. 2017;70(1):42-55.
27. Krishnaswamy A, Tuzcu EM, Kapadia SR. Integration of MDCT and fluoroscopy using C-arm computed tomography to guide structural cardiac interventions in the cardiac catheterization laboratory. Catheter Cardiovasc Interv. 2015;85(1):139-47.
28. Blair JEA, Atri P, Friedman JL, et al. Diastolic function and transcatheter aortic valve replacement. J Am Soc Echocardiogr. 2017;30(6):541-51.
29. Sato K, Kumar A, Jones BM, et al. Reversibility of cardiac function predicts outcome after transcatheter aortic valve replacement in patients with severe aortic stenosis. J Am Heart Assoc. 2017;6(7):e005798.
30. Spitzer E, Van Mieghem NM, Pibarot P, et al. Rationale and design of the Transcatheter Aortic Valve Replacement to UNload the Left ventricle in patients with ADdvanced heart failure (TAVR UNLOAD) trial. Am Heart J. 2016;182:80-8.

31. Andreini D, Pontone G, Mushtaq S, et al. Diagnostic accuracy of multidetector computed tomography coronary angiography in 325 consecutive patients referred for transcatheter aortic valve replacement. Am Heart J. 2014; 168(3):332-9.
32. Ko BS, Cameron JD, Munnur RK, et al. Noninvasive CT-derived FFR based on structural and fluid analysis. A comparison with invasive FFR for detection of functionally significant stenosis. JACC Cardiovasc Imaging. 2017;10(6): 663-73.
33. Schoenhagen P, Numburi U, Halliburton SS, et al. Three-dimensional imaging in the context of minimally invasive and transcatheter cardiovascular interventions using multi-detector computed tomography: from pre-operative planning to intra-operative guidance. Eur Heart J. 2010; 31(22):2727-40.

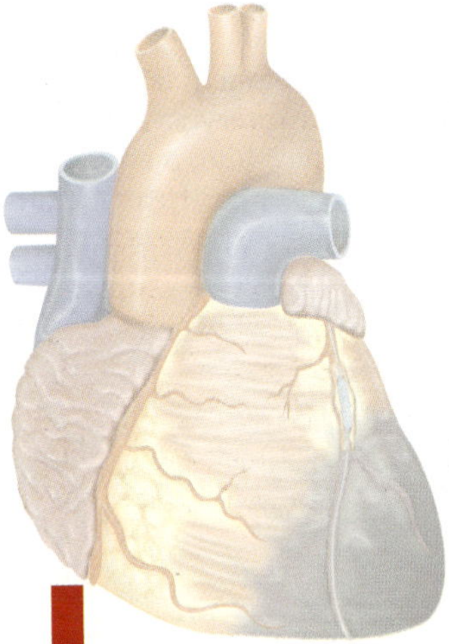

140

CHAPTER

Recent Advances in Strain Echocardiographic Analysis of Coronary Artery Disease

V Amuthan, RVA Ananth

INTRODUCTION

Echocardiography remains one of the marvels of twenty first century and is one of the most important tools in the evaluation of coronary artery disease. The 2011 appropriate use criteria for echocardiography classified use of echocardiography in the diagnosis of suspected MI as appropriate.[1] We shall review the role of echocardiography in the diagnosis and prognosis of coronary artery disease with special reference to strain by speckle-tracking echocardiography (STE).

REGIONAL WALL MOTION ANALYSIS AND STRAIN IMAGING IN CORONARY ARTERY DISEASE

Echocardiographic evidence of regional wall motion abnormality occurs prior to ECG changes and can occur within seconds of coronary arterial occlusion—as early as 12.5 seconds in studies reported.[2,3] In the emergency department, routine eyeballing usually picks up the presence of regional wall motion abnormality, which occur prior to ECG changes.[2,3] A bull's eye plot can be constructed from the recommendations of the American Society of Echocardiography where the outer ring represents the basal segments, the middle ring represents the segments at mid-papillary muscle level, and the inner ring represents the distal level.[4,5] The anterior insertion of the right ventricular wall into the left ventricle defines the border between the antero-septal and anterior segments. Starting from this point, the myocardium is subdivided into six equal segments of 60°. The apical myocardium in the 17-segment models is divided instead into four equal segments of 90°. In the 17-segment model, an additional segment (apical cap) is added in the center of the bull's eye. However, this methodology of eyeballing depends considerably on the expertise of the interpreter and shows relatively low interobserver agreement.

Regional strain is a dimensionless measurement of deformation, expressed as a fractional or percentage change from an object's original dimension. The left ventricular (LV) myocardium consists of circumferential fibers in the mid-wall layer and longitudinal fibers in the endocardial and epicardial layers, and myofibril orientation changes continuously from right-handed helix in subendocardium to left-handed helix in subepicardium. The LV function is determined by the sum of contraction and relaxation in these three layers. Speckle-tracking echocardiography (STE) is a novel technique, which has emerged as one of the best method that analyses motion and strain by tracking natural acoustic reflections and interference patterns within an ultrasonic window. The image-processing algorithm tracks user-defined regions of interest, which are comprised of blocks of approximately 20–40 pixels containing stable patterns that are described as "speckles," "markers," "patterns," "features," or "fingerprints."[6] The normal strain in the range of –20 is given a color coding of pink and abnormal dyskinesia of +20 is color-coded blue. The two-dimensional (2D) echocardiography-derived longitudinal strain is analyzed using propriety software in Quad view and bull's eye plot or the automated functional imaging (AFI). The ease with which we derive information similar to nuclear scans is really amazing. However, this wonderful technique hampered by inter-vender nonagreement has been finally settled by the Consensus document published by the EACVI/ASE/Industry Task Force to Standardize Deformation Imaging.[7]

ACUTE MYOCARDIAL INFARCTION AND IDENTIFICATION OF INFARCT-RELATED ARTERY

In patients with acute myocardial infarctions, accuracy for the prediction of global functional improvement as well as LV remodeling by 2D STE is comparable with that of late gadolinium enhancement cardiac magnetic resonance (CMR) imaging. The prediction of segmental functional improvement is noninferior using myocardial deformation analysis by 2D STE compared with of late gadolinium enhancement CMR in patients with ST-elevation myocardial infarctions (STEMI).[8] The STE can identify the regional distribution of wall motion abnormality and thus the infarct-related artery. Figure 1 is the strain bull's eye plot or AFI showing the reduced strain in anterior septum in the basal, mid-LV segments, anterior wall in the mid-left ventricular, and apical segments. Figure 2 shows the coronary angiogram in the same patient showing the totally occluded proximal left anterior descending artery. Figure 3 is from a patient with inferior wall STEMI showing the reduced strain in right coronary artery territory: inferior septum, inferior wall, and inferolateral wall. Figure 4 shows the totally occluded right coronary artery. Intervention was done in right coronary artery only. Figure 5 is from a patient with inferior wall STEMI with abnormal strain in left circumflex territory. Figure 6 shows the critical lesion in left circumflex.

ACUTE CORONARY SYNDROME AND LEFT MAIN DISEASE

The prediction of left main coronary artery disease is important in clinical diagnosis and management of patients with coronary artery disease. The STE with bull's eye AFI is useful in this regard.[8] In a study of 108 patients with left main disease and three-vessel disease, there was reduction in longitudinal peak systolic strain of basal and mid-LV segments more than the apical segments. Apex of the LV

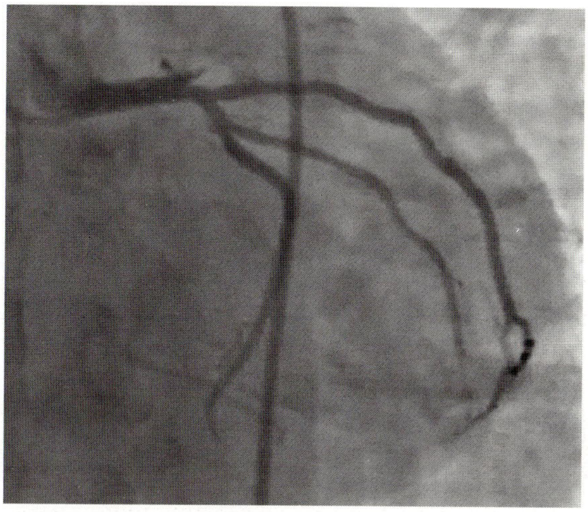

Fig. 2: Left coronary angiogram from the same patient showing totally occluded proximal LAD.

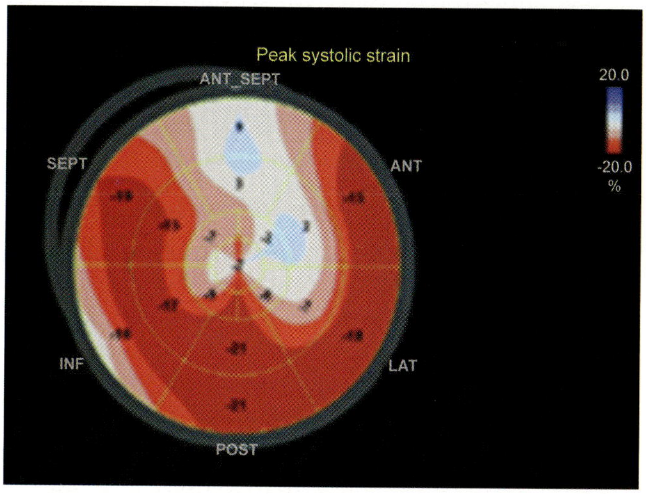

Fig. 1: Automated functional imaging from a patient with LAD occlusion.

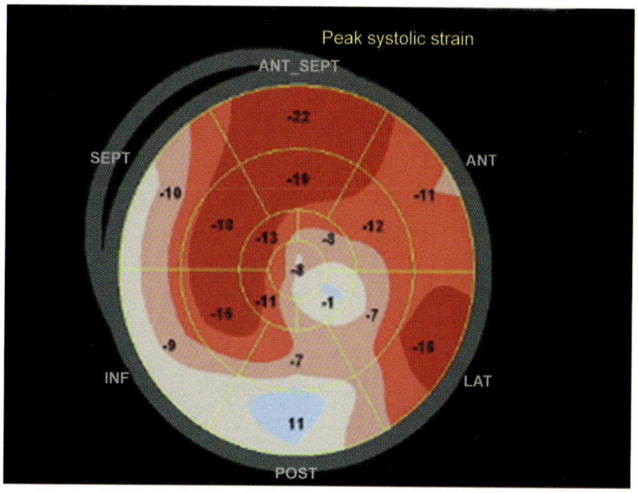

Fig. 3: Automated functional imaging from a patient with RCA occlusion.

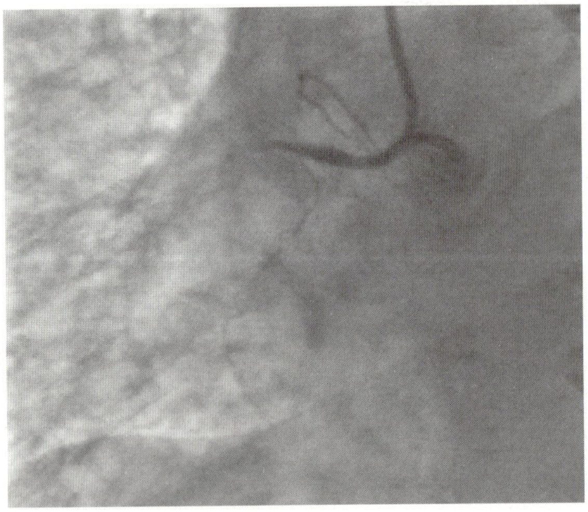

Fig. 4: Right coronary angiogram from this patient showing the total proximal occlusion of RCA.

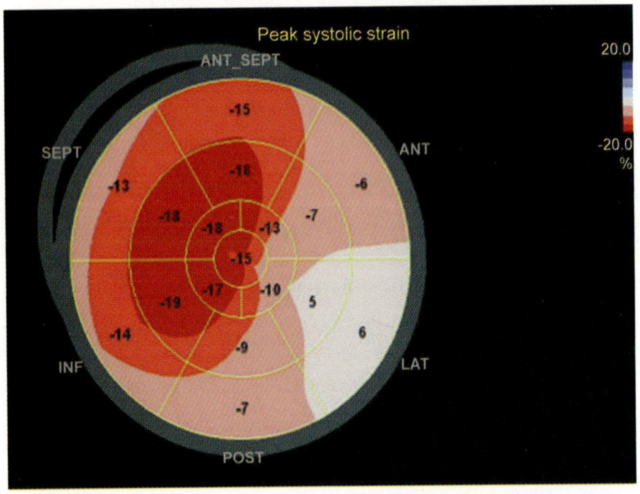

Fig. 5: Automated functional imaging from a patient with LCX obstruction.

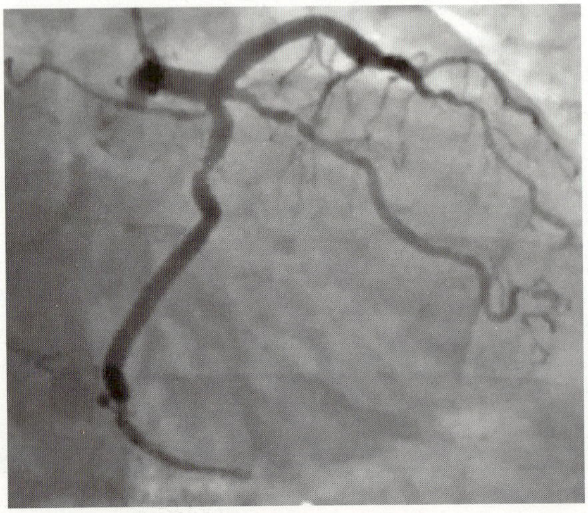

Fig. 6: Left coronary angiogram showing 90% narrowing of proximal left circumflex.

has prominent rotational motion in addition to longitudinal function, which results in less affection of this segment. The helical alignment of the LV results in longitudinal alignment in basal and mid-LV segments and circular alignment in the apex, which results in the rotational motion.[9] Figure 7 is a case example of 54-year-old gentleman who was admitted for the third time in ICCU with acute pulmonary edema and previous two normal 2D echocardiography reports. The strain analysis revealed abnormal strain in basal anterior septum, mid-LV anterior and inferior septum, and inferior and anterolateral wall and anterior wall. The left ventricular ejection fraction was 48% and global longitudinal strain (GLS) –14%. The coronary angiogram showed left main coronary artery bifurcation disease with thrombus in proximal LCX and mid-RCA disease (Fig. 8).

CHRONIC STABLE ANGINA AND EXERCISE STRESS STRAIN ECHOCARDIOGRAPHY

Stress echocardiographic sensitivity and specificity have made it a practical and reliable test to detect myocardial ischemia during rest, pharmacological stress using dobutamine and immediately after exercise. Exercise stress test is superior to pharmacologic stress test as exercise capacity is an important predictor of outcome and prognosis. Exercise echocardiography is usually performed before and immediately after peak exercise. The patient should be preferably transferred to the recombinant position and echocardiographic images should be obtained preferably with 60 seconds, before the heart rate settles down.

Regardless of the type of stress, the echocardiographic evidence of ischemia is always the same: abnormal regional motility. The visual analysis of these abnormalities requires a trained operator. This operator dependence has promoted the search for a semiautomatic method to reduce stress echo limitations and improve test accuracy. Two-dimensional echocardiography with stress strain analysis by STE along three-dimensional ejection fraction was done in a 64-year-old gentleman with diabetes and hypertension who was seen for Class III Angina. He had a positive treadmill exercise test at the first minute of stage I of Bruce protocol. The peak systolic strain AFI bull's eye plot for basal and peak exercise showed additional areas of abnormal strain in inferolateral, anterolateral, and anterior wall with fall in ejection fraction from 56% to 40% on peak stress and GLS decreased from –17% to –14% peak stress (Figs. 9 and 10). The coronary angiogram revealed triple vessel disease: diffuse calcifications in LMCA, LCX, and total cutoff of mid-RCA. Thus, strain or myocardial deformation analysis based on 2D speckle tracking allows discriminating between myocardial active and passive movements, which has resulted in a growing interest to introduce this new technique during stress echo.

CHRONIC STABLE ANGINA AND DOBUTAMINE STRESS ECHOCARDIOGRAPHY

Pharmacologic stress test is done in patients who could not exercise.[10,11] The graded dobutamine stress test consists of five 3-minute stages of infusion of 5, 10, 20, 30, and 40 mics/kg/min of infusion of dobutamine followed by intravenous injection of 0.5–2 mg atropine if there is no increase in the desired heart rate. The echocardiographic images are obtained at rest, at each stage, and during recovery. The standard end points similar to the treadmill exercise echocardiography may be followed. However, one should be aware of the potential complications of arrhythmias, such as frequent ventricular ectopics, ventricular tachycardia, and atrial fibrillation, and the test should be terminated on their presence. Dobutamine can also induce left ventricular mid-cavity and outflow tract obstruction in 10–15% of patients. Figures 11 and 12 show the results of dobutamine stress echo of a 54-year-old gentleman with diabetes who had undergone total right knee replacement 1 year back and had developed sepsis of right knee and was planned for exploration and arthrodesis. As the patient could not be assessed by Treadmill, DSE was done. The ease with which the dobutamine strain echocardiography could demonstrate the presence of coronary artery disease could be noted.

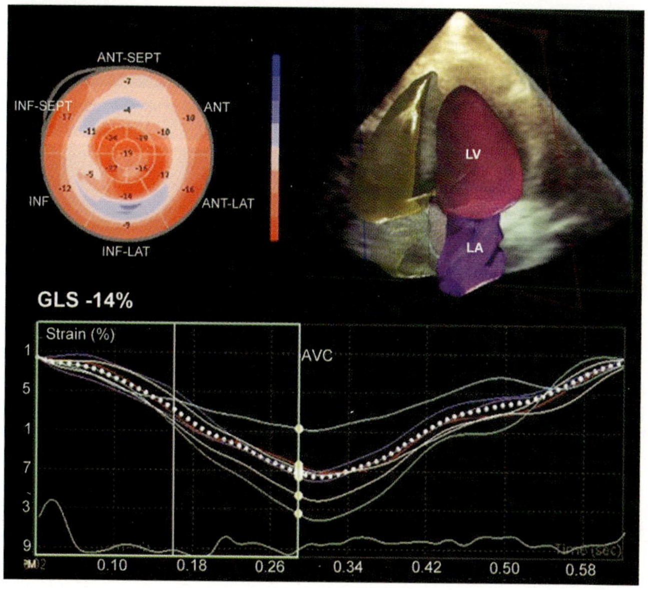

Fig. 7: Bull's eye plot of longitudinal strain imaging in a patient with left main coronary occlusion showing the abnormally reduced strain in basal and mid-LV segments associated with reduced ejection fraction.

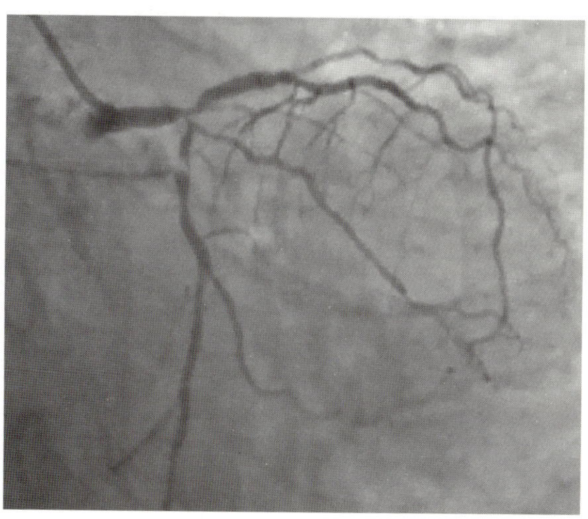

Fig. 8: Left coronary angiogram in the same patient showing tight bifurcation lesion in the left main coronary artery.

CURRENT STATUS OF THREE-DIMENSIONAL MYOCARDIAL STRAIN ESTIMATION

With developments in 3D transducer technology and improvements in hardware and software, 3D data sets with adequate temporal and spatial resolution are now possible and these 3D approaches can measure 3D strain from a multibeat acquisition with a frame rate set above 40 frames per second. The ability to estimate true 3D myocardial motion and deformation using various 3D STE approaches may provide cardiologists with a better view of regional myocardial mechanics, which may be important for diagnosis, prognosis, and therapy.[12]

LEFT VENTRICULAR TORSIONAL DEFORMATION AND SPECKLE-TRACKING ECHOCARDIOGRAPHY

Shortening and lengthening that are the basic functions of the myocardial fibers result in a systolic twist followed by a diastolic untwisting of the left ventricle due to helical orientation of the fibers. In systole, the LV apex undergoes a counter clockwise rotation about its longitudinal axis as viewed from the apex, preceded by a brief clockwise rotation due to the earlier shortening of the subendocardial fibers during isovolumic contraction. Rotation of the LV base in systole is opposite in direction compared to apical rotation, with a brief counter clockwise rotation during isovolumic contraction followed by a clockwise rotation during LV

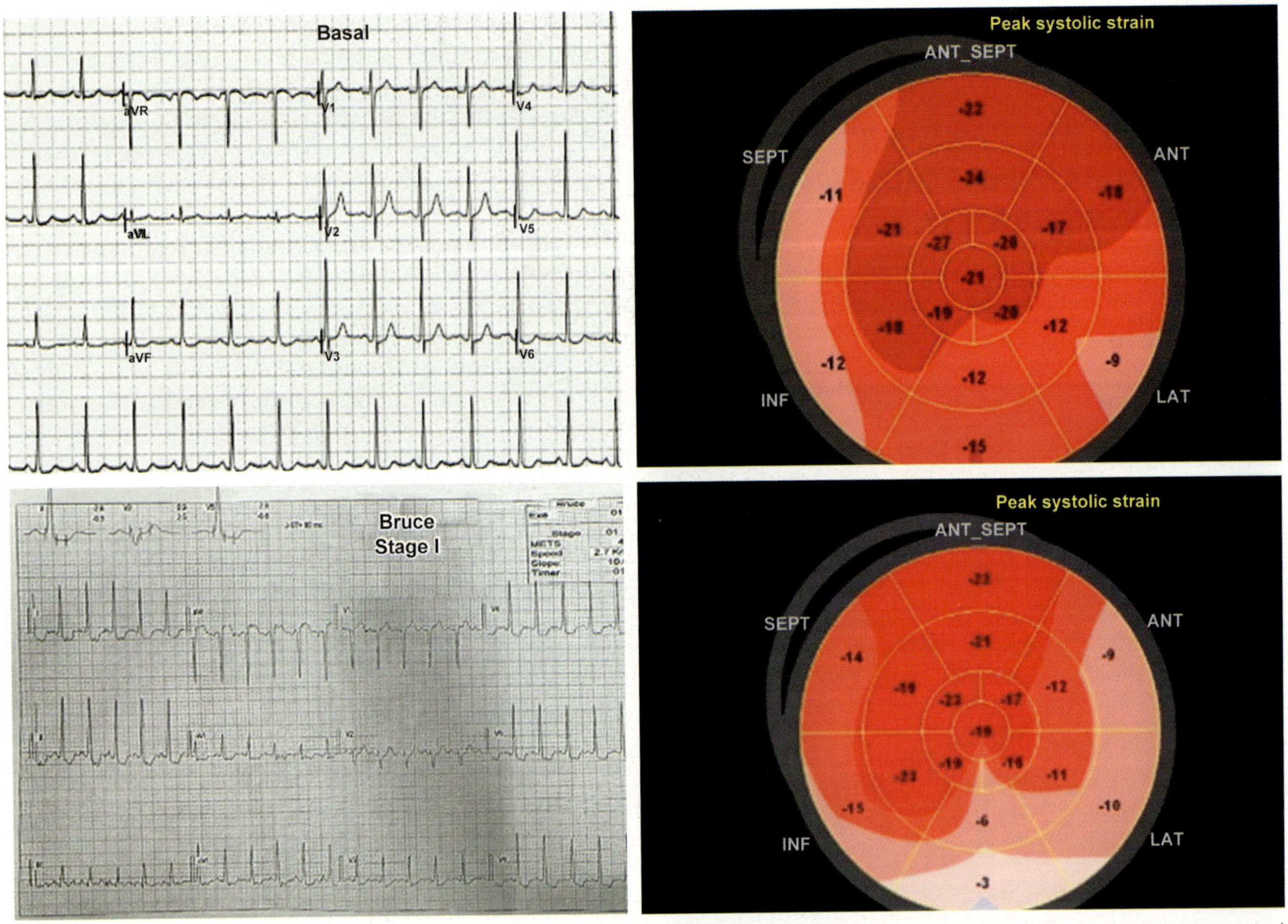

Fig. 9: Exercise stress echo: Bruce basal and Stage I peak exercise ECG and basal and immediate after exercise automated functional imaging from a patient with triple vessel disease showing the development of abnormal strain in the anterior, inferior, inferolateral, and anterolateral segments, associated with fall in ejection fraction.

ejection. This motion has been compared with that used to squeeze water out of a wet towel.[13] The main determinant of the LV twist is the apical rotation.

The complex motion of LV torsion and twist was initially studied by invasive tagging of the left ventricle by radio opaque markers or sonomicrometry and noninvasively by CMR imaging techniques. Two-dimensional and now 3D STE has emerged as an alternative noninvasive technique to assess LV rotation. Although the 2D STE correlated very well with CMR techniques, lower values for apical rotation and LV twist were reported for 2D STE due to difficulties in selection of optimal imaging planes for such computation. This is because of limited acoustic windows and oblique orientation of the heart in the patient's chest cavity and because the 2D method computes twist directly from peak rotation values from apical and basal

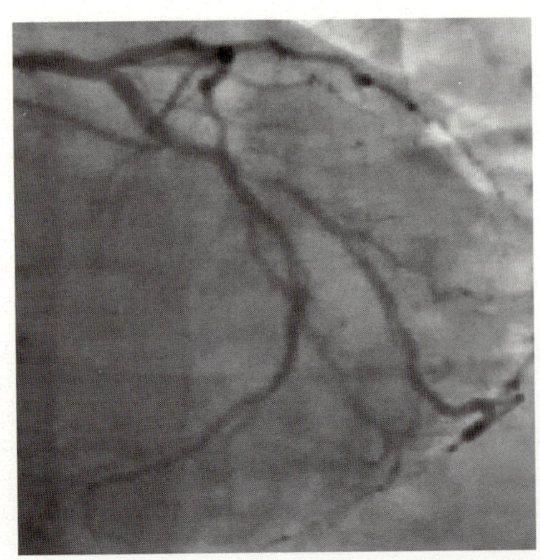

Fig. 10: LCA and RCA evidence of triple vessel disease.

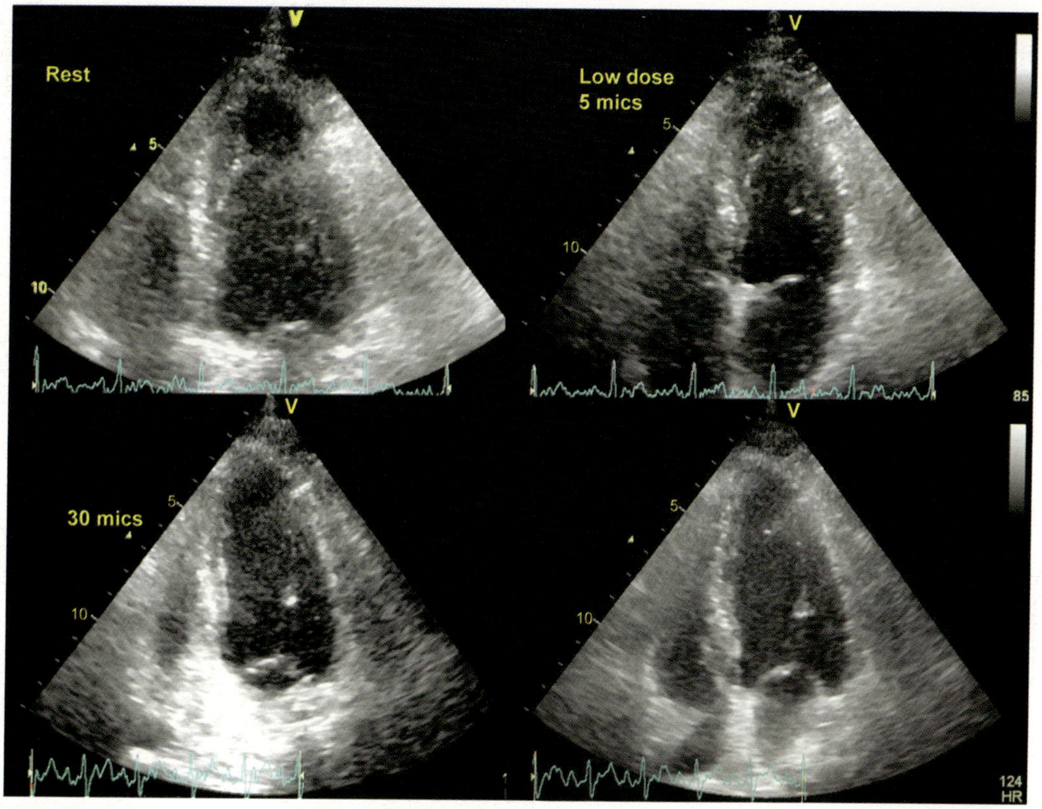

Fig. 11: Dobutamine stress echo: 2D echocardiographic four-chamber view showing basal, 5 mics/s (low dose), 30 mics/s (high dose), and during recovery. There was no regional wall motion abnormality by eye-balling.

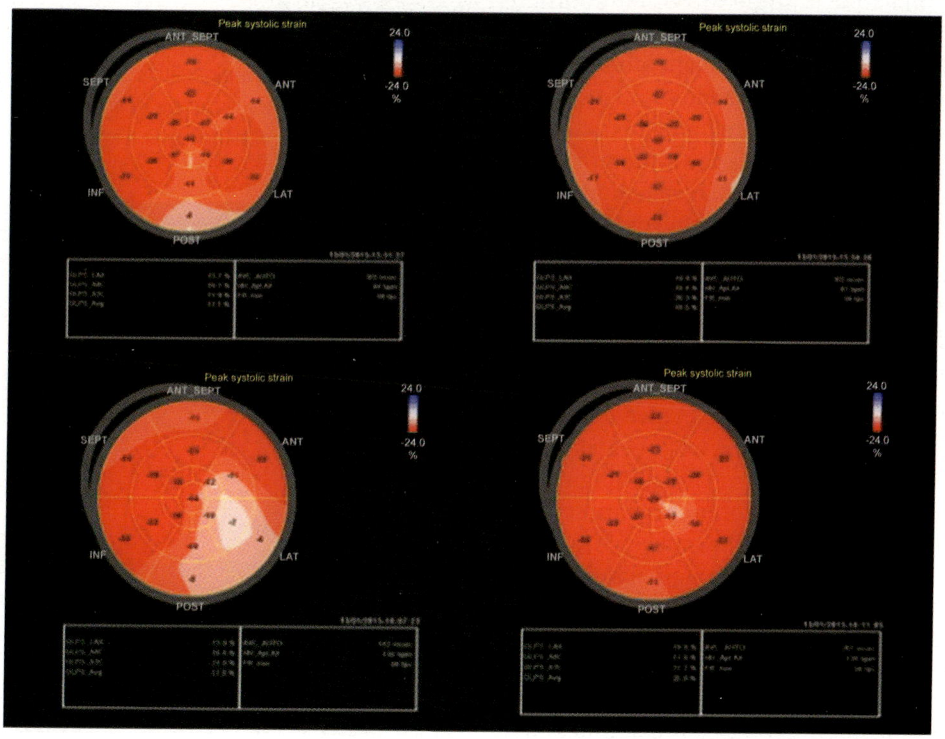

Fig 12: Dobutamine stress echo: Automated functional imaging showing basal, 5 mics/s (low dose), 30 mics/s (high dose), and during recovery showing clearly the strain abnormality during high dose and its resolution during recovery.

short-axis views, it does not reflect true torsional deformation because the images are acquired separately from entirely different cardiac cycles and rotation at each level peaks at a different time in the cardiac cycle. A recent study by Muhammad Ashraf et al., to compute LV twist from three-dimensional (3D) echocardiography concluded despite lower spatiotemporal resolution of 3D echocardiography, LV twist, and torsion can be computed accurately.[13-16]

ASSESSMENT OF MYOCARDIAL VIABILITY AND PROGNOSTICATION IN POSTMYOCARDIAL INFARCTION

In patients with STEMI and primary percutaneous interventions, the global longitudinal strain and the longitudinal strain rate of infarct-related zones were independent predictors of mortality and onset of heart failure even in the presence of normal ejection fraction.[17-19]

LV ejection fraction: The cornerstone of the prognostication and treatment schedule for STEMI echocardiographic evaluation starts with evaluation of left ventricular ejection fraction. Despite its limitations, ejection fraction has become part of the lingua franca of cardiology.[20] The evidence base for modern cardiology is so heavily based on this simple measurement that it is unlikely to disappear. The problems in calculating EF as the ratio between stroke volume and end-diastolic volume and their solutions are enumerated in Table 2. 3D imaging is available with echocardiography, MRI, and CT. The main attraction and advantage of 3D imaging is to avoid geometric assumptions when calculations of LV volumes are being obtained and to avoid errors created by cutting a 3D structure in two dimensions. The current software for 3D evaluation of LVEF is much easier and can be performed within minutes in the setting of emergency room. The sphericity index derived from 3D echocardiography (LVEDV divided by the volume of a sphere whose diameter is the LV end-diastolic long axis) is an added by-product and is the best predictor for LV dilatation.[21]

Global longitudinal strain: It has evolved as one of the most robust parameter, and this has been shown to identify subclinical LV dysfunction. Global longitudinal strain is calculated using a variety of proprietary software (EchoPAC, GE Medical Systems, Milwaukee, WI, United States; Syngo velocity vector imaging, Siemens, Mountain View, CA, United States; LV analysis, TomTec GmbH, Unterschlessheim, Germany). The GLS is well validated as a marker for the measurement of LV longitudinal deformation, which has emerged as a sensitive and specific marker to detect early and subtle myocardial dysfunction. In one of the recent meta-analysis, Kalam et al., have shown the independent prognostic significance of GLS in patients with mild-LV global impairment. The prognostic value of this information seems likely to be superior to that provided by LVEF.[15] Left ventricular GLS before discharge after ST segment–elevation myocardial infarction is independently associated with LV dilatation at follow-up.[22] In another study of 576 patients who underwent echocardiography ≤24 hours after primary percutaneous coronary intervention for STEMI, GLS, and Wall motion score index (WMSI) were comparable and both superior for early risk assessment compared with volume-based left ventricular function indicators such as LVEF and ESVI. Compared with WMSI, the advantage of GLS is the provision of a semiautomated quantitative measure.[23,24] Figure 13 shows a 70-year-old patient who had been stented in left anterior descending artery after an anterior wall myocardial infarction, 3 years before. The strain echocardiographic AFI study for myocardial viability was comparable to radionuclide study, which is shown in Figure 14.

RIGHT VENTRICULAR STRAIN

The EACVI/ASE task force consensus document has recommended the methods of performing the RV free wall strain from the RV-focused apical four-chamber view.[25] Because the RV free wall is thin, the region of interest is standardized as 5 mm. To regionalize, the RV free wall in end diastole is divided into basal, mid, and apical segments. At present, only the peak systolic strain is being studied and the average of the all the three free wall segments is recorded as the RV free wall peak systolic strain. All the six segments are recorded as RV global peak systolic strain (Fig. 15). The normal RV strain values have been published recently.[26,27]

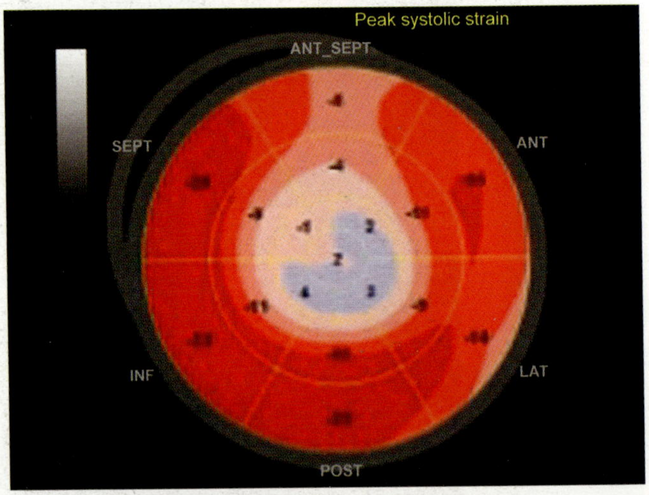

Fig. 13: Automated function imaging from a 70-year-old patient who had been stented in left anterior descending artery after an anterior wall myocardial infarction, 3 years before.

The lowest expected values for RV global strain and RV free wall strain are –17% and –19%, respectively. The RV global strain correlated with the cardiac MRI-derived RV ejection fraction in a study of patients with acute myocardial infarction and RV dysfunction.[28] RV function assessment by RV free wall peak systolic strain has a strong prognostic value in patients who undergo primary percutaneous intervention.[29]

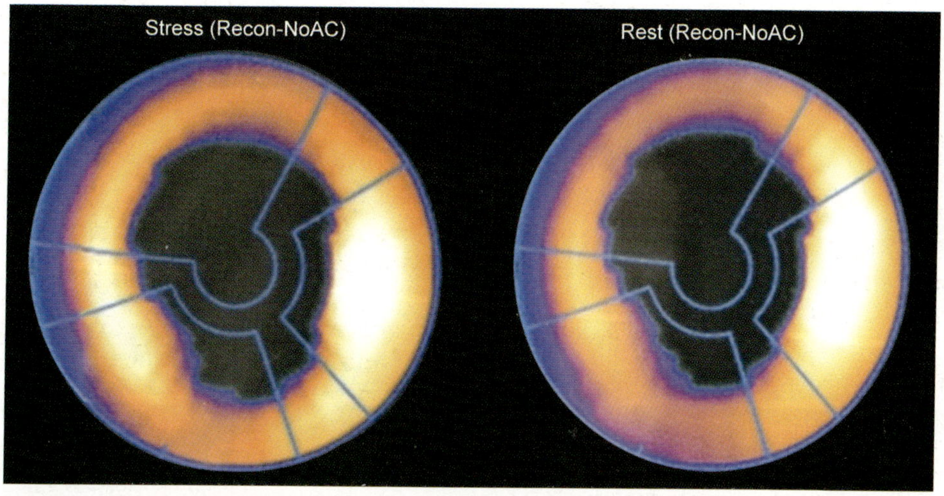

Fig. 14: Stress—rest Technetium[99] radionuclide study from the same patient showing comparable result.

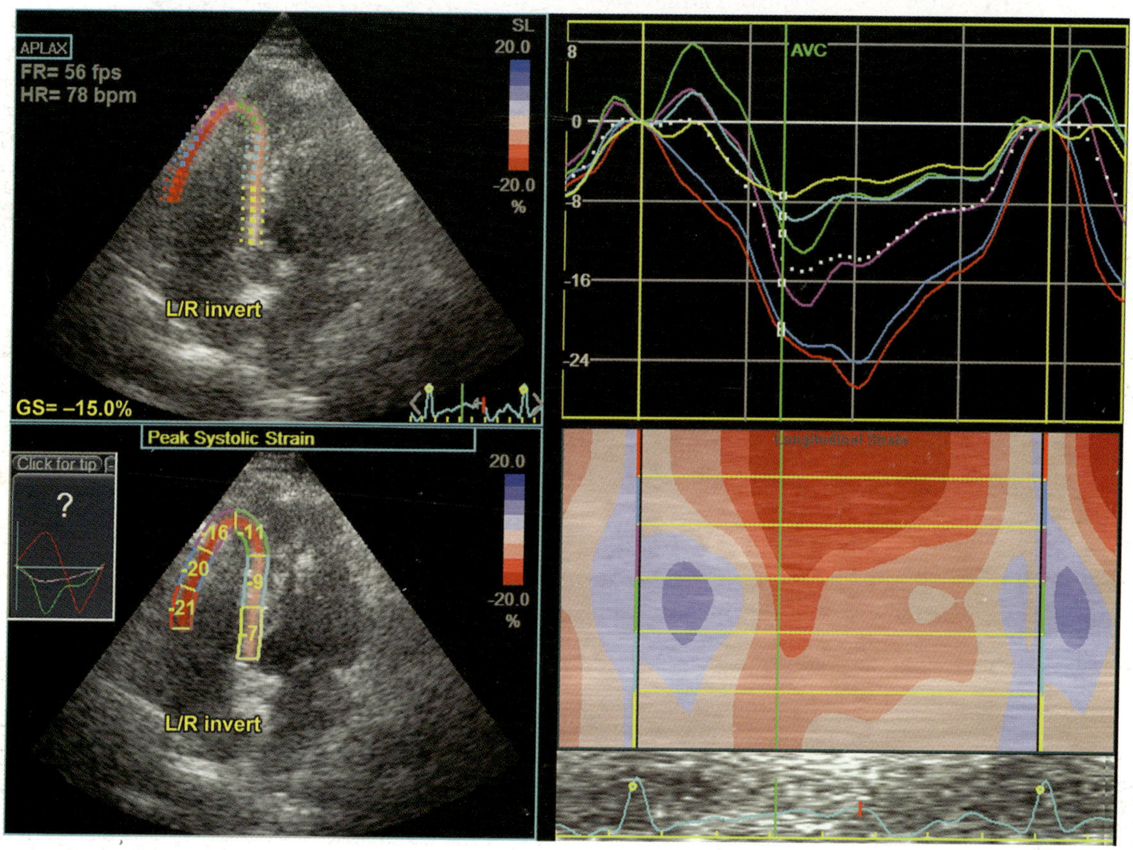

Fig. 15: RV global strain of −15 and RV free wall strain of −19% in a patient with status after drug eluting stent deployment in dominant distal left circumflex, who developed tight lesion in ostial PDA and OM4 lesion indicating abnormal RV function.

LEFT ATRIAL STRAIN

The EACVI/ASE industry task force has also published the normal standardization for deriving the left atrial global longitudinal strain.[25] The following steps may be followed. (1) The imaging of the left atrium should be done in the apical four-chamber plane without fore shortening of the left atrium. (2) The endocardium of the left atrium should be traced from one side of the mitral annulus to the other by extrapolating across the pulmonary veins and left atrial appendage. (3) The default region of interest width can be selected as 3 mm. (4) Left atrial deformation is a cyclical process divided into three phases (Figs. 16 and 17): (a) *Reservoir phase*: It starts at end diastole (Mitral

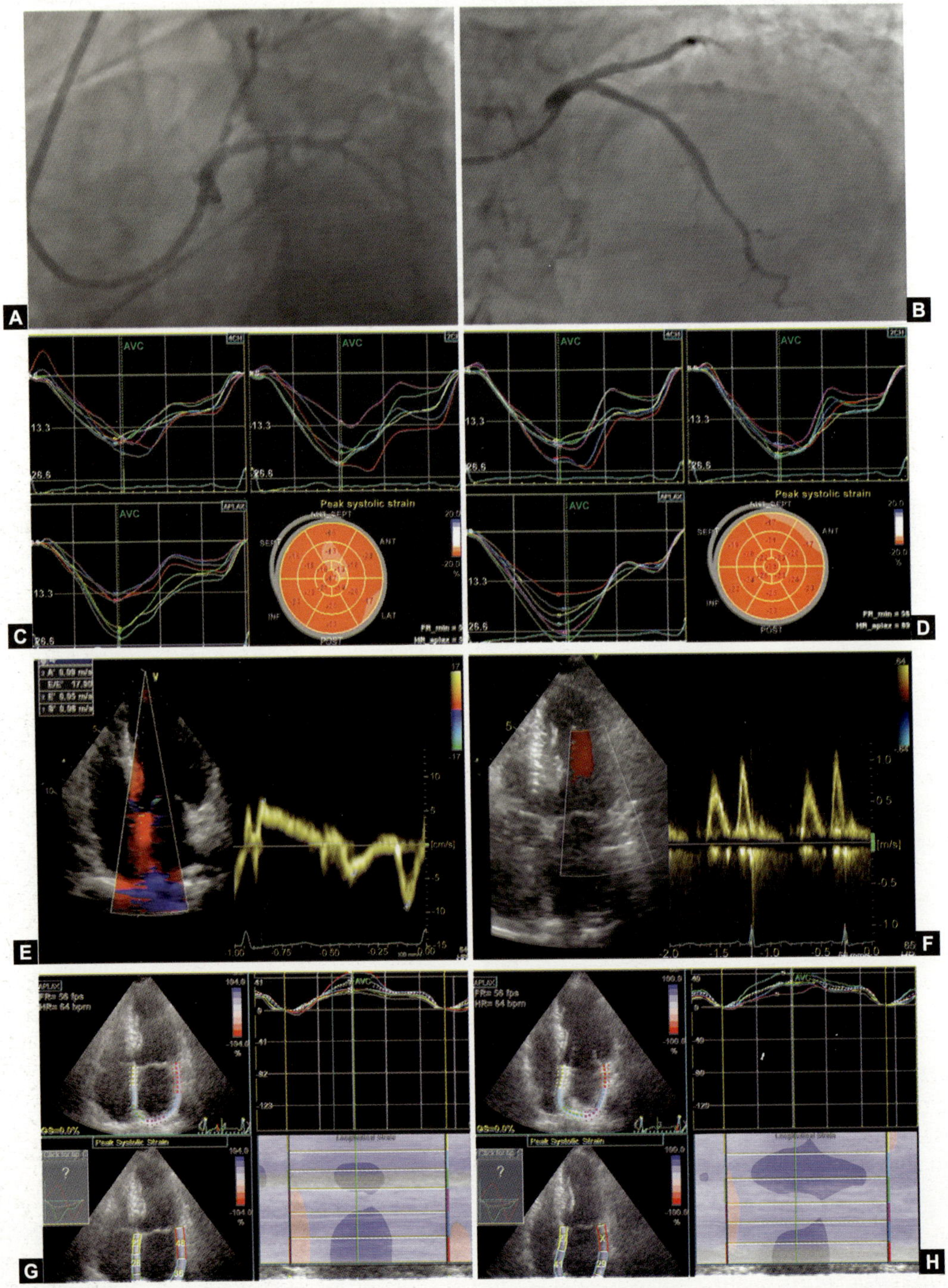

Figs. 16A to H: Diastolic stress test in a patient who had persistent Class III symptoms after left main and proximal LAD stenting 1 year back (A and B). Patient developed severe breathlessness at Stage 1 Bruce and stopped the exercise. The basal GLS (C) reduced at peak exercise (D) and the E/e′ increased from 13 to 17 (E and F). LA strain during basal (G) and immediately after exercise (H).

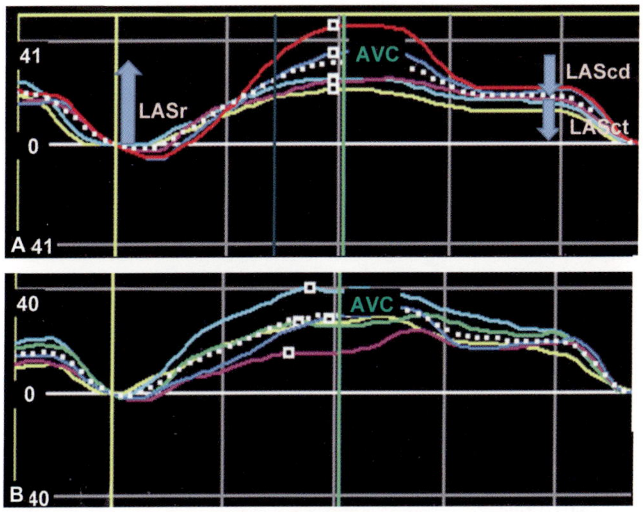

Figs. 17A and B: LA strain curves during basal (A) and immediately after exercise (B). The mean longitudinal peak systolic left atrial strain in white dotted line has to be taken for calculation. LASr, which is a positive value, is measured from strain at mitral valve opening minus the strain at end diastole "LAScd," which is a negative value, is derived by subtracting the strain at onset of atrial contraction minus the strain at opening of mitral valve "LASct," which is a negative value, is derived by subtracting the strain LV end diastole (at mitral valve closure) minus the strain at the onset of atrial contraction, in patients with sinus rhythm.

valve closure) to mitral valve opening. The strain recorded during this phase is labeled as "*LASr*," which is a positive value measured from strain at mitral valve opening minus the strain at end diastole (mitral valve closure). Reduction in LASr (Left atrial strain reservoir) was associated with impairment of all measures of left ventricular systolic and diastolic function and was related to composite outcome of death and hospitalization.[30] (b) *Conduit phase*: It starts at mitral valve opening and ends at the onset of atrial contraction in patients with sinus rhythm and ends at mitral valve closure in atrial fibrillation. The strain recorded during this phase is labeled as "*LAScd*," which is a negative value. It is derived by subtracting the strain at onset of atrial contraction minus the strain at opening of mitral valve. (c) *Contraction phase*: It occurs at the onset of atrial contraction until end diastole (mitral valve closure) in patients with sinus rhythm. The strain recorded during this phase is labeled as "*LASct*," which is a negative value. It is derived by subtracting the strain LV end diastole (at mitral valve closure) minus the strain at the onset of atrial contraction, in patients with sinus rhythm.

CONCLUSION

Two-dimensional speckle tracking has improved the accuracy of left ventricular deformation imaging and torsion dynamics. The regional and global longitudinal strain analysis of left ventricle, right ventricle, and left atrium are of immense benefit in patients with coronary artery disease and in the day-to-day practice of cardiology.

REFERENCES

1. Douglas PS, Garcia MJ, Haines DE, et al. American College of Cardiology Foundation Appropriate Use Criteria Task Force, American Society of Echocardiography, American Heart Association, American Society of Nuclear Cardiology, Heart Failure Society of America, Heart Rhythm Society, Society for Cardiovascular Angiography and Interventions, Society of Critical Care Medicine, Society of Cardiovascular Computed Tomography, Society for Cardiovascular Magnetic Resonance. J Am Coll Cardiol. 2011;57(9):1126.
2. Schinkel AFL, Bax JJ, Geleijnse ML, et al. Noninvasive evaluation of ischaemic heart disease: myocardial perfusion imaging or stress echocardiography? Eur Heart J. 2003;24(9):789-800.
3. Wohlgelernter D, Cleman M, Highman HA, et al. Regional myocardial dysfunction during coronary angioplasty: evaluation by two-dimensional echocardiography and 12 lead electrocardiography. J Am Coll Cardiol. 1986;7(6):1245.
4. Schiller NB, Shah PM, Crawford M, et al. Recommendations for quantitation of the left ventricle by two-dimensional echocardiography. American Society of Echocardiography Committee on Standards, Subcommittee on Quantitation of Two-Dimensional Echocardiograms. J Am Soc Echocardiogr. 1989;2(5):358-67.
5. Roberto ML, Badano LP, Mor-Avi V, et al. Recommendations for cardiac chamber quantification by echocardiography in adults: an update from the American Society of Echocardiography and the European Association of Cardiovascular Imaging. J Am Soc Echocardiogr. 2015;28(1):1-39.
6. Geyer H, Caracciolo G, Abe H, et al. Assessment of myocardial mechanics using speckle tracking echocardiography: Fundamentals and clinical applications. J Am Soc Echocardiogr. 2010;23(4):351-69.
7. Voigt JU, Pedrizzetti G, Lysyansky P, et al. Definitions for a common standard for 2D speckle tracking echocardiography. Consensus document of the EACVI/ASE/ Industry Task Force to Standardize Deformation Imaging. Eur Heart J Cardiovasc Imaging. 2015; 16(1):1-11.
8. Altiok E, Becker M, Koos R, et al. Myocardial deformation imaging by two-dimensional speckle-tracking echocardiography for prediction of global and segmental functional changes after acute myocardial infarction: a comparison with late gadolinium enhancement cardiac magnetic resonance. J Am Soc Echocardiogr. 2014;27(3):249-57.
9. Choi JO, Cho SW, Song YB, et al. Longitudinal 2D strain at rest predicts the presence of left main and three vessel coronary artery disease in patients without regional wall motion abnormality. Eur J Echocardiogr. 2009;10(5):695-701.
10. Bax J, Poldermans D, Elhendy A, et al. Improvement of left ventricular ejection fraction, heart failure symptoms and prognosis after revascularization in patients with chronic coronary artery disease and viable myocardium detected

by dobutamine stress echocardiography. J Am Coll Cardiol. 1999;34(1):163-9.
11. Yamada A, Luis SA, Sathianathan D, et al. Reproducibility of regional and global longitudinal strains derived from two-dimensional speckle-tracking and Doppler tissue imaging between expert and novice readers during quantitative dobutamine stress echocardiography. J Am Soc Echocardiogr. 2014;27(8):880.
12. Mannaerts HF, van der Heide JA, Kamp O, et al. Early identification of left ventricular remodelling after myocardial infarction, assessed by transthoracic 3D echocardiography. Eur Heart J. 2004;25(8):680-7.
13. Beladan CC, Călin A, Roşca M, et al. Left ventricular twist dynamics: principles and applications. Heart. 2014;100(9): 731-40.
14. Helle-Valle T, Crosby J, Edvardsen T, et al. New noninvasive method for assessment of left ventricular rotation: speckle tracking echocardiography. Circulation. 2005;112(20):3149-56.
15. Ashraf M, Myronenko A, Nguyen T, et al. Defining left ventricular apex-to-base twist mechanics computed from high-resolution 3D echocardiography: validation against sonomicrometry. JACC Cardiovasc Imaging. 2010;3(3):227-34.
16. Buckberg GD, Mahajan A, Jung B, et al. MRI myocardial motion and fiber tracking: a confirmation of knowledge from different imaging modalities. Eur J Cardiothorac Surg. 2006;29(Suppl. 1):S165-77.
17. Prastaro M, Pirozzi E, Gaibazzi N, et al. Expert review on the prognostic role of echocardiography after acute myocardial infarction. J Am Soc Echocardiogr. 2017;30(5):431.
18. Marwick TH. Methods used for the assessment of LV systolic function: common currency or tower of Babel? Heart. 2013;99(15):1078-86.
19. Park YH, Kang SJ, Song JK, et al. Prognostic value of longitudinal strain after primary reperfusion therapy in patients with anterior-wall acute myocardial infarction. J Am Soc Echocardiogr. 2008;21(3):262-7.
20. Antoni ML, Mollema SA, Delgado V, et al. Prognostic importance of strain and strain rate after acute myocardial infarction. Eur Heart J. 2010;31(13):1640-7.
21. Mollema SA, Nucifora G, Bax JJ. Prognostic value of echocardiography after acute myocardial infarction. Heart. 2009;95(21):1732-45.
22. Kashif K, Otahal P, Marwick TH. Prognostic implications of global LV dysfunction: a systematic review and meta-analysis of global longitudinal strain and ejection fraction. Heart. 2014;100:1673-80.
23. Joyce E, Hoogslag GE, Leong DP, et al. Association between left ventricular global longitudinal strain and adverse left ventricular dilatation after ST-segment–elevation myocardial infarction. Circul Cardiovasc Imaging. 2014;7(1):74-81.
24. Munk K, Andersen NH, Terkelsen CJ, et al. Global left ventricular longitudinal systolic strain for early risk assessment in patients with acute myocardial infarction treated with primary percutaneous intervention. J Am Soc Echocardiogr. 2012;25(6):644-51.
25. Badano LP, Kolias TJ, Muraru D, et al, Gerard Aurigemma Standardization of left atrial, right ventricular, and right atrial deformation imaging using two-dimensional speckle tracking echocardiography: a consensus document of the EACVI/ASE/Industry Task Force to standardize deformation imaging. Eur Heart J Cardiovasc Imaging. 2018;19(6): 591-600.
26. Morris Da, Krisper M, Nakatani S, et al. Normal range and usefulness of right ventricular systolic strain to detect subtle right ventricular systolic abnormalities in patients with heart failure: a multicentre study. Eur Heart J Cardiovasc Imaging. 2017;18(2):212-23.
27. Badano LP, Muraru D. Subclinical right ventricular dysfunction by strain analysis: refining the targets of echocardiographic imaging in systemic sclerosis. Circ Cardiovasc Imaging. 2016;9(6)
28. Lemarié J, Huttin O, Girerd N, et al. Usefulness of speckle-tracking imaging for right ventricular assessment after acute myocardial infarction: a magnetic resonance imaging/echocardiographic comparison within the relation between aldosterone and cardiac remodeling after myocardial infarction study. J Am Soc Echocardiogr. 2015;28(7):818.
29. Antoni ML, Scherptong RW, Atary JZ, et al. Prognostic value of right ventricular function in patients after acute myocardial infarction treated with primary percutaneous coronary intervention. Circ Cardiovasc Imaging. 2010;3(3): 264-71.
30. Ersbøll M, Andersen MJ, Valeur N, et al. The prognostic value of left atrial peak reservoir strain in acute myocardial infarction is dependent on left ventricular longitudinal function and left atrial size. Circ Cardiovasc Imaging. 2013;6(1):26-33.
31. Feigenbaum H. Echocardiographic chamber quantification in the era of multimodality imaging: beware of unintended consequences. J Am Soc Echocardiogr. 2015;28(7):847-50.

141

CHAPTER

Newer Advances in Computed Tomography and Magnetic Resonance Imaging in Cardiac Imaging

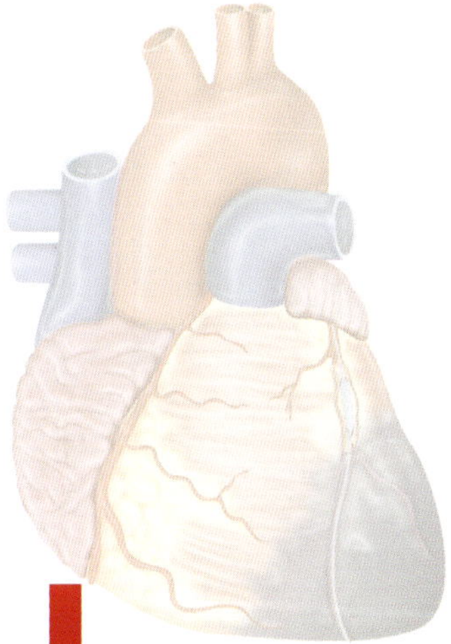

Harsh Mahajan, Suman Singhal

INTRODUCTION

All imaging technologies have undergone continual improvements since their inception so that today imaging has become essential in both clinical practice and research. In the past few decades, cardiac imaging has also undergone breathtaking advancements from single slice to multislice CT (MSCT) which started from four-slice systems in 1998 to the latest 256-slice and 320-slice CT systems. There has been development of spectral/dual-energy CT using various technologies that provide improved tissue characterization and temporal resolution compared to what is possible with a conventional CT. The MSCT helps in detecting coronary calcium deposits, assessment of degree of coronary luminal stenosis, and prediction of disease outcomes.[1-3] In addition to this, it has a potential to characterize atherosclerotic plaques, visualize coronary artery wall morphology, and identify nonstenotic plaques that may not be detected by invasive coronary angiography (ICA)[4,5] and by functional evaluation of coronary artery disease (CAD).[4] The CT coronary angiography (CTCA) helps in evaluation of stents, coronary bypass grafts, myocardial perfusion, and prediction of disease outcome. Advances in radiation dose reduction techniques such as automatic tube current modulation, ECG-based tube current modulation, automatic tube current and voltage selection, and several generations of iterative reconstruction algorithms have ensured that high-quality cardiac images can be obtained with minimal radiation.[5] Cardiovascular magnetic resonance (CMR) has undergone marked technical development and has become gold standard technique for evaluating myocardial function, quantifying myocardial volumes, and detecting myocardial scar. The CMR has the unique ability to provide detailed tissue characterization, including assessment of edema, iron overload, and diffuse myocardial fibrosis. Recent guidelines and appropriate use criteria document indications for CMR for the evaluation of congenital heart disease, heart failure, and CAD. In this review article, we are discussing newer advancements in cardiac CT—plaque imaging and functional evaluation of CAD. Newer advances and evolving CMR techniques including non-contrast T1- and T2-mapping, advances in nonbreath-hold and non-ECG-gated techniques, blood oxygen level-dependent (BOLD) imaging, and role of MR in molecular imaging are being [...] discussed.

NEW ADVANCES IN COMPUTED TOMOGRAPHY PLAQUE IMAGING

"Vulnerable plaque" is an atheromatous plaque in wall of an artery that is particularly unstable, thrombosis-prone with a high probability of undergoing rapid progression and rupture, thus becoming culprit plaque. Histopathologic examinations demonstrated that thin-cap fibroatheroma (TCFA) exhibits similar plaque morphologies as ruptured plaques.[6] The CTCA with newer technological advancements and improved submillimeter spatial resolution is able to assess plaque characteristics including identification of the "vulnerable plaque." Features associated with plaque vulnerability are positive remodeling (PR), the presence of spotty calcifications, and lower plaque density. In patients

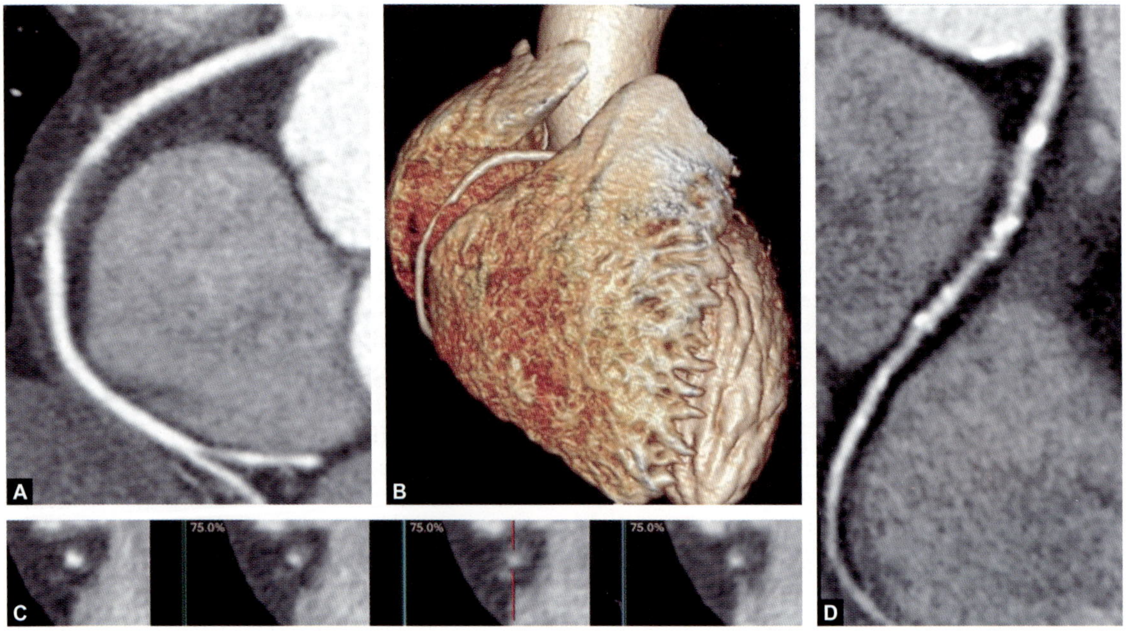

Figs. 1A to D: CT features of plaque vulnerability. (A) Curved reformatted image. (B) Volume rendered image and (C) axial sections showing LAP and PR in mid-RCA. (D) Curved reformatted image of LAD in another patient showing spotty calcification. (LAP: low attenuation plaque; CT: computed tomography; PR: positive remodeling)

with acute coronary syndrome (ACS), the combined presence of these three features allows identification of the unstable lesion with a PPV, a NPV, and an accuracy of 95, 60, and 70%, respectively.[7] Motoyama and colleagues targeted PR (defined as diameter of plaque 10% larger than reference vessel) and low attenuation plaque (LAP) [<30 Hounsfield units (HU)] as potential predictors of ACS (Figs. 1A to D). Patients with both factors had a 22.2% chance of developing ACS versus 3.7% for only one of the above and 0.5% chance if a plaque had none of the above features. The PR and/or LAP independently predicted acute coronary events HR 22.8 (95% CI, 6.9–75.2; $p < 0.001$).[8] In a study by Park et al.,[9] an association between certain atherosclerotic plaque characteristics (APCs), depicted by CTCA and the presence of ischemia by invasive functional flow reserve (FFR), was found.[9] In this study, 252 stable patients without a previous revascularization procedure were included and simultaneously evaluated by CTCA and ICA, with FFR as gold standard for functional significance. Among the CTCA obstructive (≥50% stenosis) lesions, the authors found that only one-half of them were functionally significant by FFR, and the independent predictors of ischemia were lesion length, PR (index ≥1.1), and the presence of LAP (<30 HU). The presence of two or more of these APCs was associated with 13-fold increased odds of ischemia by invasive FFR, and spotty calcification, another APC evaluated, was not an independent predictor of ischemia. Non-calcified plaques can further be classified as homogeneous or heterogeneous based on attenuation patterns. Heterogeneous plaques are characterized by at least two regions with different attenuations values, while homogeneous plaques do not have regions visually differentiable. Based on cross-sectional images, heterogeneous plaques can be divided into ones with napkin-ring sign (NRS) and ones without.[10] The NRS plaques are characterized by a low attenuation central area with a higher attenuation ring-like peripheral area.[11] Maurovich-Horvat et al. showed based on ex vivo examinations that NRS plaques have excellent specificity and low sensitivity (98.9%; 24.4%, respectively) to identify plaques with a large necrotic core, which is a key feature of rupture prone TCFAs.[12] Atherosclerotic plaque burden can also be calculated. Min et al. proposed a score system, the segment stenosis score (SSS), and the segment involvement score (SIS) to quantify plaque burden.[13] The SSS is calculated by grading all coronary segments as follows: 0, no plaque; 1, <50% stenosis; 2, 50–69% stenosis; 3, ≥70% stenosis. The SIS is the number of affected segments. Based on 1,127 patients, SSS had a hazard ratio of 1.99 (95% CI: 1.48–2.67), while SIS had a hazard ratio of 1.23 (95% CI: 1.13–1.34). Similarly, the results from the CONFIRM registry also showed SIS to be an independent predictor of major adverse events (hazard ratio: 1.22; 95% CI: 1.03–1.44).[14]

Current limitation: High image quality required, spatial resolution, LAP cutoff affected by several factors.

COMPUTED TOMOGRAPHY MYOCARDIAL PERFUSION

Myocardial perfusion imaging (CT-MPI) provides functional evaluation of CAD and hemodynamic assessment of obstructive coronary artery lesions. The major advantage of CTCA lies in a very high negative predictive value, which rules out CAD with high reliability. However, the positive predictive value of the test is not sufficiently high, ascribed to a relatively high false-positive rate. The CT assessment of myocardial perfusion is based on the distribution of iodinated contrast material during its first pass through the myocardium. Because the contrast material's distribution is determined by the arterial blood supply, myocardial perfusion defects can be identified as hypoattenuating areas containing reduced amounts of contrast material.[15] Two different approaches are available for CT-MPI: static or dynamic, static CT-MPI further be categorized into single- and dual-energy techniques. Static myocardial perfusion evaluation at rest is generally performed using CTCA image sets already obtained for the morphologic assessment of the coronary arteries; thus, no additional acquisition time or radiation is necessary. If assessment of myocardial perfusion at stress is desired, an additional acquisition during pharmacologic stress is obtained (Fig. 2). A direct comparison with single-energy myocardial perfusion image reconstructions showed the superior diagnostic performance of dual-energy iodine maps for the detection of perfusion defects using SPECT.[16] Ko et al.[17] also found the incremental diagnostic value of combined coronary CTA and CT perfusion compared with coronary CTA alone with a marked increase in sensitivity (91.8–93.5%), specificity (67.7–85.5%), PPV (73.6–88.3%), and NPV (87.5–91.4%). Dynamic CT-MPI provides a quantitative estimation of myocardial time-attenuation curves and other parameters, such as myocardial blood flow.[18] The concept of dynamic CT-MPI is based on the evaluation of multiple sequential CT datasets of myocardial attenuation levels after the injection of a contrast bolus, enabling the generation of time-attenuation curves during arrival and washout of contrast to and from the myocardium and aorta over time. Cutoff points between 75 and 78 mL/100 mL/min have been proposed as the optimal threshold values for the discrimination between significant and no significant lesions.[18] The core limitation of dynamic CT-MPI is a significantly increased radiation dose compared with static CT-MPI, as well as the need for longer breath-holding that warrants the use of further motion correction algorithms.[19,20] A recently published multicenter study (CORE320 [coronary artery evaluation using 320-row multidetector computed tomography angiography and myocardial perfusion]) has confirmed earlier findings on a larger scale. In this study, the overall performance of CT-MPI in the diagnosis of obstructive CAD was higher than that of SPECT.[21]

Current limitation: Beam-hardening artifacts, limited experience and validation, and more radiation; Dynamic MPI requires wide detector coverage.

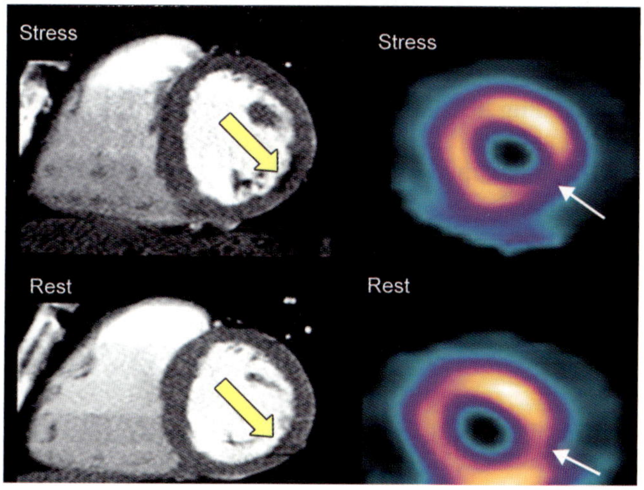

Fig. 2: CT-MPI images at rest and stress are compared with SPECT images showing a subendocardial hypoattenuating ischemic area in inferolateral wall.
(CT-MPI: computed tomography myocardial perfusion imaging)

COMPUTED TOMOGRAPHY FUNCTIONAL FLOW RESERVE

The CT-FFR is an advanced post-processing technique, performed either in offsite or onsite, where by using mathematical assumptions and modeling, computational fluid dynamic model is generated and FFR is obtained non-invasively from a routine coronary CTA. The CT-FFR technology is based on three key principles. The first is that coronary supply meets myocardial demand at rest (total resting coronary flow is relative to ventricular mass). The second is that resistance of the microcirculation at rest is inversely but not linearly proportional to the size of the feeding vessel. The third principle is that microcirculation reacts predictably to maximal hyperemic conditions in patients with normal coronary flow. On the basis of these principles, a lumped parameter model representing the resistance to flow during simulated hyperemia is applied to each coronary branch of the segmented coronary CTA model.[22] The CT-FFR was modeled for adenosine-induced hyperemia, and an CT-FFR ≤0.80 was considered to be diagnostic of lesion-specific ischemia.[23] The CT-FFR was compared to invasive FFR and had a per-vessel accuracy of 84.3%, sensitivity of 87.9%, and specificity of 82.2% in the discover FLOW trial.[24] This technique has been shown to convert 68% of CT "false positives" to true negatives and obviate the need for ICA in 61% of individuals compared to a simple CTA-based algorithm[25] Integrating CT-MPI with CT-FFR and reserving CT-MPI for intermediate CTA-FFR results also improves diagnostic performance while omitting nearly one-half of the population from CT-MPI examinations.[26]

Current limitation: Remote evaluation and dependence on high image quality.

TRANSLUMINAL ATTENUATION GRADIENT AND CORRECTED CORONARY OPACIFICATION

Computed tomography coronary angiography allows noninvasive assessment of coronary flow due to isotemporal differences in contrast attenuation between proximal and distal portions of the coronaries, especially evident in the presence of stenosis.[27,28] For a given coronary cross-section, the mean luminal contrast opacification in HU is calculated, which may be influenced by the time-density curve of the intravascular contrast agent and acquisition timing.[29] TAG is the most common method for the assessment of functional relevance of coronary stenosis based on this attenuation gradient. It is defined as the linear regression coefficient between luminal contrast attenuation (HU) and length from the ostium (cm).[28] It involves the reconstruction of cross-sections perpendicular to the centerline of the vessel at 5-mm intervals from the ostium to the distal level, where the vessel cross-sectional area falls below 2.0 mm^2. Although there is no standardization of cutoff values, still TAG decreases consistently and significantly with maximum stenosis severity on a per-vessel basis, especially in vessels with calcified lesions, as reported by Choi et al.[30] in a study including 370 coronaries from 126 patients using a 64-row MDCT scanner. Furthermore, adding TAG to the interpretation of CTCA may improve diagnostic accuracy, especially in the presence of calcified plaques.[30,31] CT scanners that are not capable of acquiring the whole heart in a single beat lack temporal uniformity for luminal contrast assessment. This temporal misalignment between subvolumes refers to differences in opacification induced by temporal changes between acquisitions of the superior versus inferior subvolumes. A proposed method to overcome this limitation is corrected contrast opacification (CCO), for which a quotient of the mean intraluminal HU in a coronary segment and the descending aorta in the same axial plane is calculated.[32] A combination of CCO with TAG has been proposed, yielding an improved discrimination of significant lesions compared with TAG alone.[33]

Current limitation: Lack of standardized cutoff values, limited data, and some conflicting results.

Further advances in coronary CT angiography in coronary artery disease and CAD-RADS are discussed in chapter on Advances in CT Coronary Angiography Evaluation in Coronary Artery Disease.

NEW ADVANCES IN MAGNETIC RESONANCE IMAGING ADVANCED TECHNIQUES FOR FIRST PERFUSION CARDIOVASCULAR MAGNETIC RESONANCE

First-pass perfusion imaging using CMR has emerged as an attractive alternative to single photon emission computed tomography MPI for the assessment of patients with suspected CAD. Perfusion is assessed using CMR by imaging the first pass of a gadolinium-based contrast agent through the myocardium during vasodilator stress. Regions that are hypoperfused have a slower uptake and lower concentration of contrast and appear as hypointense perfusion defects. With recent technical advancements, current imaging techniques typically image three short-axis myocardial slices (thickness, 8–10 mm) with an in-plane resolution of 2–3 mm for conventional methods and <2 mm for advanced high-resolution approaches typically using parallel imaging techniques or *k–t* acceleration.[34] The performance of high-resolution perfusion CMR was compared with positron emission tomography MPI in a limited study of 41 patients with CAD and demonstrated similar performance both in terms of visual analysis and in terms of quantification of perfusion reserve.[35]

Whole-heart Spatial Coverage

Most significant recent advancement in CMR is the ability to achieve improved whole-heart spatial coverage, either by extending the number of two-dimensional slices or by acquiring 3D volumetric data. Recent spiral approaches using compressed sensing have enabled whole-heart data acquisition.[36] A recent multicenter study showed excellent diagnostic performance for 3D whole-heart perfusion CMR for detection of functionally significant CAD defined by fractional flow reserve (sensitivity and specificity, 84.7% and 90.8%, respectively).[37]

Improved Imaging of Subendocardial Perfusion

Cardiovascular magnetic resonance perfusion imaging has the unique ability to resolve the differences in myocardial perfusion between subepicardial and subendocardial layers because of its potential for high spatial resolution

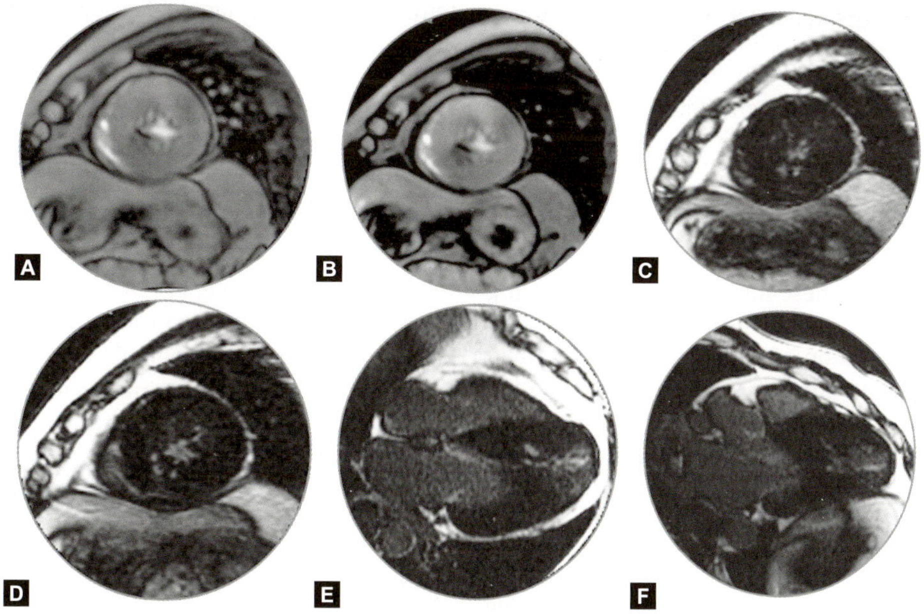

Figs. 3A to F: Patient for assessment of HOCM, FGRE-TC myocardial perfusion (rest) showing perfusion defect (A, B), 2D-MDE displaying subendocardial enhancement on delayed scans short-axis views (C, D) and four-chamber views (E, F).

ranging from 1.2 mm to 3 mm. This is relevant because the subendocardium is the most susceptible layer to ischemia and typically the earliest affected. Conventional CMR techniques, however, are limited by the so-called subendocardial dark-rim artifact (DRA) and may fall short of reliable imaging of subendocardial perfusion.[38] High-resolution (1.4 mm in-plane) perfusion CMR with Cartesian sampling, based on *k–t* BLAST, reduces the extent of DRA, and, thereby, enables accurate detection of subendocardial ischemia (Figs. 3A to F).[34]

ADVANCES IN T1-MAPPING

A range of T1-mapping techniques is available based on inversion recovery sequences. Native T1 values are from signals originating from the intracellular and extracellular compartments and reflect intrinsic differences in tissue properties. Increased native T1 values are useful in detecting acute myocardial pathologies, such as edema, infarction, and myocarditis, and subacute cardiomyopathies, such as cardiac amyloidosis, hypertrophic cardiomyopathy, and dilated cardiomyopathy, and in assessing diffuse fibrosis.[39-41] Low global myocardial T1 values have clinical utility in myocardial iron overload (siderosis)[42] and Fabry disease.[43] Native T1-mapping can also detect the increase in myocardial blood volume associated with coronary vasodilation distal to significant coronary stenoses.[44]

Gadolinium-free Cardiac Magnetic Resonance Stress T1-Mapping to Distinguish Epicardial from Microvascular Coronary Disease

Cardiac MR stress T1-mapping has shown considerable promise for the non-invasive assessment of ischemia.[44,45] Adenosine stress and rest T1-mapping can distinguish between normal, ischemic, infarcted, and remote myocardium without the need for gadolinium contrast agents as they have distinctive rest and stress T1 profiles. Normal myocardium in control subjects exhibited normal resting T1, with significant positive T1 reactivity during adenosine vasodilatory stress (6.2 ± 0.5%). In patients with CAD, infarcted myocardium showed distinctively high resting T1, differentiating it from all other myocardial tissue classes, without significant T1 reactivity (0.2 ± 1.5%). Ischemic myocardium showed mildly (but significantly) elevated resting T1 compared with normal, without significant T1 reactivity (0.2 ± 0.8%). Remote (non-ischemic/infarcted) myocardium in patients with CAD, although having normal resting T1, had a blunted T1 reactivity (3.9 ± 0.6%), possibly due to coronary microvascular dysfunction. The utility of stress T1-mapping for the detection of ischemia in more complex CAD, such as chronic total occlusion and after coronary artery bypass grafting, requires further investigation.[46]

ADVANCES IN T2-MAPPING

Myocardial edema is an important component of many disease processes that affect the myocardium including myocarditis and myocardial infarction. Prior to the widespread availability of T2-mapping pulse sequences, edema was typically imaged using dark-blood T2-weighted spin echo pulse sequences, but these sequences have several inherent limitations. Newly developed T2-mapping sequences can overcome these limitations by quantifying T2 relaxation times.[34] T2*-mapping has become well established for the detection of myocardial iron overload and predicts both the progression to heart failure and the requirement for future chelation therapy.[47]

T2*-Mapping of Myocardial Infarction

T2*-mapping in recent studies have demonstrated that hemorrhagic infarction leads to chronic iron deposition in the myocardial scar, which is associated with ongoing inflammation and monocyte infiltration.[47] In patients with chronic ischemic cardiomyopathy who subsequently received an ICD, early evidence suggests that hemorrhagic infarction and chronic iron deposition are potentially new physiological mechanisms of heart failure and arrhythmia in CAD.[48]

NONBREATH-HOLD AND NONELECTROCARDIOGRAPHIC-GATED CARDIOVASCULAR MAGNETIC RESONANCE TECHNIQUES

An active area of research in CMR is to obtain high-quality images without the need for breath-holding or ECG gating. By significantly under sampling the raw data, it is possible to perform real-time CMR without ECG gating, which provides tolerance to arrhythmias. Non-Cartesian sampling patterns are often used for real-time cine imaging because they are more time-efficient and robust to flow and motion.[34] Kellman et al.[49] developed a retrospective reconstruction method to improve temporal and spatial resolution of real-time cine by combining data acquired over multiple heartbeats using respiratory motion correction and rebinning of data.

BLOOD OXYGEN LEVEL-DEPENDENT CARDIOVASCULAR MAGNETIC RESONANCE IMAGING

In the clinical evaluation of CAD, a desirable goal is to identify functionally significant disease without recourse to physical or pharmacological stress. Blood oxygen level-dependent cardiac magnetic resonance is a technique that can detect myocardial ischemia.[50] The transition from diamagnetic oxyhemoglobin to paramagnetic deoxyhemoglobin induces T2 or T2* differences, thereby generating oxygen-dependent magnetic resonance contrast. In diseased myocardium, BOLD signal differences relative to normal myocardium may reflect not only differences of blood oxygenation, but also of vascular volume. Increased microvascular volume, with concomitant increase in the absolute quantity of hemoglobin, is expected to alter BOLD signal and thus BOLD imaging at rest can be used to detect functionally significant CAD without stress.[51]

CARDIOVASCULAR MAGNETIC RESONANCE AND MOLECULAR IMAGING

Recent studies have described the utility of CMR in characterizing coronary plaque. In a study of T1, T2, and ultrashort echo time CMR in 28 plaques from fixed post-mortem human coronary arteries, CMR demonstrated high specificity and sensitivity for detection of calcification (100% and 90%, respectively) and lipid-rich necrotic core (90% and 75%, respectively), with complete agreement in plaque histological classification in 22 of 28 cases (weighted $K = 0.6945$, $p < 0.0001$).[52] Although still experimental, this data show that CMR may be used for in vivo coronary plaque imaging in future.

CONCLUSION

Imaging will always be an integral part of clinical cardiovascular medicine. The past few decades have witnessed significant improvements in cardiovascular imaging, which is all to the benefit of better diagnosis, management, and early prevention of cardiovascular disease. With new realities in health care emphasizing quality and cost-effectiveness, future technologies in both CT and CMR will need to demonstrate value through greater efficiency and efficacy of care and/or patient outcomes.

REFERENCES

1. Nieman K, Oudkerk M, Rensing BJ, et al. Coronary angiography with multi-slice computed tomography. Lancet. 2001;357:599-603.
2. Achenbach S, Gieslar T, Ropers D, et al. Detection of coronary artery stenosis by contrast-enhanced, retrospectively electrocardiographically-gated multislice computed tomography. Circulation. 2001;103:2535-8.

3. Sun Z, Jiang W. Diagnostic value of multislice CT angiography in coronary artery disease: a meta-analysis. Eur J Radiol. 2006;60:279-86.
4. Gonçalves P, Rodríguez-Granillo GA. Functional evaluation of coronary disease by CT angiography. JACC: Cardiovasc Imaging. 2015;8(1):1.
5. Mowatt G, Cook JA, Hillis GS, et al. 64-Slice computed tomography angiography in the diagnosis and assessment of coronary artery disease: systematic review and meta-analysis. Heart. 2008;94:1386-93. 10.1136/hrt.2008.145292
6. Virmani R, Burke AP, Kolodgie FD, et al. Pathology of the thin-cap fibroatheroma: a type of vulnerable plaque. J Interv Cardiol. 2003;16:267-72. 10.1034/j.1600-0854.2003.8042.
7. Motoyama S, Kondo T, Sarai M, et al. Multislice computed tomographic characteristics of coronary lesions in acute coronary syndromes. J Am Coll Cardiol. 2007;50:319-26.
8. Motoyama S, Sarai M, Harigaya H, et al. Computed tomographic angiography characteristics of atherosclerotic plaques subsequently resulting in acute coronary syndrome. J Am Coll Cardiol. 2009;54:49-57.
9. Park HB, Heo R, OH B, et al. Atherosclerotic plaque characteristics by CT angiography identify coronary lesions that cause ischemia: a direct comparison to fractional flow reserve. J Am Coll Cardiol Img. 2015;8:1-10.
10. Maurovich-Horvat P, Hoffmann U, Vorpahl M, et al. The napkin-ring sign: CT signature of high-risk coronary plaques? JACC Cardiovasc Imaging. 2010;3:440-4. 10.1016/j.jcmg.2010.02.003
11. Maurovich-Horvat P, Ferencik M, Voros S, et al. Comprehensive plaque assessment by coronary CT angiography. Nat Rev Cardiol. 2014;11:390-402. doi:10.1038/nrcardio.2014.60
12. Maurovich-Horvat P, Schlett CL, Alkadhi H, et al. The napkin-ring sign indicates advanced atherosclerotic lesions in coronary CT angiography. JACC Cardiovasc Imaging. 2012;5:1243-52. doi:10.1016/j.jcmg.2012.03.019
13. Min JK, Shaw LJ, Devereux RB, et al. Prognostic value of multidetector coronary computed tomographic angiography for prediction of all-cause mortality. J Am Coll Cardiol. 2007;50:1161-70. doi:10.1016/j.jacc.2007.03.067
14. Hadamitzky M, Achenbach S, Al-Mallah M, et al. Optimized prognostic score for coronary computed tomographic angiography: results from the CONFIRM registry (COronary CT Angiography EvaluatioN For Clinical Outcomes: An InteRnational Multicenter Registry). J Am Coll Cardiol. 2013;62:468-76. doi:10.1016/j.jacc.2013.04.064
15. George RT, Silva C, Cordeiro MA, et al. Multidetector computed tomography myocardial per-fusion imaging during adenosine stress. J Am Coll Cardiol. 2006;48:153-60.
16. Arnoldi E, Lee YS, Ruzsics B, et al. CT detection of myocardial blood volume deficits: dual-energy CT compared with single-energy CT spectra. J Cardiovasc Comput Tomogr. 2011;5:421-29.
17. Ko SM, Choi JW, Hwang HK, et al. Diagnostic performance of combined noninvasive anatomic and functional assessment with dual-source CT and adenosine-induced stress dual-energy CT for detection of significant coronary stenosis. AJR. 2012;198:512-20.
18. Rossi A, Dharampal A, Wragg A, et al. Diagnostic performance of hyperaemic myocardial blood flow index obtained by dynamic computed tomography: does it predict functionally significant coronary lesions? Eur Heart J Cardiovasc Imaging. 2014;15:85-94.
19. Hahnken AH, Klotz E, Pietsch H, et al. Quantitative whole heart stress perfusion CT imaging as noninvasive assessment of hemodynamics in coronary artery stenosis: preliminary animal experience. Invest Radiol. 2010;45:298-305.
20. Rossi A, Merkus D, Klotz E, et al. Stress myocardial perfusion: imaging with multidetector CT. Radiology. 2014;270:25-46.
21. George RT, Mehra VC, Chen MY, et al. Myocardial CT perfusion imaging and SPECT for the diagnosis of coronary artery disease: a head-to-head comparison from the CORE320 multicenter diagnostic performance study. Radiology. 2014;272:407-16.
22. Gonçalves P, Rodríguez-Granillo GA, Spitzer E, et al. Functional evaluation of coronary disease by CT angiography. JACC: Cardiovasc Imaging. 2015;8(11):1322-35.
23. Koo BK, Erglis A, Doh JH, et al. Diagnosis of ischemia-causing coronary stenoses by noninvasive fractional flow reserve computed from coronary computed tomographic angiograms. Results from the prospective multicenter DISCOVER-FLOW (Diagnosis of Ischemia-Causing Stenoses Obtained Via Noninvasive Fractional Flow Reserve) study. J Am Coll Cardiol. 2011;58:1989-97.
24. Douglas PS, Pontone G, Hlatky MA, et al. Clinical outcomes of fractional flow reserve by computed tomographic angiography-guided diagnostic strategies vs usual care in patients with suspected coronary artery disease: The prospective longitudinal trial of FFRCT: outcome and resource impacts study. Eur Heart J. 2015;36:3359-67.
25. Min JK, Leipsic J, Pencina MJ, et al. DIagnostic accuracy of fractional flow reserve from anatomic CT angiography. JAMA. 2012;308:1237-45.
26. Coenen A, Rossi A, Lubbers MM, et al. Integrating CT myocardial perfusion and CT-FFR in the work-up of coronary artery disease. JACC: Cardiovasc Imaging. 2017;10(7):760-70.
27. Rybicki FJ, Otero HJ, Steigner ML, et al. Initial evaluation of coronary images from 320-detector row computed tomography. Int J Cardiovasc Imaging. 2008;24:535-46.
28. Steigner ML, Mitsouras D, Whitmore AG, et al. Iodinated contrast opacification gradients in normal coronary arteries imaged with prospectively ECG-gated single heart beat 320-detector row computed tomography. Circ Cardiovasc Imaging. 2010;3:179-86.
29. Loewe C, Stadler A. Computed tomography assessment of hemodynamic significance of coronary artery disease: CT perfusion, contrast gradients by coronary CTA, and fractional flow reserve review. J Thorac Imaging. 2014;29:163-72.
30. Choi JH, Min JK, Labounty TM, et al. Intracoronary transluminal attenuation gradient in coronary CT angiography for determining coronary artery stenosis. J Am Coll Cardiol Img. 2011;4:1149-57.

31. Zheng M, Wei M, Wen D, et al. Transluminal attenuation gradient in coronary computed tomography angiography for determining stenosis severity of calcified coronary artery: a primary study with dual-source CT. Eur Radiol. 2015;25:1219-28.
32. Choi JH, Koo BK, Yoon YE, et al. Diagnostic performance of intracoronary gradient-based methods by coronary computed tomography angiography for the evaluation of physiologically significant coronary artery stenoses: a validation study with fractional flow reserve. Eur Heart J Cardiovasc Imaging. 2012;13:1001-07.
33. Stuijfzand WJ, Danad I, Raijmakers PG, et al. Additional value of transluminal attenuation gradient in CT angiography to predict hemodynamic significance of coronary artery stenosis. J Am Coll Cardiol Img. 2014;7:374-86.
34. Salerno M, Sharif B, Arheden H, et al, Recent advances in cardiovascular magnetic resonance techniques and applications. Circ Cardiovascular Imaging. 2017;10(6).
35. Morton G, Chiribiri A, Ishida M, et al. Quantification of absolute myocardial perfusion in patients with coronary artery disease: comparison between cardiovascular magnetic resonance and positron emission tomography. J Am Coll Cardiol. 2012;60:1546-55.
36. Yang Y, Kramer CM, Shaw PW, et al. First-pass myocardial perfusion imaging with whole-heart coverage using L1-SPIRiT accelerated variable density spiral trajectories. Magn Reson Med. 2016;76:1375-87.
37. Manka R, Wissmann L, Gebker R, et al. Multicenter evaluation of dynamic three-dimensional magnetic resonance myocardial perfusion imaging for the detection of coronary artery disease defined by fractional flow reserve. Circ Cardiovasc Imaging. 2015;8:003061
38. Gerber BL, Raman SV, Nayak K, et al. Myocardial first-pass perfusion cardiovascular magnetic resonance: history, theory, and current state of the art. J Cardiovasc Magn Reson. 2008;10:18.
39. Taylor AJ, Salerno M, Dharmakumar R, et al. T1 mapping: basic techniques and clinical applications. JACC Cardiovasc Imaging. 2016;9:67-81.
40. Bull S, White SK, Piechnik SK, et al. Human non-contrast T1 values and correlation with histology in diffuse fibrosis. Heart. 2013;99:932-7.
41. Ferreira VM, Piechnik SK, Dall'Armellina E, et al. Non-contrast T1-mapping detects acute myocardial edema with high diagnostic accuracy: a comparison to T2-weighted cardiovascular magnetic resonance. J Cardiovasc Magn Reson. 2012;14:42.
42. Feng Y, He T, Carpenter JP, et al. In vivo comparison of myocardial T1 with T2 and T2* in thalassaemia major. J Magn Reson Imaging. 2013;38:588-93.
43. Sado DM, White SK, Piechnik SK, et al. Identification and assessment of Anderson-Fabry disease by cardiovascular magnetic resonance noncontrast myocardial T1 mapping. Circ Cardiovasc Imaging. 2013;6:392-8.
44. Liu A, Wijesurendra RS, Francis JM, et al. Adenosine stress and rest T1 mapping can differentiate between ischemic, infarcted, remote, and normal myocardium without the need for gadolinium contrast agents. JACC Cardiovasc Imaging. 2016;9:27-36.
45. Piechnik SK, Neubauer S, Ferreira VM. State-of-the-art review: stress T1 mapping-technical considerations, pitfalls and emerging clinical applications. MAGMA [E-pub ahead of print]. 2018;31(1):131-41.
46. Liu A, Wijesurendra RS, Liu JM, et al. Gadolinium-free cardiac MR stress T1-mapping to distinguish epicardial from microvascular coronary disease. J Am Coll Cardiol. March;71(9):957-68. doi:10.1016/j.jacc.2017.11.071
47. Tanner MA, Galanello R, Dessi C, et al. A randomized, placebo-controlled, double-blind trial of the effect of combined therapy with deferoxamine and deferiprone on myocardial iron in thalassemia major using cardiovascular magnetic resonance. Circulation. 2007;115:1876-84.
48. Kali A, Kumar A, Cokic I, et al. Chronic manifestation of postreperfusion intramyocardial hemorrhage as regional iron deposition: a cardiovascular magnetic resonance study with ex vivo validation. Circ Cardiovasc Imaging. 2013;6:218-28.
49. Kellman P, Chefd'hotel C, Lorenz CH, et al. High spatial and temporal resolution cardiac cine MRI from retrospective reconstruction of data acquired in real time using motion correction and resorting. Magn Reson Med. 2009;62:1557-64.
50. Friedrich MG, Karamitsos TD. Oxygenation-sensitive cardiovascular magnetic resonance. J Cardiovasc Magn Reson. 2013;15:43.
51. Lockie T, Ishida M, Perera D, et al. High-resolution magnetic resonance myocardial perfusion imaging at 3.0-Tesla to detect hemodynamically significant coronary stenoses as determined by fractional flow reserve. J Am Coll Cardiol. 2011;57:70-5.
52. Karolyi M, Seifarth H, Liew G, et al. Classification of coronary atherosclerotic plaques ex vivo with T1, T2, and ultrashort echo time CMR. J Am Coll Cardiol Img. 2013;6:466-74.
53. Cokic I, Kali A, Yang HJ, et al. Iron-sensitive cardiac magnetic resonance imaging for prediction of ventricular arrhythmia risk in patients with chronic myocardial infarction: early evidence. Circ Cardiovasc Imaging. 2015;8:e003642.

142

CHAPTER

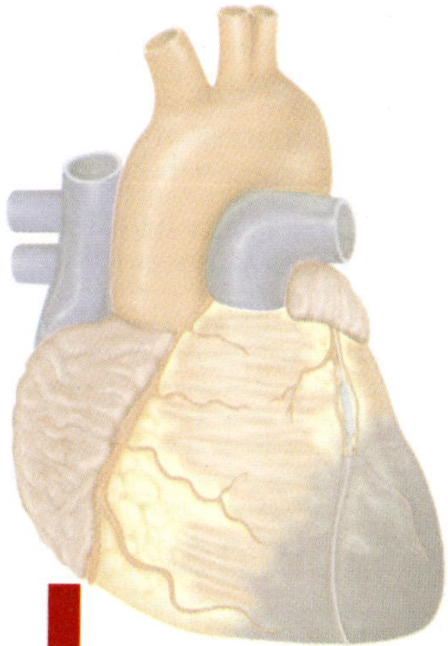

Current Concepts of Radiotracer Technology and its Future Directions

N Ramamoorthy, Meera Venkatesh

INTRODUCTION

The use of radiopharmaceuticals (RPhs) as tracers (radiotracers) for monitoring *cum* imaging organ function (or lesion) has been an important tool in many branches of medicine including cardiology. Mapping the blood flow to the myocardium (myocardial perfusion) with a suitable radiotracer has been of considerable clinical interest and was one of the very early aims of diagnostic nuclear medicine (NM) imaging. In the management of the large volume patients of coronary artery diseases (CAD) in general, and of ischemic heart disease (IHD) in particular, functional and evidence-based demonstration (by imaging) of sites of low or nil perfusion, as well as of the viability of the corresponding zone(s) of myocardium, would be unique value addition by NM. This has been the rationale for the NM approach, while such a development was initially hindered due to nonavailability of a suitable γ emitting, short-lived potassium radioisotope (RI). The discovery of thallous chloride—^{201}Tl (in mid-1970s), as a potassium mimic for tracing myocardial perfusion, due to similarity of ionic charge and size, heralded a major milestone in the history of RPh products and NM practice, and the birth of myocardial perfusion imaging (MPI) and nuclear cardiology;[1,2] the rest is history, as described below.

RADIOTRACERS FOR MYOCARDIAL PERFUSION

Thallium-201: Thallous ion is a mimic of intracellular K^+, due to similarity of ionic size and charge. The RI ^{201}Tl, with 74 hours half-life and suitable photon emission (both γ and X-rays—E□ 135 and 167 keV; 69–80 keV Hg X-rays), has been a fair-match for imaging with γ camera and SPECT. TlCl has very high myocardial extraction from the blood resulting in 3–4% of the injected dose (i.d.) of ^{201}Tl being taken up by the myocardium. There has also been an additional advantage (bonus!) of $^{201}Tl^+$, in terms of its relatively slower uptake and slower washout from "compromised but viable" myocardial tissues (ischemic areas), as compared to normal healthy myocardial cells. This helped obtain stress and rest images of myocardial perfusion, with a single injection of ^{201}TlCl and imaging twice—injection of tracer at peak exercise and imaging soon after to visualize healthy myocardial segments, and a delayed image at 3–4 hours p.i. to additionally visualize viable ischemic areas (if present). This feature of differential washout of the tracer (invariably cited as "redistribution," a misnomer) between high and low blood flow regions of myocardium clinched an important place for ^{201}Tl imaging in NM. Dose of just 50–75 MBq (about 1.5–2 mCi) was sufficient to obtain myocardial images with the then prevalent planar γ camera. With the advent of SPECT, an important change for better quality of images, the dose of ^{201}Tl was increased up to 130 MBq (3.5 mCi), and superior resolution image slices of myocardial perfusion were routinely registered and reported. Nuclear cardiology has since become a key clinical tool.[1,2]

Technetium-99m products: ^{99m}Tc (6 hours half-life; E□ 140.5 keV (89%)) was the most preferred RI for imaging in NM during 1970s and 1980s. This triggered much R&D efforts world over to develop alternates to ^{201}Tl and culminated in the development and launch of

^{99m}Tc-sestamibi (Tc(I) hexakis isonitrile monocationic complex), by a US-based company. The concept in this development was to design a moderately lipophilic, cationic complex of ^{99m}Tc to mimic the thallous ion. This was subsequently supplemented by another similar monocationic complex product, called ^{99m}Tc-tetrofosmin, launched by a company in the United Kingdom. In these cases, two separate injections of the tracer are necessary to elicit stress and rest perfusion pattern in patients. The myocardial extraction efficiency of ^{99m}Tc tracers was only 50–60% of that of ^{201}Tl. This was partly compensated by injecting larger dose of ^{99m}Tc-RPh. The phasing out of ^{201}Tl did not hence take place for a long time, and it is only since 2000, reduction in the use of ^{201}Tl occurred. The arrival of ^{99m}Tc-based products for MPI and the entry of SPECT in NM, however, took place more or less at the same time. This quickly led to MPI being done with SPECT and ^{99m}Tc products, making the image quality superior to that obtainable with $^{201}Tl^{+}$. Nearly, 40–50% of all the NM imaging done with ^{99m}Tc is for myocardium.[1-3]

PET tracers, ^{82}Rb, and $^{13}NH_3$: The use of PET tracers for MPI, including by revisiting certain "old" PET tracers, got a revival with the arrival of PET/CT in 2001, and which has become the fastest growing imaging modality since then. The high-resolution image quality offered by PET/CT, and along with better quantitation capability, further strengthened PET MPI information content.[4,5] The use of $^{82}Rb^{+}$ (K^{+} analog, obtained from ^{82}Sr-^{82}Rb RI generator) for PET imaging of myocardial perfusion, has hence increasingly attracted global attention, and more particularly after the 2008–2010 supply crisis of ^{99}Mo-^{99m}Tc (x). ^{82}Sr with a half-life of 25 days enables RI generators (available from commercial sources, e.g. Cardiogen) of shelf-life of about a month or two. Further, the 75-second half-life of ^{82}Rb is well suited for repeat imaging studies, wherever warranted, as for example, need-based physiological or pharmacological intervention procedures. The other PET tracer for MPI is ^{13}N (10-minute half-life) as $^{13}NH_4^{+}$ for MPI, but its use is limited to NM centers with access to on-site (medical) cyclotron facility.[4,5] New PET tracers for MPI are underdevelopment and evaluation, as briefly cited later in this article.

RADIOTRACERS FOR MYOCARDIAL VIABILITY

PET tracer ^{18}F-2-fluoro-2-deoxy glucose (^{18}F-FDG) for glucose metabolism: Soon after the entry of ^{18}F-FDG in NM in late 1970s, its clinical utility in cardiology was realized to show the extent of viability of the suspect segments or damaged/injured myocardium. In the period post-2001, with medical cyclotron (MC) and PET tracer such as ^{18}F-FDG becoming globally commonplace items (as evident by the 18 MC and 150+ PET/CT now in India, and nearly 1,000 lots of ^{18}F-FDG being produced per day using about 900 MC in operation globally), NM's valuable role in managing cardiac patients using ^{18}F-FDG has increased significantly, since it helps to demonstrate myocardial viability in an unequivocal manner. The blood flow starved region(s), shown with ^{99m}Tc + SPECT image, lighting up with ^{18}F-FDG on PET image, helps plan or confirm the plan, for the subsequent intervention required (or otherwise). ^{18}F-FDG tracer, proven for its high-value contributions in oncology, is being harnessed for the benefit of cardiac patients too.[4-6]

FUTURE DIRECTION—ADDITIONAL RADIOTRACERS FOR MYOCARDIAL PERFUSION

SPECT tracers: The quest for superior imaging RPh for myocardial perfusion had also led (in 1990s) to a neutral complex of ^{99m}Tc known as ^{99m}Tc-Teboroxime, which had a higher myocardial extraction than even ^{201}TlCl (and much higher than that of ^{99m}Tc-sestamibi and ^{99m}Tc-tetrofosmin). However, its fast washout feature and the finite time needed for imaging hindered its prospects for regular clinical utility at that time. Recently, a novel SPECT imaging system—called G-SPECT, multipin-hole, ultrafast system—is on the anvil, which can acquire image of a single organ in 0.5–5 minutes. The launch of this high-performance system can usher in the regular clinical use of this superior radiotracer for myocardial imaging in future.[7]

PET tracers: Several ^{18}F-labeled molecules are under investigation for MPI thanks to large-scale routine use of ^{18}F in NM (TBq (kCi) level production daily), and a few of these are in clinical trials. The important development reported for myocardial imaging is ^{18}F-flurpiridaz.[5] This compound is a structural analog of pyridaben, which is an enzyme inhibitor of mitochondrial complex 1 (MC1), a protein found primarily on myocardial cells. This product is reported to show a very high first-pass extraction fraction, which makes it promising for myocardial perfusion PET imaging.

The generator produced PET tracer ^{68}Ga (68-minute half-life, obtained from ^{68}Ge half-life 271 days) is being increasingly used in NM, mostly for its valuable role in tumor mets imaging. The availability of ^{68}Ga from long shelf-life ^{68}Ge-^{68}Ga generator is an important advantage, as it obviates the dependence on an on-site cyclotron. Another positron emitter RI Copper-64, well investigated for tumor imaging with PET, has 12.7 hours half-life (about 17% positron emission) and is attractive for daily production and distribution. Taken together with the amenability of trivalent gallium and bivalent copper for complexation by a variety of chelating moieties, concerted R&D efforts on ^{68}Ga-based and ^{64}Cu-based PET tracers for myocardial imaging are underway.[8] A much welcome development will be the availability of a new RPh product for PET imaging of myocardial perfusion in future. The superior resolution of PET images and greater quantitation capability of PET are the key drivers for this pursuit.

Harnessing quantitation advantage of PET: The role of NM imaging of myocardium can be extended to serve beyond perfusion in the management of patients with CAD/IHD by making use of the superior quantitation capability possible with PET images acquired using appropriate tracers.[5] Responding to the importance and role of absolute quantitation of myocardial flow, expressed in terms of coronary flow ratio (CFR—ratio of the myocardial blood flow at peak hyperemia to resting), in management of cardiac patients with coronary stenosis, one can derive the CFR values using tracers whose uptake is directly proportional to the blood flow. The PET tracer, ^{15}O-water (half-life 2.06 minutes), which diffuses freely across myocyte membranes, with 100% extraction fraction, would be the ideal tracer for the purpose. However, its use is limited due to practical logistics including the very short half-life. Among the other myocardial perfusion PET tracers, $^{82}Rb^{+}$ and ^{13}N-ammonia can be used, despite their nonideal myocardial extraction fractions. ^{82}Rb that can be derived from a generator has an edge over ^{13}N-ammonia and hence preferred currently for CFR estimation. ^{18}F-flurpiridaz, a product in advanced stage of clinical trial, seems set to emerge as the new tracer for similar use, as it has the required attributes, namely uptake proportional to the flow, 110-minute half-life, and low positron energy (0.635 MeV) enabling high-resolution images.

The growth in hybrid imaging using PET/CT in NM, and the availability of CT along with PET, could be an added advantage for estimation of another important parameter Fractional Flow Reserve (FFR), for management of patients with coronary stenosis. Recent advances in computational fluid dynamics, and image-based modeling, have made it possible to calculate FFR noninvasively without the need for additional imaging, modification of acquisition protocols, or administration of medication. This added possibility from PET/CT imaging can be another boost to the value addition from Nuclear (PET) Cardiology.

FUTURE DIRECTION—REVISITING RADIOTRACERS FOR MYOCARDIAL METABOLISM

Imaging fatty acid metabolism with SPECT tracer ^{123}I-FAA and PET tracer ^{18}F-FAA: A very early development in myocardial imaging involved iodine-123-labeled fatty acid analogs (FAA), as tracer of myocardial metabolism imaging. Fatty acid is a primary source of energy for myocardium, and hence, radioiodinated analogs of fatty acid derivatives (ortho/para iodo-phenyl-pentadecanoic acid (IPPA)) were attractive vector molecules for myocardial imaging.[1,2] ^{123}I (13.3-hour half-life; E□ 159 keV (84%)) is an ideal agent for imaging with γ camera and SPECT, but this could not, however, live up to its promise due to the earlier mindset that 13.3-hour half-life of ^{123}I is too short to be transported to end users from the production center. It is an irony that despite growth in the deployment of MC, and the paradigm-shift with respect to half-life of RI in use nowadays (viz. widespread distribution and use of 110-minute half-life ^{18}F), interest in production and use of ^{123}I has remained low. ^{18}F-labeled fatty acid analogs have been reported as PET tracer for myocardial metabolism imaging with limited success (e.g. 16-[^{18}F]fluoro-4-thia-palmitate).[9] It would be appropriate to revisit ^{123}I and product like IPPA for possible use with SPECT/CT in future due to the large number of MC in operation. In view of the enhanced availability of PET/CT, one can also consider using the analogous PET tracer ^{124}I-IPPA.

FUTURE DIRECTION—NONINVASIVE IMAGING OF CORONARY ARTERIAL PLAQUES?

Can there be a suitable radiotracer that will lit up the interiors of the coronary arteries, almost in the same manner as the conventional angiography shows it all? This, if and when realized, will be a phenomenal achievement, though the development of such a product and achieving the required degree of high resolution with imaging instrumentation, would pose severe challenges. Potential tracers for targeting arterial plaques have been cited in many conferences and publications.[10] PET imaging of atherosclerosis will be of great help to identify the at-risk individuals earlier in the disease process, as well as to subsequently monitor their response to therapy. Of the several PET tracers studied for imaging atherosclerosis, the commonly cited RPh is ^{18}F-FDG, while ^{11}C-choline, ^{18}F-galacto-RGD, ^{11}C-acetate, and ^{11}C-PK11195 have been tested in clinics. However, the small size of the atherosclerotic lesions in coronary arteries, in the vicinity of circulating tracer in blood, and the respiratory and cardiac movements during the image acquisition, would all lead to a high degree of uncertainty of the information derived. This may be possibly better addressed by PET/MR system, where MR can provide high spatial resolution and exquisite soft tissue contrast, to complement PET. If a simple intravenous injection of an RPh, and after physiological stress, would elicit what you can otherwise see only in a cath lab, it would be truly a game changer in NM-RPh practice. It is deemed worthwhile to aim for large concerted development efforts in this direction.

CONCLUSION

Myocardial imaging option of NM has been very useful to assess risk and guide management for cost-effective cardiac care, with the typical absorbed radiation dose from MPI study being in the range of 2–10 mSv and up to 20 mSv for dual RI study (cf. angio-CT 12 mSv; coronary angio 7–12 mSv). Emerging advances in NM-RPh, and imaging instrumentation (e.g. G-SPECT), would provide additional options for myocardial imaging in future, and at the same time, the scope to expand ongoing utilization for established indications needs to be emphasized. It is known that the use of nuclear cardiology is grossly heterogeneous across the world. There is high utilization of myocardial imaging, where cardiac-related mortality is lower, and low utilization, where such mortality is higher.[11,12] Although this is not singularly attributable to nonutilization of NM, it goes to reiterate the point that there is a definite need, as well as scope, to expand the use of nuclear cardiology for all established indications. This would include inter alia the following: for patients whose stress ECG results are equivocal; for establishing adequacy and uniformity of perfusion profile in select group of cardiac patients; for showing extent of viability, when deemed desirable or pertinent, prior to revascularization procedures, etc. One can also consider to include MPI as a part of medical fitness assessment program of personnel, who are engaged in very crucial roles and responsibilities, such as airline pilots, submarine operators, drivers involved in mass transport of public (buses, trains, etc.), volunteers wishing to take part in adventure sports, etc. The coming together of cardiologists and NM fraternity in recent years in many a forum in India (e.g. NCSI, WCCICC, GCDC, APICON) augurs well for greater professional understanding and smooth adoption of NM procedures, on needs-based and values-based manner, for the benefit of cardiac patients. This can also become a good model to emulate by several other countries.

REFERENCES

1. Schelbert HR, Current status and prospects of new radionuclides and radiopharmaceuticals for cardiovascular nuclear medicine. Semin Nucl Med. 1987;17:145-81 http://www.seminarsinnuclearmedicine.com/article/S0001-2998(87)80019-3/pdf.
2. Ramamoorthy N, Venkatesh M, Myocardial imaging products' evolution: change for the better, in cardiac imaging update 2017. Delhi: Jaypee Brothers Medical Publishers (P) Ltd.; 2017. pp. 80-4.
3. Sogbein OO, Pelletier-Galarneau M, Schindler TH, et al. New SPECT and PET radiopharmaceuticals for imaging cardiovascular disease. Hindawi Publishing Corporation; BioMed Res Int. 2014, Article ID 942960.
4. Maddahi J, Packard RR. Cardiac PET perfusion tracers: current status and future directions. Semin Nucl Med. 2014;44:333-43. http://www.ncbi.nlm.nih.gov/pmc/articles/PMC4333146/pdf/nihms657665.pdf.
5. Veeranna V, Dorbala S. Myocardial perfusion imaging with PET, PET/CT, PET/MRI: technical advances and future applications. In: Perfusion imaging in clinical practice, Chapter 22. Netherland: Wolters Kluwer; 2015. pp. 398-411.
6. Li Y, Wei Zhang W, Wu H, et al. Advanced tracers in PET imaging of cardiovascular disease. Hindawi Publishing Corporation; BioMed Res Int. 2014, Article ID 50453.
7. Breakthrough scanning technology: G-SPECT. MILabs, The Netherlands. https://www.milabs.com/breakthrough-scanning-technology-g-spect/.
8. Hsiao Y-M, Mathias CJ, Wey S-P, et al. Synthesis and biodistribution of lipophilic monocationic gallium radiopharmaceuticals derived from N,N′-bis(3-aminopropyl)-N,N′-dimethylethylenediamine: potential agents for PET myocardial imaging with 68Ga. Nucl Med Biol. 2009;36:39-45.
9. Shoup TM, Elmaleh DR, Brownell A-L, et al. Evaluation of (4-[18F]fluorophenyl) triphenylphosphonium ion. A potential myocardial blood flow agent for PET. Mol Imaging Biol. 2011;13:511-17.
10. Orbay H, Hong H, Zhang Y, et al. Positron emission tomography imaging of atherosclerosis. Theranostics. 2013;3:894-902. http://www.thno.org/v03p0894.htm.
11. International Atomic Energy Agency. Nuclear Cardiology: its role in cost effective care. IAEA Human Health Series Report 18; 2012.
12. Vitola JV. Confronting the epidemics of CVD worldwide. Vienna: IAEA Scientific Forum; 2017. https://www.iaea.org/sites/default/files/vitola-presentation190917.pdf.

Index

Page numbers followed by *b* refer to box, *f* refer to figure, *fc* refer to flowchart, and *t* refer to table.

C

D

E

F

G

H

I

M

N

O

P

S

T

W

X

Y

Z